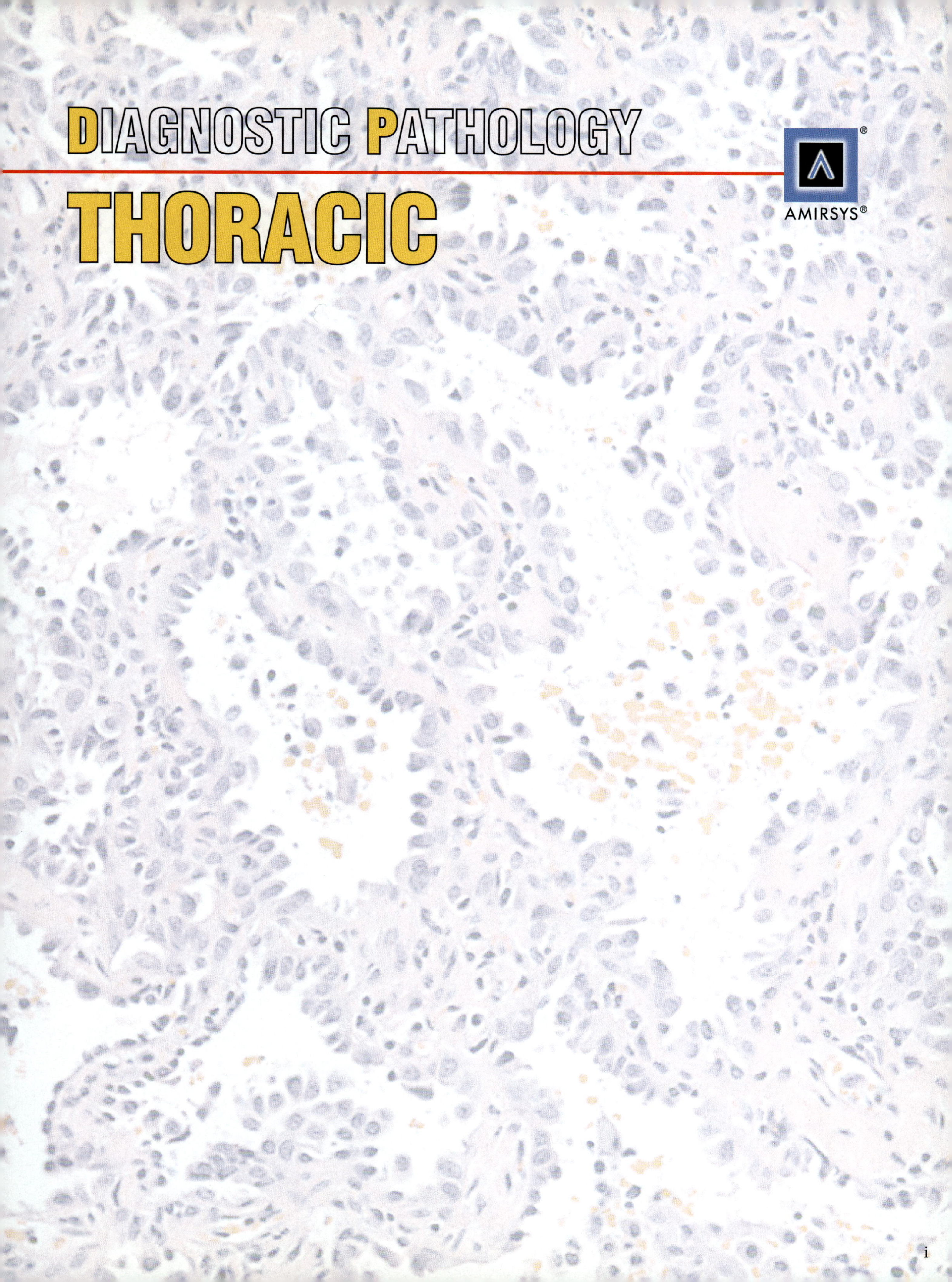

DIAGNOSTIC PATHOLOGY

THORACIC

AMIRSYS®

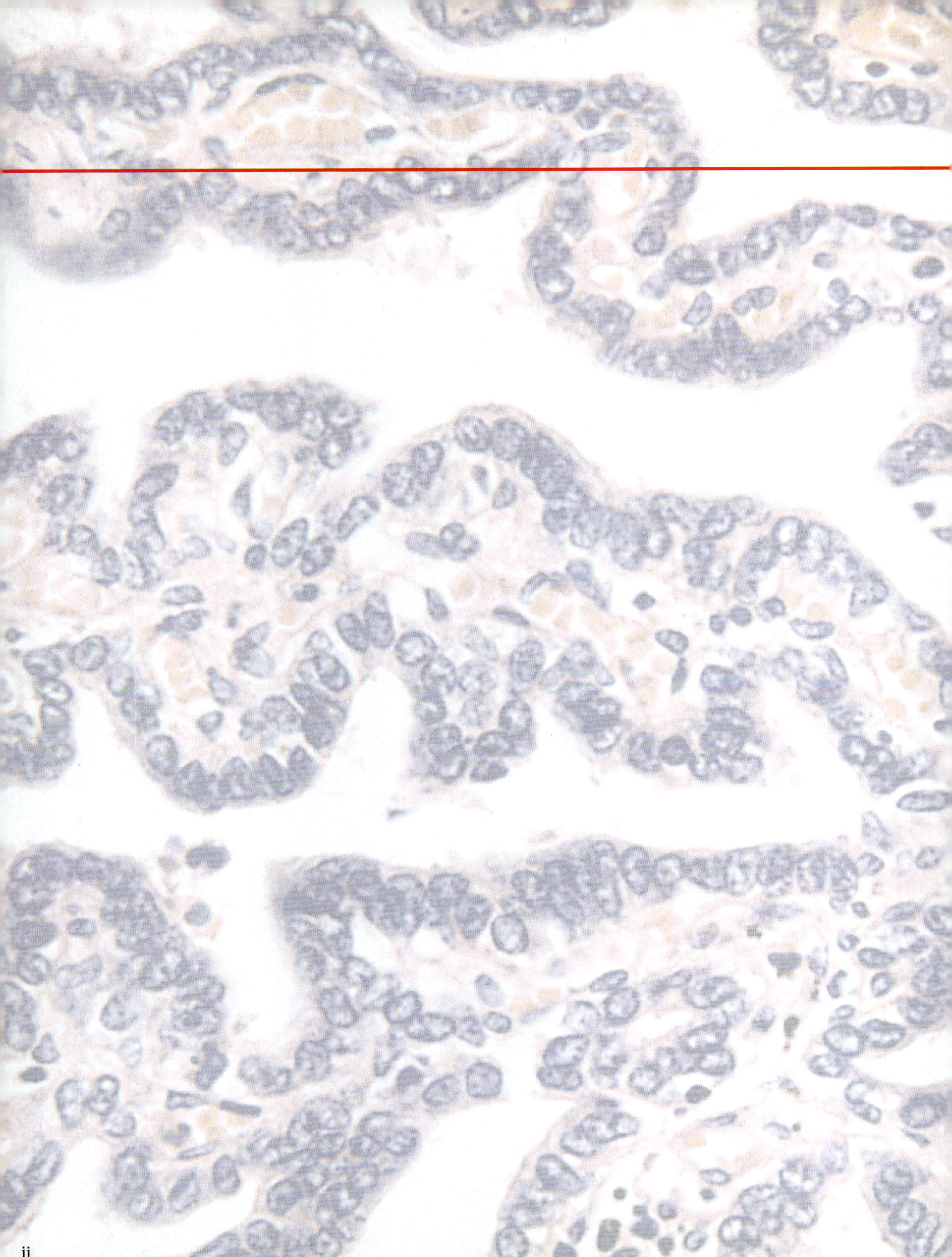

DIAGNOSTIC PATHOLOGY

THORACIC

AMIRSYS®

Saul Suster, MD
Professor and Chairman
Department of Pathology and Laboratory Medicine
Medical College of Wisconsin
Milwaukee, WI

Cesar A. Moran, MD
Professor
Department of Pathology
The University of Texas M. D. Anderson Cancer Center
Houston, TX

AMIRSYS®
Names you know. Content you trust.®

First Edition

Printed in Canada by Friesens, Altona, Manitoba, Canada

ISBN: 978-1-931884-49-5

Notice and Disclaimer

Suster, Saul.
Diagnostic pathology. Thoracic / Saul Suster, Cesar A. Moran.
p. ; cm.
Thoracic
Includes bibliographical references and index.
ISBN 978-1-931884-49-5
1. Chest--Diseases--Atlases. 2. Respiratory organs--Diseases--Atlases. I. Moran, Cesar. II. Title. III. Title: Thoracic.
[DNLM: 1. Thoracic Diseases--pathology--Atlases. 2. Diagnosis, Differential--Atlases. 3. Lung Diseases--pathology--Atlases. 4. Pleural Diseases--pathology--Atlases. WF 17]
RC941.S92 2012
616.1--dc23
2011017713

This book is dedicated to my wife, Jenny Suster, without whose support and companionship nothing would have been possible.

And to our children, Dana Deborah and David Ilan, for having made the whole journey worthwhile.

SS

To my parents, Rigoberto Moran (RIP) and Leticia Moran.

And to my wife, Susan, and daughters, Kate Leticia and Elisa Jean.

CAM

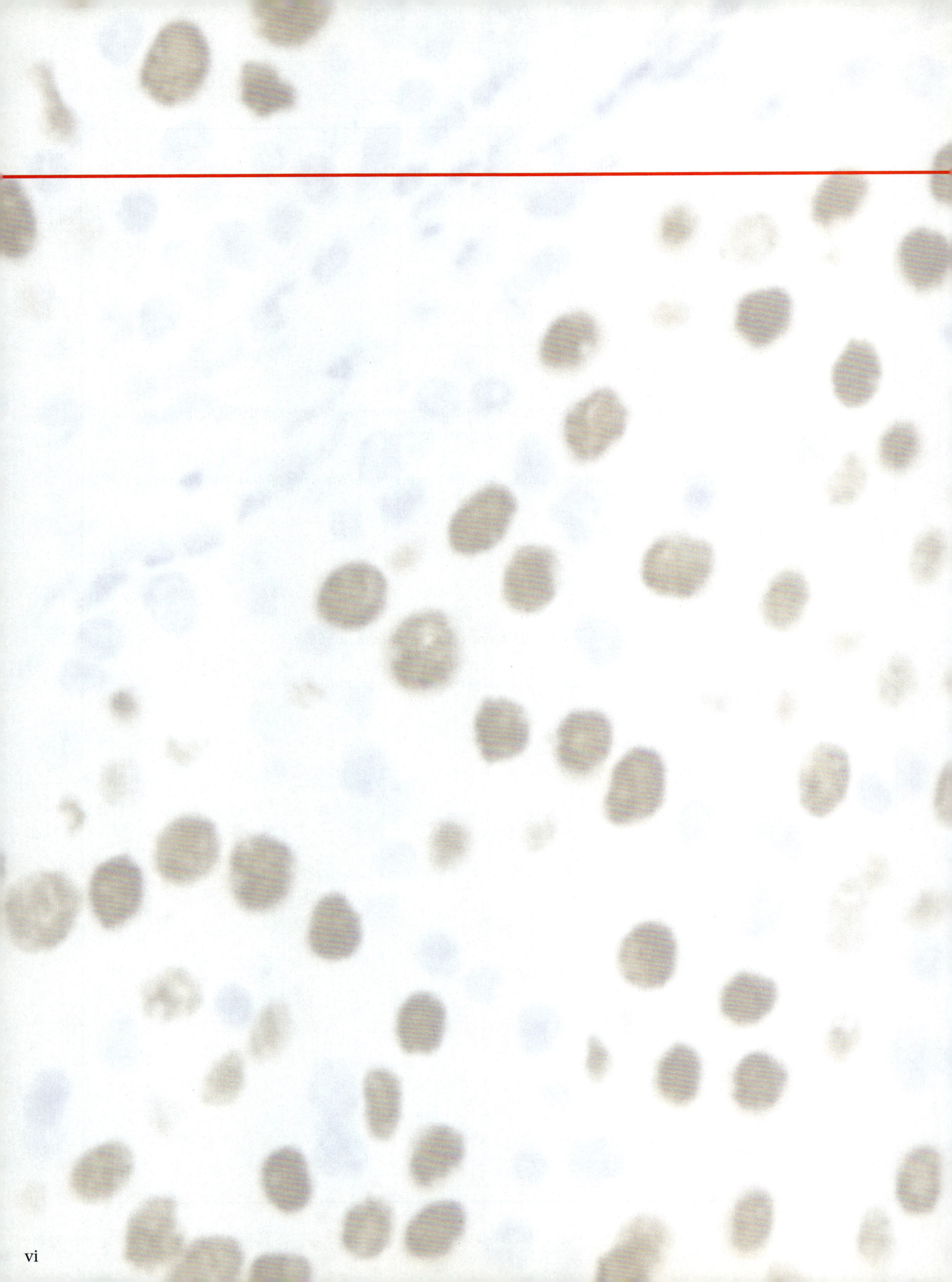

DIAGNOSTIC PATHOLOGY

THORACIC

AMIRSYS®

Amirsys, creators of the highly acclaimed radiology series Diagnostic Imaging, proudly introduces its new Diagnostic Pathology series, designed as easy-to-use reference texts for the busy practicing surgical pathologist. Written by world-renowned experts, the series will consist of 15 titles in all the crucial diagnostic areas of surgical pathology.

The newest book in this series, *Diagnostic Pathology: Thoracic*, contains approximately 850 pages of comprehensive, yet concise, descriptions of more than 165 specific diagnoses. Amirsys's pioneering bulleted format distills pertinent information to the essentials. Each chapter has the same organization providing an easy-to-read reference for making rapid, efficient, and accurate diagnoses in a busy surgical pathology practice. A highlighted Key Facts box provides the essential features of each diagnosis. Detailed sections on Terminology, Etiology/Pathogenesis, Clinical Issues, Macroscopic and Microscopic Findings, and the all important Differential Diagnoses follow so you can find the information you need in the exact same place every time.

Most importantly, every diagnosis features numerous high-quality images, including gross pathology, H&E and immunohistochemical stains, correlative radiographic images, and richly colored graphics, all of which are fully annotated to maximize their illustrative potential.

We believe that this lavishly illustrated series, with its up-to-date information and practical focus, will become the core of your reference collection. Enjoy!

Elizabeth H. Hammond, MD
Executive Editor, Pathology
Amirsys, Inc.

Paula J. Woodward, MD
President
Amirsys Publishing, Inc.

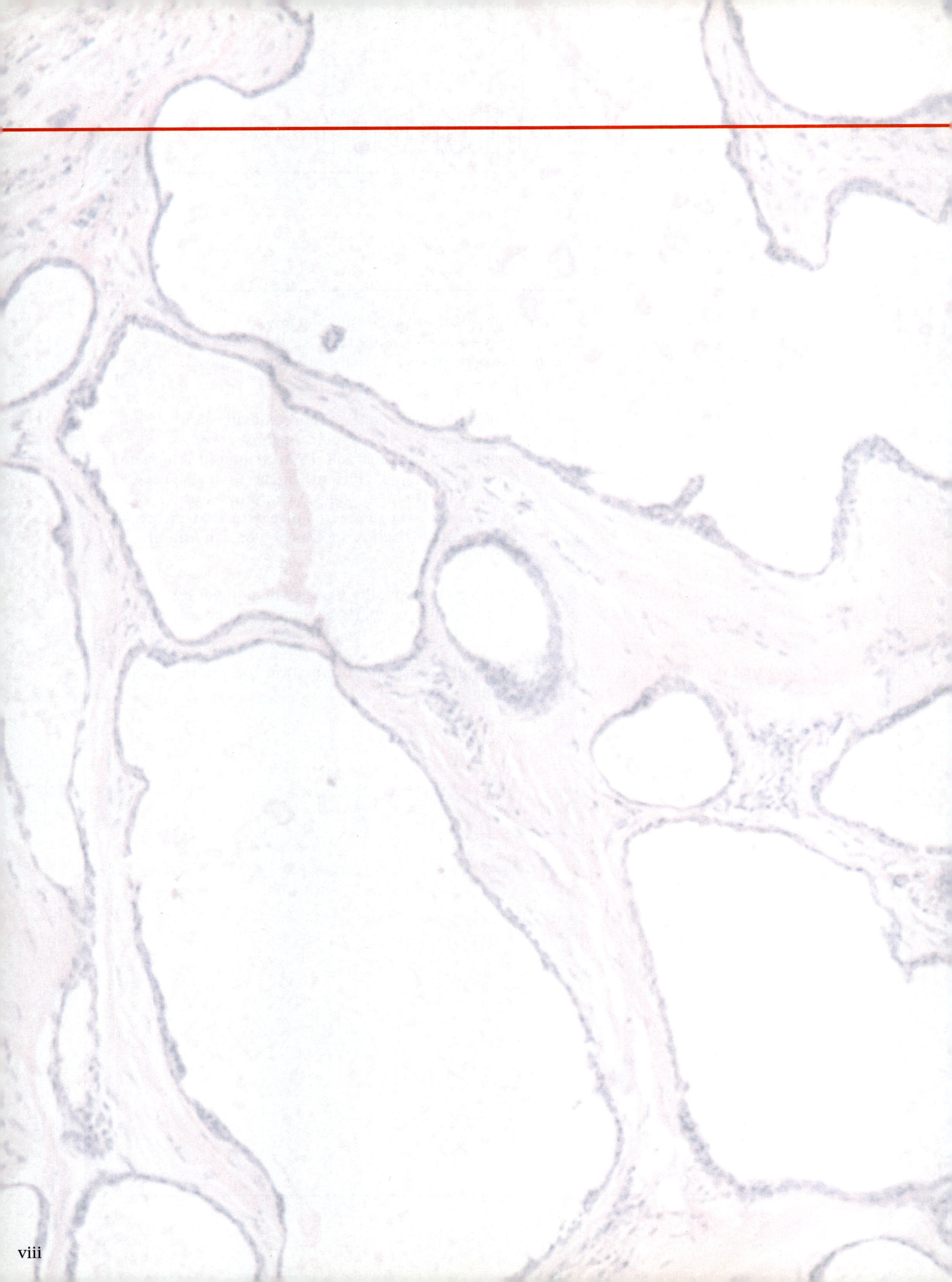

PREFACE

Thoracic pathology represents an important component of modern surgical pathology practice at most major medical centers. Although there are many excellent books and monographs on the topic, the purpose of this volume is to create a practical reference for practicing pathologists that emphasizes the visual spectrum of diseases of the chest cavity. As such, this book illustrates not only the different pathologic conditions, including unusual variations in morphology, but also features that may pose difficulties and represent pitfalls for diagnosis. The illustrations are accompanied by detailed explanations of the findings to help the reader understand subtle features that may be critical for diagnosis. Each chapter is accompanied by bulleted text that highlights the most salient and pertinent information on each subject, including a detailed list of differential diagnoses with helpful clues that orient the reader to the important differentiating points. Key facts are summarized separately in a box, and tables with pertinent information regarding immunohistochemical stains and other ancillary techniques are also provided. The user-friendly format of this book will help the reader get to the information faster and with fewer of the distractions that can result from a lengthy text.

We have endeavored to achieve a balanced perspective in the treatment of the various topics included in the book and to present the most up-to-date information available to us. However, the book draws heavily on the personal experience of the authors, and as such it may reflect a personal bias in the choice of terminology for some of the conditions described. We have tried to be all-inclusive and to present varying opinions and perspectives on controversial topics. A few topics have been left out of this volume (e.g., transplant pathology of the lung, pediatric and congenital lung diseases) because it was felt they were too sub-specialized for inclusion in a volume aimed at practicing general pathologists. It is hoped that this book will be of help to practicing surgical pathologists, as well as pathology residents and fellows in training, to quickly identify and check information that will help them resolve problems during routine signout of cases. The printed version has, as a companion, an online version that will undergo regular updates and will allow the reader enhanced access and flexibility for the use of this reference source.

We would like to thank the production team at Amirsys for the patience and support displayed during the lengthy production phase of this book. We also thank Elizabeth Hammond, MD, and Paula Woodward, MD, for their support and confidence in our ability to complete this volume. It has been our privilege to be able to share our experience with all of our colleagues.

Saul Suster, MD
Professor and Chairman
Department of Pathology and Laboratory Medicine
Medical College of Wisconsin
Milwaukee, WI

Cesar A. Moran, MD
Professor
Department of Pathology
The University of Texas M. D. Anderson Cancer Center
Houston, TX

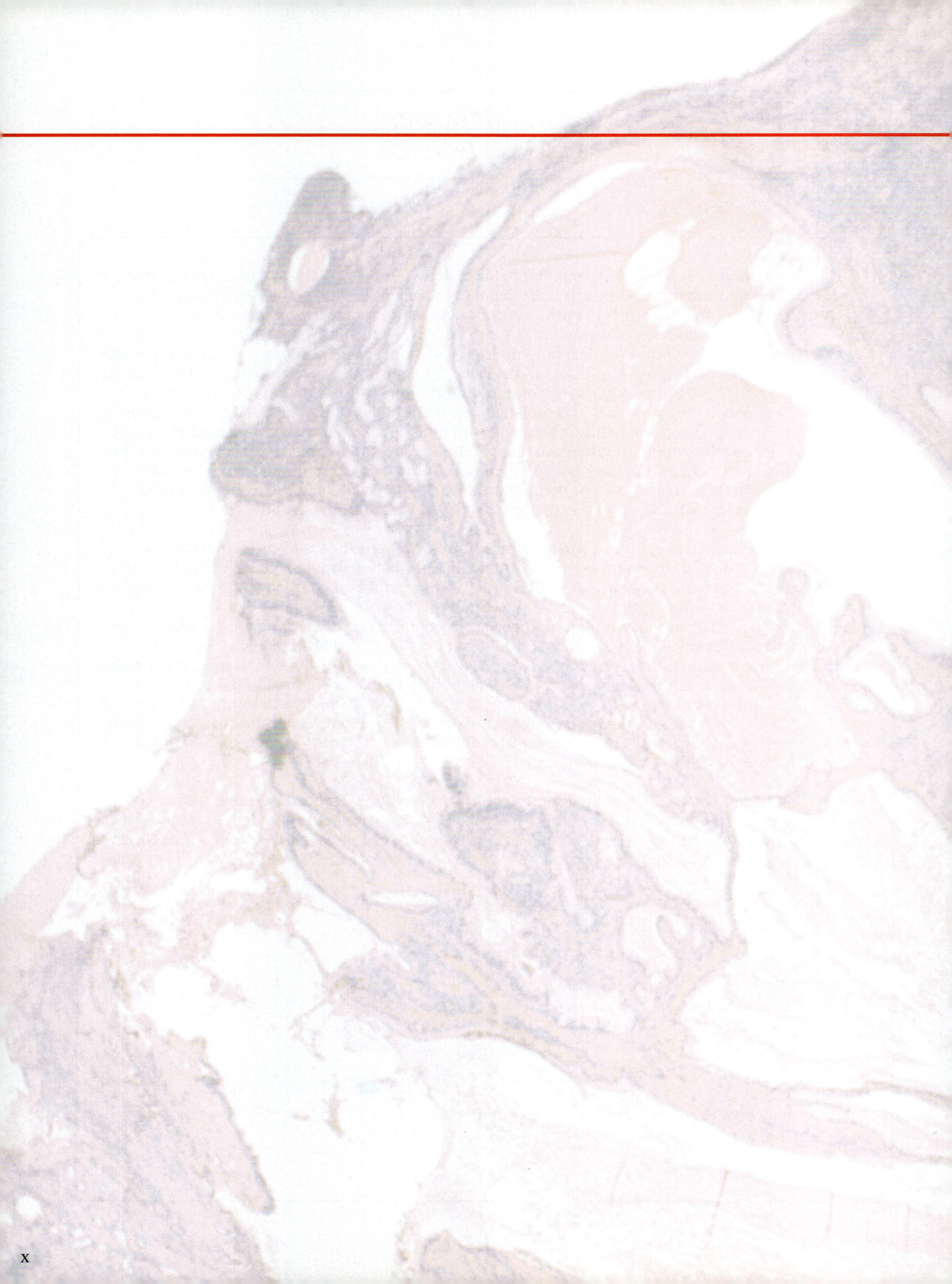

ACKNOWLEDGMENTS

Text Editing
Ashley R. Renlund, MA
Arthur G. Gelsinger, MA
Matthew R. Connelly, MA
Lorna Morring, MS
Alicia M. Moulton, BA
Rebecca L. Hutchinson, BA
Angela M. Green, BA

Image Editing
Jeffrey J. Marmorstone, BS
Lisa A. Magar, BS

Medical Text Editing
Neda Kalhor, MD

Illustrations
Lane R. Bennion, MS
Richard Coombs, MS
Laura C. Sesto, MA

Art Direction and Design
Laura C. Sesto, MA
Mirjam Ravneng

Assistant Editor
Dave L. Chance, MA

Publishing Lead
Kellie J. Heap, BA

AMIRSYS®
Names you know. Content you trust.®

SECTIONS

TABLE OF CONTENTS

PART I
Lung

SECTION 1
Neoplasms, Benign

SECTION 2
Neoplasms, Malignant, Primary

Epithelial Neoplasms

Salivary Gland-type Tumors

Mesenchymal Neoplasms

Lymphoproliferative Disorders

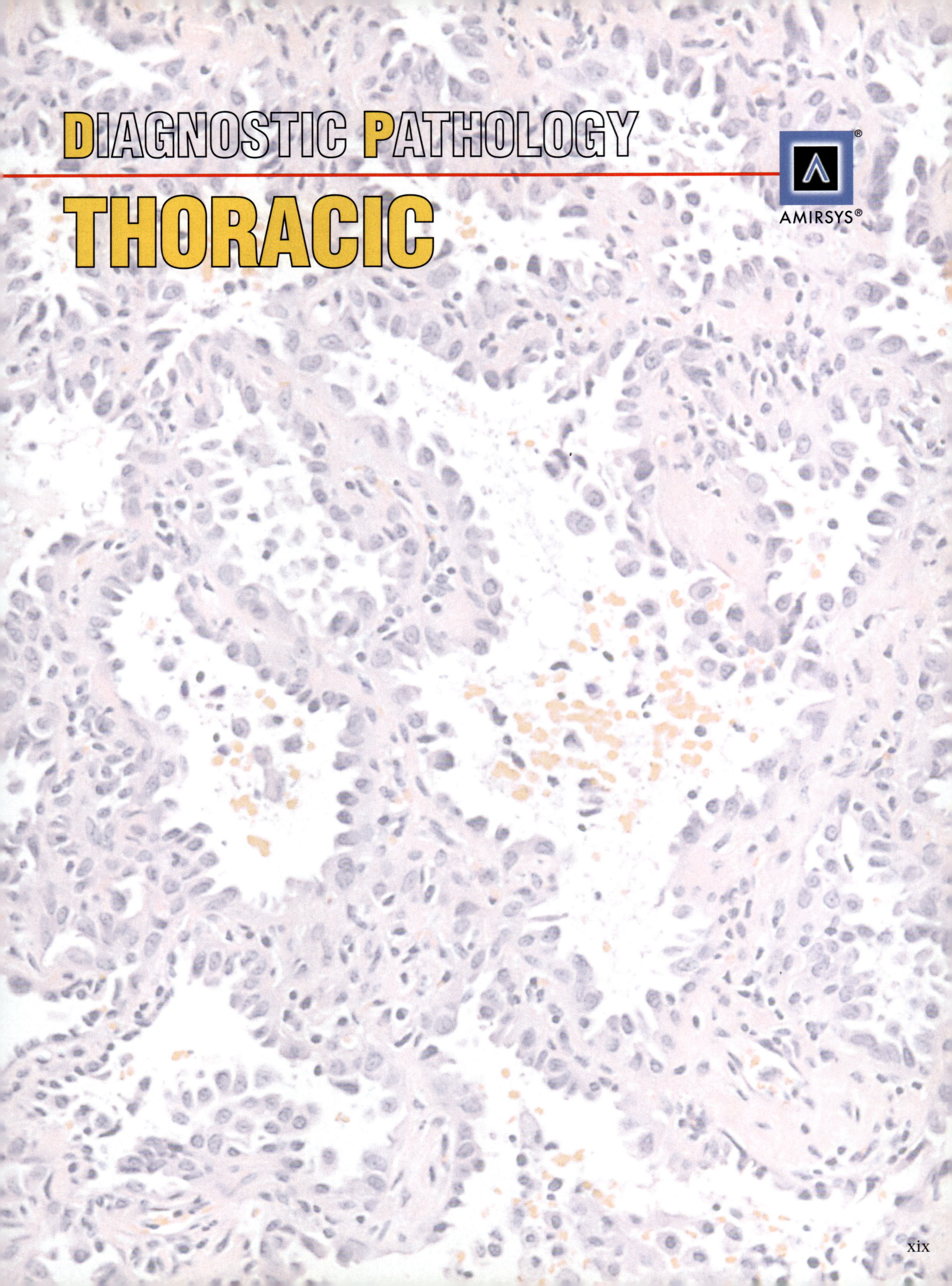

DIAGNOSTIC PATHOLOGY

THORACIC

AMIRSYS®

Other Rare Tumors and Benign Pseudotumoral Conditions

Lung Cancer Protocols

SECTION 3 Neoplasms, Metastatic

SECTION 4 Nonneoplastic and Systemic Conditions

SECTION 5 Parasitic Disorders

SECTION 6 Infectious Diseases

PART II
Pleura

SECTION 1
Neoplasms, Benign

SECTION 2
Neoplasms, Malignant, Primary

Epithelial Neoplasms

Pleural Mesothelioma Protocols

SECTION 3
Other Lesions of the Pleura

PART III
Mediastinum

SECTION 1
Neoplasms, Benign

SECTION 2
Neoplasms, Malignant, Primary

Epithelial Neoplasms

Germ Cell Tumors

Hematopoietic Malignancies

Mesenchymal Neoplasms

Sympathetic Nervous System Tumors

Other Tumors

Thymoma and Thymic Carcinoma Protocols

SECTION 3 Other Benign/Reactive Conditions

PART IV Reference

SECTION 1 Antibody Index

Neoplasms, Benign

CARTILAGINOUS HAMARTOMA

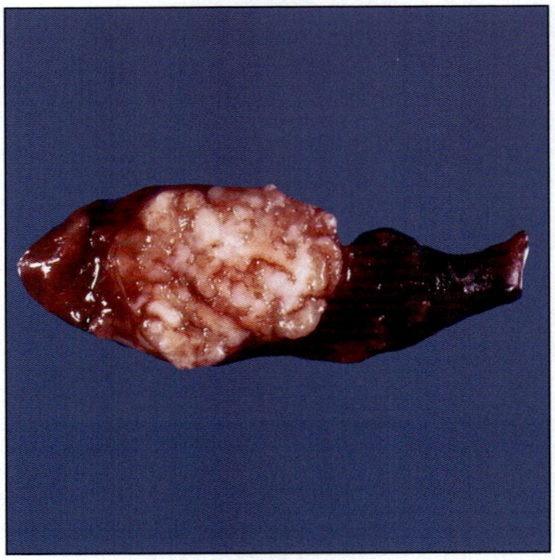

Gross photograph shows a well-circumscribed intrapulmonary tumor, slightly lobulated with a cartilaginous appearance. These features are classical for cartilaginous hamartoma.

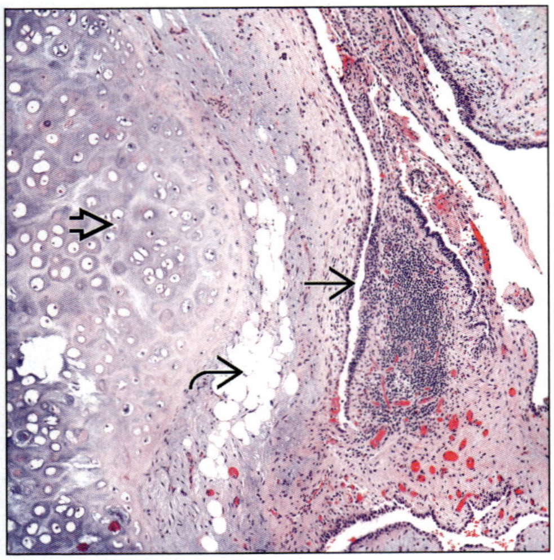

CH shows areas of well-formed cartilage ⇨, adipose tissue ⇗, and invaginated respiratory epithelium →. These features are characteristic of hamartoma.

TERMINOLOGY

Abbreviations

- Cartilaginous hamartoma (CH)

Synonyms

- Benign mesenchymoma

Definitions

- Benign mesenchymal tumor of the lung

ETIOLOGY/PATHOGENESIS

Pathogenesis

- It is not clear whether CH represents a true tumor or hamartomatous lesion
  - Thus, both terms, benign mesenchymoma and hamartoma, have been used interchangeably

CLINICAL ISSUES

Presentation

- Intrapulmonary coin lesion of variable size
- Central or peripheral tumor

Treatment

- Surgical approaches
  - Complete surgical resection

Prognosis

- Excellent prognosis; cured by simple excision

MACROSCOPIC FEATURES

General Features

- Well-circumscribed lesion
- Firm with mucoid and cartilaginous areas
- Usually solitary
- Rarely hamartomas may present as multiple intrapulmonary lesions

MICROSCOPIC PATHOLOGY

Histologic Features

- Mature cartilage
- Adipose tissue
- Myxoid stroma
- Invaginations of respiratory epithelium

Predominant Pattern/Injury Type

- Chondromyxoid

Predominant Cell/Compartment Type

- Cartilaginous

DIFFERENTIAL DIAGNOSIS

Bronchial Chondroma

- Does not show invaginations of respiratory epithelium
- Branchial chondroma rarely will show additional adipose tissue
- May be associated with other conditions, such as gastric smooth muscle tumors

Pleomorphic Adenoma (PA)

- Shows presence of epithelial component that immunophenotypically is myoepithelial
- PA in the lung rarely shows mature cartilage
- Also lacks presence of invaginations of respiratory epithelium

Chondrosarcoma, Primary or Metastatic

- Displays more cellular atypia
- Does not have admixture of adipose tissue
- Lacks presence of invaginations of respiratory epithelium
- Some cases of chondrosarcomas may arise from pre-existing hamartomas

CARTILAGINOUS HAMARTOMA

Key Facts

Terminology
- Benign mesenchymoma

Clinical Issues
- Intrapulmonary coin lesion of variable size
- Central or peripheral tumor
- Complete surgical resection
- Excellent prognosis

Macroscopic Features
- Well-circumscribed lesion
- Firm with mucoid and cartilaginous areas
- Usually a single lesion
- Rarely hamartomas may present as multiple intrapulmonary lesions

Top Differential Diagnoses
- Bronchial chondromas
  - Do not show invaginations of respiratory epithelium
  - May be associated with other conditions, such as gastric smooth muscle tumors
- Pleomorphic adenoma
  - Shows presence of epithelial component that immunophenotypically is myoepithelial
  - PA in the lung rarely will show mature cartilage
  - Also lacks presence of invaginations of respiratory epithelium
- Chondrosarcoma
  - Will display more cellular atypia
  - Does not have admixture of adipose tissue
  - Lacks presence of invaginations of respiratory epithelium

Immunohistochemistry

Antibody	Reactivity	Staining Pattern	Comment
CK-PAN	Positive	Cytoplasmic	In invaginated respiratory epithelium
S100	Positive	Nuclear	Chondroid component
EMA	Positive	Cell membrane	Respiratory epithelium
SOX9	Positive	Nuclear	Cartilage
Desmin	Positive	Cytoplasmic	In muscle component
Vimentin	Positive	Cytoplasmic	
CD34	Positive	Cytoplasmic	In vessels and adipose tissue

- In cases of metastatic disease, clinical history is the most important feature

Bronchial Lipomas
- Almost exclusively composed of adipose tissue
- Lipomas do not display areas of cartilage
- Great majority of lipomas are in central location, whereas hamartomas are more common in periphery

Bronchial Teratoma
- Teratomas show tissues from the 3 germinal layers
- Skin appendages are commonly seen in teratomas and are absent in hamartomas
- Hair and teeth are commonly seen in teratomas and are absent in hamartomas
- Teratomas are predominantly cystic, whereas hamartomas are more commonly solid tumors

DIAGNOSTIC CHECKLIST

Clinically Relevant Pathologic Features
- Cartilaginous gross appearance

Pathologic Interpretation Pearls
- Chondromyxoid tumor with invaginations of respiratory epithelium
- Mature cartilage
- Areas of ossification may be present
- Presence of adipose tissue
- Well-circumscribed tumor lesion

SELECTED REFERENCES

1. Park CM et al: Images in clinical medicine. "Popcorn" calcifications in a pulmonary chondroid hamartoma. N Engl J Med. 360(12):e17, 2009
2. de Almeida LF et al: Giant pulmonary hamartoma. J Thorac Imaging. 23(3):188-90, 2008
3. Guo W et al: Surgical treatment and outcome of pulmonary hamartoma: a retrospective study of 20-year experience. J Exp Clin Cancer Res. 27:8, 2008
4. Ozbudak IH et al: Giant cystic chondroid hamartoma of the lung. J Pediatr Surg. 43(10):1909-11, 2008
5. Kang MW et al: Multiple central endobronchial chondroid hamartoma. Ann Thorac Surg. 83(2):691-3, 2007
6. Bini A et al: Multiple chondromatous hamartomas of the lung. Interact Cardiovasc Thorac Surg. 1(2):78-80, 2002
7. van den Bosch JM et al: Mesenchymoma of the lung (so called hamartoma): a review of 154 parenchymal and endobronchial cases. Thorax. 42(10):790-3, 1987
8. Tomashefski JF Jr: Benign endobronchial mesenchymal tumors: their relationship to parenchymal pulmonary hamartomas. Am J Surg Pathol. 6(6):531-40, 1982
9. Minasian H: Uncommon pulmonary hamartomas. Thorax. 32(3):360-4, 1977
10. Ray JF 3rd et al: The coin lesion story: update 1976. Twenty years' experience with thoracotomy for 179 suspected malignant coin lesions. Chest. 70(03):332-6, 1976
11. Bateson EM: So-called hamartoma of the lung--a true neoplasm of fibrous connective tissue of the bronchi. Cancer. 31(6):1458-67, 1973

CARTILAGINOUS HAMARTOMA

Microscopic Features

__(Left)__ Peripheral areas of a CH show extensive myxoid changes ⇨ and inflammatory infiltrate ➡. The sole presence of cartilage should raise the suspicion of pulmonary hamartoma. __(Right)__ CH shows slight lobulation separated by invaginated respiratory epithelium. Note that there is not well-formed cartilage but rather myxoid change.

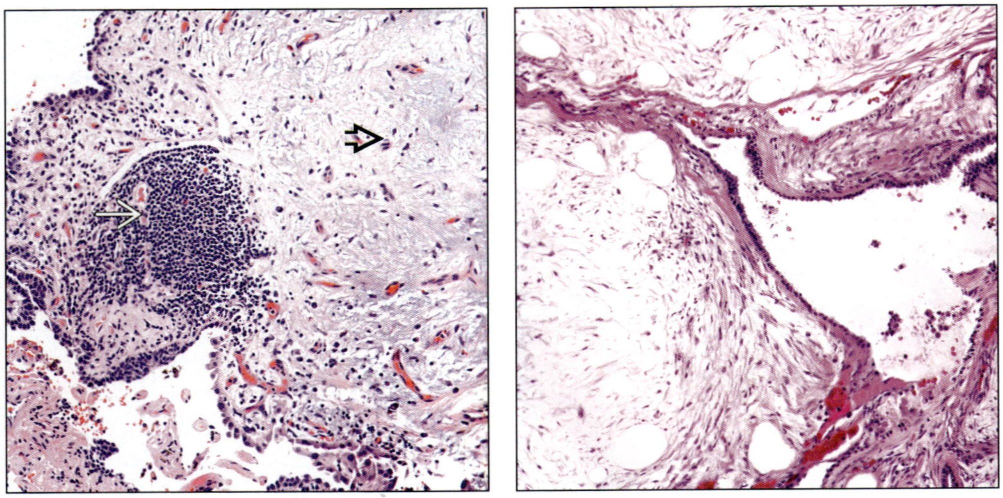

__(Left)__ CH is shown with different components in which the tumor shows predominantly mature cartilage ⇨, areas of adipose tissue ↷, and entrapped epithelial elements →. These are the classic features of a hamartoma. __(Right)__ High-power magnification shows a myxoid area in a pulmonary hamartoma. Note the spindle cell proliferation in a myxoid background. Similar features may be seen in other mesenchymal tumors.

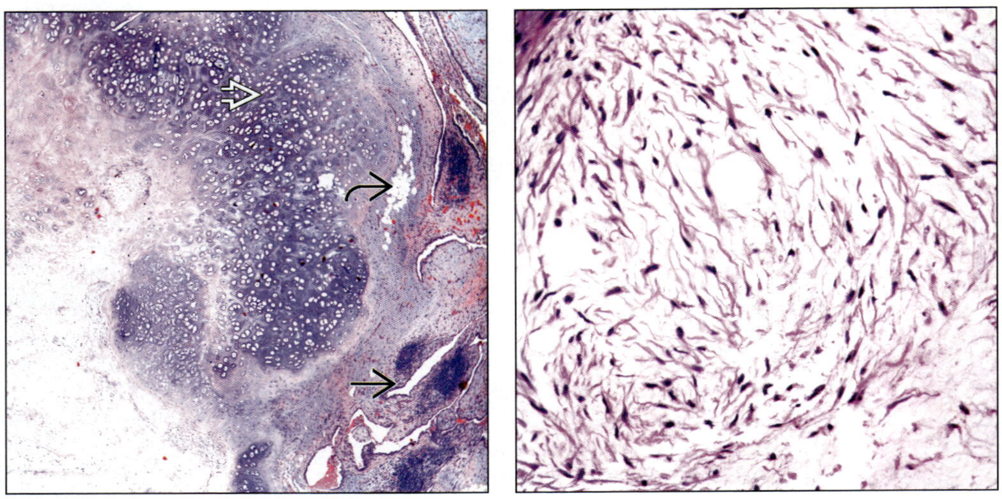

__(Left)__ Pulmonary hamartoma shows extensive areas of muscle differentiation ↷ with entrapped alveolar structures →. In some unusual cases, the presence of muscle may be more extensive with only focal areas of cartilage. __(Right)__ High-power view shows the adipose tissue component in a pulmonary hamartoma. Note the presence of mature adipose tissue with areas of myxoid change ↷ similar to that seen in true lipomatous tumors.

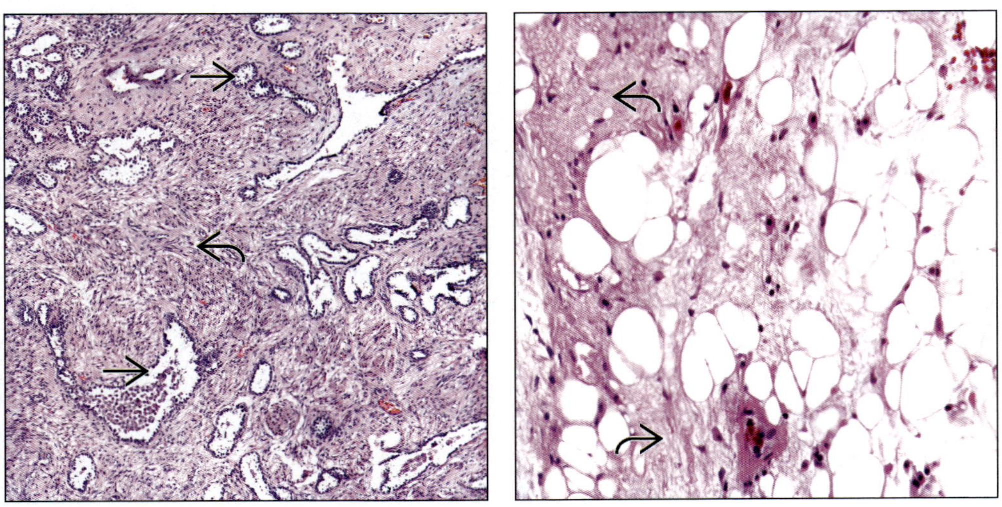

CARTILAGINOUS HAMARTOMA

Microscopic Features

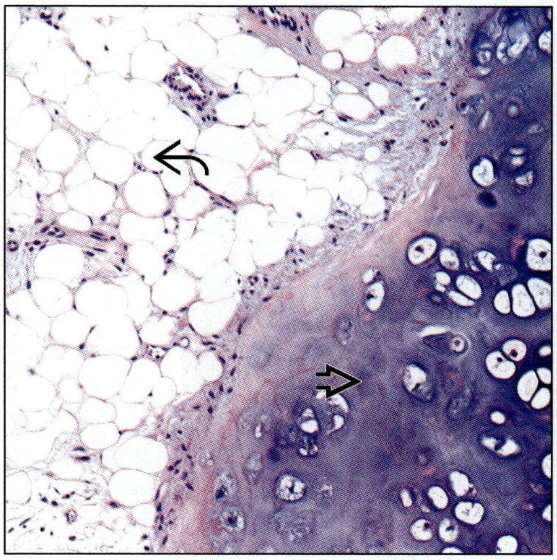

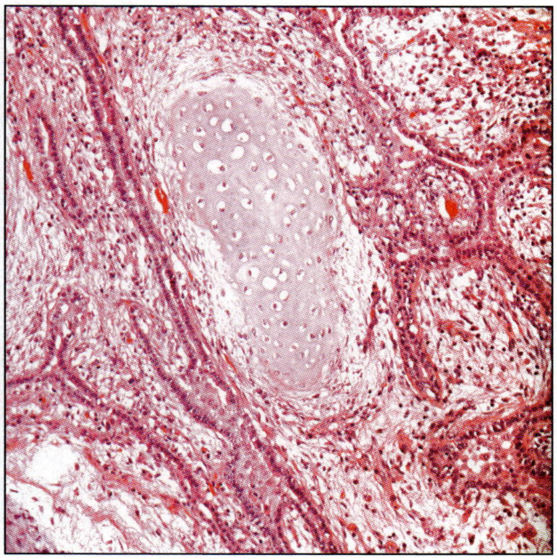

(Left) Pulmonary hamartoma shows the typical features of mature cartilaginous ⇨ and adipose tissue ↗. These 2 components may be seen in different proportions. **(Right)** Mature cartilage and compressed lung parenchyma may also be present in CH. In this case, the cartilaginous component is rather minimal, while the lesion displays more prominent epithelial invaginations with associated myxoid change in the stroma.

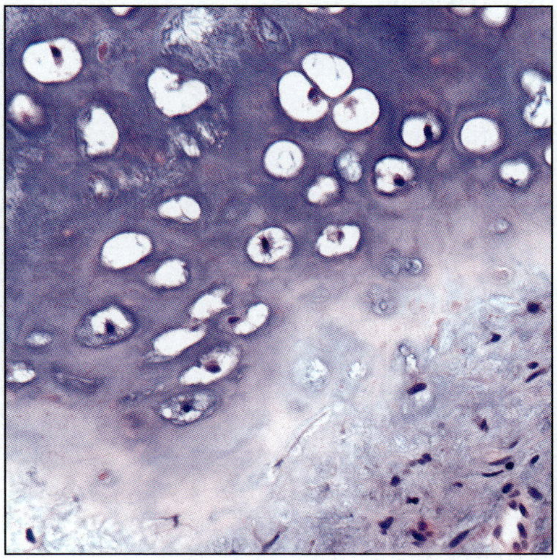

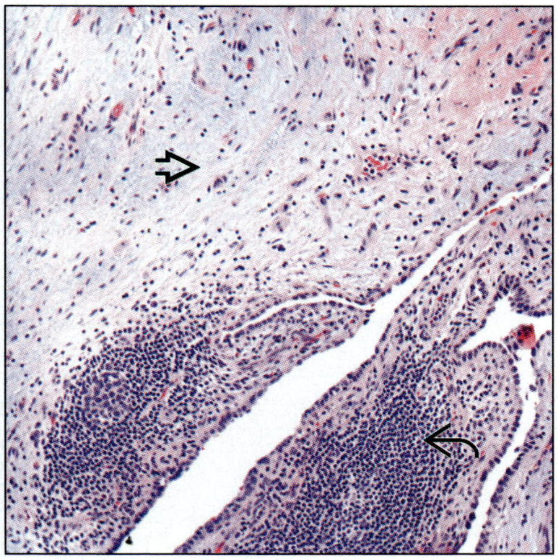

(Left) High-power view shows the cartilaginous component in a pulmonary hamartoma. Note the absence of nuclear atypia or mitotic activity, which is useful in separating these lesions from other malignant cartilaginous tumors. **(Right)** CH shows areas in which the respiratory epithelium shows inflammatory changes and lymphoid hyperplasia ↗. Note the presence of myxoid areas with an inflammatory reaction ⇨.

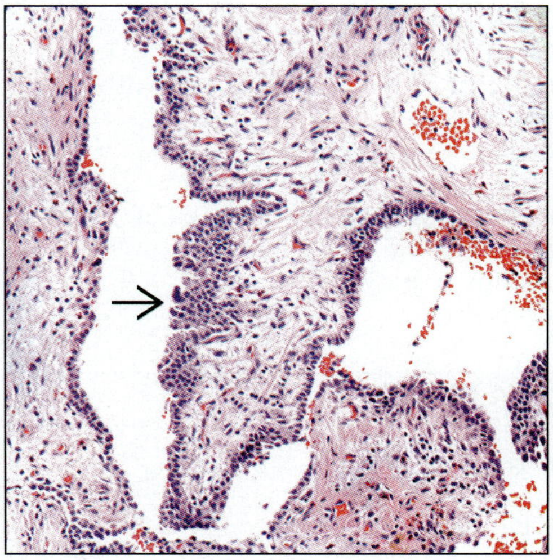

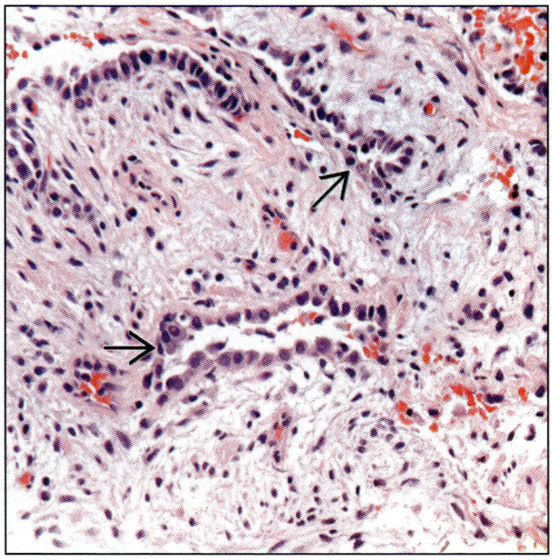

(Left) Closer view shows the entrapped epithelial component of a CH with focal hyperplastic changes →. The epithelial component associated with pulmonary hamartomas does not show any cellular atypia or dysplastic changes. **(Right)** Entrapped epithelial structures representing alveoli → admixed with focal areas of myxoid change. These changes by themselves are not diagnostic of pulmonary hamartoma as they may be seen in other conditions.

ALVEOLAR ADENOMA

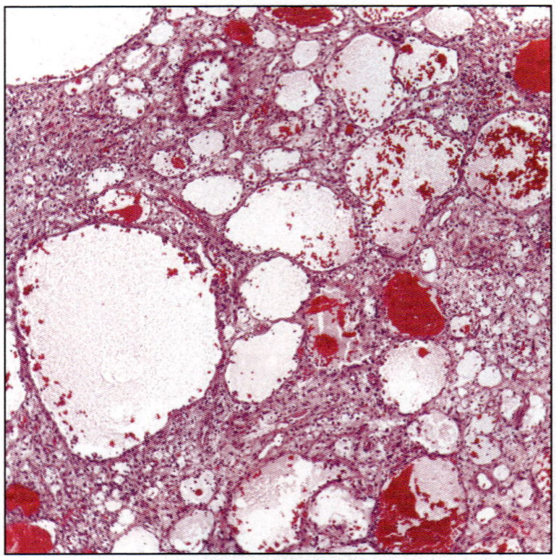

Pulmonary alveolar adenoma shows characteristic cystic areas alternating with more solid areas. The low power mimics a vascular neoplasm.

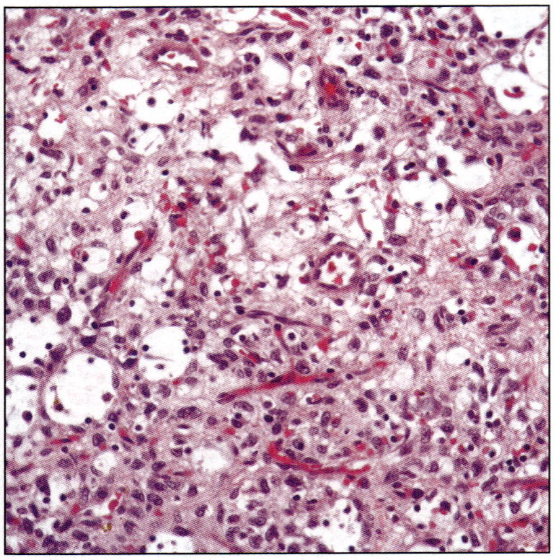

Alveolar adenoma shows a more solid proliferation in which the cells appear to have clear cytoplasm. Note the absence of cellular atypia or mitotic activity.

TERMINOLOGY

Definitions

- Benign intraparenchymal lung tumor

ETIOLOGY/PATHOGENESIS

Etiology

- Although the etiology of this tumor is not completely understood, it may originate from pneumocytes

CLINICAL ISSUES

Epidemiology

- Incidence
  - Rare tumor
- Age
  - Generally in adults
- Gender
  - No gender predilection
- Ethnicity
  - No ethnic predilection

Site

- Intrapulmonary mass

Presentation

- Cough
- Chest pain
- Asymptomatic

Treatment

- Surgical approaches
  - Lobectomy
  - Wedge resection

Prognosis

- Excellent

IMAGE FINDINGS

General Features

- Location
  - Solitary pulmonary mass

MACROSCOPIC FEATURES

General Features

- Tumors may be cystic and hemorrhagic

Size

- Tumors may vary from 1-3 cm in diameter

MICROSCOPIC PATHOLOGY

Histologic Features

- Well circumscribed
- Generally cystic appearance
- Dilated spaces of different sizes
- Clear acellular material within cystic areas
- Dilated spaces lined by medium-sized cells with hobnail appearance
- Focal areas of glandular appearance
- Alternating solid areas
- Mild inflammatory component composed of lymphocytes and plasma cells
- Absence of mitotic activity
- Absence of necrosis

ANCILLARY TESTS

Histochemistry

- PAS-diastase
  - Reactivity: Positive

ALVEOLAR ADENOMA

Key Facts

Terminology
- Benign intraparenchymal lung tumor

Etiology/Pathogenesis
- Although the etiology of this tumor is not completely understood, it may originate from pneumocytes

Clinical Issues
- General features
  - Unusual occurrence
  - Generally in adults
  - Solitary pulmonary lesion
  - Cough
  - Chest pain
- Treatment
  - Lobectomy
  - Wedge resection
- Prognosis
  - Excellent

Microscopic Pathology
- Well circumscribed
- Generally cystic appearance
- Dilated spaces of different sizes
- Clear acellular material within cystic areas
- PAS-positive material

Top Differential Diagnoses
- Adenocarcinoma
- Bronchioloalveolar carcinoma
- Lymphangioma
- Glomus tumor

Immunohistochemistry

Antibody	Reactivity	Staining Pattern	Comment
CK-PAN	Positive	Cytoplasmic	Strong diffuse staining
EMA	Positive	Cell membrane	Strong and diffuse
Surfactant	Positive	Cytoplasmic	May be focal
TTF-1	Positive	Nuclear	May be focal in some cells lining cystic spaces and in some solid areas
CD31	Negative		
CD34	Negative		
FVIIIRAg	Negative		
S100	Negative		
D2-40	Negative		
Actin-sm	Negative		

DIFFERENTIAL DIAGNOSIS

Adenocarcinoma
- Cellular atypia and mitotic activity
- More solid or glandular component

Bronchioloalveolar Carcinoma
- Displays a lepidic growth pattern
- Shows mucinous component
- It would be unusual for bronchioloalveolar carcinoma to show cystic component

Lymphangioma
- Dilated lymphatic spaces
- It would be unusual for lymphangioma to show cystic and solid components
- May show positive staining for D2-40, whereas alveolar adenoma will be negative

Glomus Tumor
- Cystic and solid areas similar to alveolar adenoma
- Strong positive staining for actin

DIAGNOSTIC CHECKLIST

Clinically Relevant Pathologic Features
- Most patients are asymptomatic

Pathologic Interpretation Pearls
- Cystic and solid areas
- Acellular material within cystic spaces
- PAS-positive material in cystic spaces
- Absence of necrosis and mitotic activity

SELECTED REFERENCES

1. Petrella F et al: Giant alveolar adenoma causing severe dyspnoea. J Thorac Oncol. 5(7):1088-90, 2010
2. Cakan A et al: Alveolar adenoma: an unusual lung tumor. Interact Cardiovasc Thorac Surg. 2(3):345-7, 2003
3. Yousem SA et al: Alveolar adenoma. Hum Pathol. 17(10):1066-71, 1986

ALVEOLAR ADENOMA

Microscopic Features

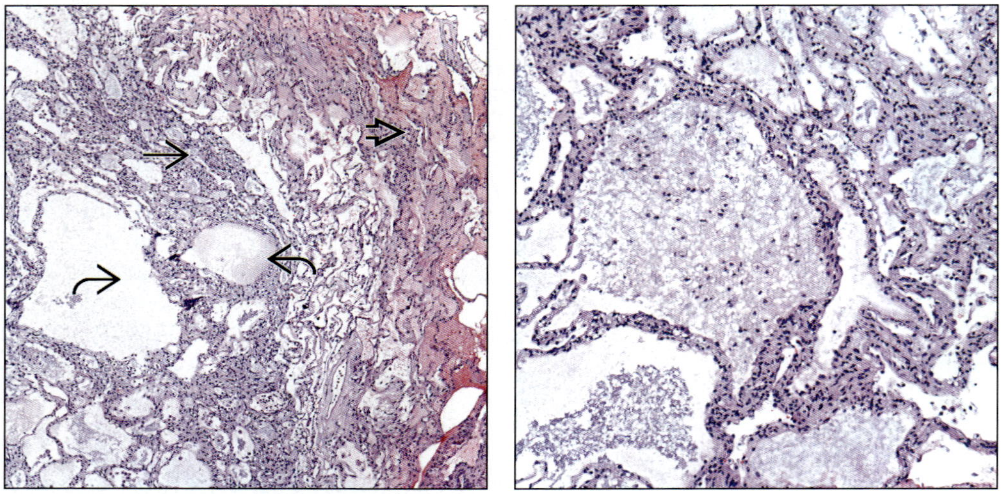

(Left) *Alveolar adenoma shows cystic areas admixed with solid areas. Note that the lesion is well circumscribed. Adjacent lung parenchyma appears to be congested.* ***(Right)*** *Cystically dilated areas in this alveolar adenoma contain clear fluid and scattered macrophages. The lining is flattened, and the appearance is that of a distended alveolar structure.*

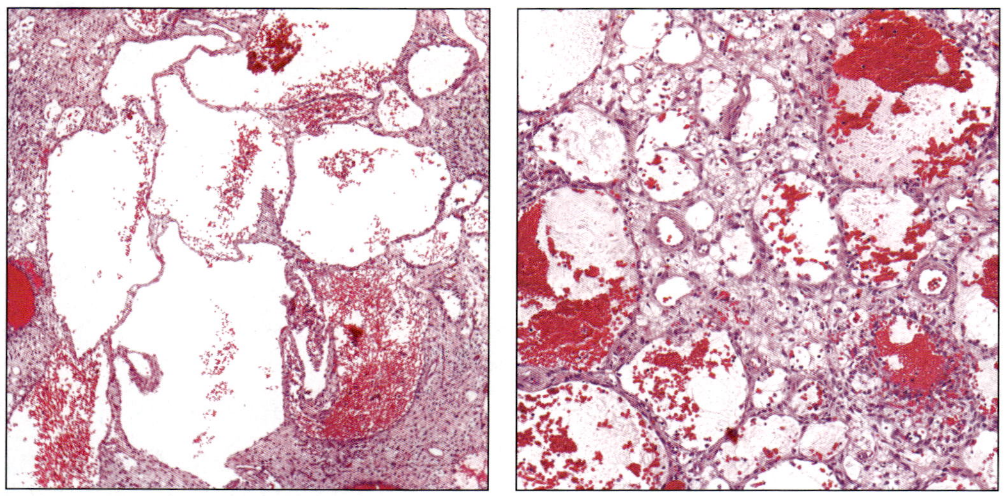

(Left) *In some areas, the cystic areas closely mimic a vascular neoplasm, and they can be confused for distended lymphatics or other vascular structures. Note that the cystic structures do not contain fluid.* ***(Right)*** *Cystically dilated areas of different sizes, some containing fresh blood, are shown. This feature can easily be confused with a hemangioma.*

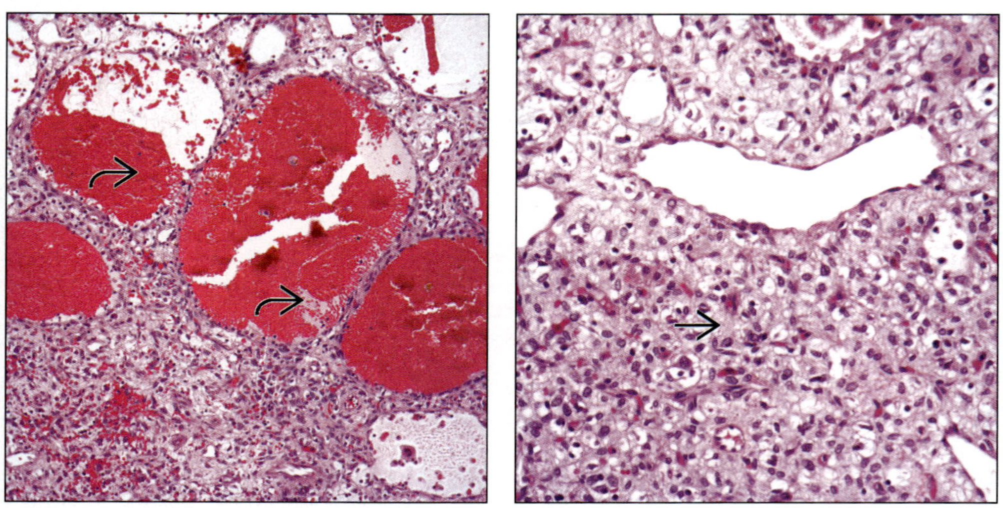

(Left) *Cystically dilated areas containing fresh blood admixed with more solid cellular proliferation are shown. However, the cystic structures are not lined by endothelial cells.* ***(Right)*** *Solid areas of an alveolar adenoma show a small cystically dilated area and a subtle hemangiopericytic appearance. In the solid component the cells appear to have clear cell cytoplasm.*

ALVEOLAR ADENOMA

Microscopic Features

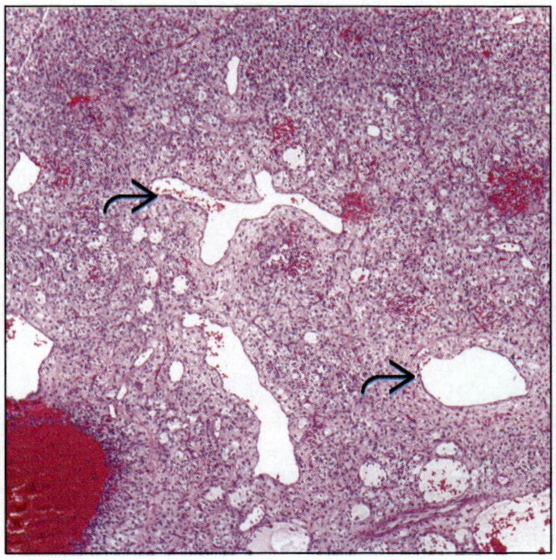

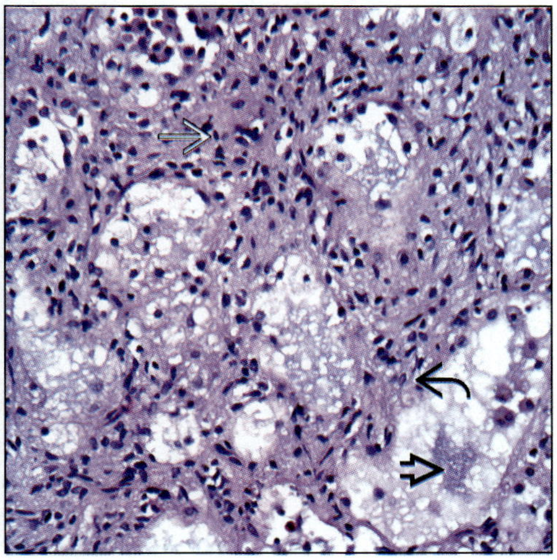

(Left) *Low-power view shows an alveolar adenoma mimicking a hemangiopericytic growth pattern. The dilated spaces → can be easily confused for vascular structures at this magnification.* ***(Right)*** *Alveolar adenoma shows more cellular areas → admixed with cystic areas →. Interestingly, the material in the lumens of the cystic areas appears to be more chondroid-like →.*

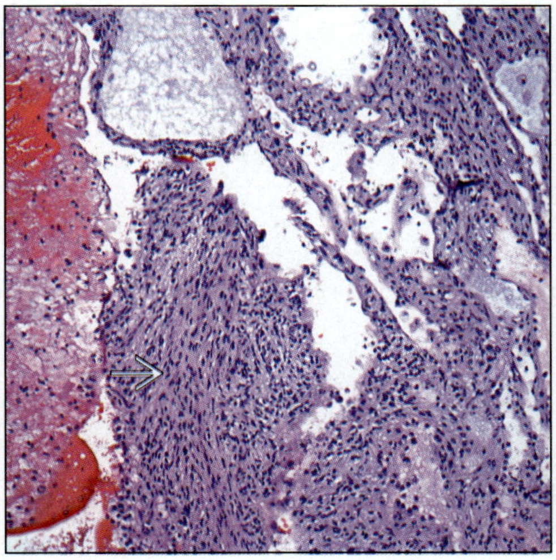

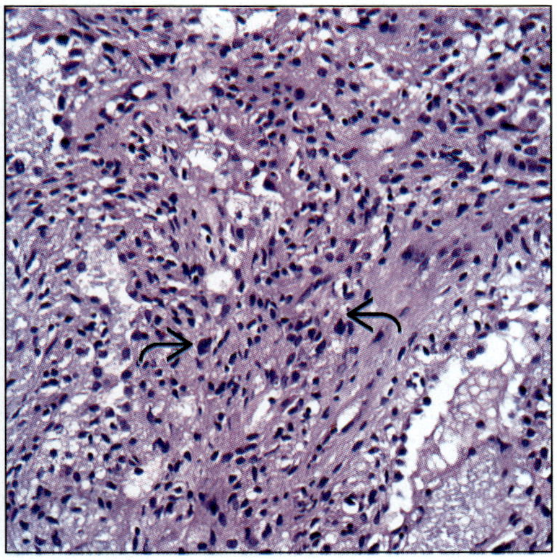

(Left) *In some focal areas, the solid component of an alveolar adenoma may take the form of a spindle cell proliferation →. However, these areas lack nuclear atypia and mitotic activity.* ***(Right)*** *Closer magnification of the solid spindle cell component, which closely mimics a neural tumor, is shown. Although there are some pyknotic nuclei →, there is no mitotic activity.*

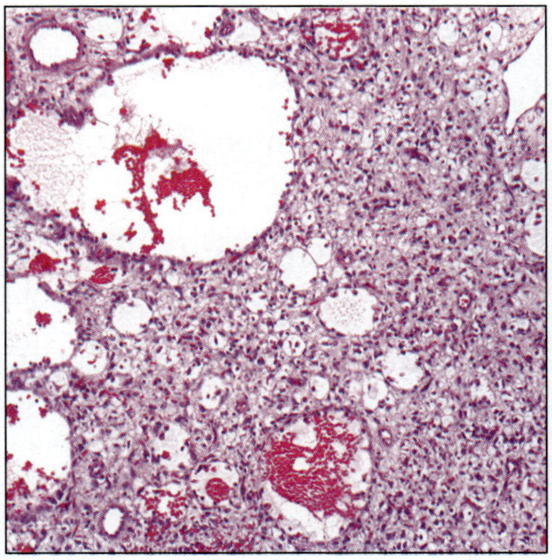

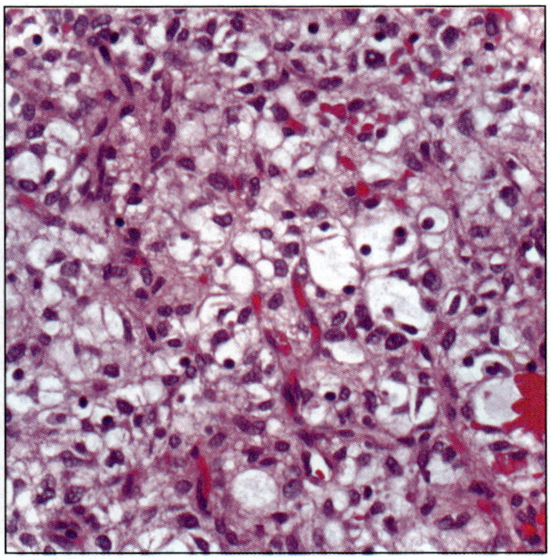

(Left) *Alveolar adenoma shows the more conventional histology consisting of cystic areas admixed with solid areas. The cystic areas contain fresh blood or clear acellular fluid.* ***(Right)*** *Solid areas in an alveolar adenoma with a clear cell appearance are shown. Note the absence of nuclear atypia and mitotic activity.*

MUCOUS GLAND ADENOMA

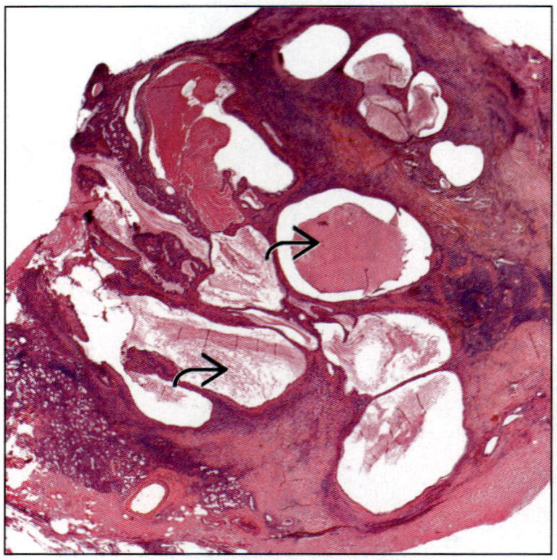

Low-power view shows a mucous gland adenoma of the lung with abnormal dilatation ⮫ of endobronchial glands.

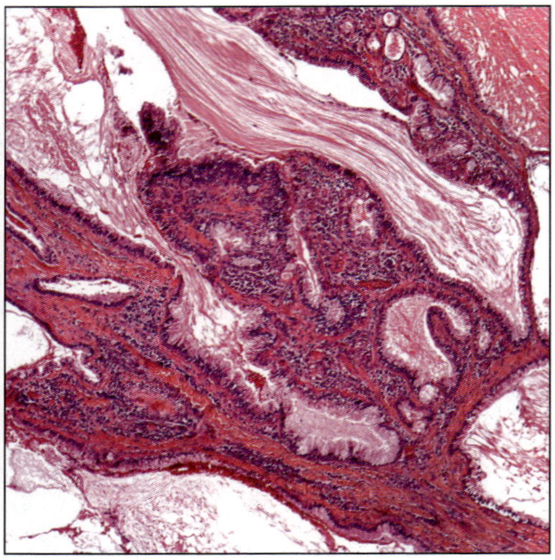

High-power view of a mucous gland adenoma shows dilated endobronchial glands displaying an absence of mitotic activity or nuclear atypia. Note the presence of mucous material in the lumen of the glands.

TERMINOLOGY

Synonyms

- Bronchial adenoma

Definitions

- Benign tumor characterized by exuberant enlargement of normal endobronchial glands filled with mucous content lying above cartilaginous plate

ETIOLOGY/PATHOGENESIS

Etiology

- Exuberant dilatation and proliferation of normal endobronchial glands with mucoid material in lumens
- Enlargement of normal endobronchial glands

CLINICAL ISSUES

Epidemiology

- Incidence
  - Rare tumors
- Age
  - May occur at any age
- Gender
  - No gender predilection

Site

- Tumor is central in endobronchial location

Presentation

- Cough
- Hemoptysis
- Chest pain
- Difficulty breathing
- Asymptomatic

Treatment

- Surgical approaches
  - Conservative surgical excision

Prognosis

- Excellent prognosis

MACROSCOPIC FEATURES

General Features

- Exophytic endobronchial tumor
- Varying tumor size from 0.8-6 cm
- Well circumscribed
- Cystic, soft, contain jelly-like material

MICROSCOPIC PATHOLOGY

Histologic Features

- Tumor does not extend beyond cartilaginous (bronchial) plate

Predominant Pattern/Injury Type

- Cystic
- Tubulo-papillary
- Tubular cysts

Predominant Cell/Compartment Type

- Epithelial, glandular

DIFFERENTIAL DIAGNOSIS

Mucoepidermoid Carcinoma

- Invades beyond cartilaginous (bronchial) plate into adjacent lung parenchyma
- May share similar histopathological features with mucous gland adenomas
- Presence of glandular proliferation of different sizes is more in favor of mucus gland adenoma

MUCOUS GLAND ADENOMA

Key Facts

Terminology
- Benign tumor characterized by exuberant enlargement of normal endobronchial glands filled with mucous content above cartilaginous plate

Etiology/Pathogenesis
- Exuberant dilatation and proliferation of normal endobronchial glands with mucoid material in lumens
- Enlargement of normal endobronchial glands

Clinical Issues
- Difficulty breathing
- Chest pain
- Cough
- Hemoptysis
- Asymptomatic
- Tumor is central in endobronchial location

Macroscopic Features
- Exophytic endobronchial tumors
- Varying tumor size from 0.8-6 cm
- Well-circumscribed tumors
- Cystic, soft, contain jelly-like material

Microscopic Pathology
- Cystic
- Tubulo-papillary
- Tubular cysts
- Epithelial, glandular
- Tumor does not extend beyond cartilaginous (bronchial) plate

Top Differential Diagnoses
- Mucoepidermoid carcinoma

Immunohistochemistry

Antibody	Reactivity	Staining Pattern	Comment
CK-PAN	Positive	Cytoplasmic	Diffuse
EMA/MUC1	Positive	Cell membrane	Diffuse
CEA-M	Positive	Cytoplasmic	Diffuse
TTF-1	Positive	Nuclear	
p63	Positive	Nuclear	In the squamous component
CK7	Positive	Cytoplasmic	
CDX-2	Negative		
CK20	Negative		

Histochemical Features of Mucous Gland Adenoma

Histochemical Stain	Result	Location
Mucicarmine	Positive	In columnar cells
D-PAS	Positive	In columnar cells
PAS	Positive	In acinar cells

Adenocarcinoma
- Nuclear pleomorphism, mitotic activity are features of adenocarcinoma
  - In bronchial adenomas, abnormal dilatation of normal endobronchial glands
  - Glandular proliferation is of different-sized glands
  - Mixture of seromucinous and dilated glandular structures is more in keeping with adenoma

DIAGNOSTIC CHECKLIST

Clinically Relevant Pathologic Features
- Gross appearance

Pathologic Interpretation Pearls
- Tumor confined between bronchial epithelium and bronchial cartilage

SELECTED REFERENCES

1. Milenković B et al: Mucous gland adenoma simulating bronchial asthma: case report and literature review. J Asthma. 44(9):789-93, 2007
2. Méjean-Lebreton F et al: [Benign salivary gland-type tumors of the bronchus: expression of high molecular weight cytokeratins.] Ann Pathol. 26(1):30-4, 2006
3. Morini F et al: Bronchial adenoma: an unusual cause of recurrent pneumonia in childhood. Ann Thorac Surg. 76(6):2085-7, 2003
4. Kwon JW et al: Mucous gland adenoma of the bronchus: CT findings in two patients. J Comput Assist Tomogr. 23(5):758-60, 1999
5. England DM et al: Truly benign "bronchial adenoma". Report of 10 cases of mucous gland adenoma with immunohistochemical and ultrastructural findings. Am J Surg Pathol. 19(8):887-99, 1995
6. Dickstein PJ et al: Bronchial mucous gland adenoma presenting as bronchogenic cyst. Pediatr Pulmonol. 16(6):370-4, 1993
7. Pass HI: Bronchial adenoma. Ann Thorac Surg. 52(5):1201-3, 1991

MUCOUS GLAND ADENOMA

Microscopic Features

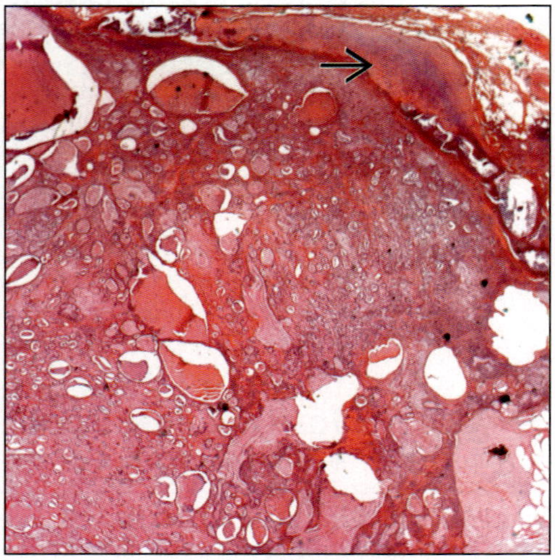
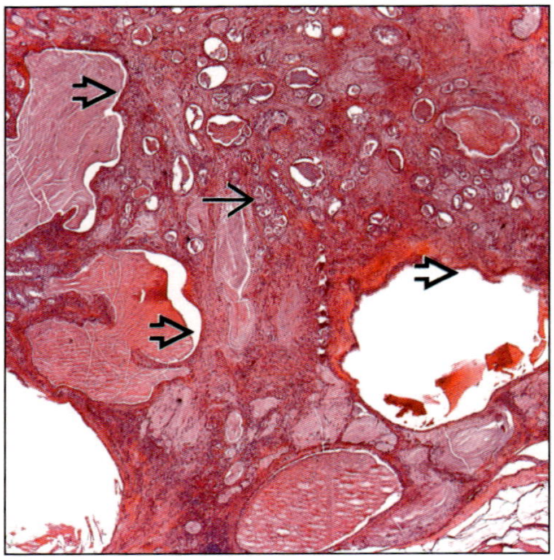

(Left) *Mucous gland adenoma shows a characteristic cystic growth pattern admixed with more solid areas. Note that the tumor does not penetrate beyond the cartilaginous (bronchial) plate* ⇒. ***(Right)*** *Mucus gland adenoma is shown with cystically dilated glands* ⇨. *The tumor also displays areas of solid proliferation adjacent to the dilated glands* ⇒. *All these changes represent enlargement of normal bronchial structures.*

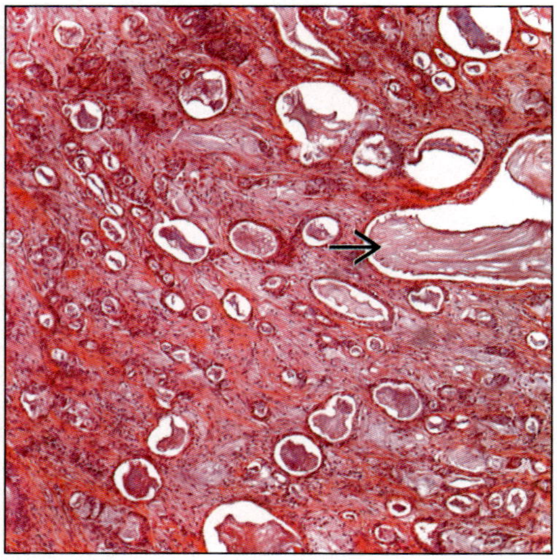
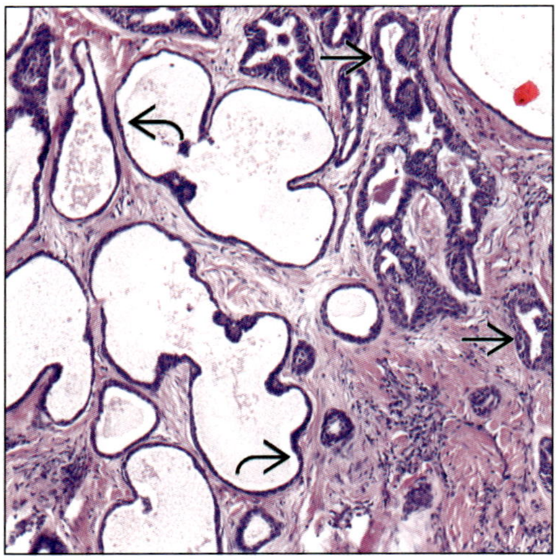

(Left) *Mucus gland adenoma is shown with small cystically dilated glands lined by squamous epithelium. More dilated glands are also present* ⇒. *This low-power view may also be seen in cases of low-grade bronchial mucoepidermoid carcinoma.* ***(Right)*** *Mucous gland adenoma shows a range of dilated glandular structures. Some glands are dilated with flattened epithelium* ↷ *while other glands are compressed and appear to be within normal limits* ⇒.

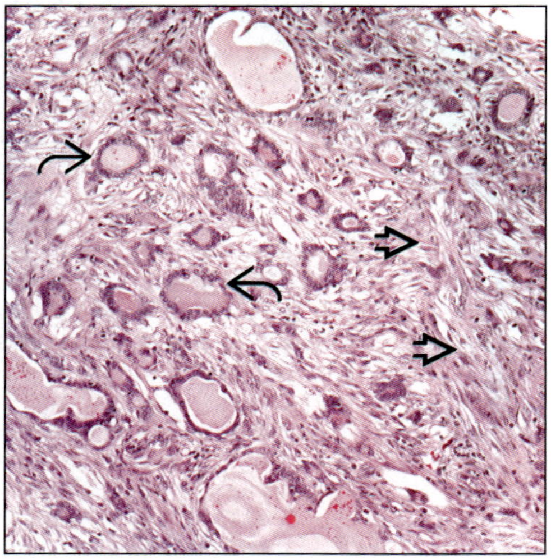
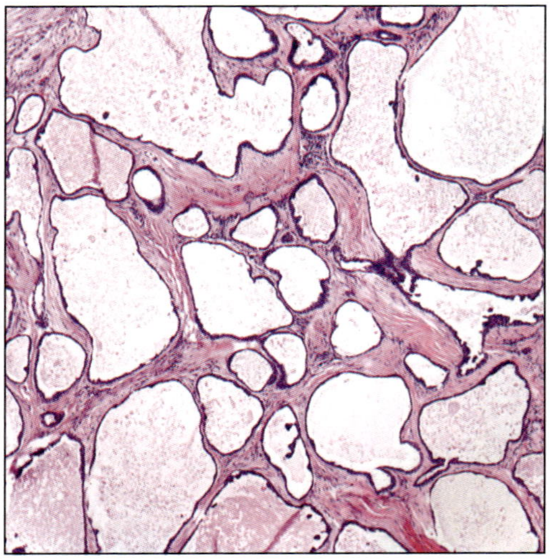

(Left) *Low-power view of a mucous gland adenoma shows a proliferation of glandular structures* ↷ *embedded in a spindle cell stroma* ⇨. *This particular pattern may also be seen in salivary gland-type tumors of the lung.* ***(Right)*** *Mucus gland adenoma is shown with dilated glands lined by flattened epithelium. Inside the glands, there is mucous secretion. The glands are separated by bands of collagenous tissue.*

MUCOUS GLAND ADENOMA

Microscopic Features

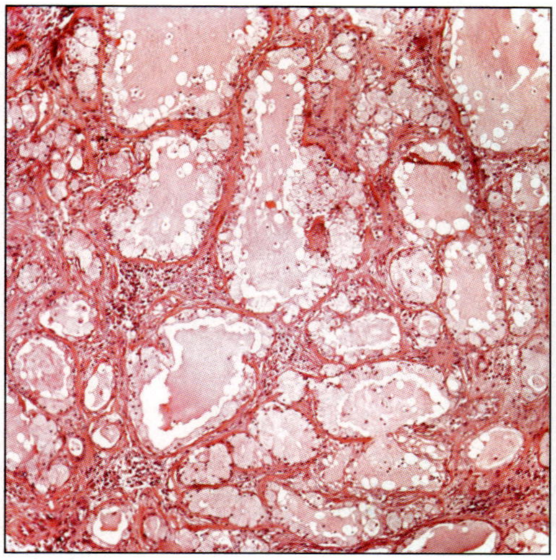
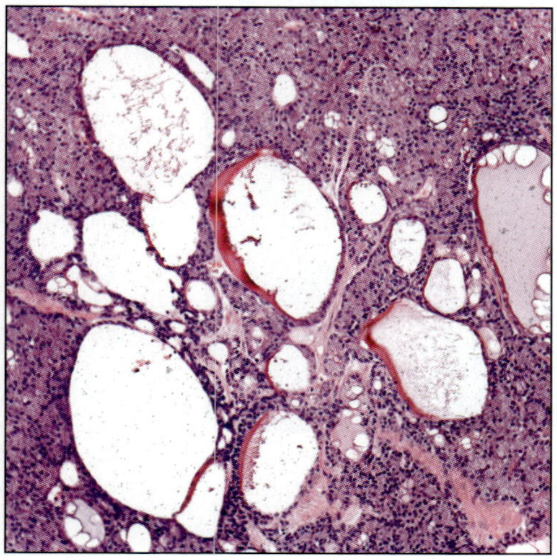

(Left) *Mucus gland adenoma shows dilated glands containing mucoid material in their lumens and lined by mucinous epithelium. This pattern may be confused with mucinous adenocarcinoma.* ***(Right)*** *Mucus gland adenoma shows dilated glands admixed with solid glandular proliferation. The solid glandular component represents an exuberant proliferation of serous endobronchial glands. No mitotic activity or nuclear atypia is present.*

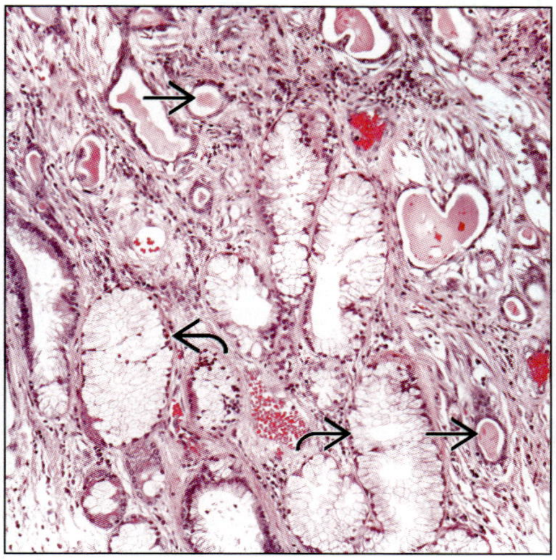
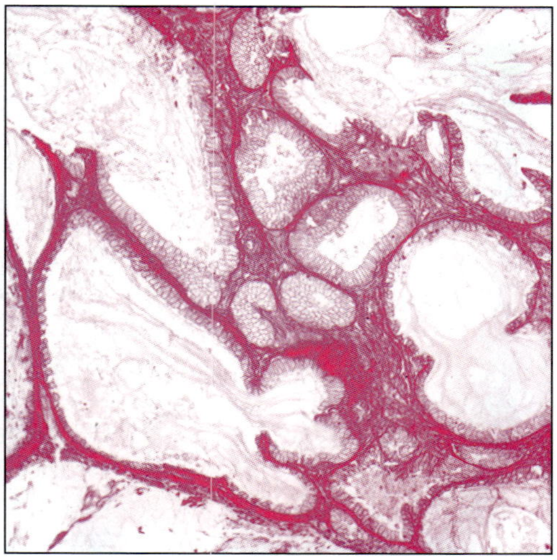

(Left) *Mucous gland adenoma shows dilated hyperplastic mucous glands adjacent to small glands. One of the characteristics of mucous gland adenoma is the presence of different sized glandular structures.* ***(Right)*** *High-power view shows mucinous glandular proliferation in a mucous gland adenoma. Note the different sizes, absence of nuclear atypia, and mitotic activity. Similar features may be seen in mucinous adenocarcinomas.*

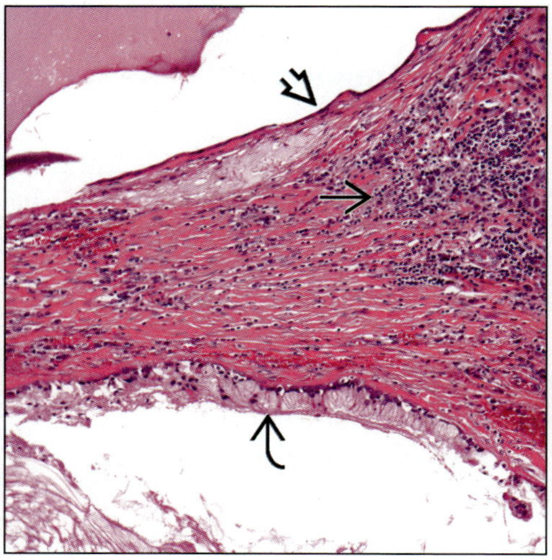
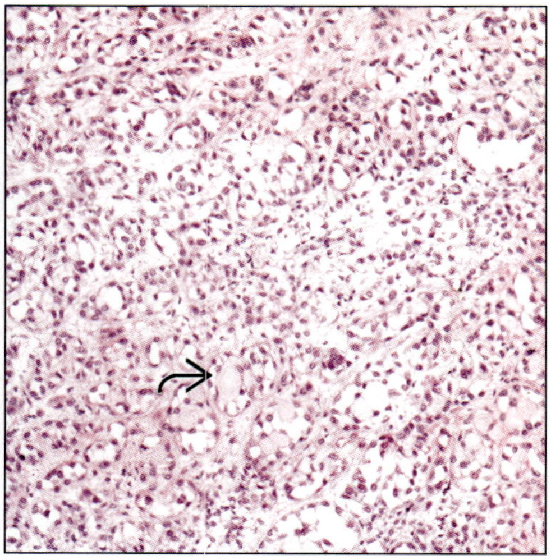

(Left) *Some mucous gland adenomas may show an extensive inflammatory reaction. Two types of glands are seen, one lined by flattened epithelium and the other by mucinous epithelium, separated by fibroconnective tissue with an inflammatory reaction.* ***(Right)*** *Mucous gland adenoma shows a solid growth pattern. This feature is unusual; however, one can still see the outline of some small glands that have coalesced to form this solid pattern.*

ENDOBRONCHIAL LIPOMA

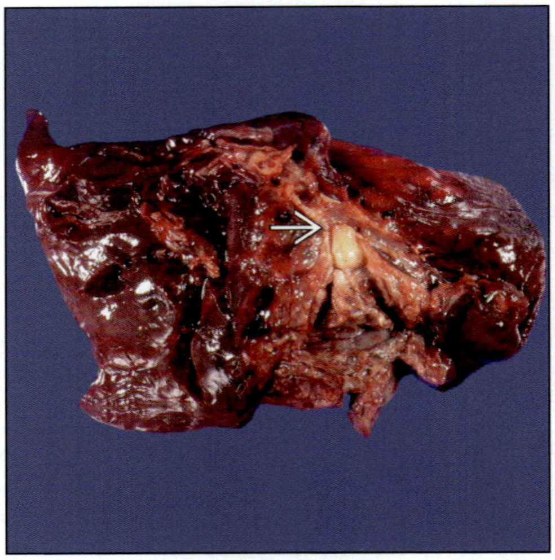

Gross photograph shows an endobronchial lipoma ➔. Note the presence of a yellow tumor mass obstructing the main pulmonary airway.

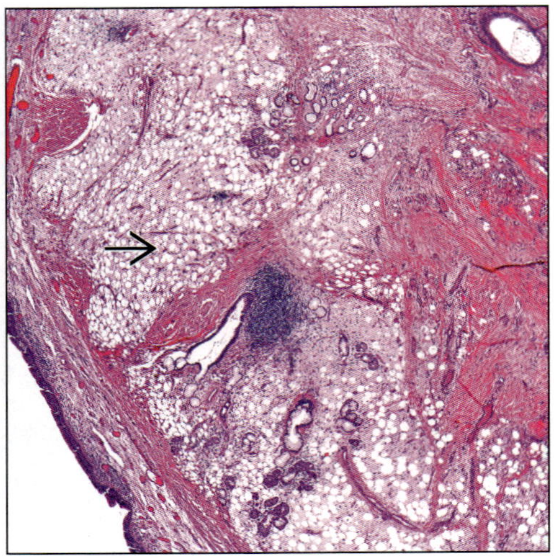

Hematoxylin & eosin low-power view shows an endobronchial lipoma. Note the presence of extensive areas of mature adipose tissue ➔.

TERMINOLOGY

Synonyms

- Lipomatous hamartoma, fibrolipoma

Definitions

- Benign mesenchymal neoplasm composed exclusively of mature adipose tissue

ETIOLOGY/PATHOGENESIS

Etiology

- These tumors are of unknown etiology
- Bronchial lipomas have been associated with obesity

CLINICAL ISSUES

Epidemiology

- Incidence
  - Bronchial lipomas are unusual tumors
- Age
  - Lipomas are more common in adults
- Gender
  - No gender predilection has been observed

Site

- Endobronchial location

Presentation

- Cough
- Shortness of breath
- Obstructive pneumonia
- Asymptomatic

Treatment

- Surgical approaches
  - Lobectomy

Prognosis

- Excellent

MACROSCOPIC FEATURES

General Features

- Well circumscribed
- Soft
- Yellowish
- Polypoid tumor obstructing bronchial lumen

Size

- Variable size between 1-5 cm in diameter

MICROSCOPIC PATHOLOGY

Histologic Features

- Mature adipose tissue
- Spindle cells
- Myxoid changes
- Absence of atypia or mitotic figures

Predominant Pattern/Injury Type

- Uniform

Predominant Cell/Compartment Type

- Adipose

DIFFERENTIAL DIAGNOSIS

Hamartoma

- Usually has presence of cartilage
- Usually has invaginations of respiratory epithelium

Mixed Tumor (Pleomorphic Adenoma)

- Usually has epithelial component
- May also have chondromyxoid areas
- Extensive areas of adipose tissue are not common in mixed tumors

Metastatic Liposarcoma

- Liposarcomas more commonly metastasize to lung parenchyma and not to endobronchial areas

ENDOBRONCHIAL LIPOMA

Key Facts

Terminology
- Synonym: Lipomatous hamartoma
- Definition: Benign mesenchymal neoplasm composed exclusively of mature adipose tissue

Clinical Issues
- Cough
- Shortness of breath
- Obstructive pneumonia
- Lipomas are more commonly seen as bronchial tumors

Macroscopic Features
- Well circumscribed
- Soft and yellowish
- Polypoid tumor obstructing bronchial lumen
- Variable size: 1-5 cm in diameter

Microscopic Pathology
- Mature adipose tissue
- Spindle cells
- Myxoid changes
- Absence of atypia or mitotic figures

Top Differential Diagnoses
- Hamartoma
  - Usually has presence of cartilage
  - Usually has invaginations of the respiratory epithelium
- Mixed tumor (pleomorphic adenoma)
  - Usually has epithelial component
  - May also have chondromyxoid areas

Immunohistochemistry

Antibody	Reactivity	Staining Pattern	Comment
S100	Positive	Nuclear	In some cases
Vimentin	Positive	Cytoplasmic	
CK-PAN	Negative		May stain entrapped normal glandular structures
EMA	Negative		May stain entrapped normal glandular structures
CD34	Negative		Positive staining in vessels and in some adipose tissue
Actin-sm	Negative		May stain entrapped vessels
HMB-45	Negative		
Actin-HHF-35	Negative		
Desmin	Negative		
Caldesmon	Negative		

- History of liposarcoma will aid in diagnosis
- Displays more cellular atypia

Angiomyolipoma
- Most angiomyolipomas in the lung are not in endobronchial location
- Commonly associated with tuberous sclerosis
- Shows presence of vessels and smooth muscle proliferation
- Immunohistochemical studies using HMB-45 and actin-sm will be useful

DIAGNOSTIC CHECKLIST

Clinically Relevant Pathologic Features
- Gross appearance

Pathologic Interpretation Pearls
- Mature adipose tissue
- Lack of atypical features
- Absence of cartilaginous component

SELECTED REFERENCES

1. Oury Bah M et al: [Endobronchial lipoma: imaging findings. A case report.] Rev Pneumol Clin. 65(1):36-9, 2009
2. Pollefliet C et al: Endobronchial lipomas: rare benign lung tumors, two case reports. J Thorac Oncol. 4(5):658-60, 2009
3. Filosso PL et al: Hemoptysis caused by an endobronchial lipoma. J Thorac Cardiovasc Surg. 135(4):954-5, 2008
4. Basoglu A et al: Endobronchial lipoma: a rare cause of bronchial occlusion. Interact Cardiovasc Thorac Surg. 3(2):263-4, 2004
5. Muraoka M et al: Endobronchial lipoma: review of 64 cases reported in Japan. Chest. 123(1):293-6, 2003
6. Rama Rao PS et al: Endobronchial lipoma. Eur J Cardiothorac Surg. 19(4):512, 2001
7. De Abajo C et al: [Endobronchial lipomas. Apropos of 4 cases.] Rev Pneumol Clin. 52(6):373-7, 1996
8. Moran CA et al: Endobronchial lipomas: a clinicopathologic study of four cases. Mod Pathol. 7(2):212-4, 1994
9. Bango A et al: Endobronchial lipomas. Respiration. 60(5):297-301, 1993
10. Peng RL et al: Endobronchial lipoma associated with lipomatosis. AJR Am J Roentgenol. 158(1):210-1, 1992
11. Nataf P et al: [Endobronchial lipomas. Apropos of 16 cases.] Rev Pneumol Clin. 45(5):203-5, 1989
12. Schraufnagel DE et al: Endobronchial lipoma. Chest. 75(1):97-9, 1979

ENDOBRONCHIAL LIPOMA

Microscopic Features

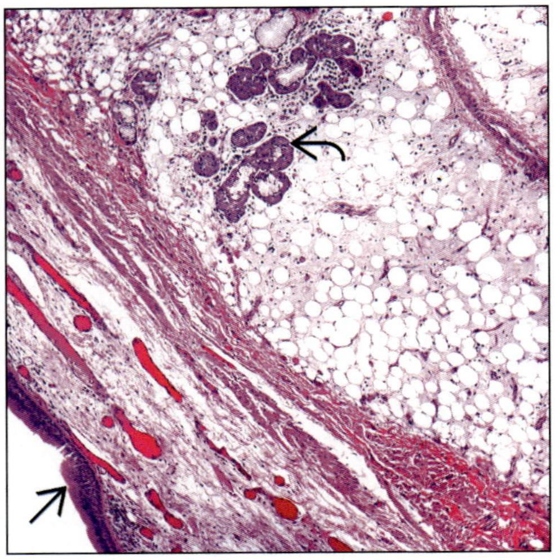

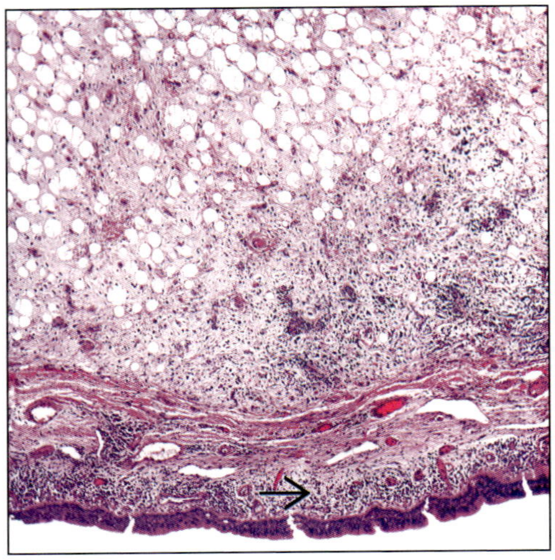

*(**Left**) Endobronchial lipoma shows mature adipose tissue and entrapped endobronchial glands →. Note that the respiratory epithelium is within normal limits, and normal endobronchial glands ↗ are present. (**Right**) Endobronchial lipoma shows inflammatory changes underneath the respiratory epithelium →. Essentially, there appears to be a cambium-like layer between normal structures and the tumor.*

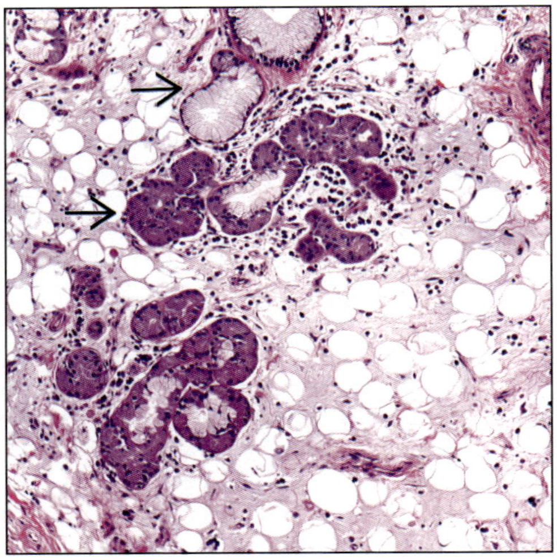

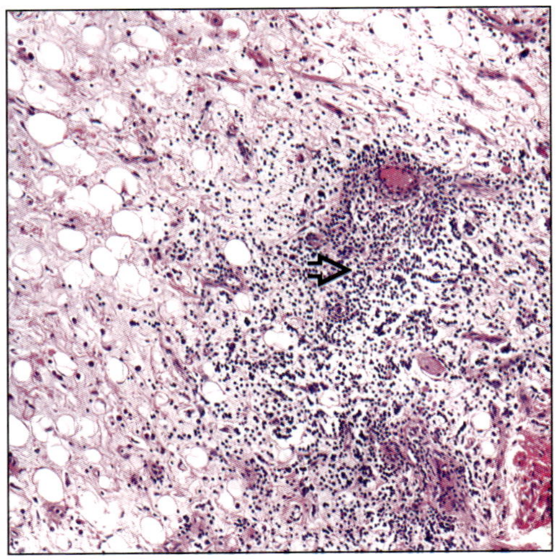

*(**Left**) High-power view shows an endobronchial lipoma with entrapped endobronchial glands →. Some glands are serous and others are mucinous; however, the tumor does not involve or destroy normal endobronchial structures. (**Right**) Endobronchial lipoma shows areas of chronic inflammation ⇨ admixed with the adipose tissue. Inflammatory changes in endobronchial lipomas are usually focal and not prominent.*

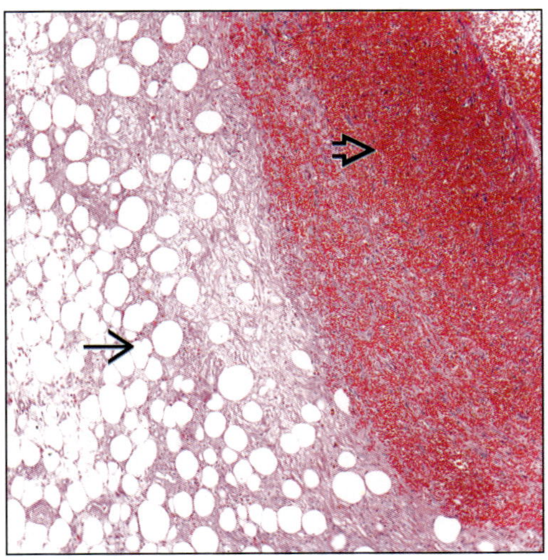

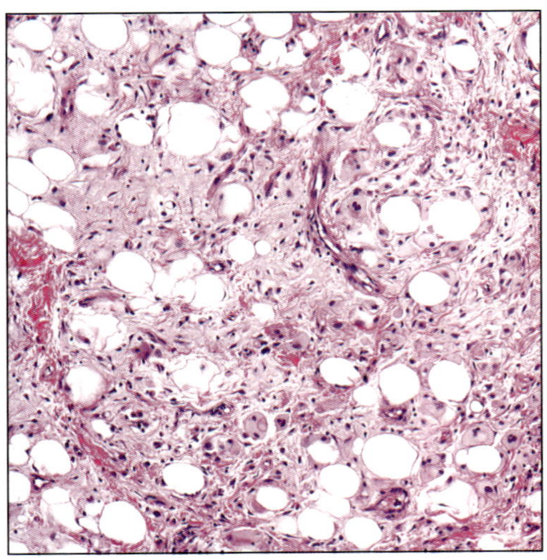

*(**Left**) Areas of hemorrhage, although unusual, can be seen in some cases of endobronchial lipomas. In this case, there is an extensive area of hemorrhage ⇨ adjacent to more conventional lipomatous areas →. (**Right**) Endobronchial lipoma shows adipose tissue with more myxoid changes and mild inflammation. The presence of myxoid changes should not be interpreted as atypical changes. Myxoid changes are invariably seen in these cases, at least focally.*

ENDOBRONCHIAL LIPOMA

Microscopic Features

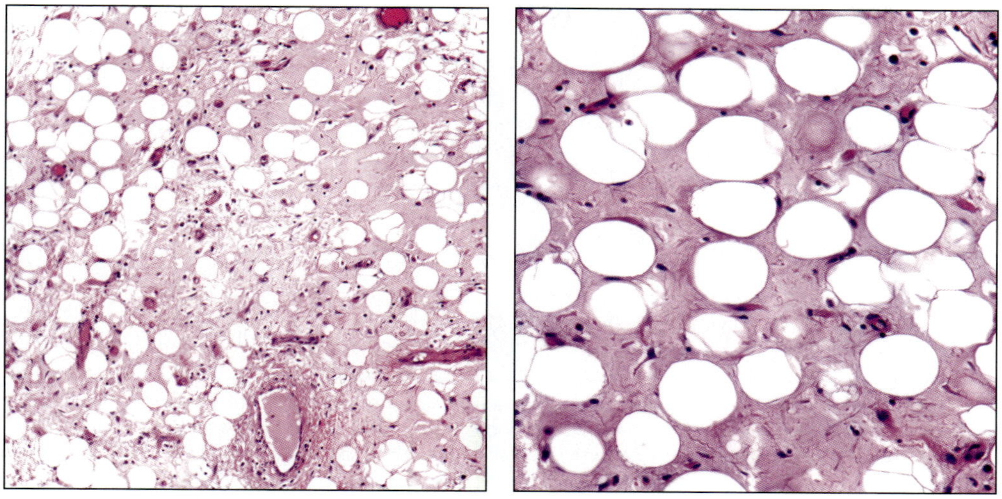

(Left) *Prominent myxoid changes and vascular proliferation are shown in an endobronchial lipoma. In this high-power view, the tumor does not display any cytological atypia.* ***(Right)*** *Higher power view shows an endobronchial lipoma with prominent myxoid changes. Pure myxoid endobronchial lipomas are rare; the majority of cases will display the presence of mature adipose tissue like that seen in lipomas of soft tissues.*

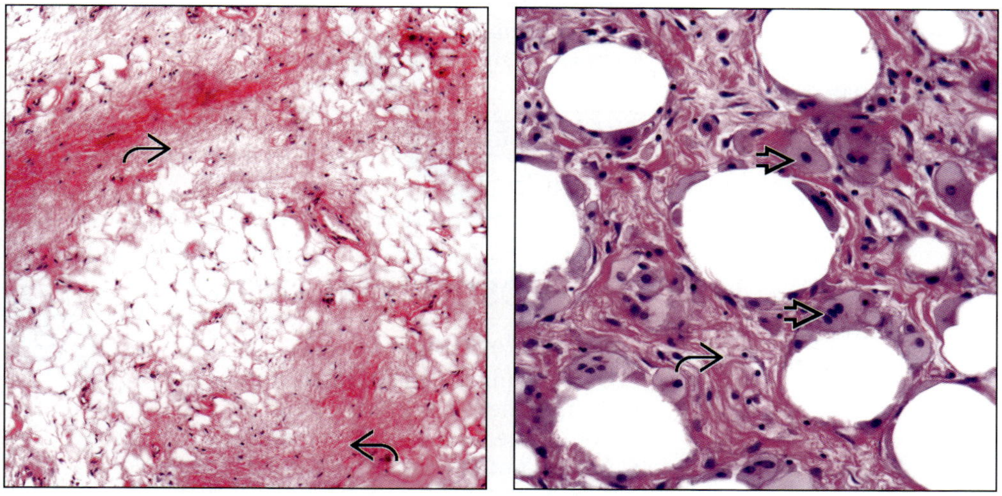

(Left) *In some cases of endobronchial lipoma, the fibrous component ↪ may be more prominent. This feature has been used in the past as the basis for the term fibrolipoma.* ***(Right)*** *In some other cases, the lipomatous component is associated not only with the fibrous component ↪ but also with numerous mucinophages ⇨.*

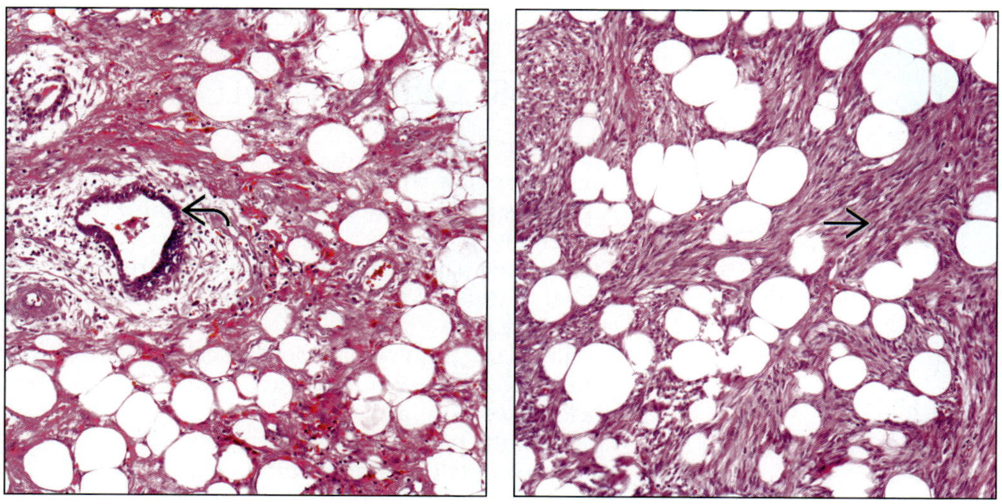

(Left) *Endobronchial fibrolipoma shows a focal area with a residual atrophic endobronchial gland ↪. The adjacent areas show more conventional features of fibrolipoma.* ***(Right)*** *In some cases of endobronchial lipomas, the tumor may also show areas of spindle cellular proliferation → similar to that described in spindle cell lipomas of soft tissues.*

PULMONARY ADENOFIBROMA/ADENOMYOMA

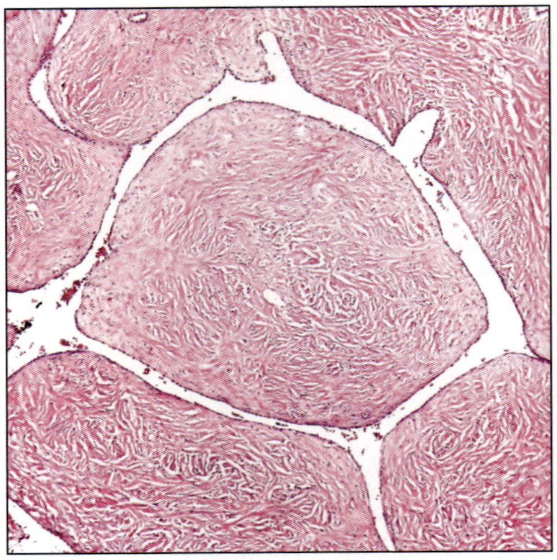

Scanning magnification of pulmonary adenofibroma shows club-like papillae lined by a single layer of simple, cuboidal epithelium. The cores of the papillae contain a bland spindle cell population.

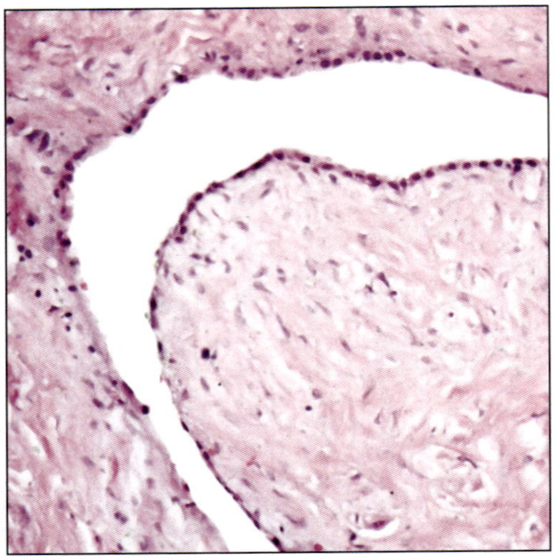

High magnification of club-like papilla in pulmonary adenofibroma shows a single layer of cuboidal epithelial cells in the periphery and bland spindle cell population in the cores embedded in collagenous stroma.

TERMINOLOGY

Abbreviations

- Pulmonary adenofibroma (PAF), pulmonary adenomyoma (PAM)

Synonyms

- Pulmonary fibroadenoma, adenofibromatous hamartoma, adenomyomatous hamartoma, fibroleiomyomatous hamartoma

Definitions

- Benign hamartomatous intrapulmonary fibroblastic or myofibroblastic proliferation that entraps glands in its growth

ETIOLOGY/PATHOGENESIS

Developmental Anomaly

- Hamartomatous origin most commonly postulated

Pathogenesis

- May also represent benign neoplastic stromal proliferation that entraps normal respiratory structures in its growth

CLINICAL ISSUES

Site

- Intraparenchymatous, well-circumscribed nodule

Presentation

- Solitary "coin" lesion
- Incidental finding on routine chest x-rays

Treatment

- Surgical approaches
  - Lobectomy or wedge resection for small, superficial lesions

Prognosis

- Benign tumor
- Cured by simple surgical excision

IMAGE FINDINGS

CT Findings

- Well-circumscribed small intraparenchymatous lesion

MACROSCOPIC FEATURES

General Features

- Well-circumscribed but unencapsulated
- Firm, rubbery tissue
- Homogeneous, tan-pink cut surface
- Tumors not in contact with pleural surface or bronchus

Size

- Usually small (1-2 cm in greatest diameter)

MICROSCOPIC PATHOLOGY

Histologic Features

- Low-power view characterized by club-shaped papillary structures lined by a layer of simple cuboidal epithelium
- Club-shaped papillae resemble papillary structures similar to those of müllerian adenofibromas of female genital tract
- Papillary structures contain spindle cells in the stroma with bland cytologic appearance devoid of mitoses or nuclear pleomorphism
- Lining of the papillary structures can also be composed of tall columnar epithelium
- Occasional gland-like spaces can be seen scattered within the lesion

PULMONARY ADENOFIBROMA/ADENOMYOMA

Key Facts

Clinical Issues
- Intraparenchymatous, well-circumscribed nodule
- Solitary "coin" lesion
- Incidental finding on routine chest x-rays

Macroscopic Features
- Well-circumscribed but unencapsulated
- Homogeneous, tan-pink cut surface
- Usually small (1-2 cm in greatest diameter)

Microscopic Pathology
- Low-power view characterized by club-shaped papillary structures lined by a layer of simple cuboidal epithelium
- Club-shaped papillae resemble papillary structures similar to those of müllerian adenofibromas of the female genital tract
- Papillary structures contain spindle cells in the stroma with bland cytologic appearance devoid of mitoses or nuclear pleomorphism
- Epithelium lining the gland-like spaces and papillae is bland and devoid of cytologic atypia
- Spindle cell stromal component is made up of bland spindle cells with no mitotic activity or nuclear pleomorphism

Ancillary Tests
- Epithelial cells lining the papillae stain positive for cytokeratins and EMA
- Spindle cells stain positive for vimentin or may be positive for vimentin and SMA
- Spindle cells are negative for CD34 and Bcl-2
- Epithelial cells lining the papillae show nuclear positivity for TTF-1

- Proportion of cellularity and spindle cells to fibrous stroma may vary from lesion to lesion

Cytologic Features
- Epithelium lining the gland-like spaces and papillae is bland and devoid of cytologic atypia
- Spindle cell stromal component is made up of bland spindle cells with no mitotic activity or nuclear pleomorphism
- Spindle stromal cells may show a fascicular pattern of growth with areas of stromal hyalinization or myxoid change

ANCILLARY TESTS

Immunohistochemistry
- Epithelial cells lining the papillae stain positive for cytokeratins and EMA
- Spindle cells stain positive for vimentin or may be positive for vimentin, SMA, and desmin
- Spindle cells are negative for CD34 and Bcl-2
- Spindle cells are negative for other differentiation markers (S100 protein, CD31, keratin, EMA, etc.)
- Epithelial cells lining the papillae show nuclear positivity for TTF-1

DIFFERENTIAL DIAGNOSIS

Cartilaginous Hamartoma
- Prominent mature cartilaginous component present
- Absence of significant spindle cell stromal component

Intrapulmonary Solitary Fibrous Tumor (SFT)
- Intrapulmonary SFT may also contain entrapped gland-like spaces at periphery of lesion
- Formation of club-like papillary structures is not a feature of SFT
- Tumor cells in SFT are positive for CD34 and Bcl-2

Biphasic Pulmonary Blastoma
- Glandular component displays more primitive appearance that resembles respiratory epithelium during weeks 8-10 of gestation
- Stromal spindle cell component is poorly differentiated and resembles sarcoma, with high mitotic index
- May show areas of hemorrhage and necrosis

Pulmonary Carcinosarcoma
- Epithelial component in carcinosarcoma is frankly malignant (adenocarcinoma or squamous cell carcinoma)
- Stromal component in carcinosarcoma is frankly malignant with nuclear pleomorphism and high mitotic activity
- Stromal component may show smooth muscle, adipose, vascular, cartilaginous, osseous, or neural differentiation

Metastases of Sarcomas to the Lung
- Metastatic sarcomas often entrap epithelial structures at their periphery, simulating adenofibroma
- Distribution of entrapped epithelial elements is at edges, not widespread and haphazard as in adenofibroma
- Spindle cell component in metastatic sarcoma is usually high grade and atypical
- Clinical history may be helpful by alerting the pathologist to a previous tumor at another location

SELECTED REFERENCES

1. Suster S et al: Pulmonary adenofibroma: report of two cases of an unusual type of hamartomatous lesion of the lung. Histopathology. 23(6):547-51, 1993
2. Gorelkin L: Fibroleiomyomatous hamartoma: a rare benign pulmonary "coin lesion". South Med J. 71(1):88-9, 1978
3. Scarff RW et al: Fibroadenoma of the lung. J Pathol Bacteriol. 56:257-59, 1944

INTRAPULMONARY SOLITARY FIBROUS TUMOR

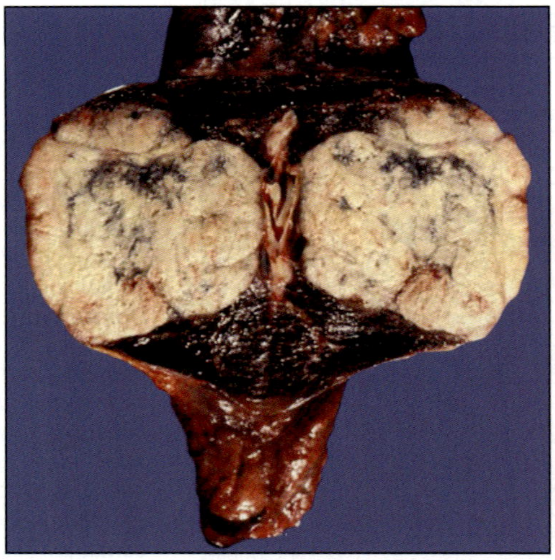

Gross appearance of an intrapulmonary solitary fibrous tumor shows a large, fleshy, bosselated tumor mass located within lung parenchyma expanding the pleura.

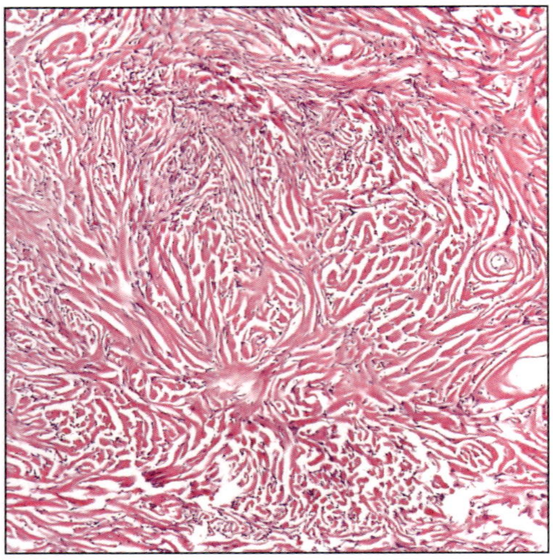

Characteristic histologic appearance of an intrapulmonary solitary fibrous tumor shows parallel arrays of rope-like collagen flanked by small, bland-appearing spindle cells.

TERMINOLOGY

Abbreviations

- Solitary fibrous tumor (SFT)

Synonyms

- Localized fibrous tumor, hemangiopericytoma, intrapulmonary fibroma, pulmonary fibrosarcoma

Definitions

- Primary intrapulmonary neoplastic proliferation of dendritic fibroblasts

CLINICAL ISSUES

Presentation

- Cough
- Chest pain
- Dyspnea
- Clubbing of fingers

Treatment

- Complete surgical excision (lobectomy) is favored approach

Prognosis

- Majority of tumors (90%) are benign and cured by complete excision
- About 10% behave aggressively (malignant solitary fibrous tumor) and can lead to death of patient

MACROSCOPIC FEATURES

General Features

- Generally well-circumscribed but unencapsulated intraparenchymatous masses
- Rubbery, whorled, tan-white cut surface
- Can show areas of hemorrhage and necrosis (malignant cases)

MICROSCOPIC PATHOLOGY

Histologic Features

- **Benign SFT**
  - Variation of growth patterns, including fascicular, storiform, hemangiopericytic, herringbone, wavy neural, and angiofibromatous
  - Frequent admixture of cellular areas with hypocellular areas of stromal sclerosis
  - Rope-like linear pattern of stromal sclerosis is highly characteristic
  - Tumors may often entrap benign bronchial structures and airspaces at lesion periphery, simulating a biphasic neoplasm
  - Usually sharp circumscription of the process from surrounding uninvolved lung parenchyma
  - High vascularity with numerous vessels of varying caliber size
- **Malignant SFT**
  - Poor circumscription and foci of infiltration of lung parenchyma and bronchial structures
  - Marked increase in cellularity and nuclear pleomorphism
  - Increased mitotic activity (> 3 per 10 high-power fields)
  - Presence of frequent atypical mitoses
  - Multinucleated malignant giant cells
  - Foci of tumor cell necrosis
  - Foci of vascular invasion

Cytologic Features

- Composed of small spindle cells without cytologic atypia in majority of cases
- Spindle cells can show wavy nuclei simulating peripheral nerve sheath tumors
- Cases with prominent stromal sclerosis can show small, round hyperchromatic nuclei devoid of cytoplasmic rims

PULMONARY ADENOFIBROMA/ADENOMYOMA

Microscopic and Immunohistochemical Features

__(Left)__ Scanning magnification of pulmonary adenofibroma shows club-like papillae with sparse spindle cell population set against a collagenous stroma. The appearance is reminiscent of müllerian-derived adenofibromas of the ovaries. __(Right)__ High magnification of pulmonary adenofibroma shows club-like papilla lined by a single layer of bland-appearing, cuboidal epithelial cells devoid of cytologic atypia. The central core of the papilla contains a sparse, bland-appearing spindle cell population.

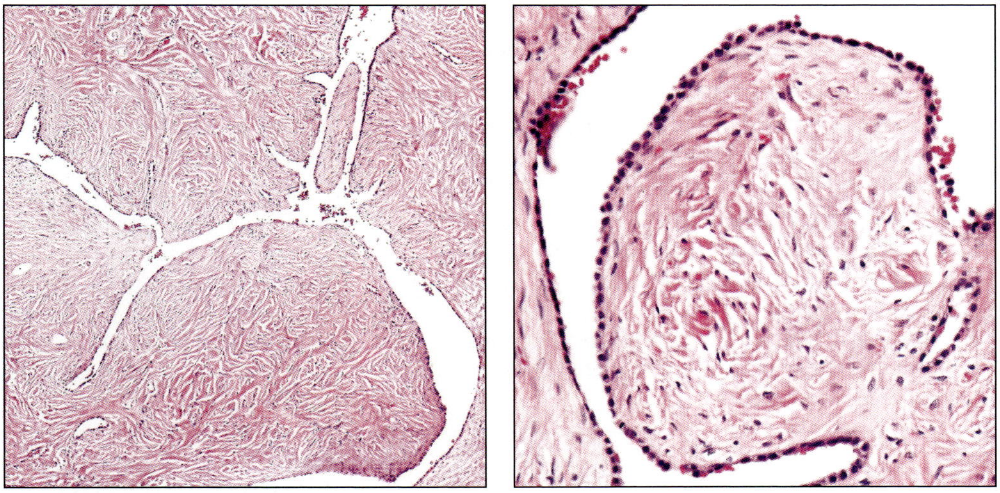

__(Left)__ Pulmonary adenofibroma shows small, entrapped gland-like spaces embedded in the stroma deep within the tumor and surrounded by a bland-appearing fibroblastic spindle cell proliferation. __(Right)__ High magnification of pulmonary adenofibroma shows a focal area of stromal hyalinization. Notice the branching glandular lumen ⮫ surrounded by a dense spindle cell population in the surrounding stroma. Cases like this can closely resemble solitary fibrous tumors of the lung.

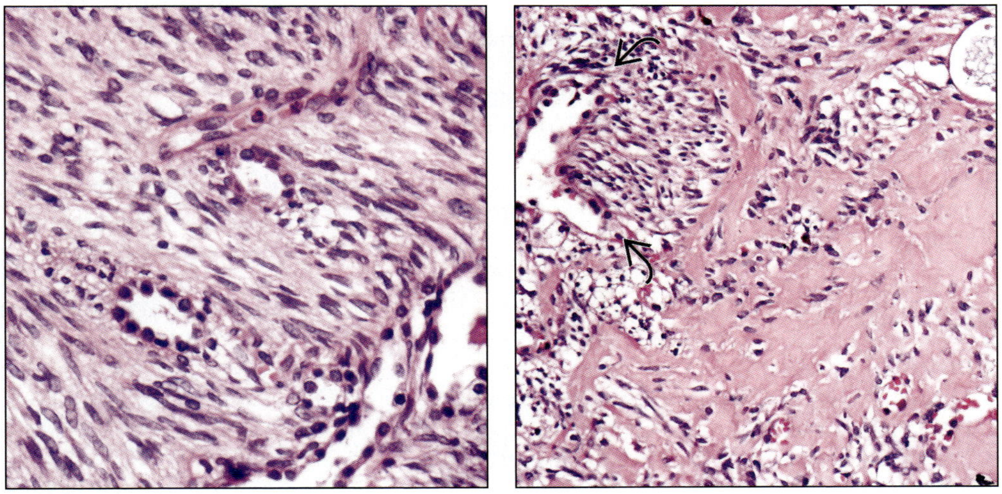

__(Left)__ Pan-cytokeratin stain in pulmonary adenofibroma decorates the tumor cells lining the abortive papilla →. Notice the complete lack of reactivity of the bland spindle cells seen in the underlying stroma. __(Right)__ Immunohistochemical staining for vimentin intermediate filaments in pulmonary adenofibroma shows strong positive staining of spindle cells in the stroma. Notice the negative staining of the epithelial cells lining the papillary structures.

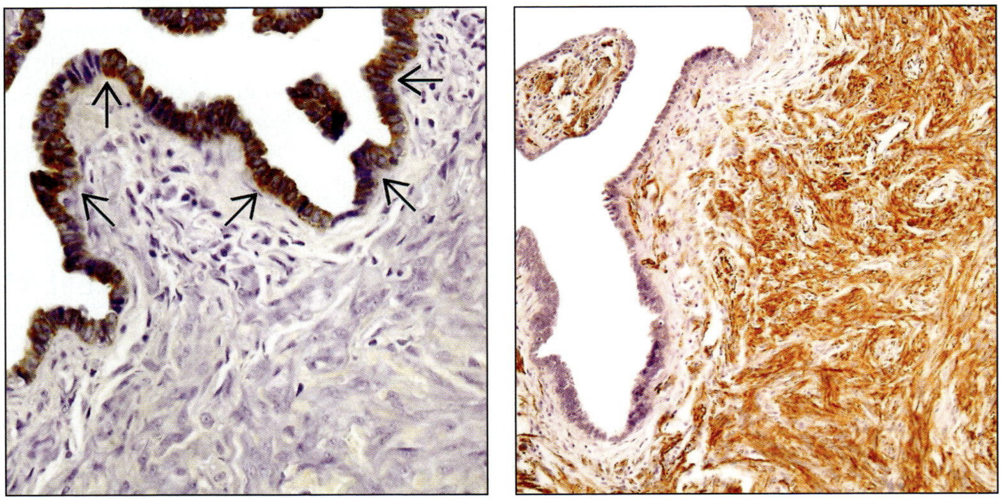

PULMONARY ADENOFIBROMA/ADENOMYOMA

Key Facts

Clinical Issues
- Intraparenchymatous, well-circumscribed nodule
- Solitary "coin" lesion
- Incidental finding on routine chest x-rays

Macroscopic Features
- Well-circumscribed but unencapsulated
- Homogeneous, tan-pink cut surface
- Usually small (1-2 cm in greatest diameter)

Microscopic Pathology
- Low-power view characterized by club-shaped papillary structures lined by a layer of simple cuboidal epithelium
- Club-shaped papillae resemble papillary structures similar to those of müllerian adenofibromas of the female genital tract
- Papillary structures contain spindle cells in the stroma with bland cytologic appearance devoid of mitoses or nuclear pleomorphism
- Epithelium lining the gland-like spaces and papillae is bland and devoid of cytologic atypia
- Spindle cell stromal component is made up of bland spindle cells with no mitotic activity or nuclear pleomorphism

Ancillary Tests
- Epithelial cells lining the papillae stain positive for cytokeratins and EMA
- Spindle cells stain positive for vimentin or may be positive for vimentin and SMA
- Spindle cells are negative for CD34 and Bcl-2
- Epithelial cells lining the papillae show nuclear positivity for TTF-1

- Proportion of cellularity and spindle cells to fibrous stroma may vary from lesion to lesion

Cytologic Features
- Epithelium lining the gland-like spaces and papillae is bland and devoid of cytologic atypia
- Spindle cell stromal component is made up of bland spindle cells with no mitotic activity or nuclear pleomorphism
- Spindle stromal cells may show a fascicular pattern of growth with areas of stromal hyalinization or myxoid change

ANCILLARY TESTS

Immunohistochemistry
- Epithelial cells lining the papillae stain positive for cytokeratins and EMA
- Spindle cells stain positive for vimentin or may be positive for vimentin, SMA, and desmin
- Spindle cells are negative for CD34 and Bcl-2
- Spindle cells are negative for other differentiation markers (S100 protein, CD31, keratin, EMA, etc.)
- Epithelial cells lining the papillae show nuclear positivity for TTF-1

DIFFERENTIAL DIAGNOSIS

Cartilaginous Hamartoma
- Prominent mature cartilaginous component present
- Absence of significant spindle cell stromal component

Intrapulmonary Solitary Fibrous Tumor (SFT)
- Intrapulmonary SFT may also contain entrapped gland-like spaces at periphery of lesion
- Formation of club-like papillary structures is not a feature of SFT
- Tumor cells in SFT are positive for CD34 and Bcl-2

Biphasic Pulmonary Blastoma
- Glandular component displays more primitive appearance that resembles respiratory epithelium during weeks 8-10 of gestation
- Stromal spindle cell component is poorly differentiated and resembles sarcoma, with high mitotic index
- May show areas of hemorrhage and necrosis

Pulmonary Carcinosarcoma
- Epithelial component in carcinosarcoma is frankly malignant (adenocarcinoma or squamous cell carcinoma)
- Stromal component in carcinosarcoma is frankly malignant with nuclear pleomorphism and high mitotic activity
- Stromal component may show smooth muscle, adipose, vascular, cartilaginous, osseous, or neural differentiation

Metastases of Sarcomas to the Lung
- Metastatic sarcomas often entrap epithelial structures at their periphery, simulating adenofibroma
- Distribution of entrapped epithelial elements is at edges, not widespread and haphazard as in adenofibroma
- Spindle cell component in metastatic sarcoma is usually high grade and atypical
- Clinical history may be helpful by alerting the pathologist to a previous tumor at another location

SELECTED REFERENCES

1. Suster S et al: Pulmonary adenofibroma: report of two cases of an unusual type of hamartomatous lesion of the lung. Histopathology. 23(6):547-51, 1993
2. Gorelkin L: Fibroleiomyomatous hamartoma: a rare benign pulmonary "coin lesion". South Med J. 71(1):88-9, 1978
3. Scarff RW et al: Fibroadenoma of the lung. J Pathol Bacteriol. 56:257-59, 1944

Microscopic and Immunohistochemical Features

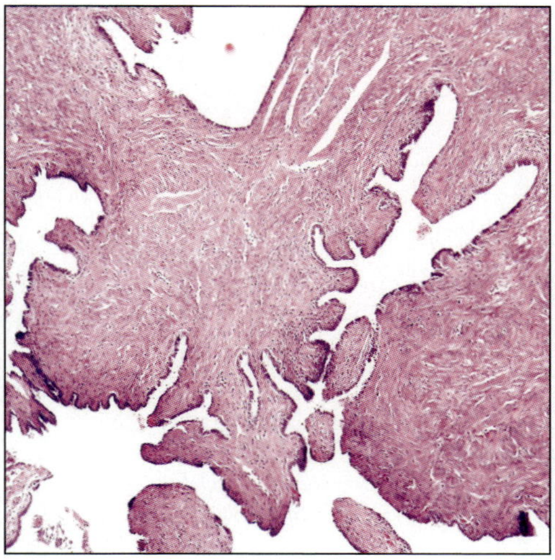

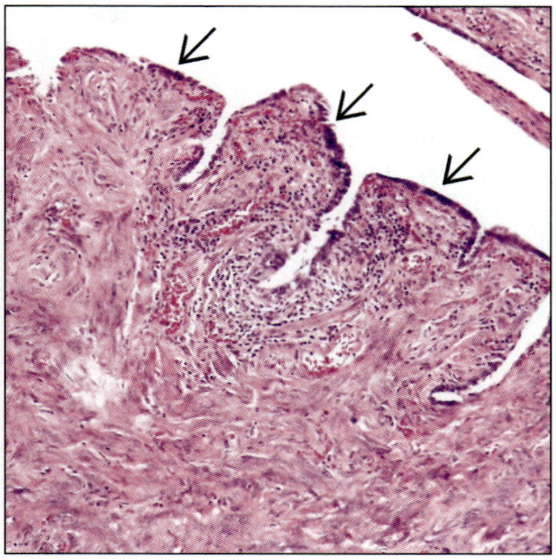

(Left) *Scanning magnification of pulmonary adenomyoma shows club-like papillary structures lined by a single layer of epithelial cells containing a cellular spindle stromal proliferation.* ***(Right)*** *High magnification of pulmonary adenomyoma shows small abortive papillae lined by a single layer of small, bland-appearing cuboidal epithelial cells* →*. The underlying stroma contains a spindle cell proliferation characterized by spindle cells with oval nuclei and abundant eosinophilic cytoplasm.*

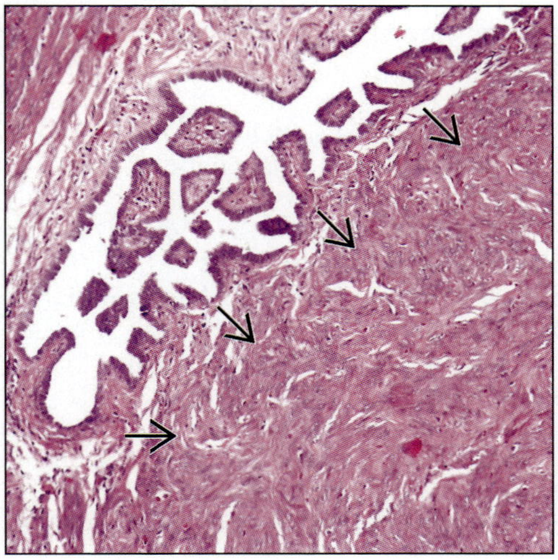

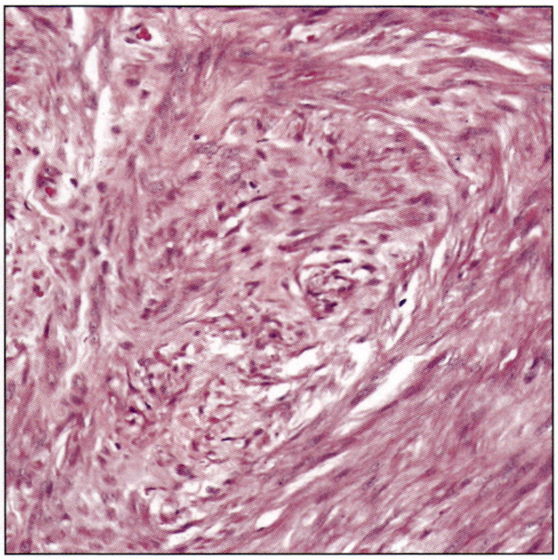

(Left) *Scanning magnification of pulmonary adenomyoma shows small, complex papillary projections into a lumen lined by a single layer of simple columnar epithelium. The stroma underneath this area shows a dense population of bland-appearing spindle cells with abundant eosinophilic cytoplasm* →*.* ***(Right)*** *High magnification of stromal component in pulmonary adenomyoma shows fascicles of bland-appearing spindle cells with abundant eosinophilic cytoplasm devoid of mitotic activity.*

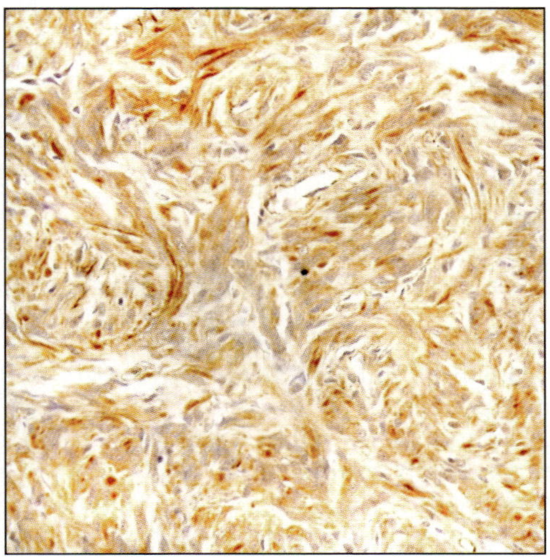

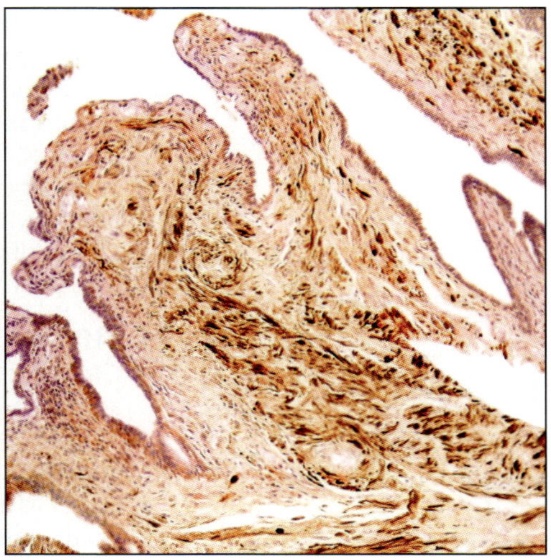

(Left) *Immunohistochemical staining of the stromal component of pulmonary adenomyoma for smooth muscle actin (SMA) shows diffuse positivity in the spindle cells.* ***(Right)*** *Immunohistochemical staining of pulmonary adenomyoma shows strong positivity of spindle cells in the stroma for desmin intermediate filaments. Notice the absence of immunohistochemical reactivity for this antibody in the thin layer of tall columnar epithelial cells lining the papillae.*

INTRAPULMONARY SOLITARY FIBROUS TUMOR

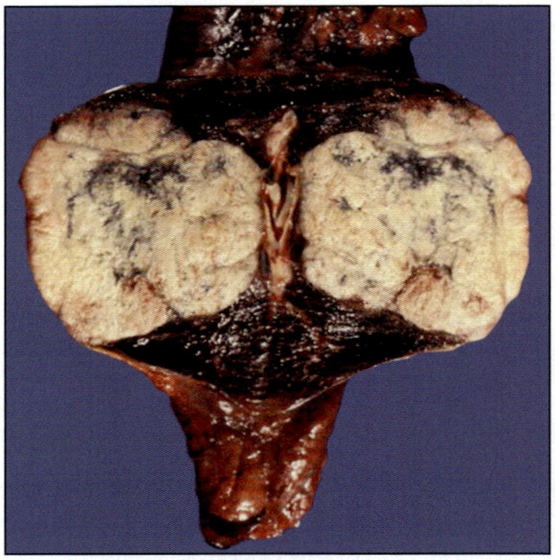

Gross appearance of an intrapulmonary solitary fibrous tumor shows a large, fleshy, bosselated tumor mass located within lung parenchyma expanding the pleura.

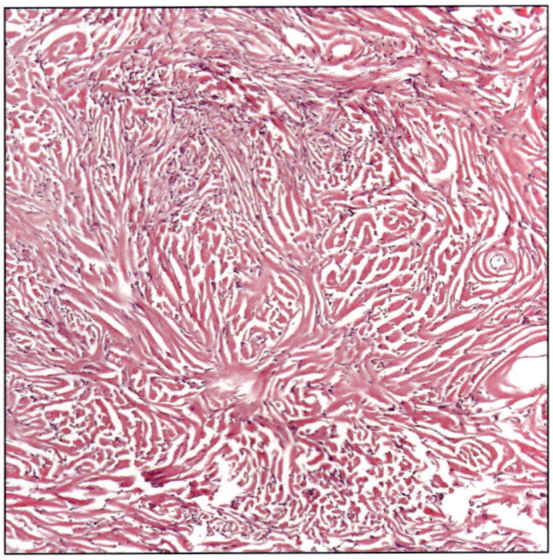

Characteristic histologic appearance of an intrapulmonary solitary fibrous tumor shows parallel arrays of rope-like collagen flanked by small, bland-appearing spindle cells.

TERMINOLOGY

Abbreviations

- Solitary fibrous tumor (SFT)

Synonyms

- Localized fibrous tumor, hemangiopericytoma, intrapulmonary fibroma, pulmonary fibrosarcoma

Definitions

- Primary intrapulmonary neoplastic proliferation of dendritic fibroblasts

CLINICAL ISSUES

Presentation

- Cough
- Chest pain
- Dyspnea
- Clubbing of fingers

Treatment

- Complete surgical excision (lobectomy) is favored approach

Prognosis

- Majority of tumors (90%) are benign and cured by complete excision
- About 10% behave aggressively (malignant solitary fibrous tumor) and can lead to death of patient

MACROSCOPIC FEATURES

General Features

- Generally well-circumscribed but unencapsulated intraparenchymatous masses
- Rubbery, whorled, tan-white cut surface
- Can show areas of hemorrhage and necrosis (malignant cases)

MICROSCOPIC PATHOLOGY

Histologic Features

- **Benign SFT**
  - Variation of growth patterns, including fascicular, storiform, hemangiopericytic, herringbone, wavy neural, and angiofibromatous
  - Frequent admixture of cellular areas with hypocellular areas of stromal sclerosis
  - Rope-like linear pattern of stromal sclerosis is highly characteristic
  - Tumors may often entrap benign bronchial structures and airspaces at lesion periphery, simulating a biphasic neoplasm
  - Usually sharp circumscription of the process from surrounding uninvolved lung parenchyma
  - High vascularity with numerous vessels of varying caliber size
- **Malignant SFT**
  - Poor circumscription and foci of infiltration of lung parenchyma and bronchial structures
  - Marked increase in cellularity and nuclear pleomorphism
  - Increased mitotic activity (> 3 per 10 high-power fields)
  - Presence of frequent atypical mitoses
  - Multinucleated malignant giant cells
  - Foci of tumor cell necrosis
  - Foci of vascular invasion

Cytologic Features

- Composed of small spindle cells without cytologic atypia in majority of cases
- Spindle cells can show wavy nuclei simulating peripheral nerve sheath tumors
- Cases with prominent stromal sclerosis can show small, round hyperchromatic nuclei devoid of cytoplasmic rims

INTRAPULMONARY SOLITARY FIBROUS TUMOR

Key Facts

Clinical Issues
- Cough
- Chest pain
- Dyspnea

Macroscopic Features
- Generally well-circumscribed but unencapsulated intraparenchymatous masses
- Rubbery, whorled, tan-white cut surface

Microscopic Pathology
- Variation of growth patterns, including fascicular, storiform, hemangiopericytic, herringbone, wavy neural, and angiofibromatous
- Frequent admixture of cellular areas with hypocellular areas of stromal sclerosis
- Rope-like linear pattern of stromal sclerosis is highly characteristic
- Tumors may often entrap benign bronchial structures and airspaces at lesion periphery, simulating a biphasic neoplasm
- Marked increase in cellularity and nuclear pleomorphism in cases undergoing malignant transformation
- Increased mitotic activity (> 3 per 10 high power fields) in malignant cases

Ancillary Tests
- Spindle cells are positive for CD34, Bcl-2, CD99, and vimentin
- Negative for cytokeratins, EMA, S100 protein, muscle markers, and melanoma-associated markers

- Cases can be highly cellular with uniform cell population simulating growth pattern of synovial sarcoma
- Malignant cases show atypical cells with enlarged nuclei, prominent nucleoli, and increased mitotic activity
- Multinucleated cells of varying types may be observed in benign and malignant cases
- Atypical, multinucleated giant cells are seen in malignant cases
- Abnormal (bizarre, tripolar, "sunburst") mitoses are seen in malignant cases

ANCILLARY TESTS

Immunohistochemistry
- Spindle cells are positive for CD34, Bcl-2, CD99, and vimentin
- Negative for cytokeratins, EMA, S100 protein, muscle markers, and melanoma-associated markers

Electron Microscopy
- Transmission
  - Spindle cells show fibroblastic features ultrastructurally
  - Cells often show fine dendritic cytoplasmic processes that attach with neighboring cells
  - No evidence of smooth muscle, neural, myofibroblastic, melanocytic, or other type of cellular differentiation

DIFFERENTIAL DIAGNOSIS

Leiomyoma
- Fascicles of spindle cells with fibrillary cytoplasm that appear to be cut at 90° angles
- Tumor cells are positive for SMA, desmin, SMMS, and calponin, and negative for CD34, CD99, and Bcl-2

Synovial Sarcoma
- Spindle cells are atypical with variable mitotic activity and very uniform appearance
- Very scant vascularity and absence of stromal fibrosis
- Tumor cells are positive for cytokeratins and EMA and negative for CD34
- Characterized by distinctive cytogenetic translocation (X;18) in > 85% of cases

DIAGNOSTIC CHECKLIST

Clinically Relevant Pathologic Features
- Histologic findings do not always correlate with prognosis
  - Some cases can metastasize and behave aggressively despite benign-appearing histologic features
  - Some cases with atypical morphologic features may behave in an indolent fashion

Pathologic Interpretation Pearls
- Variation of histologic growth patterns (i.e., fascicular, herringbone, storiform, hemangiopericytic, etc.) is frequently observed
- Alternating cellular and sclerotic areas are characteristic and often present
- High vascularity with prominent vessels with patent lumens is always seen
- Hemangiopericytic growth pattern is very common
- "Hemangiopericytoma of lung" is synonymous with intrapulmonary solitary fibrous tumor
- Increased cellularity, atypia, necrosis, and high mitotic activity are associated with aggressive or malignant behavior

SELECTED REFERENCES

1. Kouki HS et al: Solitary fibrous tumor of the lung. Gen Thorac Cardiovasc Surg. 56(5):249-51, 2008
2. Baliga M et al: Solitary fibrous tumor of the lung: a case report with a study of the aspiration biopsy, histopathology, immunohistochemistry, and autopsy findings. Diagn Cytopathol. 35(4):239-44, 2007

INTRAPULMONARY SOLITARY FIBROUS TUMOR

Common Histologic Features

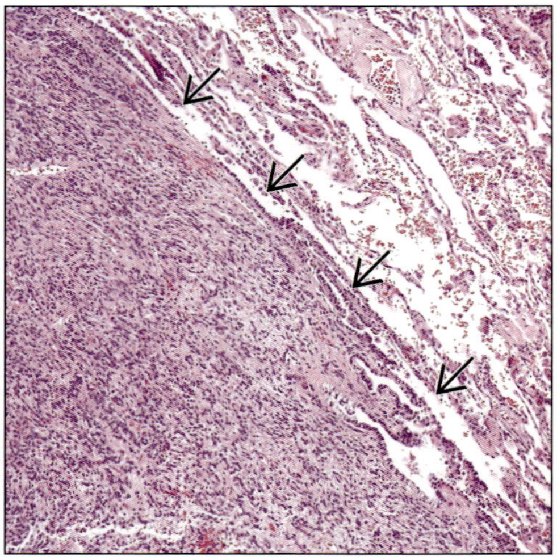
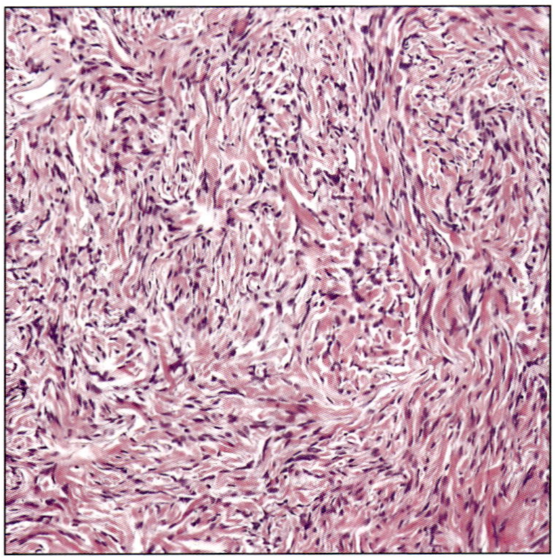

(Left) *Scanning magnification of an intrapulmonary solitary fibrous tumor shows a well-circumscribed but unencapsulated spindle cell proliferation* → *sharply separated from the surrounding lung parenchyma.* ***(Right)*** *Higher magnification of an intrapulmonary solitary fibrous tumor shows a bland spindle cell proliferation surrounded by abundant collagenous stroma. The spindle cells display a vague storiform pattern reminiscent of "fibrohistiocytic" tumors.*

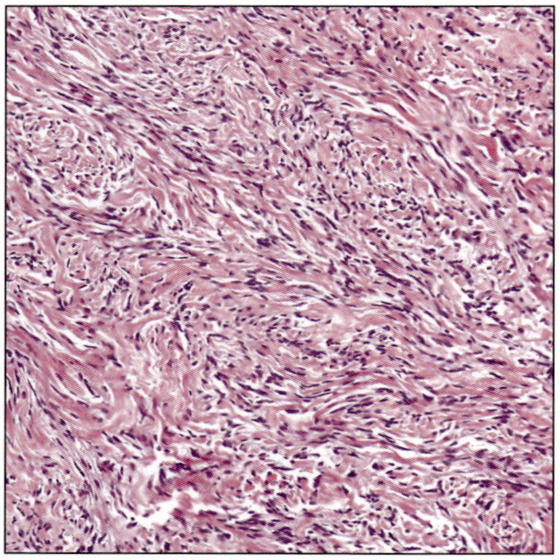
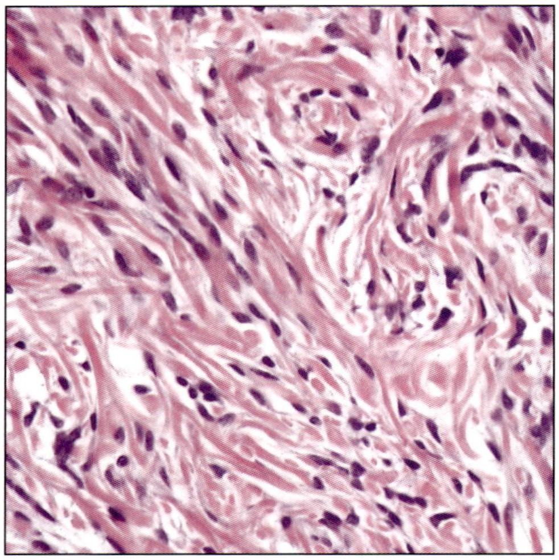

(Left) *A fascicular proliferation of spindle cells is seen in this intrapulmonary solitary fibrous tumor. The spindle cells are separated from one another by abundant collagenous matrix.* ***(Right)*** *Higher magnification of an intrapulmonary solitary fibrous tumor shows a bland-appearing population of cells lined by parallel linear strands of hyalinized, keloidal collagen adopting a rope-like configuration. This arrangement of interstitial collagen is highly distinctive for this tumor.*

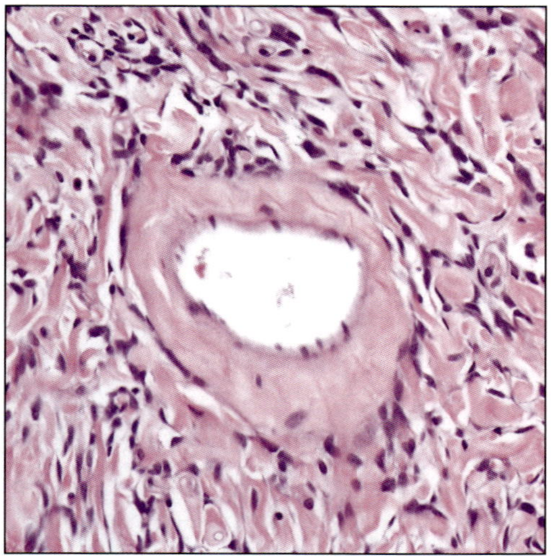
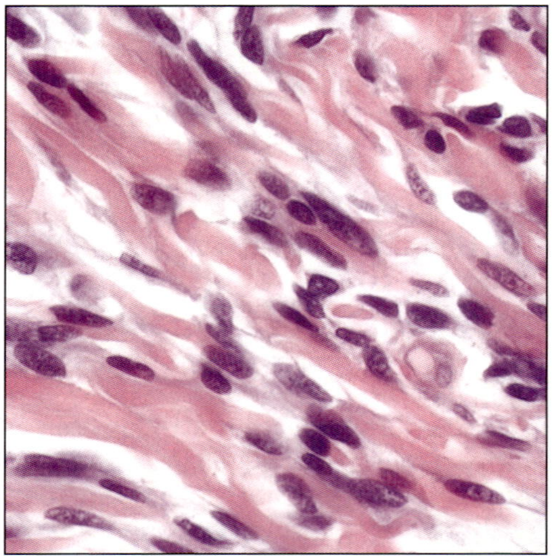

(Left) *Intrapulmonary solitary fibrous tumor shows a small-caliber vessel with prominent perivascular hyalinization. A dense vascular network with prominent perivascular hyalinization is a common feature seen in these tumors.* ***(Right)*** *High magnification of an intrapulmonary solitary fibrous tumor shows a bland-appearing population of spindle cells. The spindle cells display elongated nuclei with a dense chromatin pattern and scant rim of cytoplasm. No nucleoli or mitotic figures are seen.*

Other Histologic Features

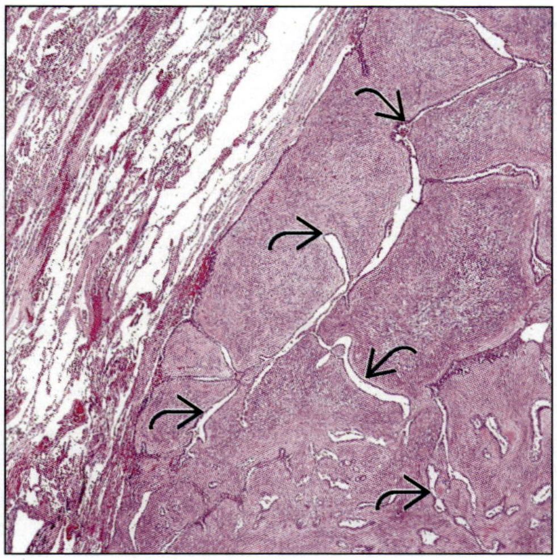
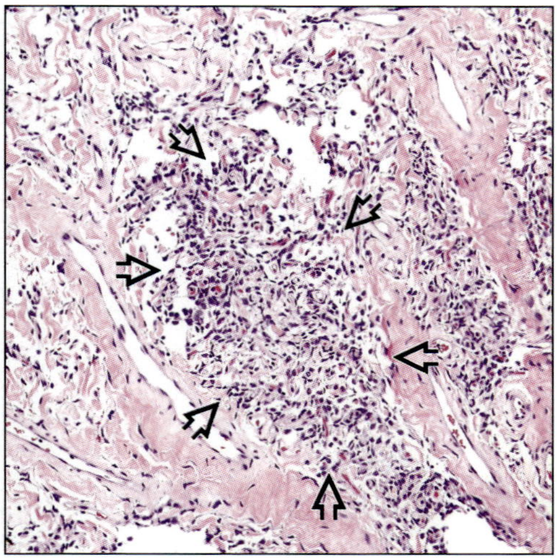

(Left) *Scanning magnification of an intrapulmonary solitary fibrous tumor shows entrapment of glandular structures and airspaces at the periphery of the tumor mass ⇨ resulting in an adenofibromatous appearance.* ***(Right)*** *Alternating hypercellular ⇨ and hypocellular areas are seen in this example of an intrapulmonary solitary fibrous tumor. Variegation in cellularity and in growth patterns is a hallmark of a solitary fibrous tumor and is often encountered in these neoplasms.*

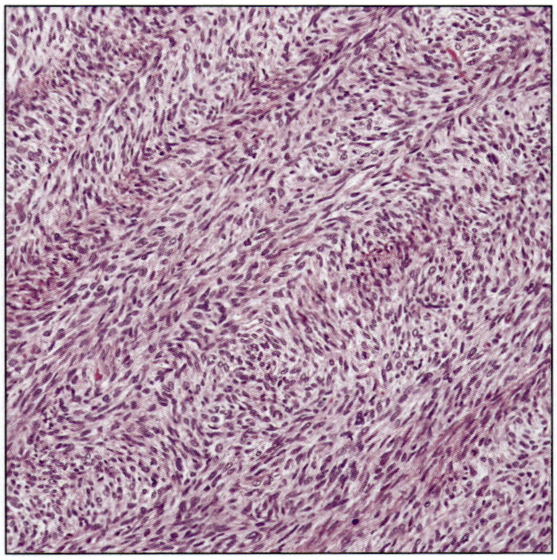
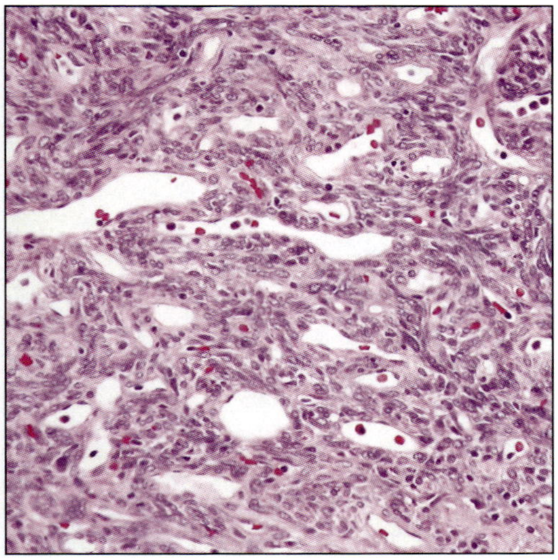

(Left) *Increased cellularity with a prominent "herringbone" pattern can often be seen in intrapulmonary solitary fibrous tumors and does not necessarily correlate with more aggressive behavior. Such tumors can be mistaken for synovial sarcoma and malignant peripheral nerve sheath tumors.* ***(Right)*** *Prominent hemangiopericytic growth pattern is seen in this intrapulmonary solitary fibrous tumor characterized by numerous small-caliber vessels with patent lumens.*

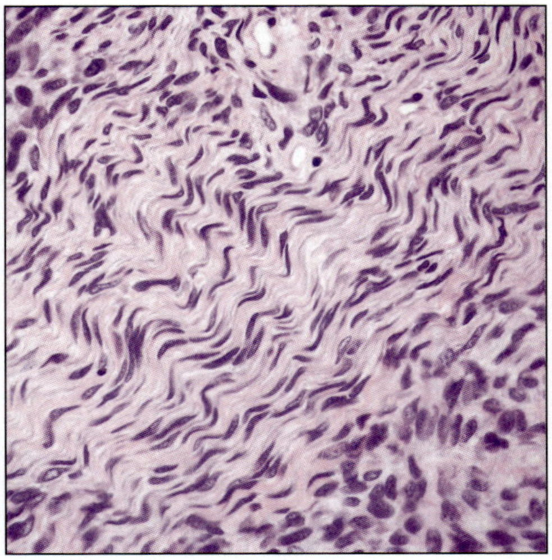
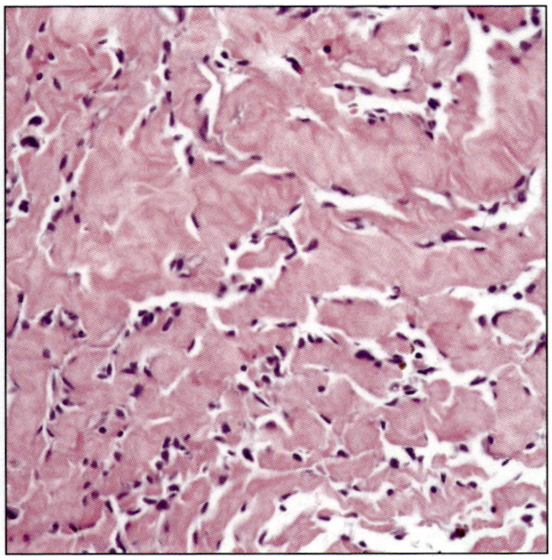

(Left) *Spindle cells with "wavy" nuclei closely reminiscent of schwannian neoplasms are seen in this example of an intrapulmonary solitary fibrous tumor. Application of immunohistochemical stains will be necessary in such cases to rule out a peripheral nerve sheath tumor.* ***(Right)*** *Extensive stromal collagenization is displayed by this intrapulmonary solitary fibrous tumor. The collagen bands are seen to compress and distort the nuclear morphology, producing small round dots.*

INTRAPULMONARY SOLITARY FIBROUS TUMOR

Cytologic and Immunohistochemical Features

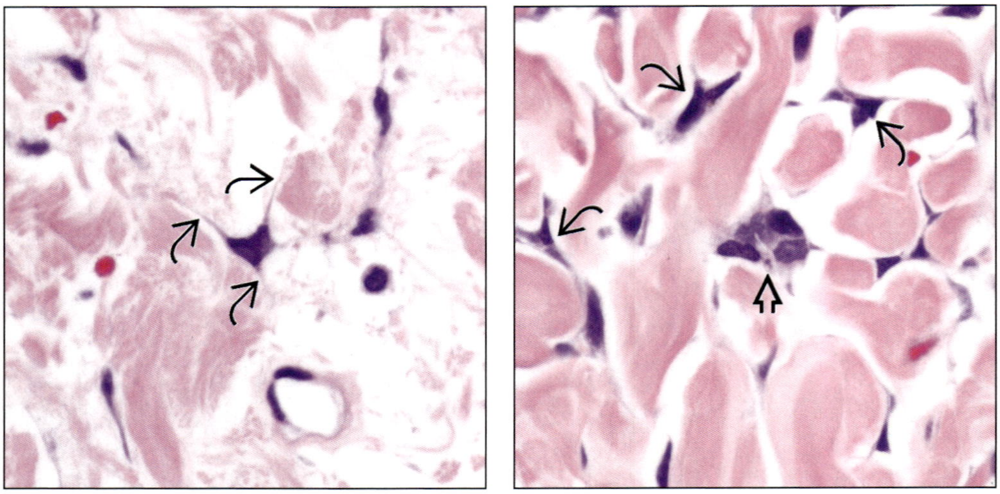

(Left) *High magnification of the sclerotic area in an intrapulmonary solitary fibrous tumor shows a stellate cell with a large, hyperchromatic nucleus and slender dendritic cytoplasmic prolongations ↷ that course along connective tissue planes and connect with neighboring cells.* ***(Right)*** *High magnification of the sclerotic area in an intrapulmonary solitary fibrous tumor shows multiple stellate dendritic cells ↷ and a multinucleated cell in the center of the field ⇨.*

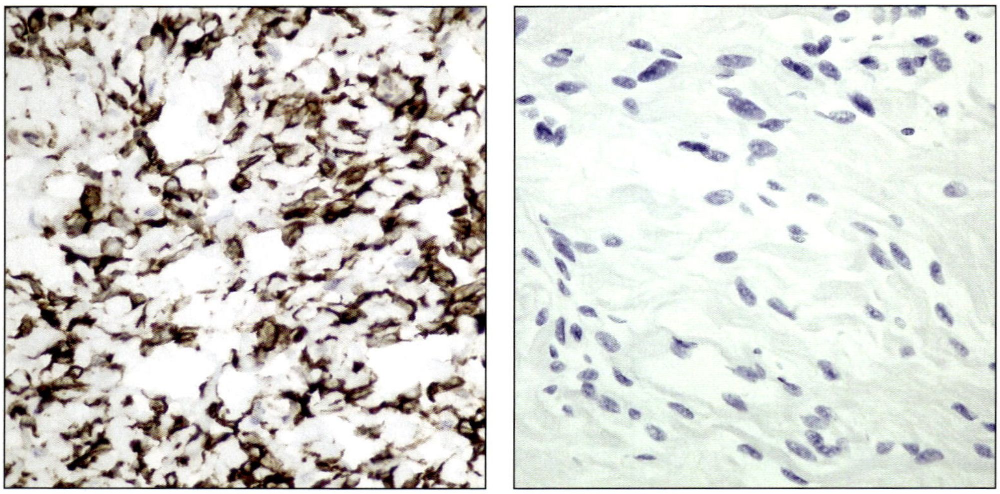

(Left) *Immunohistochemical staining for CD34 antigen in an intrapulmonary solitary fibrous tumor shows strong positivity in the spindle cells. This marker can be positive in up to 75% of cases of benign solitary fibrous tumors.* ***(Right)*** *Immunohistochemical staining for cytokeratin AE1/AE3 in intrapulmonary solitary fibrous tumor shows a negative reaction in the spindle tumor cells. Negative staining for cytokeratin is a consistent finding that helps distinguish these tumors from a sarcomatoid carcinoma.*

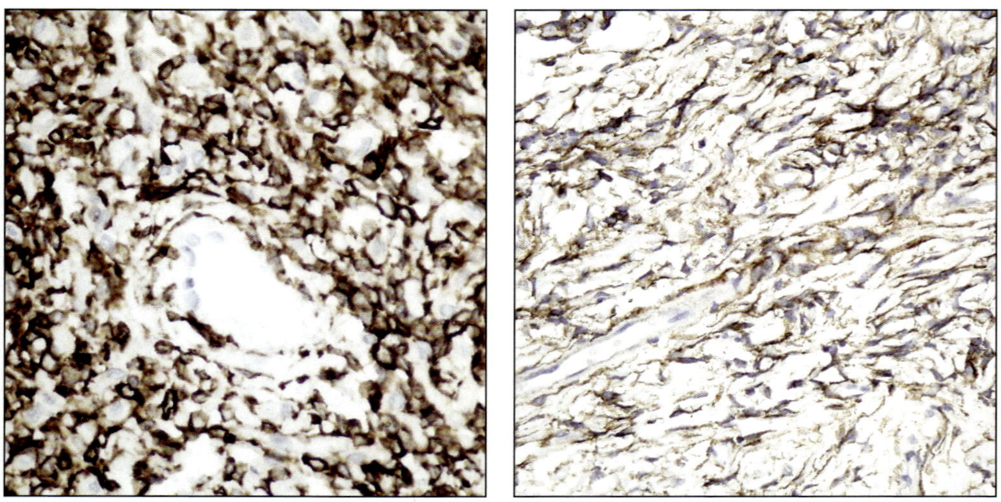

(Left) *Strong immunohistochemical staining of the spindle cells for Bcl-2 antibody is seen in this intrapulmonary solitary fibrous tumor. This marker is extremely sensitive (almost 100%) but nonspecific for these tumors.* ***(Right)*** *Immunohistochemical staining of spindle cells in an intrapulmonary solitary fibrous tumor for CD99 shows a positive reaction in the tumor cells. This is another helpful (although nonspecific) marker for the diagnosis of these tumors.*

Microscopic and Immunohistochemical Features

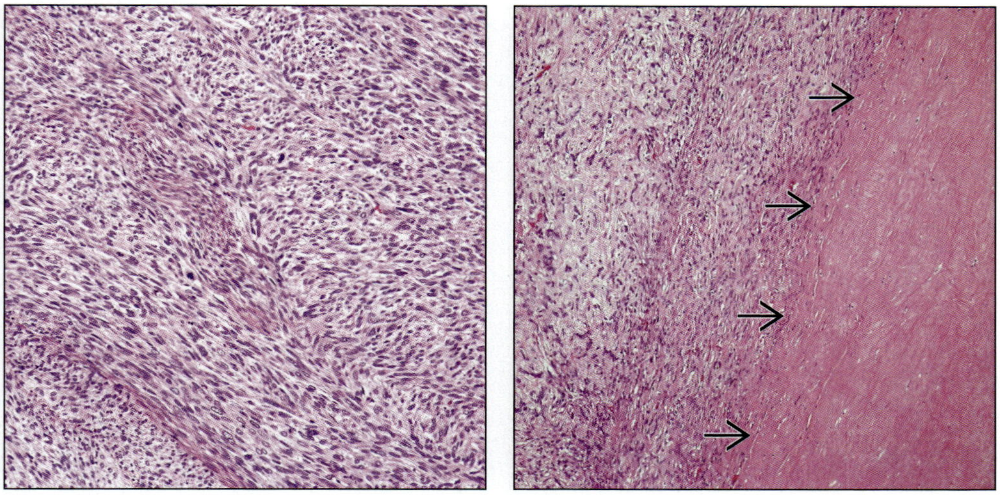

(Left) *Malignant intrapulmonary solitary fibrous tumor shows fascicles of spindle cells with a "herringbone" pattern and numerous (> 3 per 10 high power fields) mitoses. Identification of other areas displaying the conventional features of solitary fibrous tumor are necessary for diagnosis.* ***(Right)*** *Extensive area of tumor cell necrosis* → *is seen in this malignant intrapulmonary solitary fibrous tumor. Tumor cell necrosis correlates with aggressive behavior in these tumors.*

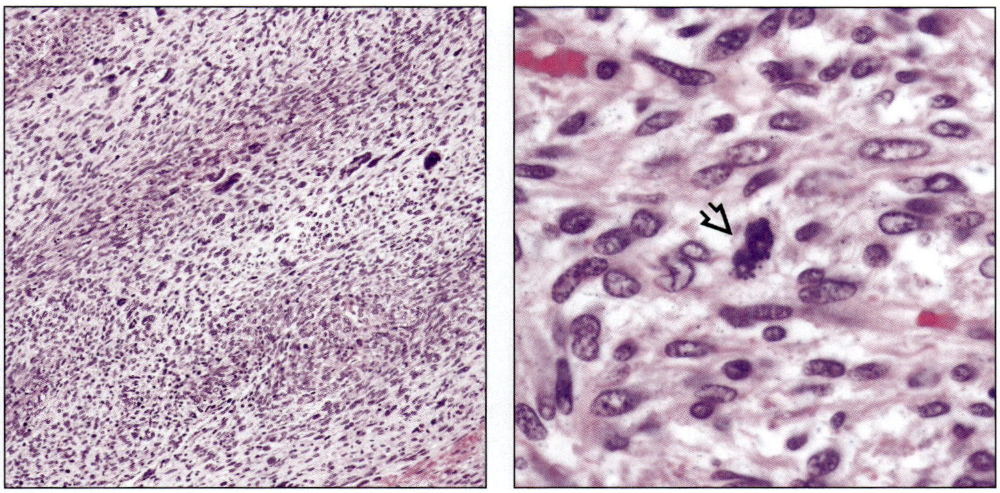

(Left) *Alternating areas of hyper- and hypocellularity are seen in this example of an intrapulmonary solitary fibrous tumor. Tumors with these features can appear indistinguishable from malignant peripheral nerve sheath tumors; electron microscopy and immunohistochemical stains will be of aid in arriving at a definitive diagnosis.* ***(Right)*** *Higher magnification from an intrapulmonary malignant solitary fibrous tumor shows an abnormal mitotic figure* ⇨.

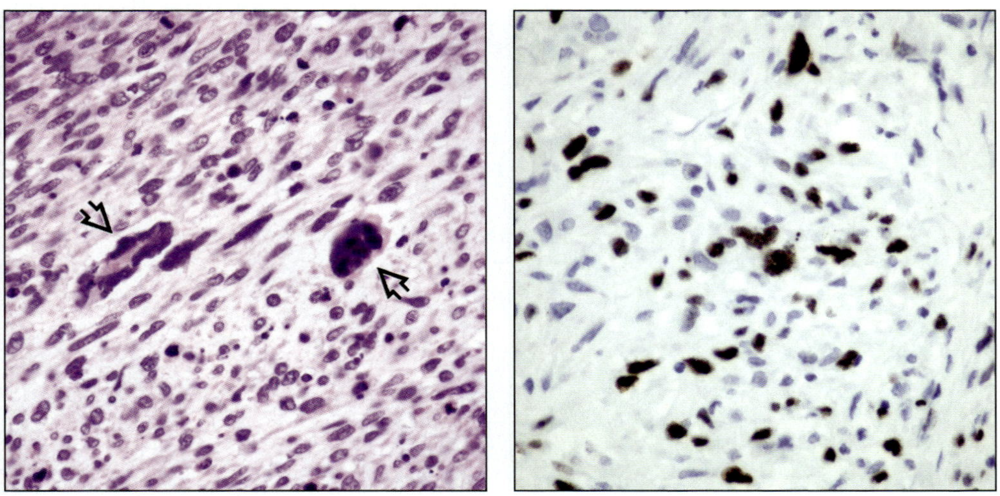

(Left) *High magnification of a metastasis of an intrapulmonary malignant SFT shows bizarre and pleomorphic tumor cells* ⇨*. The original tumor in the lung did not display this degree of cytologic atypia; however, the tumor metastasized widely after 5 years, leading to the death of the patient.* ***(Right)*** *Immunohistochemical staining of intrapulmonary SFT with Ki-67 shows numerous positive nuclei. Increased proliferative activity is associated with malignancy.*

INTRAPULMONARY SOLITARY FIBROUS TUMOR

Microscopic Features

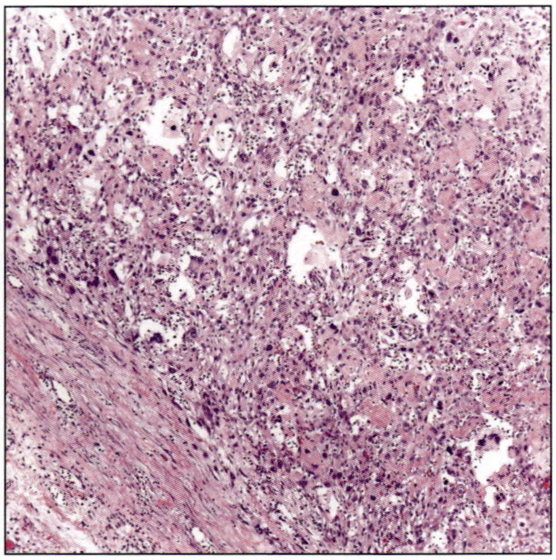

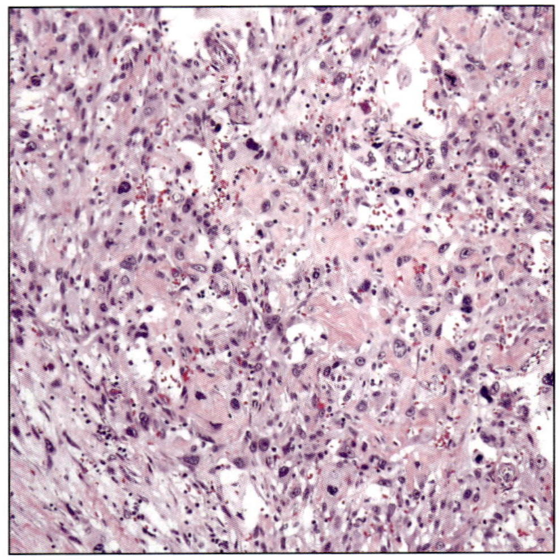

(Left) *Scanning magnification of an intrapulmonary malignant solitary fibrous tumor shows a dense population of large, pleomorphic tumor cells embedded in abundant connective tissue stroma. The histologic appearance of this tumor is indistinguishable from that of a pleomorphic high-grade sarcoma (malignant fibrous histiocytoma).* ***(Right)*** *Higher magnification of an intrapulmonary malignant solitary fibrous tumor shows sheets of large epithelioid cells embedded in abundant collagenous stroma.*

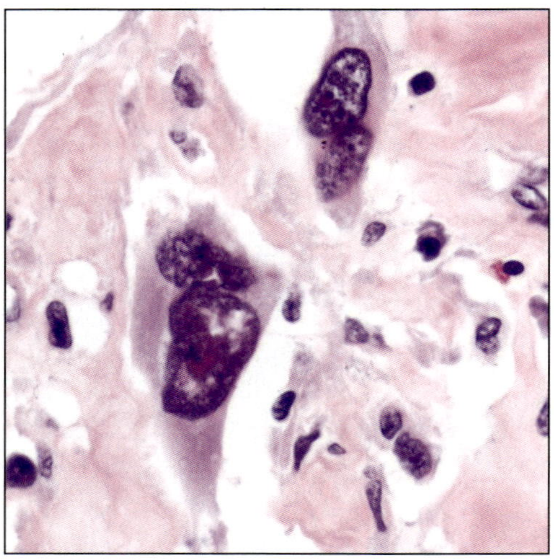

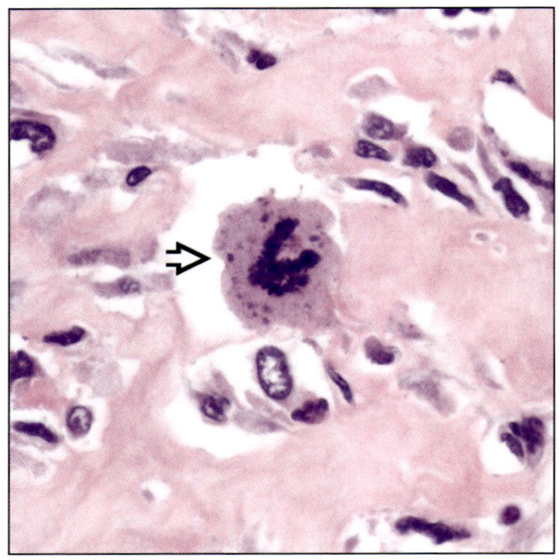

(Left) *Morphology of the tumor cells in an intrapulmonary malignant solitary fibrous tumor shows large multinucleated cells with bizarre nuclei; prominent and often multiple large, eosinophilic nucleoli; and an abundant rim of eosinophilic cytoplasm.* ***(Right)*** *High magnification of an intrapulmonary malignant solitary fibrous tumor shows an abnormal tripolar mitosis ⇨. Up to 3 normal mitoses can be seen in benign tumors, but abnormal mitoses should be worrisome for malignancy.*

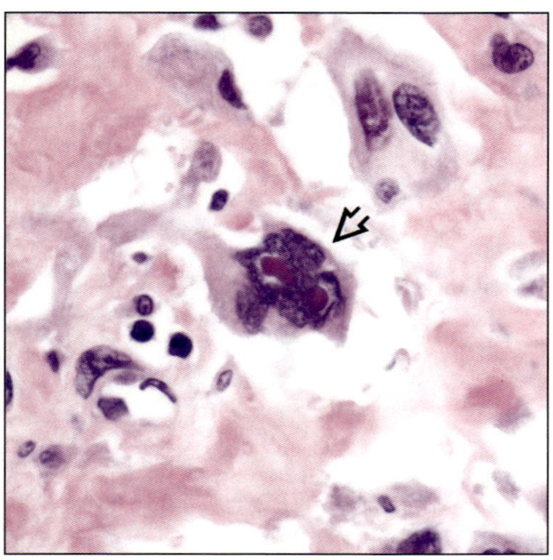

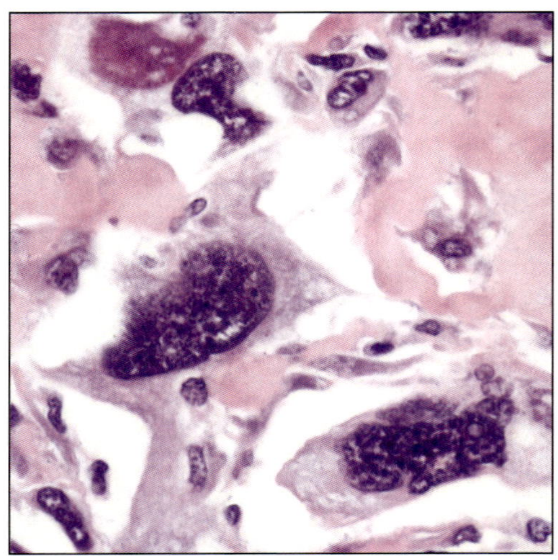

(Left) *Higher magnification of an intrapulmonary malignant solitary fibrous tumor shows a binucleated cell with prominent "owl-eyed" eosinophilic nucleoli resembling a Reed-Sternberg cell ⇨.* ***(Right)*** *Bizarre mononuclear cells with large, hyperchromatic nuclei are seen in this example of an intrapulmonary malignant solitary fibrous tumor. Tumors with these features will require extensive sampling to identify areas with more conventional features of solitary fibrous tumors.*

Microscopic Features

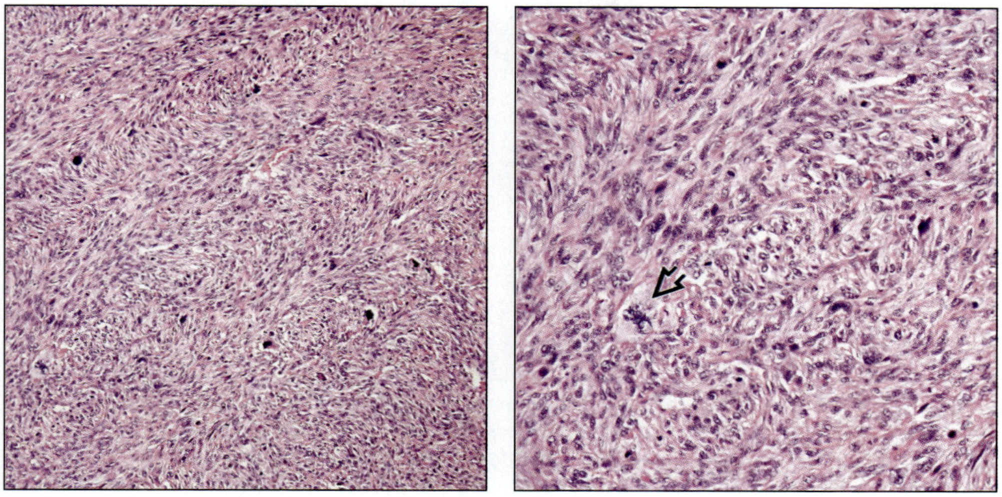

(Left) *Scanning magnification of an intrapulmonary malignant solitary fibrous tumor shows dense fascicles of atypical spindle cells containing multiple scattered pleomorphic and atypical nuclei. The histologic appearance of this tumor is essentially that of a high-grade fibrosarcoma.* ***(Right)*** *Higher magnification of an intrapulmonary malignant solitary fibrous tumor shows fascicles of atypical spindle cells with scattered mitoses. Notice the abnormal mitotic figure ⇨.*

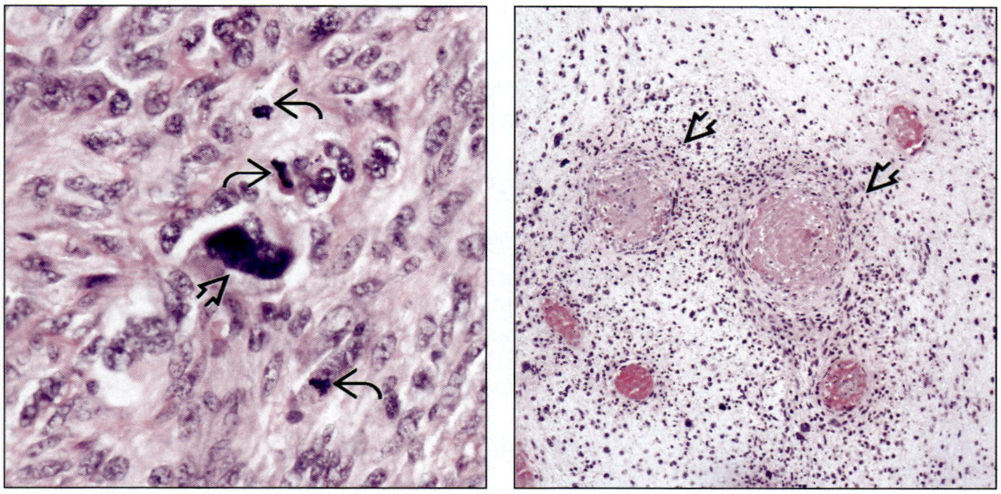

(Left) *Higher magnification of an intrapulmonary malignant solitary fibrous tumor shows atypical spindle cells with numerous mitoses (3 mitoses ↷ in this high-power field). Also notice the bizarre nucleus in the large, atypical cell in the center of the field ⇨.* ***(Right)*** *Malignant intrapulmonary solitary fibrous tumor shows an atypical cell population containing scattered bizarre tumor cells with perivascular condensation ⇨ embedded in an abundant myxoid matrix.*

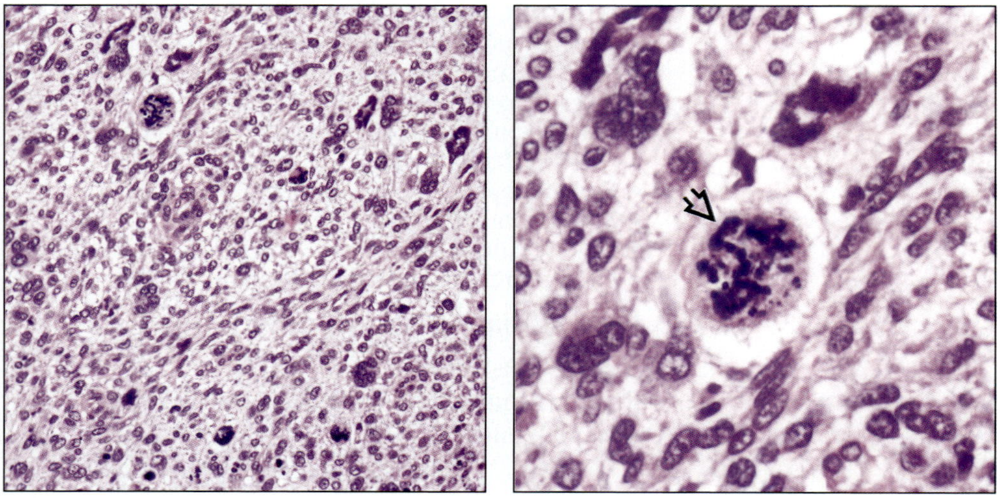

(Left) *Malignant intrapulmonary solitary fibrous tumor with prominent myxoid stroma shows a highly cellular area containing atypical spindle cells admixed with larger, bizarre cells with hyperchromatic nuclei and numerous mitoses.* ***(Right)*** *Higher magnification of a malignant intrapulmonary solitary fibrous tumor shows detail of the atypical cells. Notice that the large cell in the center ⇨ has abnormal mitosis and a "sunburst" chromatin pattern.*

GLOMUS TUMOR

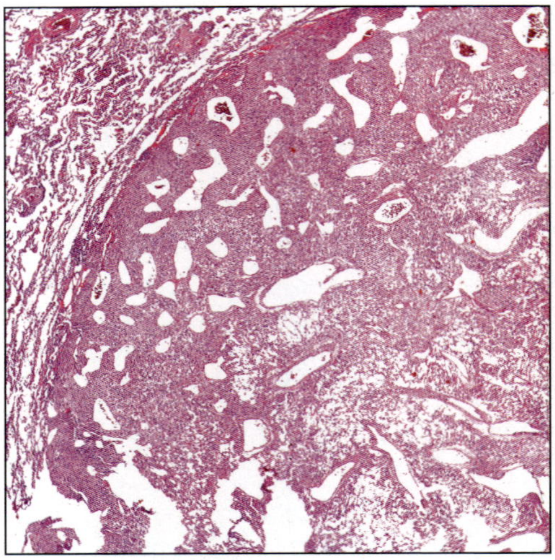

Low-power view of a primary pulmonary glomus tumor shows a well-defined tumor mass replacing normal lung parenchyma.

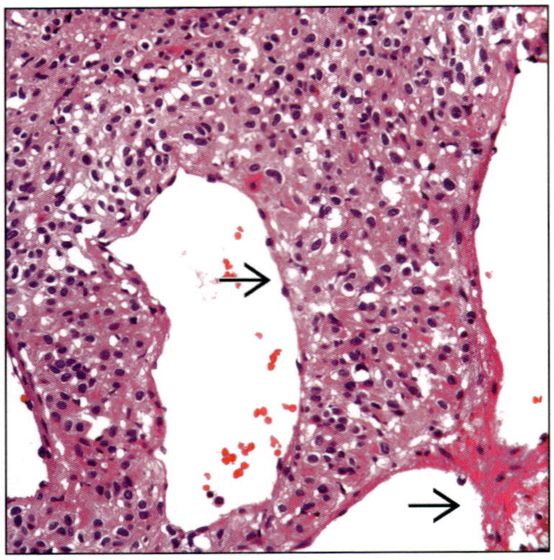

High-power view of a primary pulmonary glomus tumor shows ectatic blood vessels ⇒ and a cellular proliferation composed of medium-sized cells with clear and eosinophilic cytoplasm.

TERMINOLOGY

Synonyms

- Glomangioma, glomic tumor

Definitions

- Benign tumor with smooth muscle differentiation

ETIOLOGY/PATHOGENESIS

Etiology

- Glomus tumors are believed to originate from glomus body
- Debated whether it represents a true tumor or hyperplasia

CLINICAL ISSUES

Epidemiology

- Incidence
  - Very rare tumor in lung
- Age
  - Cases reported have been in adults
- Gender
  - No gender predilection

Presentation

- Cough
- Shortness of breath
- Asymptomatic

Treatment

- Surgical approaches
  - Complete surgical resection

Prognosis

- Excellent

IMAGE FINDINGS

General Features

- Coin lesion in intrapulmonary location
- Central tumor obstructing bronchial lumen

MACROSCOPIC FEATURES

General Features

- Well-circumscribed tumor embedded in lung parenchyma
- White to tan in color without hemorrhage &/or necrosis

Size

- May vary from 1-5 cm in diameter

MICROSCOPIC PATHOLOGY

Histologic Features

- Well-circumscribed tumor nodule
- Solid and homogeneous cellular proliferation
- Ectatic blood vessels
- Cellular proliferation with clear cytoplasm mimicking "fried-egg" appearance
- Hemangiopericytic pattern
- Mucohyaline changes
- Mitotic figures are absent
- Necrosis and hemorrhage are absent

Predominant Pattern/Injury Type

- Solid

Predominant Cell/Compartment Type

- Smooth muscle

GLOMUS TUMOR

Key Facts

Terminology
- Synonyms: Glomangioma, glomic tumor

Clinical Issues
- Cough
- Shortness of breath
- Asymptomatic

Image Findings
- Coin lesion in intrapulmonary location
- Central tumor obstructing bronchial lumen

Microscopic Pathology
- Solid and homogeneous cellular proliferation
- Ectatic blood vessels
- Cellular proliferation with clear cytoplasm mimicking "fried-egg" appearance
- Mitotic figures are absent
- Necrosis and hemorrhage are absent

Top Differential Diagnoses
- Glomangiosarcoma
  - Mitotic figures and cellular pleomorphism are most important features to separate from glomangioma
- Leiomyoma
  - Rarely displays prominent ectatic blood vessels with edema of wall
  - Both tumors may show similar immunohistochemical profile
  - Tumor cells are mostly oval or spindled
- Carcinoma
  - Displays more cellular atypia and mitotic activity
  - Shows positive staining for epithelial markers

Immunohistochemistry

Antibody	Reactivity	Staining Pattern	Comment
Vimentin	Positive	Cytoplasmic	
Actin-sm	Positive	Cytoplasmic	
Desmin	Positive	Cytoplasmic	In some cases
NSE	Positive	Cytoplasmic	In some cases
LEU-7	Positive	Cytoplasmic	In some cases
CD34	Positive	Cytoplasmic	In some cases
S100	Negative		
CK-PAN	Negative		
EMA	Negative		
Myoglobin	Negative		
HMB-45	Negative		
Chromogranin-A	Negative		

DIFFERENTIAL DIAGNOSIS

Glomangiosarcoma
- Mitotic figures and cellular pleomorphism are most important features to separate from glomangioma
- Areas of necrosis and sclerosis may be present
- In focal areas, more conventional areas of glomangioma are commonly seen

Leiomyoma
- Shows more spindle cellular proliferation
- Rarely displays prominent ectatic blood vessels
- Both tumors may show similar immunohistochemical phenotype
- Tumor cells are mostly oval or spindled

Carcinoma
- Displays more cellular atypia and mitotic activity
- Does not show strong positive reaction for actin-sm
- Shows positive staining for epithelial markers

DIAGNOSTIC CHECKLIST

Clinically Relevant Pathologic Features
- Cytoplasmic features

Pathologic Interpretation Pearls
- Cellular proliferation with clear cell changes admixed with ectatic blood vessels
- Monotonous appear of tumor cells with "fried-egg" appearance

SELECTED REFERENCES

1. Gaertner EM et al: Pulmonary and mediastinal glomus tumors--report of five cases including a pulmonary glomangiosarcoma: a clinicopathologic study with literature review. Am J Surg Pathol. 24(8):1105-14, 2000
2. Koss MN et al: Primary pulmonary glomus tumor: a clinicopathologic and immunohistochemical study of two cases. Mod Pathol. 11(3):253-8, 1998
3. Tang CK et al: Glomangioma of the lung. Am J Surg Pathol. 2(1):103-9, 1978

GLOMUS TUMOR

Microscopic Features

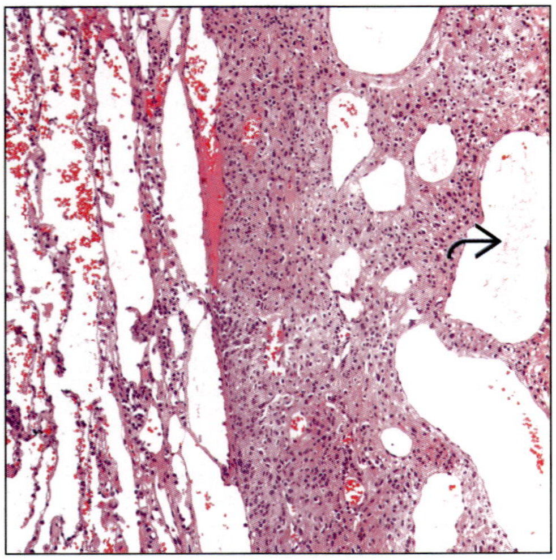
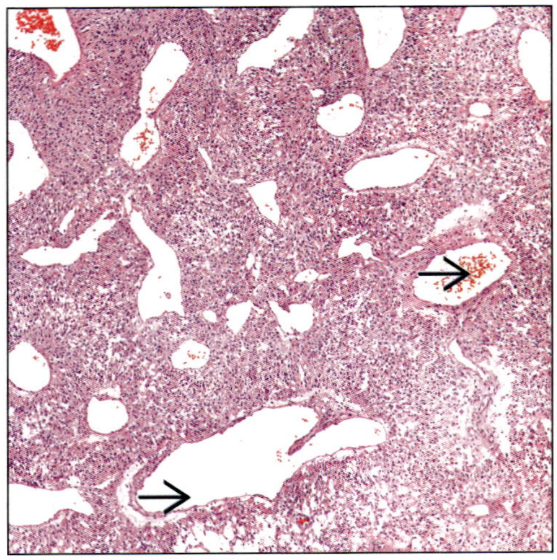

(Left) *Low-power view of a pulmonary glomus tumor shows the well-defined border of the tumor. Note that the tumor is not encapsulated and in addition, the tumor shows a rather homogeneous cellular proliferation with dilated spaces ↷.* ***(Right)*** *Pulmonary glomus tumor shows classical appearance of a cellular proliferation alternating with numerous ectatic blood vessels →, giving an appearance of a vascular neoplasm.*

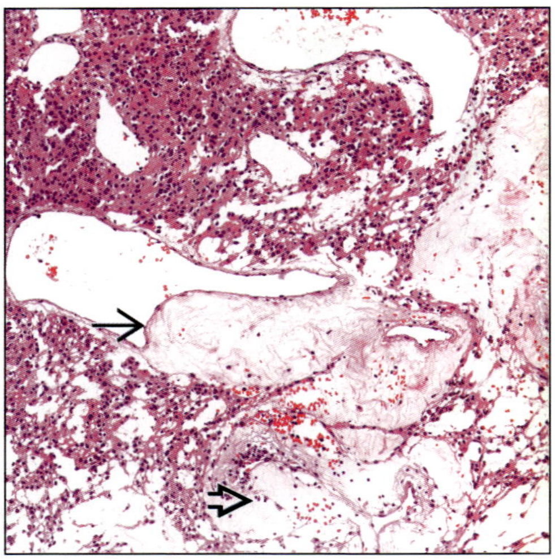
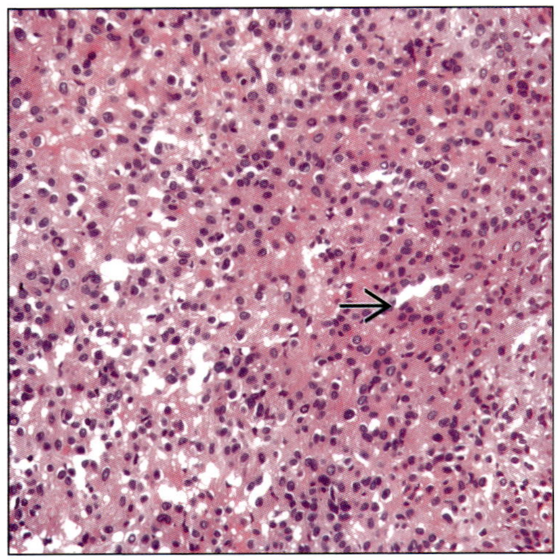

(Left) *The vessels in a pulmonary glomus tumor show prominent edematous changes in the walls →. Some of the vessels are compressed and difficult to recognize as vascular structures ⇨.* ***(Right)*** *In other areas, a glomus tumor in the lung shows a predominantly solid growth pattern with inconspicuous blood vessels →. The uniformity and bland cytologic appearance of the tumor cell population is a clue for correct diagnosis.*

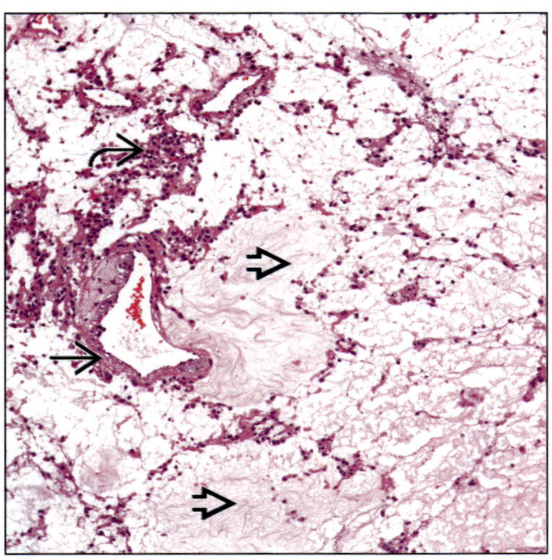
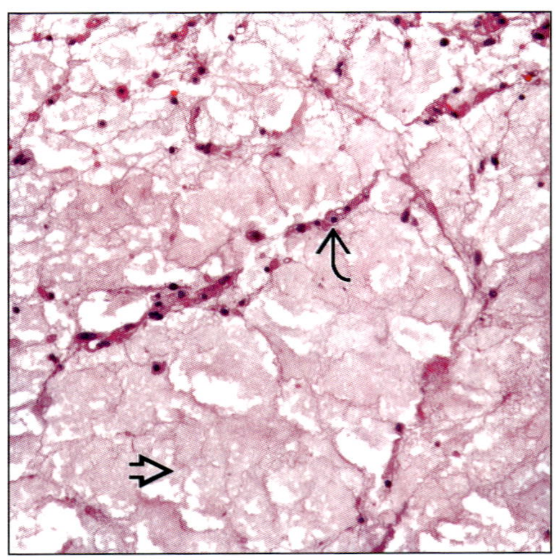

(Left) *Pulmonary glomus tumor with an extensive edematous ⇨ component distending the alveolar spaces. Still, one is able to recognize a dilated vascular structure → and cluster of tumor cells ↷.* ***(Right)*** *High-power view shows the edematous component of a pulmonary glomus tumor. Although an unusual feature, extensive edematous ⇨ areas may be seen in which the neoplastic cells can be easily missed ↷.*

Microscopic Features

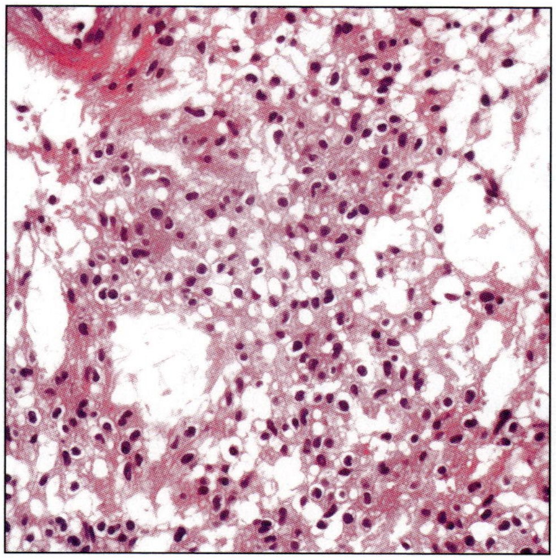
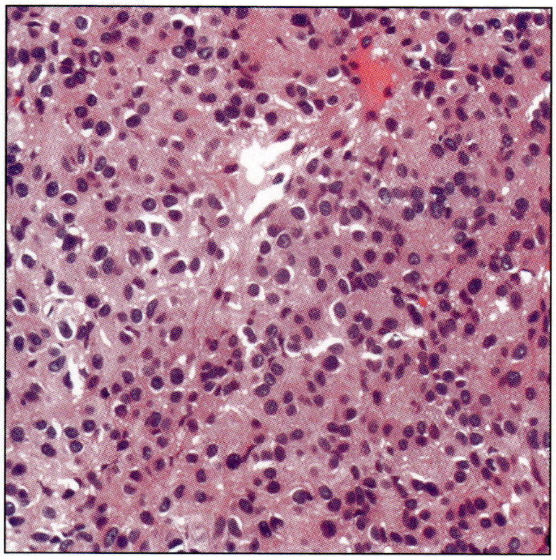

(Left) *High-power view of a pulmonary glomus tumor shows a cellular proliferation composed of medium-sized cells with clear cytoplasm and "fried egg" appearance. Note the absence of nuclear atypia or mitotic activity.* ***(Right)*** *High-power view of a more solid area of a glomus tumor shows medium-sized cells with eosinophilic cytoplasm. The round uniform cells with centrally placed dark nuclei are quite distinctive for this tumor.*

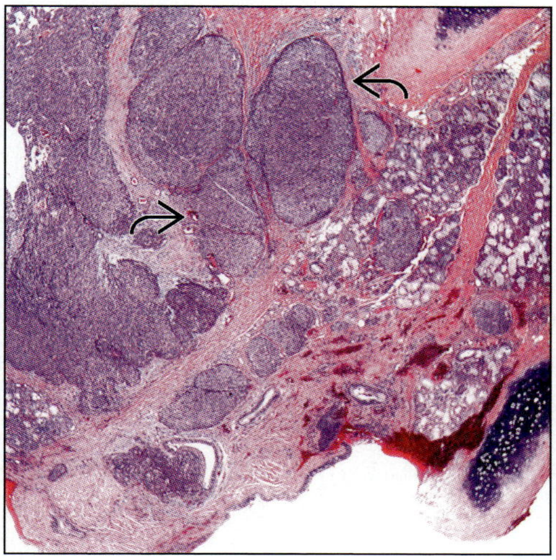
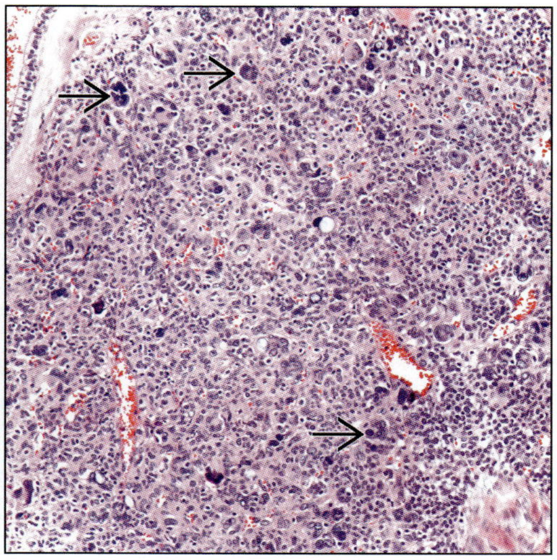

(Left) *Glomangiosarcoma shows a more haphazard growth pattern with infiltrative borders. In this case, the tumor is in a central location growing in lobules of different sizes ⤻ adjacent to a bronchus.* ***(Right)*** *Pulmonary glomangiosarcoma shows prominent nuclear atypia and multinucleated cells →. These cytologic features are not seen in the benign counterpart of a glomus tumor.*

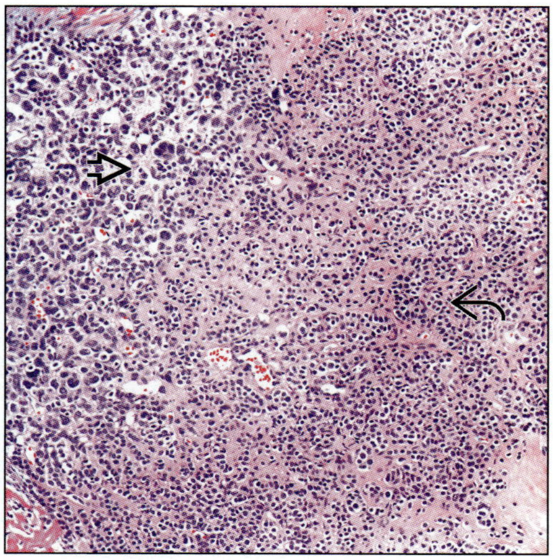
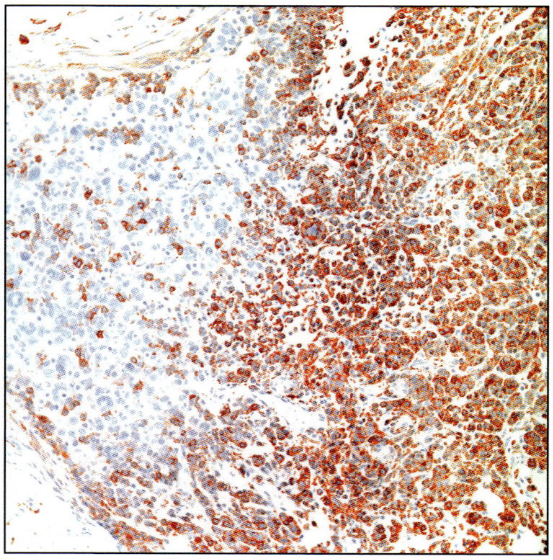

(Left) *Pulmonary glomangiosarcoma shows transitional areas with a benign glomus tumor ⤻ developing into a malignant glomus tumor (glomangiosarcoma) ⇨. This feature may be helpful in order to properly classify the tumor as glomangiosarcoma.* ***(Right)*** *Smooth muscle actin immunohistochemical stain shows a strong positive reaction in the glomus component and scattered positive cells in the glomangiosarcomatous component.*

INTRAPULMONARY THYMOMA

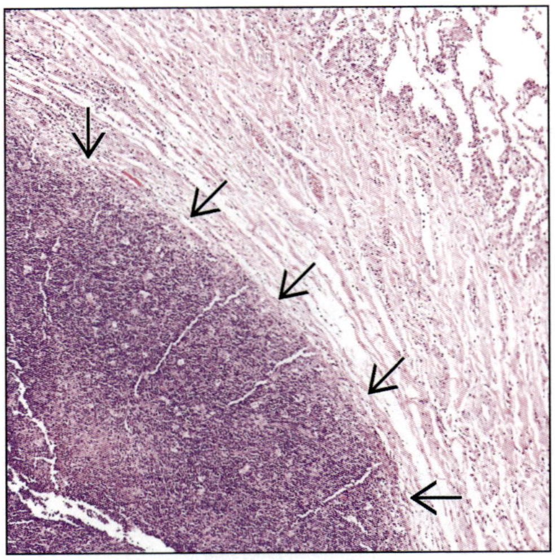

Scanning magnification of an intrapulmonary thymoma shows a well-circumscribed nodule composed of densely packed small lymphocytes ⇒ separated from the lung parenchyma by a band of connective tissue.

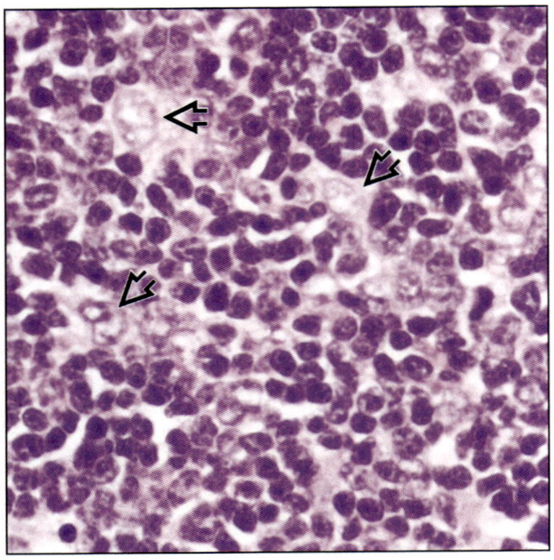

Higher magnification of an intrapulmonary thymoma shows a characteristic biphasic population of cells composed of numerous small T lymphocytes and scattered larger epithelial cells with vesicular nuclei ⇨.

TERMINOLOGY

Abbreviations

- Intrapulmonary thymoma (IPT)

Definitions

- Primary thymic epithelial neoplasm arising from embryologically displaced elements within the lung

ETIOLOGY/PATHOGENESIS

Developmental Anomaly

- Aberrant embryological development of the thymus gland in ectopic locations

CLINICAL ISSUES

Epidemiology

- Age
  - 25-77 years
- Gender
  - Female predilection (M:F = 1:7)

Site

- Intraparenchymatous location within lung parenchyma; central and peripheral
- Predilection for right lobe of lung
- May be multifocal

Presentation

- Cough
- Chest pain
- Incidental finding on chest x-ray in 50% of patients
- Not commonly associated with myasthenia gravis, aplastic anemia, or other paraneoplastic syndromes

Treatment

- Surgical approaches
  - Lobectomy

Prognosis

- Most cases cured with simple surgical excision

IMAGE FINDINGS

General Features

- Location
  - Well-circumscribed intraparenchymatous mass
- Size
  - 0.5-10 cm in greatest dimension

CT Findings

- Absence of mediastinal involvement on CT scans

MACROSCOPIC FEATURES

General Features

- Well-circumscribed tumor surrounded by normal lung parenchyma
- Gray-white, homogeneous cut surface
- May show areas of hemorrhage and cystic degeneration

MICROSCOPIC PATHOLOGY

Histologic Features

- Well-circumscribed cellular proliferation showing variable admixture of epithelial cells and lymphocytes
- **Lymphocyte-rich thymoma (WHO types B1-B2)**
  - Sheets of small lymphocytes admixed with scattered, large, pale epithelial cells with large vesicular nuclei with prominent nucleoli
  - Areas of "medullary" differentiation (lighter areas within sheets of small lymphocytes)
  - Dilated perivascular spaces
  - Lobules separated by bands of fibrous tissue on scanning magnification
- **Epithelial-rich thymoma (WHO type B3)**

INTRAPULMONARY THYMOMA

Key Facts

Clinical Issues
- Intraparenchymatous location within lung parenchyma; central and peripheral
- Incidental finding on chest x-ray in 50% of patients

Image Findings
- 0.5-10 cm in greatest dimension

Macroscopic Features
- Well-circumscribed tumor surrounded by normal lung parenchyma

Microscopic Pathology
- Well-circumscribed cellular proliferation showing various admixtures of epithelial cells and lymphocytes
  - Lymphocyte-rich thymoma (WHO types B1-B2)
  - Epithelial-rich thymoma (WHO type B3)
  - Spindle cell thymoma (WHO types A and AB)
- Epithelial cells in intrapulmonary thymomas are bland, with minimal atypia
- Tumor cells are intimately admixed with small T lymphocytes in varying proportions

Ancillary Tests
- Neoplastic epithelial cells show positive cytoplasmic staining for cytokeratins (AE1/AE3, CAM5.2, CK19)
- Neoplastic epithelial cells show strong nuclear positivity for p63
- Lymphocytes stain as immature T lymphoblasts (CD1a, CD3, TdT, and CD99 positive)
- Spindle cells are negative for mesenchymal markers of differentiation (S100 protein, SMA, desmin, CD34)
- Spindle cells may stain positive for calretinin and Bcl-2

  - Sheets of large epithelioid cells with large nuclei showing prominent chromatin pattern and nucleoli
  - Sparse population of scattered small lymphocytes admixed with epithelial cells
  - Epithelial cells show sharp cell borders with areas of early or abortive squamous differentiation
  - Abundant perivascular spaces
- **Spindle cell thymoma (WHO types A and AB)**
  - Sheets of oval to spindle cells with minimal or no cytologic atypia or mitotic activity
  - Spindle cells may adopt fascicular, storiform, herringbone, or hemangiopericytic growth pattern
  - Sparse population of small lymphocytes admixed with spindle cells
  - Spindle cells may be seen surrounding occasional gland-like spaces

Cytologic Features
- Epithelial cells in most intrapulmonary thymomas are bland, with minimal atypia
- Tumor cells are intimately admixed with small T lymphocytes in varying proportions

ANCILLARY TESTS

Immunohistochemistry
- Neoplastic epithelial cells show positive cytoplasmic staining for cytokeratins (AE1/AE3, CAM5.2, CK19)
- Neoplastic epithelial cells show strong nuclear positivity for p63
- Lymphocytes stain as immature T lymphoblasts (CD1a, TdT, and CD99 positive)
- Spindle cells are negative for mesenchymal markers of differentiation (S100 protein, SMA, desmin, CD34)

DIFFERENTIAL DIAGNOSIS

Lymphoblastic Lymphoma
- Sheets of lymphocytes with "starry sky" appearance can be seen in both
- Positivity of small lymphocytes for TdT, CD3, and CD99 can be seen in both
- Lymphoma will be negative for cytokeratin stains
- Molecular studies will not show any gene rearrangements of T-cell receptors in thymoma

Well-differentiated Squamous Cell Carcinoma
- Sheets of epidermoid-appearing cells with sharp cell borders can be seen in both
- Squamous cell carcinoma shows more prominent keratinization and cytologic atypia
- Lymphocytes in squamous cell carcinoma are of B-cell type rather than T-lymphocytes
- Lobulation and perivascular spaces favor thymoma over squamous cell carcinoma

Sarcomatoid (Spindle Cell) Carcinoma
- Usually shows more pronounced cytologic atypia and mitotic activity than spindle cell thymoma
- Lacks immature T-lymphocytic component
- Negative for p63

Intrapulmonary Solitary Fibrous Tumor (Hemangiopericytoma)
- Prominent hemangiopericytic growth pattern can be seen in both
- Tumor cells are negative for cytokeratin stains and p63 and positive for CD34 and Bcl-2

SELECTED REFERENCES

1. Myers PO et al: Primary intrapulmonary thymoma: a systematic review. Eur J Surg Oncol. 33(10):1137-41, 2007
2. Moran CA et al: Primary intrapulmonary thymoma. A clinicopathologic and immunohistochemical study of eight cases. Am J Surg Pathol. 19(3):304-12, 1995
3. James CL et al: Intrapulmonary thymoma. Histopathology. 21(2):175-7, 1992
4. Fukayama M et al: Pulmonary and pleural thymoma. Diagnostic application of lymphocyte markers to the thymoma of unusual site. Am J Clin Pathol. 89(5):617-21, 1988

INTRAPULMONARY THYMOMA

Lymphocyte-rich and Spindle Cell Thymoma

(Left) *Scanning magnification of intrapulmonary thymoma, lymphocyte-rich type (WHO B1) shows a dense population of small lymphoid cells sharply separated from the surrounding lung parenchyma by a thin fibrous capsule* ➔. ***(Right)*** *Higher magnification of an intrapulmonary lymphocyte-rich thymoma shows a large cell with a vesicular nucleus and prominent eosinophilic nucleolus* ⇨ *corresponding to a neoplastic thymic epithelial cell. Notice the large number of surrounding small lymphocytes.*

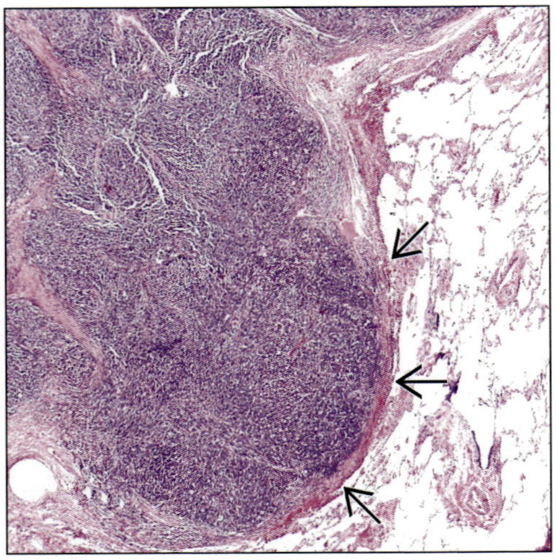

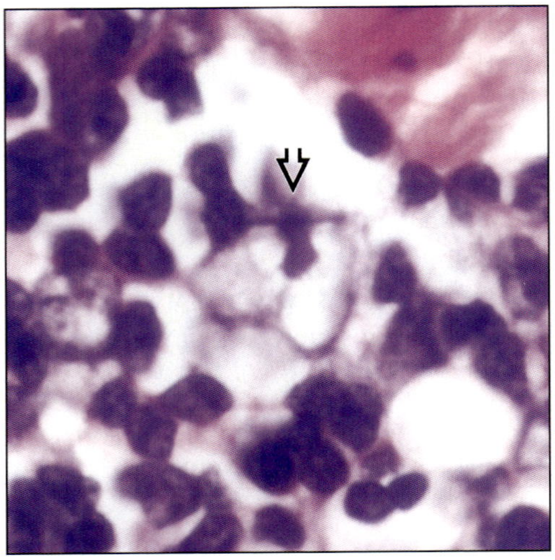

(Left) *Example of an intrapulmonary thymoma of lymphoepithelial type (WHO B2) shows an approximately even admixture of small lymphocytes and neoplastic thymic epithelial cells.* ***(Right)*** *Immunohistochemical staining of a lymphocyte-rich intrapulmonary thymoma for cytokeratin AE1/AE3 shows scattered keratin-positive (dark brown) cells corresponding to the neoplastic thymic epithelial cells. Notice the abundance of nonreactive small lymphocytes in the background.*

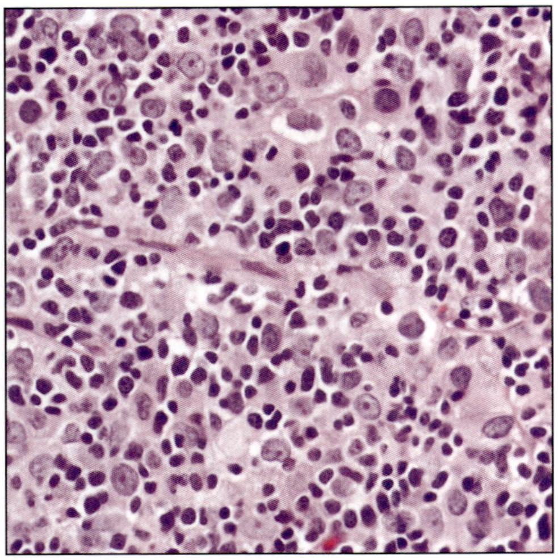

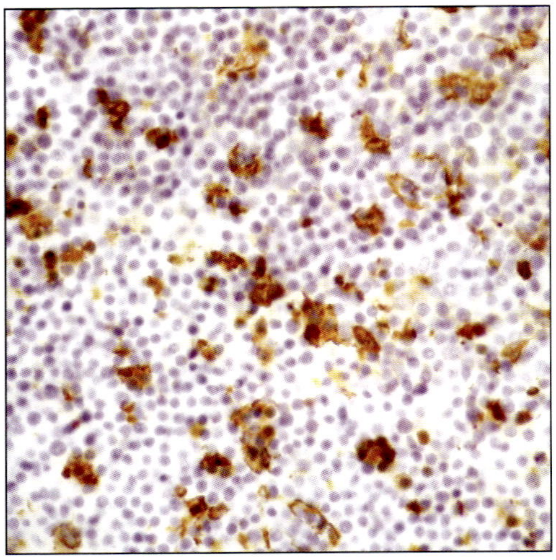

(Left) *Intrapulmonary spindle cell thymoma is composed of cells with slender nuclei with a scattered chromatin pattern and a scant rim of amphophilic cytoplasm. Notice the absence of small lymphocytes, cytologic atypia, or mitotic activity.* ***(Right)*** *Immunohistochemical staining of an intrapulmonary spindle cell thymoma for p63 antigen shows nuclear positivity in the spindle cells. p63 is a sensitive (although nonspecific) marker for thymic epithelial cells.*

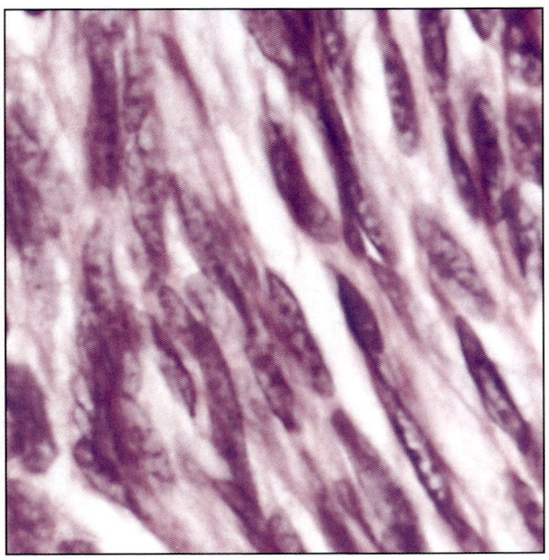

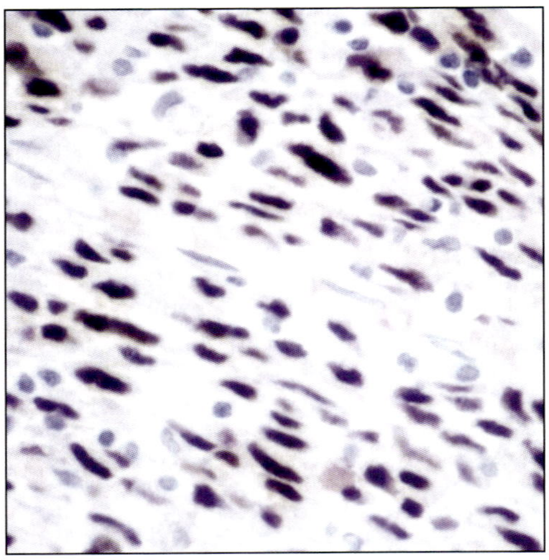

Atypical Thymoma (WHO B3)

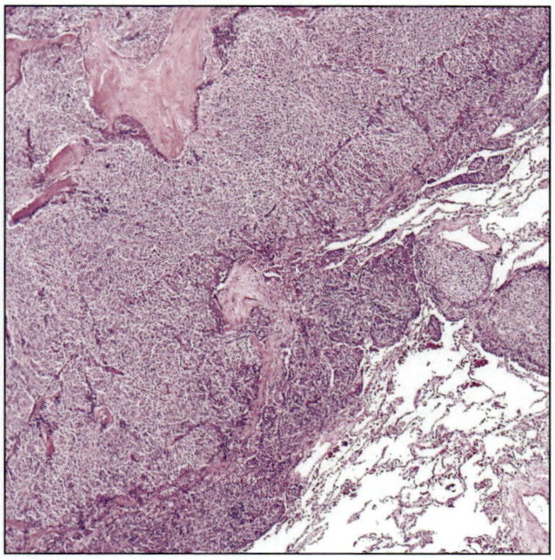
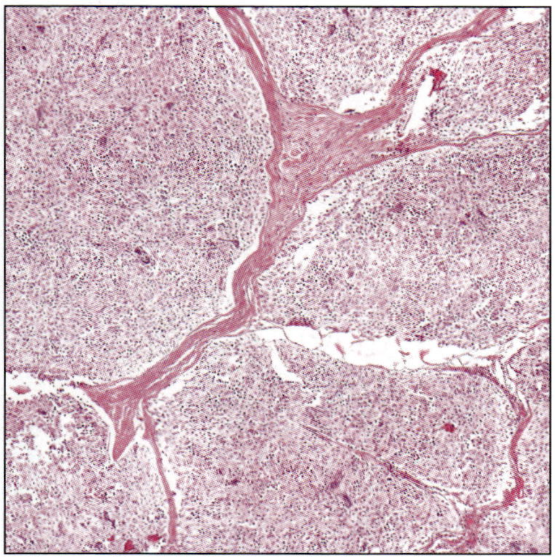

(Left) *Scanning magnification of an intrapulmonary atypical thymoma (WHO B3) shows sheets of large epithelioid cells separated from the surrounding lung parenchyma.* ***(Right)*** *Intrapulmonary atypical thymoma shows striking lobulation with large nodules of epithelial cells separated by broad bands of fibrous connective tissue. Preservation of the lobular architecture is one of the organotypical features of the thymus that distinguishes atypical thymoma (WHO B3).*

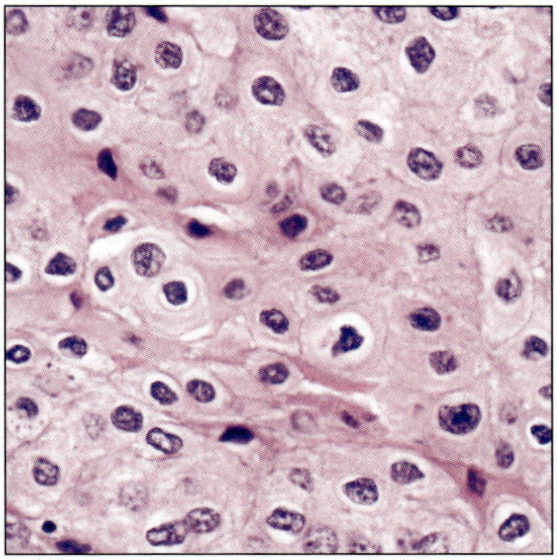
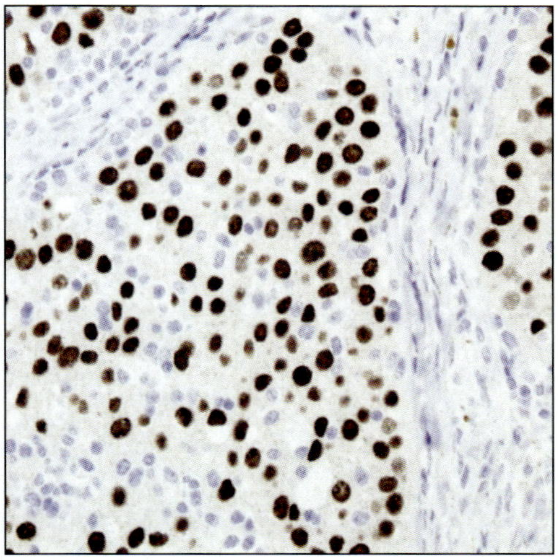

(Left) *High magnification of an intrapulmonary atypical thymoma shows sheets of round to polygonal epithelial cells with round to oval nuclei surrounded by an ample rim of eosinophilic cytoplasm with sharp cell borders. The sharp cell borders give the tumor a distinctive "squamoid" appearance.* ***(Right)*** *Immunohistochemical staining of intrapulmonary atypical thymoma with p63 antibody shows strong nuclear positivity of the tumor cells for this marker.*

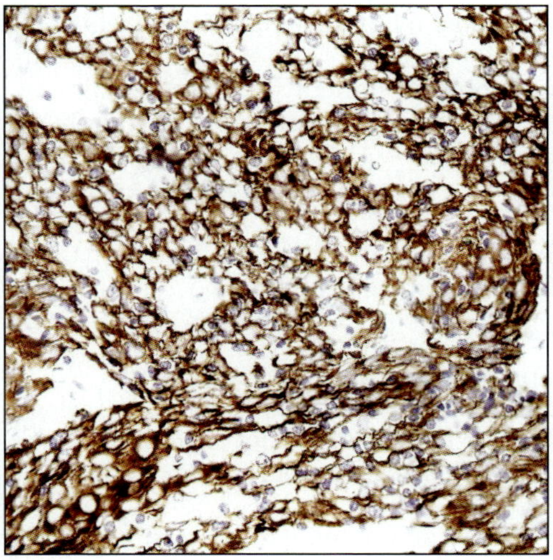
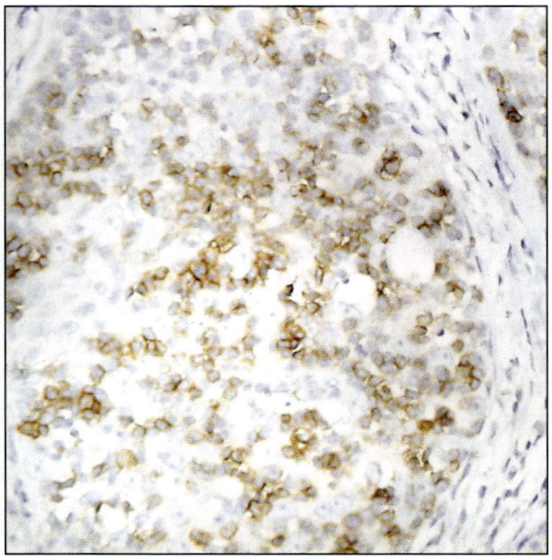

(Left) *Immunohistochemical staining of intrapulmonary atypical thymoma with broad-spectrum keratin (AE1/AE3) shows strong cytoplasmic positivity of the tumor cells.* ***(Right)*** *Immunohistochemical staining of intrapulmonary atypical thymoma with CD1a shows a few scattered positive small lymphocytes in the background. The demonstration of CD1a or TdT-positive immature T lymphoblasts admixed with the epithelial cells supports the thymic derivation of the tumor.*

PULMONARY PARAGANGLIOMA

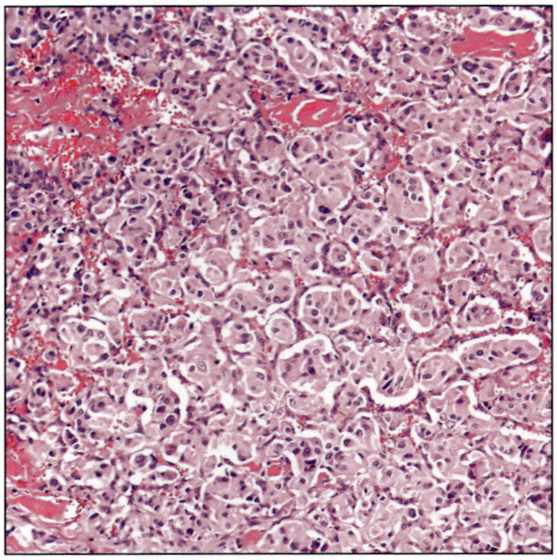

Scanning magnification of pulmonary paraganglioma shows characteristic neuroendocrine architecture (zellballen pattern) of these tumors composed of discrete "nests" of epithelioid cells.

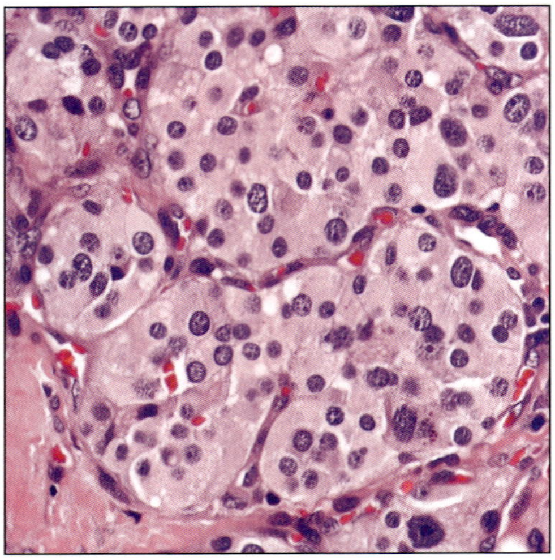

Higher magnification of pulmonary paraganglioma shows a population of tumor cells with round nuclei and a stippled chromatin pattern that is surrounded by an ample rim of eosinophilic cytoplasm.

TERMINOLOGY

Synonyms

- Pulmonary chemodectoma, extraadrenal paraganglioma

Definitions

- Primary neuroendocrine lung neoplasm derived from ectopic paraganglionic elements

CLINICAL ISSUES

Epidemiology

- Incidence
  - Extremely rare tumor in pulmonary location
- Age
  - Middle-aged adults (40-50 years of age)
- Gender
  - Male predominance

Presentation

- Solitary, peripheral "coin" lesion
- Central, endobronchial lesion
- Endocrine symptoms
  - Hypertension
  - Increased serum norepinephrine
  - Cushing syndrome
- Endobronchial lesion may present with obstructive symptoms
  - Cough
  - Wheezing
  - Dyspnea
  - Stridor

Treatment

- Surgical excision

Prognosis

- Majority of reported cases have been benign

MACROSCOPIC FEATURES

General Features

- Well-circumscribed intraparenchymatous nodule
- Smooth, well-circumscribed endobronchial lesion

Size

- 1-3 cm in greatest diameter

Cut Surface

- Smooth, homogeneous, and well circumscribed
- Tan-brown to pink
- Highly vascularized; rarely may show hemorrhage

MICROSCOPIC PATHOLOGY

Histologic Features

- Principal feature is "endocrine" or "organoid" growth pattern
- Most common pattern of growth is discrete nests of tumor cells separated by fibrovascular septa (zellballen pattern)
- Rare cases may show prominent stromal sclerosis
- Foci of necrosis or vascular invasion are only rarely encountered
- Stroma may be very vascularized with large, ectatic vessels
- Trabecular, microacinar, or ribbon-like growth patterns are distinctively rare in paraganglioma

Cytologic Features

- Large round or polygonal cells with abundant eosinophilic cytoplasm
- Large round cells with abundant clear cytoplasm
- Elongated cells with spindle nuclei and abundant cytoplasm
- Oncocytic cells with abundant granular eosinophilic cytoplasm
- Cell nuclei are generally small and contain inconspicuous nucleoli

Key Facts

Clinical Issues
- Extremely rare tumor in pulmonary location
- Solitary, peripheral "coin" lesion
- Central, endobronchial lesion

Microscopic Pathology
- Principal feature is "endocrine" or "organoid" growth pattern
- Most common pattern of growth is discrete nests of tumor cells separated by fibrovascular septa (zellballen pattern)
- Large round or polygonal cells with abundant eosinophilic cytoplasm
- Large round cells with abundant clear cytoplasm
- Elongated cells with spindle nuclei and abundant cytoplasm
- Oncocytic cells with abundant granular eosinophilic cytoplasm
- Foci containing cells with macronuclei or bizarre nuclei but devoid of mitotic activity are common

Ancillary Tests
- Strong positivity of tumor cells for neuroendocrine-associated markers, including chromogranin, synaptophysin, and CD56
- S100 protein-positive sustentacular cells are seen surrounding the tumor cell "nests"

Diagnostic Checklist
- Histologic features are notoriously unreliable for predicting biologic behavior
- Most common differential diagnosis is with pulmonary "carcinoid" tumor

- Foci containing cells with macronuclei or bizarre nuclei but devoid of mitotic activity are common
- Mitoses are rare and usually normal
- Intranuclear cytoplasmic inclusions ("pseudoinclusions") can be occasionally identified
- Large cells with abundant cytoplasm and large nuclei resembling ganglion cells can also be occasionally seen

ANCILLARY TESTS

Frozen Sections
- Immersion of fresh tissue in Bouin fixative or other picric acid-containing solution will characteristically turn the specimen brown

Immunohistochemistry
- Strong positivity of tumor cells for neuroendocrine-associated markers, including chromogranin, synaptophysin, and CD56
- S100 protein-positive sustentacular cells are seen surrounding the tumor cell nests
- Tumor cells contain neurofilament-type intermediate filaments, but these may be difficult to demonstrate by immunohistochemistry
- Other peptides that may be expressed by the tumor cells include ACTH, VIP, leu- or met-enkephalins, and calcitonin

Electron Microscopy
- Transmission
  - Large cells containing abundant cytoplasmic dense-core neurosecretory granules
    - Dense-core granules are characterized by eccentric halos that impart them with a blister-like appearance

DIFFERENTIAL DIAGNOSIS

Well-differentiated Neuroendocrine Carcinoma (Carcinoid Tumor)
- Tumor cells are universally positive for cytokeratins
- S100 protein-positive sustentacular cells may also be present in carcinoid tumors
- Microacinar, trabecular, or ribbon-like growth patterns favor a diagnosis of carcinoid tumor

Metastatic Paraganglioma to the Lung
- Rare event; clinical history of previous tumor is the only reliable means for making this diagnosis

DIAGNOSTIC CHECKLIST

Clinically Relevant Pathologic Features
- Histologic features are notoriously unreliable for predicting biologic behavior
- Diagnosis of malignancy is established based on the documentation of metastases
- Most common differential diagnosis is with pulmonary "carcinoid" tumor

Pathologic Interpretation Pearls
- Nuclear pleomorphism and macronucleoli are frequent and characteristic findings that do not correlate with clinical behavior
- Presence of trabecular growth pattern, ribbons, or festoons are indicative of a carcinoid tumor rather than paraganglioma
- Strong cytokeratin positivity in the tumor cells generally rules out a diagnosis of paraganglioma in a neuroendocrine neoplasm
- Well-developed population of S100 protein-positive sustentacular cells around tumor cell nests generally favors a diagnosis of paraganglioma

SELECTED REFERENCES

1. Shibahara J et al: Primary pulmonary paraganglioma: report of a functioning case with immunohistochemical and ultrastructural study. Am J Surg Pathol. 28(6):825-9, 2004
2. Cerilli LA et al: Neuroendocrine neoplasms of the lung. Am J Clin Pathol. 116 Suppl:S65-96, 2001

PULMONARY PARAGANGLIOMA

Histologic Growth Patterns

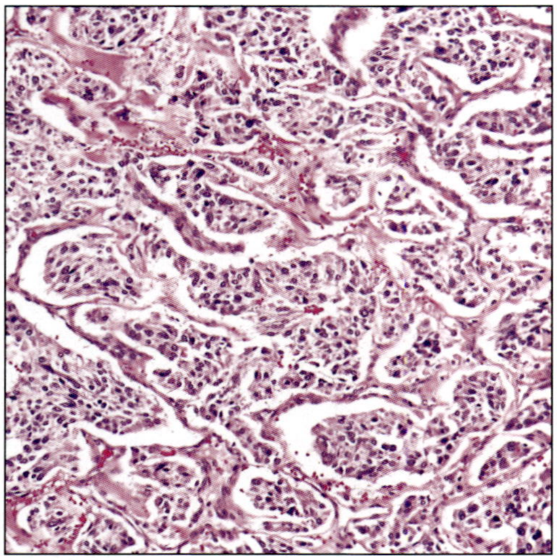

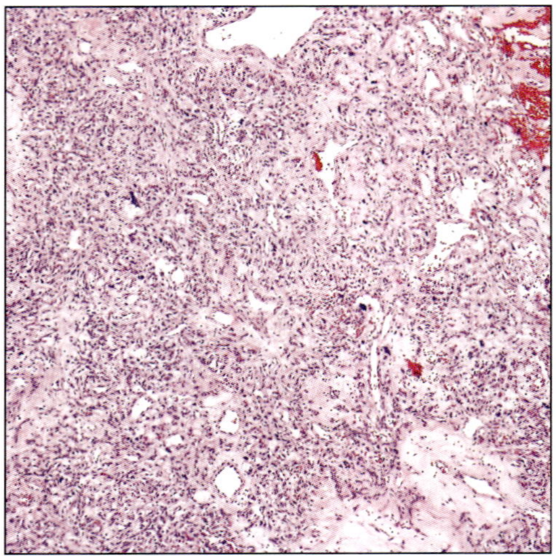

(Left) *"Organoid" growth pattern is the most typical appearance of a pulmonary paraganglioma and is characterized by well-defined nests of relatively uniform tumor cells surrounded by delicate fibrovascular septae (zellballen pattern).* ***(Right)*** *A more diffuse, sheet-like growth pattern can occasionally be observed in pulmonary paraganglioma and is caused by the confluence of the nests of tumor cells. Other areas in the same tumor, however, display the characteristic zellballen pattern.*

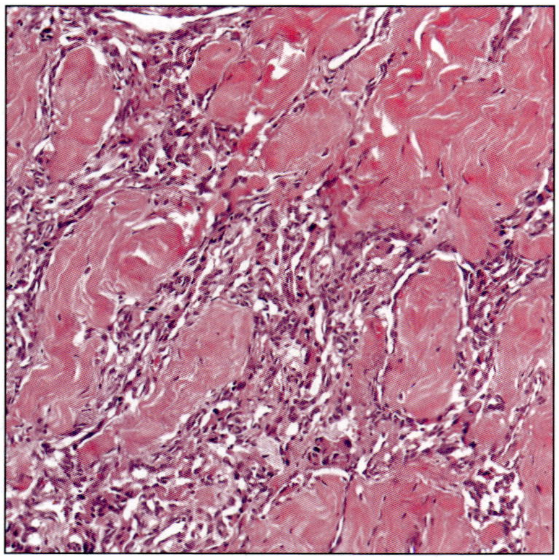

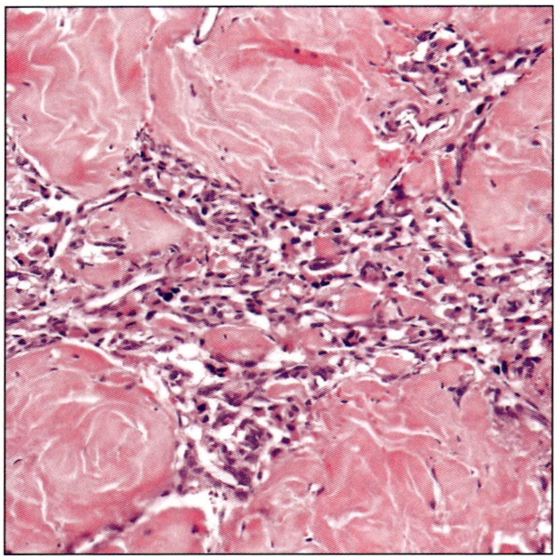

(Left) *Stromal sclerosis is another feature that may sometimes be observed in pulmonary paraganglioma. It is characterized by heavy deposits of dense collagen in the stroma surrounding the nests of tumor cells.* ***(Right)*** *Higher magnification of pulmonary paraganglioma with stromal sclerosis shows heavy deposits of hyalinized collagen circumscribing residual islands of tumor cells. The tumor cells in such cases tend to become distorted and often adopt an oval or spindled appearance.*

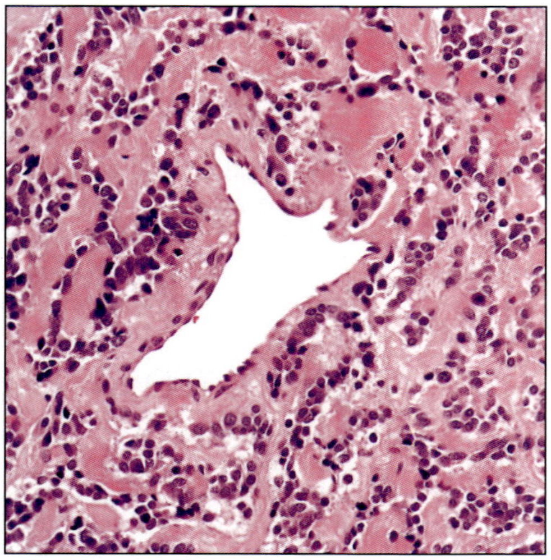

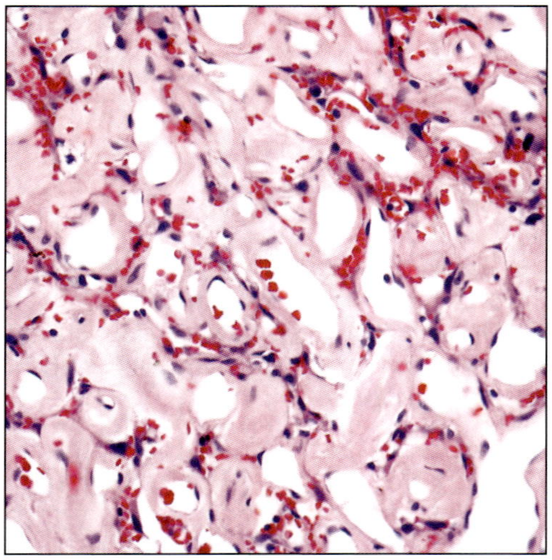

(Left) *Perivascular "targetoid" arrangement of tumor cells may be seen in pulmonary paraganglioma. The tumor cells tend to become arranged concentrically around the lumen of the vessel walls and to aggregate in small clusters that are separated by collagenized stroma.* ***(Right)*** *Perivascular hyalinization and stromal sclerosis is another feature that can be observed focally in many paragangliomas as an expression of degenerative or involuting changes within the tumor.*

PULMONARY PARAGANGLIOMA

Cytologic Features

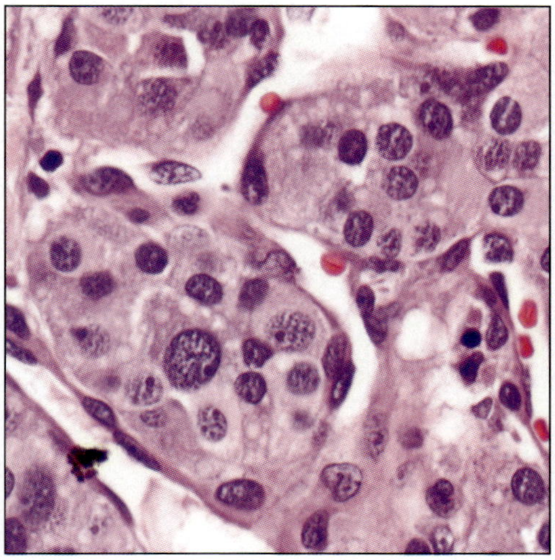
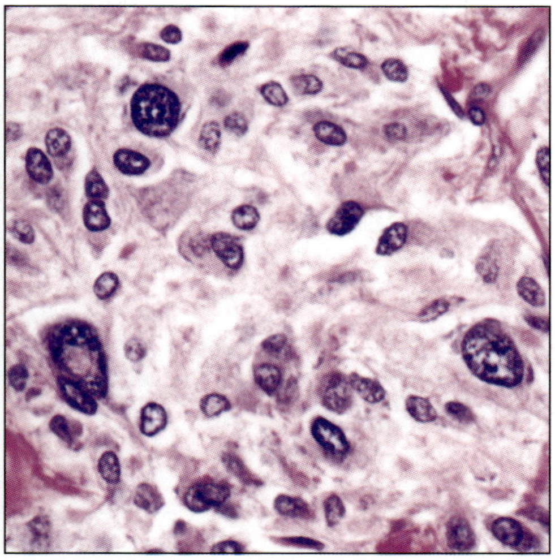

(Left) *Characteristic histology of pulmonary paraganglioma shows cells with round nuclei showing a dispersed chromatin pattern surrounded by an ample rim of granular, eosinophilic cytoplasm.* ***(Right)*** *High magnification of pulmonary paraganglioma shows nucleomegaly, with a few markedly enlarged, hyperchromatic nuclei. The presence of these atypical nuclei in the absence of significant or abnormal mitotic activity has no prognostic significance.*

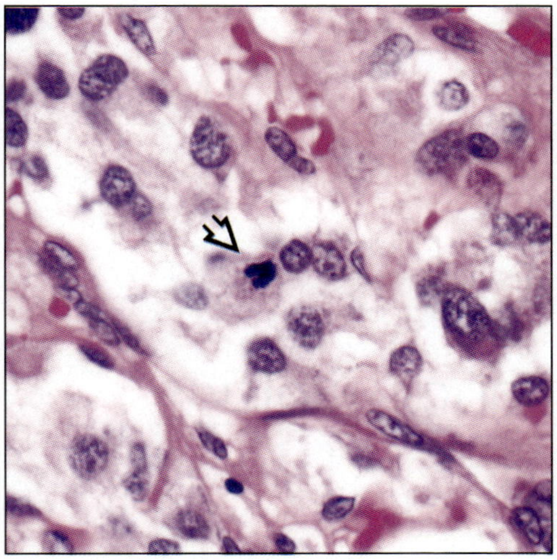
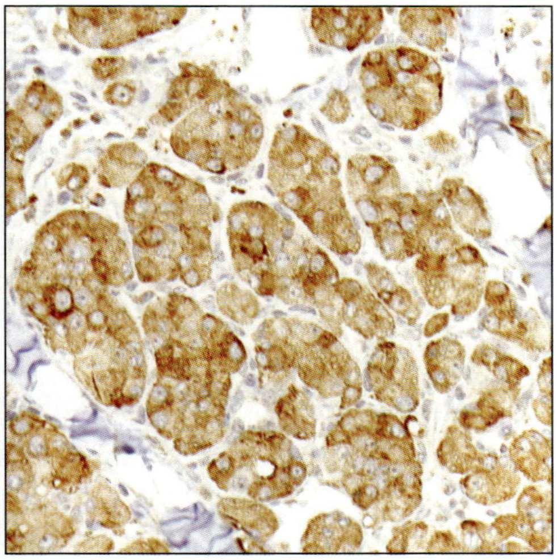

(Left) *An isolated mitotic figure is seen in the center of the field ➢ in this pulmonary paraganglioma. Rare mitoses can be observed in otherwise benign paragangliomas, and this feature does not necessarily correlate with a more aggressive clinical behavior.* ***(Right)*** *Chromogranin stain in pulmonary paraganglioma shows diffuse cytoplasmic positivity. Unlike other "neuroendocrine" neoplasms, paragangliomas are almost always negative for cytokeratin stains.*

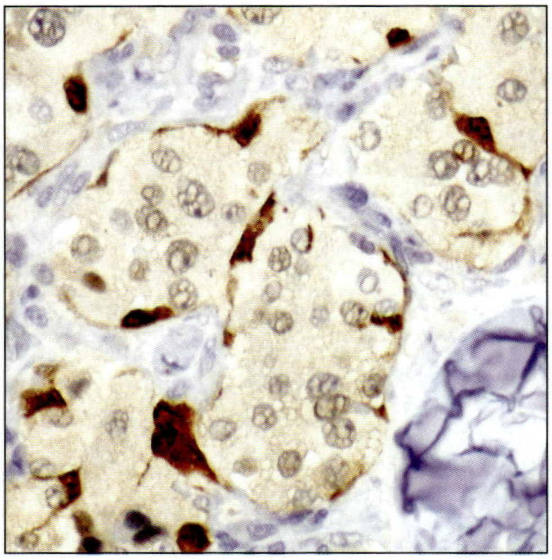
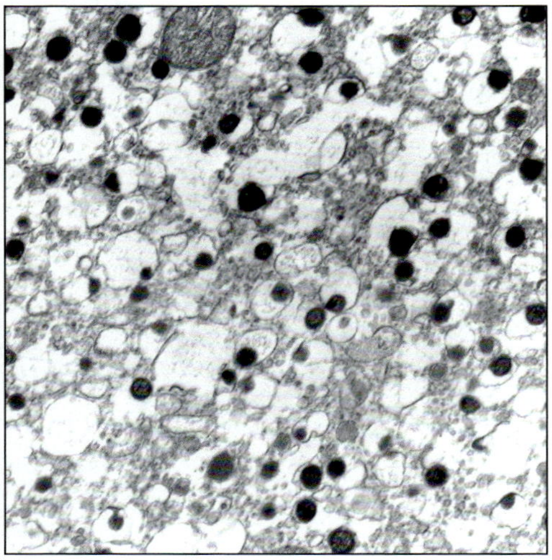

(Left) *Immunohistochemical staining of pulmonary paraganglioma for S100 protein shows a network of "sustentacular" S100(+) tumor cells surrounding the tumor cell "nests."* ***(Right)*** *Ultrastructural appearance of a tumor cell in pulmonary paraganglioma shows multiple membrane-bound, dense-core neurosecretory cytoplasmic granules. Notice the blister-like appearance of the granules caused by retraction of the membranes and eccentric location of the dense cores.*

PULMONARY MENINGIOMA

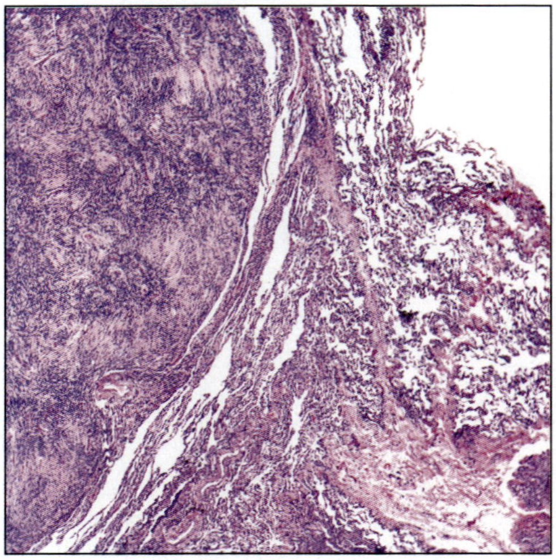

Hematoxylin & eosin section shows a well-circumscribed intraparenchymal tumor replacing the normal lung parenchyma.

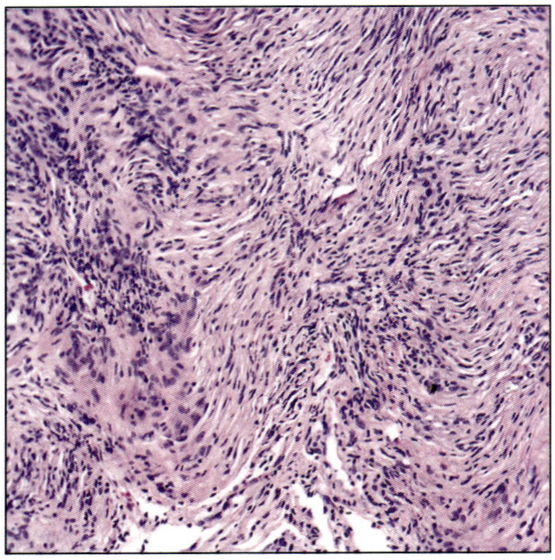

Hematoxylin & eosin section shows a mixture of spindle and oval cells. Note the absence of mitotic activity &/or hemorrhage. The tumor shows bland cytology.

TERMINOLOGY

Definitions

- Primary intrapulmonary meningothelial neoplasm

ETIOLOGY/PATHOGENESIS

Etiology

- Previous meningothelial-like nodules
- In cases where pulmonary meningioma is associated with other small lesions of same histology
- Pluripotential cells
- Cells capable of undergoing differentiation toward meningothelial cells
- Heterotopic embryonic rests
- Possible ectopic neuroectodermal tissue in lung

CLINICAL ISSUES

Epidemiology

- Incidence
  - Primary pulmonary meningiomas are exceedingly rare
  - Only a few short series of cases have been reported
- Age
  - More common in adults
- Gender
  - No gender predilection for pulmonary meningiomas

Presentation

- Asymptomatic
- Cough
- Chest pain
- Shortness of breath

Treatment

- Surgical approaches
  - Lobectomy
  - Wedge excision in small tumors

Prognosis

- Generally excellent prognosis
- Aggressive behavior in malignant tumors

MACROSCOPIC FEATURES

General Features

- Varying tumor size: 1-6 cm
- Well-circumscribed tumor lesion
- Cut surface is white and homogeneous

MICROSCOPIC PATHOLOGY

Histologic Features

- Presence of psammoma bodies
- Whorled pattern of growth
- Spindle cells arranged in vague storiform pattern
- Focal areas with presence of foamy macrophages
- Mixture of meningothelial "transitional" and spindle cells

Predominant Pattern/Injury Type

- Whorled

Predominant Cell/Compartment Type

- Meningothelial
- Spindle

DIFFERENTIAL DIAGNOSIS

Well-differentiated Neuroendocrine Carcinoma (Carcinoid)

- Carcinoid usually does not show characteristic whorled pattern
- Presence of psammoma bodies would be unusual for carcinoid tumors

Key Facts

Terminology
- Primary intrapulmonary meningothelial neoplasm

Clinical Issues
- Cough
- Asymptomatic
- Lobectomy
- Wedge excision in small tumors
- Good prognosis in conventional cases
- Aggressive behavior in malignant tumors

Macroscopic Features
- Varying tumor size: 1-6 cm
- Well-circumscribed

Microscopic Pathology
- Spindle (fibrous meningioma)
- Meningothelial (transitional meningioma)
- Presence of psammoma bodies
- Whorled pattern
- Spindle cells arranged in vague storiform pattern

Ancillary Tests
- EMA
- KERATIN-PAN
- CD34
- TTF-1

Top Differential Diagnoses
- Well-differentiated neuroendocrine carcinoma (carcinoid)
- Malignant meningioma
- Meningothelial-like nodule
- Meningotheliomatosis

Immunohistochemistry

Antibody	Reactivity	Staining Pattern	Comment
EMA/MUC1	Positive	Cell membrane	Diffuse
CK-PAN	Positive	Cytoplasmic	Focal in few cases
TTF-1	Positive	Nuclear	In some cases
Vimentin	Positive		
CK5/6	Negative		
CD34	Negative		May show focal positive staining in fibrous meningiomas
Bcl-2	Negative		

- Presence of mixed histologies of spindle and transitional cells is not characteristic of carcinoid tumors
- Meningiomas are negative for neuroendocrine markers while carcinoid tumors are positive

Malignant Meningioma
- Increased mitotic activity &/or presence of necrosis and hemorrhage
- Similar immunophenotype as conventional pulmonary meningioma

Meningothelial-like Nodule
- Usually < 5 mm and may represent incidental finding
- Histology of both lesions is similar
- Similar immunophenotype as conventional pulmonary meningioma

Meningotheliomatosis
- Characterized by multiple small tumors
- Tumor nodules are < 5 cm in diameter
- Similar immunophenotype as conventional pulmonary meningioma

DIAGNOSTIC CHECKLIST

Pathologic Interpretation Pearls
- Whorled pattern
- Spindle cell pattern
- Mixed spindle and transitional pattern
- Psammoma bodies
- Lack of mitotic activity
- Lack of necrosis
- Usually tumor < 3 cm in diameter

GRADING

Malignant Meningioma
- Presence of increased mitotic activity &/or necrosis and hemorrhage

SELECTED REFERENCES

1. Incarbone M et al: Primary pulmonary meningioma: report of a case and review of the literature. Lung Cancer. 62(3):401-7, 2008
2. Meirelles GS et al: Primary pulmonary meningioma manifesting as a solitary pulmonary nodule with a false-positive PET scan. J Thorac Imaging. 21(3):225-7, 2006
3. van der Meij JJ et al: Primary pulmonary malignant meningioma. Ann Thorac Surg. 80(4):1523-5, 2005
4. Prayson RA et al: Primary pulmonary malignant meningioma. Am J Surg Pathol. 23(6):722-6, 1999
5. Moran CA et al: Primary intrapulmonary meningiomas. A clinicopathologic and immunohistochemical study of ten cases. Cancer. 78(11):2328-33, 1996

PULMONARY MENINGIOMA

Microscopic Features

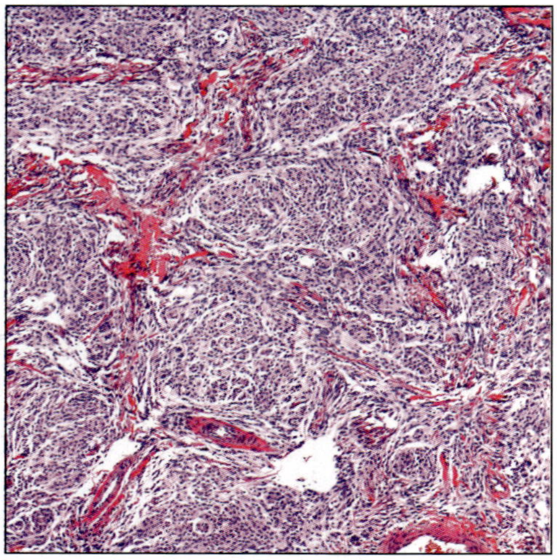
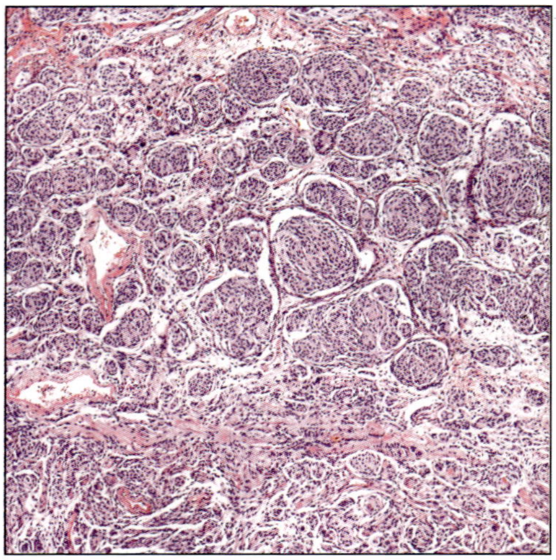

(Left) *Hematoxylin & eosin section shows a vague nested pattern separated in some areas by fibrocollagenous tissue. The tumor shows a homogeneous growth pattern without areas of necrosis or hemorrhage.* ***(Right)*** *Hematoxylin & eosin section shows a characteristic whorled pattern of growth. Tumor cells are separated in small nests by thin fibrocollagenous tissue. The cellular proliferation is fairly homogeneous. Areas of necrosis are absent.*

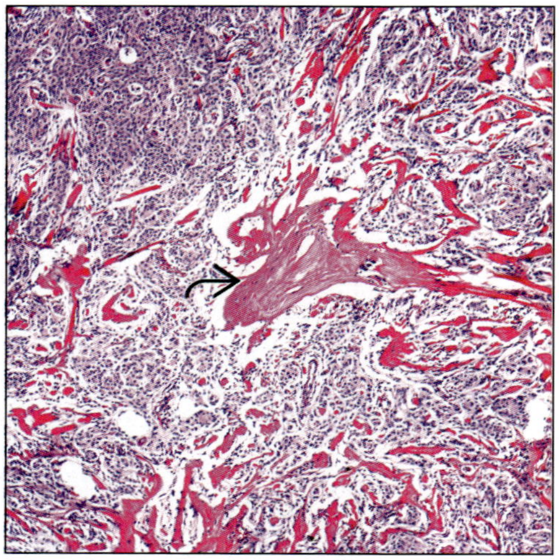
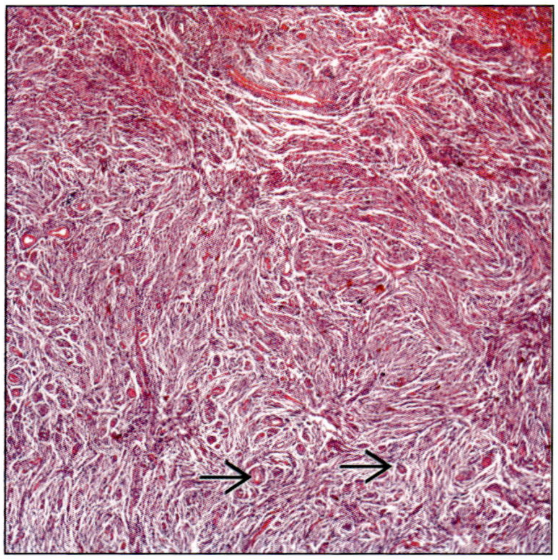

(Left) *This pulmonary meningioma shows extensive areas of collagenization ↷, which can be misinterpreted for true mesenchymal neoplasms. Such areas are uncommon and are more often seen in fibrous meningiomas.* ***(Right)*** *Hematoxylin & eosin section shows a more prominent spindle cell component with a proliferation of small ectatic vessels →. This growth pattern may suggest a true mesenchymal tumor. Still, nuclear atypia and mitotic activity are absent.*

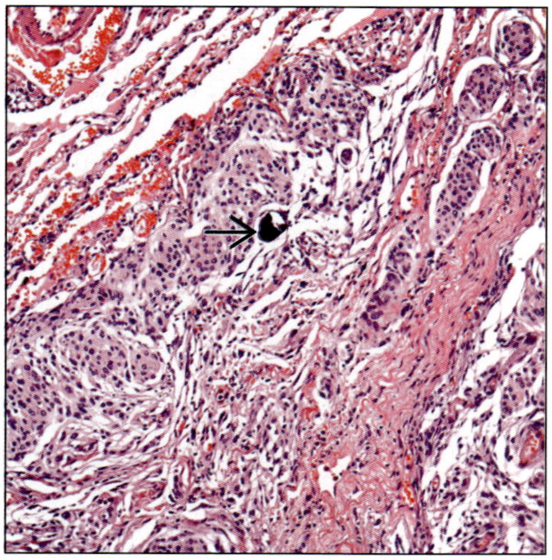
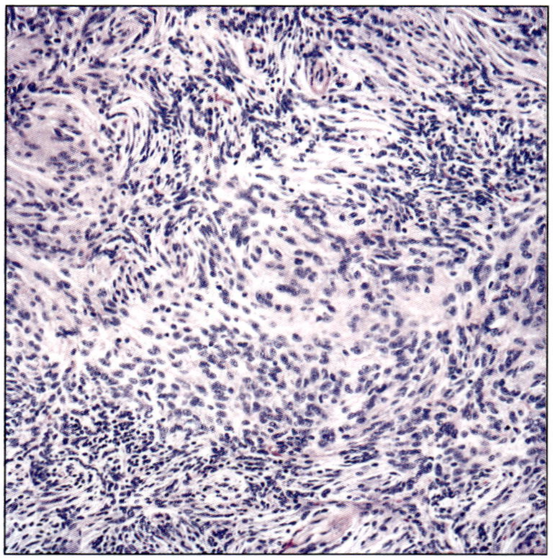

(Left) *Hematoxylin & eosin section shows a characteristic whorled pattern with presence of psammoma bodies → toward the periphery of the tumor. In some cases, the presence of these calcifications may be focal or numerous.* ***(Right)*** *Hematoxylin & eosin section shows a high-power view of an intrapulmonary meningioma with a homogeneous growth pattern composed of rather small oval cells. Note the absence of mitotic activity or nuclear pleomorphism.*

Microscopic Features

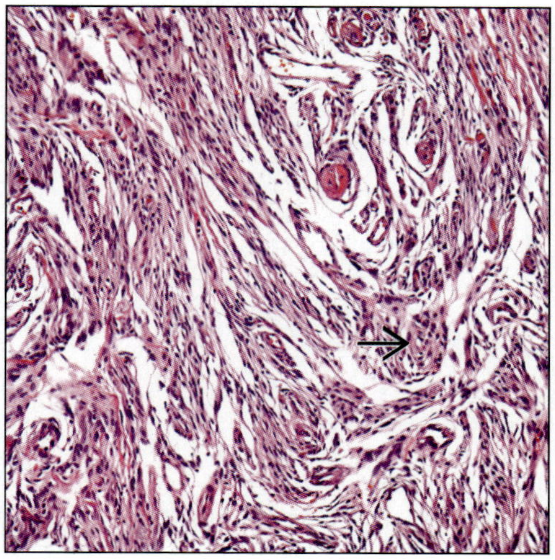

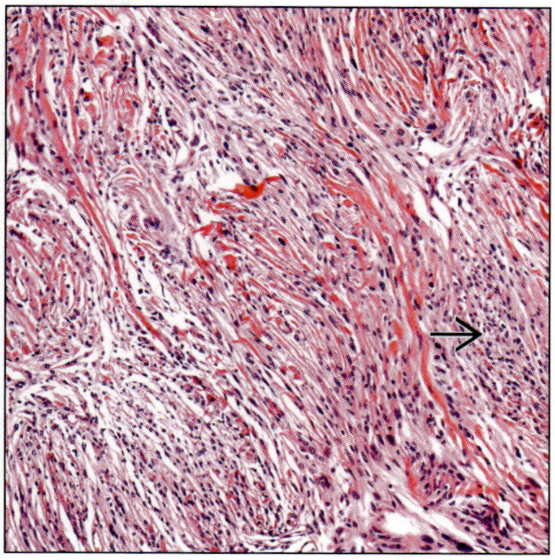

(Left) *Hematoxylin & eosin section shows a fibrous meningioma composed of spindle cells arranged in a vague storiform pattern. In some focal areas, it is still possible to identify transitional areas →.* ***(Right)*** *Hematoxylin & eosin section shows a fibrous meningioma composed of spindle cells admixed with collagen fibers. Note the absence of nuclear atypia or mitotic activity. Still, in some areas, a hint of more conventional transitional areas is visible →.*

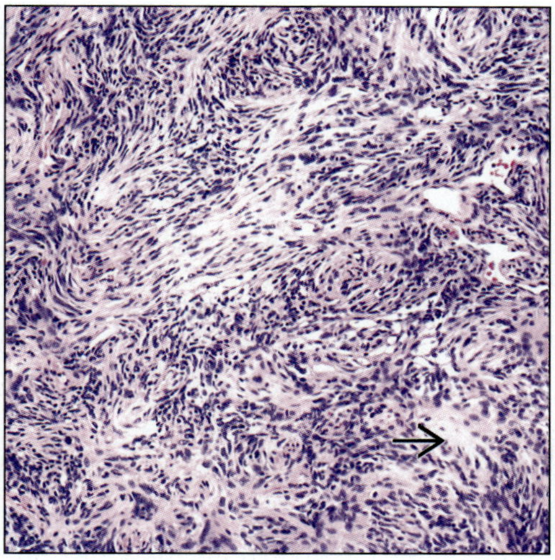

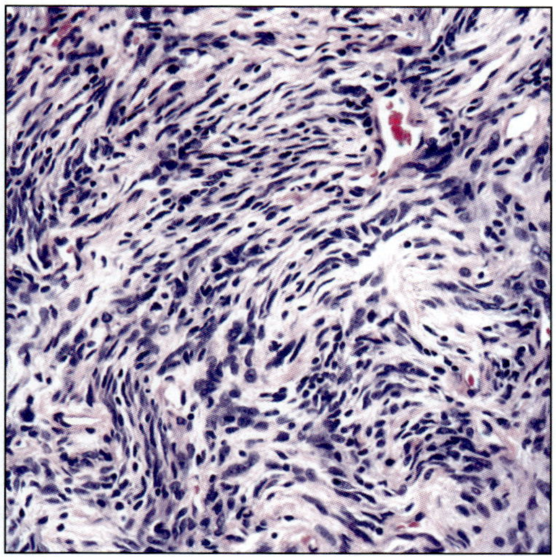

(Left) *Hematoxylin & eosin section shows a fibrous meningioma with focal areas of transitional meningioma and a characteristic whorled pattern →. The pattern is reminiscent of a neural tumor.* ***(Right)*** *Hematoxylin & eosin section shows a high-power view of a fibrous meningioma that displays a pattern reminiscent of a neural tumor. The cellular proliferation is homogeneous and lacks mitotic activity and nuclear atypia.*

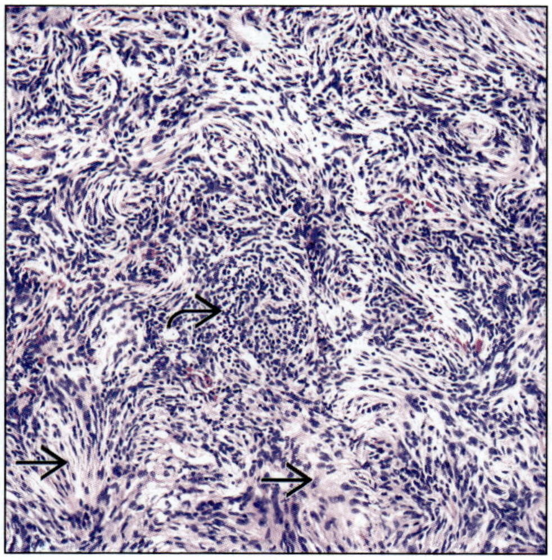

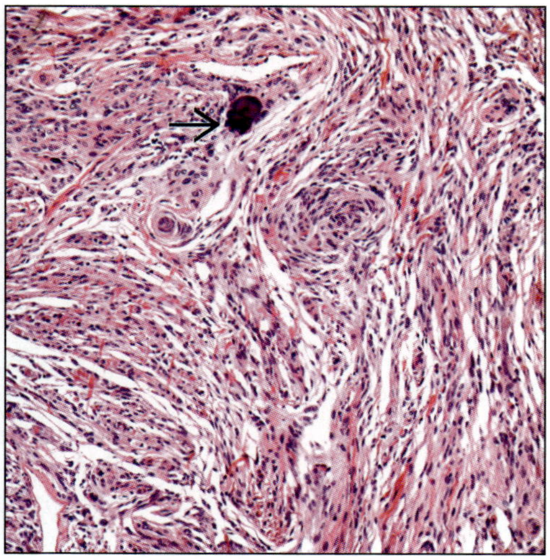

(Left) *Pulmonary meningioma with a spindle cell proliferation is admixed with inflammatory reaction composed mainly of lymphocytes ↷. These features may be misleading for an inflammatory reaction; however, more conventional areas → are also present.* ***(Right)*** *H&E toward the periphery of a fibrous meningioma shows more conventional areas of transitional meningioma with presence of psammoma bodies →. These areas are classic for the diagnosis of pulmonary meningioma.*

MINUTE MENINGOTHELIAL-LIKE NODULE

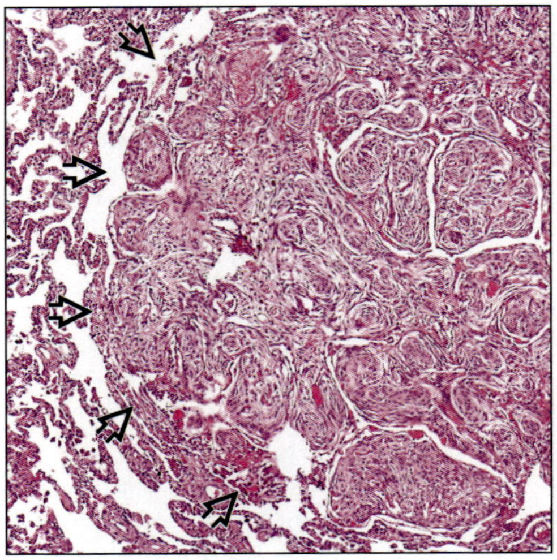

Scanning magnification of a minute pulmonary meningothelial-like nodule shows well-circumscribed proliferation of epithelioid cells that are sharply separated from the surrounding lung parenchyma ⇨.

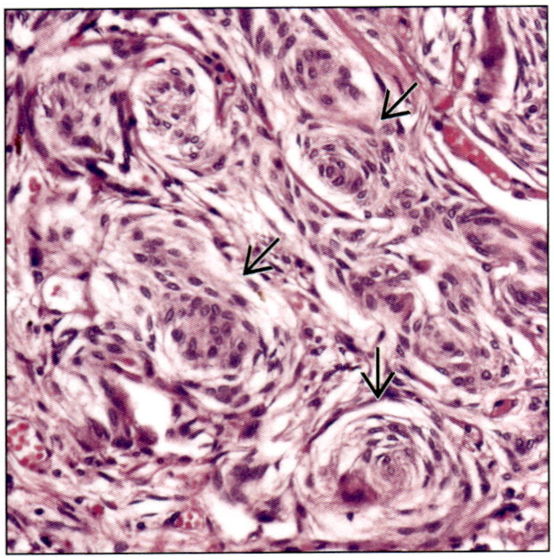

High magnification of minute pulmonary meningothelial-like nodule shows clusters and islands of round to oval cells with abundant eosinophilic cytoplasm displaying characteristic "whorling" effect →.

TERMINOLOGY

Abbreviations

- Minute meningothelial-like nodules (MMN)

Synonyms

- Minute pulmonary chemodectoma

Definitions

- Small intrapulmonary nodules composed of cells bearing histologic, immunohistochemical, and ultrastructural features of meningothelial cells

ETIOLOGY/PATHOGENESIS

Developmental Anomaly

- Believed to arise from rests displaced in the lung during embryogenesis
- Distributed interstitially alongside small veins
- Often found in association with pulmonary thromboemboli

Pathogenesis

- May result from clonal expansion as shown by amplification of the X-chromosome-linked human androgen receptor gene (HUMARA assay)

CLINICAL ISSUES

Epidemiology

- Incidence
  - Found in about 7% of surgically resected lungs
- Age
  - 30-75 years (mean = 61 years)
- Gender
  - Female predilection (M:F = 1:2)

Presentation

- Usually asymptomatic
- Found incidentally in lungs resected for other reasons, particularly lung adenocarcinoma
- May present with progressive shortness of breath
- Can present with diffuse, symptomatic, bilateral interstitial lung infiltrates (diffuse pulmonary meningotheliomatosis)

Prognosis

- Lesions most often represent an incidental finding of no clinical significance
- There is currently no known treatment for rare symptomatic, diffuse, and bilateral cases (diffuse pulmonary meningotheliomatosis)

IMAGE FINDINGS

CT Findings

- Can present as randomly distributed micronodules on thin section CT

MACROSCOPIC FEATURES

General Features

- Usually an incidental microscopic finding

Size

- 1-3 mm
- In rare instances, may reach up to 1 cm in greatest diameter

MICROSCOPIC PATHOLOGY

Histologic Features

- Ill-defined, focal accumulation of oval or epithelioid cells in pulmonary interstitium
- Oval or epithelioid cells tend to focally adopt a "whorled" appearance
- Lesions may be microscopic (1-2 mm) or measure up to 1 cm in diameter

Key Facts

Clinical Issues
- Usually asymptomatic
- Can present with diffuse, symptomatic bilateral interstitial lung infiltrates (diffuse pulmonary meningotheliomatosis)
- Lesions most often represent an incidental finding of no clinical significance

Image Findings
- Can present as randomly distributed micronodules on thin section CT

Microscopic Pathology
- Ill-defined, focal accumulation of oval or epithelioid cells in pulmonary interstitium
- Oval or epithelioid cells tend to focally adopt a whorled appearance
- Lesions may be microscopic (1-2 mm) or measure up to 1 cm in diameter
- Lesions may be seen in close proximity of vessels
- Cells are oval or epithelioid and surrounded by an ample rim of eosinophilic cytoplasm with indistinct cell borders
- Cells contain small, centrally placed nuclei devoid of mitotic activity
- Nuclei may contain intranuclear cytoplasmic inclusions

Ancillary Tests
- Tumor cells are positive for vimentin and EMA
- Cells contain long, branching, interdigitating cytoplasmic cell processes joined by numerous desmosomes

- Lesions may be seen in close proximity of vessels

Cytologic Features
- Cells are oval or epithelioid and surrounded by an ample rim of eosinophilic cytoplasm with indistinct cell borders
- Cells contain small, centrally placed nuclei devoid of mitotic activity
- Nuclei may contain intranuclear cytoplasmic inclusions

ANCILLARY TESTS

Immunohistochemistry
- Tumor cells are positive for vimentin and EMA
- Tumor cells may also react with antibodies to progesterone receptors
- Tumor cells are generally negative for neuroendocrine markers, S100 protein, cytokeratins, and other differentiation markers

Electron Microscopy
- Cells contain long, branching, interdigitating cytoplasmic cell processes joined by numerous desmosomes
- Cells contain no evidence of neurosecretory granules

Mutational Analysis
- Loss of heterozygosity affecting up to 3 genomic loci has been demonstrated in up to 25% of single case reports studied
- Loss of heterozygosity affecting multiple loci (> 7) has been demonstrated in cases with multiple disseminated lesions

DIFFERENTIAL DIAGNOSIS

Neuroendocrine Pulmonary "Tumorlet"
- Cells tend to be round with "salt and pepper" nuclear chromatin pattern
- Pulmonary tumorlet does not display whorling pattern of growth
- Cells are positive for chromogranin and synaptophysin and negative for EMA

Lymphangioleiomyomatosis (LAM)
- Spindle cells usually have a rim of clear cytoplasm
- Spindle cells usually line the walls of dilated cysts
- Spindle cells are positive for HMB-45 and negative for EMA

Metastatic Carcinoma
- Usually shows striking lymphangitic rather than interstitial distribution
- Marked cytologic atypia, nuclear pleomorphism, and mitotic activity
- Strong cytokeratin positivity

SELECTED REFERENCES

1. Mizutani E et al: Minute pulmonary meningothelial-like nodules: clinicopathologic analysis of 121 patients. Hum Pathol. 40(5):678-82, 2009
2. Suster S et al: Diffuse pulmonary meningotheliomatosis. Am J Surg Pathol. 31(4):624-31, 2007
3. Ionescu DN et al: Pulmonary meningothelial-like nodules: a genotypic comparison with meningiomas. Am J Surg Pathol. 28(2):207-14, 2004
4. Kuroki M et al: Minute pulmonary meningothelial-like nodules: high-resolution computed tomography and pathologic correlations. J Thorac Imaging. 17(3):227-9, 2002
5. Sellami D et al: Minute pulmonary meningothelial-like nodules: thin-section CT appearance. J Comput Assist Tomogr. 25(2):311-3, 2001
6. Niho S et al: Immunohistochemical and clonal analysis of minute pulmonary meningothelial-like nodules. Hum Pathol. 30(4):425-9, 1999
7. Gaffey MJ et al: Minute pulmonary meningothelial-like nodules. A clinicopathologic study of so-called minute pulmonary chemodectoma. Am J Surg Pathol. 12(3):167-75, 1988

MINUTE MENINGOTHELIAL-LIKE NODULE

Histologic Features

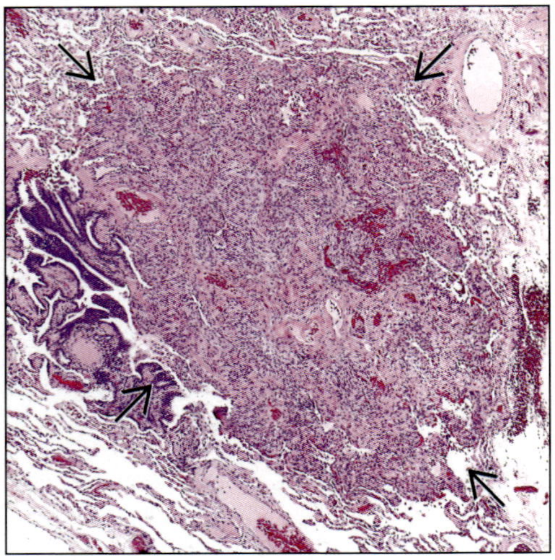

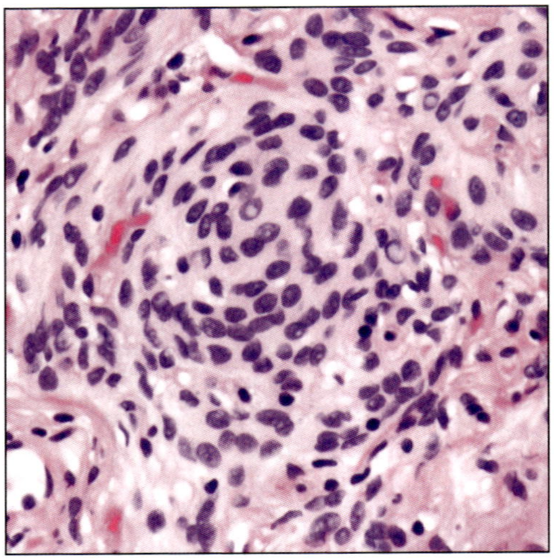

(Left) *Scanning magnification of a minute pulmonary meningothelial-like nodule shows a discrete, well-circumscribed area of consolidation adjacent to a small bronchiole that is sharply delineated from surrounding pulmonary parenchyma ⇒.* ***(Right)*** *Higher magnification of a minute pulmonary meningothelial-like nodule shows a cluster of oval epithelioid cells with an indistinct rim of eosinophilic cytoplasm adopting a concentric arrangement ("whorling") of the tumor cells.*

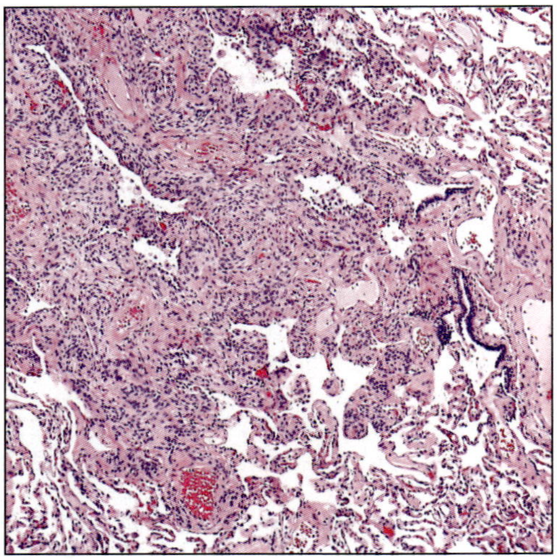

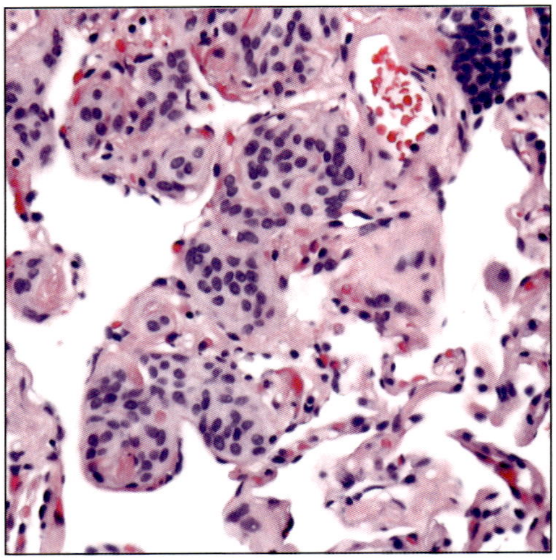

(Left) *Minute pulmonary meningothelial-like nodule shows thickening of alveolar septae by the proliferating meningothelial cells with compression of the airspaces and cuffing of small vessels by tumor cells.* ***(Right)*** *Higher magnification of a minute pulmonary meningothelial-like nodule shows small clusters of oval cells with abundant eosinophilic cytoplasm located in the interstitium of the alveolar septae. The cells closely resemble the pia-arachnoid cells in the brain.*

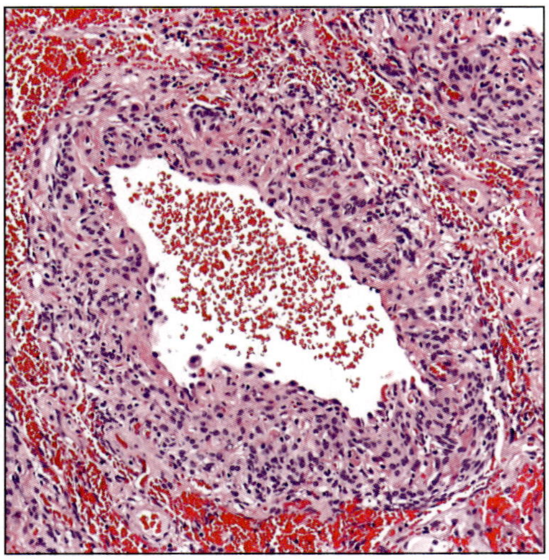

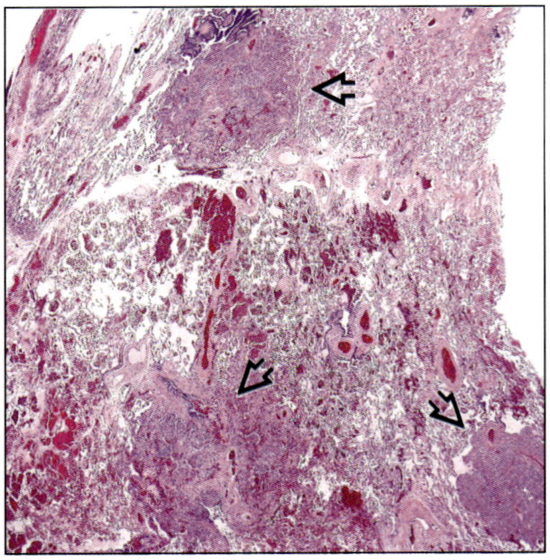

(Left) *Minute pulmonary meningothelial-like nodule shows distinct perivascular distribution with concentric arrangement of the meningothelial cells around the lumen of a dilated, medium-sized blood vessel.* ***(Right)*** *Diffuse pulmonary meningotheliomatosis shows multiple small, discrete nodules composed of clusters of meningothelial cells scattered throughout the lung parenchyma ⇨. The lesions in this condition are usually diffuse, bilateral, and symptomatic.*

MINUTE MENINGOTHELIAL-LIKE NODULE

Cytologic and Immunohistochemical Features

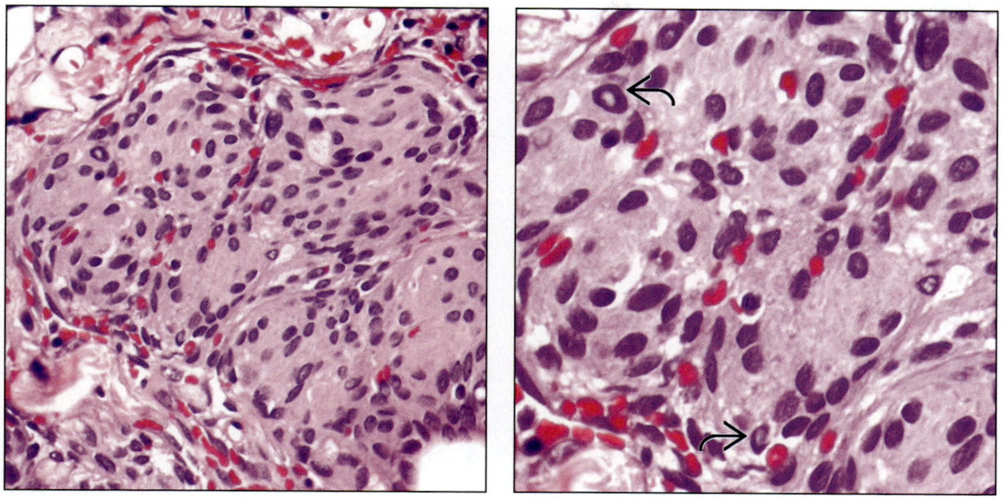

(Left) *Minute pulmonary meningothelial-like nodule shows small aggregates of uniform, oval to spindle cells. The cells in these nodules are indistinguishable from those seen in intracranial meningiomas.* ***(Right)*** *Higher magnification of a minute pulmonary meningothelial-like nodule shows cells with oval nuclei and a dense chromatin pattern surrounded by an indistinct rim of eosinophilic cytoplasm. Occasional intranuclear cytoplasmic inclusions are seen* ↪.

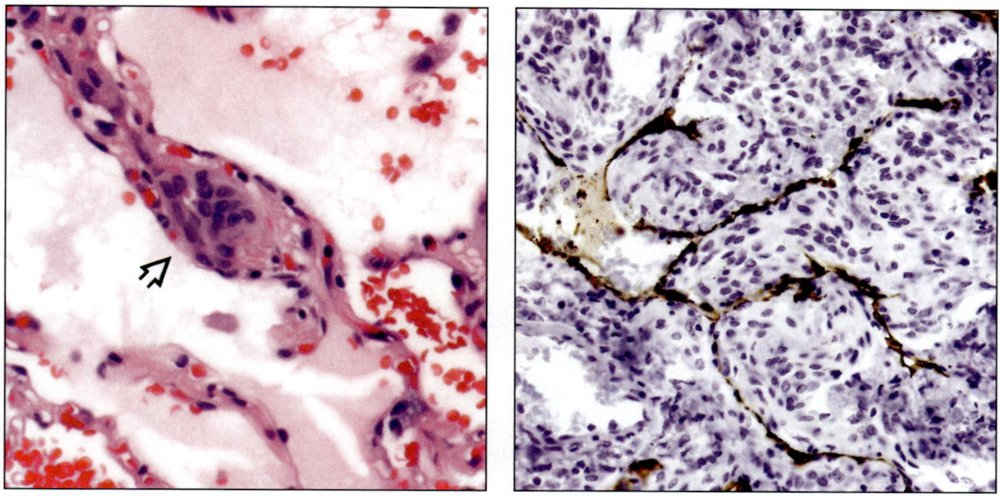

(Left) *High magnification shows an isolated focus of a minute pulmonary meningothelial lesion involving the alveolar wall* ⇨. *The cluster of meningothelial cells is minute and composed of about a dozen cells that form a tight cluster that expands and dilates the alveolar septum.* ***(Right)*** *Immunohistochemical staining of a minute pulmonary meningothelial nodule shows a continuous layer of cytokeratin-positive alveolar cells lining collapsed alveolar walls.*

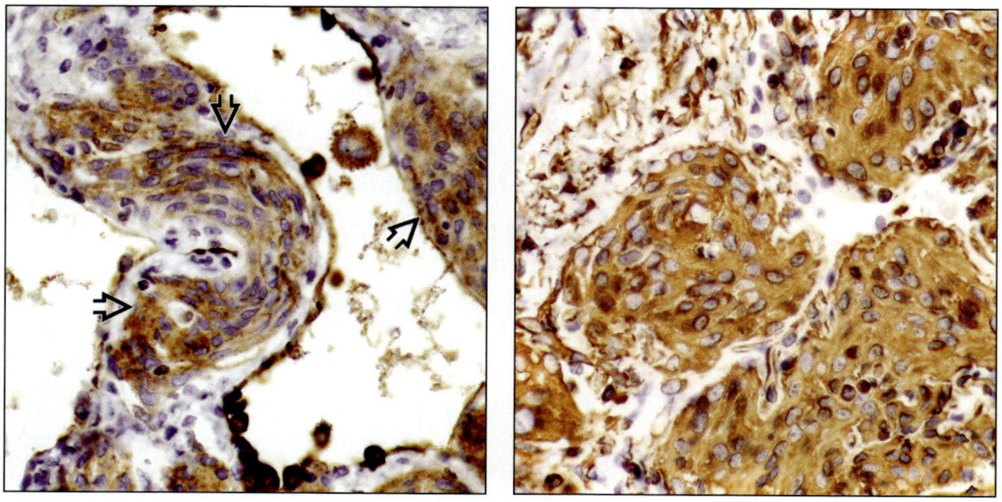

(Left) *Immunohistochemical staining of a minute pulmonary meningothelial-like nodule for EMA shows positive staining of alveolar cells lining the airspaces as well as strong positivity of the spindle and oval cells lying within the interstitium for this antibody* ⇨. ***(Right)*** *Immunohistochemical staining of a small pulmonary meningothelial-like nodule shows strong, positive cytoplasmic staining of the clusters of meningothelial cells with vimentin antibodies.*

GRANULAR CELL TUMOR

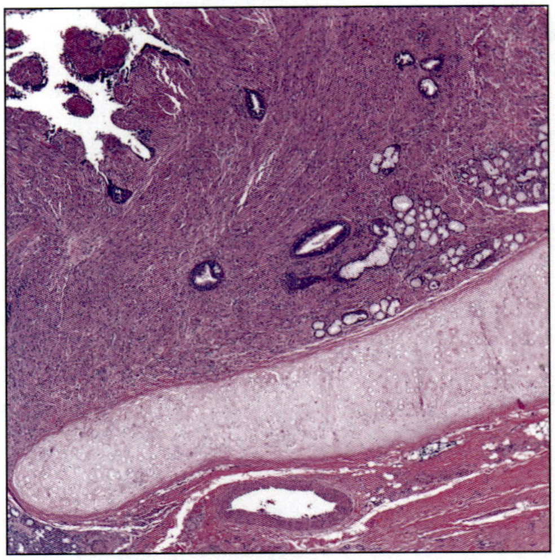

Low-power view shows a granular cell tumor growing in an endobronchial location. Note the homogeneous pattern of growth.

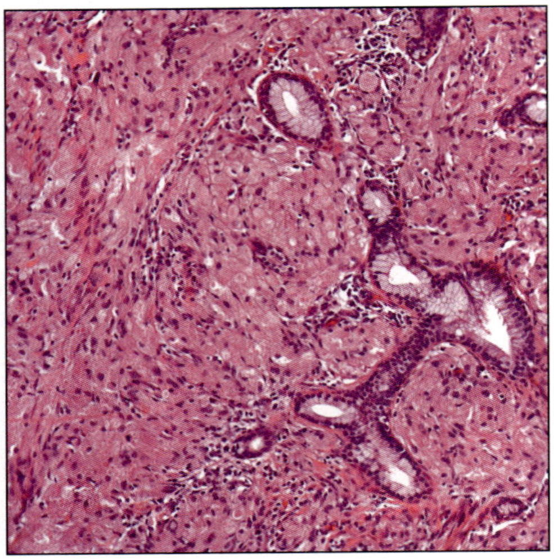

High-power view of a granular cell tumor shows the characteristic granular cytoplasm with a small round nucleus. No necrosis or mitotic activity is present.

TERMINOLOGY

Abbreviations

- Granular cell tumor (GCT)

Synonyms

- Myoblastoma

Definitions

- Benign neoplasm composed of medium-sized cells with prominent granular cytoplasm
- Malignant counterpart shows similar histology but with nuclear atypia and mitotic activity

ETIOLOGY/PATHOGENESIS

Etiology

- Uncertain histogenesis
  - Recently a neural origin has been suggested

CLINICAL ISSUES

Presentation

- Cough
- Dyspnea
- Hemoptysis
- Wheezing
- Asymptomatic

Treatment

- Surgical approaches
  - Complete surgical resection

Prognosis

- Excellent in benign cases
- Malignant granular cell tumor behaves aggressively

MACROSCOPIC FEATURES

General Features

- Central tumor, often endobronchial
- Tumors are firm and tan in color
- Size of tumors varies from 1-5 cm in diameter
- Polypoid tumor obstructing airway
- Coin lesion, less common
- Necrosis &/or hemorrhage are signs of aggressive behavior

MICROSCOPIC PATHOLOGY

Histologic Features

- In benign tumors
  - Medium-sized cells
  - Small nuclei with inconspicuous nucleoli
  - Absence of mitotic activity
  - Absence of hemorrhage or necrosis
  - Infiltration in peribronchial lymph nodes may be seen
- In malignant tumors
  - Necrosis and hemorrhage are commonly seen
  - Medium-sized cells with round nuclei and prominent nucleoli
  - Mitotic figures commonly encountered

Predominant Pattern/Injury Type

- Circumscribed

Predominant Cell/Compartment Type

- Granular

ANCILLARY TESTS

Histochemistry

- Periodic acid-Schiff
  - Reactivity: Positive
  - Staining pattern

GRANULAR CELL TUMOR

Key Facts

Terminology
- Granular cell tumor (GCT)
  - Benign neoplasm composed of medium-sized cells with prominent granular cytoplasm
  - Malignant counterpart shows similar histology but with nuclear atypia and mitotic activity
- Synonym: Myoblastoma

Etiology/Pathogenesis
- More recently suggested as a neural origin for these tumors
  - Still no universal agreement
- Uncertain histogenesis

Clinical Issues
- Complete surgical resection
- Excellent in benign cases
- Malignant granular cell tumor behaves aggressively

Macroscopic Features
- Central tumor, often endobronchial
- Size of tumors varies from 1-5 cm in diameter

Ancillary Tests
- Periodic acid-Schiff
- Positive

Top Differential Diagnoses
- Melanoma
  - HMB-45 and Melan-A are negative in GCT
- Neurogenic sarcoma
- Carcinoma
  - Carcinomas generally show positive staining for epithelial markers (keratins, EMA) while GCTs are negative

Immunohistochemistry

Antibody	Reactivity	Staining Pattern	Comment
S100	Positive	Cytoplasmic	Strong
NSE	Positive	Cytoplasmic	Although positive, it is not specific
Actin-sm	Positive	Cytoplasmic	May be positive, thus the notion of muscle origin
LEU-7	Positive	Cytoplasmic	Variable intensity
Cathespin-B	Positive	Cytoplasmic	In some cases
Vimentin	Positive	Cytoplasmic	Although positive, it is not specific
Chymotrypsin	Positive	Cytoplasmic	In some cases with variable staining intensity
CK-PAN	Negative		
EMA/MUC1	Negative		
Desmin	Negative		
CEA-M	Negative		
GFAP	Negative		
Chromogranin-A	Negative		
NFP	Negative		

- Cytoplasmic

DIFFERENTIAL DIAGNOSIS

Melanoma
- Cellular pleomorphism is more common in melanomas
- HMB-45 and Melan-A negative in GCT

Neurogenic Sarcoma
- In cases of malignant granular cell tumor
  - Presence of cells with granular cytoplasm is more characteristic of granular cell tumor
  - GCT shows strong positive reaction for S100 protein while that pattern of staining would be unusual for neurogenic sarcoma

Carcinoma with Oncocytic Cytoplasm
- Generally show positive staining for epithelial markers (keratin, EMA) while GCT are negative
- Negative for S100 protein

DIAGNOSTIC CHECKLIST

Clinically Relevant Pathologic Features
- Cytoplasmic features
- Mitotic rate

Pathologic Interpretation Pearls
- Granular cellular proliferation with absence of mitotic activity and nuclear atypia

SELECTED REFERENCES

1. Jiang M et al: Pulmonary malignant granular cell tumor. World J Surg Oncol. 1(1):22, 2003
2. Ordóñez NG: Granular cell tumor: a review and update. Adv Anat Pathol. 6(4):186-203, 1999
3. Deavers M et al: Granular cell tumors of the lung. Clinicopathologic study of 20 cases. Am J Surg Pathol. 19(6):627-35, 1995
4. Lack EE et al: Granular cell tumor: a clinicopathologic study of 110 patients. J Surg Oncol. 13(4):301-16, 1980

GRANULAR CELL TUMOR

Microscopic Features

(Left) *Granular cell tumor is seen with small clusters of tumor cells just beneath the respiratory epithelium. No epithelial component is present in the tumor.* ***(Right)*** *Granular cell tumor is growing focally in a polypoid fashion. Still, one can identify intact respiratory epithelium ⇨ and also some uninvolved bronchial glands → scattered amongst the tumor.*

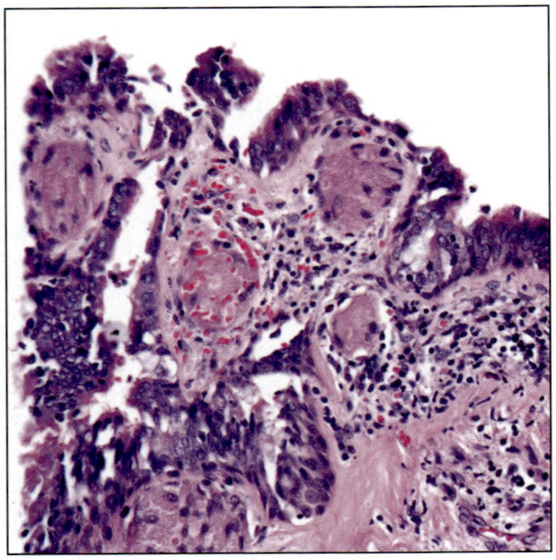

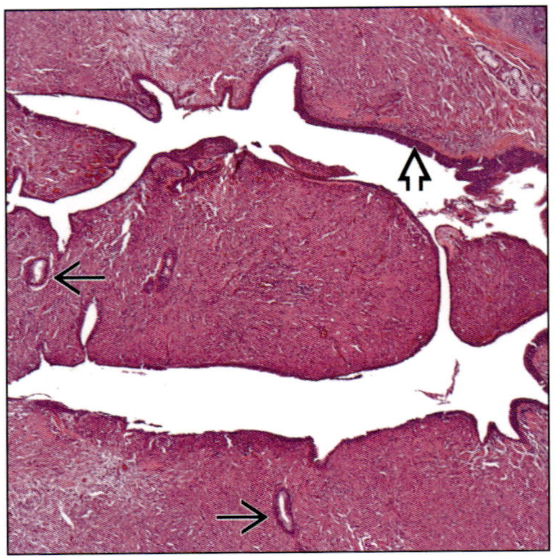

(Left) *Granular cell tumor of the lung shows a mixture of normal endobronchial glands ➡ and granular cells ↶. It is important to note that the tumor does not destroy the normal endobronchial glands.* ***(Right)*** *Extensive areas of hemorrhage and islands of granular cell tumor are shown. The appearance is that of a neuroid neoplasm, and the cells have light eosinophilic to clear cytoplasm.*

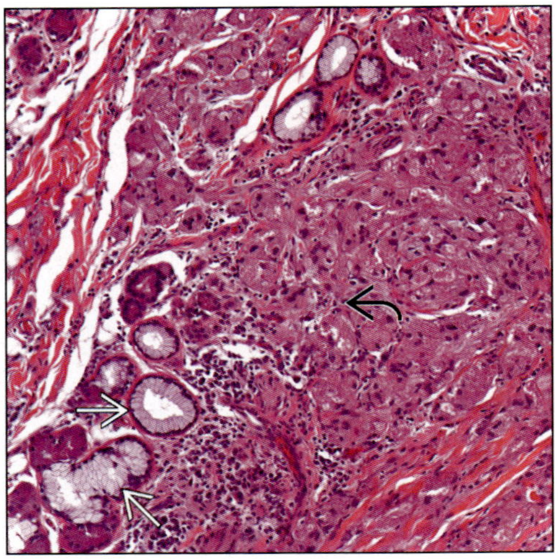

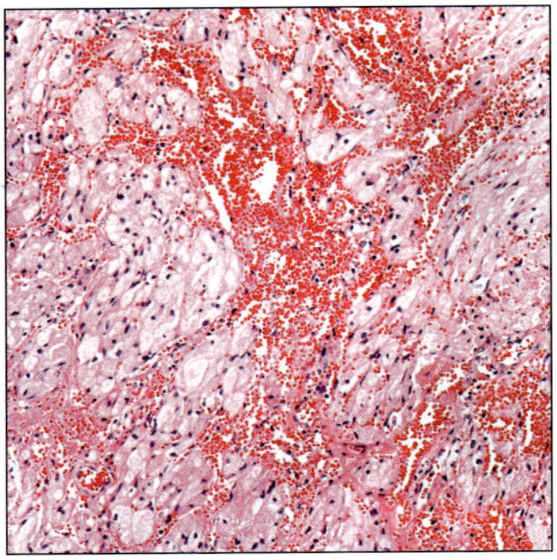

(Left) *Granular cell tumor is seen growing in cords dissecting strands of fibroconnective tissue. In addition, focal metaplastic bone formation is present →.* ***(Right)*** *Granular cell tumor shows perineural involvement →. This feature is unusual and should not be considered a feature of malignancy. Notice that the cellular proliferation does not show features of atypia.*

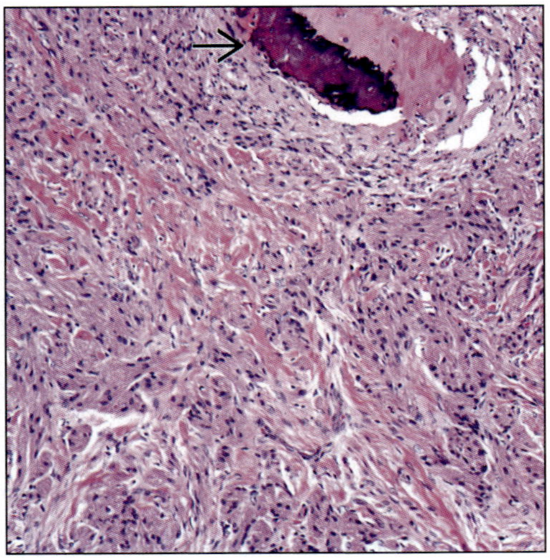

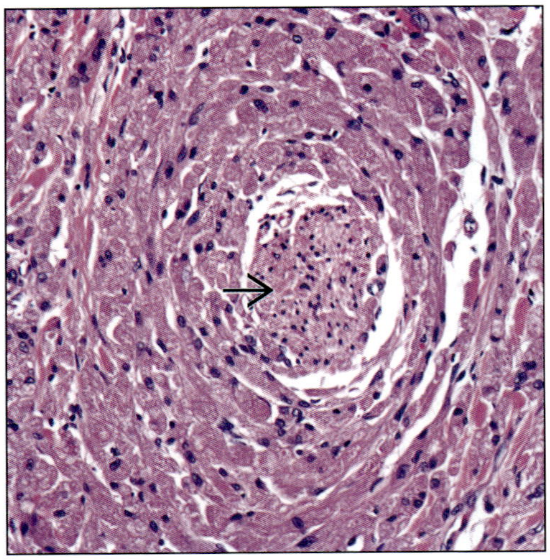

Microscopic Features

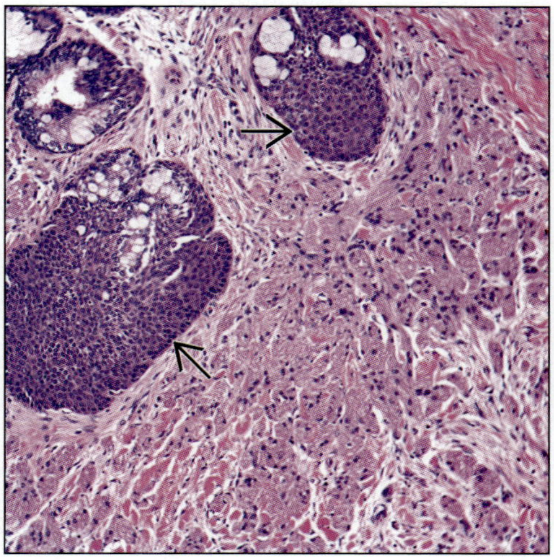
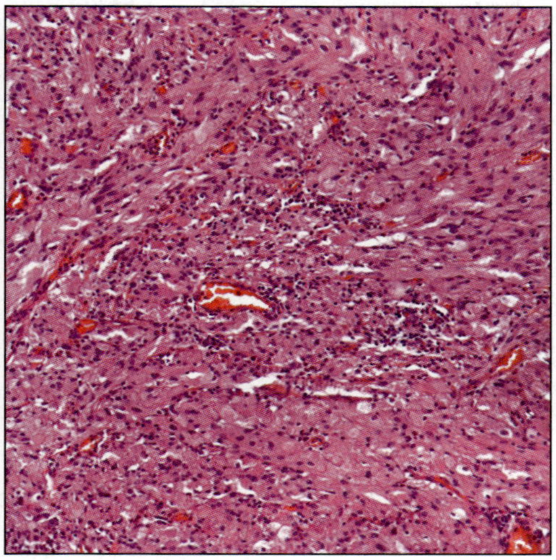

(Left) *Granular cell tumor growing along bronchial glands with squamous metaplasia →. One important feature of a GCT is the pattern of growth with sparing of the bronchial glands.* ***(Right)*** *GCT shows focal inflammatory changes. In general, inflammatory changes are not common in GCTs. Most GCTs are fairly uniform tumors with a monotonous, homogeneous appearance.*

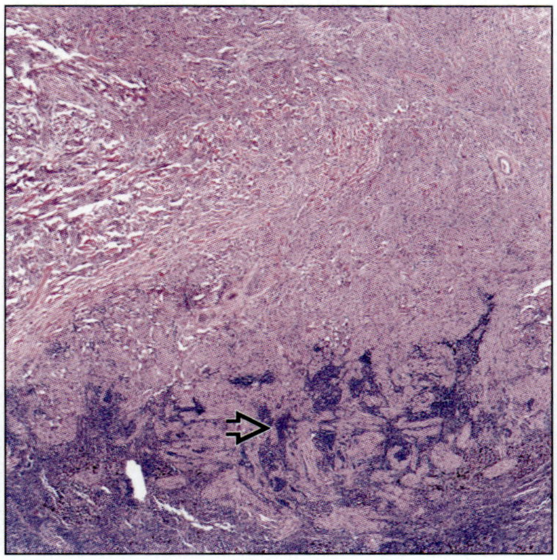
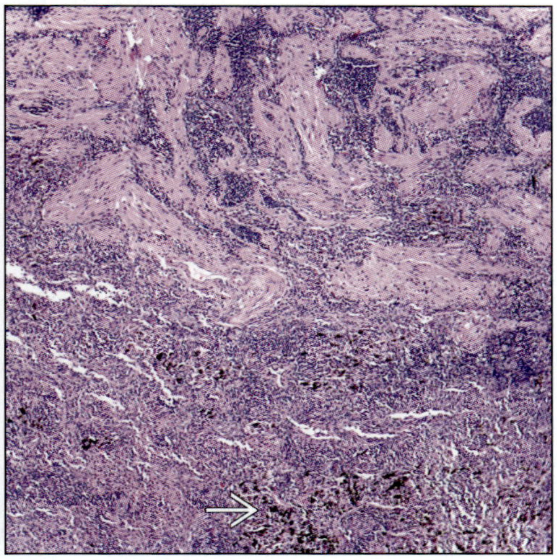

(Left) *Ill-defined GCT is shown growing adjacent to lymphoid tissue →. Granular cell tumors characteristically are not encapsulated and many times have infiltrative borders.* ***(Right)*** *Closer view shows a GCT infiltrating a lymph node. This feature, although rare, occurs in some otherwise benign cases due to the ill-defined borders of the tumor. Note the presence of anthracotic pigment in the lymph node →.*

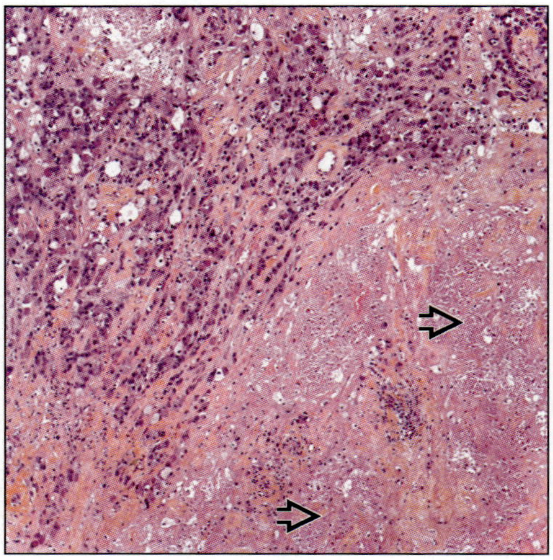
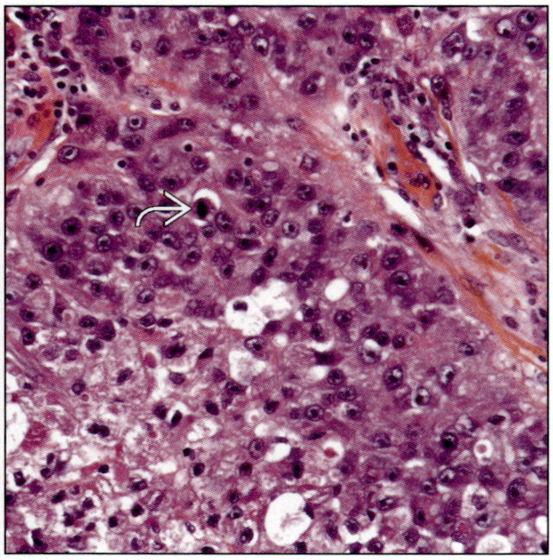

(Left) *Malignant granular cell tumor shows extensive areas of necrosis →. The presence of necrosis is generally a sign of aggressiveness. In addition, such a feature should prompt a closer examination of the cellular proliferation.* ***(Right)*** *Hematoxylin & eosin shows a malignant granular cell tumor in which the cytologic atypia is marked. In addition, mitotic figures are easily identifiable →. These features are the ones that separate benign from malignant tumors.*

SCLEROSING HEMANGIOMA (PNEUMOCYTOMA)

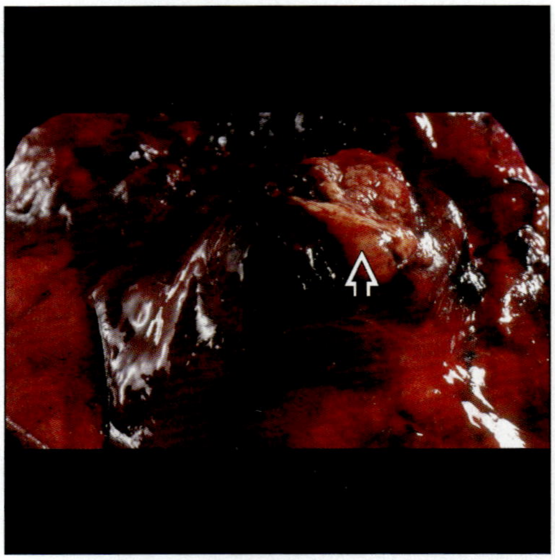

Gross photograph of sclerosing hemangioma shows a well-circumscribed intrapulmonary tumor mass. The tumor has been bisected and shows a fleshy, focally hemorrhagic surface.

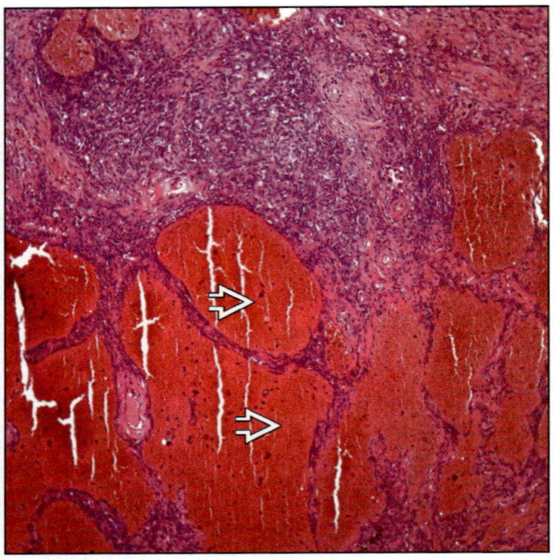

Sclerosing hemangioma shows dilated vascular spaces filled with blood, giving the appearance of a true vascular tumor.

TERMINOLOGY

Abbreviations
- Sclerosing hemangioma (SH)

Synonyms
- Pneumocytoma

Definitions
- Benign neoplasm of pneumocyte derivation

ETIOLOGY/PATHOGENESIS

Histogenesis
- Tumor appears to have pneumocytic differentiation, yet histogenesis remains unclear

CLINICAL ISSUES

Epidemiology
- Incidence
  - Tumor of rare occurrence
- Age
  - 4th or 5th decade of life
- Gender
  - More common among women

Presentation
- Asymptomatic
- Cough
- Chest pain
- Hemoptysis

Treatment
- Surgical approaches
  - Complete surgical resection

Prognosis
- Excellent
- In unusual cases, tumor metastasizes to lymph nodes

MACROSCOPIC FEATURES

General Features
- Well-circumscribed but not encapsulated
  - More often peripheral tumor; rarely central location

Size
- 1-8 cm in diameter

MICROSCOPIC PATHOLOGY

Histologic Features
- Solid
- Papillary
- Sclerotic
- Hemorrhagic
- Combination of patterns often present in same tumor

Cytologic Features
- Small cells with hobnail nuclei lining papillary structures
- Monotonous population of round/polyclonal cells with clear cytoplasm in solid areas

DIFFERENTIAL DIAGNOSIS

Papillary Carcinoma
- Marked nuclear atypia &/or increased mitotic activity
- Presence of biphasic cellular population is characteristic of SH
- Carcinoma and SH show positive staining for similar markers, including keratin and TTF-1
- Increased proliferative activity (↑ Ki-67 stain)

Mesothelioma
- Would be unusual for mesothelioma to present with intrapulmonary mass
- Generally negative for TTF-1
- SH may show different growth patterns in same tumor

SCLEROSING HEMANGIOMA (PNEUMOCYTOMA)

Key Facts

Terminology
- Pneumocytoma

Etiology/Pathogenesis
- Tumor appears to have pneumocytic differentiation, yet histogenesis remains unclear

Clinical Issues
- Incidence
  - More common among women
  - Tumor is more common in 4th and 5th decade of life

Macroscopic Features
- Well-circumscribed but not encapsulated
  - More often peripheral tumor
  - Rarely central tumor

Microscopic Pathology
- Biphasic
- Solid
- Papillary
- Sclerotic
- Hemorrhagic
- Combination of patterns more often present in same tumor

Top Differential Diagnoses
- Papillary carcinoma
  - SH lacks nuclear atypia &/or increased mitotic activity
  - Presence of biphasic cellular population characteristic of SH

Immunohistochemistry

Antibody	Reactivity	Staining Pattern	Comment
EMA/MUC1	Positive	Cytoplasmic	Stromal and cuboidal cells
TTF-1	Positive	Nuclear	Stromal and cuboidal cells
CK-PAN	Positive	Cytoplasmic	Weak and focal in stromal cells
KERATIN-LMW	Positive	Cytoplasmic	Stromal cells and cuboidal cells
CK7	Positive	Cytoplasmic	Stromal cell and cuboidal cells
Clara cell antigen	Positive	Cytoplasmic	Cuboidal cells
SURFACTANT	Positive	Cytoplasmic	Cuboidal cells
S100	Positive	Cytoplasmic	In some cases
CEA-M	Positive	Cytoplasmic	In some cases
CD31	Negative		
CD34	Negative		
Desmin	Negative		

- Calretinin and CK5/6 are usually negative in SH and positive in mesotheliomas

Inflammatory Pseudotumor (IPT)
- Usually shows presence of prominent inflammatory component based on plasma cells
- Generally negative for TTF-1
- Presence of dual cell population seen in SH is not present in IPT
- ALK1 may be seen positive in IPT and negative in SH

Metastatic Papillary Carcinoma of Thyroid
- Both thyroid carcinoma and SH show positive staining for TTF-1
- SH is negative for thyroglobulin, while thyroid carcinoma is positive
- History of thyroid neoplasm or thyroid mass is very helpful

DIAGNOSTIC CHECKLIST

Pathologic Interpretation Pearls
- Biphasic cellular proliferation composed of cuboidal cells and stromal ("pale") cells

SELECTED REFERENCES

1. Khoury JD et al: Cystic sclerosing haemangioma of the lung. Histopathology. 43(3):239-43, 2003
2. Devouassoux-Shisheboran M et al: A clinicopathologic study of 100 cases of pulmonary sclerosing hemangioma with immunohistochemical studies: TTF-1 is expressed in both round and surface cells, suggesting an origin from primitive respiratory epithelium. Am J Surg Pathol. 24(7):906-16, 2000
3. Shimosato Y: Lung tumors of uncertain histogenesis. Semin Diagn Pathol. 12(2):185-92, 1995
4. Moran CA et al: Sclerosing hemangioma of the lung. Granulomatous variant. Arch Pathol Lab Med. 118(10):1028-30, 1994
5. Katzenstein AL et al: Sclerosing hemangioma of the lung: a clinicopathologic study of 51 cases. Am J Surg Pathol. 4(4):343-56, 1980
6. Kennedy A: "Sclerosing haemangioma" of the lung: an alternative view of its development. J Clin Pathol. 26(10):792-9, 1973
7. Liebow AA et al: Sclerosing hemangioma (histiocytoma, xanthoma) of the lung. Cancer. 9(1):53-75, 1956

SCLEROSING HEMANGIOMA (PNEUMOCYTOMA)

Microscopic Features

(Left) *SH shows a prominent papillary growth pattern, giving the appearance of a true papillary neoplasm. This feature may be extensive in some cases; however, it would be unusual for SH to have exclusively this pattern of growth.* ***(Right)*** *Solid cellular proliferation is shown with only focal ectatic vessels and areas of sclerosis. Most cases of SH will display a combination of different growth patterns.*

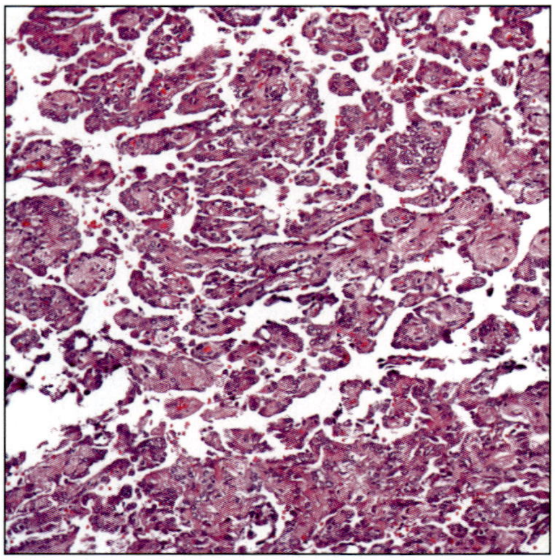

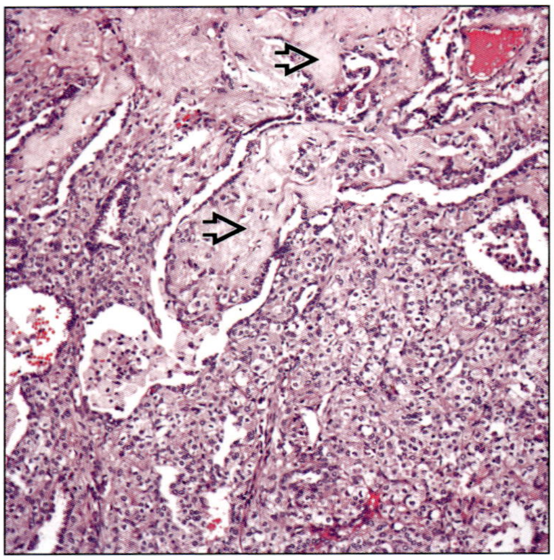

(Left) *Sclerosing hemangioma shows prominent sclerotic changes with dilated vascular spaces. Note the presence of a more subtle cellular proliferation. This histological feature may make the diagnosis of SH more difficult.* ***(Right)*** *Sclerosing hemangioma shows a combination of hemorrhagic areas mimicking a vascular tumor, focal sclerotic areas, and solid cellular proliferation.*

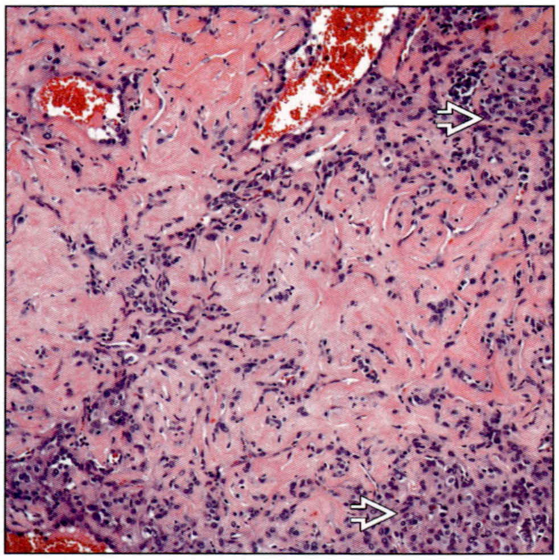

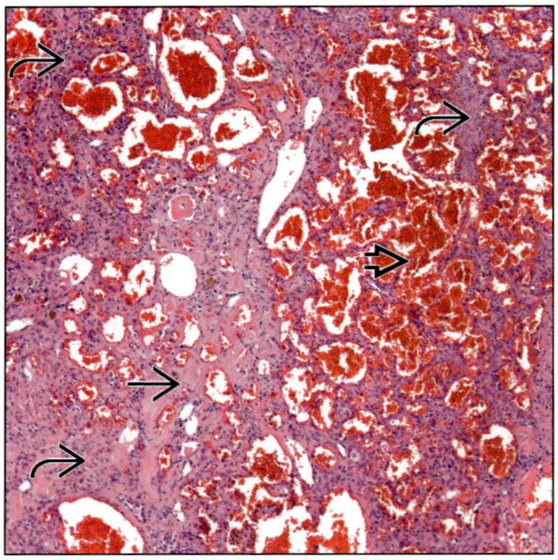

(Left) *Sclerosing hemangioma shows a prominent solid cellular proliferation with focal entrapment of adipose tissue. There is no evidence of necrosis, nuclear atypia, &/ or mitotic activity.* ***(Right)*** *Sclerosing hemangioma shows the 2 classic types of cells: Low cuboidal in the surface and the so-called "pale" or stromal cells, which are round to oval.*

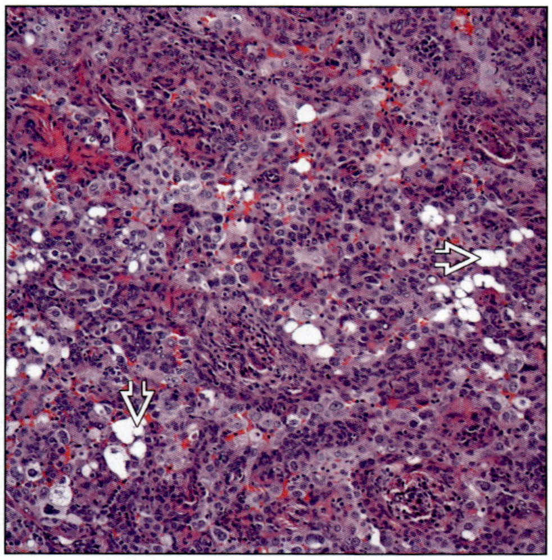

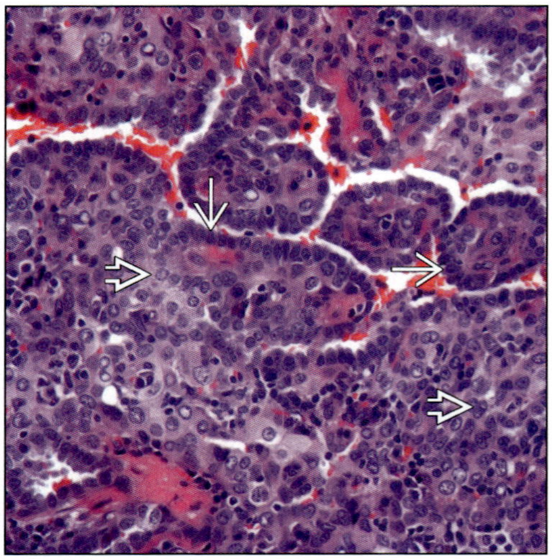

Microscopic Features

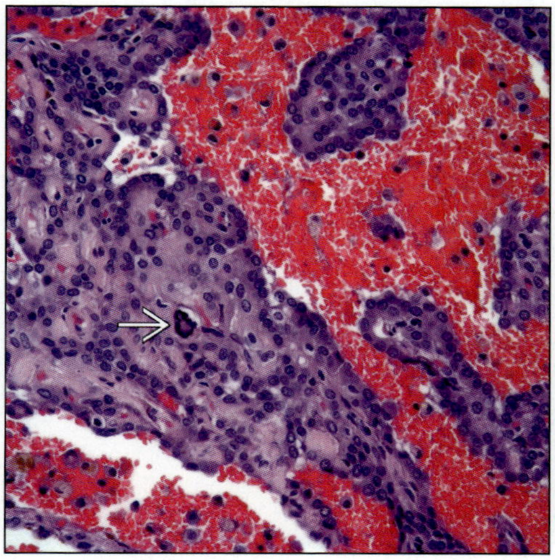

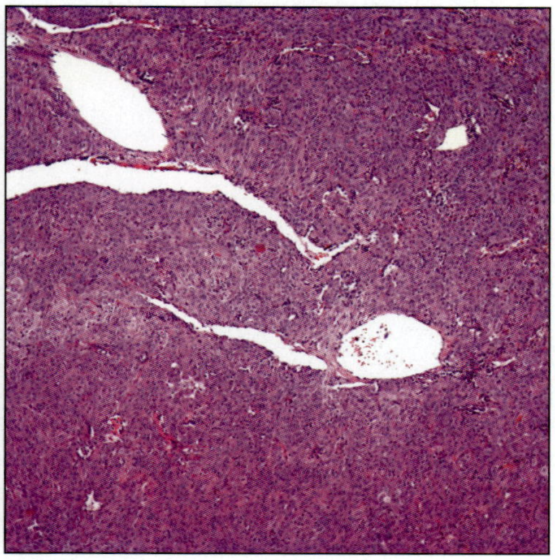

(Left) *Sclerosing hemangioma shows a vague papillary growth pattern admixed with hemorrhagic areas. A single psammoma body is also present* ➔*.* ***(Right)*** *Sclerosing hemangioma shows a solid growth pattern with only focal dilated vascular spaces. Usually SH will show a combination of at least 2 different growth patterns.*

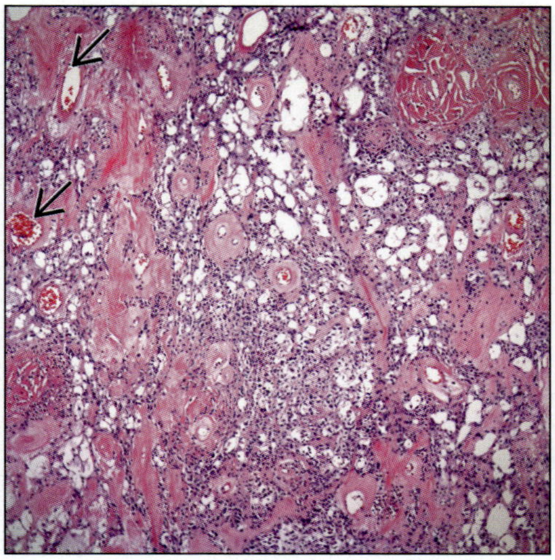

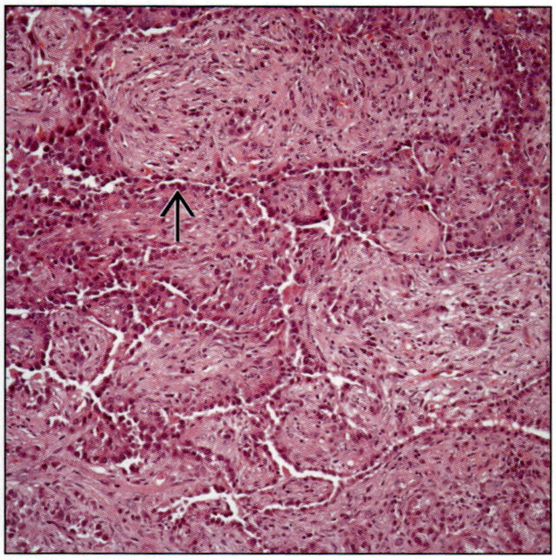

(Left) *Sclerosing hemangioma shows extensive areas of sclerosis admixed with solid stromal cells. Note the presence of dilated "true" vessels* ➔*.* ***(Right)*** *In this sclerosing hemangioma, prominent surface low cuboidal cells lining the papillary infolding* ➔ *are shown. The stromal or "pale" cells are not prominent and are embedded in the sclerotic areas.*

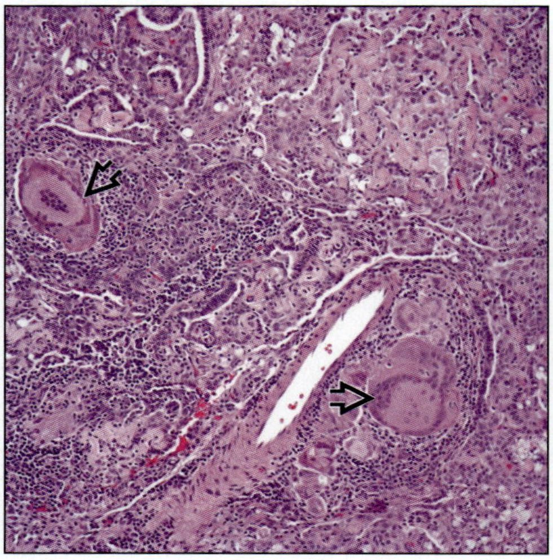

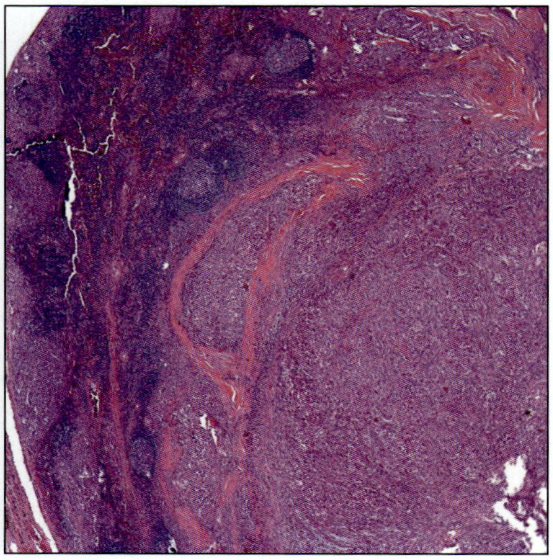

(Left) *Sclerosing hemangioma shows prominent multinucleated giant cells* ➔ *and adjacent inflammatory reaction, giving the appearance of a granulomatous process. These features are unusual in sclerosing hemangiomas.* ***(Right)*** *Lymph node is shown with metastatic sclerosing hemangioma. Although this tumor is considered benign, some unusual cases will metastasize to hilar lymph nodes.*

CLEAR CELL "SUGAR" TUMOR (PEComa)

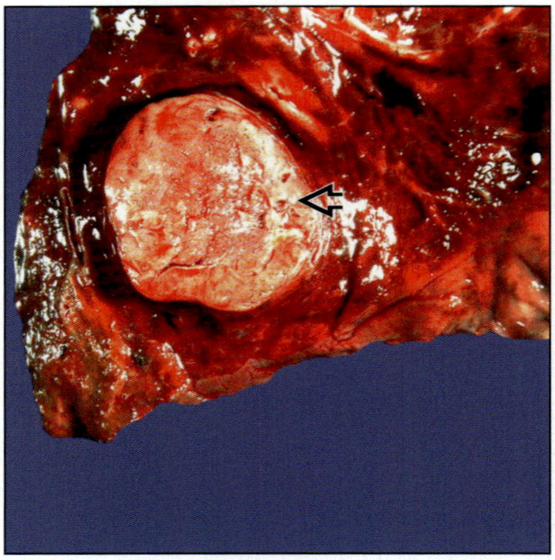

Gross photograph shows a well-circumscribed intrapulmonary clear cell "sugar" tumor ⮚. The cut surface is homogeneous and light tan.

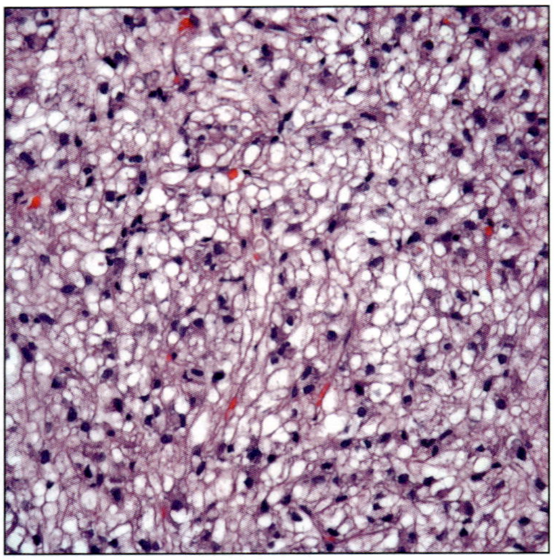

Sugar tumor is seen with prominent clear cell proliferation. Note the absence of cellular atypia, necrosis, and mitotic activity.

TERMINOLOGY

Synonyms

- Clear cell tumor

Definitions

- Benign intrapulmonary neoplasm with prominent clear cells

ETIOLOGY/PATHOGENESIS

Etiology

- Recently sugar tumor has been regarded as part of the family of tumors designated as PEComas
- Myo-melanocytic differentiation

CLINICAL ISSUES

Epidemiology

- Age
  - Although tumor is more common in adults, it has been reported in children
- Gender
  - No gender predilection

Presentation

- Asymptomatic
- Fever
- Anemia
- Pneumonia
- Elevated platelet count
- Elevated erythrocyte sedimentation rate
- Hemoptysis (rarely)
- History of tuberous sclerosis

Treatment

- Surgical approaches
  - Complete surgical resection

Prognosis

- Excellent

MACROSCOPIC FEATURES

General Features

- Peripheral tumor
- Well circumscribed but not encapsulated
- Tan to pink in color
- 1-7 cm in diameter

MICROSCOPIC PATHOLOGY

Histologic Features

- Sheets of clear cells with dilated vascular spaces
- Absence of nuclear atypia
- Absence of necrosis &/or hemorrhage
- Absence of mitotic activity
- Occasionally cells may adopt a spindle cell appearance

Predominant Pattern/Injury Type

- Sheets

Predominant Cell/Compartment Type

- Clear

ANCILLARY TESTS

Histochemistry

- Periodic acid-Schiff
  - Reactivity: Positive
  - Staining pattern
    - Cytoplasmic

DIFFERENTIAL DIAGNOSIS

Clear Cell Carcinoma, Primary or Metastatic

- Renal cell carcinoma

CLEAR CELL "SUGAR" TUMOR (PEComa)

Key Facts

Terminology
- Benign intrapulmonary neoplasm with prominent clear cells

Etiology/Pathogenesis
- Myo-melanocytic differentiation (PEComa)

Clinical Issues
- Although tumor is more common in adults, it has been reported in children
- No gender predilection
- Asymptomatic

Macroscopic Features
- Peripheral tumor
- 1-7 cm in diameter

Microscopic Pathology
- Sheets of clear cells with dilated vascular spaces

Ancillary Tests
- Periodic acid-Schiff
- Positive

Top Differential Diagnoses
- Clear cell carcinoma, primary or metastatic
  - Sugar tumor is negative for epithelial markers
  - Sugar tumor lacks nuclear atypia &/or mitotic activity

Diagnostic Checklist
- Clear cells with abundant dilated vascular vessels mimicking hemangiopericytoma

Immunohistochemistry

Antibody	Reactivity	Staining Pattern	Comment
CD34	Positive	Cytoplasmic	It may be only focal
S100	Positive	Cytoplasmic	Some cases may be negative
CD1a	Positive	Cytoplasmic	A good number of cases are negative
HMB-45	Positive	Cytoplasmic	In cytoplasm of clear cells, but may be negative in spindle cells
HMB-50	Positive	Cytoplasmic	Focal positivity in some cases
NSE	Positive	Cytoplasmic	Not specific for clear cell tumors
FXIIIA	Positive	Cytoplasmic	In some cases but not specific
Cathespin-B	Positive	Cytoplasmic	In some cases but not specific
CK-PAN	Negative		
EMA/MUC1	Negative		

Histochemical Features of Sugar Tumor of Lung

Histochemical Stain	Reactivity	Comment
PAS	Positive	Glycogen content
D-PAS	Negative	Negative for intracellular mucin
Mucicarmine	Negative	Negative for intracellular mucin

  - History of or presence of renal tumor
  - Will display more cytologic atypia and mitotic figures
  - Will show positive staining for epithelial markers (keratin, EMA)
- Clear cell carcinoma of thyroid origin
  - History of or presence of thyroid tumor
  - Thyroid carcinoma will show positive staining for thyroid hormones and epithelial markers
- Lung clear cell carcinoma
  - Will display more cellular atypia and mitotic activity
  - Lung carcinomas are positive for epithelial markers

DIAGNOSTIC CHECKLIST

Clinically Relevant Pathologic Features
- Cytoplasmic features

Pathologic Interpretation Pearls
- Clear cells with abundant dilated vascular vessels, mimicking hemangiopericytoma

SELECTED REFERENCES

1. Gaffey MJ et al: Clear cell tumor of the lung. Immunohistochemical and ultrastructural evidence of melanogenesis. Am J Surg Pathol. 15(7):644-53, 1991
2. Liebow AA et al: Benign clear cell ("sugar") tumors of the lung. Yale J Biol Med. 43(4-5):213-22, 1971

CLEAR CELL "SUGAR" TUMOR (PEComa)

Imaging and Microscopic Features

(Left) *Radiograph shows a well-defined intrapulmonary mass ➔ (so-called coin lesion).* ***(Right)*** *Sugar tumor shows a homogeneous cellular proliferation composed of cells with light eosinophilic or clear cytoplasm. Note the absence of necrosis &/or hemorrhage. The tumor cell population is quite monotonous and grows forming solid sheets of cells.*

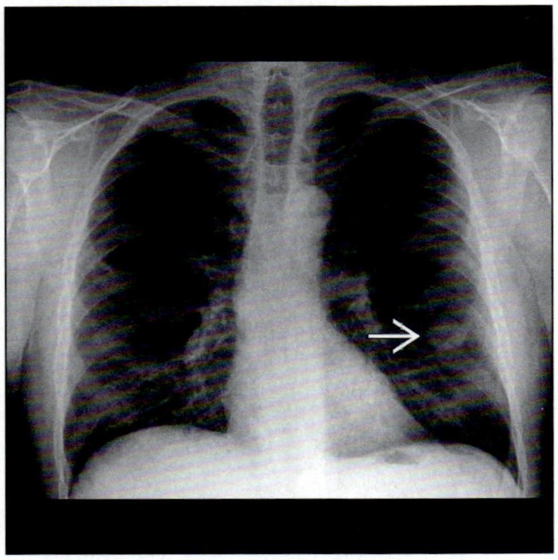

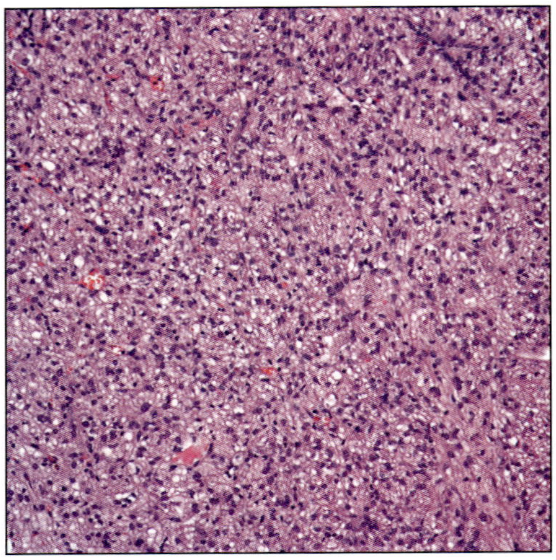

(Left) *Sugar tumor shows round cells with clear cytoplasm admixed with spindle cells with a vague storiform pattern →. This pattern may be confused for a mesenchymal neoplasm.* ***(Right)*** *Hematoxylin & eosin shows a sugar tumor with focal areas of hemorrhage toward the periphery of the tumor. Uninvolved lung parenchyma is still present ⇨. These areas do not represent tumor hemorrhage but rather ectatic vascular spaces with pools of red cells.*

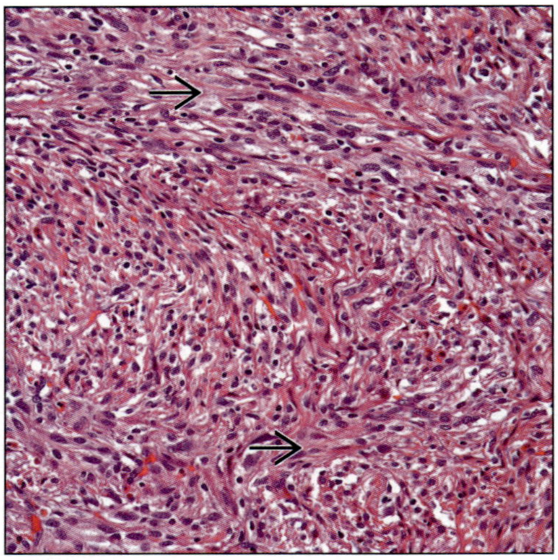

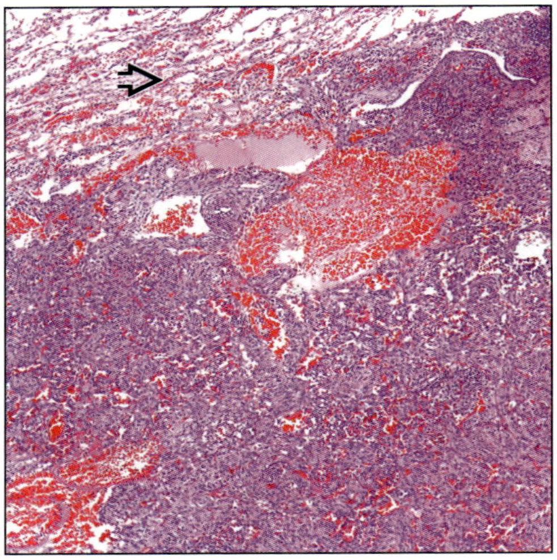

(Left) *Clear cell tumor is seen with prominent ectatic vessels, possibly mimicking a vascular tumor. However, even at this magnification one can appreciate the presence of cells with clear cytoplasm.* ***(Right)*** *Close view of the clear cell proliferation around an ectatic blood vessel. The tumor does not show cellular atypia or mitotic activity. A discrete vascular network is present.*

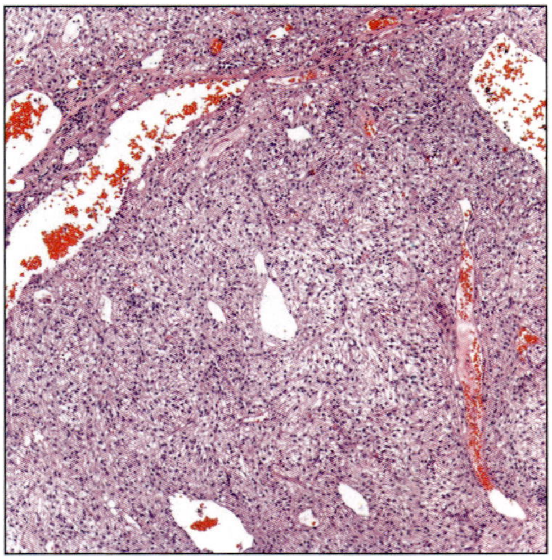

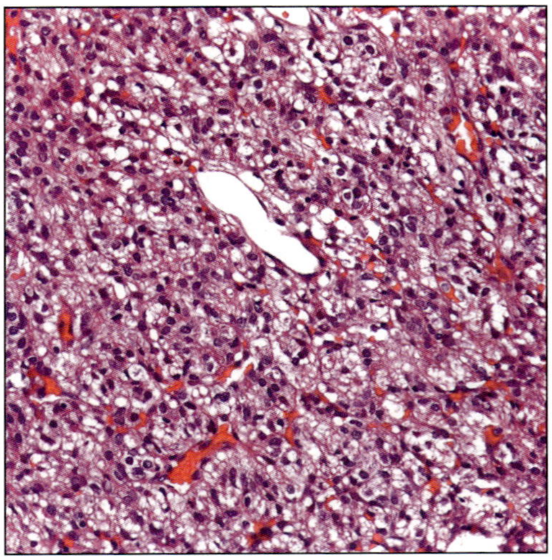

Microscopic Features

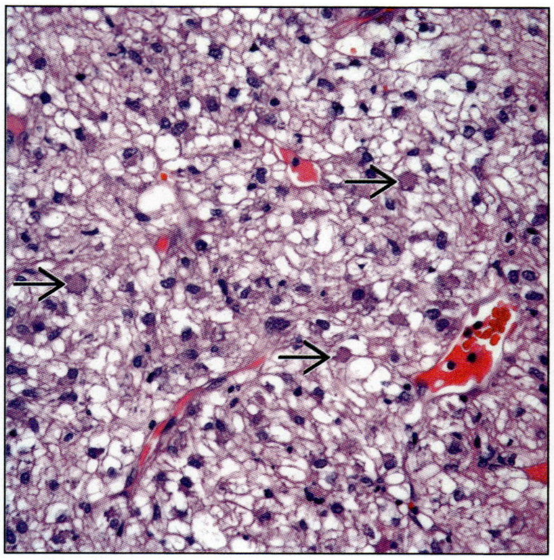

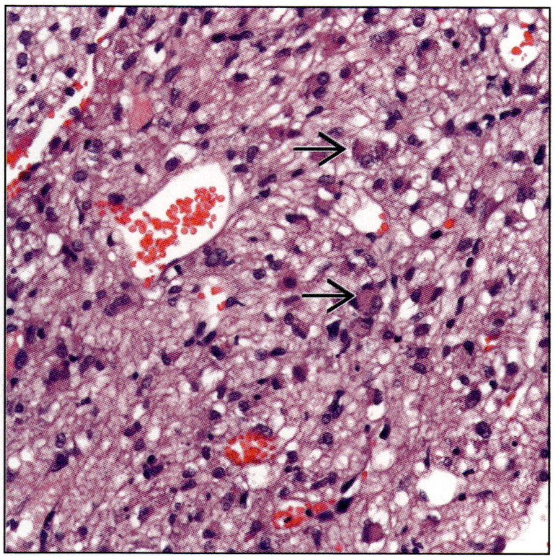

(Left) *Clear cell proliferation with ganglion-like cells* → *gives the appearance of a neuroid neoplasm. These features, although not very conspicuous, are often seen in many cases.* ***(Right)*** *Hematoxylin & eosin shows numerous ganglion-like cells* → *and fewer cells with clear cytoplasm and a fibrillary-like background. This appearance can be mistaken for a neural tumor.*

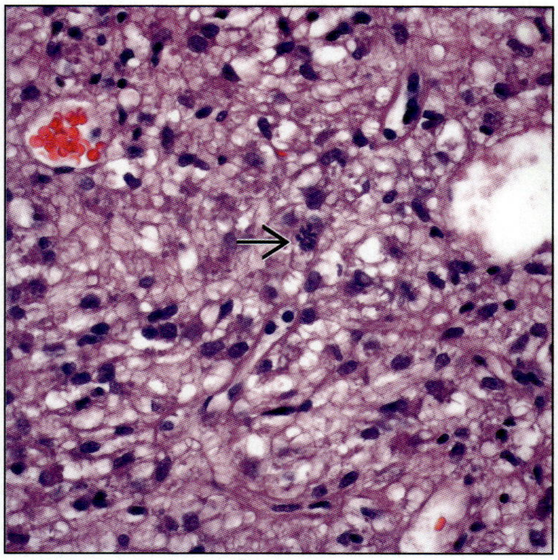

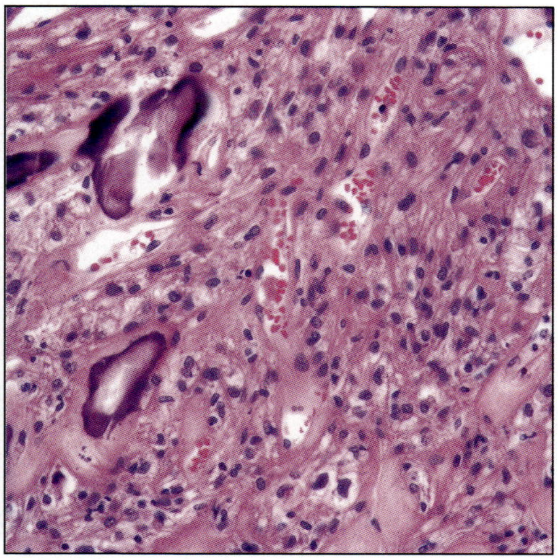

(Left) *Sugar tumor with clear cell proliferation. Note the presence of a mitotic figure* →*. In a few cases, one may observe occasional mitotic figures; however, that is not a common feature.* ***(Right)*** *Hematoxylin & eosin shows a sugar tumor with focal areas of calcifications admixed with clear and spindle cells. This pattern can be easily confused for a true vascular tumor, such as a glomus tumor.*

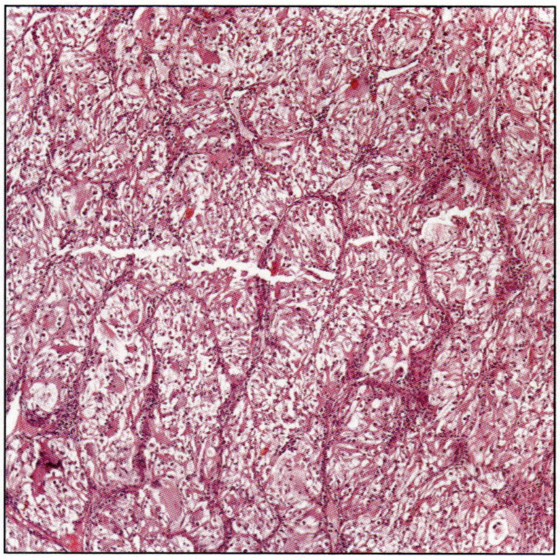

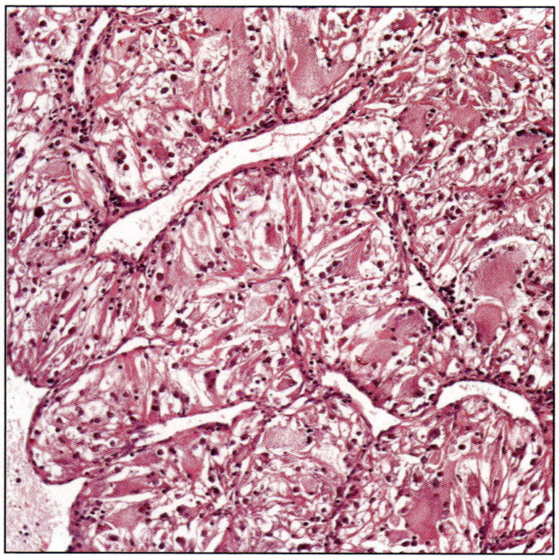

(Left) *Clear cell tumor is seen with a prominent nested pattern resembling a neuroendocrine neoplasm. In small biopsies, the use of immunohistochemistry to properly rule out a neuroendocrine tumor needs to be done.* ***(Right)*** *Clear cell tumor is seen with numerous so-called spider cells, which are another feature of sugar tumors. In addition, this pattern may be seen in paragangliomas, thus the need for a careful evaluation.*

Neoplasms, Malignant, Primary

Epithelial Neoplasms

Salivary Gland-type Tumors

Mesenchymal Neoplasms

Lymphoproliferative Disorders

Other Rare Tumors and Benign Pseudotumoral Conditions

Lung Cancer Protocols

OVERVIEW OF MALIGNANT EPITHELIAL NEOPLASMS OF THE LUNG

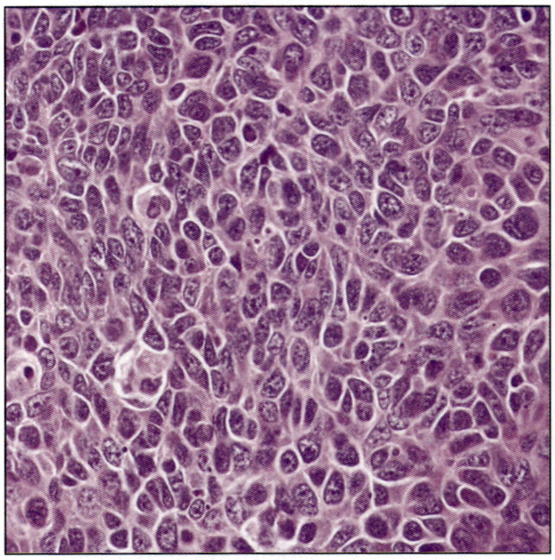

Poorly differentiated non-small cell carcinoma of the lung shows sheets of large, atypical cells with large nuclei and prominent nucleoli and without evidence of glandular or squamous differentiation.

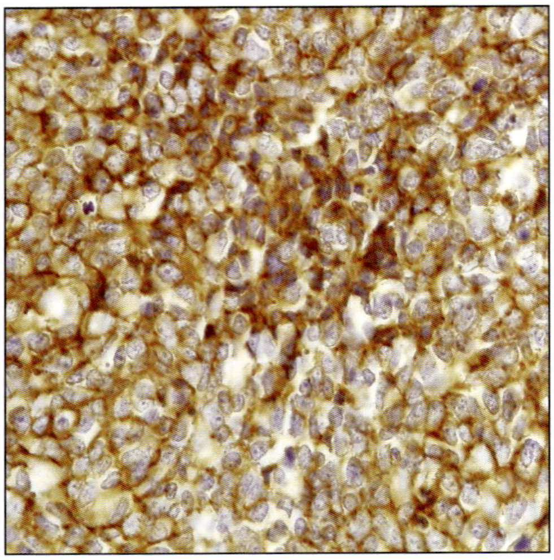

Immunohistochemical staining for cytokeratin AE1/AE3 in poorly differentiated non-small cell carcinoma of the lung shows strong positivity of the tumor cells for this antibody.

TERMINOLOGY

Definitions

- Neoplastic process showing histological, immunohistochemical, or ultrastructural evidence of epithelial differentiation

Principles of Classification

- Classification of lung carcinoma, which constitutes the vast majority of primary lung cancers based on clinical implications
  - Small cell carcinoma (SCC)
    - Rapidly growing tumors that have metastasized early and widely to distant organs at time of initial diagnosis
    - Respond well to chemo- and radiotherapy
    - Are generally not considered good surgical candidates
  - Non-small cell lung carcinoma (NSCLC)
    - Tends to be slower growing and of lesser stage at time of diagnosis
    - When in lower stages (I-II), considered good surgical candidates
- Histopathologic classification of lung cancer according to lines of differentiation
  - Bronchogenic carcinoma
    - Squamous cell carcinoma
    - Adenocarcinoma
    - Large cell/anaplastic carcinoma
    - Neuroendocrine carcinoma (carcinoid, atypical carcinoid, and small cell carcinoma)
  - Bronchial gland (salivary-type) tumors
    - Adenoid cystic carcinoma
    - Mucoepidermoid carcinoma
    - Epimyoepithelial carcinoma
  - Mixed epithelial-mesenchymal tumors
    - Carcinosarcoma
    - Pulmonary blastoma

EPIDEMIOLOGY

Age Range

- 40-70 years of age

Gender

- More common in men (M:F = 3:1)

Incidence

- Lung cancer is one of the most common malignant neoplasms worldwide
- Lung cancer accounts for approximately 12% of all new cancers and 18% of all cancer deaths
- Areas of highest incidence and mortality include Europe, North America, Australia, and South America
- Certain populations are at increased risk (African-Americans, Maoris in New Zealand)

ETIOLOGY/PATHOGENESIS

Pathogenesis

- Tobacco smoke is the major predisposing factor for development of lung cancer
  - Smokers experience an 8-15x increased risk for developing lung cancer than nonsmokers
  - Risk is directly proportional to number of cigarettes smoked per day and duration of smoking
- Occupational exposure is also strongly associated with development of lung cancer
  - Asbestos exposure is associated with increased risk for development of lung cancer
  - Ionizing radiation exposure is another factor involved in development of lung cancer
  - Urban air pollution is a risk factor for lung cancer with an excess risk in the order of 50%

Lung Cancer Protocols

OVERVIEW OF MALIGNANT EPITHELIAL NEOPLASMS OF THE LUNG

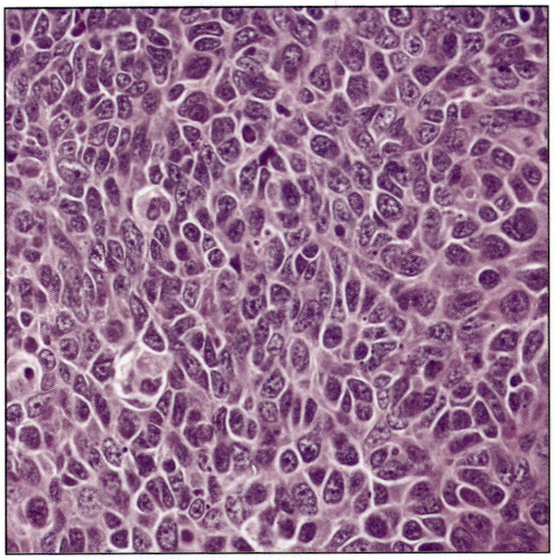

Poorly differentiated non-small cell carcinoma of the lung shows sheets of large, atypical cells with large nuclei and prominent nucleoli and without evidence of glandular or squamous differentiation.

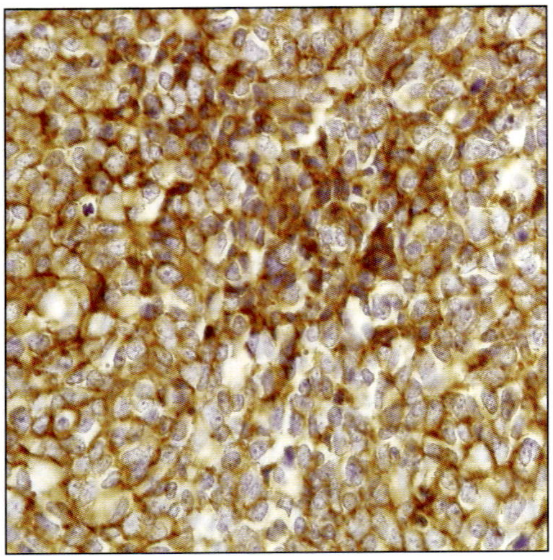

Immunohistochemical staining for cytokeratin AE1/AE3 in poorly differentiated non-small cell carcinoma of the lung shows strong positivity of the tumor cells for this antibody.

TERMINOLOGY

Definitions

- Neoplastic process showing histological, immunohistochemical, or ultrastructural evidence of epithelial differentiation

Principles of Classification

- Classification of lung carcinoma, which constitutes the vast majority of primary lung cancers based on clinical implications
  - Small cell carcinoma (SCC)
    - Rapidly growing tumors that have metastasized early and widely to distant organs at time of initial diagnosis
    - Respond well to chemo- and radiotherapy
    - Are generally not considered good surgical candidates
  - Non-small cell lung carcinoma (NSCLC)
    - Tends to be slower growing and of lesser stage at time of diagnosis
    - When in lower stages (I-II), considered good surgical candidates
- Histopathologic classification of lung cancer according to lines of differentiation
  - Bronchogenic carcinoma
    - Squamous cell carcinoma
    - Adenocarcinoma
    - Large cell/anaplastic carcinoma
    - Neuroendocrine carcinoma (carcinoid, atypical carcinoid, and small cell carcinoma)
  - Bronchial gland (salivary-type) tumors
    - Adenoid cystic carcinoma
    - Mucoepidermoid carcinoma
    - Epimyoepithelial carcinoma
  - Mixed epithelial-mesenchymal tumors
    - Carcinosarcoma
    - Pulmonary blastoma

EPIDEMIOLOGY

Age Range

- 40-70 years of age

Gender

- More common in men (M:F = 3:1)

Incidence

- Lung cancer is one of the most common malignant neoplasms worldwide
- Lung cancer accounts for approximately 12% of all new cancers and 18% of all cancer deaths
- Areas of highest incidence and mortality include Europe, North America, Australia, and South America
- Certain populations are at increased risk (African-Americans, Maoris in New Zealand)

ETIOLOGY/PATHOGENESIS

Pathogenesis

- Tobacco smoke is the major predisposing factor for development of lung cancer
  - Smokers experience an 8-15x increased risk for developing lung cancer than nonsmokers
  - Risk is directly proportional to number of cigarettes smoked per day and duration of smoking
- Occupational exposure is also strongly associated with development of lung cancer
  - Asbestos exposure is associated with increased risk for development of lung cancer
  - Ionizing radiation exposure is another factor involved in development of lung cancer
  - Urban air pollution is a risk factor for lung cancer with an excess risk in the order of 50%

OVERVIEW OF MALIGNANT EPITHELIAL NEOPLASMS OF THE LUNG

CLINICAL IMPLICATIONS

Clinical Presentation

- Progressive shortness of breath
- Cough
- Chest pain
- Hemoptysis
- Pleural effusion
- Paraneoplastic symptoms
  - Ectopic secretion of peptide hormones: ACTH, ADH, etc.
  - Neurologic symptoms: Sensory abnormalities, autoimmune neuropathies, encephalomyelitis
  - Eaton-Lambert myasthenic syndrome
  - Hypercalcemia due to production of parathormone-like substance associated with squamous cell carcinoma
  - Clubbing of fingers (hypertrophic pulmonary osteoarthropathy)
  - Carcinoid syndrome due to serotonin production by neuroendocrine carcinomas

MICROSCOPIC FINDINGS

General Features

- Histologic examination remains the mainstay of classification and diagnosis
- Bronchogenic carcinoma is characterized by recapitulating normal structures of tracheobronchial tree
  - Adenocarcinomas form glands and may be well, moderately, and poorly differentiated
    - Subtypes of adenocarcinoma include acinar, papillary, solid, signet-ring, bronchoalveolar, mucinous, fetal, and clear cell type
  - Squamous cell carcinoma recapitulates pavemented epithelium of squamous mucosa and may be well to poorly differentiated
    - Subtypes include keratinizing, papillary, small cell, lymphoepithelioma-like, basaloid, spindle (sarcomatoid), and clear cell
  - Large cell/anaplastic carcinomas are poorly differentiated tumors without evidence of squamous or glandular differentiation
    - Subtypes include pleomorphic, anaplastic, clear cell, giant cell, sarcomatoid, and rhabdoid
  - Neuroendocrine carcinomas show evidence of neuroendocrine differentiation by histology, immunohistochemistry, or ultrastructurally
    - Subtypes include well differentiated ("carcinoid"), moderately differentiated ("atypical carcinoid"), and poorly differentiated (small cell carcinoma)

Immunohistochemical Features

- Markers associated with lung adenocarcinoma include TTF-1, NAPSIN-A, CK7, CEA, and MOC-31
- Markers associated with squamous cell carcinoma include CK7, CK5/6, MOC-31, and p63
- Markers associated with neuroendocrine carcinomas include CK7, chromogranin, synaptophysin, CD56, and CD57

Ultrastructural Features

- Organelles associated with adenocarcinomas include zymogen granules, microvilli, and intracellular lumens
- Organelles associated with squamous cell carcinomas include tonofilaments and well-developed desmosome-type intercellular junctions
- Organelles associated with neuroendocrine neoplasms include dense-core, membrane-bound neurosecretory intracytoplasmic granules

Genetic and Molecular Alterations

- Genetic changes frequent in all major histologic types
  - *TP53* mutations are detected in up to 50% of NSCLC and in over 70% of SCC
  - Inactivation of the pathway encoding the retinoblastoma gene, *RB1* (13q11), leading to loss of Rb protein expression
  - Loss of heterozygosity (LOH) on chromosome 3p is detectable in up to 80% of NSCLC and SCC
  - Hypermethylation of the cyclin-dependent kinase inhibitor p16 is seen in up to 50% of all lung cancers
  - Loss of heterozygosity (LOH) of the fragile histidine triad (*FHIT*) gene on chromosome 3p14.2 occurs in 40-70% of all lung cancers
- Genetic changes specific for some histologic types
  - *KRAS* mutation (12p21) is found in 30-50% of all lung adenocarcinomas
  - Amplification of MYC (8q21-23) is common in small cell neuroendocrine carcinomas
  - *EGFR* mutations are present in NSCLC
  - *LKB1* mutations occur more commonly in lung adenocarcinoma and large cell carcinoma
  - *ALK* gene rearrangements leading to *EML4-ALK* fusion has been detected preferentially in adenocarcinomas

SELECTED REFERENCES

1. Lim EH et al: Using whole genome amplification (WGA) of low-volume biopsies to assess the prognostic role of EGFR, KRAS, p53, and CMET mutations in advanced-stage non-small cell lung cancer (NSCLC). J Thorac Oncol. 4(1):12-21, 2009
2. Alberg AJ et al: Epidemiology of lung cancer: ACCP evidence-based clinical practice guidelines (2nd edition). Chest. 132(3 Suppl):29S-55S, 2007
3. Jemal A et al: Cancer statistics, 2007. CA Cancer J Clin. 57(1):43-66, 2007
4. Pan H et al: Loss of heterozygosity patterns provide fingerprints for genetic heterogeneity in multistep cancer progression of tobacco smoke-induced non-small cell lung cancer. Cancer Res. 65(5):1664-9, 2005
5. Shigematsu H et al: Clinical and biological features associated with epidermal growth factor receptor gene mutations in lung cancers. J Natl Cancer Inst. 97(5):339-46, 2005
6. Sanchez-Cespedes M et al: Chromosomal alterations in lung adenocarcinoma from smokers and nonsmokers. Cancer Res. 61(4):1309-13, 2001
7. Gealy R et al: Comparison of mutations in the p53 and K-ras genes in lung carcinomas from smoking and nonsmoking women. Cancer Epidemiol Biomarkers Prev. 8(4 Pt 1):297-302, 1999

ADENOCARCINOMA

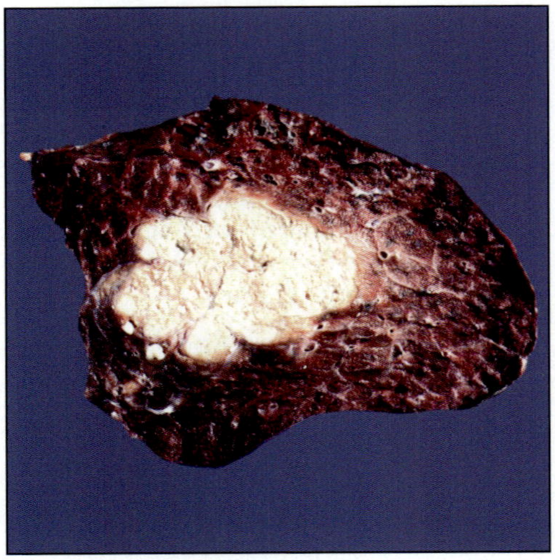

Gross photograph shows a peripherally located lung adenocarcinoma. The mass is relatively well demarcated but not encapsulated. It is tan and nodular.

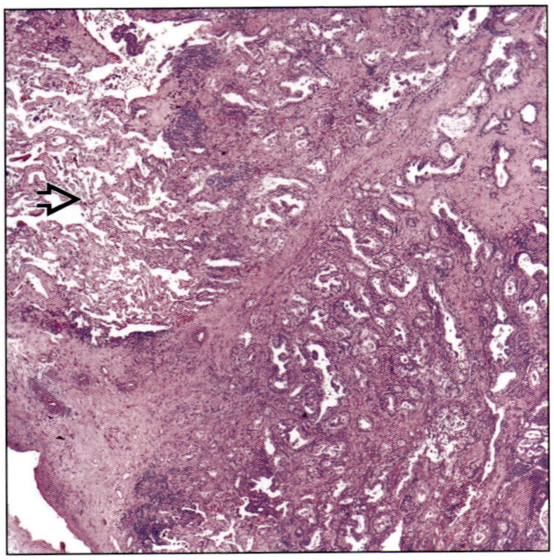

Well-differentiated adenocarcinoma destroying normal lung parenchyma. Note the contrast with normal lung parenchyma ➢.

TERMINOLOGY

Abbreviations

- Adenocarcinoma (AdenoCa)

Definitions

- Malignant epithelial neoplasm with glandular differentiation

ETIOLOGY/PATHOGENESIS

Environmental Exposure

- Close association with tobacco use

Etiology

- Tumor probably originates from endobronchial glands

CLINICAL ISSUES

Epidemiology

- Incidence
  - In last decade, adenocarcinomas have become more prevalent than any other non-small cell carcinoma
  - Currently is most common non-small cell carcinoma
- Age
  - Although more common in adults, adenocarcinomas also occur in younger individuals
  - Adenocarcinomas are more common in 6th and 7th decades of life

Presentation

- Cough
- Weight loss
- Difficulty breathing
- Chest pain
- Cushing syndrome
- Superior vena cava syndrome
- Pancoast syndrome
- Hemoptysis

Treatment

- Surgical approaches
  - Segmentectomy, lobectomy, pneumonectomy
- Adjuvant therapy
  - Chemotherapy, radiation therapy, or both
  - Cases positive for epidermal growth factor receptor (*EGFR*) mutation may receive different treatment

Prognosis

- Depends on stage at time of diagnosis
- Patients with carcinomas positive for EGFR mutation may have better prognosis
- It is also possible that tumors with better differentiated histology have more favorable outcome
- It may also be related to other pulmonary function factors as well as other medical conditions

MACROSCOPIC FEATURES

General Features

- Peripheral or central tumors
  - Tumors may show necrosis &/or hemorrhage
  - Homogeneous tan surface
  - Well-circumscribed but not encapsulated

Sections to Be Submitted

- Tumor in relation to pleural surface
  - Pleural involvement crucial for staging tumors < 3 cm in size

Size

- Varying size from 0.6 cm to > 10 cm

MICROSCOPIC PATHOLOGY

Histologic Features

- Malignant glandular component

Key Facts

Terminology
- Malignant epithelial neoplasm with glandular differentiation

Etiology/Pathogenesis
- Close association with tobacco smoking

Clinical Issues
- Cough
- Weight loss
- Chest pain
- Difficulty breathing

Macroscopic Features
- Peripheral or central tumors
- Varying size from 0.6 cm to > 10 cm

Microscopic Pathology
- Acinar
- Solid
- Papillary

Ancillary Tests
- EGFR by FISH
- Analysis of exons 18, 19, 20, and 21

Top Differential Diagnoses
- Adenocarcinoma from extrathoracic origin
- Atypical adenomatous hyperplasia (AAH)
- Adenoid cystic carcinoma (ACC)
- Fetal adenocarcinoma (monophasic pulmonary blastoma)
- Papillary carcinoma of thyroid origin

Predominant Pattern/Injury Type
- Acinar
- Solid
- Papillary
- Mixed

Predominant Cell/Compartment Type
- Epithelial

True Papillary Carcinoma
- Should be composed of at least 75% true papillae with fibrovascular cores
- This particular pattern is believed to be more aggressive
- Lymph node metastases in this pattern are commonly seen
- TTF-1(+) and thyroglobulin(-)

Papillary Carcinoma with Morular Component
- Similar criteria to true papillary carcinoma
- Presence of morular component in alveolar spaces
- "Morules" are of different sizes and always in intraalveolar location
- TTF-1(+) and thyroglobulin(-)

Micropapillary Carcinoma
- Composed of small micropapillae without fibrovascular cords
- This pattern is often seen in combination with true papillary carcinoma
- TTF-1(+) and thyroglobulin(-)

Hepatoid Adenocarcinoma
- Composed of cords of neoplastic cells resembling hepatic parenchyma
- This pattern is commonly placed among large cell carcinomas of lung
- TTF-1 may show focal positive staining

Warthin-like Adenocarcinoma
- Prominent lymphoid component similar to tumors in salivary gland
- Some cases of mucoepidermoid carcinoma may also display similar features
- Glandular proliferation with cells producing mucin embedded in inflammatory background
- TTF-1 may show positive staining

Adenomatoid Tumor-like Adenocarcinoma
- Bland appearance similar to true adenomatoid tumor
- In some cases, can be confused with so-called alveolar adenoma
- TTF-1 and keratin 7 positive

ANCILLARY TESTS

Histochemistry
- Mucicarmine
  - Reactivity: Positive
  - Staining pattern
    - Cytoplasmic
- PAS-diastase
  - Reactivity: Positive
  - Staining pattern
    - Cytoplasmic

EGFR by Fluorescent In Situ Hybridization (FISH)
- Analysis of exons 18, 19, 20, and 21

DIFFERENTIAL DIAGNOSIS

Adenocarcinoma from Extrathoracic Origin
- Immunohistochemistry positive for TTF-1; keratin 7 would favor lung origin in vast majority of cases

Atypical Adenomatous Hyperplasia (AAH)
- Lesion ≤ 0.5 cm in diameter
- Shares similar histological features with BAC

Adenoid Cystic Carcinoma (ACC)
- Shows characteristic double layer-forming glands

ADENOCARCINOMA

Immunohistochemistry			
Antibody	**Reactivity**	**Staining Pattern**	**Comment**
CEA-M	Positive	Cytoplasmic	
TTF-1	Positive	Nuclear	Often negative in mucinous tumors
CD15	Positive	Cytoplasmic	Often negative in poorly differentiated tumors
MOC-31	Positive	Cytoplasmic	Some mesotheliomas may show focal positive staining
CK-PAN	Positive	Cytoplasmic	
CK7	Positive	Cytoplasmic	
SURFACTANT	Positive	Cytoplasmic	Negative in many cases of primary lung origin
CDX-2	Positive		
EpCAM/BER-EP4/ CD326	Positive	Cell membrane	Some mesotheliomas are positive
NAPSIN-A	Positive	Cell membrane	Positive in most well-differentiated tumors
PRP	Negative		
Mammaglobin	Negative		
ERP	Negative		Some lung adenocarcinomas may be positive
CK20	Negative		Some lung adenocarcinomas may show weak positive staining

- Immunohistochemical studies show myoepithelial differentiation

Fetal Adenocarcinoma (Monophasic Pulmonary Blastoma)

- Presence of morules and embryonic-type glandular structures
- Presence of cytoplasmic mucin content in favor of AdenoCa

Papillary Carcinoma of Thyroid Origin

- Histologically tumors with papillary pattern may show similar histological features
- Positive TTF-1 and negative staining for thyroglobulin favors primary lung cancer

DIAGNOSTIC CHECKLIST

Pathologic Interpretation Pearls

- Size of lesion will separate carcinoma from AAH
- Cases designated as AAH are under 5 mm in diameter

GRADING

Low Grade

- Well-differentiated adenocarcinoma composed of easily identifiable glandular structures & arranged in back-to-back arrangement
- Absence of necrosis, increased mitotic activity, and nuclear atypia
- Glandular tumoral structures may be separated by extensive areas of collagenization

Intermediate Grade

- Moderately differentiated adenocarcinoma composed of identifiable glands
- Tumor may show more nuclear atypia and mitotic activity
- Glandular structures may show more disarray

High Grade

- Poorly differentiated adenocarcinoma may show solid areas with ↑ mitotic activity and nuclear atypia
- Necrosis and hemorrhage may be present

SELECTED REFERENCES

1. Wahbah M et al: Changing trends in the distribution of the histologic types of lung cancer: a review of 4,439 cases. Ann Diagn Pathol. 11(2):89-96, 2007
2. Moran CA: Pulmonary adenocarcinoma: the expanding spectrum of histologic variants. Arch Pathol Lab Med. 130(7):958-62, 2006
3. Prudkin L et al: Epidermal growth factor receptor abnormalities in lung cancer. Pathogenetic and clinical implications. Ann Diagn Pathol. 10(5):306-15, 2006
4. Moran CA et al: Papillary lung carcinoma with prominent "morular" component. Am J Clin Pathol. 122(1):106-9, 2004
5. Amin MB et al: Micropapillary component in lung adenocarcinoma: a distinctive histologic feature with possible prognostic significance. Am J Surg Pathol. 26(3):358-64, 2002
6. Arnould L et al: Hepatoid adenocarcinoma of the lung: report of a case of an unusual alpha-fetoprotein-producing lung tumor. Am J Surg Pathol. 21(9):1113-8, 1997
7. Silver SA et al: True papillary carcinoma of the lung: a distinct clinicopathologic entity. Am J Surg Pathol. 21(1):43-51, 1997
8. Rosado-de-Christenson ML et al: Bronchogenic carcinoma: radiologic-pathologic correlation. Radiographics. 14(2):429-46; quiz 447-8, 1994
9. Haque AK: Pathology of carcinoma of lung: an update on current concepts. J Thorac Imaging. 7(1):9-20, 1991
10. Ishikura H et al: Hepatoid adenocarcinoma: a distinctive histological subtype of alpha-fetoprotein-producing lung carcinoma. Virchows Arch A Pathol Anat Histopathol. 417(1):73-80, 1990

ADENOCARCINOMA

Microscopic Features

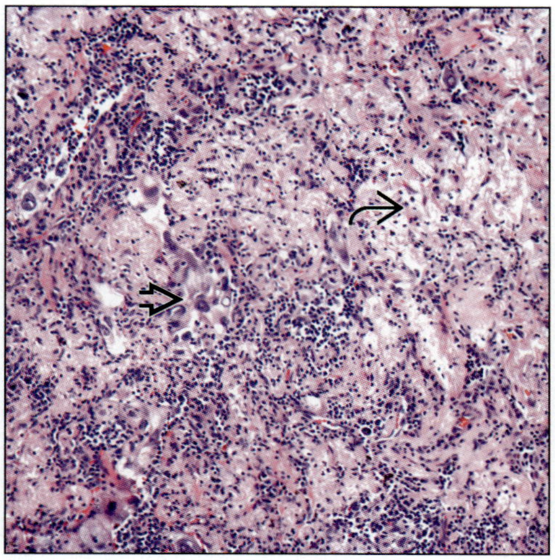
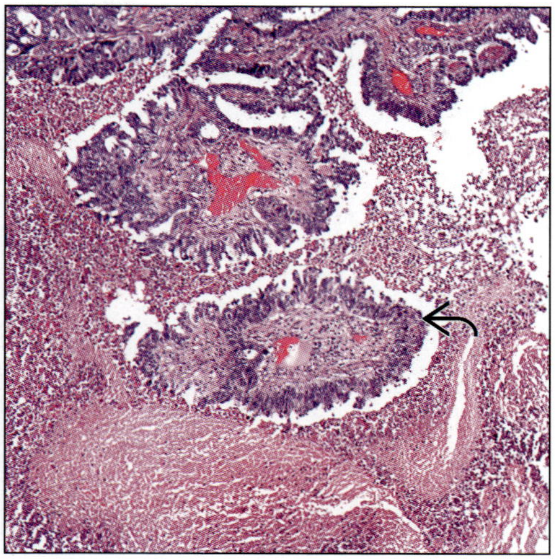

(Left) *Adenocarcinoma shows extensive areas of scarring → and inflammatory reaction. Note the presence of a cluster of malignant cells ⇨ embedded in extensive areas of collagenization.* **(Right)** *Adenocarcinoma is seen with malignant glands → floating in areas of extensive necrosis. No residual lung parenchyma is present.*

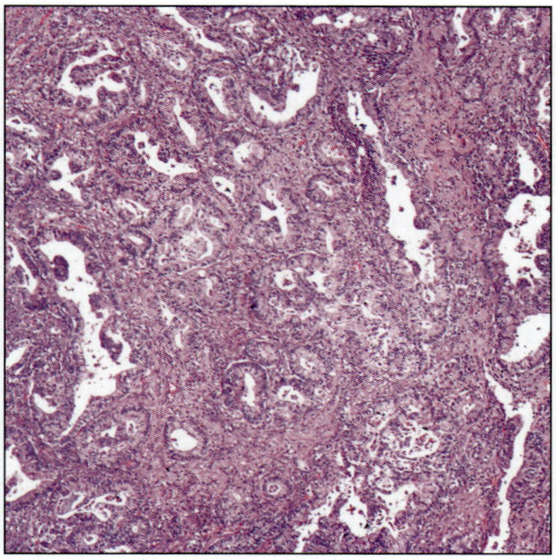
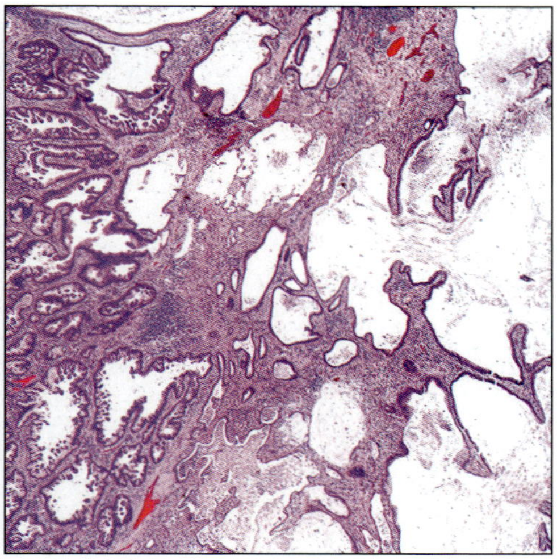

(Left) *Adenocarcinoma with an acinar pattern of growth. The neoplastic glandular proliferation is composed of glands of different sizes in a back-to-back arrangement.* **(Right)** *Adenocarcinoma in which a nonmucinous component merges with a mucinous component shows cystic changes, while the nonmucinous component reveals a more acinar component.*

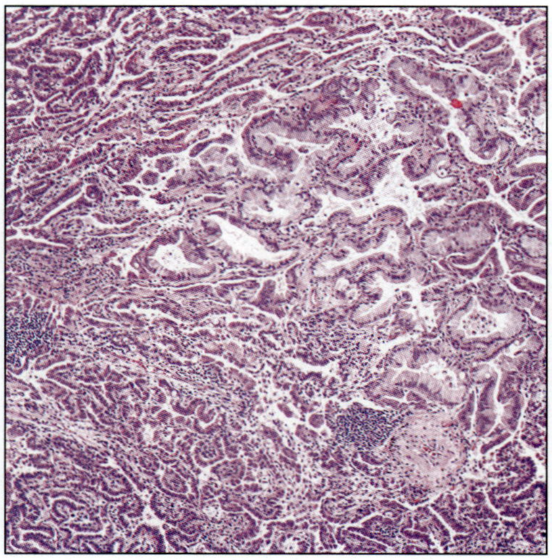
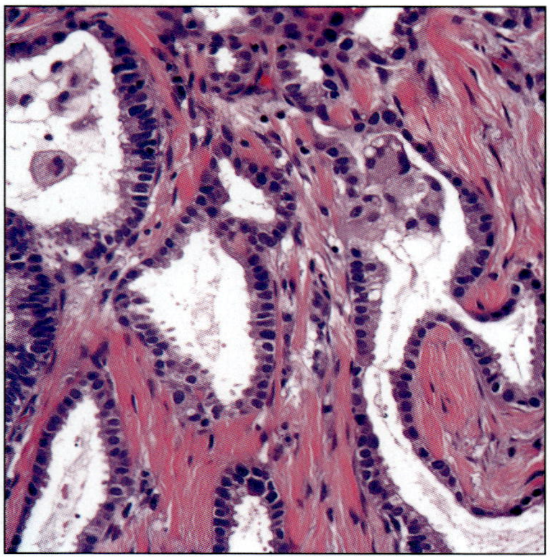

(Left) *Adenocarcinoma shows predominantly a nonmucinous type of glandular epithelium. In focal areas, a nonmucinous type of glandular proliferation merges with glands composed of a mucinous type of epithelium. This component may often be rather subtle.* **(Right)** *High-power view of a well-differentiated adenocarcinoma is composed of malignant glands with low cuboidal epithelium.*

Microscopic Features

*(**Left**) High-power view shows a well-differentiated adenocarcinoma with an acinar growth pattern. The glands are irregular with nuclear atypia and scattered mitotic figures. (**Right**) Adenocarcinoma with prominent inflammatory changes ⮚. These changes may be very extensive or may form abscess areas within the tumor.*

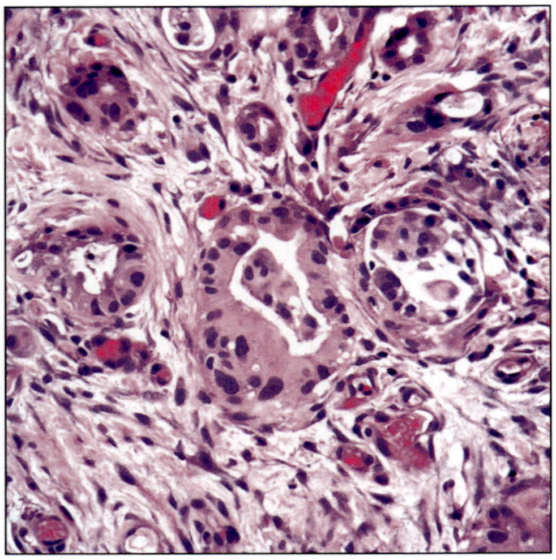

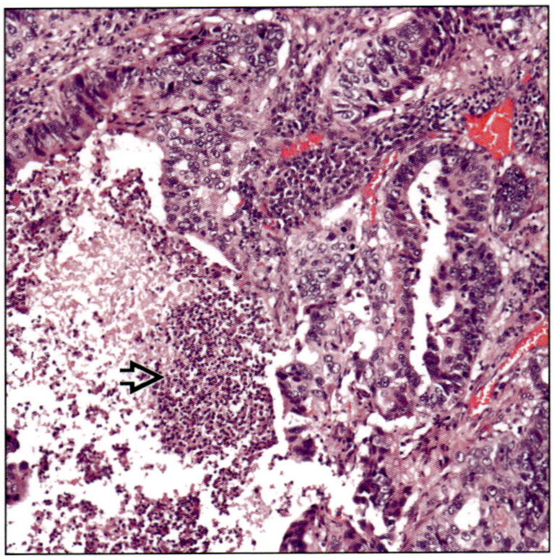

*(**Left**) Well-differentiated adenocarcinoma with an acinar growth pattern is composed of small glandular proliferation of different sizes. The glands are arranged in a haphazard pattern with fibrotic and inflammatory reaction. (**Right**) Moderately differentiated adenocarcinoma displays easily recognizable glandular structures of different sizes. The glands are separated by an inflammatory reaction. Some of the glands are collapsed and show more nuclear atypia.*

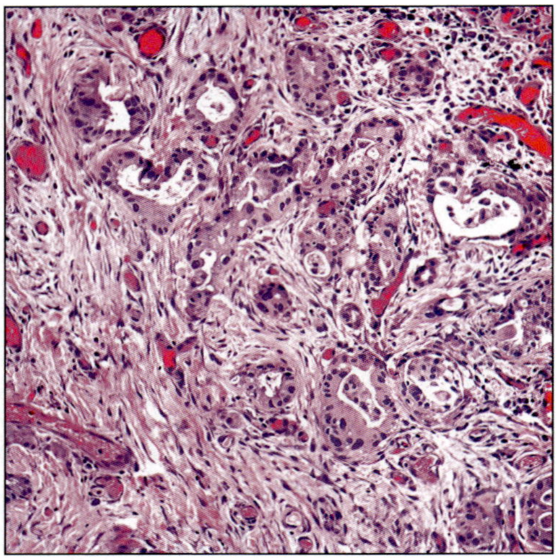

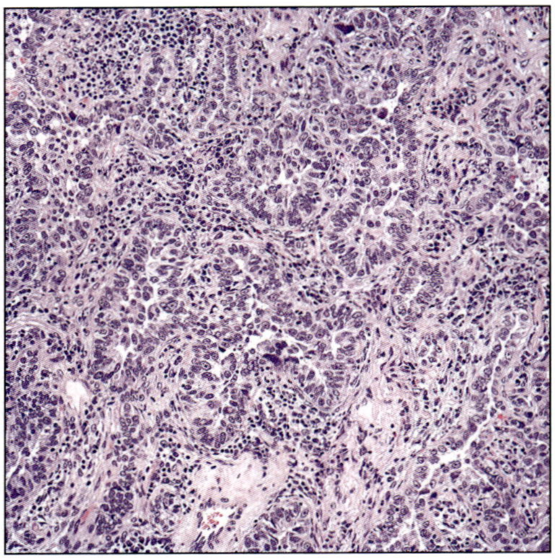

*(**Left**) Moderately differentiated adenocarcinoma shows the malignant glandular proliferation admixed with areas of fibrosis and inflammatory reaction. (**Right**) High-power view shows a moderately differentiated adenocarcinoma revealing glandular structures with more nuclear atypia and mitotic activity. The glands have a vague enteric type of differentiation, mimicking a metastasis from colonic origin.*

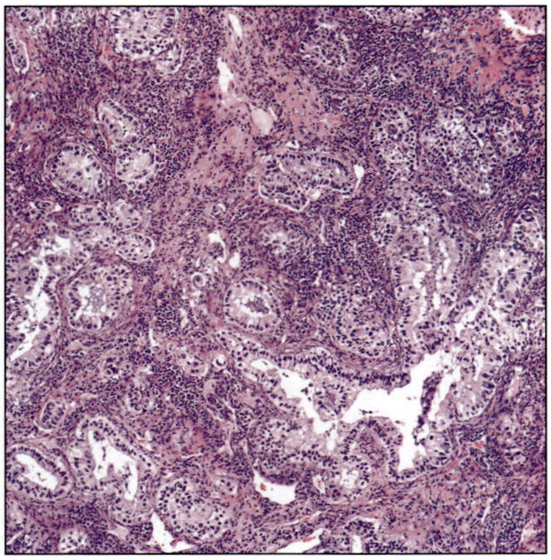

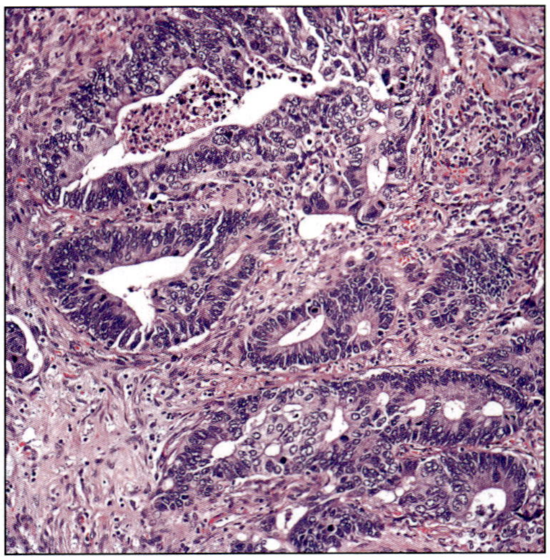

ADENOCARCINOMA

Microscopic and Gross Features

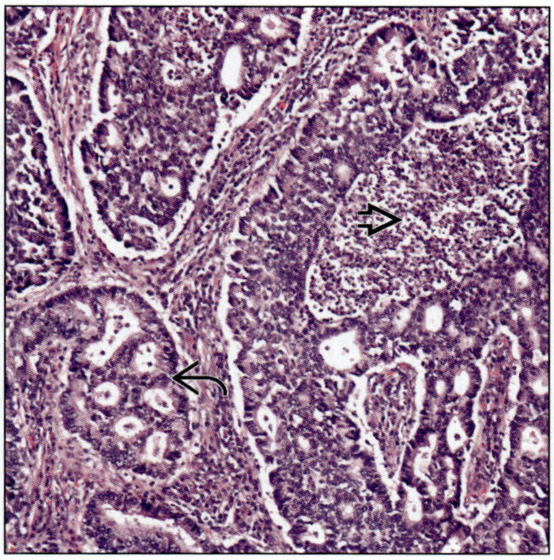
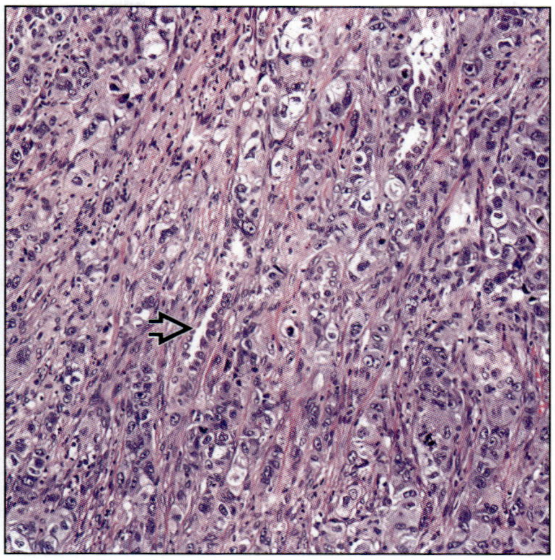

(Left) *Adenocarcinoma with comedo-like necrosis → and acinar pattern →. The pattern has a vague neuroendocrine morphology, while in some areas it shows conventional glandular differentiation.* ***(Right)*** *Intermediate-power view of a poorly differentiated adenocarcinoma with vague glandular formation → is shown. The presence of glandular differentiation in some poorly differentiated adenocarcinomas may be focal.*

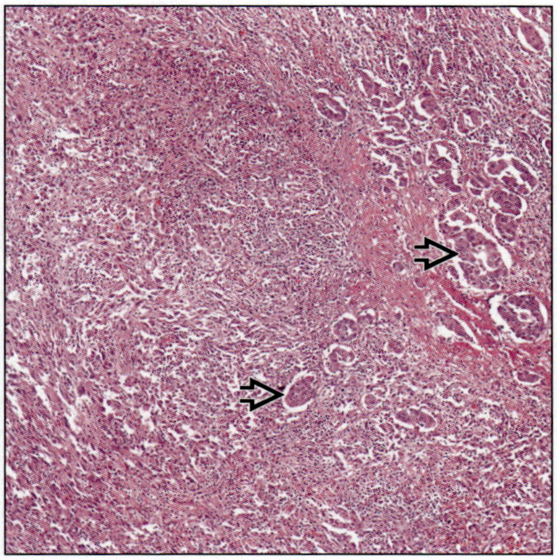
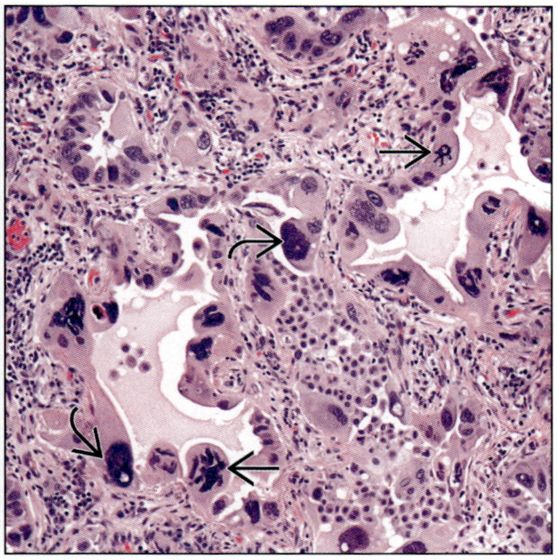

(Left) *Poorly differentiated adenocarcinoma with only focal glandular differentiation →. Most of the tumor has a predominantly solid growth pattern.* ***(Right)*** *Adenocarcinoma with the presence of numerous multinucleated giant cells →. Note the presence of atypical bizarre mitotic figures →.*

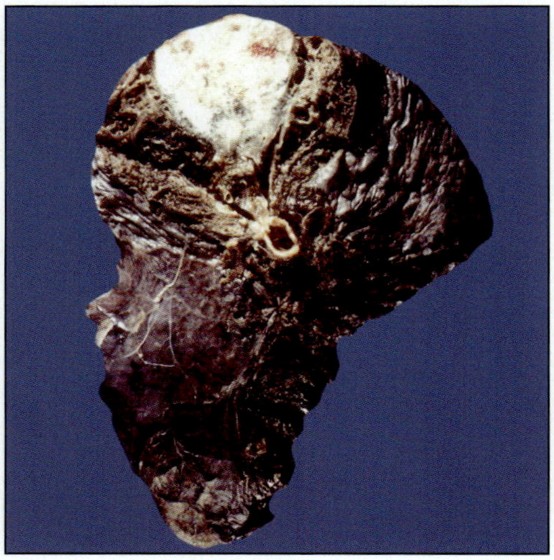
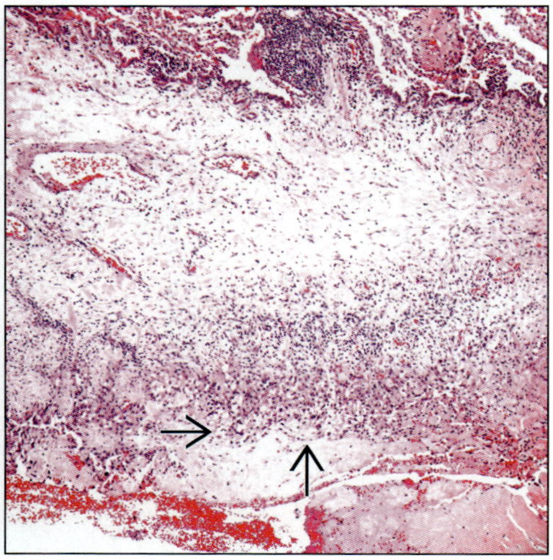

(Left) *Gross photograph shows an adenocarcinoma grossly involving the pleural surface. This feature is highly important in tumors less than 3 cm in order to properly establish a pathological stage.* ***(Right)*** *Adenocarcinoma → involving the pleural surface. This particular feature is highly important in tumors less than 3 cm in which pleural involvement will upgrade the pathologic staging of the tumor to a higher level (T2).*

ADENOCARCINOMA

Microscopic and Gross Features

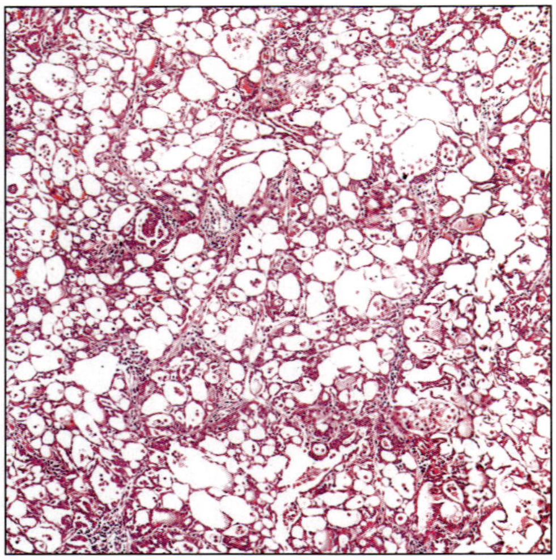

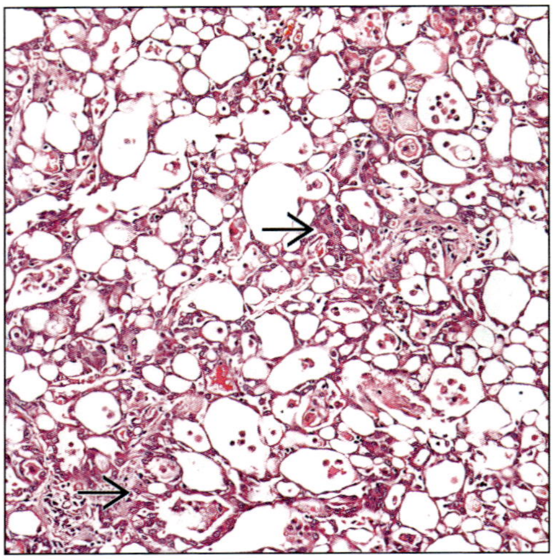

(Left) *An unusual pattern of growth in adenocarcinoma. This pattern mimics an adenomatoid tumor due to the presence of bland cystic-like areas admixed with cords of malignant cells.* ***(Right)*** *Adenomatoid-like adenocarcinoma of the lung. Note the presence of cystic-like areas admixed with more solid groups of neoplastic cells ⇒.*

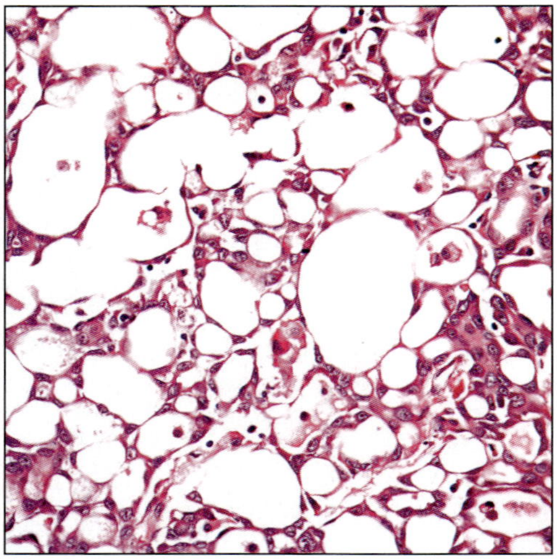

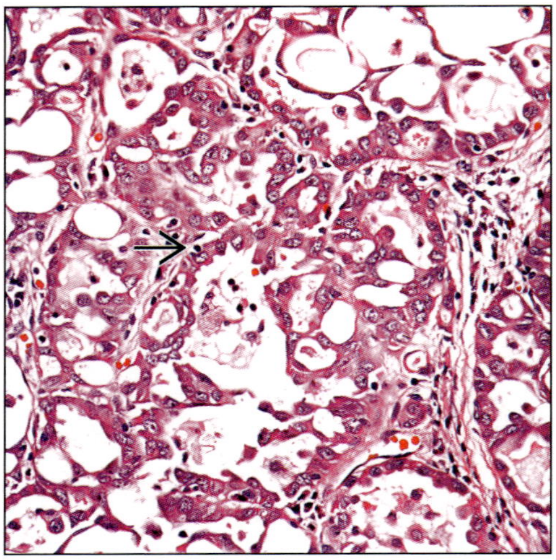

(Left) *High-power view shows an adenomatoid tumor-like adenocarcinoma. The cells have a bland appearance with absence of marked nuclear atypia and mitotic activity.* ***(Right)*** *High-power view shows an adenomatoid tumor-like adenocarcinoma. Note the presence of a more glandular component, nuclear atypia, and rare mitotic figures ⇒. These areas are more in keeping with a "garden variety" adenocarcinoma.*

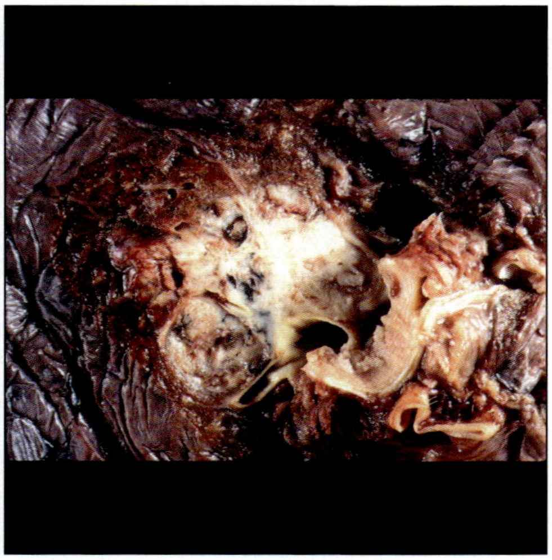

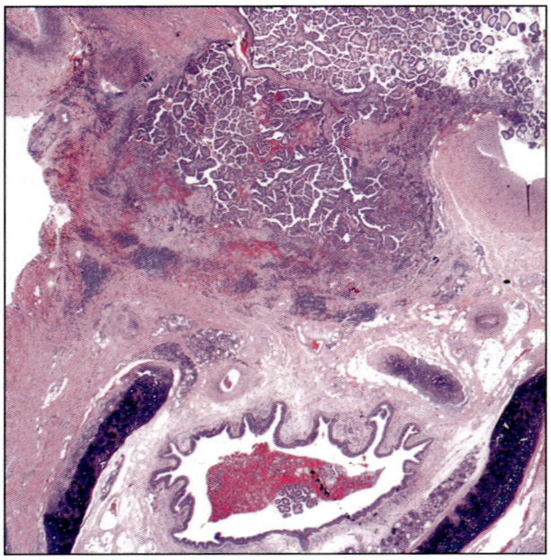

(Left) *Gross photograph shows centrally located pulmonary adenocarcinoma. The tumor is tan with irregular borders involving the airway.* ***(Right)*** *Low-power view shows a central adenocarcinoma with prominent papillary features. True papillary carcinoma of the lung should be composed of at least a 75% papillary component.*

ADENOCARCINOMA

Variant Microscopic Features

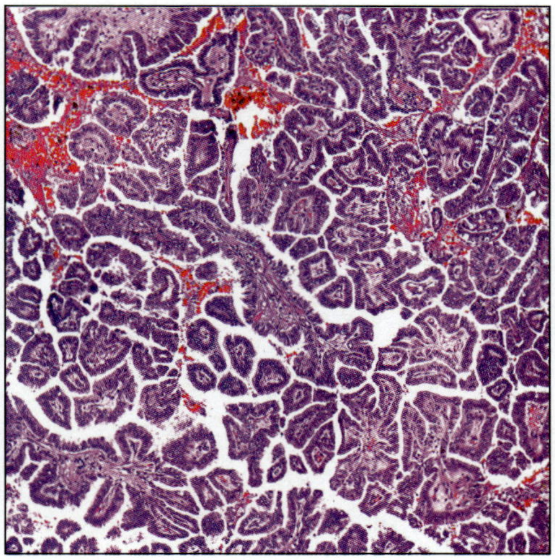

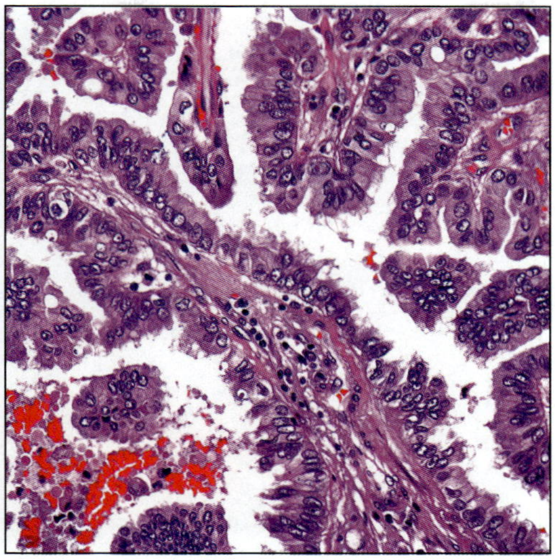

*(**Left**) True papillary carcinoma of the lung. Note the predominant papillary pattern of growth of this neoplasm. In such a tumor, one may consider the possibility of metastatic papillary neoplasms of extrathoracic origin, such as thyroid carcinoma. (**Right**) High-power view shows a true papillary carcinoma of the lung; note the presence of true papillae. The nuclear characteristics of this tumor may mimic those seen in thyroid carcinomas.*

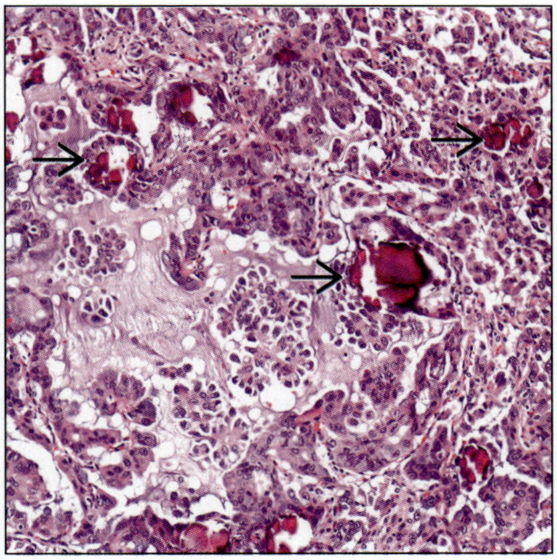

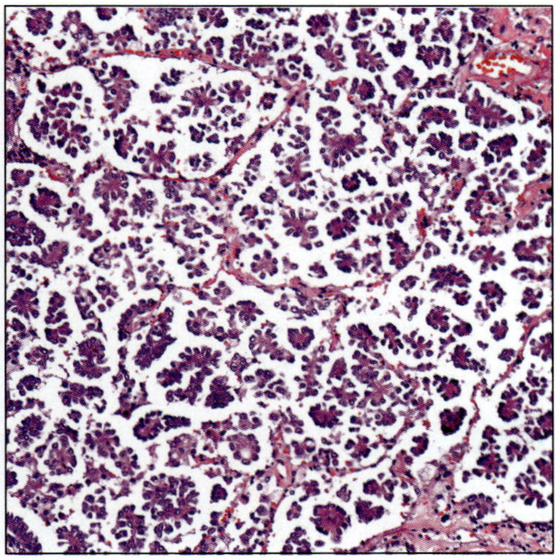

*(**Left**) High-power magnification shows a papillary carcinoma of the lung with numerous psammoma bodies → similar to those seen in papillary thyroid carcinomas. (**Right**) Micropapillary adenocarcinoma of the lung. Note the presence of the micropapillae filling the alveolar spaces, most of them without any connection to the alveolar lining.*

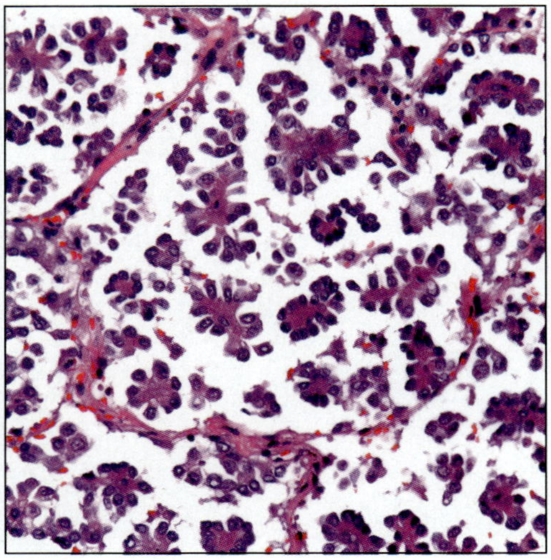

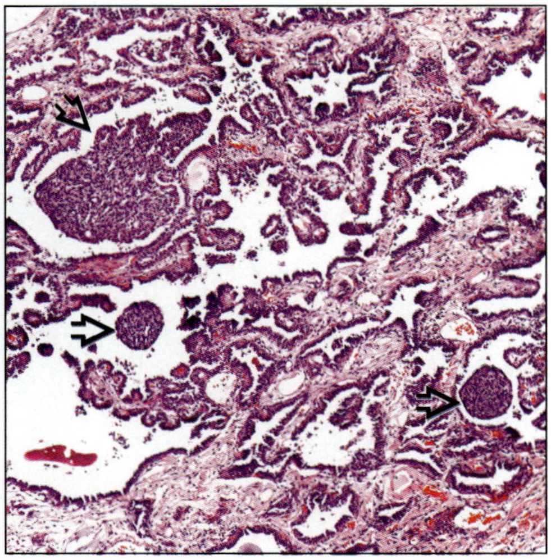

*(**Left**) High-power view shows a micropapillary adenocarcinoma of the lung. Note that the micropapillae filling the alveolar spaces are devoid of fibrovascular cord, contrary to true papillae. (**Right**) Pulmonary papillary adenocarcinoma shows the presence of a "morular" component floating in the alveolar spaces ⇨. This tumor has been designated as papillary adenocarcinoma with a morular component.*

ADENOCARCINOMA

Variant Microscopic Features

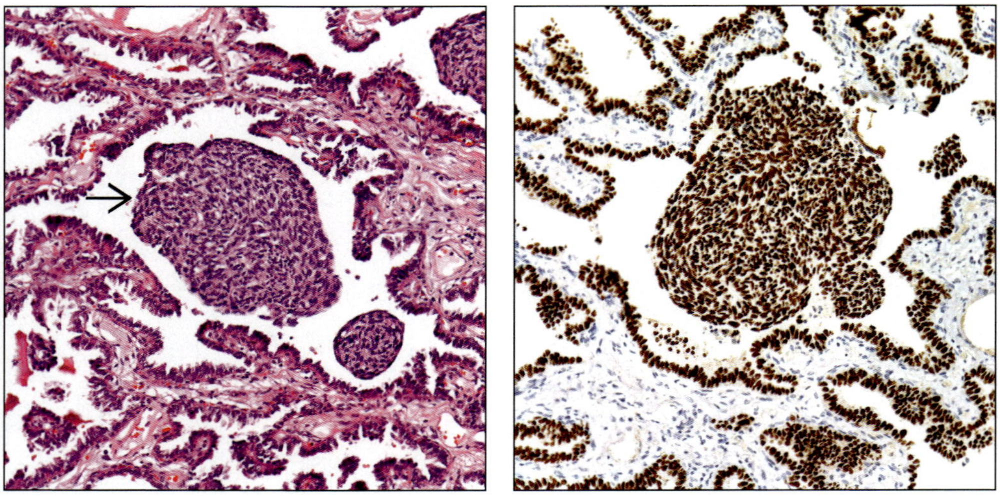

(Left) *High-magnification view shows a papillary adenocarcinoma with morular component. Note the presence of the "morules" → within the alveolar spaces, in contrast to those seen in monophasic blastomas, which are in the interstitium at the base of the glands.* ***(Right)*** *Immunohistochemical stain for TTF-1 with strong nuclear staining in the "morular" component of the tumor is shown. Note that adjacent neoplastic glands are also positive.*

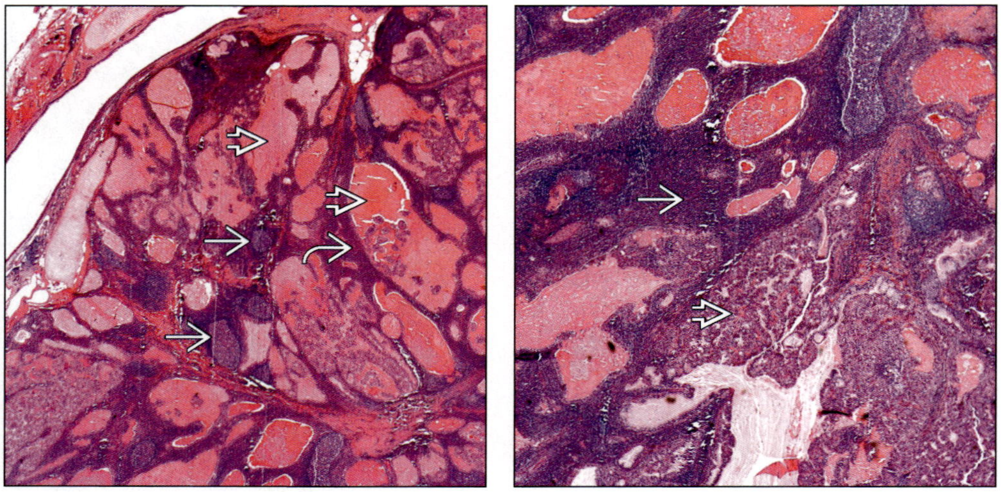

(Left) *Adenocarcinoma of the lung with a Warthin-like appearance. The tumor is centrally located and exhibits the presence of a marked inflammatory reaction →, intraluminal exudate →, and germinal centers →.* ***(Right)*** *Intermediate magnification shows the Warthin-like appearance of this pulmonary adenocarcinoma of the lung. Note the separation between the malignant component → and the inflammatory reaction →.*

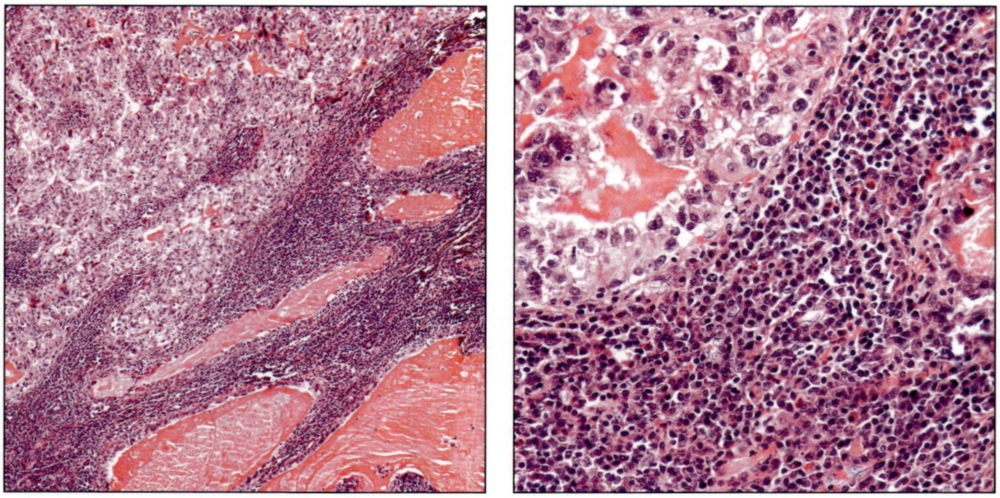

(Left) *High-power view shows a Warthin-like adenocarcinoma of the lung, in which the epithelial malignant component exhibits features more in keeping with a conventional adenocarcinoma. Note that the adjacent areas have an inflammatory exudate.* ***(Right)*** *High-power view of the neoplastic glandular elements is composed of tall columnar epithelium and nuclei displaced toward the luminal surface. An adjacent inflammatory component is present.*

Variant Microscopic Features

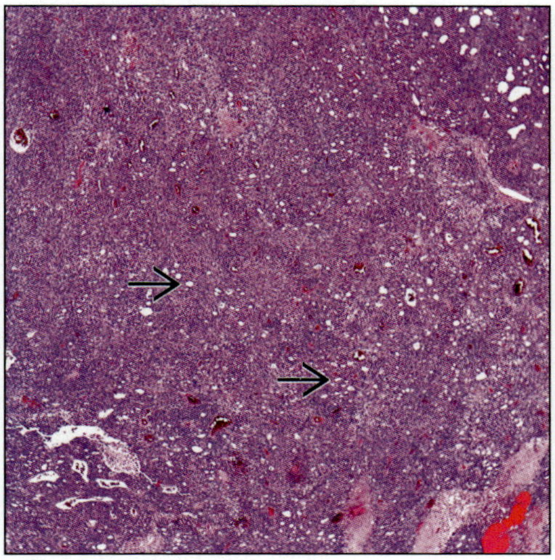

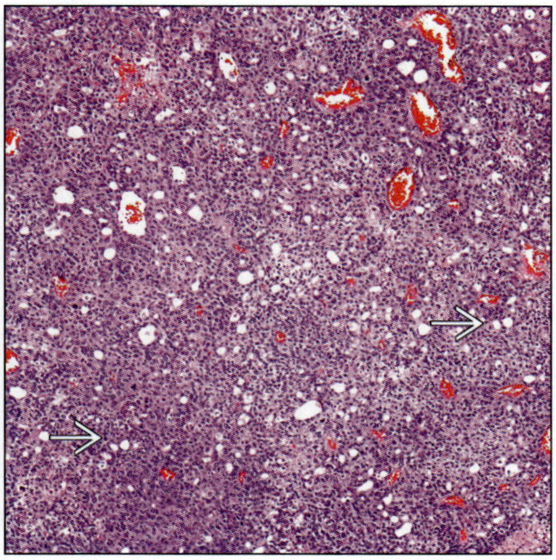

(Left) *Solid sheets of neoplastic cells of a hepatoid adenocarcinoma of the lung. The tumor is essentially composed of neoplastic cells mimicking hepatic parenchyma. Note the presence of "empty spaces" mimicking fat droplets* →. ***(Right)*** *Intermediate-power view shows a hepatoid adenocarcinoma of the lung. The sheets of neoplastic cells admixed with fat droplet-like areas* → *impart a hepatic-like look to this neoplasm.*

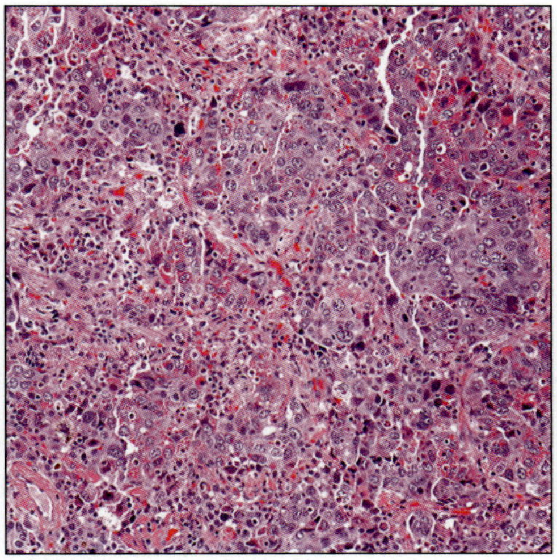

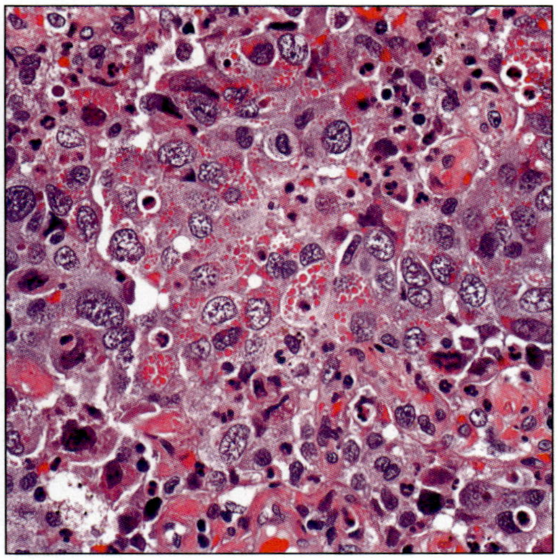

(Left) *Hepatoid adenocarcinoma of the lung with numerous intra- and extracellular hyaline globules. Still, the tumor forms glandular structures.* ***(Right)*** *High-power view shows a hepatoid adenocarcinoma of the lung, revealing neoplastic cells with moderate amounts of eosinophilic cytoplasm, round nuclei, and some cells with prominent nucleoli. Also note the presence of hyaline globules.*

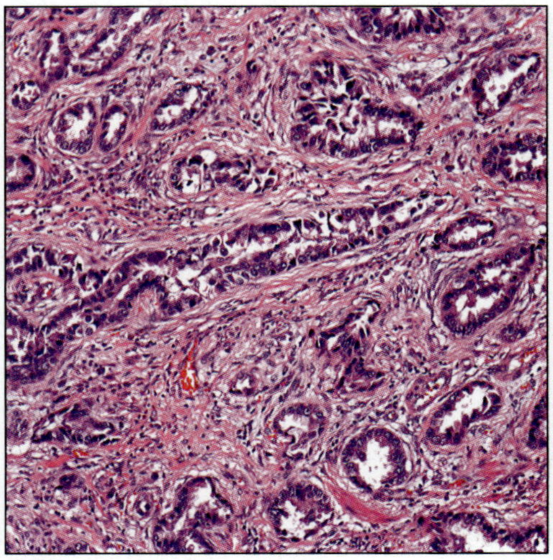

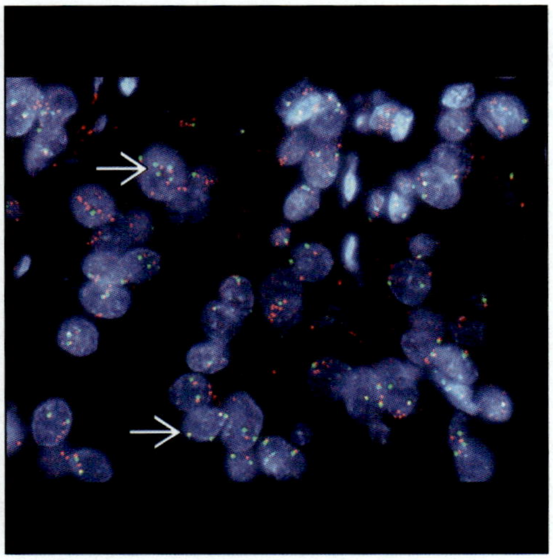

(Left) *Primary pulmonary adenocarcinoma in which FISH studies were available is shown. It is important to note that there is not a particular histopathologic growth pattern that can be correlated with mutational analysis.* ***(Right)*** *FISH shows gene amplification of the characteristic EGFR mutation in a pulmonary adenocarcinoma* →.

BRONCHIOLOALVEOLAR CELL CARCINOMA

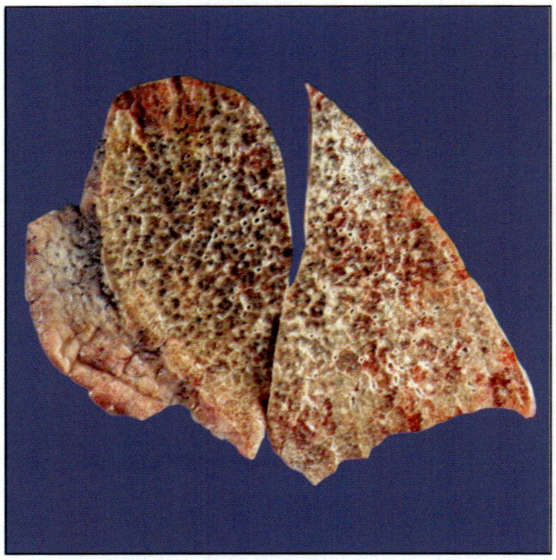

Gross photograph shows multiple small pulmonary nodules of different sizes. This represents the multinodular pattern of bronchioloalveolar cell carcinoma.

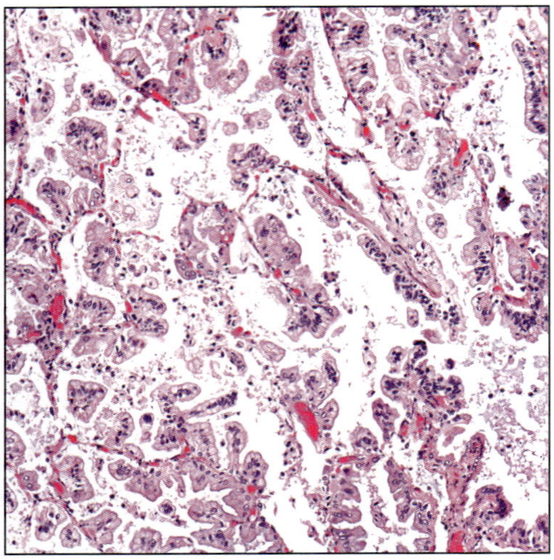

Bronchioloalveolar carcinoma shows a lepidic growth pattern. Note the absence of tumor infiltrating the interstitium. However, absence of pleural invasion must also be excluded for this diagnosis.

TERMINOLOGY

Abbreviations

- Bronchioloalveolar cell carcinoma (BAC)

Synonyms

- Adenocarcinoma in situ, adenocarcinoma with bronchioloalveolar pattern

Definitions

- Well-differentiated adenocarcinoma
- Lesion with relatively bland cytologic features that arises in periphery of lung and spreads along the walls of distal air spaces
- Subset of adenocarcinoma common and distinctive enough to warrant separation from other subtypes
- Adenocarcinoma with BAC pattern
  - No evidence of stromal, vascular, or pleural invasion
  - Essentially, current definition is similar to that of in situ adenocarcinoma

ETIOLOGY/PATHOGENESIS

Environmental Exposure

- BAC appears not to be associated with tobacco use

CLINICAL ISSUES

Epidemiology

- Incidence
  - Incidence of true BAC is not high and may represent less than 10% of all carcinomas of lung
- Age
  - Tumor can occur at any age

Presentation

- Cough
- Chest pain
- Shortness of breath
- Bronchorrhea

Treatment

- Surgical approaches
  - Wedge resection, lobectomy, or pneumonectomy

Prognosis

- As currently defined, BAC tumors of 2 cm or less are expected to do well
- In those tumors that are multifocal, prognosis may not be as good

MACROSCOPIC FEATURES

General Features

- Localized tumor mass: Usually < 3 cm in diameter
- Multinodular pattern: Extensive areas of lung parenchyma are involved in miliary fashion
- Diffuse pattern: No distinct tumor mass or nodule is present
  - Lung parenchyma appears congested, mimicking lobar pneumonia

MICROSCOPIC PATHOLOGY

Histologic Features

- Conventional type
  - Tumor cells are small and dark with hyperchromatic nuclei and scant cytoplasm
  - Tumor cells display prominent hobnail appearance and are devoid of nucleoli or mitotic figures
- Mucinous type
  - Tumor cells are tall columnar and contain abundant mucinous cytoplasm

Predominant Pattern/Injury Type

- Circumscribed
- Mucinous
- Diffuse

BRONCHIOLOALVEOLAR CELL CARCINOMA

Key Facts

Terminology
- Bronchioloalveolar cell carcinoma (BAC)
  - Adenocarcinoma with BAC pattern and no evidence of stromal, vascular, or pleural invasion
  - Essentially, current definition is that of in situ adenocarcinoma

Etiology/Pathogenesis
- BAC appears not to be associated with tobacco smoking

Macroscopic Features
- Localized tumor mass: Usually < 3 cm in diameter
- Multinodular pattern: Extensive areas of lung parenchyma are involved in miliary fashion
- Diffuse pattern: No distinct tumor mass or nodule is present
  - Lung parenchyma appears congested, mimicking pneumonia

Top Differential Diagnoses
- Atypical adenomatous hyperplasia (AAH)
  - Tumor nodule of < 0.5 cm in greatest dimension
- Metastatic adenocarcinoma
  - Good clinical history and physical examination
  - Immunohistochemical studies may be helpful in determining primary site
- Invasive adenocarcinoma
  - By definition, BAC is a tumor with no lymphatic, pleural, or interstitial invasion
  - Complete examination of tumor is required in order to rule out invasion
  - Presence of lymph node involvement rules out diagnosis of BAC

Immunohistochemistry

Antibody	Reactivity	Staining Pattern	Comment
KERATIN-LMW	Positive	Cytoplasmic	
CEA-M	Positive	Cytoplasmic	Helpful in both mucinous and nonmucinous tumors
CK7	Positive	Cytoplasmic	
TTF-1	Positive	Nuclear	In some mucinous cases, stain may be negative
CK20	Negative		May show focal positive staining in tumor cells in some cases
CDX-2	Negative		May show focal positive staining in tumor cells in some mucinous tumors
GCDFP-15	Negative		

DIFFERENTIAL DIAGNOSIS

Atypical Adenomatous Hyperplasia (AAH)
- Tumor nodule < 0.5 cm in greatest dimension
- Histology very similar to BAC

Metastatic Adenocarcinoma
- Past or present history of adenocarcinoma outside of thoracic cavity
- Immunohistochemical studies may be helpful in determining primary site

Pulmonary Invasive Adenocarcinoma
- BAC lacks presence of vascular, lymphatic, pleural, or interstitial involvement by tumor cells

DIAGNOSTIC CHECKLIST

Clinically Relevant Pathologic Features
- Noninvasive pattern
- Diagnosis of BAC cannot be achieved in biopsy specimens
- Histopathological examination of entire tumor is required for diagnosis of BAC
- Lymph node sampling is required to properly rule out metastatic disease

Pathologic Interpretation Pearls
- Extensive pools of mucin
- Alveolar wall lined by neoplastic cells
- Absence of pleural invasion
- Absence of interstitial invasion

SELECTED REFERENCES

1. Hajdu SI: The story of bronchioloalveolar carcinoma. Ann Clin Lab Sci. 35(3):336-8, 2005
2. Travis WD et al: Tumours of the lung, pleura, thymus, and heart. Pathology & Genetics: World Health Organization (WHO). Lyon: IARC Press. 38, 2004
3. Sidhu GS et al: The concept of bronchioloalveolar cell adenocarcinoma: redefinition, a critique of the 1999 WHO classification, and an ultrastructural analysis of 155 cases. Int J Surg Pathol. 11(2):89-99, 2003
4. Colby TV et al: Tumors of the lower respiratory tract. Atlas of Tumor Pathology: Armed Forces Institute of Pathology (AFIP). (13):203, 1995
5. Daly RC et al: Bronchoalveolar carcinoma: factors affecting survival. Ann Thorac Surg. 51(3):368-76; discussion 376-7, 1991
6. Manning JT Jr et al: Bronchioloalveolar carcinoma: The significance of two histopathologic types. Cancer. 54(3):525-34, 1984
7. Carter D et al: Tumors of the lower respiratory tract. Armed Forces Institute of Pathology (AFIP). (17):127, 1980
8. Liebow AA: Bronchiolo-alveolar carcinoma. Adv Intern Med. 10:329-58, 1960

BRONCHIOLOALVEOLAR CELL CARCINOMA

Microscopic Features

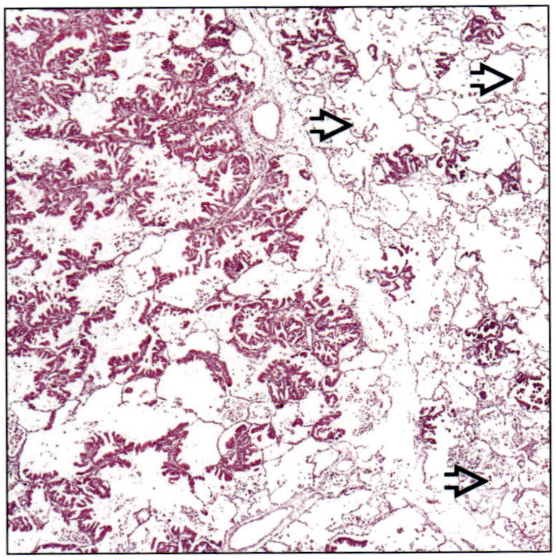

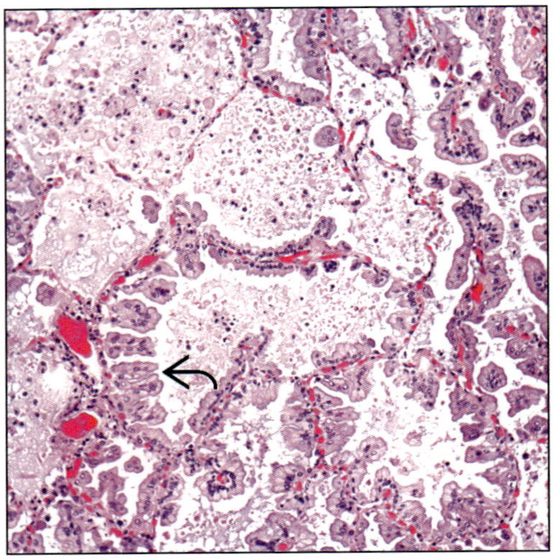

(Left) *Predominantly alveolar pattern in bronchioloalveolar cell carcinoma is shown, in which malignant cells line the alveolar walls. Also note the presence of areas of normal lung parenchyma* ⇨. ***(Right)*** *Bronchioloalveolar cell carcinoma shows a classical pattern of lepidic growth. Note the presence of neoplastic cells lining the alveolar wall* ⇨. *Still, one is able to follow the "normal" architecture of the lung parenchyma.*

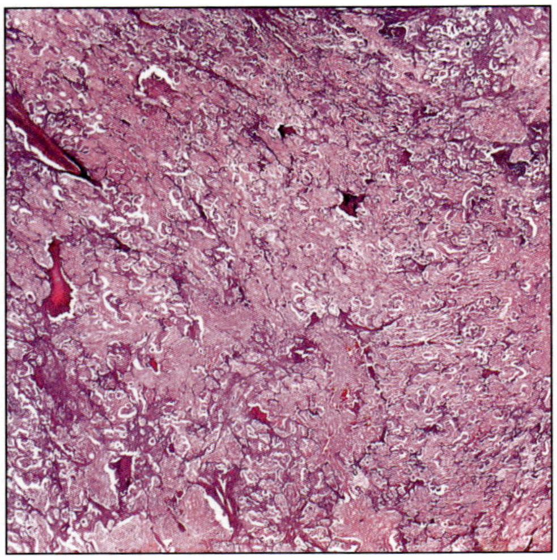

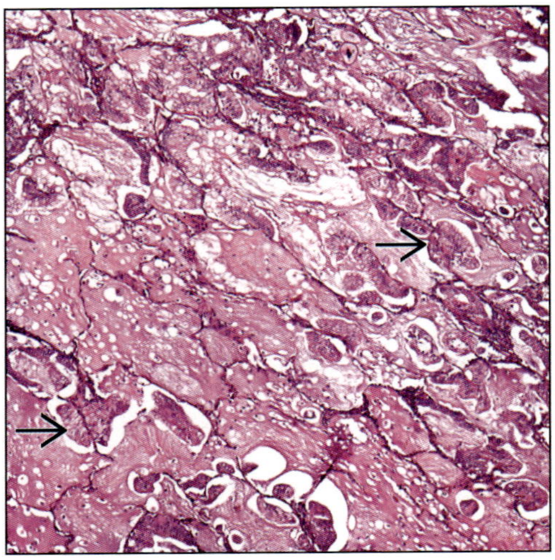

(Left) *Bronchioloalveolar cell carcinoma shows extensive areas of lung parenchyma replaced with proteinaceous fluid filling the alveolar spaces. This pattern represents the so-called pneumonic pattern of bronchioloalveolar cell carcinoma.* ***(Right)*** *Pneumonic pattern of bronchioloalveolar cell carcinoma in which the alveoli are filled with edematous fluid is shown here with only focal areas of alveoli replaced by mucinous epithelium* →.

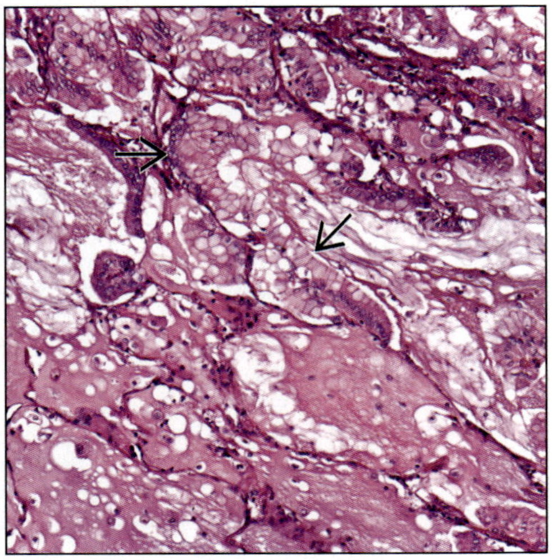

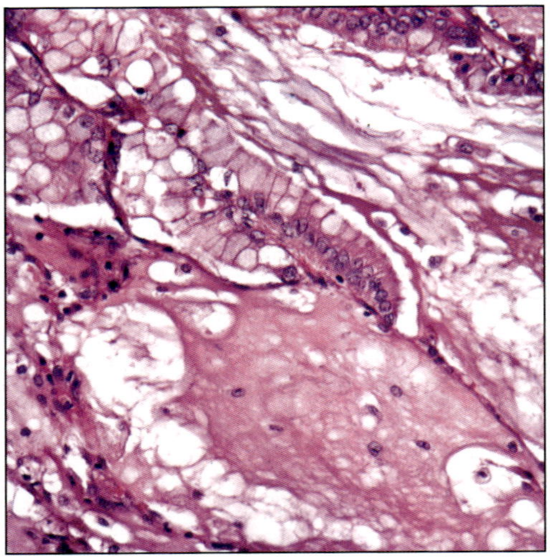

(Left) *Closer view shows the pneumonic variant of bronchioloalveolar cell carcinoma. Note the presence of mucinous epithelium replacing the alveolar lining* →. ***(Right)*** *Mucinous type of epithelium replacing the alveolar lining. The mucinous epithelium is composed of columnar cells with nuclei displaced toward the base. No cellular atypia or mitotic activity is present.*

BRONCHIOLOALVEOLAR CELL CARCINOMA

Microscopic Features

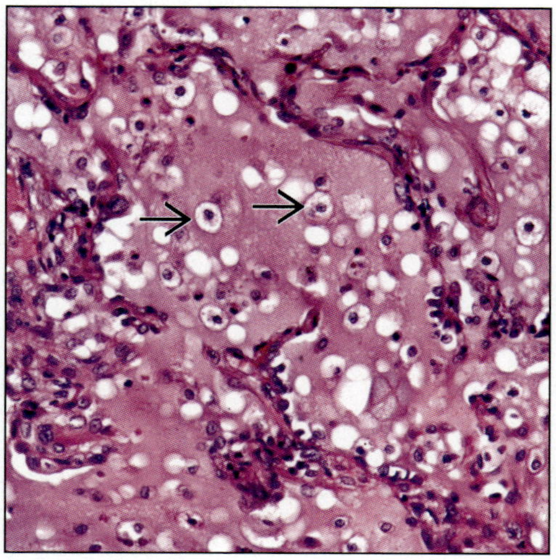

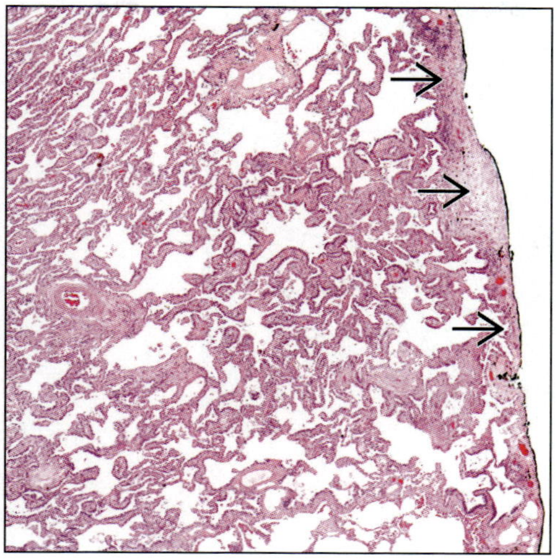

(Left) *Adjacent areas of normal lung parenchyma in a pneumonic type of bronchioloalveolar cell carcinoma. The alveoli are filled with fluid and numerous floating macrophages →.* ***(Right)*** *Nodular (nonmucinous) pattern of bronchioloalveolar cell carcinoma is shown. The tumor is in a subpleural location without pleural → or interstitial involvement.*

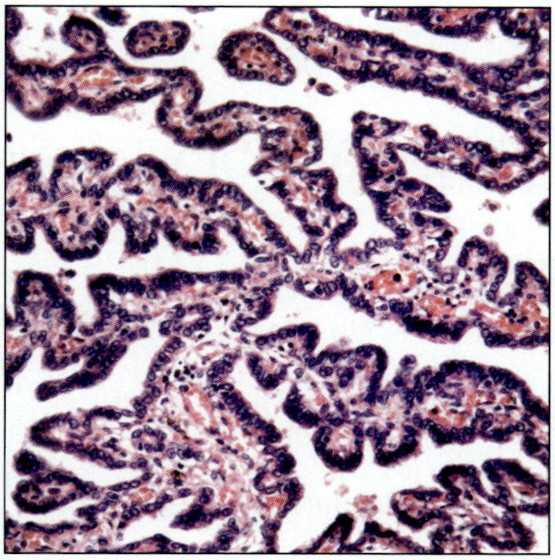

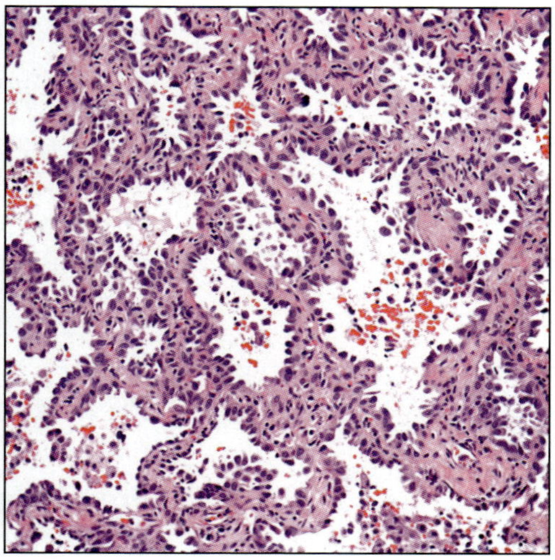

(Left) *Bronchioloalveolar cell carcinoma is seen composed of cellular proliferation lining the alveolar walls. The cells are low to flat cuboidal with pyknotic nuclei and an absence of mitotic activity or nuclear atypia. Note the lack of interstitial involvement.* ***(Right)*** *Bronchioloalveolar cell carcinoma in which the alveolar walls are lined by cells displaying more nuclear atypia. However, the tumor cells do not show mitotic activity.*

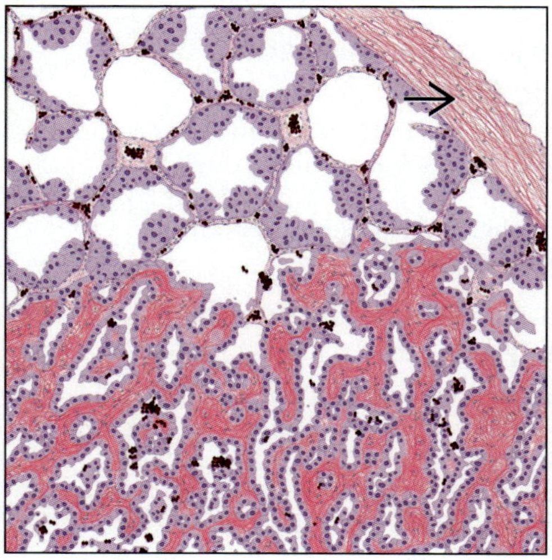

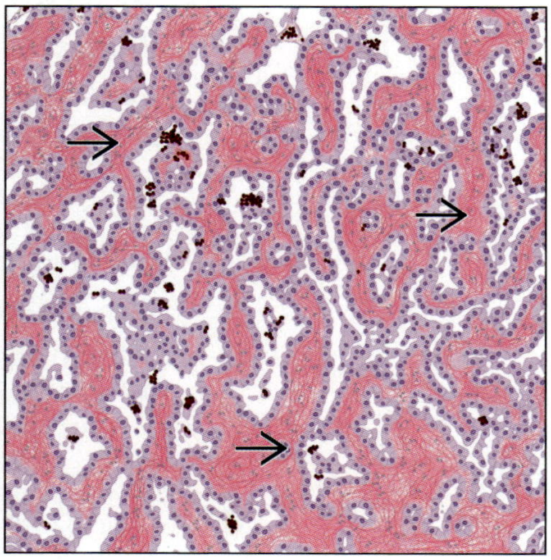

(Left) *Illustration of a bronchioloalveolar cell carcinoma highlights the absence of pleural involvement by the tumor →. This is an important criterion for the diagnosis of BAC.* ***(Right)*** *Illustration of bronchioloalveolar cell carcinoma demonstrates bronchioloalveolar proliferation with an absence of tumor cells in the interstitium →. This is another important feature in the current criteria for the diagnosis of BAC.*

MUCINOUS ("COLLOID") CARCINOMA

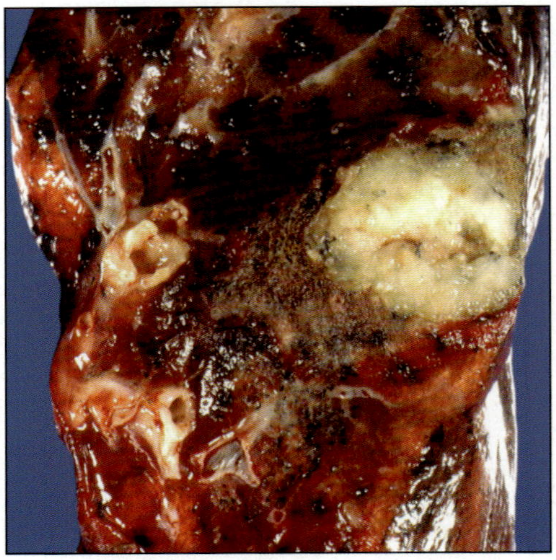

Gross photograph of mucinous carcinoma shows a well-defined subpleural tumor with a mucoid consistency. No evidence of necrosis or hemorrhage is present.

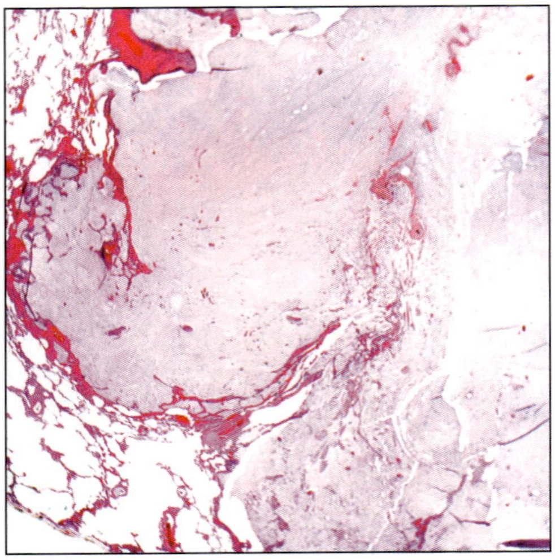

Lung parenchyma is replaced by extensive areas of mucoid material that destroy alveolar walls. This presentation may mimic a benign mucinous cyst.

TERMINOLOGY

Synonyms

- Mucinous cystadenoma, mucinous cystic tumor, multilocular cystic carcinoma, mucinous cystic tumor of borderline malignancy

Definitions

- Epithelial neoplasm with extensive mucin production

CLINICAL ISSUES

Epidemiology

- Incidence
  - Pure colloid carcinomas of the lung are rare
- Age
  - Colloid carcinomas are more common in adult patients
- Gender
  - No gender predilection

Presentation

- Cough
- Chest pain
- Shortness of breath
- Asymptomatic

Treatment

- Surgical approaches
  - Lobectomy

Prognosis

- Depends on staging at time of diagnosis

MACROSCOPIC FEATURES

General Features

- Well-defined tumor mass
- Mucoid consistency
- Cystic changes may be present

Size

- Varies from 1 to > 10 cm

MICROSCOPIC PATHOLOGY

Histologic Features

- Extensive areas of mucin deposition
- Alveolar wall lined with mucinous epithelium
- Single cells or clusters of cells are seen floating in the mucin

Predominant Pattern/Injury Type

- Mucinous

Predominant Cell/Compartment Type

- Epithelial

DIFFERENTIAL DIAGNOSIS

Metastatic Mucinous Carcinoma of Extrathoracic Origin

- Clinical history of or clinical evaluation for colonic, ovarian, breast, or urachal carcinoma will be important
- Immunohistochemical studies important in determining primary site

Bronchioloalveolar Carcinoma (BAC), Mucinous Variant

- In BAC, lepidic growth pattern is characteristic feature in which alveolar lining is substituted by mucinous type of epithelium
- BAC commonly will diffusely involve the entire lung or extensive areas of it
- Immunohistochemical features of BAC and colloid carcinoma may be similar

MUCINOUS ("COLLOID") CARCINOMA

Key Facts

Terminology
- Mucinous cystadenoma, mucinous cystic tumor, multilocular cystic carcinoma, mucinous cystic tumor of borderline malignancy

Macroscopic Features
- Well-defined tumor mass with mucoid consistency, solid &/or cystic
- Varies from 1 to > 10 cm

Microscopic Pathology
- Extensive areas of mucinous deposition
- Alveolar wall lined with mucinous epithelium
- Single cells or clusters of cells embedded in mucin

Ancillary Tests
- TTF-1 nuclear positivity (may be negative in some cases)
- CK7 cytoplasmic positivity
- CK20 negative (may be positive in some cases)
- CDX2 negative (may be positive in some cases)

Top Differential Diagnoses
- Metastatic mucinous carcinoma of extrathoracic origin
  - Clinical history of or clinical evaluation for colonic, ovarian, breast, or urachal carcinoma will be important
  - Immunohistochemical studies important in determining primary site

Diagnostic Checklist
- Extensive mucin
- Alveolar wall lined with mucinous epithelium

Immunohistochemistry

Antibody	Reactivity	Staining Pattern	Comment
TTF-1	Positive	Nuclear	May be negative in many cases
CK7	Positive	Cytoplasmic	Staining may be as strong as in solid adenocarcinomas
CEA-M	Positive	Cytoplasmic	
CK-PAN	Positive	Cytoplasmic	
CK20	Negative		May be positive in a fair number of cases
CDX-2	Negative		May be positive in some colloid carcinomas
GCDFP-15	Negative		
PR	Negative		

Histochemical Features of Colloid Carcinoma

Histochemical Stain	Result	Comment
Mucicarmine	Strongly positive	In intracellular as well as extracellular areas
D-PAS	Positive	Also in intracellular and extracellular areas
PAS	Negative	

DIAGNOSTIC CHECKLIST

Clinically Relevant Pathologic Features
- Gross appearance

Pathologic Interpretation Pearls
- Extensive mucin
- Alveolar wall lined with mucinous epithelium

GRADING

Colloid Carcinoma
- Considered low-grade malignant neoplasm
- Behavior determined by pathological staging at time of diagnosis

SELECTED REFERENCES

1. Bacha D et al: A pulmonary mucinous cystic tumour of borderline malignancy. Pathologica. 100(3):189-91, 2008
2. Maeda R et al: Primary pulmonary mucinous (colloid) adenocarcinoma. Gen Thorac Cardiovasc Surg. 56(4):195-8, 2008
3. Moran CA: Pulmonary adenocarcinoma: the expanding spectrum of histologic variants. Arch Pathol Lab Med. 130(7):958-62, 2006
4. Türüt H et al: Primary pulmonary mucinous adenocarcinoma in a 15-year-old boy. Eur J Cardiothorac Surg. 29(5):851-3, 2006
5. Brownlee NA et al: Mucinous (colloid) adenocarcinoma of the lung. Arch Pathol Lab Med. 129(1):121-2, 2005
6. Okimasa S et al: Mucinous (colloid) adenocarcinoma. Jpn J Thorac Cardiovasc Surg. 53(6):305-8, 2005
7. Jayaram G et al: Mucinous carcinoma (colloid carcinoma) of the lung diagnosed by fine needle aspiration cytology: a case report. Malays J Pathol. 25(1):63-8, 2003
8. Moran CA. Mucin-rich tumors of the lung. Adv Anat Pathol. 2(5):299-305, 1995
9. Moran CA et al: Mucinous (so-called colloid) carcinomas of lung. Mod Pathol. 5(6):634-8, 1992
10. Graeme-Cook F et al: Pulmonary mucinous cystic tumors of borderline malignancy. Hum Pathol. 22(2):185-90, 1991

MUCINOUS ("COLLOID") CARCINOMA

Microscopic Features

*(**Left**) In this lung parenchyma replaced by mucoid material, note the cyst-like appearance of the tumor destroying normal alveolar parenchyma. This feature can be incorrectly assumed to indicate a benign cystadenoma. (**Right**) Extensive mucoid material destroying normal alveolated parenchyma. Note that the alveolar wall is being replaced by mucinous epithelium ⇨.*

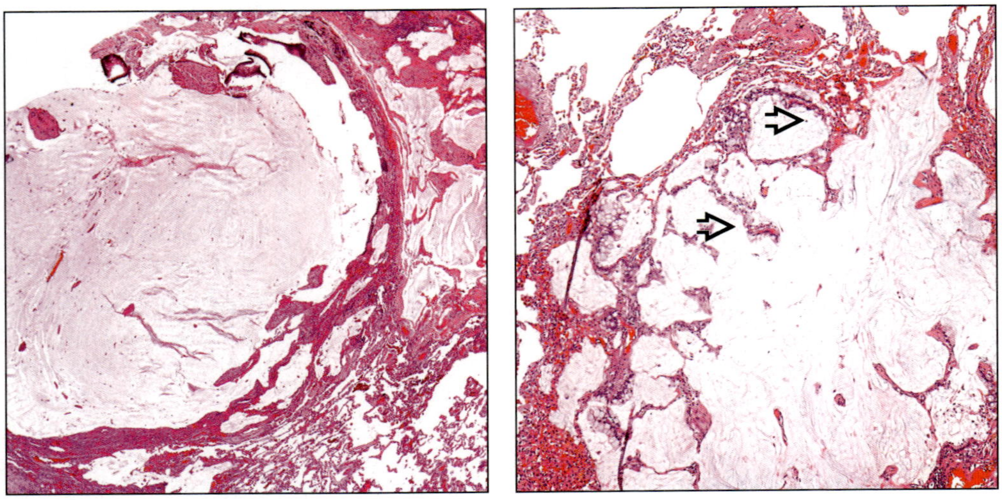

*(**Left**) Alveolated parenchyma is destroyed by large amounts of mucoid material. Note the focal areas in which the alveolar walls remain intact; they are lined by mucinous epithelium ⇨. (**Right**) Several areas in which the alveolar wall is being replaced by a mucinous type of epithelium ↷ are shown. However, one important feature is the breakdown of alveolar walls with partial replacement by mucinous epithelium.*

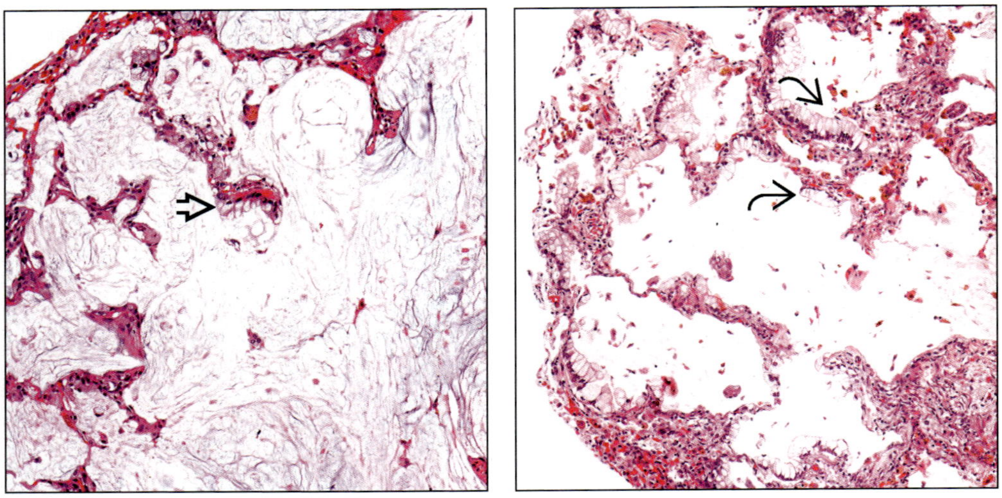

*(**Left**) Cystic areas are seen in which there is an obvious mucinous epithelial lining. In addition, there are adjacent areas of fibrosis with inflammatory changes. (**Right**) Closer view shows the mucinous type of epithelium of a cystic structure containing large amounts of mucinous material. In addition, there are many pigmented macrophages ↷, whose appearance contrasts with that of the mucinous cells.*

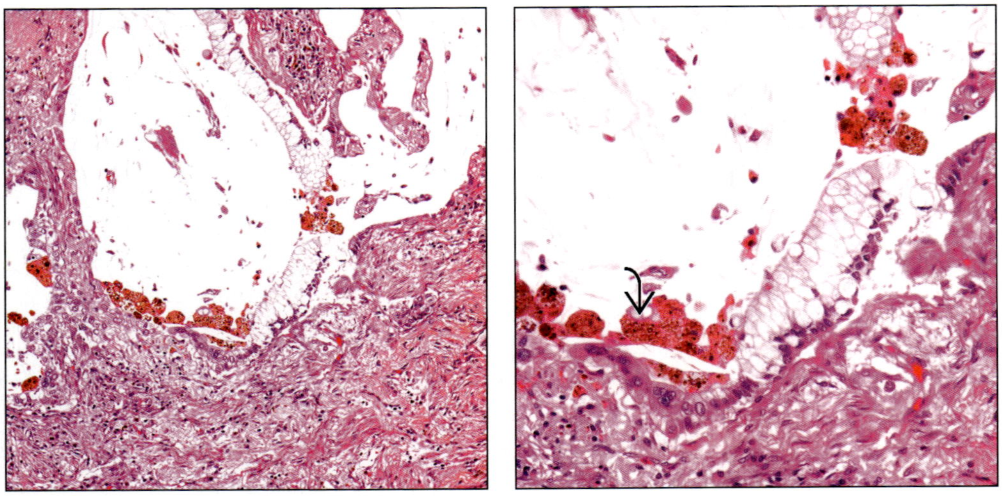

MUCINOUS ("COLLOID") CARCINOMA

Microscopic Features

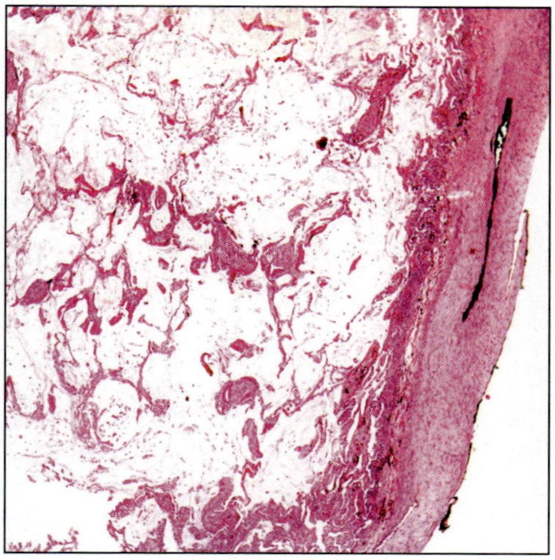

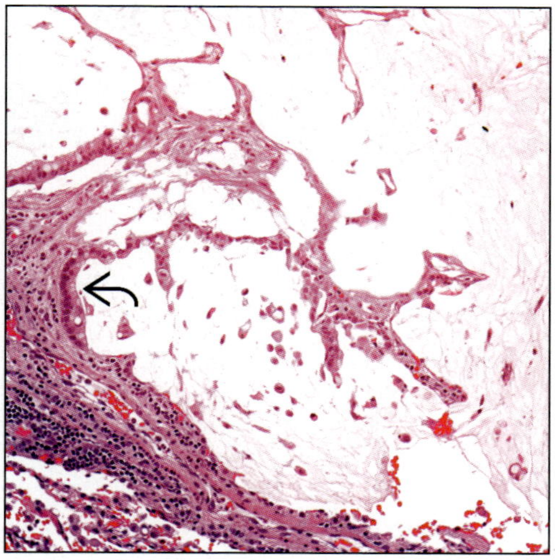

(Left) *Colloid carcinoma in subpleural location. The pleura appears to be thickened and inflamed. Colloid carcinomas rarely show pleural involvement.* ***(Right)*** *Colloid carcinoma of the lung shows extensive mucoid material with only focal areas in which the alveolar wall is lined by mucinous-secreting epithelium ↶. This feature may be very subtle.*

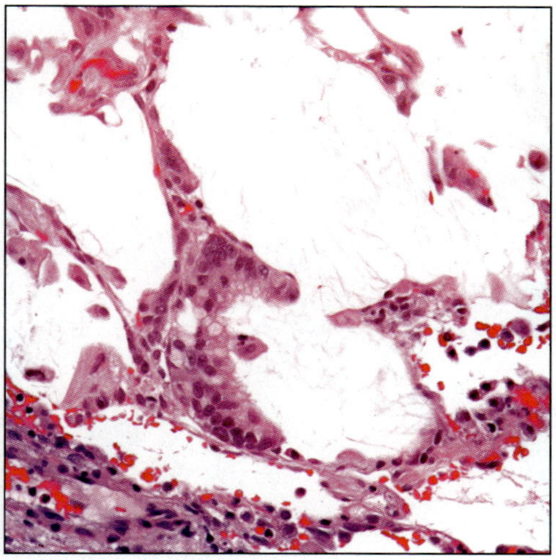

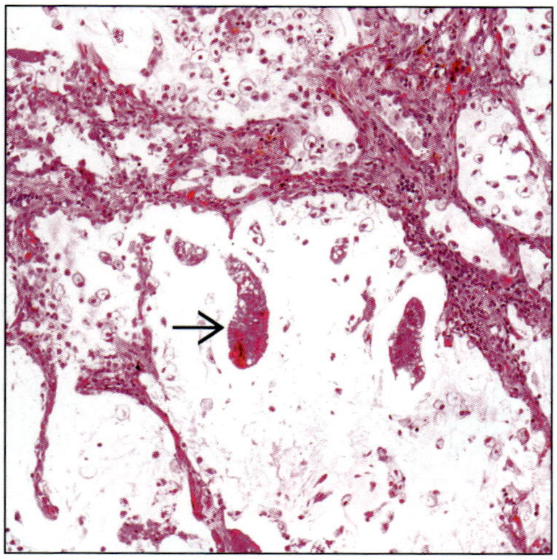

(Left) *High-power view shows the mucinous epithelium lining the alveolar wall. There is loss of polarization with nuclear atypia. However, mitotic activity is not present.* ***(Right)*** *Extensive pools of mucin are seen with only a focus containing a detached fragment of mucinous epithelium →. The remaining portion of the alveolated parenchyma appears inflamed.*

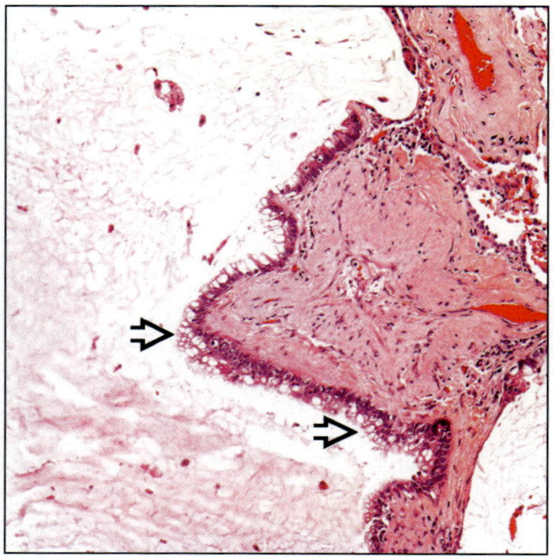

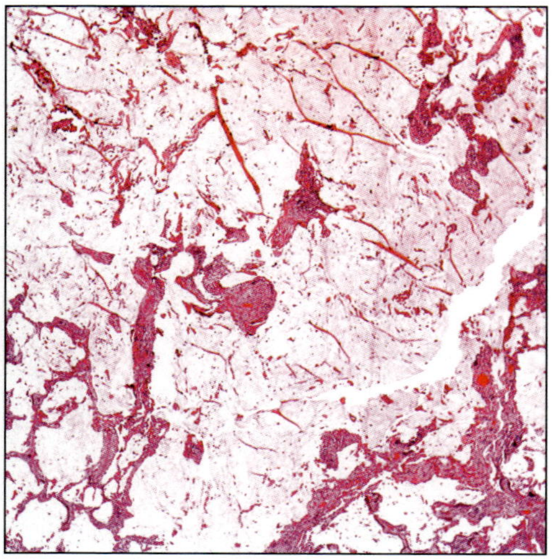

(Left) *A predominantly cystic neoplasm is seen in which the walls of the cysts are lined by a mucinous type of epithelium ⇒. The walls of this cyst are fibrotic and inflamed.* ***(Right)*** *Extensive areas of mucin deposition give the false impression of a benign obstructive process. However, the presence of extensive areas of mucinous material should raise the suspicion of a colloid carcinoma.*

MUCINOUS ("COLLOID") CARCINOMA

Microscopic Features

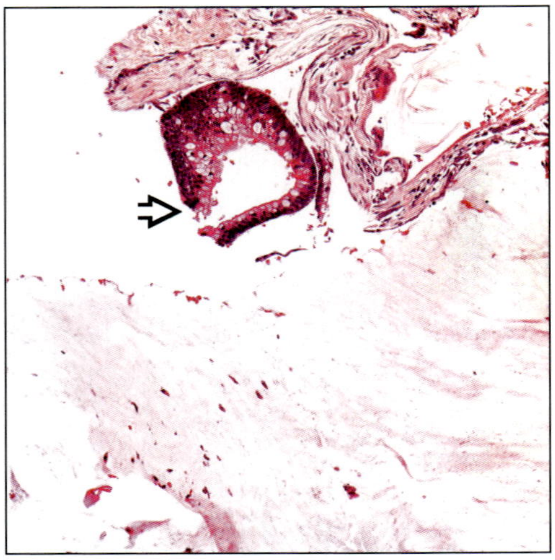
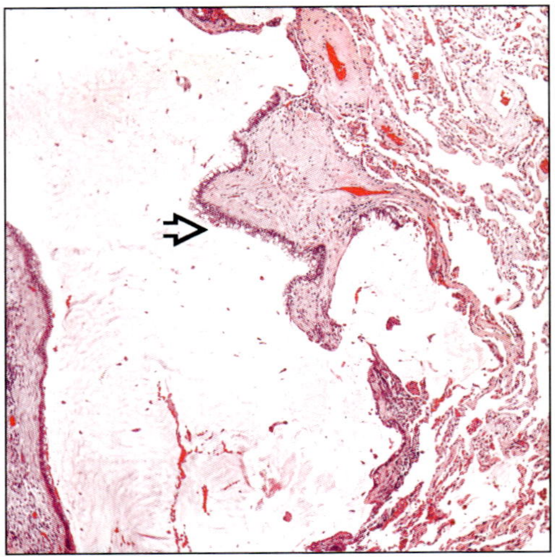

(Left) *Hematoxylin & eosin shows only a focus of mucinous type of epithelium ⇨. Extensive mucinous material is also present. The appearance may mimic a metastasis from gastrointestinal origin.* ***(Right)*** *Hematoxylin & eosin shows a cystic tumor with normal-appearing adjacent lung parenchyma. This appearance may give a false impression of bronchiectasis; however, note the presence of the mucinous type of epithelium ⇨.*

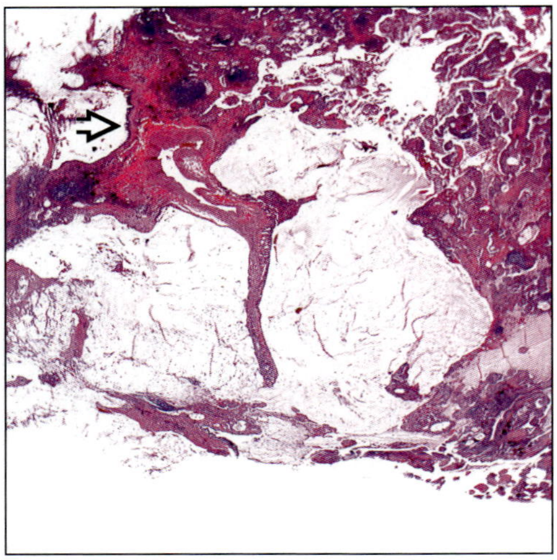
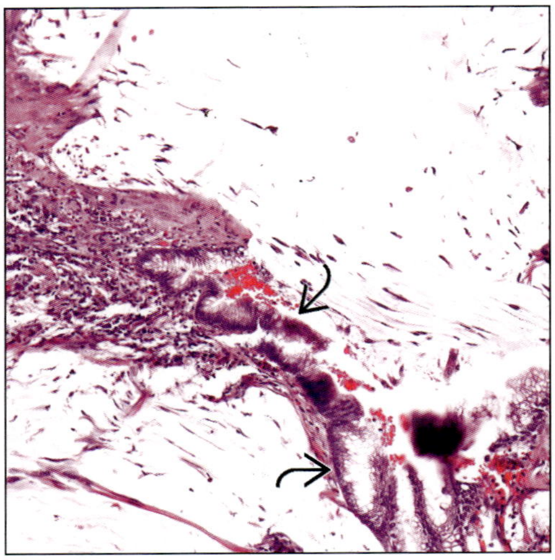

(Left) *Hematoxylin & eosin shows colloid carcinoma that is predominantly cystic, not the presence of cystic structures with extensive mucinous deposition. Note the presence of mucinous type of epithelium in one of the upper cysts ⇨.* ***(Right)*** *Hematoxylin & eosin shows extensive mucinous component with areas with prominent mucinous epithelium ↷. This feature may be found only focally in these tumors.*

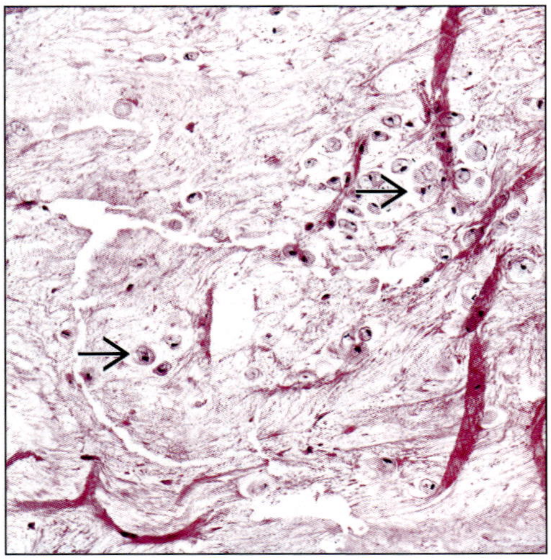
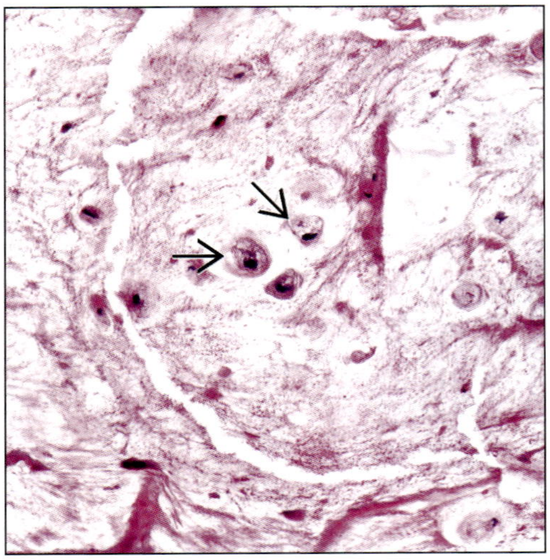

(Left) *Hematoxylin & eosin shows only extensive mucinous deposition. However, one can still see the presence of single neoplastic cells →.* ***(Right)*** *Hematoxylin & eosin shows a closer view of single neoplastic cells floating in pools of mucin →. This feature alone may also be seen in cases of signet ring cell carcinomas of the lung or in metastatic mucinous carcinomas from extrathoracic origin.*

MUCINOUS ("COLLOID") CARCINOMA

Microscopic Features

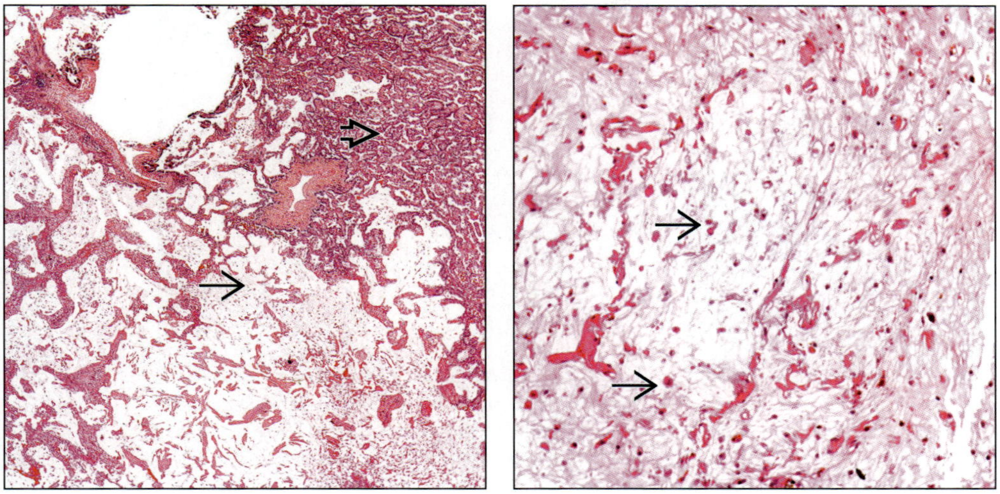

(Left) *Hematoxylin & eosin shows focal transitional areas of colloid carcinoma → with more conventional areas of solid adenocarcinoma ⇨. This feature is seen in only a minority of cases of colloid carcinomas.* ***(Right)*** *Hematoxylin & eosin shows extensive areas of mucoid material with many mucinophages →. No neoplastic cells are present in this area. This feature may be misinterpreted as a pneumonic process.*

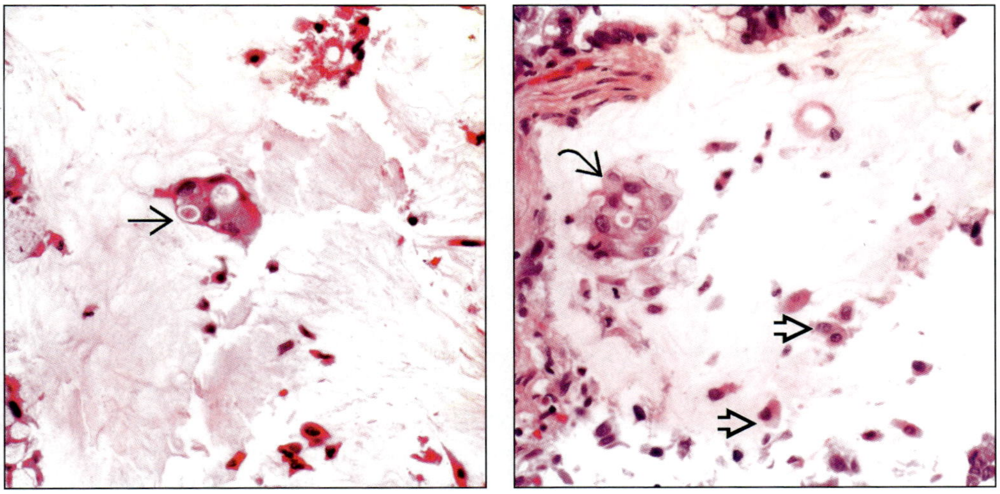

(Left) *Hematoxylin & eosin shows a single cluster of neoplastic cells → floating in extensive areas of mucin. In some cases, this is a common occurrence.* ***(Right)*** *Hematoxylin & eosin shows a focus of neoplastic cells ↷ in association with many mucinophages ⇨. In cases in which one is not sure of the epithelial nature of the cellular proliferation, the use of immunohistochemical studies is helpful.*

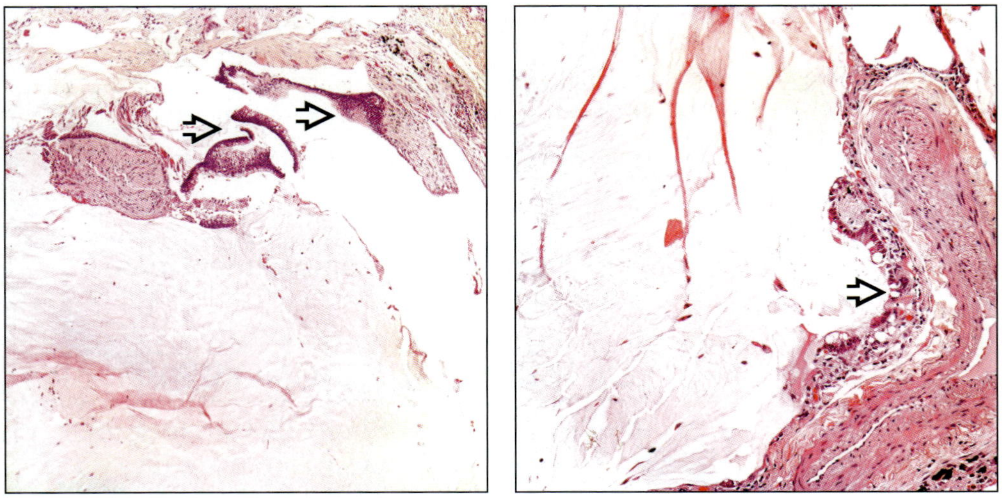

(Left) *Hematoxylin & eosin shows a predominantly cystic tumor with extensive areas of mucin and only a focal area of the mucinous type of epithelium ⇨. This feature has also been misinterpreted as a mucinous cystadenoma.* ***(Right)*** *Hematoxylin & eosin shows a predominantly cystic tumor in which only a focal area of a cystic wall is lined by mucinous type of epithelium ⇨. This feature is the one that has been used to also call these tumors "cystic mucinous tumors."*

SIGNET RING CELL CARCINOMA

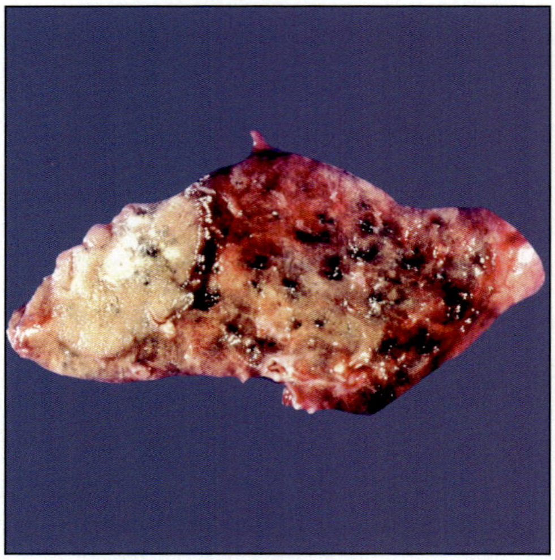

Gross photograph shows a signet ring cell carcinoma. The mass is well defined but not encapsulated. The surface is tan and fairly homogeneous.

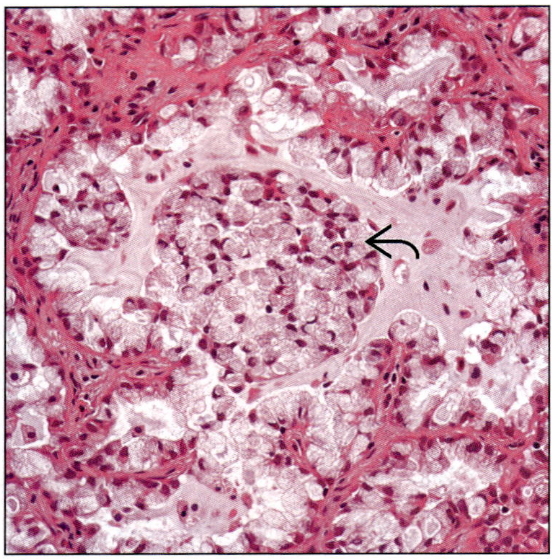

Signet ring cell carcinoma of the lung shows a classical acinar growth pattern with numerous malignant cells ➔ floating in a mucoid material.

TERMINOLOGY

Synonyms

- Adenocarcinoma with signet ring cells

Definitions

- Non-small cell carcinoma with signet ring cells similar to those described in gastrointestinal tract

ETIOLOGY/PATHOGENESIS

Etiology

- Signet ring cell carcinoma appears to be closely related to bronchial cell-type adenocarcinoma
- Bronchial glands may be the site of origin for these tumors

CLINICAL ISSUES

Epidemiology

- Incidence
  - Primary signet ring cell carcinomas of lung are rare
  - There is no definitive data on the epidemiology of this tumor
- Age
  - Individuals between 30-70 years old
  - Like conventional adenocarcinomas, signet ring cell carcinomas are more common in 6th and 7th decades of life
- Gender
  - No gender predilection

Site

- No apparent predilection for any side or any lung segment

Presentation

- Chest pain
- Shortness of breath
- Cough
- Weight loss

Treatment

- Surgical approaches
  - Lobectomy
- Adjuvant therapy
  - Chemotherapy and radiation therapy depending on clinical and pathological staging

Prognosis

- Aggressive behavior

MACROSCOPIC FEATURES

General Features

- 1 to > 5 cm in greatest dimension
- May have central or peripheral location
- Soft consistency, light tan, ± hemorrhage &/or necrosis

MICROSCOPIC PATHOLOGY

Histologic Features

- Tumor should be at least 75% signet cell component

Predominant Pattern/Injury Type

- Acinar
- Diffuse

Predominant Cell/Compartment Type

- Epithelial

DIFFERENTIAL DIAGNOSIS

Metastatic Signet Ring Cell Carcinoma

- Gastrointestinal, breast, and ovarian origin
  - Use of immunohistochemical stains is highly important in determining primary site

SIGNET RING CELL CARCINOMA

Key Facts

Terminology
- Synonym: Adenocarcinoma with signet ring cells
- Definition
  - Non-small cell carcinoma with signet ring cells similar to those described in gastrointestinal tract

Clinical Issues
- Symptoms
  - Chest pain
  - Shortness of breath
  - Weight loss
  - Cough
- Treatment
  - Lobectomy
  - Chemotherapy &/or radiation depending on clinical setting
- Prognosis
  - Aggressive behavior

Macroscopic Features
- 1 to > 5 cm in greatest dimension
- May have central or peripheral location

Microscopic Pathology
- Tumor should be at least 75% signet cell component
- Predominant pattern/injury type
  - Acinar
  - Diffuse

Top Differential Diagnoses
- Metastatic signet ring cell carcinoma
  - Gastrointestinal, breast, and ovarian origin

Immunohistochemistry

Antibody	Reactivity	Staining Pattern	Comment
CK8/18/CAM5.2	Positive	Cytoplasmic	Strong reaction in majority of cases
CK7	Positive	Cytoplasmic	Strong reaction in majority of cases
TTF-1	Positive	Nuclear	May be focal in some cases
CEA-M	Positive	Cytoplasmic	Strong reaction in majority of cases
CD15	Positive	Cytoplasmic	May show only focal positivity
EMA	Positive	Cell membrane	May be weak positive reaction
CK20	Negative		
CDX-2	Negative		
GCDFP-15	Negative		
ERP	Negative		
PRP	Negative		
Mammaglobin	Negative		
CK5/6	Negative		
p63	Negative		
Molecular Studies			
ALK1	Positive		Some cases of mucinous carcinomas including signet ring cell carcinomas of the lung may show ALK1 positivity by FISH or PCR

Histochemical Features of Signet Ring Cell Carcinomas of the Lung

Histochemical Stain	Result
Mucicarmine	Strong positive reaction for intracellular mucin
D-PAS	Positive reaction for intracellular mucin
PAS	Focal areas containing intracellular glycogen

DIAGNOSTIC CHECKLIST

Pathologic Interpretation Pearls
- Signet ring cell component

SELECTED REFERENCES

1. Moran CA: Pulmonary adenocarcinoma: the expanding spectrum of histologic variants. Arch Pathol Lab Med. 130(7):958-62, 2006
2. Castro CY et al: Primary signet ring cell adenocarcinomas of the lung: a clinicopathological study of 15 cases. Histopathology. 39(4):397-401, 2001

SIGNET RING CELL CARCINOMA

Microscopic Features

(Left) *Signet ring cell carcinoma destroys normal lung parenchyma with extensive areas of proteinaceous fluid filling some of the alveolar spaces. In addition, clusters of neoplastic cells are also present and fill alveolar spaces* ➔*.* ***(Right)*** *Neoplastic cellular proliferation of round to oval cells is shown with clear cytoplasm and small nuclei in signet ring cell carcinoma of the lung. Fibrous collagen bands separate acini of neoplastic cells.*

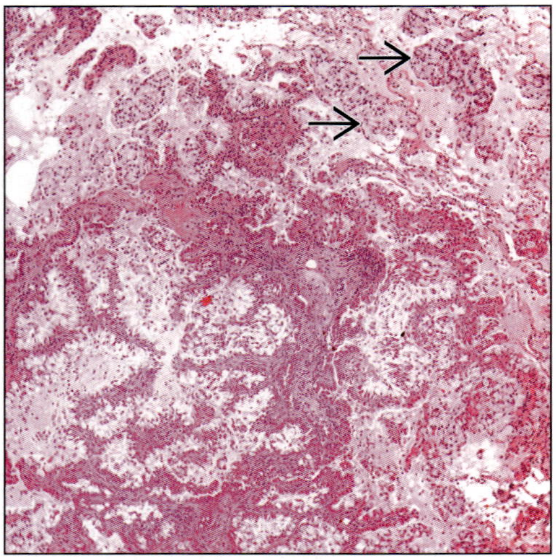

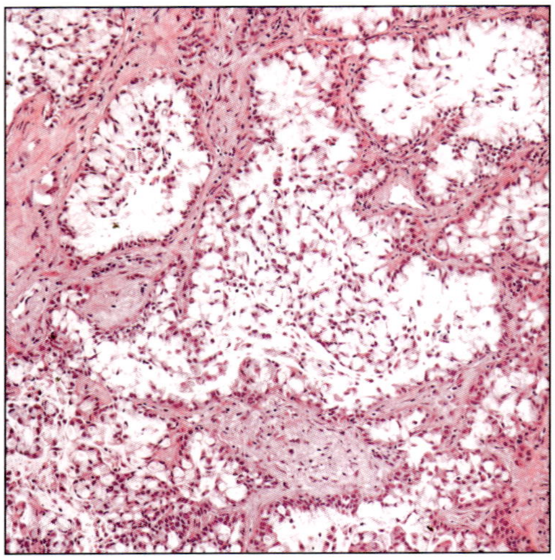

(Left) *Clusters of neoplastic cells fill alveolar spaces* ➔ *in signet ring cell carcinoma of the lung. Note the presence of extensive areas of proteinaceous fluid filling the alveolar spaces* ⇨*.* ***(Right)*** *Signet ring cell carcinoma is shown with a predominantly solid growth pattern. However, even at this magnification, one can still identify signet ring cells.*

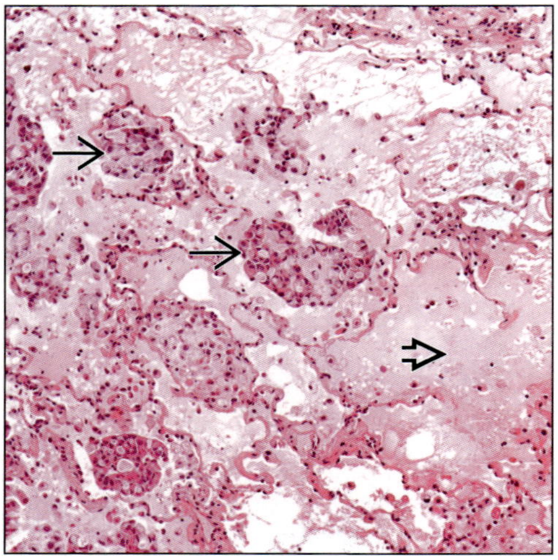

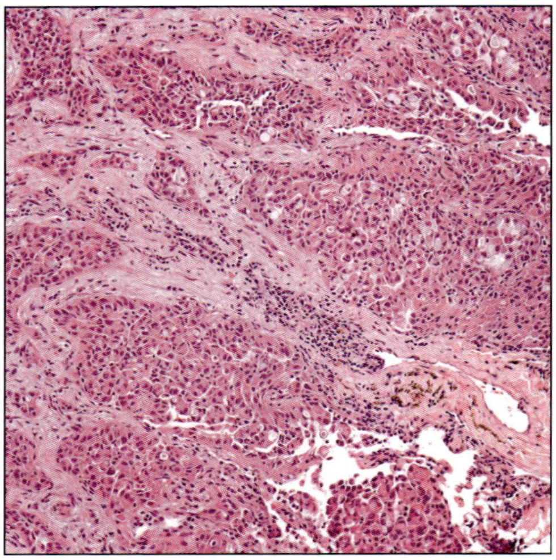

(Left) *High-power view shows a solid component of a signet ring cell carcinoma of the lung. Note the presence of numerous signet ring cells* ➔ *admixed with more conventional neoplastic cells.* ***(Right)*** *High-power view of a signet ring cell carcinoma is shown. Note the presence of the classical morphological features of signet ring cells, essentially round to oval cells, clear cytoplasm, and nuclei displaced toward the periphery* ➔*.*

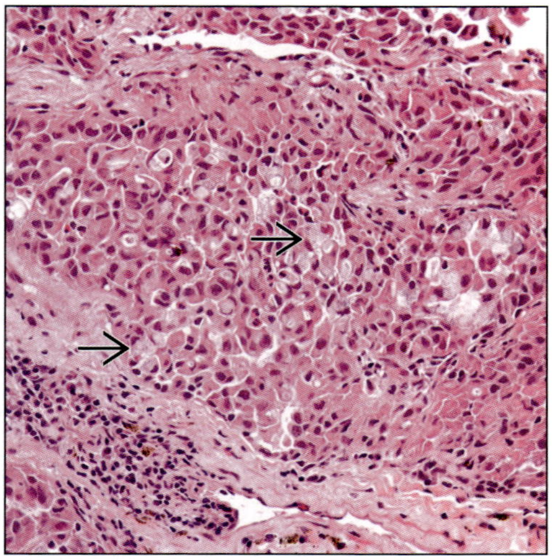

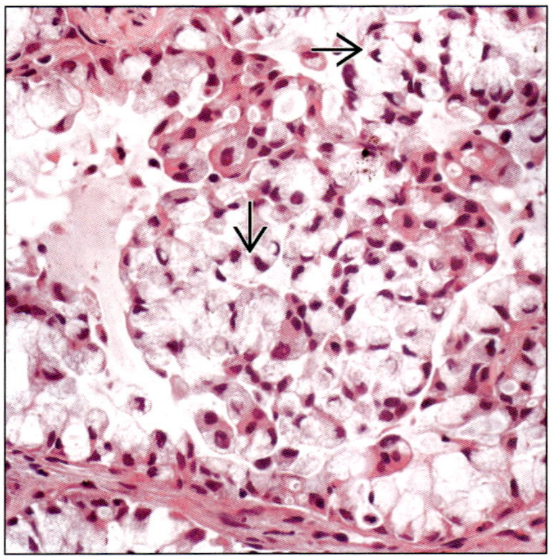

Microscopic Features

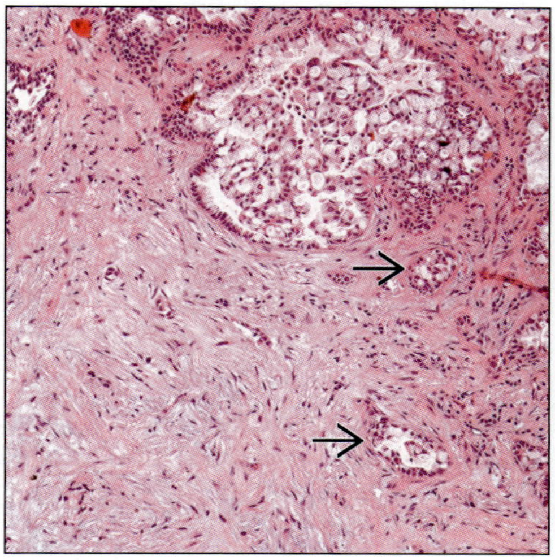
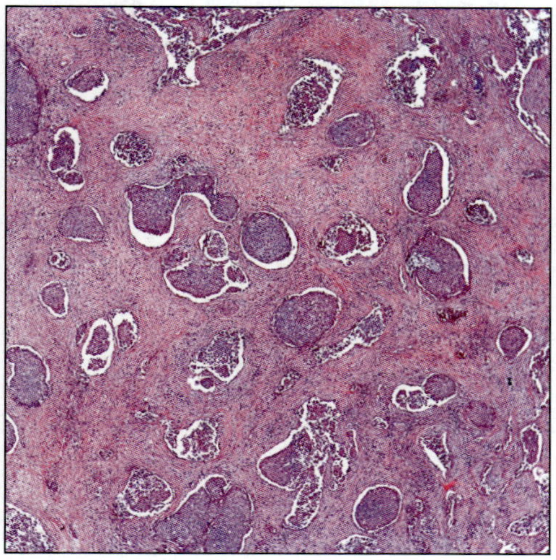

*(**Left**) Signet ring cell carcinoma is shown with acinar growth pattern and extensive areas of hyalinization. In some areas, neoplastic acini are dissecting the fibrocollagenous tissue →. (**Right**) Signet ring cell carcinoma is shown with a nodular type of growth pattern. The nodules are separated by extensive areas of fibrocollagenous stroma, mimicking extensive lymphatic permeation.*

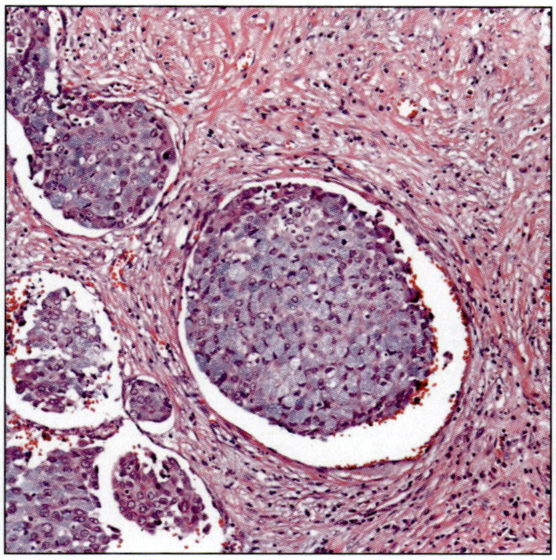
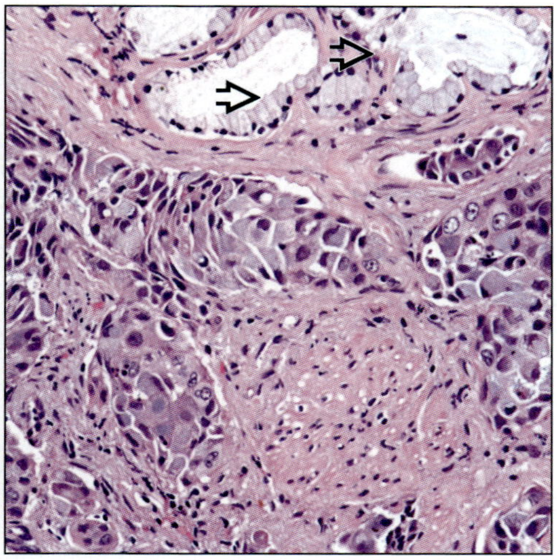

*(**Left**) High-power view shows a signet ring cell carcinoma with retraction artifact from areas of fibrocollagenous stroma. This type of extensive collagenization is rather unusual in signet ring cell carcinomas. (**Right**) Signet ring cell carcinoma with diffuse growth pattern is seen adjacent to normal submucosal glands ⇨.*

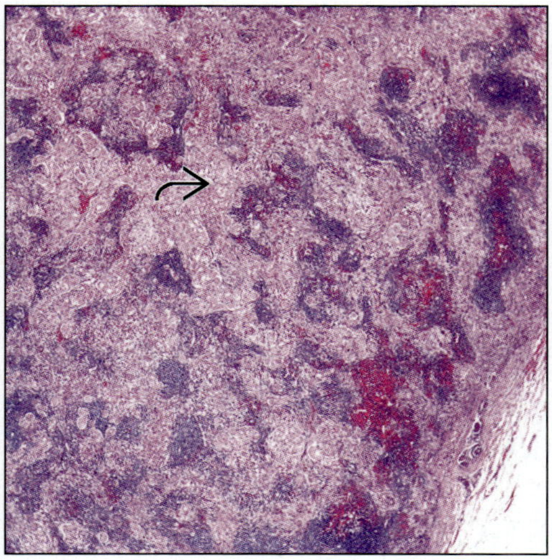
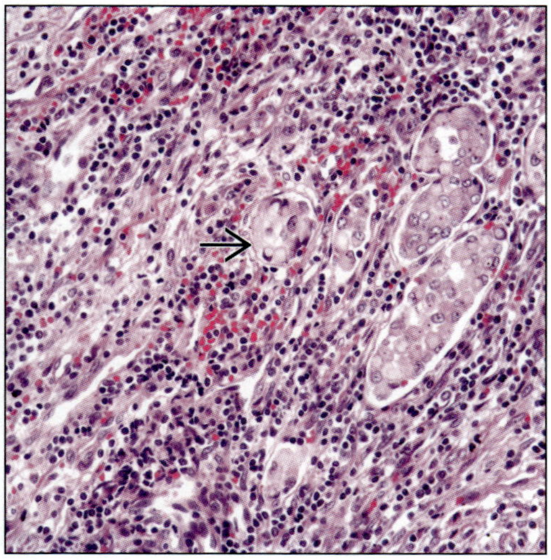

*(**Left**) Low-power magnification of lymph node is shown with metastatic signet ring cell carcinoma ↪. The tumor is destroying extensive areas of nodal normal architecture. (**Right**) High-power view of the neoplastic cells is shown infiltrating nodal tissue. Note the presence of the preserved signet ring cell morphology at this metastatic site →.*

ENDOMETRIOID-LIKE CARCINOMA

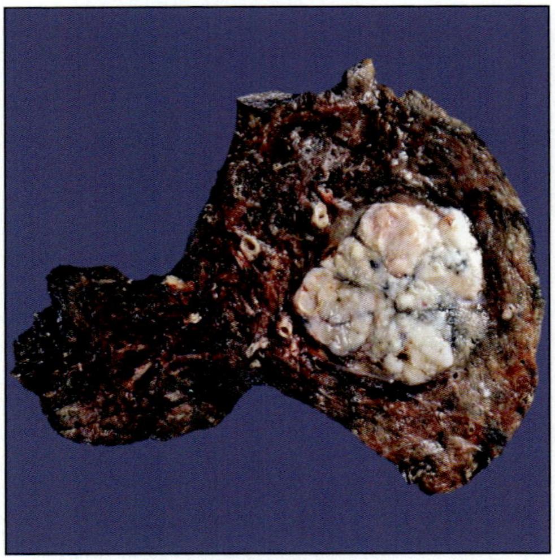

Gross photograph of an endometrioid-like carcinoma of the lung shows a well-circumscribed but not encapsulated mass. The tumor is light tan and slightly lobulated.

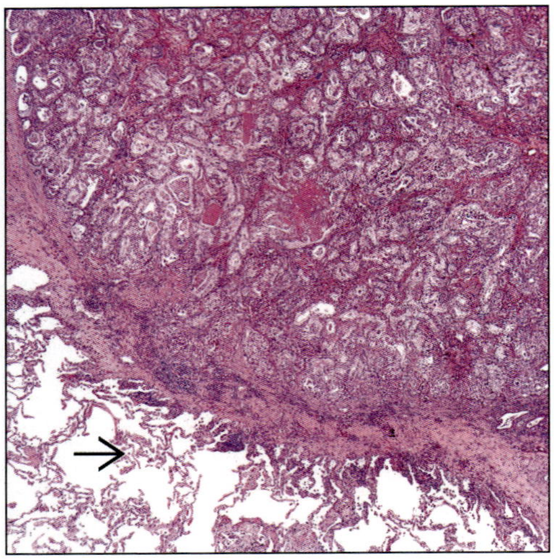

Endometrioid adenocarcinoma shows a malignant glandular proliferation destroying lung parenchyma. Note the tumor mass is well circumscribed and a rim of normal lung parenchyma is present ➔.

TERMINOLOGY

Synonyms
- Endometrioid adenocarcinoma

Definitions
- Malignant epithelial neoplasms that mimics secretory endometrium

CLINICAL ISSUES

Presentation
- Cough
- Hemoptysis
- Difficulty breathing
- Chest pain

Treatment
- Surgical approaches
  - Lobectomy or pneumonectomy
- Adjuvant therapy
  - Radiation or chemotherapy depending on clinical stage

Prognosis
- Depends on clinical and pathological stage

MACROSCOPIC FEATURES

General Features
- Tumor mass is light tan to brown
- From 1 cm to > 10 cm in greatest diameter
- Hemorrhage or necrosis may be seen
- Tumor may be central or peripheral

MICROSCOPIC PATHOLOGY

Histologic Features
- Glands composed of cells with clear cytoplasm mimicking secretory phase of endometrium
- Absence of morular component
- Neoplastic cells with intracellular mucin

Predominant Pattern/Injury Type
- Glandular

Predominant Cell/Compartment Type
- Epithelial, glandular

DIFFERENTIAL DIAGNOSIS

Pulmonary Blastoma
- Endometrioid adenocarcinoma
  - Lacks morular component between glandular structures
  - Lacks primitive glands that recapitulate lung development of approximately weeks 11-16
  - Shows intracellular mucin while blastoma lacks it

Metastatic Endometrioid Adenocarcinoma from Gynecologic Primary
- Differential diagnosis more important in female patients
- Clinical history &/or complete physical examination are of utmost importance
- Use of immunohistochemical stains may help in some cases
- TTF-1 may be positive in a small number of primary endometrial adenocarcinomas

DIAGNOSTIC CHECKLIST

Clinically Relevant Pathologic Features
- Metastatic distribution

ENDOMETRIOID-LIKE CARCINOMA

Key Facts

Terminology
- Malignant epithelial neoplasms with features mimicking secretory endometrium

Clinical Issues
- Symptoms
  - Cough
  - Dyspnea
  - Hemoptysis
  - Chest pain
- Prognosis
  - Depends on clinical and pathological stage
- Treatment options
  - Lobectomy or pneumonectomy
  - Radiation &/or chemotherapy depending on clinical stage

Top Differential Diagnoses
- Pulmonary blastoma: Endometrioid adenocarcinoma
  - Lacks morular component between glandular structures
  - Lacks primitive glands that recapitulate lung development of approximately weeks 11-16
  - Shows intracellular mucin while blastoma lacks it
- Metastatic endometrioid adenocarcinoma from gynecologic primary
  - Differential diagnosis more important in female patients
  - Clinical history &/or complete physical examination → correct interpretation
  - Use of immunohistochemical stains may help in some cases

Immunohistochemistry

Antibody	Reactivity	Staining Pattern	Comment
TTF-1	Positive	Nuclear	Some cases of uterine adenocarcinoma may also show positive nuclear staining
KERATIN-LMW	Positive	Cytoplasmic	In glandular structures
MOC-31	Positive	Cytoplasmic	In glandular component
EpCAM/BER-EP4/ CD326	Positive	Cell membrane	
CK7	Positive	Cytoplasmic	Strongly positive
CEA-M	Positive	Cytoplasmic	
TAG72	Positive	Cytoplasmic	May show weak positive reaction
WT1	Positive	Nuclear	May be positive or negative
CA125	Negative		May be positive in some lung adenocarcinomas
ER	Negative		Focal weak positive staining may be seen
PR	Negative		
p63	Negative		

Histochemical Features of Endometrioid Adenocarcinoma of the Lung

Histochemical Stain	Result	Comment
Mucicarmine	Positive	Intracellular mucin
D-PAS	Positive	Intracellular mucin
PAS	Positive	In cells containing glycogen

Pathologic Interpretation Pearls
- Malignant glands similar to those seen in menstrual phase of secretory endometrium
- Back to back glandular proliferation
- Presence of intracellular mucin
- Absence of morules

SELECTED REFERENCES

1. Longo M et al: Fetal adenocarcinoma of the lung in a 25-year-old woman. J Thorac Oncol. 3(4):441-3, 2008
2. Siami K et al: Thyroid transcription factor-1 expression in endometrial and endocervical adenocarcinomas. Am J Surg Pathol. 31(11):1759-63, 2007
3. Adluri RK et al: Pulmonary blastoma--a rare tumor with variable presentation. Eur J Cardiothorac Surg. 29(2):236-9, 2006
4. Harada T et al: Pulmonary blastoma within bronchioloalveolar cell carcinoma. Respirology. 11(3):339-42, 2006
5. Steinhauer JR et al: 'Secretory endometrioid-like' adenocarcinoma of the lung. Histopathology. 47(2):219-20, 2005

ENDOMETRIOID-LIKE CARCINOMA

Microscopic Features

*(**Left**) Endometrioid adenocarcinoma of the lung shows a malignant glandular proliferation. Even at this magnification, it is possible to observe the clear cytoplasm. (**Right**) Closer view of the malignant glandular component shows focal areas in which the glands contain intraluminal mucinous material ↷, while most of the glands have an empty lumen.*

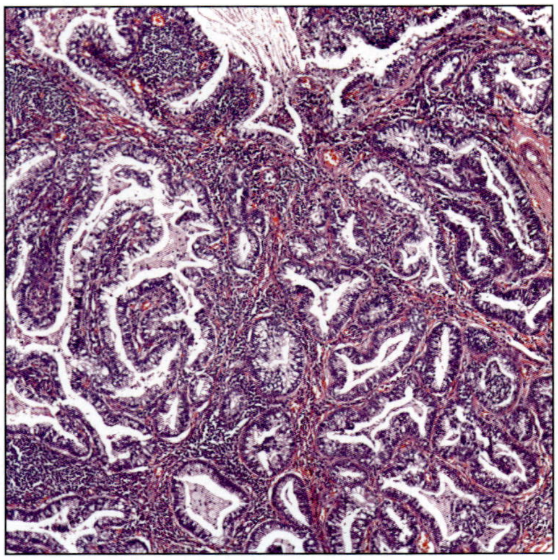

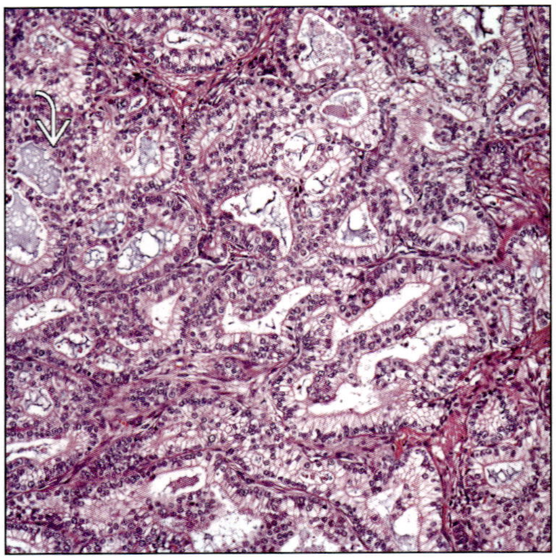

*(**Left**) Areas of necrosis → are present in endometrioid adenocarcinoma; however, extensive areas of necrosis are not a common feature in this type of neoplasm. (**Right**) Malignant glands filled with foamy macrophages ↗ are probably due to obstruction. However, the basic histology of the endometrioid-like adenocarcinoma is still present.*

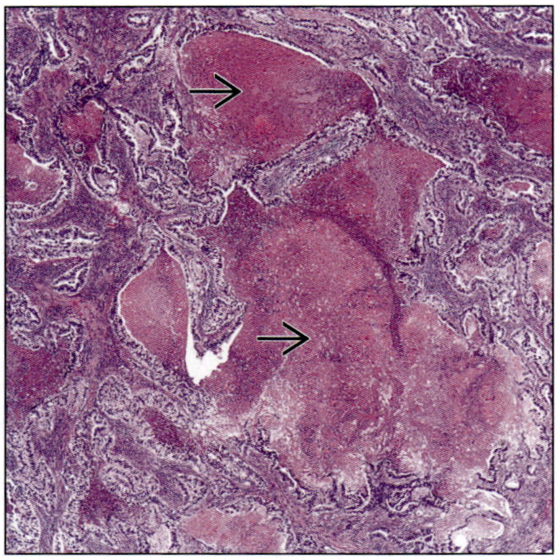

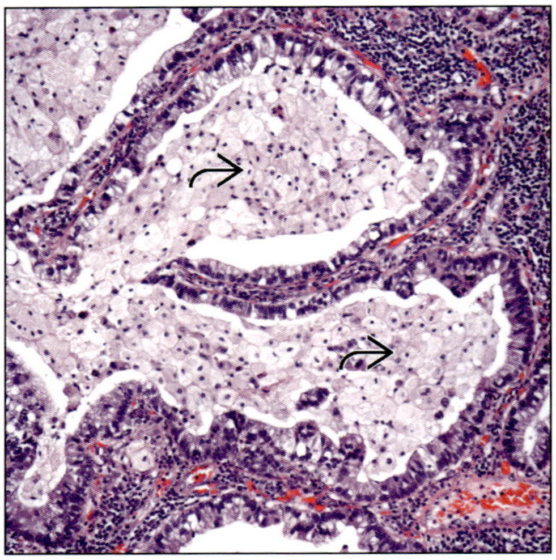

*(**Left**) Endometrioid adenocarcinoma shows a malignant glandular proliferation in which the malignant glands are separated by thin fibroconnective tissue. A focal area with more extensive fibrosis is also present ⇨. (**Right**) Endometrioid adenocarcinoma shows a malignant glandular proliferation separated by thin bands of fibroconnective tissue and focal inflammatory change ↗.*

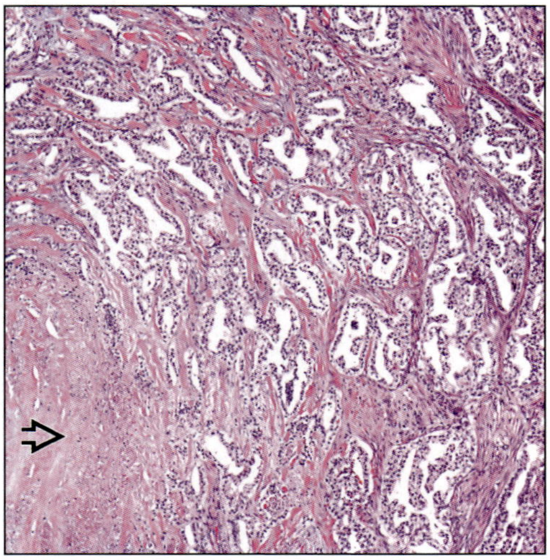

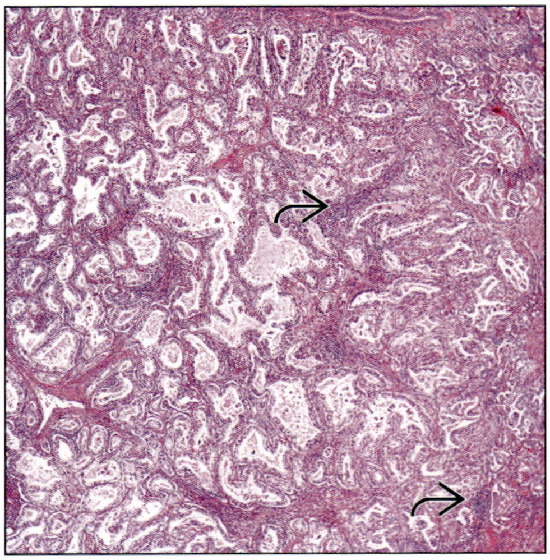

Microscopic Features

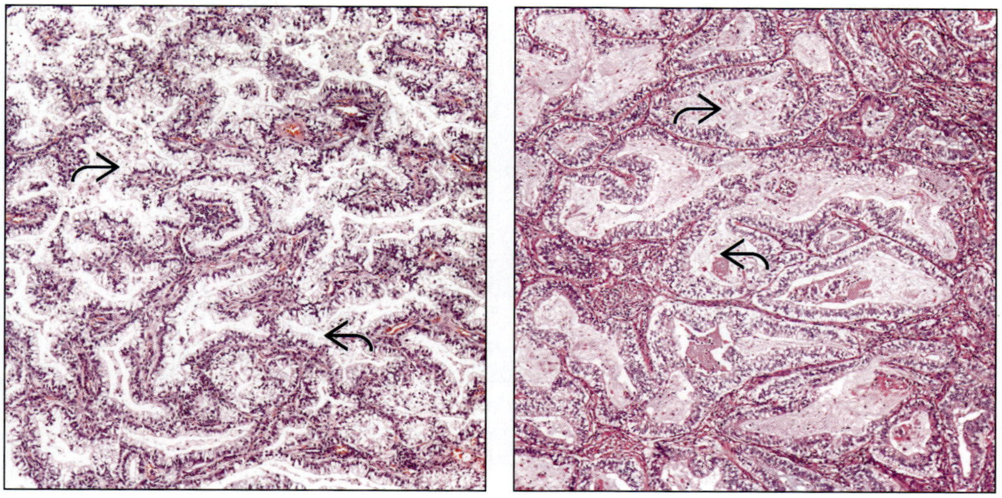

*(**Left**) Malignant glandular proliferation is shown in which the glands are composed of cells with prominent clear cytoplasm and basally located nuclei ↪. Note the lack of cytologic atypia or increased mitotic activity. (**Right**) Endometrioid adenocarcinoma shows glands filled with acellular material ↪. Note the presence of malignant glands of different sizes and tumor cells with clear cytoplasm.*

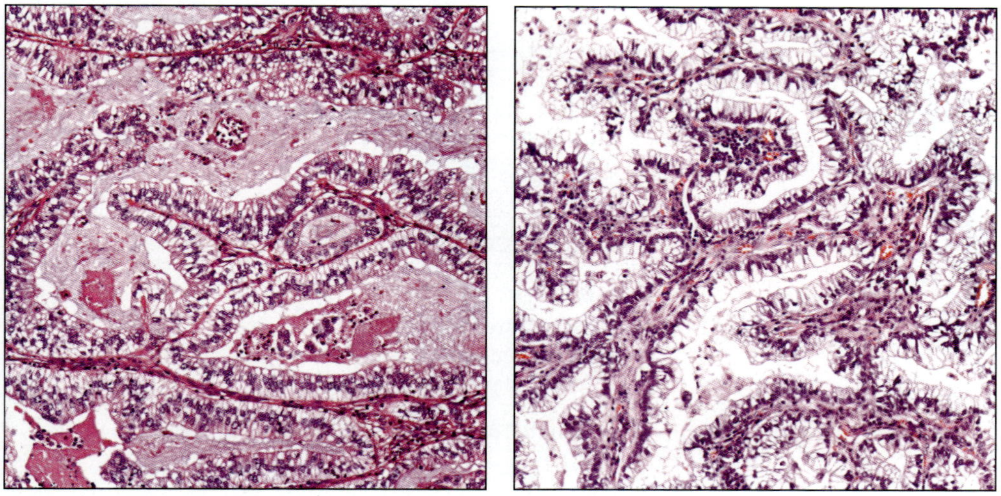

*(**Left**) Higher magnification view of the cellular component of endometrioid adenocarcinoma mimics the secretory phase of the menstrual endometrium. (**Right**) Closer view shows malignant glands with only moderate nuclear atypia and rare mitotic figures. Note the absence of a "morular" component.*

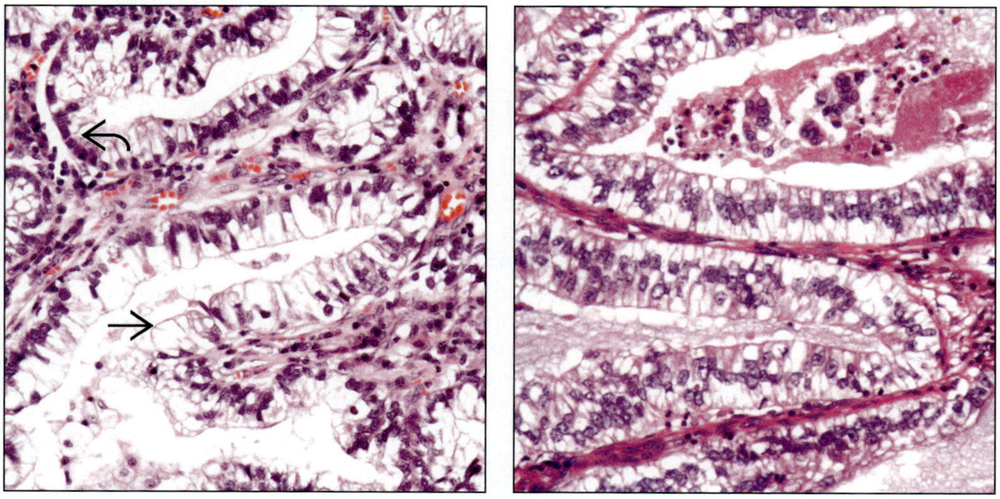

*(**Left**) Higher magnification of the glandular component shows basal location of the nucleus ↪ and clear cytoplasm →. Mitotic figures are rare. (**Right**) Higher magnification of the cellular component shows the "piano keys" appearance, similar to that described in the secretory phase of the menstrual endometrium.*

SQUAMOUS CELL CARCINOMA

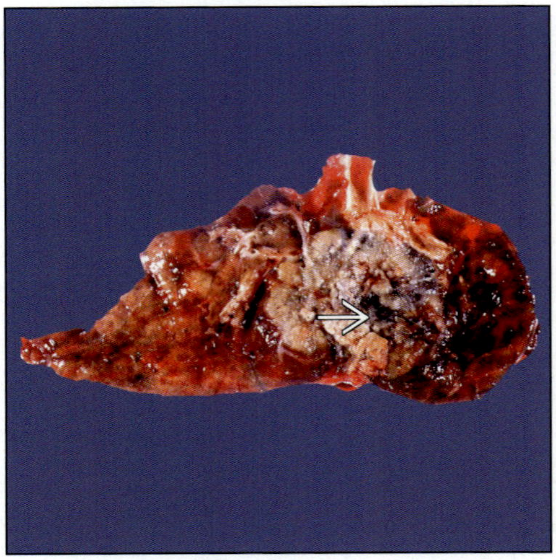

Gross photograph of squamous cell carcinoma of the lung shows a centrally located large neoplasm. The tumor has a soft consistency and focal areas of necrosis ➡.

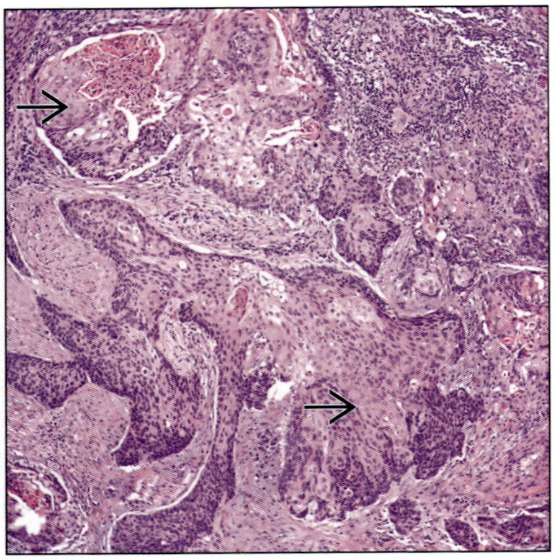

Keratinizing well-differentiated squamous cell carcinoma. Note the presence of keratin formation, characteristic of well-differentiated tumors ➡.

TERMINOLOGY

Synonyms

- Epidermoid carcinoma

Definitions

- Malignant epithelial neoplasm with squamous (epidermoid) differentiation

ETIOLOGY/PATHOGENESIS

Environmental Exposure

- Associated with tobacco smoke

CLINICAL ISSUES

Presentation

- Cough
- Shortness of breath
- Hemoptysis
- Chest pain

Treatment

- Surgical approaches
  - Wedge resection
  - Lobectomy
  - Pneumonectomy
- Radiation
  - Chemotherapy or radiation therapy

Prognosis

- Depends on stage at time of diagnosis

MACROSCOPIC FEATURES

General Features

- Central or peripheral tumors
- White or light brown in color with homogeneous cut surface
- Cut surface may show areas of hemorrhage &/or necrosis
- Tumors may be predominantly cystic
- Tumor size may vary from 2 cm to > 10 cm in diameter

MICROSCOPIC PATHOLOGY

Histologic Features

- Keratinization
- Keratin pearls
- Intercellular bridges

Predominant Pattern/Injury Type

- Solid
- Cystic
- Spindled

Predominant Cell/Compartment Type

- Epithelial, squamous

DIFFERENTIAL DIAGNOSIS

Small Cell Carcinoma

- In cases of small cell variant of squamous cell carcinoma, the presence of an in situ squamous component will be helpful for diagnosis
- Chromatin pattern of small cell carcinoma ("salt and pepper") not present in small cell variant of squamous cell carcinoma
- May show positive staining for neuroendocrine markers and TTF-1

Sarcoma

- May identify residual focal areas of squamous differentiation in spindle cell variant of squamous cell carcinoma

SQUAMOUS CELL CARCINOMA

Key Facts

Terminology
- Malignant epithelial neoplasm with squamous (epidermoid) differentiation

Macroscopic Features
- Central or peripheral tumors
- White or light brown in color with homogeneous cut surface; cut surface may show areas of hemorrhage &/ or necrosis
- Tumors may be predominantly cystic
- Tumor size may vary from 2 cm to > 10 cm in diameter

Microscopic Pathology
- Solid
- Cystic
- Spindled

Top Differential Diagnoses
- Small cell carcinoma
  - In cases of small cell variant of squamous cell carcinoma, may be able to identify in situ squamous component
  - Chromatin pattern of small cell carcinoma, "salt and pepper," not present in small cell variant of squamous cell carcinoma
- Sarcoma
  - In spindle cell variant of squamous cell carcinoma, may identify residual focal areas of squamous differentiation
- Large cell neuroendocrine carcinoma
  - In cases of basaloid squamous cell carcinoma, large cell neuroendocrine carcinoma may enter the differential diagnosis

Immunohistochemistry

Antibody	Reactivity	Staining Pattern	Comment
CK5/6	Positive	Cytoplasmic	May also be positive in mesotheliomas
p63	Positive	Nuclear	May be positive in other types of carcinomas
KERATIN-LMW	Positive	Cytoplasmic	Not specific for squamous cell carcinoma
Vimentin	Positive	Cytoplasmic	May also be positive in nonepithelial tumors
CD117	Positive	Cytoplasmic	In some cases
Synaptophysin	Negative	Nuclear & cytoplasmic	Some cases may show focal positive staining
Chromogranin-A	Negative		

- Immunohistochemical markers for mesenchymal origin may prove useful

Large Cell Neuroendocrine Carcinoma
- In cases of basaloid squamous cell carcinoma, large cell neuroendocrine carcinoma may enter the differential diagnosis
- Basaloid squamous cell carcinoma is negative for neuroendocrine markers
- Immunomarkers for neuroendocrine origin will show positive staining

DIAGNOSTIC CHECKLIST

Pathologic Interpretation Pearls
- Presence of keratinization, keratin pearls, &/or intercellular bridges

GRADING

Well-differentiated Squamous Cell Carcinoma
- Tumor shows obvious keratinization, and at high-power view, intercellular bridges are apparent

Moderately Differentiated Squamous Cell Carcinoma
- Tumors show more cellular and nuclear atypia
  - Keratinization is not obvious

Poorly Differentiated Squamous Cell Carcinoma
- Sheets of tumor cells with only focal keratinization, high mitotic activity, and prominent cellular and nuclear atypia

In Situ Squamous Cell Carcinoma
- Tumor is limited to bronchial mucosa, full thickness

SELECTED REFERENCES

1. Pelosi G et al: CD117 immunoreactivity in stage I adenocarcinoma and squamous cell carcinoma of the lung: relevance to prognosis in a subset of adenocarcinoma patients. Mod Pathol. 17(6):711-21, 2004
2. Pelosi G et al: p63 immunoreactivity in lung cancer: yet another player in the development of squamous cell carcinomas? J Pathol. 198(1):100-9, 2002
3. Suster S et al: Spindle cell squamous carcinoma of the lung. Immunocytochemical and ultrastructural study of a case. Histopathology. 11(8):871-8, 1987
4. Sherwin RP et al: Exophytic endobronchial carcinoma. J Thorac Cardiovasc Surg. 43:716-30, 1962

SQUAMOUS CELL CARCINOMA

Microscopic Features

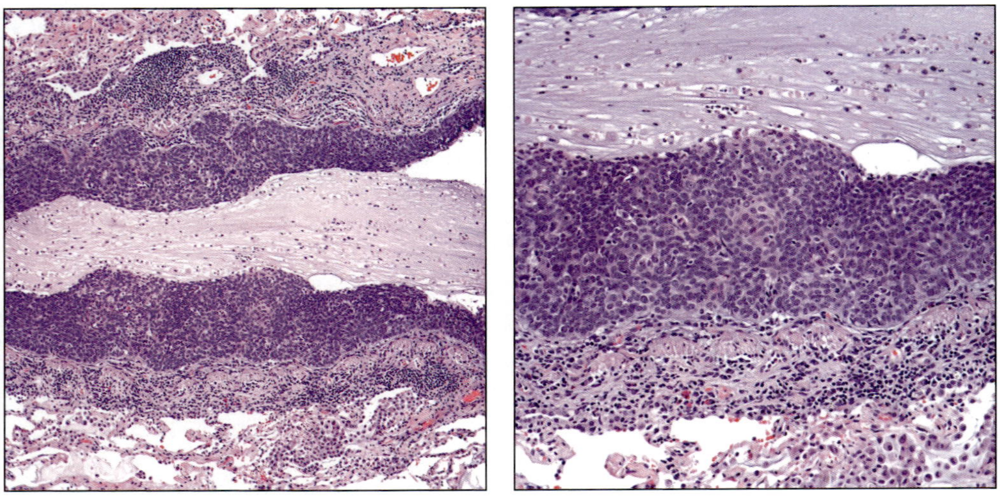

(Left) *In situ bronchial squamous cell carcinoma shows bronchial mucosa completely replaced (full thickness) by neoplastic cells. Note the lack of invasion into adjacent lung parenchyma.* ***(Right)*** *Full thickness of the bronchial mucosa replaced by a neoplastic cellular proliferation characteristic of in situ squamous cell carcinoma shows mild inflammatory reaction adjacent to the neoplastic cells.*

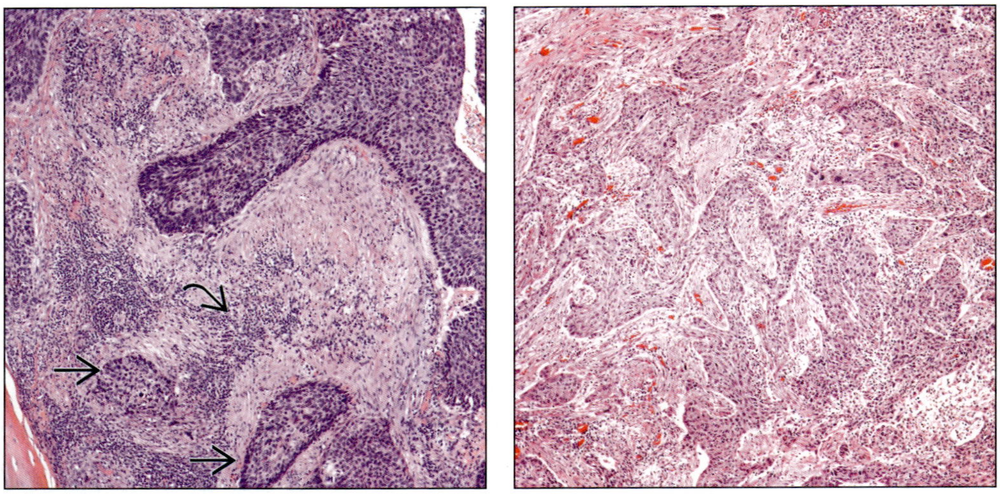

(Left) *Predominantly in situ squamous cell carcinoma with focal areas of minimally invasive tumor. Tumor islands of squamous cell carcinoma* ➔ *are admixed with an inflammatory reaction* ⤻*.* ***(Right)*** *Moderately differentiated squamous cell carcinoma. The tumor does not show marked keratinization, but the growth pattern is typical of squamous cell carcinoma. Cellular and nuclear atypia are present.*

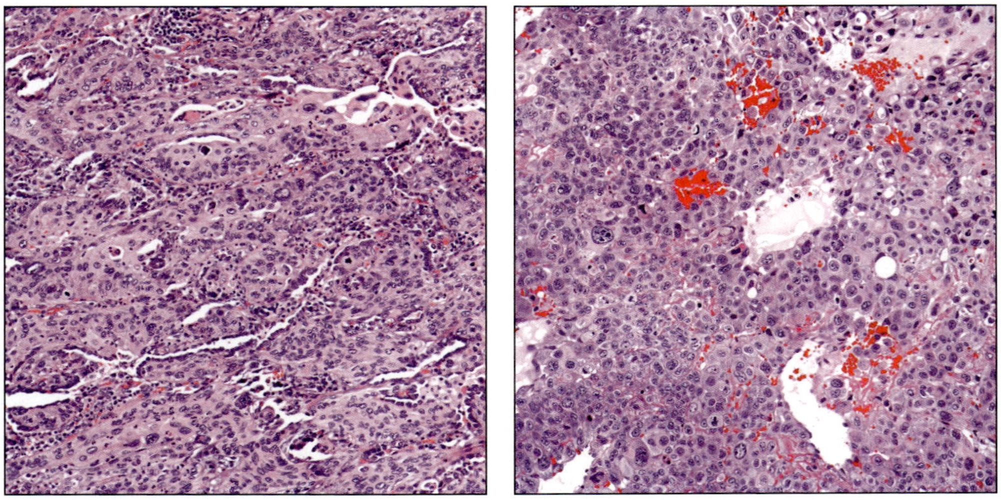

(Left) *Poorly differentiated squamous cell carcinoma growing in cords of neoplastic cells. Note the presence of marked cellular and nuclear atypia. Mitotic figures are present.* ***(Right)*** *Sheets of neoplastic cells with focal perivascular arrangement are seen in this example of poorly differentiated squamous cell carcinoma. The tumor shows only focal single cell keratinization.*

Microscopic Features

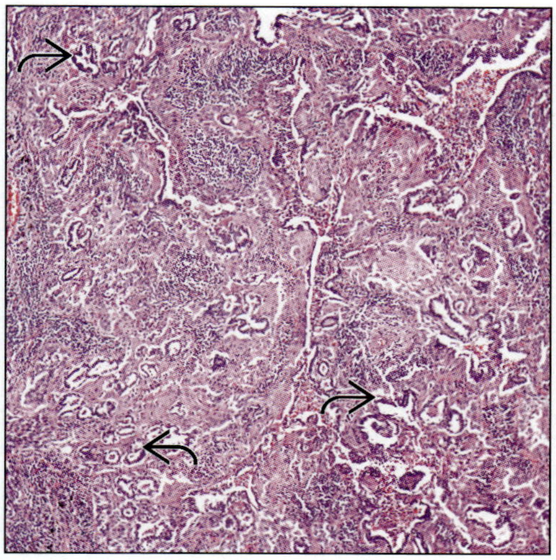
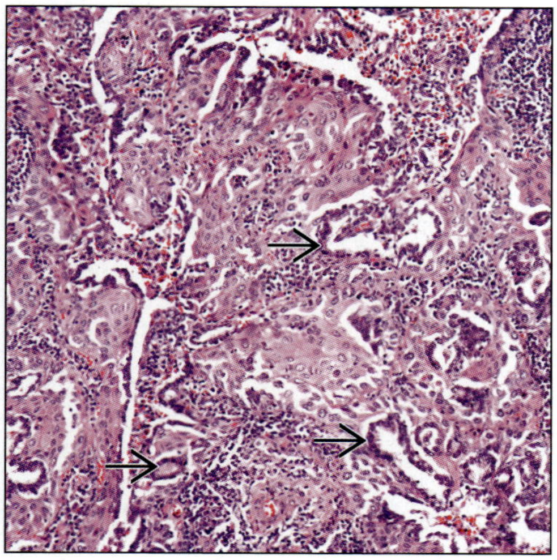

(Left) *Pseudoglandular appearance of a squamous cell carcinoma, so-called adenoid-like squamous cell carcinoma. Note the presence of glandular structures ⮫ that can be confused for adenocarcinoma.* ***(Right)*** *Adenoid-like squamous cell carcinoma. Note the entrapped alveolar structures, which impart a pseudoglandular appearance →.*

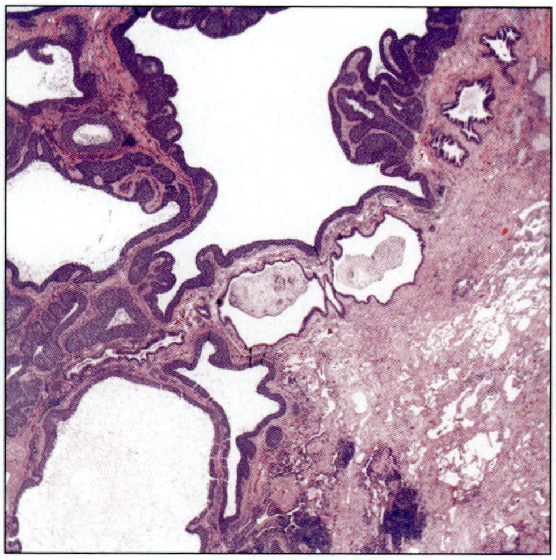
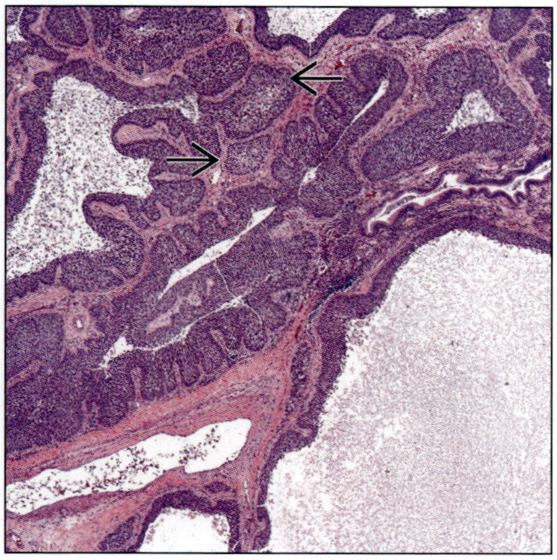

(Left) *Predominantly cystic squamous cell carcinoma. At this magnification, the tumor appears to be an in situ carcinoma due its cystic nature. This histological pattern is unusual and commonly associated with areas of necrosis.* ***(Right)*** *Cystic squamous cell carcinoma in which there are unequivocal areas of invasion →. This particular pattern is rather unusual in primary lung neoplasms.*

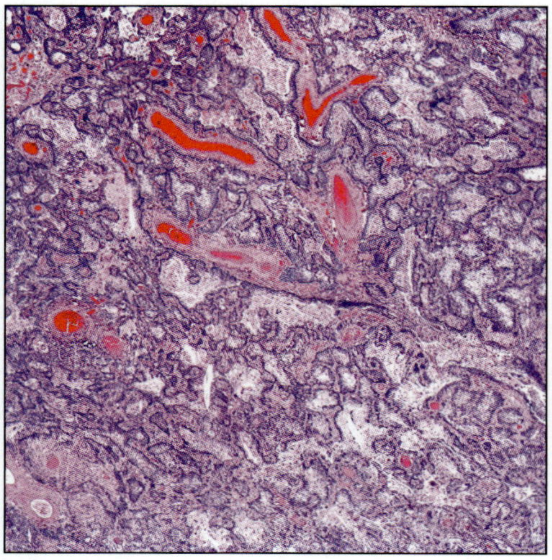
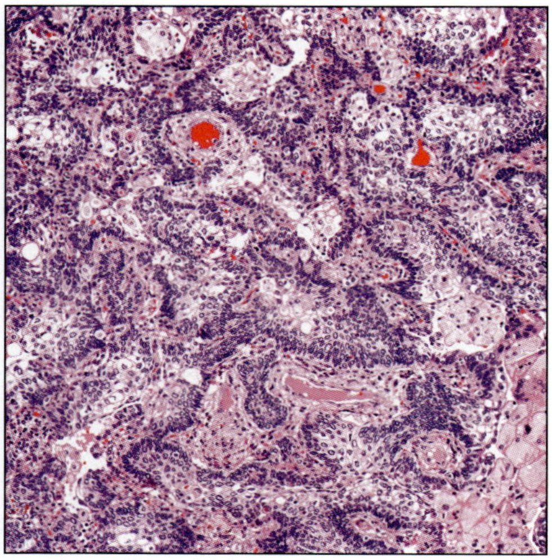

(Left) *Squamous cell carcinoma with a prominent ameloblastoma-like pattern. The tumor grows in a manner similar to those tumors occurring in the jaw. Also note the presence of prominent clear cell changes.* ***(Right)*** *Ameloblastoma-like squamous cell carcinoma. Note the presence of focal keratinization, clear cells with squamous differentiation, and mild to moderate cellular or nuclear atypia.*

SQUAMOUS CELL CARCINOMA

Microscopic Features

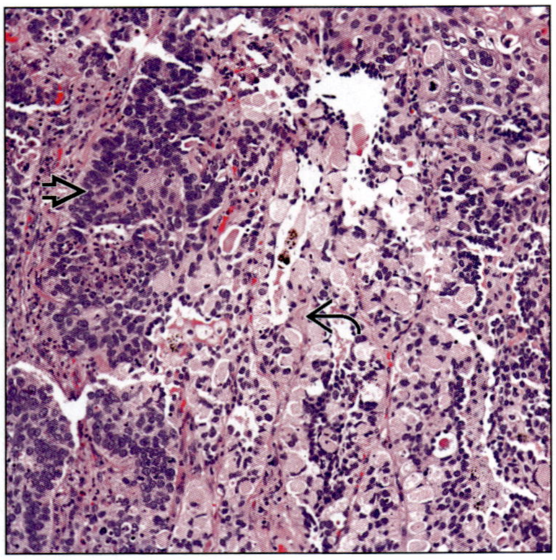

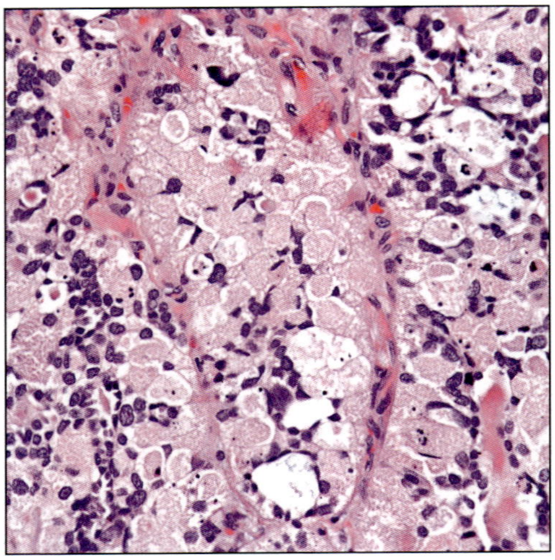

(Left) *Squamous cell carcinoma with granular-like changes. Note the presence of conventional areas of squamous cell carcinoma ⇨ transitioning into larger cells with granular-like changes ↷.* ***(Right)*** *High magnification of the granular cell variant of squamous cell carcinoma. High-power view shows cells with prominent granular cytoplasm. No mitotic activity or nuclear atypia are present.*

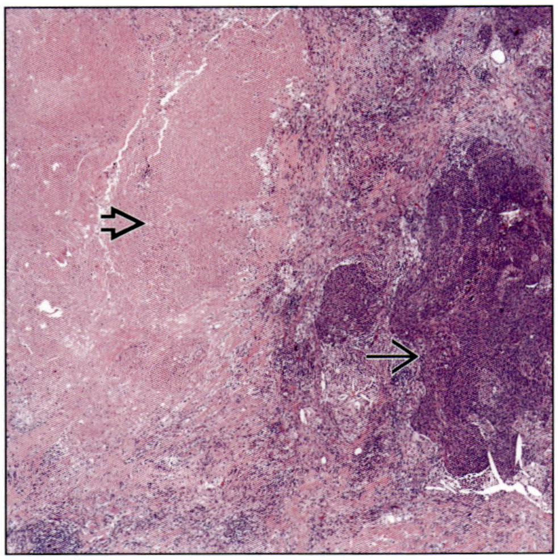

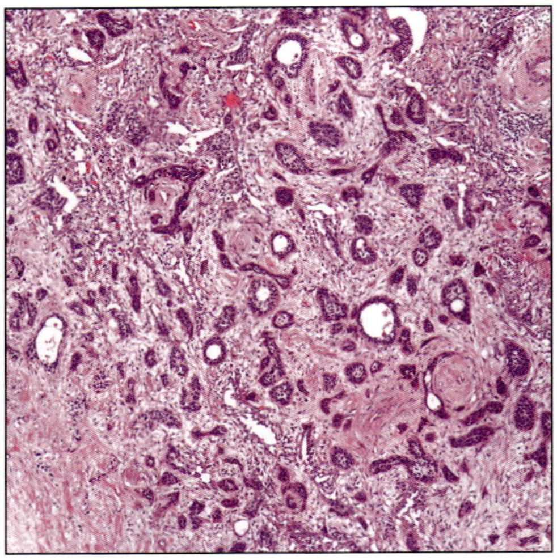

(Left) *Moderately differentiated squamous cell carcinoma → with extensive areas of necrosis ⇨. In some cases, the presence of viable tumor may be only focal.* ***(Right)*** *Squamous cell carcinoma with a predominantly syringomatous-like growth pattern. This growth pattern mimics that of adnexal skin tumors. This pattern is similar to the so-called microcystic squamous cell carcinoma of the skin.*

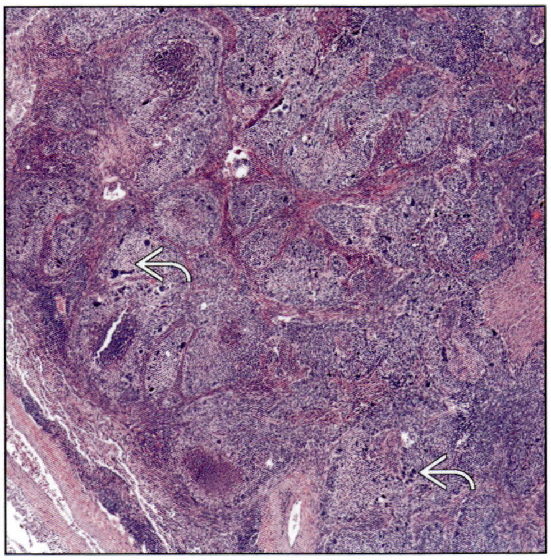

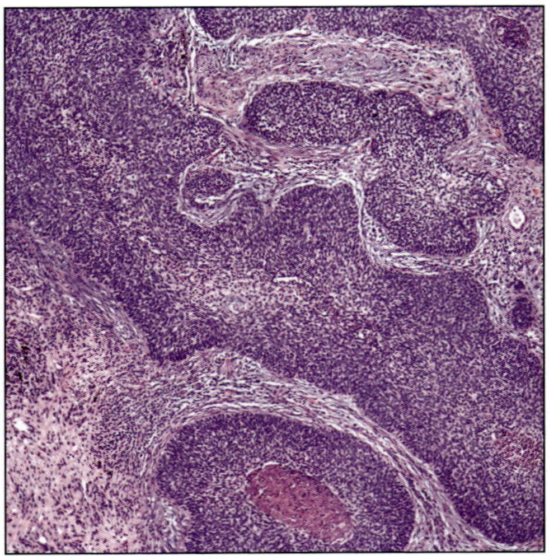

(Left) *Basaloid growth pattern in squamous cell carcinoma. The tumor shows marked cellular atypia and areas of necrosis. Scattered large atypical cells ↶ are seen admixed with the basaloid tumor cells.* ***(Right)*** *High-power view of a basaloid squamous cell carcinoma. The tumor recapitulates the similar pattern of the adnexal basal cell carcinoma of the skin.*

Microscopic Features

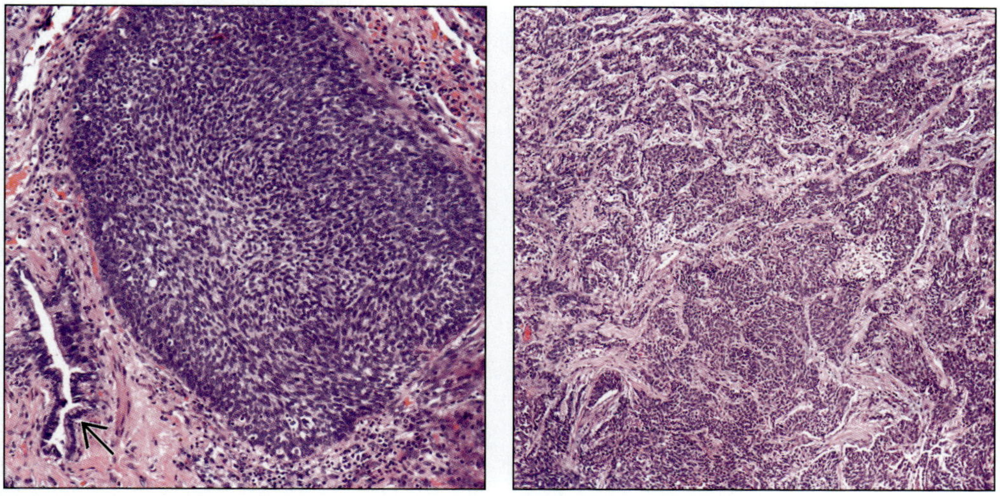

(Left) *Higher magnification of a basaloid squamous cell carcinoma shows vague squamoid differentiation and prominent basaloid growth with palisading of the nuclei. Note the adjacent normal airway* →. ***(Right)*** *Poorly differentiated squamous cell carcinoma with a growth pattern mimicking neuroendocrine neoplasms, the so-called small cell variant of squamous cell carcinoma.*

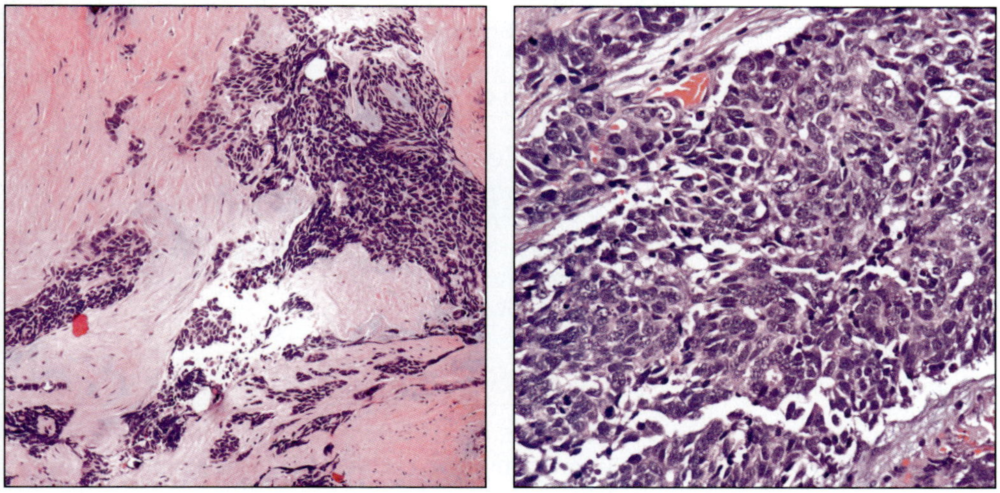

(Left) *So-called small cell variant of squamous cell carcinoma. The tumor shows a neoplastic cellular proliferation composed of rather smaller cells in a pattern that mimics small cell carcinoma.* ***(Right)*** *High-power view of the small cell variant of squamous cell carcinoma. Note the presence of cells with scant cytoplasm; however, the presence of nucleoli is more in keeping with a non-small cell carcinoma.*

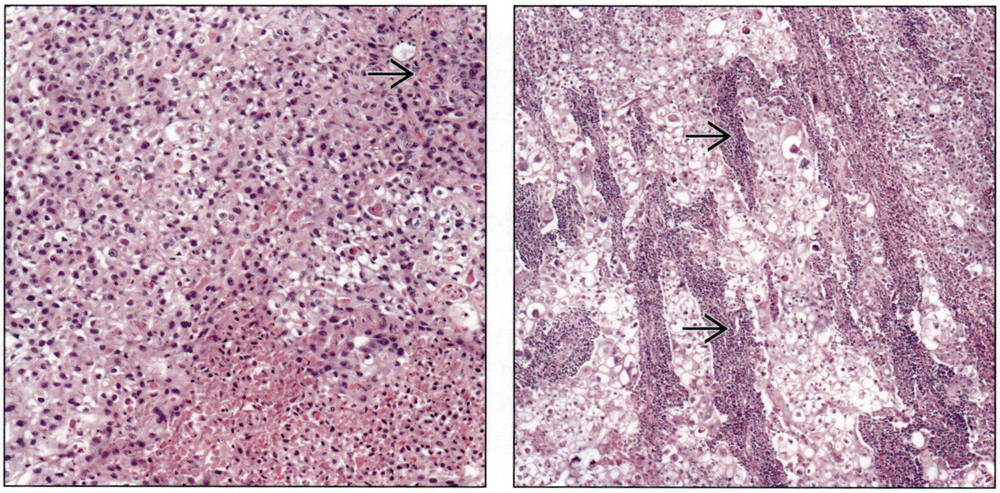

(Left) *Poorly differentiated squamous cell carcinoma with extensive necrosis and clear cell features. Note the presence of single-cell keratinization* →. ***(Right)*** *High-power view of a squamous cell carcinoma with clear cell features. Note the presence of cellular and nuclear atypia and the presence of an admixed inflammatory response* →.

SPINDLE CELL (SARCOMATOID) CARCINOMA

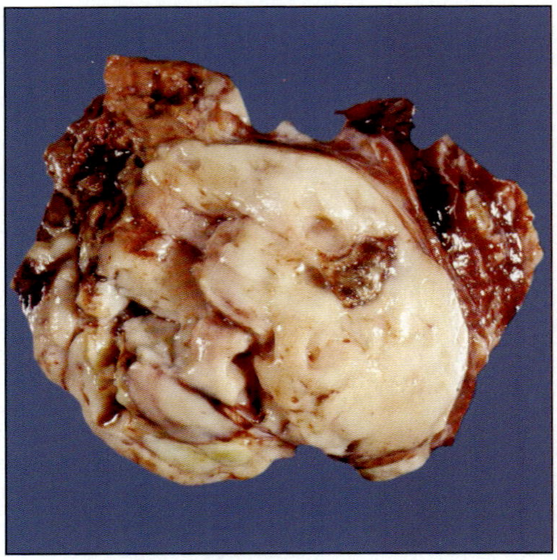

Gross photograph shows an intrapulmonary large mass that is white, firm, and well circumscribed. The cut surface is smooth and homogeneous.

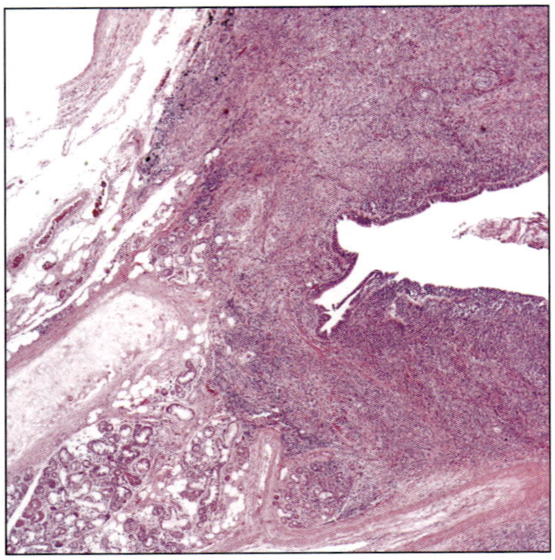

Centrally located spindle cell (sarcomatoid) carcinoma shows a tumor with solid and diffuse malignant cellular proliferation.

TERMINOLOGY

Synonyms

- Carcinoma with pseudosarcomatous component, pseudosarcomatous carcinoma, spindle cell carcinoma

Definitions

- Malignant epithelial neoplasm composed of spindle cells

ETIOLOGY/PATHOGENESIS

Etiology

- Sarcomatoid carcinomas may represent poorly differentiated squamous cell carcinomas

CLINICAL ISSUES

Epidemiology

- Incidence
  - Sarcomatoid carcinomas account for a small percentage of primary lung neoplasms
- Age
  - Similar to other non-small cell carcinomas
- Gender
  - No gender predilection

Presentation

- Cough
- Chest pain
- Hemoptysis
- Difficulty breathing

Treatment

- Surgical approaches
  - Lobectomy or pneumonectomy
- Adjuvant therapy
  - Chemotherapy &/or radiation therapy

Prognosis

- Depends on stage at time of diagnosis

MACROSCOPIC FEATURES

General Features

- Central or peripheral tumors
- 2 to > 10 cm in diameter
- Firm, light tan, and well-circumscribed but not encapsulated
- Areas of necrosis may be seen

MICROSCOPIC PATHOLOGY

Histologic Features

- Tumor composed exclusively of malignant spindle cells
- In some cases, focal areas of classic squamous cell carcinoma may be seen

Predominant Pattern/Injury Type

- Sarcomatoid

Predominant Cell/Compartment Type

- Epithelial

DIFFERENTIAL DIAGNOSIS

Pleomorphic Carcinoma (PC)

- In addition to spindle cell component, PC should have presence of multinucleated giant cells
- PC and sarcomatoid carcinoma share similar immunohistochemical profile

Leiomyosarcoma

- Sarcomatoid carcinomas
  - Negative staining for
    - Desmin
    - Caldesmon

SPINDLE CELL (SARCOMATOID) CARCINOMA

Key Facts

Terminology
- Carcinoma with pseudosarcomatous component, pseudosarcomatous carcinoma, spindle cell carcinoma

Clinical Issues
- Cough
- Chest pain
- Hemoptysis

Macroscopic Features
- Central or peripheral tumors
- 2 to > 10 cm in diameter
- Firm, light tan, and well-circumscribed but not encapsulated
- Areas of necrosis may be seen

Microscopic Pathology
- Tumor composed exclusively of malignant spindle cells

Top Differential Diagnoses
- Pleomorphic carcinoma (PC)
  - In addition to spindle cell component, PC should have presence of multinucleated giant cells
- Leiomyosarcoma: Sarcomatoid carcinoma
  - Should have negative staining for desmin, caldesmon, or SMA
  - May show focal areas of squamous differentiation
- Malignant fibrous histiocytoma
  - Absence of immunoreactivity for epithelial markers

Immunohistochemistry

Antibody	Reactivity	Staining Pattern	Comment
KERATIN-LMW	Positive	Cytoplasmic	
EMA/MUC1	Positive	Cell membrane	
CK5/6	Positive	Cytoplasmic	In some cases
Vimentin	Positive	Cytoplasmic	
CD15	Positive	Cytoplasmic	Focally positive in some cases
NSE	Negative		
Actin-sm	Negative		May be focally positive in some cases
Desmin	Negative		
Caldesmon	Negative		
MYOD1	Negative		
CD31	Negative		
S100	Negative		
Calretinin	Negative		In some cases, focal positive staining may be seen
CEA-M	Negative		
Chromogranin-A	Negative		
p63	Negative		Focally positive in some cases
TTF-1	Negative		In some cases, focal positive staining may be seen

    - Smooth muscle actin (SMA)
  - May show focal areas of squamous differentiation

Malignant Fibrous Histiocytoma
- Absence of immunoreactivity for epithelial markers

DIAGNOSTIC CHECKLIST

Pathologic Interpretation Pearls
- Tumor composed exclusively of malignant spindle cells

SELECTED REFERENCES

1. Chhatwani L et al: Adjuvant treatment of resected lung cancer. Proc Am Thorac Soc. 6(2):194-200, 2009
2. Rossi G et al: A reevaluation of the clinical significance of histological subtyping of non--small-cell lung carcinoma: diagnostic algorithms in the era of personalized treatments. Int J Surg Pathol. 17(3):206-18, 2009
3. Stinchcombe TE et al: Current treatments for advanced stage non-small cell lung cancer. Proc Am Thorac Soc. 6(2):233-41, 2009
4. Ro JY et al: Sarcomatoid carcinoma of the lung. Immunohistochemical and ultrastructural studies of 14 cases. Cancer. 69(2):376-86, 1992
5. Matsui K et al: Spindle cell carcinoma of the lung. A clinicopathologic study of three cases. Cancer. 67(9):2361-7, 1991
6. Humphrey PA et al: Pulmonary carcinomas with a sarcomatoid element: an immunocytochemical and ultrastructural analysis. Hum Pathol. 19(2):155-65, 1988
7. Suster S et al: Spindle cell squamous carcinoma of the lung. Immunocytochemical and ultrastructural study of a case. Histopathology. 11(8):871-8, 1987

Microscopic Features

*(**Left**) Sarcomatoid carcinoma ⮳ of the lung shows a tumor that is well circumscribed but not encapsulated. Note that toward the periphery there is the presence of normal lung parenchyma ⇨. (**Right**) Sarcomatoid squamous cell carcinoma shows malignant spindle cell proliferation composed of elongated cells with marked nuclear atypia. Note the presence of a residual normal endobronchial gland ⇨.*

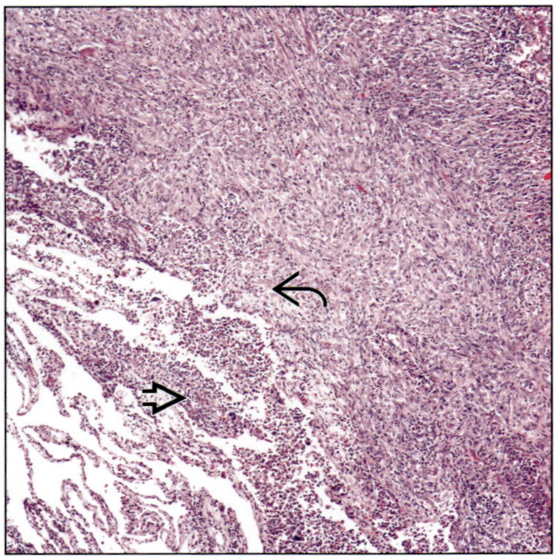

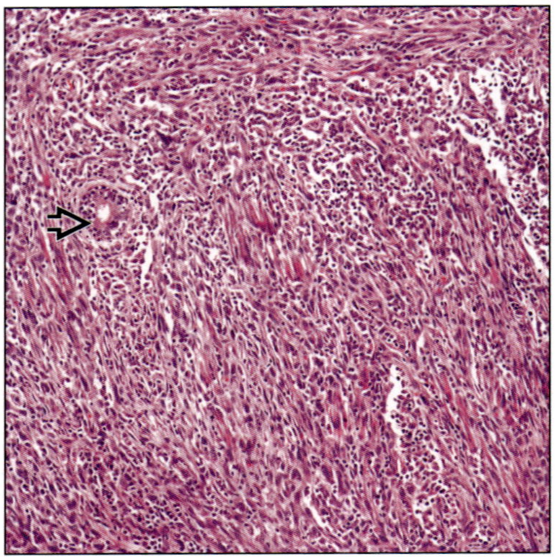

*(**Left**) Malignant spindle cell proliferation in a sarcomatoid squamous cell carcinoma of the lung is admixed with an inflammatory component composed of lymphocytes and plasma cells →. (**Right**) Malignant spindle cell proliferation with residual dilated alveolar structures →. It is important to recognize these entrapped structures and not interpret them as part of the tumor, which may lead to the erroneous diagnosis of a biphasic neoplasm.*

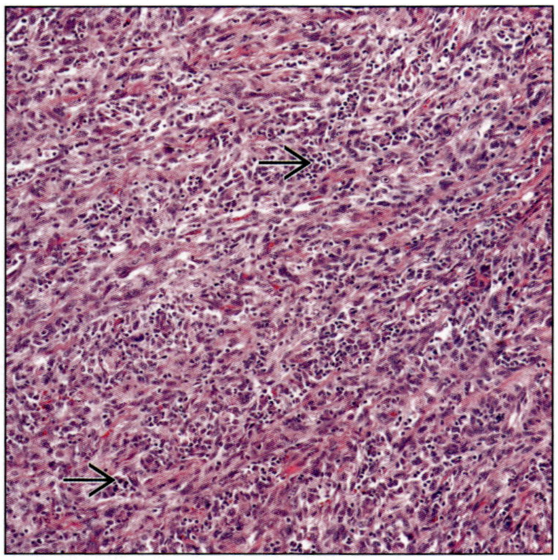

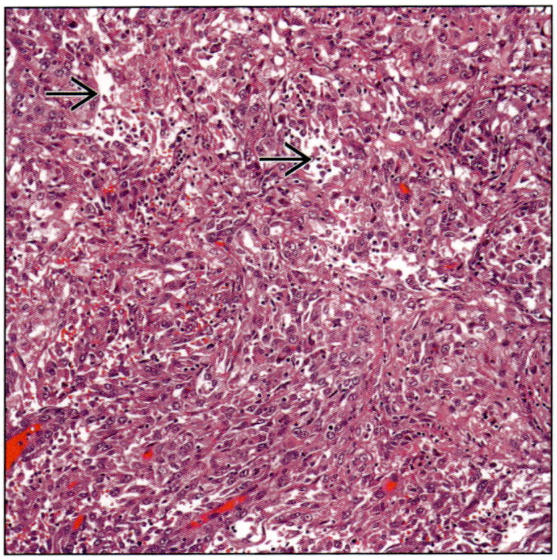

*(**Left**) Extensive presence of abundant red cells deposited in dilated spaces mimics a vascular neoplasm in sarcomatoid squamous cell carcinoma of the lung. Note the presence of a malignant spindle cell component admixed with the red cells. (**Right**) Malignant spindle cell proliferation composed of elongated cells with atypical nuclei and some cells with prominent nucleoli, admixed with red cells ⮳ and dilated vascular spaces →, mimics a vascular neoplasm.*

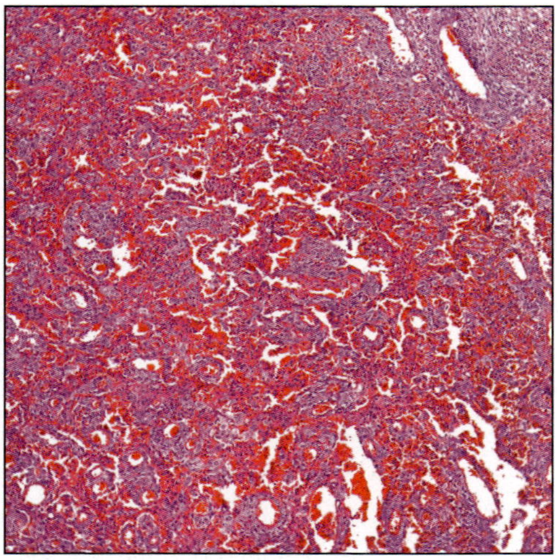

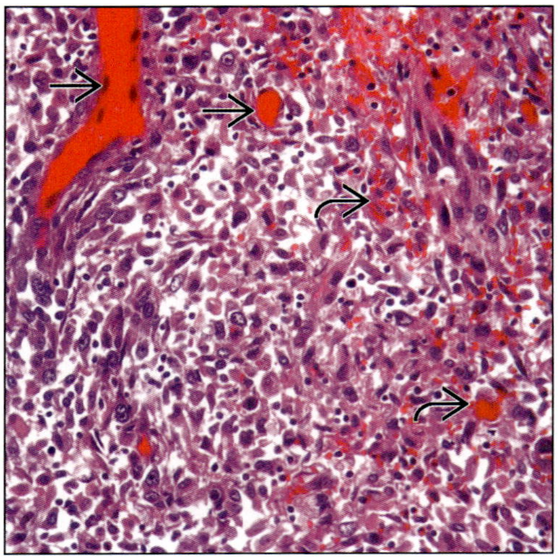

SPINDLE CELL (SARCOMATOID) CARCINOMA

Microscopic Features

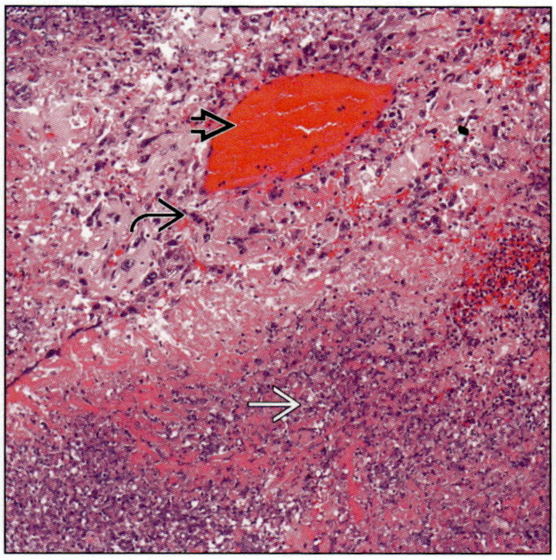
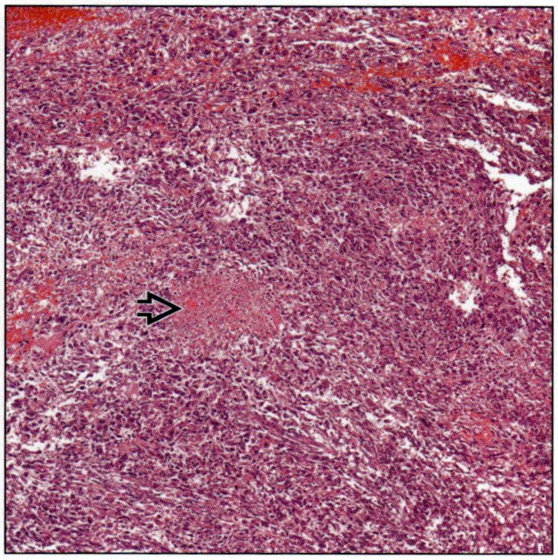

(Left) *Dilated vascular space ⇨ surrounded by malignant spindle cells ↪ and extensive necrosis ➡ are seen in this sarcomatoid squamous cell carcinoma of the lung. This pattern can easily imitate a vascular neoplasm.* ***(Right)*** *Malignant spindle cell proliferation without any specific growth pattern and focal areas of necrosis ⇨. A similar feature may be seen in other poorly differentiated carcinomas of the lung.*

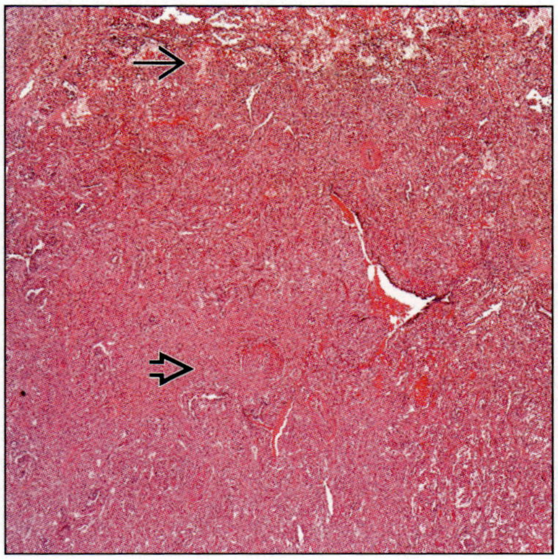
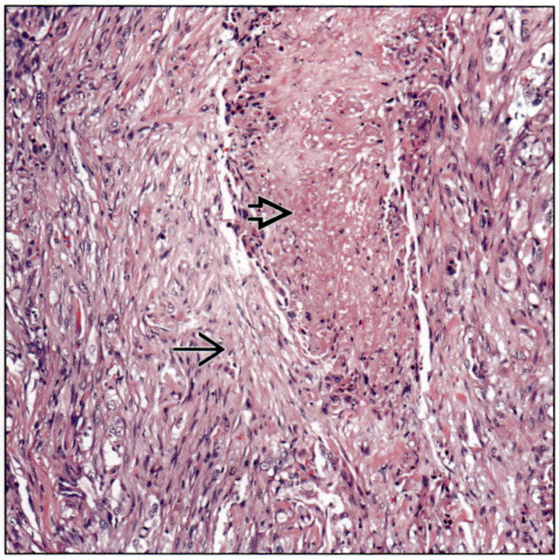

(Left) *Malignant spindle cell proliferation ⇨ clearly delineated from normal lung parenchyma → is seen in a sarcomatoid squamous cell carcinoma. However, at this power, this growth pattern can be confused with an organizing pneumonia.* ***(Right)*** *Sarcomatoid carcinoma shows a neoplastic proliferation of elongated cells → admixed with areas of necrosis ⇨. The latter is a common feature in these tumors.*

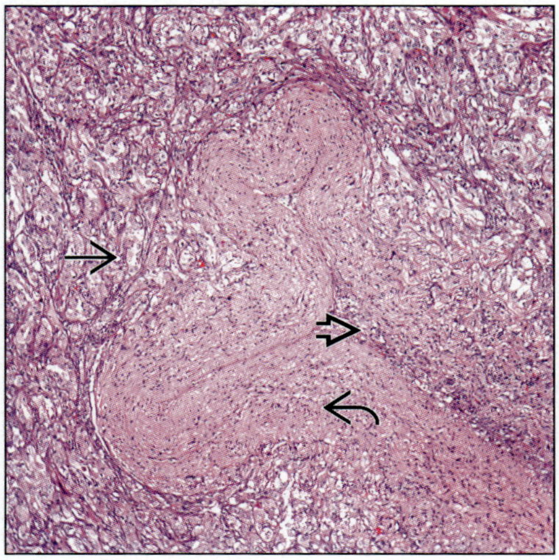
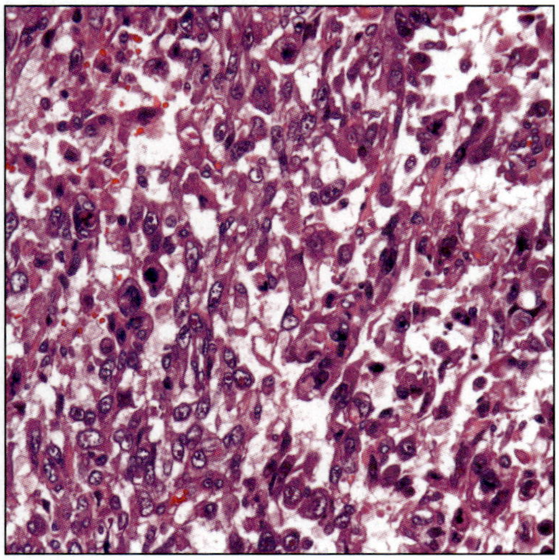

(Left) *Sarcomatoid carcinoma → involving and compressing a large vessel ↪. There is vascular permeation ⇨ of the tumor.* ***(Right)*** *Higher magnification of the spindle cell component in a sarcomatoid squamous cell carcinoma of the lung shows marked cellular and nuclear atypia.*

LYMPHOEPITHELIOMA-LIKE CARCINOMA

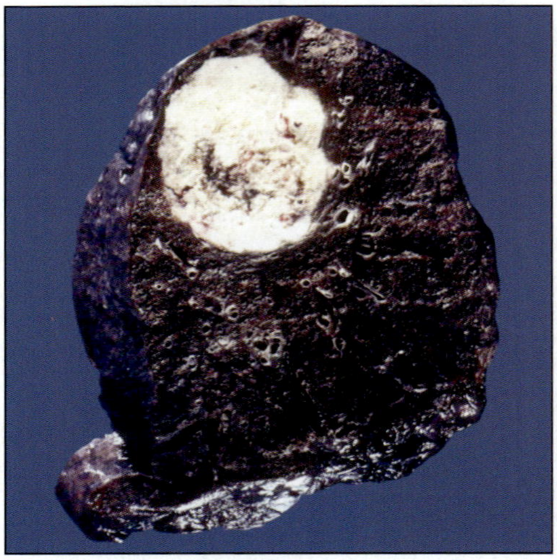

Gross photograph of a lymphoepithelial-like carcinoma shows a well-circumscribed intrapulmonary mass with focal central necrosis. The tumor has a peripheral subpleural location.

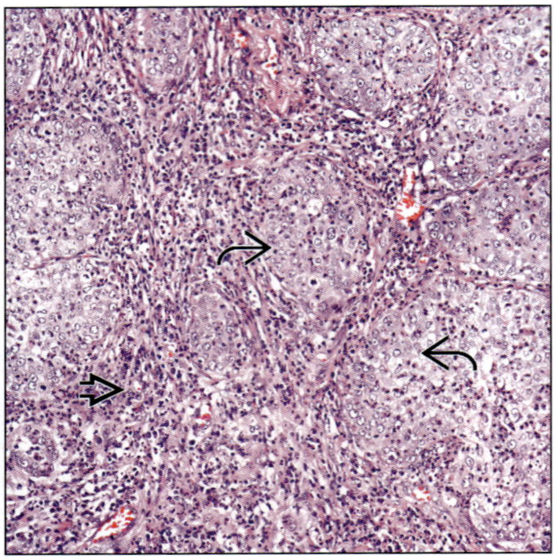

LELC of the lung shows the classic appearance of clusters of neoplastic cells ⮫ surrounded by a prominent inflammatory background ⇨.

TERMINOLOGY

Abbreviations

- Lymphoepithelioma-like carcinoma (LELC)

Definitions

- Malignant epithelial neoplasm with prominent inflammatory component

ETIOLOGY/PATHOGENESIS

Environmental Exposure

- Appears not to be related to tobacco smoke

Infectious Agents

- Closely associated with Epstein-Barr virus (EBV) infection
- More common in people of Asian background though also described in Caucasians

CLINICAL ISSUES

Presentation

- Cough
- Hemoptysis
- Difficulty breathing
- Chest pain
- Weight loss

Treatment

- Surgical approaches
  - Lobectomy
- Adjuvant therapy
  - Chemotherapy or radiation therapy may be used depending on stage

Prognosis

- Depends on stage at time of diagnosis

MACROSCOPIC FEATURES

General Features

- Tumor may be in central or peripheral location
- Essentially indistinguishable from other non-small cell carcinomas
- Necrosis is common finding

Size

- Tumors may vary in size and may be > 10 cm

MICROSCOPIC PATHOLOGY

Histologic Features

- Large epithelial cells with scant cytoplasm and vesicular nuclei
- Lobulated pattern of growth
- Cells with round to oval nuclei and prominent nucleoli
- Nuclear atypia and increased mitotic activity
- Prominent inflammatory background
- Lymphocytes and plasma cells easily identified
- EBER studies are positive in tumor cells

Predominant Pattern/Injury Type

- Mixed
- Inflammatory

Predominant Cell/Compartment Type

- Epithelial

DIFFERENTIAL DIAGNOSIS

Metastatic Nasopharyngeal Carcinoma

- Identical histological features to counterpart in head and neck
- Clinical history &/or physical examination play important role in determining primary site
- Immunohistochemical features may be similar

LYMPHOEPITHELIOMA-LIKE CARCINOMA

Key Facts

Terminology
- Lymphoepithelioma-like carcinoma (LELC)
  - Malignant epithelial neoplasm with prominent inflammatory component

Etiology/Pathogenesis
- Appears not to be related to tobacco smoke
- Closely associated with Epstein-Barr virus (EBV) infection
- More common in people of Asian background though also described in Caucasians

Microscopic Pathology
- Inflammatory
- Epithelial
- Malignant epithelial component embedded in inflammatory background composed predominantly of lymphocytes and plasma cells

Top Differential Diagnoses
- Metastatic nasopharyngeal carcinoma
  - Identical histological features to counterpart in head and neck
  - Clinical history &/or physical examination play important role in determining primary site
- Large cell carcinoma
  - Presence of prominent inflammatory component should raise suspicion of LELC

Diagnostic Checklist
- Histological features similar to nasopharyngeal carcinoma (Schmincke tumor)

Immunohistochemistry

Antibody	Reactivity	Staining Pattern	Comment
KERATIN-LMW	Positive	Cytoplasmic	
EMA/MUC1	Positive	Cell membrane	
Bcl-2	Positive	Cytoplasmic	Inflammatory component
p53	Positive	Cytoplasmic	
CD15	Positive	Cytoplasmic	Inflammatory component
CK8/18/CAM5.2	Positive	Cytoplasmic	
CK7	Positive	Cytoplasmic	
TTF-1	Negative		Focal positive nuclear staining is found in some cases

In Situ Hybridization

Probe	Type	Result	Interpretation	Comment
EBER	FISH	Positive	Cell membrane	In epithelial component as well as in inflammatory component

Large Cell Carcinoma
- Presence of prominent inflammatory component should raise suspicion of LELC
- Will display sheets of large neoplastic cells with prominent nucleoli
- Extensive areas of necrosis &/or hemorrhage commonly seen

DIAGNOSTIC CHECKLIST

Pathologic Interpretation Pearls
- Histological features similar to nasopharyngeal carcinoma (Schmincke tumor)
- Prominent inflammatory background
- Lymphocytes and plasma cells easily identified
- Histological features of large cell carcinoma
- EBER positive

SELECTED REFERENCES

1. Hoxworth JM et al: Lymphoepithelioma-like carcinoma of the lung: radiologic features of an uncommon primary pulmonary neoplasm. AJR Am J Roentgenol. 186(5):1294-9, 2006
2. Ho JC et al: Lymphoepithelioma-like carcinoma of the lung: experience with ten cases. Int J Tuberc Lung Dis. 8(7):890-5, 2004
3. Kobayashi M et al: Pulmonary lymphoepithelioma-like carcinoma: predominant infiltration of tumor-associated cytotoxic T lymphocytes might represent the enhanced tumor immunity. Intern Med. 43(4):323-6, 2004
4. Han AJ et al: Lymphoepithelioma-like carcinoma of the lung with a better prognosis. A clinicopathologic study of 32 cases. Am J Clin Pathol. 115(6):841-50, 2001
5. Chan JK et al: Primary lymphoepithelioma-like carcinoma of the lung. A clinicopathologic study of 11 cases. Cancer. 76(3):413-22, 1995
6. Gal AA et al: Detection of Epstein-Barr virus in lymphoepithelioma-like carcinoma of the lung. Mod Pathol. 4(2):264-8, 1991
7. Bégin LR et al: Epstein-Barr virus related lymphoepithelioma-like carcinoma of lung. J Surg Oncol. 36(4):280-3, 1987

LYMPHOEPITHELIOMA-LIKE CARCINOMA

Microscopic Features

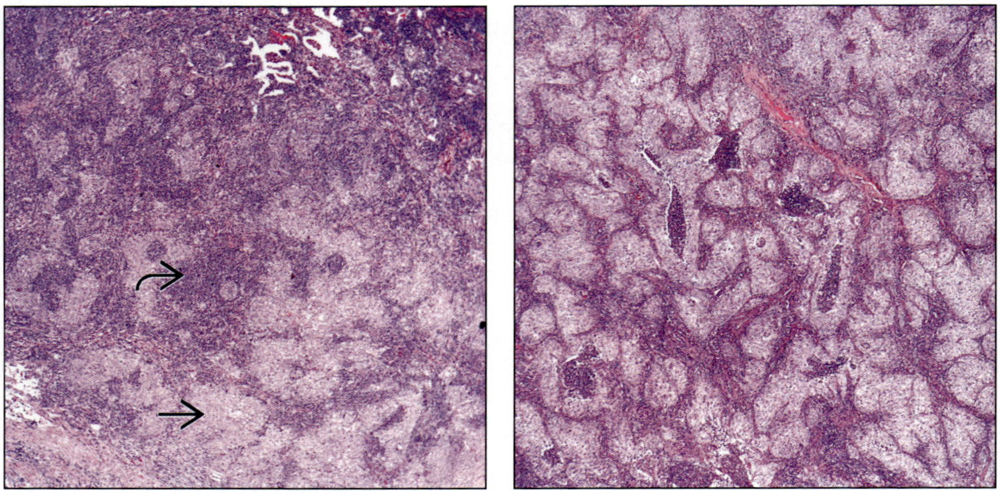

(Left) *Malignant epithelial cells → surrounded by prominent inflammatory background ↷. At this magnification, one can easily miss the malignant epithelial component as a reactive process.* ***(Right)*** *Malignant epithelial cells growing in a vague micro-acinar pattern. At this higher magnification, the difference between the epithelial and the inflammatory component is easily demonstrated.*

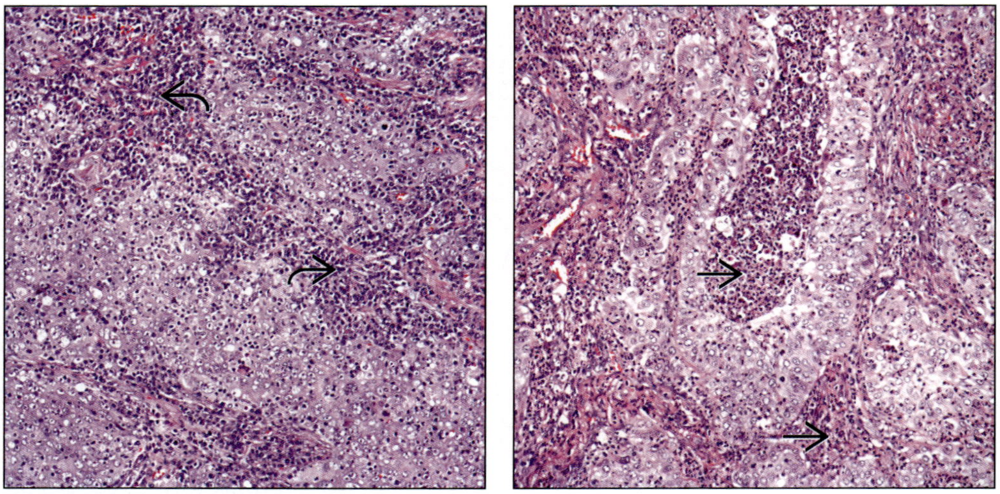

(Left) *LELC of the lung shows sheets of neoplastic cells growing in a rather nonspecific growth pattern. However, important to note is the presence of a marked inflammatory background ↷.* ***(Right)*** *Malignant epithelial cells in a vague pseudoglandular arrangement. Note the presence of inflammatory cells, predominantly lymphocytes →, in the lumen of this pseudogland mimicking comedo-like necrosis.*

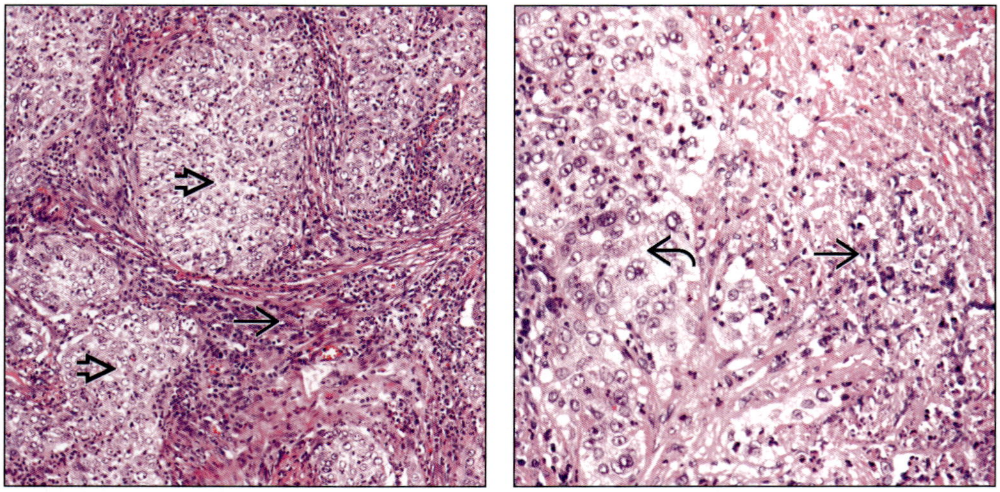

(Left) *Islands of malignant epithelial cells ⇨ of different sizes are separated by fibroconnective tissue with a prominent inflammatory background →.* ***(Right)*** *Despite the presence of a prominent inflammatory background, extensive areas of necrosis are not that common in LELC. However, in some cases, focal areas of necrosis → may obscure the neoplastic process ↷.*

Microscopic Features

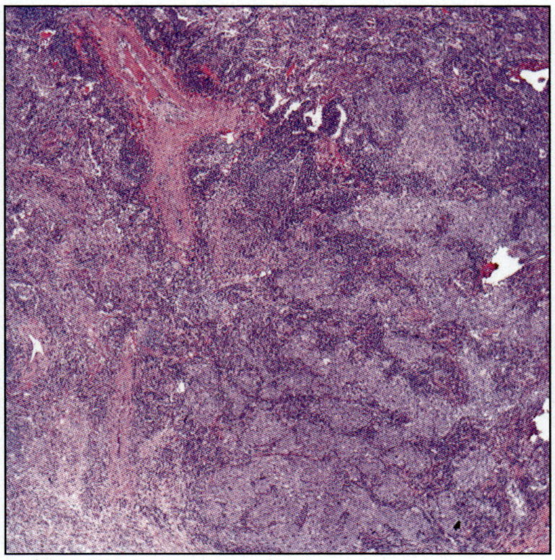

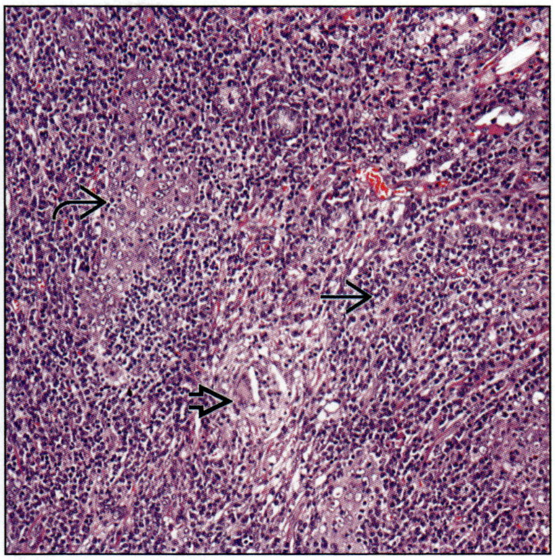

(Left) *Mixture of islands of malignant cells admixed with a prominent inflammatory background are seen, probably representing an organizing pneumonia associated with the tumor.* ***(Right)*** *A cluster of neoplastic cells is admixed with a marked inflammatory background. The inflammatory background is marked by the presence of giant cells.*

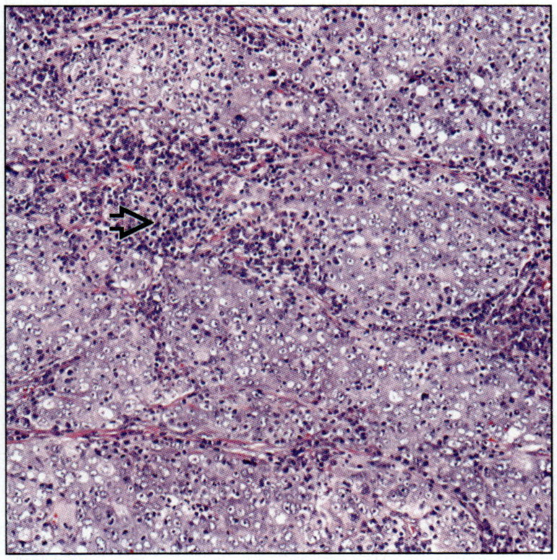

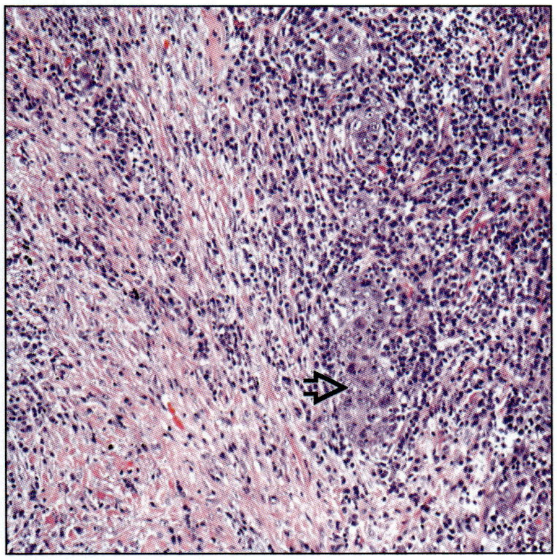

(Left) *Discrete inflammatory background in LELC. The neoplastic component does not show any particular growth pattern.* ***(Right)*** *Predominantly inflammatory component is seen in this LELC. Note the presence of small islands of neoplastic cells. In some cases in which the inflammatory component is marked, the neoplastic process may be missed.*

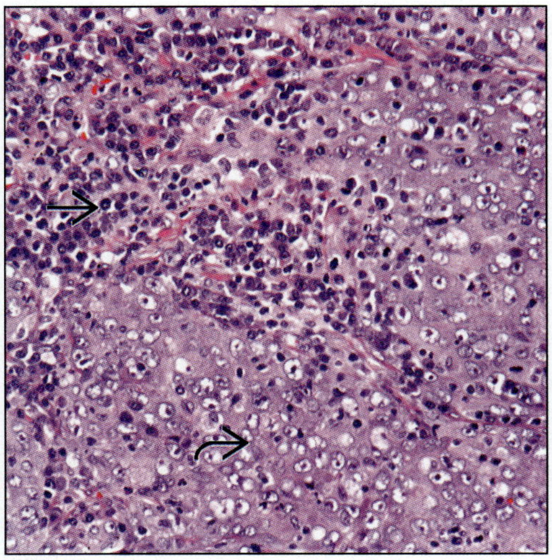

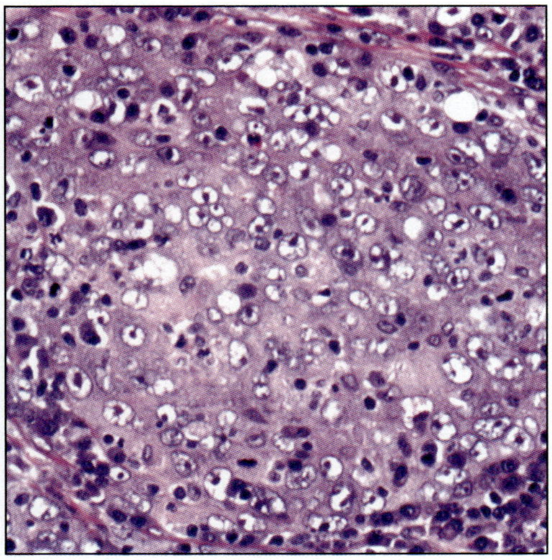

(Left) *Higher magnification of an LELC of the lung shows the 2 components in more detail, clearly highlighting the epithelial component from the inflammatory component.* ***(Right)*** *High-power view of the epithelial neoplastic component in LELC of the lung. The cells are round to oval with indistinct cell membranes, ample cytoplasm, round to oval nuclei, and prominent nucleoli.*

POORLY DIFFERENTIATED SQUAMOUS CARCINOMA, SMALL CELL VARIANT

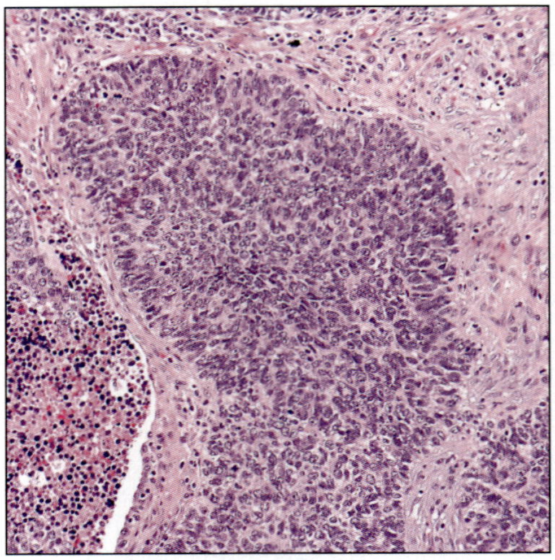

Scanning magnification of small cell variant of poorly differentiated squamous cell carcinoma of the lung shows an island of small tumor cells with peripheral palisading of nuclei.

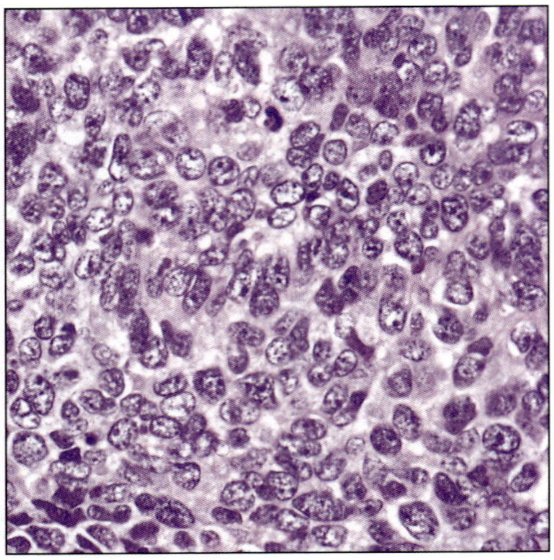

High magnification of small cell variant of poorly differentiated squamous cell carcinoma of the lung shows monotonous round tumor cells with hyperchromatic nuclei and a scant rim of cytoplasm.

TERMINOLOGY

Definitions

- Poorly differentiated squamous cell carcinoma exhibiting small cell morphology and lacking overt features of squamous differentiation

CLINICAL ISSUES

Presentation

- Cough
- Chest pain
- Weight loss
- History of cigarette smoking

Treatment

- Options, risks, complications
  - Treatment by surgery, chemotherapy, or radiation depends on stage and grade at presentation
- Surgical approaches
  - Lobectomy and lymph node dissection
- Adjuvant therapy
  - Combination chemotherapy for advanced stages

Prognosis

- Depends on grade and stage at presentation; generally poor

IMAGE FINDINGS

General Features

- Best diagnostic clue
  - Peripheral spiculated pulmonary nodule in a smoker
  - Hilar and mediastinal lymphadenopathy
  - Bronchial stenosis and associated atelectasis

MACROSCOPIC FEATURES

General Features

- Well-circumscribed, tan-white mass
- Foci of hemorrhage and necrosis
- Intraparenchymatous; unrelated to major bronchi

Sections to Be Submitted

- 1 section per cm of largest tumor diameter

Size

- 4-5 cm

MICROSCOPIC PATHOLOGY

Histologic Features

- Islands, sheets, and cords of monotonous small, hyperchromatic tumor cells
- Tumor cell islands may display prominent basaloid peripheral palisading of nuclei
- Tumor cell islands may show prominent central, comedo-like areas of necrosis
- Tumor cell cords and islands may be separated by prominent desmoplastic stroma with lymphoid cell infiltrates
- Tumor cell islands may be separated by geographic, irregular areas of necrosis
- Tumors can show evidence of vascular and perineural invasion

Cytologic Features

- Cells have large, hyperchromatic nuclei with dense chromatin pattern and prominent nucleoli
- Cells can be round, polygonal, or ovoid and display a conspicuous rim of cytoplasm with distinct cell borders
- Tumors may show scattered single-cell keratinization or abortive foci of squamous differentiation
- Tumors can display high mitotic activity (> 10 mitoses per 10 HPF)

POORLY DIFFERENTIATED SQUAMOUS CARCINOMA, SMALL CELL VARIANT

Key Facts

Clinical Issues

- Cough
- History of cigarette smoking
- Treatment by surgery, chemotherapy, or radiation depends on stage and grade at presentation

Image Findings

- Peripheral spiculated pulmonary nodule in a smoker

Microscopic Pathology

- Islands, sheets, and cords of monotonous small, hyperchromatic tumor cells
- Tumor cell islands may display prominent basaloid peripheral palisading of nuclei
- Cells have large, hyperchromatic nuclei with dense chromatin pattern and prominent nucleoli
- Cells can be round, polygonal, or ovoid and display a conspicuous rim of cytoplasm with distinct cell borders
- Tumor cells are positive for broad-spectrum cytokeratin and MOC31
- Tumor cells are weakly and focally positive for CK7
- Tumor cells are uniformly negative for neuroendocrine markers including chromogranin-A, synaptophysin, CD56, and NSE
- Tumor cells are negative for TTF-1, CK20, and CEA

Diagnostic Checklist

- Possibility of metastasis from a basaloid-squamous cell carcinoma of the oral cavity or head and neck region should always be ruled out 1st

ANCILLARY TESTS

Immunohistochemistry

- Tumor cells
  - Positive for broad-spectrum cytokeratin and MOC31
  - Weakly and focally positive for CK7
  - Uniformly negative for neuroendocrine markers including chromogranin-A, synaptophysin, CD56, and NSE
  - Negative for TTF-1, CK20, and CEA
  - May display p63 nuclear staining, which is usually restricted to periphery of basaloid tumor islands

Electron Microscopy

- Tumor cells contain desmosomes and tonofilaments
- Tumor cells do not display cytoplasmic dense-core neurosecretory granules

DIFFERENTIAL DIAGNOSIS

Small Cell Neuroendocrine Carcinoma

- Nuclei show "smudged" nuclear chromatin pattern with little nuclear detail and small or inconspicuous nucleoli
- Only scant rim of cytoplasm surrounding nuclei
- Stains positive for neuroendocrine markers (chromogranin, synaptophysin, CD56, and NSE)
- Shows strong, dot-like paranuclear positivity for CK7

Moderately Differentiated Neuroendocrine Carcinoma ("Atypical Carcinoid")

- Morphologically, may be virtually indistinguishable from small cell variant of squamous cell carcinoma
- Strong positivity for neuroendocrine markers (chromogranin-A, synaptophysin, CD56, and NSE)

Large Cell Neuroendocrine Carcinoma

- Morphologically, large cell neuroendocrine carcinoma may be indistinguishable from small cell variant of squamous cell carcinoma
- Most important feature is positivity for neuroendocrine markers (chromogranin, synaptophysin, CD56, and NSE)

Combined Small Cell Carcinoma

- Shows admixture of small cell neuroendocrine carcinoma and squamous cell carcinoma
- Small cell component will express neuroendocrine markers by immunohistochemistry

Metastasis from Basaloid-Squamous Cell Carcinoma of Head and Neck

- Morphologically may be indistinguishable from small cell variant of pulmonary squamous cell carcinoma
- Immunohistochemical features will be indistinguishable from small cell variant of pulmonary squamous cell carcinoma
- Obtaining a clinical history of previous tumor in the oral cavity or head and neck region is indispensable for diagnosis

DIAGNOSTIC CHECKLIST

Clinically Relevant Pathologic Features

- Tumors have similar biologic behavior as conventional squamous cell carcinoma and should not be mistaken for small cell neuroendocrine carcinoma
- Possibility of metastasis from a basaloid-squamous cell carcinoma of the oral cavity or head and neck region should always be ruled out 1st

SELECTED REFERENCES

1. Hammar S: The use of electron microscopy and immunohistochemistry in the diagnosis and understanding of lung neoplasms. Clin Lab Med. 7(1):1-30, 1987
2. Churg A et al: Small cell squamous and mixed small cell squamous--small cell anaplastic carcinomas of the lung. Am J Surg Pathol. 4(3):255-63, 1980

POORLY DIFFERENTIATED SQUAMOUS CARCINOMA, SMALL CELL VARIANT

General Histologic Features

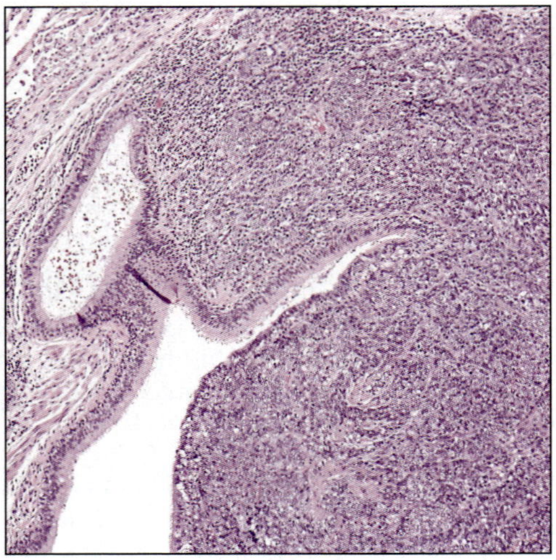
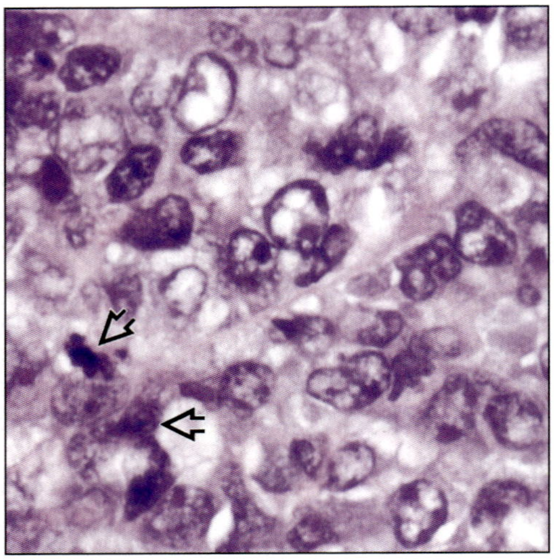

(Left) *Scanning magnification of small cell variant of poorly differentiated squamous cell carcinoma of the lung shows solid sheets of monotonous tumor cells arising from a subsegmental bronchus.* ***(Right)*** *High magnification of small cell variant of poorly differentiated squamous cell carcinoma of the lung shows sheets of tumor cells with round, often vesicular nuclei, prominent nucleoli, and a scant rim of amphophilic cytoplasm. The tumor shows scattered mitotic figures ➢.*

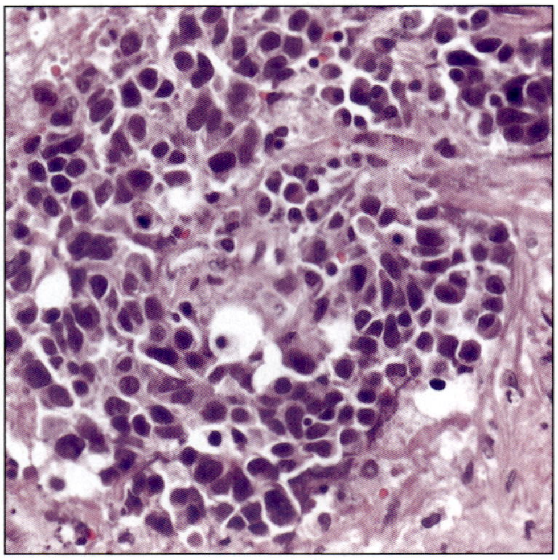
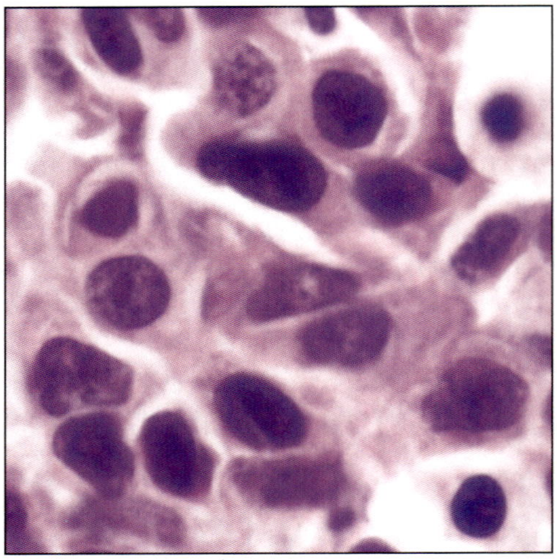

(Left) *High magnification of small cell variant of poorly differentiated squamous cell carcinoma of the lung shows an island of monotonous, relatively small tumor cells without obvious features of keratinization but with large, hyperchromatic nuclei showing abundant eosinophilic cytoplasm.* ***(Right)*** *Higher magnification of small cell variant of poorly differentiated squamous cell carcinoma shows round to oval nuclei with dense chromatin, occasional prominent nucleoli, and abundant cytoplasm.*

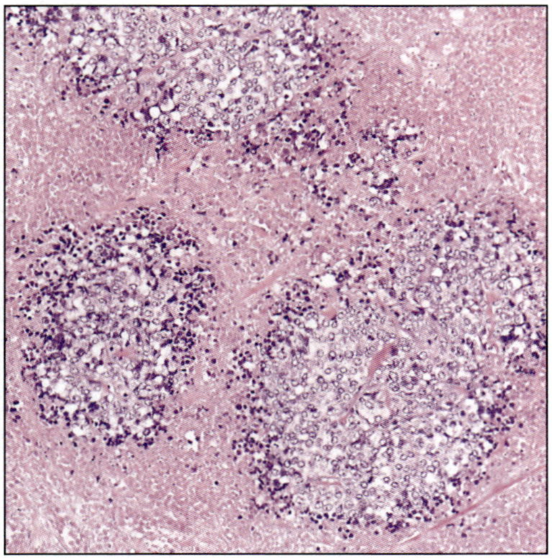
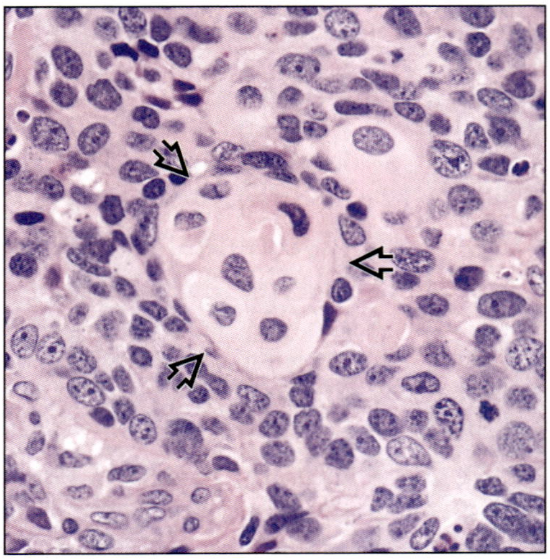

(Left) *Small cell variant of poorly differentiated squamous cell carcinoma of the lung shows perivascular tumor islands surrounded by irregular, geographic areas of necrosis.* ***(Right)*** *Small cell variant of poorly differentiated squamous cell carcinoma of the lung shows sheets of small tumor cells surrounding a central focus displaying features of abortive squamous differentiation ➢, which contains larger cells with more abundant cytoplasm, sharp cell borders, and cell moulding.*

Histologic Growth Patterns

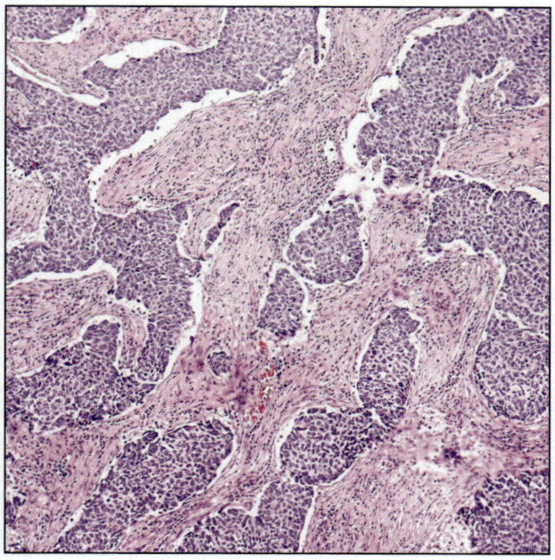
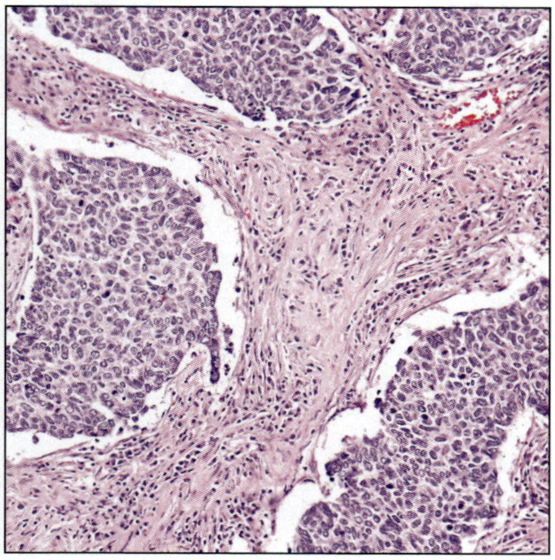

(Left) *Scanning magnification of small cell variant of poorly differentiated squamous cell carcinoma of the lung shows cords and islands of tumor cells separated by abundant desmoplastic stroma. Tumors with these features can be mistaken for large cell neuroendocrine carcinoma and atypical carcinoid.* ***(Right)*** *Higher magnification of small cell variant of poorly differentiated squamous cell carcinoma of the lung shows collagenized stroma with chronic inflammation.*

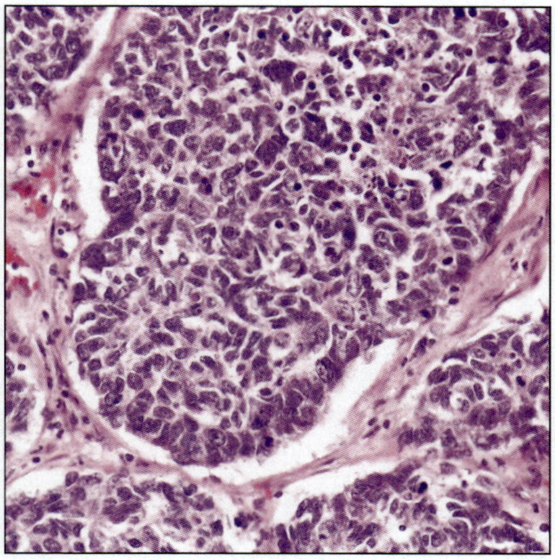
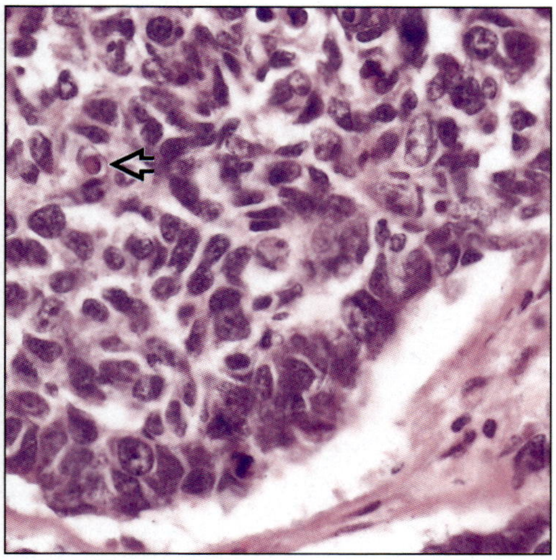

(Left) *Small cell variant of poorly differentiated squamous cell carcinoma of the lung shows a basaloid tumor cell island composed of monotonous proliferation of relatively small tumor cells with peripheral palisading of nuclei.* ***(Right)*** *Higher magnification of small cell variant of poorly differentiated squamous cell carcinoma of the lung highlights a primitive-appearing tumor cell population with scattered mitoses and occasional foci of single-cell keratinization ⇨.*

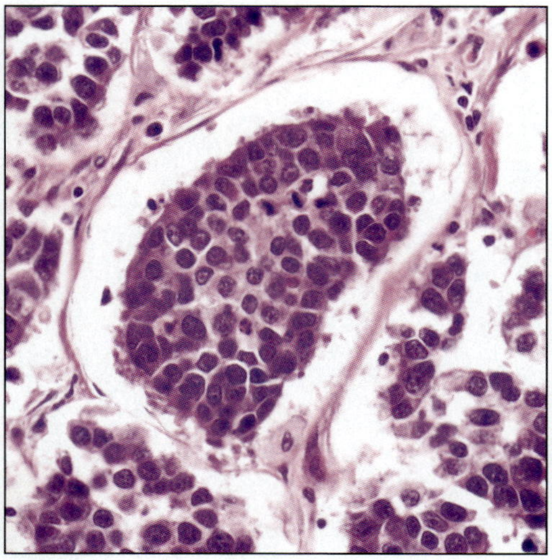
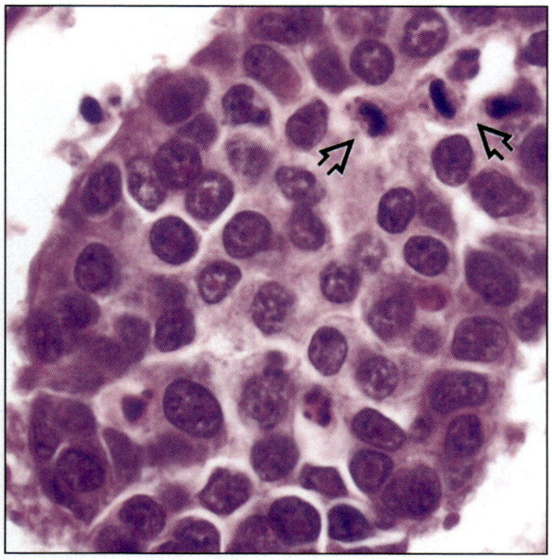

(Left) *Small islands of monotonous tumor cells are seen in the small cell variant of poorly differentiated squamous cell carcinoma of the lung infiltrating into adjacent alveolar spaces at the edges of the tumor.* ***(Right)*** *Higher magnification of a tumor cell island in small cell variant of poorly differentiated squamous cell carcinoma of the lung shows cells with hyperchromatic nuclei, prominent nucleoli, and abundant cytoplasm. Notice the cell moulding and the scattered mitoses ⇨.*

POORLY DIFFERENTIATED SQUAMOUS CARCINOMA, SMALL CELL VARIANT

Histologic Growth Patterns

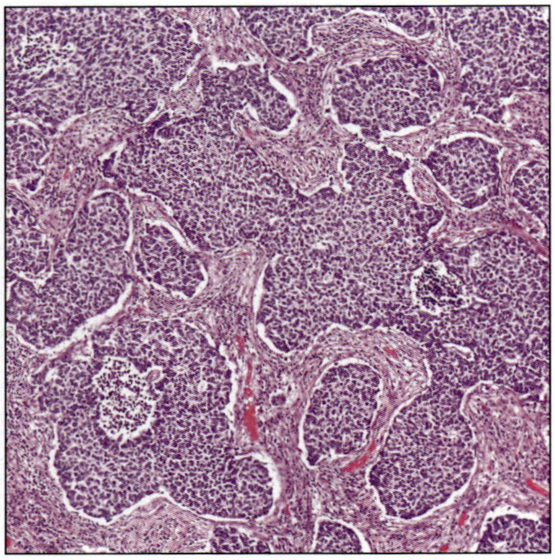

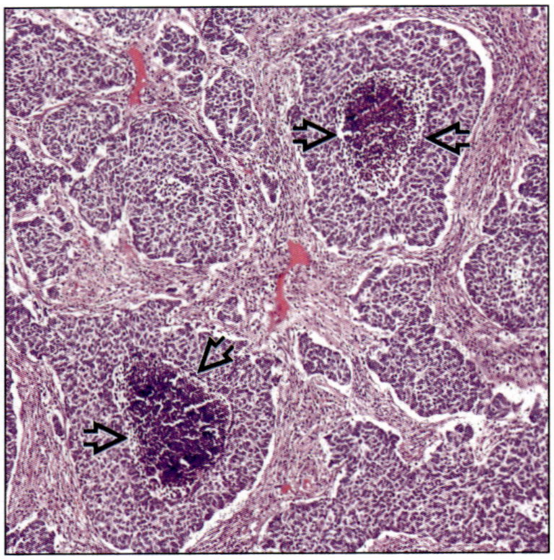

(Left) *Scanning magnification of small cell variant of poorly differentiated squamous cell carcinoma of the lung shows islands of small tumor cells separated by abundant desmoplastic stroma.* **(Right)** *Scanning magnification of small cell variant of poorly differentiated squamous cell carcinoma of the lung shows tumor cell islands separated by desmoplastic stroma. Notice the foci of comedo-like central necrosis displayed in 2 of the tumor cell islands ⇨.*

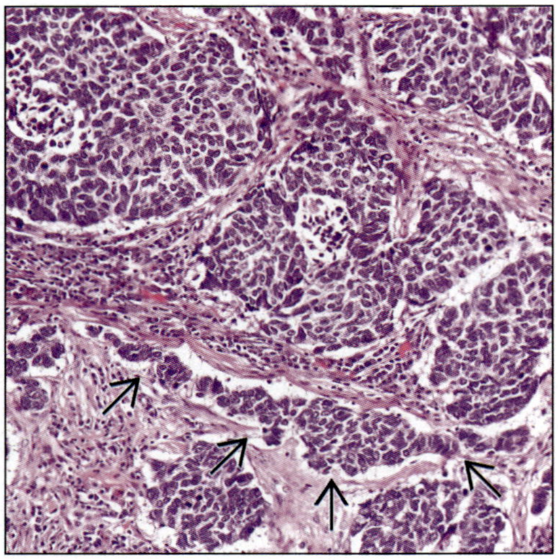

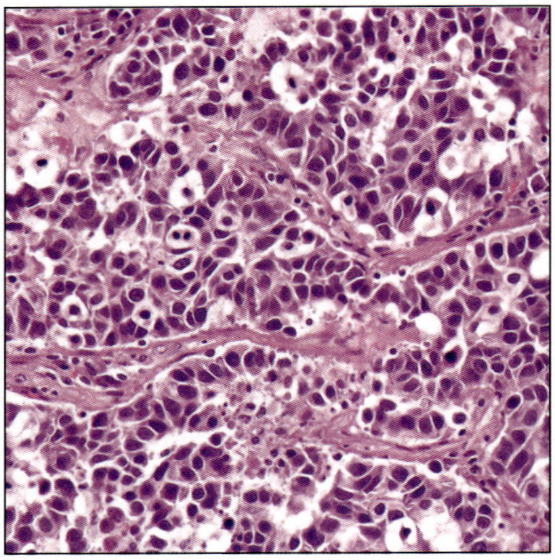

(Left) *Scanning magnification of small cell variant of poorly differentiated squamous cell carcinoma of the lung shows basaloid islands of monotonous tumor cells along with cord-like trabecular formation →.* **(Right)** *Small cell variant of a poorly differentiated squamous cell carcinoma of the lung shows a trabecular growth pattern with cord-like strands of monotonous small round tumor cells with hyperchromatic nuclei and abundant cytoplasm, closely simulating a neuroendocrine carcinoma.*

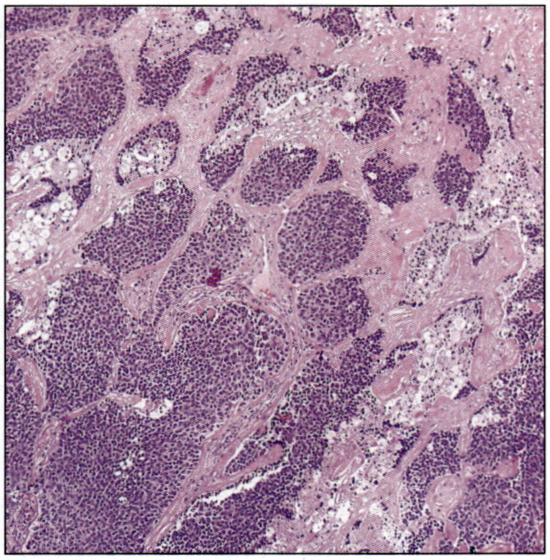

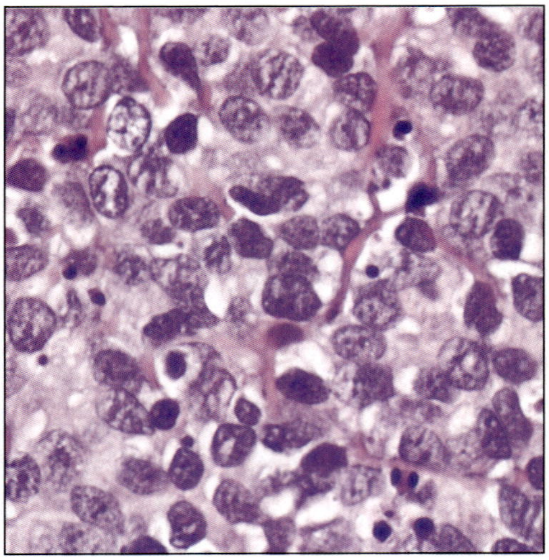

(Left) *Scanning magnification of a small cell variant of poorly differentiated squamous cell carcinoma of the lung shows small islands of uniform tumor cells separated by hyalinized connective tissue stroma.* **(Right)** *Higher magnification from an island of tumor cells in the small cell variant of poorly differentiated squamous cell carcinoma of the lung shows a primitive population of small tumor cells with hyperchromatic nuclei and a moderate rim of cytoplasm.*

Immunohistochemical Staining

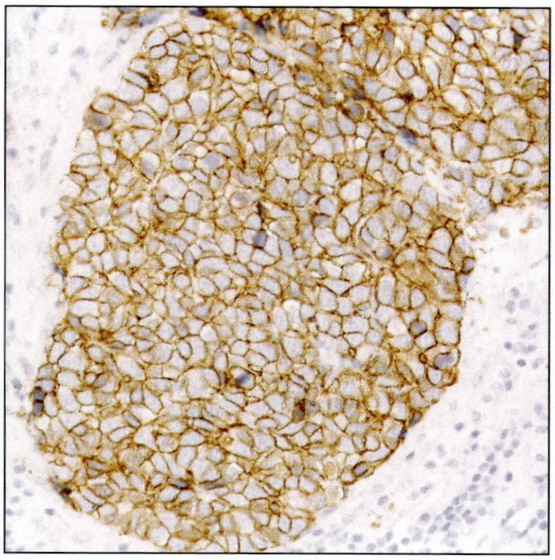

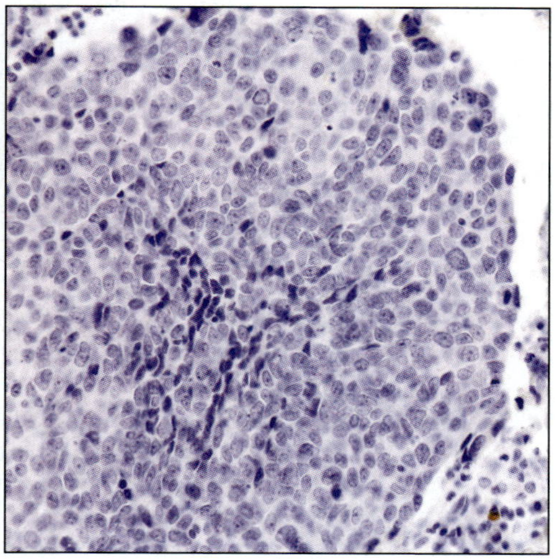

(Left) *Immunohistochemical staining for cytokeratin AE1/AE3 in the small cell variant of poorly differentiated squamous cell carcinoma of the lung shows strong positivity of the tumor cells for this antigen.* ***(Right)*** *Immunohistochemical staining for chromogranin-A in a small cell variant of poorly differentiated squamous cell carcinoma of the lung shows a negative reaction. Other neuroendocrine markers such as synaptophysin, CD56, and NSE are also negative.*

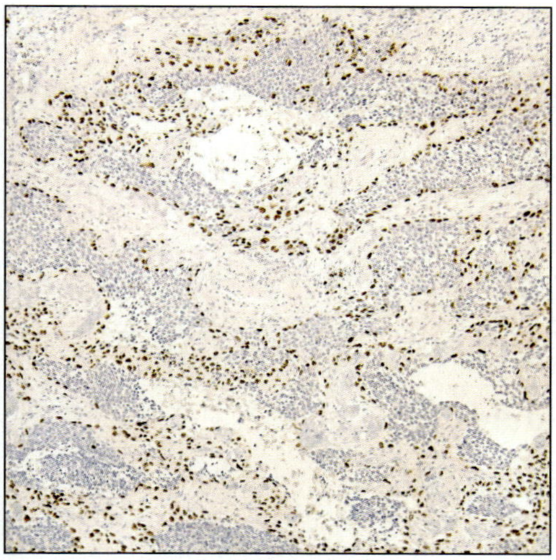

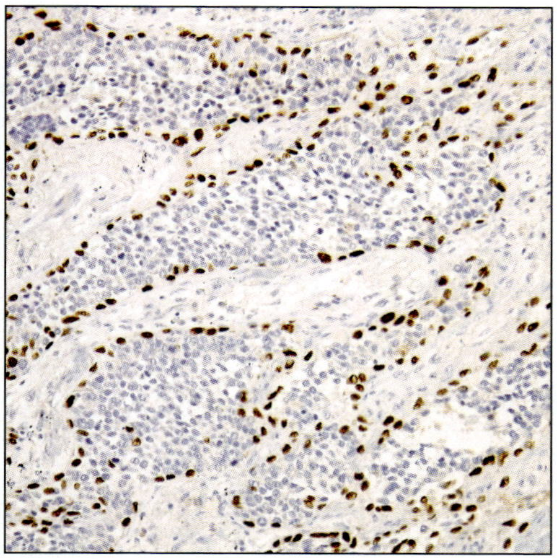

(Left) *Immunohistochemical staining for p63 in a small cell variant of poorly differentiated squamous cell carcinoma of the lung with prominent basaloid features shows a distinctive pattern of staining restricted to the periphery of the basaloid islands.* ***(Right)*** *Higher magnification of immunohistochemical staining of a small cell variant of poorly differentiated squamous cell carcinoma shows nuclear staining with p63 only in the periphery of the tumor cell islands.*

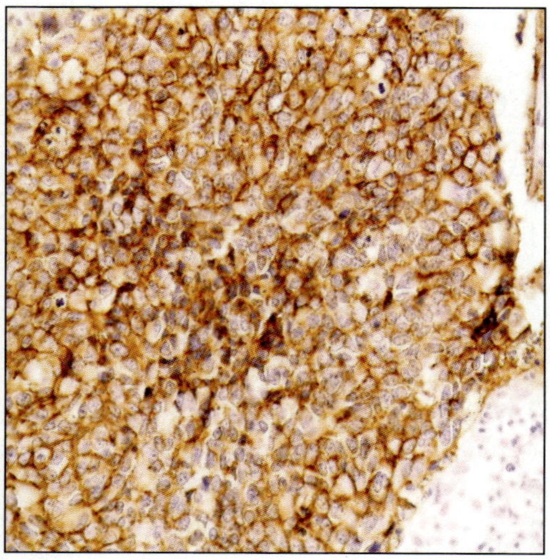

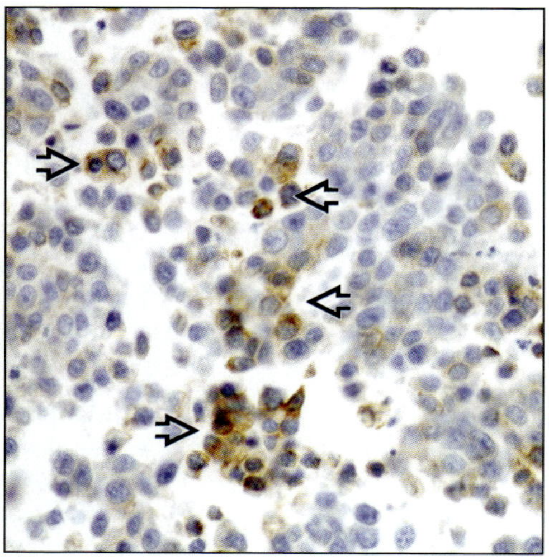

(Left) *Immunohistochemical staining of a small cell variant of poorly differentiated squamous cell carcinoma of the lung for MOC31 shows strong positivity of the tumor cells for this marker.* ***(Right)*** *Immunohistochemical staining of a small cell variant of poorly differentiated squamous cell carcinoma of the lung for CK7 shows focal, weak positivity of the tumor cells for this antigen ⇨. Staining for CK7 is usually weak and focal in these tumors.*

LARGE CELL (ANAPLASTIC) CARCINOMA

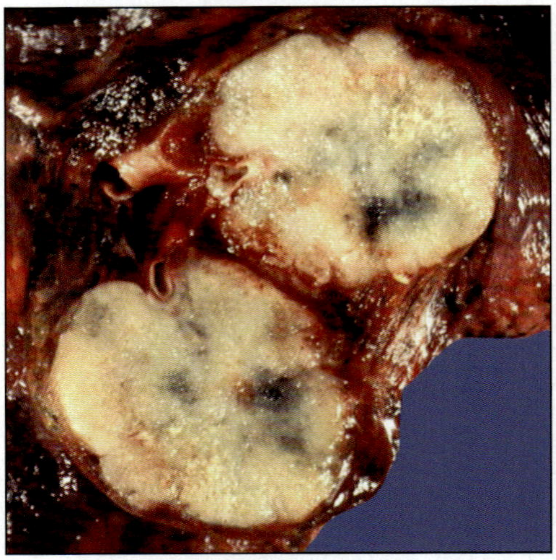

Cut surface shows gross appearance of large cell (anaplastic) carcinoma of the lung characterized by a large, well-circumscribed, tan-cream tumor with foci of hemorrhage and necrosis.

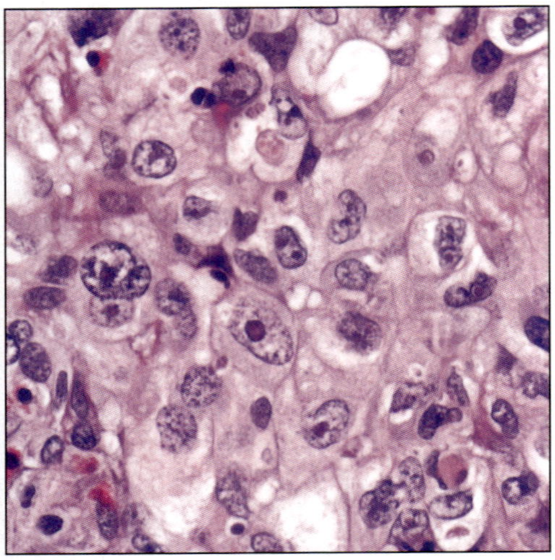

Histologic appearance of large cell (anaplastic) carcinoma of the lung shows sheets of large tumor cells without evidence of glandular or squamous differentiation.

TERMINOLOGY

Synonyms

- Pleomorphic carcinoma, giant cell carcinoma, rhabdoid carcinoma, large cell undifferentiated carcinoma

Definitions

- Malignant epithelial neoplasm of the lung displaying large cell or anaplastic morphology with no specific histologic features of differentiation

ETIOLOGY/PATHOGENESIS

Etiology

- Originates from a putative primitive progenitor cell capable of multidirectional differentiation

CLINICAL ISSUES

Epidemiology

- Incidence
  - Accounts for approximately 8-10% of all lung cancers
  - Most commonly seen in smokers
- Age
  - Adults from 50-70 years old (average: 60 years)
- Gender
  - Male predilection

Presentation

- Cough
- Chest pain
- Dyspnea

Treatment

- Surgical approaches
  - Surgical excision is recommended for stage I tumors
- Adjuvant therapy
  - Adjuvant chemotherapy is indicated for stage II tumors
- Radiation
  - Radiotherapy has also been employed in stage I and II tumors
  - Combination chemotherapy combined with radiation is employed for stage III tumors

Prognosis

- Generally poor prognosis with short survival

IMAGE FINDINGS

General Features

- Location
  - Periphery of lungs
- Size
  - Generally large (> 5 cm in greatest diameter)
- Morphology
  - Subpleural mass with invasion of pleura, chest wall, or adjacent structures

MACROSCOPIC FEATURES

General Features

- Large, well-circumscribed tumor mass with soft, tan-white tissue that bulges above cut surface
- Frequent areas of hemorrhage and necrosis

MICROSCOPIC PATHOLOGY

Histologic Features

- Neoplastic population is composed of large tumor cells without histologic evidence of glandular or squamous differentiation
  - Variegated histology with different growth patterns
- **Large cell carcinoma, NOS**

LARGE CELL (ANAPLASTIC) CARCINOMA

Key Facts

Clinical Issues
- Cough
- Chest pain
- Dyspnea
- Generally poor prognosis with short survival
- Most commonly seen in smokers

Image Findings
- Periphery of lungs
- Generally large (> 5 cm in greatest diameter)

Microscopic Pathology
- Neoplastic population is composed of large tumor cells without histologic evidence of glandular or squamous differentiation
- Variegated histology with different growth patterns, including
  - Large cell carcinoma, NOS
  - Giant cell carcinoma
  - Clear cell carcinoma
  - Large cell carcinoma with "rhabdoid" features
- Tumor cells are usually very large and measure 3-4x the size of a normal histiocyte
- Nuclei are enlarged and may be multilobated or multinucleated
- Frequent mitotic figures with abnormal mitoses
- Lymphoid cell emperipolesis
- Syncytiotrophoblastic-like tumor cells

Ancillary Tests
- Most cases are positive for broad-spectrum keratin and low-molecular weight cytokeratins (CAM5.2)
- Tumor cells are negative for neuroendocrine markers (chromogranin, synaptophysin, CD56)

  - Sheets of large tumor cells with vesicular chromatin, prominent nucleoli, and abundant rim of cytoplasm
  - May display discohesive growth pattern that resembles a sarcoma (e.g., malignant fibrous histiocytoma, pleomorphic subtype)
  - May be accompanied by abundant inflammatory cell infiltrate in the stroma admixed with tumor cells ("inflammatory" subtype)
  - May display prominent engulfment of lymphoid cells (emperipolesis) by tumor cells
- **Giant cell carcinoma**
  - Sheets of large, pleomorphic tumor cells that are often multilobated and display prominent multinucleation
  - Tumor cells may resemble syncytiotrophoblastic tumor cells of choriocarcinoma
  - Pleomorphic tumor cells may secrete β-HCG
- **Clear cell carcinoma**
  - Tumor composed of sheets of large tumor cells with abundant clear cytoplasm
  - No histologic evidence of glandular or squamous differentiation
  - May show abortive features of glandular or squamous differentiation ultrastructurally
- **Large cell carcinoma with "rhabdoid" features**
  - Sheets of large, atypical tumor cells displaying large eosinophilic cytoplasmic inclusions
  - Eosinophilic inclusions may displace nucleus to periphery of cell
  - Eosinophilic inclusions contain admixture of cytokeratin and vimentin intermediate filaments

Cytologic Features
- Tumor cells are usually very large and measure 2-4x the size of a normal histiocyte
- Nuclei are enlarged and may be multilobated or multinucleated
- Frequent mitotic figures with abnormal mitoses
- Tumor cell emperipolesis
- Syncytiotrophoblastic-like tumor cells

ANCILLARY TESTS

Immunohistochemistry
- Most cases are positive for broad-spectrum keratin and low-molecular weight cytokeratins (CAM5.2)
- Tumor cells are negative for neuroendocrine markers (chromogranin, synaptophysin, CD56)
- Pleomorphic tumor cells may be positive for β-HCG

DIFFERENTIAL DIAGNOSIS

Pleomorphic High-Grade Sarcoma (MFH)
- Discohesive population of pleomorphic tumor cells
- Strong vimentin positivity; absence of reactivity for epithelial markers
  - Rare cases of MFH may show focally aberrant expression of cytokeratin

Metastasis of Anaplastic Carcinoma from Other Organs
- Anaplastic carcinoma of pancreas, thyroid, bladder, and stomach can metastasize to lungs
- Clinical history and imaging studies are indispensable to rule out a metastasis

Metastasis of Choriocarcinoma from Genital Tract
- Mixture of cyto- and syncytiotrophoblastic cells set against heavily hemorrhagic background
- History of gonadal or retroperitoneal tumor is indispensable for diagnosis

SELECTED REFERENCES

1. Hanagiri T et al: Results of surgical resection for patients with large cell carcinoma of the lung. Int J Surg. 8(5):391-4, 2010
2. Nagashio R et al: Significant high expression of cytokeratins 7, 8, 18, 19 in pulmonary large cell neuroendocrine carcinomas, compared to small cell lung carcinomas. Pathol Int. 60(2):71-7, 2010

LARGE CELL (ANAPLASTIC) CARCINOMA

Histologic Features

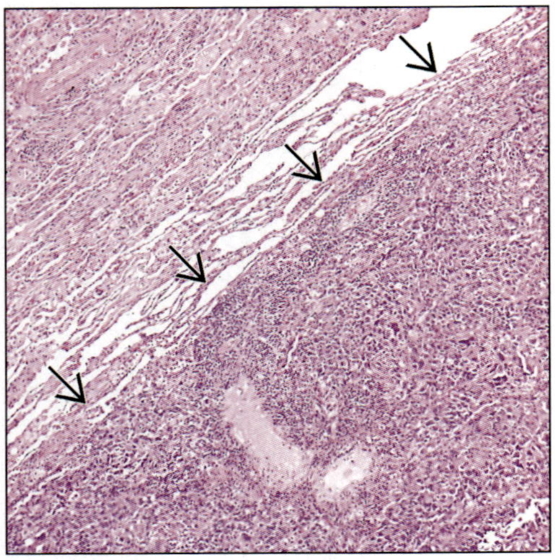
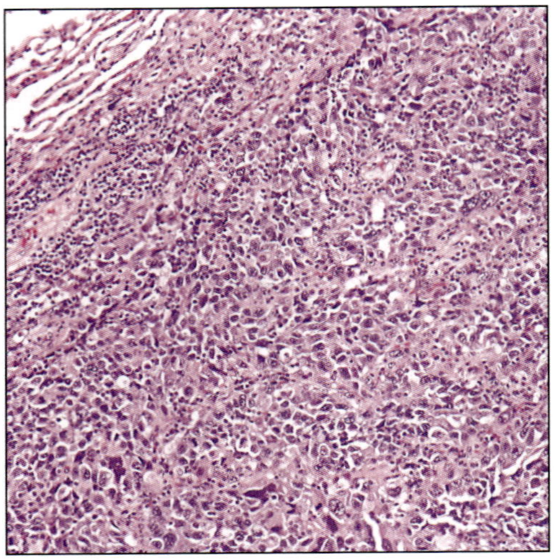

(Left) *Scanning magnification of large cell (anaplastic) carcinoma of the lung shows a well-circumscribed but unencapsulated tumor cell population sharply separated from the surrounding lung parenchyma* ⇒. ***(Right)*** *Large cell (anaplastic) carcinoma of the lung shows sheets of large, anaplastic tumor cells in a haphazard arrangement without any evidence of gland formation or squamous differentiation. Tumors like this may resemble malignant lymphoma or pleomorphic sarcoma.*

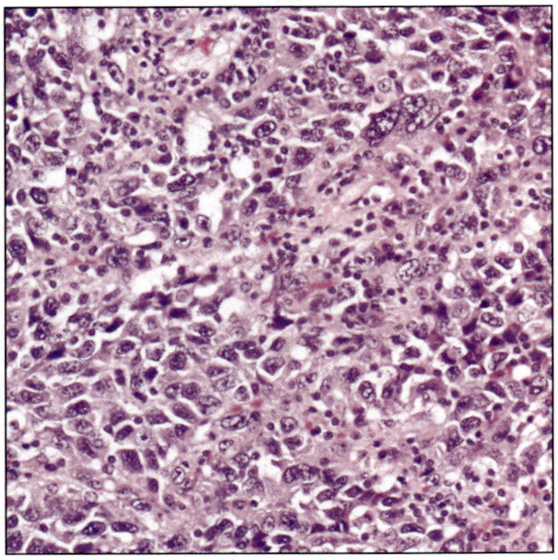
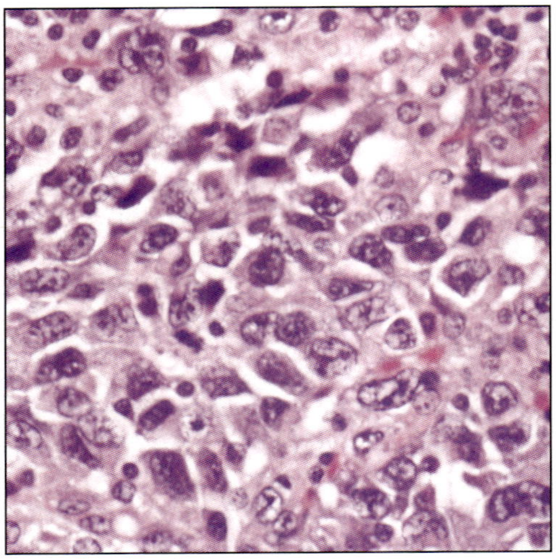

(Left) *Higher magnification of large cell (anaplastic) carcinoma of the lung shows sheets of large tumor cells without any supportive stroma. The discohesive appearance of the tumor cells can suggest a variety of alternate diagnoses due to the total absence of any distinctive features of differentiation.* ***(Right)*** *High magnification of large cell (anaplastic) carcinoma of the lung shows anaplastic tumor cells with enlarged, hyperchromatic nuclei and prominent nucleoli.*

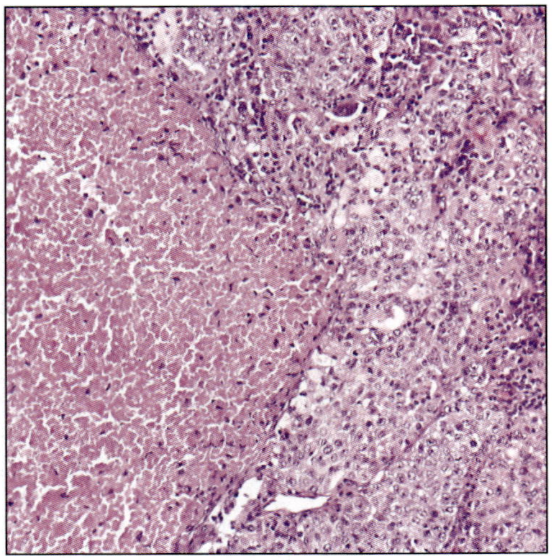
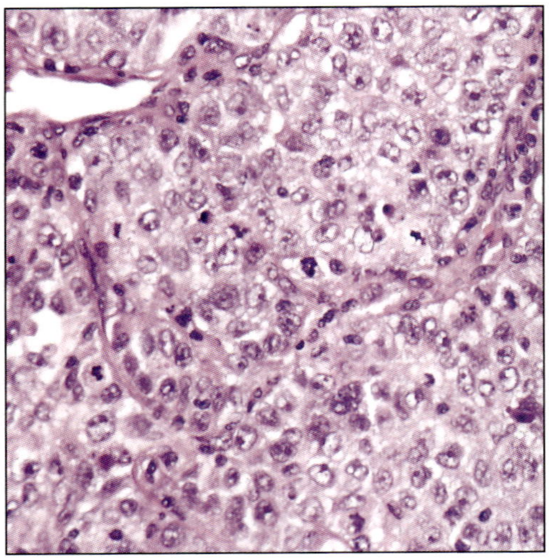

(Left) *Scanning magnification of large cell (anaplastic) carcinoma of the lung shows extensive areas of tumor necrosis (left) and sheets of large tumor cells without any apparent features of differentiation.* ***(Right)*** *High magnification of large cell (anaplastic) carcinoma of the lung shows sheets of large, atypical tumor cells with large vesicular nuclei, prominent nucleoli, and frequent mitotic figures. The sheet-like pattern of growth can simulate a diffuse large cell lymphoma.*

LARGE CELL (ANAPLASTIC) CARCINOMA

Histologic and Immunohistochemical Features

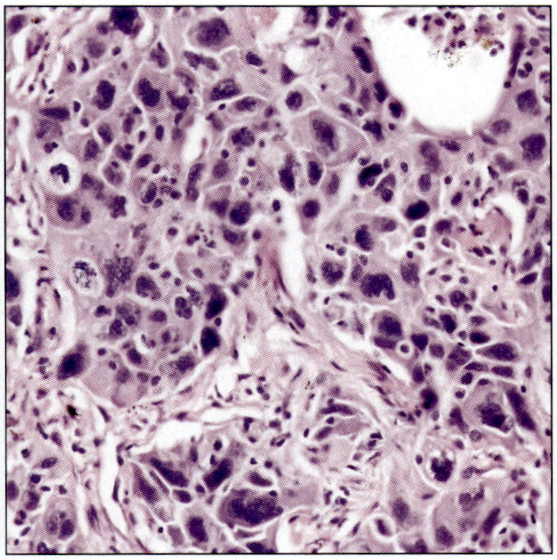

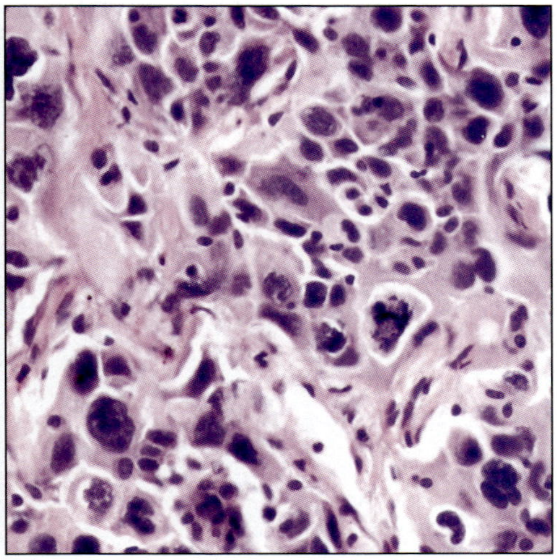

(Left) *Scanning magnification of large cell (anaplastic) carcinoma of the lung shows islands of large tumor cells with bizarre nuclei and numerous mitoses. The islands of tumor cells are separated by scant fibrovascular stroma.* ***(Right)*** *Higher magnification of large cell (anaplastic) carcinoma of the lung shows bizarre nuclear morphology with enlarged, hyperchromatic nuclei and occasional multinucleated tumor cells. There is no evidence of glandular or squamous differentiation.*

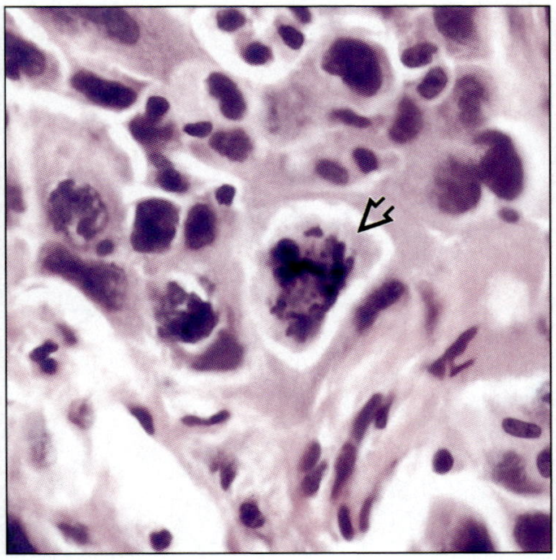

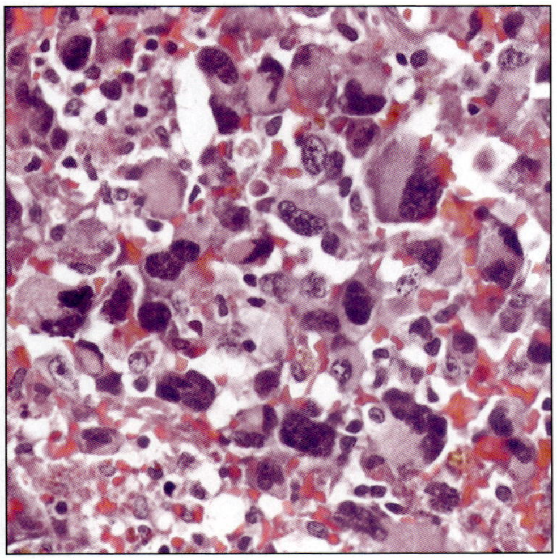

(Left) *High magnification in large cell (anaplastic) carcinoma of the lung shows bizarre tumor cells with enlarged, hyperchromatic nuclei and an indistinct rim of eosinophilic cytoplasm. Notice the abnormal mitotic figure in the center* ⇨*.* ***(Right)*** *Large cell (anaplastic) carcinoma of the lung shows a discohesive population of large, bizarre tumor cells devoid of any supporting stroma. Notice the abundance of red blood cells scattered in the background and a few scant small lymphocytes.*

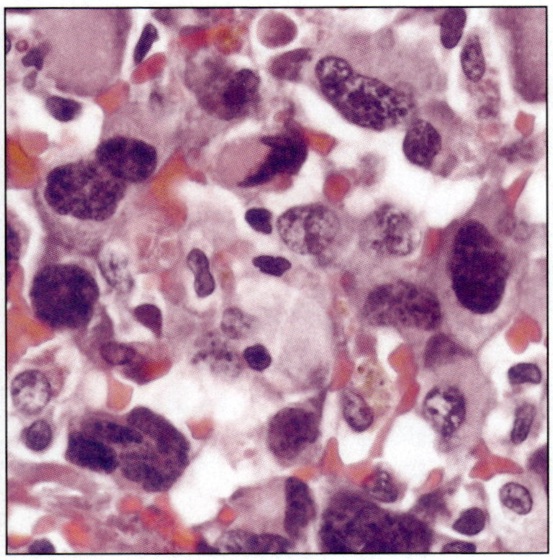

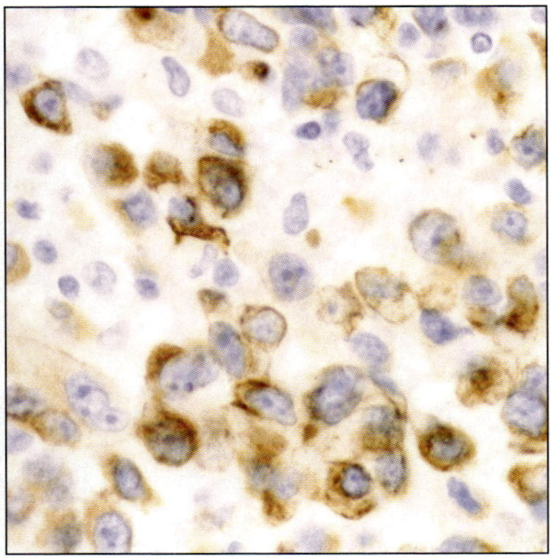

(Left) *Higher magnification of large cell (anaplastic) carcinoma of the lung shows large, bizarre tumor cells with abnormally shaped, hyperchromatic nuclei with large, often multiple eosinophilic nucleoli and a scant rim of eosinophilic cytoplasm.* ***(Right)*** *Immunohistochemical staining of large cell (anaplastic) carcinoma of the lung for cytokeratin AE1/AE3 (broad-spectrum keratin) shows strong cytoplasmic positivity in a large number of the tumor cells for this antibody.*

LARGE CELL (ANAPLASTIC) CARCINOMA

Pleomorphic Histology

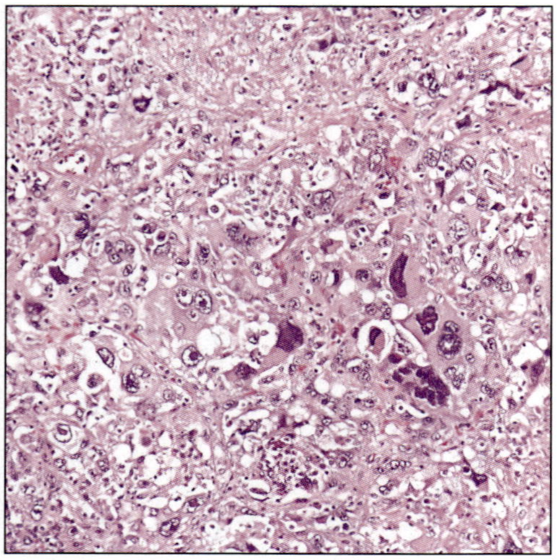

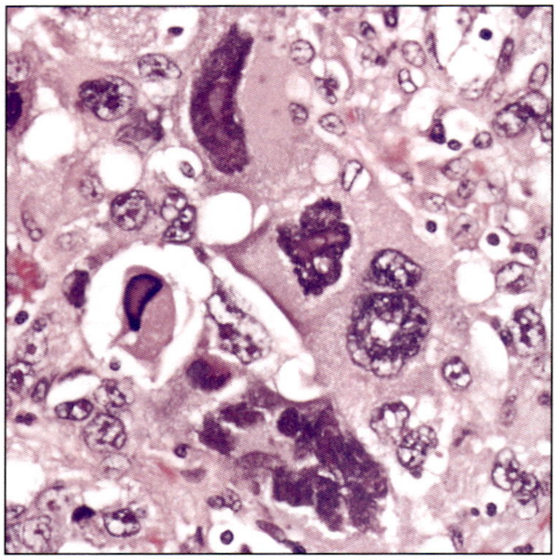

*(**Left**) Scanning magnification of large cell (anaplastic) carcinoma of the lung shows numerous bizarre tumor cells, somewhat reminiscent of syncytiotrophoblastic cells in choriocarcinoma. (**Right**) Choriocarcinoma-like appearance of large cell (anaplastic) carcinoma of the lung shows tumor cells with bizarre nuclei and multinucleated forms reminiscent of syncytiotrophoblastic tumor cells. These cells can stain positive with antibodies to β-HCG.*

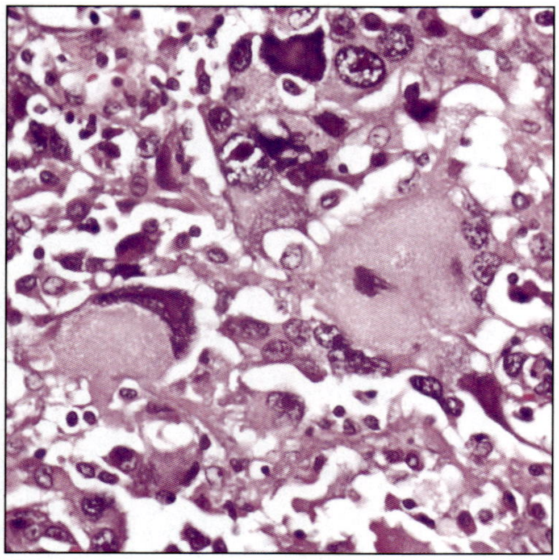

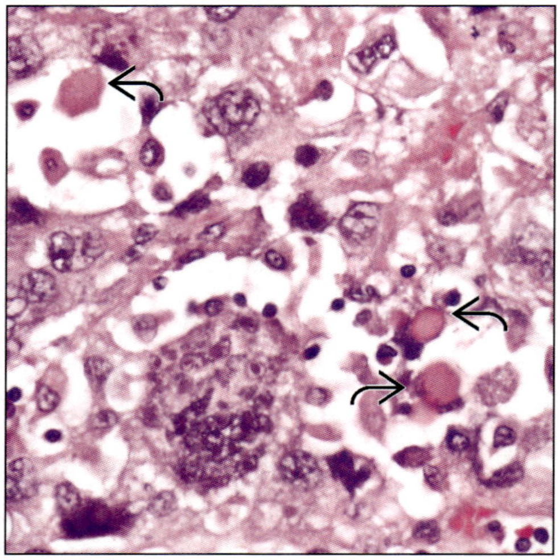

*(**Left**) Large cell (anaplastic) carcinoma of the lung shows bizarre tumor cells with abundant, finely granular, and sometimes vacuolated cytoplasm reminiscent of tumor cells seen in "fibrohistiocytic" malignant neoplasms. Tumors with these features can be easily mistaken for malignant fibrous histiocytoma. (**Right**) Large cell (anaplastic) carcinoma of the lung shows dense, eosinophilic hyaline globules ↪ scattered in between tumor cells in the interstitium.*

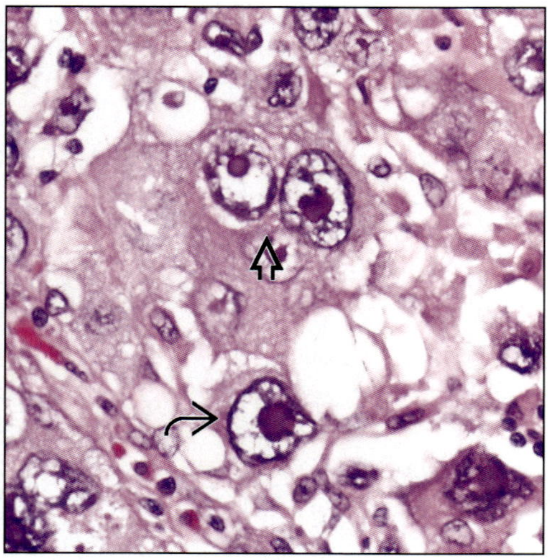

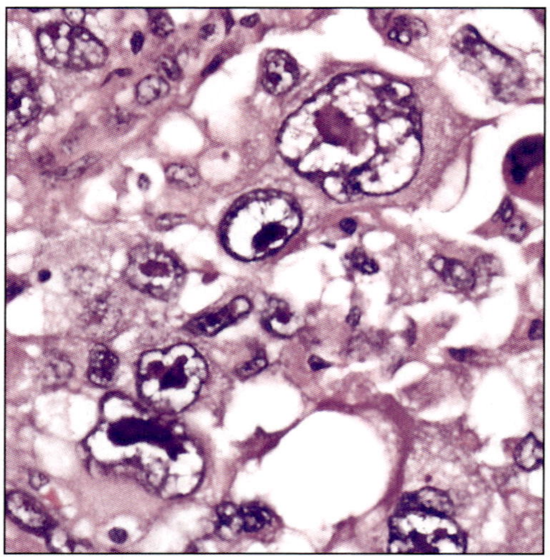

*(**Left**) High magnification of large cell (anaplastic) carcinoma of the lung shows Reed-Sternberg-like tumor cells. Notice the binucleated form at the top ⇨ displaying double nuclei with "owl-eyed" nucleoli and the mononuclear type ↪ showing a single enlarged nucleus with a prominent eosinophilic nucleolus. (**Right**) Large cell (anaplastic) carcinoma of lung shows bizarre cells with deeply eosinophilic macronucleoli. Cases like this can be confused with Hodgkin disease.*

LARGE CELL (ANAPLASTIC) CARCINOMA

"Inflammatory" Variant

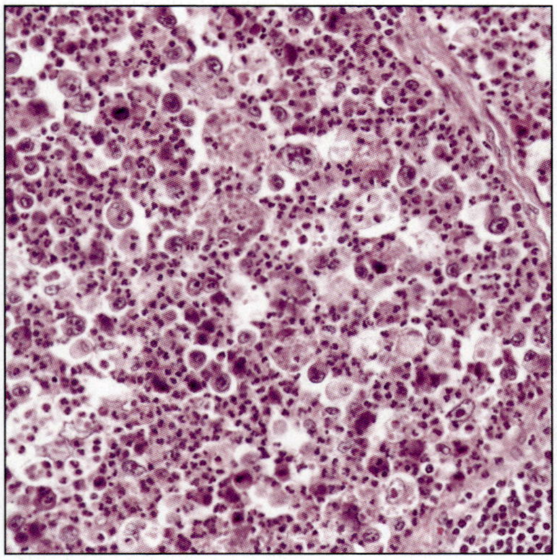

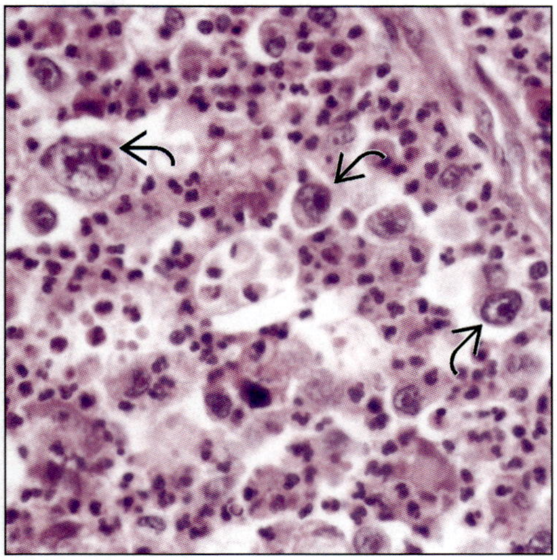

(Left) *Scanning magnification of large cell (anaplastic) carcinoma, "inflammatory variant," shows sheets of polymorphonuclear leukocytes admixed with scattered larger cells. The overall appearance on scanning magnification is that of an abscess.* ***(Right)*** *Higher magnification of "inflammatory variant" of large cell (anaplastic) carcinoma of the lung shows numerous polymorphonuclear leukocytes with only a few scattered larger, atypical cells in the background ↷.*

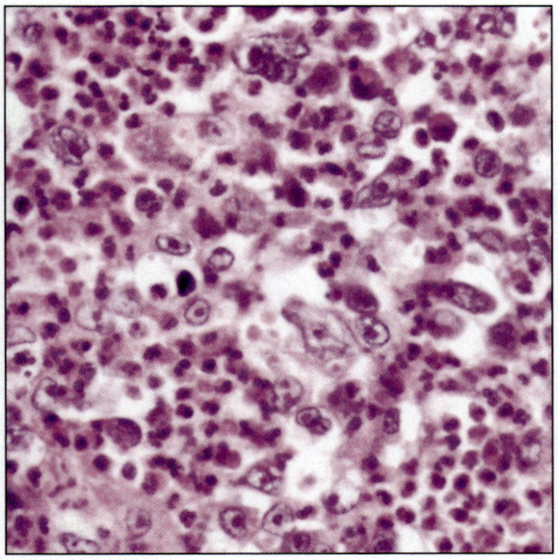

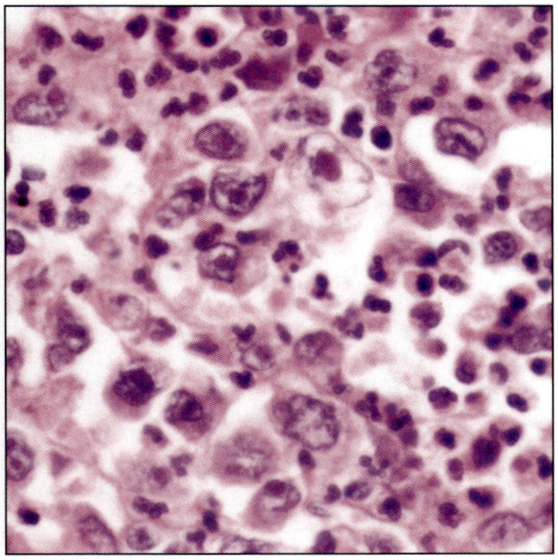

(Left) *Inflammatory type of large cell (anaplastic) carcinoma of the lung shows a discohesive population of atypical mononuclear cells surrounded by abundant polymorphonuclear leukocytes. Tumors with this appearance can be easily mistaken for inflammatory malignant fibrous histiocytoma.* ***(Right)*** *Higher magnification of "inflammatory-type" large cell (anaplastic) carcinoma of the lung shows atypical cells with vesicular nuclei and prominent nucleoli.*

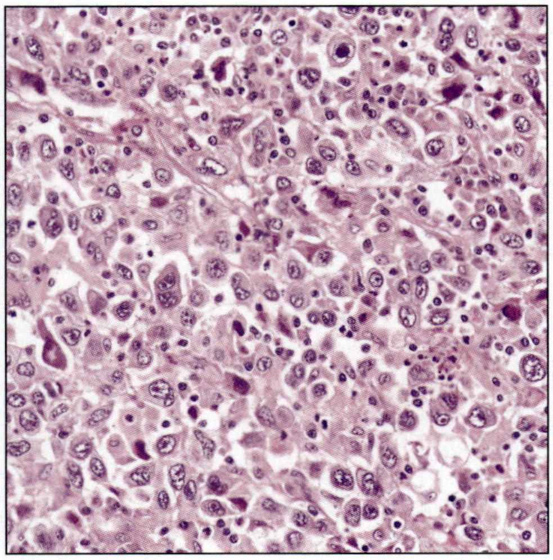

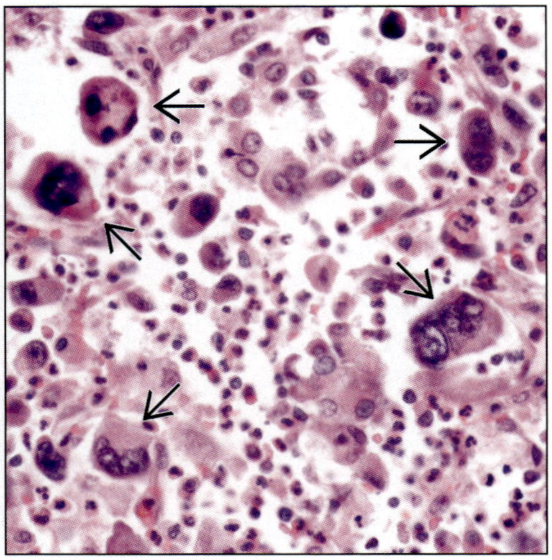

(Left) *Scanning magnification of "inflammatory-type" large cell (anaplastic) carcinoma of the lung shows sheets of large, atypical cells separated by inflammatory cells. The number of atypical cells is much larger and predominates over the inflammatory elements in this example.* ***(Right)*** *Higher magnification of large cell (anaplastic) carcinoma of the lung, "inflammatory type," shows an abundance of eosinophils and small lymphocytes scattered in between the large, atypical cells →.*

LARGE CELL (ANAPLASTIC) CARCINOMA

"Rhabdoid" Type

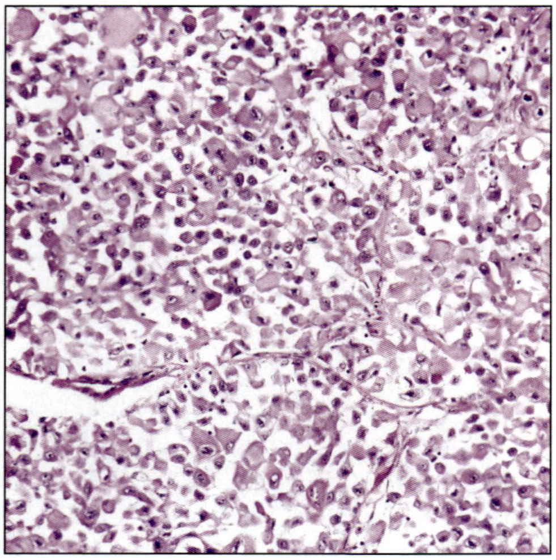

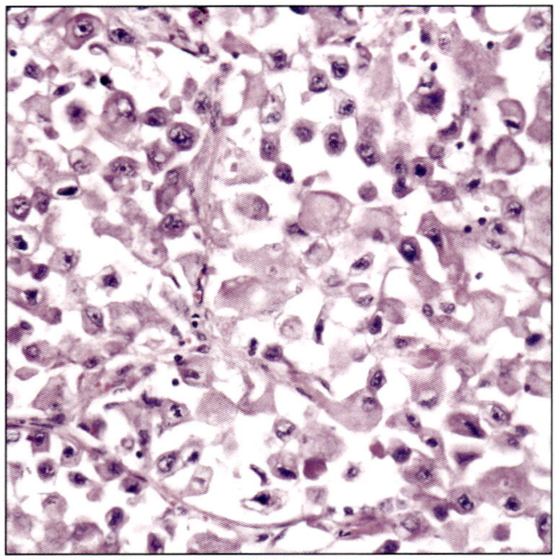

(Left) *Scanning magnification of large cell (anaplastic) carcinoma of the lung shows sheets of cells containing large, paranuclear, dense eosinophilic cytoplasmic inclusions simulating "rhabdoid" cells.* ***(Right)*** *Large cell (anaplastic) carcinoma of the lung shows cells with large, densely eosinophilic cytoplasmic inclusions. Tumors with these features can resemble the so-called rhabdoid tumors of the kidney and other organs, rhabdomyosarcoma and metastatic malignant melanoma.*

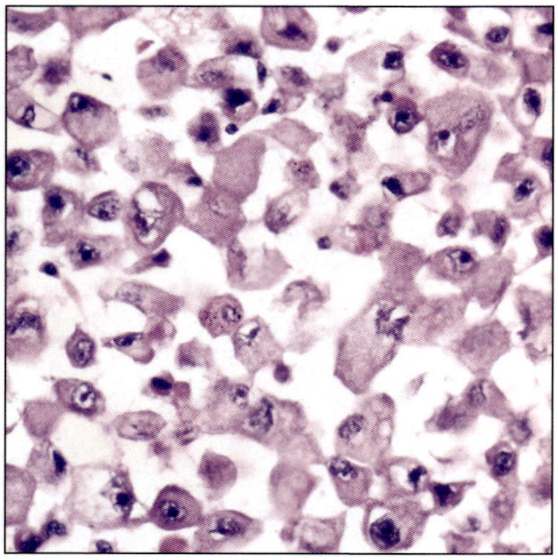

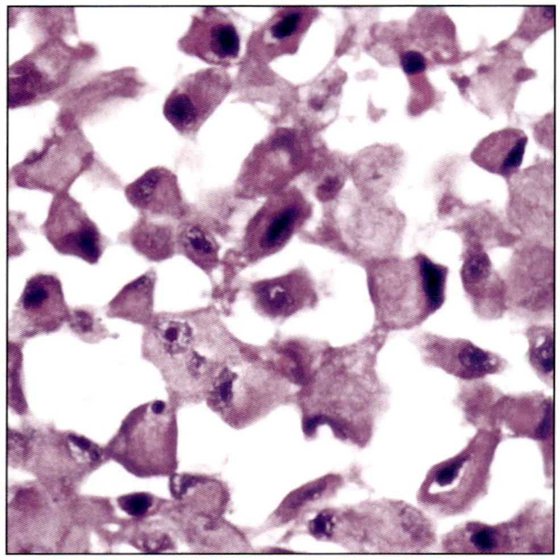

(Left) *Large cell (anaplastic) carcinoma of the lung composed of large, discohesive tumor cells with eccentric globular, eosinophilic cytoplasmic inclusions simulating "rhabdoid" cells.* ***(Right)*** *Higher magnification of large cell (anaplastic) carcinoma of the lung with rhabdoid appearance shows large cells with eccentric eosinophilic cytoplasmic inclusions. The dense cytoplasmic inclusions display abundant intermediate filaments by electron microscopy and are positive for cytokeratin.*

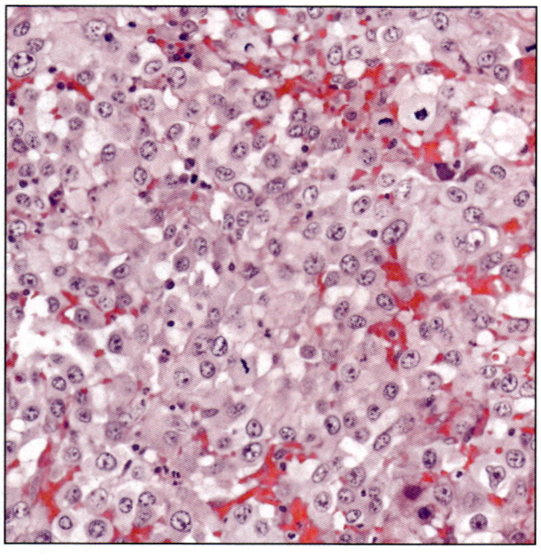

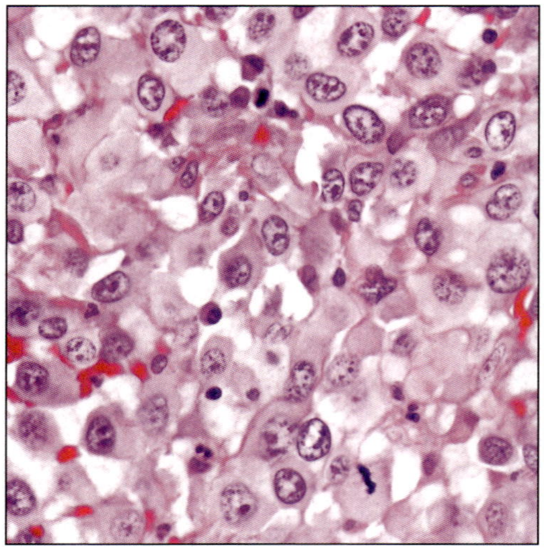

(Left) *Scanning magnification of large cell (anaplastic) carcinoma of the lung displays sheets of uniform tumor cells with dense eosinophilic cytoplasmic inclusions imparting them with a "rhabdoid" appearance.* ***(Right)*** *Higher magnification of large cell (anaplastic) carcinoma of the lung shows large, atypical cells containing dense, eosinophilic cytoplasmic inclusions. Use of immunohistochemical stains will be necessary in a case like this to distinguish the tumor from a metastasis.*

LARGE CELL (ANAPLASTIC) CARCINOMA

Clear Cell Type

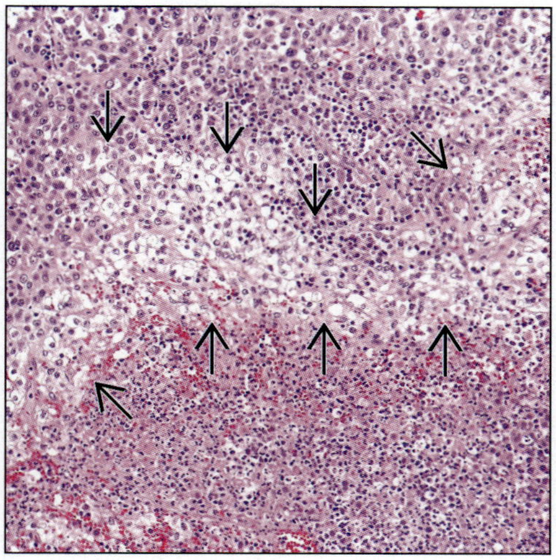
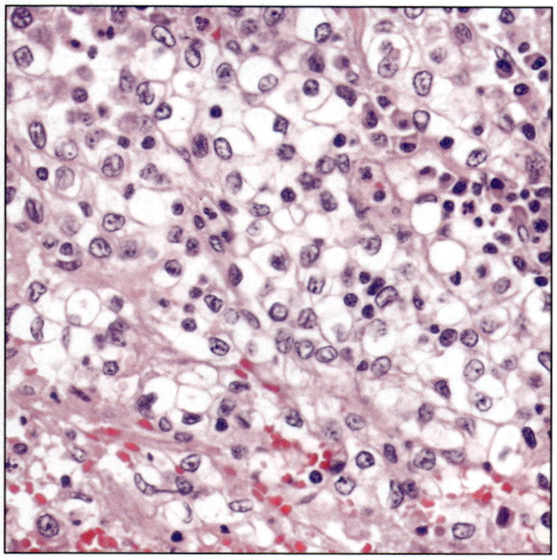

(Left) *Scanning magnification of large cell (anaplastic) carcinoma of the lung shows transition between cells with abundant eosinophilic cytoplasm (top) and cells with clear cytoplasm* ➔. ***(Right)*** *Large cell (anaplastic) carcinoma of the lung shows sheets of large cells with abundant clear cytoplasm. Notice inflammatory cells admixed with the tumor cells. Tumors like this must be distinguished from metastases of clear cell carcinoma from other organs.*

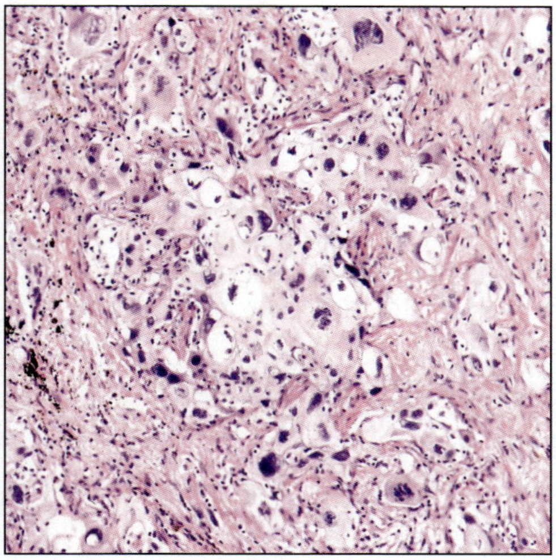
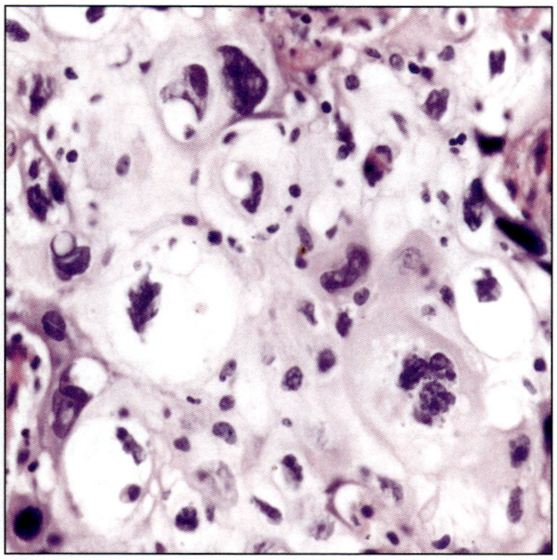

(Left) *Scanning magnification of large cell (anaplastic) carcinoma of the lung shows bizarre tumor cells with abundant clear cytoplasm. The islands of tumor cells are embedded in abundant fibrous stroma.* ***(Right)*** *Higher magnification of large cell (anaplastic) carcinoma of the lung, clear cell type, shows large, atypical tumor cells with bizarre nuclei surrounded by an ample rim of clear cytoplasm. The nuclear morphology in this example is quite pleomorphic and atypical.*

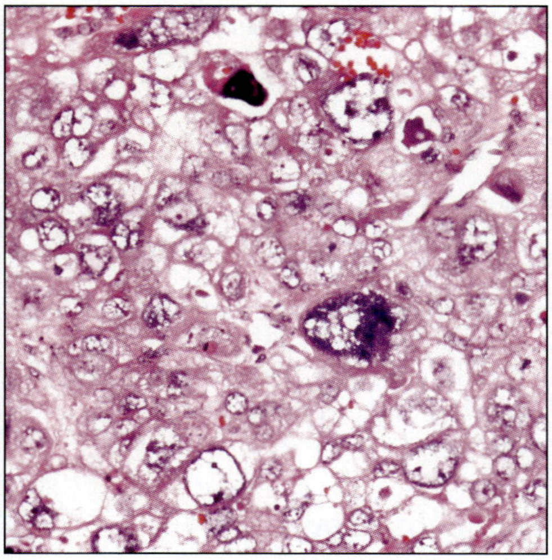
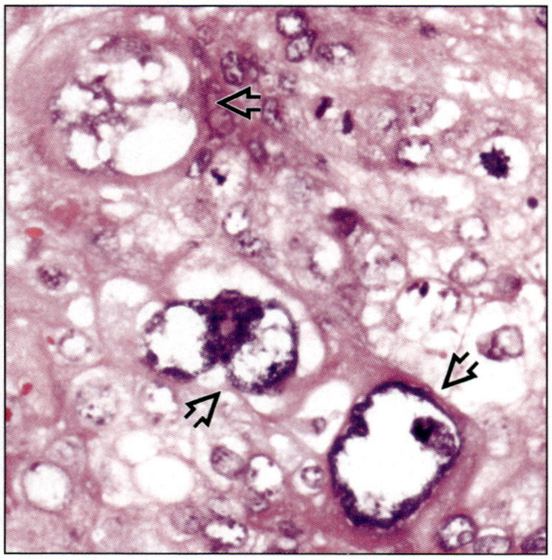

(Left) *Scanning magnification of large cell (anaplastic) carcinoma of the lung shows sheets of large, bizarre tumor cells with atypical nuclei with vesicular chromatin pattern and abundant clear cytoplasm.* ***(Right)*** *Higher magnification of large cell (anaplastic) carcinoma of the lung shows bizarre, atypical cells with abundant clear or lightly eosinophilic cytoplasm. Notice the large, bizarre cells with vesicular nuclei and multinucleated forms* ⇨.

PLEOMORPHIC CARCINOMA

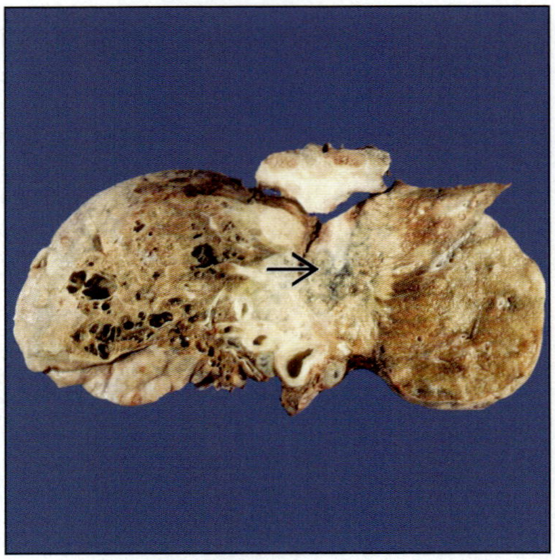

Gross photograph of pleomorphic carcinoma of the lung shows a large centrally located malignant neoplasm. The tumor shows a smooth cut surface and focal necrosis ➔.

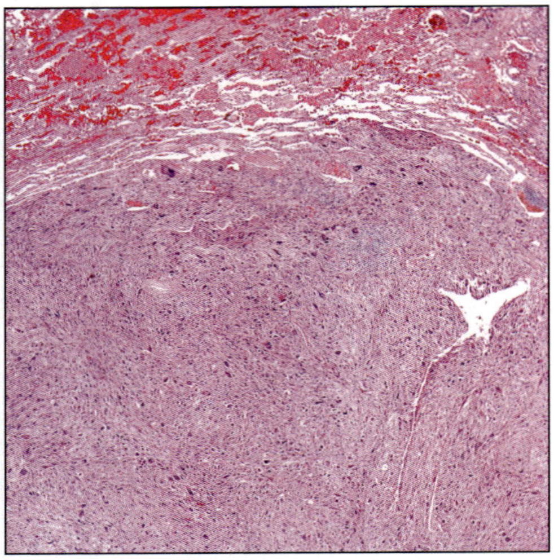

Pleomorphic carcinoma of the lung shows a cellular proliferation composed of spindle and large multinucleated giant cells. The tumor appears well circumscribed but not encapsulated.

TERMINOLOGY

Abbreviations

- Pleomorphic carcinoma (PC)

Synonyms

- Giant cell carcinoma, carcinoma with giant cells, carcinoma with pseudosarcomatous stroma, pseudosarcomatous carcinoma, metaplastic carcinoma

Definitions

- Malignant epithelial neoplasm composed of spindle and multinucleated giant cells in different proportions

ETIOLOGY/PATHOGENESIS

Etiology

- PC may represent a genetically distinct type of malignancy separate from squamous cell carcinoma and adenocarcinoma

CLINICAL ISSUES

Presentation

- Asymptomatic
- Chest pain
- Hemoptysis
- Cough

Treatment

- Surgical approaches
  - Lobectomy or pneumonectomy
- Adjuvant therapy
  - Chemotherapy or radiation therapy depending on clinical setting

Prognosis

- Depends on stage at diagnosis
- Majority of cases are in advanced clinical stages
- Prognosis is poor

MACROSCOPIC FEATURES

General Features

- Central or peripheral
- Varying size but generally large tumors
- Well circumscribed but not encapsulated
- Light tan with homogeneous cut surface
  - Areas of necrosis &/or hemorrhage may be seen

MICROSCOPIC PATHOLOGY

Histologic Features

- Mixture of 2 distinct components, spindle and giant cells

Predominant Pattern/Injury Type

- Sarcomatoid

Predominant Cell/Compartment Type

- Epithelial

DIFFERENTIAL DIAGNOSIS

Malignant Fibrous Histiocytoma (MFH)

- Touton-type giant cells in MFH; multinucleated malignant cells in PC
- Areas of squamous cell carcinoma or adenocarcinoma in most cases of PC
- Studies using keratin antibodies helpful as sarcomatoid component may show keratin expression
  - MFH may also show focal positive staining for keratin

Pulmonary Leiomyosarcoma

- Immunohistochemistry studies for desmin, caldesmon, and SMA generally negative in PC cases while positive in leiomyosarcomas

PLEOMORPHIC CARCINOMA

Key Facts

Terminology

- Malignant epithelial neoplasm composed of spindle and multinucleated giant cells in different proportions

Etiology/Pathogenesis

- PC may represent a genetically distinct type of malignancy separate from squamous and adenocarcinoma

Clinical Issues

- Symptoms
  - Chest pain
  - Hemoptysis
  - Cough
- Prognosis
  - Majority of cases are in advanced clinical stages
  - Prognosis is poor
- Lobectomy or pneumonectomy
- Chemotherapy or radiation therapy depending on clinical setting

Microscopic Pathology

- Mixture of 2 distinct components, sarcomatoid and giant cells

Top Differential Diagnoses

- Malignant fibrous histiocytoma (MFH)
- Pulmonary leiomyosarcoma
- Sarcomatoid carcinoma
- Metastatic choriocarcinoma

Immunohistochemistry

Antibody	Reactivity	Staining Pattern	Comment
KERATIN-LMW	Positive	Cytoplasmic	May be only focal positive staining
EMA/MUC1	Positive	Cell membrane	May be negative in many cases
Vimentin	Positive	Cytoplasmic	Nonspecific
Actin-HHF-35	Positive	Cytoplasmic	Focal in spindle cell component
CD68	Positive	Cytoplasmic	Focal in spindle cell component
Desmin	Negative		
MYOD1	Negative		
Myoglobin	Negative		
Caldesmon	Negative		
CD31	Negative		

- Presence of multinucleated giant cell component is not a common feature, even in cases of high-grade leiomyosarcoma
- Most pulmonary leiomyosarcomas are confined to lung, while PC is commonly in advanced clinical stage

Sarcomatoid Carcinoma

- Though sarcomatoid carcinoma and PC are often coded under same category, PC has sarcomatoid component in association with multinucleated giant cells
- Sarcomatoid carcinoma shows only spindle cell component
- Both tumors share similar immunohistochemical profile

Metastatic Choriocarcinoma

- History of previous germ cell tumor is important
- Choriocarcinomas would show presence of cyto- and syncytiotrophoblastic components
- Areas of necrosis and hemorrhage admixed with tumors cells are more common in choriocarcinomas
- Immunohistochemical stains for hCG are more commonly and strongly positive in choriocarcinoma
- Some cases of PC may show positive staining for hCG

DIAGNOSTIC CHECKLIST

Pathologic Interpretation Pearls

- Mixture of malignant spindle cell components in association with malignant multinucleated giant cells

SELECTED REFERENCES

1. Toba H et al: [Surgically treated pleomorphic carcinoma of the lung.] Kyobu Geka. 62(3):202-6, 2009
2. Mochizuki T et al: Pleomorphic carcinoma of the lung: clinicopathologic characteristics of 70 cases. Am J Surg Pathol. 32(11):1727-35, 2008
3. Hirano H et al: Pulmonary pleomorphic carcinoma producing hCG. Pathol Int. 57(10):698-702, 2007
4. Yamamoto S et al: Clinicopathological investigation of pulmonary pleomorphic carcinoma. Eur J Cardiothorac Surg. 32(6):873-6, 2007
5. Yuki T et al: Pleomorphic carcinoma of the lung: a surgical outcome. J Thorac Cardiovasc Surg. 134(2):399-404, 2007
6. Przygodzki RM et al: Pleomorphic (giant and spindle cell) carcinoma is genetically distinct from adenocarcinoma and squamous cell carcinoma by K-ras-2 and p53 analysis. Am J Clin Pathol. 106(4):487-92, 1996
7. Fishback NF et al: Pleomorphic (spindle/giant cell) carcinoma of the lung. A clinicopathologic correlation of 78 cases. Cancer. 73(12):2936-45, 1994

PLEOMORPHIC CARCINOMA

Microscopic Features

(Left) *PC demonstrates classic histopathologic features of combined spindle and giant cell components arranged in a haphazard fashion. Note the presence of residual bronchial cartilage* ⇨. ***(Right)*** *PC shows conventional features of a mixture of giant and spindle cells* ⇨. *The tumor is sparing the normal endobronchial mucinous glands* ↪.

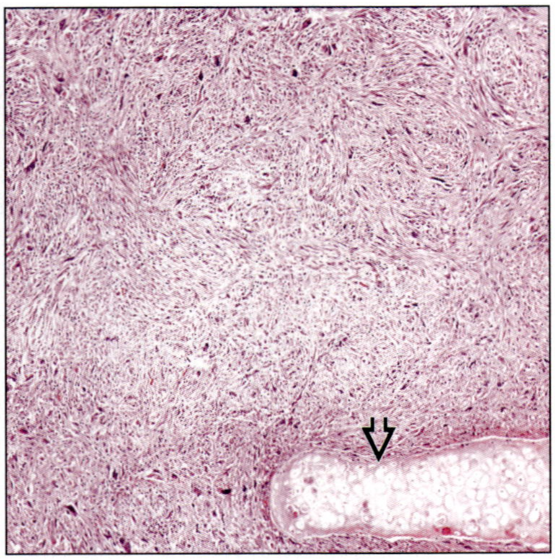

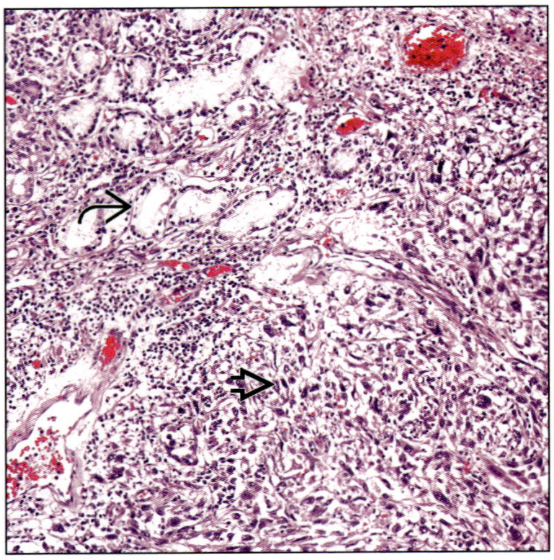

(Left) *PC demonstrates extensive areas of spindle and giant cell components admixed with dilated vascular spaces and mild inflammatory response.* ***(Right)*** *PC is shown with extensive areas of necrosis* ➡. *Note that in this particular illustration, the epithelial component shows multinucleated giant cells* → *but not the spindle cell component.*

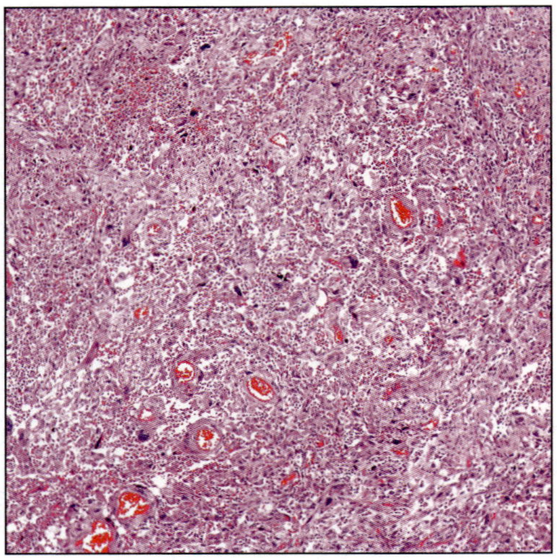

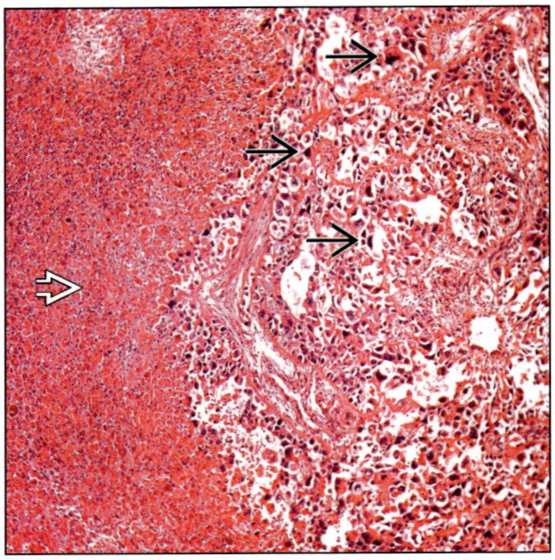

(Left) *Numerous malignant giant cells admixed with spindle cells and acute inflammation* → *are present in this PC. This growth pattern may be seen in pulmonary sarcomas.* ***(Right)*** *High-power view of a PC shows large cells, some of them multinucleated* ⇨ *with bizarre nuclei. Mitotic activity is present* ↪. *These features are commonly seen in pulmonary PC.*

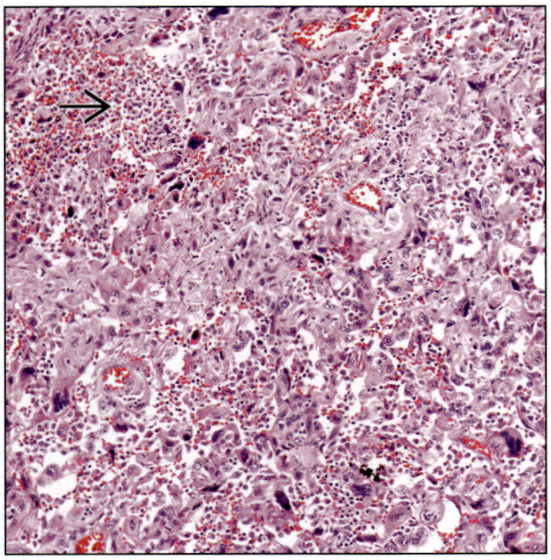

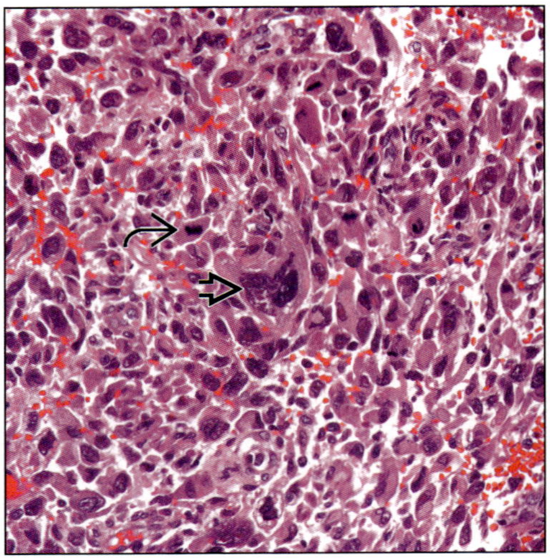

Microscopic Features

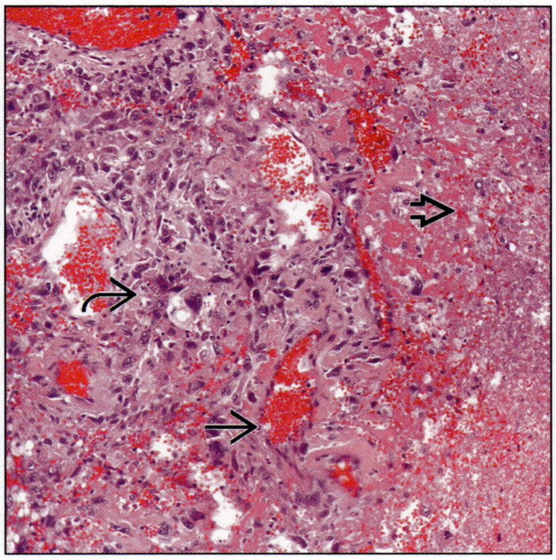
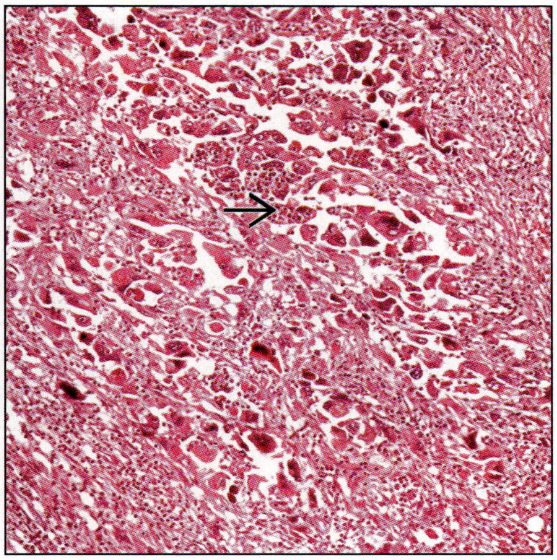

(Left) *Pulmonary PC shows extensive necrosis ⇨ and ectatic vessels →, which could mimic a vascular neoplasm. However, the neoplastic cellular proliferation shows a mixture of multinucleated giant cells and spindle cells ↷.* ***(Right)*** *Higher magnification shows a multinucleated malignant cell component admixed with an acute inflammatory component →.*

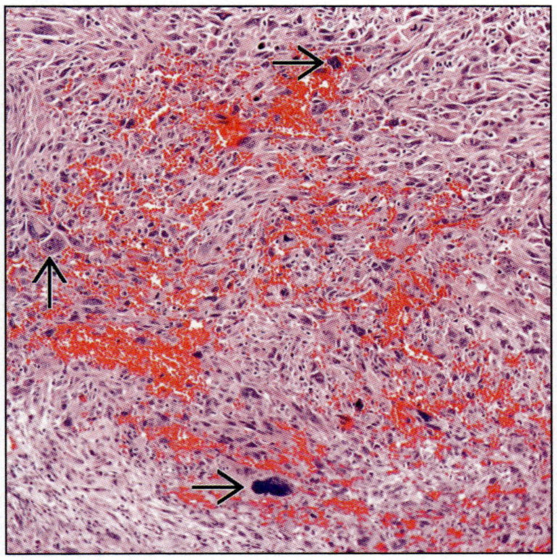
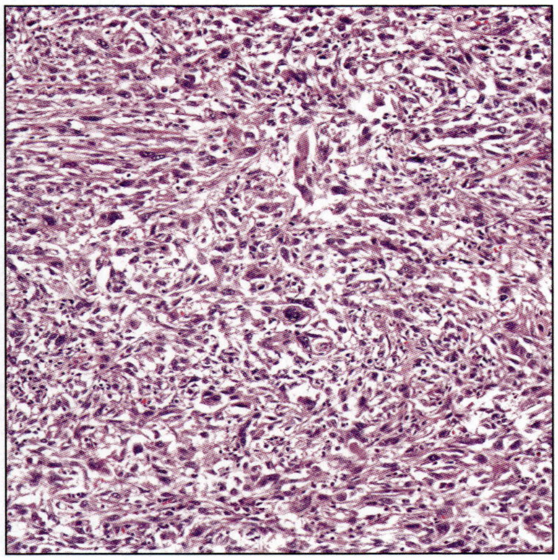

(Left) *H&E shows PC with a malignant spindle cell component admixed with numerous multinucleated giant cells → and extensive areas of extravasated red cells, mimicking a vascular neoplasm.* ***(Right)*** *In some cases of pulmonary PC, the spindle cell proliferation combined with giant cells closely mimics a true sarcoma, such as a malignant fibrous histiocytoma (MFH).*

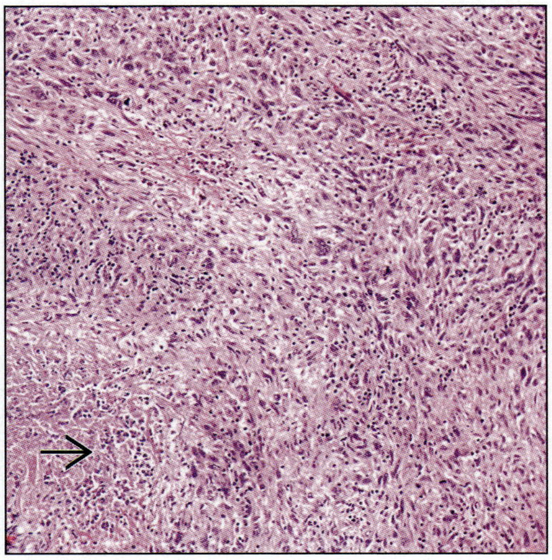
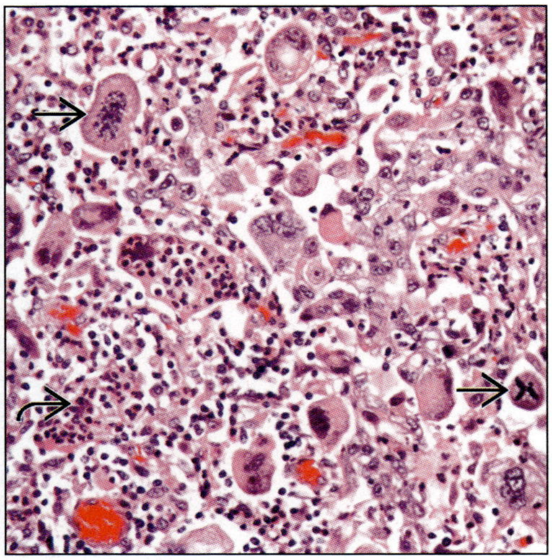

(Left) *PC is shown with a predominantly spindle cell component and an inconspicuous giant cell component. Areas of necrosis are present →, while the spindle cell component mimics a sarcomatous growth pattern.* ***(Right)*** *Numerous malignant multinucleated giant cells in PC are shown. Note the presence of atypical mitotic figures ↷. An acute inflammatory component is also present →.*

NEUROENDOCRINE CARCINOMA (INCLUDING SMALL CELL CARCINOMA)

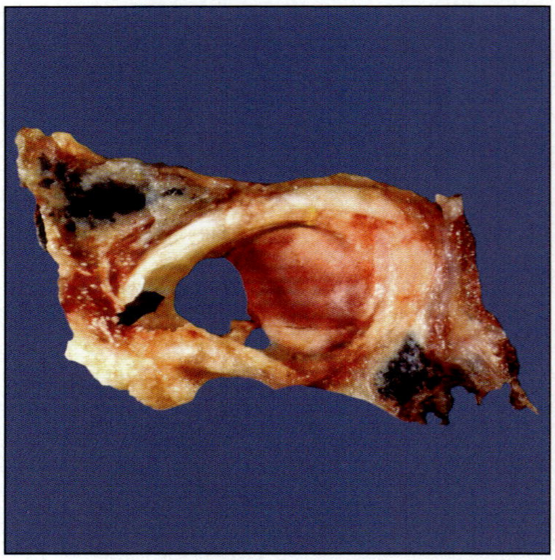

Gross photograph of neuroendocrine carcinoma shows an endobronchial tumor obstructing approximately 50% of the bronchial lumen.

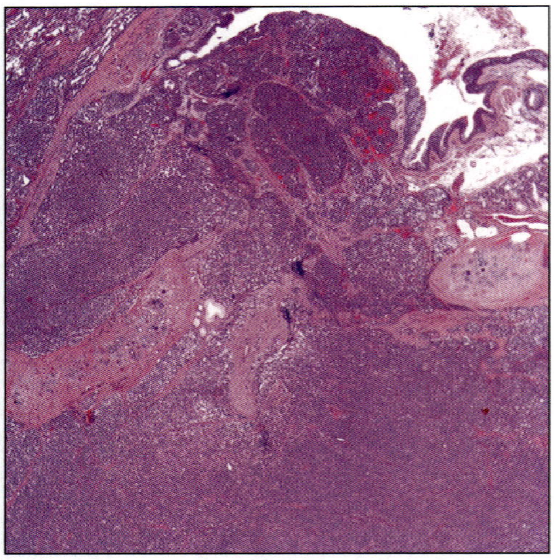

Low-power view of a low-grade endobronchial neuroendocrine carcinoma (carcinoid tumor). Note the organized pattern of growth.

TERMINOLOGY

Abbreviations

- Typical carcinoid (TC), atypical carcinoid (AT), small cell neuroendocrine carcinoma (SCNEC), large cell neuroendocrine carcinoma (LCNEC)

Synonyms

- Carcinoid tumor, atypical carcinoid, small cell carcinoma

Definitions

- Spectrum of neoplasms ranging from low- to high-grade malignancy showing neuroendocrine differentiation

ETIOLOGY/PATHOGENESIS

Etiology

- Tumor is thought to be derived from Kulchitsky cells

CLINICAL ISSUES

Presentation

- Cough
- Incidental finding
- Hemoptysis
- Paraneoplastic syndromes
- Chest pain
- Weight loss
- Dyspnea

Treatment

- Surgical approaches
  - Low- and intermediate-grade tumor
- Adjuvant therapy
  - High-grade tumors

Prognosis

- Low-grade neoplasms
  - Survival rate at 5 years: > 75%
- Intermediate-grade neoplasms
  - Survival rate at 5 years: ~ 50%
- High-grade neoplasms
  - Survival rate at 5 years: May be < 5%

MACROSCOPIC FEATURES

General Features

- Endobronchial or intraparenchymal tumor
- High-grade tumor may show extensive areas of necrosis

Size

- 0.5 to > 10 cm in diameter

MICROSCOPIC PATHOLOGY

Histologic Features

- Low-grade tumors
  - < 3 Mitotic figures per 10 HPF
  - Necrosis is absent
- Intermediate-grade tumors
  - 3-10 mitotic figures per 10 HPF
  - Comedo-like necrosis
- High-grade tumors
  - > 10 Mitotic figures per 10 HPF
  - Necrosis is present
- Large cell neuroendocrine carcinoma requires neuroendocrine pattern and positive staining with neuroendocrine markers (chromogranin-A, synaptophysin, CD56)
  - Cells with prominent nucleoli
  - Neuroendocrine markers must be positive
  - Electron microscopic studies show neurosecretory granules

NEUROENDOCRINE CARCINOMA (INCLUDING SMALL CELL CARCINOMA)

Key Facts

Terminology
- Spectrum of neoplasms ranging from low- to high-grade malignancy

Clinical Issues
- Paraneoplastic syndromes

Macroscopic Features
- Endobronchial or intraparenchymal tumor
- 0.5 to > 10 cm in diameter

Microscopic Pathology
- Neuroendocrine pattern, mitotic activity, necrosis
- Low-grade tumors: < 2 mitotic figures per 10 HPF; absence of necrosis
- Intermediate-grade tumor: 3-10 mitotic figures per 10 HPF; comedo-like necrosis
- High-grade tumors: > 10 mitotic figures per 10 HPF; necrosis is present
- Large cell neuroendocrine carcinoma requires neuroendocrine pattern and positive staining with neuroendocrine markers (chromogranin-A, synaptophysin, CD56)
- In small cell carcinoma, mitotic count of > 10 per 10 HPF applies only to resected specimens, not biopsy material

Ancillary Tests
- Chromogranin-A
- Synaptophysin
- CD56

Diagnostic Checklist
- Mitotic rate

  - Comedo-like necrosis
- Small cell carcinoma
  - Miotic figures > 10 per 10 HPF applies only to resected specimens
  - Neuroendocrine markers are not required for diagnosis

Predominant Pattern/Injury Type
- Nesting
- Diffuse
- Mucinous
- Glandular

Predominant Cell/Compartment Type
- Oncocytic
- Spindle
- Melanocytic
- Epithelial, neuroendocrine
- Clear

DIFFERENTIAL DIAGNOSIS

Low-Grade Neuroendocrine Carcinoma
- < 3 mitotic figures and absence of necrosis
- Well-organized growth pattern

Intermediate-Grade Neuroendocrine Carcinoma
- Mitotic activity from 3-9 per 10 HPF and necrosis
- Often a combination of well-organized nested pattern and diffuse pattern of growth

High-Grade Neuroendocrine Carcinoma
- > 10 mitotic figures per 10 HPF, necrosis &/or hemorrhage (in resected specimens)
- Positive neuroendocrine markers (synaptophysin, chromogranin-B, &/or CD56) in cases of large cell neuroendocrine carcinoma
- In cases of small cell carcinoma, neuroendocrine markers may be negative

Carcinoid Tumorlet
- These tumors are usually < 5 mm in diameter
- Tumorlets and carcinoid tumors share same immunophenotype

Metastatic Neuroendocrine Carcinoma of Extrathoracic Origin
- Clinical history of previous tumor is of utmost importance
- Immunohistochemical study for TTF-1 may be helpful

Pulmonary Paraganglioma
- Paragangliomas and neuroendocrine tumors show positive staining for neuroendocrine markers
- Paragangliomas are usually negative for keratin
- Paragangliomas generally do not show mitotic activity
- Paragangliomas usually show cells with macronuclei

Large Cell Carcinoma
- Large cell neuroendocrine carcinoma must show neuroendocrine pattern and positive neuroendocrine markers

Large Cell Carcinoma with Neuroendocrine Differentiation
- Histology is that of conventional non-small cell carcinoma with positive neuroendocrine markers

Large Cell Carcinoma with Neuroendocrine Pattern
- Tumors show neuroendocrine histologic pattern but negative staining for neuroendocrine markers

DIAGNOSTIC CHECKLIST

Clinically Relevant Pathologic Features
- Mitotic rate

Pathologic Interpretation Pearls
- Neuroendocrine pattern
- Rosettes
- Necrosis

NEUROENDOCRINE CARCINOMA (INCLUDING SMALL CELL CARCINOMA)

Immunohistochemistry

Antibody	Reactivity	Staining Pattern	Comment
Chromogranin-A	Positive	Cytoplasmic	Strongly positive but not global
Synaptophysin	Positive	Cytoplasmic	Diffuse positive staining
CD56	Positive	Cytoplasmic	Diffuse staining
KERATIN-LMW	Positive	Cytoplasmic	Diffuse staining
TTF-1	Positive	Nuclear	In most cases
CD57	Positive	Cytoplasmic	In some cases
Bombesin	Positive	Cytoplasmic	In some cases
LEU-7	Positive	Cytoplasmic	In some cases
CK7	Positive	Cytoplasmic	Diffuse positive staining
CDX-2	Negative		

Molecular Features of Neuroendocrine Carcinomas

Study	Result
11q deletion	Well-differentiated and moderately differentiated carcinomas
10q and 13q losses	Well-differentiated and moderately differentiated carcinomas
3q gain	Small cell carcinoma
10q - 16q - 17p deletions	High-grade neuroendocrine carcinomas
LOH at 3p14.2-p21.3	More common in moderately differentiated carcinomas
RB gene	Well-differentiated and moderately differentiated carcinomas

- Mitotic activity
- Positive neuroendocrine markers in large cell neuroendocrine carcinoma

GRADING

Low-Grade Neuroendocrine Carcinoma (Carcinoid Tumor)

- Tumors with < 3 mitoses per 10 HPF and no necrosis

Intermediate-Grade Neuroendocrine Carcinoma (Atypical Carcinoid)

- Tumors with ≥ 3 but > 10 per 10 HPF and necrosis

High-Grade Neuroendocrine Carcinoma

- Small cell carcinoma
- Large cell neuroendocrine carcinoma
  - For large cell neuroendocrine carcinoma, neuroendocrine markers must be positive

SELECTED REFERENCES

1. Moran CA et al: Neuroendocrine carcinomas of the lung: a critical analysis. Am J Clin Pathol. 131(2):206-21, 2009
2. Segawa Y et al: Immunohistochemical detection of neuroendocrine differentiation in non-small-cell lung cancer and its clinical implications. J Cancer Res Clin Oncol. 135(8):1055-9, 2009
3. Di Fabio R et al: Paraneoplastic neuromuscular disease in lung large cell neuroendocrine carcinoma. Can J Neurol Sci. 35(4):516-8, 2008
4. Dörffel Y et al: Neuroendocrine tumors: characterization with contrast-enhanced ultrasonography. Ultraschall Med. 29(5):506-14, 2008
5. García-Yuste M et al: Neuroendocrine tumors of the lung. Curr Opin Oncol. 20(2):148-54, 2008
6. Gustafsson BI et al: Bronchopulmonary neuroendocrine tumors. Cancer. 113(1):5-21, 2008
7. Namwongprom S et al: Correlation of chromogranin A levels and somatostatin receptor scintigraphy findings in the evaluation of metastases in carcinoid tumors. Ann Nucl Med. 22(4):237-43, 2008
8. Pinchot SN et al: Carcinoid tumors. Oncologist. 13(12):1255-69, 2008
9. Sica G et al: Immunohistochemical expression of estrogen and progesterone receptors in primary pulmonary neuroendocrine tumors. Arch Pathol Lab Med. 132(12):1889-95, 2008
10. Thomas R et al: Clinico-pathologic study of pulmonary carcinoid tumours--a retrospective analysis and review of literature. Respir Med. 102(11):1611-4, 2008
11. Tschernatsch M et al: Paraneoplastic neurological syndromes in patients with carcinoid. Eur J Neurol. 15(12):1390-4, 2008
12. Yao JC et al: One hundred years after "carcinoid": epidemiology of and prognostic factors for neuroendocrine tumors in 35,825 cases in the United States. J Clin Oncol. 26(18):3063-72, 2008
13. Moran CA et al: Neuroendocrine carcinomas (carcinoid, atypical carcinoid, small cell carcinoma, and large cell neuroendocrine carcinoma): current concepts. Hematol Oncol Clin North Am. 21(3):395-407; vii, 2007
14. Cerilli LA et al: Neuroendocrine neoplasms of the lung. Am J Clin Pathol. 116 Suppl:S65-96, 2001
15. Travis WD et al: Survival analysis of 200 pulmonary neuroendocrine tumors with clarification of criteria for atypical carcinoid and its separation from typical carcinoid. Am J Surg Pathol. 22(8):934-44, 1998
16. Dresler CM et al: Clinical-pathologic analysis of 40 patients with large cell neuroendocrine carcinoma of the lung. Ann Thorac Surg. 63(1):180-5, 1997
17. Arrigoni MG et al: Atypical carcinoid tumors of the lung. J Thorac Cardiovasc Surg. 64(3):413-21, 1972

NEUROENDOCRINE CARCINOMA (INCLUDING SMALL CELL CARCINOMA)

Low-Grade NE Carcinoma (Carcinoid Tumor)

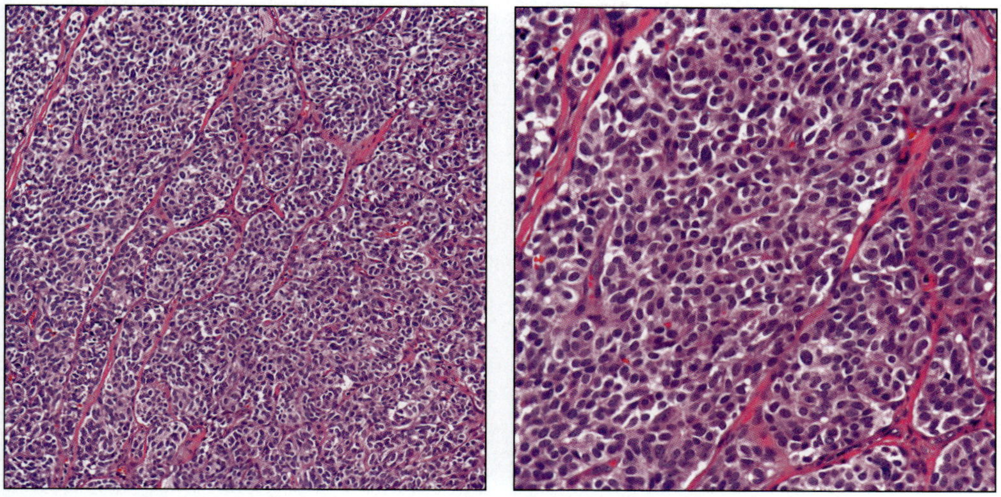

(Left) *Nesting pattern in a low-grade neuroendocrine carcinoma. Note the well-organized growth and the delicate bands of fibroconnective tissue separating the nests of tumor cells.* ***(Right)*** *Homogeneous cellular proliferation without nuclear atypia, necrosis, or hemorrhage. Notice the well-organized pattern of growth, which is one important parameter in low-grade neuroendocrine lung tumors.*

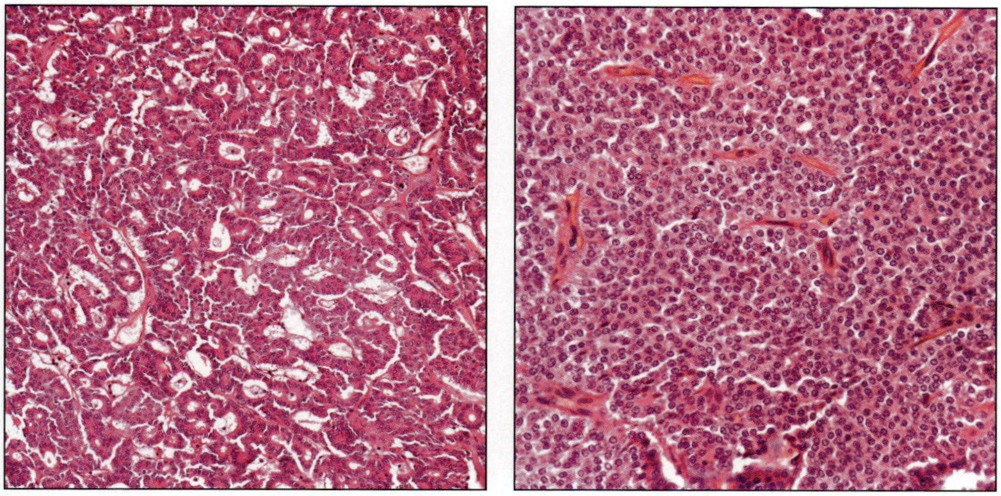

(Left) *Tubular (glandular) pattern of a low-grade neuroendocrine carcinoma. This glandular pattern at low-power view may mimic adenocarcinoma.* ***(Right)*** *Sheets of cells with a homogeneous pattern in a low-grade neuroendocrine carcinoma. Note the absence of necrosis &/or hemorrhage. These features are highly important in low-grade tumors in helping to separate them from higher grade tumors.*

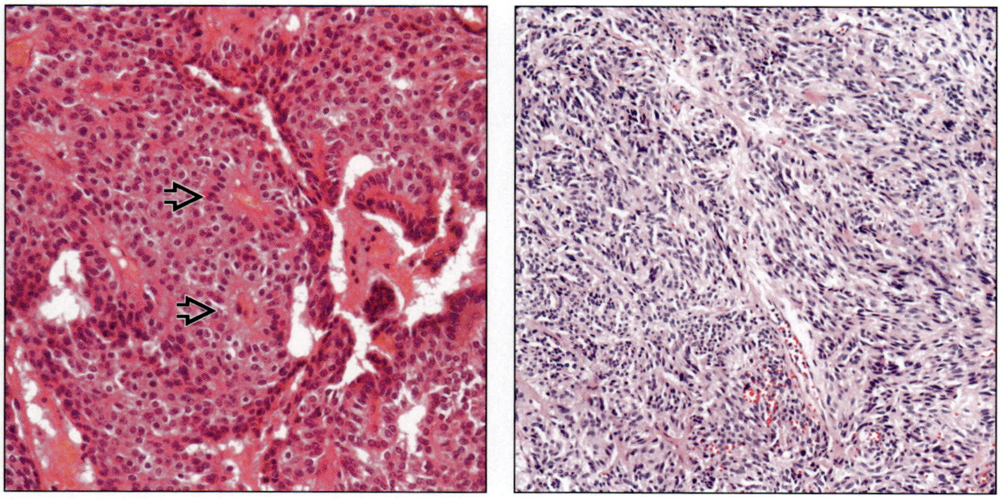

(Left) *Presence of rosettes* ➩ *in a well-differentiated neuroendocrine carcinoma. Also important to note is the absence of mitotic activity &/or necrosis.* ***(Right)*** *Low-grade NE carcinoma with prominent spindle cell growth pattern. The tumor does not show necrosis, hemorrhage, or mitotic activity, which are not features of low-grade tumors.*

NEUROENDOCRINE CARCINOMA (INCLUDING SMALL CELL CARCINOMA)

Low-Grade NE Carcinoma (Carcinoid Tumor)

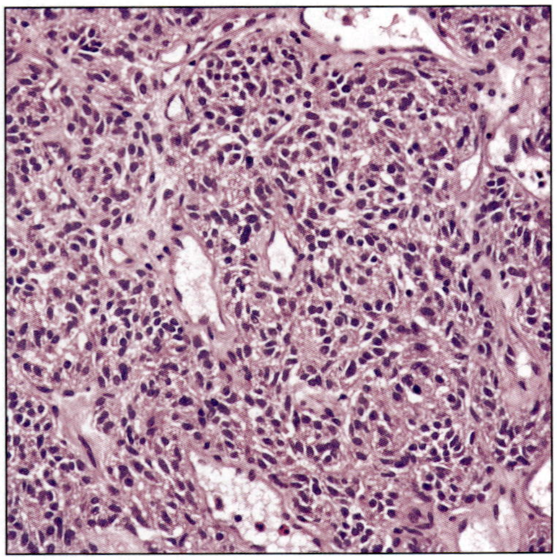

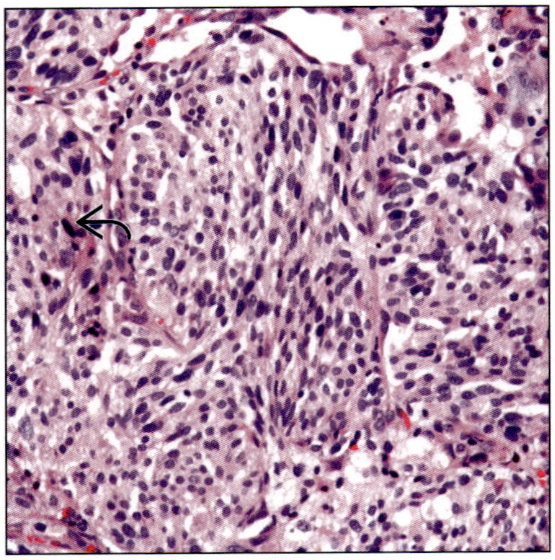

(Left) *Spindle cells around ectatic vessels in a manner mimicking hemangiopericytoma. However, the homogeneity of nuclei and the light eosinophilic cytoplasm are more in keeping with a neuroendocrine tumor.* ***(Right)*** *High-power magnification of a low-grade spindle cell neuroendocrine carcinoma (carcinoid tumor). Note the absence of mitotic activity or marked nuclear pleomorphism. Scattered apoptotic cells are present →.*

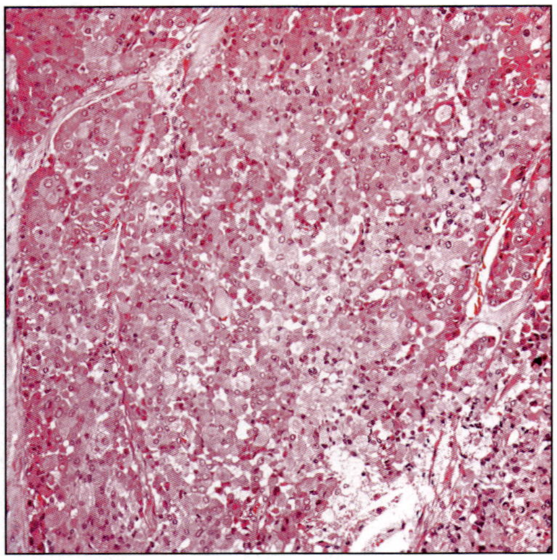

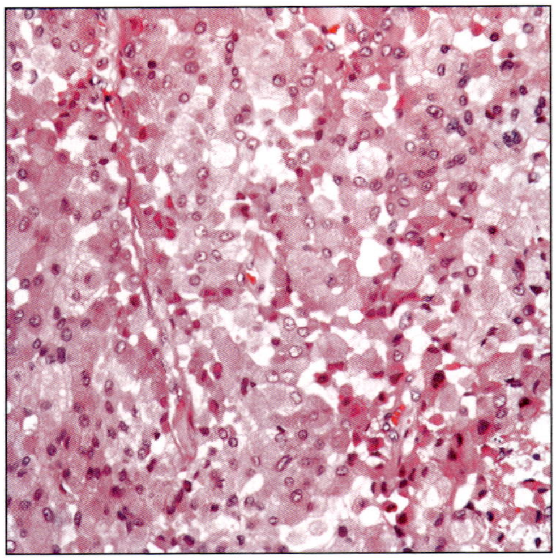

(Left) *Oncocytic variant of well-differentiated neuroendocrine carcinoma of the lung on hematoxylin & eosin shows sheets of oncocytic cells with a homogeneous appearance. Note the absence of nuclear atypia, necrosis, &/or mitotic activity.* ***(Right)*** *Hematoxylin & eosin shows oncocytic cells without mitotic activity. The cytoplasm of the cells is brightly eosinophilic, and the nuclei are homogeneous. In some cells, nucleoli are easily identifiable.*

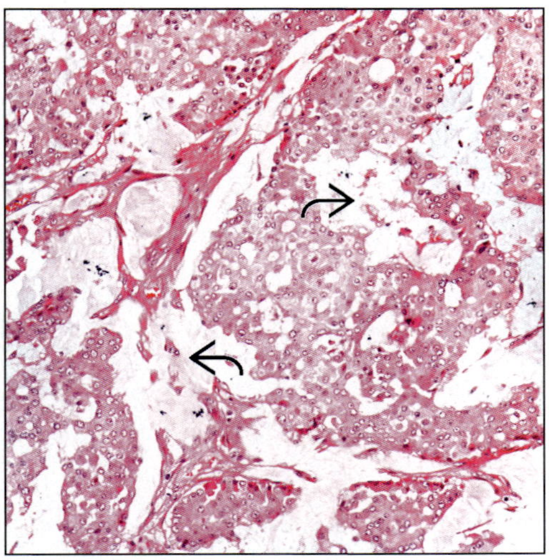

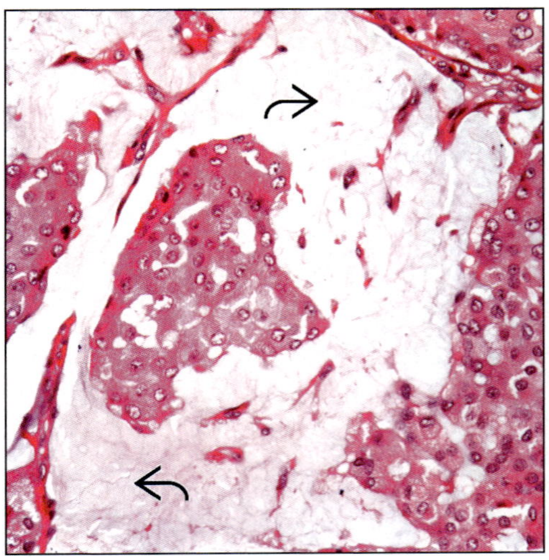

(Left) *Neuroendocrine carcinoma, low grade with presence of abundant mucoid material →. In addition, the tumor shows oncocytic features. Mucinous neuroendocrine carcinomas of the lung are rare.* ***(Right)*** *High-power magnification of a mucinous neuroendocrine carcinoma. Note that there is no mitotic activity or marked nuclear atypia. The presence of mucoid material → is unusual and may be mistaken for a metastatic mucinous carcinoma.*

NEUROENDOCRINE CARCINOMA (INCLUDING SMALL CELL CARCINOMA)

Low-Grade NE Carcinoma (Carcinoid Tumor)

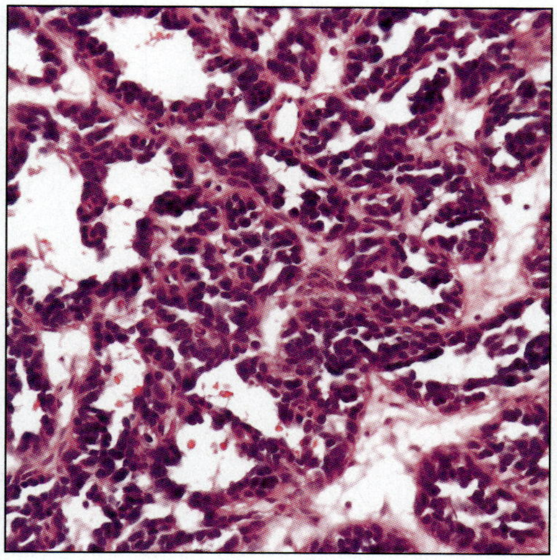
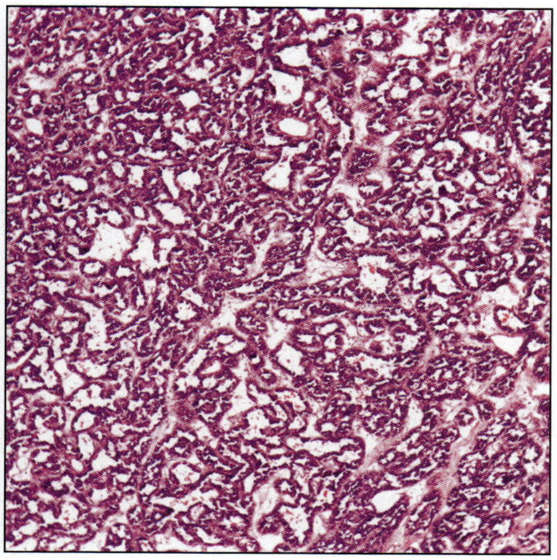

(Left) *Well-differentiated neuroendocrine carcinoma shows glands composed of rather small cells without mitotic activity. This glandular architecture may be erroneously interpreted as adenocarcinoma. Thus, a careful cytological examination of the neoplastic cells is important.* ***(Right)*** *Glandular pattern of a low-grade neuroendocrine carcinoma. This complex architecture may mimic a well-differentiated adenocarcinoma.*

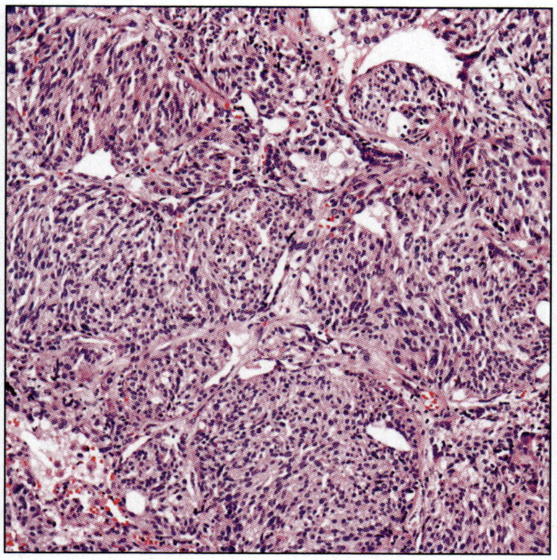
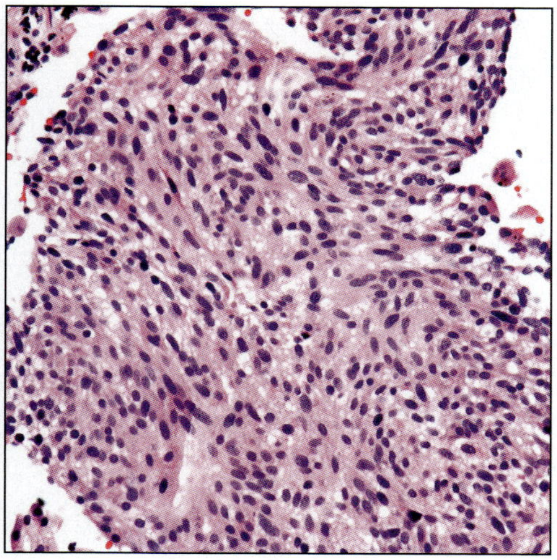

(Left) *Well-differentiated neuroendocrine carcinoma shows subtle nesting pattern with spindle cell proliferation. This architectural pattern may be misinterpreted as sarcoma or other neoplasms of neuroectodermal origin, such as melanomas.* ***(Right)*** *Spindle cells without nuclear atypia or mitotic activity. The pattern of growth mimics a neural neoplasm. A spindle cell pattern may also be seen in higher grade tumors.*

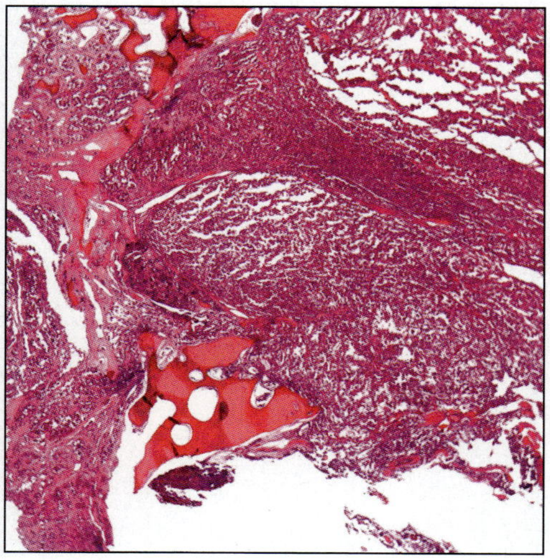
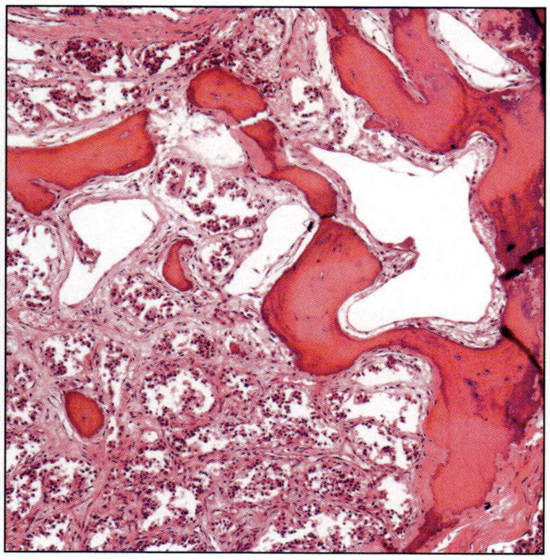

(Left) *Low-grade neuroendocrine carcinoma is shown with areas of metaplastic bone formation. Bone formation in neuroendocrine carcinomas is rare. This metaplastic change is rarely extensive.* ***(Right)*** *Closer view of the metaplastic bone formation in neuroendocrine carcinoma. Note the presence of a pseudoglandular arrangement of the neoplastic neuroendocrine cells.*

NEUROENDOCRINE CARCINOMA (INCLUDING SMALL CELL CARCINOMA)

Intermediate-Grade NE Carcinoma (Atypical Carcinoid)

*(**Left**) Gross pathology of bronchial neuroendocrine carcinoma. Note the presence of focal areas of hemorrhage and necrosis ➔. Such features should raise the suspicion of a higher grade neoplasm and require extensive sampling. (**Right**) Intermediate-grade tumor with sheets of neoplastic cells without any particular architecture. Note that the surface epithelium is intact and the tumor does not reach the respiratory epithelium →.*

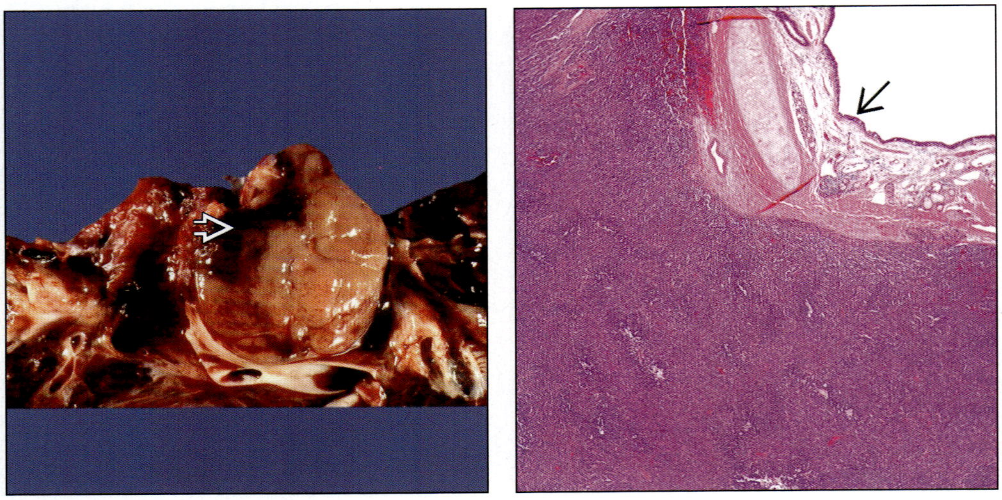

*(**Left**) Easily identifiable areas of comedo-like necrosis ➔ typical of intermediate-grade neuroendocrine carcinomas. Note the presence of nested and diffuse growth patterns, which are commonly seen in intermediate-grade tumors. (**Right**) Solid sheets and comedo-like necrotic areas characteristic of intermediate-grade neuroendocrine carcinoma. These features are very typical of intermediate-grade tumors.*

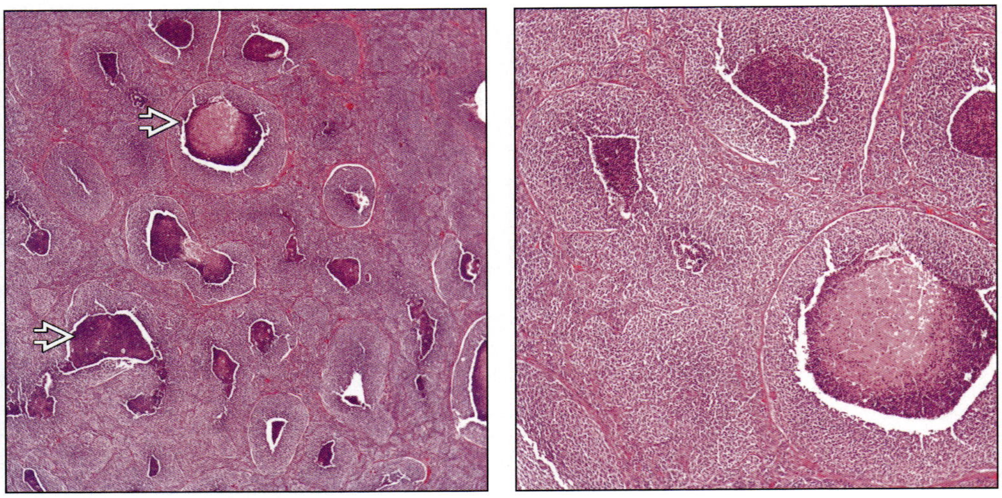

*(**Left**) Intermediate-grade neuroendocrine carcinoma with a diffuse pattern of growth and discrete areas of necrosis →. The presence of areas of diffuse growth pattern should raise the suspicion of intermediate-grade tumors. (**Right**) Closer view of areas of necrosis → in association with neoplastic neuroendocrine cells with vague nesting pattern ➔ are seen in this example of moderately differentiated neuroendocrine carcinoma.*

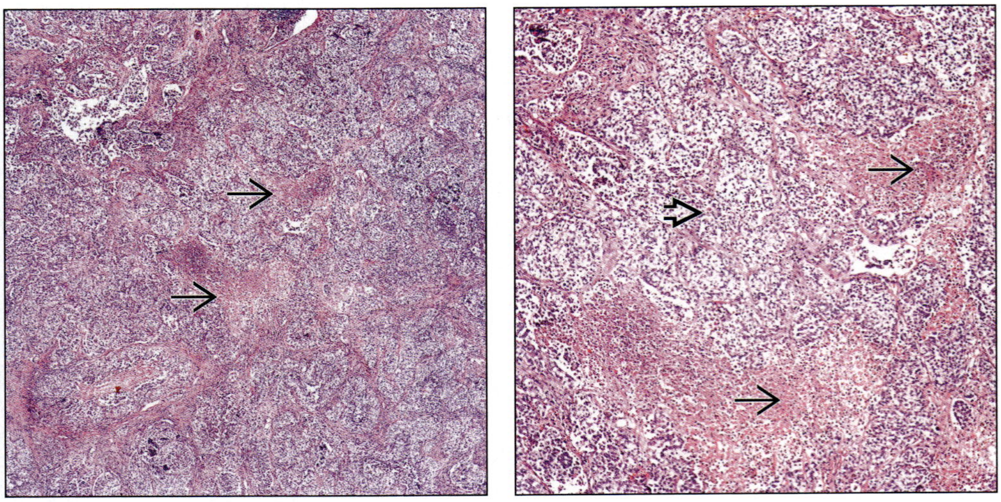

Intermediate-Grade NE Carcinoma (Atypical Carcinoid)

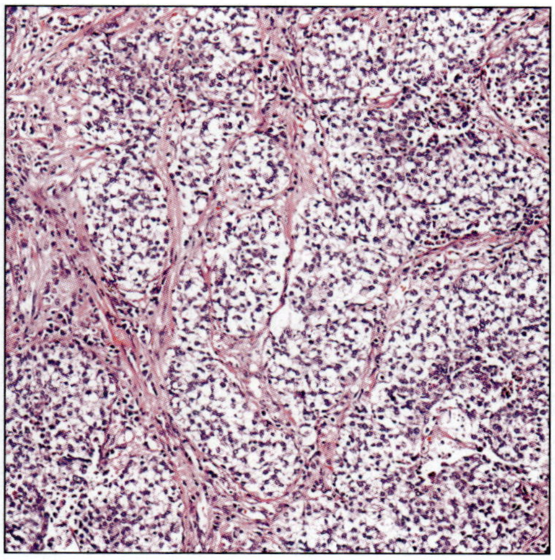
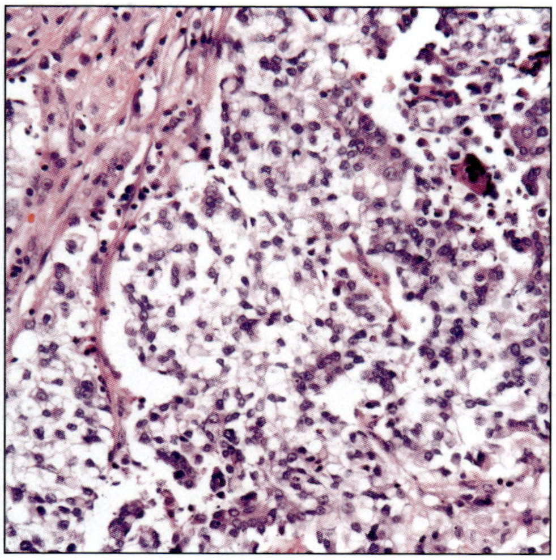

(Left) *AC shows the characteristic nesting growth pattern of neuroendocrine carcinoma; however, the neoplastic cellular proliferation is composed of clear cells. The presence of extensive areas of clear cell change in neuroendocrine carcinomas is rare.* ***(Right)*** *A closer view shows neuroendocrine cellular proliferation composed predominantly of clear cells with small round and homogeneous nuclei. Nucleoli are inconspicuous.*

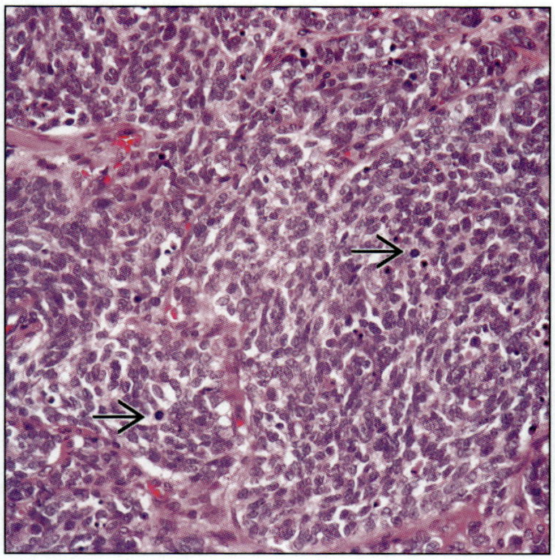
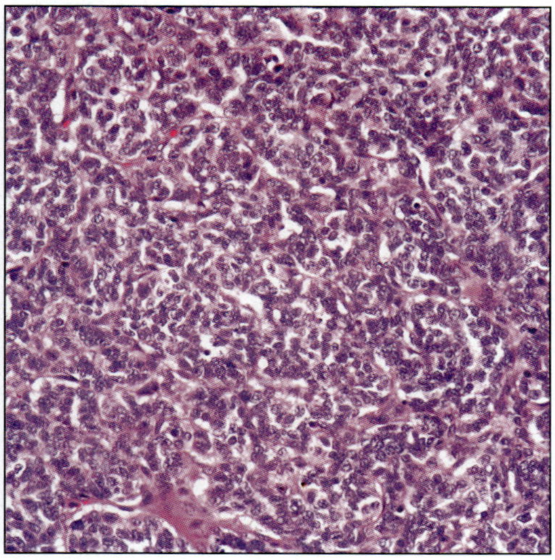

(Left) *Spindle cell neuroendocrine carcinoma with easily identifiable mitotic figures →. The mitotic count in neuroendocrine carcinoma is the most important feature in the classification of these tumors.* ***(Right)*** *Sheets of neoplastic cells in a disorganized pattern of growth. Nuclear atypia is evident and should prompt the search for mitotic activity.*

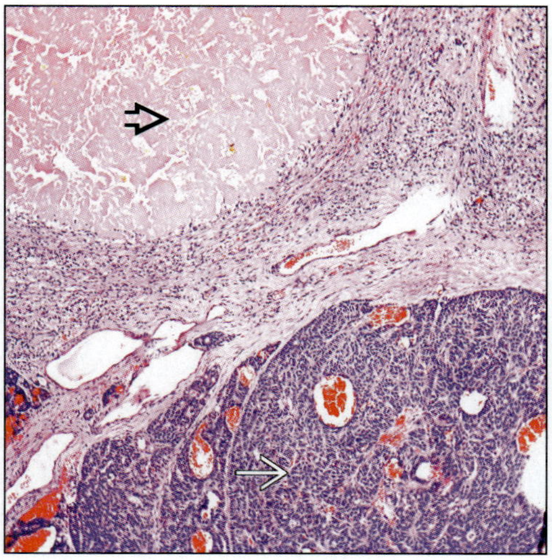
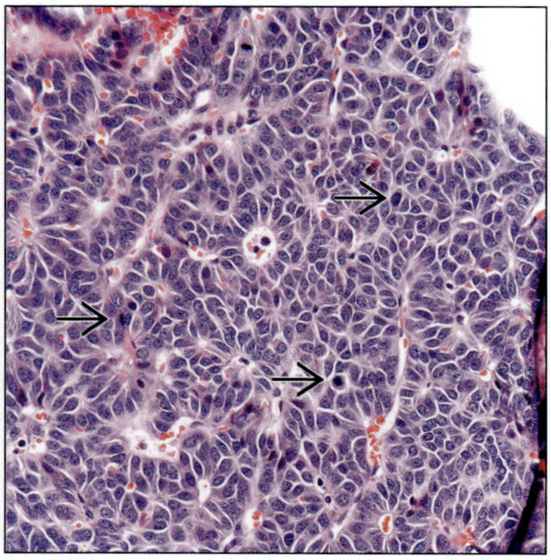

(Left) *Moderately differentiated neuroendocrine carcinoma shows extensive areas of necrosis ⇨ with areas of viable tumor ➡. It is very important to separate tumor necrosis from other possible causes of necrosis, such as necrosis secondary to needle biopsy.* ***(Right)*** *Well-organized pattern with rosettes and easily identifiable mitotic figures →. Although the pattern is fairly organized, the presence of mitotic figures is the most important criterion for grading these tumors.*

NEUROENDOCRINE CARCINOMA (INCLUDING SMALL CELL CARCINOMA)

High-Grade NE Carcinoma, Small Cell Type

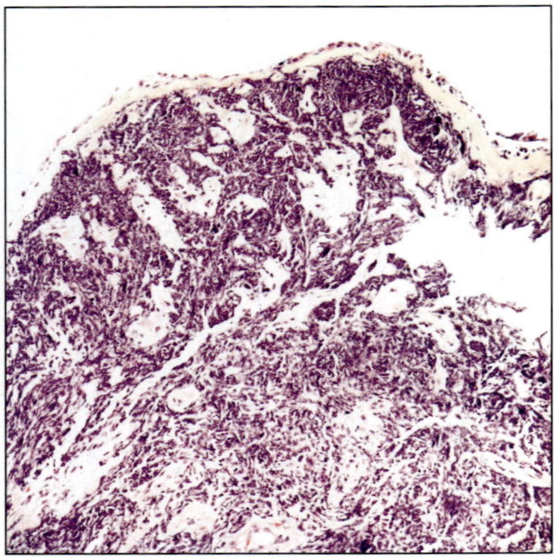

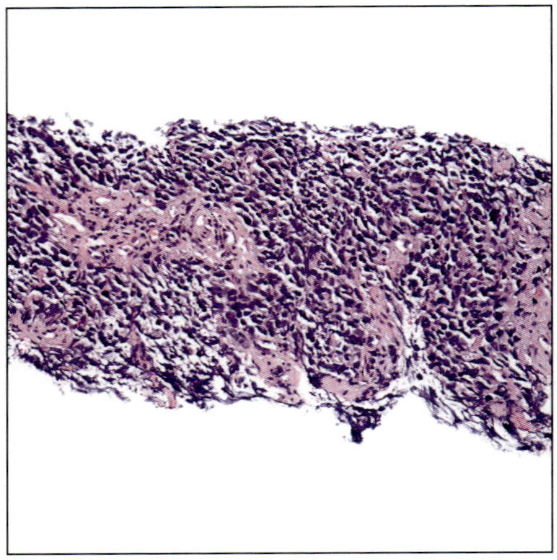

(Left) *Transbronchial biopsy specimen of small cell carcinoma with prominent crush artifact. The presence of crush artifact appears to be more commonly seen in transbronchial biopsies than in core needle biopsies.* ***(Right)*** *Core biopsy specimen of a small cell carcinoma. Note the preservation of tumor cells and the lack of crush artifact. The preservation of tumor cells is often better with this method.*

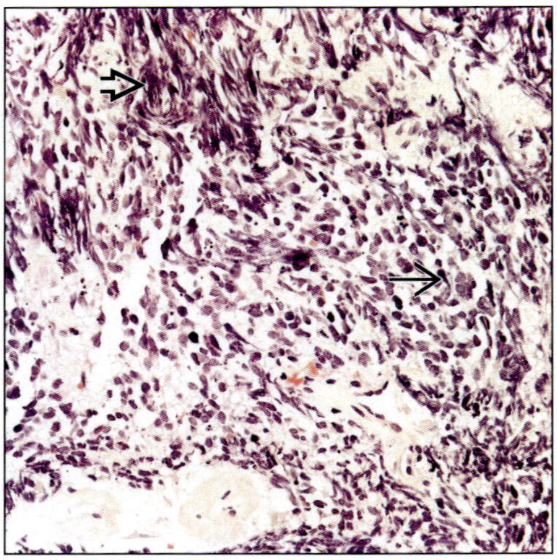

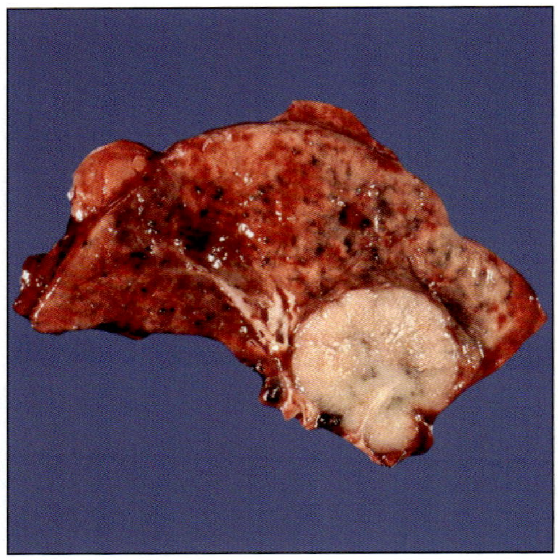

(Left) *Typical features of small cell carcinoma. Note the viable areas of tumor cells ⇨ and the crush artifact ▷. The mitotic count may not be high in a biopsy specimen, making precise categorization difficult in small samples.* ***(Right)*** *Gross photograph shows an intrapulmonary mass. The tumor is well circumscribed with a tan homogeneous cut surface. No areas of necrosis or hemorrhage are apparent.*

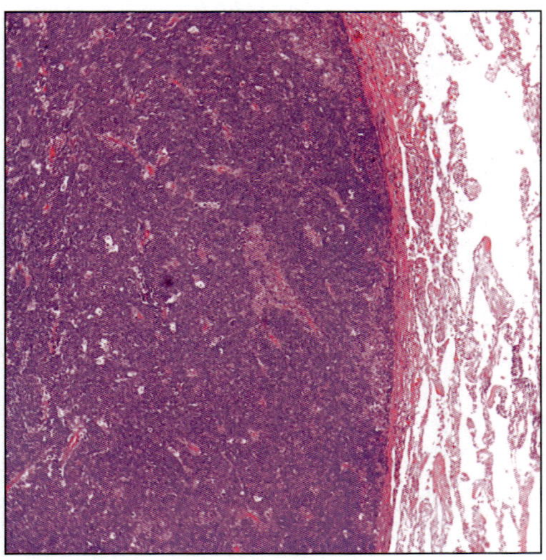

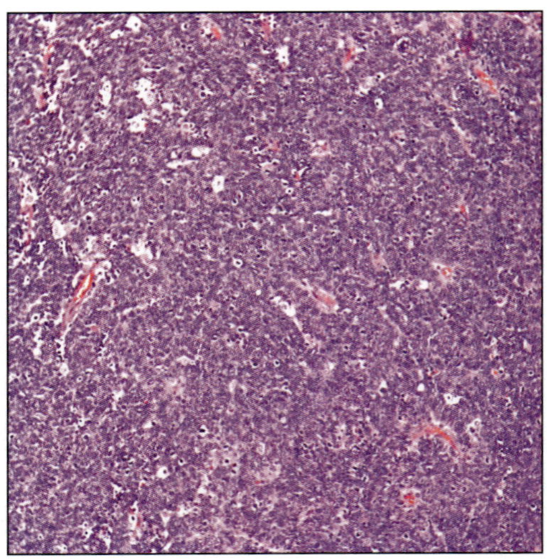

(Left) *Small cell carcinoma with diffuse sheets of tumor cells. At this magnification, it is virtually impossible to unequivocally appreciate the small cell nature of the neoplasm.* ***(Right)*** *Sheets of neoplastic cells with obvious nuclear atypia, mitotic figures, and disorganized pattern of growth are seen in this high-grade neuroendocrine carcinoma.*

NEUROENDOCRINE CARCINOMA (INCLUDING SMALL CELL CARCINOMA)

High-Grade NE Carcinoma, Small Cell Type

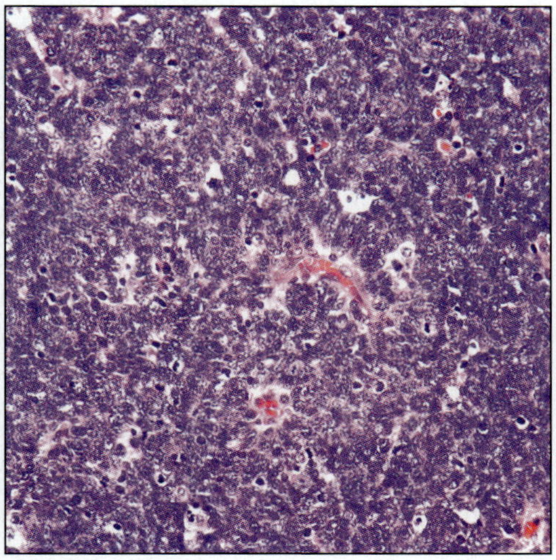
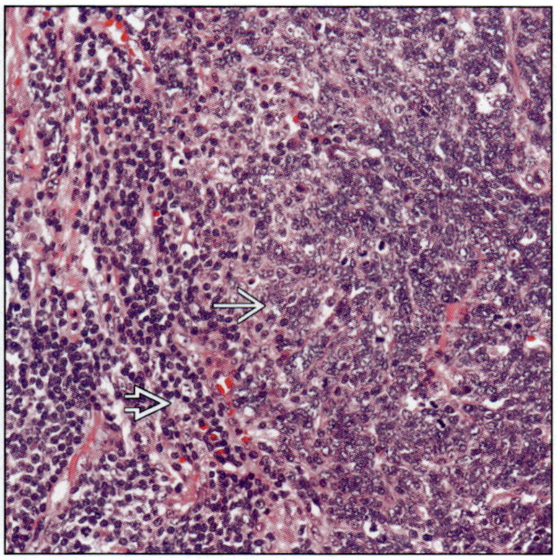

(Left) *Predominantly solid pattern of growth of neoplastic cells with high mitotic activity and prominent nuclear atypia.* ***(Right)*** *Solid pattern of neoplastic cells* ➔ *admixed with numerous inflammatory cells, predominantly lymphocytes* ⇨*. In some cases, the inflammatory response may be very prominent. It is unusual to see this type of feature in small cell carcinomas.*

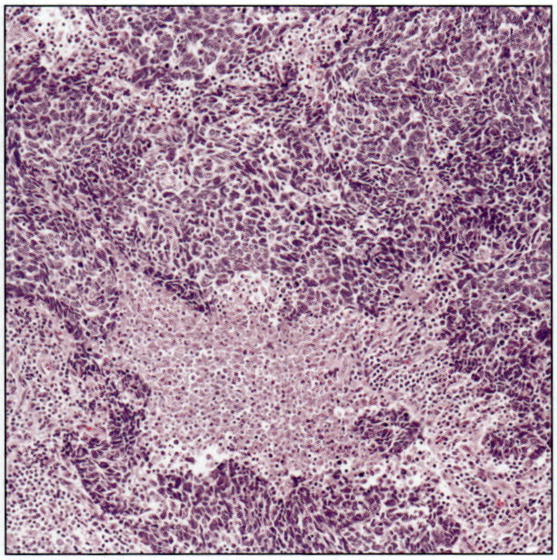
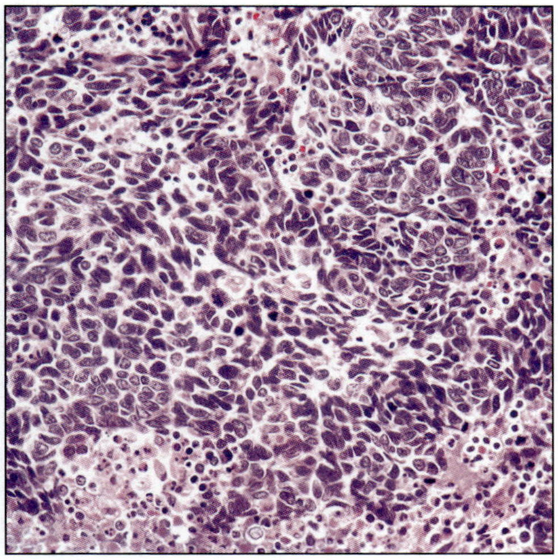

(Left) *High-grade neuroendocrine carcinoma with extensive necrosis and sheets of neoplastic cells with a vague basaloid pattern.* ***(Right)*** *Closer view of neoplastic cells in a high-grade neuroendocrine carcinoma. Note the absence of nucleoli, which is an important characteristic of these tumors. The features of small cell carcinomas in resected specimens may show better preservation than in biopsy specimens.*

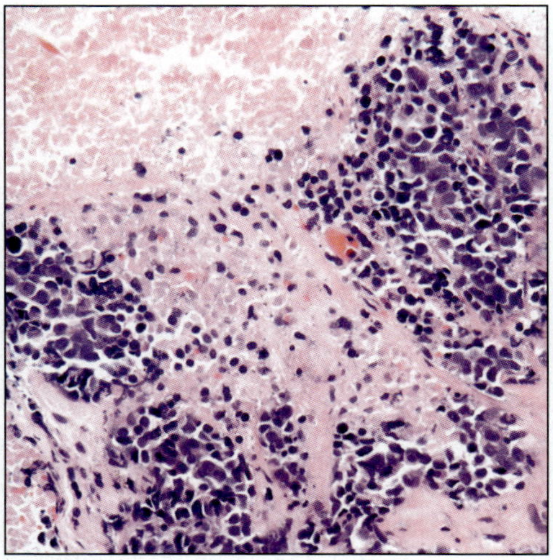
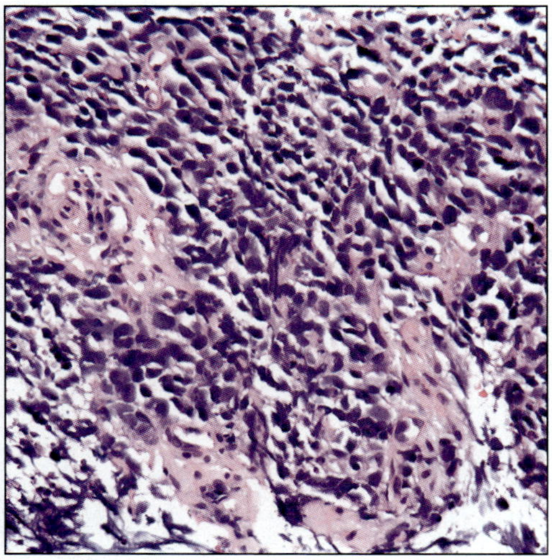

(Left) *Extensive necrosis and clusters of neoplastic cells. The tumor cytology is that of small cells with scant cytoplasm and inconspicuous nucleoli. Often the presence of extensive areas of necrosis is more commonly seen in high-grade tumors.* ***(Right)*** *Classic small cell morphology of small cells with nuclear molding and prominent atypia. However, in this illustration, the presence of mitoses is not marked.*

NEUROENDOCRINE CARCINOMA (INCLUDING SMALL CELL CARCINOMA)

High-Grade NE Carcinoma, Large Cell Type

__(Left)__ Gross photograph shows a large intrapulmonary mass of irregular borders and focal areas of necrosis. The macroscopic characteristics of large cell neuroendocrine carcinoma are not any different from other non-small cell carcinomas. __(Right)__ Large cell neuroendocrine carcinoma. Note the well-circumscribed tumor mass destroying normal lung parenchyma. Even at this magnification one can still see a nested pattern ⇨.

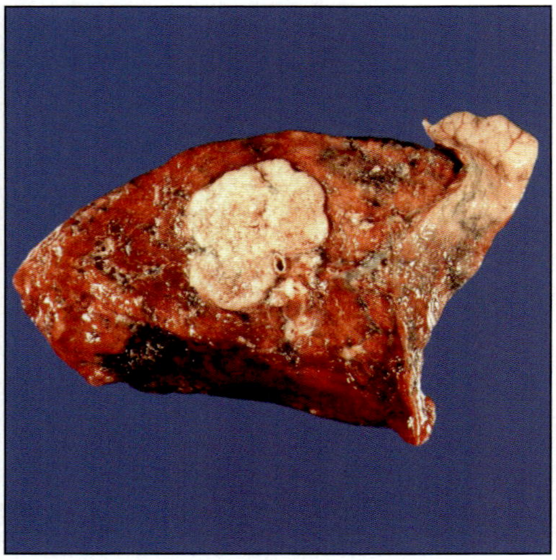

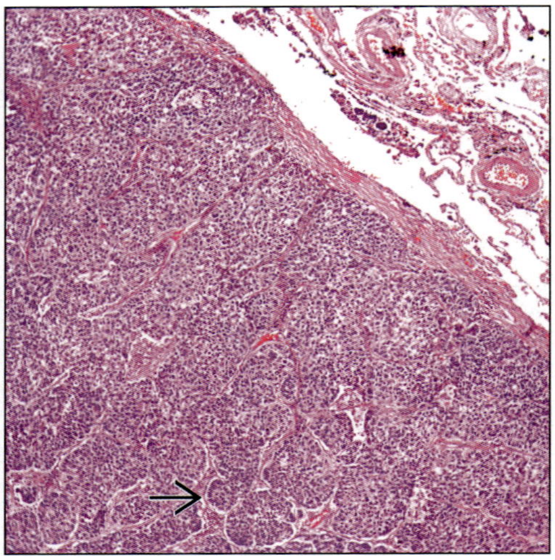

__(Left)__ Large cell neuroendocrine carcinoma with areas of comedo-like necrosis. The rest of the tumor shows a more basaloid growth pattern. This type of pattern is fairly common in large cell neuroendocrine carcinomas. __(Right)__ Large cell neuroendocrine carcinoma with a vague nested pattern. Most of the tumor is arranged in ribbons or trabeculae of neoplastic cells.

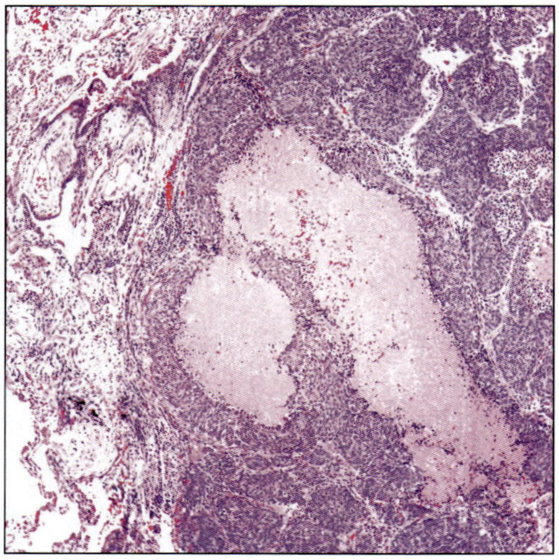

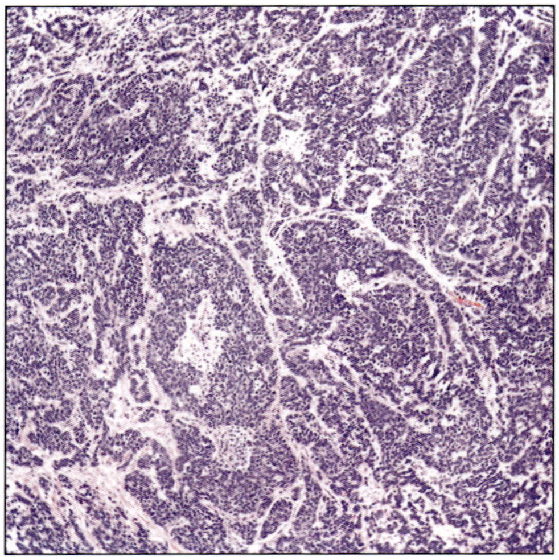

__(Left)__ Large cell neuroendocrine carcinoma with basaloid features. Note the nuclear palisading and the presence of an inflammatory component in the fibroconnective tissue. __(Right)__ Closer view of the large cell neuroendocrine carcinoma, displaying larger cells with round nuclei, light eosinophilic cytoplasm, and prominent nucleoli. Essentially the morphology is that of large cell carcinoma with positive neuroendocrine markers.

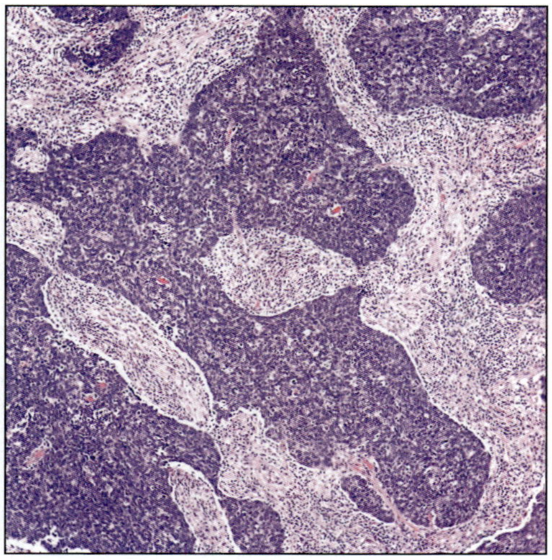

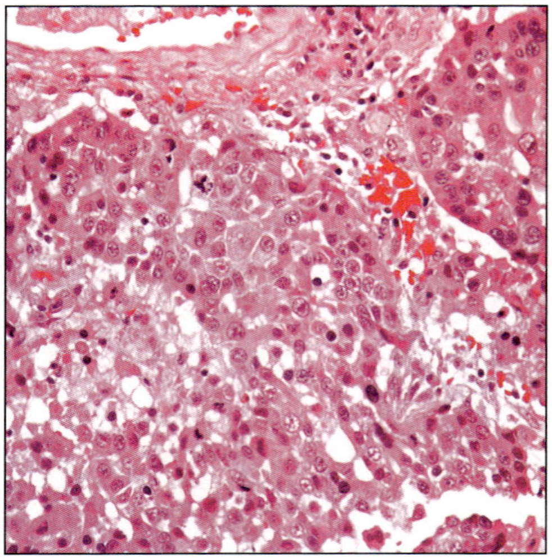

High-Grade NE Carcinoma, Large Cell Type

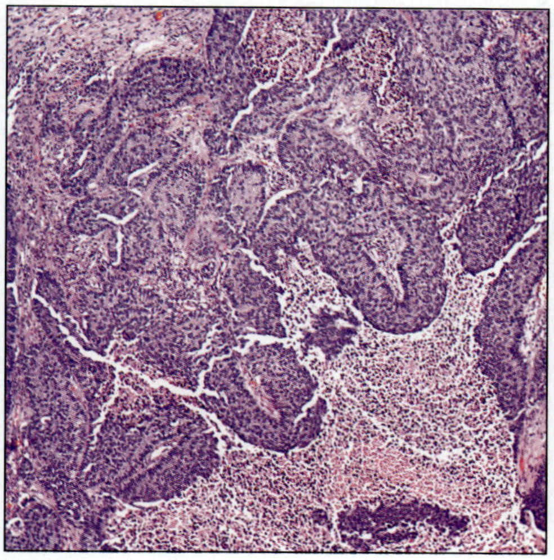

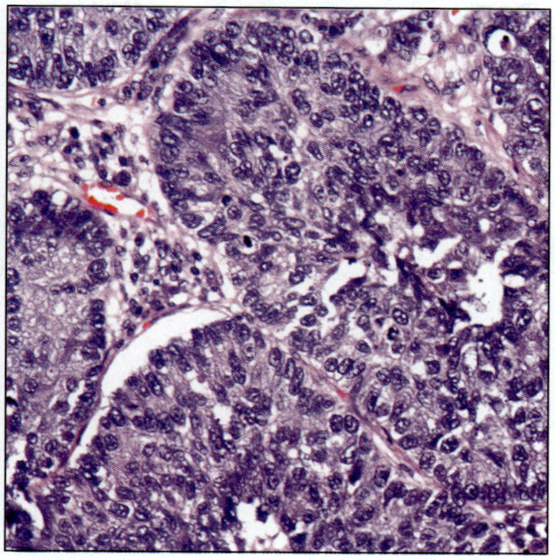

(Left) *Large cell neuroendocrine carcinoma with necrosis and organoid pattern of growth. This pattern, however, may be seen in tumors that do not show positive neuroendocrine markers.* ***(Right)*** *Closer view of neoplastic cells displaying nuclear atypia and prominent nucleoli. However, it is the positive staining for neuroendocrine markers that confirms the diagnosis of large cell neuroendocrine carcinoma.*

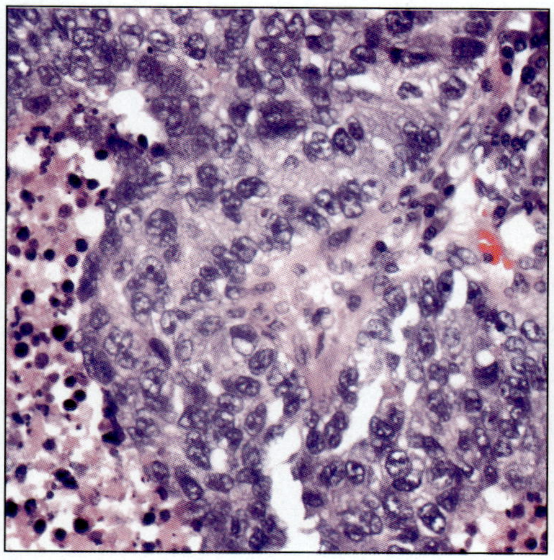

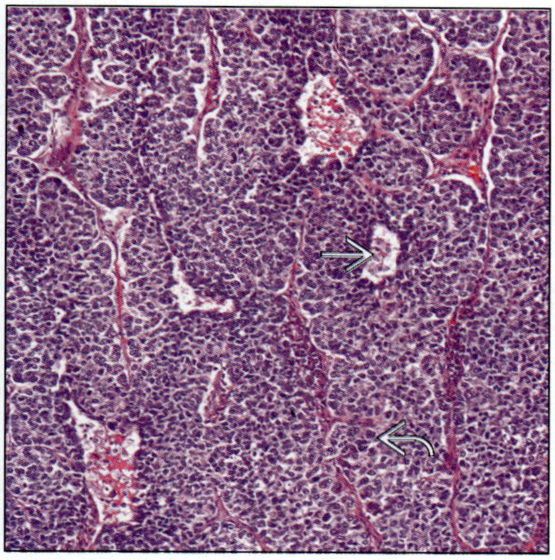

(Left) *High-power view of larger cells with ample cytoplasm, round nuclei, and prominent nucleoli. These features are those of a non-small cell carcinoma.* ***(Right)*** *High-grade neuroendocrine carcinoma with more conventional nesting pattern and absence of obvious necrosis. In some focal areas, there is a hint of comedo-like necrosis* ➔ *and the presence of larger pleomorphic cells* ↪.

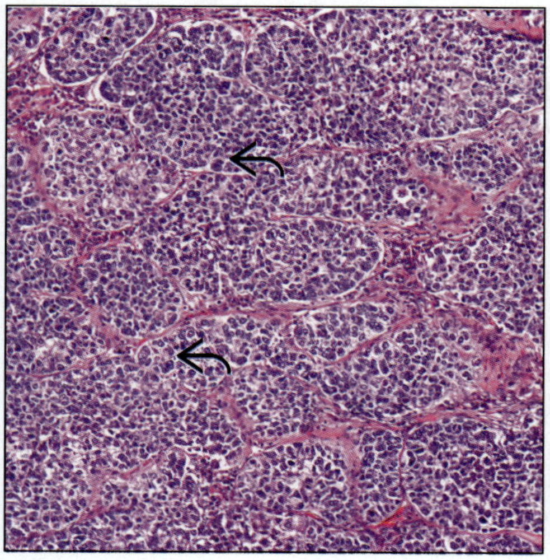

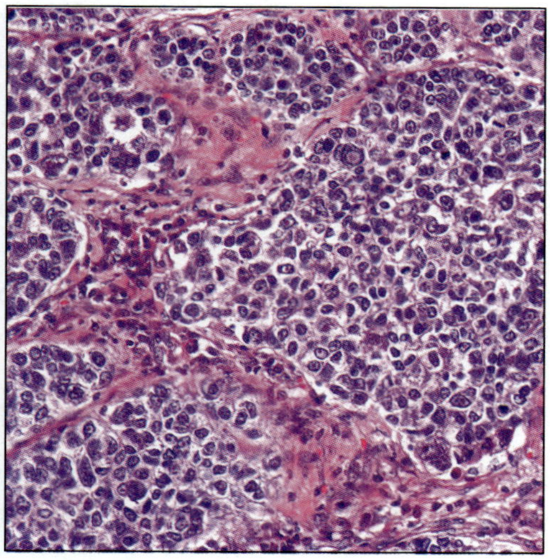

(Left) *High-grade neuroendocrine carcinoma is shown with a very organized pattern of growth. Necrosis is absent; however, note the presence of marked nuclear atypia* ↪*, which should raise the suspicion of a higher grade neoplasm.* ***(Right)*** *High-grade neuroendocrine carcinoma shows the classic characteristics of prominent nuclear atypia and increased mitotic activity; however, necrosis is absent.*

CARCINOSARCOMA

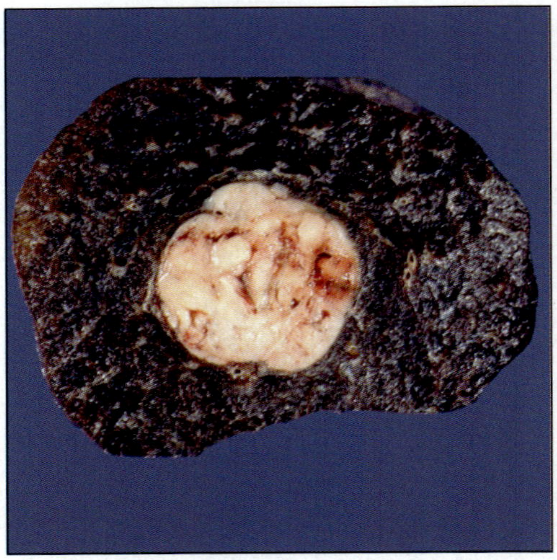

Gross photograph of pulmonary carcinosarcoma shows a well-circumscribed, light tan, fleshy intrapulmonary mass. Note the absence of necrosis and hemorrhage.

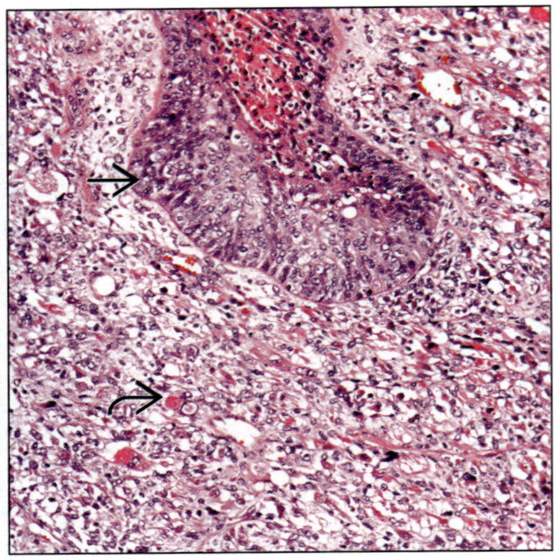

Primary carcinosarcoma of the lung shows classical features of squamous cell carcinoma ⇒ and rhabdomyosarcoma ⇒.

TERMINOLOGY

Abbreviations

- Carcinosarcoma (CSC)

Definitions

- Malignant biphasic neoplasm composed of malignant epithelial and malignant mesenchymal components

ETIOLOGY/PATHOGENESIS

Environmental Exposure

- Carcinosarcomas have been linked to tobacco smoke

Etiology

- Collision tumor
- Composite tumor
- Tumor derived from stem cells with multiple differentiation
- Biphasic sarcomatoid carcinomas

CLINICAL ISSUES

Epidemiology

- Incidence
  - More common in men than women

Site

- May be central or peripheral

Presentation

- Cough
- Dyspnea
- Hemoptysis
- Chest pain
- Weight loss
- Obstructive pneumonia

Treatment

- Surgical approaches
  - Complete resection
- Adjuvant therapy
  - No definitive specific treatment

Prognosis

- Poor

MACROSCOPIC FEATURES

General Features

- Central tumors may grow in polypoid fashion, obstructing airway
- Peripheral tumors may reach large size
- Areas of necrosis &/or hemorrhage are common

Size

- 2 cm to > 10 cm in diameter

MICROSCOPIC PATHOLOGY

Histologic Features

- Presence of conventional carcinoma (any type) with sarcoma (any type)
- Squamous cell carcinoma is most common epithelial component

Predominant Pattern/Injury Type

- Biphasic

Predominant Cell/Compartment Type

- Epithelial, biphasic, or mixed

DIFFERENTIAL DIAGNOSIS

Carcinoma

- In small biopsy specimen where only epithelial component is present

CARCINOSARCOMA

Key Facts

Terminology

- Malignant biphasic neoplasm composed of malignant epithelial and malignant mesenchymal components

Etiology/Pathogenesis

- Carcinosarcomas have been linked to tobacco use

Clinical Issues

- More common in men than women
- May be central or peripheral

Macroscopic Features

- Central tumors may grow in polypoid fashion, obstructing airways
- Peripheral tumors may reach large size
- Areas of necrosis &/or hemorrhage are common
- 2 cm to > 10 cm in diameter

Microscopic Pathology

- Biphasic
- Presence of conventional carcinoma (any type) with sarcoma (any type)
- Squamous cell carcinoma is most common epithelial component
- Epithelial, biphasic, or mixed

Top Differential Diagnoses

- Carcinoma
  - In small biopsy specimen where only epithelial component is present
- Sarcoma
  - In small biopsy specimen where only sarcomatous component is present

Immunohistochemistry

Antibody	Reactivity	Staining Pattern	Comment
EMA/MUC1	Positive	Cell membrane	In epithelial component
CK5/6	Positive	Cytoplasmic	In epithelial component (squamous cell)
CK-PAN	Positive	Cytoplasmic	In epithelial component
CEA-M	Positive	Cytoplasmic	In epithelial component (adenocarcinoma)
Desmin	Positive	Cytoplasmic	In sarcomatous component (muscle differentiation)
MYOD1	Positive	Cytoplasmic	In sarcomatous component (muscle differentiation)
CD31	Positive	Cytoplasmic	If vascular differentiation (angiosarcoma)
CD34	Positive	Cytoplasmic	If vascular differentiation (angiosarcoma)
S100	Positive	Cytoplasmic	Chondroid component
SOX2	Positive	Nuclear	Chondroid component
Myoglobin	Positive	Cytoplasmic	Muscle differentiation

- In larger specimens, presence of mixed population epithelial/mesenchymal will lead to correct interpretation

Sarcoma

- In small biopsies if only component is mesenchymal
- In larger specimens, presence of any heterologous sarcomatous component in association with carcinoma is diagnostic

DIAGNOSTIC CHECKLIST

Clinically Relevant Pathologic Features

- Tissue distribution

Pathologic Interpretation Pearls

- Combined tumor with carcinoma and sarcomatous elements

SELECTED REFERENCES

1. Pardo J et al: Primary mixed squamous carcinoma and osteosarcoma (carcinosarcomas) of the lung have a CGH mapping similar to primitive squamous carcinomas and osteosarcomas. Diagn Mol Pathol. 17(3):151-8, 2008
2. Mito A et al: [Case of pulmonary carcinosarcoma and a summary of 17 cases reported in Japan.] Nihon Kokyuki Gakkai Zasshi. 42(8):749-54, 2004
3. Aurello P et al: Squamocellular carcinoma and chondrosarcoma: a true pulmonary carcinosarcoma. Report of a case. Anticancer Res. 23(3C):3073-6, 2003
4. Petrov DB et al: Primary pulmonary sarcomas and carcinosarcomas--postoperative results and comparative survival analysis. Eur J Cardiothorac Surg. 23(4):461-6, 2003
5. Rossi G et al: Pulmonary carcinomas with pleomorphic, sarcomatoid, or sarcomatous elements: a clinicopathologic and immunohistochemical study of 75 cases. Am J Surg Pathol. 27(3):311-24, 2003
6. Koss MN et al: Carcinosarcomas of the lung: a clinicopathologic study of 66 patients. Am J Surg Pathol. 23(12):1514-26, 1999
7. Nappi O et al: Biphasic and monophasic sarcomatoid carcinomas of the lung. A reappraisal of 'carcinosarcomas' and 'spindle-cell carcinomas'. Am J Clin Pathol. 102(3):331-40, 1994
8. Davis MP et al: Carcinosarcoma of the lung: Mayo Clinic experience and response to chemotherapy. Mayo Clin Proc. 59(9):598-603, 1984

CARCINOSARCOMA

Microscopic Features

*(**Left**) This low-power view shows a mixed cellular composition. Note the presence of eroded superficial epithelium →. This is a centrally located carcinosarcoma. (**Right**) Carcinosarcoma shows discrete merging between malignant epithelial → and malignant mesenchymal components ⇨. In a cursory review, this tumor can be misdiagnosed as conventional carcinoma.*

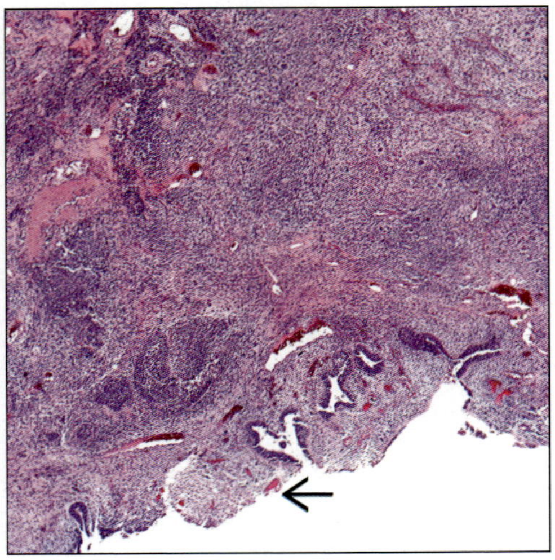

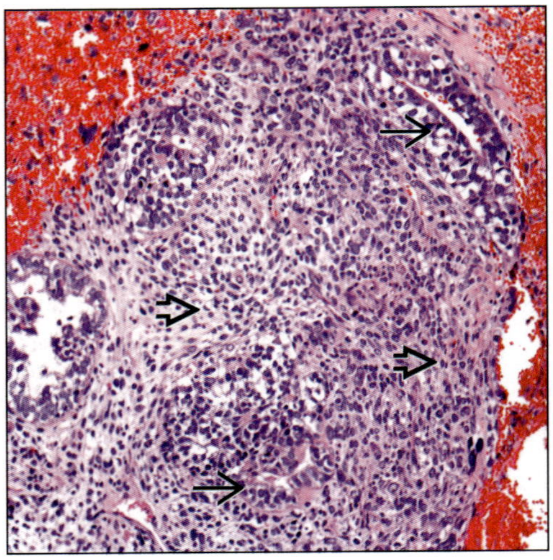

*(**Left**) Carcinosarcoma with predominant sarcomatous elements. The sarcoma component of this tumor is of the high-grade type. In some cases, the use of immunohistochemistry may facilitate the identification of the specific sarcomatous component. (**Right**) Carcinosarcoma is shown in which there is myogenic differentiation in the form of rhabdomyosarcoma. In some cases, the merging of epithelial and mesenchymal components may not be so obvious.*

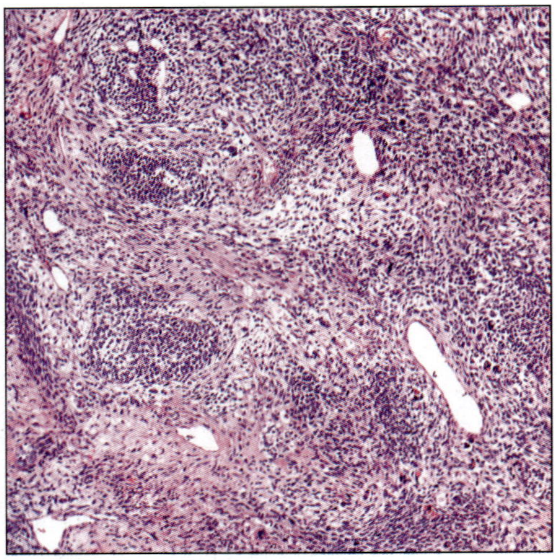

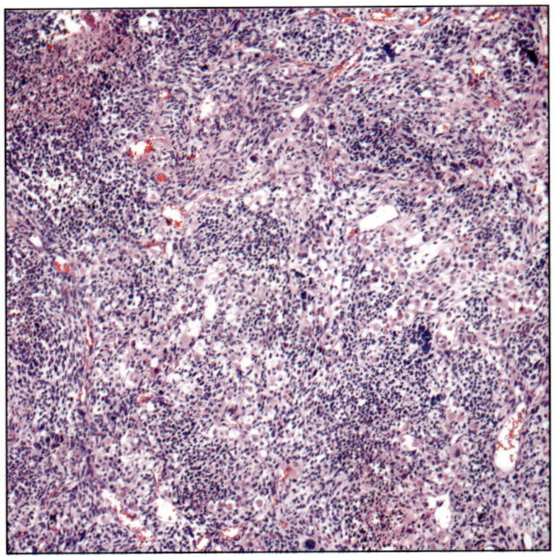

*(**Left**) Carcinosarcoma is shown in which the malignant component is of glandular type ⇨, while the sarcomatous component is rather undifferentiated →. (**Right**) Carcinosarcoma is seen with an easily identifiable squamous cell carcinoma ⇨ admixed with areas of high-grade sarcomatous component →. Squamous cell carcinoma is one of the most common components of carcinosarcoma.*

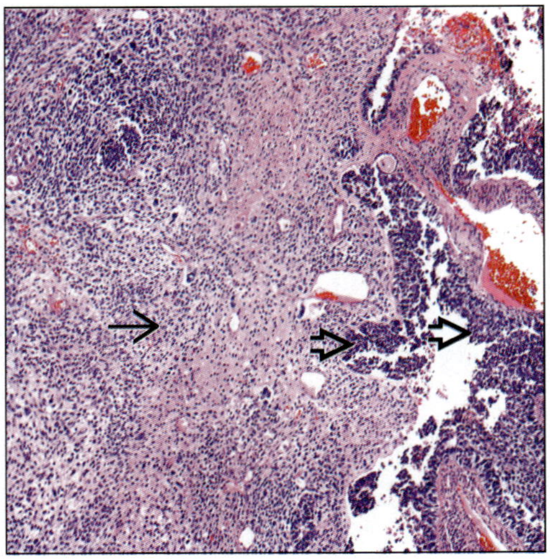

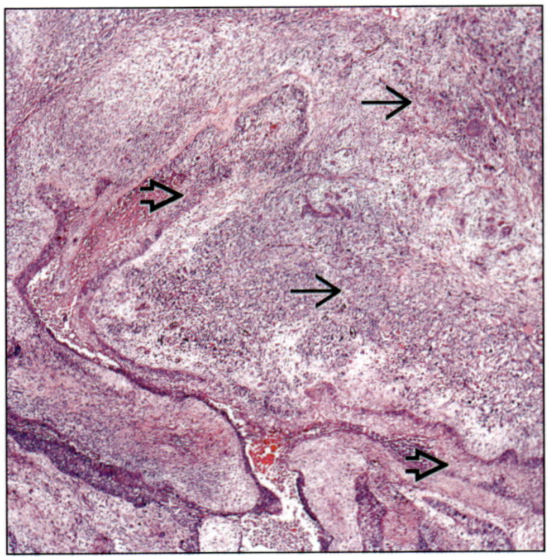

Microscopic Features

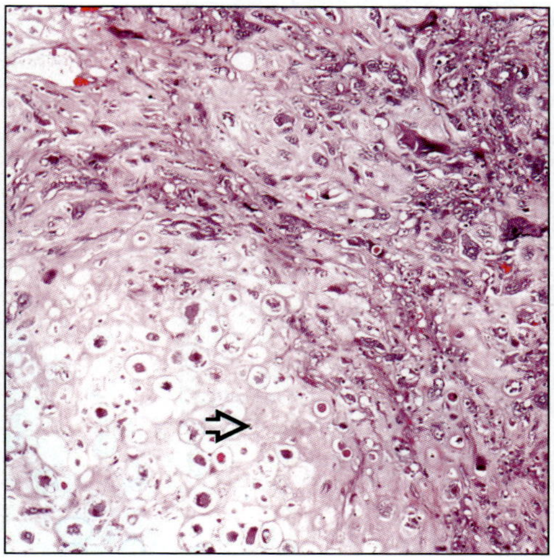

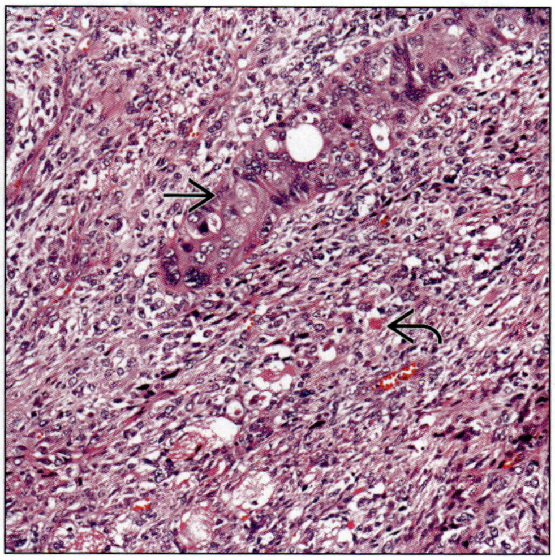

(Left) *Carcinosarcoma with a high-grade chondrosarcoma ⇨ as the mesenchymal component. In this image, the presence of an epithelial component is not obvious, and cases like this require extensive sampling to demonstrate its presence.* ***(Right)*** *In some cases of carcinosarcoma, the mesenchymal component may be more extensive than the epithelial component. In this illustration, the rhabdomyosarcoma is more prominent ↷ than the squamous cell carcinoma →.*

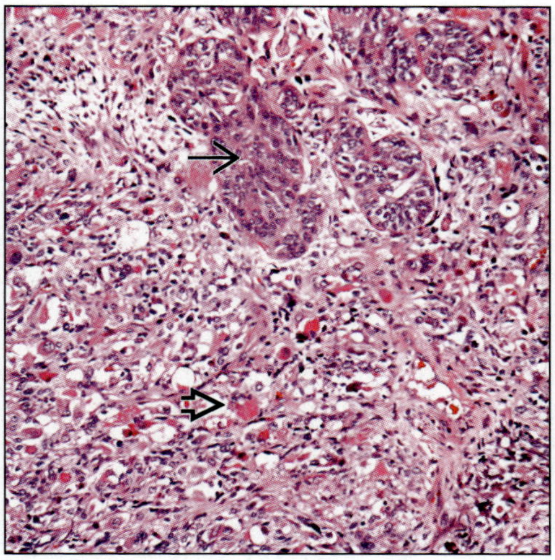

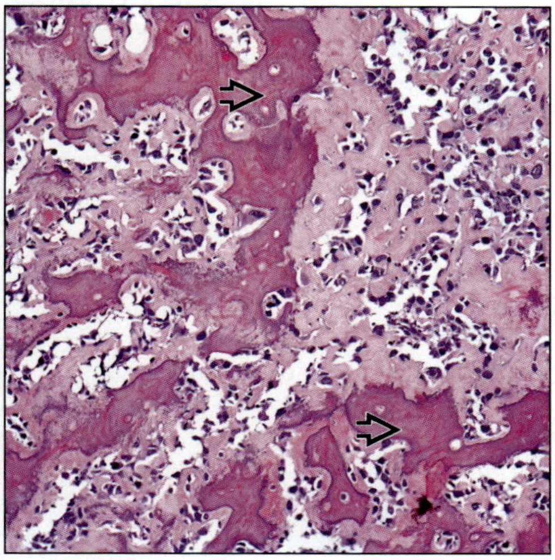

(Left) *Predominantly rhabdomyosarcomatous component ⇨ is seen with only focal areas of a malignant epithelial component (squamous cell carcinoma) →. In seen here, the epithelial component may be a minor component in some cases.* ***(Right)*** *Carcinosarcoma is shown in which the mesenchymal component is composed of osteosarcoma. Note presence of bone formation ⇨. Essentially any sarcomatous component may be present in carcinosarcomas of the lung.*

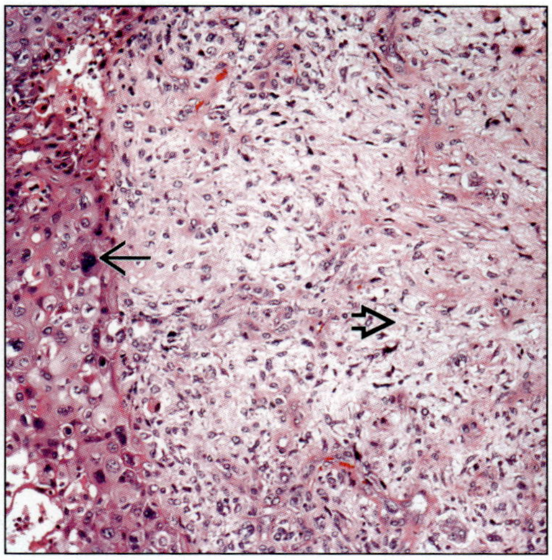

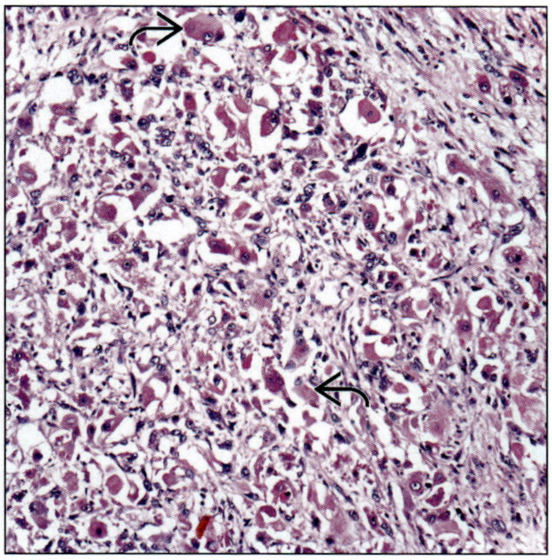

(Left) *Carcinosarcoma with squamous cell carcinoma → as well as a sarcomatous component with myxoid and vascular features ⇨. In some cases of carcinosarcoma, the light microscopy may not be helpful to differentiate the specific type of sarcoma.* ***(Right)*** *Classic rhabdomyosarcoma with numerous rhabdomyoblasts ↷ as a component of a carcinosarcoma. In some tumors, the epithelial component may be minor.*

PULMONARY BLASTOMA

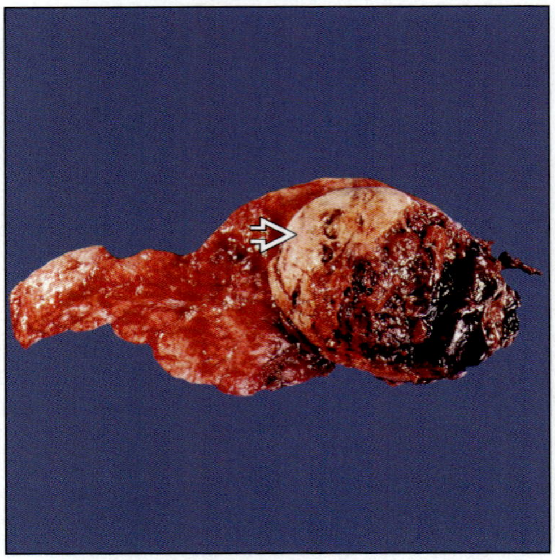

Gross photograph of pulmonary blastoma shows an intrapulmonary mass with areas of hemorrhage and necrosis. The tumor in the more viable areas appears light tan in color ➡.

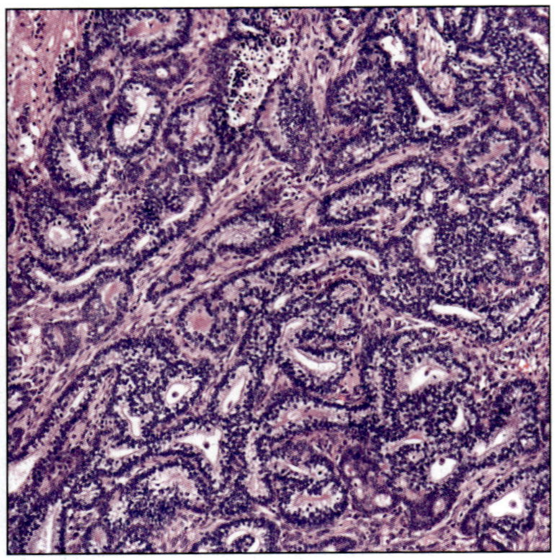

PB shows a complex glandular proliferation with a back-to-back arrangement with little intervening stromal tissue.

TERMINOLOGY

Abbreviations

- Pulmonary blastoma (PB)

Synonyms

- Well-differentiated fetal adenocarcinoma
- Pulmonary embryoma

Definitions

- PB monophasic type (well-differentiated fetal adenocarcinoma)
  - Glandular component recapitulates embryonic development of lung
- PB biphasic type
  - Composed of epithelial glandular component and sarcomatous elements

CLINICAL ISSUES

Epidemiology

- Incidence
  - Rare tumor that may account for < 1% of all pulmonary neoplasms
- Age
  - Tumor is more common in adults

Presentation

- Cough
- Hemoptysis
- Chest pain
- Asymptomatic

Treatment

- Surgical approaches
  - Complete surgical resection
- Adjuvant therapy
  - No specific treatment

Prognosis

- Monophasic pulmonary blastomas have better prognosis
- Biphasic pulmonary blastomas behave more aggressively
- Tumor size (> 5 cm) linked with poor prognosis

MACROSCOPIC FEATURES

General Features

- Central or peripheral tumor
- Well-circumscribed but not encapsulated
- Homogeneous or slightly lobulated cut surface
- Tan in color ± areas of necrosis &/or hemorrhage
- Tumor size varies from 1-20 cm in diameter

MICROSCOPIC PATHOLOGY

Histologic Features

- Glandular component mimics embryologic development of lung between 11-18 weeks
- Presence of morules (squamoid foci)

Predominant Pattern/Injury Type

- Glandular
- Biphasic

Predominant Cell/Compartment Type

- Epithelial, glandular
- Epithelial, biphasic or mixed

DIFFERENTIAL DIAGNOSIS

Adenocarcinoma

- Glandular proliferation of PB recapitulates embryologic development of lung (weeks 11-18)
- Adenocarcinoma will lack presence of morules
- Absence of intracellular mucin in PB

PULMONARY BLASTOMA

Key Facts

Terminology
- Synonyms: Well-differentiated fetal adenocarcinoma, pulmonary embryoma
- PB monophasic type (well-differentiated fetal adenocarcinoma): Glandular component recapitulates embryonic development of lung
- PB biphasic type: Composed of epithelial glandular component and sarcomatous elements

Clinical Issues
- Monophasic pulmonary blastomas have better prognosis
- Biphasic pulmonary blastomas behave more aggressively
- Tumor size (> 5 cm) linked with poor prognosis

Microscopic Pathology
- Glandular component mimics embryologic development of lung between weeks 11-18
- Presence of morules

Top Differential Diagnoses
- Adenocarcinoma
  - Absence of intracellular mucin in PB
  - In carcinosarcoma, glandular epithelial component will not show embryonic features of glandular component of PB
- Pleuropulmonary blastoma
  - Epithelial component is benign
  - Tumor is pleural-based rather than intraparenchymatous

Immunohistochemistry

Antibody	Reactivity	Staining Pattern	Comment
TTF-1	Positive	Nuclear	In majority of cases in glandular component
KERATIN-LMW	Positive	Cytoplasmic	In glandular component
EMA/MUC1	Positive	Cell membrane	In glandular component
CEA-M	Positive	Cytoplasmic	In glandular component
Chromogranin-A	Positive	Cytoplasmic	Morules only
p53	Positive	Cytoplasmic	
Desmin	Positive	Cytoplasmic	In muscle component
SOX2	Positive	Nuclear	Chondroid component
Myoglobin	Positive	Cytoplasmic	Rhabdomyosarcomatous component

Histochemical Features of Pulmonary Blastomas

Histochemical Stain	Result	Comment
Mucicarmine	Negative for intracellular mucin	May show positive staining in intraluminal areas
D-PAS	Negative for intracellular mucin	
PAS	Positive for intracellular glycogen	

Carcinosarcoma
- Most commonly has squamous cell carcinoma as epithelial component
- Glandular epithelial component will not show embryonic features of glandular component of PB
- Absence of morules

Pleuropulmonary Blastoma
- Tumor of children
- Epithelial component is benign
- Usually is cystic tumor based on the pleura

DIAGNOSTIC CHECKLIST

Clinically Relevant Pathologic Features
- Age distribution

Pathologic Interpretation Pearls
- Glandular proliferation with morular component mimicking embryonic development of lung between weeks 11-18

SELECTED REFERENCES

1. Berho M et al: Malignant mixed epithelial/mesenchymal neoplasms of the lung. Semin Diagn Pathol. 12(2):123-39, 1995
2. Koss MN et al: Pulmonary blastomas. Cancer. 67(9):2368-81, 1991
3. Nakatani Y et al: Pulmonary endodermal tumor resembling fetal lung: a clinicopathologic study of five cases with immunohistochemical and ultrastructural characterization. Hum Pathol. 21(11):1097-107, 1990
4. Kodama T et al: Six cases of well-differentiated adenocarcinoma simulating fetal lung tubules in pseudoglandular stage. Comparison with pulmonary blastoma. Am J Surg Pathol. 8(10):735-44, 1984

PULMONARY BLASTOMA

Microscopic Features

*(**Left**) Normal lung parenchyma of an embryo is shown between the 11th and 18th weeks. The resemblance to the monophasic pulmonary blastoma is marked, thus the designation of fetal-type adenocarcinoma. (**Right**) Monophasic pulmonary blastoma is composed of anastomosing glands of different sizes with the classic supranuclear vacuole.*

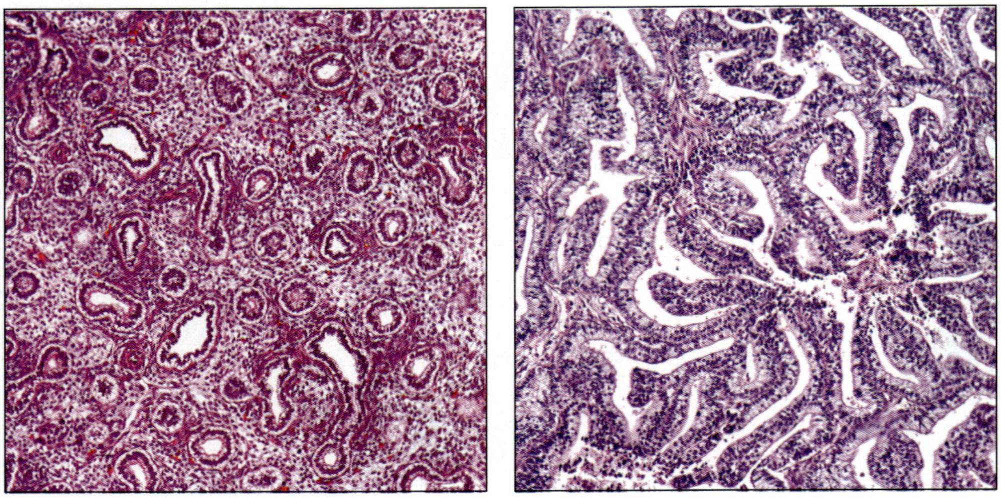

*(**Left**) Higher magnification shows a monophasic pulmonary blastoma formed by glands with nuclei displaced toward the base and supranuclear vacuoles. This arrangement mimics endometrioid-like carcinomas. Also note the presence of the minimal stromal component →. (**Right**) Monophasic pulmonary blastoma is shown with the classical glandular arrangement and focal squamous morule formation ⇨.*

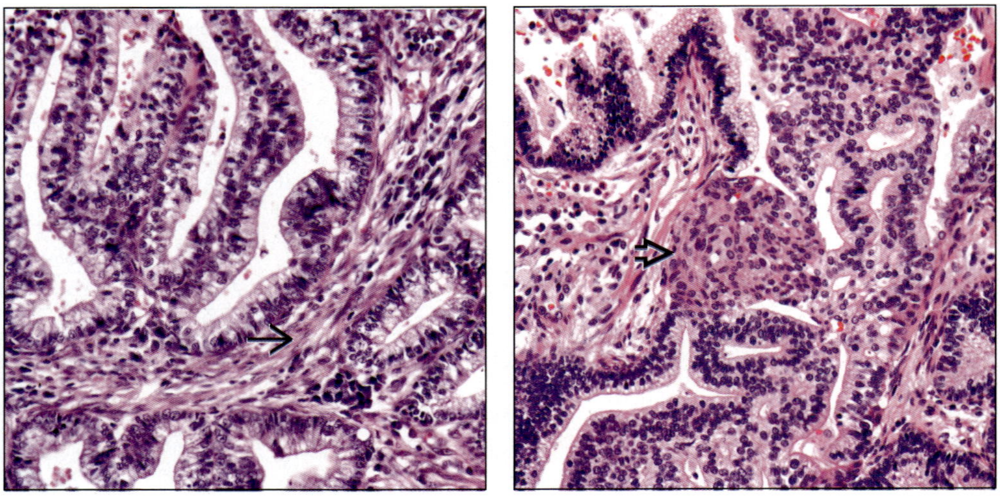

*(**Left**) Low-power view of a monophasic pulmonary blastoma with comedo-like necrosis and a vague cribriform-like pattern. (**Right**) Monophasic pulmonary blastoma is shown in which the glandular proliferation is present within the alveolar spaces in an alveolar-like type of invasion. Note the presence of more nuclear atypia and mitotic activity.*

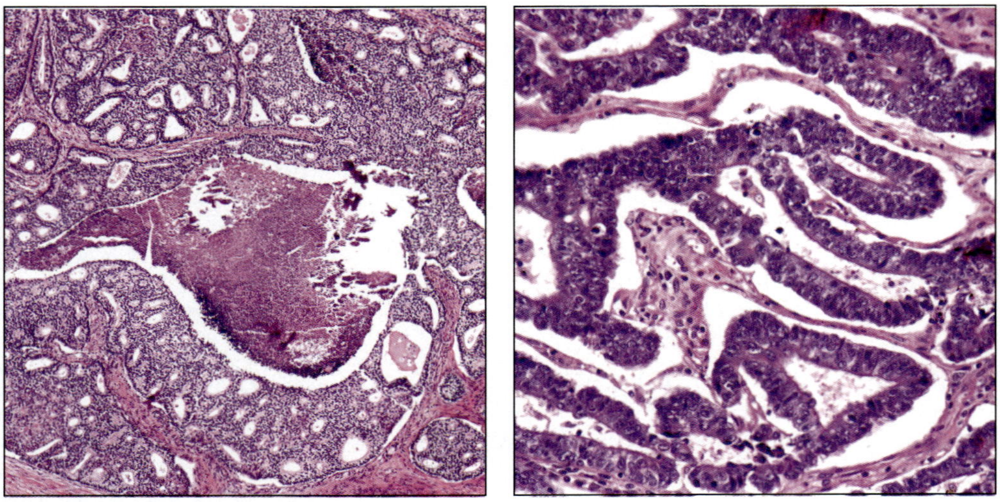

Microscopic Features

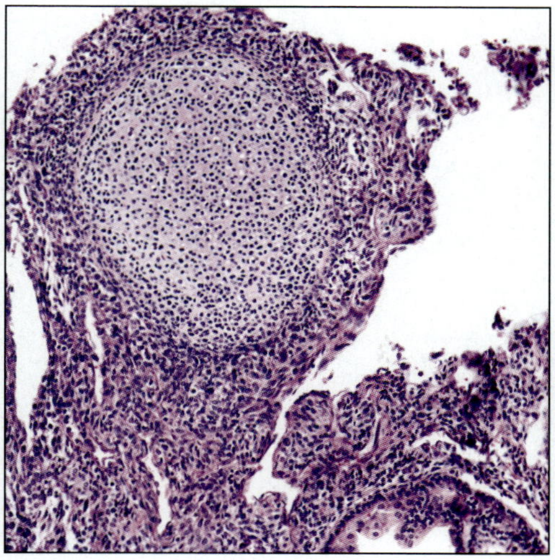
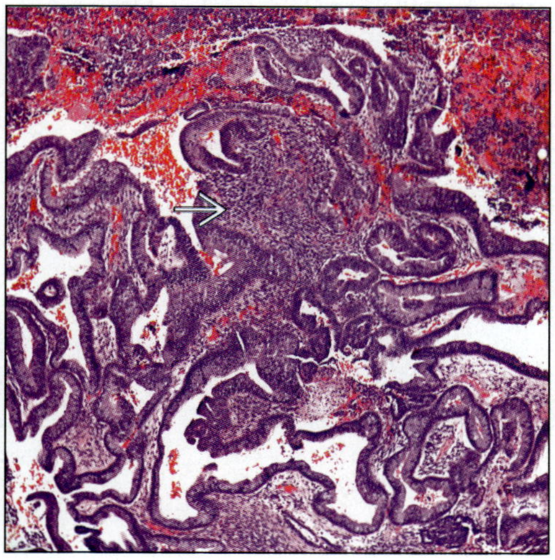

(Left) Monophasic pulmonary blastoma is shown with a focal area of cartilage. This feature may be confused for a carcinosarcoma or with a biphasic tumor. Although rare, this feature can occur in monophasic tumors. *(Right)* Biphasic pulmonary blastoma shows a complex glandular arrangement with dilated glands. Within the glandular structures there is subtle spindle cell proliferation ➔.

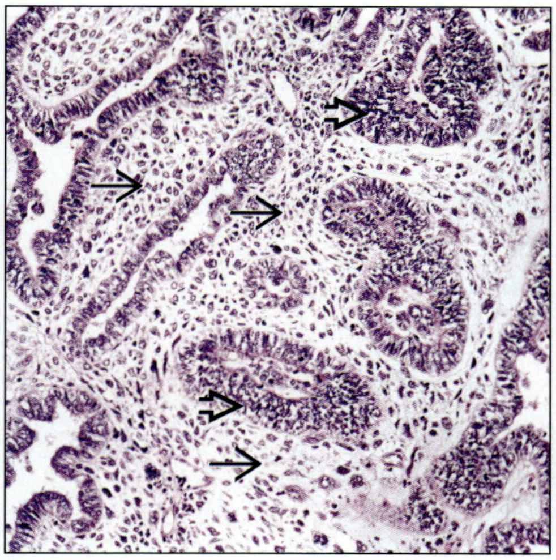
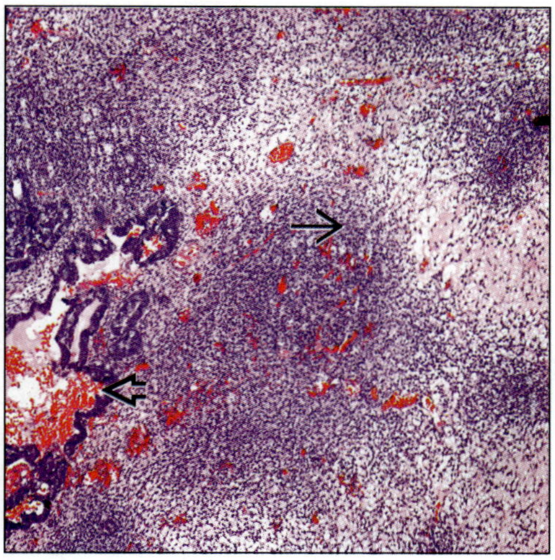

(Left) Closer view shows a biphasic pulmonary blastoma with 2 components: A glandular malignant epithelial component ⇨ and a malignant mesenchymal component →. *(Right)* Biphasic pulmonary blastoma is shown with a prominent malignant mesenchymal component → and only small areas of epithelial glandular elements ⇨.

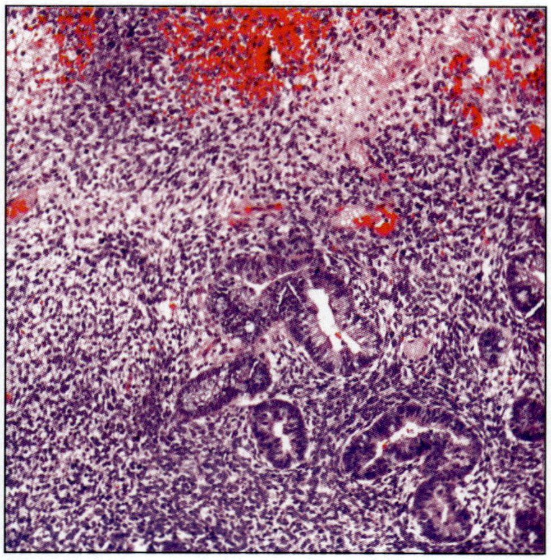
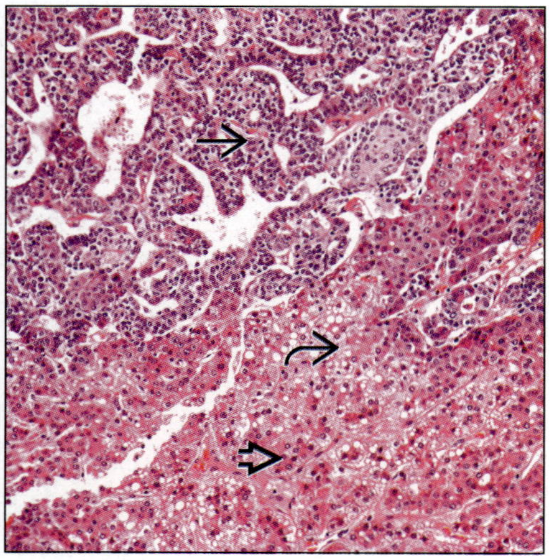

(Left) Higher magnification of a biphasic pulmonary blastoma is shown with glandular and mesenchymal components. *(Right)* Pulmonary blastoma → is shown with a hepatocellular carcinomatous component ⇨. In the hepatocellular component, note the areas that can be construed as fat droplets ↷. This is an unusual feature that only occasionally may be seen in these tumors.

ADENOID CYSTIC CARCINOMA

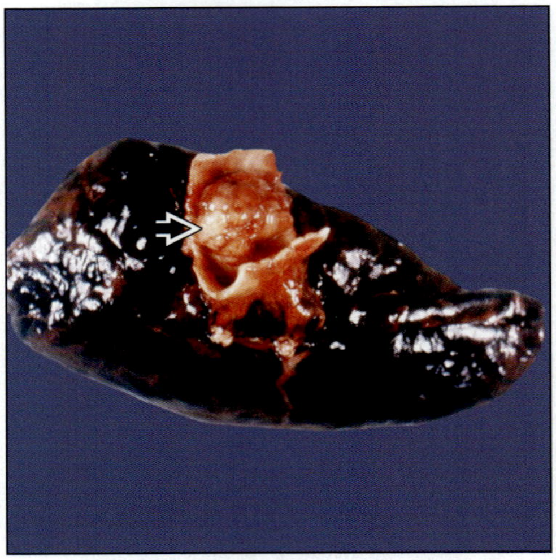

Gross photograph of adenoid cystic carcinoma shows a polypoid endobronchial tumor mass ➡ obstructing most of the bronchial lumen.

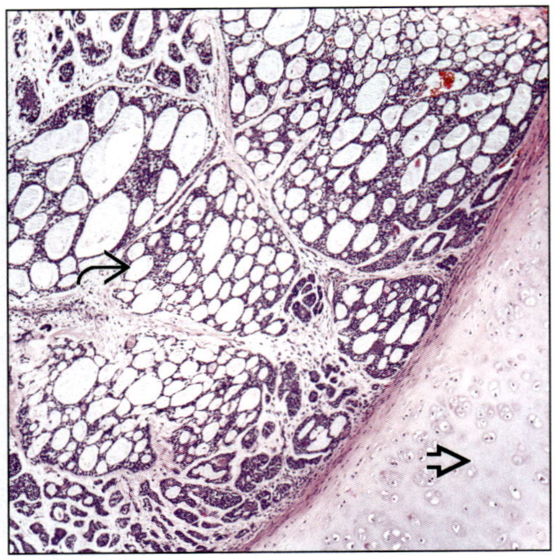

Adenoid cystic carcinoma shows conventional cylindromatous growth pattern. Note the presence of bronchial cartilage ➡ and the tumor obliterating normal lung parenchyma ↗.

TERMINOLOGY

Synonyms

- Cylindroma
  - Old term for this tumor related to the common cribriform growth pattern

Definitions

- Epithelial neoplasm similar to that occurring in salivary glands

ETIOLOGY/PATHOGENESIS

Etiology

- Tumor may originate from endobronchial glands
- Rare in parenchymal location

CLINICAL ISSUES

Epidemiology

- Incidence
  - 2nd most common salivary gland type tumor of the lung after mucoepidermoid carcinoma
- Age
  - Tumor appears to be more common in adults

Presentation

- Cough
- Hemoptysis
- Shortness of breath
- Chest pain

Treatment

- Surgical approaches
  - Lobectomy or pneumonectomy

Prognosis

- Slow-growth tumor
- May follow aggressive behavior with metastasis
- Recurrences are common

MACROSCOPIC FEATURES

General Features

- Endobronchial tumor
- Submucosal mass, which may penetrate bronchial wall

Size

- 1-3 cm in greatest dimension

MICROSCOPIC PATHOLOGY

Histologic Features

- Cylindromatous or cribriform growth pattern
- Spaces within mass represent pseudocysts rather than glands
- Spaces result from compression of cords of cell coursing through myxoid stroma
- Solid areas lack luminal structures and may show peripheral palisading
- True mucin-producing glands may be seen but are extremely rare
- Perineural invasion is common as in salivary gland tumor of same type

Predominant Pattern/Injury Type

- Cylindromatous
- Solid
- Tubular

Predominant Cell/Compartment Type

- Epithelial

ANCILLARY TESTS

Histochemistry

- Periodic acid-Schiff
  - Reactivity: Positive

ADENOID CYSTIC CARCINOMA

Key Facts

Terminology
- Epithelial neoplasm similar to that occurring in salivary glands

Clinical Issues
- Presentation
  - Cough, hemoptysis, dyspnea, chest pain
- Treatment
  - Lobectomy or pneumonectomy
- Pathogenesis
  - May follow aggressive behavior with metastasis

Macroscopic Features
- Endobronchial tumor
- Submucosal mass, which may penetrate bronchial wall

Microscopic Pathology
- Most common pattern cribriform with spaces within mass represent pseudocysts rather than glands
- Perineural invasion is common as in salivary gland tumor of same type

Ancillary Tests
- Immunohistochemical stains confirm immunophenotype of myoepithelial cells: Positive with CK-PAN, actin-sm, and vimentin

Top Differential Diagnoses
- Adenocarcinoma

Diagnostic Checklist
- Glands are composed of 2 rows of cells surrounding pseudocystic spaces

Immunohistochemistry

Antibody	Reactivity	Staining Pattern	Comment
CK-PAN	Positive	Cytoplasmic	Tumor cells uniformly positive
Actin-sm	Positive	Cytoplasmic	Many, but not all, cells show staining, emphasizing the dual nature of this tumor
S100	Positive	Nuclear	Usually only focal positive
Vimentin	Positive	Cytoplasmic	Uniform tumor cell staining

  - Staining pattern
    - Stromal matrix
  - PAS will also stain mucinous material within gland lumina of true glands when they are seen
- Alcian blue
  - Reactivity: Positive
  - Staining pattern
    - Stromal matrix

DIFFERENTIAL DIAGNOSIS

Adenocarcinoma
- Presence of cylindromatous pattern and myoepithelial immunophenotype is more in keeping with adenoid cystic carcinoma
  - Adenocarcinomas do not show tumor cell staining with actin-sm or S100
- May have obvious mucin positivity and common true glands

Metastatic Adenoid Cystic Carcinoma
- Appearance is identical
- History of extrapulmonary adenoid cystic carcinoma

Mucoepidermoid Carcinoma
- Endobronchial mass
- Admixture of mucin-secreting cells, squamous cells, and intermediate cells in various proportions

DIAGNOSTIC CHECKLIST

Pathologic Interpretation Pearls
- Glands are composed of 2 rows of cells
- Cribriform pattern is most common
- Immunophenotype different from adenocarcinomas
  - Uniform staining of tumor cells with vimentin, actin-sm, and focal staining with S100
- Perineural invasion common

STAGING

Clinical Follow-Up
- Staging at time of diagnosis appears to be the most important parameter in predicting prognosis

SELECTED REFERENCES

1. Moran CA: Primary salivary gland-type tumors of the lung. Semin Diagn Pathol. 12(2):106-22, 1995
2. Moran CA et al: Primary adenoid cystic carcinoma of the lung. A clinicopathologic and immunohistochemical study of 16 cases. Cancer. 73(5):1390-7, 1994
3. Nomori H et al: Adenoid cystic carcinoma of the trachea and main-stem bronchus. A clinical, histopathologic, and immunohistochemical study. J Thorac Cardiovasc Surg. 96(2):271-7, 1988

ADENOID CYSTIC CARCINOMA

Microscopic Features

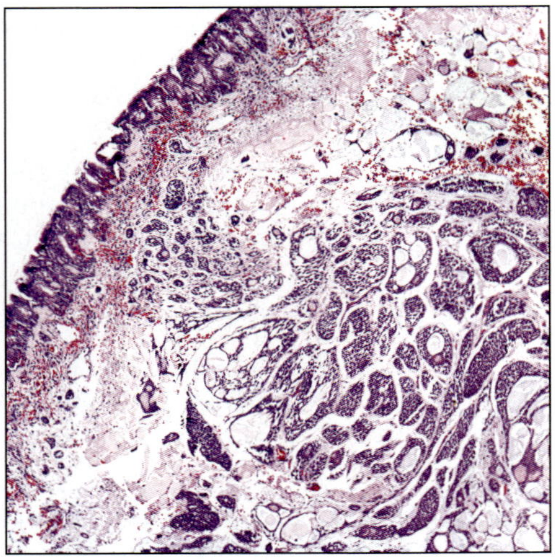

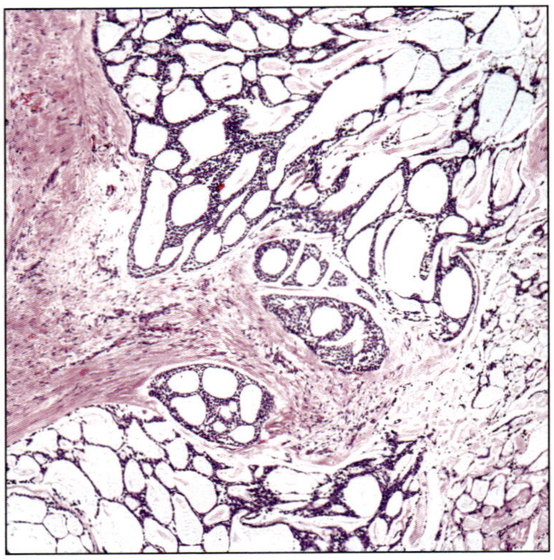

(Left) *Adenoid cystic carcinoma shows conventional cylindromatous pattern. Note the presence of uninvolved respiratory epithelium which appears to be within normal limits.* ***(Right)*** *The cylindromatous variant of adenoid cystic carcinoma is the most common. The tumor is composed of islands of tumor cells separated by fibroconnective tissue that show a striking cribriform architecture.*

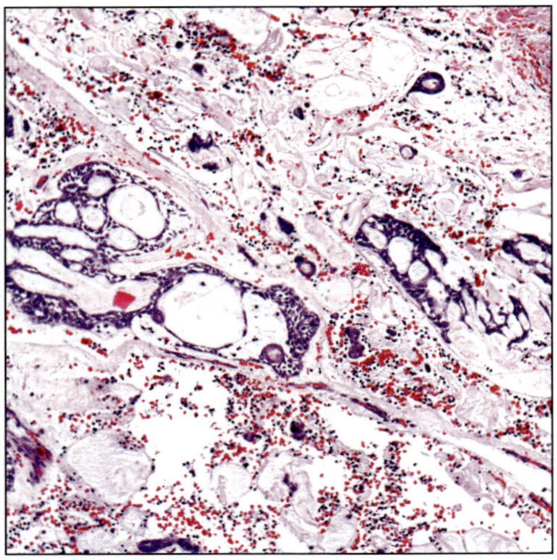

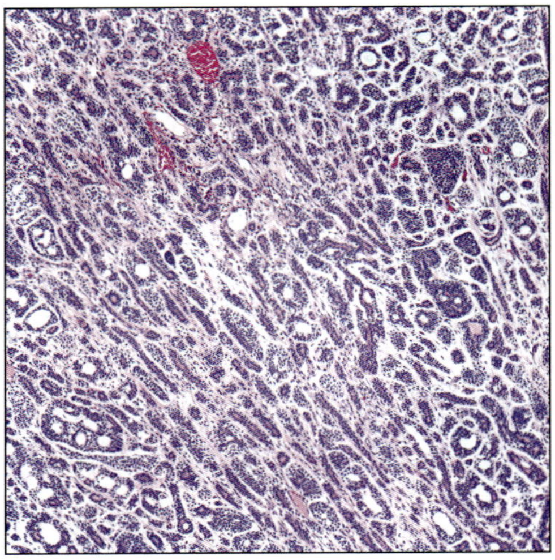

(Left) *In some areas, the islands of tumor cells are embedded in edematous stroma. However, the characteristic features are still preserved in the epithelial component.* ***(Right)*** *In other areas, the glandular proliferation may show prominent compression of the glandular structures making it difficult to recognize the cylindromatous pattern of growth.*

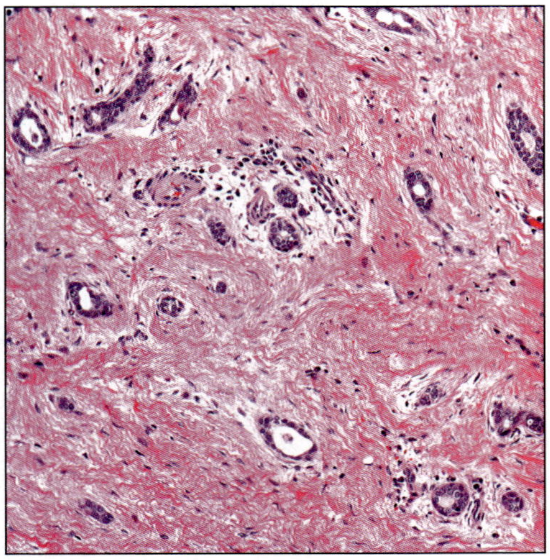

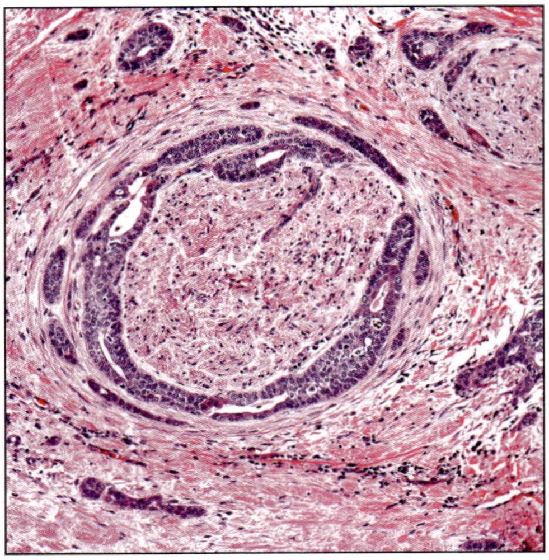

(Left) *Extensive areas of collagenization with only scattered areas of tumor cells. This type of pattern can also be seen in pleomorphic adenomas (mixed tumors).* ***(Right)*** *Prominent perineural invasion is present in these tumors and is an important feature that may aid in the diagnosis of adenoid cystic carcinoma.*

ADENOID CYSTIC CARCINOMA

Microscopic Features

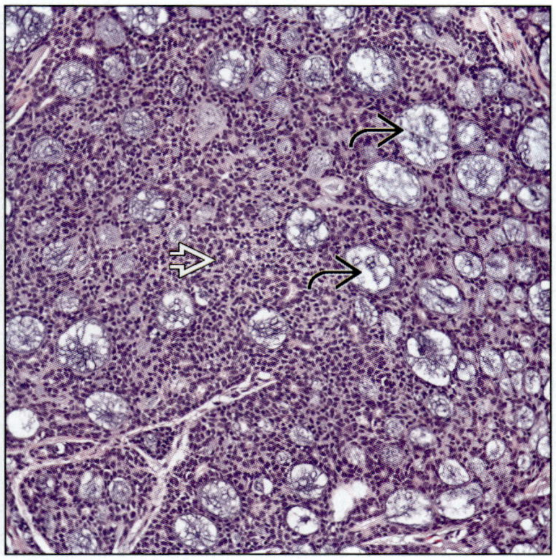
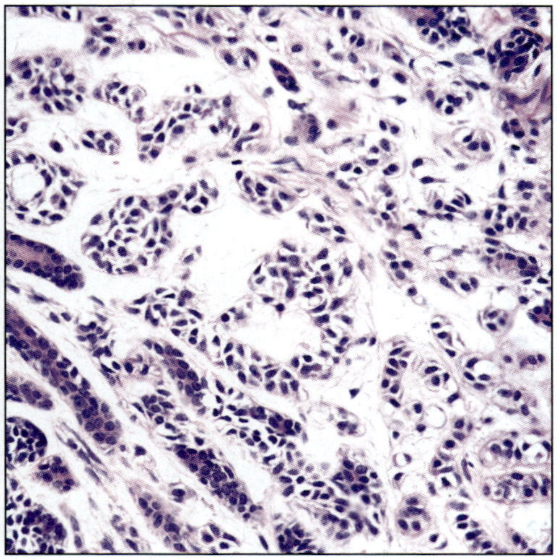

***(Left)** Adenoid cystic carcinoma shows areas of solid cellular proliferation* ➡ *and cystic structures* ↪ *containing mucoid material. This feature is common in these tumors. **(Right)** Some cases of adenoid cystic carcinoma may show prominent clear cell changes. In some cases, the proliferation is similar to that seen in epithelial-myoepithelial carcinoma.*

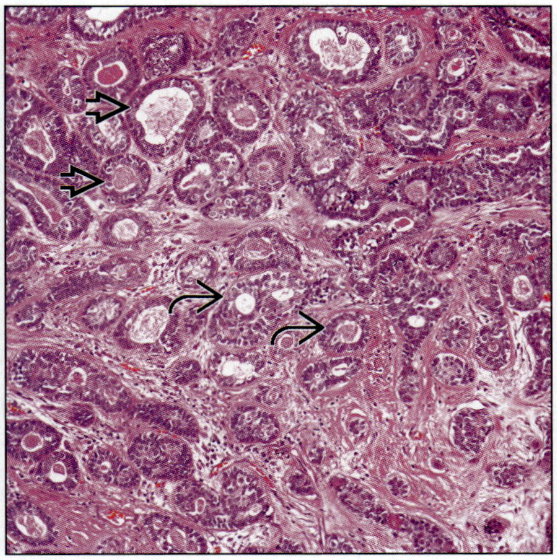
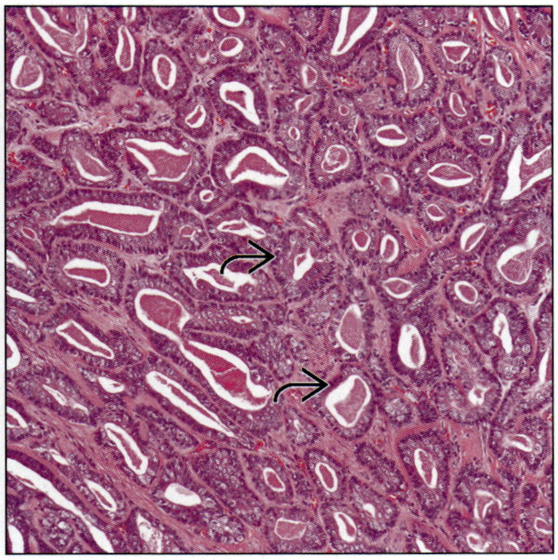

***(Left)** Tubular variant* ⇨ *of adenoid cystic carcinoma merging with more conventional areas* ↪*. It is common to see 2 growth patterns in the same tumor. **(Right)** Tubular growth pattern of adenoid cystic carcinoma shows a proliferation of glandular structures* ↪*, which closely mimic a conventional adenocarcinoma.*

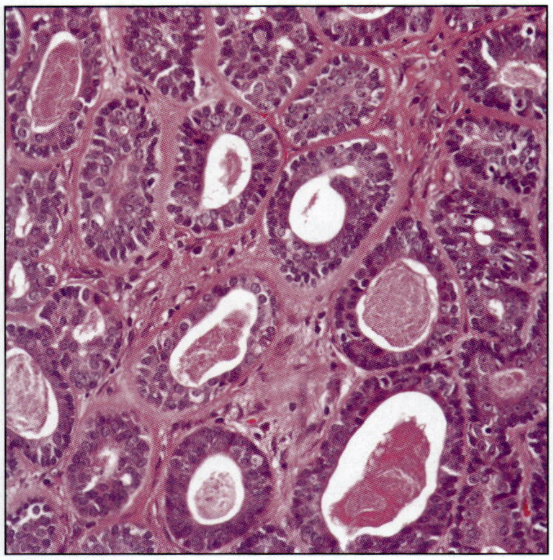
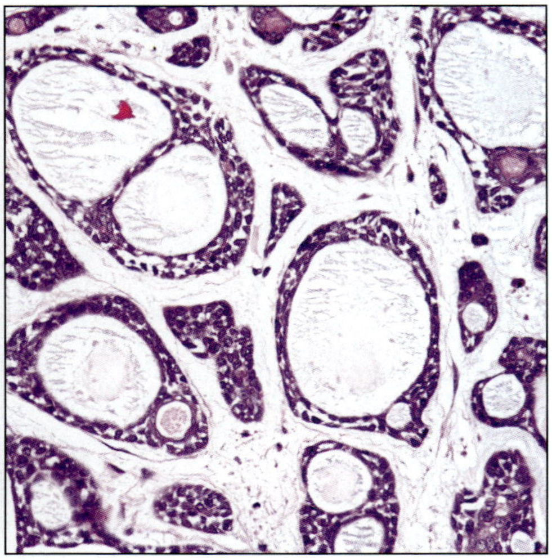

***(Left)** Higher magnification of the neoplasm shows that these glandular structures are similar to the more conventional pattern of this tumor. The glands are composed of 2 rows of cells. Mitotic activity is not present. **(Right)** The cylindromatous variant of adenoid cystic carcinoma shows that the glands are also composed of 2 rows of cells and contain mucoid material. Mitotic activity is also absent.*

ADENOID CYSTIC CARCINOMA

Microscopic Features

*(**Left**) Although not common, the presence of necrosis ↪ may be encountered focally in cases of adenoid cystic carcinoma. Extensive areas of necrosis are not common in these tumors. (**Right**) In some cases of adenoid cystic carcinoma, the tumor may display cords of neoplastic cells embedded in a fibroblastic stroma, giving the impression of a biphasic neoplasm.*

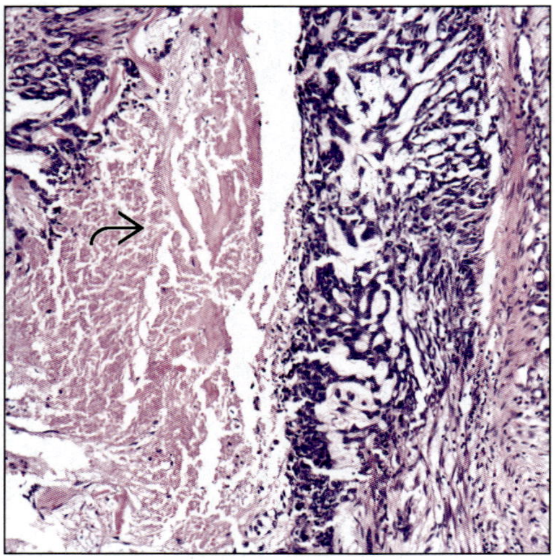

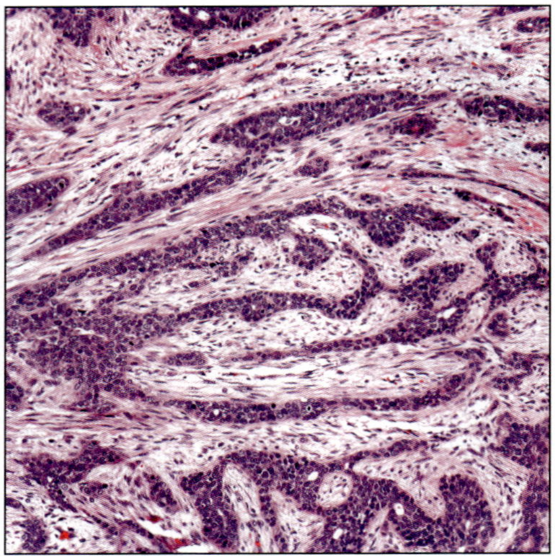

*(**Left**) Hematoxylin & eosin shows an adenoid cystic carcinoma with a prominent tubular component and clear cells ➔. Also note the presence of a hyalinized stroma ↪ separating islands of tumor cells. (**Right**) Hematoxylin & eosin shows a classic histology of an adenoid cystic carcinoma with clusters of clear cells →. The presence of clear cells suggest sebaceous differentiation. This feature is unusual in adenoid cystic carcinomas of the lung.*

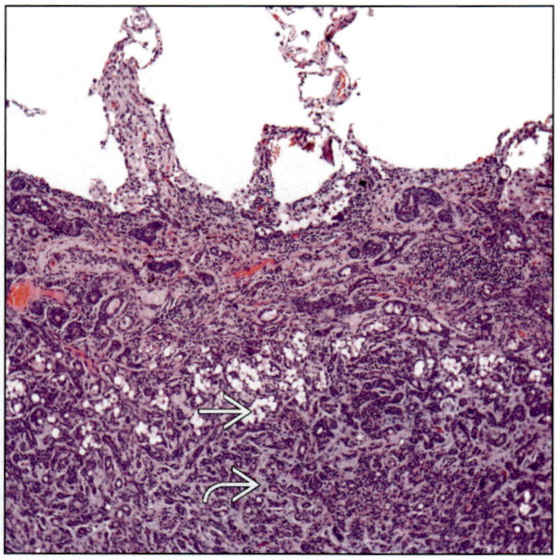

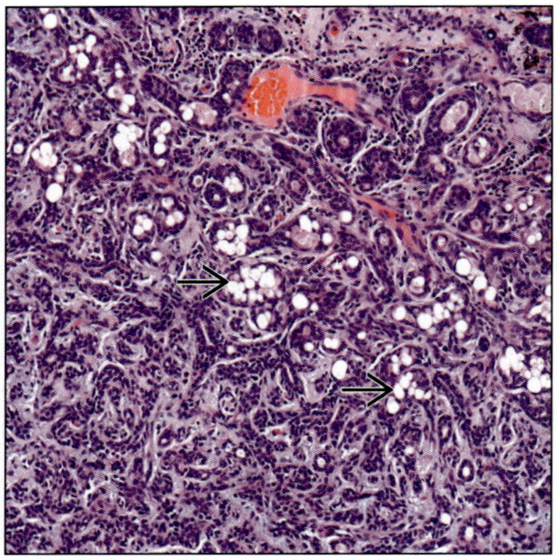

*(**Left**) Hematoxylin & eosin shows conventional growth pattern of adenoid cystic carcinoma with a clear cell component dissecting fibrocollagenous stroma. This feature requires careful attention in determining the extent of invasion by the tumor. (**Right**) Hematoxylin & eosin shows higher magnification of the clear cells, which represent sebaceous differentiation in adenoid cystic carcinoma. Cytoplasm appears to contain lipid inclusions.*

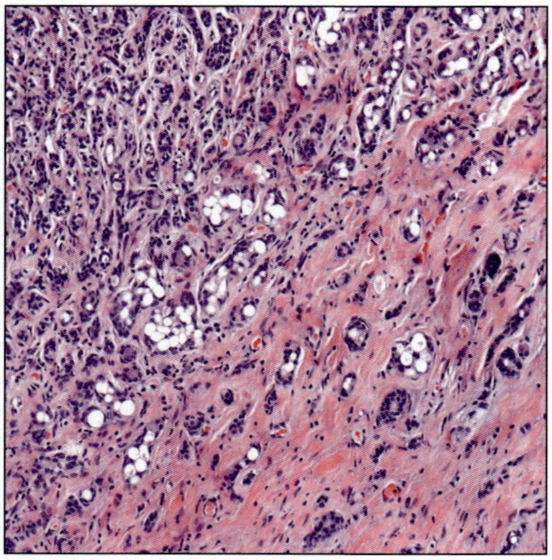

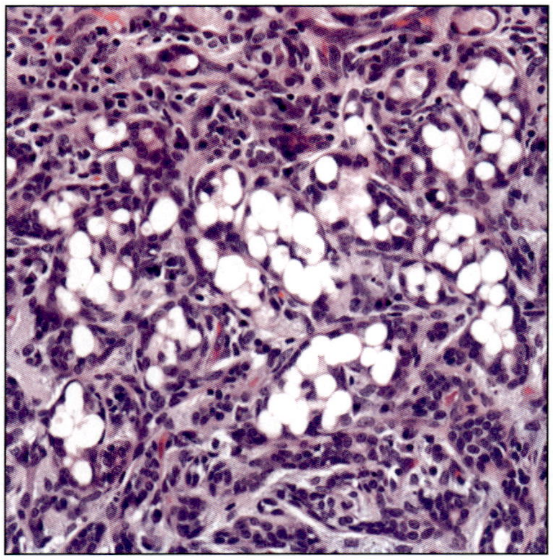

ADENOID CYSTIC CARCINOMA

Microscopic Features

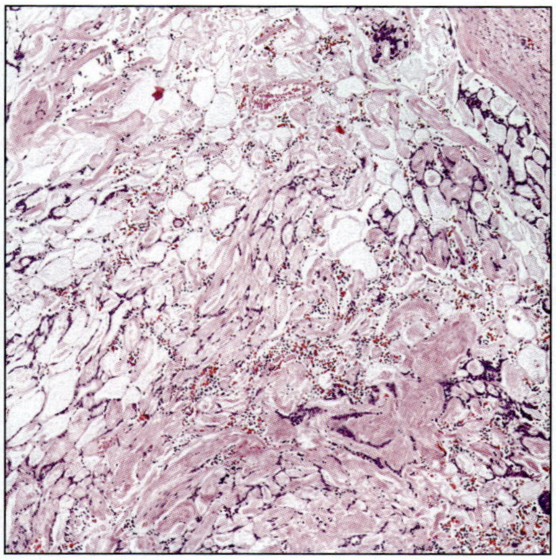
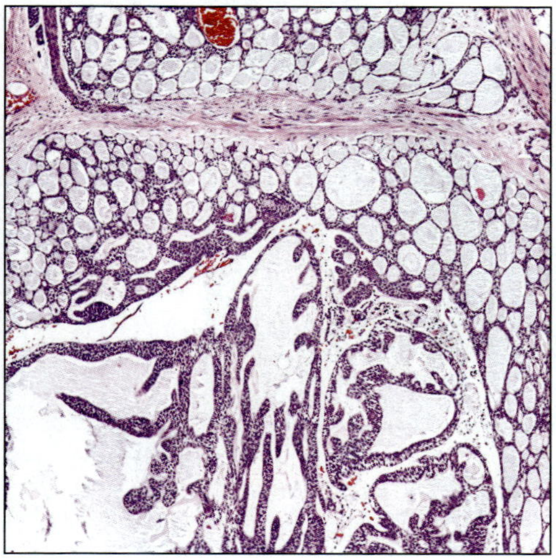

*(**Left**) Adenoid cystic carcinoma with extensive areas of hyalinization. This type of growth pattern is uncommon in the lung and can make the diagnosis difficult. Primary pleomorphic adenomas of the lung may show similar features. (**Right**) Adenoid cystic carcinoma is seen with focal presence of larger cysts and adjacent classic growth pattern. The presence of large cystic structures is uncommon and, when alone, can make the diagnosis difficult.*

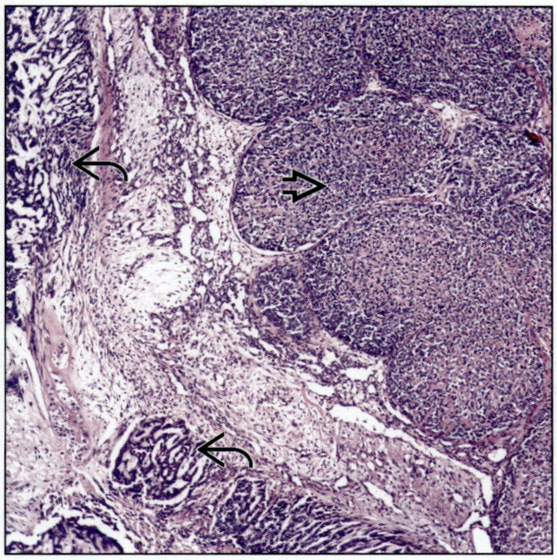
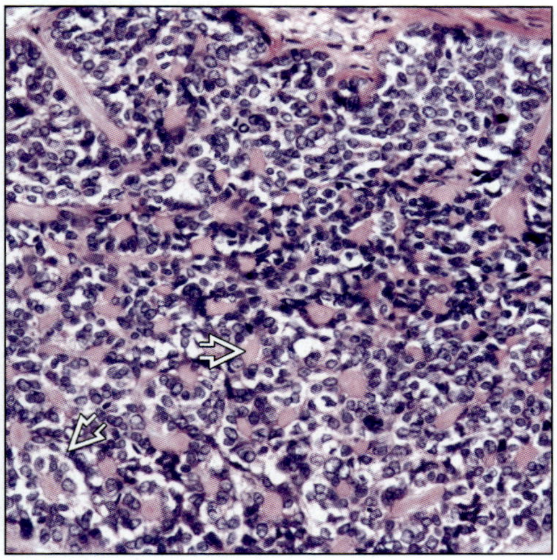

*(**Left**) Extensive areas of solid variant of adenoid cystic carcinoma are separated by fibrocollagenous tissue from more conventional areas of this tumor. (**Right**) Higher magnification of a solid area in which one can still identify a remnant of tubular structures. These structures may also be confused for pseudorosettes and for a neuroendocrine tumor.*

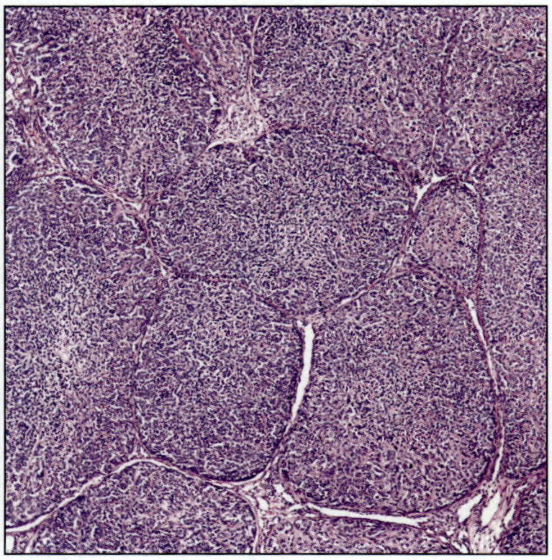
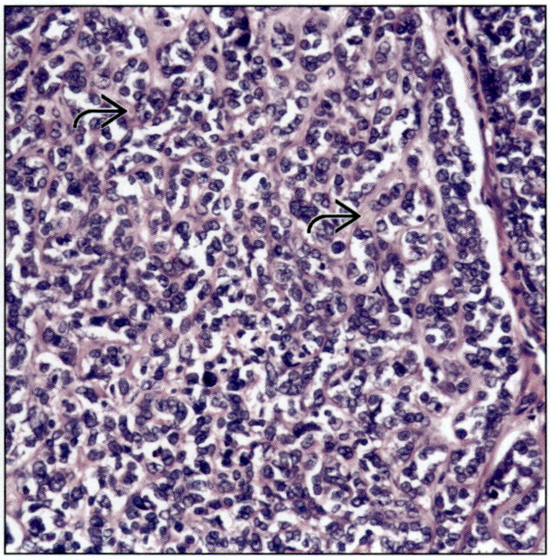

*(**Left**) Solid growth pattern with a vague lobular appearance. Fortunately, even in cases with an extensive solid pattern, the tumor may also show focal areas of the conventional pattern. (**Right**) Higher magnification shows a cellular proliferation with moderate nuclear atypia and the presence of a basement membrane, which gives the appearance of amyloid deposition.*

MUCOEPIDERMOID CARCINOMA

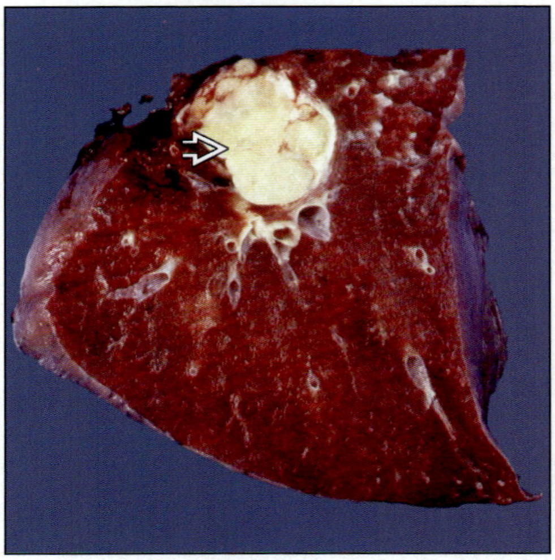

Gross photograph shows a well-circumscribed, yellowish, central tumor mass ➡. Usually, low-grade mucoepidermoid carcinomas of the lung are central tumors.

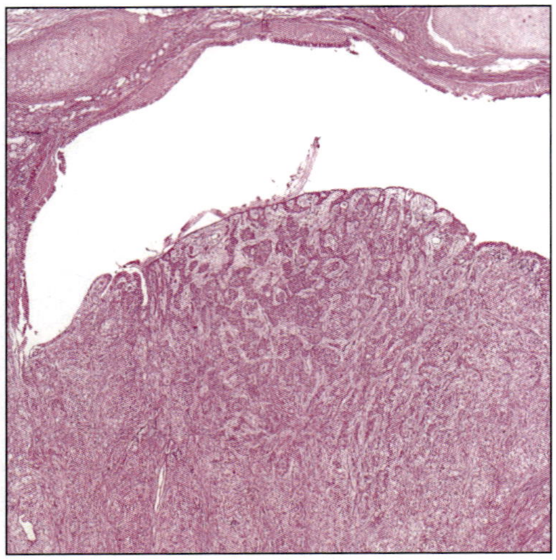

Panoramic view of a low-grade MEC in an endobronchial location. The tumor is growing in a polypoid fashion, obstructing the bronchial lumen.

TERMINOLOGY

Abbreviations

- Mucoepidermoid carcinoma (MEC)

Synonyms

- Mucoepidermoid tumor

Definitions

- Epithelial neoplasm composed of epidermoid cells admixed with mucus-secreting cells (mucocytes)

ETIOLOGY/PATHOGENESIS

Incidence

- Tumor more common in adults but has been reported in children

CLINICAL ISSUES

Presentation

- Cough
- Shortness of breath
- Hemoptysis

Treatment

- Surgical approaches
  - Complete surgical resection, usually lobectomy

Prognosis

- Prognosis depends on grading of neoplasm
  - Low-grade tumors, completely resected: Very good
  - High-grade tumors may require additional medical treatment in addition to surgical resection

MACROSCOPIC FEATURES

General Features

- Tumor more common in central location than in periphery of lung
  - MEC is usually an endobronchial tumor

Size

- 1-5 cm in greatest dimension

MICROSCOPIC PATHOLOGY

Histologic Features

- Epidermoid component without keratinization
  - Clear cells (intermediate cells)
  - Mucous-producing cells (mucocytes)
  - Lack of nuclear atypia or high mitotic activity

Predominant Pattern/Injury Type

- Solid
- Cystic

Predominant Cell/Compartment Type

- Epithelial

DIFFERENTIAL DIAGNOSIS

Lymphoepithelioma-like Carcinoma

- Usually shows increased mitotic activity and cellular atypia
- Characteristically has inflammatory stroma composed of lymphocytes and plasma cells
- Does not show the presence of mucocytes or low-grade areas of MEC

Adenosquamous Carcinoma

- Shows conventional areas of adenocarcinoma and squamous cell carcinoma

MUCOEPIDERMOID CARCINOMA

Key Facts

Terminology
- Epithelial neoplasm composed of epidermoid and clear cells admixed with mucus-secreting cells (mucocytes)

Clinical Issues
- Prognosis
  - Depends on grading of tumor
  - For low-grade tumors, prognosis is very good
  - For high-grade tumors, additional medical treatment may be necessary
- Symptoms
  - Cough
  - Shortness of breath
  - Hemoptysis

Macroscopic Features
- MEC usually an endobronchial tumor

Microscopic Pathology
- Epidermoid component without keratinization
- Clear cells (intermediate cells)
- Mucous-producing cells (mucocytes)
- Lack of nuclear atypia or high mitotic activity

Top Differential Diagnoses
- Lymphoepithelioma-like carcinoma
- Adenosquamous carcinoma
- Squamous cell carcinoma

Diagnostic Checklist
- MEC generally does not show areas of keratinization
- Epidermoid cells admixed with mucous cells

Immunohistochemistry

Antibody	Reactivity	Staining Pattern	Comment
AE1/AE3	Positive	Cytoplasmic	Positive in any epithelial neoplasm
CK-LMW-NOS	Positive	Cytoplasmic	Positive in any epithelial neoplasm
CK5/6	Positive	Cytoplasmic	Positive in epidermoid component
CEA-M	Positive	Cytoplasmic	May be negative in some cases
p63	Positive	Nuclear	In epidermoid component
Vimentin	Negative		

Histochemical Features of Mucoepidermoid Carcinoma of the Lung

Histochemical Stain	Result
Mucicarmine	Positive
D-PAS	Positive
PAS	Positive

- Mucoepidermoid carcinoma shows only epidermoid component without keratinization

Squamous Cell Carcinoma
- In a small biopsy, it may be difficult or impossible to separate both of these entities
  - Lack of keratinization and presence of mucocytes admixed with epidermoid cells will favor MEC
  - Presence of squamous cell carcinoma in situ would favor squamous cell carcinoma

Mucous Gland Adenoma
- Does not invade beyond cartilaginous bronchial tissue

DIAGNOSTIC CHECKLIST

Clinically Relevant Pathologic Features
- Gross appearance
  - Central tumor obstructing bronchial lumen

Pathologic Interpretation Pearls
- MEC generally does not show areas of keratinization
  - Epidermoid cell admixed with mucous cells

GRADING

Low-Grade MEC
- Low-grade tumor characterized by epidermoid component with mucus-producing cells without increased mitotic activity, nuclear pleomorphism, necrosis, or hemorrhage

High-Grade MEC
- High-grade tumors characterized by epidermoid component with areas of nuclear pleomorphism, mitotic activity, necrosis, or hemorrhage

SELECTED REFERENCES

1. Vadasz P et al: Mucoepidermoid bronchial tumors: a review of 34 operated cases. Eur J Cardiothorac Surg. 17(5):566-9, 2000
2. Moran CA: Primary salivary gland-type tumors of the lung. Semin Diagn Pathol. 12(2):106-22, 1995
3. Yousem SA et al: Mucoepidermoid tumors of the lung. Cancer. 60(6):1346-52, 1987

MUCOEPIDERMOID CARCINOMA

Microscopic Features

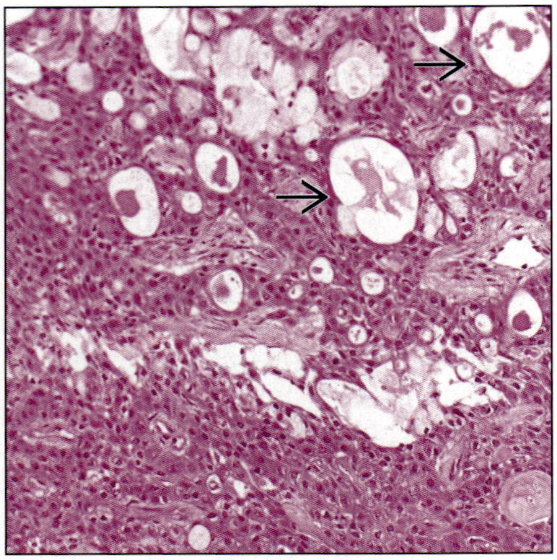

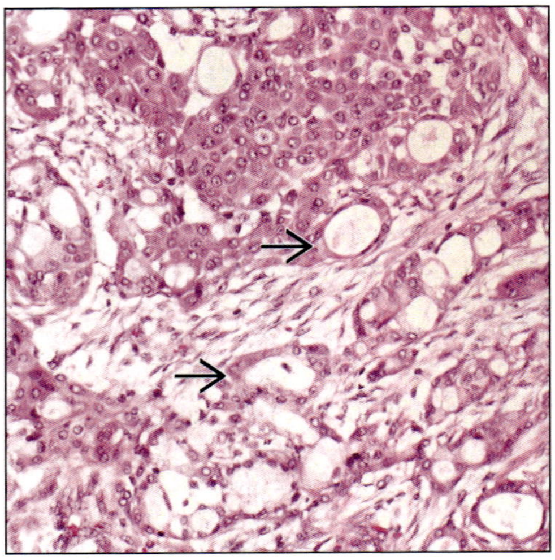

(Left) *Solid sheets of nonkeratinizing cells admixed with cystic spaces* → *containing acellular material in their lumens. The presence of solid and cystic areas is commonly seen in low-grade tumors.* ***(Right)*** *MEC shows a solid, epidermoid, nonkeratinizing cellular component and a pseudoglandular component* →*. One important feature in these tumors is the lack of keratinization.*

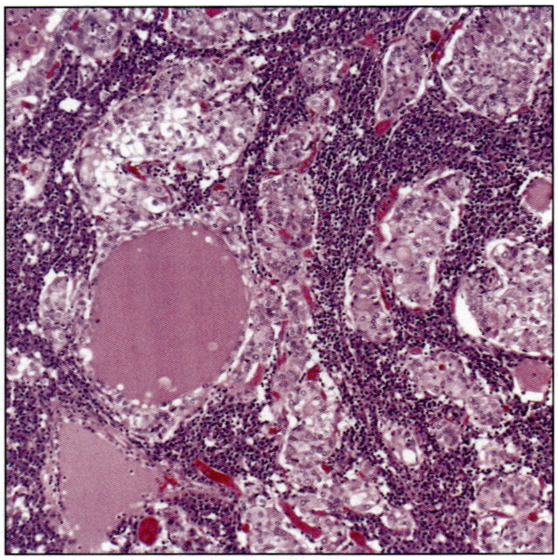

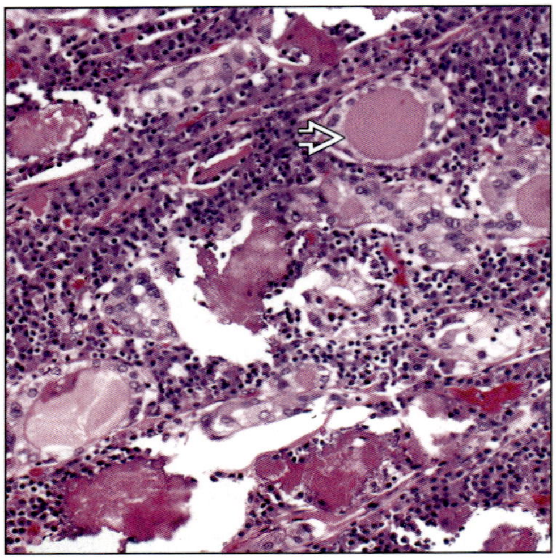

(Left) *Pseudoglandular structures with marked chronic inflammation, namely plasma cells. The presence of inflammatory changes in mucoepidermoid carcinoma is not common and may pose problems in the interpretation.* ***(Right)*** *Pseudoglandular pattern with acellular intraluminal material* ➡ *and prominent inflammatory background. At this magnification, it is possible to distinguish both epithelial and inflammatory components.*

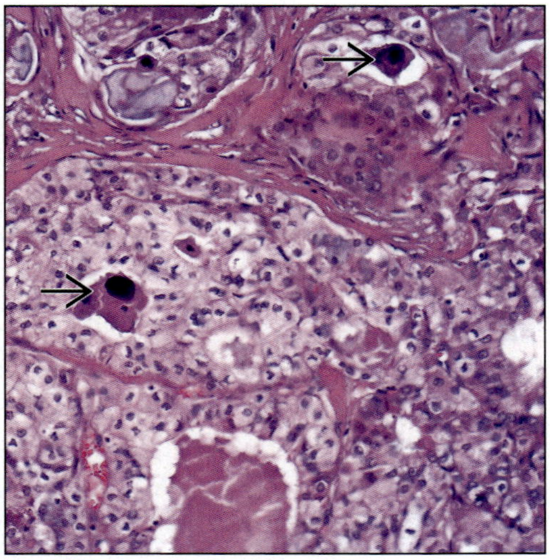

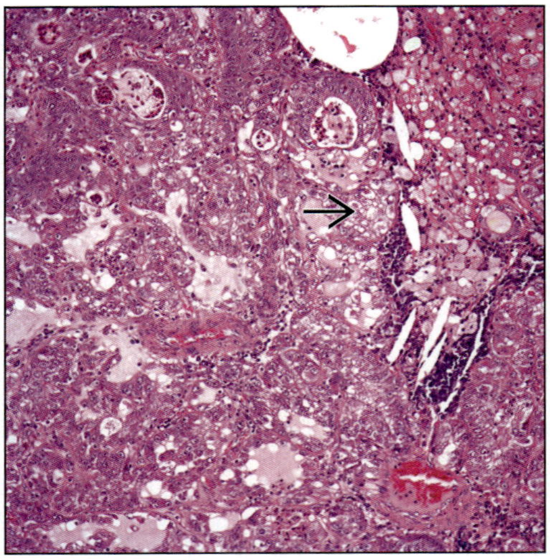

(Left) *Pseudoglandular epithelial component with numerous intraluminal calcifications* →*. The presence of these calcifications is more commonly seen in tumors with inflammatory changes.* ***(Right)*** *Pseudoglandular proliferation with numerous clear (intermediate) cells* →*. This may represent a pitfall in diagnosis as similar features may be seen in non-small cell carcinomas with clear cell changes.*

MUCOEPIDERMOID CARCINOMA

Microscopic Features

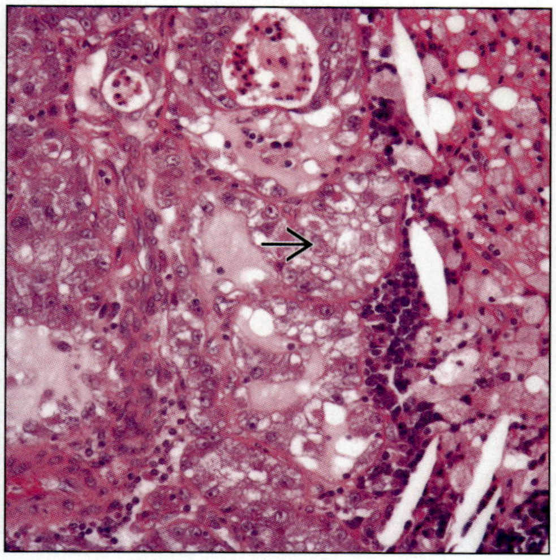
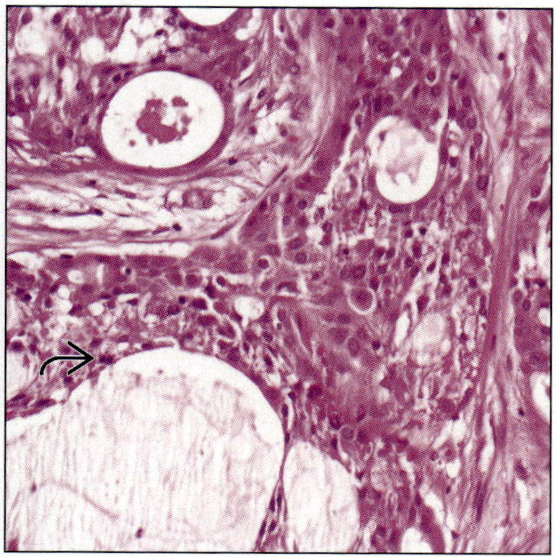

(Left) *Mucoepidermoid carcinoma shows clear (intermediate) → cells admixed with inflammatory cells. Note the absence of nuclear atypia and mitotic activity. More importantly, there is no keratinization or true glandular differentiation.* ***(Right)*** *Epidermoid component with cystic structures admixed with mucous-producing cells (mucocytes) ↪. This growth pattern is diagnostic of mucoepidermoid carcinoma.*

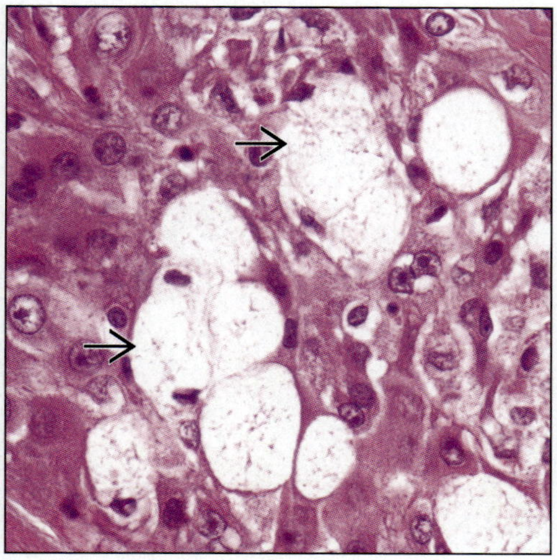
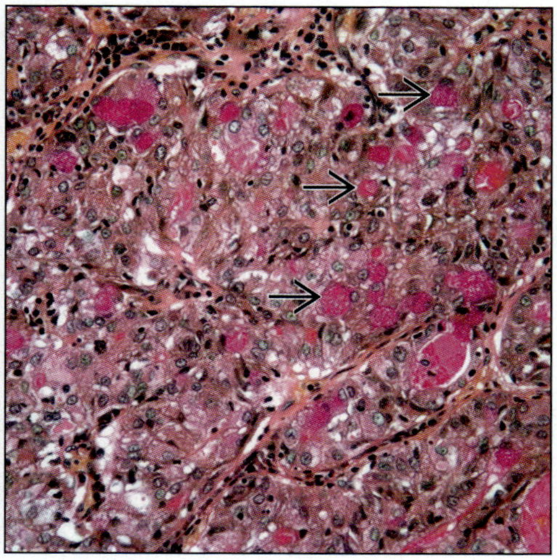

(Left) *Epidermoid nonkeratinizing cellular component admixed with mucocytes →. The mucus-producing cells are bland and nonneoplastic, and their presence is essential for the diagnosis.* ***(Right)*** *Mucicarmine stain shows abundant mucin-producing cells (mucocytes) →. The use of histochemical stains to demonstrate the presence of mucin is helpful in these cases. In some cases, it may not be as florid as depicted here.*

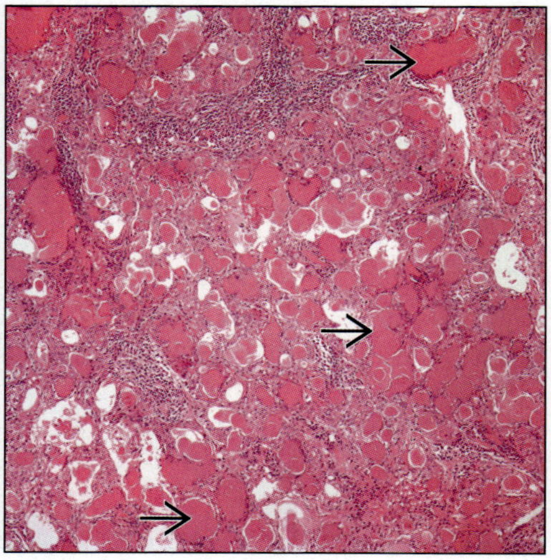
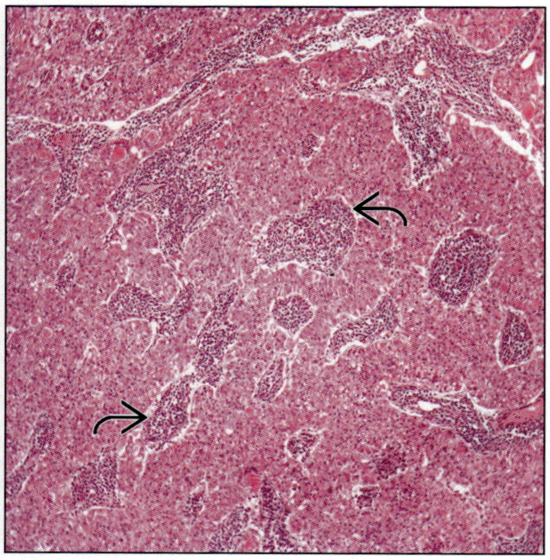

(Left) *Low-grade MEC is shown with prominent amorphous material in the lumens of the cystic structures →.* ***(Right)*** *Low-grade MEC is shown with a more solid epithelial component arranged in trabeculae. Interestingly, the solid sheets of neoplastic cells have an oncocytic-like appearance. Note the discrete areas of inflammatory reaction ↪. Oncocytic change is very rare in mucoepidermoid carcinoma of the lung.*

MUCOEPIDERMOID CARCINOMA

Microscopic Features

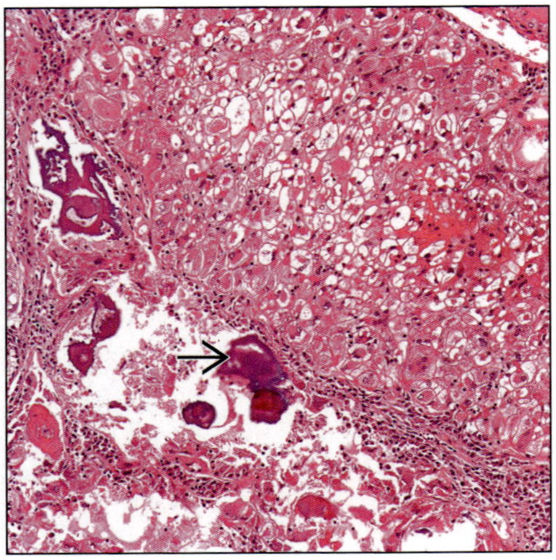

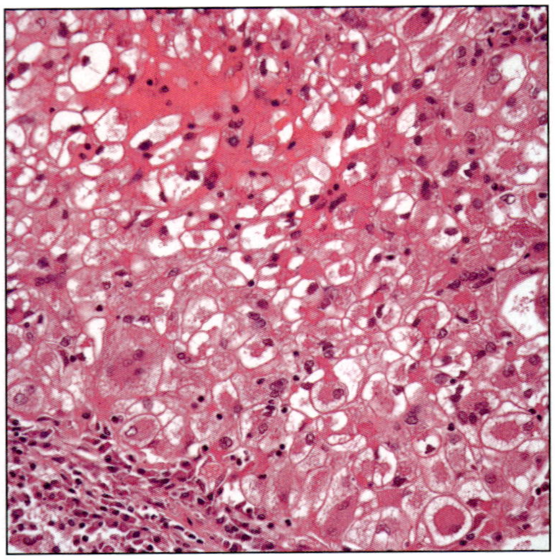

(Left) *Low-grade MEC with prominent clear cells and adjacent calcifications →. Similar features may also be seen in non-small cell carcinomas with clear cell features.* ***(Right)*** *Higher magnification of the clear cell component is shown in a low-grade MEC. Note the absence of nuclear atypia, mitotic activity, and keratinization. Some cells have an oncocytic appearance.*

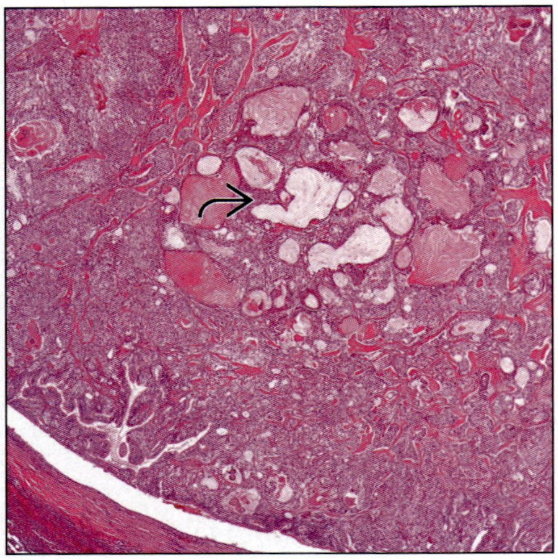

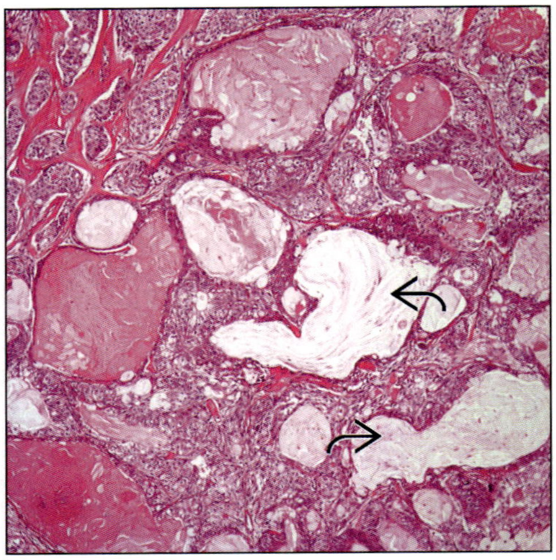

(Left) *Low-grade MEC with extensive solid component and focal cystic structures →. In cases in which the solid component is prominent, the diagnosis may pose more difficulties.* ***(Right)*** *Cystic structures → in a low-grade MEC are shown with numerous mucocytes and presence of intraluminal mucin. This high-power view shows the classical feature of these tumors.*

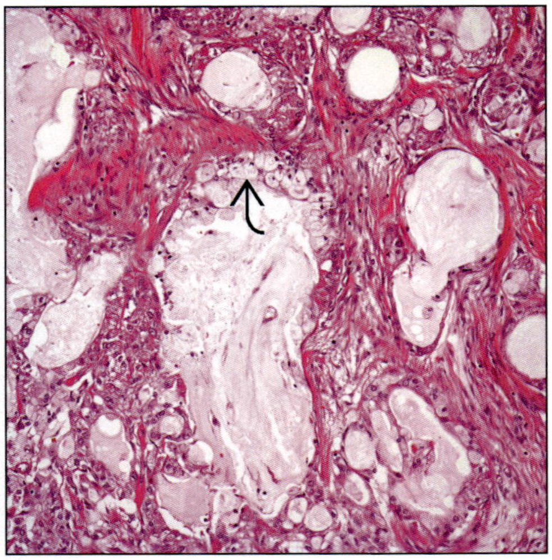

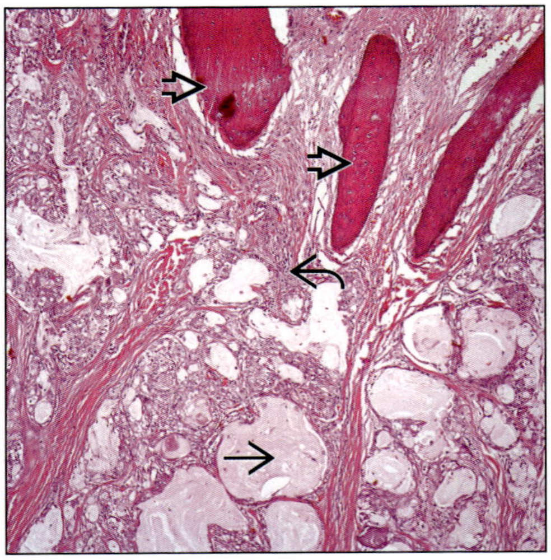

(Left) *Higher magnification shows mucin-producing cells lining cystic structures →. Similar features may also be seen in cases of mucous gland adenomas of the bronchus.* ***(Right)*** *Low-grade MEC shows the classical admixture of mucous cells and intraluminal mucus → alongside a solid cellular component → and areas of ossification →. Ossification is not a common feature of MEC.*

Microscopic Features

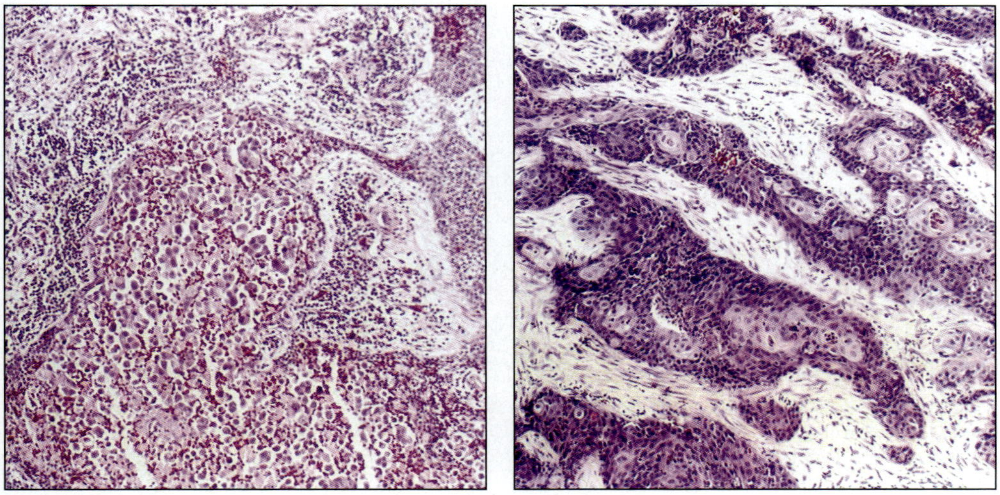

(Left) *High-grade mucoepidermoid carcinoma shows solid epithelial proliferation with marked atypical features admixed with necrosis. These features by themselves can be seen in cases of non-small cell carcinomas.* ***(Right)*** *Solid epidermoid component with cellular atypia arranged in a trabecular growth pattern. These features in the right context are diagnostic of high-grade MEC. Note the absence of the solid/cystic growth pattern present in low-grade tumors.*

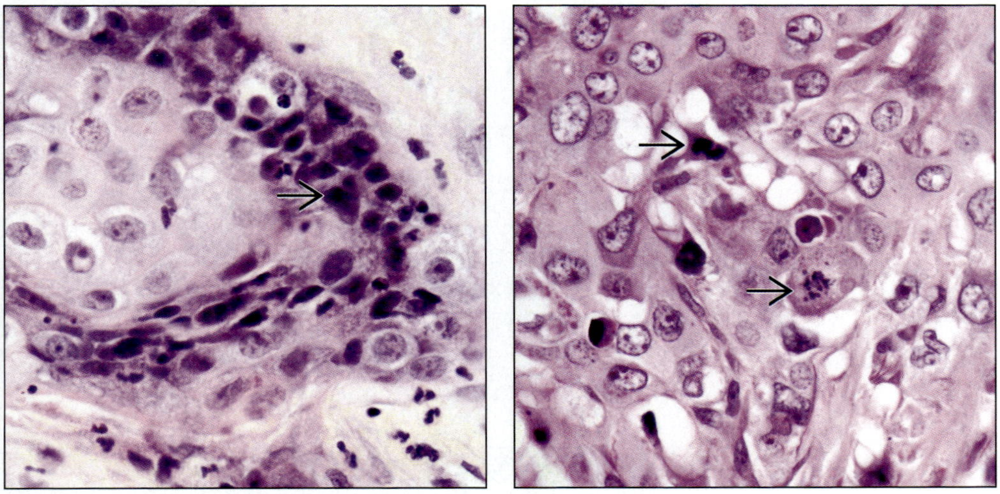

(Left) *Higher magnification of a high-grade MEC. Note the prominent nuclear atypia* →*. This histopathological feature may also be seen in ordinary cases of squamous cell carcinoma of the lung.* ***(Right)*** *High-grade MEC with an atypical epithelial, nonkeratinizing cellular proliferation with marked nuclear atypia and mitosis* →*. These features alone are diagnostic of high-grade MEC.*

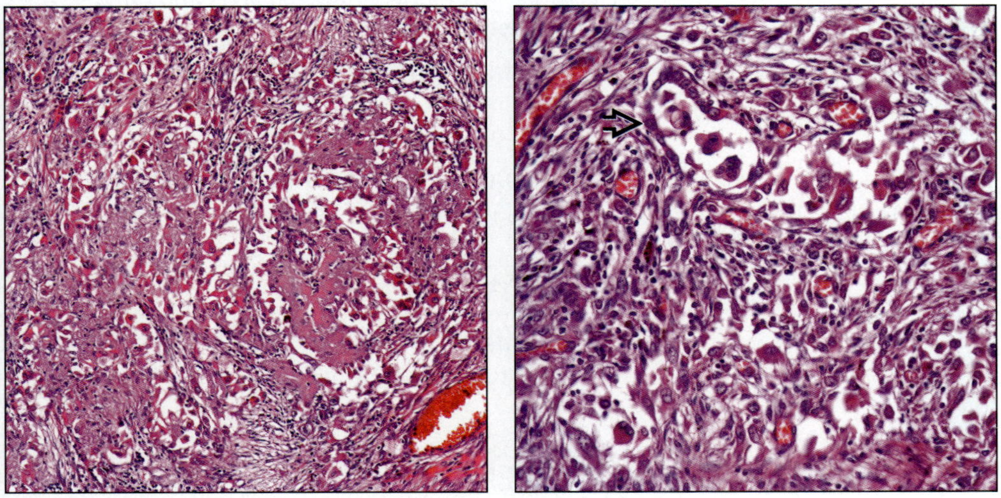

(Left) *High-grade MEC is shown with focal fibrinoid material admixed with a prominent atypical cellular proliferation. These features should be carefully analyzed for the diagnosis of high-grade MEC.* ***(Right)*** *High-grade MEC is shown with marked cellular atypia and focal spindle cell component. Note the presence of remnants of cystic epithelial structures* ⇨*. The presence of nuclear atypia and mitotic activity are features of high-grade MEC.*

EPI-MYOEPITHELIAL CARCINOMA

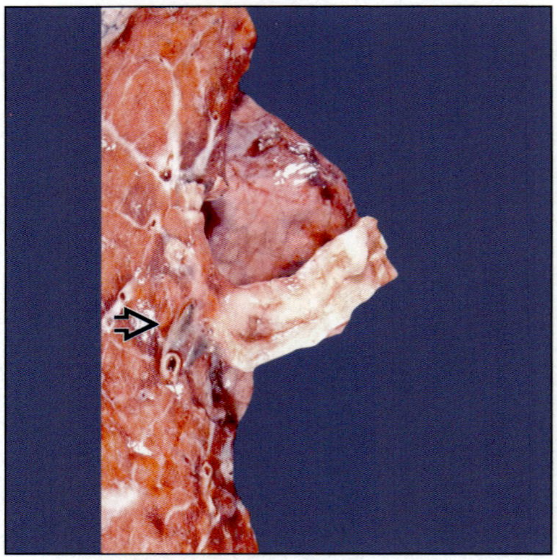

Gross photograph of epi-myoepithelial carcinoma shows an endobronchial tumor ⇨ obstructing most of the lumen. Note the infiltrative nature of the tumor.

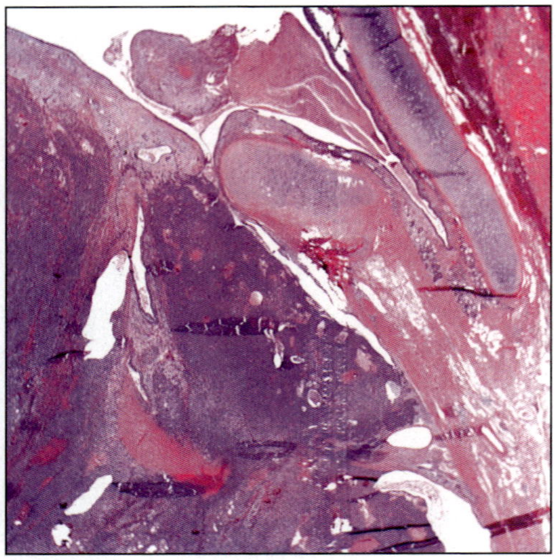

Panoramic view shows epi-myoepithelial carcinoma with a solid and tubular pattern. This low-power view can be seen in other tumors of salivary gland origin.

TERMINOLOGY

Abbreviations

- Epi-myoepithelial carcinoma (EMC)

Synonyms

- Adenomyoepithelioma
- Epithelial-myoepithelial tumor
- Epithelial-myoepithelial tumor of unknown malignant potential
- Pneumocytic adenomyoepithelioma

Definitions

- Salivary gland-type tumor with epithelial and myoepithelial component

ETIOLOGY/PATHOGENESIS

Etiology

- Origin of this tumor similar to other tumors of salivary gland type; may be from endobronchial glands

CLINICAL ISSUES

Epidemiology

- Incidence
  - Unusual occurrence as primary lung neoplasm
  - No more than 15-20 cases reported in literature

Site

- Invariably a central tumor

Presentation

- Cough
- Shortness of breath
- Hemoptysis
- Fever

Treatment

- Surgical approaches
  - Lobectomy
  - Pneumonectomy

Prognosis

- Good
- Tumor has potential to metastasize

MACROSCOPIC FEATURES

General Features

- Endobronchial tumor
- Rare tumor

Size

- 2.5-5 cm in greatest dimension

MICROSCOPIC PATHOLOGY

Histologic Features

- Glandular with inner epithelial layer and outer myoepithelial layer

Predominant Pattern/Injury Type

- Tubular
- Solid

Predominant Cell/Compartment Type

- Epithelial, glandular

ANCILLARY TESTS

Immunohistochemistry

- Can highlight inner epithelial and outer myoepithelial layers

DIFFERENTIAL DIAGNOSIS

Adenoid Cystic Carcinoma

- In small biopsies

EPI-MYOEPITHELIAL CARCINOMA

Key Facts

Terminology
- Adenomyoepithelioma, epithelial-myoepithelial tumor, epithelial-myoepithelial tumor of unknown malignant potential, pneumocytic adenomyoepithelioma

Clinical Issues
- Cough
- Chest pain
- Hemoptysis

Macroscopic Features
- Endobronchial tumor
- 2.5-5 cm in greatest dimension

Microscopic Pathology
- Tubular
- Epithelial, glandular
- Glandular with inner epithelial layer and outer myoepithelial layer
- Solid

Ancillary Tests
- CK-PAN
- S100

Top Differential Diagnoses
- Adenoid cystic carcinoma
- Mixed tumor (pleomorphic adenoma)
- Adenocarcinoma

Diagnostic Checklist
- Tubular structures with inner epithelial layer and outer layer of clear myoepithelial cells

Immunohistochemistry

Antibody	Reactivity	Staining Pattern	Comment
CK-PAN	Positive	Cytoplasmic	
S100	Positive	Nuclear & cytoplasmic	Focally and weakly
Actin-sm	Positive	Cytoplasmic	Stains only myoepithelial cells
TTF-1	Positive	Nuclear	In some cases
Vimentin	Positive	Cytoplasmic	

  - Very difficult or impossible to differentiate
  - Both tumors show myoepithelial differentiation
  - Cylindromatous pattern is more common in adenoid cystic carcinoma
- In resected specimens
  - Presence of bi-layer of cells forming glandular component is more common in adenoid cystic carcinoma
  - Areas of cylindromatous pattern is more common in adenoid cystic carcinoma
  - Presence of intraglandular mucoid material is more common in adenoid cystic carcinoma
  - Presence of glandular structures with internal layer (epithelial) and external layers of clear cells (myoepithelial cells) is classic for EMC

Mixed Tumor (Pleomorphic Adenoma)
- EMC lacks presence of mesenchymal components
  - Cartilage
  - Bone
  - Prominent chondromyxoid background
- Bi-layer showing inner epithelial + outer clear cell layer of myoepithelial cells is characteristic of P-EMC

Adenocarcinoma
- No bilayer of epithelial and myoepithelial cells
- Tumor cells may or may not be arranged in glands
- Tumor cells may have malignant cytological features

DIAGNOSTIC CHECKLIST

Pathologic Interpretation Pearls
- Tubular structures with inner epithelial layer and outer layer of clear myoepithelial cells

GRADING

Low-Grade Carcinoma
- Tumor lacks marked nuclear atypia or increased mitotic activity
- Lymph node metastasis has been described

SELECTED REFERENCES

1. Nguyen CV et al: Pulmonary epithelial-myoepithelial carcinoma: a clinicopathologic and immunohistochemical study of 5 cases. Hum Pathol. 40(3):366-73, 2009
2. Chang T et al: Pneumocytic adenomyoepithelioma: a distinctive lung tumor with epithelial, myoepithelial, and pneumocytic differentiation. Am J Surg Pathol. 31(4):562-8, 2007
3. Chao TY et al: Bronchial epithelial-myoepithelial carcinoma. Ann Thorac Surg. 83(2):689-91, 2007
4. Muslimani AA et al: Recurrent bronchial epithelial-myoepithelial carcinoma after local therapy. Clin Lung Cancer. 8(6):386-8, 2007
5. Fulford LG et al: Epithelial-myoepithelial carcinomas of the bronchus. Am J Surg Pathol. 25(12):1508-14, 2001
6. Wilson RW et al: Epithelial-myoepithelial carcinoma of the lung: immunohistochemical and ultrastructural observations and review of the literature. Hum Pathol. 28(5):631-5, 1997

EPI-MYOEPITHELIAL CARCINOMA

Microscopic Features

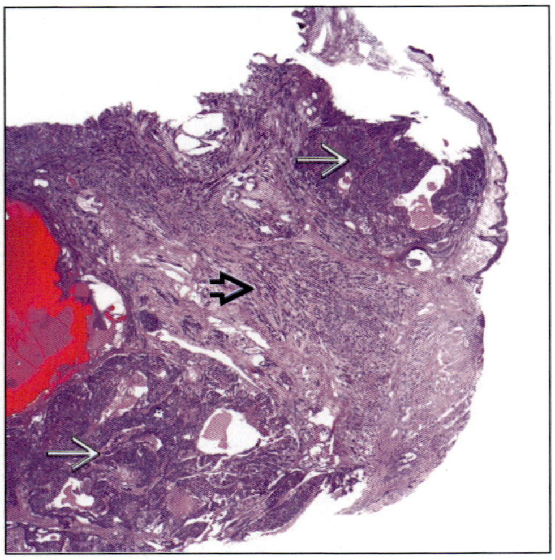

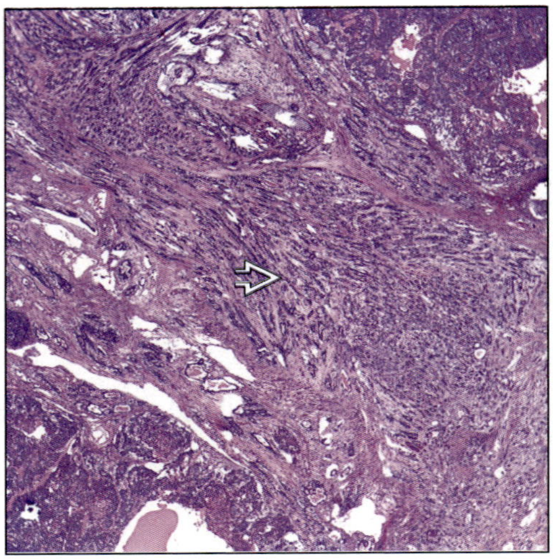

(Left) *Epi-myoepithelial carcinoma of lung shows solid areas → admixed with a glandular component → and focal areas of hemorrhage. This low-power view can be easily confused with conventional adenocarcinoma.* ***(Right)*** *Streaming of tubular structures →. Adjacent tumor areas show a more glandular appearance. The presence of a bi-layer glandular proliferation should suggest the differential diagnosis of EMC.*

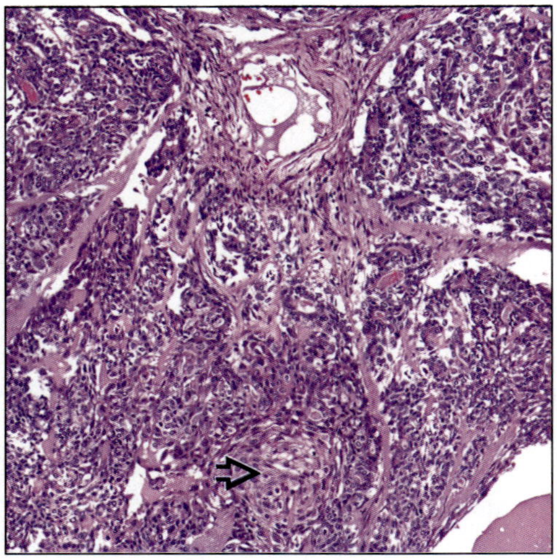

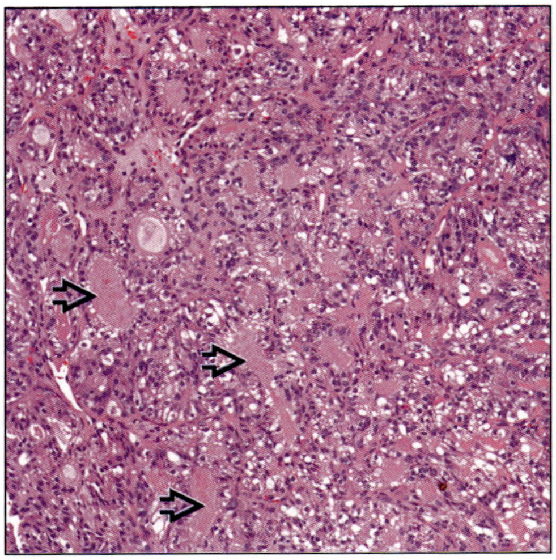

(Left) *EMC with solid component and focal squamous morules →. Although the presence of morules would suggest blastoma, the glandular component of EMC would be unusual in cases of pulmonary blastoma.* ***(Right)*** *Tubular structures with amorphous acellular material in the lumen of glands →. Even at this magnification, one can identify clear cells. This pattern may also be seen in cases of adenoid cystic carcinoma.*

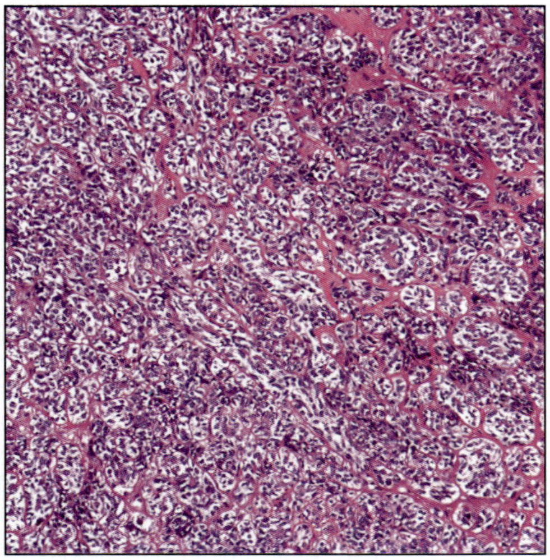

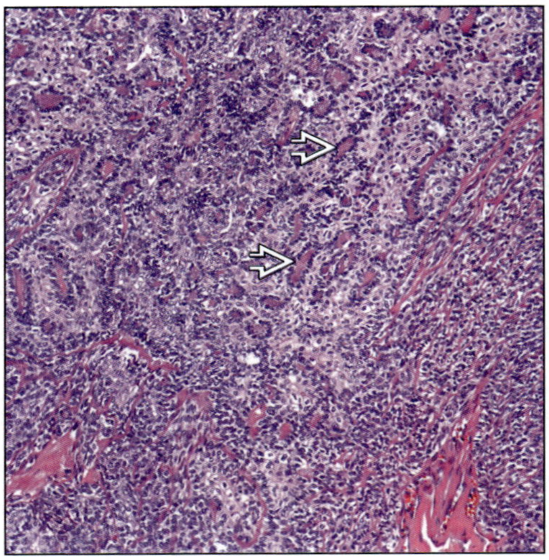

(Left) *Proliferation of clear myoepithelial cells separated by a thin fibrocollagenous material. This pattern of predominant clear myoepithelial cells also suggests the possibility of pure myoepithelial carcinoma.* ***(Right)*** *Tubular structures with prominent epithelial component →. Although the appearance is that of a glandular proliferation, the "glands" are composed of 2 cell populations.*

Microscopic Features

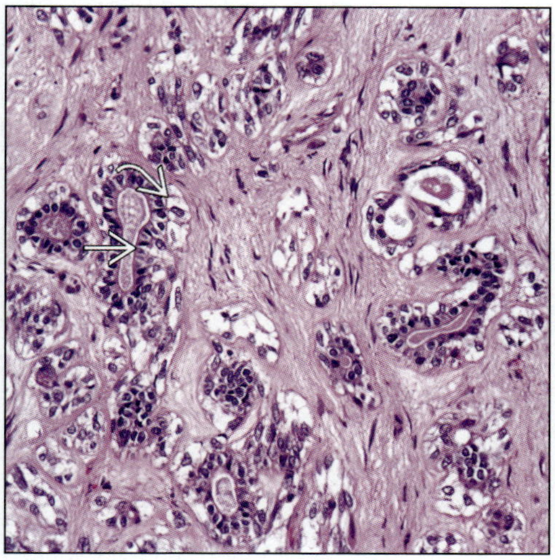
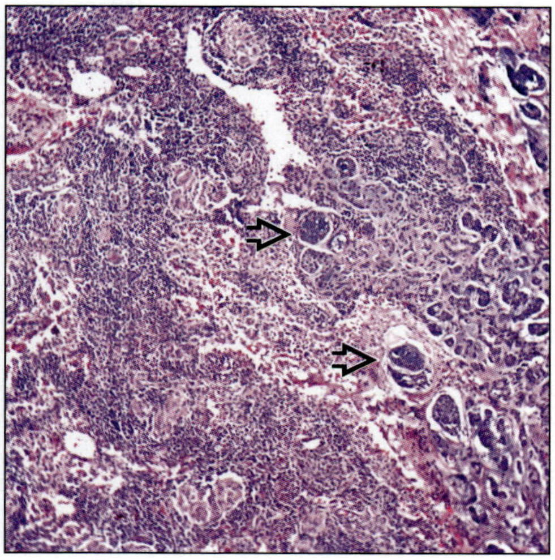

(Left) *Epi-myoepithelial carcinoma shows classical tubular structures with dual epithelial ➔ and clear cell myoepithelial components ➔. This pattern is classical for the diagnosis of EMC.* ***(Right)*** *Metastatic EMC in a lymph node ⇨. This feature is rarely seen in EMC and should be carefully evaluated in all those cases in which lymph nodes are available for histological examination.*

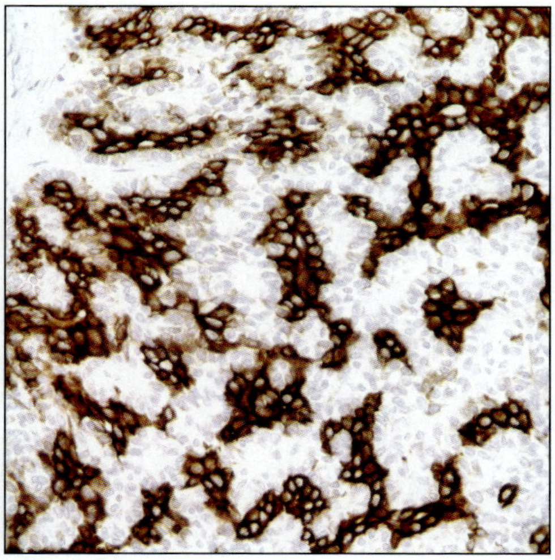
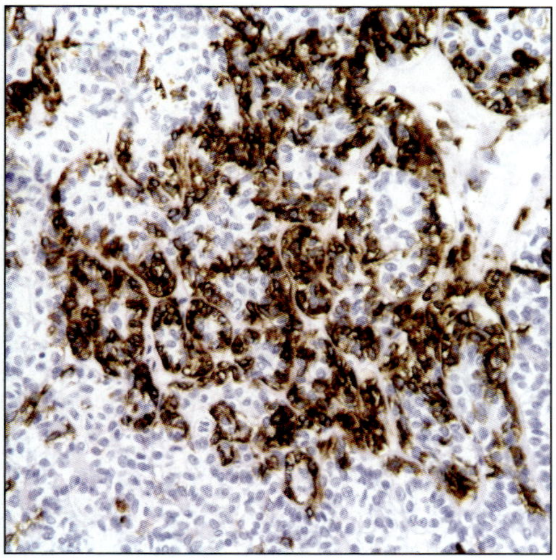

(Left) *CK-PAN shows a strong positive reaction in the epithelial component. It is important to recognize that this staining pattern is not necessarily pathognomonic of EMC.* ***(Right)*** *Actin-sm shows strong positive reaction in the myoepithelial component. As with CK-PAN, this is not specific for EMC.*

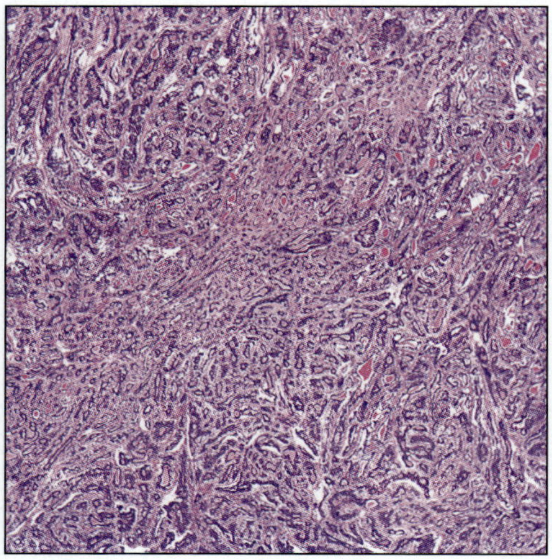
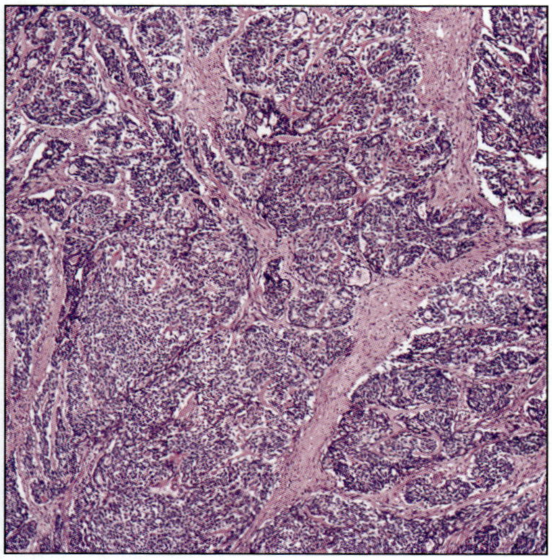

(Left) *EMC is shown growing in a more disorganized pattern of tubular structures of different sizes admixed with some solid components. A similar pattern may be seen in cases of adenoid cystic carcinoma.* ***(Right)*** *EMC with a more solid growth pattern with bands of fibroconnective tissue. This image may also be seen in adenoid cystic carcinoma. Closer examination in these cases will show the typical features of EMC.*

EPI-MYOEPITHELIAL CARCINOMA

Microscopic Features

(Left) *Solid component in an EMC, in which one can still identify small tubular structures →.* ***(Right)*** *Clusters of tubular structures are separated by thin fibroconnective tissue. In some tubular structures one can identify a dual cellular proliferation. The identification of glands with a double layer of cells is important in establishing the diagnosis of EMC. Immunohistochemical stains will be of help in identifying the myoepithelial component.*

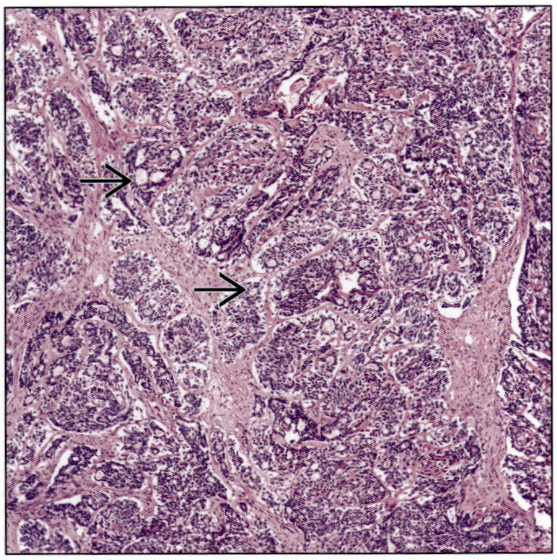

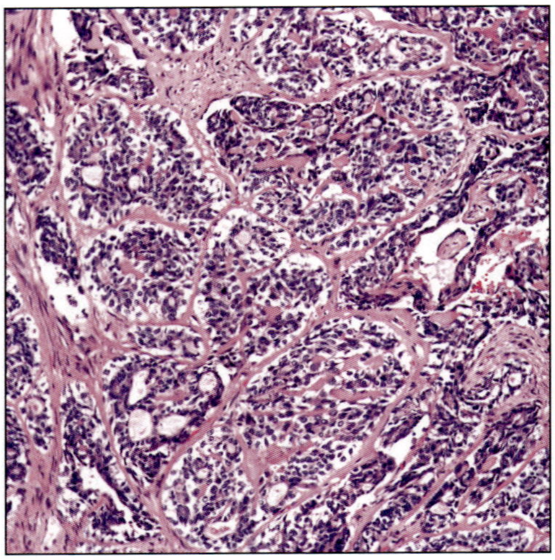

(Left) *EMC is shown with foci of squamous metaplasia. This histopathological finding may be more marked in some areas ⇨. However, this component is not extensive enough to suggest the possibility of a collision tumor.* ***(Right)*** *Marked hyalinization with only a few groups of tubular structures in EMC. Still, the basic cellular component for the diagnosis of EMC is present.*

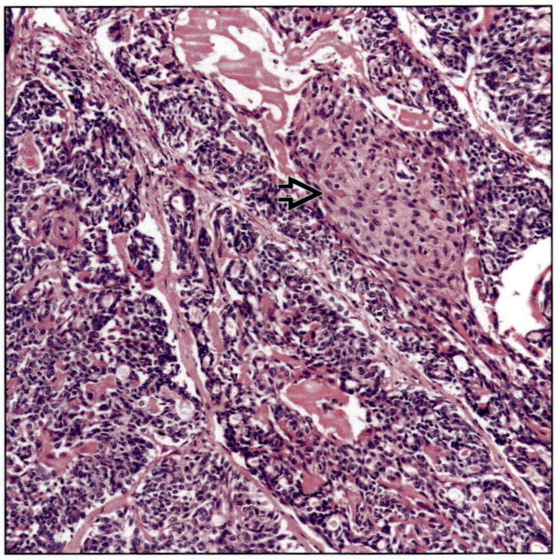

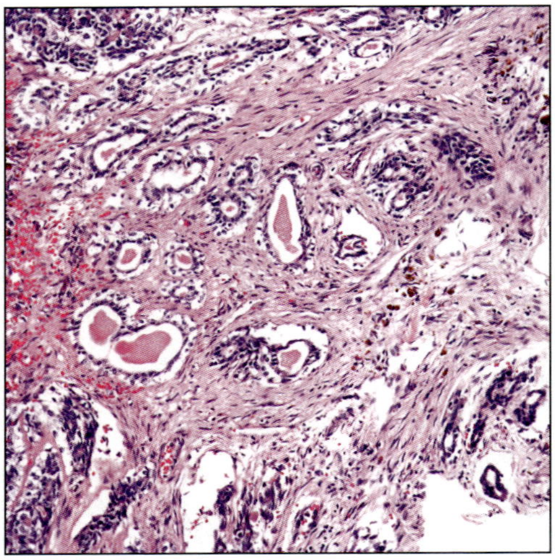

(Left) *Focal fibrinoid necrosis in EMC. Note the presence of the characteristic tubular structures around the fibrinoid areas of necrosis. This fibrinoid necrosis may be secondary to previous biopsy.* ***(Right)*** *Classical myoepithelial proliferation is composed of rather small cells with round to oval nuclei and absent nucleoli. Small residual tubular structures are still present →. Note the absence of increased mitotic activity.*

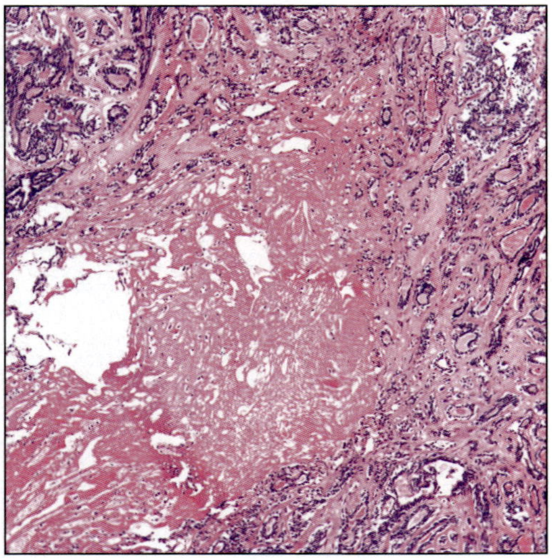

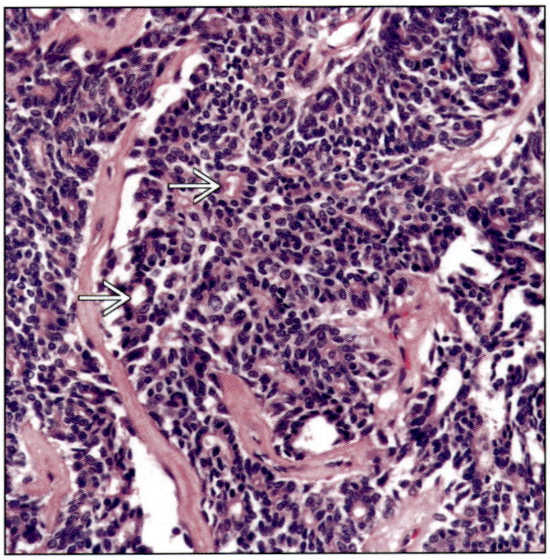

Microscopic Features

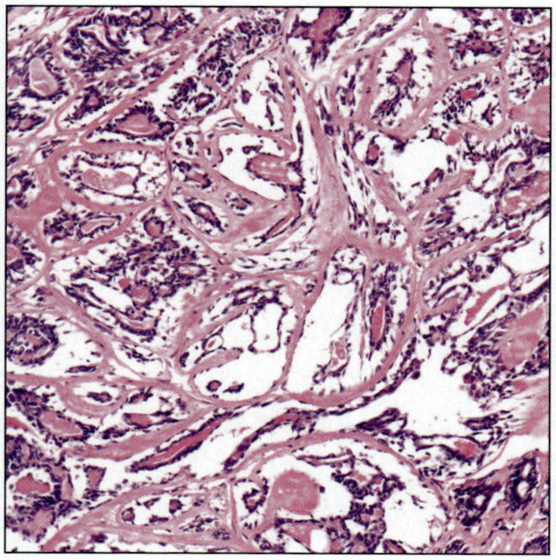

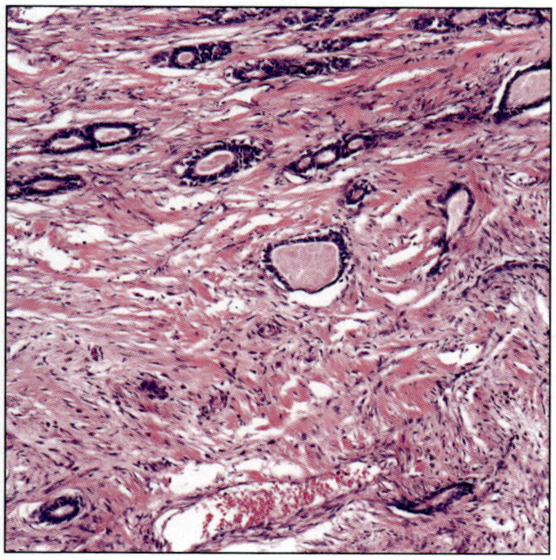

(Left) *Epi-myoepithelial carcinoma of the lung shows marked hyalinization of the stroma separating tubular structures. Note the dual cellular population of the tubular structures.* ***(Right)*** *Residual tubular structures are seen dissecting fibroconnective tissue. Although the basic component for the diagnosis of EMC is present, in small biopsies, an unequivocal diagnosis may be more difficult.*

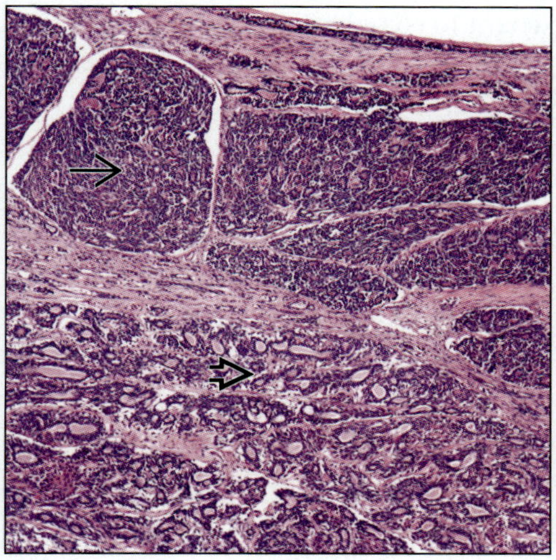

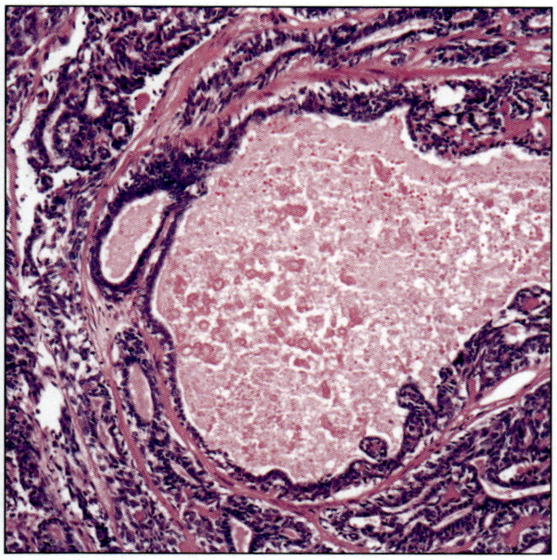

(Left) *Hematoxylin & eosin shows clear demarcation of a solid* → *component and the more characteristic tubular component* ⇨*. In resected specimens, the diagnosis may be more apparent while in small biopsies with sampling of only solid areas, the diagnosis may be much more difficult.* ***(Right)*** *Hematoxylin & eosin shows focal cystic areas in EMC. Note the classic tubular growth pattern around the cystic component. These large cystic changes are unusual in EMC.*

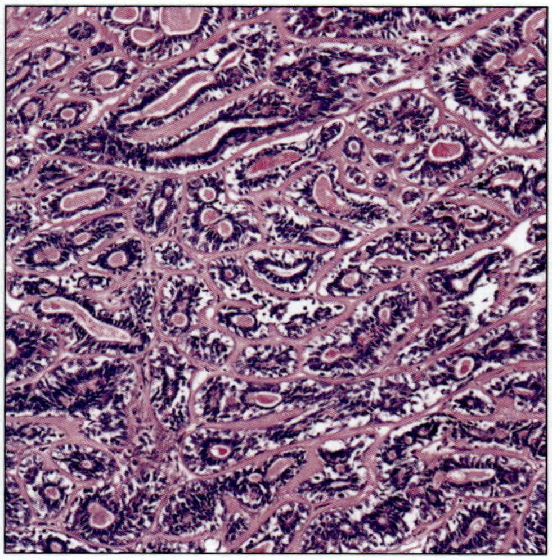

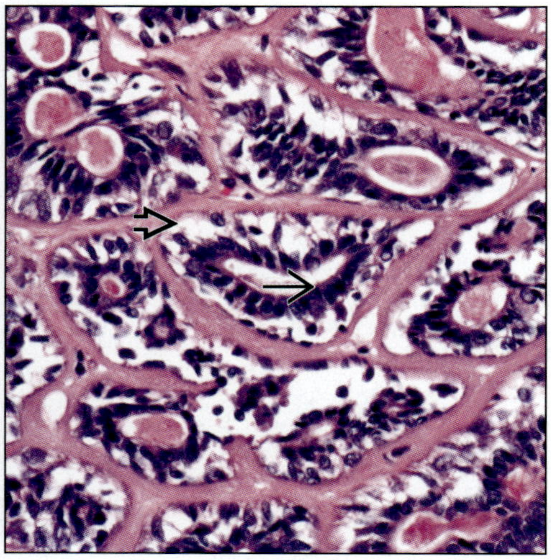

(Left) *Hematoxylin & eosin shows the characteristic growth pattern of EMC, tubular structures lined by a dual cell population. This is the classical histology of EMC.* ***(Right)*** *Higher magnification of the tubular structures shows an epithelial component* → *and a clear cell outer myoepithelial component* ⇨ *in this classical example of epi-myoepithelial carcinoma of the lung.*

ACINIC CELL CARCINOMA

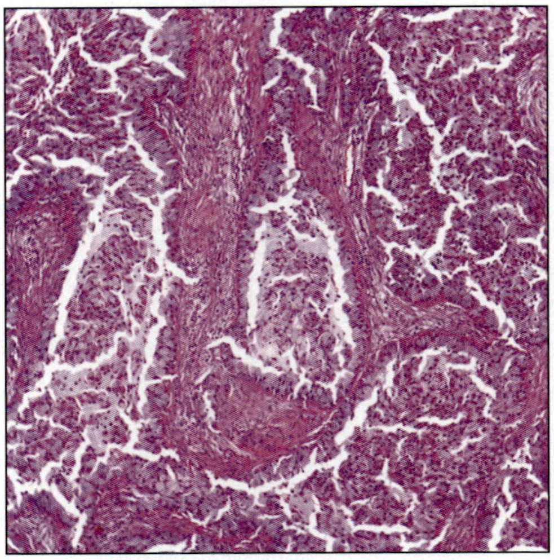

Acinic cell carcinoma of the lung with acinar pattern is shown. Note the presence of bands of fibroconnective tissue, giving the appearance of a lobulated neoplasm.

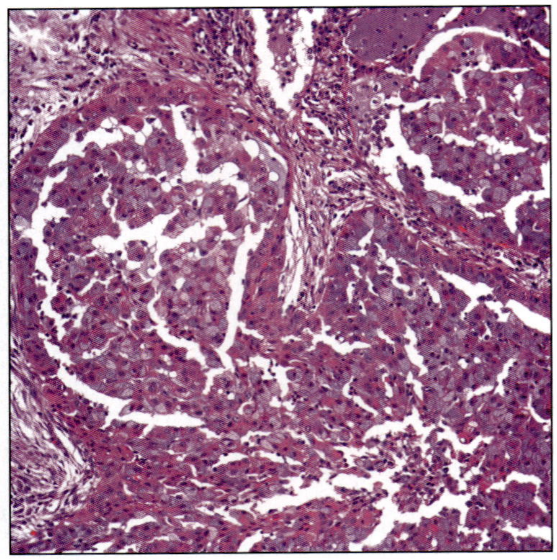

Acinic cell carcinoma of lung showing a vague glandular appearance and composed of medium-sized cells with ample granular cytoplasm. Note the absence of nuclear atypia or mitotic activity.

TERMINOLOGY

Synonyms

- Fechner tumor

Definitions

- Epithelial neoplasm similar to that in salivary glands

CLINICAL ISSUES

Presentation

- Chest pain
- Shortness of breath
- Cough
- Asymptomatic

Treatment

- Surgical approaches
  - Lobectomy

Prognosis

- Good in majority of cases
  - Tumor may follow aggressive behavior with metastasis

MACROSCOPIC FEATURES

General Features

- Intraparenchymal mass
- Tumor is well demarcated but not encapsulated
- Necrosis and hemorrhage are not common

Size

- Usually tumors measure 1-5 cm in greatest dimension

MICROSCOPIC PATHOLOGY

Histologic Features

- Large cells with abundant granular cytoplasm
- Signet ring-like cell appearance
- Low mitotic count to complete absence of mitotic activity
- Absence of nuclear atypia
- Absence of necrosis &/or hemorrhage

Predominant Pattern/Injury Type

- Acinar
- Cystic
- Organoid

Predominant Cell/Compartment Type

- Epithelial

DIFFERENTIAL DIAGNOSIS

Adenocarcinoma

- Will show more nuclear atypia and mitotic figures
- Will show positive cytoplasmic staining for mucin with D-PAS and mucicarmine
- Cells in acinic cell carcinoma are larger with abundant granular cytoplasm
- Acinic cell carcinoma will show by EM the characteristic dark electron-dense zymogen granules
  - Shows strong positive cytoplasmic reaction with PAS

Oncocytic Variant of Neuroendocrine Carcinoma

- Acinic cell carcinoma negative for neuroendocrine markers
- By electron microscopy, neuroendocrine carcinoma will display neurosecretory granules
  - May show mitotic activity and necrosis

Metastatic Acinic Cell Carcinoma

- Previous history of acinic cell carcinoma of head and neck region is crucial in establishing primary site

ACINIC CELL CARCINOMA

Key Facts

Terminology
- Fechner tumor
- Epithelial neoplasm similar to that in salivary glands

Clinical Issues
- Cough
- Chest Pain
- Asymptomatic

Macroscopic Features
- Necrosis and hemorrhage are not common
- Tumor is well demarcated but not encapsulated
- Intraparenchymal mass
- Usually the tumors measure from 1-5 cm in greatest dimension

Top Differential Diagnoses
- Adenocarcinoma
  - Shows positive cytoplasmic staining for mucin content with D-PAS and mucicarmine
  - Shows more nuclear atypia and mitotic figures
- Oncocytic variant of neuroendocrine carcinoma
  - Acinic cell carcinoma negative for neuroendocrine markers
- Metastatic acinic cell carcinoma
  - Previous history of acinic cell carcinoma of the head and neck region is crucial in establishing primary site

Diagnostic Checklist
- Granular cytoplasm brightly positive for PAS
- EM: Electron-dense zymogen granules

Immunohistochemistry

Antibody	Reactivity	Staining Pattern	Comment
KERATIN-LMW	Positive	Cytoplasmic	In all cases
Amylase	Positive	Cytoplasmic	Only in some cases
Chymotrypsin	Positive	Cytoplasmic	Only in some cases
EMA	Positive	Cell membrane	
TTF-1	Positive	Nuclear	Not in all cases
CK7	Positive	Cytoplasmic	
CK20	Negative		
CDX-2	Negative		

Histochemical Features of Acinic Cell Carcinomas of Lung

Histochemical Stain	Reactivity	Comment
PAS	Strongly positive	
Mucicarmine	Negative	Focal cytoplasmic mucin positive cells may be seen
D-PAS	Negative	

DIAGNOSTIC CHECKLIST

Clinically Relevant Pathologic Features
- EM: Electron-dense zymogen granules

Pathologic Interpretation Pearls
- Granular cytoplasm brightly positive for PAS
- Signet ring-like cells
- Low mitotic activity
- Oncocytic features
- Papillocystic features

SELECTED REFERENCES

1. Chuah KL et al: Recurrence of pulmonary acinic cell carcinoma. Arch Pathol Lab Med. 130(7):932-3, 2006
2. Sabaratnam RM et al: Acinic cell carcinoma: an unusual cause of bronchial obstruction in a child. Pediatr Dev Pathol. 7(5):521-6, 2004
3. Watanabe K et al: Fine-needle aspiration cytology of bronchial acinic cell carcinoma: a case report. Diagn Cytopathol. 30(5):359-61, 2004
4. Lee HY et al: Primary acinic cell carcinoma of the lung with lymph node metastasis. Arch Pathol Lab Med. 127(4):e216-9, 2003
5. Rodriguez J et al: Combined typical carcinoid and acinic cell tumor of the lung: a heretofore unreported occurrence. Hum Pathol. 34(10):1061-5, 2003
6. Ukoha OO et al: Acinic cell carcinoma of the lung with metastasis to lymph nodes. Chest. 115(2):591-5, 1999
7. Moran CA: Primary salivary gland-type tumors of the lung. Semin Diagn Pathol. 12(2):106-22, 1995
8. Moran CA et al: Acinic cell carcinoma of the lung ("Fechner tumor"). A clinicopathologic, immunohistochemical, and ultrastructural study of five cases. Am J Surg Pathol. 16(11):1039-50, 1992
9. Fechner RE et al: Acinic cell tumor of the lung. A histologic and ultrastructural study. Cancer. 29(2):501-8, 1972

ACINIC CELL CARCINOMA

Microscopic Features

*(**Left**) Acinar pattern of acinic cell carcinoma of the lung shows tumor nests separated by thin bands of fibroconnective tissue. (**Right**) Acinar proliferation of large neoplastic cells with ample granular cytoplasm and small nuclei displaced toward the periphery of the cells is seen in acinic cell carcinoma of the lung. Note the absence of mitotic activity and nuclear atypia.*

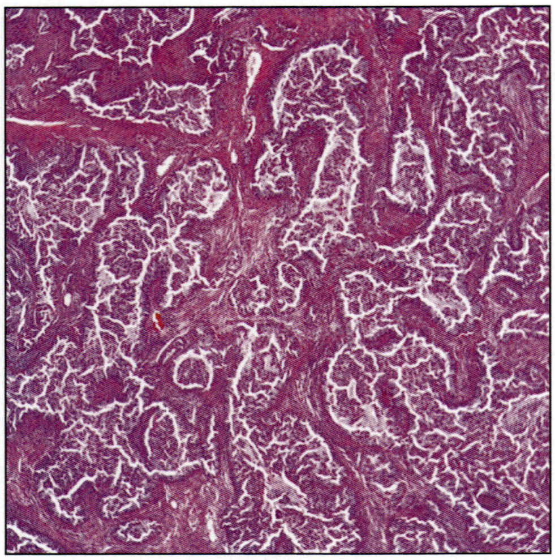

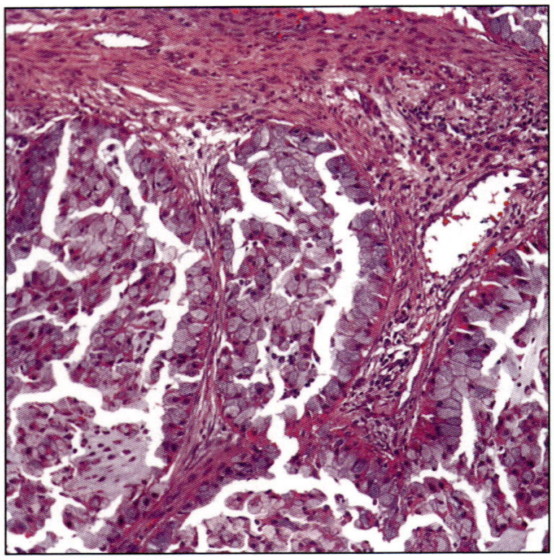

*(**Left**) High-power view of the cytologic features of acinic cell carcinoma shows large cells with eccentric nuclei, abundant cytoplasm, and inconspicuous nucleoli. Some of the cells may be confused with signet ring cells. (**Right**) Acinic cell carcinoma of the lung shows neoplastic cells floating in alveolar spaces ↪, giving the appearance of a pneumonic type of neoplasm.*

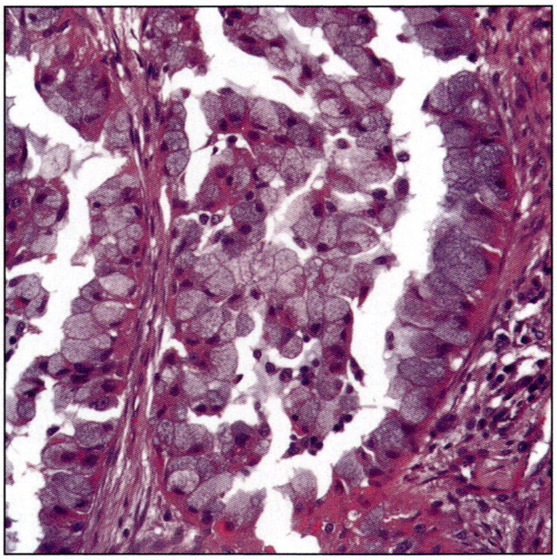

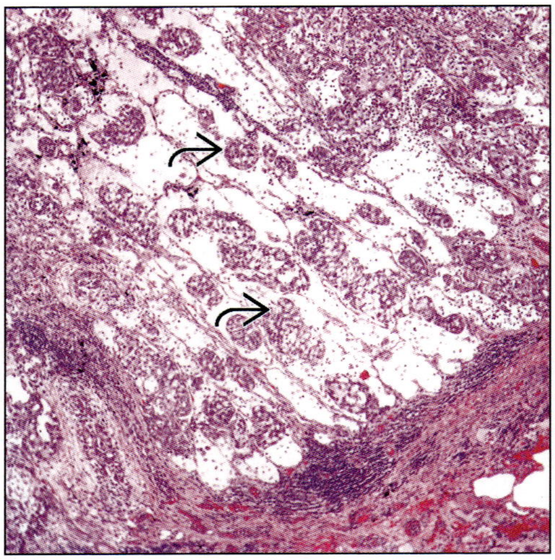

*(**Left**) High magnification of acinic cell carcinoma of the lung shows neoplastic cells with abundant clear cytoplasm and nuclei displaced toward the periphery of the cells. This appearance can be easily confused with a signet ring cell carcinoma of the lung. (**Right**) Acinic cell carcinoma composed of cells with clear cytoplasm. The cells arranged in an acinar pattern appear to be dissecting fibroconnective tissue stroma.*

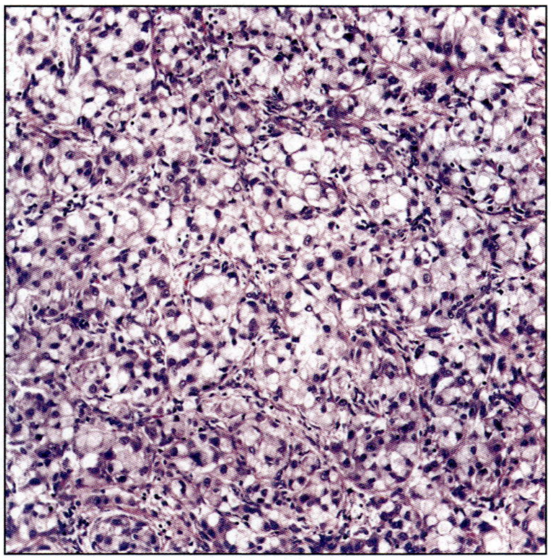

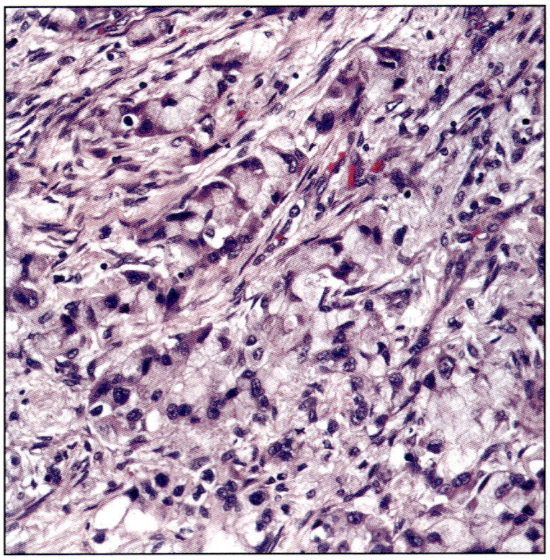

ACINIC CELL CARCINOMA

Microscopic Features

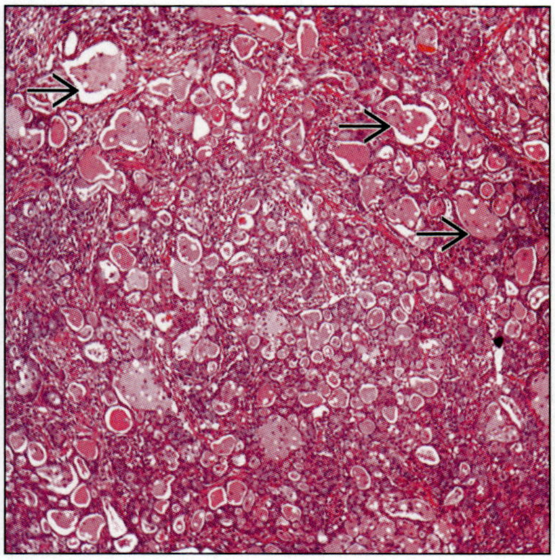
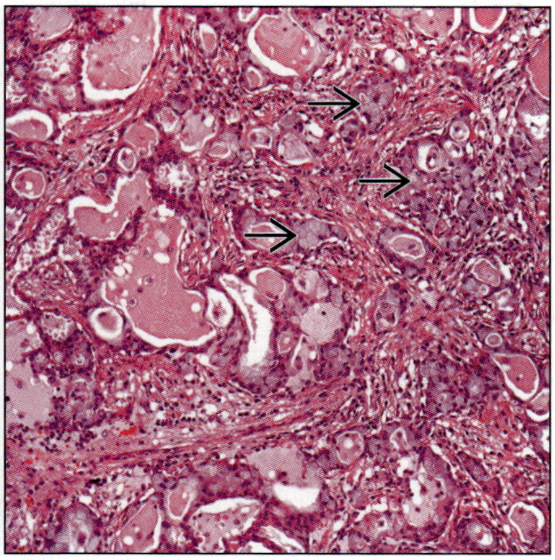

(Left) *Low-power view of acinic cell carcinoma shows a microcystic pattern* → *and focal solid acinar pattern. This low-power appearance can be seen in some other tumors of salivary gland type, such as mucoepidermoid carcinomas.* ***(Right)*** *Higher magnification shows cystic areas lined by neoplastic cells with abundant granular cytoplasm* →*. Different from mucoepidermoid carcinomas that have mucin-producing epithelial cells, in acinic cell carcinoma, the cells contain glycogen.*

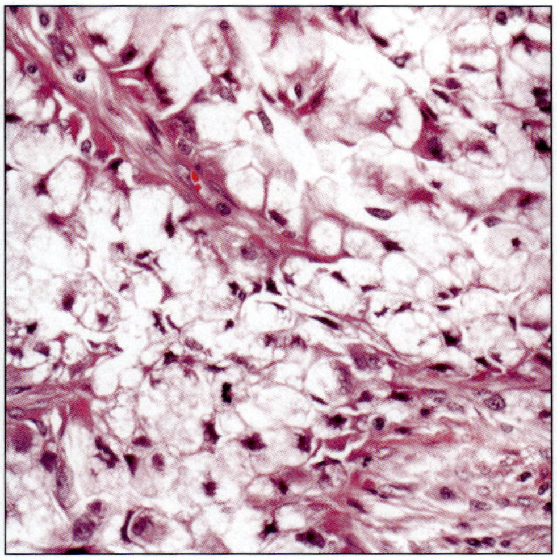
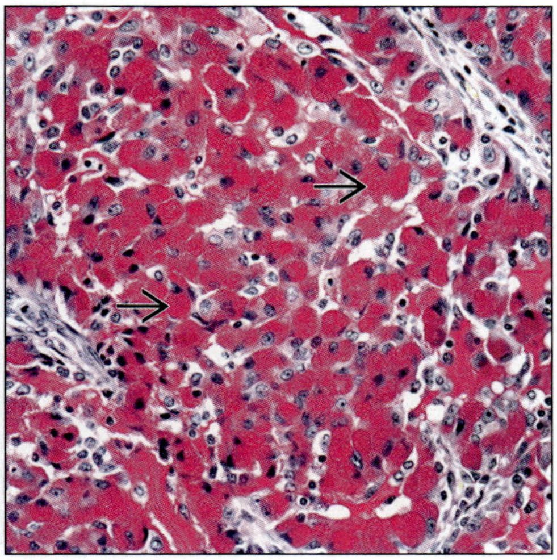

(Left) *Acinic cell carcinoma shows cells with clear cytoplasm and nuclei displaced toward the periphery. This appearance may mimic a signet ring cell carcinoma of either lung or gastrointestinal origin. Note the absence of marked nuclear atypia or mitotic activity.* ***(Right)*** *PAS stain before diastase digestion shows acinic cell carcinoma with strong positive cytoplasmic reaction* →*. This is one of the most important features of acinic cell carcinoma.*

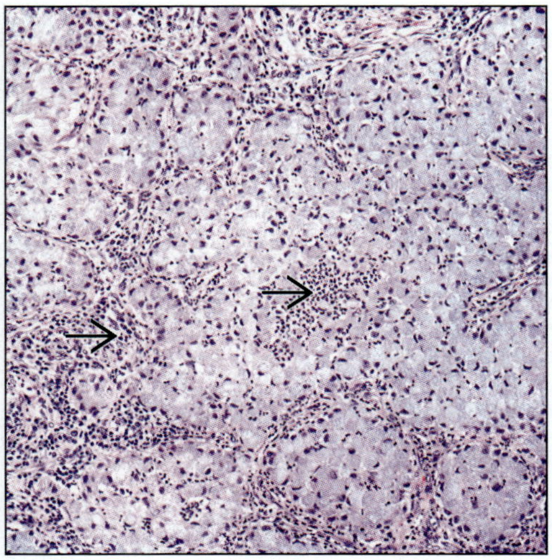
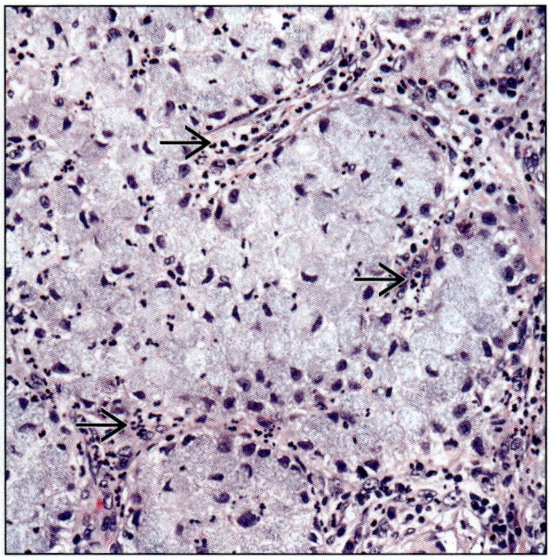

(Left) *Acinic cell carcinoma of the lung shows a classical acinar component. Note the presence of neoplastic cells admixed with an inflammatory component* →*.* ***(Right)*** *Higher magnification shows a classical cellular component of acinic cell carcinoma admixed with an acute inflammatory infiltrate* →*. Note the presence of tumor cells with granular cytoplasm and the absence of mitotic figures or nuclear atypia.*

ACINIC CELL CARCINOMA

Microscopic Features

(Left) *Acinic cell carcinoma of the lung in a central location is seen. The tumor is in an endobronchial location but is not obstructing the bronchial lumen. In addition, note the prominent oncocytic changes and nested pattern.* ***(Right)*** *Acinic cell carcinoma is seen with a prominent nested pattern of growth with an oncocytic cellular proliferation. This appearance is similar to that of neuroendocrine carcinomas of the lung.*

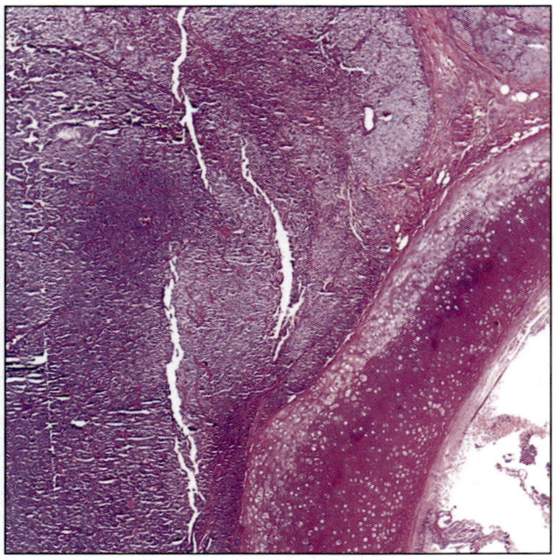

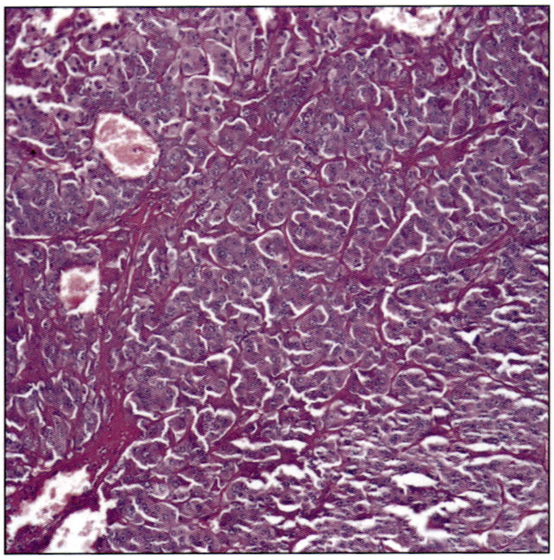

(Left) *High-power view shows a homogeneous cellular proliferation with round nuclei, oncocytic cytoplasm, and ample granular cytoplasm. Note the absence of necrosis and mitotic activity. Similar features may also be seen in conventional neuroendocrine carcinomas of the lung.* ***(Right)*** *TEM shows numerous electron-dense zymogen granules, a chief characteristic of acinic cell carcinoma ⇨. This feature alone is diagnostic of acinic cell carcinoma.*

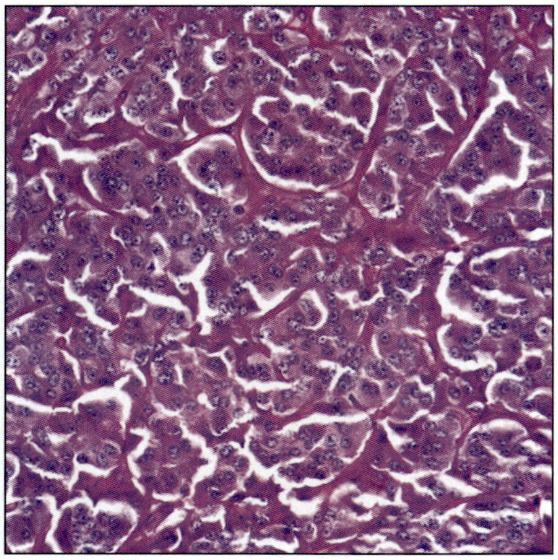

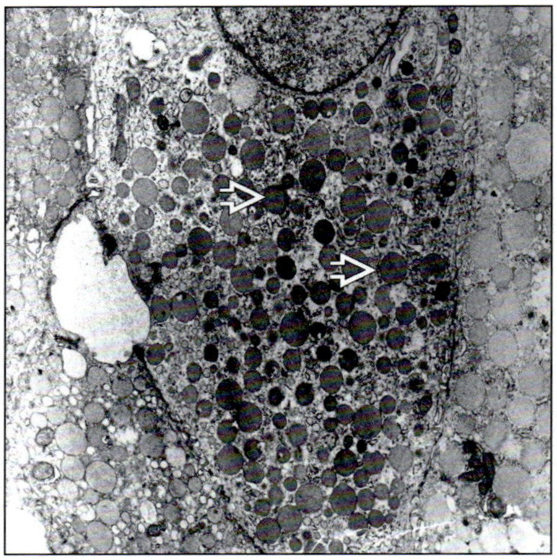

(Left) *Acinic cell carcinoma of the lung shows a more mixed type of histology. The neoplastic cellular proliferation is composed of clear and oncocytic cells. This pattern is not that common in these tumors.* ***(Right)*** *Higher magnification shows the admixture of clear and oncocytic cells in acinic cell carcinoma. Note the absence of nuclear atypia or mitotic activity. Still, the cytoplasm of the clear cells is granular, which raises the diagnosis of acinic cell carcinoma.*

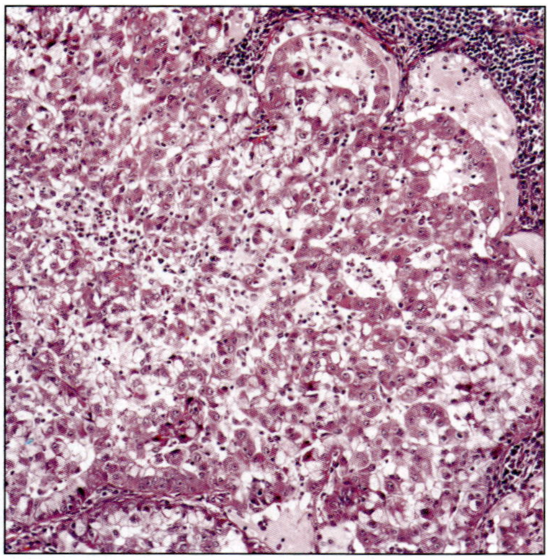

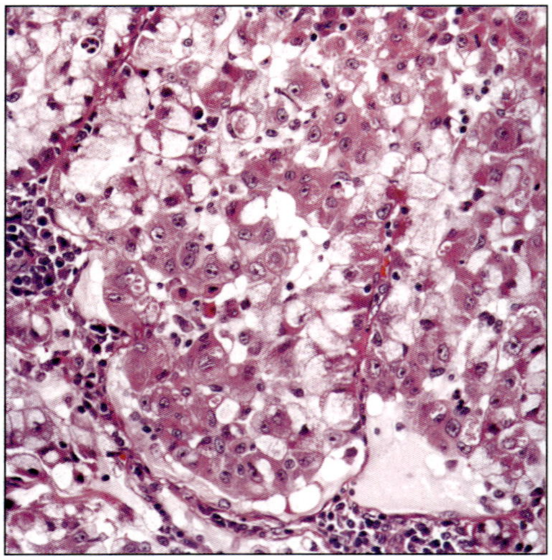

Microscopic Features

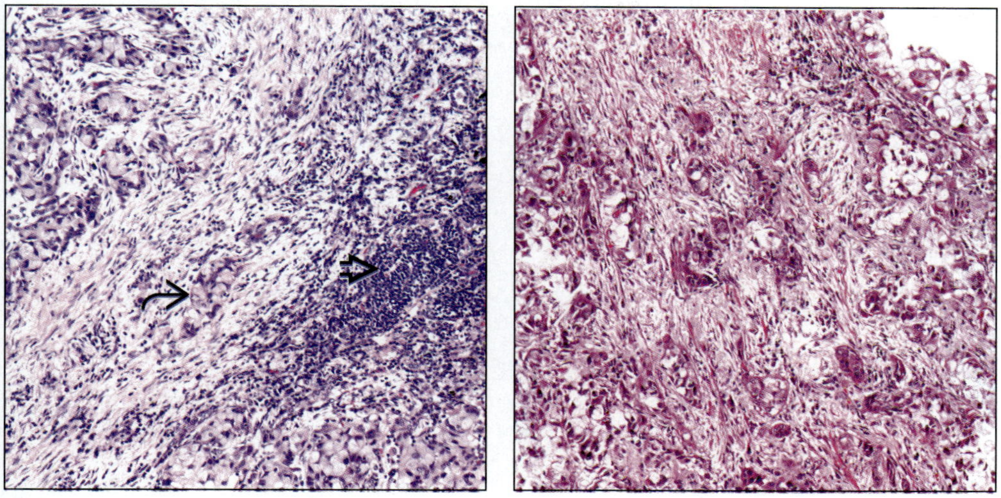

(Left) *Clusters of neoplastic cells dissecting fibroconnective tissue ↷. Adjacent tissue shows inflammatory changes, namely, the presence of lymphocytes ⇨.* ***(Right)*** *Acinic cell carcinoma of the lung shows a focal solid component admixed with more conventional features. A cursory review of similar areas may be mistaken for conventional adenocarcinoma.*

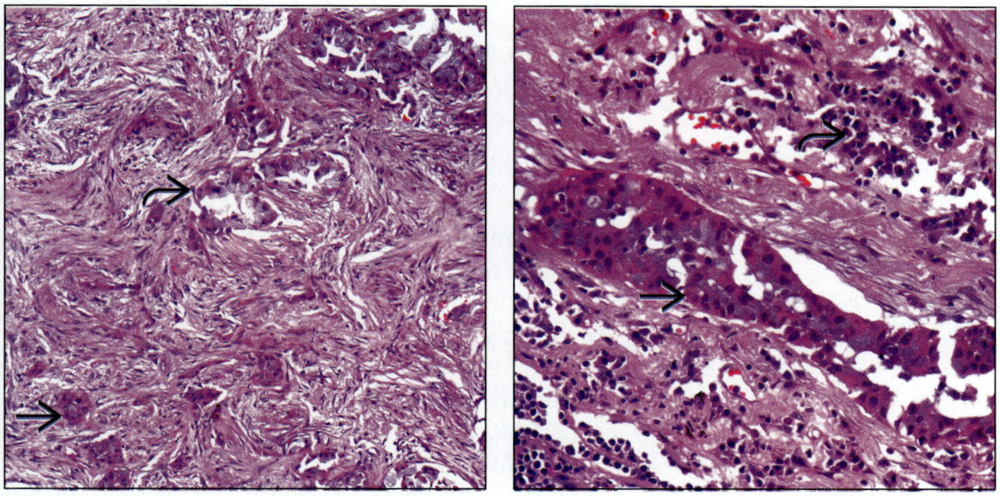

(Left) *In some cases of acinic cell carcinoma, there are areas of fibrosis in which one is able to identify glandular structures ↷ or small clusters of neoplastic cells →.* ***(Right)*** *An isolated island of neoplastic cells is embedded in fibroconnective tissue →. Adjacent tissue shows chronic inflammatory changes with presence of numerous plasma cells ↷.*

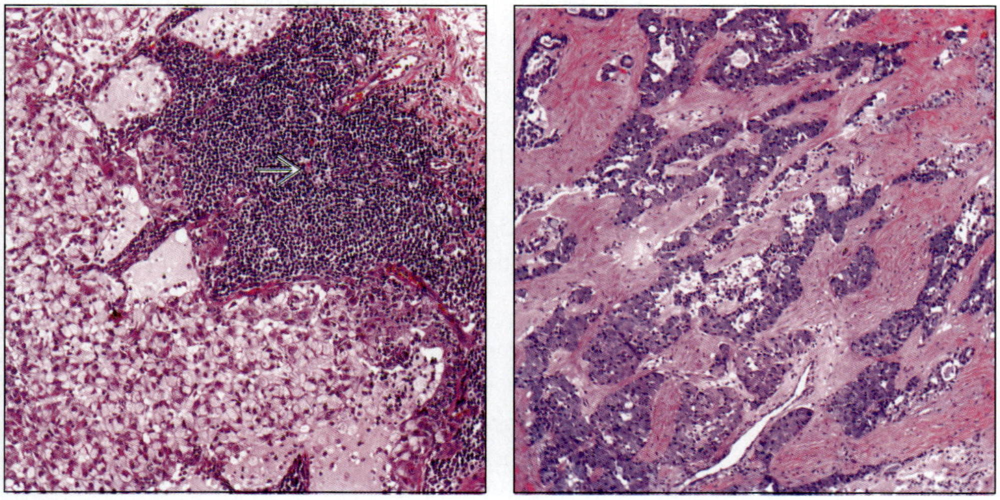

(Left) *In some cases of acinic cell carcinoma, the tumor may show lymphoid aggregates ➡ intermixed with the neoplastic cellular proliferation.* ***(Right)*** *Acinic cell carcinoma of the lung shows neoplastic cells arranged in cords and trabeculae dissecting areas of fibrocollagenous tissue. This pattern can also be seen in the conventional type of pulmonary adenocarcinoma.*

MIXED TUMOR

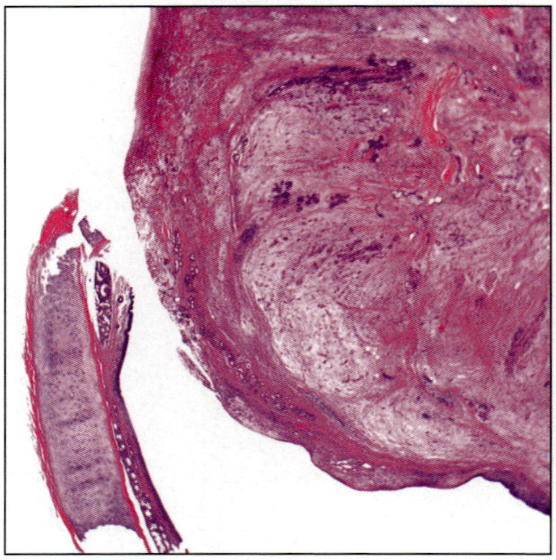

Panoramic view of a benign mixed tumor. Note the central location, as the tumor is growing just beneath the bronchial mucosa.

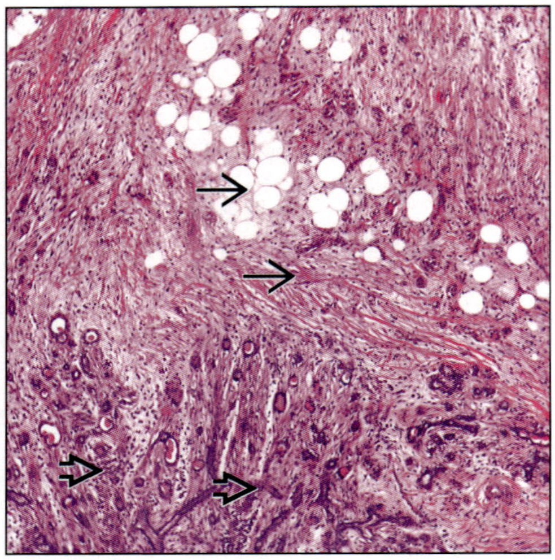

Benign mixed tumor is seen with a mixture of epithelial elements ⮚ and mesenchymal elements →.

TERMINOLOGY

Abbreviations

- Mixed tumor (MT)

Synonyms

- Pleomorphic adenoma (PA)

Definitions

- Biphasic neoplasm with epithelial/myoepithelial and mesenchymal differentiation

CLINICAL ISSUES

Presentation

- Cough
- Incidental finding
- Hemoptysis

Treatment

- Surgical approaches
  - Lobectomy

Prognosis

- Excellent for benign tumor
- Malignant mixed tumors may need additional therapy

MACROSCOPIC FEATURES

General Features

- Endobronchial tumor

Size

- 1-5 cm in greatest dimension

MICROSCOPIC PATHOLOGY

Histologic Features

- Presence of chondromyxoid background with focal cartilage admixed with epithelial component

Predominant Pattern/Injury Type

- Biphasic

Predominant Cell/Compartment Type

- Epithelial, biphasic, or mixed

DIFFERENTIAL DIAGNOSIS

Non-Small Cell Carcinoma

- In small biopsy with only well-differentiated epithelial component sampled
  - In resected specimens, diagnosis should not pose a problem

Epi-myoepithelial Carcinoma

- Both tumors show myoepithelial component
- Epithelial myoepithelial carcinoma does not show presence of cartilage or other heterologous elements
- Glandular component of inner layer of epithelial cells and outer layer of myoepithelial cells is characteristic of epithelial-myoepithelial carcinoma

Mucoepidermoid Carcinoma

- Issue in small biopsy with only epithelial component sampled
- In resected specimens, diagnosis is not a problem
- Mucoepidermoid carcinomas show presence of mucus-producing and intermediate cells

Carcinosarcoma

- Carcinosarcomas will show presence of malignant mesenchymal and malignant epithelial components

MIXED TUMOR

Key Facts

Terminology
- Synonym: Pleomorphic adenoma (PA)
- Biphasic neoplasm with epithelial/myoepithelial and mesenchymal differentiation

Clinical Issues
- Symptoms
  - Cough
  - Dyspnea
  - Chest pain
  - Hemoptysis
- Prognosis
  - Excellent for benign tumors
  - Malignant mixed tumors may need additional therapy

Macroscopic Features
- Endobronchial tumor
- 1-5 cm in greatest dimension

Ancillary Tests
- GFAP
- CK-PAN
- S100
- Actin-sm

Top Differential Diagnoses
- Non-small cell carcinoma
- Epithelial/myoepithelial carcinoma
- Mucoepidermoid carcinoma
- Carcinosarcoma
- Pulmonary hamartoma

Immunohistochemistry

Antibody	Reactivity	Staining Pattern	Comment
CK-PAN	Positive	Cytoplasmic	
S100	Positive	Nuclear & cytoplasmic	
Actin-sm	Positive	Cytoplasmic	
GFAP	Positive	Nuclear & cytoplasmic	Only in a small number of cases
EMA	Positive	Cell membrane	In epithelial component
CD34	Positive	Cytoplasmic	In vessels and adipose tissue
Vimentin	Positive	Cytoplasmic	
Actin-HHF-35	Positive	Cytoplasmic	
SOX9	Positive	Nuclear	In cartilaginous areas

Pulmonary Hamartoma
- Most hamartomas will show prominent cartilaginous component and invaginations of epithelium
- Hamartomas do not show presence of myoepithelial cellular proliferation

DIAGNOSTIC CHECKLIST

Clinically Relevant Pathologic Features
- Tissue distribution

Pathologic Interpretation Pearls
- Presence of epithelial/myoepithelial cells admixed with chondromyxoid or cartilaginous areas

GRADING

Benign Mixed Tumors
- Components are mature elements without atypical histological features

Malignant Mixed Tumor (Ex-Pleomorphic Adenoma)
- Malignant mixed tumors will display conventional malignant components either in epithelial or mesenchymal component

SELECTED REFERENCES

1. Kamiyoshihara M et al: Pleomorphic adenoma of the main bronchus in an adult treated using a wedge bronchiectomy. Gen Thorac Cardiovasc Surg. 57(1):43-5, 2009
2. Fitchett J et al: A rare case of primary pleomorphic adenoma in main bronchus. Ann Thorac Surg. 86(3):1025-6, 2008
3. Méjean-Lebreton F et al: [Benign salivary gland-type tumors of the bronchus: expression of high molecular weight cytokeratins.] Ann Pathol. 26(1):30-4, 2006
4. Ang KL et al: Primary pulmonary pleomorphic adenoma. An immunohistochemical study and review of the literature. Arch Pathol Lab Med. 127(5):621-2, 2003
5. Raja V et al: Unusual presentations of uncommon tumors: case 1. Benign metastasizing pleomorphic adenoma. J Clin Oncol. 20(9):2400-3, 2002
6. Takeuchi E et al: A case of pleomorphic adenoma of the lung with multiple distant metastases--observations on its oncogene and tumor suppressor gene expression. Anticancer Res. 18(3B):2015 -20, 1998
7. Moran CA: Primary salivary gland-type tumors of the lung. Semin Diagn Pathol. 12(2):106-22, 1995
8. Moran CA et al: Benign and malignant salivary gland-type mixed tumors of the lung. Clinicopathologic and immunohistochemical study of eight cases. Cancer. 73(10):2481-90, 1994
9. Hayes MM et al: Malignant mixed tumor of bronchus: a biphasic neoplasm of epithelial and myoepithelial cells. Mod Pathol. 6(1):85-8, 1993

MIXED TUMOR

Microscopic Features

(Left) *Benign mixed tumor with prominent chondromyxoid background and remnants of epithelial elements. The identification of embedded epithelial elements is an important feature in these tumors.* ***(Right)*** *Epithelial cells embedded in an acellular chondromyxoid background. Note the discrete vascular proliferation. The presence of mature cartilage in these tumors in the lung is rare.*

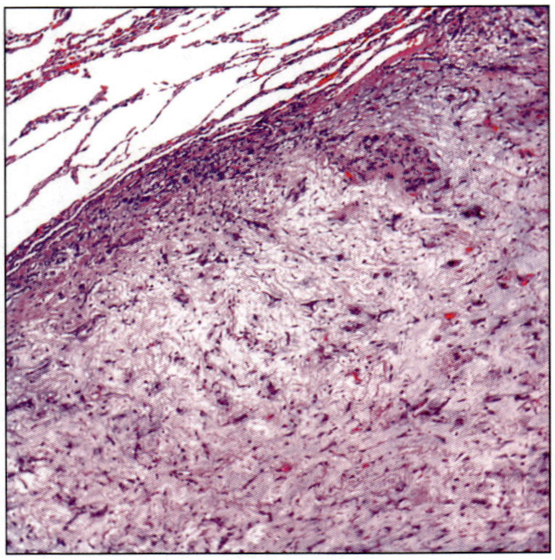

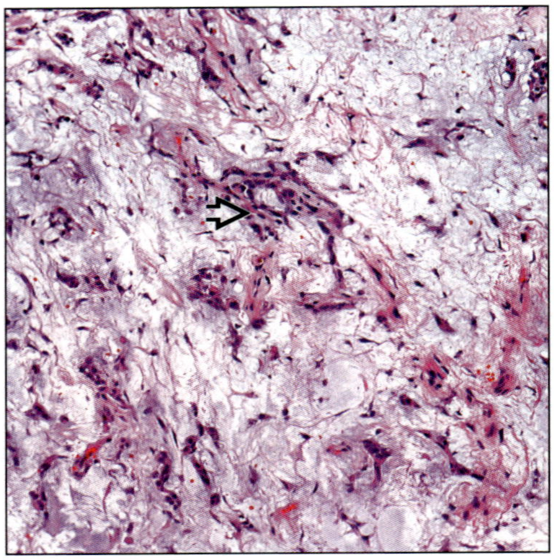

(Left) *Epithelial/myoepithelial proliferation admixed with hypocellular areas. This growth pattern may mimic a benign vascular tumor due to the compressed appearance of the epithelial component.* ***(Right)*** *Disorganized epithelial/myoepithelial cellular proliferation embedded in a myxoid matrix. In addition, there is a discrete vascular component.*

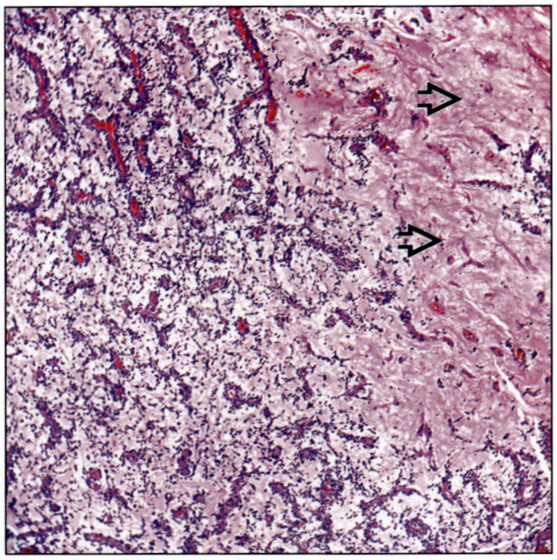

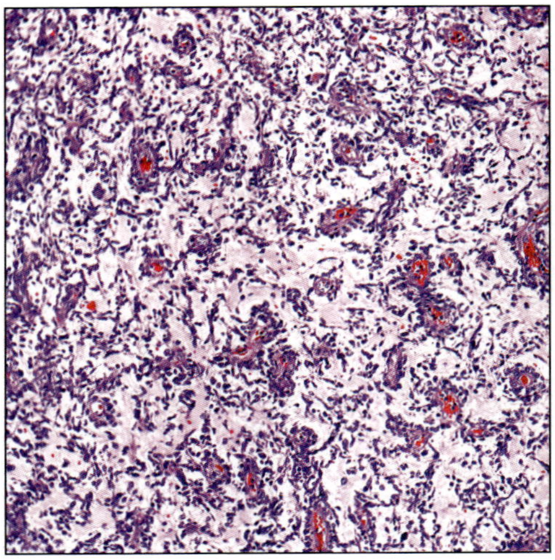

(Left) *Mixed tumor of the lung shows chondromyxoid background, epithelial proliferation, and squamous keratinization.* ***(Right)*** *Tubular structures are seen embedded in a fibrocollagenous background. The tubular structures show dual cell layer; similar features may be seen in epithelial/myoepithelial carcinoma.*

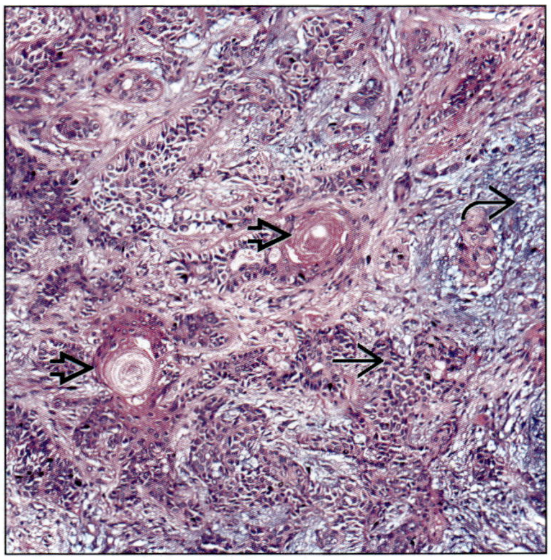

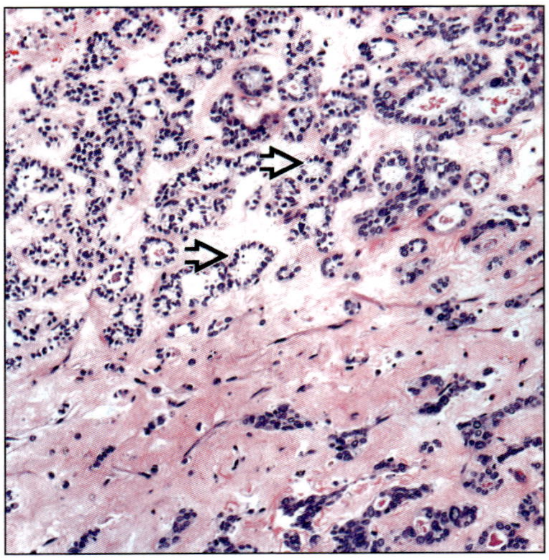

MIXED TUMOR

Microscopic Features

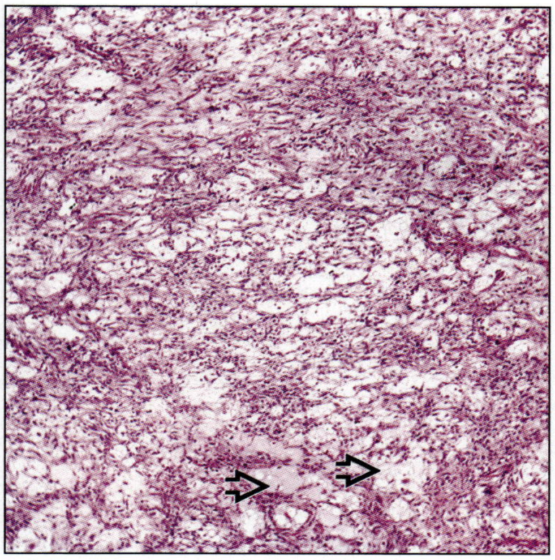
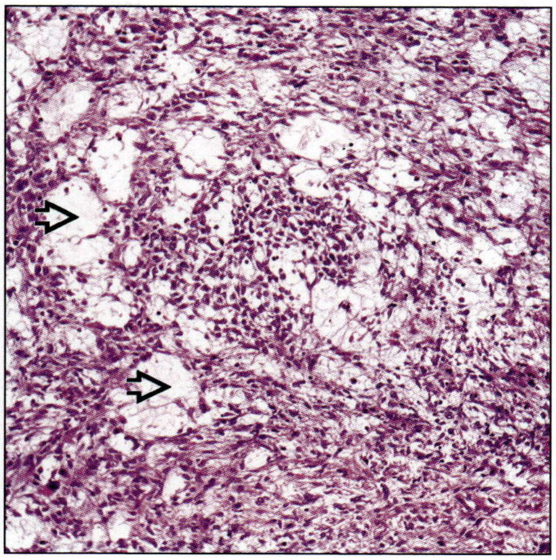

(Left) *Hypercellular myoepithelial areas with minimal myxoid component. The presence of solid areas in many cases raises the suspicion of malignant transformation.* ***(Right)*** *Closer view of myoepithelial cells and myxoid component. Note the absence of nuclear atypia, mitotic activity, necrosis &/or hemorrhage.*

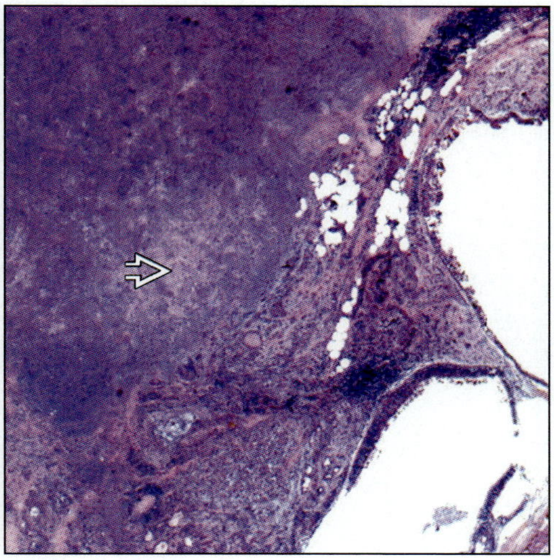
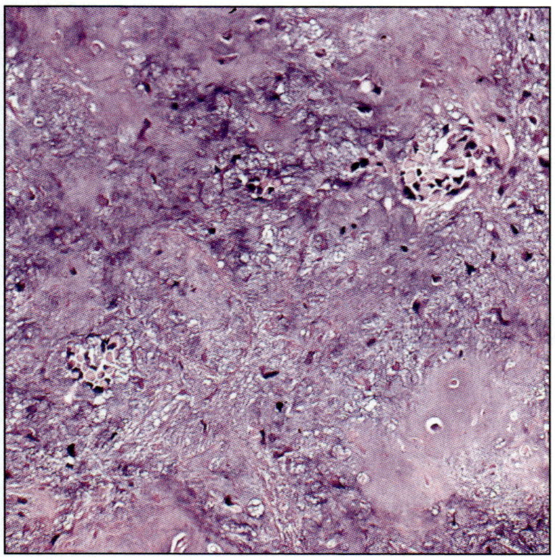

(Left) *Mixed tumor with prominent cartilaginous component and focal cystic changes. The presence of well-formed mature cartilage in mixed tumors of the lung is not common.* ***(Right)*** *Prominent chondromyxoid stroma with low cellular epithelial component. Note the absence of nuclear atypia in both components. Such features are in keeping with a mixed (pleomorphic) adenoma.*

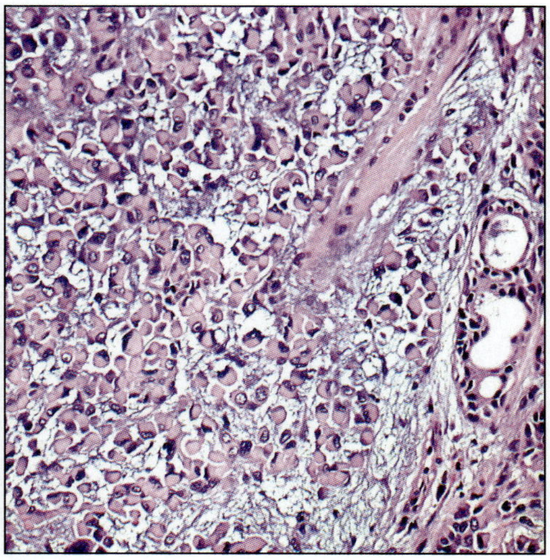
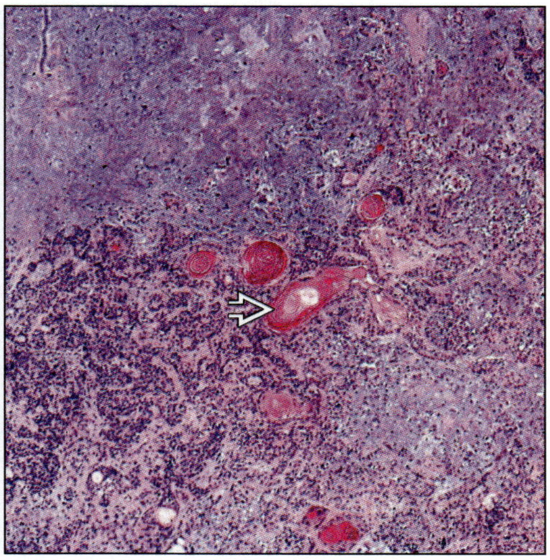

(Left) *Benign mixed tumor with prominent plasmacytoid cellular component and myxoid background. This is another unusual feature for this tumor in the lung, and it can be confused for another type of neoplasm.* ***(Right)*** *Benign mixed tumor with epithelial and chondromyxoid component and areas of squamous metaplasia. Although these features are commonly seen in salivary gland tumors, they are not common in the lung.*

MIXED TUMOR

Microscopic Features

*(**Left**) Benign mixed tumor is shown with a mixture of different epithelial and mesenchymal elements. In this low-power view, the tumor can be easily interpreted as a hamartoma of the lung. (**Right**) Benign mixed tumor with epithelial component ⇨ resembles adnexal structures. Areas of hyalinized tissue are also present → admixed with some inflammatory reaction.*

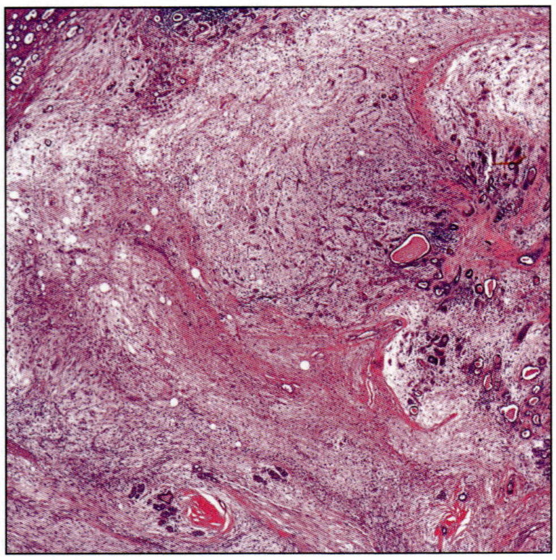

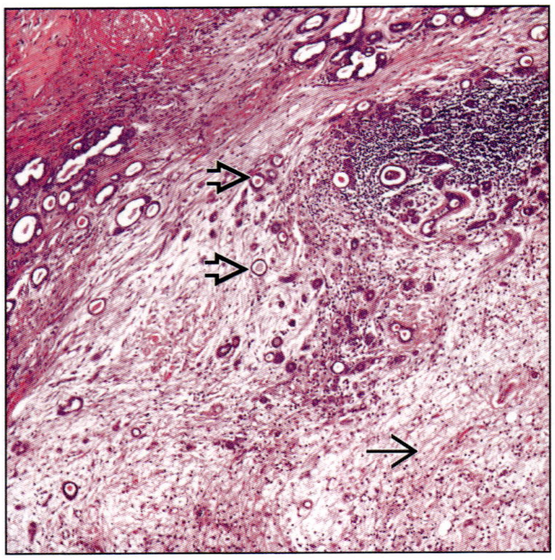

*(**Left**) Benign mixed tumor with a combination of myxoid, epithelial, and focal cartilaginous → elements is shown. These features should raise the suspicion of a primary mixed tumor of the lung. (**Right**) Benign mixed tumor shows a more epithelial component toward the periphery of the tumor, while toward the center of the lesion, the tumor appears to be less cellular and more myxoid.*

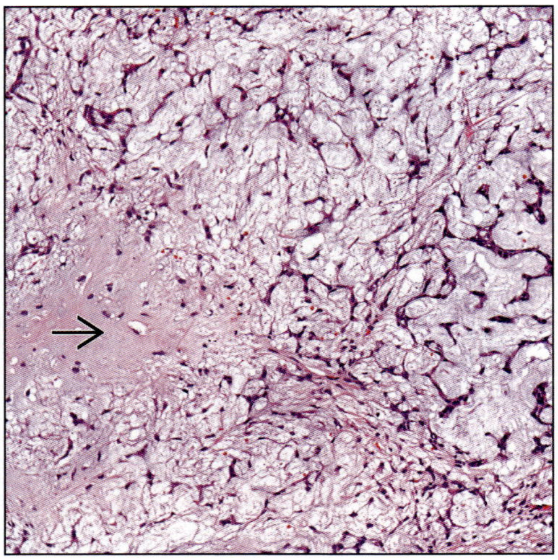

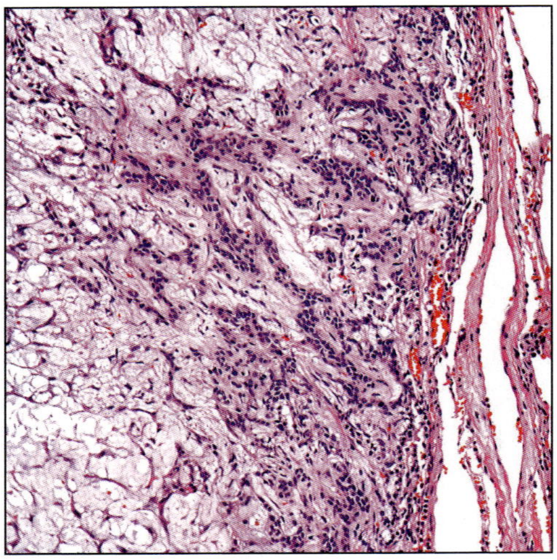

*(**Left**) Focal cystic areas are shown admixed with epithelial and myxoid elements in a benign mixed tumor. Such invaginations of epithelium are commonly seen in pulmonary hamartomas. However, in this case the cellular proliferation would be unusual for that lesion. (**Right**) Benign mixed tumor with more characteristic epithelial component admixed with myxoid background. The epithelial component ⇨ is represented by the classic myoepithelial proliferation.*

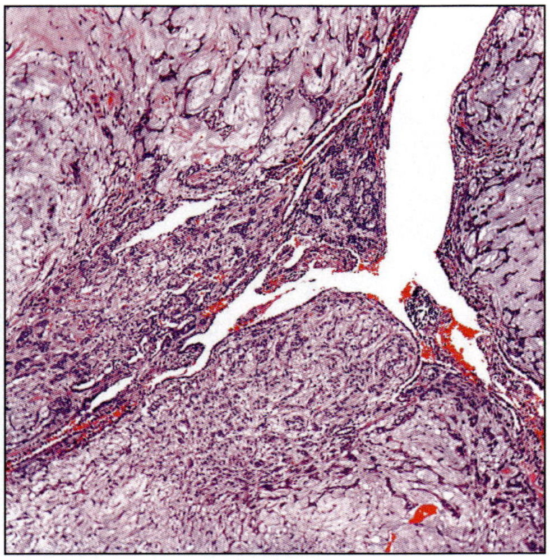

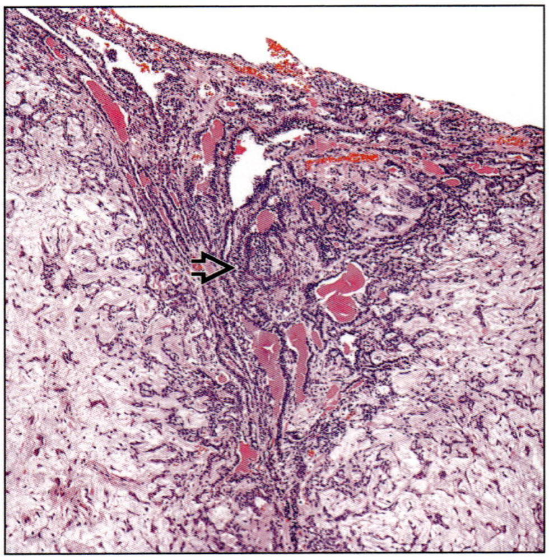

MIXED TUMOR

Microscopic Features

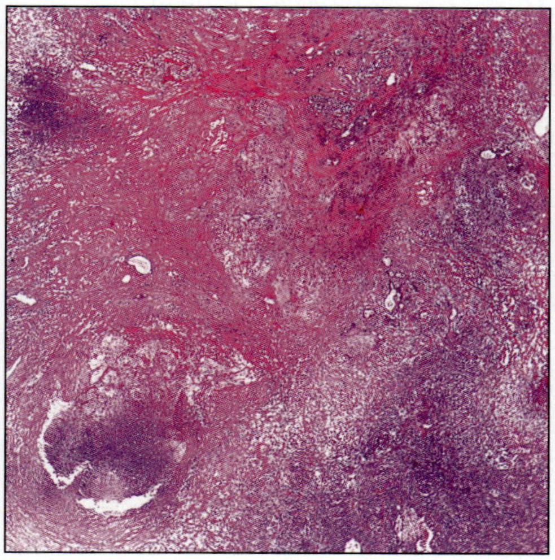

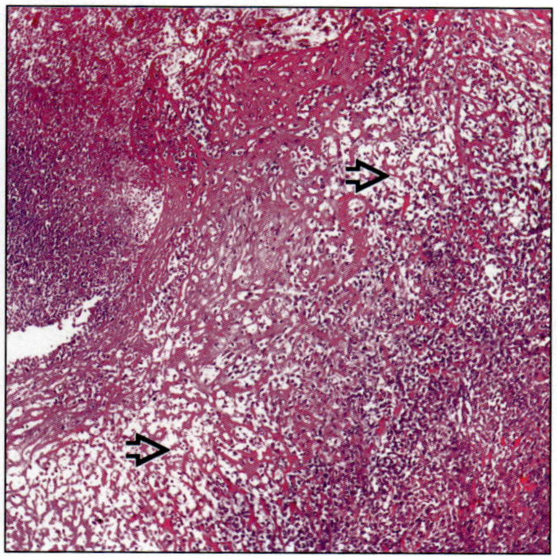

(Left) *Hypercellular areas are admixed with necrosis in malignant mixed tumor. The presence of necrosis should raise the suspicion of a malignant change, and careful review of the histology should be performed.* ***(Right)*** *Areas of necrosis and fibrinoid changes are admixed with clear myoepithelial cells ➾ in a malignant mixed tumor. Note the disorganized growth of the tumor in comparison to the benign counterpart.*

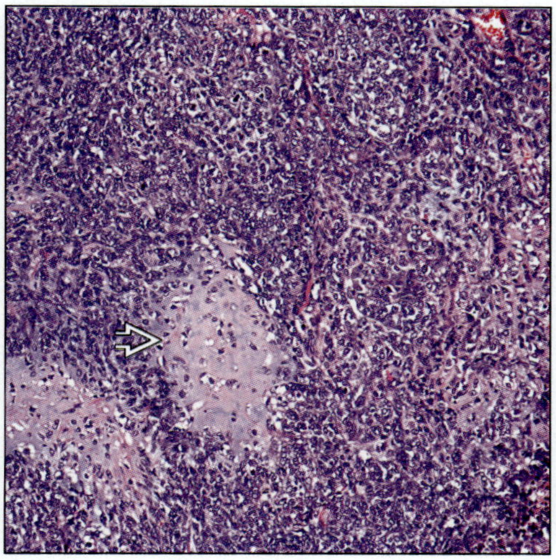

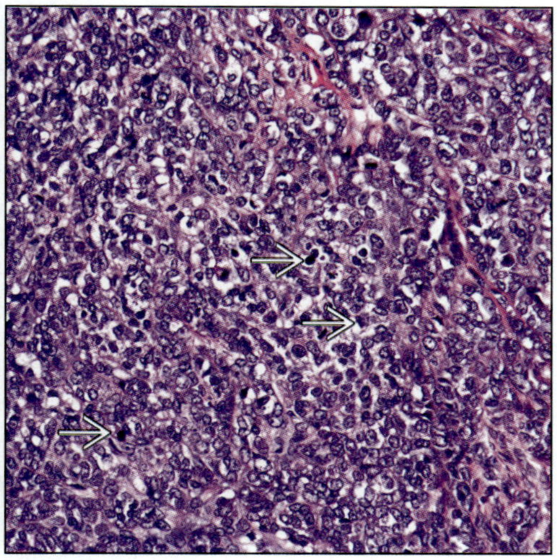

(Left) *Malignant mixed tumor is shown with a focal residual cartilaginous component ➾. The presence of cartilage and an undifferentiated epithelial malignant tumor raise the possibility of carcinosarcoma; however, the cartilage does not show malignant features.* ***(Right)*** *Malignant mixed tumor with hypercellular areas is shown. Note the presence of nuclear atypia and mitotic figures ➔. This feature by itself is not diagnostic of malignant mixed tumor.*

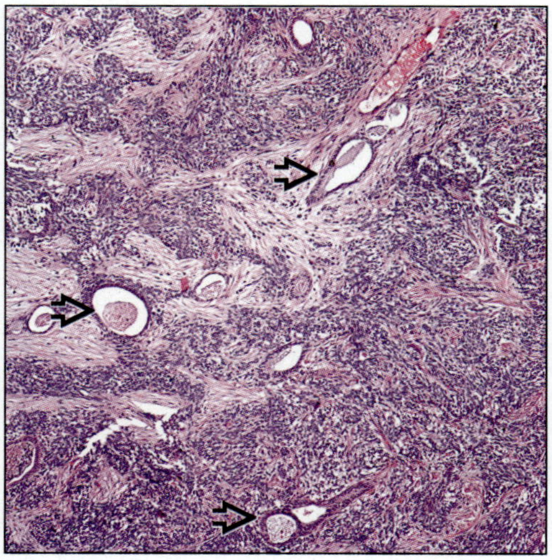

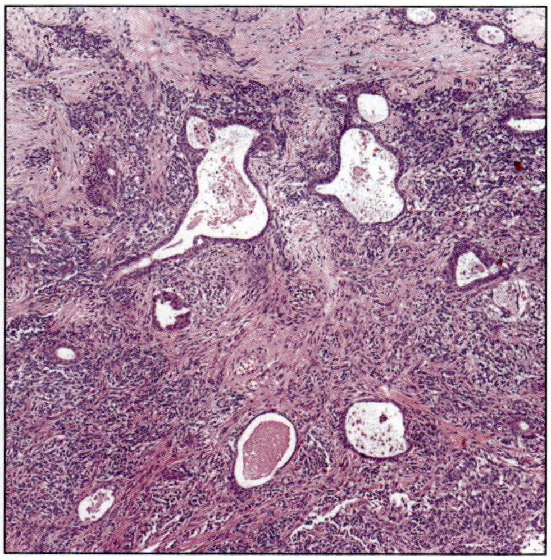

(Left) *Malignant mixed tumor with areas resembling the benign counterpart, namely the presence of cystic epithelial elements ➾. The presence of areas of benign mixed tumor is important in the diagnosis of malignant mixed tumors.* ***(Right)*** *Malignant mixed tumor with cystic epithelial elements resembling benign mixed tumor. Note the adjacent atypical cellular proliferation in keeping with a malignant component.*

INTRAPULMONARY SYNOVIAL SARCOMA

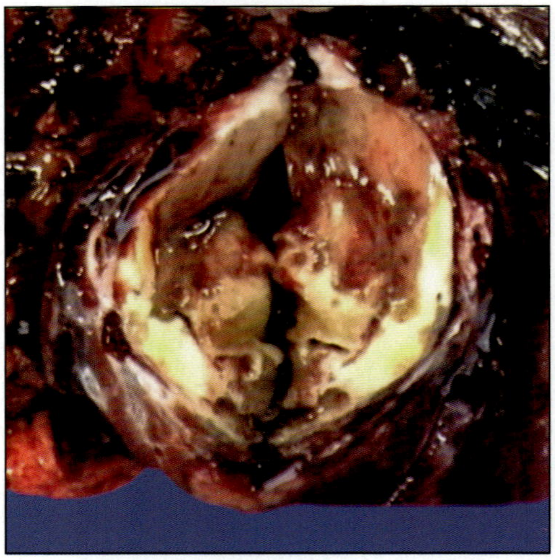

Gross appearance of primary synovial sarcoma of the lung shows well-circumscribed, intraparenchymatous tumor mass with areas of necrosis and glistening homogeneous gray-white cut surface.

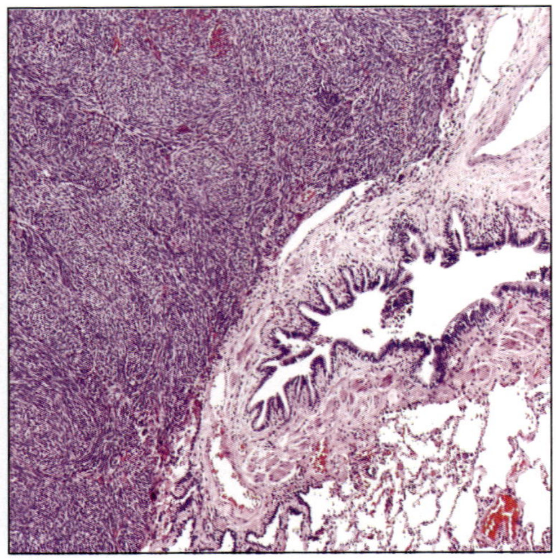

Histologic appearance of synovial sarcoma of the lung on scanning magnification shows a solid tumor composed of sheets of spindle cells that is sharply circumscribed from the surrounding lung parenchyma.

TERMINOLOGY

Definitions

- Primary pulmonary malignant neoplasm characterized by a spindle cell morphology and displaying features of epithelial differentiation

CLINICAL ISSUES

Epidemiology

- Incidence
  - Rare (< 1% of all lung neoplasms)
- Age
  - Children to adults (mean age = 38 years)
- Gender
  - Slight predilection for women

Presentation

- Chest pain
- Shortness of breath
- Cough
- Hemoptysis
- May be asymptomatic and represent an incidental finding on chest x-ray

Treatment

- Surgical approaches
  - Complete surgical excision is treatment of choice
- Adjuvant therapy
  - Combination chemotherapy is indicated in advanced cases

Prognosis

- Similar behavior as synovial sarcoma in peripheral soft tissue locations
- Aggressive behavior with frequent recurrences and metastases
- Metastases are to bone, central nervous system, liver, and skin
- > 50% of patients die of tumor within 5-7 years after diagnosis

MACROSCOPIC FEATURES

General Features

- Well-circumscribed, unencapsulated, solitary mass within lung parenchyma
- Tan-white to gray, rubbery to gelatinous cut surface
- Hemorrhage and necrosis
- May show prominent cystic changes
- Most often found in the periphery of the lung
- Some tumors may be present endobronchially in central locations

Sections to Be Submitted

- At least 1 section per centimeter of greatest tumor diameter

Size

- 1-20 cm (median size = 4 cm)

MICROSCOPIC PATHOLOGY

Histologic Features

- Majority of tumors in the lung are of the monophasic spindle cell type
- Fascicles of monotonous atypical spindle cells with variety of growth patterns
  - Herringbone pattern
  - Hemangiopericytic growth pattern
  - Storiform growth pattern
  - Neural-like palisading growth pattern
- Some tumors may show prominent myxoid stromal changes
- Areas of hemorrhage and necrosis
- Foci of stromal hyalinization with bony metaplasia
- Areas of vascular invasion

Key Facts

Clinical Issues
- Chest pain
- Shortness of breath
- Cough
- Aggressive behavior with frequent recurrences and metastases

Macroscopic Features
- Well-circumscribed, unencapsulated, solitary mass within lung parenchyma
- Tan-white to gray, rubbery to gelatinous cut surface

Microscopic Pathology
- Fascicles of monotonous atypical spindle cells with variety of growth patterns
  - Herringbone pattern
  - Hemangiopericytic growth pattern
  - Storiform growth pattern
  - Neural-like palisading growth pattern
- Tumor cells may display epithelioid morphology, with round nuclei surrounded by scant eosinophilic cytoplasm

Ancillary Tests
- Tumor cells show focal (spotty) cytoplasmic positivity for cytokeratins (AE1/AE3, CAM5.2, CK8/18, CK19)
- Tumor cells show focal (spotty) positivity for EMA
- Tumor cells consistently show diffuse and strong positivity for Bcl-2 oncogene
- Majority of cases (> 80%) show characteristic t(X;18) translocation
- Fusion products include *SYT/SSX1*, *SYT/SSX2*, and *SYT/SSX4*

Cytologic Features
- Monotonous population of atypical spindle cells with dense chromatin pattern and scant cytoplasm
- Striking absence of intervening stroma supporting the tumor cells
- Tumor cells may display epithelioid morphology, with round nuclei surrounded by scant eosinophilic cytoplasm
- Variable mitotic activity (range = 2-20 mitoses per 10 high power fields)

ANCILLARY TESTS

Immunohistochemistry
- Tumor cells show
  - Focal (spotty) cytoplasmic positivity for cytokeratins (AE1/AE3, CAM5.2, CK8/18, CK19)
  - Focal (spotty) positivity for EMA
  - Diffuse and strong positivity for Bcl-2
  - Positivity for CD99
  - May be positive for S100 protein, calponin, calretinin, HBME-1, and CD117

Cytogenetics
- Majority of cases (> 80%) show characteristic (X;18)(p11;q11) translocation

Molecular Genetics
- FISH and RT-PCR are useful for detecting the fusion protein of the translocation in formalin-fixed paraffin-embedded tissues
- Fusion products include *SYT/SSX1*, *SYT/SSX2*, and *SYT/SSX4*

DIFFERENTIAL DIAGNOSIS

Intrapulmonary Solitary Fibrous Tumor (SFT)
- Areas of stromal sclerosis and dense, linear, rope-like collagen deposition is a common feature in SFT
- Tumors cells in SFT are generally positive for CD34 and negative for cytokeratins and EMA
- Not associated with any cytogenetic abnormality (i.e., they are negative for the X;18 translocation)

Malignant Peripheral Nerve Sheath Tumor (MPNST)
- Pattern of expression of S100 protein may overlap with synovial sarcoma
- May also show focal expression of cytokeratins, EMA, and Bcl-2
- Generally negative for t(X;18)
- Distinctive, long, interdigitating cytoplasmic processes by electron microscopy

Metastasis of Synovial Sarcoma from Peripheral Soft Tissues
- Lung is 2nd most common site of metastasis from synovial sarcoma of soft tissue
- Existence of a primary source outside the lungs needs to always be ruled out clinically

DIAGNOSTIC CHECKLIST

Pathologic Interpretation Pearls
- Tumor is characterized by striking uniformity of the spindle cells
- Nuclear pleomorphism, bizarre nuclear forms, and abnormal mitoses are usually lacking

SELECTED REFERENCES

1. Hartel PH et al: Primary pulmonary and mediastinal synovial sarcoma: a clinicopathologic study of 60 cases and comparison with five prior series. Mod Pathol. 20(7):760-9, 2007
2. Suster S et al: Expression of bcl-2 oncoprotein in benign and malignant spindle cell tumors of soft tissue, skin, serosal surfaces, and gastrointestinal tract. Am J Surg Pathol. 22(7):863-72, 1998
3. Zeren H et al: Primary pulmonary sarcomas with features of monophasic synovial sarcoma: a clinicopathological, immunohistochemical, and ultrastructural study of 25 cases. Hum Pathol. 26(5):474-80, 1995

INTRAPULMONARY SYNOVIAL SARCOMA

Common Histologic Features

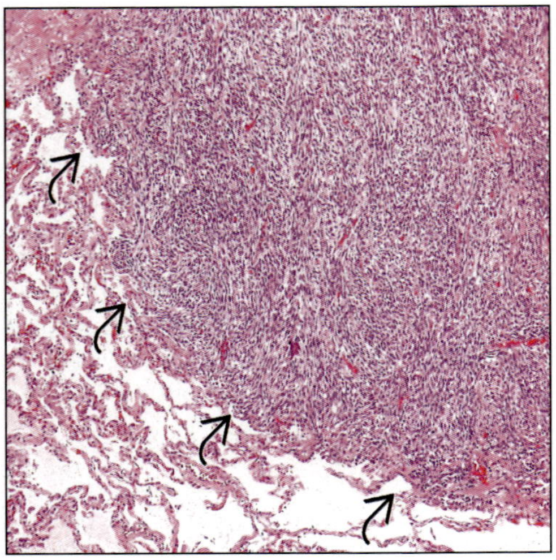

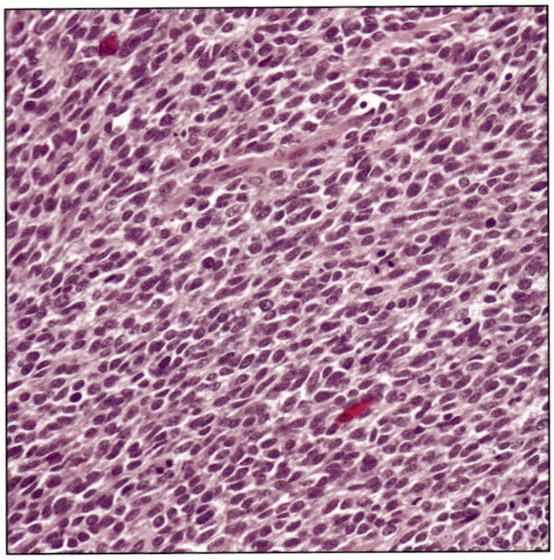

(Left) *Scanning magnification of a pulmonary synovial sarcoma shows a well-circumscribed tumor nodule composed of a uniform population of atypical spindle cells. Notice the absence of a capsule and sharp circumscription from the surrounding pulmonary parenchyma →.* ***(Right)*** *Scanning magnification of intrapulmonary synovial sarcoma shows monotonous sheets of uniform, atypical spindle cells with very little intervening stroma. Hardly any vessels can be discerned in this field.*

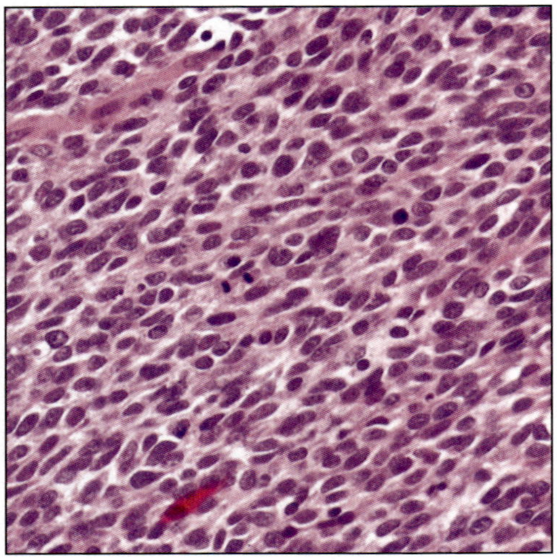

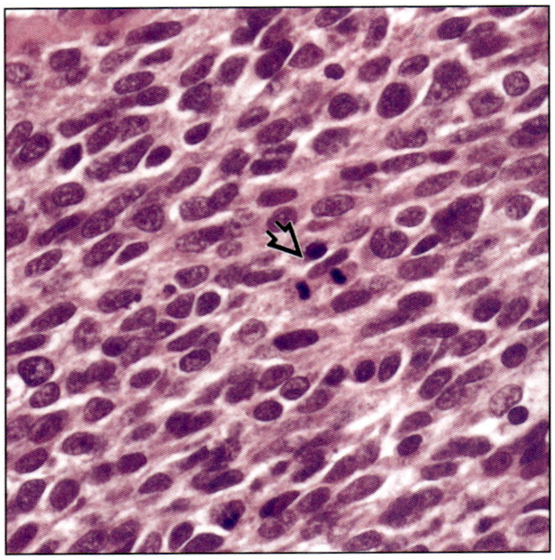

(Left) *Intrapulmonary synovial sarcoma shows sheets of monotonous tumor cells with oval nuclei and a dense chromatin pattern; there are also a few scattered mitotic figures. Mitotic activity can vary from very minimal (1-2 mitoses per 10 high power fields) to high (> 10 mitoses per 10 high power fields) in these tumors.* ***(Right)*** *Higher magnification of intrapulmonary synovial sarcoma shows a population of atypical spindle cells with hyperchromatic nuclei. Notice a mitotic figure in the center →.*

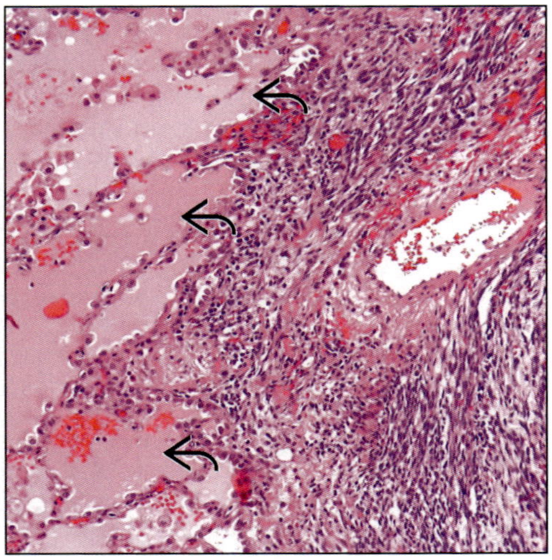

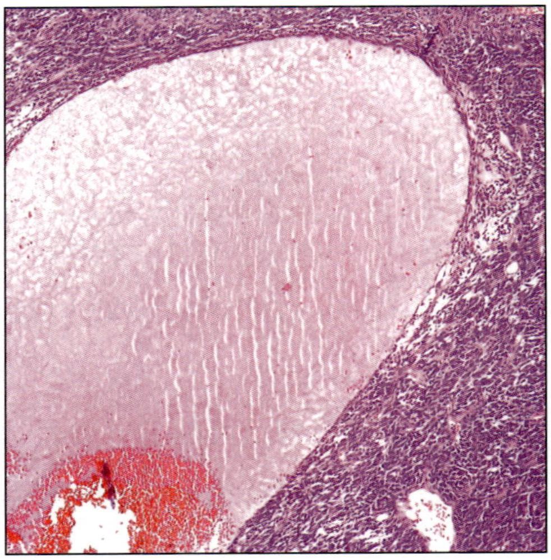

(Left) *Interphase between intrapulmonary synovial sarcoma (right) and adjacent lung parenchyma with pulmonary edema → is shown. The neoplastic spindle cell population appears to end abruptly and does not infiltrate along the alveolar septa.* ***(Right)*** *Scanning magnification of an intrapulmonary synovial sarcoma shows prominent cystic changes involving the tumor. The cysts can coalesce and lead to extensive cystic degeneration that can be appreciated grossly as well as on imaging studies.*

Histologic Features

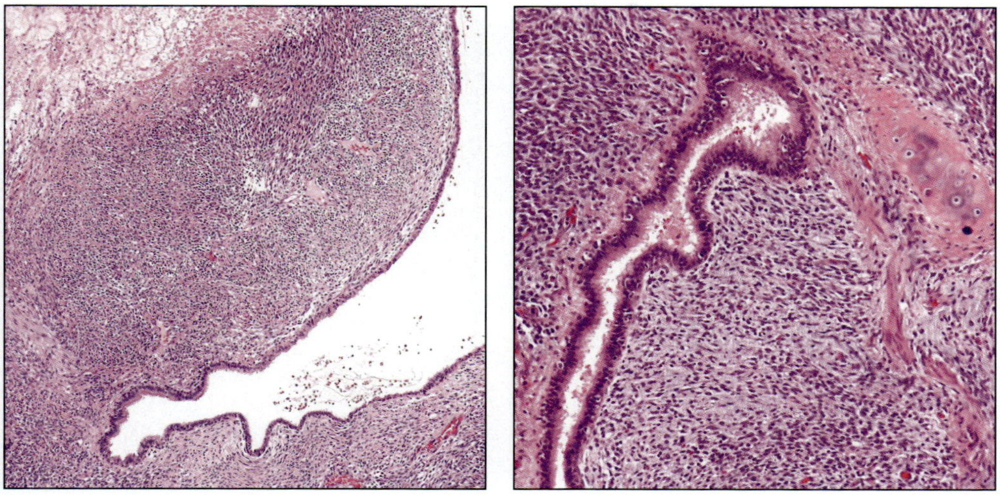

(Left) *Scanning magnification of intrapulmonary synovial sarcoma shows endobronchial growth with polypoid protrusion into the bronchial lumen. Such tumors can ulcerate and bleed, causing hemoptysis.* ***(Right)*** *Pulmonary synovial sarcoma shows entrapment and destruction of the wall of a bronchus. Areas displaying these features can be misinterpreted for a biphasic malignant neoplasm, such as carcinosarcoma. The entrapped glandular elements, however, are normal.*

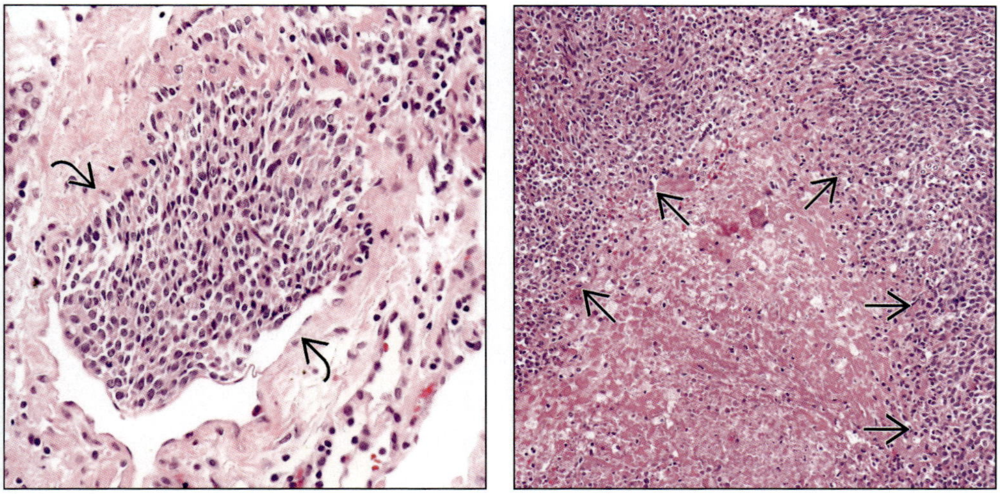

(Left) *Intrapulmonary synovial sarcoma shows a focus of vascular invasion in the lung parenchyma. Notice the tumor thrombus attached to the wall and protruding into and distorting the vessel lumen ⮫.* ***(Right)*** *Area of coagulative necrosis in pulmonary synovial sarcoma shows extensive necrotic debris (center) flanked by a residual viable tumor cell population ➔. Intrapulmonary synovial sarcoma can often be accompanied by extensive intratumoral cell necrosis.*

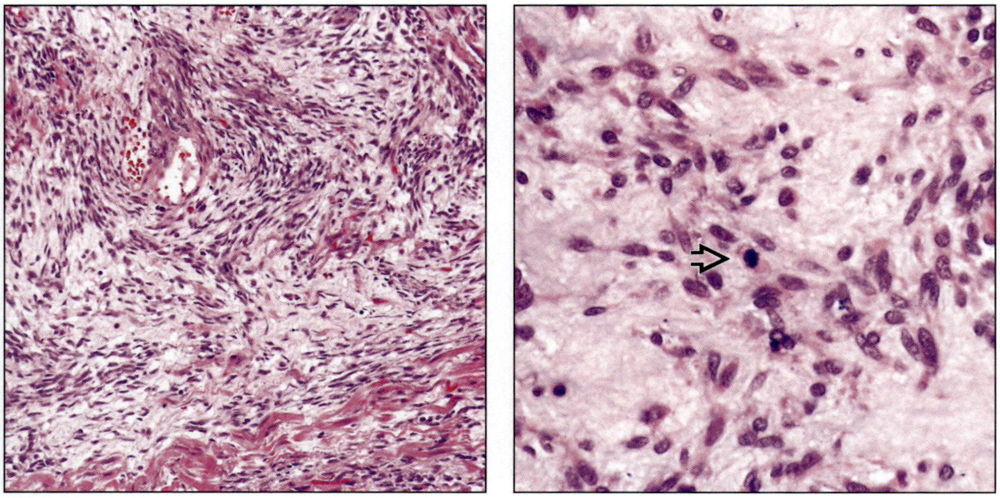

(Left) *Prominent myxoid stromal changes are seen in this intrapulmonary synovial sarcoma. Tumors with these features can be mistaken for nerve sheath neoplasms, metastases of myxofibrosarcoma, and other myxoid tumors.* ***(Right)*** *Higher magnification of pulmonary synovial sarcoma with myxoid changes shows spindle cell population embedded in abundant myxoid matrix. The spindle cells are monotonous and display similar features to other synovial sarcomas, including mitoses ⇨.*

INTRAPULMONARY SYNOVIAL SARCOMA

Histologic Growth Patterns

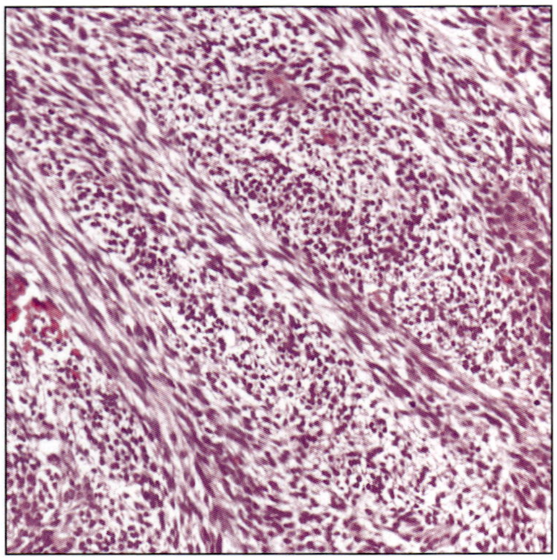

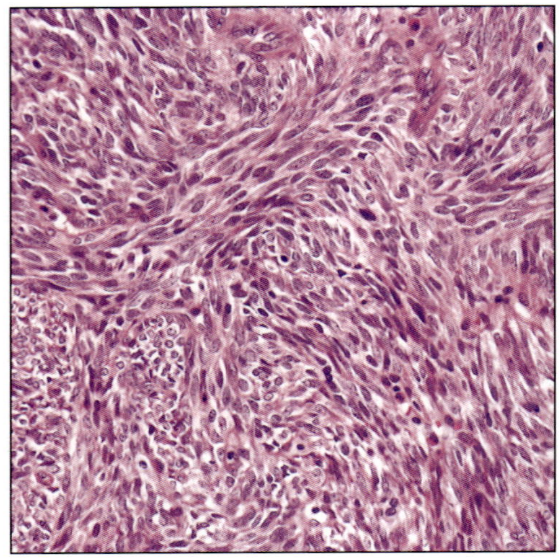

(Left) *Scanning magnification of pulmonary synovial sarcoma shows a "herringbone" growth pattern with fascicles of tumor cells intersecting at acute angles. This appearance can be indistinguishable from a malignant peripheral nerve sheath tumor.* ***(Right)*** *Intrapulmonary synovial sarcoma shows a storiform pattern of growth. Tumors displaying these features are commonly mistaken for "fibrohistiocytic" neoplasms such as malignant fibrous histiocytoma.*

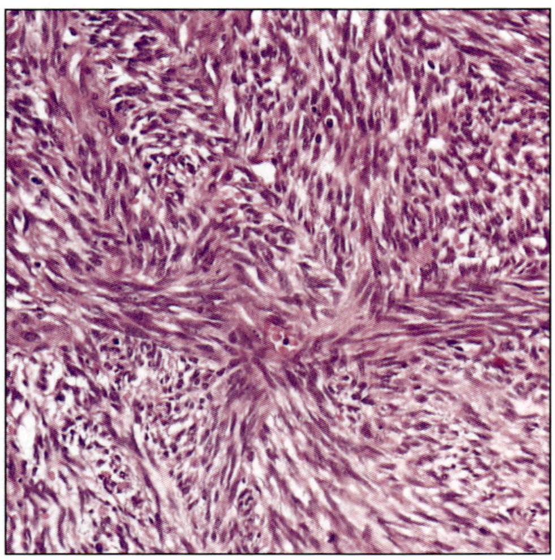

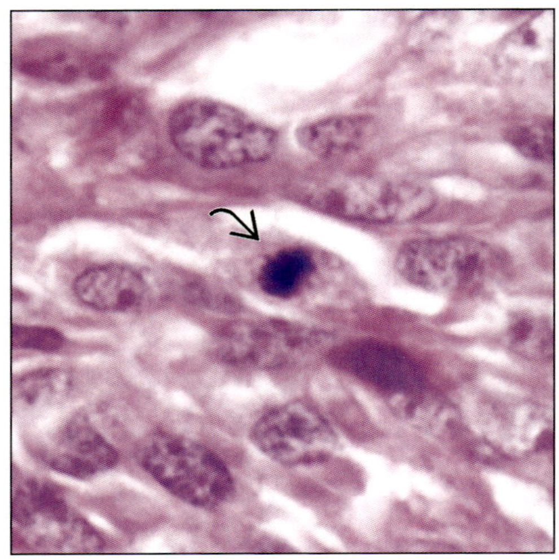

(Left) *Monophasic synovial sarcoma of the lung shows a striking storiform growth pattern reminiscent of malignant fibrous histiocytoma, dermatofibrosarcoma protuberans, and other "fibrohistiocytic" tumors.* ***(Right)*** *Higher magnification of pulmonary synovial sarcoma with storiform pattern shows cells with uniform spindle-shaped nuclei with scant cytoplasm. The nuclei of the cells show vesicular chromatin with occasional small nucleoli. Notice the mitotic figure in the center ➔.*

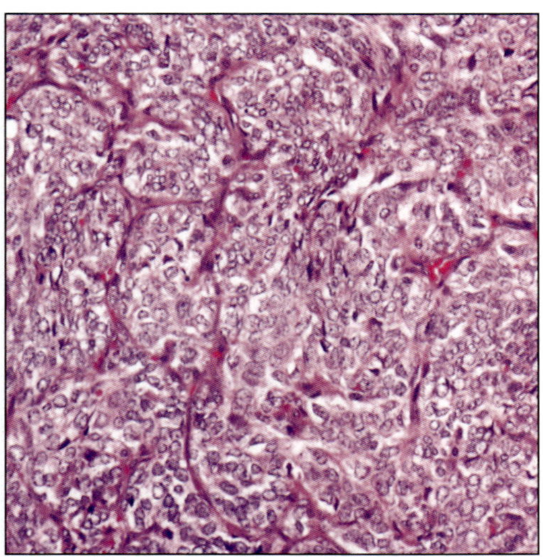

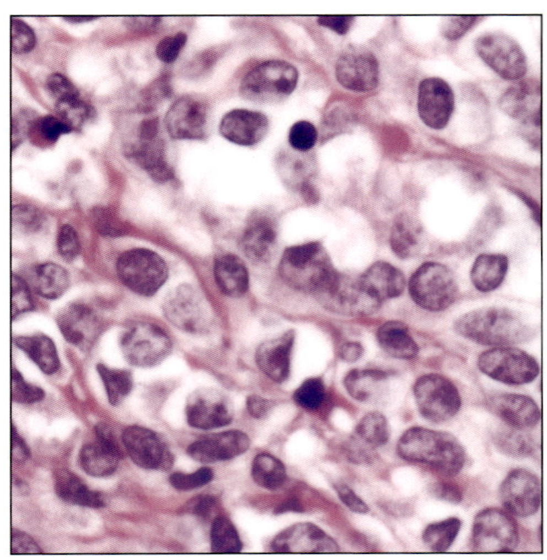

(Left) *Pulmonary synovial sarcoma shows a nested pattern of growth characterized by discrete round islands of tumor cells separated by thin fibrovascular septa. Tumors with these features can be easily mistaken for metastases of amelanotic malignant melanoma to the lung.* ***(Right)*** *Higher magnification of pulmonary synovial sarcoma shows uniform round nuclei with a scant rim of lightly eosinophilic to amphophilic cytoplasm. Tumors with these features are classed as "poorly differentiated."*

Growth Patterns and Immunohistochemistry

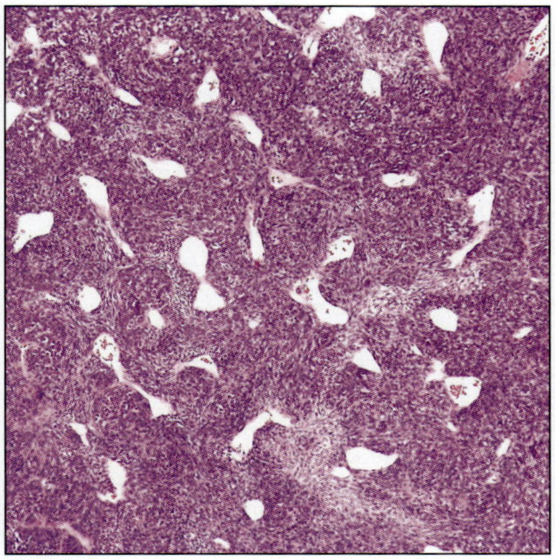

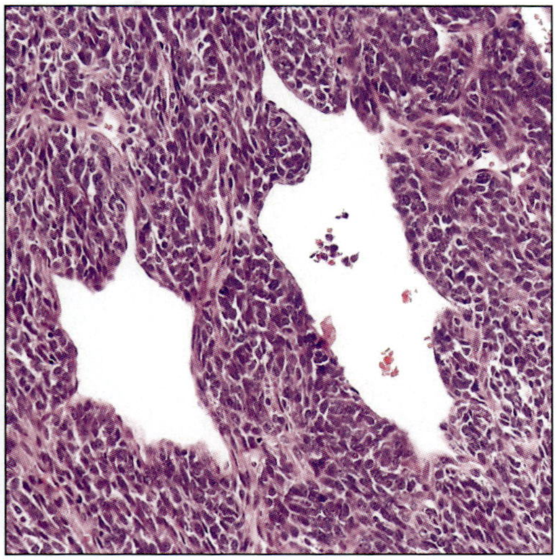

(Left) *Scanning magnification of intrapulmonary synovial sarcoma shows a striking hemangiopericytomatous growth pattern characterized by multiple small branching vessels with open lumens.* ***(Right)*** *Higher magnification of intrapulmonary synovial sarcoma with a hemangiopericytic growth pattern shows 2 small vessels with irregular contours and open lumens. Tumors with these features have been misdiagnosed in the past as pulmonary hemangiopericytoma.*

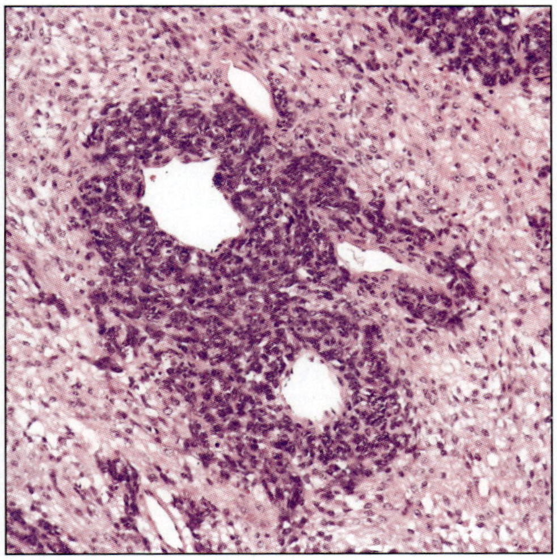

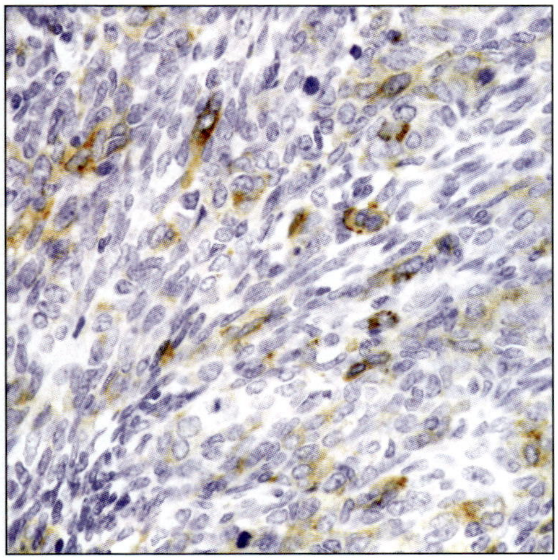

(Left) *Pulmonary synovial sarcoma shows perivascular cuffing of small vessels by tumor cells surrounded by abundant tumor cell necrosis.* ***(Right)*** *Characteristic pattern of staining in synovial sarcoma for cytokeratin broad-spectrum stain (cytokeratin AE1/AE3) shows spotty staining of isolated, scattered tumor cells with this antibody. Some cases may show complete absence of cytokeratin staining, and multiple tissue blocks may need to be evaluated to identify focal positivity.*

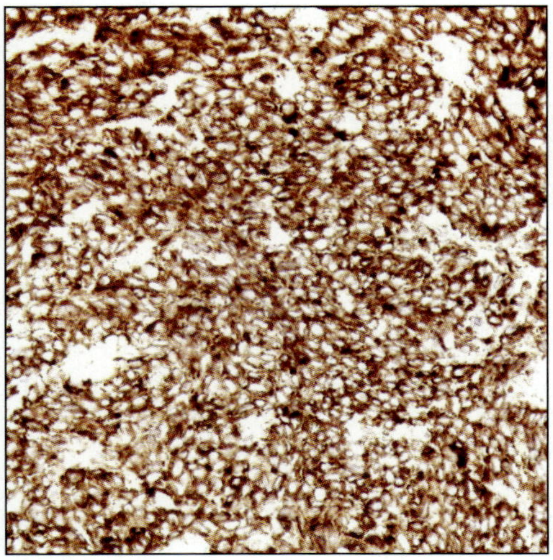

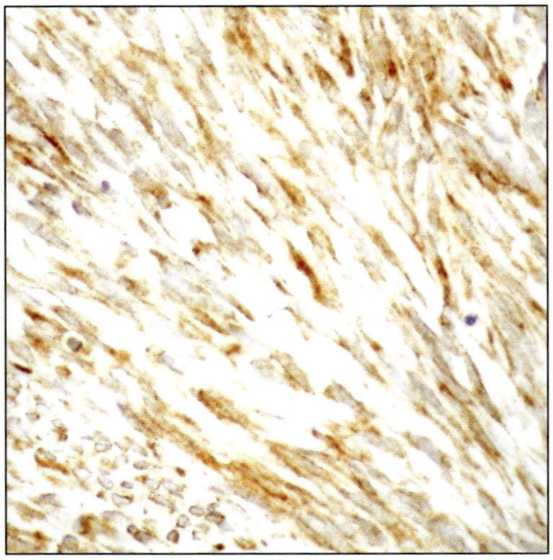

(Left) *Immunohistochemical staining of pulmonary synovial sarcoma for Bcl-2 oncogene shows a strong pattern of positivity. Virtually all the tumor cells show strong cytoplasmic positivity, a highly characteristic finding in synovial sarcoma.* ***(Right)*** *Immunohistochemical staining in pulmonary synovial sarcoma for epithelial membrane antigen (EMA) shows scattered positive cells. Positivity for this antigen can be just as spotty and weak as for cytokeratin.*

LEIOMYOSARCOMA

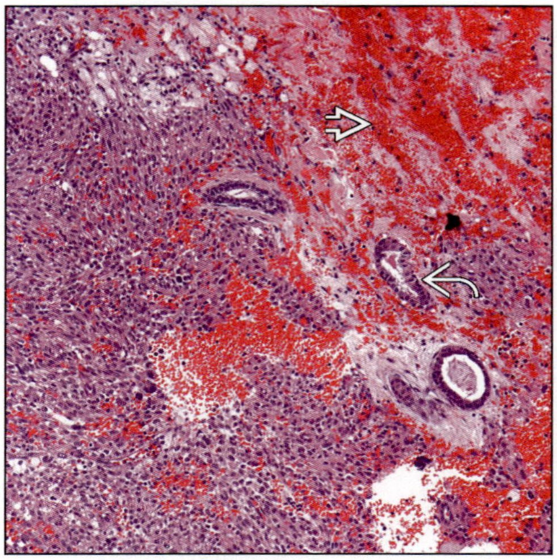

Pulmonary leiomyosarcoma shows a spindle cell proliferation composed with cells with eosinophilic cytoplasm. Areas of hemorrhage ➡ and entrapped epithelial structures ➡ are present.

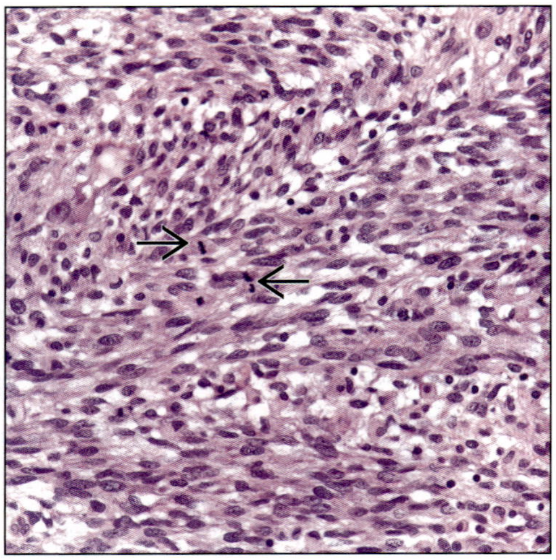

Higher magnification of a LMS shows a distinct fascicular growth pattern with moderate nuclear atypia and numerous mitotic figures ➡.

TERMINOLOGY

Abbreviations

- Pulmonary leiomyosarcoma (LMS)

Definitions

- Malignant mesenchymal neoplasm of smooth muscle origin

CLINICAL ISSUES

Epidemiology

- Incidence
  - Represents < 1% of all malignant neoplasms of lung
- Age
  - Has been described in any age group from newborns to adult patients
- Gender
  - No predilection for any gender

Presentation

- Cough
- Hemoptysis
- Chest pain
- Shortness of breath
- Weight loss
- Asymptomatic

Treatment

- Surgical approaches
  - Lobectomy or pneumonectomy
- Adjuvant therapy
  - Chemo-radiation may be used in some cases

Prognosis

- Depends on tumor differentiation and clinical staging
- Widespread metastatic disease can occur
- Some patients may follow aggressive course with death in < 24 months

MACROSCOPIC FEATURES

General Features

- Well-circumscribed tumors
- Endobronchial or peripheral
- Cut surface is white and firm
- Areas of hemorrhage and necrosis may be present

Size

- Tumor varies in size from 1 cm to > 10 cm in diameter

MICROSCOPIC PATHOLOGY

Histologic Features

- Spindle cell proliferation of elongated cells with cigar-shaped nuclei

Predominant Pattern/Injury Type

- Sarcomatoid

Predominant Cell/Compartment Type

- Myoid

DIFFERENTIAL DIAGNOSIS

Hemangiopericytoma

- Does not usually display marked cellular pleomorphism
- Shows negative staining for muscle markers

Monophasic Synovial Sarcoma

- Usually shows more cohesive spindle cell proliferation
- Generally shows negative results with muscle markers
- Usually shows positive staining for keratin, EMA/MUC1, and Bcl-2

Solitary Fibrous Tumor

- Usually shows positive staining for CD34 and Bcl-2
- Displays negative staining for muscle markers

LEIOMYOSARCOMA

Key Facts

Clinical Issues

- Incidence
  - Represents < 1% of all malignant neoplasms of lung
  - Described in any age group from newborns to adults
- Symptoms
  - Cough
  - Hemoptysis
  - Chest pain
  - Dyspnea
  - Weight loss
  - Asymptomatic

Macroscopic Features

- Endobronchial or peripheral
- Areas of hemorrhage and necrosis may be present
- Tumors vary in size from 1 to > 10 cm in diameter

Top Differential Diagnoses

- Hemangiopericytoma
  - Usually does not display marked cellular pleomorphisms
  - Shows negative staining for muscle markers
- Monophasic synovial sarcoma
  - Usually shows a more cohesive spindle cell proliferation
  - Generally shows negative results with muscle markers
  - Usually shows positive staining for keratin, EMA/MUC1, and Bcl-2
- Solitary fibrous tumor
  - Usually shows positive staining for CD34 and Bcl-2
  - Displays negative staining for muscle markers

Immunohistochemistry

Antibody	Reactivity	Staining Pattern	Comment
Actin-HHF-35	Positive	Cytoplasmic	
Desmin	Positive	Cytoplasmic	May be negative in high-grade tumors
Caldesmon	Positive	Cytoplasmic	May be negative in high-grade tumors
Actin-sm	Positive	Cytoplasmic	
CK-PAN	Negative		May be focally positive in low-grade tumors
EMA	Negative		
CD34	Negative		
Bcl-2	Negative		
S100	Negative		

- Usually displays different growth pattern in same tumor

DIAGNOSTIC CHECKLIST

Clinically Relevant Pathologic Features

- Mitotic rate

Pathologic Interpretation Pearls

- Spindle cell proliferation with variable mitotic activity and presence or absence of necrosis &/or hemorrhage

GRADING

Low Grade

- Mild cytologic atypia
- Miotic figures: 1-3 per 10 HPF
- Necrosis and hemorrhage are absent
- Spindle fascicular growth pattern

Intermediate Grade

- Fascicular growth pattern
- Cytologic atypia is present but not marked
- Hypercellular areas
- Mitotic figures: 3-8 per 10 HPF
- Necrosis and hemorrhage are absent

High Grade

- Fascicular and solid growth patterns
  - Hemangiopericytic or storiform growth pattern may be present
- Necrosis &/or hemorrhage are present
- Cellular pleomorphism is obvious
- Mitotic figures: > 8 per 10 HPF
- Atypical mitotic figures may be seen

SELECTED REFERENCES

1. Moran CA et al: Primary leiomyosarcomas of the lung: a clinicopathologic and immunohistochemical study of 18 cases. Mod Pathol. 10(2):121-8, 1997
2. Jimenez JF et al: Primary bronchopulmonary leiomyosarcoma in childhood. Arch Pathol Lab Med. 110(4):348-51, 1986
3. Guccion JG et al: Bronchopulmonary leiomyosarcoma and fibrosarcoma. A study of 32 cases and review of the literature. Cancer. 30(3):836-47, 1972

LEIOMYOSARCOMA

Gross and Microscopic Features

(Left) Pulmonary leiomyosarcoma shows a large intraparenchymal tumor. The tumor is hemorrhagic, and although close to the main airway, it does not appear to obstruct it. *(Right)* Pulmonary leiomyosarcoma with its classical growth pattern composed of fascicles of cells with elongated nuclei. At this power, one cannot identify the presence of mitotic activity or necrosis.

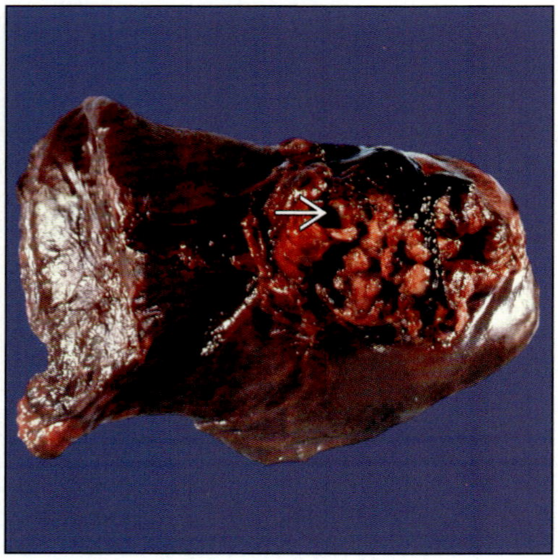

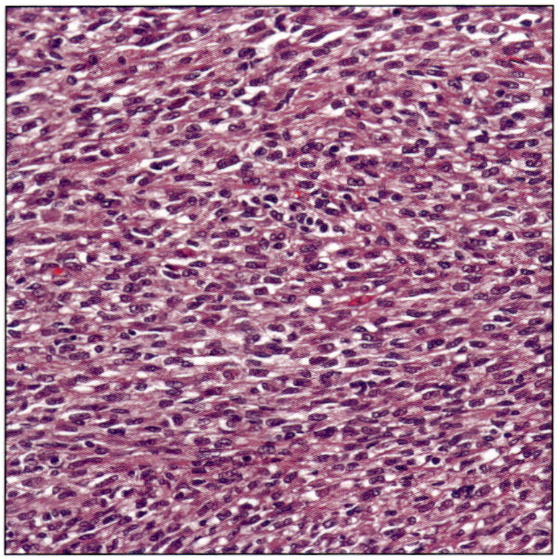

(Left) Leiomyosarcoma with extensive areas of necrosis. The finding of necrosis and mitotic activity are features of high-grade sarcoma. *(Right)* Leiomyosarcoma show dilated vessels reminiscent of hemangiopericytoma (HPC). HPC features may be commonly seen in leiomyosarcomas.

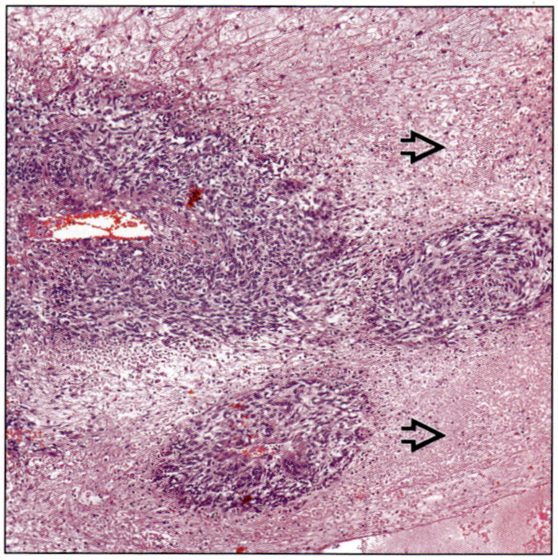

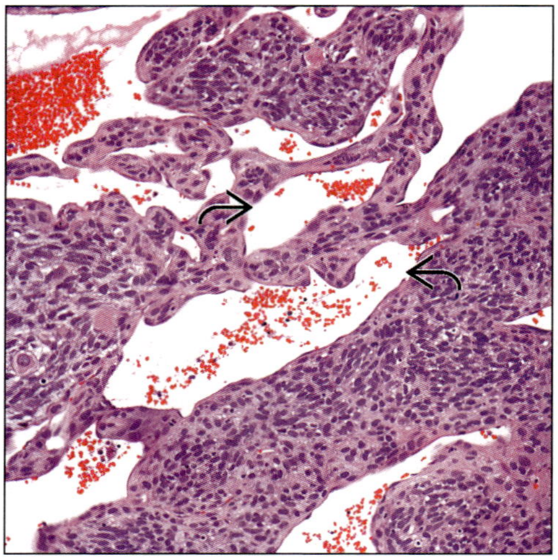

(Left) Intermediate-grade pulmonary leiomyosarcoma shows a fascicular growth pattern with spindle cells with moderate amounts of eosinophilic cytoplasm and a more epithelioid appearance. *(Right)* Intermediate-grade pulmonary leiomyosarcoma shows an epithelioid appearance with collections of foamy macrophages and a mild inflammatory reaction.

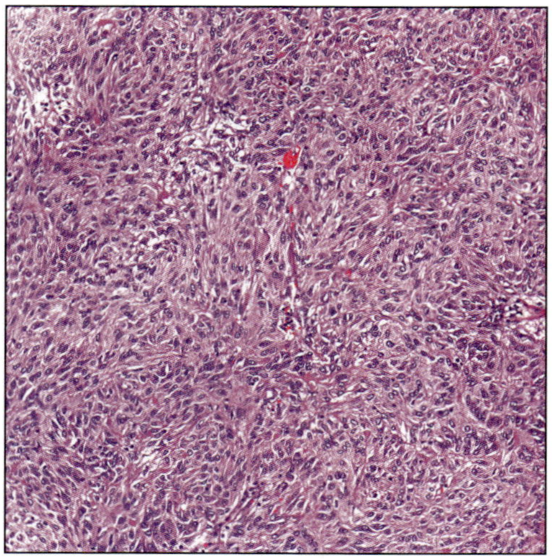

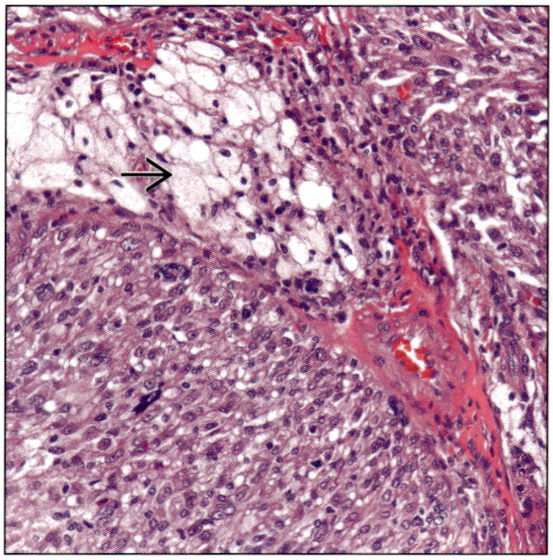

Microscopic Features

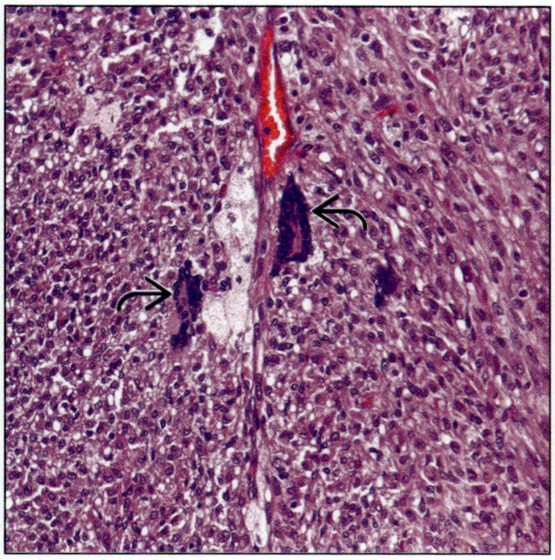
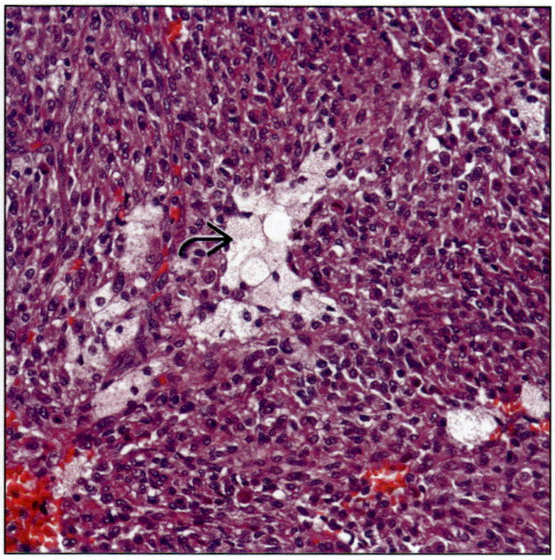

(Left) *Intermediate-grade pulmonary leiomyosarcoma is shown with a cluster of multinucleated giant cells. Note that the multinucleated giant cells do not show nuclear atypia or mitotic activity. This is an unusual feature in these tumors.* ***(Right)*** *Leiomyosarcoma with small collections of foamy macrophages. Such a finding may be seen not only in smooth muscle tumors but also in an inflammatory pseudotumor of lung.*

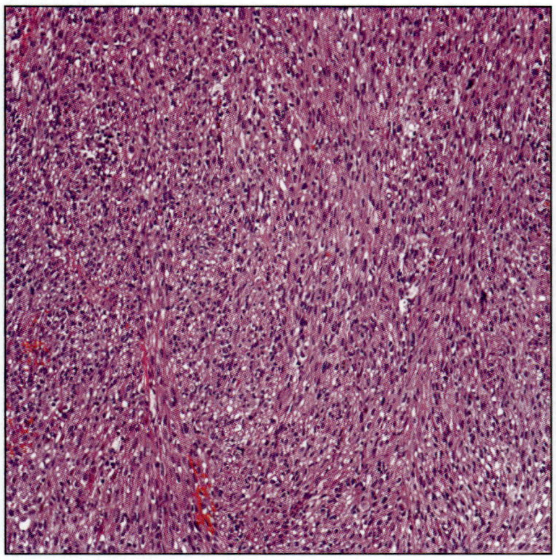
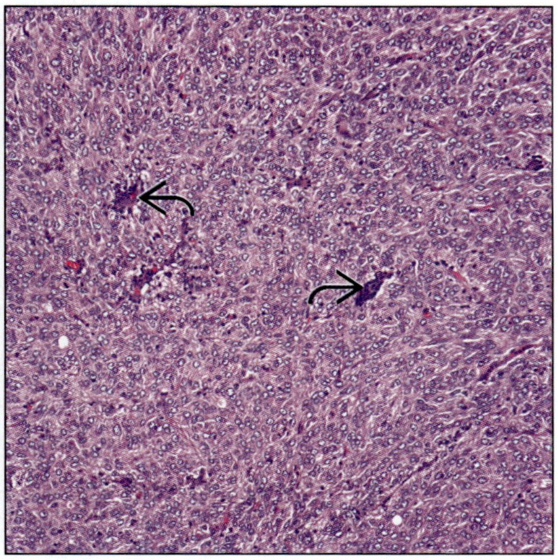

(Left) *Leiomyosarcoma shows conventional features of a spindle cellular proliferation with cigar-shaped nuclei and mild nuclear atypia. The finding of mitotic activity is important for proper classification.* ***(Right)*** *Leiomyosarcoma with clusters of inflammatory cells. Note the epithelioid appearance of the tumor in contrast to the conventional spindle cellular proliferation.*

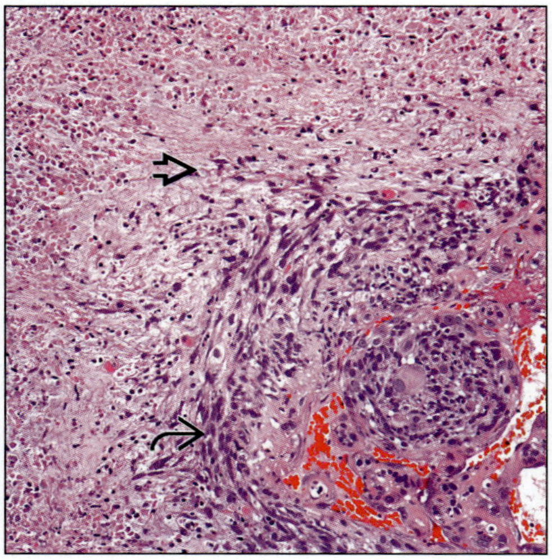
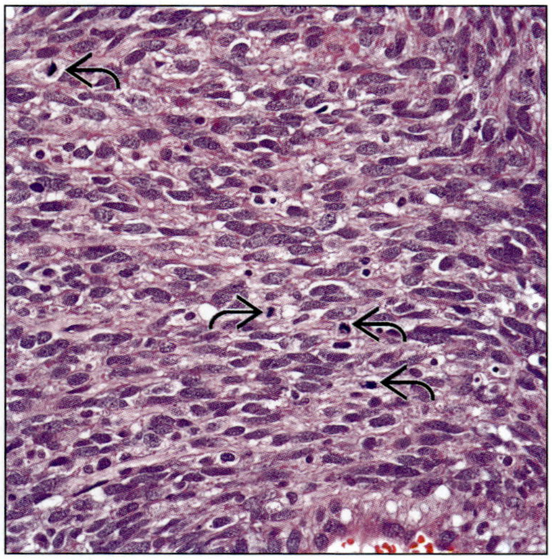

(Left) *High-grade leiomyosarcoma shows alternating areas of a pleomorphic spindle cell proliferation and areas of necrosis. These features are important for proper classification.* ***(Right)*** *High-grade leiomyosarcoma shows numerous mitotic figures. Usually, mitotic figures are easily identifiable in high-grade tumors.*

NEUROGENIC SARCOMA (MALIGNANT PERIPHERAL NERVE SHEATH TUMOR)

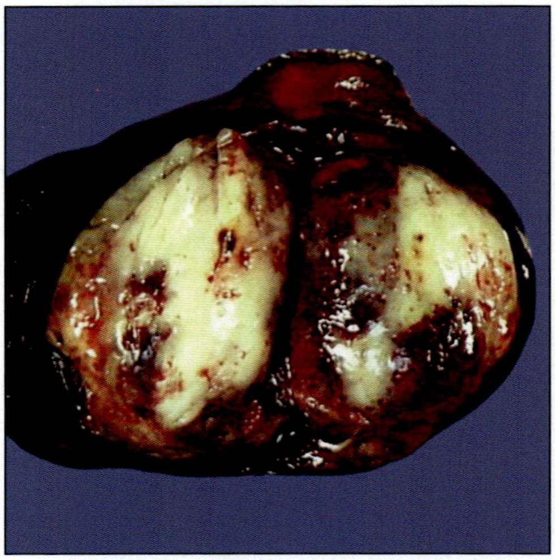

Gross appearance of primary neurogenic sarcoma of the lung in a resected specimen shows a fleshy, well-circumscribed tumor mass with extensive areas of hemorrhage and a glistening cut surface.

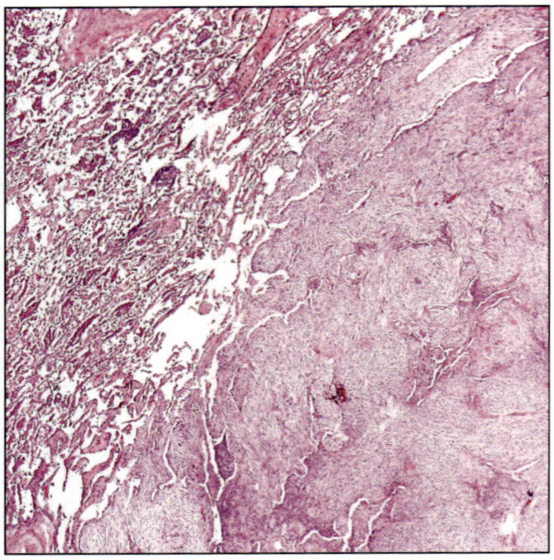

Neurogenic sarcoma of the lung shows well-circumscribed spindle cell tumor in lung parenchyma. Clinical history and special stains are required to separate this from other primary and metastatic tumors.

TERMINOLOGY

Synonyms

- Malignant peripheral nerve sheath tumor
- Malignant schwannoma

Definitions

- Primary malignant lung neoplasm showing evidence of peripheral nerve sheath differentiation

CLINICAL ISSUES

Epidemiology

- Incidence
  - Extremely rare tumor
  - Often associated with neurofibromatosis
- Age
  - Affects all age groups
  - Most frequent in young adults and middle-aged patients (30-50 years of age)
- Gender
  - No sex predilection

Presentation

- Large intraparenchymatous mass
  - Tumors may be central or peripheral
  - Tumors may arise in endobronchial location
- Shortness of breath
- Cough
- Chest pain
- Small peripheral tumors may be asymptomatic and discovered incidentally

Treatment

- Surgical approaches
  - Surgical excision
- Adjuvant therapy
  - Chemotherapy and radiation therapy may be employed for advanced or unresectable cases

Prognosis

- Aggressive behavior with recurrences and metastases
- Usually rapidly progressive course with fatal outcome

MACROSCOPIC FEATURES

General Features

- Large, fleshy, gray-white, lobulated tumor
- May be partially encapsulated
- Frequent hemorrhage and necrosis

Sections to Be Submitted

- Submit at least 1 section per centimeter of largest tumor diameter

Size

- Usually large (> 5 cm in greatest dimension)

MICROSCOPIC PATHOLOGY

Histologic Features

- Fascicular atypical spindle cell proliferation
- Frequent "herringbone" pattern of growth
- Alternating hyper- and hypocellular areas
- Well-developed storiform pattern can be sometimes observed
- Perivascular pattern of growth with extensive intervening areas of necrosis
- Prominent myxoid stromal changes
- Frequent areas of cystic degeneration, hemorrhage, and necrosis
- Heterologous elements may be present including bone, cartilage, and benign glandular inclusions
- Rhabdomyoblastic differentiation may be present (malignant "triton" tumor)
- Tumor may entrap benign respiratory epithelium at the periphery of the lesion, simulating a biphasic neoplasm

NEUROGENIC SARCOMA (MALIGNANT PERIPHERAL NERVE SHEATH TUMOR)

Key Facts

Clinical Issues
- Extremely rare tumor
- Often associated with neurofibromatosis
- Tumors may be central or peripheral
- Tumors may arise in endobronchial location
- Aggressive behavior with recurrences and metastases

Microscopic Pathology
- Fascicular atypical spindle cell proliferation
- Frequent "herringbone" pattern of growth
- Alternating hyper- and hypocellular areas
- Rhabdomyoblastic differentiation may be present (malignant "triton" tumor)
- Frequent areas of cystic degeneration, hemorrhage, and necrosis
- Prominent myxoid stromal changes

Ancillary Tests
- S100 protein is of limited utility for diagnosis because expression is lost or only focal in malignant neural neoplasms
- Immunohistochemical staining has very low specificity for diagnosis of neurogenic sarcoma
- Shows complex interdigitating cytoplasmic processes covered by basal lamina material on EM

Diagnostic Checklist
- Immunohistochemical staining may be of very limited value for diagnosis in neurogenic sarcoma
- 2 most reliable features for establishing diagnosis are a history of neurofibromatosis and ultrastructural findings

Cytologic Features
- Tumor cells may be spindle or epithelioid
- Spindle cells show enlarged, wavy nuclei with increased chromatin pattern and prominent nucleoli
- Mitotic activity can be pronounced (> 10 mitoses per 10 high-power fields)
- Epithelioid cells are large, round, or polygonal and contain hyperchromatic nuclei surrounded by abundant cytoplasm
- Malignant "triton" tumor contains foci of small, round, or spindle rhabdomyoblasts with hyperchromatic nuclei and eccentric pink cytoplasm

ANCILLARY TESTS

Immunohistochemistry
- S100 protein is of limited utility for diagnosis because expression is lost or only focal in malignant neural neoplasms
- Neurofilaments, nerve growth factor receptor (NGFR), CD57, and other neural-associated markers may be positive but are not distinctive
- In rare cases, focal positivity for keratin or EMA may be observed
- Rhabdomyoblastic elements in malignant "triton" tumors stain strongly with desmin, MYOD1, and myogenin
- Immunohistochemical staining has very low specificity for the diagnosis of neurogenic sarcoma
- Immunohistochemical staining is important in the context of ruling out alternate diagnostic possibilities

Cytogenetics
- No specific translocation or genetic profile has been demonstrated so far

Electron Microscopy
- Shows complex interdigitating cytoplasmic processes covered by basal lamina material
- Extracellular matrix contains long-spacing collagen (so-called Luse bodies)

DIFFERENTIAL DIAGNOSIS

Monophasic Synovial Sarcoma
- Also shows fascicular growth with prominent "herringbone" pattern
- Usually displays prominent "hemangiopericytic" growth pattern not seen in neurogenic sarcoma
- Can be positive for S100 protein in up to 30% of cases
- Focally positive for cytokeratin and EMA and strongly positive for Bcl-2 and CD99
- Does not display long, slender, and interdigitating cytoplasmic process by electron microscopy
- Associated in > 85% of cases with SYT cytogenetic translocation; t(X;18)

Solitary Fibrous Tumor
- Morphology may be indistinguishable from that of neurogenic sarcoma
- May also show fascicular growth with prominent "herringbone" pattern
- Shows immunohistochemical reactivity for CD34, Bcl-2, and CD99
- Does not display interdigitating cytoplasmic processes by electron microscopy

DIAGNOSTIC CHECKLIST

Pathologic Interpretation Pearls
- Immunohistochemical staining may be of very limited value for diagnosis in neurogenic sarcoma
- 2 most reliable features for establishing diagnosis are a history of neurofibromatosis and ultrastructural findings

SELECTED REFERENCES

1. Uchiyama M et al: Primary pulmonary malignant schwannoma with extension to the tracheal carina. J Thorac Cardiovasc Surg. 133(1):265-7, 2007
2. Bartley TD et al: Intrapulmonary neurogenic tumors. J Thorac Cardiovasc Surg. 50:114-23, 1965

NEUROGENIC SARCOMA (MALIGNANT PERIPHERAL NERVE SHEATH TUMOR)

Growth Patterns

(Left) *Scanning magnification of malignant peripheral nerve sheath tumor of the lung (neurogenic sarcoma) shows a fascicular pattern of growth. Notice the sharp circumscription of the tumor from the surrounding lung parenchyma with absence of a capsule.* ***(Right)*** *High magnification of neurogenic sarcoma of the lung with fascicular growth pattern shows atypical spindle cells with scattered mitoses. Notice the entrapped gland-like airspaces at the periphery of the lesion simulating a biphasic neoplasm →.*

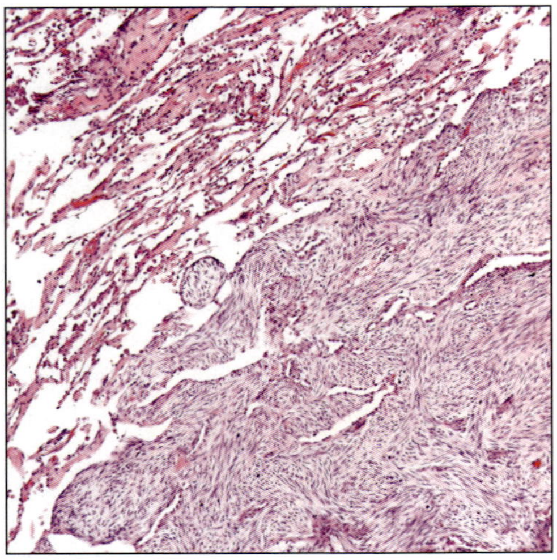

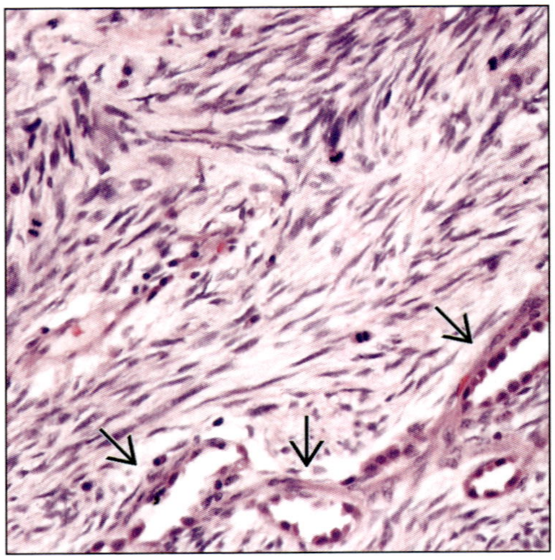

(Left) *Scanning magnification of neurogenic sarcoma of the lung shows a characteristic appearance with dark (hypercellular) zones ↪ alternating with lighter (hypocellular) areas.* ***(Right)*** *Neurogenic sarcoma of the lung shows palisading of spindle tumor cells reminiscent of Verocay bodies (Antoni type A pattern). This very unusual feature is rarely seen in these tumors. It is mostly observed only in the very well-differentiated examples of these lesions.*

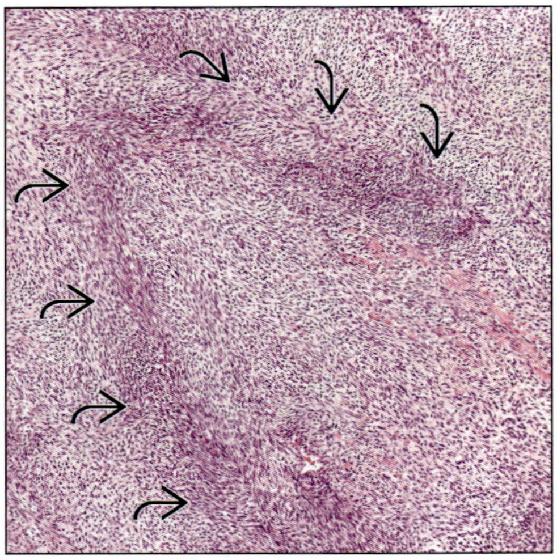

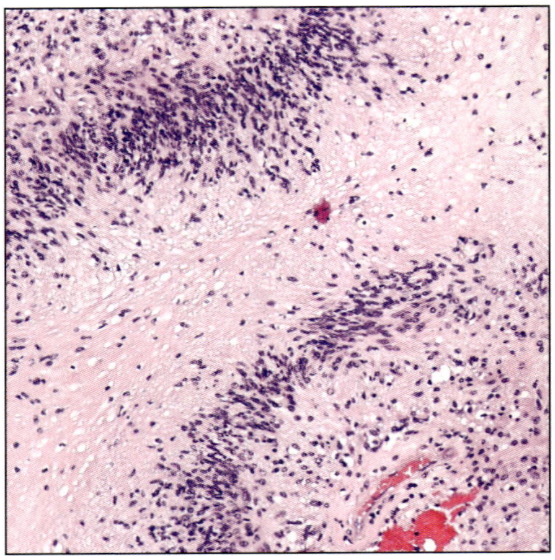

(Left) *Scanning magnification of a malignant peripheral nerve sheath tumor (neurogenic sarcoma) of the lung shows a striking "herringbone" pattern of growth that simulates a fibrosarcoma.* ***(Right)*** *Scanning magnification of neurogenic sarcoma of the lung shows a striking peritheliomatous growth pattern resulting in "balls" of tumor cells surrounding small vessels ⇨. The "balls" of tumor cells are characteristically surrounded by extensive intervening areas of necrosis.*

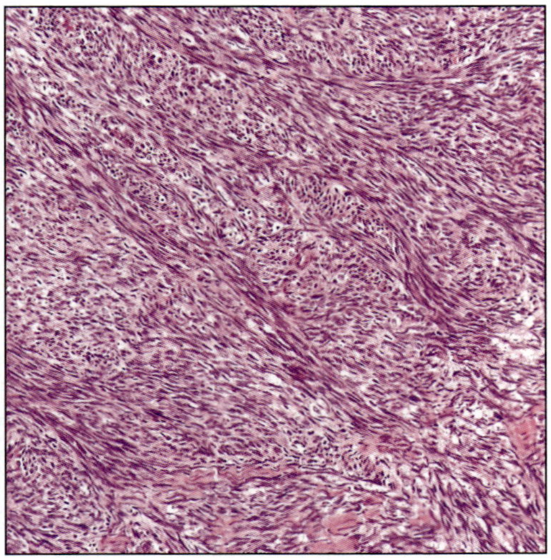

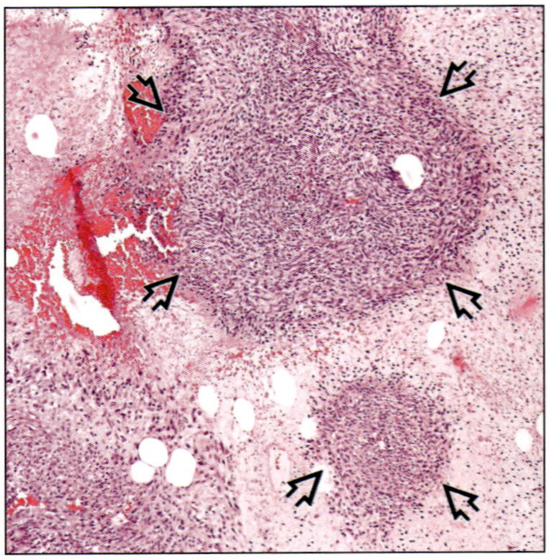

Cytologic Features

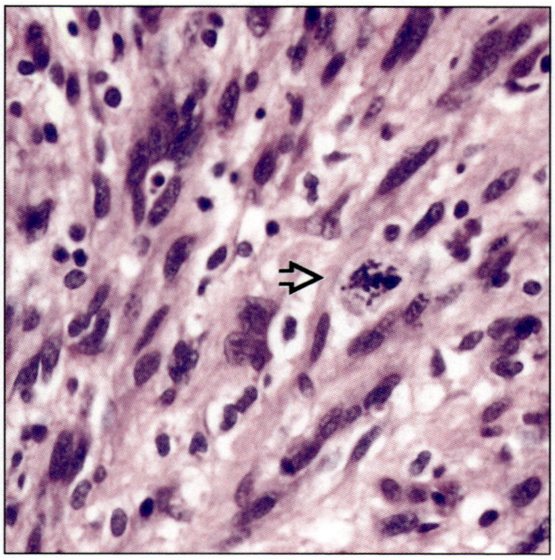

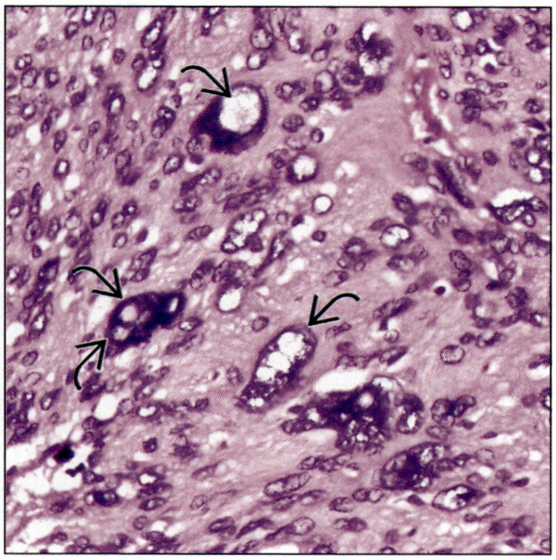

(Left) *High magnification of malignant peripheral nerve sheath tumor of the lung shows atypical spindle cell population with scattered abnormal mitoses ⇨. Notice the inflammatory cell infiltrate in the background stroma.* ***(Right)*** *Malignant peripheral nerve sheath tumor of the lung shows spindle cell population with marked nuclear pleomorphism. Notice large, hyperchromatic tumor cells displaying intranuclear cytoplasmic inclusions (nuclear pseudoinclusions) ↷.*

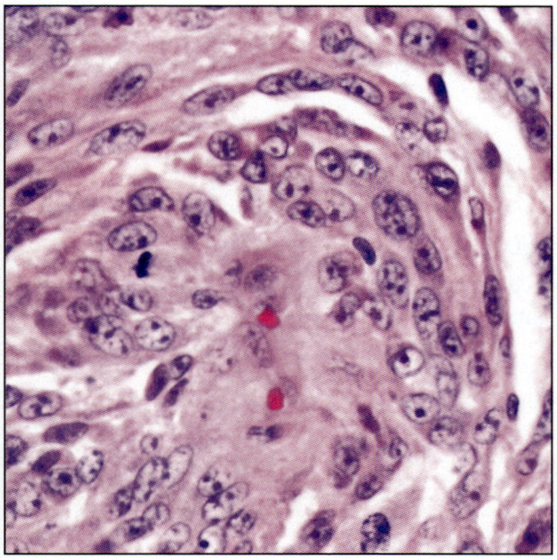

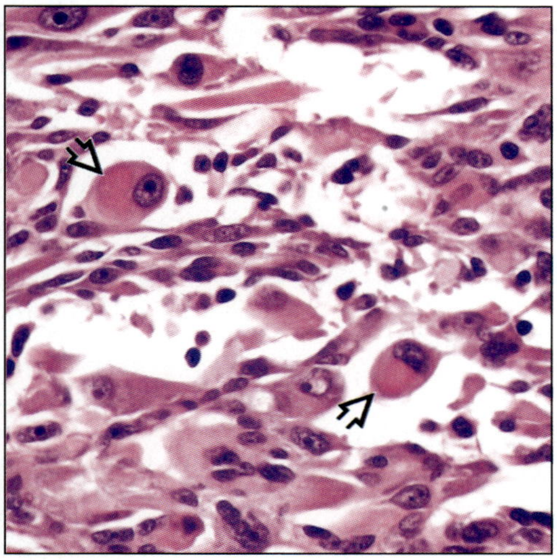

(Left) *Epithelioid variant of malignant peripheral nerve sheath tumor of the lung shows cells with round nuclei containing prominent eosinophilic nucleoli and surrounded by an abundant rim of eosinophilic cytoplasm.* ***(Right)*** *Malignant peripheral nerve sheath tumor of the lung with rhabdomyoblastic differentiation (malignant "triton" tumor) shows scattered large rhabdomyoblastic cells with eccentric nuclei and abundant pink cytoplasm ⇨.*

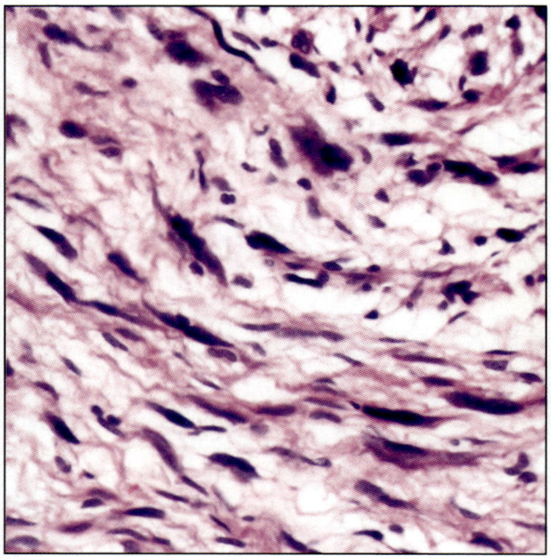

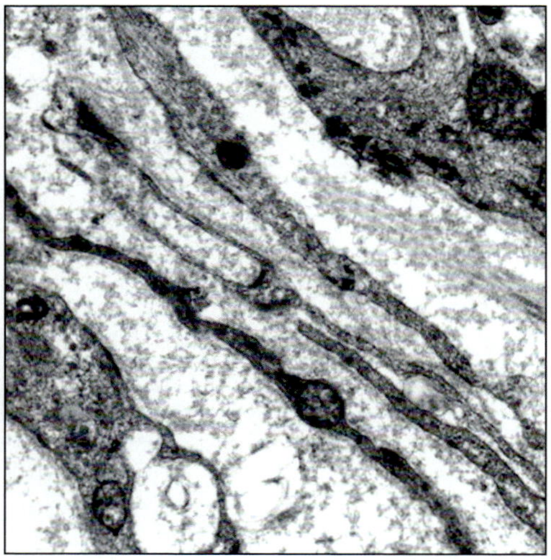

(Left) *Malignant peripheral nerve sheath tumor of lung shows atypical spindle cell population with "wavy" nuclei. Notice the abundant, lightly myxoid background matrix.* ***(Right)*** *Ultrastructural appearance of malignant peripheral nerve sheath tumor of the lung shows long, slender cytoplasmic prolongations that intertwine with one another and are partially covered by a thin layer of basal lamina material. This feature is distinctive for these tumors and a helpful adjunct for diagnosis.*

OSTEOSARCOMA

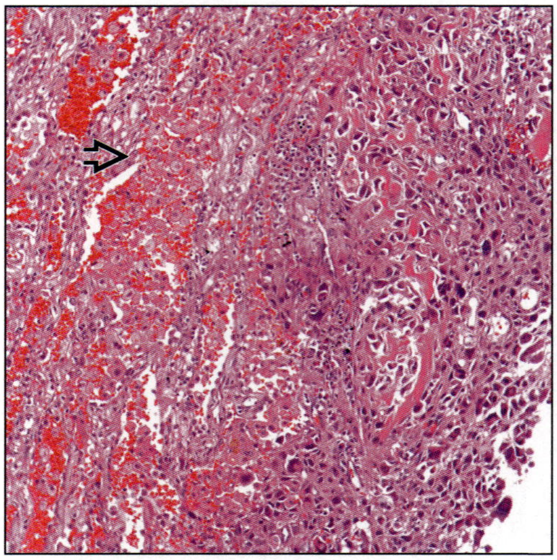

Primary pulmonary osteosarcoma shows a pleomorphic cellular proliferation with numerous multinucleated giant cells of the osteoclast type. Note the presence of uninvolved lung parenchyma ⮚.

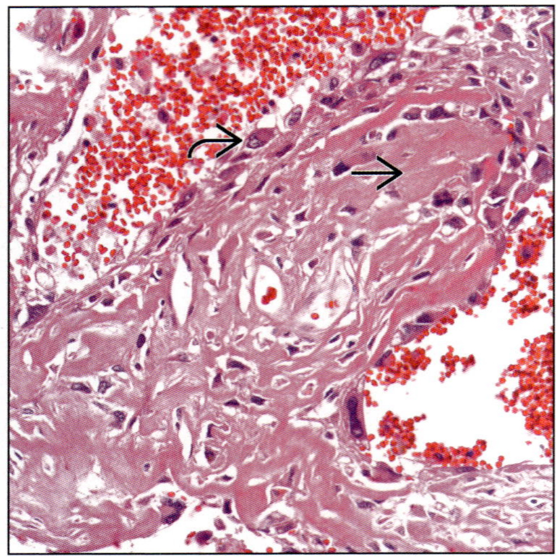

High-power view of an osteosarcoma shows osteoid deposition → and a rim of neoplastic cells ↗.

TERMINOLOGY

Synonyms
- Osteogenic sarcoma

Definitions
- Malignant mesenchymal neoplasm with osseous differentiation

CLINICAL ISSUES

Epidemiology
- Incidence
  - Osteosarcomas of lung are exceedingly rare with < 30 cases reported in the literature
- Age
  - Osteosarcomas of lung appear to be more common in 5th and 6th decades of life
- Gender
  - No gender predilection

Presentation
- Cough
- Shortness of breath
- Chest pain
- Hemoptysis
- Asymptomatic

Laboratory Tests
- In most cases of pulmonary osteosarcoma, levels of alkaline phosphatase are normal

Treatment
- Surgical approaches
  - Lobectomy or pneumonectomy
- Adjuvant therapy
  - Chemo-radiation is questionable
- There is no specific treatment

Prognosis
- Poor survival
- Death may occur within 12 months after initial diagnosis

MACROSCOPIC FEATURES

General Features
- Well-defined tumor
- Solid, "rock-hard"

Size
- Varies from 4 to > 10 cm in diameter

MICROSCOPIC PATHOLOGY

Histologic Features
- Malignant spindle cell proliferation
- Osteoid formation
- Osteoclast giant cells
- Mitotic activity
- Cartilaginous component may be present

Predominant Pattern/Injury Type
- Ossification

Predominant Cell/Compartment Type
- Spindle

DIFFERENTIAL DIAGNOSIS

Bronchial Chondroma
- May show ossification in center of lesion
- Does not show osteoid formation
- Will not display cellular atypia &/or mitotic activity

Carcinosarcoma
- Displays epithelial component

OSTEOSARCOMA

Key Facts

Terminology
- Malignant mesenchymal neoplasm with osseous differentiation

Clinical Issues
- Incidence
  - Osteosarcomas of lung are exceedingly rare with > 30 cases reported
  - Pulmonary osteosarcomas appear to be more common in 5th and 6th decades of life
- Symptoms
  - Cough
  - Dyspnea
  - Chest pain
  - Hemoptysis
  - Asymptomatic
- Laboratory findings
  - In most cases of pulmonary osteosarcoma, levels of alkaline phosphatase are normal
- Treatment and prognosis
  - No specific treatment
  - Poor survival
  - Death may occur within 12 months after initial diagnosis

Top Differential Diagnoses
- Bronchial chondroma
  - May show ossification in center of lesion
- Chondrosarcomas
  - Does not show osteoid formation
  - Does not display cellular atypia &/or mitotic activity
- Carcinosarcoma
  - Displays epithelial component

Immunohistochemistry

Antibody	Reactivity	Staining Pattern	Comment
Osteonectin	Positive	Cytoplasmic	May be only focal
S100	Positive	Nuclear	In chondroid areas
SOX9	Positive	Nuclear	In chondroid areas
Vimentin	Positive	Cytoplasmic	
Osteopontin	Negative		
CK-PAN	Negative		Will stain only entrapped pulmonary parenchyma
Desmin	Negative		
Actin-HHF-35	Negative		
MYOD1	Negative		
Myoglobin	Negative		
Myogenin	Negative		

- In majority of carcinosarcomas, osteoid component is only focal

Chondrosarcoma
- Does not show osteoid formation

Hamartoma
- Displays more benign cartilaginous component
- Shows presence of invaginations of respiratory epithelium
- Lacks presence of osteoid

Poorly Differentiated Carcinomas (Non-Small Cell Type)
- In some carcinomas, presence of prominent basal lamina may be confused with osteoid
- Carcinomas will show positive staining for epithelial markers

DIAGNOSTIC CHECKLIST

Clinically Relevant Pathologic Features
- Gross appearance

Pathologic Interpretation Pearls
- Osteoid formation

SELECTED REFERENCES

1. Shenjere P et al: Primary pulmonary osteosarcoma: a report of 4 cases and a review of the literature. Int J Surg Pathol. 19(2):225-9, 2011
2. Karfis EA et al: Primary extraosseous osteosarcoma of the lung. Acta Oncol. 49(1):114-6, 2010
3. Niimi R et al: Primary osteosarcoma of the lung: a case report and review of the literature. Med Oncol. 25(2):251-5, 2008
4. Yamazaki K et al: Primary osteosarcoma of the lung: a case report. Ann Thorac Cardiovasc Surg. 12(2):126-8, 2006
5. Kadowaki T et al: Two cases of primary pulmonary osteosarcoma. Intern Med. 44(6):632-7, 2005
6. Chapman AD et al: Primary pulmonary osteosarcoma: case report and molecular analysis. Cancer. 91(4):779-84, 2001
7. Wagner MS et al: Primary chondroblastic osteosarcoma of the lung. Sarcoma. 3(3-4):193-5, 1999
8. Loose JH et al: Primary osteosarcoma of the lung. Report of two cases and review of the literature. J Thorac Cardiovasc Surg. 100(6):867-73, 1990
9. Colby TV et al: Primary osteosarcoma of the lung. A reappraisal following immunohistologic study. Arch Pathol Lab Med. 113(10):1147-50, 1989

OSTEOSARCOMA

Microscopic Features

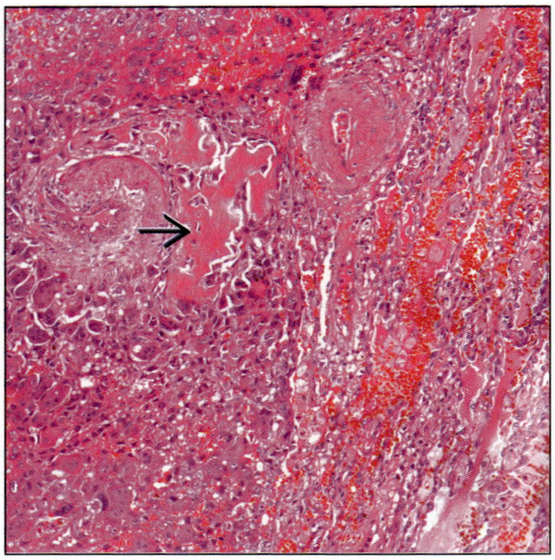
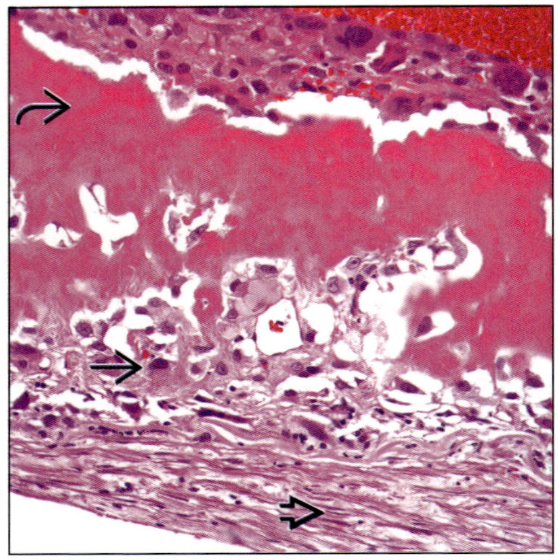

*(**Left**) In this pulmonary osteosarcoma with adjacent lung parenchyma, note that the tumor is not encapsulated but rather shows ill-defined borders. In addition, note the presence of osteoid formation ⇒ admixed with the neoplastic cellular proliferation. (**Right**) Osteosarcoma with extensive osteoid deposition ↷. The tumor is in a subpleural location ⇨. Numerous malignant cells are also present ⇒.*

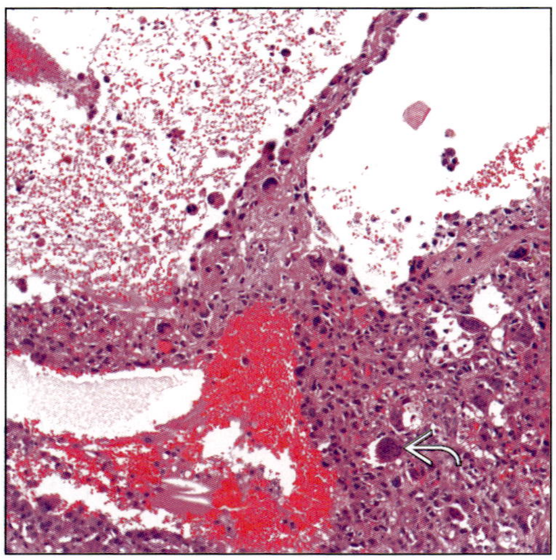
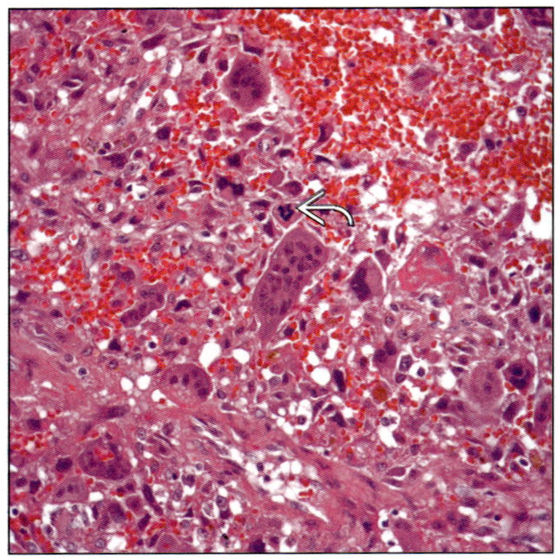

*(**Left**) Osteosarcoma with cystic changes. Note the presence of numerous osteoclast-type giant cells ↶ admixed with blood and other mononuclear cells. (**Right**) High-power view of the cellular composition of an osteosarcoma shows numerous osteoclast-type giant cells admixed with atypical mononuclear cells, some of them showing atypical mitotic figures ➘.*

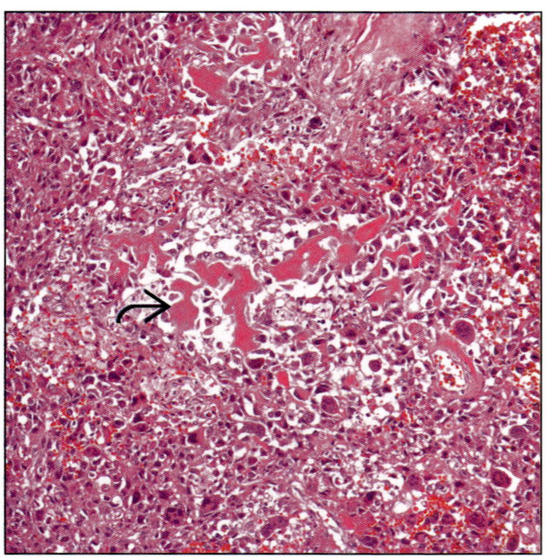
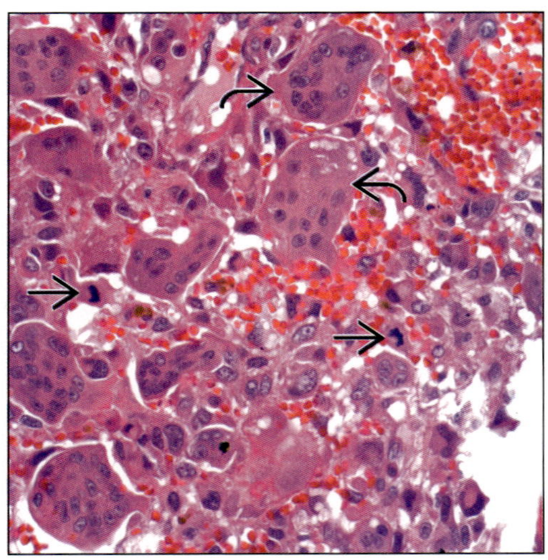

*(**Left**) In some cases of osteosarcoma, the presence of osteoid may be only minimal ↷. The presence of osteoid is highly important to make the diagnosis of osteosarcoma. (**Right**) Higher magnification of areas composed predominantly of multinucleated giant cells ↷, which do not show mitotic activity. However, adjacent mononuclear cells show mitotic activity ⇒.*

Microscopic Features

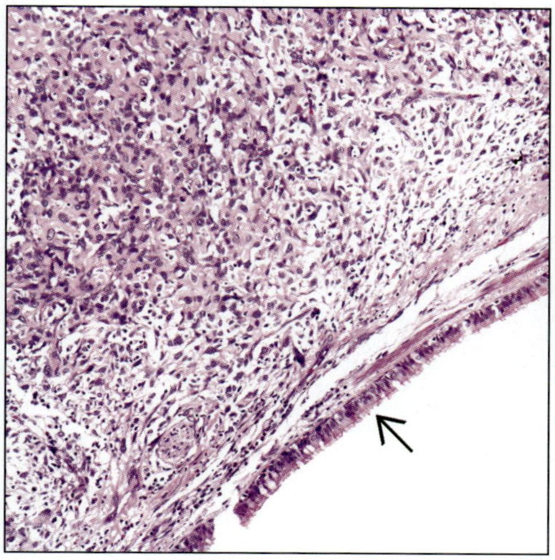

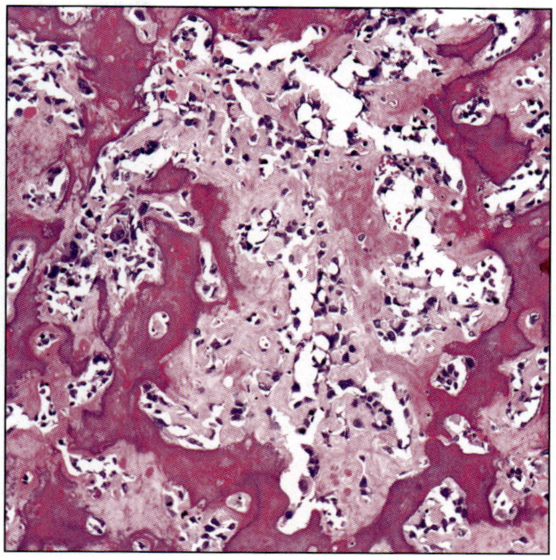

***(Left)** Low-power view of an osteosarcoma of the lung shows a tumor growing beneath the bronchial epithelium →. In this type of tumor, no in situ component is found. **(Right)** In some other cases of osteosarcoma, the presence of ossification is more apparent and easily identifiable. It is crucial to properly sample these tumors in order to rule out epithelial components.*

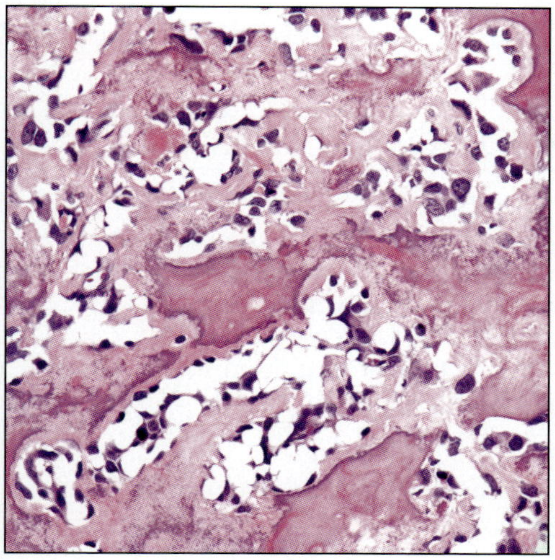

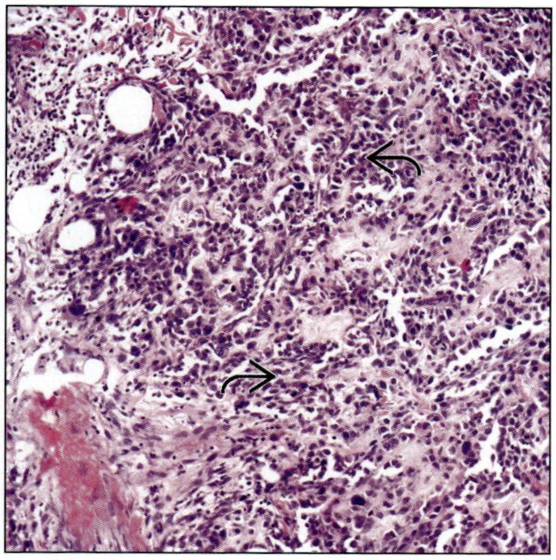

***(Left)** Higher magnification shows a neoplastic cellular proliferation composed of rather small cells with indistinct cell borders, inconspicuous nucleoli, and an absence of mitotic activity. Note the presence of obvious osteoid formation. **(Right)** In cases in which osteoid is not easily identifiable, the tumor can be easily misdiagnosed for another sarcoma or epithelial malignancy. In this illustration, the tumor cells appear epithelial ↗.*

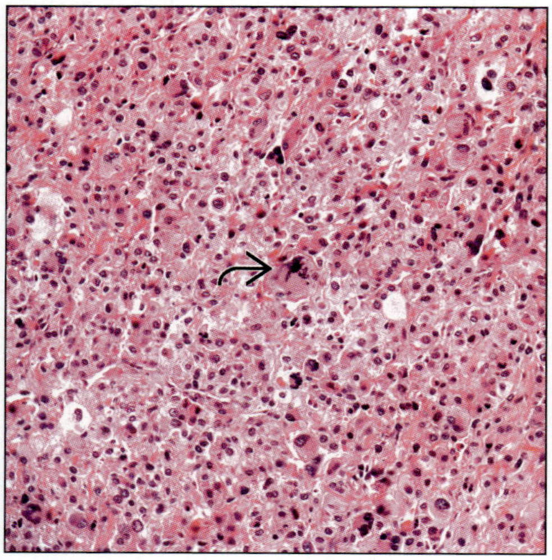

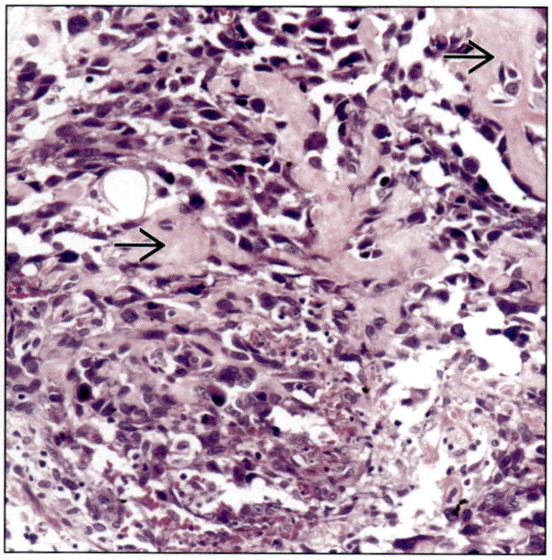

***(Left)** This neoplastic cellular proliferation can be easily confused with an epithelial tumor. The cells show nuclear pleomorphism with atypical mitotic figures ↗, but osteoid is not present. **(Right)** In some other cases, the neoplastic cellular proliferation shows spindle cell features mimicking some other type of spindle cell sarcoma. However, the presence of osteoid → should raise the possibility of osteosarcoma.*

CHRONDROSARCOMA

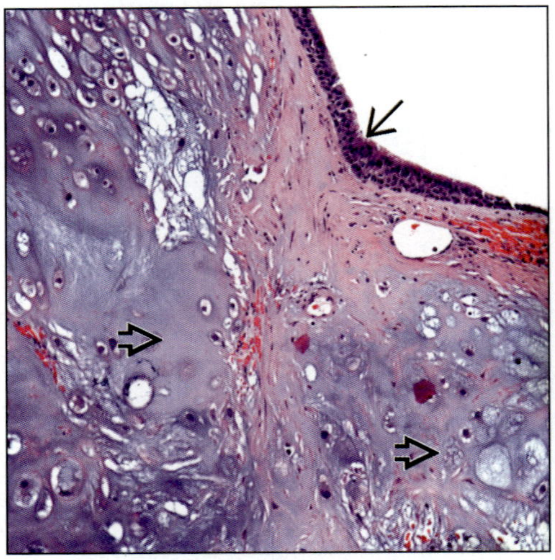

Low-power view of a pulmonary chondrosarcoma shows the tumor ⇨ growing beneath the bronchial epithelium →. The respiratory epithelium is not involved.

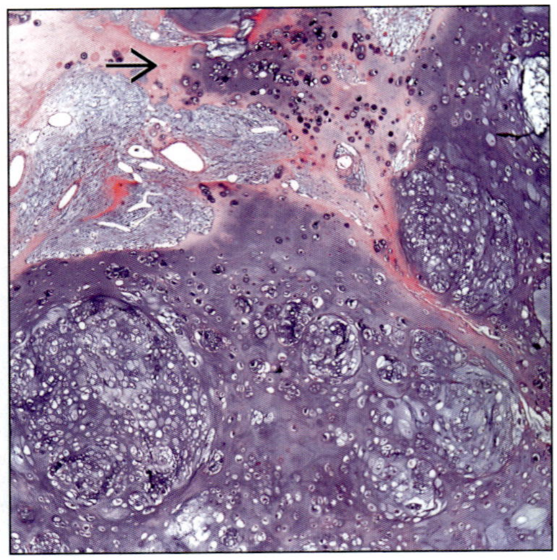

Disorganized growth pattern with lobulation is seen and at the center, with focal early ossification →. The areas of ossification should not be interpreted as an osteosarcomatous component.

TERMINOLOGY

Definitions

- Malignant mesenchymal neoplasm with cartilaginous differentiation

CLINICAL ISSUES

Epidemiology

- Incidence
  - Primary chondrosarcomas of lung are exceedingly rare
- Age
  - Primary chondrosarcomas of lung are more common in 6th and 7th decades of life
- Gender
  - No gender predilection

Site

- Primary chondrosarcomas in lung can be either central or peripheral

Presentation

- Shortness of breath
- Hemoptysis
- Cough
- Bronchial obstruction
- Asymptomatic

Treatment

- Surgical approaches
  - Lobectomy
  - Sleeve resection
  - Pneumonectomy
- Adjuvant therapy
  - Chemo-radiation is questionable

Prognosis

- Central tumors may have less aggressive behavior
- Peripheral tumors may follow more aggressive behavior
- Survival is poor

MACROSCOPIC FEATURES

General Features

- Tumor may obliterate bronchial lumen in central tumors
- Peripheral tumors are usually larger
- Well-delineated tumors
- White with slightly lobulated appearance
- Hard or mucoid consistency

Size

- Varies from 1-2 cm to > 10 cm in diameter

MICROSCOPIC PATHOLOGY

Histologic Features

- Atypical cartilage
- Chondromyxoid
- Myxoid
- Mesenchymal

Predominant Pattern/Injury Type

- Chondromyxoid

Predominant Cell/Compartment Type

- Cartilaginous

DIFFERENTIAL DIAGNOSIS

Hamartoma

- Shows invagination of respiratory epithelium
- Generally shows cartilage mixed with adipose tissue
- Would not show marked atypia &/or mitotic activity

CHRONDROSARCOMA

Key Facts

Terminology
- Malignant mesenchymal neoplasm with cartilaginous differentiation

Clinical Issues
- Incidence
  - Primary chondrosarcomas of lung are exceedingly rare
  - More common in 6th and 7th decades of life
  - Can be either central or peripheral tumors
- Symptoms
  - Shortness of breath
  - Hemoptysis
  - Cough
  - Bronchial obstruction

Microscopic Pathology
- Atypical cartilage
- Chondromyxoid
- Myxoid
- Mesenchymal

Top Differential Diagnoses
- Hamartoma shows invagination of respiratory epithelium
  - Shows mixed areas with adipose tissue
- Carcinoma is a consideration in cases of mesenchymal chondrosarcoma
  - Shows positive staining with epithelial markers
- Mixed tumor may also show other types of tissues
- Carcinosarcoma should show evidence of epithelial component

Immunohistochemistry

Antibody	Reactivity	Staining Pattern	Comment
SOX9	Positive	Nuclear	May be seen in other noncartilaginous tumors
S100	Positive	Nuclear	May be positive in neural crest-derived tumors
CK-PAN	Negative		Positive staining should raise possibility of carcinosarcoma
CD34	Negative		
Desmin	Negative		May raise possibility of muscle neoplasm
Actin-HHF-35	Negative		
MYOD1	Negative		
EMA	Negative		

Carcinoma
- Is a consideration in cases of mesenchymal chondrosarcoma
- Shows positive staining with epithelial markers
- Generally would show more nuclear atypia and mitotic activity

Mixed Tumor (Pleomorphic Adenoma)
- Shows presence of associated epithelial component
- May also show other types of tissues
- Mixed tumors in lung usually do not show atypical cartilaginous component
- Mixed tumors would display myoepithelial differentiation

Carcinosarcoma
- Should show evidence of epithelial component
  - Squamous cell carcinoma
  - Adenocarcinoma
  - Large cell carcinoma

Metastatic Chondrosarcoma
- Clinical history is most important feature
- May show more than 1 pulmonary lesion in lung
- May show bilateral distribution

DIAGNOSTIC CHECKLIST

Clinically Relevant Pathologic Features
- Gross appearance

Pathologic Interpretation Pearls
- Cartilaginous tumor with atypia

SELECTED REFERENCES

1. Steurer S et al: Dedifferentiated chondrosarcoma of the lung: case report and review of the literature. Clin Lung Cancer. 8(7):439-42, 2007
2. Huang HY et al: Primary mesenchymal chondrosarcoma of the lung. Ann Thorac Surg. 73(6):1960-2, 2002
3. Hayashi T et al: Primary chondrosarcoma of the lung. A clinicopathologic study. Cancer. 72(1):69-74, 1993
4. Jazy FK et al: Primary chondrosarcoma of the lung. A report of two cases. Clin Oncol. 10(3):273-9, 1984
5. Yellin A et al: Chondrosarcoma of the bronchus. Chest. 84(2):224-6, 1983
6. Sun CC et al: Primary chondrosarcoma of the lung. Cancer. 50(9):1864-6, 1982
7. Morgan AD et al: Primary chondrosarcoma of the lung. Case report and review of the literature. J Thorac Cardiovasc Surg. 64(3):460-6, 1972
8. Rees GM: Primary chondrosarcoma of lung. Thorax. 25(3):366-71, 1970

CHRONDROSARCOMA

Microscopic Features

(Left) *Low-power view of a low-grade pulmonary chondrosarcoma shows a good comparison between neoplastic cartilage* → *and normal bronchial cartilage* ⇨. *The tumor is obliterating the bronchial lumen.* ***(Right)*** *Primary chondrosarcoma of the lung is shown with myxoid features* ⇨ *and the presence of osteoclast-like giant cells* →. *This finding may also suggest the possibility of metastatic osteogenic sarcoma.*

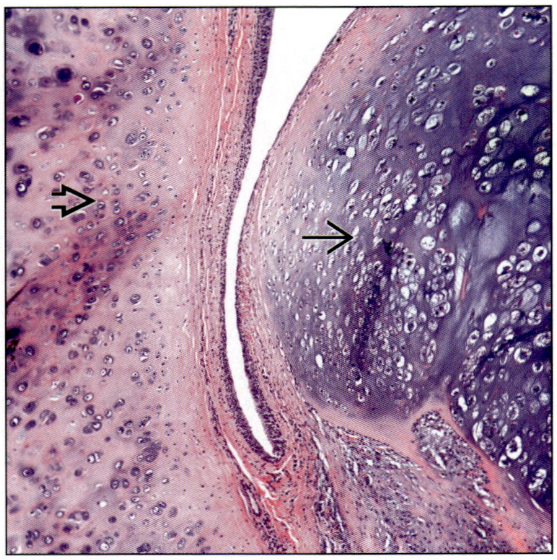

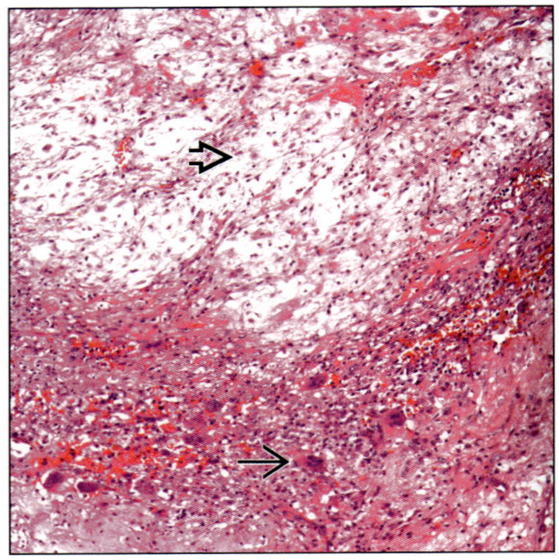

(Left) *Bronchial chondrosarcoma shows neoplastic cells embedded in a myxoid background. Even at this magnification, one can observe prominent nuclear atypia.* ***(Right)*** *High-power magnification shows prominent nuclear atypia and binucleated atypical cells* ↷.

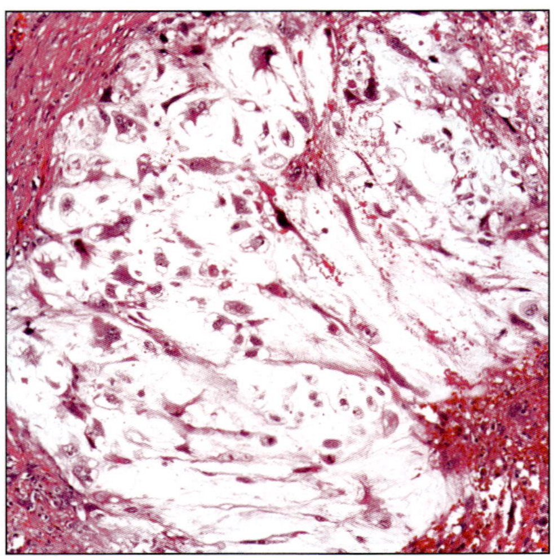

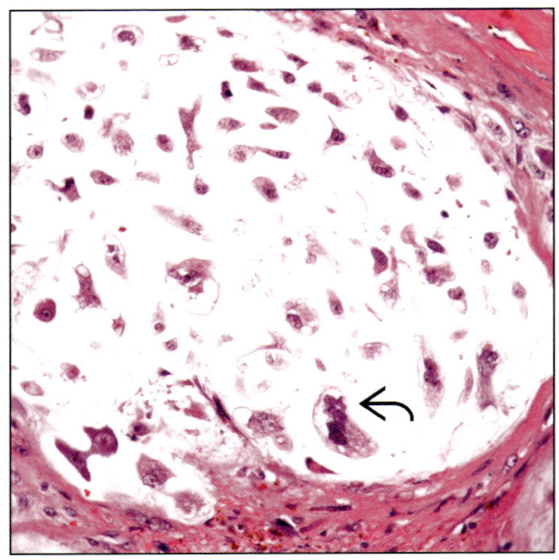

(Left) *Myxoid chondrosarcoma shows sheets of neoplastic cells without a particular growth pattern. This cellular proliferation can be easily confused for an epithelial neoplasm.* ***(Right)*** *High-power view of a primary myxoid chondrosarcoma of the lung shows a neoplastic cellular proliferation with more nuclear atypia and scattered mitotic figures* →.

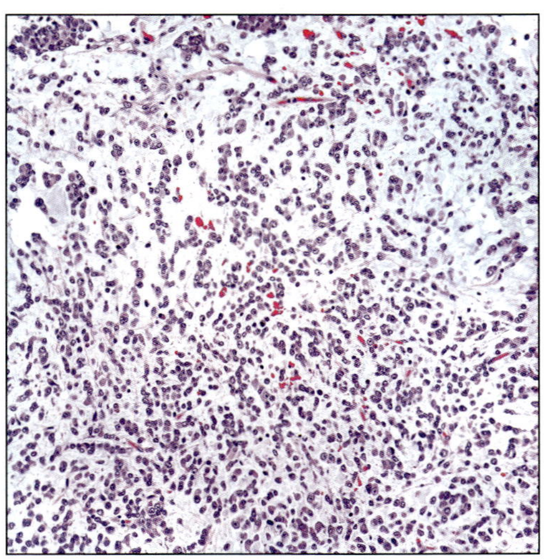

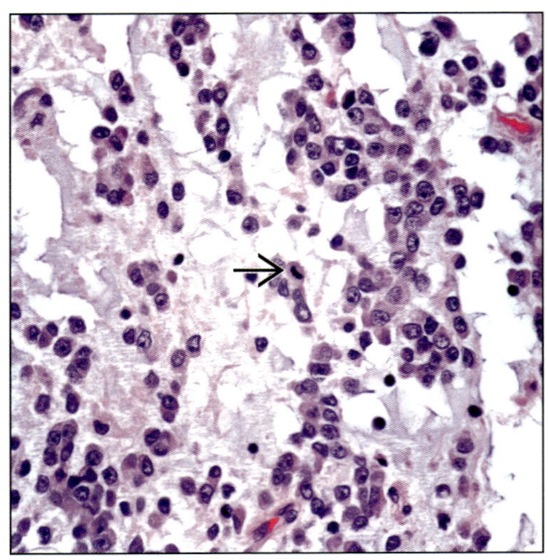

Microscopic Features

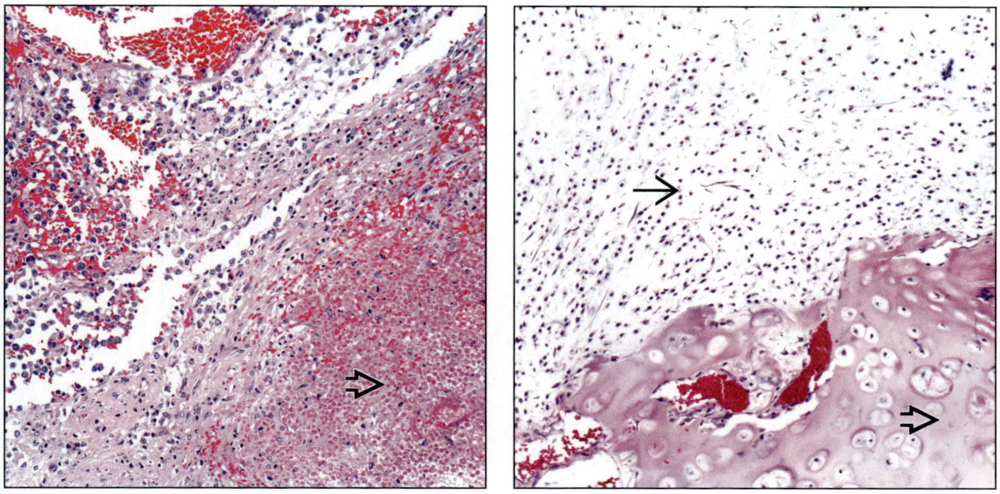

(Left) *Extensive areas of necrosis may be seen in unusual cases ⇨; however, necrosis is usually absent in low-grade tumors. Its presence usually indicates a high-grade tumor.* ***(Right)*** *Low-grade bronchial chondrosarcoma contrasts between the normal bronchial cartilage ⇨ and the neoplastic cartilage →.*

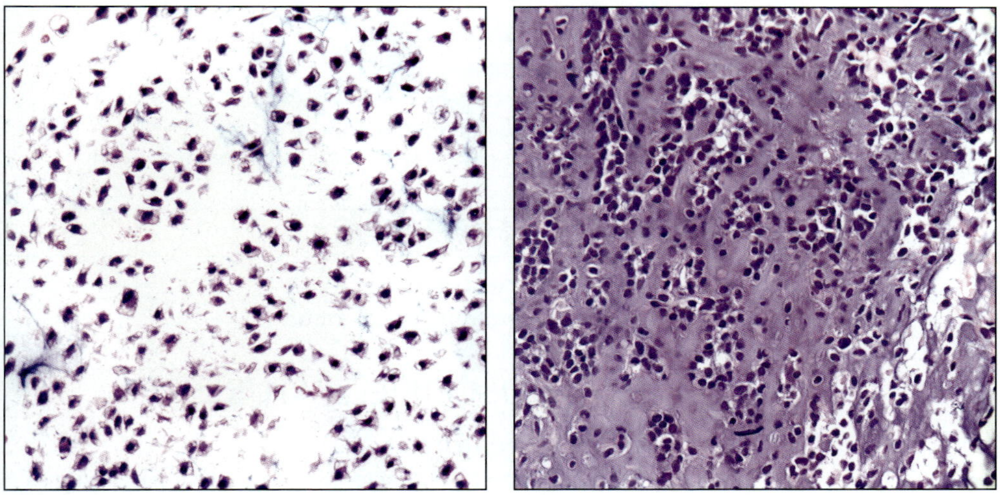

(Left) *High-power view of a low-grade chondrosarcoma shows an atypical cartilaginous proliferation; however, no mitotic activity is present.* ***(Right)*** *Low-power view of a primary pulmonary malignant neoplasm is composed of rather small cells embedded in a chondromyxoid background. These features are typical of mesenchymal chondrosarcoma. This pattern can be easily confused with a neuroendocrine carcinoma.*

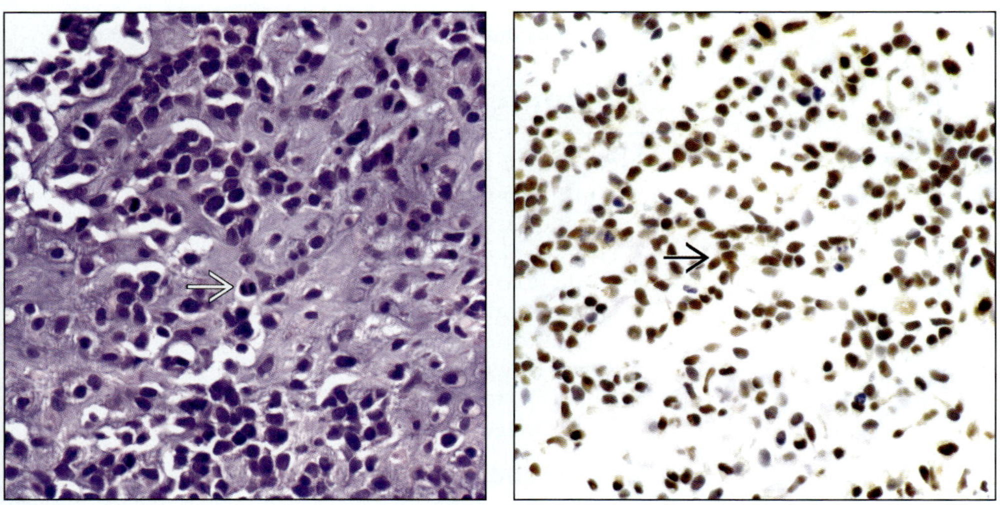

(Left) *High-power view of a primary mesenchymal chondrosarcoma of the lung shows a neoplastic cellular proliferation composed of small cells. Mitotic figures are easily identified ➡.* ***(Right)*** *SOX9 immunostain in a mesenchymal chondrosarcoma of the lung shows strong nuclear staining → in tumor cells. In cases with this type of morphology, the use of immunostains is important for proper classification of the tumor.*

EPITHELIOID HEMANGIOENDOTHELIOMA

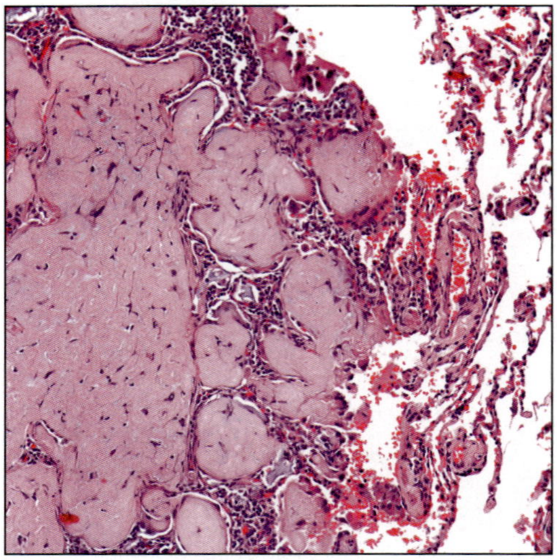

Classical presentation of epithelioid hemangioendothelioma in the lung. Note the presence of a nodule replacing lung parenchyma and infiltrating alveolar spaces.

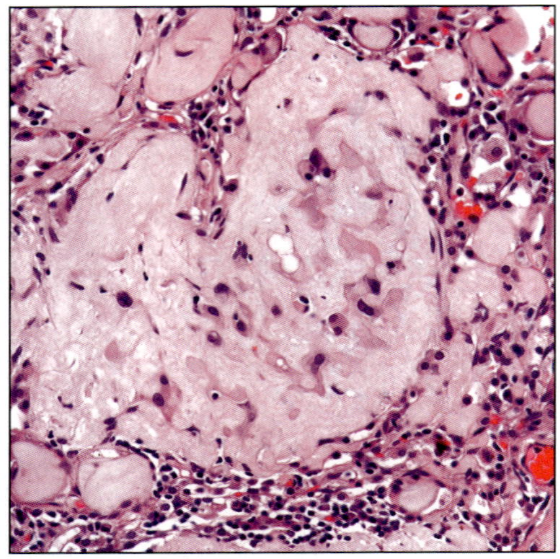

High magnification of epithelioid hemangioendothelioma shows a chondromyxoid background with scattered epithelioid cells embedded in the stroma.

TERMINOLOGY

Abbreviations

- Epithelioid hemangioendothelioma (EH)

Synonyms

- Intravascular bronchioloalveolar tumor (IVBT)

Definitions

- Vascular neoplasm of low- to intermediate-grade malignancy

ETIOLOGY/PATHOGENESIS

Etiology

- Vascular origin from precursor mesenchymal cells

CLINICAL ISSUES

Epidemiology

- Incidence
  - Tumor is unusual in lung
- Age
  - Appears to be more common in young adults; however, age may range from 7-72 years old
- Gender
  - More common in women

Site

- Usually bilateral pulmonary infiltrates

Presentation

- Cough
- Shortness of breath
- Pleuritic pain
- Asymptomatic

Treatment

- There is no specific treatment
- Radiation and chemotherapy can be attempted
- Steroids have been tried

Prognosis

- Unpredictable
- Spontaneous regression can occur
- Protracted course may follow
- Aggressive course with fatal outcome may occur

IMAGE FINDINGS

General Features

- Bilateral pulmonary infiltrates

MACROSCOPIC FEATURES

General Features

- Multiple nodules replacing normal lung parenchyma
- Nodules are soft or may be mucoid in consistency

Size

- Nodules may measure from a few mm to 2-3 cm

MICROSCOPIC PATHOLOGY

Histologic Features

- Multiple pulmonary nodules
- Nodules in different phases of development
- Prominent chondromyxoid background
- Epithelioid cells embedded in chondromyxoid background
- Low mitotic count
- Signet ring cell-like cellular appearance
- Cluster of tumor cells in polypoid intraalveolar pattern
- Extravasated red cells

Predominant Pattern/Injury Type

- Chondromyxoid

EPITHELIOID HEMANGIOENDOTHELIOMA

Key Facts

Terminology
- Epithelioid hemangioendothelioma (EH)
- Synonym: Intravascular bronchioloalveolar tumor (IVBT)

Clinical Issues
- Incidence
  - Unusual tumor in lung
  - Appears to be more common in young adults; age range: 7-72 years
  - More common in women
- Symptoms
  - Cough
  - Dyspnea
  - Pleuritic pain
  - Asymptomatic
- Presentation
  - Bilateral pulmonary infiltrates
- Treatment
  - There is no specific treatment

Top Differential Diagnoses
- Angiosarcoma
  - Usually shows high mitotic count
  - May also show areas of necrosis
  - Shows more nuclear atypia
- Metastatic carcinoma
  - Shows positive staining for epithelial markers (keratins and EMA/MUC1)
  - Negative for vascular markers (FVIIIRAg, CD31, and CD34)
- Metastatic chordoma
  - Also negative for vascular markers (CD31, CD34)
  - Negative history of chordoma elsewhere

Immunohistochemistry

Antibody	Reactivity	Staining Pattern	Comment
CD31	Positive	Cytoplasmic	
CD34	Positive	Cytoplasmic	
FVIIIRAg	Positive	Cytoplasmic	
ERP	Positive	Nuclear	In some cases only
PRP	Positive	Nuclear	In some cases only
CK-PAN	Positive	Cytoplasmic	Can be positive in many cases

Predominant Cell/Compartment Type
- Epithelioid

DIFFERENTIAL DIAGNOSIS

Angiosarcoma
- Usually shows high mitotic count
- May also show areas of necrosis
- Shows more nuclear atypia

Metastatic Carcinoma
- Shows positive staining for epithelial markers (keratins and EMA/MUC1)
- Negative for vascular markers (FVIIIRAg, CD31, and CD34)

Metastatic Chordoma
- Also negative for vascular markers (CD31, CD34)
- Negative history of chordoma elsewhere

DIAGNOSTIC CHECKLIST

Clinically Relevant Pathologic Features
- Gross appearance

Pathologic Interpretation Pearls
- Chondromyxoid background
- Multiple nodules
- Low mitotic count
- Positive staining for vascular markers

SELECTED REFERENCES

1. Schwartz A et al: [Sclerosing intravascular bronchiolo-alveolar tumor.] Rev Mal Respir. 9(2):219-22, 1992
2. Yousem SA et al: Unusual thoracic manifestations of epithelioid hemangioendothelioma. Arch Pathol Lab Med. 111(5):459-63, 1987
3. Weiss SW et al: Epithelioid hemangioendothelioma and related lesions. Semin Diagn Pathol. 3(4):259-87, 1986
4. Dail DH et al: Intravascular, bronchiolar, and alveolar tumor of the lung (IVBAT). An analysis of twenty cases of a peculiar sclerosing endothelial tumor. Cancer. 51(3):452-64, 1983
5. Bhagavan BS et al: Intravascular bronchiolo-alveolar tumor (IVBAT): A low-grade sclerosing epithelioid angiosarcoma of lung. Am J Surg Pathol. 6(1):41-52, 1982
6. Weiss SW et al: Epithelioid hemangioendothelioma: a vascular tumor often mistaken for a carcinoma. Cancer. 50(5):970-81, 1982
7. Weldon-Linne CM et al: Angiogenic nature of the "intravascular bronchioloalveolar tumor" of the lung: an electron microscopic study. Arch Pathol Lab Med. 105(4):174-9, 1981
8. Corrin B et al: Histogenesis of the so-called "intravascular bronchioloalveolar tumour". J Pathol. 128(3):163-7, 1979

EPITHELIOID HEMANGIOENDOTHELIOMA

Microscopic Features

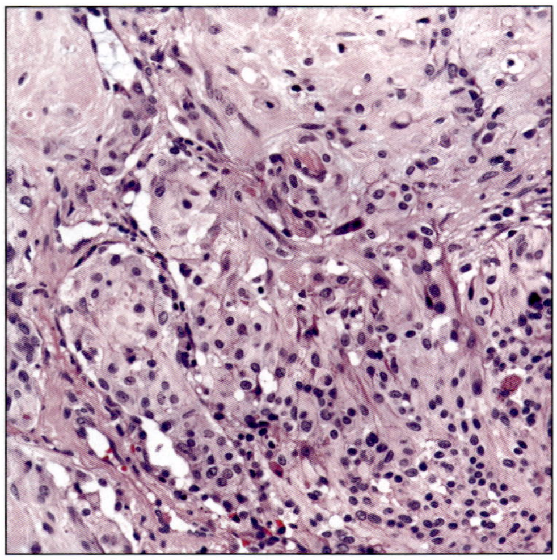

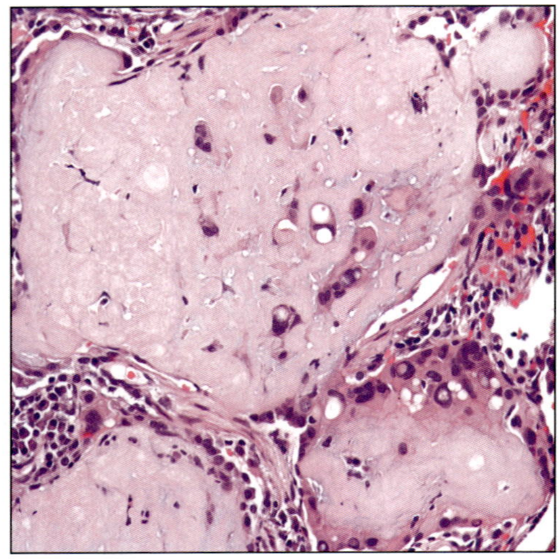

(Left) *This epithelioid hemangioendothelioma shows more cellular areas in which the chondromyxoid background is not that apparent. This growth pattern may be seen in other nonvascular tumors of the lung.* ***(Right)*** *High-power view of epithelioid hemangioendothelioma of the lung shows clusters of epithelioid cells embedded in a hyalinized acellular stroma. The epithelioid cells do not show nuclear atypia or mitotic activity.*

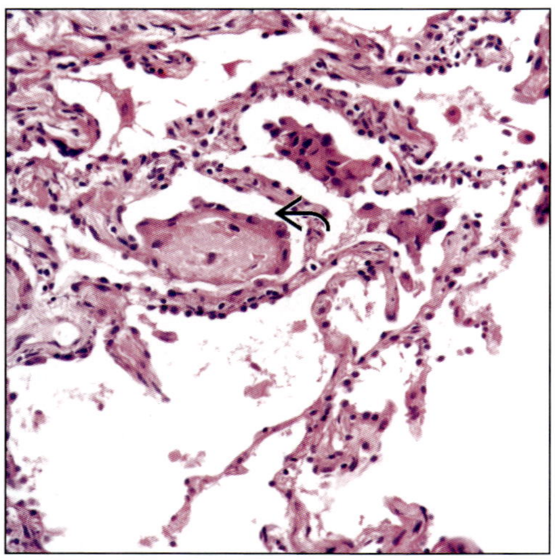

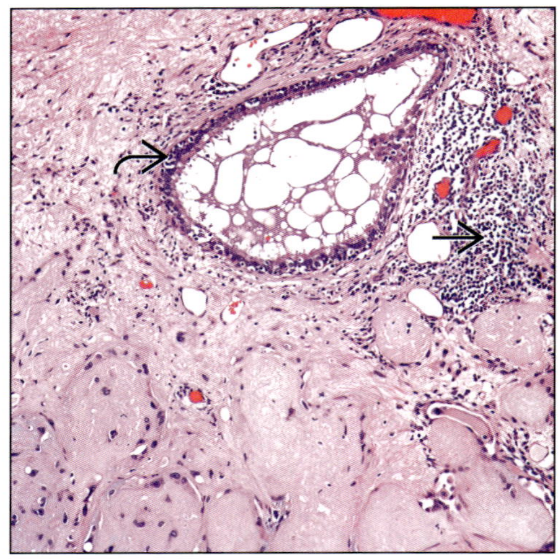

(Left) *Epithelioid hemangioendothelioma of the lung shows a polypoid tumor nodule filling an alveolar space. This histological feature gave rise to the initial interpretation of EH as an intravascular bronchioloalveolar tumor (IVBAT).* ***(Right)*** *EH of the lung shows extensive hyalinized areas with low cellularity. In addition, there is an entrapped epithelial structure, which may suggest a biphasic neoplasm. Note the adjacent inflammatory infiltrate.*

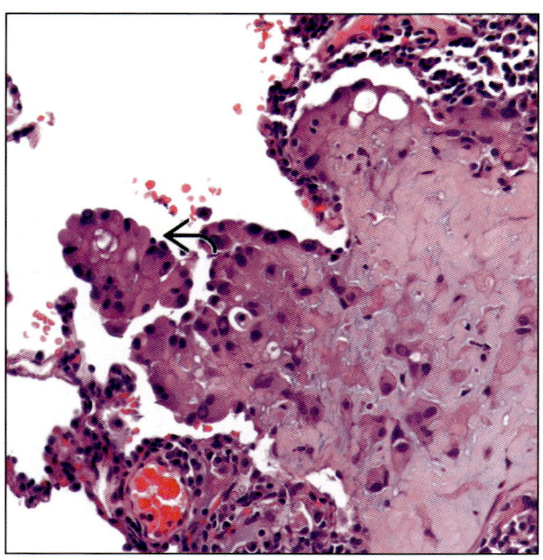

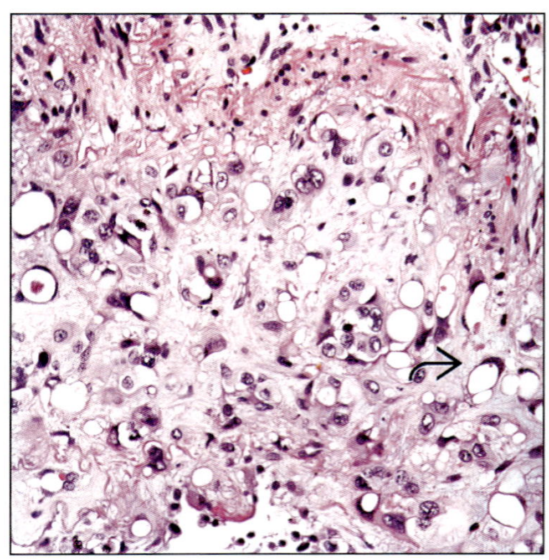

(Left) *In some areas, epithelioid hemangioendothelioma may appear as forming papillary structures as illustrated in this case. However, note the chondromyxoid background that is characteristic of EH.* ***(Right)*** *This epithelioid hemangioendothelioma shows more cellular areas, some of the cells resembling signet ring cells. Thus, this tumor may easily be confused for a true epithelial malignancy.*

EPITHELIOID HEMANGIOENDOTHELIOMA

Microscopic Features

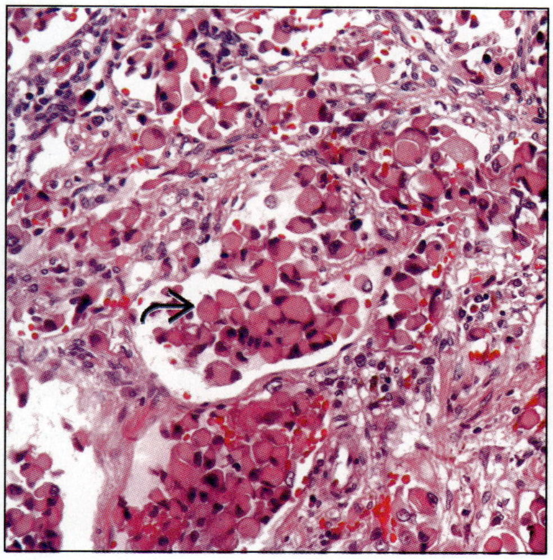

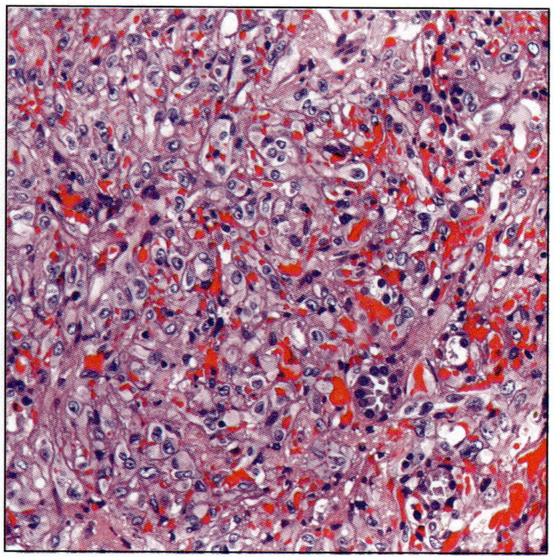

(Left) *Epithelioid hemangioendothelioma of the lung shows cells with features of rhabdoid cells. This histologic feature may be easily confused for a metastatic sarcoma or carcinoma of the lung.* ***(Right)*** *EH of the lung is shown predominantly composed of spindle cells and extravasated red cells. Note the solid growth pattern and the absence of hyalinized areas.*

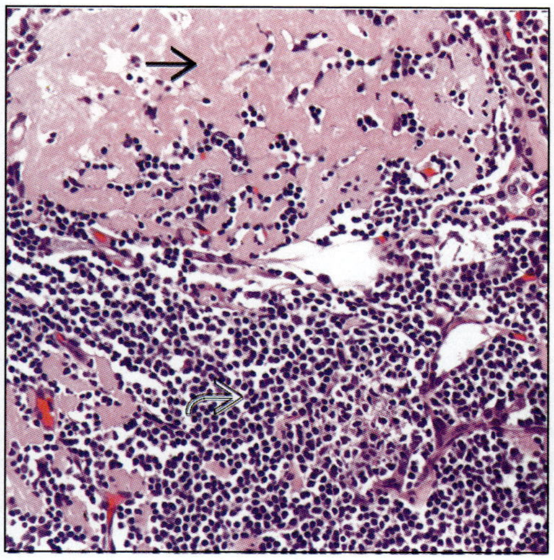

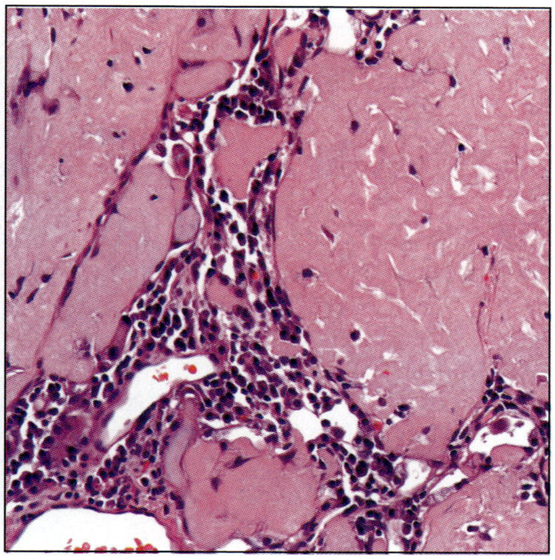

(Left) *High-power view shows a prominent hyalinized area in an EH of lung. In addition, an inflammatory infiltrate is also present. This feature may also be confused with cases of amyloid deposition in the lung.* ***(Right)*** *High magnification shows the presence of plasma cells adjacent to areas of markedly amorphous material closely mimicking amyloid deposition.*

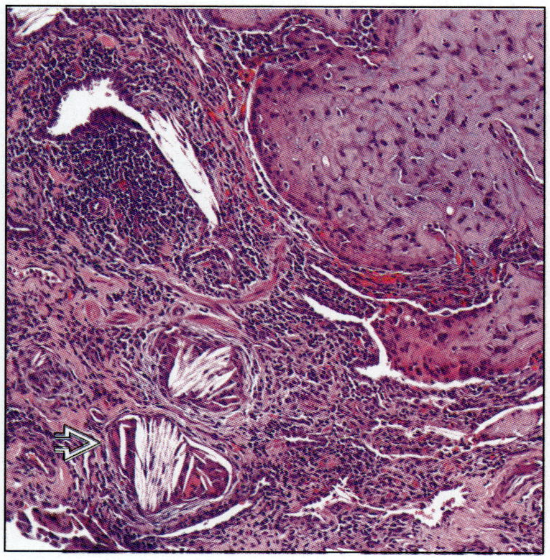

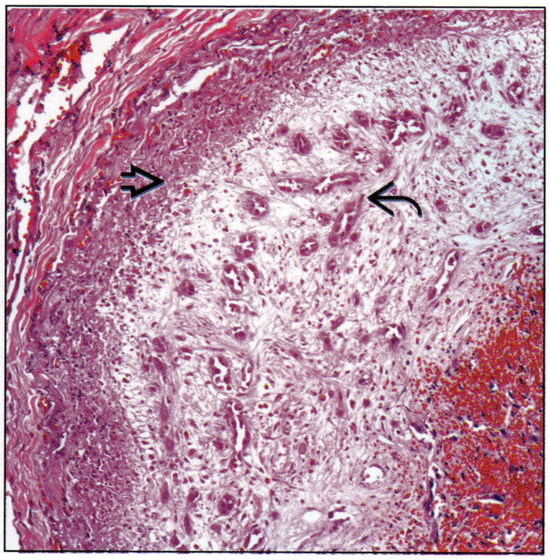

(Left) *The inflammatory changes present in EH of the lung may include cholesterol cleft granulomas and chronic inflammatory cells, namely plasma cells.* ***(Right)*** *In some unusual cases, EH may involve pulmonary vessels. The cellular proliferation is actually forming gland-like structures that may be confused with an adenocarcinoma.*

ANGIOSARCOMA

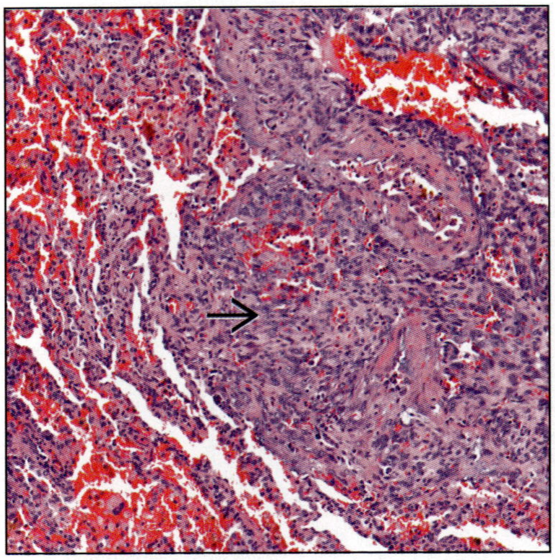

Primary angiosarcoma of the lung shows a spindle cellular proliferation ⇒ replacing lung parenchyma. One is still able to observe extravasated red cells.

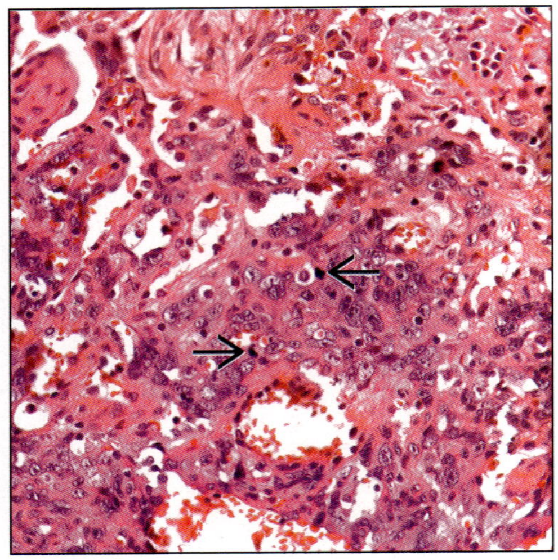

High-power view of a pulmonary angiosarcoma shows prominent nuclear atypia and increased mitotic activity ⇒.

TERMINOLOGY

Synonyms

- Hemangiosarcoma

Definitions

- Malignant vascular neoplasm

ETIOLOGY/PATHOGENESIS

Environmental Exposure

- Some cases have been linked to radiation and others to farming

CLINICAL ISSUES

Epidemiology

- Incidence
  - It is estimated that angiosarcomas account for 0.02% of all lung tumors
- Age
  - Tumor occurs in any age group
- Gender
  - No predilection

Presentation

- Shortness of breath
- Hemoptysis
- Pulmonary hemorrhage
- Chest pain

Treatment

- Surgical approaches
  - Lobectomy
  - Chemotherapy
  - Radiation

Prognosis

- Poor
- Widespread metastasis

MACROSCOPIC FEATURES

General Features

- Single or multiple pulmonary nodules
- Ill-defined tumor nodule
- Hemorrhagic tumor nodule

Size

- Varies from 1 to > 5 cm in diameter

MICROSCOPIC PATHOLOGY

Histologic Features

- Epithelioid malignant cells forming vascular channels
- Walls of vessels lined with hobnail-like cells
- Miotic figures are common
- Spindle cell component
- Areas of hemorrhage
- Areas of necrosis

Predominant Pattern/Injury Type

- Hemorrhagic

Predominant Cell/Compartment Type

- Epithelioid

DIFFERENTIAL DIAGNOSIS

Epithelioid Hemangioendothelioma

- Does not show increased mitotic activity
- Extensive areas of necrosis are not a component
- Characteristically shows chondromyxoid background
- Shares similar immunophenotype with angiosarcoma

Carcinoma

- Shows negative staining with vascular markers

Key Facts

Terminology
- Hemangiosarcoma

Clinical Issues
- Symptomatology
  - Shortness of breath
  - Hemoptysis
  - Frank pulmonary hemorrhage

Macroscopic Features
- Single or multiple pulmonary nodules

Microscopic Pathology
- Epithelioid malignant cells forming vascular channels
- Walls of vessels lined with hobnail-like cells
- Miotic figures are common
- Areas of hemorrhage
- Areas of necrosis

Top Differential Diagnoses
- Epithelioid hemangioendothelioma
  - Lacks increased mitotic activity
  - Extensive areas of necrosis are not a feature
  - Characteristically shows chondromyxoid background
  - Shares similar immunophenotype with angiosarcoma
- Carcinoma
  - Carcinoma will show negative staining with vascular markers
- Metastatic angiosarcoma
  - Clinical history is most important feature
  - Primary and metastatic angiosarcoma may share similar presentation

Immunohistochemistry

Antibody	Reactivity	Staining Pattern	Comment
CD31	Positive	Cytoplasmic	In the vascular component
CD34	Positive	Cytoplasmic	In the vascular component
ULEX-1	Positive	Cytoplasmic	In the vascular component
FVIIIRAg	Positive	Cytoplasmic	
CK-PAN	Negative	Cytoplasmic	May be positive in rare cases
S100	Negative		
Desmin	Negative		
CEA-M	Negative		
Actin-HHF-35	Negative		
EMA	Negative		

Metastatic Angiosarcoma
- Clinical history is most important feature
- Primary and metastatic angiosarcoma may share similar presentation

DIAGNOSTIC CHECKLIST

Clinically Relevant Pathologic Features
- Gross appearance

Pathologic Interpretation Pearls
- Epithelioid or spindle cell neoplasm with vascular differentiation

SELECTED REFERENCES

1. Wilson R et al: Complete radiographic response of primary pulmonary angiosarcomas following gemcitabine and taxotere. Lung Cancer. 61(1):131-6, 2008
2. Herrak L et al: [Primary pulmonary angiosarcoma.] Rev Mal Respir. 24(1):73-6, 2007
3. Saint-Blancard P et al: [Three-year survival after treatment of a primary pulmonary angiosarcoma.] Rev Pneumol Clin. 63(1):55-8, 2007
4. Patsios D et al: Epithelioid angiosarcoma of the lung: a rare late complication of Lucite plombage. Br J Radiol. 79(943):e36-9, 2006
5. Bouhaouala MH et al: [Primary pulmonary angiosarcoma.] Rev Pneumol Clin. 61(2):115-8, 2005
6. Lund L et al: Epithelioid angiosarcoma involving the lungs. Arch Pathol Lab Med. 129(1):e7-10, 2005
7. Pandit SA et al: Primary angiosarcoma of the lung. Ann Diagn Pathol. 9(5):302-4, 2005
8. Engelke C et al: Pulmonary haemangiosarcoma with main pulmonary artery thrombosis imitating subacute pulmonary embolism with infarction. Br J Radiol. 77(919):623-5, 2004
9. López L et al: [Persistent hemoptysis secondary to extensive epithelioid angiosarcoma.] Arch Bronconeumol. 40(4):188-90, 2004
10. Sheppard MN et al: Primary epithelioid angiosarcoma of the lung presenting as pulmonary hemorrhage. Hum Pathol. 28(3):383-5, 1997
11. Segal SL et al: Angiosarcoma presenting as diffuse alveolar hemorrhage. Chest. 94(1):214-6, 1988
12. Palvio DH et al: Primary angiosarcoma of the lung presenting as intractable hemoptysis. Thorac Cardiovasc Surg. 35(2):105-7, 1987
13. Yousem SA: Angiosarcoma presenting in the lung. Arch Pathol Lab Med. 110(2):112-5, 1986

ANGIOSARCOMA

Microscopic Features

(Left) *Pulmonary angiosarcoma with prominent papillary-like architecture. This feature is unusual and can be confused with other more common primary lung tumors.* ***(Right)*** *High magnification shows papillary-like structures lined by a neoplastic cellular proliferation composed of rather small cells. Mitotic activity is not prominent.*

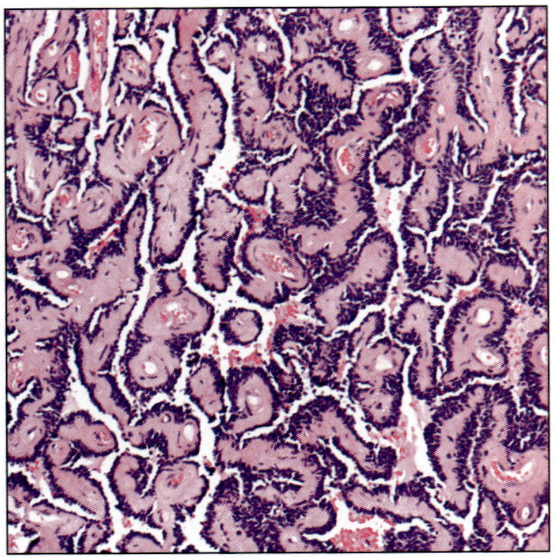

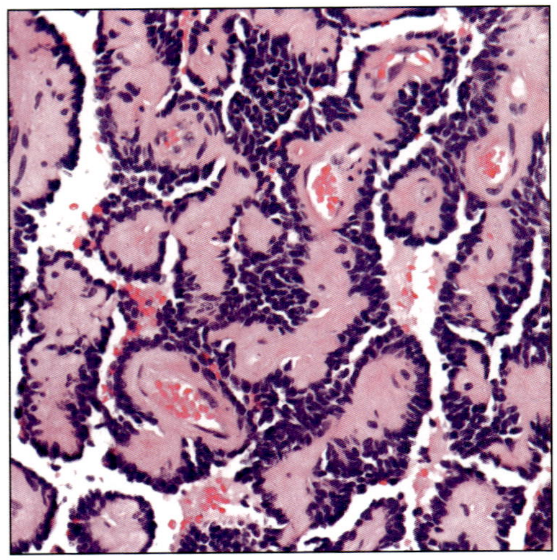

(Left) *Angiosarcoma ↷ is seen involving a large pulmonary vessel ⇨. Although unusual, such a feature may aid in the diagnosis of angiosarcoma.* ***(Right)*** *Low-power view of a pulmonary angiosarcoma shows the classical pattern of dilated vascular spaces replaced by tumoral cells ↷ mixed with fresh blood →.*

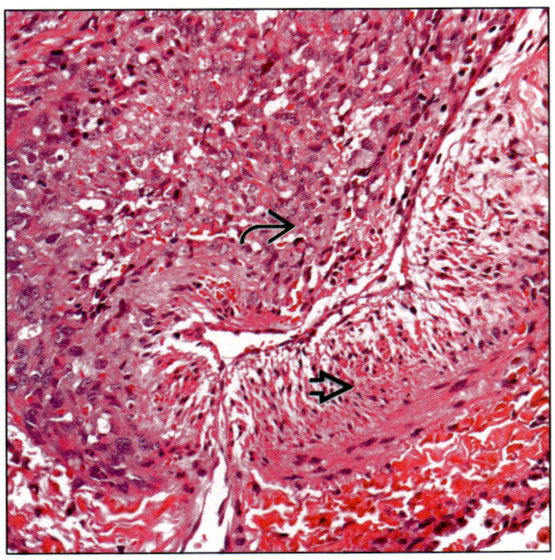

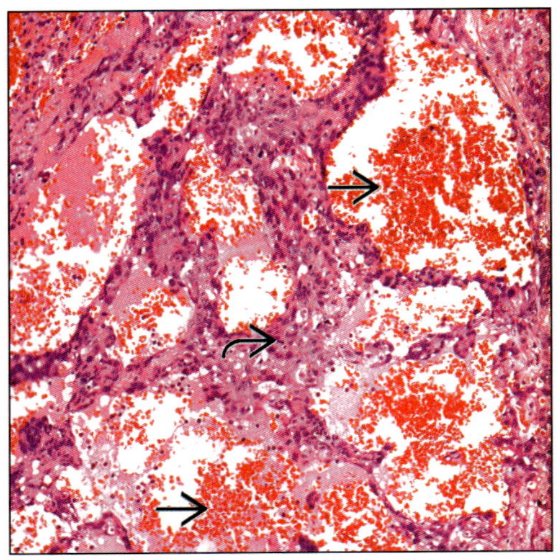

(Left) *More conventional areas of angiosarcoma show the typical vascular proliferation with flattened endothelial cells. Marked nuclear atypia and mitotic activity are not present.* ***(Right)*** *Angiosarcoma with solid areas. This histological feature may be confused for an epithelial tumor, namely, neuroendocrine carcinoma.*

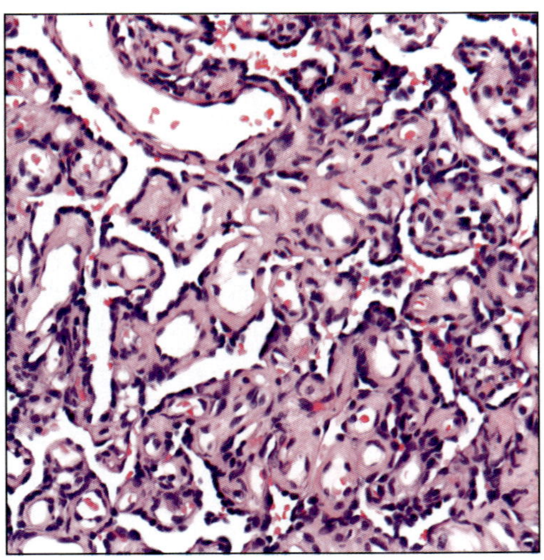

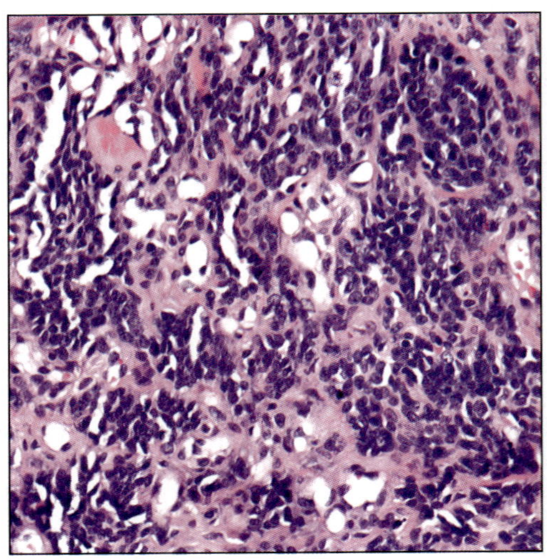

Microscopic Features

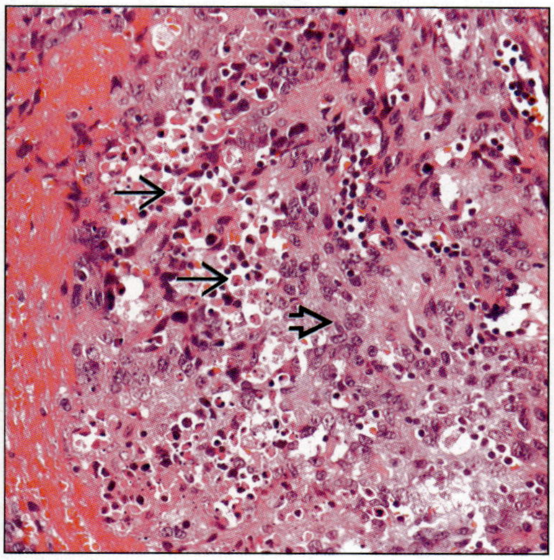
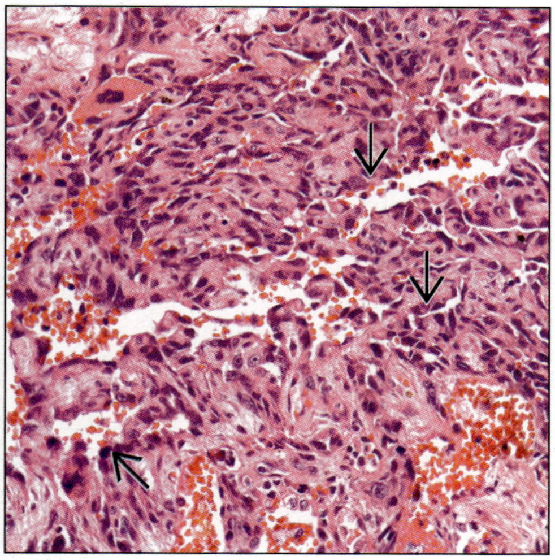

(Left) Pulmonary angiosarcoma shows single-cell necrosis ⇨ and solid areas composed of oval medium-sized cells ⇨. Similar features may be seen in high-grade carcinomas of the lung. The vascular nature of the tumor is not apparent in this growth pattern. **(Right)** Pulmonary angiosarcoma shows vasoformative areas ⇨ and prominent nuclear atypia. The presence of vasoformative areas should alert one of the possibility of angiosarcoma. Vascular markers should be helpful.

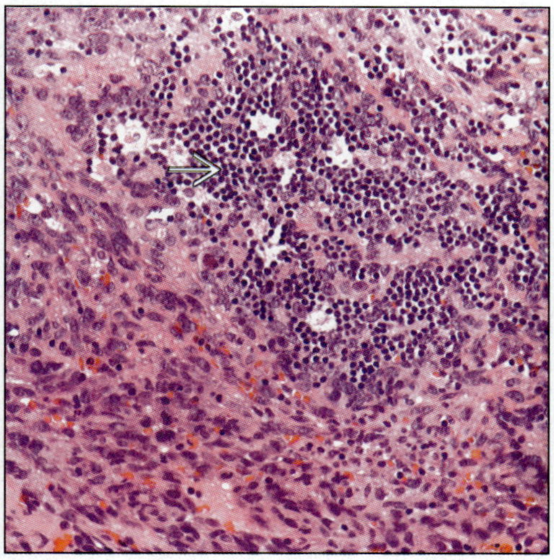
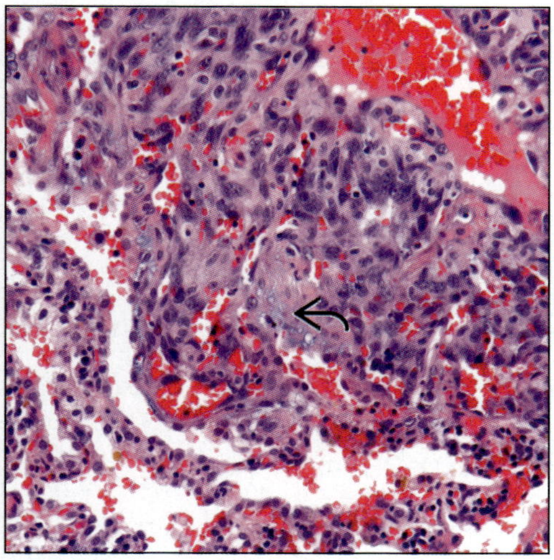

(Left) Pulmonary angiosarcoma with prominent spindle cell features and focal areas of inflammatory infiltrate ➡. The presence of inflammatory changes associated with angiosarcoma is not common, except in areas of necrosis. **(Right)** This angiosarcoma is composed of spindle cells with only focal areas that show some myxoid change ⇨, which may raise the possibility of hemangioendothelioma.

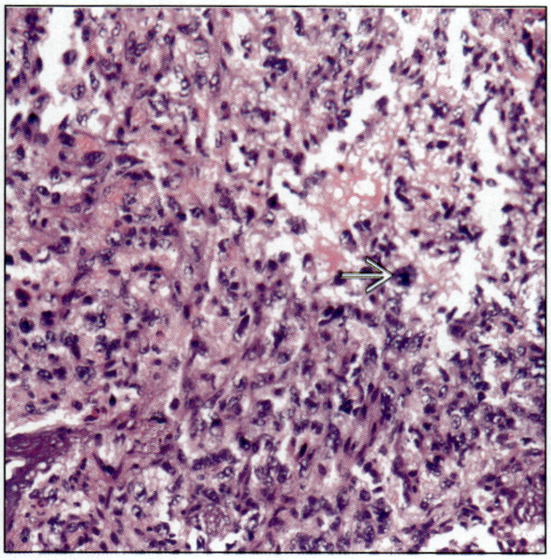
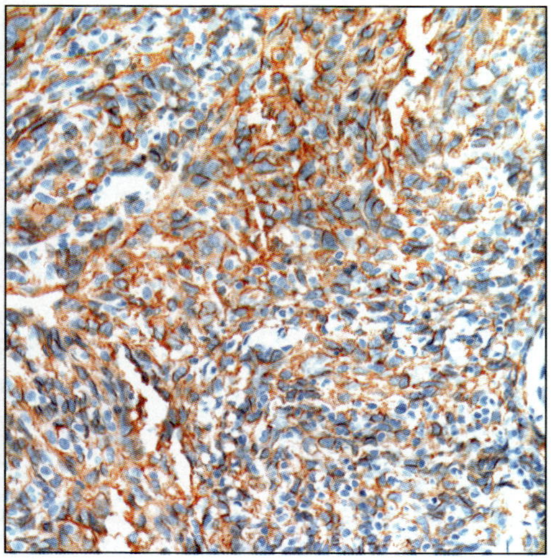

(Left) High-power view of a pulmonary angiosarcoma shows prominent nuclear atypia and atypical mitotic figures ➡. These features are more in keeping with a high-grade angiosarcoma. **(Right)** CD31 immunohistochemical stain shows positive staining in tumor cells in a pulmonary angiosarcoma. The use of immunohistochemical vascular markers is important to exclude other primary epithelial or mesenchymal tumors of the lung.

KAPOSI SARCOMA

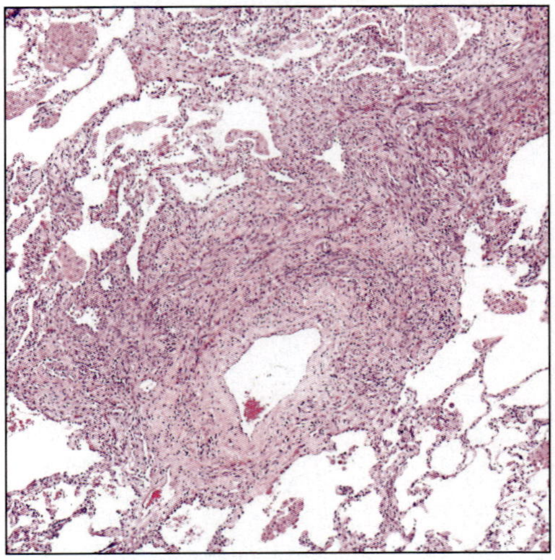

Scanning magnification in pulmonary involvement by Kaposi sarcoma shows characteristic perivascular distribution of the atypical spindle cell proliferation extending into adjoining alveolar septa.

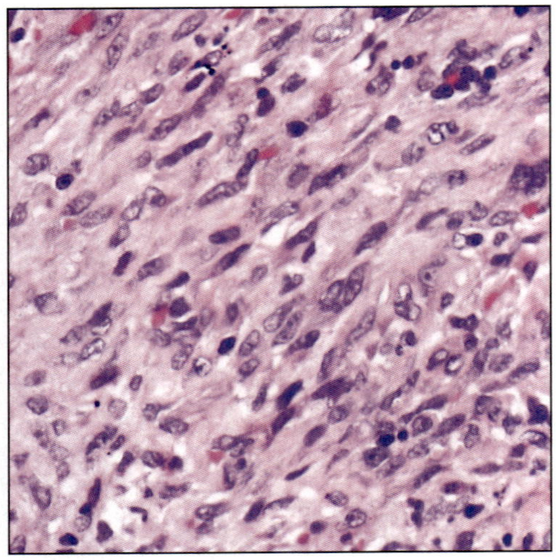

Higher magnification of pulmonary Kaposi sarcoma shows dense atypical spindle cell proliferation admixed with a few scattered inflammatory cells. Notice the scattered red blood cells in the interstitium.

TERMINOLOGY

Abbreviations

- Kaposi sarcoma (KS)

Definitions

- Low-grade spindle cell sarcoma derived from vascular endothelial cells

ETIOLOGY/PATHOGENESIS

Pathogenesis

- Commonly associated with HIV infection in patients with AIDS
- Associated with human herpes virus 8 (HHV-8) infection

CLINICAL ISSUES

Epidemiology

- Incidence
  - High incidence in homosexual men and intravenous drug abusers with AIDS
  - May also affect immunosuppressed patients and transplant patients
- Age
  - 20-40 years of age

Presentation

- Cough
- Dyspnea
- Hemoptysis

Treatment

- Adjuvant therapy
  - Combination chemotherapy (doxorubicin, bleomycin, and vincristine)
- Radiation
  - Only used for palliation in advanced cases
- Antiviral compounds
  - Zidovudine, interferon, and other antiviral compounds

Prognosis

- Poor prognosis; most patients die within 2 years of diagnosis
- Median survival is slightly better for responders to chemotherapy

IMAGE FINDINGS

General Features

- Bilateral interstitial infiltrates with ill-defined nodularity
- Discrete, localized intraparenchymatous mass that may be associated with a bronchus
- Mediastinal lymphadenopathy
- Bilateral pleural effusion

MACROSCOPIC FEATURES

General Features

- Ill-defined, bluish-red intraparenchymatous nodules

MICROSCOPIC PATHOLOGY

Histologic Features

- Lesions follow intrapulmonary fibrous septa with perivascular and peribronchial distribution
- Monotonous spindle cell proliferation with fascicular growth pattern intersecting at right angles
- Frequent anastomosing and slit-like vascular spaces containing abundant extravasated red blood cells
- Abundant deposition of hemosiderin pigment in stroma

Cytologic Features

- Spindle cells show mild to moderate cytologic atypia

KAPOSI SARCOMA

Key Facts

Etiology/Pathogenesis
- Commonly associated with HIV infection in patients with AIDS
- Associated with human herpes virus 8 (HHV-8) infection

Clinical Issues
- High incidence in homosexual men and intravenous drug abusers with AIDS
- May also affect immunosuppressed patients and transplant patients
- Cough
- Dyspnea
- Hemoptysis
- 20-40 years of age

Image Findings
- Bilateral interstitial infiltrates with ill-defined nodularity
- Discrete, localized intraparenchymatous mass that may be associated with a bronchus

Microscopic Pathology
- Monotonous spindle cell proliferation with fascicular growth pattern intersecting at right angles
- Frequent anastomosing and slit-like vascular spaces containing abundant extravasated red blood cells
- Spindle cells show mild to moderate cytologic atypia

Ancillary Tests
- Spindle tumor cells are positive for CD34 and CD31
- Tumor cells show strong nuclear positivity for HHV8 antibody

- Cell nuclei are hyperchromatic and may show occasional small nucleoli
- Scattered mitoses are commonly present
- Dense extracellular hyaline globules may be seen scattered in interstitium
- Spindle cell population may be admixed with inflammatory cell elements, including small lymphocytes, plasma cells, and histiocytes

ANCILLARY TESTS

Immunohistochemistry
- Spindle tumor cells are positive for CD34 and CD31
- Tumor cells are usually negative for FVIIIRAg
- Tumor cells show strong nuclear positivity for HHV8 antibody
- Nuclear transcription factor, FLI1, is also positive though not specific

Cytogenetics
- Random chromosomal aberrations have been reported, including gain of 8q and 1q and loss of 3p
- Rearrangements of 7q22, 8p11, 13q11, and 19q13

Molecular Genetics
- Comparative genomic hybridization studies have shown recurrent gains at 11q13
- Amplification studies have identified target genes *FGF4* and *FGF3*, and rearrangements of *KRAS2* and *TP53*

DIFFERENTIAL DIAGNOSIS

Leiomyosarcoma
- Fascicular spindle cell proliferation of cells displaying blunt ends and intracytoplasmic vacuoles
- Commonly present as large intraparenchymatous tumors rather than as multiple small nodules
- Tumor cells are negative for vascular markers and show strong positivity for muscle markers (desmin, actin, h-caldesmon, calponin, etc.)
- Spindle cells contain abundant cytoplasmic microfilaments with focal densities on electron microscopy

Fibrosarcoma
- Fascicular spindle cell proliferation with prominent stromal sclerosis
- Commonly presents as large intraparenchymatous tumor rather than as multiple small nodules
- Tumor cells are negative for vascular markers (CD31, CD34) and only stain positive for vimentin

Synovial Sarcoma
- Fascicular spindle cell proliferation composed of monotonous atypical spindle cells with scant stroma
- May show prominent hemangiopericytic growth pattern but lacks abundance of anastomosing small vessels and extravasated red blood cells
- Commonly presents as large intraparenchymatous tumor rather than as multiple small nodules
- Tumor cells are positive for cytokeratin, EMA, Bcl-2, and CD99 and negative for vascular markers (CD31, CD34)

DIAGNOSTIC CHECKLIST

Clinically Relevant Pathologic Features
- Multifocality and bilaterality of lesions with interstitial pattern of distribution in HIV(+) patients

Pathologic Interpretation Pearls
- Ill-defined nodular lesions composed of spindle cell fascicles with abundant extravasated red blood cells
- Presence of scattered hyalin globules admixed with spindle cells

SELECTED REFERENCES

1. Weissferdt A et al: Primary vascular tumors of the lungs: a review. Ann Diagn Pathol. 14(4):296-308, 2010
2. Garay SM et al: Pulmonary manifestations of Kaposi's sarcoma. 1987. Chest. 136(5 Suppl):e30, 2009

KAPOSI SARCOMA

Histologic Features

*(**Left**) Scanning magnification of a pulmonary lesion in Kaposi sarcoma shows perivascular distribution of the process. There is a dense spindle cell proliferation concentrically surrounding the entire wall of a small-caliber vessel ⇨. (**Right**) Higher magnification of a pulmonary lesion in Kaposi sarcoma shows dense perivascular spindle cell proliferation → that is sharply circumscribed and separated from the surrounding uninvolved lung parenchyma.*

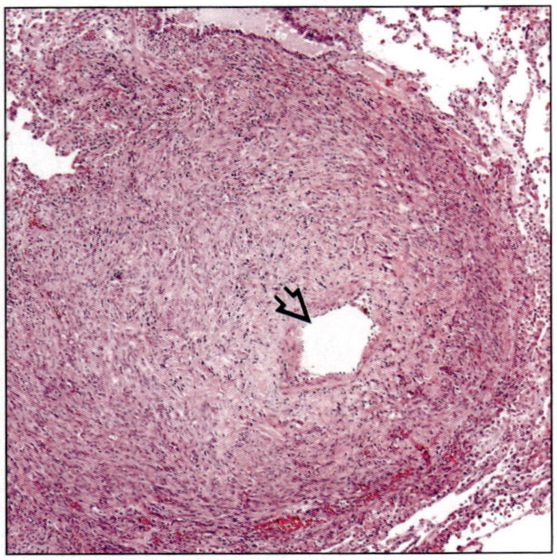

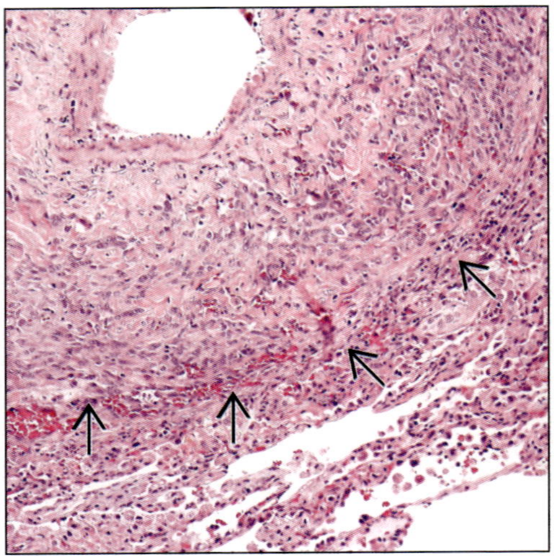

*(**Left**) Pulmonary lesion in Kaposi sarcoma shows fascicles of spindle cells containing a few scattered mitotic figures. There are numerous extravasated red blood cells scattered in the interstitium. The presence of these extravasated red blood cells should raise the possibility of Kaposi sarcoma in the differential diagnosis. (**Right**) Higher magnification of a pulmonary lesion in Kaposi sarcoma shows spindle cell proliferation abutting the wall of a bronchiole →.*

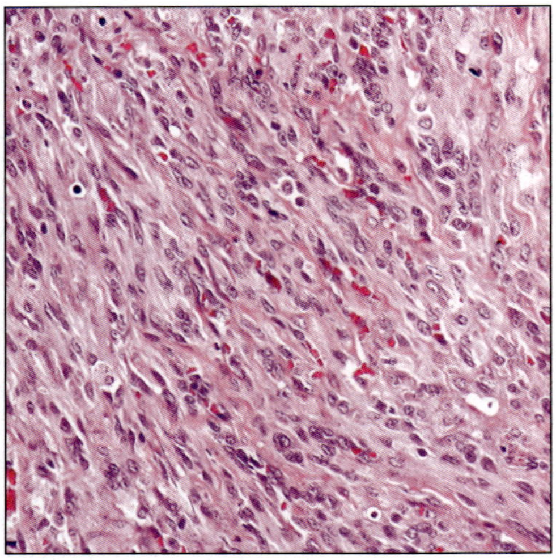

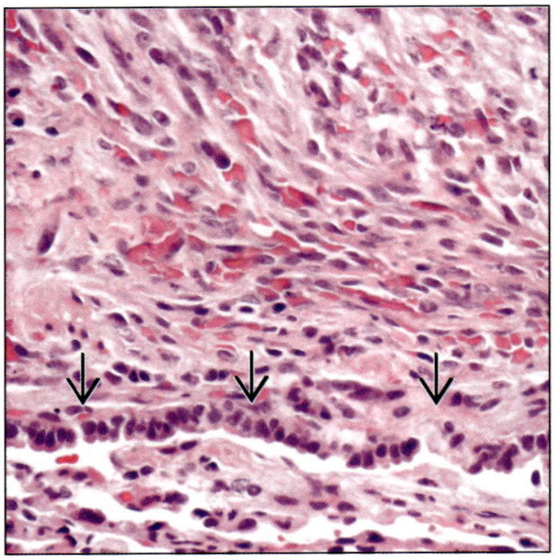

*(**Left**) High magnification of a pulmonary lesion in Kaposi sarcoma shows atypical spindle cell proliferation surrounding ectatic vascular spaces and vascular slits. The cells show scattered mitoses and occasional scattered extravasated red blood cells. (**Right**) High magnification in a pulmonary lesion of Kaposi sarcoma shows spindle cell proliferation displaying mild cytologic atypia with scattered nuclear chromatin and small eosinophilic nucleoli. Notice the single mitotic figure ⇨.*

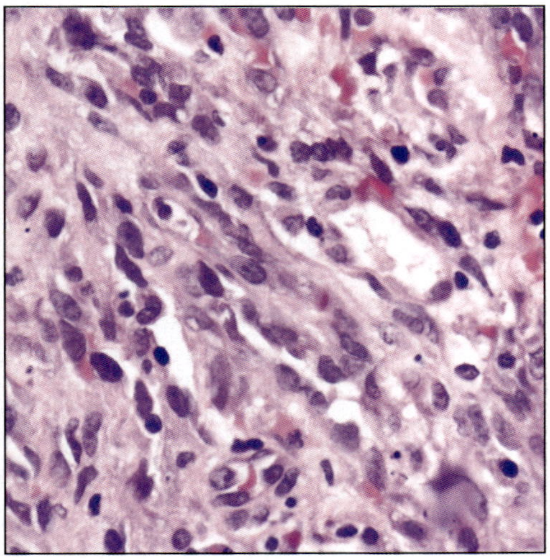

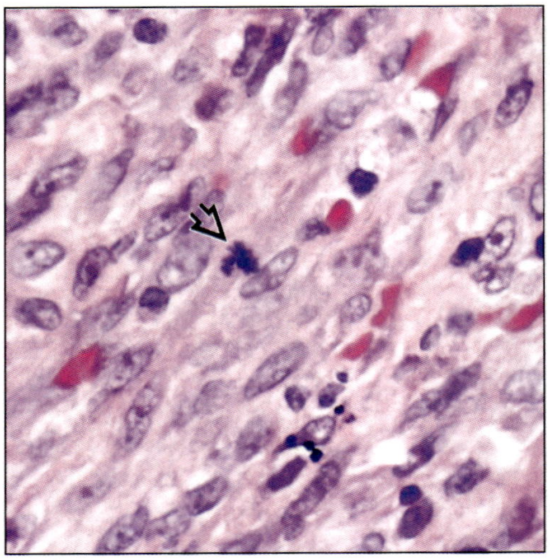

Histologic Features

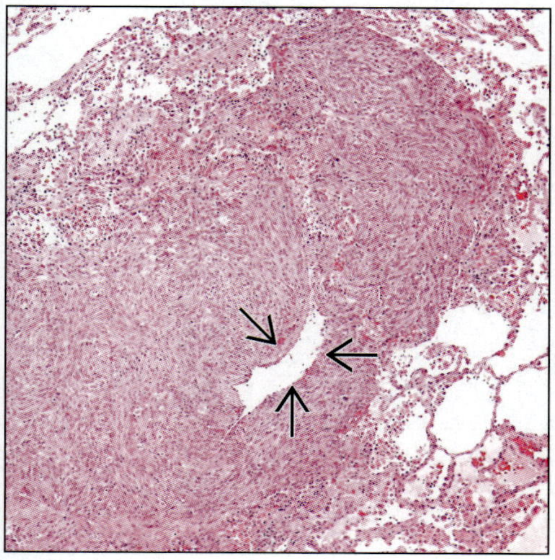

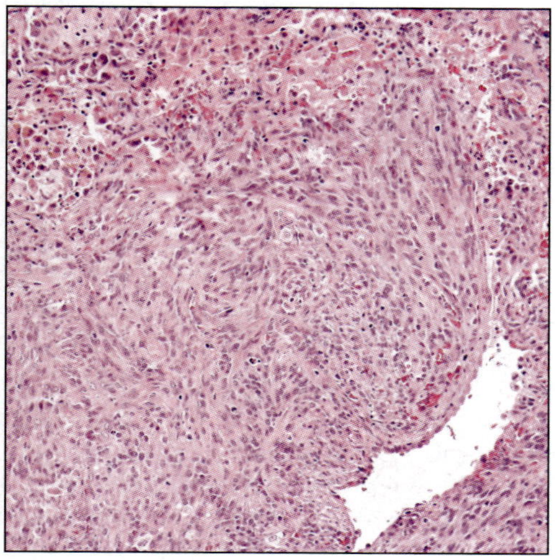

(Left) Scanning magnification of a pulmonary lesion in Kaposi sarcoma shows perivascular proliferation forming a well-defined tumor nodule replacing the lung parenchyma. Notice the small dilated vessel → in the center of the nodule. *(Right)* Higher magnification of a pulmonary lesion in Kaposi sarcoma shows dense perivascular cellular proliferation composed of fascicles of spindle cells with minimal cytologic atypia that intersect at 90° angles.

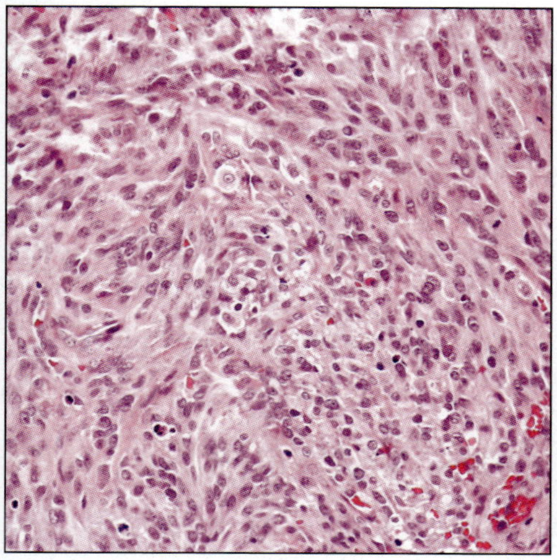

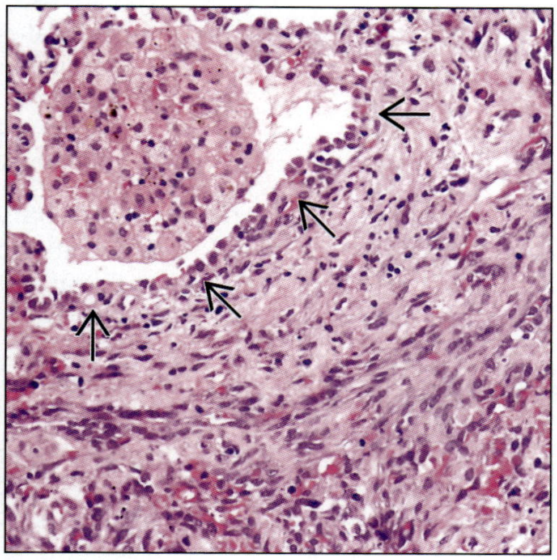

(Left) High magnification of a pulmonary lesion in Kaposi sarcoma shows dense spindle cell proliferation forming fascicles that intersect at right angles. This histologic appearance can be mistaken for a benign or malignant smooth muscle proliferation (i.e., leiomyoma, low-grade leiomyosarcoma). *(Right)* High magnification of a pulmonary lesion in Kaposi sarcoma shows spindle cell proliferation with minimal atypia and extravasated red blood cells surrounding a dilated airspace →.

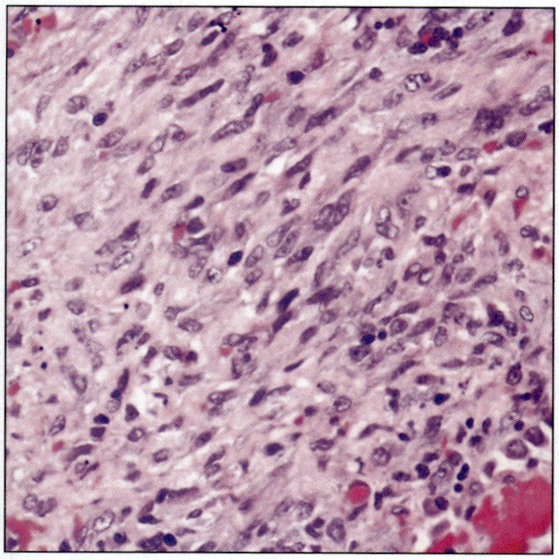

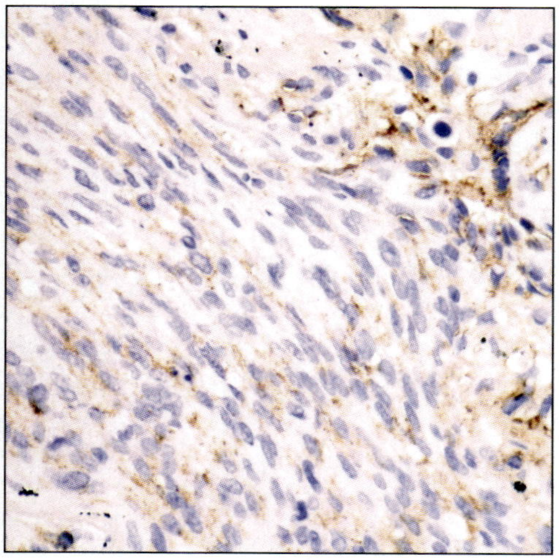

(Left) Higher magnification of a pulmonary lesion in Kaposi sarcoma shows a dense spindle cell population showing oval to spindled nuclei with minimal cytologic atypia. This histologic appearance can be mistaken for other types of low-grade spindle cell neoplasms. *(Right)* Immunohistochemical staining of a pulmonary lesion of Kaposi sarcoma for the vascular endothelial-related marker, CD31, shows faint positivity in many of the proliferating spindle cells.

PULMONARY ARTERY SARCOMA

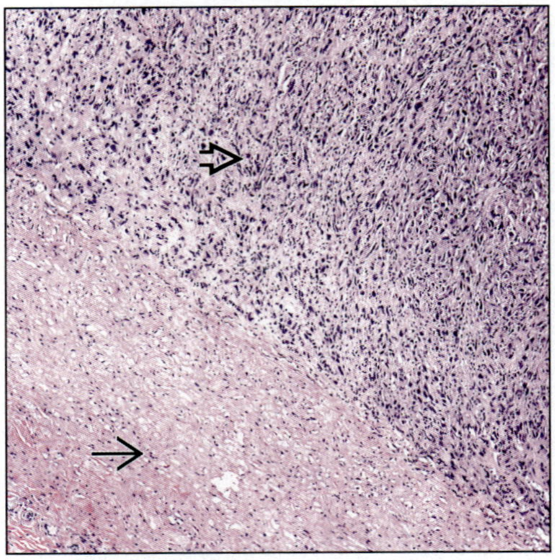

Pulmonary artery sarcoma shows a high-grade sarcoma ⇨ in close association with the wall of the pulmonary artery ⇨. Identification of the pulmonary vessel is essential for the diagnosis.

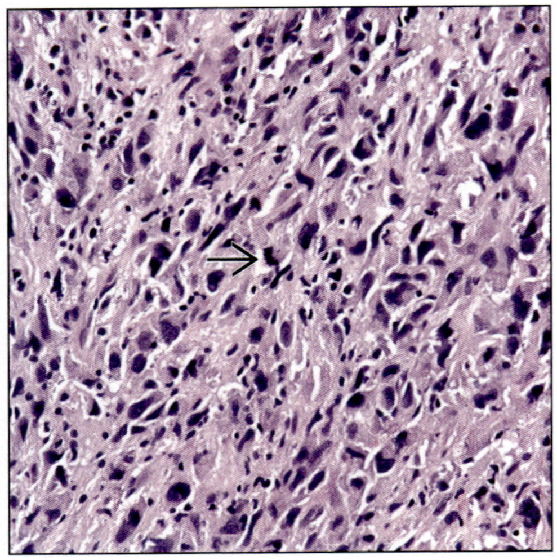

High-grade sarcoma shows extensive areas of pleomorphic cells and atypical mitotic figures ⇨. In many cases, the type of sarcoma is unclassified.

TERMINOLOGY

Abbreviations

- Pulmonary artery sarcoma (PAS)

Synonyms

- Intimal sarcoma

Definitions

- Malignant mesenchymal tumor originating from wall of pulmonary trunk

ETIOLOGY/PATHOGENESIS

Etiology

- Has been suggested to arises from pluripotential cells
- Most probably arises from pulmonary trunk

CLINICAL ISSUES

Epidemiology

- Incidence
  - Rare tumors that represent < 1% of all malignant mesenchymal tumors of lung
- Age
  - Usually occurs in adults
- Gender
  - No gender predilection has been observed in these tumors

Presentation

- Cough
- Chest pain
- Shortness of breath
- Fatigue
- Syncope
- Often confused for other medical conditions, such as pulmonary hypertension, pneumonia, or asthma

Treatment

- Surgical approaches
  - Lobectomy or pneumonectomy
- Adjuvant therapy
  - Chemotherapy &/or radiation may be of use depending on type of sarcoma

Prognosis

- Intrathoracic metastasis may occur in 50% of patients
- Extrathoracic metastasis may occur in about 15% of patients
- Death may occur in a period of 12 months after initial diagnosis

MACROSCOPIC FEATURES

General Features

- Tumor obliterating lumen of artery
- Identification of pulmonary trunk
- Identification of pulmonary artery
- Polypoid tumor in intraluminal location

Sections to Be Submitted

- Tangential sections to properly evaluate arterial wall

Size

- Tumors vary in size up to > 5 cm in diameter

MICROSCOPIC PATHOLOGY

Histologic Features

- Varied mesenchymal differentiation
  - Angiosarcoma
  - Rhabdomyosarcoma
  - Chondrosarcoma
  - Osteosarcoma
  - Leiomyosarcoma

PULMONARY ARTERY SARCOMA

Key Facts

Terminology
- Synonym: Intimal sarcoma
- Malignant mesenchymal tumor originating from wall of pulmonary trunk

Clinical Issues
- Cough
- Chest pain
- Shortness of breath
- Fatigue
- Syncope

Macroscopic Features
- Most important characteristic is that tumor must be attached to pulmonary artery

Microscopic Pathology
- Varied mesenchymal differentiation
- Angiosarcoma
- Rhabdomyosarcoma
- Chondrosarcoma
- Osteosarcoma
- Leiomyosarcoma

Top Differential Diagnoses
- Metastatic sarcoma
  - Clinical history of extrathoracic tumor should lead toward correct interpretation
- Primary intrapulmonary sarcoma
  - Identification of tumor into lumen of pulmonary artery is hallmark of this tumor

Diagnostic Checklist
- Gross appearance
- Wide spectrum of sarcomatous differentiation

Immunohistochemistry

Antibody	Reactivity	Staining Pattern	Comment
CD31	Positive	Cytoplasmic	If vascular differentiation
CD34	Positive	Cytoplasmic	If vascular differentiation
Myoglobin	Positive	Cytoplasmic	If rhabdomyosarcoma is present
MYOD1	Positive	Cytoplasmic	If rhabdomyosarcoma is present
Desmin	Positive	Cytoplasmic	If muscle differentiation
Muscle specific actin	Positive	Cytoplasmic	If muscle differentiation
S100	Positive	Nuclear	If chondroid differentiation
SOX9	Positive	Nuclear	If chondroid differentiation

Predominant Pattern/Injury Type
- Spindled

Predominant Cell/Compartment Type
- Arterial intima

DIFFERENTIAL DIAGNOSIS

Metastatic Sarcoma
- Clinical history of extrathoracic tumor should lead to correct interpretation

Primary Intrapulmonary Sarcoma
- Identification of tumor growing into lumen of pulmonary artery is hallmark of this tumor

DIAGNOSTIC CHECKLIST

Clinically Relevant Pathologic Features
- Gross appearance

Pathologic Interpretation Pearls
- Tumor obliterating lumen of vessel
- Polypoid tumor protruding into arterial lumen
- Wide spectrum of sarcomatous differentiation

SELECTED REFERENCES

1. Shehatha J et al: Surgical management of extensive pulmonary artery sarcoma. Ann Thorac Surg. 87(4):1269-71, 2009
2. Singla Long S et al: CT features of pulmonary artery sarcoma: critical aid to a challenging diagnosis. Emerg Radiol. Epub ahead of print, 2009
3. Huo L et al: Pulmonary artery sarcoma: a clinicopathologic and immunohistochemical study of 12 cases. Am J Clin Pathol. 125(3):419-24, 2006
4. Huo L et al: Pulmonary artery angiosarcoma: a clinicopathologic and radiological correlation. Ann Diagn Pathol. 9(4):209-14, 2005
5. Okuno T et al: Leiomyosarcoma of the pulmonary vein. Pathol Int. 50(10):839-46, 2000
6. Goldblum JR et al: Epithelioid angiosarcoma of the pulmonary artery. Hum Pathol. 26(11):1275-7, 1995
7. Kimura I et al: Primary osteogenic sarcoma of pulmonary artery. Jpn J Med. 29(1):32-7, 1990
8. Baker PB et al: Pulmonary artery sarcomas. A review and report of a case. Arch Pathol Lab Med. 109(1):35-9, 1985
9. Pain JA et al: Primary leiomyosarcoma of the pulmonary artery. Eur J Respir Dis. 65(2):139-43, 1984

PULMONARY ARTERY SARCOMA

Gross and Microscopic Features

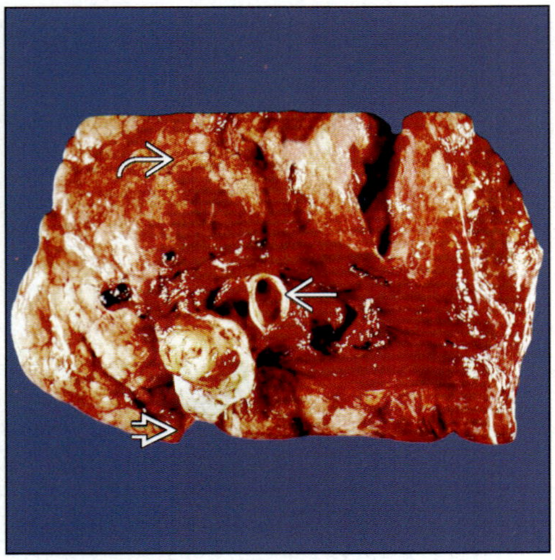

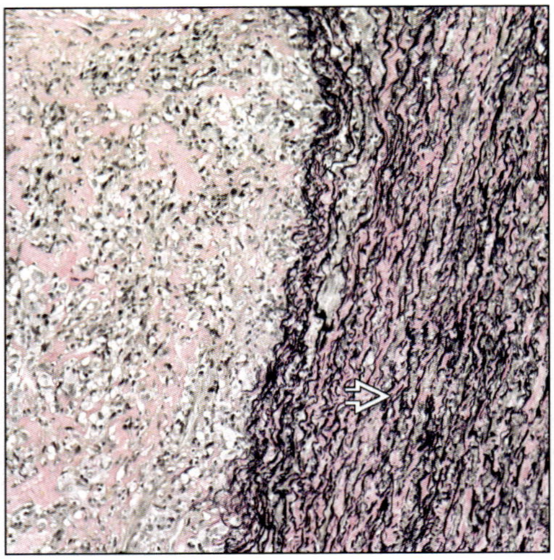

(Left) *Gross photograph shows a primary pulmonary artery sarcoma. It is important to properly identify the vessel with intraluminal tumor, the main airway should be patent and with no evidence of tumor. The remaining pulmonary parenchyma is congested but essentially within normal limits.* ***(Right)*** *In many cases of pulmonary artery sarcoma, special stains, such as elastic stains, may help in the identification of a pulmonary vessel.*

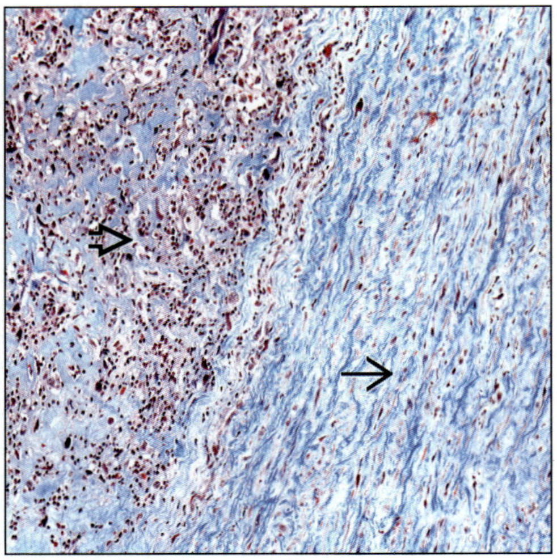

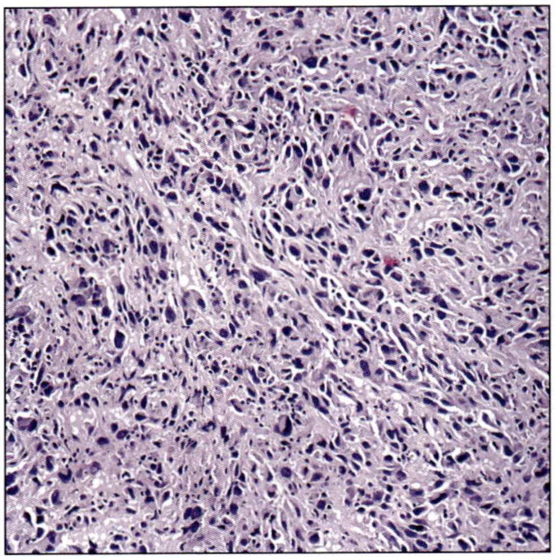

(Left) *Other histochemical stains that may help in separating a tumor from a pulmonary vessel is the Masson stain, which in this illustration clearly separates both components, tumor and vessel.* ***(Right)*** *Undifferentiated high-grade sarcoma shows numerous large and multinucleated cells. In some cases, even with the use of immunohistochemistry, no specific differentiation is encountered.*

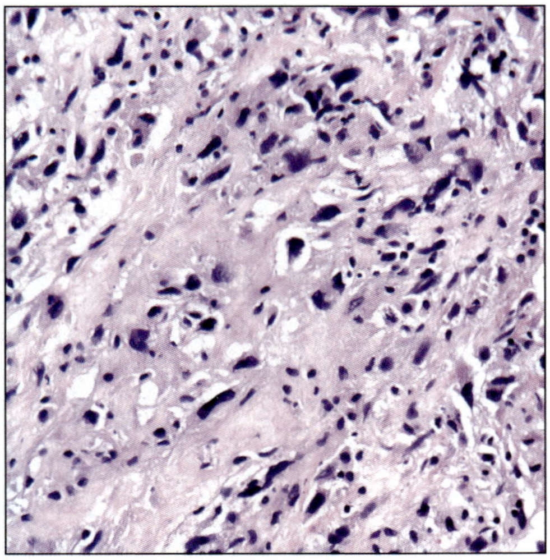

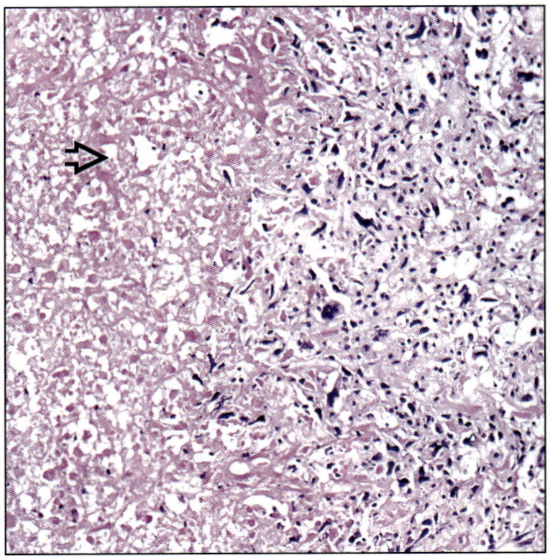

(Left) *Higher magnification shows the presence of spindle and multinucleated cells typical of high-grade sarcomas.* ***(Right)*** *One additional feature that is commonly encountered in cases of pulmonary artery sarcoma is the presence of necrosis. This feature is more common in high-grade sarcomas.*

Microscopic Features

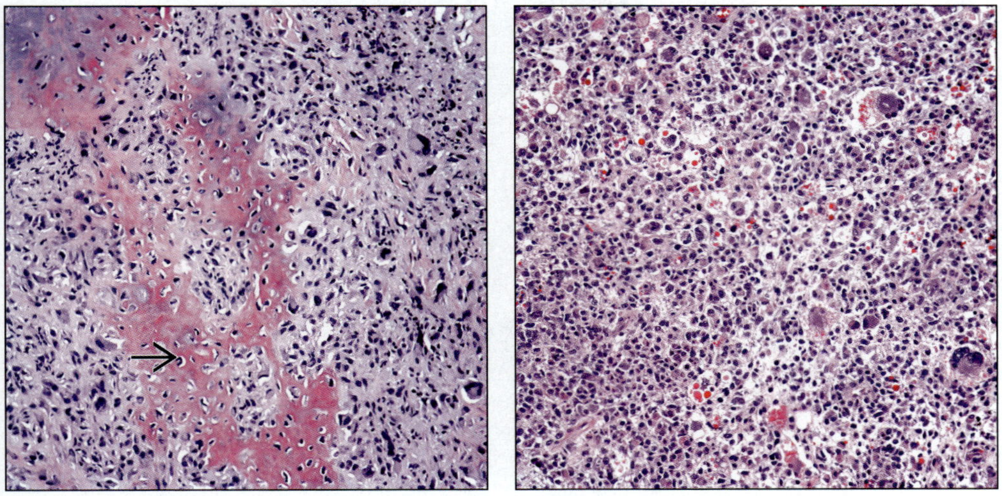

(Left) *High-grade pulmonary artery sarcoma shows osteosarcomatous differentiation. Note the presence of osteoid formation* →. ***(Right)*** *High-grade pulmonary artery sarcoma shows a mixture of multinucleated giant cells and mononuclear malignant cells. This is a common feature of undifferentiated high-grade sarcomas.*

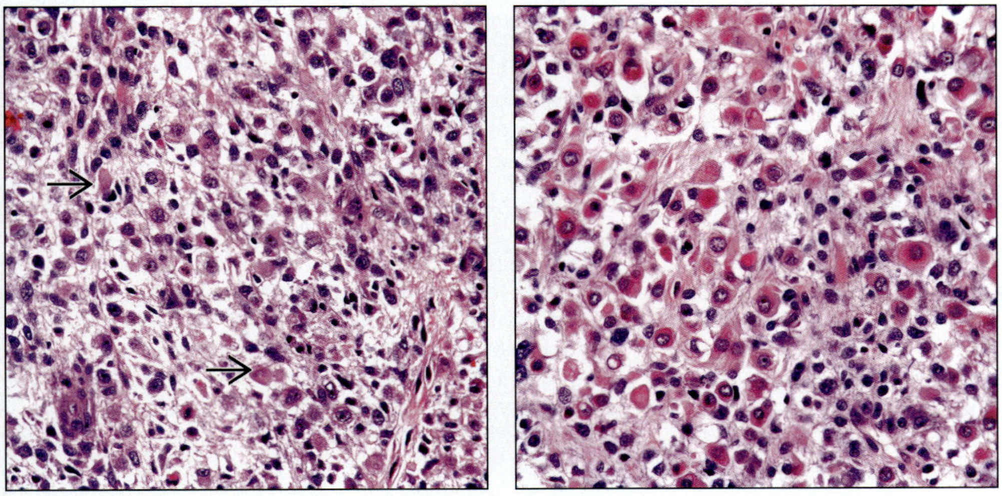

(Left) *Pulmonary artery sarcoma shows rhabdomyosarcomatous differentiation. The cells are oval, and numerous rhabdomyoblastic cells are also present* →. ***(Right)*** *Closer view of a rhabdomyosarcoma arising in the pulmonary artery. This differentiation is not uncommon among the different types of sarcomas that may arise from the pulmonary artery.*

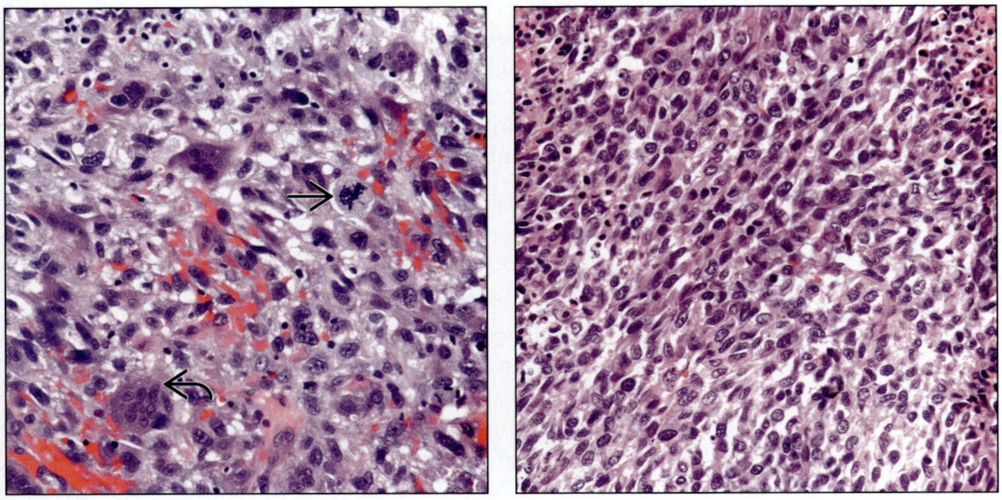

(Left) *High-power view of a pulmonary artery sarcoma is shown with a pleomorphic cellular proliferation. Note the presence of osteoclast-like multinucleated giant cells* ↩ *and the presence of atypical mitotic figures* →. ***(Right)*** *High-power view of a pulmonary artery sarcoma displays a spindle cellular proliferation admixed with mitotic figures. The features highly suggest a neurogenic sarcoma.*

PULMONARY BALT HYPERPLASIA

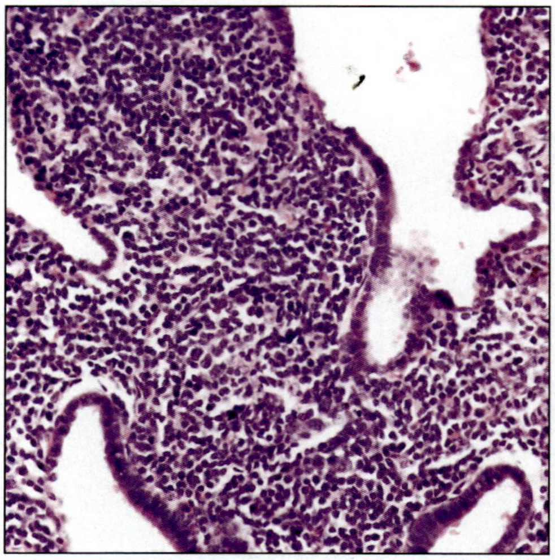

Diffuse BALT hyperplasia of the lung shows massively distended alveolar septa occupied by a population of small lymphoid cells.

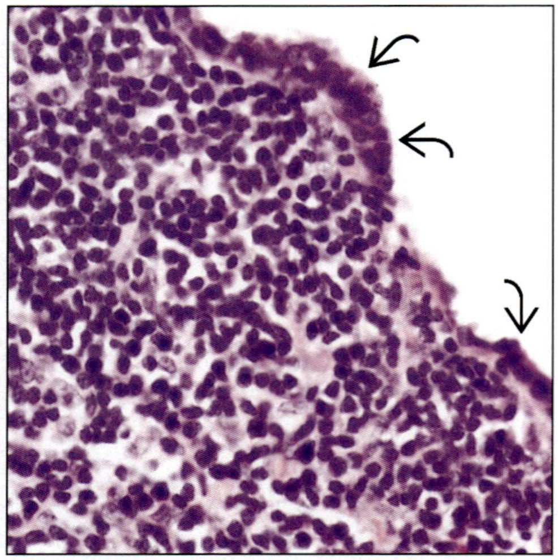

Higher magnification of diffuse BALT hyperplasia shows a dense population of small lymphoid cells abutting the respiratory lining mucosa ⇒.

TERMINOLOGY

Synonyms

- Pseudolymphoma, nodular lymphoid hyperplasia, lymphoid interstitial pneumonia

Definitions

- Polyclonal proliferation of small lymphocytes arising within lung parenchyma

ETIOLOGY/PATHOGENESIS

Pathogenesis

- Commonly associated with underlying autoimmune disorders such as Sjögren syndrome, rheumatoid arthritis, and collagen vascular diseases
- Associated with viral infection, including HIV and Epstein-Barr virus
- Associated with immunodeficiency, including common variable immunodeficiency, AIDS, and bone marrow transplants
- Idiopathic

CLINICAL ISSUES

Epidemiology

- Age
  - Adults 40-70 years of age (average = 50)
  - Diffuse form of the disease is more common in children
- Gender
  - Female predilection

Presentation

- Cough
- Dyspnea
- Asymptomatic; discovered incidentally
- Dysproteinemia (hypergammaglobulinemia in 90% of patients)
- May be associated with generalized lymphadenopathy or hepatosplenomegaly

Treatment

- Surgical excision for localized lesions
- Steroid therapy for diffuse lesions

Prognosis

- Variable course depending on extent and progression of disease
- Complete resolution is most common outcome
- Diffuse cases may progress to end-stage pulmonary fibrosis with "honeycombing" of lung parenchyma
- Diffuse cases may progress to diffuse lymphocytic lymphoma (MALT-lymphoma)
- Death may ensue due to comorbid conditions, superinfection, or renal failure

IMAGE FINDINGS

General Features

- Best diagnostic clue
  - Thin-walled cysts and centrilobular nodules
- Location
  - Basilar interstitial thickening in adults with Sjögren syndrome

Radiographic Findings

- Diffuse interstitial thickening, predominantly basilar
- Multiple nodular pulmonary opacities, often with air bronchograms (more common in AIDS patients)

CT Findings

- High-resolution CT scan shows nonspecific ground-glass opacities or consolidation
- Small (2-4 mm) centrilobular and subpleural nodules in lymphatic distribution
- Thin-walled cysts ranging from 1-30 mm in diameter (most characteristic finding)

PULMONARY BALT HYPERPLASIA

Key Facts

Terminology
- Polyclonal proliferation of small lymphocytes arising within lung parenchyma

Etiology/Pathogenesis
- Commonly associated with underlying autoimmune disorders such as Sjögren syndrome, rheumatoid arthritis, and collagen vascular diseases
- Associated with viral infection, including HIV and Epstein-Barr virus
- Associated with immunodeficiency, including common variable immunodeficiency, AIDS, and bone marrow transplants

Clinical Issues
- Mostly asymptomatic; discovered incidentally

Microscopic Pathology
- **Nodular lymphoid hyperplasia (nodular BALT hyperplasia)**
  - Multiple coalescent enlarged follicles showing prominent germinal centers
  - Interfollicular lymphoplasmacytosis
- **Follicular bronchiolitis**
  - Discrete accumulations of small lymphoid aggregates in peribronchiolar location
  - Sparing of alveolar septa by lymphoid infiltrates
- **Diffuse lymphoid (BALT) hyperplasia (diffuse interstitial pneumonia)**
  - Predominantly interstitial proliferation of small lymphocytes distending alveolar septa
  - Process is generally bilateral and diffuse

MICROSCOPIC PATHOLOGY

Histologic Features
- **Nodular lymphoid hyperplasia (nodular BALT hyperplasia)**
  - Multiple coalescent enlarged follicles show prominent germinal centers
  - Interfollicular lymphoplasmacytosis
  - Hyperplastic follicles display prominent polarity
  - Well-demarcated follicle mantle zones contain cytologically bland small lymphocytes
  - Lymphoid process does not extend along alveolar septa or into alveolar walls
- **Follicular bronchiolitis**
  - Discrete accumulations of small lymphoid aggregates in peribronchiolar location
  - Sparing of alveolar septa by lymphoid infiltrates
  - Considered the small airway equivalent of nodular lymphoid hyperplasia
- **Diffuse lymphoid (BALT) hyperplasia (diffuse interstitial pneumonia)**
  - Predominantly interstitial proliferation of small lymphocytes distending alveolar walls
  - Occasional residual germinal centers may be seen
  - Process is generally bilateral and diffuse

Cytologic Features
- Lymphoid cell population in nodular lymphoid hyperplasia and follicular bronchiolitis consists of polyclonal B lymphocytes and plasma cells
- Lymphoid cell population in diffuse lymphoid hyperplasia is composed primarily of small T cells admixed with polyclonal B lymphocytes

ANCILLARY TESTS

Immunohistochemistry
- **Nodular lymphoid hyperplasia**
  - Polyclonal pattern of light chain expression in small lymphocytes and plasma cells
  - CD5(-), CD10(-), CD23(-)
  - CD21 highlights dendritic cell network in germinal centers
- **Diffuse lymphoid hyperplasia**
  - Polyclonal population of small B lymphocytes and plasma cells
  - Abundance of small T lymphocytes in interstitial infiltrates
  - Cases occurring in the context of AIDS will show immunoreactivity for the p21 protein of HIV

Molecular Genetics
- Absence of clonality or gene rearrangements by molecular studies

DIFFERENTIAL DIAGNOSIS

MALT Lymphoma (Primary Pulmonary Marginal Zone Lymphoma)
- Diffuse proliferation of monoclonal small B lymphocytes showing kappa or lambda light chain restriction
- Colonization of germinal centers by marginal zone lymphocytes
- Formation of lymphoepithelial lesions
- Demonstration of t(11;18) (AP12/MALT1) translocation

SELECTED REFERENCES

1. Bégueret H et al: Primary lung small B-cell lymphoma versus lymphoid hyperplasia: evaluation of diagnostic criteria in 26 cases. Am J Surg Pathol. 26(1):76-81, 2002
2. Nicholson AG: Lymphocytic interstitial pneumonia and other lymphoproliferative disorders in the lung. Semin Respir Crit Care Med. 22(4):409-22, 2001
3. Abbondanzo SL et al: Nodular lymphoid hyperplasia of the lung: a clinicopathologic study of 14 cases. Am J Surg Pathol. 24(4):587-97, 2000
4. Koch JS et al: Bronchus-associated lymphoid tissue hyperplasia of the lung. AJR Am J Roentgenol. 168(4):1044, 1997

PULMONARY BALT HYPERPLASIA

Nodular BALT Hyperplasia/Follicular Bronchiolitis

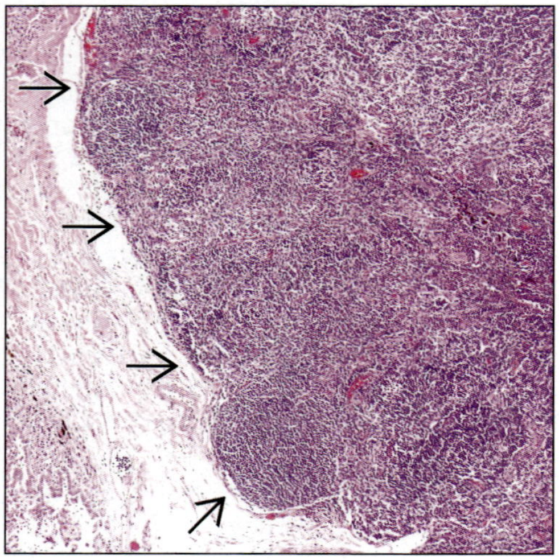
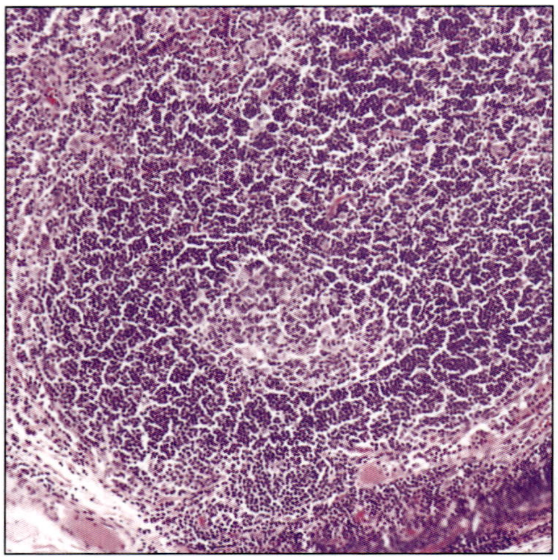

(Left) *Scanning magnification of nodular BALT hyperplasia of the lung shows a well-delineated area of consolidation → separated from the surrounding lung parenchyma. The area of consolidation is composed of numerous small lymphoid cells with scattered reactive follicles.* ***(Right)*** *Higher magnification of nodular BALT hyperplasia shows an enlarged lymphoid follicle with a germinal center. The lymphoid cell population in this case was shown to be polyclonal.*

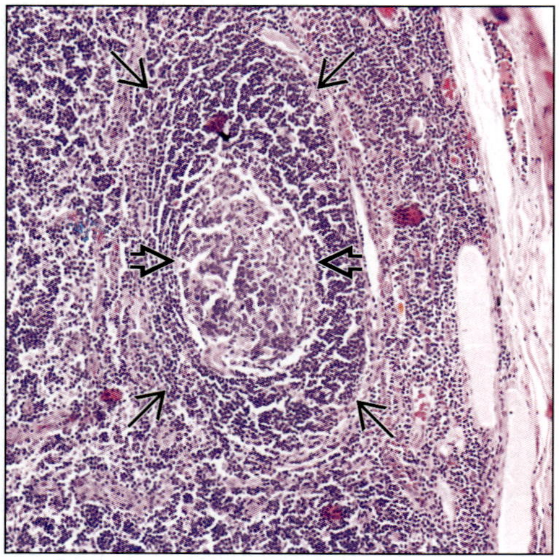
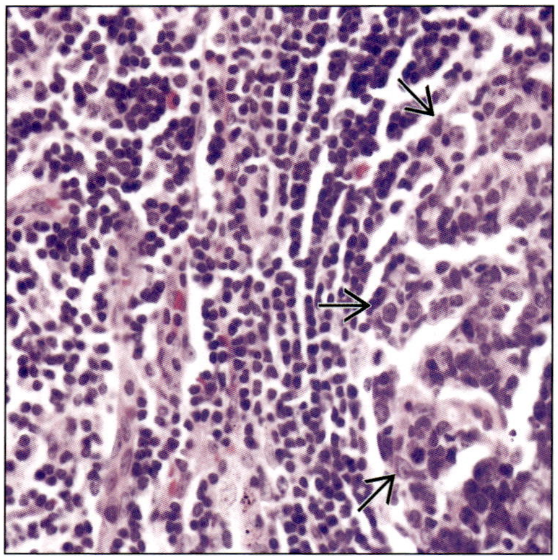

(Left) *Scanning magnification in nodular BALT hyperplasia shows a lymphoid follicle → with a reactive germinal center ⇨. The lymphoid follicle shows good "polarization"; i.e., the mantle zone surrounding the germinal center is not uniformly enlarged.* ***(Right)*** *Higher magnification from nodular BALT hyperplasia shows a portion of a germinal center → adjacent to an expanded interfollicular area that contains polyclonal small lymphocytes and plasma cells.*

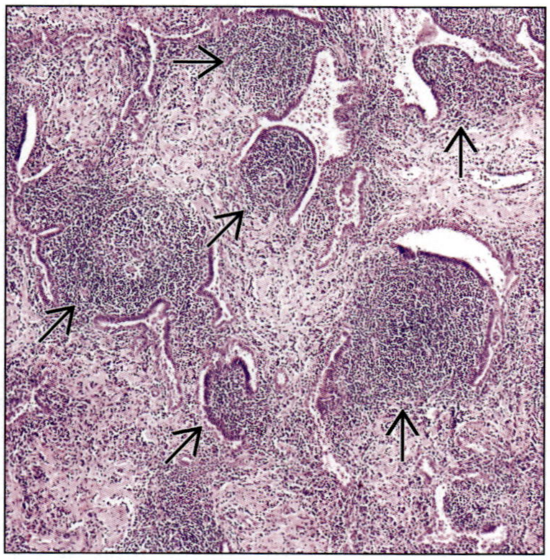
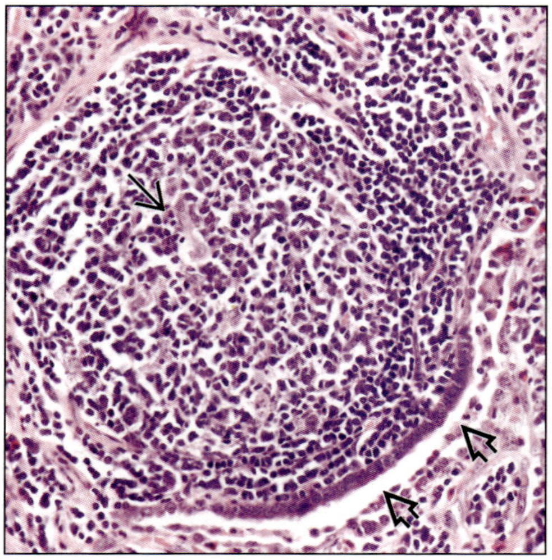

(Left) *Scanning magnification of follicular bronchiolitis shows the discrete accumulation of small lymphoid aggregates in a peribronchiolar location →. Notice the sparing of the alveolar septa by the lymphoid infiltrates.* ***(Right)*** *Higher magnification of follicular bronchiolitis shows a well-formed lymphoid aggregate compressing the lumen of a small bronchiole ⇨. The follicle shows the presence of an immature germinal center in the center of the follicle →.*

Diffuse BALT Hyperplasia

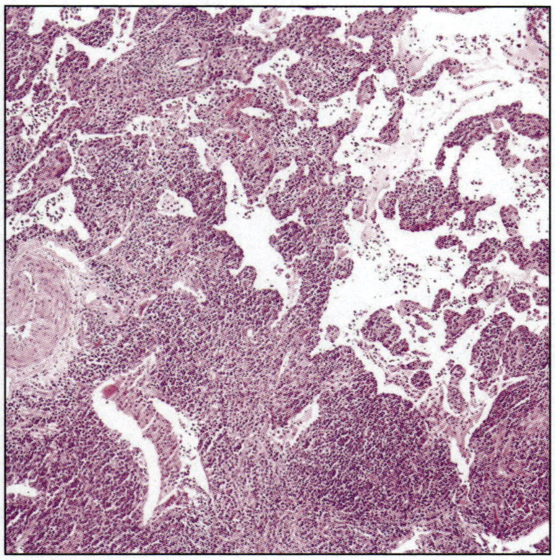
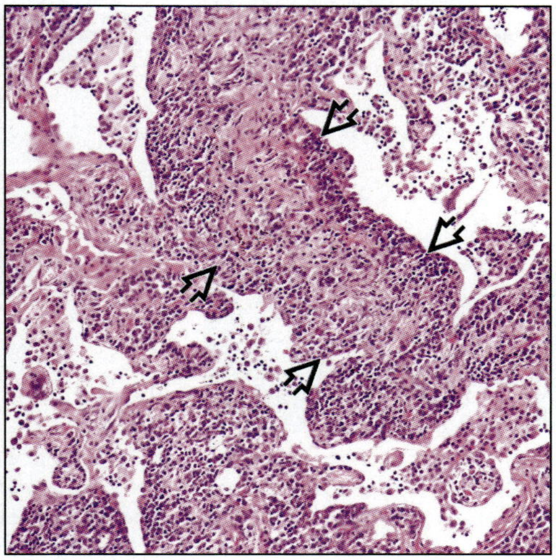

(Left) *Scanning magnification of diffuse BALT hyperplasia (lymphoid interstitial pneumonia) shows expansion of the alveolar septa by a diffuse infiltrate primarily composed of small lymphoid cells.* ***(Right)*** *Higher magnification of diffuse BALT hyperplasia of the lung (lymphoid interstitial pneumonia) shows widening of the alveolar septa ⇨ by a dense lymphoid cell population. The underlying epithelial lining of the alveolar wall remains preserved and intact.*

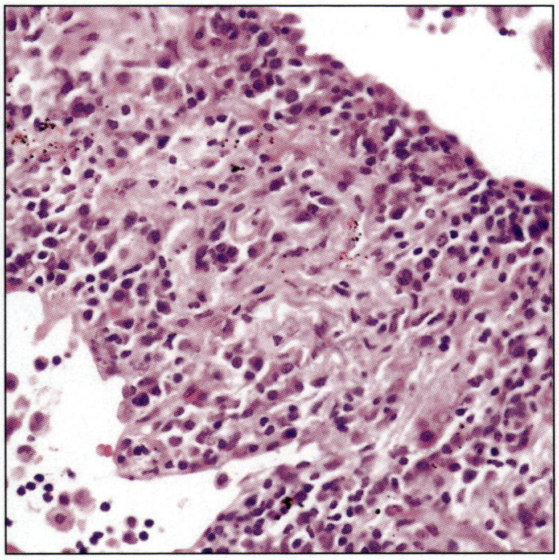
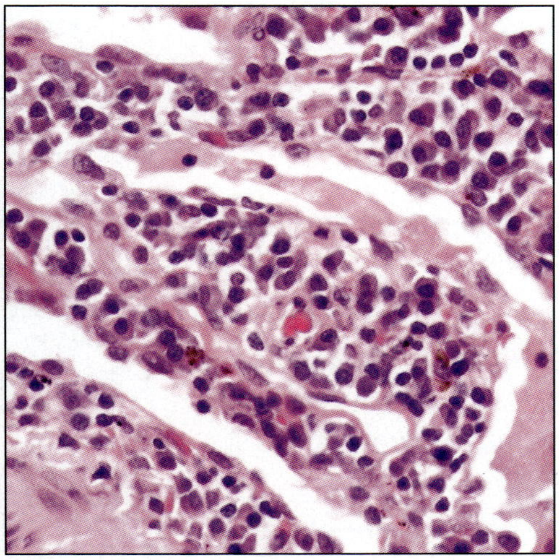

(Left) *Higher magnification of diffuse BALT hyperplasia of the lung (lymphoid interstitial pneumonia) shows expansion of the alveolar wall by a mononuclear population of lymphoid cells, including small lymphocytes, plasma cells, and histiocytes. No atypical cells are seen in the infiltrate.* ***(Right)*** *Higher magnification of diffuse BALT hyperplasia (lymphoid interstitial pneumonia) shows a dense polyclonal population of small lymphocytes admixed with plasma cells.*

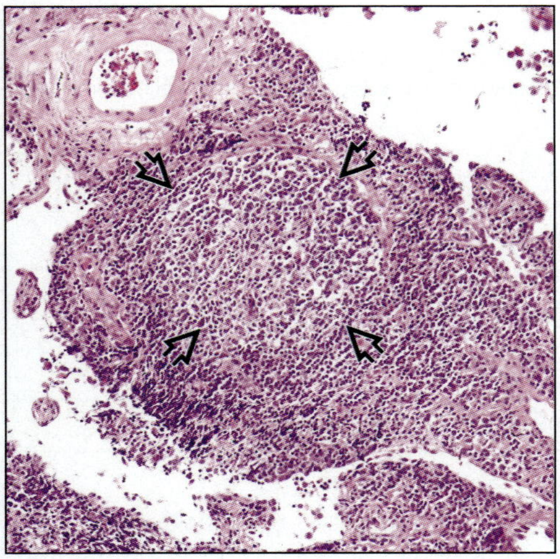
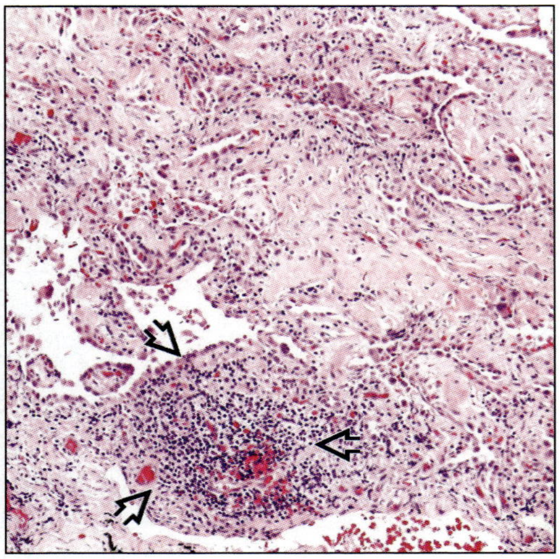

(Left) *Diffuse BALT hyperplasia (lymphoid interstitial pneumonia) of the lung shows widening of alveolar septa displaying a prominent lymphoid follicle ⇨. Cases showing these features can overlap with follicular bronchiolitis but are distinguished by the diffuse nature of the lymphoid infiltrates.* ***(Right)*** *Diffuse BALT hyperplasia (lymphoid interstitial pneumonia) in an advanced stage shows prominent interstitial fibrosis with only 1 small, abortive residual follicle present ⇨.*

PULMONARY BALT LYMPHOMA

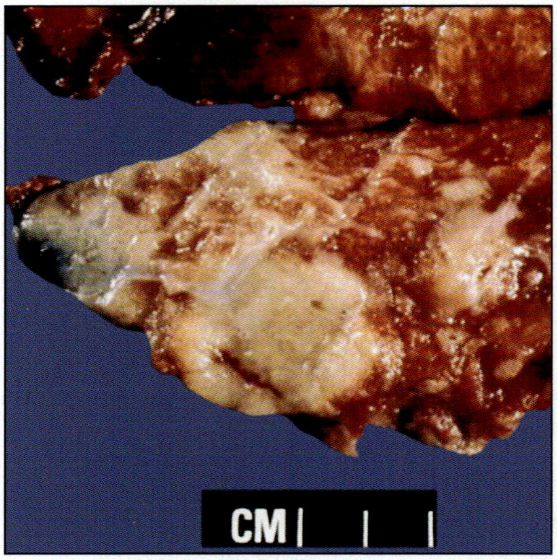

Gross appearance of BALT lymphoma of the lung shows nodular, ill-defined, coalescent areas of lung parenchyma replaced by tan-white, homogeneous, rubbery tissue.

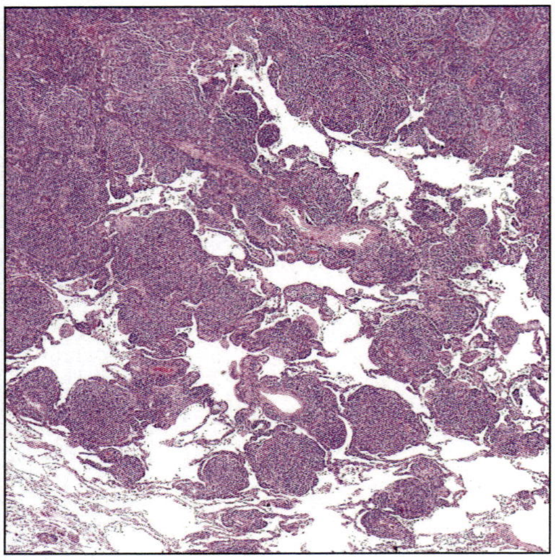

Characteristic histologic appearance of pulmonary BALT lymphoma shows expansion of alveolar septa by a monotonous population of small lymphoid cells with lymphangitic distribution.

TERMINOLOGY

Synonyms

- Marginal zone B-cell lymphoma of mucosa-associated lymphoid tissue (MALT) type

Definitions

- Monoclonal proliferation of small lymphocytes arising from marginal zone of B-cell follicles

ETIOLOGY/PATHOGENESIS

Etiology

- Thought to arise secondary to inflammatory and autoimmune processes

CLINICAL ISSUES

Epidemiology

- Incidence
  - Accounts for approximately 80% of primary lung lymphomas
  - Accounts for < 0.5% of all primary lung neoplasms
- Age
  - Most common from 50-70 years of age
  - Can occur in younger patients with underlying immunosuppression

Presentation

- Most common presentation is solitary mass on routine imaging studies
- May be localized or diffuse
- Most patients are asymptomatic
- Some patients may present with symptoms of cough, dyspnea, and chest pain

Treatment

- Surgical approaches
  - Surgical excision achieves excellent results in localized, resectable tumors
- Adjuvant therapy
  - Indicated in patients with diffuse or bilateral involvement
- Other options
  - Elderly patients with asymptomatic lesions may be clinically followed without therapy

Prognosis

- Favorable prognosis; 5-year survival in approximately 85-95%
- Small proportion of cases may progress to diffuse large B-cell lymphoma

IMAGE FINDINGS

General Features

- Location
  - Tumors are typically peripheral in location
- Morphology
  - May present as single, solitary nodule or as diffuse bilateral disease mimicking diffuse interstitial pneumonia

CT Findings

- High-resolution computerized tomographs (HRCT) show multiple solitary masses or alveolar opacities
- HRCT may also show airway dilatation, positive angiogram signs, and ground-glass shadowing at margins

MACROSCOPIC FEATURES

Cut Surface

- Tan-white, fleshy, homogeneous rubbery tissue
- Involved area of lung parenchyma can be nodular and well circumscribed or diffuse

PULMONARY BALT LYMPHOMA

Key Facts

Clinical Issues
- Most common presentation is solitary mass on routine imaging studies
- Most patients are asymptomatic
- Favorable prognosis; 5-year survival in approximately 85-95%

Image Findings
- May present as single, solitary nodule or as diffuse bilateral disease mimicking diffuse interstitial pneumonia

Microscopic Pathology
- Diffuse lymphoid infiltrates composed of small lymphocytes admixed with reactive lymphoid follicles
- Reactive lymphoid follicles may show extensive infiltration by marginal zone lymphocytes (follicular colonization)
- Infiltration of underlying epithelial structures forming "lymphoepithelial" lesions is characteristic
- Cytomorphology of neoplastic small lymphocytes is variable and includes centrocytic cells, plasmacytoid cells, and monocytoid cells

Ancillary Tests
- Neoplastic cells are positive for CD19, CD20, CD79a, and Bcl-2
- Tumor cells are negative for CD5, CD10, CD23, Bcl-1, and Bcl-6
- t(11;18)(q21;q21) is most common genetic abnormality (encountered in about 50% of cases)

MICROSCOPIC PATHOLOGY

Histologic Features
- Diffuse lymphoid infiltrates composed of small lymphocytes admixed with reactive lymphoid follicles
- Reactive lymphoid follicles may show extensive infiltration by marginal zone lymphocytes (follicular colonization)
- Infiltration of underlying epithelial structures forming "lymphoepithelial" lesions is characteristic
- Scattered larger, immunoblastic cells may be seen admixed with small lymphoid cell infiltrate
- Lymphangitic distribution characteristically observed at edges of lesions
- Stromal hyalinization and fibrosis may be seen in advanced lesions

Cytologic Features
- Cytomorphology of neoplastic small lymphocytes is variable and includes
  - Small lymphocytes with minimal nuclear irregularities resembling germinal center centrocytes
  - Plasmacytoid small lymphocytes
  - "Monocytoid" B-lymphocytes showing clear perinuclear hues and ample cytoplasm

ANCILLARY TESTS

Immunohistochemistry
- Neoplastic cells are positive for CD19, CD20, CD79a, Bcl-2, and Bcl-10
- Tumor cells are negative for CD5, CD10, CD23, Bcl-1, and Bcl-6
- Cytokeratin stains may be helpful to highlight lymphoepithelial lesions
- Light chain restriction for kappa/lambda can be demonstrated in paraffin sections only in minority of cases
- Stains for follicular dendritic cells such as CD21, CD23, and CD35 can highlight reactive follicles disrupted by neoplastic cells

Cytogenetics
- t(11;18)(q21;q21) is most common genetic abnormality (encountered in about 50% of cases)
- t(1;14) and (14;18) or trisomy 3 and 18 may also occur

Molecular Genetics
- t(11;18) translocation produces a fusion protein involving *API2* and *MALT1* genes and can be detected by expression of Bcl-10

PCR
- Clonal immunoglobulin heavy chain rearrangements are identified in majority of cases, even in absence of light chain restriction

DIFFERENTIAL DIAGNOSIS

Nodular Lymphoid Hyperplasia
- Composed of polyclonal population of lymphoid cells without lymphoepithelial lesions
- Lymphocytes do not show light chain restriction or heavy chain gene rearrangements by PCR

Diffuse Lymphoid Hyperplasia (Lymphocytic Interstitial Pneumonia)
- Interstitial lymphocytes in diffuse lymphoid hyperplasia stain as CD3(+) T cells
- B cells in diffuse lymphoid hyperplasia do not show light chain restriction or heavy chain gene rearrangements

SELECTED REFERENCES

1. Okabe M et al: API2-MALT1 fusion defines a distinctive clinicopathologic subtype in pulmonary extranodal marginal zone B-cell lymphoma of mucosa-associated lymphoid tissue. Am J Pathol. 162(4):1113-22, 2003
2. Kurtin PJ et al: Pathologic and clinical features of primary pulmonary extranodal marginal zone B-cell lymphoma of MALT type. Am J Surg Pathol. 25(8):997-1008, 2001

Histologic Features

(Left) Scanning magnification of BALT lymphoma of the lung (pulmonary marginal zone B-cell lymphoma) shows sheets of small lymphocytes expanding alveolar septa and forming a tumor nodule. The histologic appearance of this lesion can be indistinguishable from diffuse BALT hyperplasia. ***(Right)*** *Scanning magnification of BALT lymphoma of the lung shows a lymphangitic type of distribution, with small nodules* → *composed of lymphoid cells distributed along the course of the lymphatic vessels.*

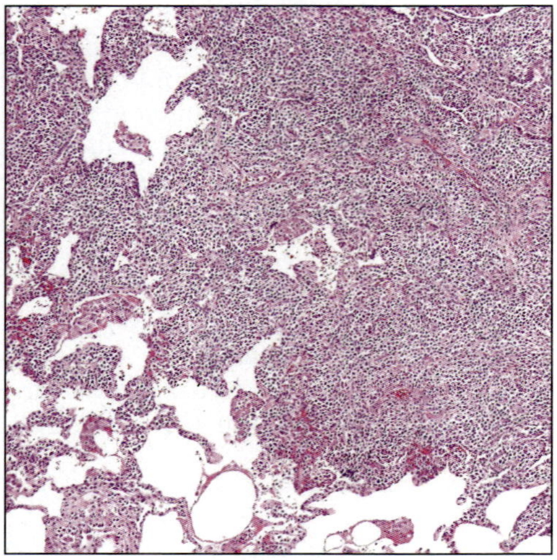

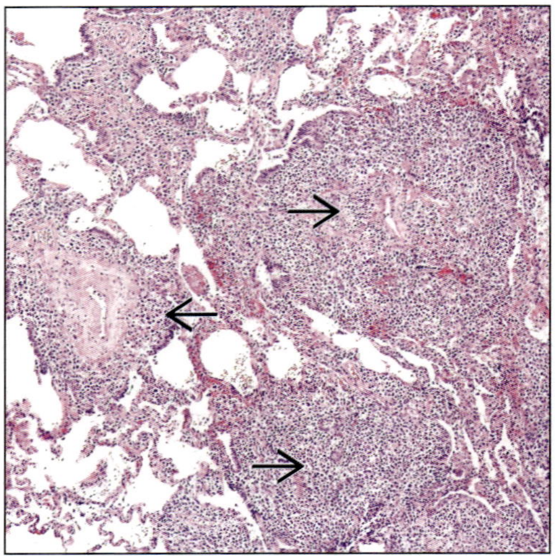

(Left) *Scanning magnification of BALT lymphoma of the lung (marginal zone B-cell lymphoma) shows involvement of a bronchus with destruction of the bronchial cartilage and a few residual hyperplastic lymphoid follicles* ⇨. ***(Right)*** *BALT lymphoma of the lung shows a residual hyperplastic lymphoid follicle with a reactive germinal center surrounded by monotonous interfollicular proliferation of small lymphocytes. Note abundant tingible-body macrophages* → *within the germinal center.*

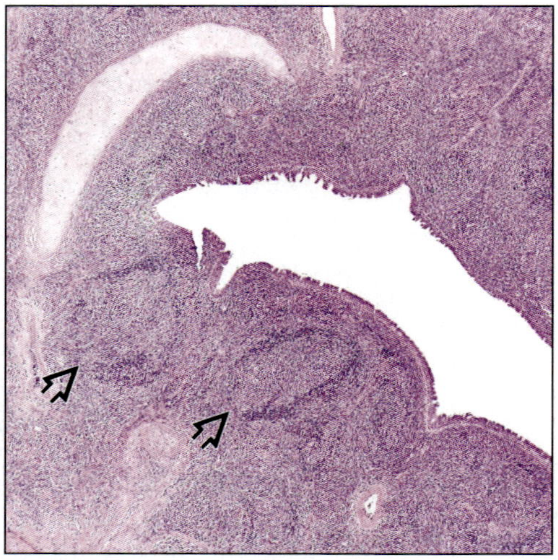

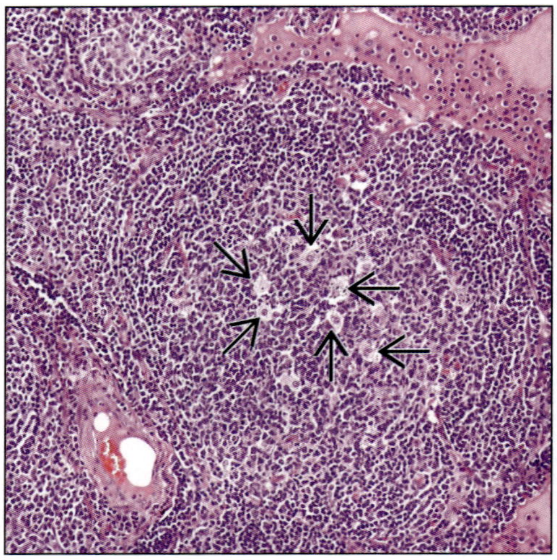

(Left) *Scanning magnification of diffuse BALT lymphoma of the lung shows a dense small lymphocytic proliferation distributed around a bronchial lumen* → *and displaying vague nodularity.* ***(Right)*** *Higher magnification of pulmonary BALT lymphoma (marginal zone B-cell lymphoma) shows a partially effaced lymphoid follicle with a burned-out, residual germinal center showing irregular infiltration by small marginal zone lymphocytes* →*. This process is known as "colonization" of follicles.*

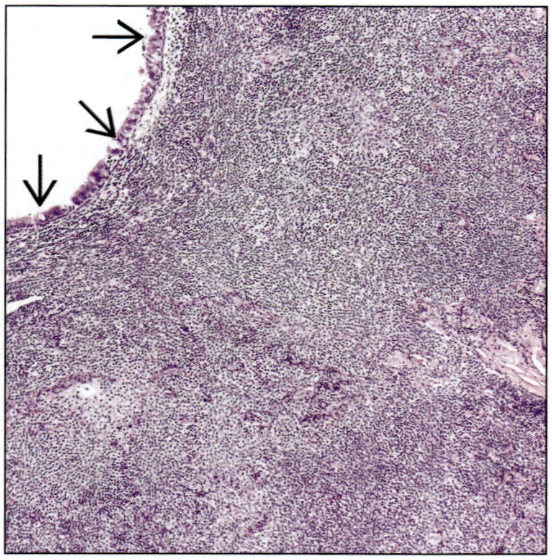

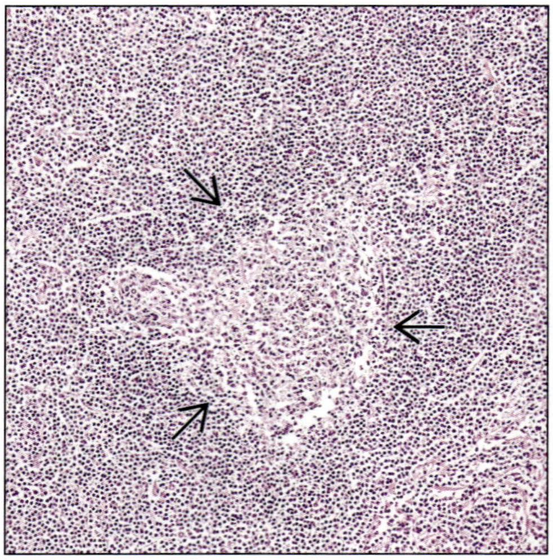

Lymphoepithelial Lesions

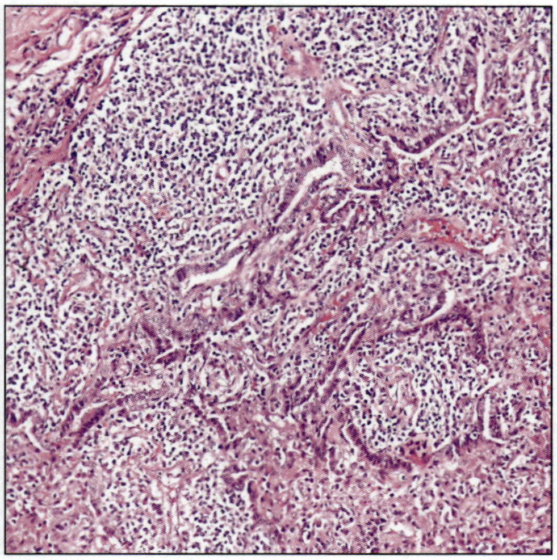

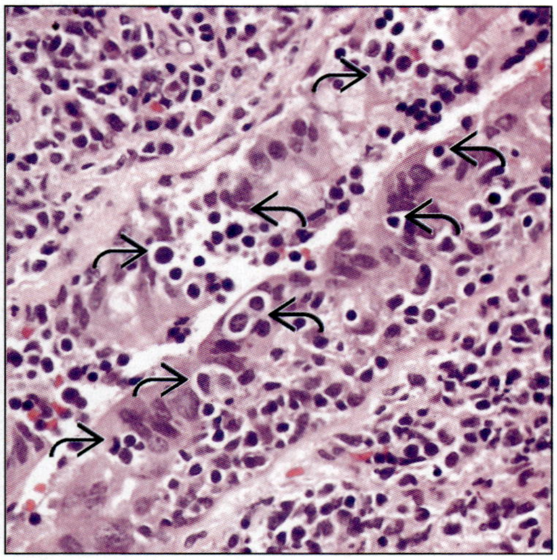

(Left) *Pulmonary BALT lymphoma (marginal zone B-cell lymphoma) shows multiple entrapped airspaces showing irregular infiltration of the mucosa by small lymphocytes.* ***(Right)*** *Higher magnification of pulmonary BALT lymphoma (marginal zone B-cell lymphoma) shows numerous lymphocytes expanding and replacing the epithelial lining in an airspace ➔. The infiltrate is mononuclear, as opposed to infiltration by neutrophils and eosinophils in acute bronchitis and bronchiolitis.*

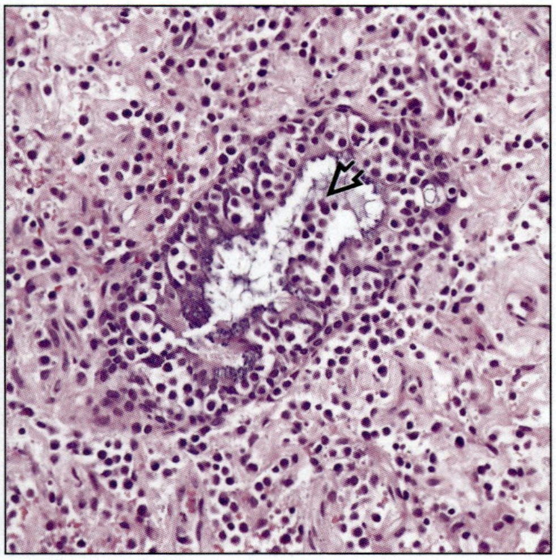

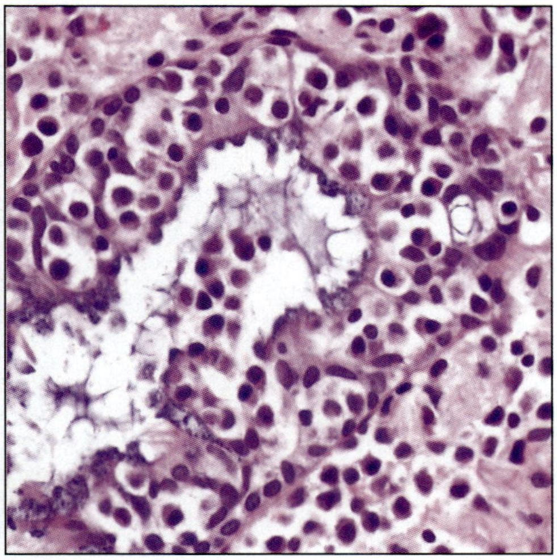

(Left) *Pulmonary BALT lymphoma (marginal zone B-cell lymphoma) shows a small airspace infiltrated by small lymphocytes. There is distortion of the bronchiolar lumen, and some of the small lymphocytes are seen to be spilling into the lumen ➔.* ***(Right)*** *Higher magnification of a pulmonary BALT lymphoma shows a well-developed lymphoepithelial lesion. The wall of this bronchiole has been almost entirely replaced by the infiltrating small lymphocytes, some of which appear plasmacytoid.*

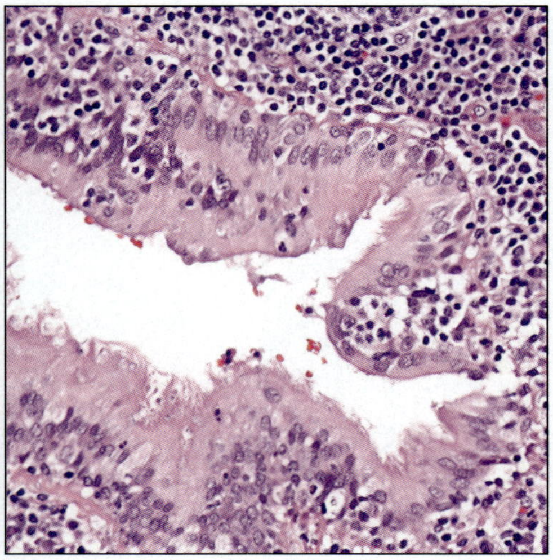

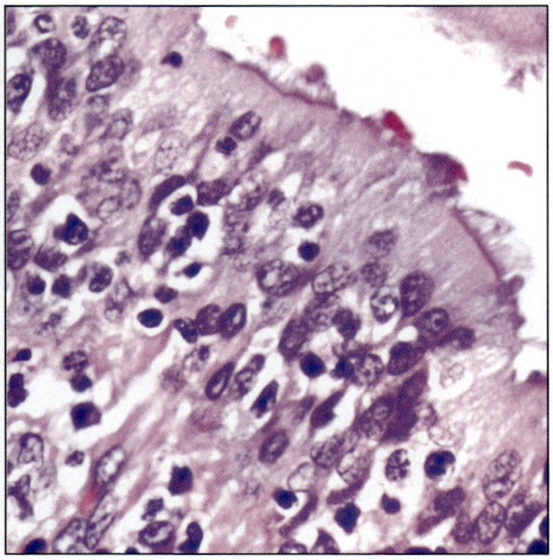

(Left) *Pulmonary BALT lymphoma shows a bronchiole with infiltration by small lymphocytes leading to the creation of a lymphoepithelial lesion. The respiratory mucosa displays a moth-eaten appearance resulting from the infiltrating lymphocytes.* ***(Right)*** *High magnification of a pulmonary BALT lymphoma (marginal zone B-cell lymphoma) shows close detail of a lymphoepithelial lesion, with tall columnar respiratory mucosa harboring a mononuclear cell population.*

PULMONARY BALT LYMPHOMA

Other Histologic Features

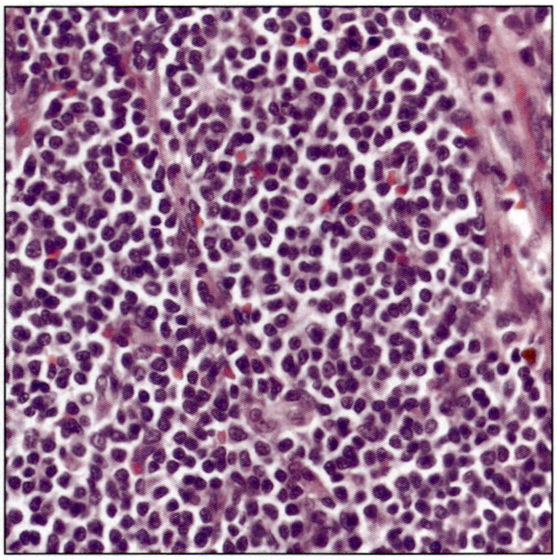
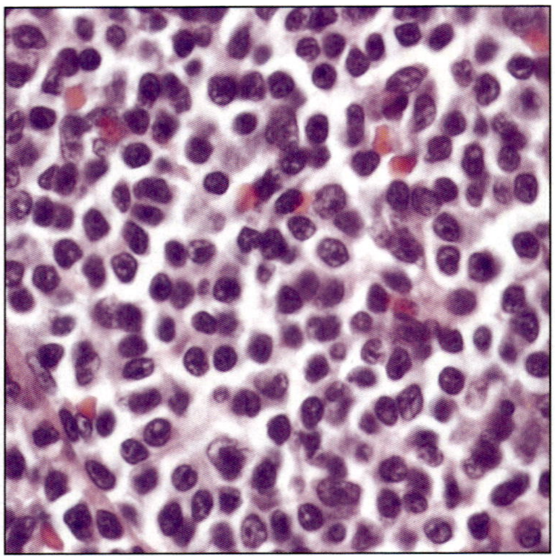

*(**Left**) Pulmonary BALT lymphoma (marginal zone B-cell lymphoma) shows a monotonous population of small B lymphocytes that resemble germinal center centrocytes. The infiltrate is very similar to that seen in small lymphocytic lymphoma/CLL, but the cells are negative for CD5, CD10, and Bcl-6. (**Right**) Higher magnification of pulmonary BALT lymphoma (marginal zone B-cell lymphoma) shows a monotonous population of small lymphocytes with minimal nuclear irregularities.*

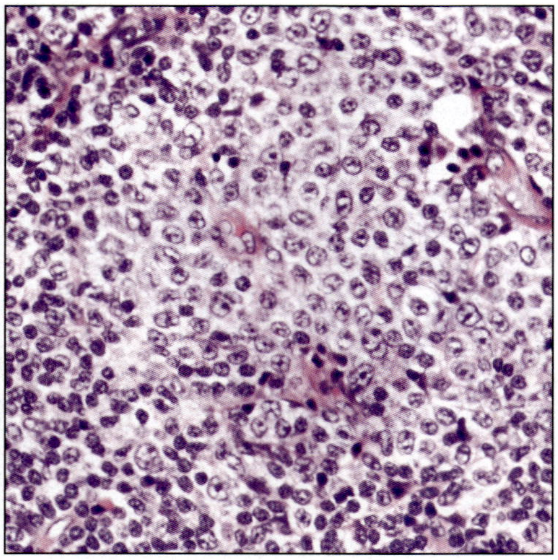
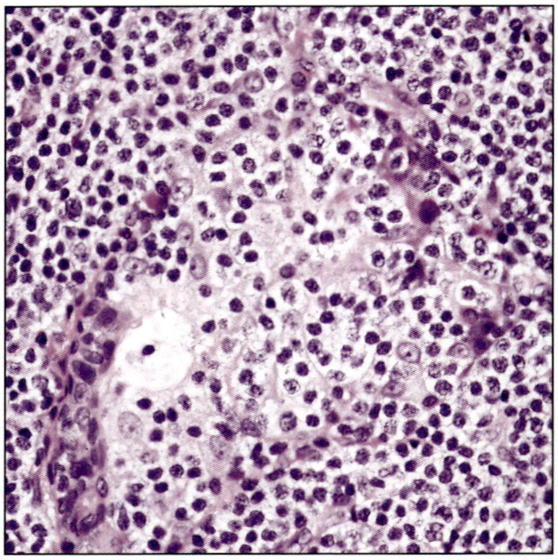

*(**Left**) Pulmonary BALT lymphoma shows a monotonous population of small lymphocytes with a striking monocytoid appearance. The cells appear less crowded than in conventional small lymphocytic lymphoma because of more abundant cytoplasm. (**Right**) Higher magnification of monocytoid marginal zone B cells in pulmonary BALT lymphoma shows clear perinuclear halos. These cells are positive for Bcl-2, in contrast to reactive monocytoid B cells, which are negative.*

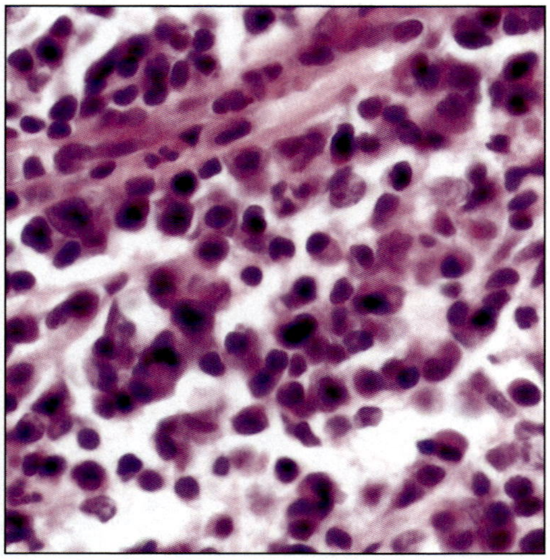
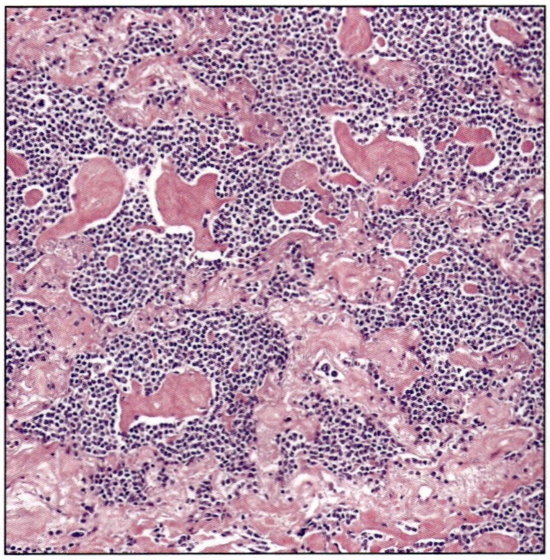

*(**Left**) Pulmonary BALT lymphoma (marginal zone B-cell lymphoma) shows a population of small lymphocytes with plasmacytoid features. Plasmacytic differentiation can be a prominent feature in these tumors that may lead to confusion with plasmacytoma. (**Right**) Pulmonary BALT lymphoma shows prominent stromal sclerosis. This phenomenon is often present in advanced and late lesions. Some tumors with plasmacytic differentiation can also display deposition of stromal amyloid.*

Immunohistochemical Features

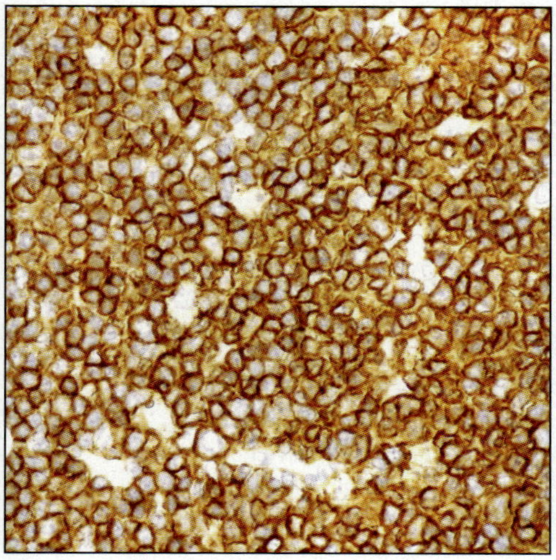

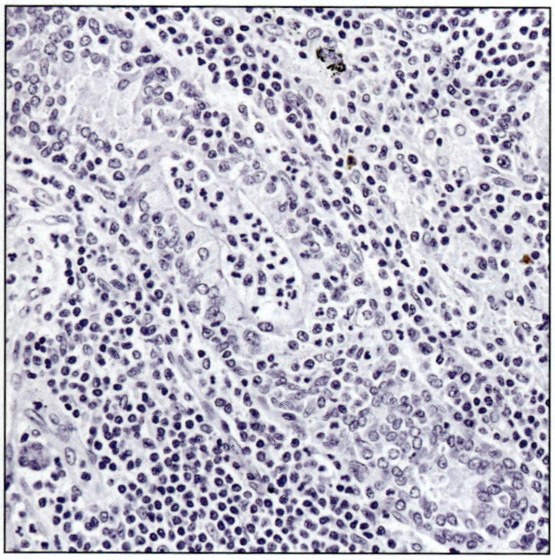

(Left) *Immunohistochemical staining of pulmonary BALT lymphoma (marginal zone B-cell lymphoma) for CD20 shows strong positivity of the tumor cells for this marker. The tumor cells in BALT lymphoma are also positive for the pan-B-cell marker, CD79a.* ***(Right)*** *Immunohistochemical staining of a lymphoepithelial lesion in pulmonary BALT lymphoma for CD5 shows negative staining of the infiltrating lymphocytes, distinguishing it from small lymphocytic lymphoma/CLL.*

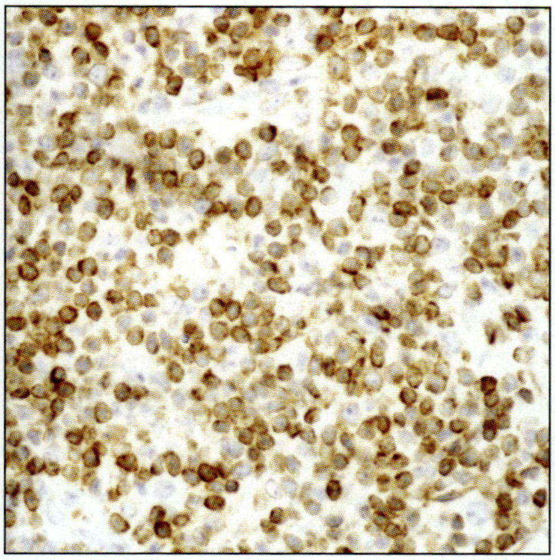

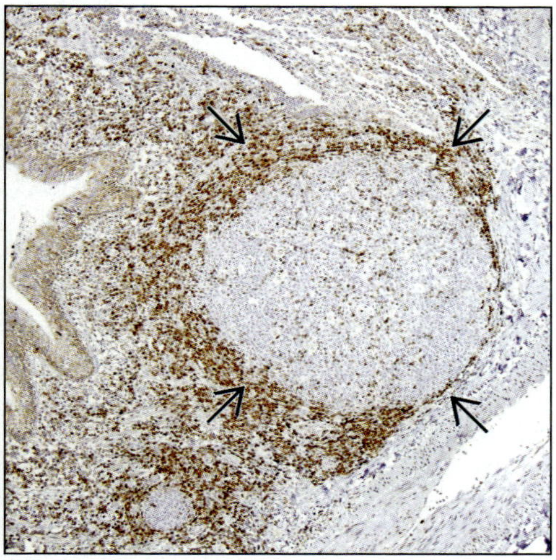

(Left) *Immunohistochemical staining of pulmonary BALT lymphoma (marginal zone B-cell lymphoma) for the Bcl-2 oncogene shows cytoplasmic positivity in the neoplastic lymphoid cells.* ***(Right)*** *Immunohistochemical staining of pulmonary BALT lymphoma (marginal zone B-cell lymphoma) for Bcl-2 shows a rim of positive small lymphocytes surrounding a lymphoid follicle ➔ with a few scattered Bcl-2 positive lymphoid cells percolating into the follicle (follicular colonization).*

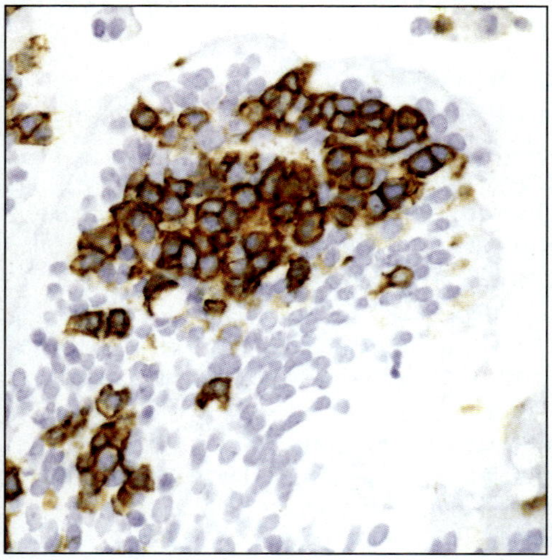

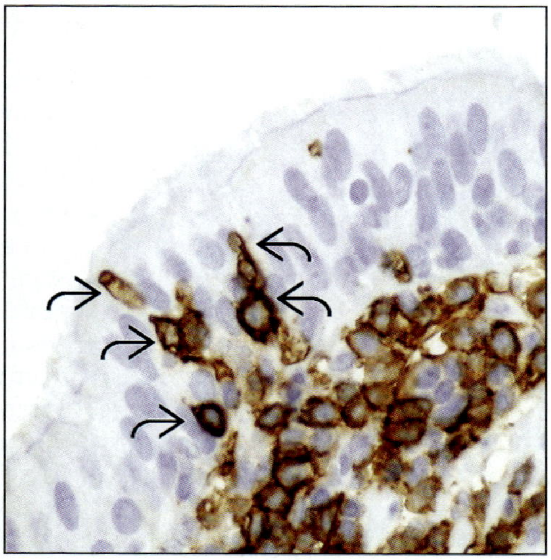

(Left) *Immunohistochemical staining of lymphoepithelial lesion in pulmonary BALT lymphoma (marginal zone B-cell lymphoma) shows numerous cells displaying strong positivity for CD20 percolating between the epithelial cells.* ***(Right)*** *Higher magnification of immunohistochemical staining with CD20 in lymphoepithelial lesion from a patient with pulmonary BALT lymphoma shows strongly positive small lymphocytes percolating in between the bronchial epithelial cells ➔.*

DIFFUSE LARGE CELL LYMPHOMA

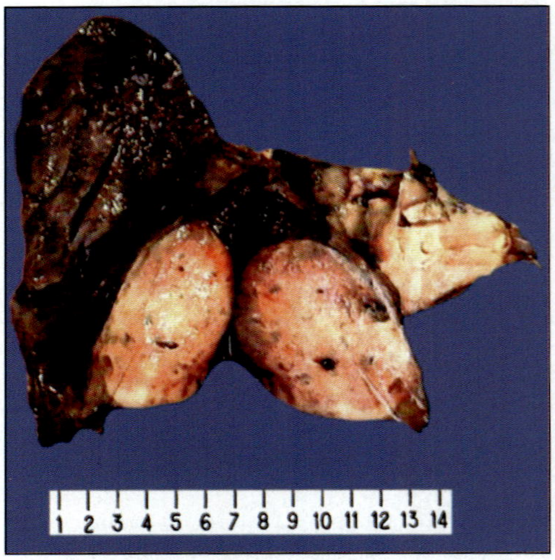

Gross appearance of diffuse large B-cell lymphoma of the lung on cut section shows a well-circumscribed tan-white nodule that is extensively replacing the lung parenchyma.

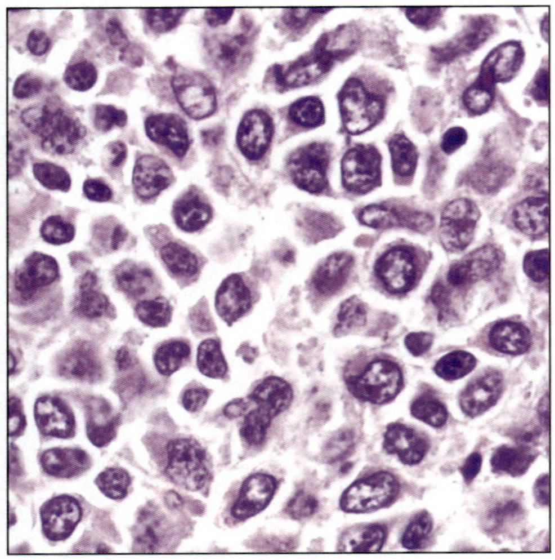

Histological appearance of diffuse large B-cell lymphoma of the lung shows a population of large lymphoid cells that are at least the same size as or larger than histiocytes.

TERMINOLOGY

Abbreviations

- Diffuse large cell lymphoma (DLCL)

Definitions

- Diffuse proliferation of large lymphoid cells with nuclei exceeding the size of a normal macrophage

ETIOLOGY/PATHOGENESIS

Etiology

- Can occur as complication of immunosuppression
- May arise from progressive transformation of preexisting low-grade MALT lymphoma

CLINICAL ISSUES

Epidemiology

- Incidence
  - Represents 10-20% of all pulmonary lymphomas
- Age
  - Adults from 50-70 years of age

Site

- Usually peripheral in location

Presentation

- Cough
- Dyspnea
- Fever and night sweats

Treatment

- Adjuvant therapy
  - Standard combination chemotherapy for DLCL

Prognosis

- 5-year survival with aggressive treatment has been reported in up to 60% of patients

IMAGE FINDINGS

Radiographic Findings

- Chest x-rays show multiple or single opacity

MACROSCOPIC FEATURES

General Features

- Well-circumscribed, tan-white tumor mass with rubbery cut surface

MICROSCOPIC PATHOLOGY

Histologic Features

- Sheets of large lymphoid cells with irregularly shaped, vesicular nuclei and prominent nucleoli
- Areas of low-grade MALT-type lymphoma may be present focally
- Tumors show a sharp interface with surrounding lung parenchyma

Cytologic Features

- Can show variable cytomorphology depending on cell type involved
  - **Diffuse large B-cell lymphoma (DLBCL)**
    - Large cells with enlarged nuclei displaying coarse chromatin pattern and prominent single nucleoli
    - Some tumors may show polylobated nuclei and multinucleated cells
    - Frequent mitotic figures & areas of tumor necrosis
    - Destruction of underlying structures and lung parenchyma
  - **B-immunoblastic lymphoma (BIL)**
    - Large nuclei containing single, large eosinophilic nucleoli, thick cell membranes, and abundant rim of cytoplasm
    - Destruction of underlying structures and lung parenchyma

DIFFUSE LARGE CELL LYMPHOMA

Key Facts

Etiology/Pathogenesis
- May arise from progressive transformation of preexisting low-grade MALT lymphoma

Clinical Issues
- Adults from 50-70 years of age
- Usually peripheral in location

Microscopic Pathology
- Sheets of large lymphoid cells with irregularly shaped, vesicular nuclei and prominent nucleoli
- Areas of low-grade MALT-type lymphoma may be present focally
- Tumors show a sharp interface with surrounding lung parenchyma
- Can show variable cytomorphology depending on cell type involved
  - Diffuse large B-cell lymphoma
  - B-immunoblastic lymphoma
  - Anaplastic large cell lymphoma
  - Peripheral T-cell lymphoma

Ancillary Tests
- Diffuse large B-cell lymphoma and B-immunoblastic lymphoma
  - Positive for CD20, CD79a, and kappa/lambda light chain restriction
- Anaplastic large cell lymphoma (ALCL)
  - Strong paranuclear and membrane staining with CD30 and pan-T-cell antigens
  - Positivity for ALK1 in subset of cases
- Peripheral T-cell lymphoma (PTCL)
  - Positive for pan-T-cell markers (CD3, CD45RO)

    - Frequent areas of necrosis and high mitotic activity
  - **Anaplastic large cell lymphoma (ALCL)**
    - Most commonly of T-cell type (although a subset of ALCL may be of B-cell type)
    - Sheets of large, bizarre tumor cells with pleomorphic nuclei and abundant cytoplasm
    - Cells may resemble Reed-Sternberg cells or metastatic carcinoma cells
    - "Horseshoe" or kidney-shaped nuclei are characteristic of ALCL
  - **Peripheral T-cell lymphoma (PTCL)**
    - Admixture of large and medium-sized atypical lymphocytes with prominent nuclear convolutions and nuclear hyperchromasia
    - Hypervascularity and eosinophilic infiltration often accompany the tumor cell population

ANCILLARY TESTS

Immunohistochemistry
- **DLBCL and BIL**
  - Tumor cells are positive for CD20 and CD79a and show kappa/lambda light chain restriction
- **ALCL**
  - Strong paranuclear (Golgi zone) and membrane staining with CD30
  - Positivity of tumor cells for ALK1 in some cases
  - Positivity of tumor cells for pan-T-cell antigens (CD3, CD45RO)
  - Some cases may be positive for pan-B-cell antigens, such as CD20
- **PTCL**
  - Positive for pan-T-cell markers (CD3, CD45RO)
  - Variable reactivity for CD2, CD5, and CD7

Molecular Genetics
- Clonal gene rearrangements of immunoglobulin heavy chain can be demonstrated by PCR in DLBCL
- Demonstration of t(2;5) chromosomal translocation in ALCL
- Demonstration of clonal gene rearrangement of *TCR* genes in PTCL

DIFFERENTIAL DIAGNOSIS

Primary or Metastatic Poorly Differentiated/ Anaplastic Carcinoma
- Sheets of large atypical cells with discohesive growth pattern that can mimic ALCL
- Positivity of tumor cells for epithelial markers (i.e., low molecular weight cytokeratins, EMA, MOC31)

Metastatic Malignant Melanoma
- Sheets or nests of large, atypical tumor cells with prominent nucleoli and abundant cytoplasm
- Tumor cells are strongly positive for S100 protein and other melanoma-associated markers (HMB45, Melan-A, tyrosinase)
  - Caveat: Melanoma cells can be positive for cytokeratins, CEA, and EMA in some cases

Lymphoepithelioma-like Carcinoma
- Sheets of large atypical cells with scant cytoplasm and prominent nucleoli that can resemble DLCL
- Syncytial growth pattern with dense stromal lymphoid cell infiltrates are characteristic
- Strong positivity for cytokeratins and negative staining for lymphoid markers
  - Caveat: Some lymphoepithelioma-like carcinomas can be positive for CD30

SELECTED REFERENCES

1. Rush WL et al: Primary anaplastic large cell lymphoma of the lung: a clinicopathologic study of five patients. Mod Pathol. 13(12):1285-92, 2000
2. Koss MN: Pulmonary lymphoid disorders. Semin Diagn Pathol. 12(2):158-71, 1995
3. Weiss LM et al: Non-Hodgkin's lymphomas of the lung. A study of 19 cases emphasizing the utility of frozen section immunologic studies in differential diagnosis. Am J Surg Pathol. 9(7):480-90, 1985

DIFFUSE LARGE CELL LYMPHOMA

Diffuse Large B-cell Lymphoma

(Left) *Scanning magnification of diffuse large B-cell lymphoma of the lung shows a monotonous tumor cell population composed of sheets of large lymphoid cells that are sharply circumscribed from the surrounding uninvolved lung parenchyma* ➔. ***(Right)*** *Diffuse large B-cell lymphoma of the lung shows sheets of large lymphoid cells growing with a discohesive growth pattern. The differential diagnosis in these cases includes anaplastic carcinoma and round cell sarcomas.*

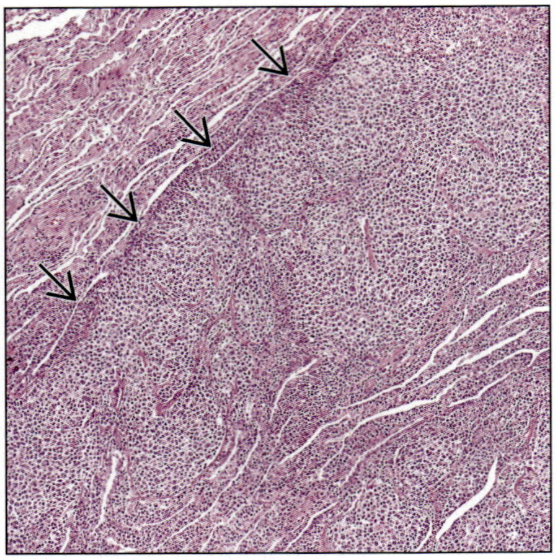

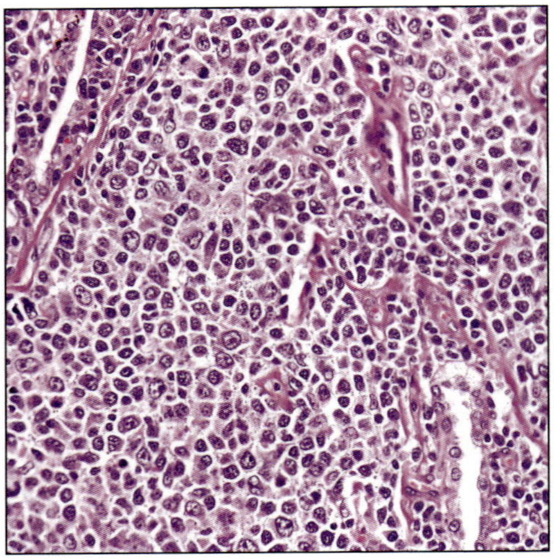

(Left) *Higher magnification of diffuse large B-cell lymphoma of the lung shows a monotonous population composed of sheets of discohesive large lymphoid cells with large nuclei and abundant cytoplasm.* ***(Right)*** *Diffuse large B-cell lymphoma of the lung shows entrapment of a small airspace* ↪ *by the tumor. Notice that the atypical lymphoid cell population neither infiltrates the epithelial structures nor damages the epithelial lining of the entrapped airspace.*

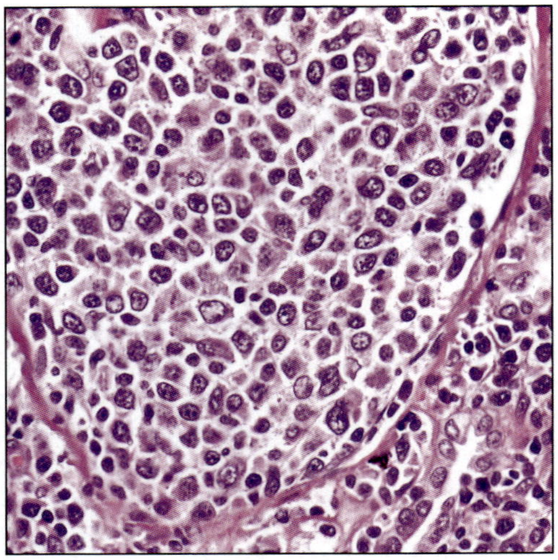

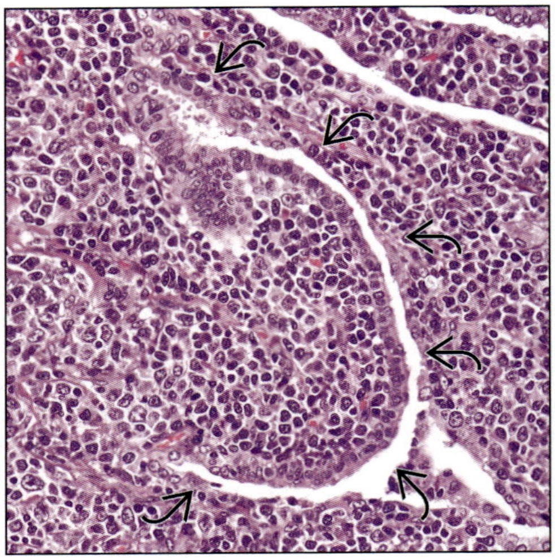

(Left) *Higher magnification of diffuse large B-cell lymphoma of the lung shows cells with enlarged nuclei that are at least the size of a normal macrophage with prominent eosinophilic nucleoli and a scant rim of amphophilic cytoplasm.* ***(Right)*** *Immunohistochemical staining of diffuse large B-cell lymphoma of the lung with the pan-B-cell marker CD20 shows strong positivity of the tumor cells for this antigen. The tumor cells will also react with antibodies to CD79a and CD45.*

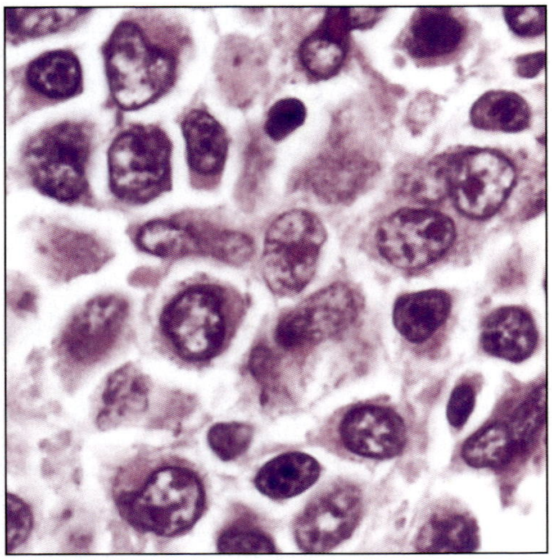

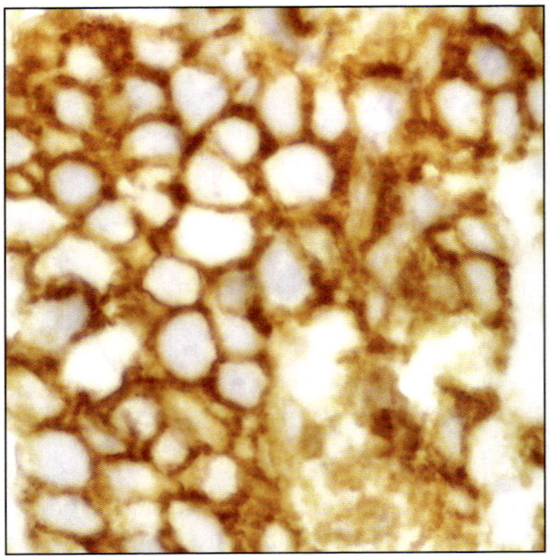

Diffuse Large B-cell Lymphoma

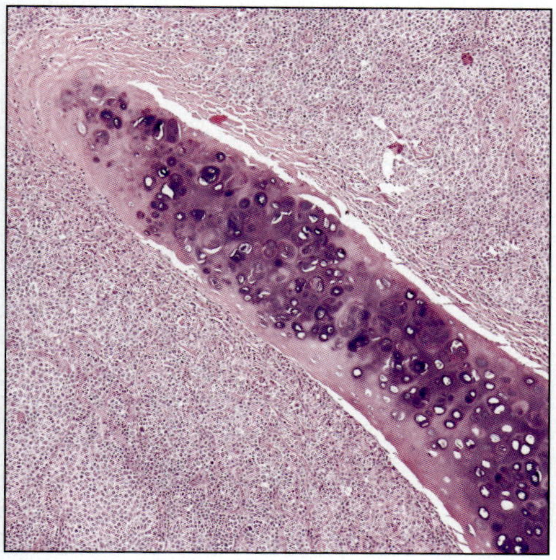

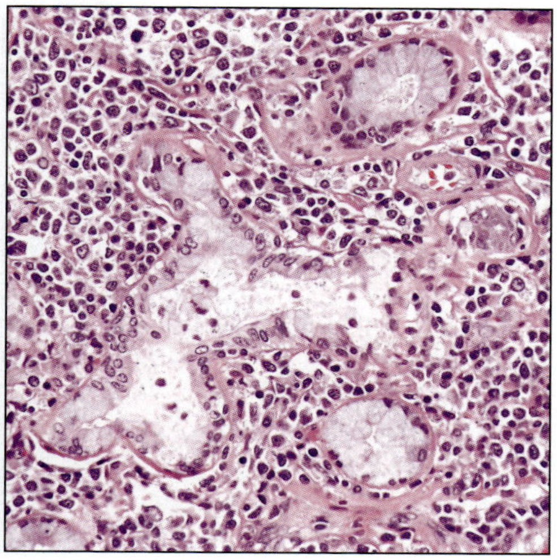

(Left) *Scanning magnification of diffuse large B-cell lymphoma of the lung shows infiltration and destruction of bronchial cartilage by the tumor. On rare occasions, the tumors can display an endobronchial location with prominent occlusion of the lumen.* ***(Right)*** *Diffuse large B-cell lymphoma of the lung shows entrapment of bronchial glands by the tumor. The tumor cells in this case were strongly positive for pan-B-cell markers, including CD20 and CD79a.*

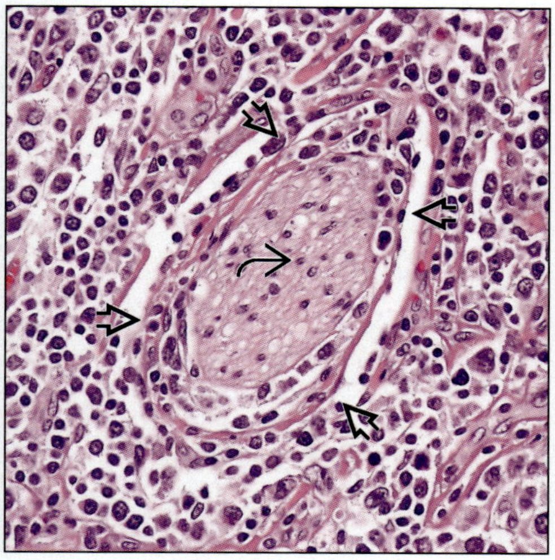

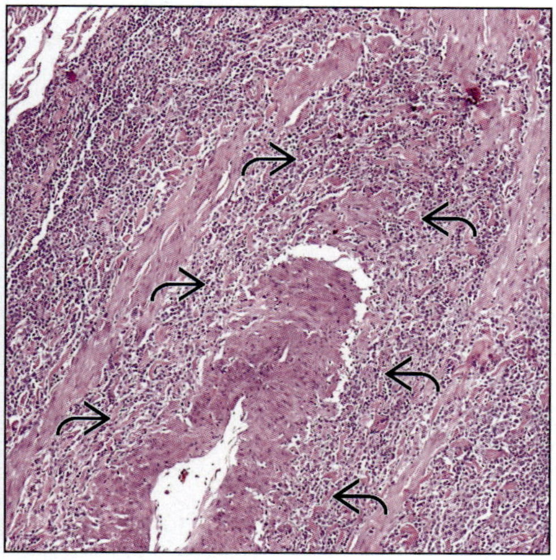

(Left) *Diffuse large B-cell lymphoma of the lung shows a focus of perineural invasion ➩. The perineurial sheath of the small nerve ↷ in the center is infiltrated by the large, atypical lymphocytes.* ***(Right)*** *Diffuse large B-cell lymphoma of the lung shows perivascular infiltration by the tumor. The tumor cells are seen to splay and replace the media in this large-caliber vessel ↷. Cases like these need to be distinguished from lymphomatoid granulomatosis.*

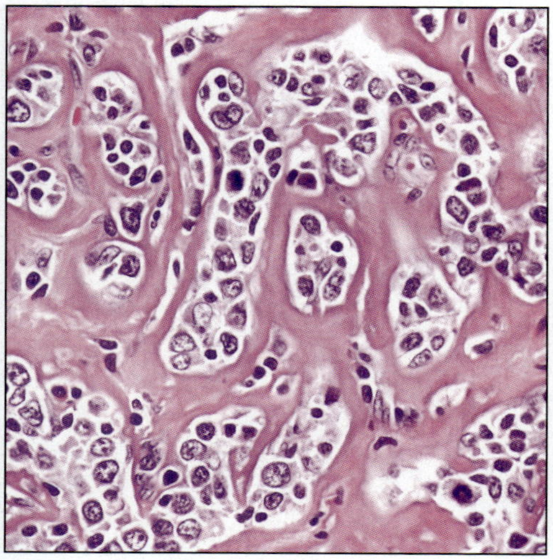

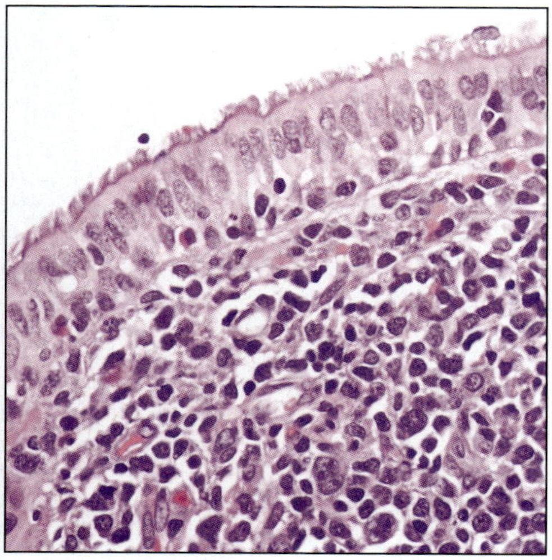

(Left) *Diffuse large B-cell lymphoma of the lung shows an unusual pattern of stromal hyalinization resulting in compartmentalization of tumor cells into small "nests" simulating carcinoma. This histologic appearance is very similar to that observed in primary diffuse large cell lymphomas of the mediastinum.* ***(Right)*** *Diffuse large B-cell lymphoma of the lung shows lymphoid cell infiltrate distributed underneath the bronchial mucosa, which does not infiltrate it.*

DIFFUSE LARGE CELL LYMPHOMA

Large Cell Immunoblastic Lymphoma

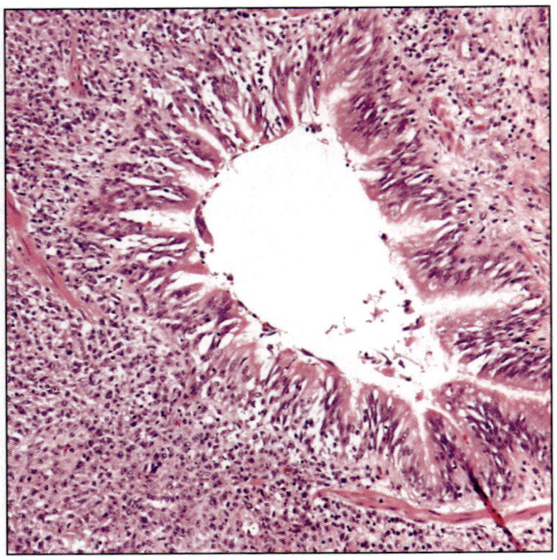

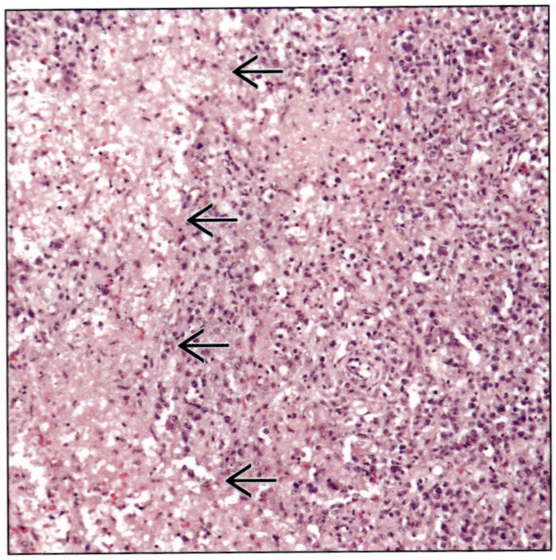

(Left) *Large cell immunoblastic lymphoma of the lung shows entrapment of an airspace by a dense, homogeneous population of large, atypical lymphoid cells.* ***(Right)*** *Immunoblastic large cell lymphoma involving the lung shows prominent areas of necrosis ⇒ surrounded by a diffuse atypical large lymphoid cell population. Immunoblastic lymphomas are high-grade malignancies that are often accompanied by extensive areas of tumor cell necrosis.*

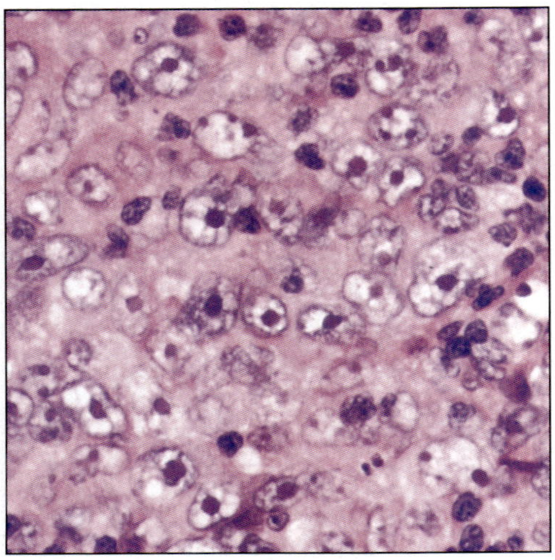

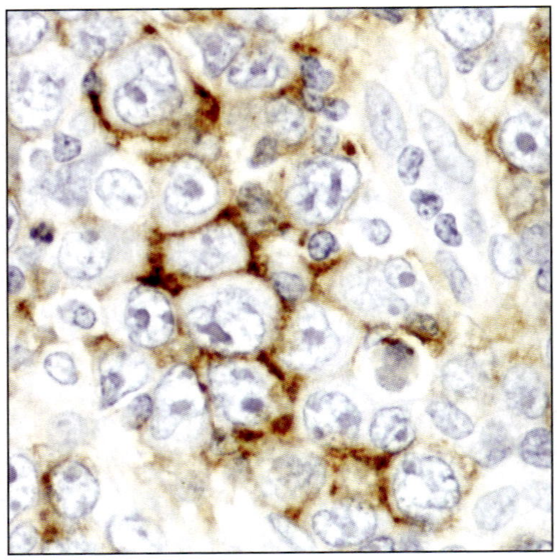

(Left) *Higher magnification of diffuse large B-cell lymphoma of the lung with immunoblastic features shows large tumor cells with large, vesicular nuclei and prominent eosinophilic nucleoli. The cells also contain abundant eosinophilic cytoplasm.* ***(Right)*** *Immunohistochemical staining of large immunoblastic lymphoma of the lung for CD20 shows positive staining in the large tumor cells. Stains for T-cell markers, CD30, and ALK1 were negative in this tumor.*

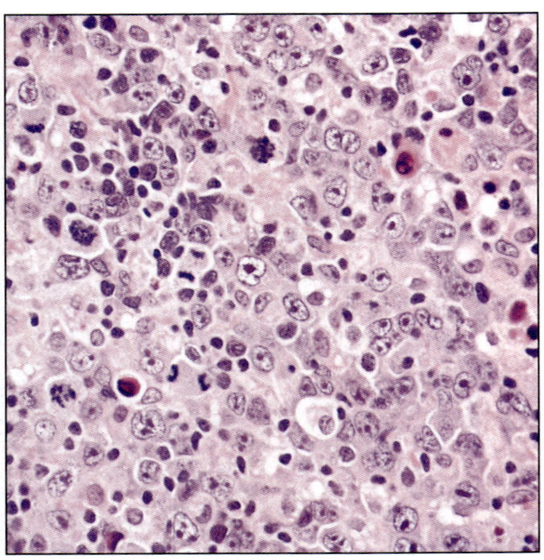

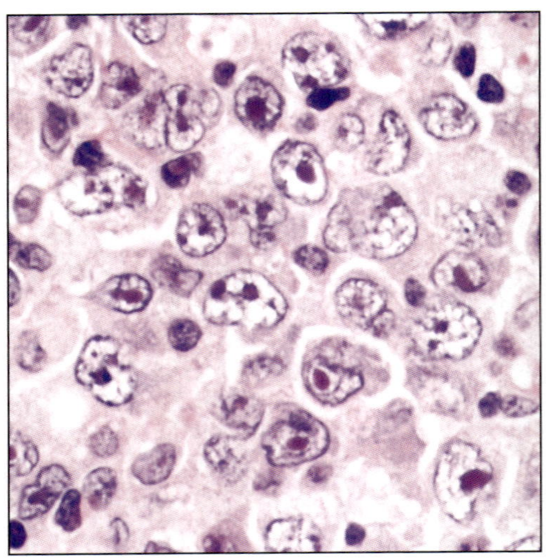

(Left) *Diffuse large B-cell lymphoma of the lung (immunoblastic type) shows sheets of large mononuclear cells with enlarged nuclei containing prominent nucleoli and surrounded by an abundant rim of cytoplasm.* ***(Right)*** *Higher magnification of immunoblastic large cell lymphoma of the lung shows large mononuclear cells with enlarged nuclei containing prominent eosinophilic nucleoli and abundant cytoplasm. These tumors are generally positive for CD20 and other pan-B-cell antigens.*

Anaplastic Large Cell Lymphoma

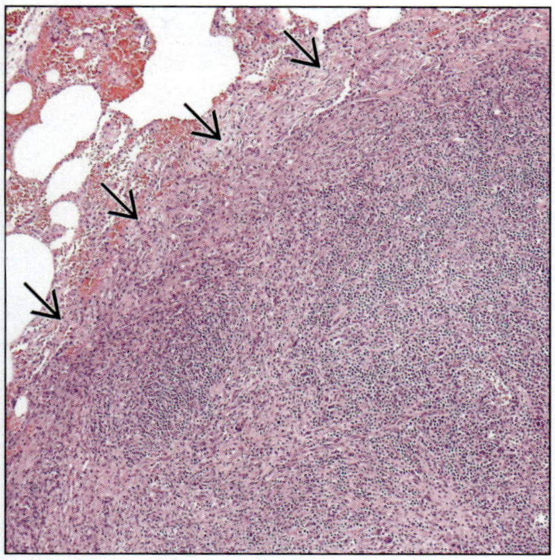
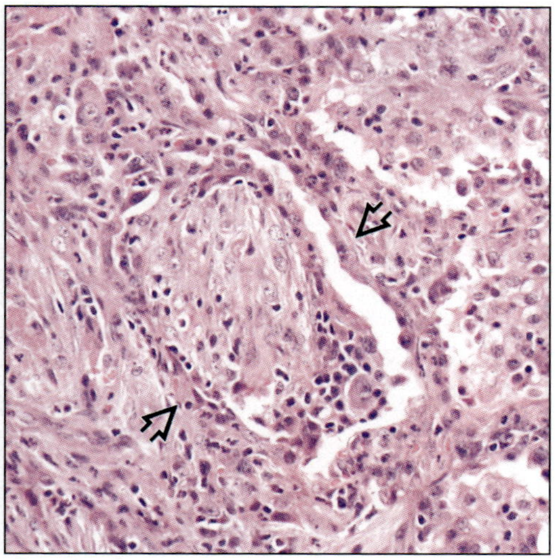

(Left) *Scanning magnification of anaplastic large cell lymphoma of the lung shows a well-circumscribed neoplastic population of cells composed of sheets of large, discohesive tumor cells. The tumor is sharply demarcated from the surrounding pulmonary parenchyma* →. ***(Right)*** *Higher magnification of an anaplastic large cell lymphoma of the lung shows entrapment of airspaces within the tumor with plugging of alveolar spaces* ⇨ *by large, atypical tumor cells.*

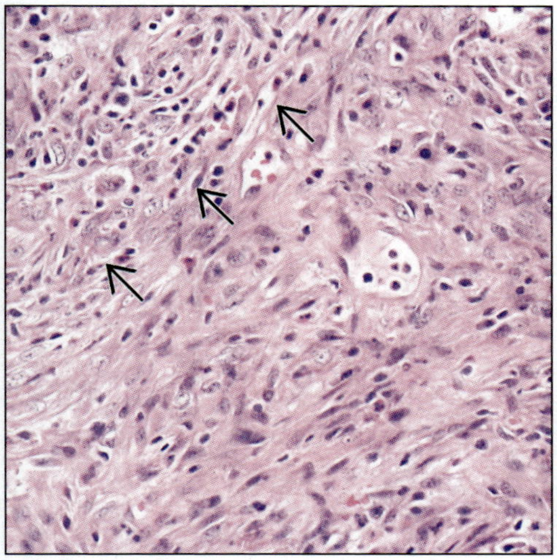
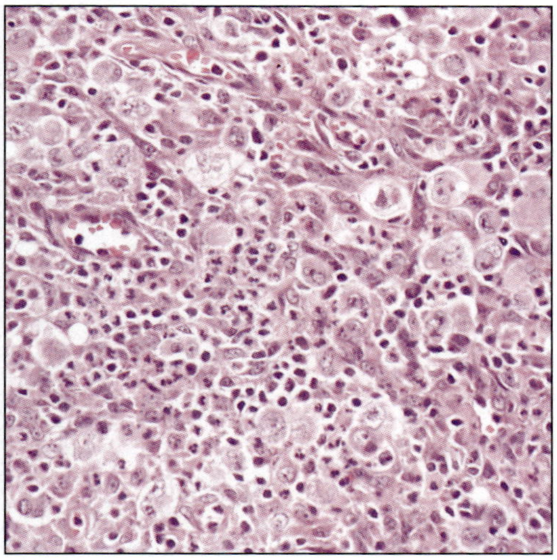

(Left) *Higher magnification of anaplastic large cell lymphoma of the lung shows large atypical cells with abundant cytoplasm and epithelioid morphology* → *blending with atypical spindle cell proliferation (lower right). Sarcomatoid appearance is an unusual feature of these tumors.* ***(Right)*** *Higher magnification of an anaplastic large cell lymphoma shows a mixed population composed of scattered small lymphocytes admixed with larger, round epithelioid cells.*

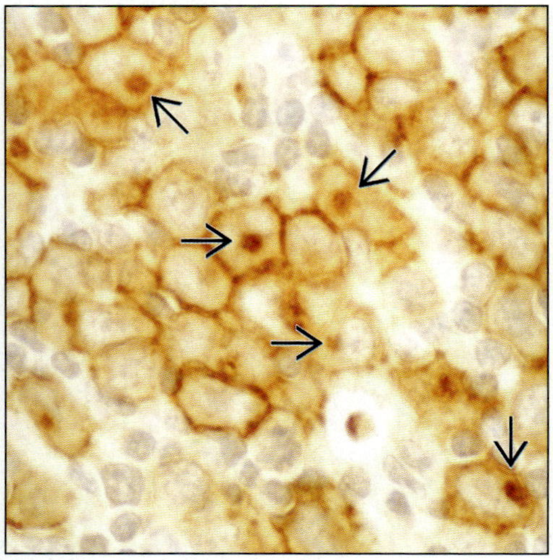
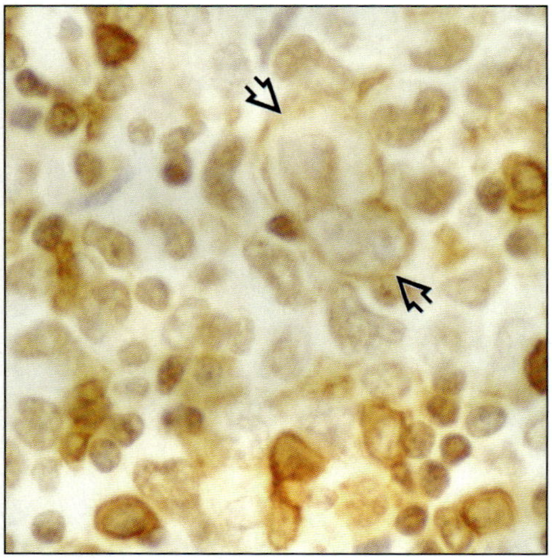

(Left) *Immunohistochemical staining of anaplastic large cell lymphoma of the lung with CD30 antibody shows strong membranous and paranuclear (Golgi zone, dot-like)* → *staining in the large tumor cells.* ***(Right)*** *Immunohistochemical staining of an anaplastic large cell lymphoma of the lung with CD45RO (UCHL-1) pan-T-cell marker shows positivity of a few scattered small lymphocytes and also membrane positivity in the large, atypical lymphoid cells* ⇨.

DIFFUSE LARGE CELL LYMPHOMA

Anaplastic Large Cell Lymphoma

(Left) *Scanning magnification of an anaplastic large cell lymphoma of the lung shows a neoplastic population composed of sheets of large, atypical cells with bizarre nuclei admixed with scattered small lymphocytes.* ***(Right)*** *Characteristic histology of anaplastic large cell lymphoma of the lung shows large atypical cells with enlarged nuclei adopting a kidney-shaped or "horseshoe" configuration ➢. This type of cell is highly distinctive (hallmark cell) for this tumor.*

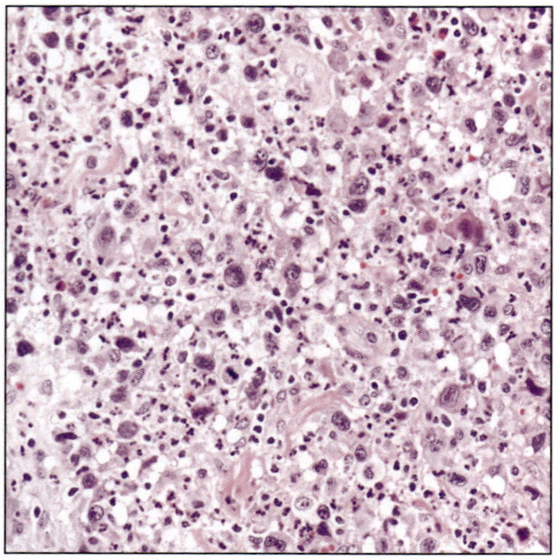

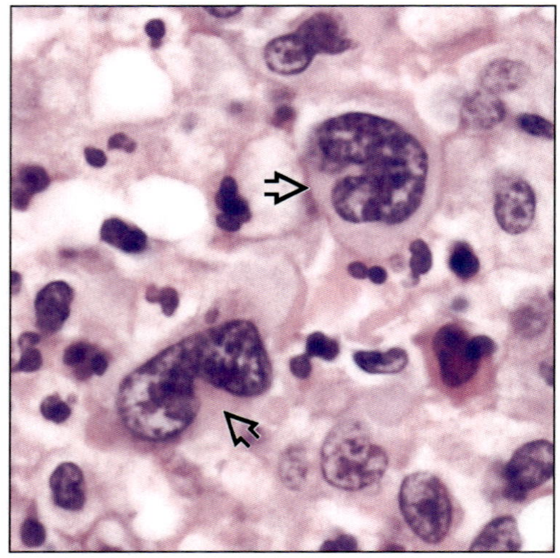

(Left) *Higher magnification of an anaplastic large cell lymphoma of the lung shows bizarre multinucleated tumor cells with multiple overlapping nuclei with prominent eosinophilic nucleoli resembling a Reed-Sternberg cell.* ***(Right)*** *Higher magnification in an anaplastic large cell lymphoma of the lung shows a Reed-Sternberg-like binucleated cell with prominent eosinophilic nucleoli ➢. Cases like this can be difficult to distinguish from Hodgkin lymphoma.*

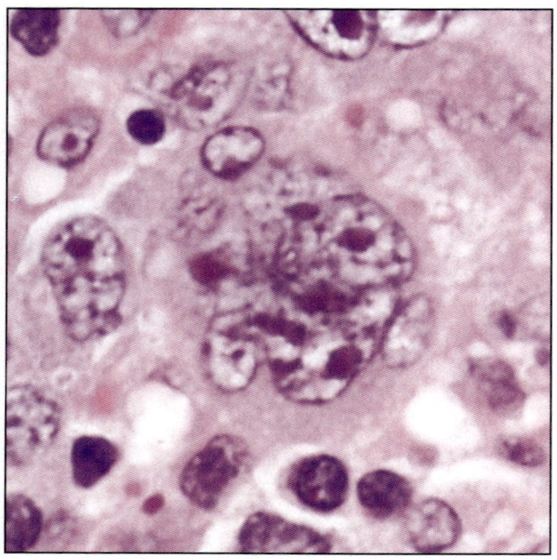

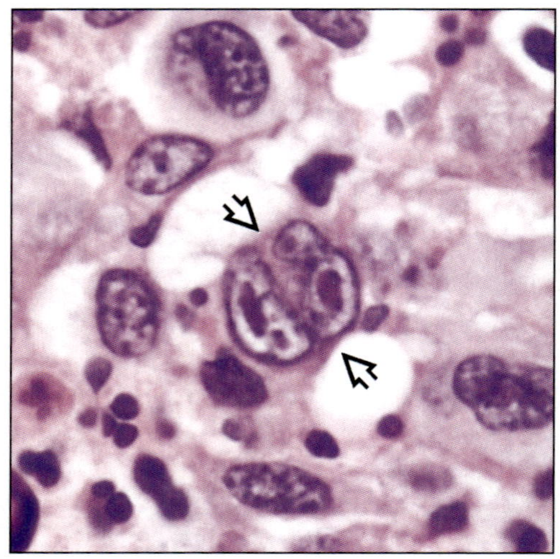

(Left) *Immunohistochemical staining of an anaplastic large cell lymphoma for CD30 antibody shows strong membranous and dot-like, paranuclear cytoplasmic staining in the large, atypical tumor cells.* ***(Right)*** *Immunohistochemical staining of an anaplastic large cell lymphoma for CD20 shows scattered positive small lymphocytes. Notice, however, that the large atypical cells in the background are negative →. These tumors can stain positive for ALK1 and for pan-T-cell markers.*

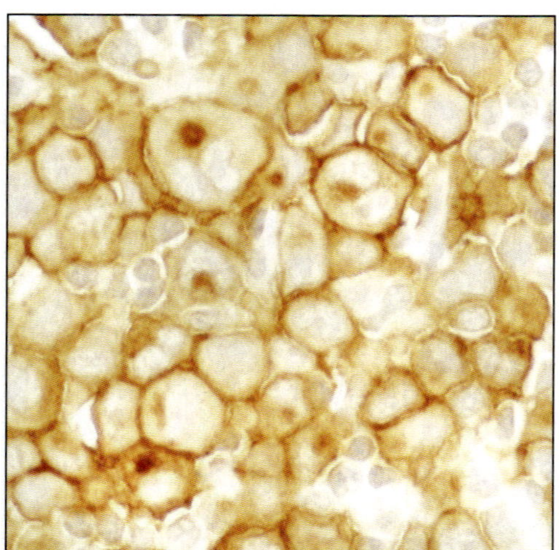

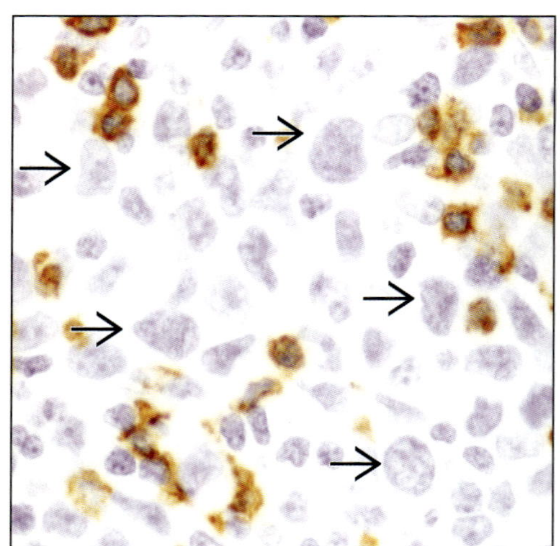

Peripheral T-cell Lymphoma

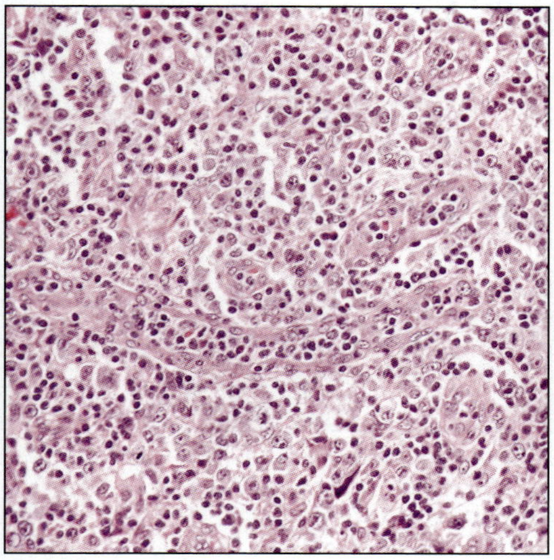

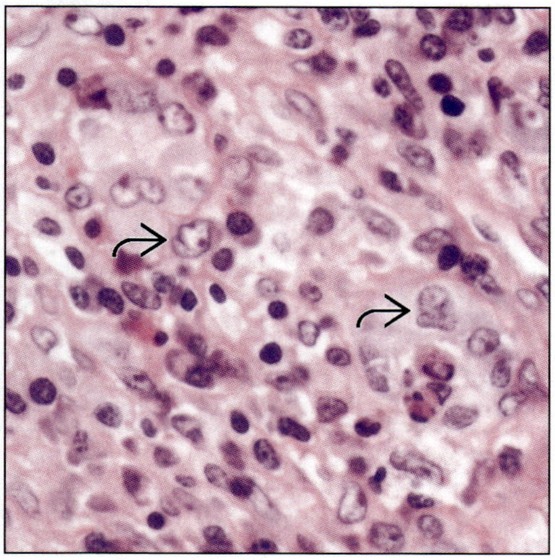

(Left) *Peripheral T-cell lymphoma of the lung shows sheets of lymphoid cells composed of a mixed population, including small lymphocytes, plasma cells, eosinophils, and scattered large, atypical lymphocytes. Notice prominent stromal hypervascularity.* ***(Right)*** *Higher magnification of a pulmonary peripheral T-cell lymphoma shows a mixed population of cells including small lymphocytes, plasma cells, eosinophils, and scattered, large, atypical lymphoid cells with convoluted nuclei ➚.*

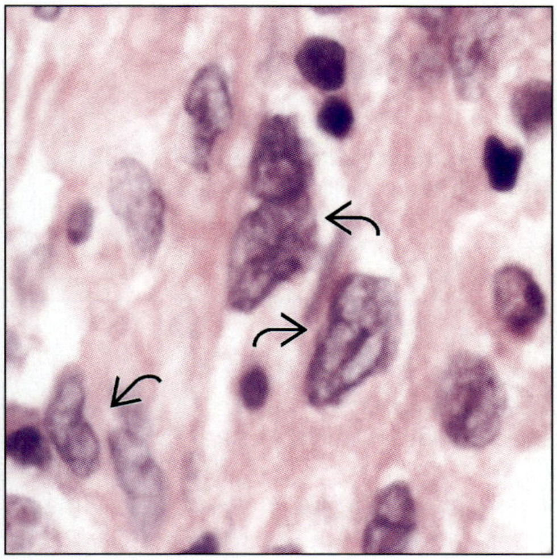

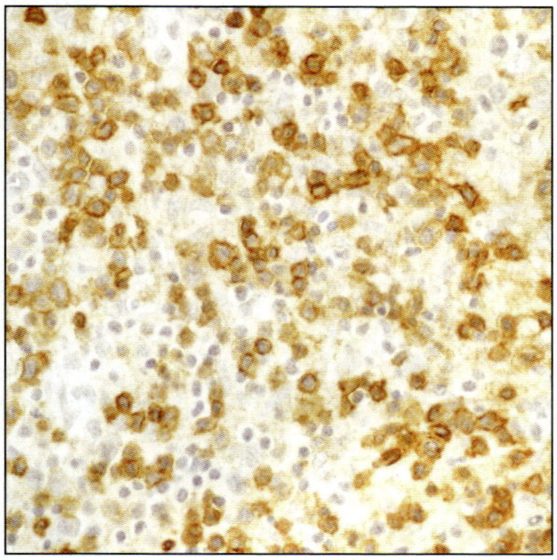

(Left) *Higher magnification of a pulmonary peripheral T-cell lymphoma shows atypical lymphoid cells ➚ with enlarged nuclei displaying irregular nuclear contours with a scant rim of amphophilic cytoplasm.* ***(Right)*** *Immunohistochemical staining of pulmonary peripheral T-cell lymphoma with a pan-T-cell marker (CD45RO [UCHL-1]) shows strong positive staining of the atypical T lymphocytes and negative staining in the smaller B cells scattered in the background.*

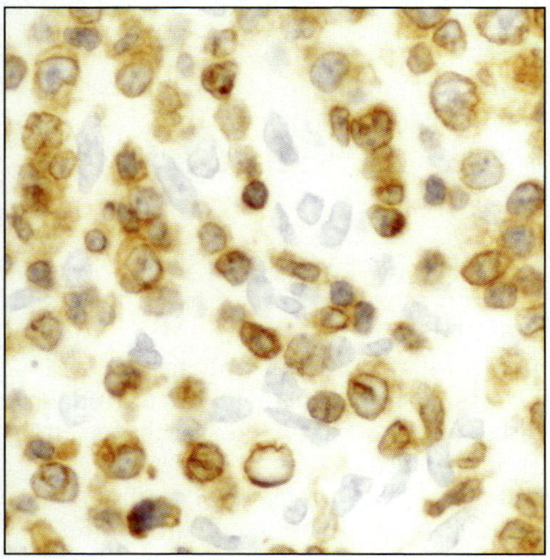

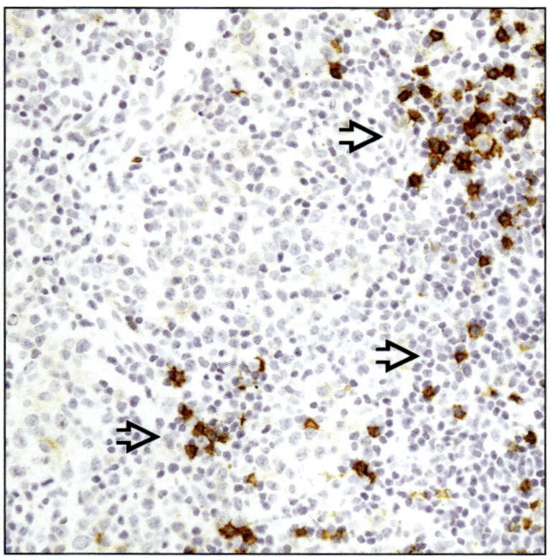

(Left) *Immunohistochemical staining of pulmonary peripheral T-cell lymphoma for CD3 antibody shows numerous positive cells with enlarged, irregular nuclei. Notice that the smaller, normal B lymphocytes in the background are negative.* ***(Right)*** *Immunohistochemical staining of pulmonary peripheral T-cell lymphoma with antibodies for the pan-B-cell marker (CD20) shows a few scattered positive cells ⇨. The larger, neoplastic T cells seen in the background are negative.*

HODGKIN LYMPHOMA

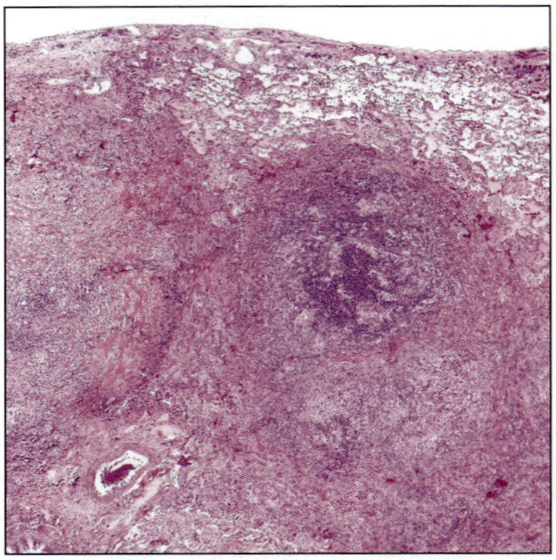

Multiple tumor nodules are seen in this lung involved with Hodgkin lymphoma. The infiltrate is composed of a mixed population of lymphocytes, plasma cells, eosinophils, and scattered large atypical cells.

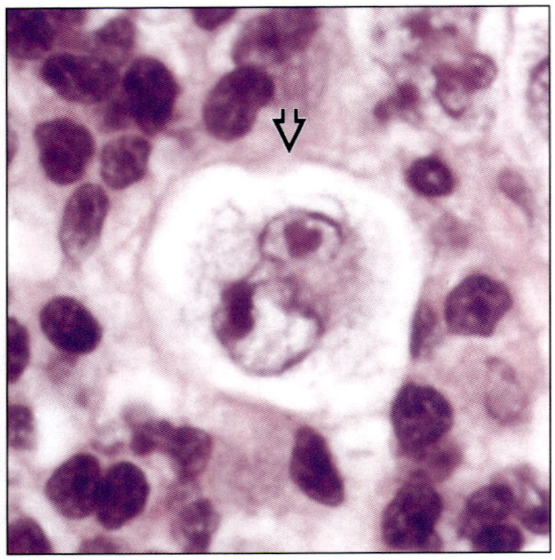

High magnification of a pulmonary nodule in Hodgkin lymphoma shows a characteristic binucleated Reed-Sternberg cell with double nuclei and prominent "owl-eyed" eosinophilic nucleoli ⊳.

TERMINOLOGY

Abbreviations

- Hodgkin lymphoma (HL)

Synonyms

- Hodgkin disease

Definitions

- Lymphoid neoplasm composed of scattered mononuclear and multinucleated atypical lymphoid cells amid a mixed lymphoreticular infiltrate

ETIOLOGY/PATHOGENESIS

Pathogenesis

- Epstein-Barr virus (EBV) has been claimed to play a role in subset of cases
- EBV infection may be cofactor in the genetic cascade of events leading to development of HL
- Neoplastic cells are derived from mature B cells at the germinal center stage of differentiation in > 98% of cases

CLINICAL ISSUES

Epidemiology

- Incidence
  - HL arising primarily in lungs is extremely rare
  - Pulmonary involvement is most often seen in course of regional or systemic dissemination
- Age
  - Bimodal age distribution with peak incidences between 20-30 years and 60-80 years

Presentation

- Night sweats
- Mediastinal, cervical, or supraclavicular lymphadenopathy

Treatment

- Adjuvant therapy
  - Combination chemotherapy

Prognosis

- Primary extranodal pulmonary HL tends to follow more aggressive behavior than nodal-based HL

IMAGE FINDINGS

General Features

- Morphology
  - Single or multiple nodules
  - Bilateral reticulonodular infiltrates are seen less frequently
  - Absence of associated lymphadenopathy in primary lung cases

MACROSCOPIC FEATURES

General Features

- Well-circumscribed gray-white masses with areas of consolidation of lung parenchyma
- Nodules may be single or multiple and randomly distributed

MICROSCOPIC PATHOLOGY

Histologic Features

- Pulmonary involvement in HL has only been described for classic form of disease (classical Hodgkin)
- Majority of cases are of nodular sclerosis subtype and rest are of mixed cellularity
- Nodules consist of varying numbers of lymphocytes, plasma cells, and eosinophils admixed with scattered Reed-Sternberg cells
- Nodules may sometimes show central areas of necrosis

HODGKIN LYMPHOMA

Key Facts

Clinical Issues

- HL arising primarily in lungs is extremely rare
- Pulmonary involvement is most often seen in course of regional or systemic dissemination
- Night sweats
- Mediastinal, cervical, or supraclavicular lymphadenopathy

Microscopic Pathology

- Majority of cases are of nodular sclerosis subtype and rest are of mixed cellularity
- Nodules consist of varying numbers of lymphocytes, plasma cells, and eosinophils admixed with scattered Reed-Sternberg cells
- Neoplastic cells are represented by transformed atypical lymphocytes (Hodgkin cells and Reed-Sternberg cells)
- Hodgkin cells (HC) are large, mononuclear cells with large nucleus containing single prominent eosinophilic nucleolus
- Reed-Sternberg cells (RSC) are bi- or multinucleated cells containing prominent eosinophilic nucleoli
- Neoplastic cells always represent minority of infiltrate (0.1-10% of cells in infiltrate)

Ancillary Tests

- Reed-Sternberg cells and their variants show strong membranous and paranuclear (Golgi zone) positivity for CD30 and CD15
- Reed-Sternberg cells shows weak positivity for Pax-5 and can express EBV-encoded LMP-1
- Reed-Sternberg cells are negative for CD45, CD79a, and, in a majority of cases, CD20

- Process can also involve bronchial wall with destruction of cartilaginous plate
- Small epithelioid granulomas and foci of bronchopneumonia may be seen at periphery of nodules

Cytologic Features

- Neoplastic cells are represented by transformed atypical lymphocytes (Hodgkin cells and Reed-Sternberg cells)
- Hodgkin cells (HC) are large, mononuclear cells with large nuclei containing single prominent eosinophilic nucleoli
- Reed-Sternberg cells (RSC) are bi- or multinucleated cells containing prominent eosinophilic nucleoli
- Cells with condensed cytoplasm and large pyknotic basophilic nuclei are known as "mummy" cells
- Reed-Sternberg cells in nodular sclerosis subtype surrounded by clear halo (retraction artifact) are known as "lacunar" cells
- Hodgkin and Reed-Sternberg cells may vary from very scant and difficult to find to abundant in a given lesion
- Neoplastic cells always represent minority of infiltrate (0.1-10% of cells in infiltrate)
- Background infiltrate is polymorphous and composed of small lymphocytes, plasma cells, eosinophils, and histiocytes

ANCILLARY TESTS

Immunohistochemistry

- Reed-Sternberg cells and their variants show strong membranous and paranuclear (Golgi zone) positivity for CD30 and CD15
- Reed-Sternberg cells are negative for CD45, CD79a, and, in a majority of cases, CD20
- Reed-Sternberg cells shows weak positivity for Pax-5 and can express EBV-encoded LMP-1

In Situ Hybridization

- EBV-infected Reed-Sternberg cells show strong expression of EBER in their nuclei by in situ hybridization

Molecular Genetics

- Reed-Sternberg cells contain clonal immunoglobulin (*Ig*) gene rearrangements in > 98% of cases
- Minority of cases (< 2%) may show *TCR* gene rearrangements (T-cell receptor rearrangements)

DIFFERENTIAL DIAGNOSIS

Anaplastic Large Cell Lymphoma (ALCL)

- Sheets of anaplastic tumor cells resembling Reed-Sternberg cells in which anaplastic cells predominate
- Majority of ALCL are of T-cell lineage and express ALK1 and T-cell markers
- ALK negative ALCL may be difficult to distinguish from HL, but it consistently demonstrates T-cell receptor (*TCR*) gene rearrangements

Lymphomatoid Granulomatosis (LYG)

- LYG may show similar histologic appearance to HL with scattered large atypical cells against mixed inflammatory background
- Atypical cells in LYG are CD20(+) and EBER(+) and do not stain for CD15 or CD30

SELECTED REFERENCES

1. Rodriguez J et al: Hodgkin lymphoma presenting with exclusive or preponderant pulmonary involvement: a clinicopathologic study of 5 new cases. Ann Diagn Pathol. 10(2):83-8, 2006
2. Costa MB et al: Histologic patterns of lung infiltration of B-cell, T-cell, and Hodgkin lymphomas. Am J Clin Pathol. 121(5):718-26, 2004

HODGKIN LYMPHOMA

Histologic and Cytologic Features

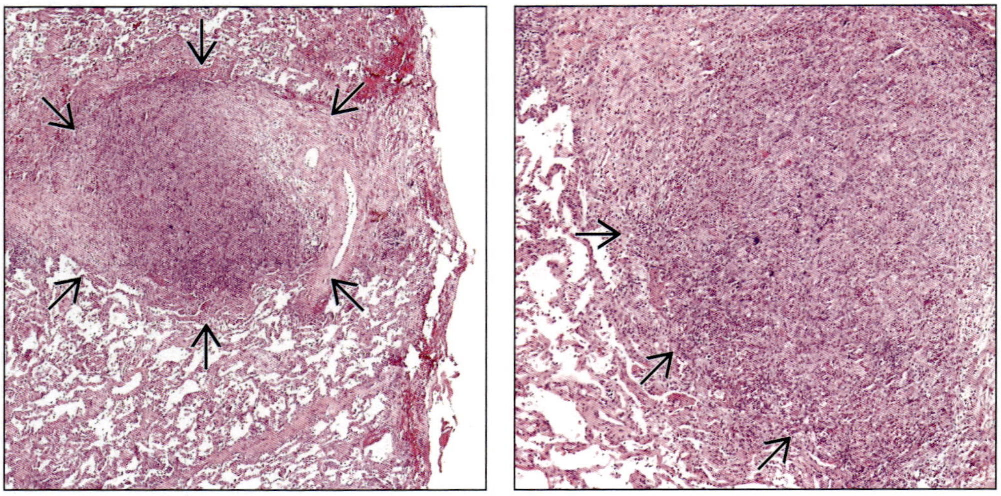

(Left) *Scanning magnification of Hodgkin lymphoma involving the lung shows a well-defined solid nodule in a subpleural location* → *surrounded by normal-appearing pulmonary parenchyma.* ***(Right)*** *Lung involvement in Hodgkin lymphoma shows a well-defined area of condensation of pulmonary parenchyma* →*. The differential diagnosis for lesions with this morphology incudes diffuse large cell lymphoma, anaplastic large cell lymphoma, and lymphomatoid granulomatosis.*

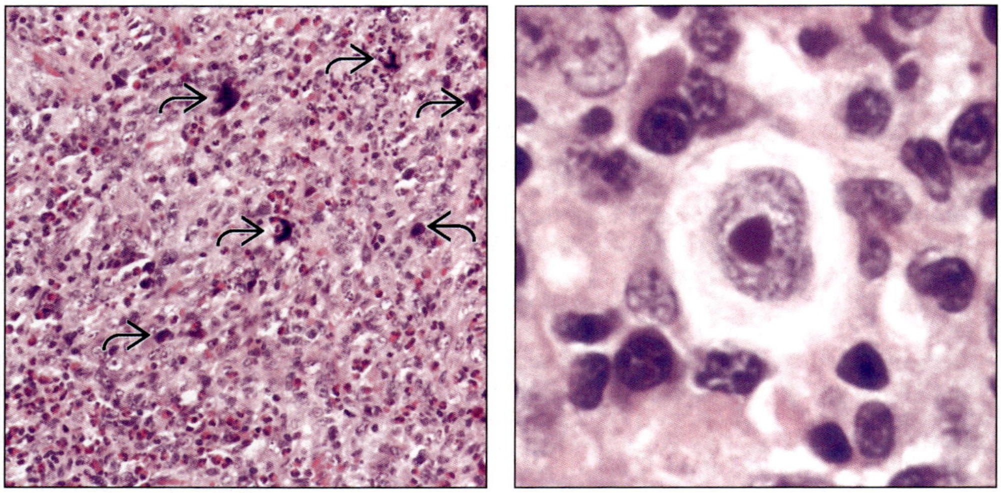

(Left) *Higher magnification of a pulmonary nodule in a patient with Hodgkin lymphoma shows a mixed cell population containing small lymphocytes, plasma cells, eosinophils, and histiocytes as well as scattered larger lymphoid cells. Some of the larger cells show pyknotic nuclei (so-called "mummy" cells)* ↪*.* ***(Right)*** *Higher magnification of a lung nodule involved with Hodgkin lymphoma shows a large mononuclear cell with a prominent eosinophilic nucleolus (so-called Hodgkin cell).*

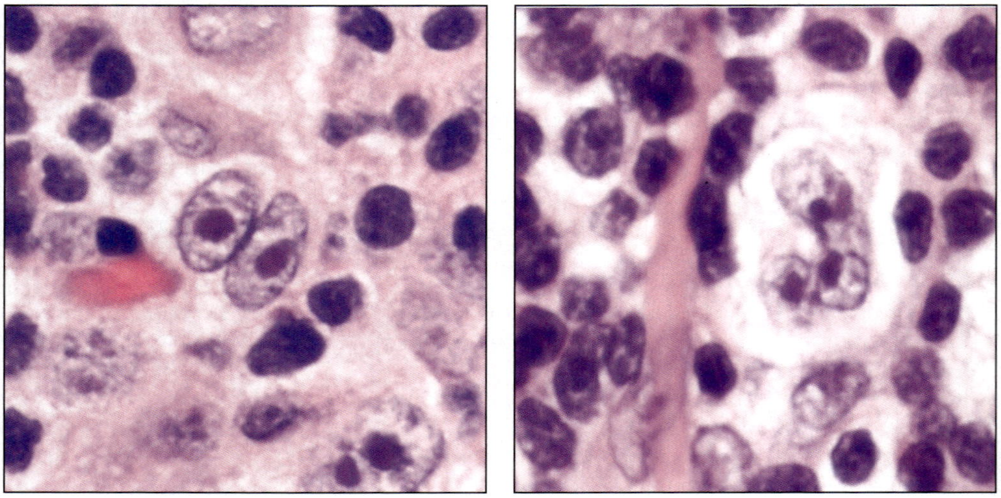

(Left) *Higher magnification of a lung nodule involved with Hodgkin lymphoma shows a classical binucleated Reed-Sternberg cell with the characteristic "owl-eyed" eosinophilic nucleoli. Mononuclear Hodgkin cells and bi- or multinucleated Reed-Sternberg cells are the neoplastic proliferating cells in Hodgkin lymphoma.* ***(Right)*** *High magnification of a lung nodule in Hodgkin lymphoma shows a multinucleated Reed-Sternberg cell with 3 nuclei containing prominent eosinophilic nucleoli.*

Histologic and Immunohistochemical Features

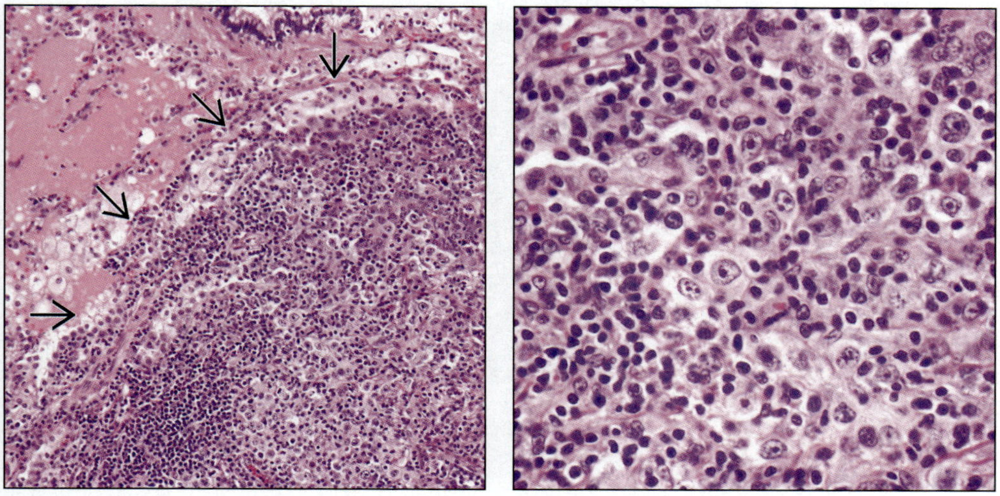

(Left) *Scanning magnification of a lung lesion in a patient with Hodgkin lymphoma shows a well-circumscribed area of parenchymal condensation → surrounded by normal lung parenchyma with intraalveolar edema fluid.* ***(Right)*** *Higher magnification from a lung nodule with HL shows a mixed population of inflammatory cells including small lymphocytes, plasma cells, histiocytes, and eosinophils admixed with scattered larger lymphoid cells with prominent nucleoli (Hodgkin cells).*

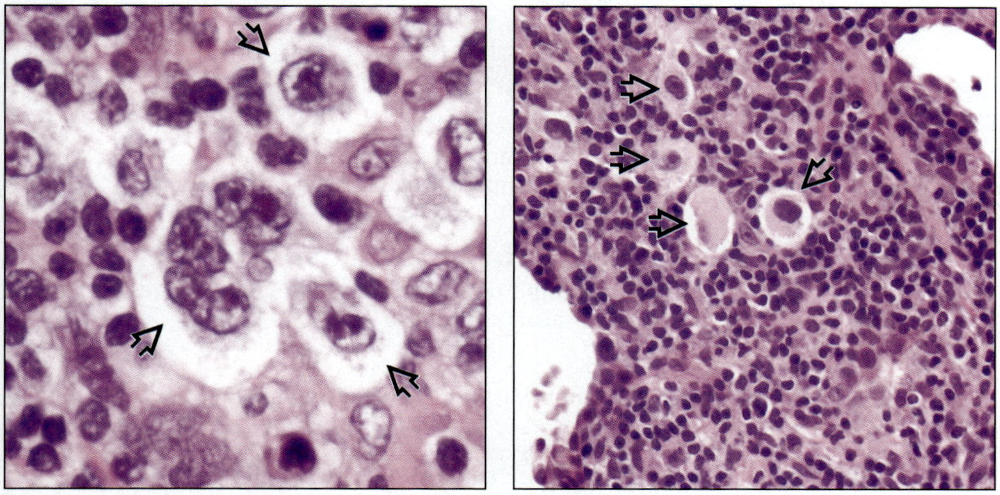

(Left) *Higher magnification of a lung nodule in a patient with Hodgkin lymphoma shows large mononuclear and multinucleated atypical cells. Bi- and multinucleated Reed-Sternberg cells in the nodular sclerosis subtype are designated "lacunar" cells due to their clear perinuclear clearing ⇨.* ***(Right)*** *Hodgkin lymphoma involving the lung shows an interstitial pattern of spread with widening of the intraalveolar septa by a mixed population of lymphoid cells containing a few Hodgkin cells ⇨.*

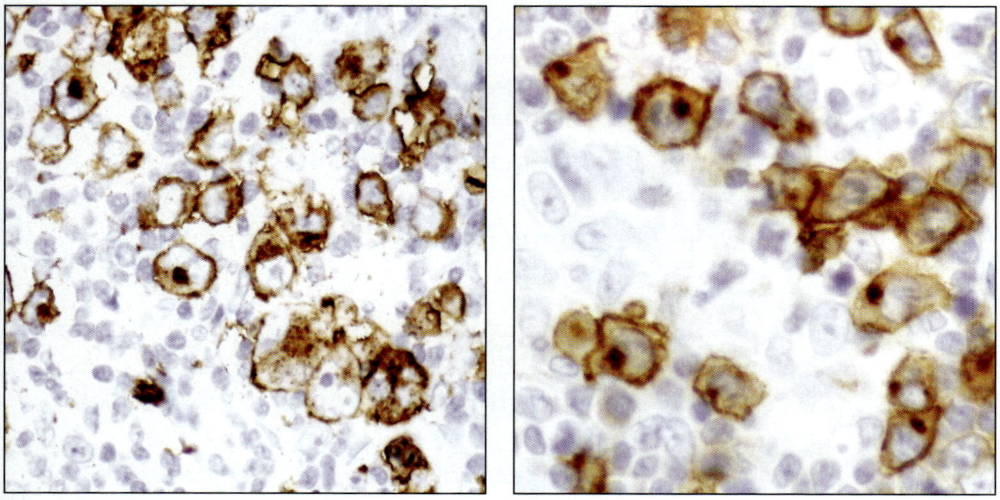

(Left) *Immunohistochemical staining of pulmonary Hodgkin lymphoma with CD30 shows positive membrane and paranuclear (Golgi zone) positivity in Reed-Sternberg cells. This antibody is expressed in 100% of cases in HL.* ***(Right)*** *Immunohistochemical staining of pulmonary Hodgkin lymphoma for CD15 shows membrane and paranuclear (Golgi zone) positivity in the large atypical cells. CD15 stains these cells less frequently than CD30 (only in about 65% of cases).*

PLASMACYTOMA

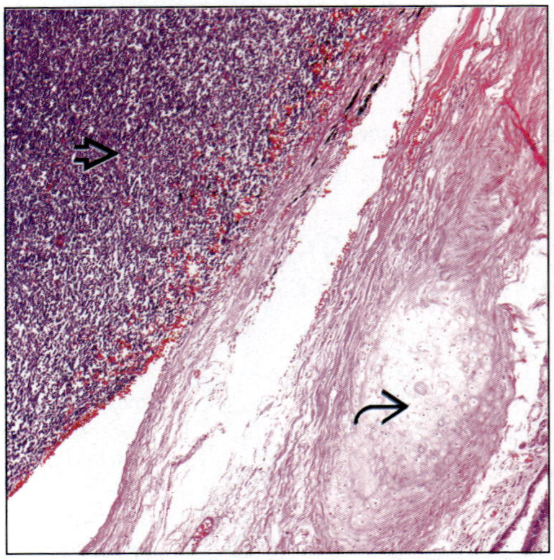

Pulmonary plasmacytoma shows destruction of the lung parenchyma by a homogeneous neoplastic cellular proliferation ⇒. Note the bronchial cartilage that is without invasion ↗.

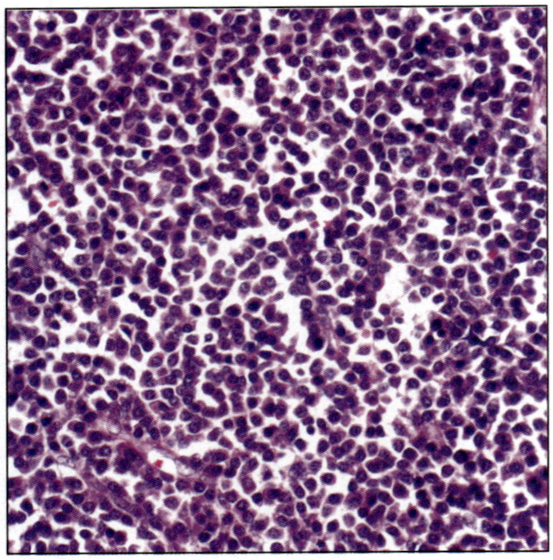

Closer view at the neoplastic cellular proliferation composed exclusively of atypical plasma cells. There is no special growth pattern.

TERMINOLOGY

Definitions

- Malignant neoplasm composed of proliferation of monoclonal plasma cells

ETIOLOGY/PATHOGENESIS

Etiology

- Plasma cell dyscrasia

CLINICAL ISSUES

Epidemiology

- Incidence
  - Primary plasmacytomas in lung are rare
  - Represent approximately 5% of all extramedullary plasmacytomas
- Age
  - Described essentially in adults
    - Usually from 50-80 years old
- Gender
  - No gender predilection for these tumors

Presentation

- Cough
- Shortness of breath
- Hemoptysis
- Multiple myeloma
- Asymptomatic

Treatment

- Surgical approaches
  - Pneumonectomy
  - Lobectomy

Prognosis

- 2-year survival rate approximately 66%
- 5-year survival rate approximately 40%
- Good possibility for long-term survival

MACROSCOPIC FEATURES

General Features

- Hilar or parenchymal mass
- Well circumscribed and firm
- Yellowish to gray in color

Sections to Be Submitted

- It is important to submit hilar lymph nodes as they may also be involved

Size

- Tumors vary from 2-8 cm in diameter

MICROSCOPIC PATHOLOGY

Histologic Features

- Diffuse plasma cell proliferation
- Plasma cell with Dutcher bodies
- Vague nested pattern
- Focal angiectatic areas
- Monoclonal gammopathy

Predominant Pattern/Injury Type

- Diffuse

Predominant Cell/Compartment Type

- Plasma cell

DIFFERENTIAL DIAGNOSIS

Inflammatory Pseudotumor, Plasma Cell Type

- Plasma cell proliferation in plasmacytomas is monoclonal
- In inflammatory pseudotumor, plasma cells are usually admixed with spindle myofibroblastic cells

PLASMACYTOMA

Key Facts

Clinical Issues
- Incidence
  - Primary plasmacytomas of lung are rare
  - May represent approximately 5% of all extramedullary plasmacytomas
  - Tumor has been described essentially in adults
- Symptoms
  - Cough
  - Hemoptysis
  - Dyspnea
  - Multiple myeloma
  - Asymptomatic
- Prognosis
  - 2-year survival rate approximately 66%
  - 5-year survival rate approximately 40%

Macroscopic Features
- Hilar or parenchymal mass
- Tumors vary from 2-8 cm in diameter
- It is important to submit hilar lymph nodes as they may also be involved

Microscopic Pathology
- Diffuse plasma cell proliferation
- Vague nested pattern
- Focal angiectatic areas
- Monoclonal gammopathy
- Plasma cell with Dutcher bodies

Top Differential Diagnoses
- Inflammatory pseudotumor, plasma cell type
- Carcinoma
- Malignant lymphoma with plasmacytoid features

Immunohistochemistry

Antibody	Reactivity	Staining Pattern	Comment
CD138	Positive	Cytoplasmic	
CD20	Positive		May be positive in some cases
Kappa or Lambda	Positive	Cytoplasmic	Monoclonal gammopathy
EMA	Positive	Cell membrane	In some cases
CD45	Positive	Cytoplasmic	In some cases

Pneumonia
- Infiltrate is mixture of plasma cells and polymorphonuclear leukocytes
- No monoclonality in pneumonia

Carcinoma
- Presence of plasma cell differentiation is important to establish proper diagnosis
- Use of immunohistochemical studies will lead to correct interpretation

Malignant Lymphoma with Plasmacytoid Features
- Plasmacytomas will have exclusive plasma cell proliferation
- Use of markers of plasma cells may be of help
- Possible association with multiple myeloma may be of help

DIAGNOSTIC CHECKLIST

Clinically Relevant Pathologic Features
- Age distribution

Pathologic Interpretation Pearls
- Plasma cell proliferation
- Monoclonal gammopathy

SELECTED REFERENCES

1. Huwer H et al: Solitary pulmonary plasmacytoma: report of two cases. Med Oncol. 27(1):59-61, 2010
2. Goździuk K et al: A rare case of solitary plasmacytoma mimicking a primary lung tumor. Ann Thorac Surg. 87(4):e25-6, 2009
3. Shaikh G et al: Primary pulmonary plasmacytoma. J Clin Oncol. 26(18):3089-91, 2008
4. Thoennissen NH et al: Solitary plasmacytoma of the lung with coexisting sarcoid-like lesions. Ann Hematol. 87(5):417-20, 2008
5. Yang F et al: [Solitary plasmacytoma: a clinicopathologic and immunophenotypic analysis of 43 cases.] Sichuan Da Xue Xue Bao Yi Xue Ban. 37(1):93-6, 144, 2006
6. Marisavljevic D et al: Plasmacytoma of the lung: an indolent disease resistant to conventional myeloma treatment: report of a case. Med Oncol. 22(2):207-10, 2005
7. Niitsu N et al: Primary pulmonary plasmacytoma involving bilateral lungs and marked hypergammaglobulinemia: differentiation from extranodal marginal zone B-cell lymphoma of mucosa-associated lymphoid tissue. Leuk Res. 29(11):1361-4, 2005
8. Edelstein E et al: Primary solitary endobronchial plasmacytoma. Ann Thorac Surg. 78(4):1448-9, 2004
9. Koss MN et al: Pulmonary plasmacytomas: a clinicopathologic and immunohistochemical study of five cases. Ann Diagn Pathol. 2(1):1-11, 1998

PLASMACYTOMA

Microscopic Features

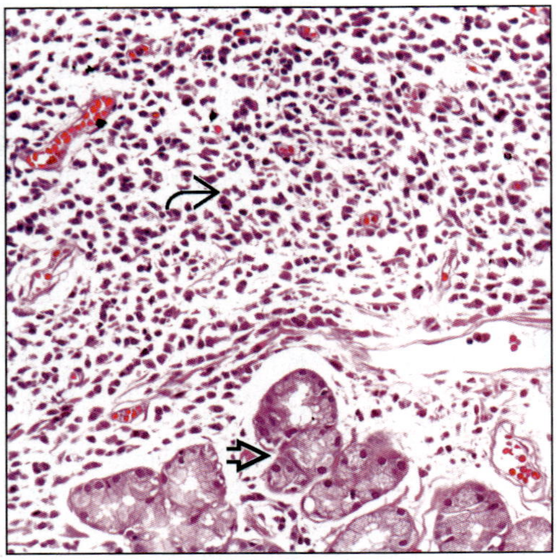
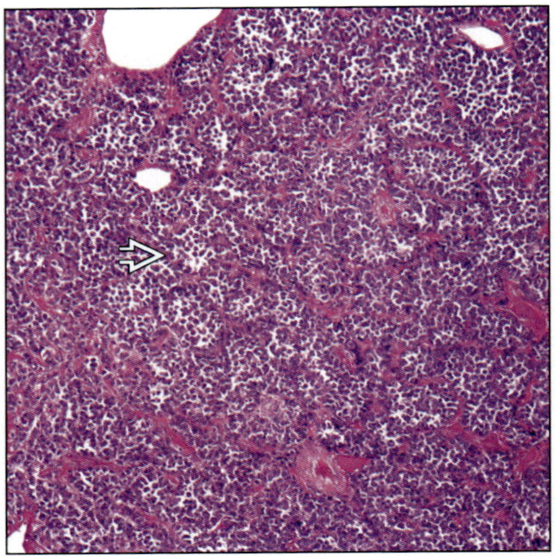

(Left) *Pulmonary plasmacytoma shows sheets of plasma cells. Endobronchial glands are present; however, these glands are not infiltrated by the plasmacytic proliferation.* ***(Right)*** *Pulmonary plasmacytoma shows a subtle nesting pattern that can be seen in other more common tumors of the lung, mainly neuroendocrine carcinomas. The tumor cells, however, are entirely composed of mature plasma cells.*

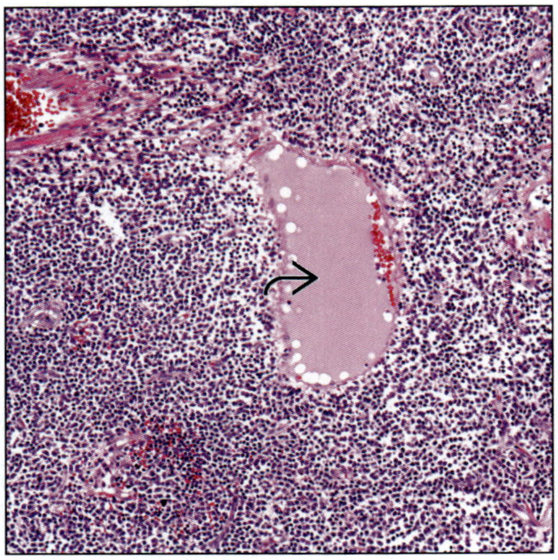
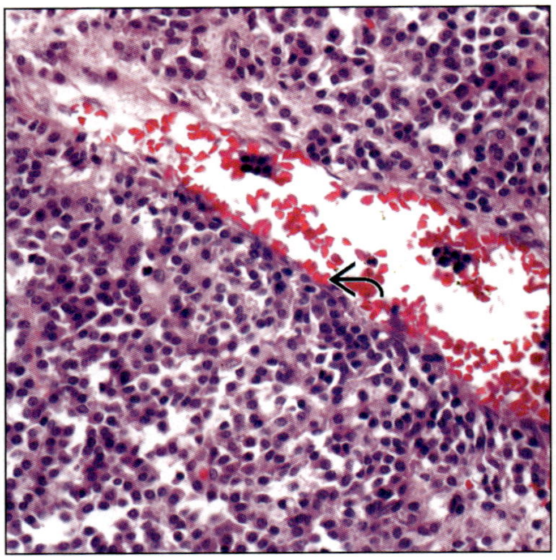

(Left) *Pulmonary plasmacytoma shows sheets of neoplastic cells around a pulmonary vessel containing edematous fluid in its lumen.* ***(Right)*** *In other areas, the pulmonary vessels can show extensive neoplastic cellular proliferation involving the endothelial cells and forming a neoplastic vasculitis.*

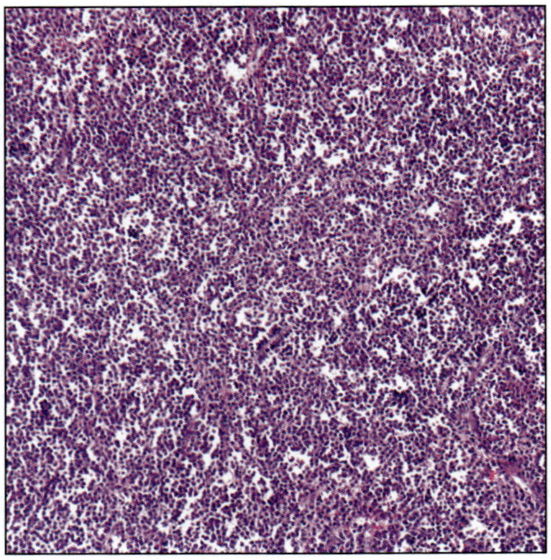
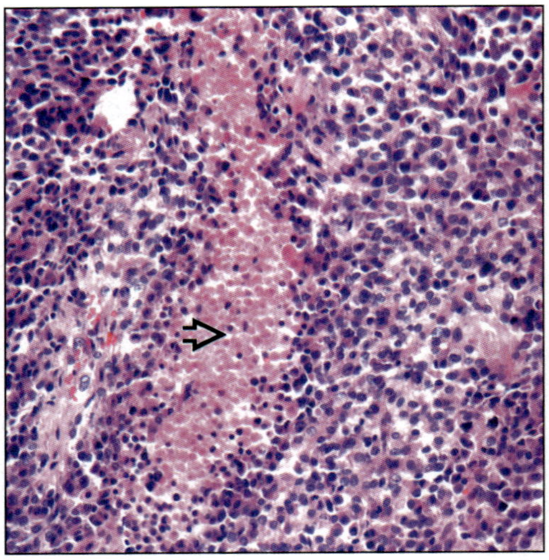

(Left) *The predominant feature of pulmonary plasmacytoma is a neoplastic homogeneous cellular proliferation growing in sheets. No definitive growth pattern is present in this case.* ***(Right)*** *In some cases of pulmonary plasmacytomas, there may be focal areas of necrosis. However, such a finding is not common in plasmacytomas of the lung.*

PLASMACYTOMA

Microscopic Features

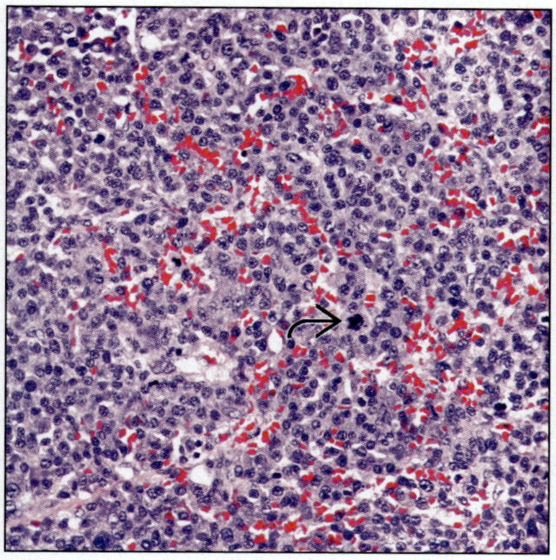

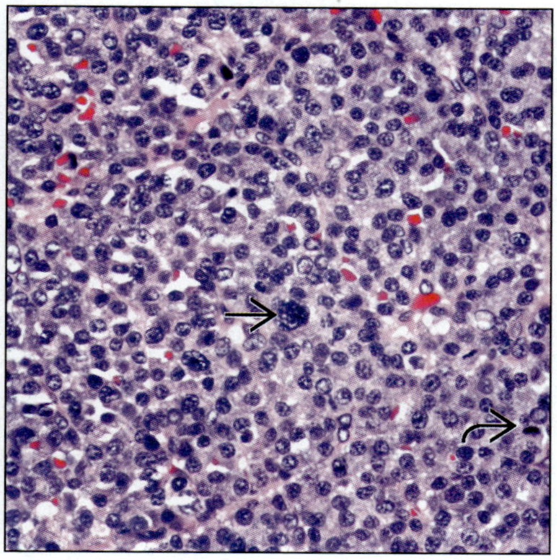

(Left) *High-power view of a less differentiated plasmacytoma of the lung is shown. Note the presence of nuclear atypia and easily identifiable mitotic figures, some of them atypical* ↪. ***(Right)*** *High-power view of a plasmacytoma of the lung is shown with a fairly homogeneous cellular proliferation and scattered multinucleated giant cells* →. *Rare mitotic figures are also present* ↪.

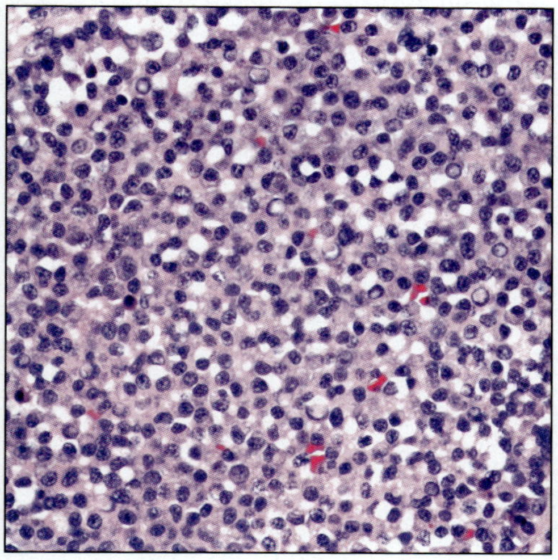

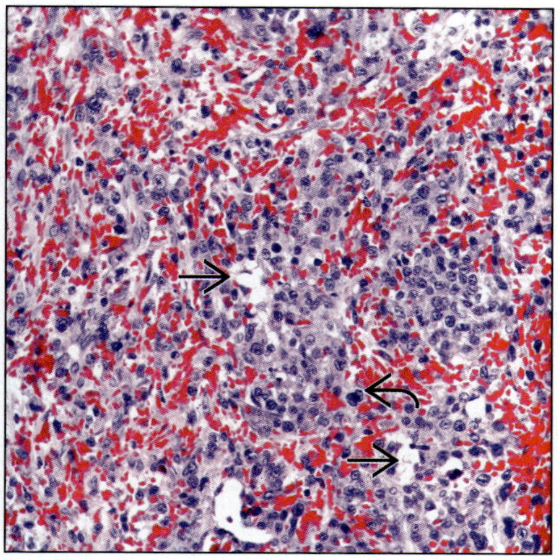

(Left) *High-power view shows the classical features of a pulmonary plasmacytoma with an atypical plasma cell proliferation, some of them containing Dutcher bodies.* ***(Right)*** *High-power view of a plasmacytoma of the lung is shown with unusual features of hemorrhage and pseudoglands* →. *Note the presence of nuclear pleomorphism* ↪ *even at this magnification.*

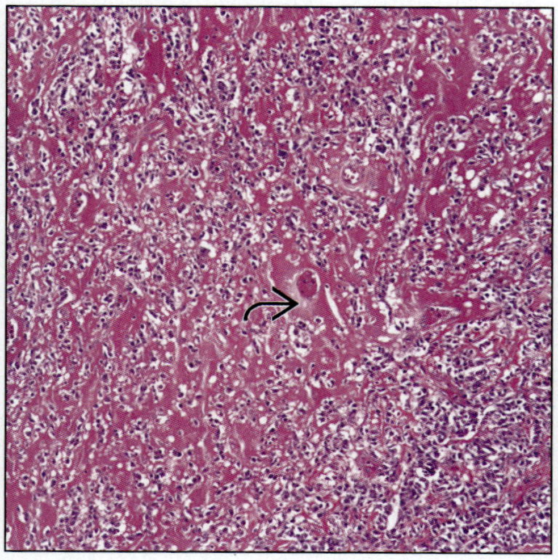

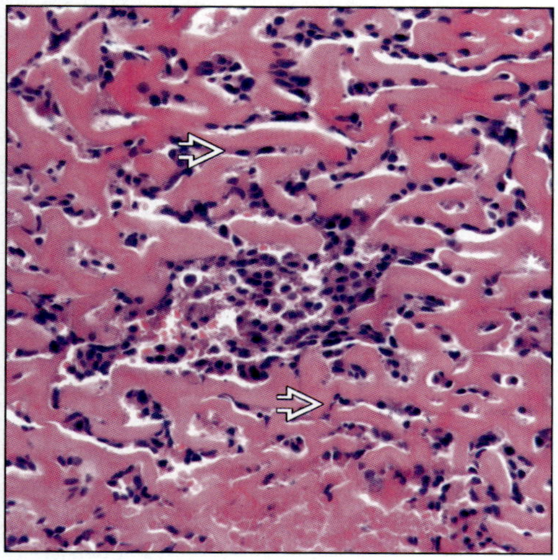

(Left) *Some cases of plasmacytoma may also show extensive areas of collagen deposition* ↪, *which may be easily confused for amyloid.* ***(Right)*** *In some cases, the presence of marked collagen fibers* ⇨ *can be so extensive that the tumor can be easily missed or misinterpreted for an inflammatory reaction.*

LYMPHOMATOID GRANULOMATOSIS

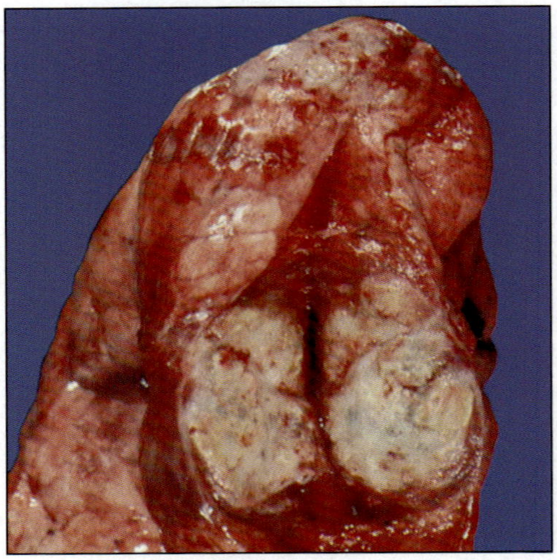

Cut surface of the lung in a patient with lymphomatoid granulomatosis shows a well-circumscribed, gray-white fleshy nodule with areas of necrosis.

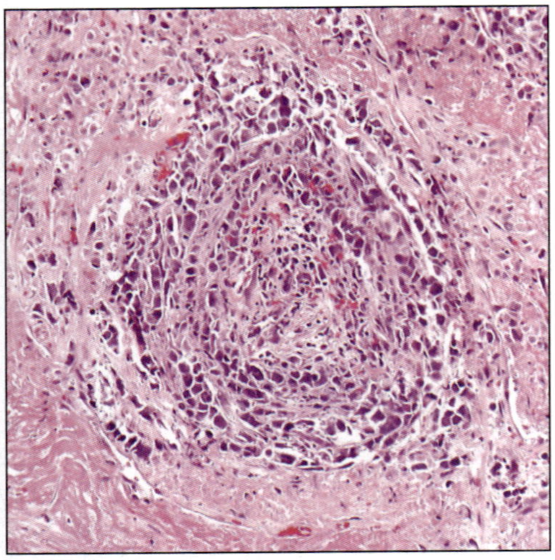

Histologic appearance of a lymphomatoid granulomatosis shows the concentric arrangement of atypical lymphoid cells around a vessel wall.

TERMINOLOGY

Abbreviations

- Lymphomatoid granulomatosis (LYG)

Synonyms

- Angiocentric immunoproliferative lesion

Definitions

- Angiocentric lymphoproliferative disorder composed of Epstein-Barr-infected B cells admixed with reactive T cells

ETIOLOGY/PATHOGENESIS

Pathogenesis

- Epstein-Barr-driven lymphoproliferative disorder arising in background of immune deficiency

CLINICAL ISSUES

Epidemiology

- Incidence
  - Rare disorder
  - Most commonly occurs in immunosuppressed patients
  - Seen in association with AIDS, transplants, or Wiskott-Aldrich syndrome
- Age
  - Most common in middle-aged adults
  - Can also occur in young adults and children

Presentation

- Cough
- Dyspnea

Laboratory Tests

- Impaired in vitro responsiveness to mitogens
- Diminished humoral and cell-mediated responsiveness to Epstein-Barr virus
- Decrease in total T cells, CD4 and CD8 lymphocytes

Natural History

- Disease is most often confined to lung but can involve other organs, including
  - Skin
  - Central nervous system
  - Kidney
- Some cases may progress to diffuse large B-cell lymphoma
- LYG is associated with up to 70% mortality, but some cases may regress spontaneously

Treatment

- Adjuvant therapy
  - Combination chemotherapy and corticosteroids
  - Rituximab
- Antiviral agents
  - Interferon has contributed to remission in some patients

IMAGE FINDINGS

Radiographic Findings

- Multiple bilateral and peripheral nodular opacities ± cavitation
- May also present with diffuse reticulonodular infiltrates or with a solitary mass

MACROSCOPIC FEATURES

General Features

- Well-circumscribed tumor mass with homogeneous gray-white cut section
- Lesions frequently contain central areas of necrosis

LYMPHOMATOID GRANULOMATOSIS

Key Facts

Terminology
- Angiocentric lymphoproliferative disorder composed of Epstein-Barr-infected B cells admixed with reactive T cells

Clinical Issues
- Cough
- Dyspnea

Microscopic Pathology
- Sheets of mixed, polymorphous atypical lymphoreticular infiltrates with destruction of lung parenchyma and extensive areas of necrosis
- Most salient feature is prominent angiocentricity of atypical lymphoid cells, with concentric arrangement of lymphoid cells replacing the intima and media
- Atypical lymphoid cells may be large and mononuclear or binucleated, resembling Reed-Sternberg cells
- LYG is subdivided into 3 grades based on number of large, EBV-positive cells in the infiltrate
- Atypical lymphoid cells may be large, mononuclear or binucleated, resembling Reed-Sternberg cells

Ancillary Tests
- Bulk of infiltrate is composed of reactive small CD2(+), CD3(+), CD4(+) T-helper lymphocytes
- Larger, atypical cells are positive for CD20 and CD79a
- Large, atypical cells are positive for EBV-latent membrane protein
- Large atypical cells react positively for EBV-encoded ribonucleotides (EBER) by in situ hybridization technique

MICROSCOPIC PATHOLOGY

Histologic Features
- Sheets of mixed, polymorphous atypical lymphoreticular infiltrates with destruction of lung parenchyma and extensive areas of necrosis
- Most salient feature is prominent angiocentricity of atypical lymphoid cells
  - Transmural infiltration of small and medium-sized vessels by atypical lymphocytes
  - Concentric arrangement of lymphoid cells replacing media and intima of vessels

Cytologic Features
- Infiltrate is polymorphous and contains abundant small lymphocytes, plasma cells, histiocytes, and scattered atypical lymphoid cells
- Atypical lymphoid cells may be large and mononuclear or binucleated, resembling Reed-Sternberg cells
- LYG is subdivided into 3 grades based on number of large, EBV-positive cells in the infiltrate
  - Grade I: Small lymphocytes predominate, and large, EBV-positive B-lymphocytes are scarce (< 5% of infiltrate)
  - Grade II: Large, EBV-positive B-lymphocytes are increased and account for 5-20% of lymphoid infiltrate
  - Grade III: Large, EBV-positive B-lymphocytes predominate, and lesion resembles a diffuse large-cell lymphoma

ANCILLARY TESTS

Immunohistochemistry
- Bulk of infiltrate is composed of reactive small CD2(+), CD3(+), CD4(+) T-helper lymphocytes
- Larger, atypical cells are positive for CD20 and CD79a
- Large, atypical cells are positive for EBV-latent membrane protein

In Situ Hybridization
- Large atypical cells react positively for EBV-encoded ribonucleotides (EBER) by in situ hybridization technique

DIFFERENTIAL DIAGNOSIS

Wegener Granulomatosis
- Lesions are characterized by neutrophil-rich areas of necrosis and true granulomas with multinucleated histiocytic giant cells
- Infiltrate is devoid of large, atypical CD20(+) B cells and EBER-positive lymphocytes

Hodgkin Lymphoma (HL)
- HL lesions rarely display angiocentric distribution of lymphoid infiltrates
- Large atypical cells are positive for CD30 and CD15 and negative for CD20 and CD79a

T-cell-rich B-cell Lymphoma (TcRBCL)
- TcRBCL has similar cell population as LYG but without tumoral necrosis and angiocentricity
- Large atypical B cells are negative for EBV

DIAGNOSTIC CHECKLIST

Pathologic Interpretation Pearls
- Term "granulomatosis" is a misnomer; granulomas and giant cells are not a feature of the process

SELECTED REFERENCES

1. Katzenstein AL et al: Lymphomatoid granulomatosis: insights gained over 4 decades. Am J Surg Pathol. 34(12):e35-48, 2010
2. Myers JL et al: Lymphomatoid granulomatosis. Evidence of immunophenotypic diversity and relationship to Epstein-Barr virus infection. Am J Surg Pathol. 19(11):1300-12, 1995

LYMPHOMATOID GRANULOMATOSIS

Histologic Features

(Left) *Scanning magnification in a patient with pulmonary lymphomatoid granulomatosis shows that the dense, well-circumscribed proliferation of lymphoid cells is sharply separated from the surrounding lung parenchyma ⇒. Notice the entrapment of airspaces within the lesion ⇒.* ***(Right)*** *Higher magnification of a lung lesion in lymphomatoid granulomatosis shows entrapped normal airspaces surrounded by dense lymphoid cell infiltrate admixed with plasma cells and histiocytes.*

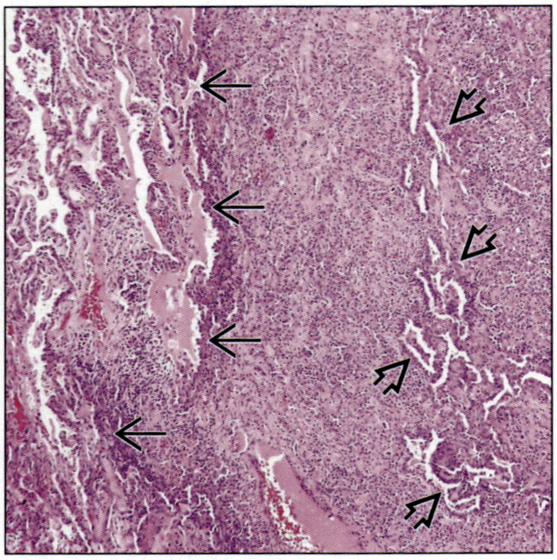
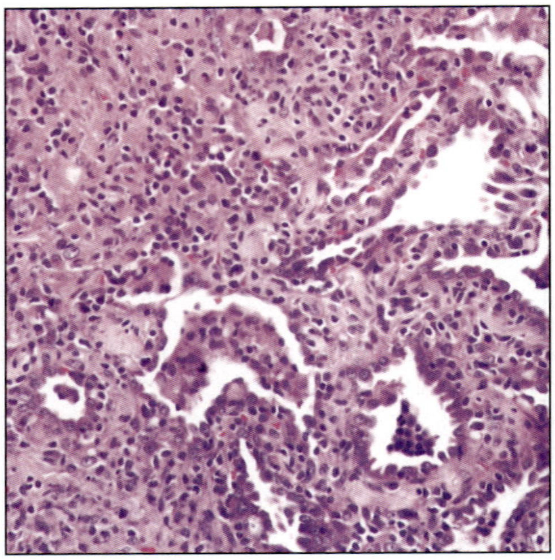

(Left) *Scanning magnification of a pulmonary lesion in lymphomatoid granulomatosis shows an extensive area of tumor cell necrosis ⇒. The bottom half of the field shows dense infiltration by a pleomorphic cell population containing large, atypical lymphocytes admixed with small lymphocytes.* ***(Right)*** *Higher magnification of a pulmonary lesion in lymphomatoid granulomatosis shows concentric infiltration of the wall of a small vessel within the lung parenchyma by atypical lymphocytes.*

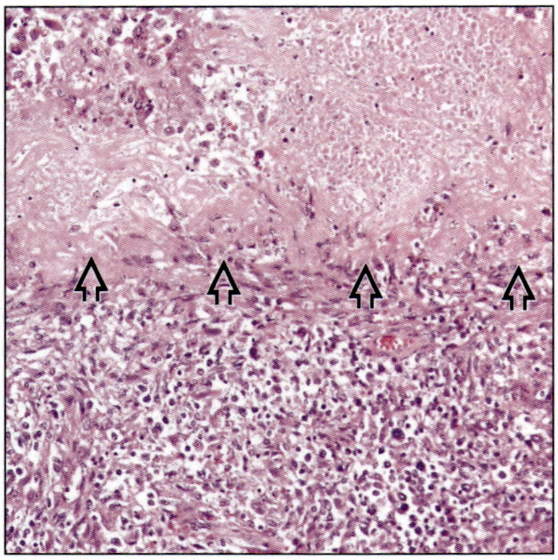
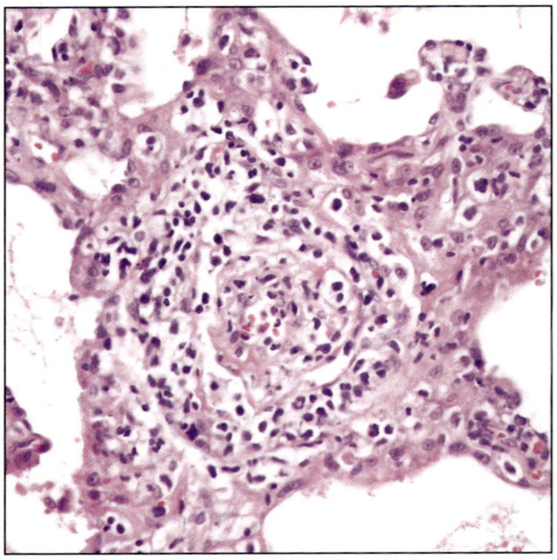

(Left) *Scanning magnification of a pulmonary lesion of lymphomatoid granulomatosis shows a large-caliber vessel with complete replacement and destruction of the adventitia and the media by a dense lymphoid cell population ⇒. The top portion of the field is also populated by a similar atypical lymphoid cell population.* ***(Right)*** *Pulmonary lesion in a patient with lymphomatoid granulomatosis shows transmural infiltration of a small-caliber vessel wall by the lymphoid cell population.*

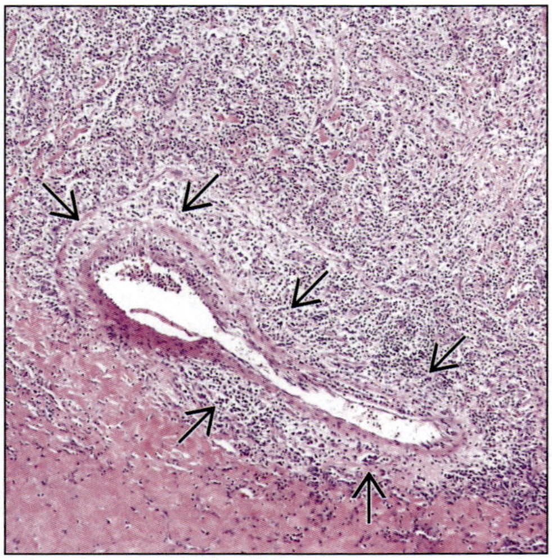
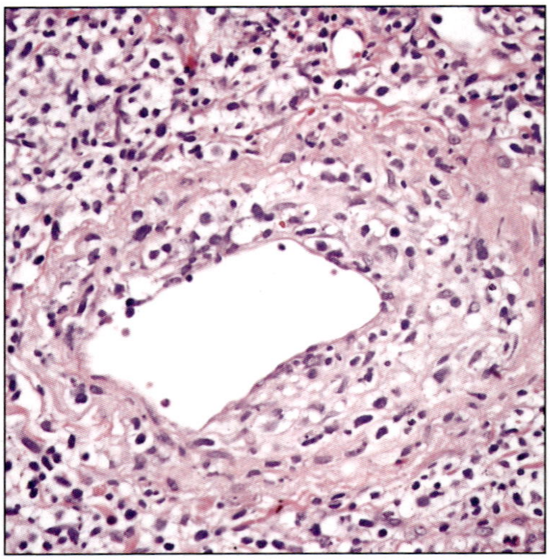

Angiocentric Pattern of Infiltration

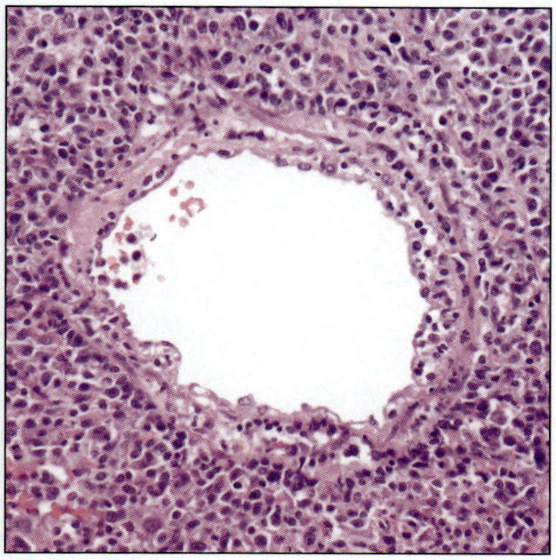

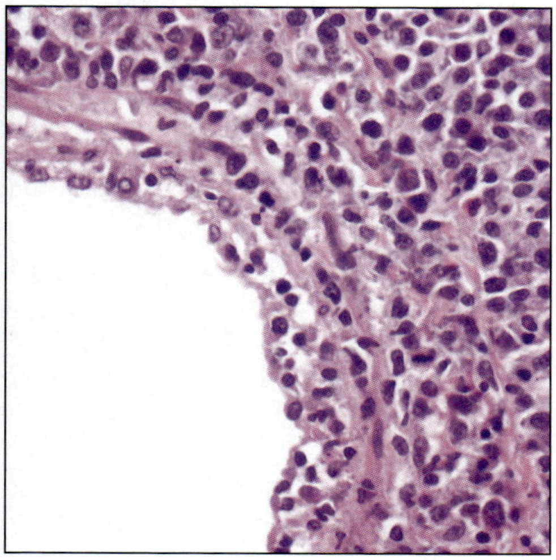

(Left) *Distinctive angiocentric pattern of infiltration of lymphoid cells in the wall of a small-caliber vessel in lymphomatoid granulomatosis shows a concentric linear arrangement of lymphocytes along the circumference of the vessel wall.* ***(Right)*** *Higher magnification of a small-caliber vessel in lymphomatoid granulomatosis shows a concentric, linear arrangement of the lymphocytes in the vessel wall with an "onion skin" distribution.*

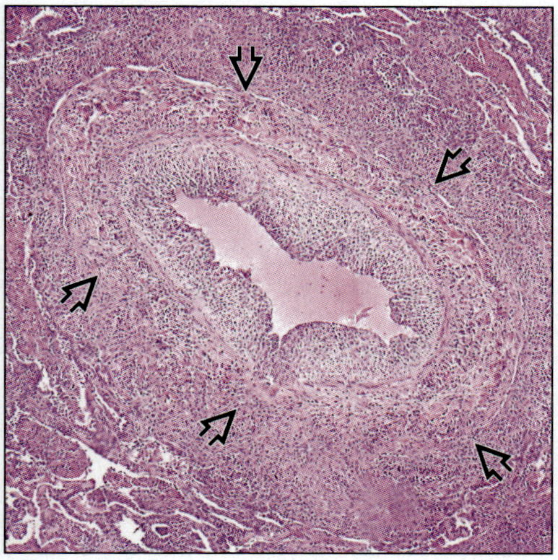

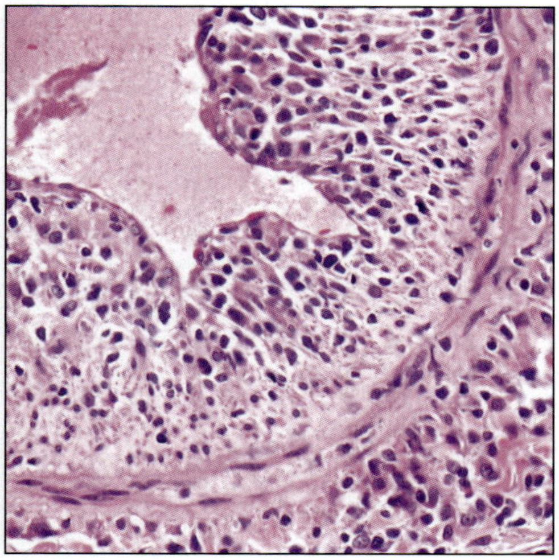

(Left) *Vessel wall in pulmonary lymphomatoid granulomatosis shows complete obliteration and replacement by sheets of lymphocytes invading the intima, media, and adventitia ⊳.* ***(Right)*** *Higher magnification of the wall of a middle-caliber vessel in a patient with pulmonary lymphomatoid granulomatosis shows complete replacement of the media and intima by dense lymphoid cell infiltrate. The lymphoid cell infiltrate is polymorphous and contains atypical lymphocytes.*

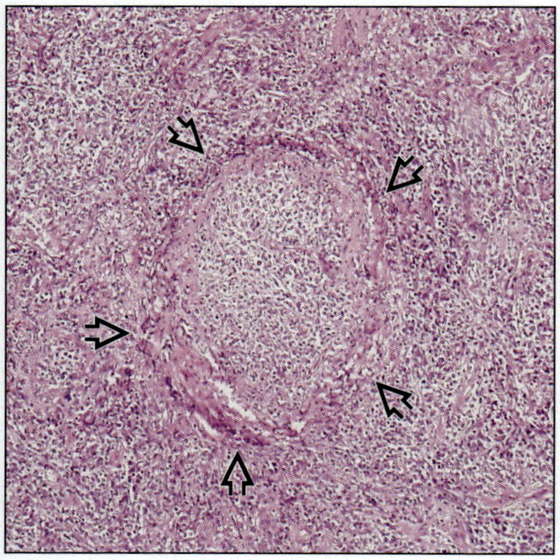

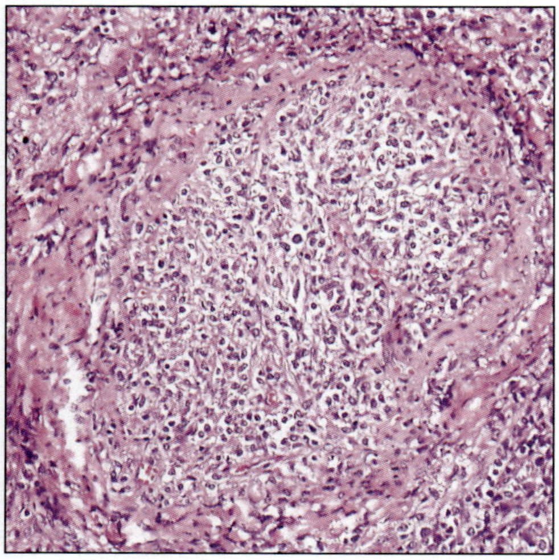

(Left) *Scanning magnification in lymphomatoid granulomatosis of the lung shows a discrete, well-circumscribed nodular area ⊳ corresponding to a small vessel that has been completely replaced by dense atypical lymphoid cell infiltration.* ***(Right)*** *Higher magnification shows an area in pulmonary lymphomatoid granulomatosis containing a small blood vessel that has been completely replaced by the atypical lymphoid infiltrate. Notice that the lumen of the vessel has been completely obliterated.*

Histologic Grades

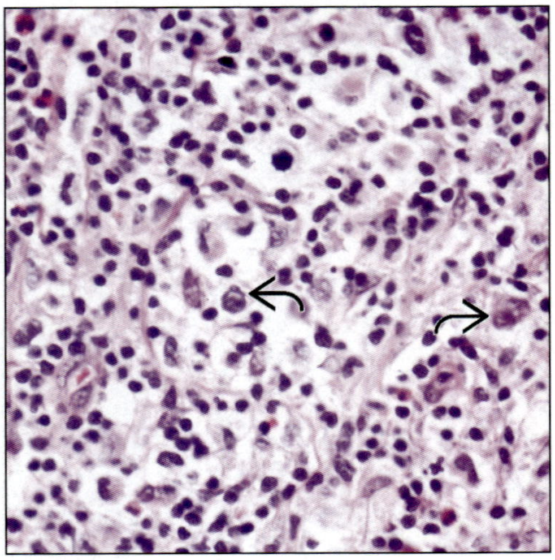
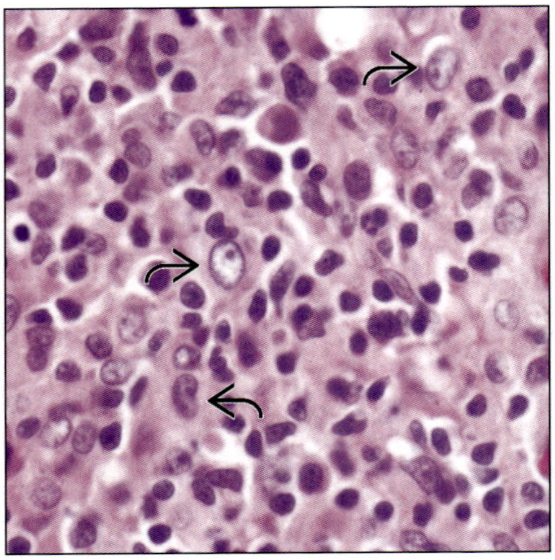

(Left) *Grade I lesion in lymphomatoid granulomatosis of the lung shows a polymorphous lymphoid cell population composed predominantly of small, round lymphocytes admixed with a few scattered, larger, atypical lymphoid cells (curved arrow).* ***(Right)*** *Higher magnification in grade I lymphomatoid granulomatosis of the lung shows an abundance of normal-appearing small lymphocytes admixed with a few scattered larger atypical lymphoid cells (curved arrow).*

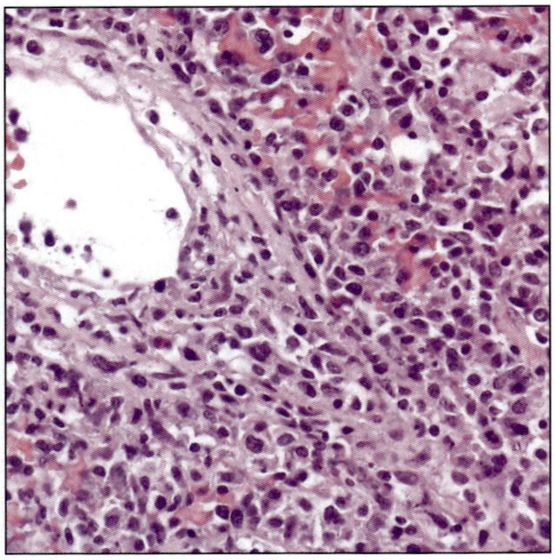
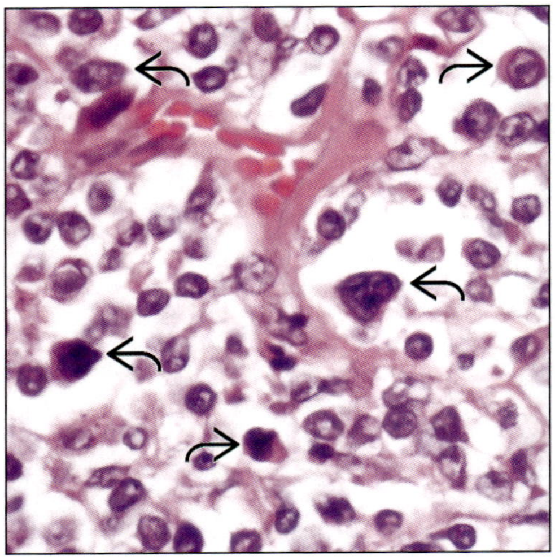

(Left) *Grade II lesion in lymphomatoid granulomatosis of the lung shows a dense lymphoid cell population with an increased number of large, atypical lymphoid cells admixed with numerous small, round normal-appearing lymphocytes.* ***(Right)*** *Higher magnification of grade II lesion in lymphomatoid granulomatosis of the lung shows large atypical lymphoid cells (curved arrow) admixed with small lymphocytes. The small lymphocytes correspond to helper T cells, and the larger lymphocytes are EBV positive.*

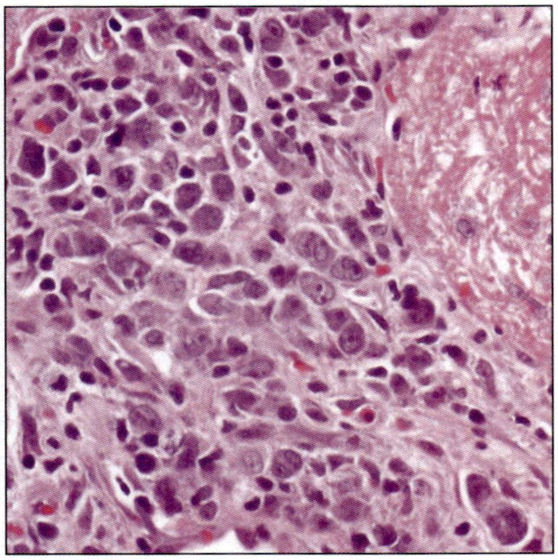
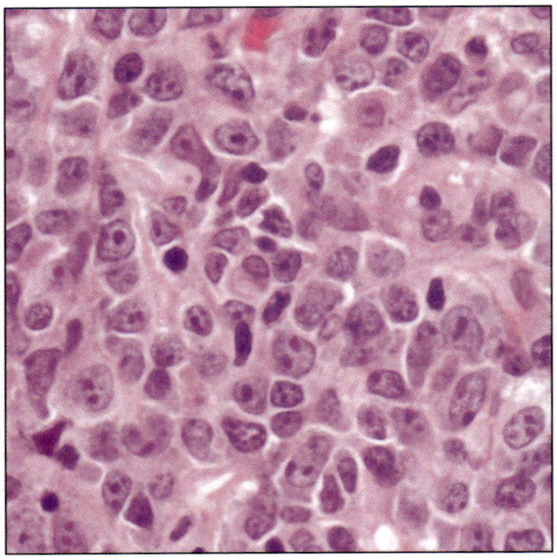

(Left) *Grade III lesion in lymphomatoid granulomatosis of the lung shows a dense population of atypical lymphoid cells with enlarged nuclei and prominent nucleoli admixed with a small number of small lymphocytes. The histologic appearance is indistinguishable from a diffuse large B-cell lymphoma.* ***(Right)*** *Higher magnification in grade III lesion of lymphomatoid granulomatosis of the lung shows sheets of large, atypical lymphocytes with very few small lymphocytes.*

Immunohistochemical and In Situ Hybridization Features

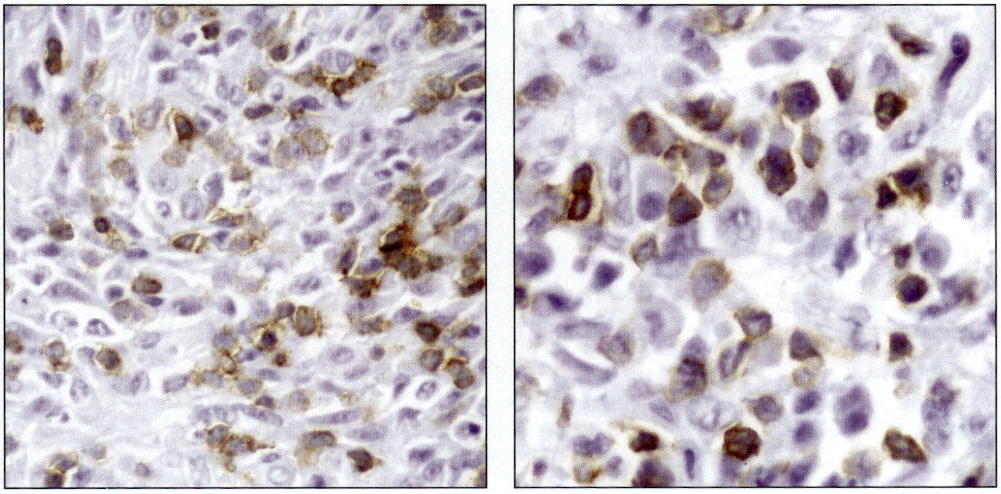

(Left) *Immunohistochemical staining for CD3 antigen in lymphomatoid granulomatosis of the lung shows numerous positive small lymphocytes admixed with larger atypical cells.* ***(Right)*** *Immunohistochemical staining of small lymphocytes in LYG of the lung for CD4 antigen identifies these cells as helper T cells. The neoplastic cells in this condition are actually the larger, atypical EBV positive, CD20 positive B-lymphocytes.*

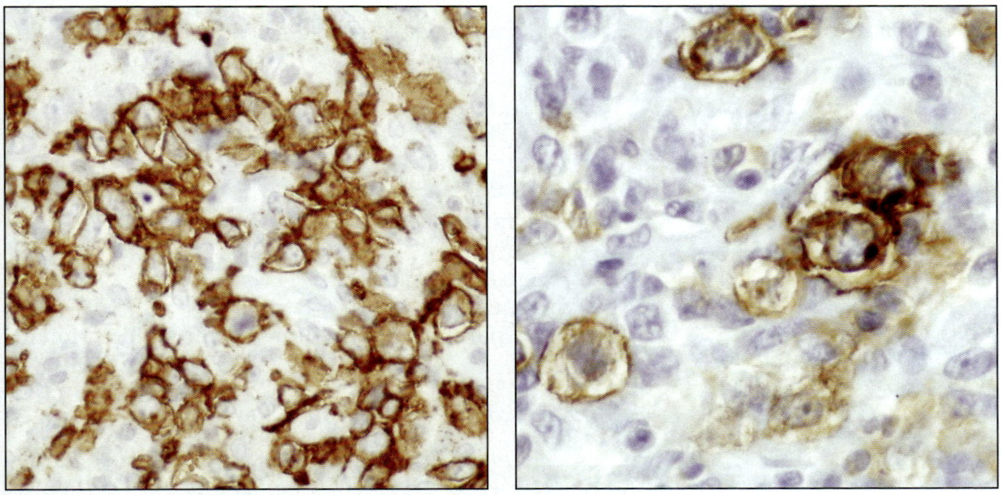

(Left) *Immunohistochemical staining for CD20 (pan-B-cell antigen) in lymphomatoid granulomatosis of the lung shows numerous large atypical cells with cytoplasmic positivity. The smaller lymphocytes scattered in the background correspond to helper T lymphocytes.* ***(Right)*** *Immunohistochemical staining for the pan-B-cell marker, CD79a, shows strong positivity in the large atypical cells and a negative reaction in the smaller T-lymphocytes in the background.*

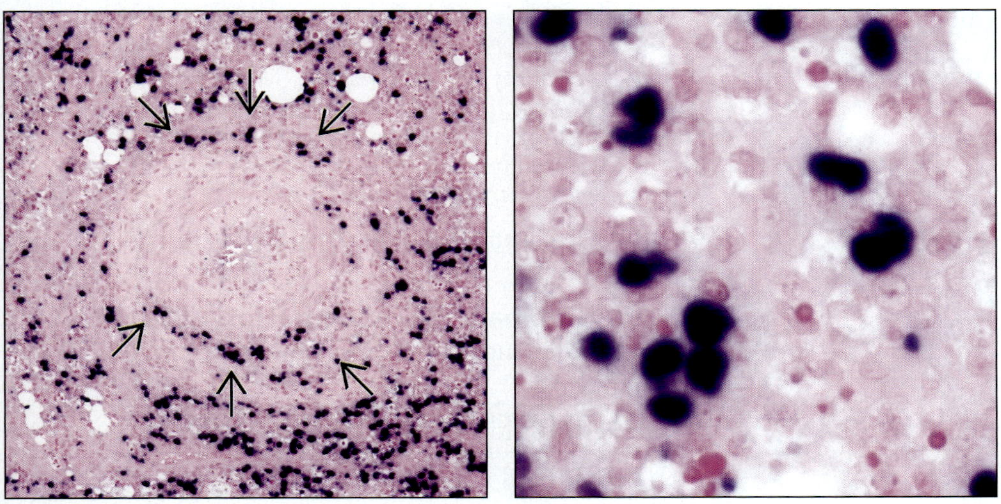

(Left) *In situ hybridization assay for the Epstein-Barr virus encoded RNA (EBER) shows scattered positive cells infiltrating a vessel wall* → *and the areas surrounding it. The number of EBER-positive cells (dark blue dots) in relation to the smaller, polymorphous lymphoid cells in the background form the basis for the histologic grading of these tumors.* ***(Right)*** *Higher magnification shows positive EBER in situ hybridization in lymphomatoid granulomatosis of the lung.*

GANGLIONEUROBLASTOMA

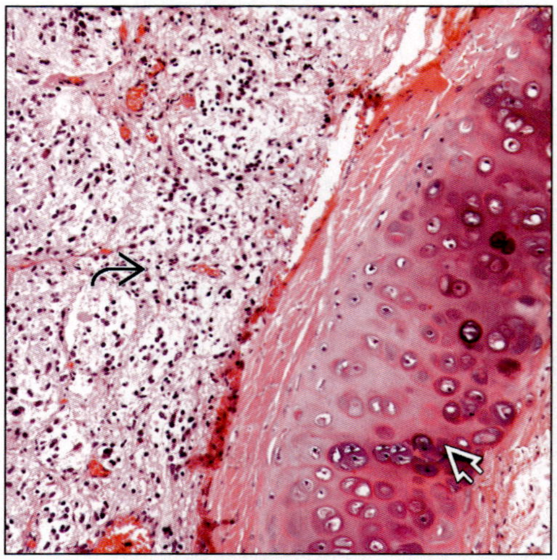

Bronchial ganglioneuroblastoma shows normal bronchial cartilage ➡ and a neoplastic cellular proliferation composed of small cells ➡ embedded in an eosinophilic background.

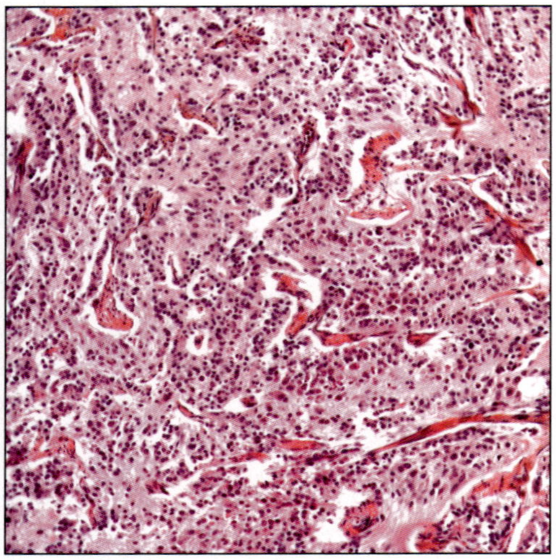

Ganglioneuroblastoma shows a classic small cell proliferation embedded in neutrophil-rich stroma. Thin strands of fibroconnective tissue are also present.

TERMINOLOGY

Abbreviations

- Pulmonary ganglioneuroblastoma (GNB)

Definitions

- Malignant neoplasm of neural origin

ETIOLOGY/PATHOGENESIS

Etiology

- Although etiology of these tumors is unknown, it is possible that they may arise from residual neural tissue in lung

CLINICAL ISSUES

Epidemiology

- Incidence
  - GNBs are exceedingly rare tumors in lung
- Age
  - Cases described have been in adults
- Gender
  - No apparent gender predilection

Presentation

- Cough
- Multiple endocrine neoplasia (MEN)
- Gastric ulcers
- Hypercalcemia
- Asymptomatic

Treatment

- Surgical approaches
  - Lobectomy or pneumonectomy
- Adjuvant therapy
  - Questionable additional therapy

Prognosis

- Difficult to evaluate due to limited number of cases reported

MACROSCOPIC FEATURES

General Features

- Well circumscribed
- Tan to white
- Homogeneous cut surface
- Intraparenchymal tumor
- Peribronchial tumor impinging into bronchial lumen

Size

- Variable size from 1-5 cm in diameter

MICROSCOPIC PATHOLOGY

Histologic Features

- Small cell proliferation
- Neuropil
- Nuclear atypia
- Mitotic activity
- Larger cells with prominent nucleoli
- Cystic changes
- Necrosis &/or hemorrhage

Predominant Pattern/Injury Type

- Diffuse

Predominant Cell/Compartment Type

- Nervous, neural

DIFFERENTIAL DIAGNOSIS

Small Cell Carcinoma

- Carcinoma will display positive staining for keratin
- Does not show the presence of neuropil

GANGLIONEUROBLASTOMA

Key Facts

Terminology
- P-GNB

Clinical Issues
- Incidence
  - GNBs are exceedingly rare tumors in the lung
  - Cases described have been in adult patients
  - There is no gender predilection
- Symptoms
  - Cough
  - Hypercalcemia
  - Gastric ulcers
  - Multiple endocrine neoplasia
  - Asymptomatic

Macroscopic Features
- Intraparenchymal tumor
- Peribronchial tumor impinging into bronchial lumen

Microscopic Pathology
- Small cell proliferation
- Neuropil
- Larger cells with prominent nucleoli
- Necrosis &/or hemorrhage

Top Differential Diagnoses
- Small cell carcinoma
  - Carcinoma will display positive staining for keratin
- Neuroendocrine carcinoma (carcinoid tumor)
  - GNB is negative for neuroendocrine markers
- Rhabdomyosarcoma
  - GNB is negative for muscle markers
- Melanoma
  - GNB is negative for mart-1 &/or HMB-45

Immunohistochemistry

Antibody	Reactivity	Staining Pattern	Comment
S100	Positive	Cytoplasmic	May be only focal
NFP	Positive	Cytoplasmic	May be focal staining only
NSE	Positive	Cytoplasmic	Strong positive staining but not specific
NeuroD1	Positive		In some cases
GFAP	Negative		
CK-PAN	Negative		May be positive in entrapped lung parenchyma
Chromogranin-A	Negative		
Myoglobin	Negative		
Desmin	Negative		
CEA-M	Negative		

- Ganglion differentiation is not present in small cell carcinomas

Neuroendocrine Carcinoma (Carcinoid Tumor)
- GNB is negative for neuroendocrine markers
- Presence of nested or trabecular growth pattern with presence of rosettes are not features of GNB

Rhabdomyosarcoma
- GNB is negative for muscle markers
- May show more pleomorphic features with increased cellular atypia and mitotic activity
- Presence of rhabdomyoblast is not a feature of GNB

Melanoma
- GNB is negative for mart-1 &/or HMB-45
- Although melanoma may have wide range of different growth patterns, it would be unusual to show presence of neuropil

DIAGNOSTIC CHECKLIST

Clinically Relevant Pathologic Features
- Nuclear features

Pathologic Interpretation Pearls
- Proliferation of small cells embedded in neuropil
- Admixture of larger cells with prominent nucleoli

SELECTED REFERENCES

1. Freeman JK et al: Combined carcinoid tumor and ganglioneuroblastoma of the lung: a case report. Int J Surg Pathol. 9(2):169-73, 2001
2. Hochholzer L et al: Primary pulmonary ganglioneuroblastoma: a clinicopathologic and immunohistochemical study of two cases. Ann Diagn Pathol. 2(3):154-8, 1998
3. Shields TW et al: Neurogenic tumors of the thorax. Surg Clin North Am. 68(3):645-68, 1988
4. Cooney TP: Primary pulmonary ganglioneuroblastoma in an adult: maturation, involution and the immune response. Histopathology. 5(4):451-63, 1981
5. Reed JC et al: Neural tumors of the thorax: subject review from the AFIP. Radiology. 126(1):9-17, 1978

GANGLIONEUROBLASTOMA

Microscopic Features

*(**Left**) Low-power view of a primary pulmonary ganglioneuroblastoma shows a neoplasm rich in neuropil →. Note the demarcation of the tumor just beneath the bronchial cartilage ↪. Also note that the bronchial lumen is not obstructed ⇨. (**Right**) Toward the periphery of a pulmonary ganglioneuroblastoma, one is able to identify lung parenchyma ⇨. Note that the tumor → is not encapsulated.*

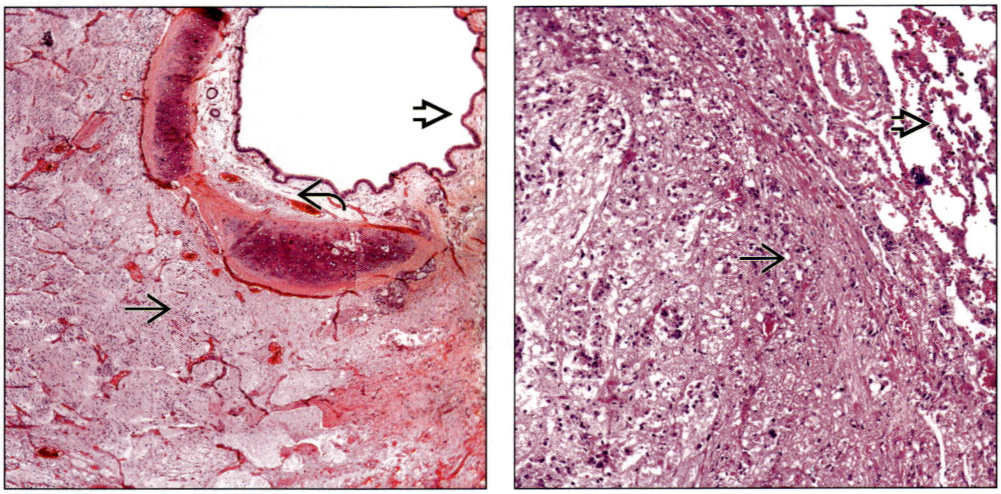

*(**Left**) Primary ganglioneuroblastoma of lung shows classical features of a small cellular proliferation embedded in a background of eosinophilic acellular material (neuropil) and focal calcification →. There are also dilated vascular spaces admixed with the tumor ↪. (**Right**) In some cases of pulmonary GNB, the presence of neuropil → can be extensive, making an unequivocal diagnosis of malignancy difficult. However, the presence of neutrophils should suggest a neural tumor.*

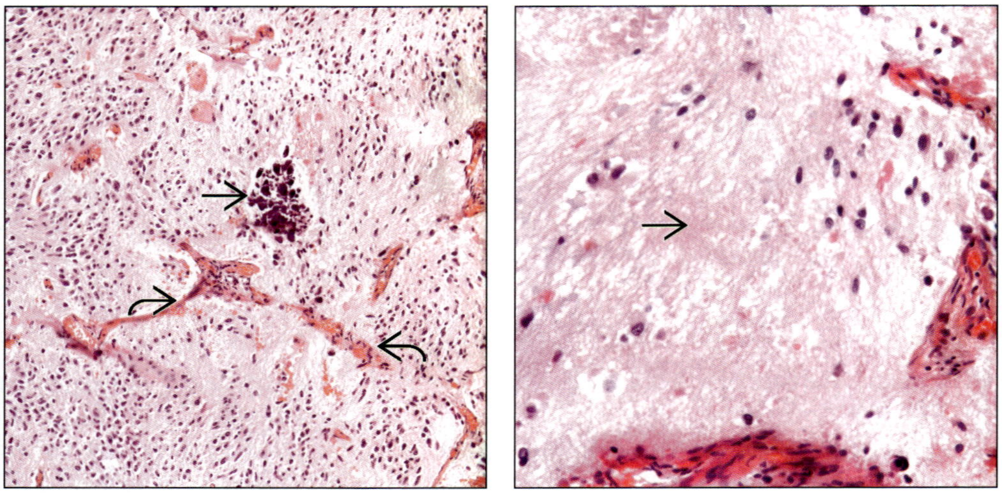

*(**Left**) Ganglioneuroblastoma shows alternating areas of hypo- → and hypercellularity ↪. These features are classic for this tumor. (**Right**) High-power view of a ganglioneuroblastoma shows small cells with scant cytoplasm, indistinct cell borders, and absence of mitotic activity. The neoplastic cellular proliferation is embedded in neuropil.*

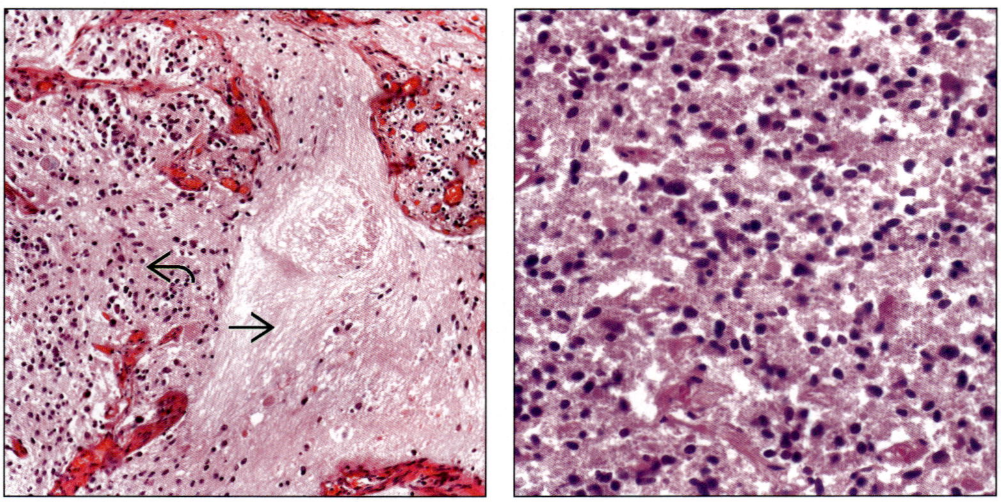

Microscopic Features

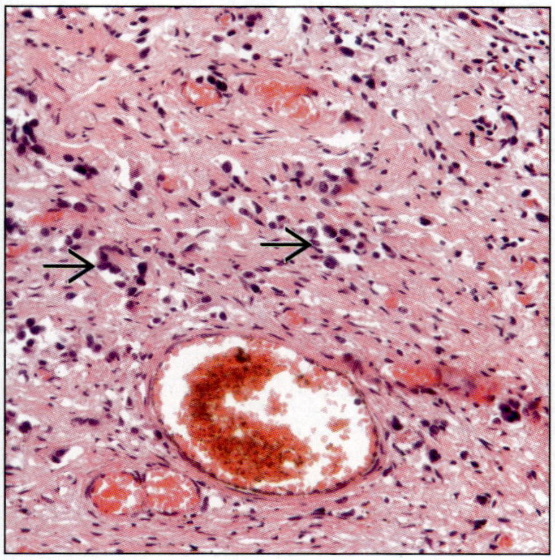

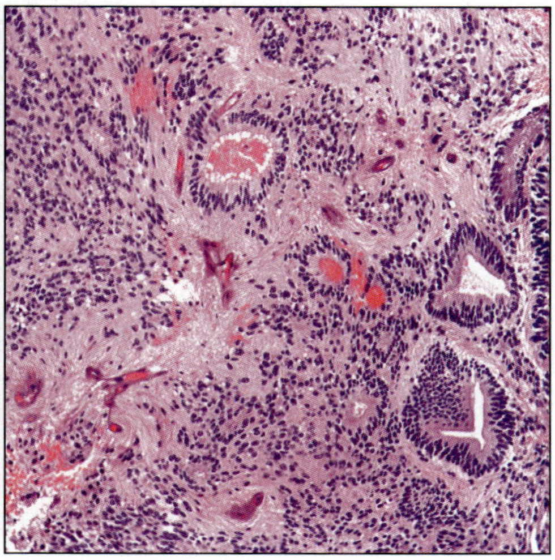

(Left) *Pulmonary ganglioneuroblastoma shows penetration of tumor cells → in areas of pulmonary fibrosis. This type of growth pattern can be easily confused with a small cell carcinoma.* ***(Right)*** *Classical case of ganglioneuroblastoma shows neural-like tubules, rosette formation, and small cellular proliferation embedded in neuropil.*

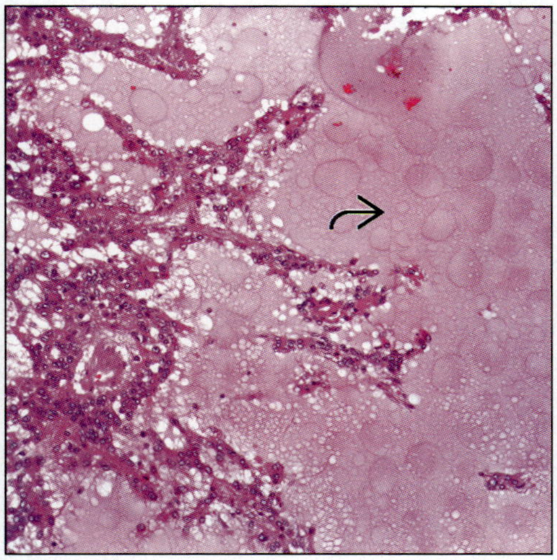

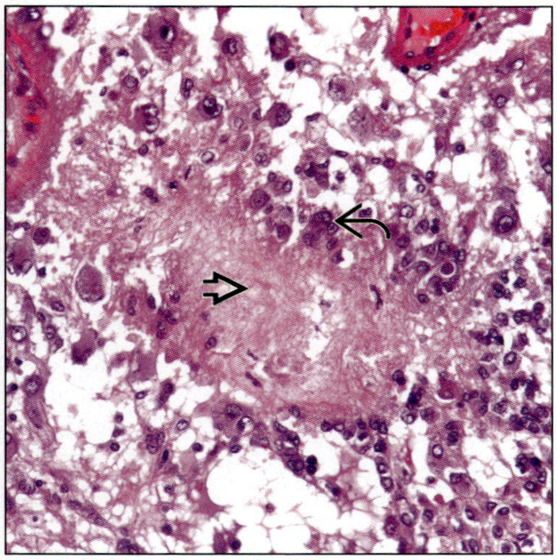

(Left) *In some areas, the neoplastic cells are admixed with edematous fluid ↷, which should not be interpreted as neutrophil.* ***(Right)*** *In contrast to the previous image, the presence of neuropil ⇨ is diagnostic of ganglioneuroblastoma. Note the presence of atypical cells around the neuropil ↷.*

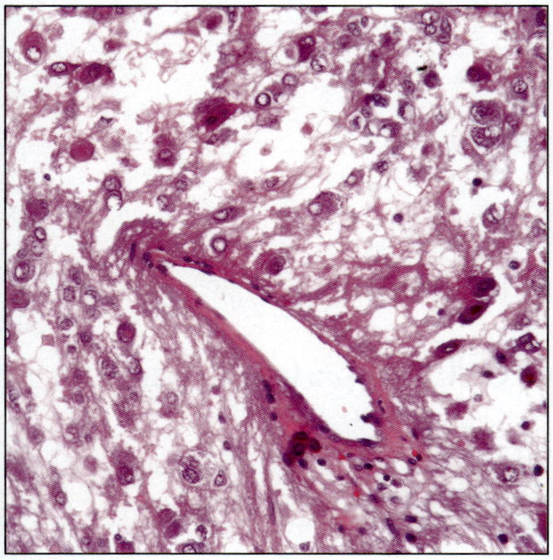

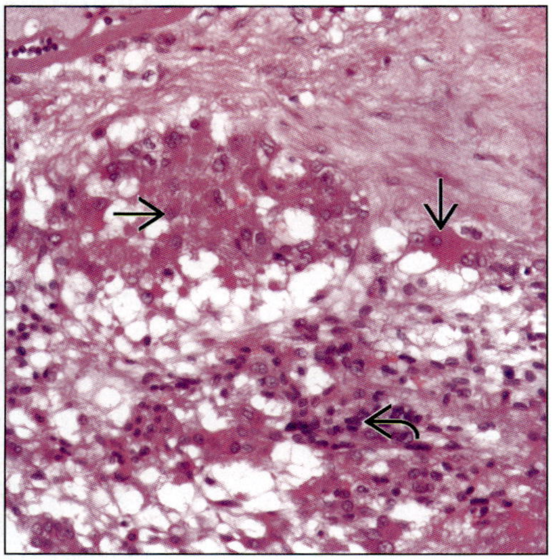

(Left) *In some cases, the neoplastic cells have a tendency to be around vessels. However, note that the intima of the vessel is not involved.* ***(Right)*** *Primary pulmonary ganglioneuroblastoma shows 2 populations of cells. One is composed of larger cells with prominent nucleoli and abundant eosinophilic cytoplasm →, and the other is composed of smaller cells with indistinct cell borders ↷.*

BRONCHIAL MALIGNANT MELANOMA

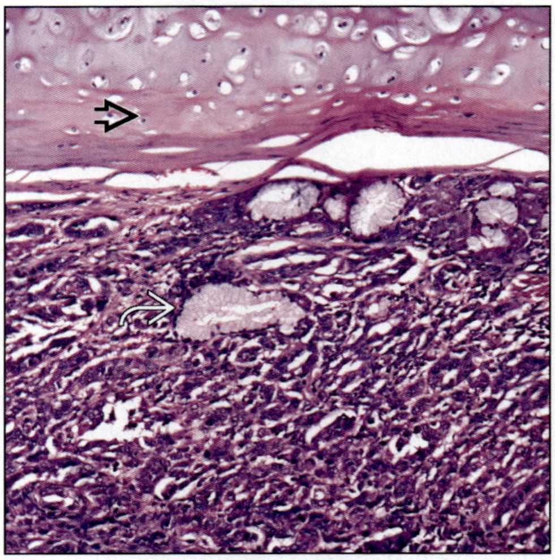

Primary bronchial melanoma involving full thickness of the bronchial epithelium. Note the presence of residual endobronchial glandular structures ➡ as well as bronchial cartilage ⇨.

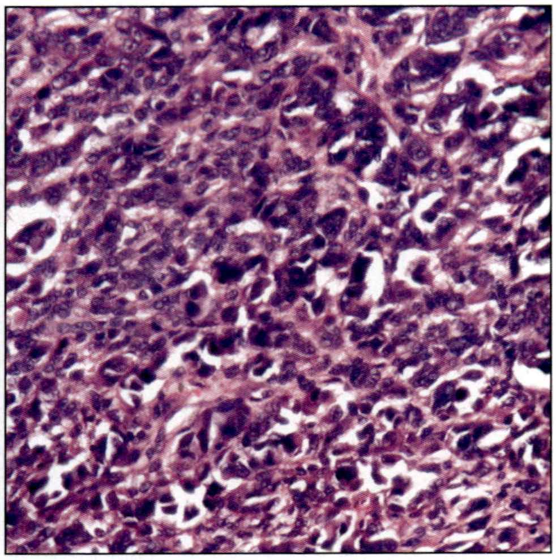

High-power view of a bronchial malignant melanoma shows prominent nuclear atypia and mitotic activity. Cellular pleomorphism is a common feature of bronchial melanoma

TERMINOLOGY

Synonyms

- Pulmonary malignant melanoma

Definitions

- Malignant neoplasm of possible neural crest derivation

ETIOLOGY/PATHOGENESIS

Etiology

- No specific etiology for these tumors when they occur in the lung

CLINICAL ISSUES

Epidemiology

- Incidence
  - Estimated that primary pulmonary melanomas represent approximately 0.01% of all lung neoplasms
- Age
  - More common in adults in 6th decade of life
- Gender
  - No gender predilection

Presentation

- Cough
- Shortness of breath
- Chest pain
- Hemoptysis
- Fever

Endoscopic Findings

- Possible pigmented lesion

Treatment

- Surgical approaches
  - Lobectomy or pneumonectomy
- Adjuvant therapy
  - Probable chemotherapy

Prognosis

- Variable
  - Death within 30 months after initial diagnosis
  - Possible survival at 5 years of 40%

MACROSCOPIC FEATURES

General Features

- Well-defined tumor mass
- Pigment
- Homogeneous surface
- Areas of necrosis &/or hemorrhage may be seen
- Polypoid bronchial mass in some cases

MICROSCOPIC PATHOLOGY

Histologic Features

- Nested pattern
- Spindle cell pattern
- Pigmented lesion
- Cells with prominent nucleoli
- Pseudonuclear inclusion
- Mitotically active
- Hemorrhage &/or necrosis

Predominant Pattern/Injury Type

- Nesting

Predominant Cell/Compartment Type

- Epithelioid

DIFFERENTIAL DIAGNOSIS

Carcinoma

- Will show negative staining for S100 protein, HMB-45, &/or mart-1

BRONCHIAL MALIGNANT MELANOMA

Key Facts

Clinical Issues

- Incidence
  - Approximately 0.01% of all lung neoplasms
  - More common in adults in 6th decade of life
- Symptoms
  - Cough
  - Dyspnea
  - Chest pain hemoptysis
  - Fever
- Endoscopic findings
  - Possible pigmented lesion

Microscopic Pathology

- Nested pattern
- Spindle cell pattern
- Pigmented lesion

Top Differential Diagnoses

- Carcinoma
  - Will show negative staining for S100 protein, HMB-45, &/or mart-1
- Neuroendocrine carcinoma
  - Melanomas are generally negative for neuroendocrine markers, i.e., chromogranin-A and synaptophysin
- Neurogenic sarcoma
  - S100 may show positive staining in both tumors
  - Negative for HMB-45 and mart-1
- Metastatic melanoma
  - Clinical history is most important and reliable way to determine primary site
  - Ocular evaluation is highly important

Immunohistochemistry

Antibody	Reactivity	Staining Pattern	Comment
S100	Positive	Cytoplasmic	May be focal
HMB-45	Positive	Cytoplasmic	May not be positive in spindle cell tumors
Mart-1	Positive	Cytoplasmic	
CEA-M	Negative		May be positive in some cases
CK-PAN	Negative		
Chromogranin-A	Negative		
EMA	Negative		
CD34	Negative		

- Melanomas and carcinomas may share positive staining for CEA-M

Neuroendocrine Carcinoma

- Melanomas are generally negative for neuroendocrine markers, i.e., chromogranin-A and synaptophysin
- Neuroendocrine carcinomas may show positive staining for S100 protein in sustentacular cells

Neurogenic Sarcoma

- S100 may show positive staining in both tumors
- Negative for HMB-45 and mart-1

Metastatic Melanoma

- Clinical history is most important and reliable way to determine primary site
- Ocular evaluation is highly important

DIAGNOSTIC CHECKLIST

Clinically Relevant Pathologic Features

- Metastatic distribution

Pathologic Interpretation Pearls

- Pigmented tumor composed of larger cells with prominent nucleoli or spindle cells

SELECTED REFERENCES

1. de Wilt JH et al: Isolated melanoma in the lung where there is no known primary site: metastatic disease or primary lung tumour? Melanoma Res. 15(6):531-7, 2005
2. Filosso PL et al: Primary malignant melanoma of the bronchus intermedius. J Thorac Cardiovasc Surg. 126(4):1215-7, 2003
3. Wöckel W et al: [Primary bronchial malignant melanoma.] Pathologe. 19(4):299-304, 1998
4. Wilson RW et al: Primary melanoma of the lung: a clinicopathologic and immunohistochemical study of eight cases. Am J Surg Pathol. 21(10):1196-202, 1997
5. Farrell DJ et al: Primary malignant melanoma of the bronchus. Thorax. 51(2):223-4, 1996
6. Barzó P et al: [Primary malignant melanoma of the lung and lower respiratory tract.] Orv Hetil. 135(5):245-9, 1994
7. Pasquini E et al: Primary bronchial malignant melanoma. A case report. Pathologica. 86(5):546-8, 1994
8. Plavsic BM et al: Melanoma metastatic to the bronchus: radiologic features in two patients. J Thorac Imaging. 9(2):67-70, 1994
9. Littman CD: Metastatic melanoma mimicking primary bronchial melanoma. Histopathology. 18(6):561-3, 1991
10. Jennings TA et al: Primary malignant melanoma of the lower respiratory tract. Report of a case and literature review. Am J Clin Pathol. 94(5):649-55, 1990
11. Santos F et al: Primary bronchopulmonary malignant melanoma. Case report. Scand J Thorac Cardiovasc Surg. 21(2):187-9, 1987

Microscopic Features

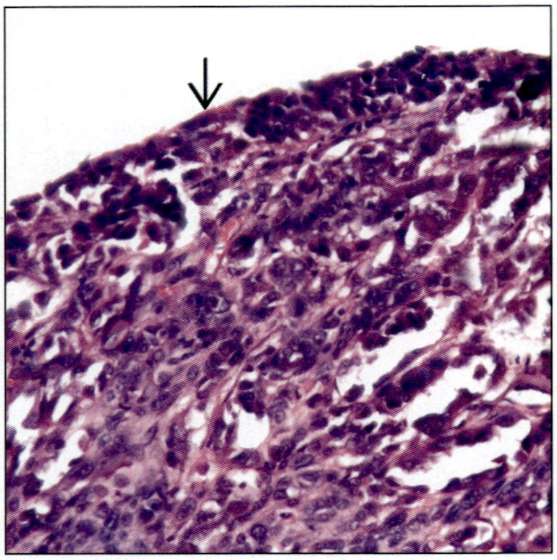

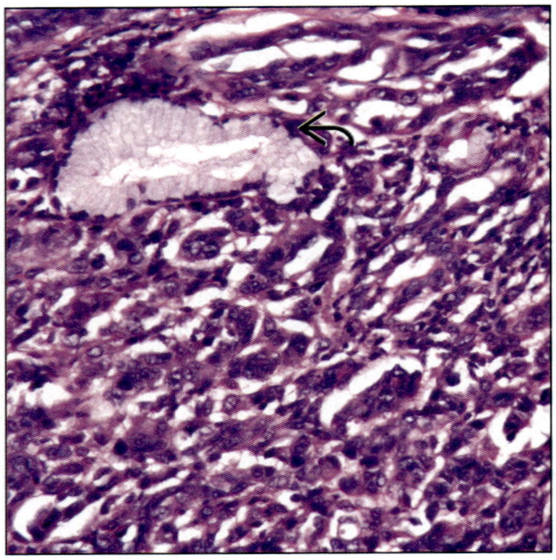

*(**Left**) Low-power view of a bronchial melanoma shows in situ changes in the surface epithelium. It is still possible to see some residual respiratory epithelium ⇒ in the surface, which is helpful in cases of primary bronchial melanoma. (**Right**) Endobronchial glands ↪ are spared by a primary bronchial melanoma. This is an unusual feature as the tumor has a tendency to obliterate normal structures.*

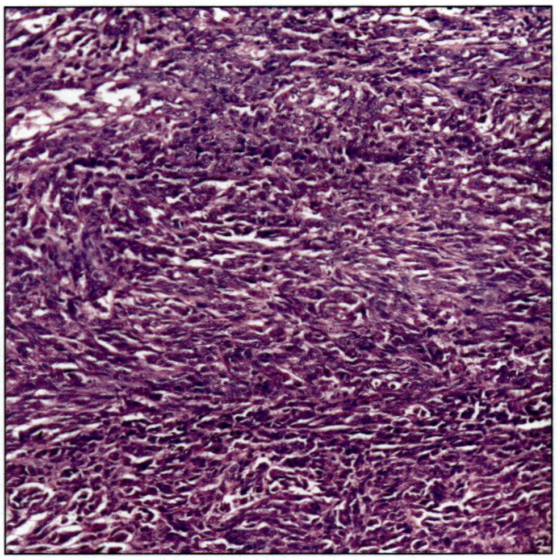

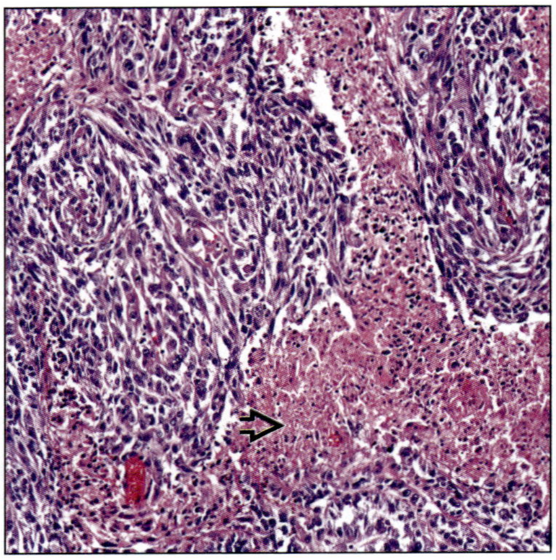

*(**Left**) Bronchial melanoma shows admixture of spindle and epithelioid cells. Both components show prominent nuclear atypia. This growth pattern may be seen in other primary malignant neoplasms of epithelial or mesenchymal origin. (**Right**) Spindle cell melanoma with areas of necrosis ⇨. The presence of necrosis can be either focal or extensive.*

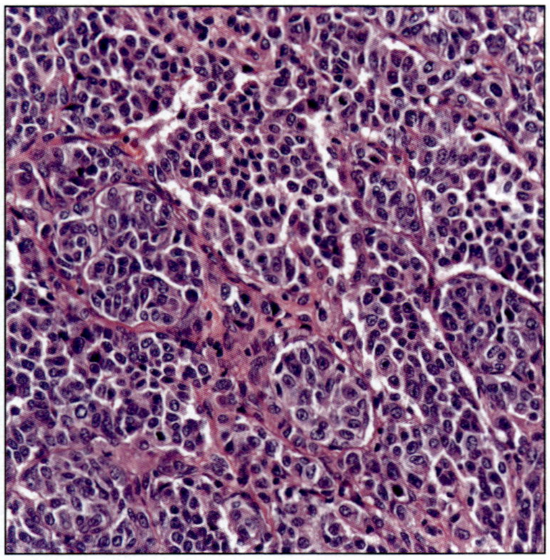

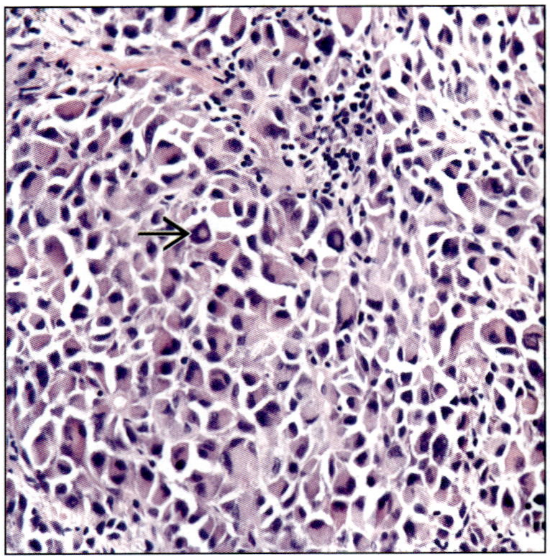

*(**Left**) Melanoma showing a nested pattern is composed of epithelioid cells closely mimicking a high-grade neuroendocrine carcinoma. Melanin pigment is absent. (**Right**) Higher magnification of the rhabdoid-like features of a bronchial melanoma shows displacement of the nuclei toward the periphery. Some of the cells show intranuclear inclusions ⇒. Similar features may be seen in rhabdoid carcinomas of the lung.*

BRONCHIAL MALIGNANT MELANOMA

Microscopic Features

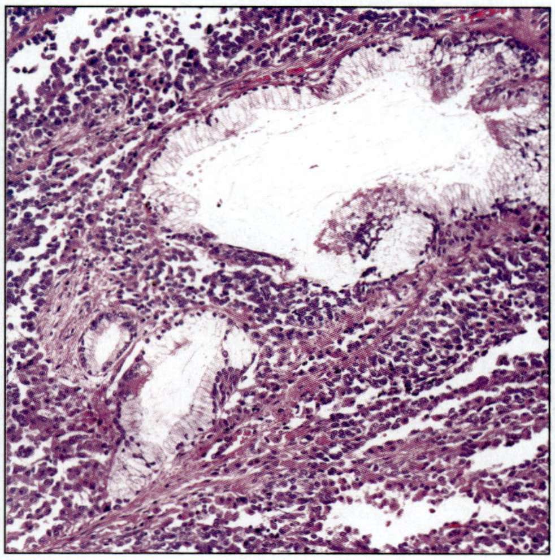

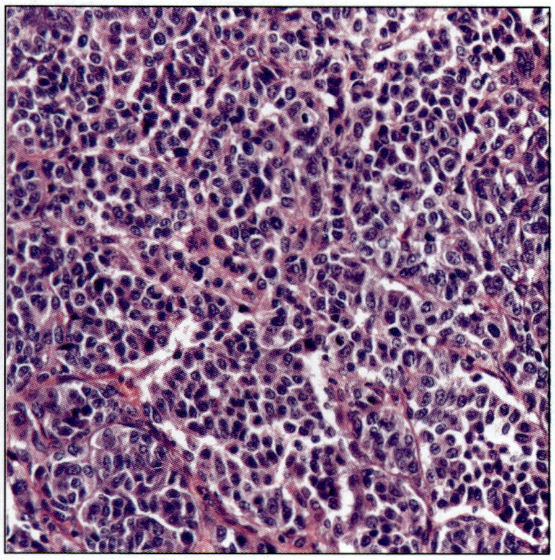

(Left) *Mucous endobronchial glands are dilated and surrounded by a rather small cellular proliferation, mimicking a neuroendocrine carcinoma.* ***(Right)*** *High-power view of a bronchial melanoma with cellular features reminiscent of a neuroendocrine carcinoma. This growth pattern can be easily misdiagnosed for carcinoid tumor. However, the use of immunohistochemical studies may lead to the correct interpretation.*

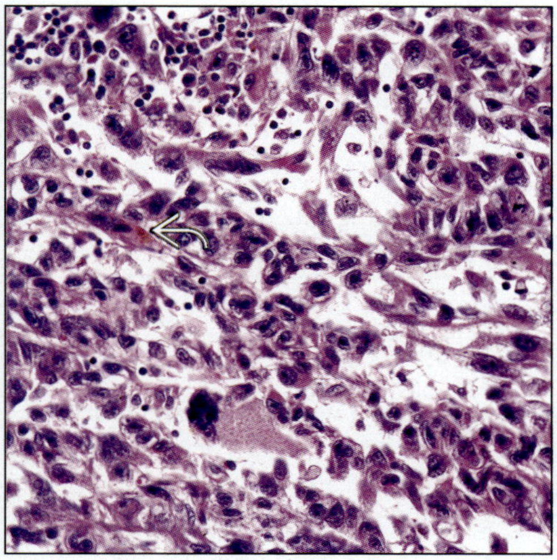

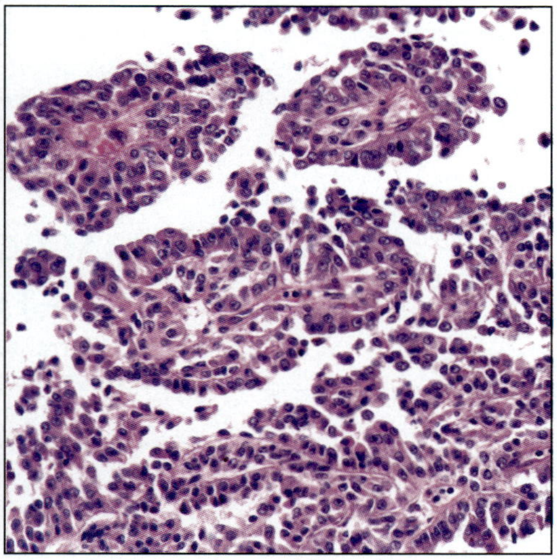

(Left) *Spindle cell melanoma with scattered multinucleated giant cells. Note the subtle presence of intracellular melanin ↪. In some tumors, melanin can be absent or only minimally present.* ***(Right)*** *High-power view shows the papillary-like structures of a bronchial malignant melanoma, which are composed of rather small cells with round nuclei and oncocytic cytoplasm. Similar features may be seen in primary lung carcinomas.*

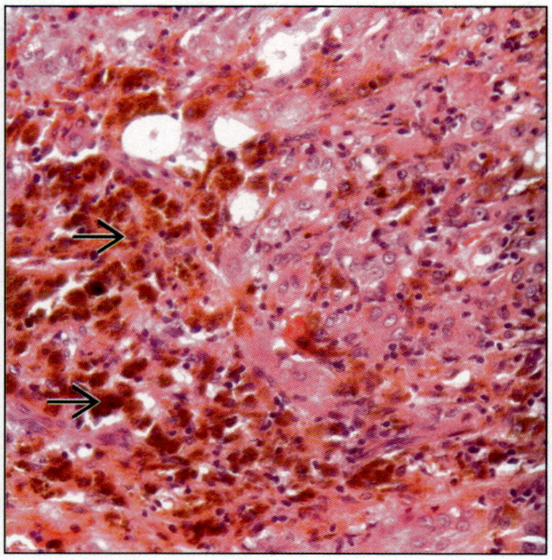

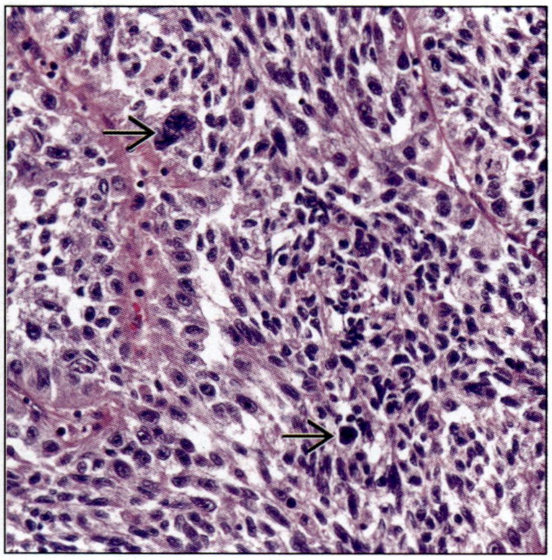

(Left) *Bronchial malignant melanoma shows epithelioid features and extensive areas of melanin pigment →. The use of histochemical stains for melanin may be helpful to separate melanin from iron pigment.* ***(Right)*** *High-power view of a bronchial melanoma shows prominent spindle cell features and scattered multinucleated giant cells →. Melanomas in the lung, like those in the skin, may show variability in their growth patterns.*

INFLAMMATORY PSEUDOTUMOR

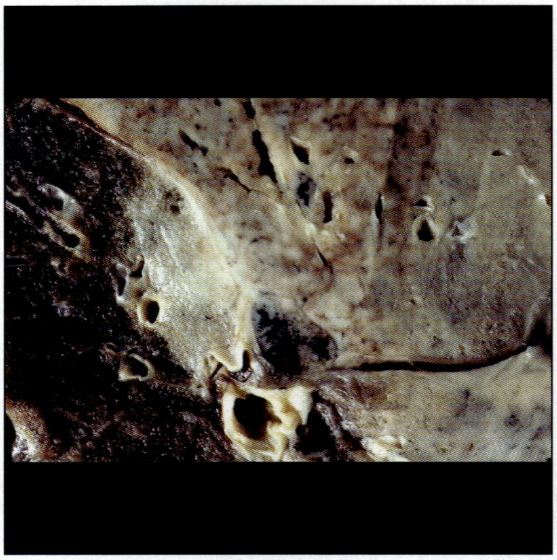

Gross photograph shows an ill-defined tumor mass growing along vascular and bronchial structures. The tumor is grayish in color and does not show areas of necrosis &/or hemorrhage.

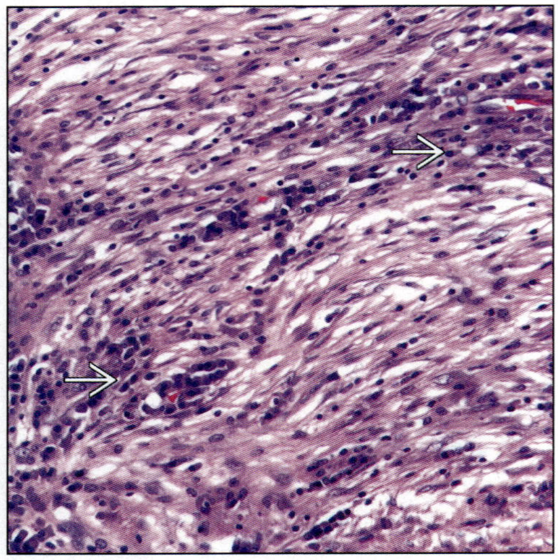

Spindle cell proliferation is seen admixed with inflammatory cells ➡. Note that the spindle cells do not show mitotic activity or cellular pleomorphism.

TERMINOLOGY

Abbreviations

- Inflammatory pseudotumor (IPT)

Synonyms

- Myofibroblastic tumor

Definitions

- Benign neoplasm of uncertain histogenesis

ETIOLOGY/PATHOGENESIS

Etiology

- Considerable debate whether IPT represents true tumor or inflammatory reaction
- Some cases may be associated to HHV-8
- Clonality has been demonstrated in some cases
- Uncertain histogenesis

CLINICAL ISSUES

Epidemiology

- Incidence
  - Tumor more common in individuals < 40 years old

Site

- Central tumor in endobronchial location
- Peripheral tumor

Presentation

- Cough
- Fever
- Chest pain
- Asymptomatic

Treatment

- Surgical approaches
  - Complete surgical resection
  - Spontaneous regression has been documented

Prognosis

- Good
- Recurrence if not completely resected
- Plasma cell variant appears to follow a less aggressive course
- Fibrohistiocytic variant appears to be more aggressive

MACROSCOPIC FEATURES

General Features

- Central tumor may grow in polypoid fashion, obstructing airway
- Peripheral tumors are larger with yellowish color
- Extrapulmonary involvement may be seen in some cases

Size

- Tumors vary in size from 1-10 cm in diameter

MICROSCOPIC PATHOLOGY

Histologic Features

- Marked plasma cell component
- Presence of Russel bodies
- Plasma cell proliferation admixed with spindle myofibroblastic cells
- Predominant fibrohistiocytic spindle cell proliferation
- Mitotic activity rare but occasional mitoses may be seen

Predominant Pattern/Injury Type

- Mixed

Predominant Cell/Compartment Type

- Histiocyte/macrophage
- Plasma cell

Key Facts

Terminology
- Myofibroblastic tumor

Etiology/Pathogenesis
- Some cases linked to HHV-8
- Clonality demonstrated in some cases

Clinical Issues
- Tumor more common in young individuals < 40 years old

Macroscopic Features
- Central tumor may grow in polypoid fashion, obstructing airway
- Peripheral tumors are larger with yellowish color
- Extrapulmonary involvement may be seen in some cases
- Tumors vary in size from 1-10 cm in diameter

Microscopic Pathology
- Plasma cell variant
- Fibrohistiocytic variant

Top Differential Diagnoses
- Plasmacytoma
  - Plasma cells in IPT are polyclonal
- Sarcoma
  - IPT fibrohistiocytic variant does not show nuclear atypia or increased mitotic activity

Diagnostic Checklist
- Plasma cell admixed with spindle fibroblastic proliferation
- Spindle cell fibrohistiocytic proliferation lacking nuclear atypia and increased mitotic activity

Immunohistochemistry

Antibody	Reactivity	Staining Pattern	Comment
ALK1	Positive	Cytoplasmic	30-40% of cases
Actin-sm	Positive	Cytoplasmic	
Vimentin	Positive	Cytoplasmic	
κ light chain	Positive	Cytoplasmic	Polyclonal
Kappa or Lambda	Positive	Cytoplasmic	Polyclonal
CK-PAN	Positive	Cytoplasmic	Focal in some cases
p80	Positive	Cytoplasmic	In approximately 30%

DIFFERENTIAL DIAGNOSIS

Plasmacytoma
- Plasma cells in IPT are polyclonal
- Generally in plasmacytomas, plasma cell proliferation is not mixed with spindle myofibroblastic cells
- Dutcher bodies are common in plasmacytomas

Sarcoma
- IPT fibrohistiocytic variant does not show marked nuclear atypia or increased mitotic activity
- Immunohistochemical studies will be useful to determine cell type involved

Sarcomatoid Carcinoma of Lung
- Spindle cell (myofibroblastic) proliferation in IPT lacks marked nuclear atypia &/or increased mitotic activity
- Immunohistochemical studies for epithelial markers, such as keratins and EMA, may show strong positive reaction in sarcomatoid carcinoma
- Presence of inflammatory component composed mainly of plasma cells would be unusual for sarcomatoid carcinoma

DIAGNOSTIC CHECKLIST

Pathologic Interpretation Pearls
- Plasma cell admixed with spindle fibroblastic proliferation
- Spindle cell fibrohistiocytic proliferation lack nuclear atypia and increased mitotic activity

SELECTED REFERENCES

1. Takeda S et al: Clinical spectrum of pulmonary inflammatory myofibroblastic tumor. Interact Cardiovasc Thorac Surg. 7(4):629-33, 2008
2. Moran CA et al: Unusual non-neoplastic lesions of the lung. Semin Diagn Pathol. 24(3):199-208, 2007
3. Kobashi Y et al: Inflammatory pseudotumor of the lung: clinicopathological analysis in seven adult patients. Int J Clin Oncol. 11(6):461-6, 2006
4. Checrallah A et al: [Inflammatory pseudotumors of the lung with spontaneous regression.] J Med Liban. 53(4):229-33, 2005
5. Cerfolio RJ et al: Inflammatory pseudotumors of the lung. Ann Thorac Surg. 67(4):933-6, 1999
6. Su LD et al: Inflammatory myofibroblastic tumor: cytogenetic evidence supporting clonal origin. Mod Pathol. 11(4):364-8, 1998
7. Gal AA et al: Prognostic factors in pulmonary fibrohistiocytic lesions. Cancer. 73(7):1817-24, 1994
8. Spencer H: The pulmonary plasma cell/histiocytoma complex. Histopathology. 8(6):903-16, 1984
9. Bahadori M et al: Plasma cell granulomas of the lung. Cancer. 31(1):191-208, 1973

INFLAMMATORY PSEUDOTUMOR

Microscopic Features

(Left) *Bronchial inflammatory pseudotumor is seen obliterating most of the bronchial lumen. This is a fairly common presentation of IPT.* ***(Right)*** *Inflammatory pseudotumor is shown in an endobronchial location. The epithelial surface is eroded, and there is a spindle cell proliferation admixed with areas of hemorrhage. Note the preservation of endobronchial glandular structures.*

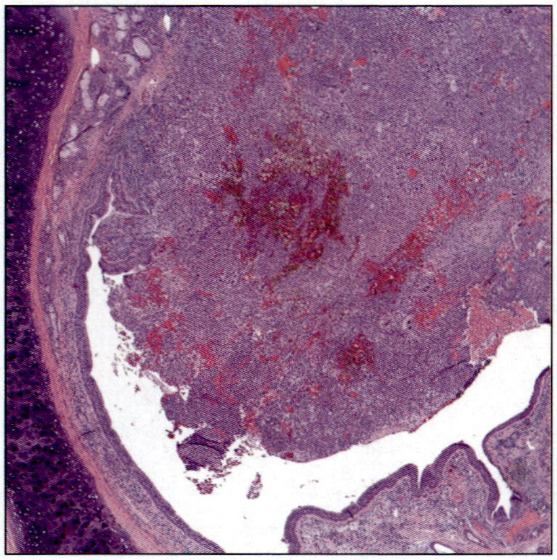

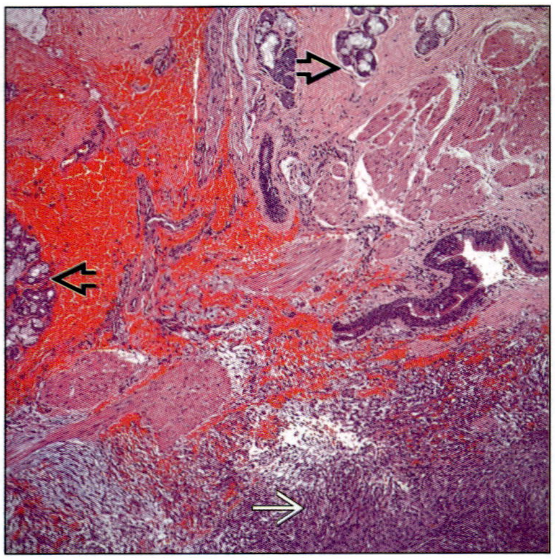

(Left) *Inflammatory pseudotumor fibrohistiocytic type with focal multinucleated giant cells (Touton type) is admixed with spindle cells. This feature although helpful is not commonly seen in these cases.* ***(Right)*** *Spindle fibrohistiocytic proliferation is admixed with large foamy macrophages. This is a helpful hint in the diagnosis of inflammatory pseudotumor. Note the absence of cellular atypia or mitotic activity.*

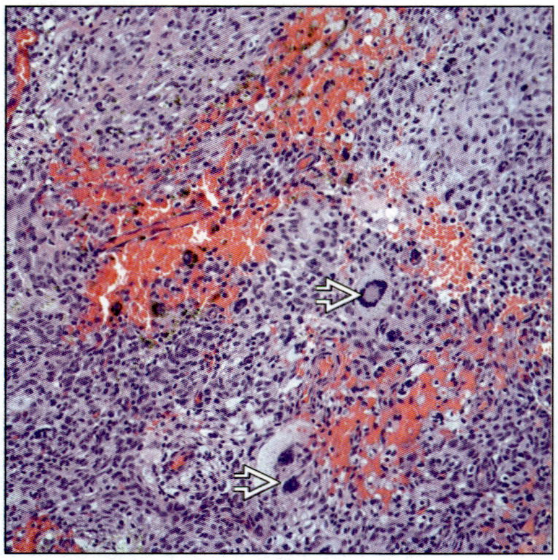

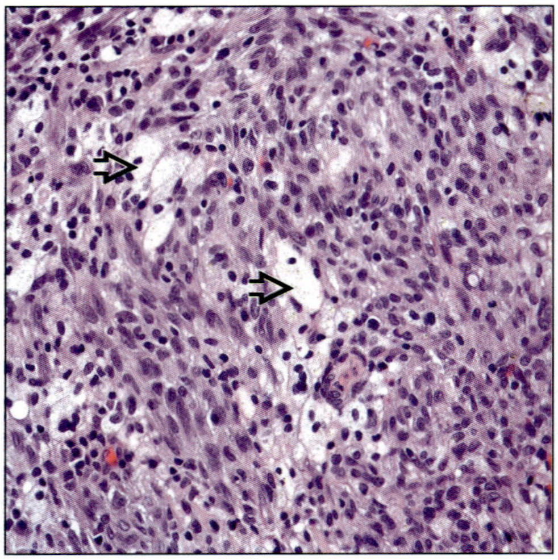

(Left) *Inflammatory pseudotumor of the fibrohistiocytic type is seen with numerous giant cells (Touton type), solid histiocytic proliferation, and foamy macrophages.* ***(Right)*** *Spindle cell proliferation is admixed with clusters of xanthomatous cells. This is a commonly seen feature in an inflammatory pseudotumor and these features are seen invariably in the majority of cases.*

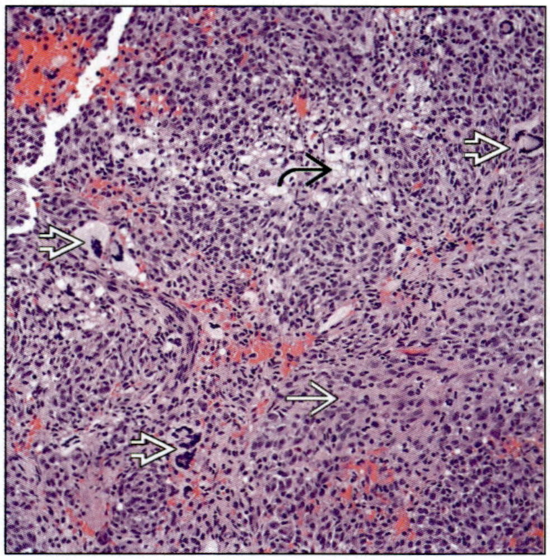

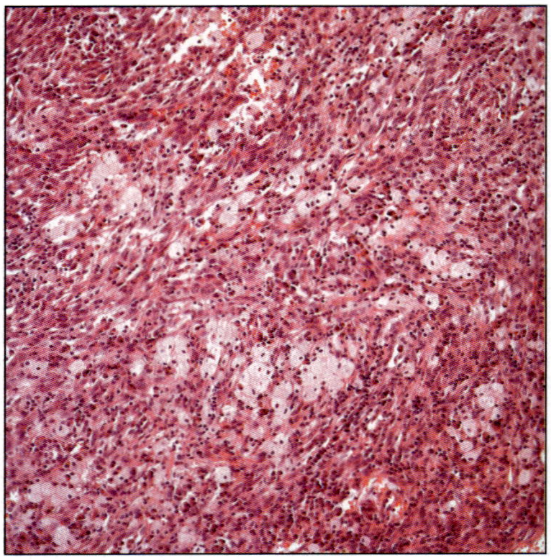

Microscopic Features

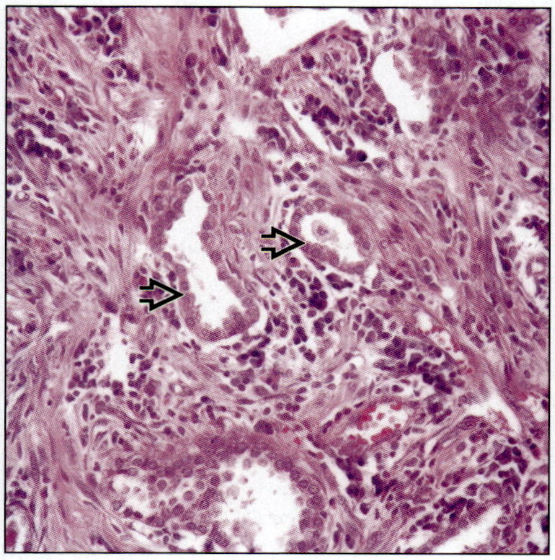

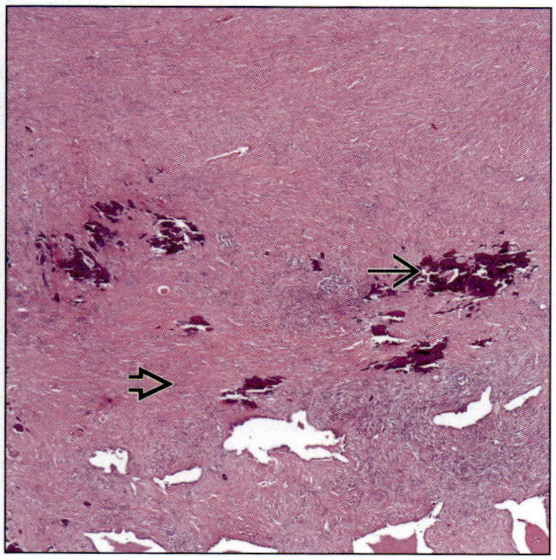

(Left) Hematoxylin & eosin shows an inflammatory pseudotumor, plasma cell type, with entrapped alveoli ⇨, fibrosis, and inflammation. These histological features are nondiagnostic of IPT but may be seen adjacent to the main tumoral lesion. *(Right)* Extensive areas of hyalinization ⇨ and focal calcification → are seen in an inflammatory pseudotumor, plasma cell type. This feature may make the diagnosis of inflammatory pseudotumor difficult to establish.

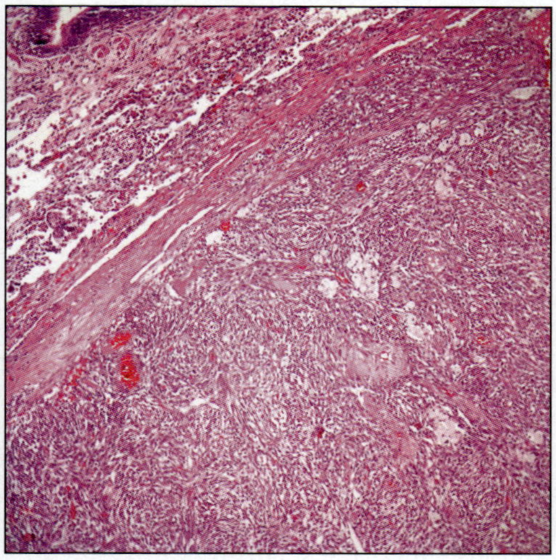

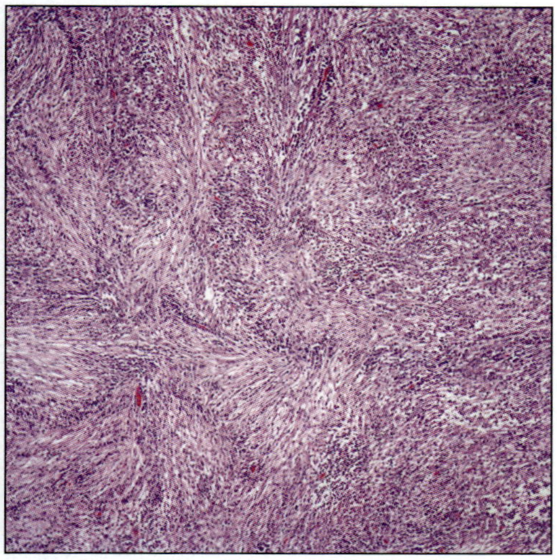

(Left) A well-circumscribed but unencapsulated inflammatory pseudotumor is seen in the periphery of the lung parenchyma. *(Right)* Low-power view of an inflammatory pseudotumor shows a vague storiform pattern. The tumor is composed of a spindle cell fibroblastic proliferation admixed with inflammatory cells, namely plasma cells. This is a common occurrence in these tumors.

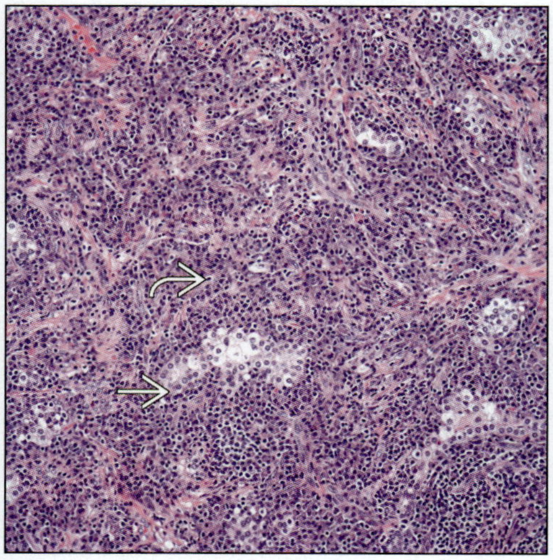

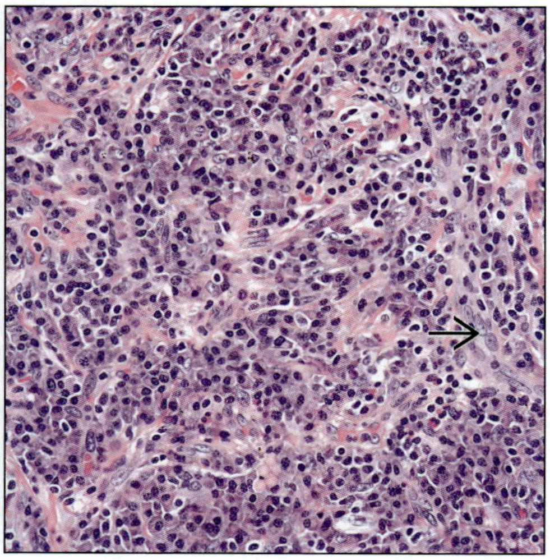

(Left) Inflammatory pseudotumor, plasma cell type, shows increased plasma cells ↷ with scattered entrapped alveolar structures →. This pattern may be easily confused for a pneumonic process. *(Right)* Hematoxylin & eosin shows marked presence of plasma cells with only scattered fibroblasts →. This pattern would also suggest a plasma cell proliferation, thus the importance of using clonality studies to rule out the diagnosis of plasmacytoma.

IgG4 SCLEROSING LUNG DISEASE

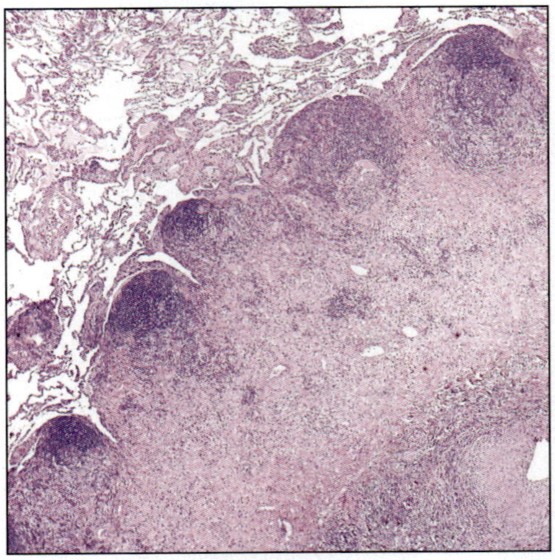

IgG4 sclerosing lung disease shows a nodular, well-circumscribed area of lung parenchyma with prominent stromal sclerosis and reactive lymphoid follicles in the periphery.

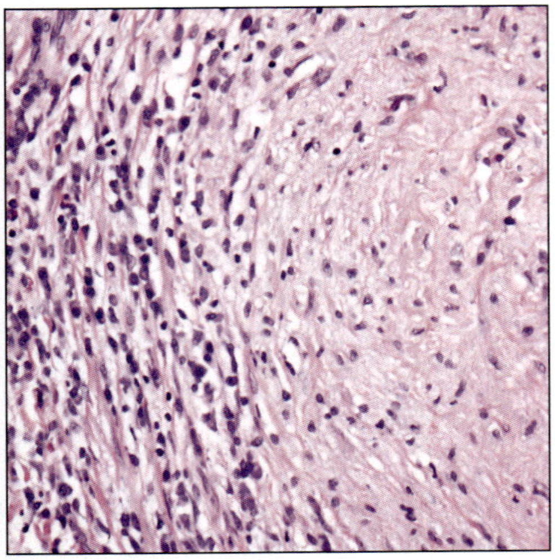

Higher magnification from an area of stromal sclerosis in IgG4 sclerosing disease of the lung shows dense infiltrate composed of plasma cells admixed with the sclerotic stroma.

TERMINOLOGY

Definitions

- Systemic disease of unknown etiology characterized by elevated production of IgG4(+) plasma cells and tissue stromal sclerosis

ETIOLOGY/PATHOGENESIS

Pathogenesis

- Unknown, but an autoimmune mechanism or hypersensitivity reaction has been postulated
- Circulating autoantibodies are present in many patients
- May be associated with other autoimmune disorders, e.g., Sjögren syndrome

CLINICAL ISSUES

Epidemiology

- Age
  - Middle-aged and elderly patients
- Gender
  - Male predominance

Presentation

- Asymptomatic incidental finding in chest x-ray
- Cough
- Hemoptysis
- Dyspnea
- Pleural effusion

Natural History

- Slowly progressive disease with involvement of multiple sites over a period of years with elevation of serum titers of IgG4
- Most commonly involved sites include pancreas, hepatobiliary tract, salivary gland, orbit, and lymph nodes
- Prototype of disease is so-called autoimmune pancreatitis
- May involve almost any other organ site in body
- Benign clinical course with good response to steroids
- Some cases may evolve to malignant lymphoma or may be associated with development of carcinoma

Prognosis

- Excellent response to steroid therapy

MICROSCOPIC PATHOLOGY

Histologic Features

- 3 histologic patterns of involvement are recognized in lung
  - **Inflammatory pseudotumor-like**
    - Solid, nodular growth pattern characterized by well-circumscribed area of sclerosis admixed with lymphocytes and plasma cells
    - Lesions closely resemble "inflammatory myofibroblastic tumor" and "inflammatory pseudotumor" of lung
    - Fibrosis is mostly paucicellular, with few myofibroblasts
  - **Bronchovascular pattern of involvement**
    - Lymphoplasmacytic infiltration and fibrosis centered around bronchovascular bundles with lymphangitic distribution
    - Expansion along interlobular septa and pleura with paucicellular fibrosis
  - **Interstitial fibrosis-like**
    - Diffuse interstitial lymphoplasmacytic infiltrates and fibrosis involving alveolar septa
    - Pattern closely resembles lymphocytic interstitial pneumonia (LIP) or cellular nonspecific interstitial pneumonia (NSIP)
    - Fibrosis is mostly paucicellular, with few myofibroblasts

IgG4 SCLEROSING LUNG DISEASE

Key Facts

Terminology
- Systemic disease of unknown etiology characterized by elevated production of IgG4(+) plasma cells and tissue stromal sclerosis

Clinical Issues
- Slowly progressive disease with involvement of multiple sites over a period of years with elevation of serum titers of IgG4
- Most commonly involved sites include pancreas, hepatobiliary tract, salivary gland, orbit, and lymph nodes

Microscopic Pathology
- 3 histologic patterns of involvement are recognized in lung: Inflammatory pseudotumor-like, bronchovascular, and interstitial fibrosis-like
- Inflammatory infiltrate is composed of small lymphocytes and mature plasma cells admixed with stromal fibrosis
- Eosinophils are commonly present accompanying inflammatory infiltrates
- Lymphoid follicles may be present in 50% of cases
- Prominent vascular component characterized by endothelialitis of veins and arteries with narrowing and obliteration of vascular lumen

Ancillary Tests
- Increased number of IgG4(+) plasma cells in tissue sections (> 50 per 10 HPF, with IgG4/IgG ratio of > 40%)
- Raised serum level of IgG4 (> 135 mg/dL) is commonly seen but is not essential for diagnosis

  - Prominent vascular involvement may closely resemble lymphomatoid granulomatosis, grade I

Cytologic Features
- Inflammatory infiltrate is composed of small lymphocytes and mature plasma cells admixed with stromal fibrosis
- Eosinophils are commonly present accompanying inflammatory infiltrates
- Lymphoid follicles may be present in 50% of cases
- Prominent vascular component characterized by endothelialitis of veins and arteries with narrowing and obliteration of vascular lumen
- Prominent histiocytes with emperipolesis reminiscent of Rosai-Dorfman disease may be seen
- Nonnecrotizing epithelioid granulomas may be noted in some cases

ANCILLARY TESTS

Immunohistochemistry
- Increased number of IgG4(+) plasma cells in tissue sections (> 50 per 10 HPF, with IgG4/IgG ratio of > 40%)

Serologic Testing
- Raised serum level of IgG4 (> 135 mg/dL) is commonly seen but is not essential for diagnosis

DIFFERENTIAL DIAGNOSIS

Inflammatory Pseudotumor/Inflammatory Myofibroblastic Tumor
- Prominent myofibroblastic component, which is usually not present in IgG4(+) sclerosing disease
- Inflammatory myofibroblastic tumor is generally ALK1(+), unlike IgG4(+) sclerosing disease, which is always negative
- Inflammatory pseudotumor/myofibroblastic tumor is negative for IgG4(+) plasma cells

Lymphoid Interstitial Pneumonia/ Nonspecific Interstitial Pneumonia
- Does not show increase of IgG4(+) plasma cells in interstitial infiltrates
- Absence of prominent vascular involvement with endothelialitis

Rosai-Dorfman Disease
- Contains dense lymphoplasmacytic infiltrates admixed with prominent histiocytic proliferation with emperipolesis
- Rosai-Dorfman disease may contain numerous IgG4(+) plasma cells
- Histiocytes in Rosai-Dorfman disease are always S100 positive, unlike those in IgG4(+) sclerosing disease, which are negative

Lymphomatoid Granulomatosis, Grade I
- Dense lymphoplasmacytic interstitial infiltrates with prominent vascular involvement
- Proliferating cells are strongly EBV(+) by EBER in situ hybridization, while plasma cells in IgG4(+) disease are negative for EBER

SELECTED REFERENCES

1. Shigemitsu H et al: IgG4-related interstitial lung disease: a new and evolving concept. Curr Opin Pulm Med. 15(5):513-6, 2009
2. Yamamoto H et al: Inflammatory myofibroblastic tumor versus IgG4-related sclerosing disease and inflammatory pseudotumor: a comparative clinicopathologic study. Am J Surg Pathol. 33(9):1330-40, 2009
3. Zen Y et al: IgG4-related lung and pleural disease: a clinicopathologic study of 21 cases. Am J Surg Pathol. 33(12):1886-93, 2009
4. Yamashita K et al: Lung involvement in IgG4-related lymphoplasmacytic vasculitis and interstitial fibrosis: report of 3 cases and review of the literature. Am J Surg Pathol. 32(11):1620-6, 2008

IgG4 SCLEROSING LUNG DISEASE

Patterns of Growth

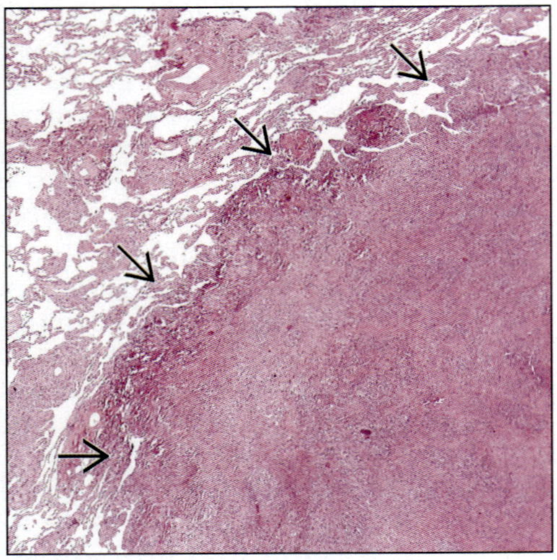

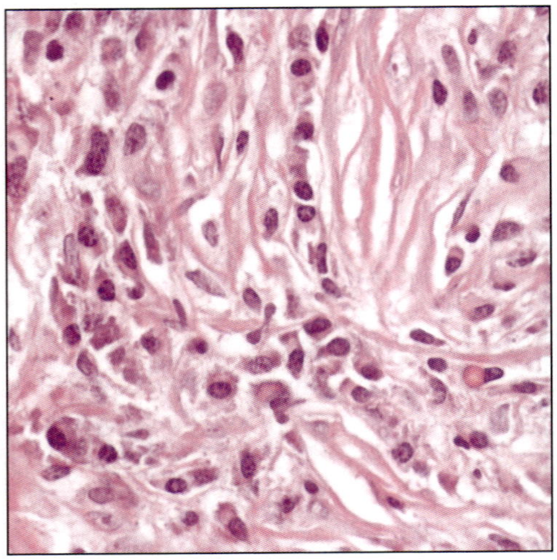

(Left) *Scanning magnification of inflammatory pseudotumor-like IgG4(+) sclerosing lung disease shows a well-circumscribed intraparenchymatous lung nodule* → *that is sharply separated from the surrounding lung parenchyma.* ***(Right)*** *Higher magnification from inflammatory pseudotumor-like IgG4(+) sclerosing lung disease shows a population of mature plasma cells set against a collagenous stroma. The fibrosis in these cases is paucicellular with scattered myofibroblasts.*

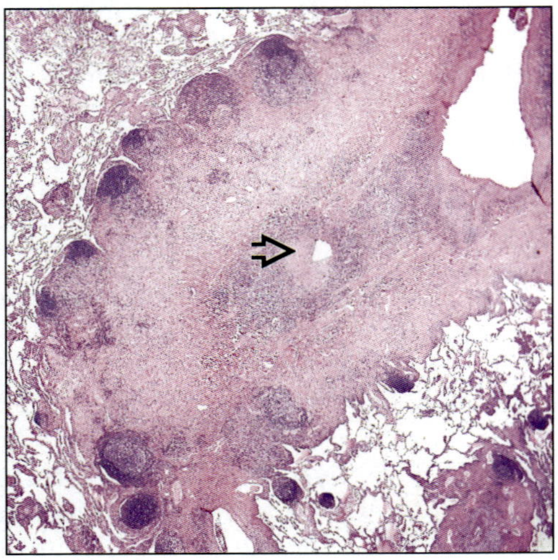

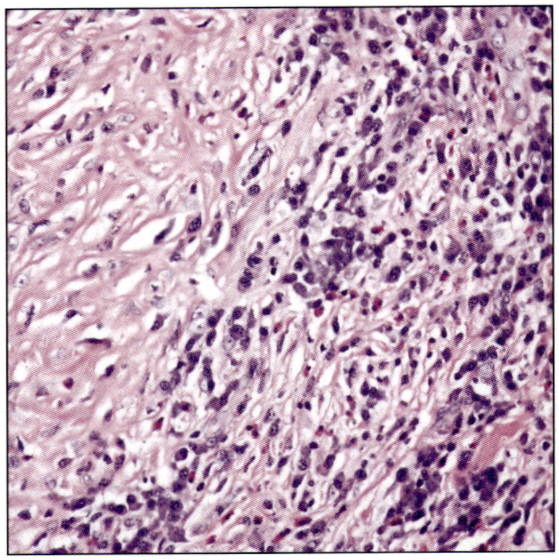

(Left) *Bronchovascular pattern of involvement of the lung in IgG4(+) sclerosing lung disease shows an area of fibrosis surrounded by multiple lymphoid follicles at the periphery and following the distribution of bronchovascular bundles. Note the sclerosed vessel* ⇨ *in the center of the field.* ***(Right)*** *Higher magnification of bronchovascular pattern of involvement in IgG4(+) sclerosing lung disease shows dense lymphoplasmacytic infiltrates with scattered eosinophils surrounding an area of sclerosis.*

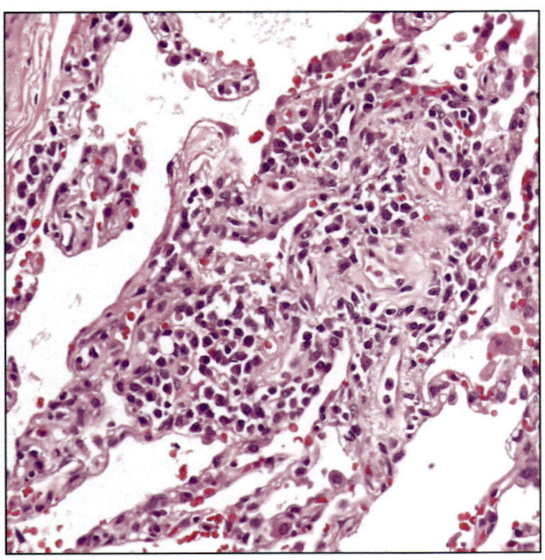

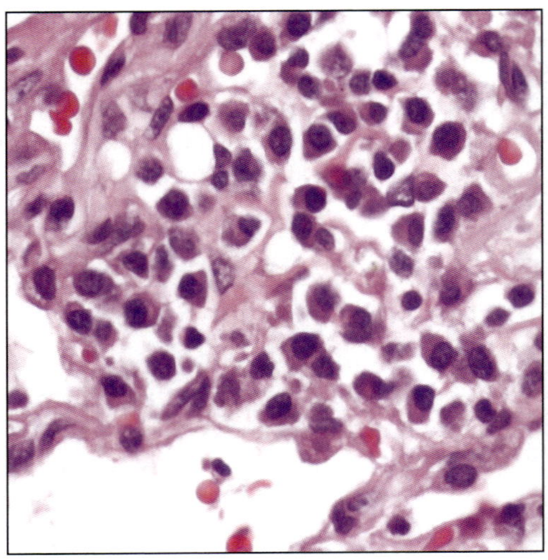

(Left) *Pattern of interstitial pneumonia in IgG4 sclerosing lung disease is characterized by expansion of alveolar septa by dense lymphoplasmacytic infiltrates with obliterative vascular changes. Lesions showing this growth pattern can be confused for the cellular form of nonspecific interstitial pneumonia (NSIP), lymphoid interstitial pneumonia, or grade I lymphomatoid granulomatosis.* ***(Right)*** *Higher magnification of an interstitial pattern in IgG4 sclerosing lung disease shows dense plasmacytic infiltration of the alveolar wall.*

Histologic Features and Special Stains

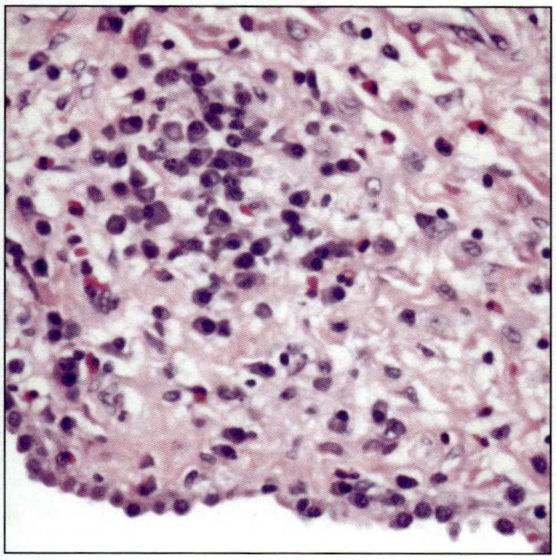

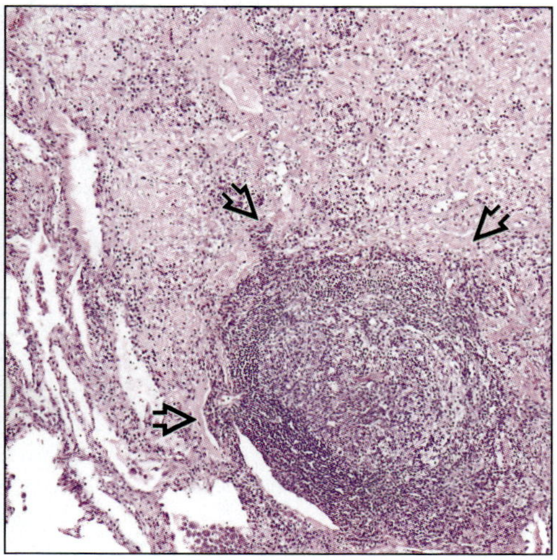

*(**Left**) Characteristic changes in IgG4 sclerosing lung disease include paucicellular stromal fibrosis and a lymphoplasmacellular inflammatory infiltrate that may harbor a prominent eosinophilic component. (**Right**) Reactive lymphoid follicles ⇨ are present in about 50% of cases of IgG4(+) sclerosing lung disease. Lymphoid follicles may be abundant. In some instances, the follicles may display features of progressive transformation of germinal centers or Castleman disease.*

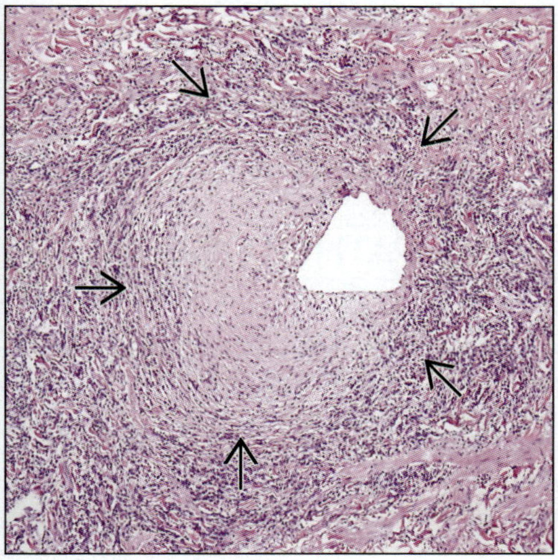

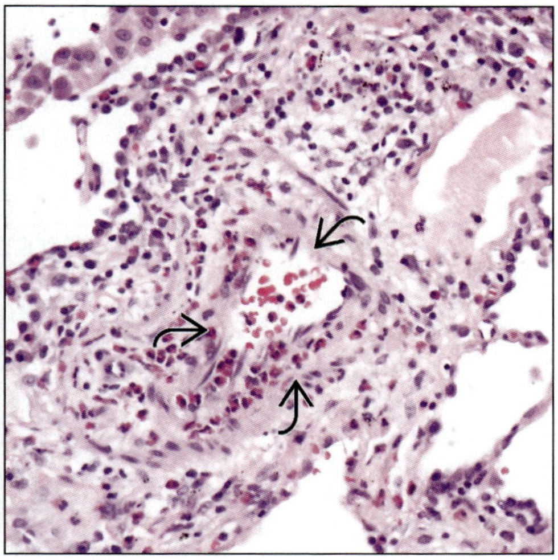

*(**Left**) Scanning magnification of lung in IgG4(+) sclerosing lung disease shows narrowing of the lumen of a mid-caliber vessel by concentric sclerosis and inflammation ⇨. Obliterative vascular changes are a common finding in IgG4(+) sclerosing disease of the lung and tend to affect both the veins and arteries. (**Right**) Small vessel in the interstitium of the lung in a patient with IgG4(+) sclerosing lung disease shows prominent endothelialitis ⇨.*

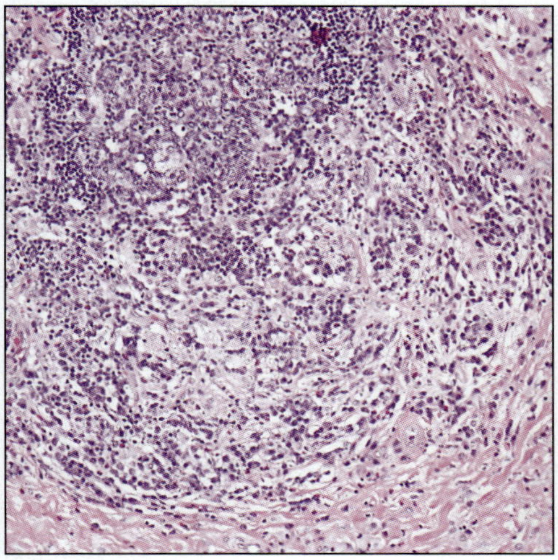

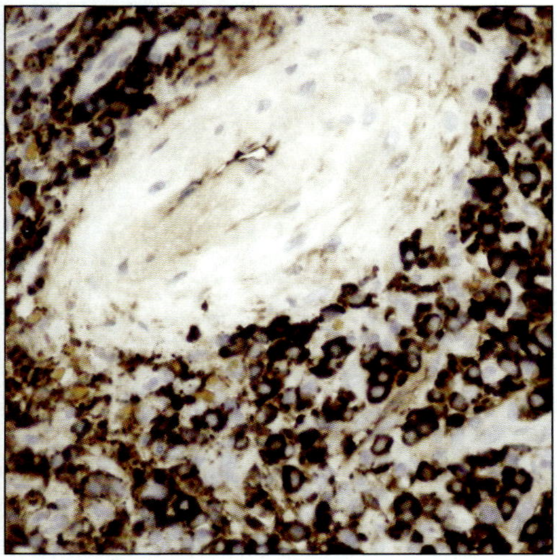

*(**Left**) IgG4(+) sclerosing lung disease shows an area with lymphoplasmacellular inflammatory infiltrates admixed with abundant histiocytes showing emperipolesis. Such areas can be closely reminiscent of Rosai-Dorfman disease. (**Right**) Immunohistochemical staining for IgG4 shows numerous plasma cells with strong cytoplasmic positivity in IgG4(+) sclerosing lung disease. There should be > 50 IgG4(+) plasma cells per 10 HPF, with an IgG4/IgG ratio of > 40%.*

JUVENILE XANTHOGRANULOMA

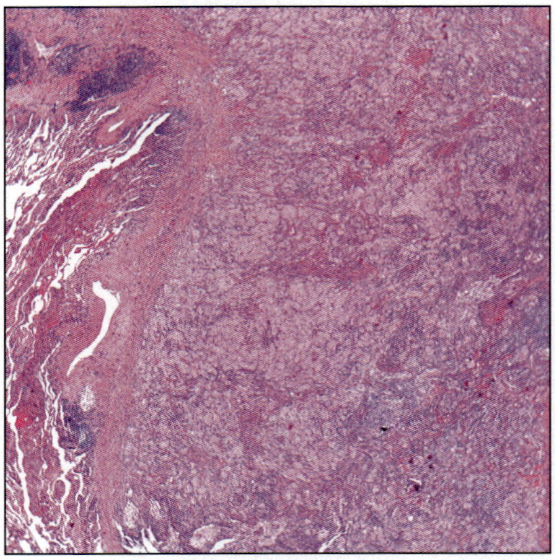

Low-power view of a JXG shows replacement of the lung parenchyma by a histiocytic proliferation admixed with inflammatory infiltrate.

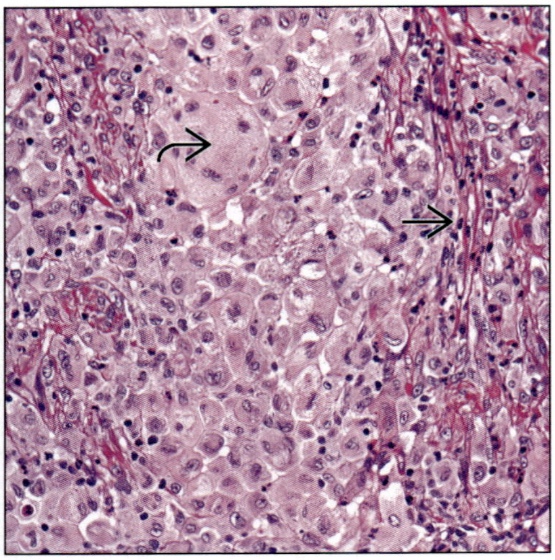

High-power view of the histiocytic proliferation shows large histiocytes ➩ with round nuclei and prominent nucleoli. A subtle inflammatory infiltrate is also present ➔.

TERMINOLOGY

Abbreviations

- Pulmonary juvenile xanthogranuloma (JXG)

Definitions

- Non-Langerhans histiocytic lesion

ETIOLOGY/PATHOGENESIS

Etiology

- Contrary to other histiocytic lesions, cell of origin for JXG is unknown
  - Plasmacytoid monocyte has been speculated as possible origin for JXG

CLINICAL ISSUES

Presentation

- Bilateral or unilateral involvement of lung parenchyma
- Multiple pulmonary lesions
- Rarely, lesion will be single
- Dermal involvement is common
- Involvement of other organ systems may occur

Treatment

- Surgical approaches
  - Complete surgical resection, if that can be accomplished

Prognosis

- Due to rarity of this lesion in lung, it is difficult to unequivocally determine prognosis
- May be determined by extent of the process

MACROSCOPIC FEATURES

General Features

- Tumor mass can range in size from 1-3 cm
- Well circumscribed but not encapsulated
- Soft and tan or yellowish in color

MICROSCOPIC PATHOLOGY

Histologic Features

- Cellular proliferation destroying lung parenchyma
- Histiocytic proliferation composed of small to medium-sized histiocytes
- Histocytes admixed with inflammatory infiltrate composed of lymphocytes and plasma cells
- Multinucleated giant cells may be present but scattered
- Absence of nuclear atypia or mitotic activity

DIFFERENTIAL DIAGNOSIS

Langerhans Cell Histiocytosis (LCH)

- Lesions in LCH may vary from cellular to fibrotic
- Presence of large number of eosinophils is more common in LCH
- Histiocytes have characteristic "grooving" of nucleus
- LCH lesions have characteristic "Medusa's head," which is not present in JXG
- Usually associated with diffuse interstitial pneumonia-like reaction in adjacent lung parenchyma
- Positive for CD1a and S100

Rosai-Dorfman (R-D) Disease of Lung

- Histiocytes in R-D disease are large with prominent nucleoli
- Enteropoiesis is characteristic of R-D disease
- Presence of prominent plasma cell component is more in favor of R-D disease

JUVENILE XANTHOGRANULOMA

Key Facts

Terminology
- Abbreviation:
  - Pulmonary juvenile xanthogranuloma (JXG)
- Definition
  - Non-Langerhans histiocytic lesion

Etiology/Pathogenesis
- Contrary to other histiocytic lesions, cell of origin for JXG is unknown
  - Plasmacytoid monocyte has been speculated as possible origin for JXG

Clinical Issues
- Presentation
  - Bilateral or unilateral involvement of lung parenchyma
  - Multiple pulmonary lesions
  - Rarely, lesion will be single
  - Dermal involvement is common
  - Involvement of other organ systems may occur

Microscopic Pathology
- Cellular proliferation destroying lung parenchyma
- Histocytes admixed with inflammatory infiltrate composed of lymphocytes and plasma cells
- Multinucleated giant cells may be present but scattered
- Absence of nuclear atypia or mitotic activity

Top Differential Diagnoses
- Langerhans cell histiocytosis (LCH)
- Rosai-Dorfman disease of lung
- Erdheim-Chester disease

Immunohistochemistry

Antibody	Reactivity	Staining Pattern	Comment
CD68	Positive	Cytoplasmic	Global and strong
FXIIIA	Positive	Cytoplasmic	May be focal
CD45	Positive	Cytoplasmic	In the lymphocytic component
HLA-DR	Positive	Cytoplasmic	May be focal
S100	Positive	Cytoplasmic	May be focal
CD4	Positive	Cytoplasmic	May be focal
CD1a	Negative		
CD3	Negative		
CD21	Negative		
CD34	Negative		
CD35	Negative		

- Would be unusual for R-D disease to show presence of multinucleated giant cells
- S100 is strongly positive
- Usually a single mass in lung

Erdheim-Chester (E-C) Disease
- Histiocytic proliferation in E-C disease characteristically follows septum and pleura
- Histiocytes in E-C disease are rather smaller
- Characteristically involves bones in symmetrical fashion
- S100 protein may show variable staining
- May share similar immunophenotype with JXG

Malacoplakia of Lung
- Generally shows histiocytic proliferation admixed with plasma cells
- Presence of Michaelis-Gutmann bodies is characteristic of malacoplakia
  - Iron and von Kossa stains highlight Michaelis-Gutmann bodies
- S100 protein is negative
- CD68 highlights histiocytic proliferation

Mycobacterial Infection
- Special stains for acid-fast bacilli show presence of organisms in histiocytes
- Mycobacterial infections would show negative results for factor XIIIa and HLA-DR

SELECTED REFERENCES

1. Bakir B et al: Atypical lung involvement in a patient with systemic juvenile xanthogranuloma. Pediatr Radiol. 37(3):325-7, 2007
2. Snijders D et al: Case for diagnosis: 4-month-old infant with increasing cough, hemoptysis, and anemia. Pediatr Pulmonol. 42(9):844-6, 2007
3. Cauro F et al: [Cerebellar, pulmonary and cutaneous localizations of juvenile xanthogranuloma.] Ann Dermatol Venereol. 129(3):307-10, 2002
4. Guthrie JA et al: Case report: juvenile xanthogranuloma with pulmonary, subcutaneous and hepatic involvement. Clin Radiol. 49(7):498-500, 1994
5. Gupta AK et al: Juvenile xanthogranuloma with pulmonary lesions. Pediatr Radiol. 18(1):70, 1988

JUVENILE XANTHOGRANULOMA

Microscopic Features

*(**Left**) Low-power view of a JXG shows an airway that is uninvolved by the histiocytic proliferation, even though some histiocytes are present within the lumen of the airway. Adjacent lung parenchyma shows inflammatory changes. (**Right**) In some cases of JXG, the histocytic proliferation destroys not only lung parenchyma but also airway structures. In this particular case, there is only residual bronchial epithelium .*

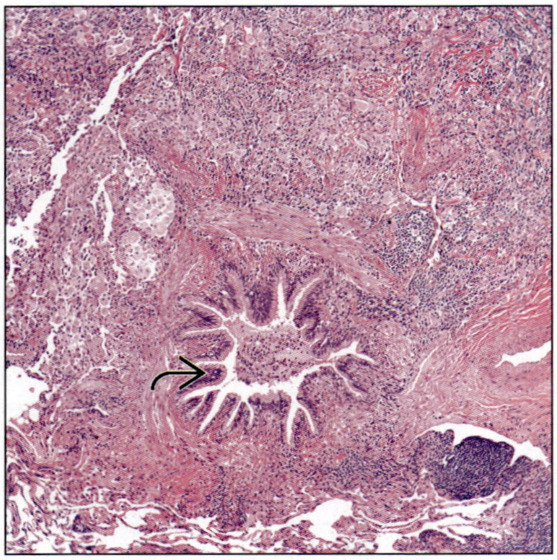

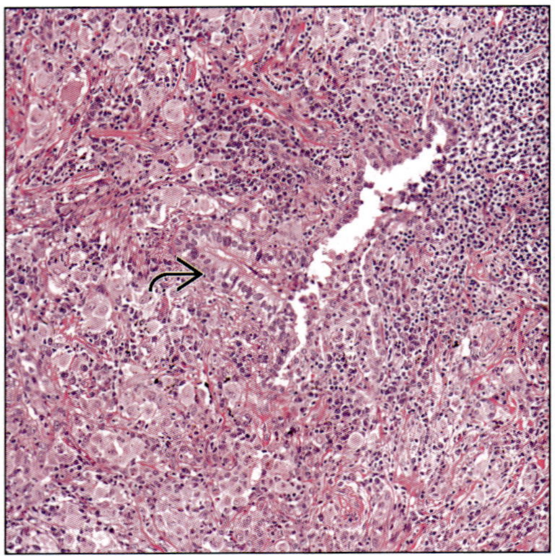

*(**Left**) Although the majority of cases of JXG consist of well-circumscribed lesions, they are not encapsulated. The histiocytic proliferation involves alveolar spaces , as can be seen in this case. (**Right**) In some other cases of JXG, the lesion appears to be well delimited by fibrocollagenous tissue . However, note that the histiocytic proliferation goes beyond that boundary into the lung parenchyma proper.*

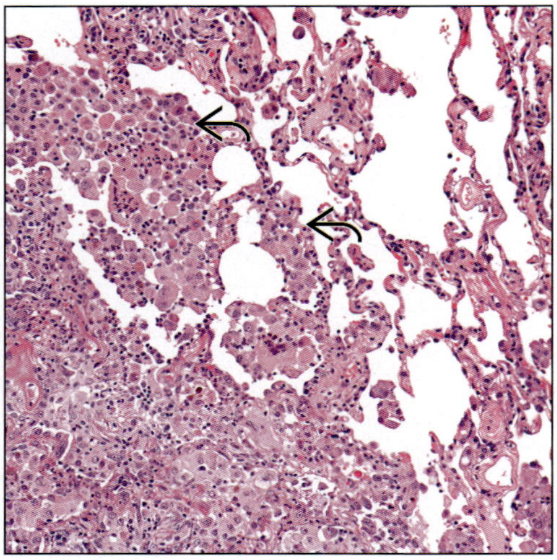

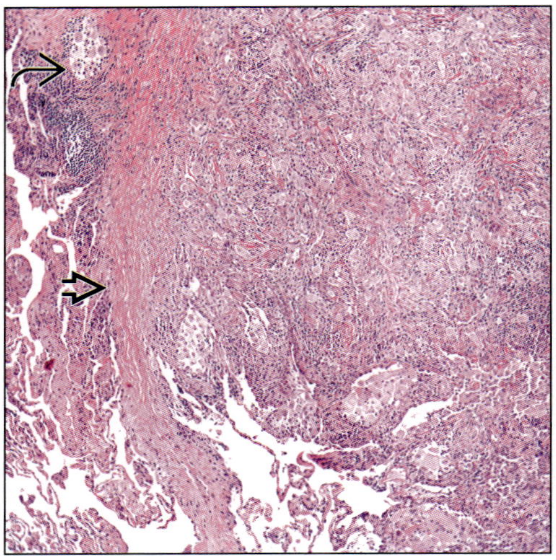

*(**Left**) Extensive areas of fibrosis with an inflammatory reaction composed of lymphocytes, plasma cells, and eosinophils are commonly seen in association with the histocytic proliferation, which can be scanty and subtle . (**Right**) Extensive areas of collagen deposition admixed with plasma cells, lymphocytes, and multinucleated histocytes are common features of JXG. However, similar features may also be seen in other types of histiocytosis.*

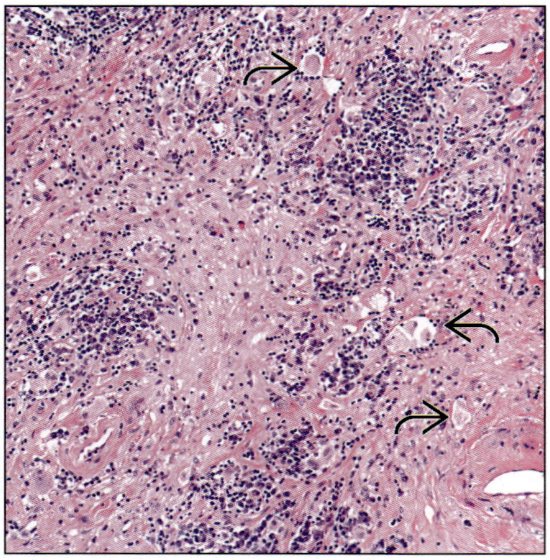

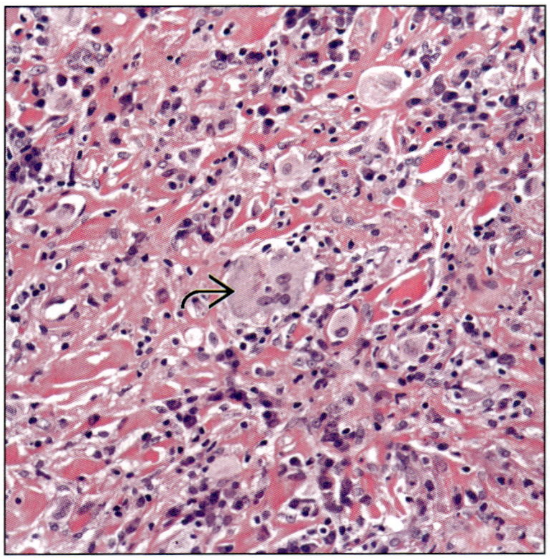

Microscopic Features

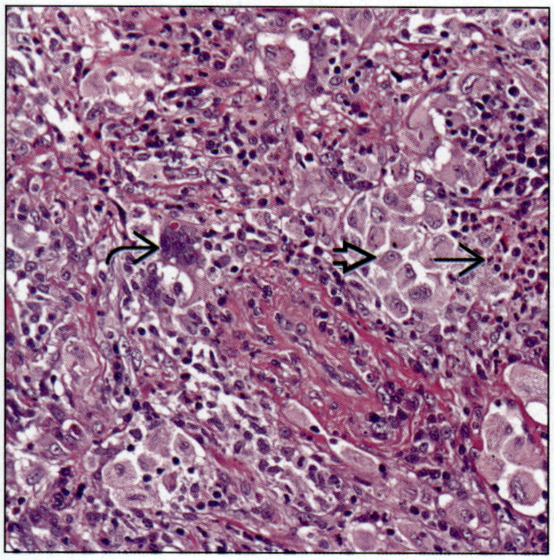

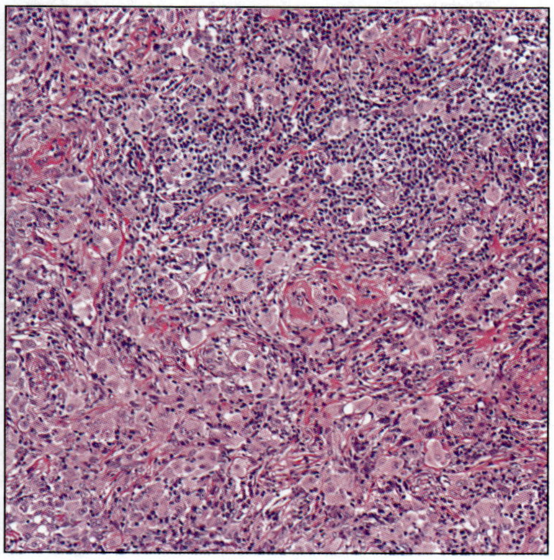

(Left) *Extensive histiocytic proliferation → with minimal inflammatory infiltrate → is shown. Note the presence of multinucleated giant cells → admixed with histiocytic proliferation.* ***(Right)*** *In other cases of JXG, the inflammatory infiltrate can be marked. The presence of this inflammatory infiltrate, composed mainly of plasma cells and lymphocytes, may also be observed in other types of histiocytosis.*

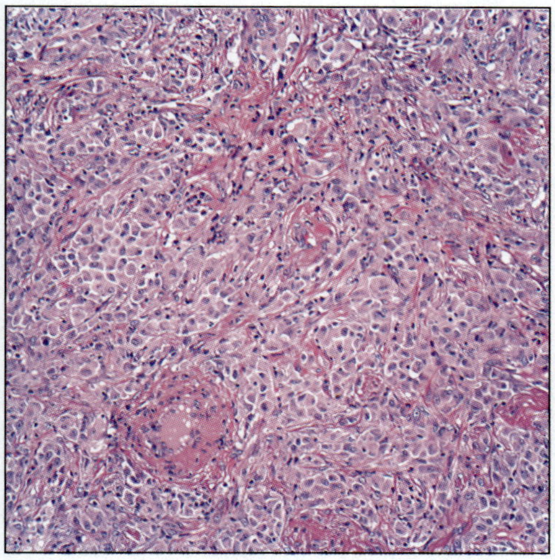

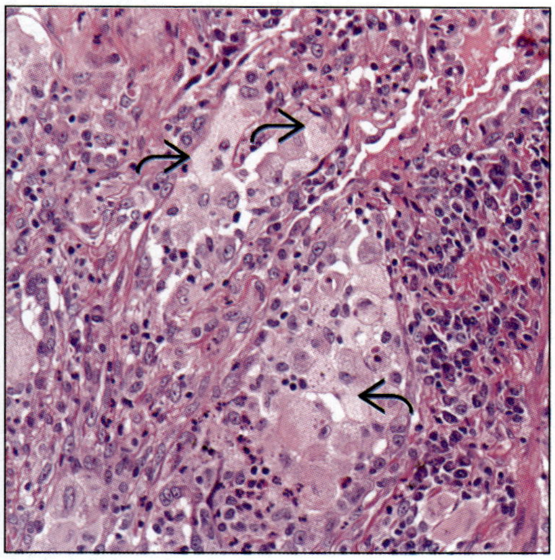

(Left) *JXG shows a more solid proliferation of histiocytes with only minimal inflammatory reaction. This type of proliferation can also be easily confused for a malignant neoplasm.* ***(Right)*** *High-power view of the histiocytic proliferation of JXG shows large histiocytes with round nuclei and prominent nucleoli. Note the ample cytoplasm of the histiocytes with more classical features of xanthomatous change →.*

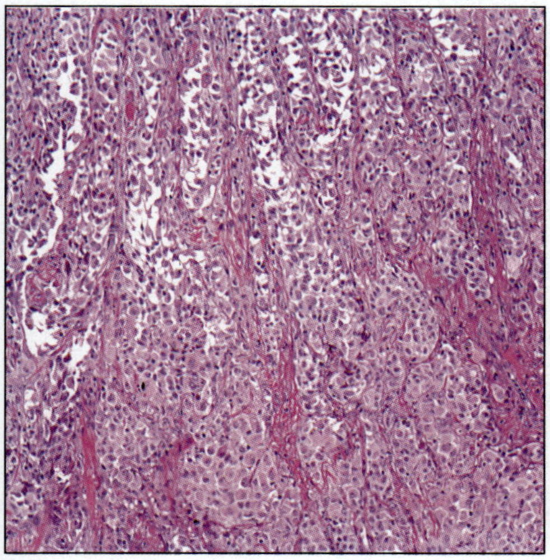

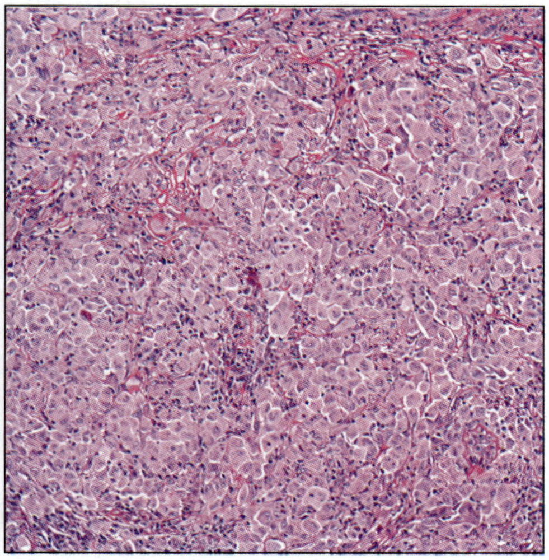

(Left) *In some cases of JXG, the histiocytic proliferation appears to actually show a subtle nested pattern. Similar features may be seen in some malignant neoplasms.* ***(Right)*** *In other cases of JXG, the histiocytic proliferation is rather solid and composed of large histiocytes but without evidence of mitotic activity &/or nuclear atypia. Note that in this particular illustration, the inflammatory reaction is minimal.*

HYALINIZING GRANULOMA

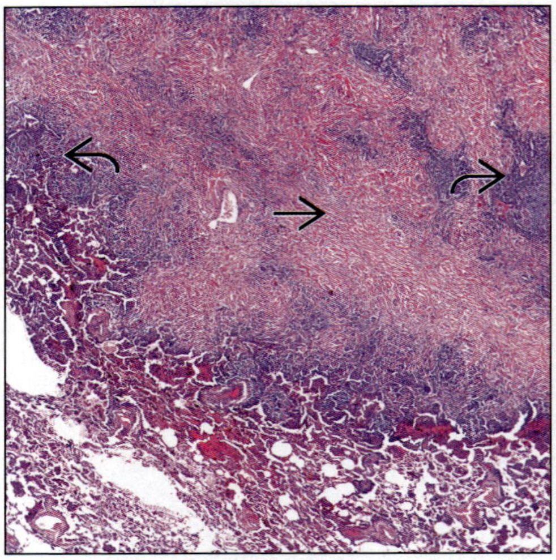

Low-power view of a hyalinizing granuloma of the lung is shown. Note the extensive fibrocollagenous tissue deposition → accompanied by an inflammatory reaction ↪.

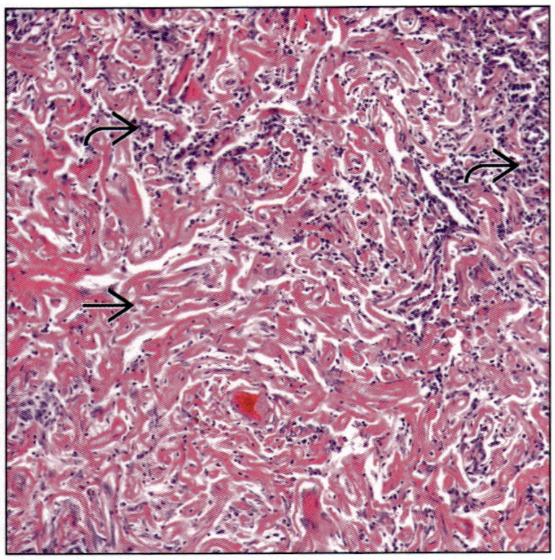

High-power magnification shows dense fibrocollagenous tissue →, rather acellular, and accompanied by an inflammatory reaction ↪.

TERMINOLOGY

Abbreviations

- Pulmonary hyalinizing granuloma (PHG)

Definitions

- Benign reactive process, probably inflammatory or autoimmune

ETIOLOGY/PATHOGENESIS

Etiology

- Unusual condition of unknown etiology
- May have autoimmune origin

Associated Conditions

- PHG may be associated with conditions with similar histological features, including
  - Retroperitoneal fibrosis
  - Sclerosing mediastinitis

CLINICAL ISSUES

Epidemiology

- Incidence
  - Rare occurrence
- Age
  - Any age group, but more common in middle-aged adults
- Gender
  - No gender predilection

Presentation

- Cough
- Dyspnea
- Chest pain
- Fever
- Asymptomatic

Laboratory Tests

- Antinuclear antibodies may be positive
- Rheumatoid factor may be positive
- Coombs positive hemolytic anemia may be positive

Treatment

- Surgical approaches
  - Complete surgical resection

Prognosis

- Good

IMAGE FINDINGS

General Features

- Single or multiple pulmonary nodules

MACROSCOPIC FEATURES

General Features

- Nodules are firm and light tan in color

Size

- Vary from 1 cm to > 10 cm in diameter

MICROSCOPIC PATHOLOGY

Histologic Features

- Prominent, dense, fibrocollagenous deposition
- Inflammatory reaction, mainly lymphocytes and plasma cells
- Dilatation of vascular spaces
- Focal calcification may be present

DIFFERENTIAL DIAGNOSIS

Amyloid Tumor

- Usually shows presence of giant cells

HYALINIZING GRANULOMA

Key Facts

Etiology/Pathogenesis
- Unusual condition of unknown origin
- May have autoimmune origin
- PHG may be associated with conditions with similar histological features, including
  - Retroperitoneal fibrosis
  - Sclerosing mediastinitis

Clinical Issues
- Epidemiology
  - Rare occurrence
  - Any age group, but more common in middle-aged adults
- Symptoms
  - Cough
  - Dyspnea
  - Chest pain
  - Fever
- Laboratory findings
  - Antinuclear antibodies
  - Rheumatoid factor may be positive
  - Coombs positive hemolithic anemia may be positive

Microscopic Pathology
- Prominent, dense, fibrocollagenous deposition
- Inflammatory reaction
- Dilatation of vascular spaces
- Focal calcification may be present

Top Differential Diagnoses
- Amyloid tumor
- Intrapulmonary solitary fibrous tumor (SFT)
- Inflammatory pseudotumor, plasma cell type (IP)

Immunohistochemistry

Antibody	Reactivity	Staining Pattern	Comment
Collagen IV	Positive	Stromal matrix	In some cases
CK-PAN	Negative		May stain entrapped alveolar or bronchial epithelium
CD34	Negative		May stain entrapped vascular structures
Bcl-2	Negative		May stain some inflammatory cells (lymphocytes)

Histochemical Features of Pulmonary Hyalinizing Granuloma

Stain	Result
Trichrome	Positive staining in collagen fibers
PAS	Highlights collagen fibers
Congo red	Negative
Mucicarmine	Negative

- Congo red is generally positive
- Amorphous material is usually acellular with no inflammatory reaction

Intrapulmonary Solitary Fibrous Tumor (SFT)
- Spindle cellular proliferation usually present
- Shows hemangiopericytic growth pattern
- Presence of an inflammatory reaction would be unusual
- Immunohistochemical studies for CD34 and Bcl-2 are commonly positive

Inflammatory Pseudotumor, Plasma Cell Type (IP)
- Marked presence of plasma cells with collections of foamy macrophages
- Likely shows positive staining for smooth muscle actin &/or ALK

Pulmonary Scar
- Scarring is usually not as extensive as in PHG
- In scars, the matrix is more of the fibroelastotic type

DIAGNOSTIC CHECKLIST

Pathologic Interpretation Pearls
- Dense fibrocollagenous tissue
- Inflammatory reaction

SELECTED REFERENCES

1. Young AS et al: Pulmonary hyalinizing granuloma and retroperitoneal fibrosis in an adolescent. Pediatr Radiol. 37(1):91-5, 2007
2. Yousem SA et al: Pulmonary hyalinizing granuloma. Am J Clin Pathol. 87(1):1-6, 1987
3. Engleman P et al: Pulmonary hyalinizing granuloma. Am Rev Respir Dis. 115(6):997-1008, 1977

HYALINIZING GRANULOMA

Microscopic Features

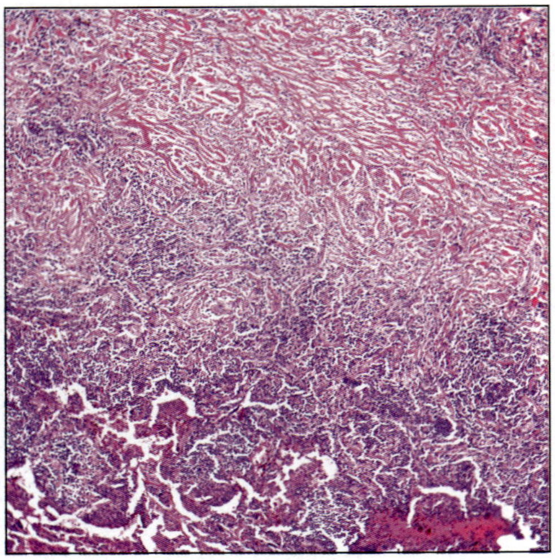
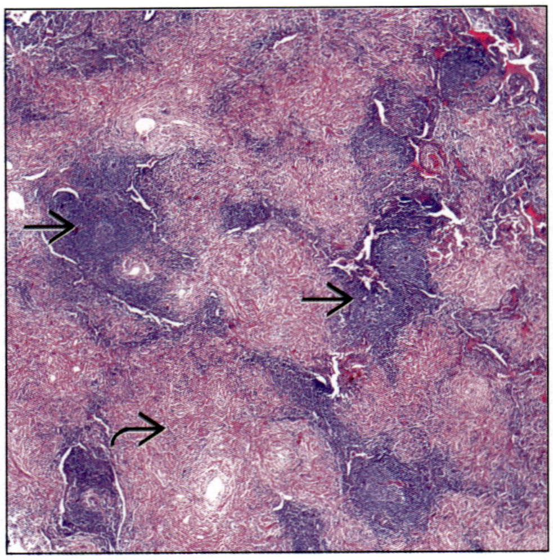

(Left) *Hyalinizing granuloma of the lung shows the classical histopathological features of dense fibrocollagenous tissue and inflammatory reaction. Note that the lesion is not encapsulated and appears to penetrate into alveolar tissue.* ***(Right)*** *Extensive hyalinization ↪ with marked inflammatory reaction → is shown. At this power, the morphological features would suggest a granulomatous reaction; however, the presence of granulomas would be unusual for this condition.*

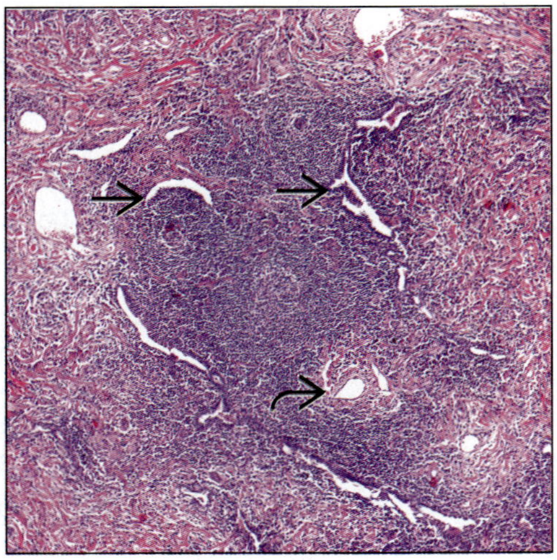
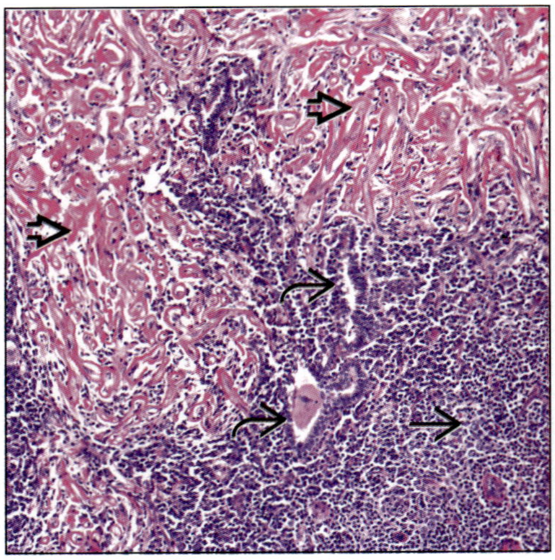

(Left) *In some areas of hyalinizing granuloma where there are marked inflammatory changes, there may be entrapped vessels ↪ giving the appearance of vasculitis. Note also the presence of entrapped airway structures →.* ***(Right)*** *Closer magnification demonstrates the presence of hyalinization represented by dense collagen fibers ⇨ and a marked inflammatory component composed mainly of lymphocytes →. Note the entrapped airway structures ↪.*

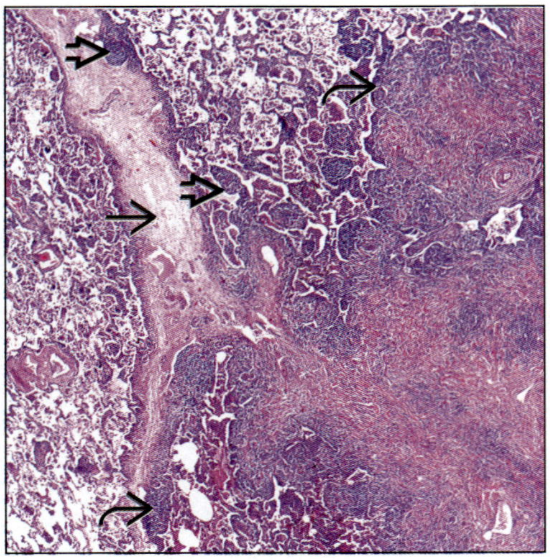
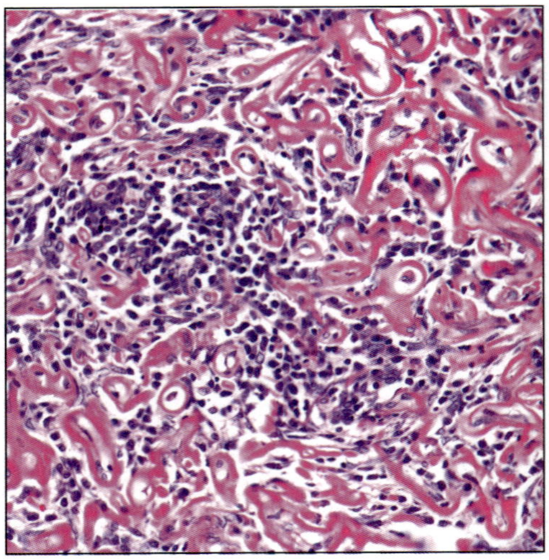

(Left) *Hyalinizing granuloma shows pushing borders ↪ into the "normal" lung parenchyma, which shows thickening of the pulmonary septum →. In addition, the inflammatory component is also present in focal areas in the pulmonary parenchyma ⇨.* ***(Right)*** *Higher magnification shows the acellular fibrocollagen admixed with inflammatory cells, mainly plasma cells. At this magnification, these features may also be shared by other tumoral conditions, including solitary fibrous tumor.*

Microscopic Features

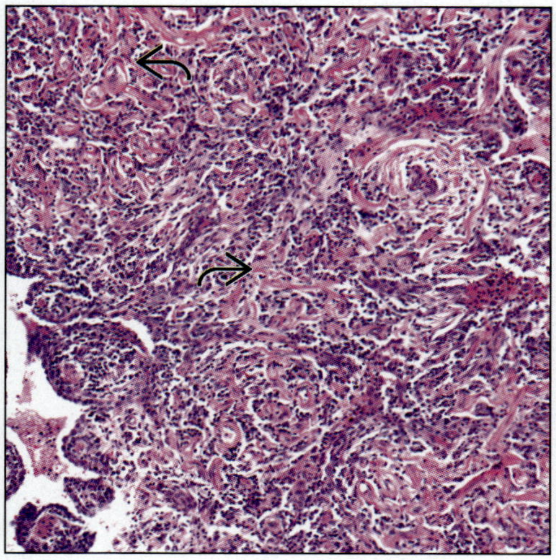

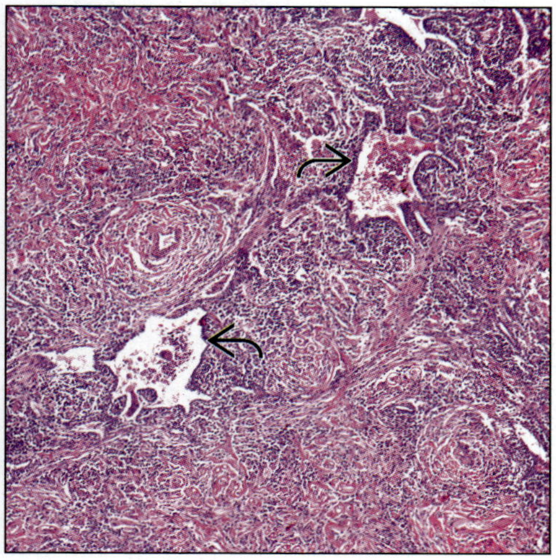

(Left) *In some areas of hyalinizing granuloma, the typical features may not be as easily identifiable. In this illustration, the presence of fibrocollagen is rather subtle* → *and the inflammatory component is also marked.* ***(Right)*** *In some areas of hyalinizing granuloma, the process appears to be involving and destroying airway structures* →*. The typical features of the process are apparent and should not be mistaken for a simple nonspecific inflammatory process.*

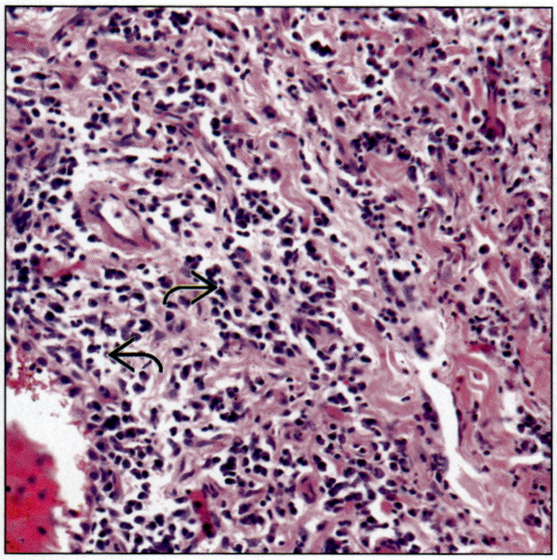

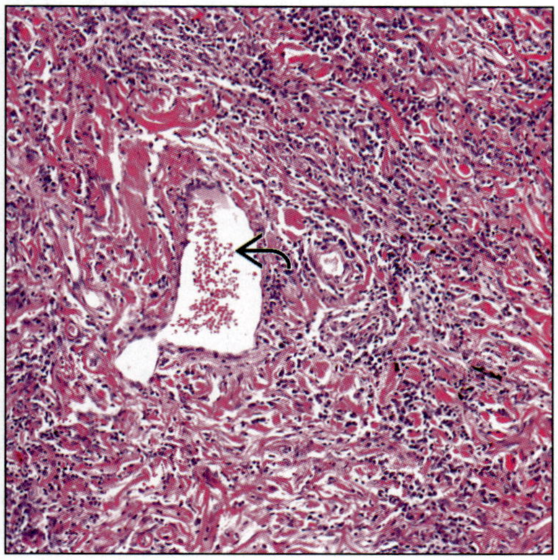

(Left) *Marked inflammatory reaction* → *composed of mature plasma cells and lymphocytes dissecting fibrocollagen is shown. However, these changes are nonspecific and cannot be construed as diagnostic for hyalinizing granuloma.* ***(Right)*** *Extensive hyalinization with inflammatory reaction and an ectatic large vessel* → *is shown. These changes can be easily associated with tumoral conditions such as solitary fibrous tumors or involvement of the lung by sclerosing mediastinitis.*

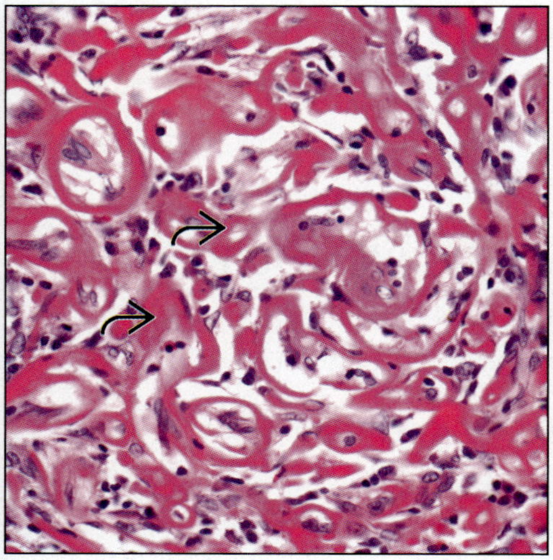

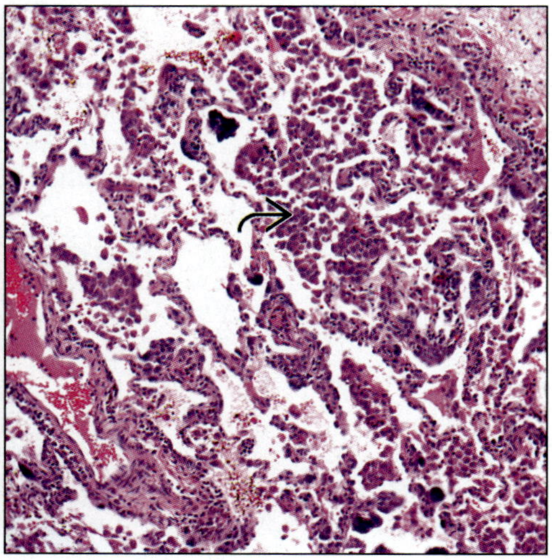

(Left) *Higher magnification of a hyalinizing granuloma of the lung shows the classical fibrocollagen* → *that in some respects mimics the "ropy" collagen that is described in solitary fibrous tumor.* ***(Right)*** *Uninvolved section of the lung parenchyma shows collections of intraalveolar pigmented macrophages* → *as well as inflammatory cells. These are common features observed in the adjacent lung parenchyma.*

AMYLOID TUMOR

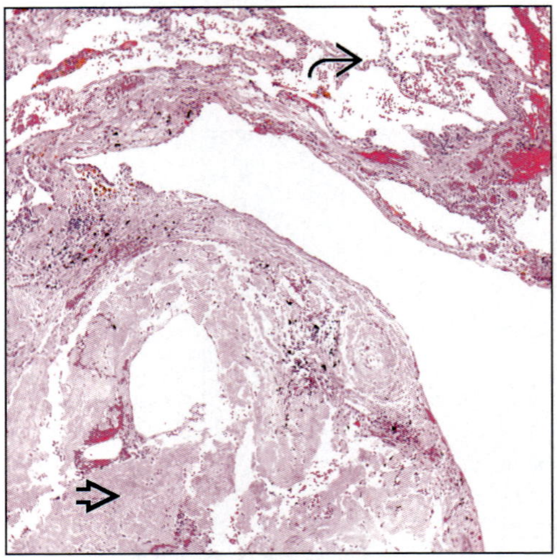

Low-power view of a pulmonary amyloid tumor shows dense amorphous material replacing normal lung parenchyma ⇨. Adjacent lung parenchyma appears to be within normal limits ↗.

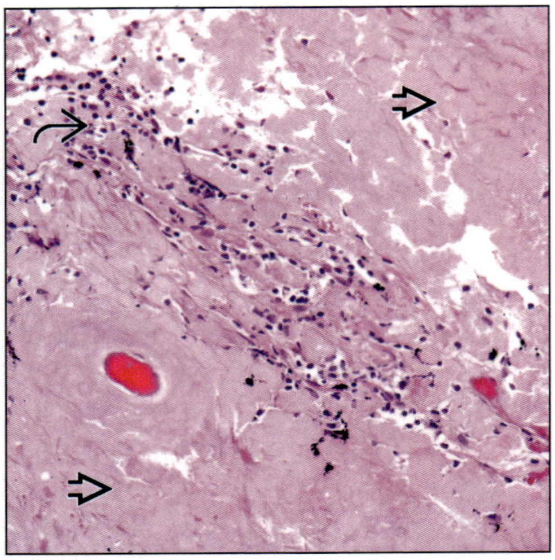

High-power view of a pulmonary amyloid tumor shows dense amorphous acellular material ⇨ with only focal areas of inflammatory reaction ↗. These features are classic for an amyloid tumor.

TERMINOLOGY

Synonyms

- Amyloidoma

Definitions

- Pulmonary mass composed of amyloid without evidence of systemic disease

ETIOLOGY/PATHOGENESIS

Etiology

- Specific cause to account for presence of amyloid in lung without systemic disease is unknown
  - Speculated to be related to
    - Light chain immunoglobulin
    - Plasma cells

Associated Conditions

- Waldenström macroglobulinemia
- Systemic amyloidosis
- Multiple myeloma
- Familial neuropathy
- Niemann-Pick disease
- Gaucher disease

CLINICAL ISSUES

Epidemiology

- Incidence
  - Rare occurrence
- Age
  - Predominantly in adults
- Gender
  - No gender predilection
- Ethnicity
  - No apparent ethnic predilection

Presentation

- Cough
- Chest pain
- Dyspnea
- Sjögren syndrome

Laboratory Tests

- Potassium permanganate oxidation technique appears to separate amyloid type AA from other forms of amyloid

Treatment

- Surgical approaches
  - Surgical resection of tumor mass by wedge resection or lobectomy

Prognosis

- It will depend on any possible associated condition

MACROSCOPIC FEATURES

General Features

- Single or multiple pulmonary nodules
- Soft and well circumscribed
- Size can range from 1 cm to > 10 cm in diameter
- Light tan in color

MICROSCOPIC PATHOLOGY

Histologic Features

- There are essentially 2 patterns in which the lung may be affected
  - Interstitial and diffuse pattern
  - Nodular
- Acellular amorphous eosinophilic material destroying lung parenchyma
- Subtle inflammatory infiltrate predominantly in periphery
- Numerous multinucleated giant cells

Key Facts

Terminology
- Synonym
  - Amyloidoma
- Definition
  - Pulmonary mass composed of amyloid without evidence of systemic disease

Etiology/Pathogenesis
- Specific cause to account for presence of amyloid in lung without systemic disease unknown; speculated to be related to
  - Light chain immunoglobulin
  - Plasma cells
- Associated conditions
  - Waldenström macroglobulinemia
  - Systemic amyloidosis
  - Multiple myeloma
  - Familial neuropathy
  - Niemann-Pick disease
  - Gaucher disease

Clinical Issues
- Rare occurrence
- Predominantly in adults
- Laboratory tests
  - Potassium permanganate oxidation technique appears to separate amyloid type AA from other types

Top Differential Diagnoses
- Hyalinizing granuloma of lung
- Intrapulmonary solitary fibrous tumor

Histochemical Features of Amyloid Tumor

Stain	Comment
Congo red	Apple green reaction under polarized light
Trichrome	May show some presence of collagen fiber under polarized light
Gomori methenamine silver	Negative
PAS	Negative
Mucicarmine	Negative

- Focal areas of ossification may be present

DIFFERENTIAL DIAGNOSIS

Pulmonary Scar
- Negative staining for Congo red amyloid stain
- Does not show subtle inflammatory reaction
- Multinucleated giant cells are generally absent in pulmonary scar

Hyalinizing Granuloma of Lung
- Negative for Congo red
- Dense ropy fibrocollagen
- Does not show presence of multinucleated giant cells

PCP Pneumonia
- Stains brightly with silver stains
- Negative for Congo red stain

Intrapulmonary Solitary Fibrous Tumor
- Negative staining for Congo red amyloid stain
- Likely shows hemangiopericytic pattern
- Multinucleated giant cells would be unusual feature for solitary fibrous tumor

DIAGNOSTIC CHECKLIST

Clinically Relevant Pathologic Features
- Some cases may be associated with MALT lymphoma of lung

Pathologic Interpretation Pearls
- Amorphous acellular material
- Subtle inflammatory infiltrate in periphery
- Presence of multinucleated giant cells

SELECTED REFERENCES

1. Calatayud J et al: Nodular pulmonary amyloidosis in a patient with rheumatoid arthritis. Clin Rheumatol. 26(10):1797-8, 2007
2. Mori S et al: Early rheumatoid arthritis in a patient with Sjögren's syndrome and pulmonary nodular amyloidosis: clinical implication of early limited use of infliximab. Mod Rheumatol. 17(6):500-6, 2007
3. Satani T et al: Amyloid deposition in primary pulmonary marginal zone B-cell lymphoma of mucosa-associated lymphoid tissue. Pathol Int. 57(11):746-50, 2007
4. Suzuki H et al: Three cases of the nodular pulmonary amyloidosis with a longterm observation. Intern Med. 45(5):283-6, 2006
5. Tokunaga T et al: Nodular pulmonary amyloidosis. Jpn J Thorac Cardiovasc Surg. 54(9):399-401, 2006
6. Dacic S et al: Nodular amyloidoma and primary pulmonary lymphoma with amyloid production: a differential diagnostic problem. Mod Pathol. 13(9):934-40, 2000

AMYLOID TUMOR

Microscopic Features

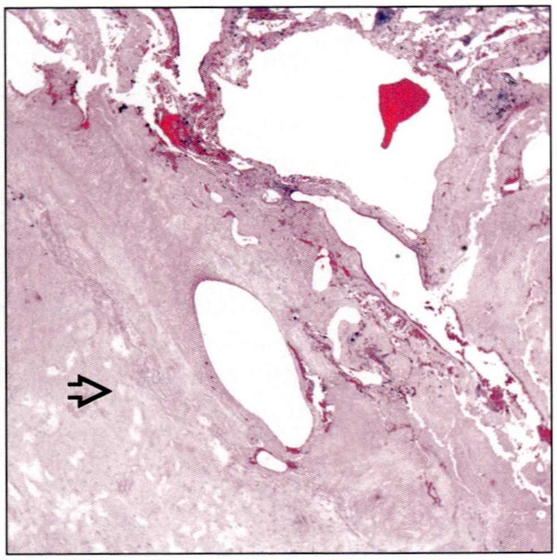

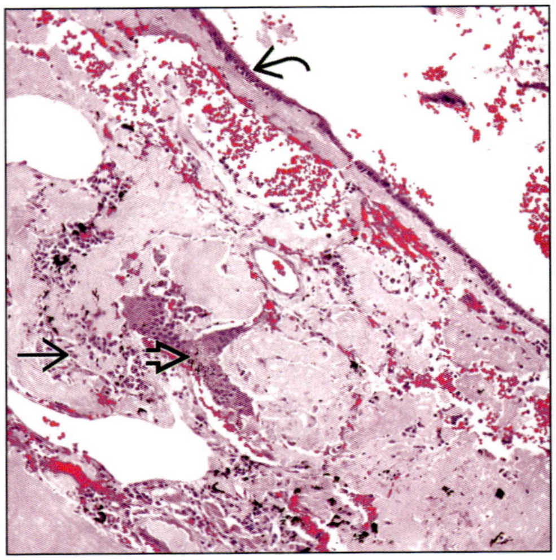

(Left) *Low-power view of a pulmonary amyloid tumor shows the classical features of amorphous acellular material* ⇨ *replacing lung parenchyma. At this magnification, this can be easily mistaken for fibrinous material or scarring of the lung parenchyma.* ***(Right)*** *Pulmonary amyloid tumor shows conventional histological features. Important to note is the presence of a residual airway* ↷*, an inflammatory reaction* →*, and the accumulation of macrophages* ⇨*.*

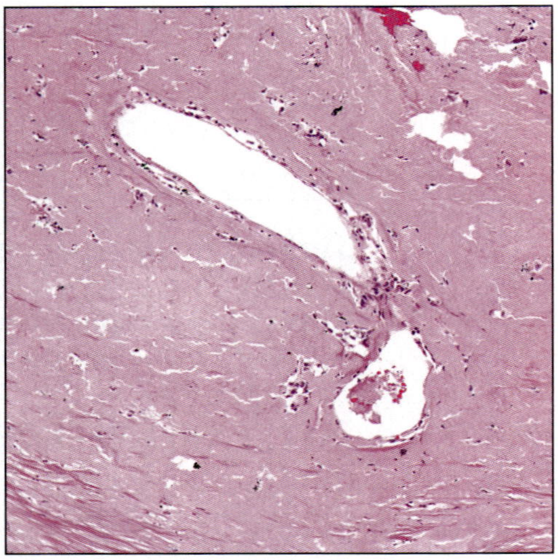

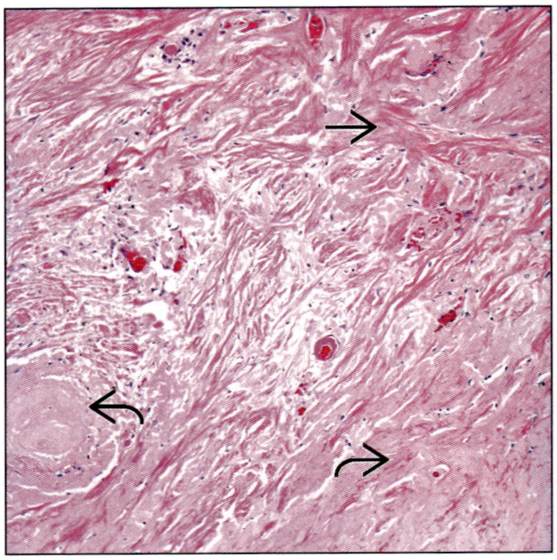

(Left) *Pulmonary amyloid tumor shows ectatic vessels and minimal inflammatory reaction. These features may be misleading for other conditions, including solitary fibrous tumor of hyalinizing granuloma of the lung.* ***(Right)*** *In some cases of amyloid tumor of the lung, the amorphous acellular material may be associated with areas of collagenization, which makes the distinction of the 2 very difficult. Amyloid* ↷ *and collagen* → *are both depicted here.*

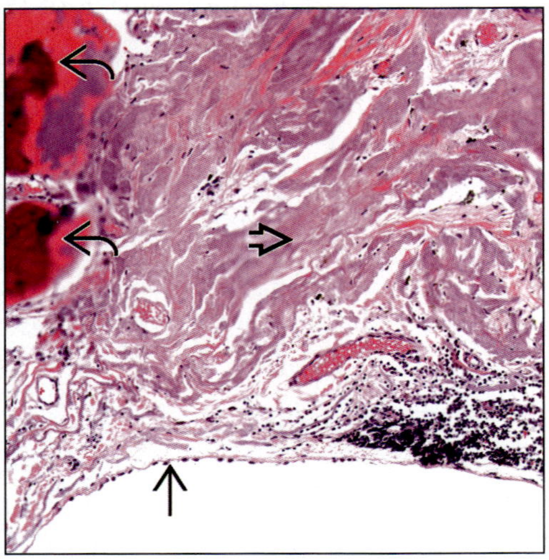

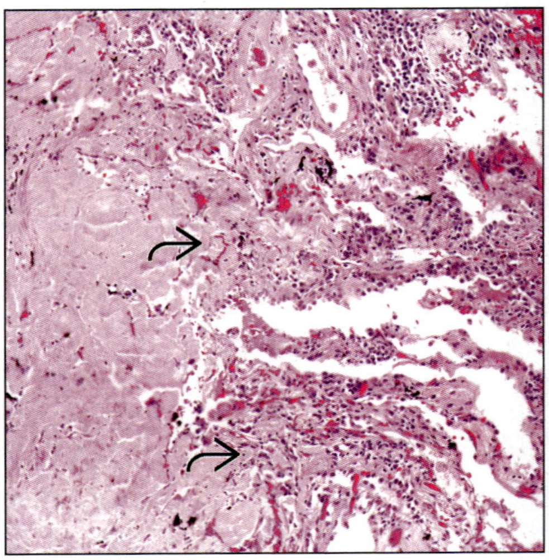

(Left) *In many cases of pulmonary amyloid tumor, the nodule is in a subpleural location; note the residual mesothelial lining* →*. In addition, the amyloid looks denser* ⇨ *with areas of ossification* ↷*.* ***(Right)*** *Although most cases of pulmonary amyloid are characterized by the presence of well-demarcated nodules, in some cases, it is possible to identify areas in which such demarcation is not well defined and the amyloid* ↷ *transitions subtly into normal lung parenchyma.*

Microscopic Features

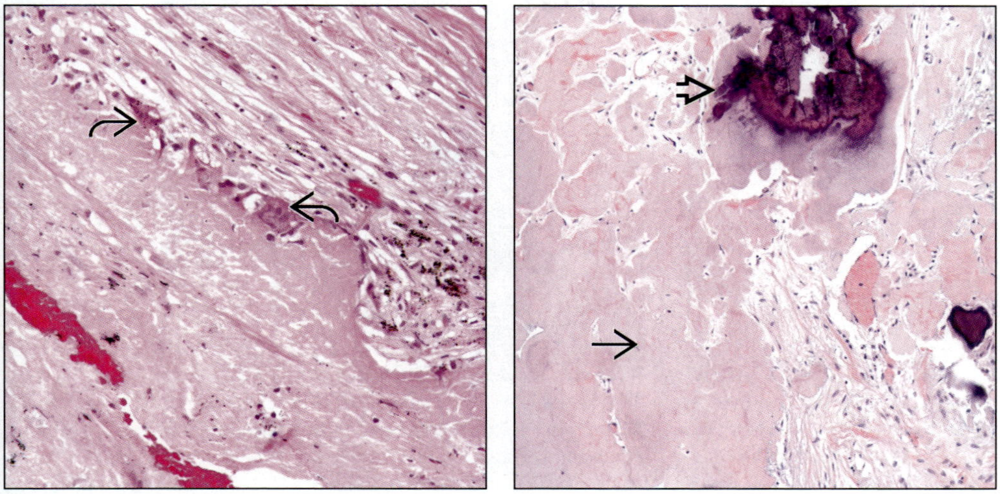

(Left) *The presence of multinucleated giant cells ↪ at the periphery of the pulmonary nodule is a common feature of pulmonary amyloid tumor.* ***(Right)*** *In addition, a pulmonary amyloid tumor may also show areas of calcification ➩ admixed with the dense amorphous acellular material →.*

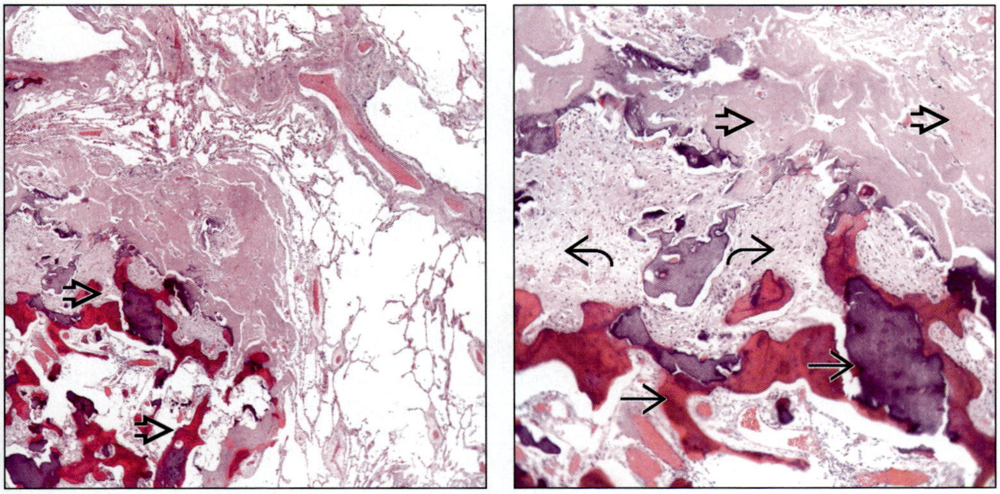

(Left) *In some cases, the presence of extensive areas of ossification ➩ can make the diagnosis of pulmonary amyloid tumor more challenging as the ossification may interfere with the identification of amyloid.* ***(Right)*** *Higher magnification shows the presence of ossification → and calcification with reactive inflammatory changes ↪. Adjacent to those changes, it is possible to identify the presence of amyloid ➩.*

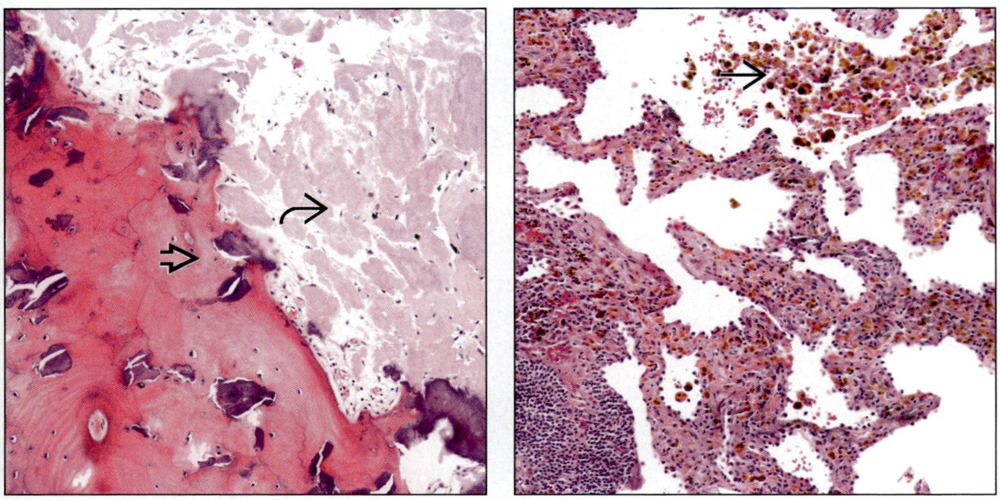

(Left) *High-power view shows transitional areas between ossification ➩ and amyloid deposition ↪. Although easily identifiable on conventional stains, the use of Congo red stain may facilitate the identification of amyloid in difficult cases.* ***(Right)*** *The changes observed in the adjacent lung parenchyma in cases of pulmonary amyloid tumor include the presence of a desquamative interstitial pneumonitis-like reaction. Note the presence of pigmented intraalveolar macrophages →.*

METASTATIC/DENDRIFORM CALCIFICATION

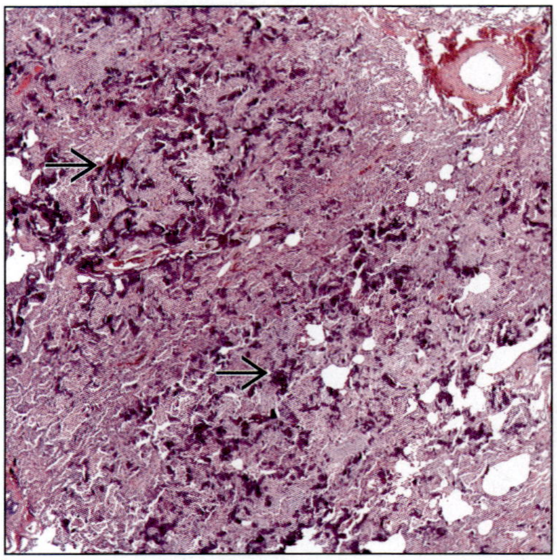

Low-power view of a section of lung shows extensive presence of calcified material ➡ in a haphazard pattern. The calcific material is deposited within the lung interstitium.

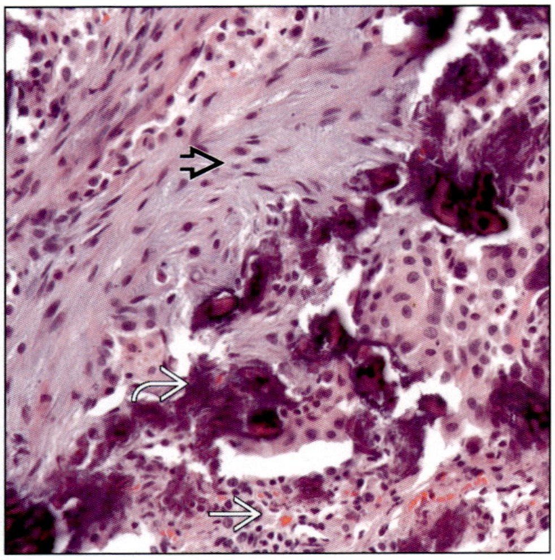

High-power view of the presence of calcific material ➡ admixed with minimal inflammation ➡ and focal fibroblastic component ➡. Note the absence of cellular atypia.

TERMINOLOGY

Synonyms

- Metastatic calcification, dendritic calcification

Definitions

- Nonneoplastic condition characterized by deposition of calcified material in the lung parenchyma

ETIOLOGY/PATHOGENESIS

Etiology

- This condition may appear in response to different clinical conditions that may include
  - Epithelial malignancies
  - Lymphoproliferative disorders
  - Post-transplant
  - Renal failure

Pathophysiology

- Exact mechanism to account for the occurrence of this disorder is not known
- Serum level of calcium and phosphates may play a role in its development

CLINICAL ISSUES

Epidemiology

- Incidence
  - Difficult to estimate since the disorder is secondary to different clinical conditions
- Age
  - Can occur in any age group
- Gender
  - No gender predilection
- Ethnicity
  - No ethnic predilection

Site

- Lung parenchyma

Laboratory Tests

- Serum levels of calcium and phosphates may be altered

Natural History

- Develops as a secondary process from diverse clinical conditions
- Process may not be limited to the pulmonary system

Treatment

- Surgical approaches
  - Patients usually require surgical resection of the portion of the lung affected

Prognosis

- Depends on the underlying condition
- From the strict point of view of calcified deposits in the lung parenchyma, prognosis depends on the extent of the process

IMAGE FINDINGS

General Features

- Bilateral
- Dense
- Asymmetrical

Other Studies

- Dual-energy digital radiography appears to be more sensitive modality

MACROSCOPIC FEATURES

General Features

- Lung parenchyma appears congested and gritty
- Cut surface may be hard in consistency

Key Facts

Terminology
- Nonneoplastic condition characterized by the deposition of calcified material in the lung parenchyma

Etiology/Pathogenesis
- This condition may appear in response to different clinical conditions that may include
  - Epithelial malignancies
  - Lymphoproliferative disorders
  - Post-transplant
  - Renal failure
- Pathophysiology
  - Exact mechanism to account for the occurrence of metastatic calcification is not known
  - Serum levels of calcium and phosphates may play a role

Clinical Issues
- Prognosis
  - Depends on the underlying condition
  - Depends on the extent of the process in the lung

Microscopic Pathology
- Calcified material may follow some specific pattern of involvement of the lung parenchyma
  - Interstitium
  - Around the bronchial wall
  - Around the airway
  - Usually follows the alveolar outlines

Diagnostic Checklist
- Pattern of distribution
- Clinical history of an associated condition

MICROSCOPIC PATHOLOGY

Histologic Features
- Haphazard distribution of calcified material in the lung parenchyma
- Calcified material may follow some specific pattern of involvement of the lung parenchyma
  - Interstitial deposition
  - Around the bronchial wall
  - Around the airway
  - Calcified material usually follows the outlines of the alveoli
- No cytologic atypia or mitotic activity is present
- No osteoid material is present
- Fibroblast-like intraalveolar proliferation

DIFFERENTIAL DIAGNOSIS

Metastatic Osteogenic Sarcoma
- Clinical history of bone tumor is of utmost importance
- Shows presence of areas of osteoid
- Shows areas of cytologic atypia and mitotic activity
- Shows calcified material destroying lung parenchyma

Dystrophic Calcification
- Histological features may be very similar
- Does not require previous tissue injury
  - Dendriform calcification requires previous tissue injury

Pulmonary Chondroma
- Shows areas of cartilage
- Pattern of calcification outlining alveoli is not the pattern of chondromas
- Chondromas are usually lung nodules or masses without diffuse distribution

Alveolar Microlithiasis
- Pattern of distribution is predominantly intraalveolar
- No preexisting condition accounts for the process
- In general, microlithiasis is not associated with serum abnormalities of calcium or phosphates

DIAGNOSTIC CHECKLIST

Clinically Relevant Pathologic Features
- Pattern of distribution
- Clinical history of an associated condition

Pathologic Interpretation Pearls
- Calcified material following the alveolar outlines
- Absent cellular atypia or mitotic activity

SELECTED REFERENCES

1. Crippa C et al: Pulmonary calciphylaxis and metastatic calcification with acute respiratory failure in multiple myeloma. J Clin Oncol. 28(9):e133-5, 2010
2. Thurley PD et al: Case report: Rapidly progressive metastatic pulmonary calcification: evolution of changes on CT. Br J Radiol. 82(980):e155-9, 2009
3. Yasuo M et al: Progressive pulmonary calcification after successful renal transplantation. Intern Med. 47(3):161-4, 2008
4. Moran CA et al: Unusual non-neoplastic lesions of the lung. Semin Diagn Pathol. 24(3):199-208, 2007
5. Li YJ et al: Fulminant pulmonary calciphylaxis and metastatic calcification causing acute respiratory failure in a uremic patient. Am J Kidney Dis. 47(4):e47-53, 2006
6. Oikonomou A et al: Metastatic pulmonary calcification in acute myeloid leukemia. Leuk Lymphoma. 47(4):759-61, 2006
7. Guermazi A et al: Imaging of diffuse metastatic and dystrophic pulmonary calcification in children after haematopoietic stem cell transplantation. Br J Radiol. 78(932):708-13, 2005
8. Kobayashi T et al: A case of metastatic pulmonary calcification after transient acute renal failure. Radiat Med. 23(6):435-8, 2005

METASTATIC/DENDRIFORM CALCIFICATION

Microscopic Features

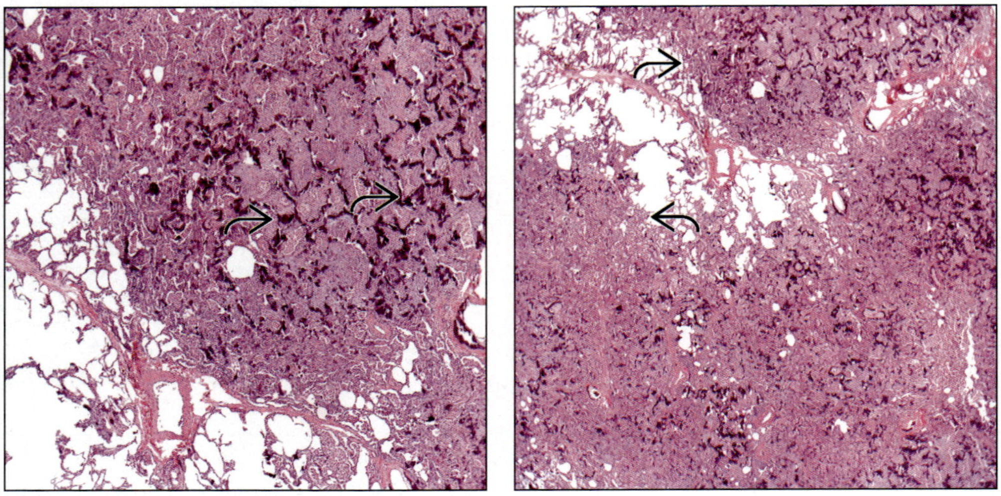

(Left) *Low-power view of a section of lung shows extensive deposition of calcified material in a manner mimicking a neoplastic process. Portions of the lung parenchyma are replaced by the presence of calcifications* ↪. ***(Right)*** *In some cases, the pattern may appear to be forming tumor nodules* ↪ *with very little intervening normal lung parenchyma. The deposition of calcified material can be very extensive, replacing lung parenchyma and thus mimicking a malignant process.*

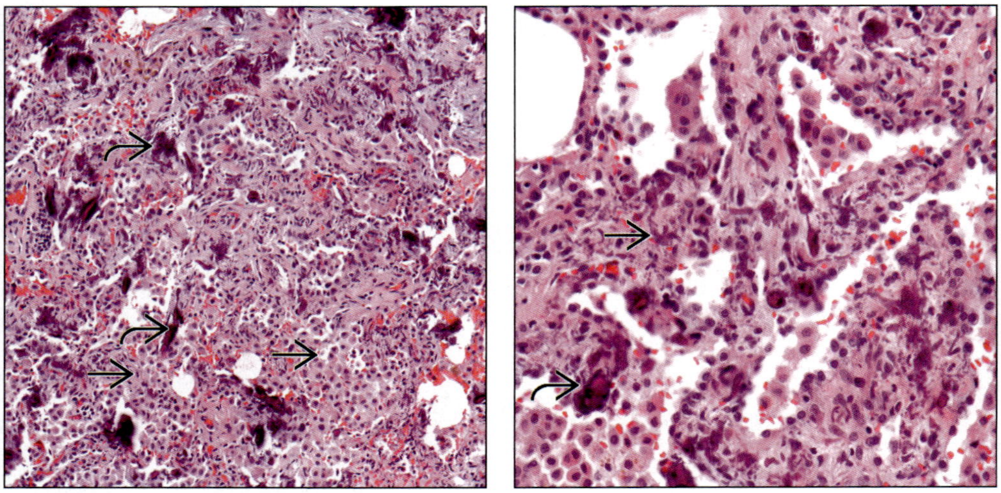

(Left) *In some cases, the presence of calcified material* ↪ *is more subtle and can be easily disregarded as simple calcification of the lung parenchyma. Note the presence of a more cellular component* →. ***(Right)*** *High-power view shows calcified material* ↪ *predominantly deposited in the lung interstitium. In some areas, the calcified material is much more difficult to recognize as it appears to be more dust-like* →.

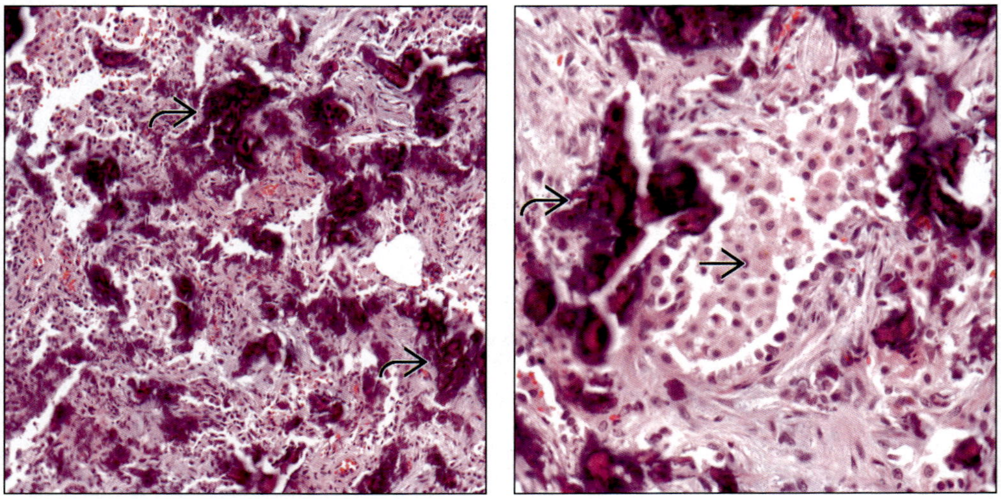

(Left) *The presence of calcified material is obvious* ↪ *in cases like this one. However, note that the calcifications are more in the interstitium than within alveolar spaces. It is also important to note the absence of cellular atypia.* ***(Right)*** *A close-up view shows the calcifications* ↪*, which are admixed with collections of histiocytes* → *and minimal or absent inflammatory response.*

METASTATIC/DENDRIFORM CALCIFICATION

Microscopic Features

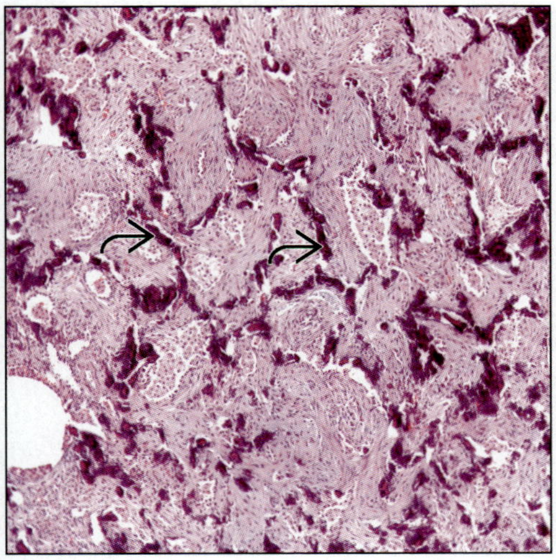

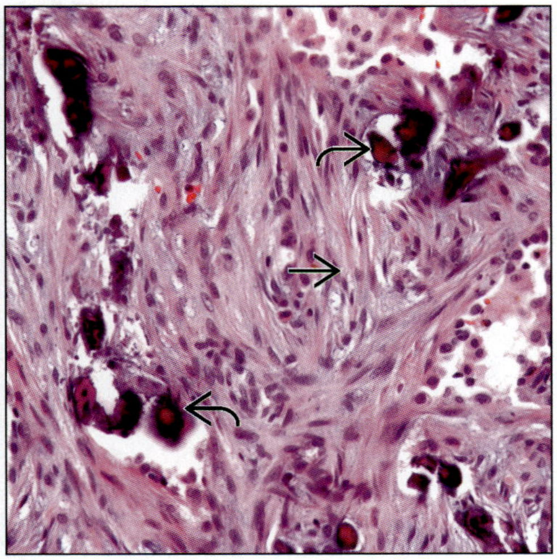

(Left) *Low-power view of a section of lung shows calcifications almost following the normal outlines of the alveolar architecture. This pattern is very common in this type of process and is an important feature for diagnosis.* ***(Right)*** *Higher magnification shows areas of calcification admixed with areas of a fibroblastic proliferation. This combination is rather common and should not be interpreted for a malignant process.*

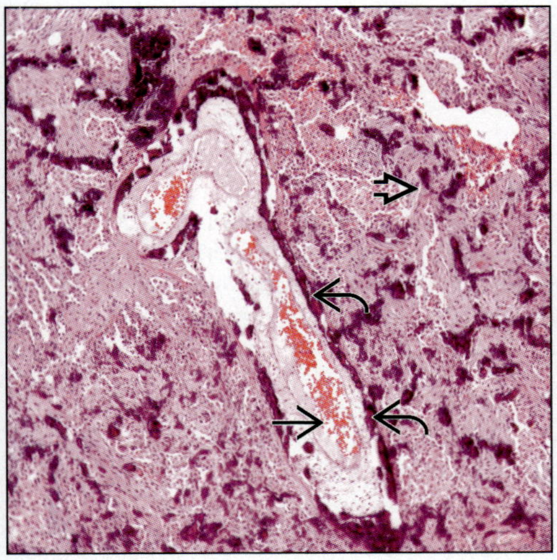

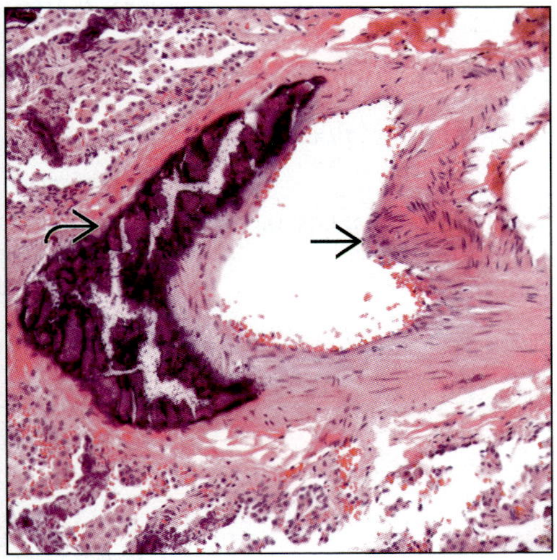

(Left) *Another important feature of dendriform calcification is the presence of calcific material around vascular structures. Also note that there are more calcifications involving the lung parenchyma.* ***(Right)*** *The presence of calcified material around vessels can be marked, resembling ossification. In this particular case, note the presence of a dilated vessel and the obvious calcification in its wall.*

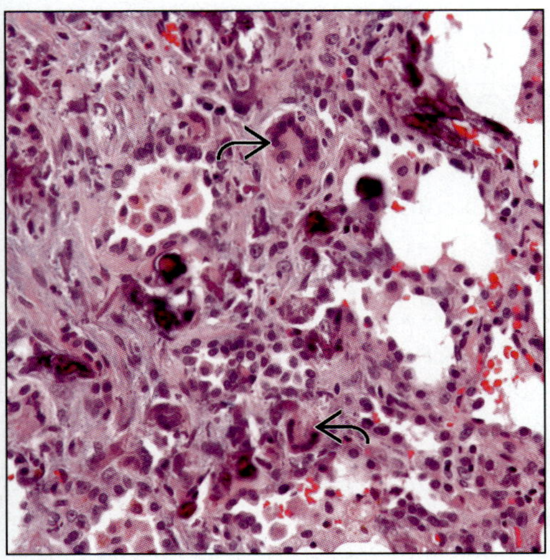

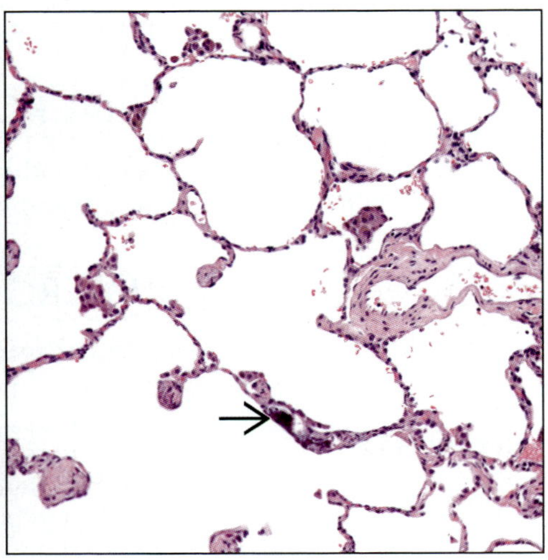

(Left) *In some unusual conditions, the calcified material may be admixed with an inflammatory reaction and also the presence of multinucleated giant cells. Such change may be secondary to the presence of the foreign material, which, in this case, is calcium.* ***(Right)*** *Even in areas of "normal" lung parenchyma, the presence of calcification may be very subtle, to the point of missing it. In this case, note the presence of calcified material within the interstitium.*

PARAFFINOMA (LIPOID PNEUMONIA)

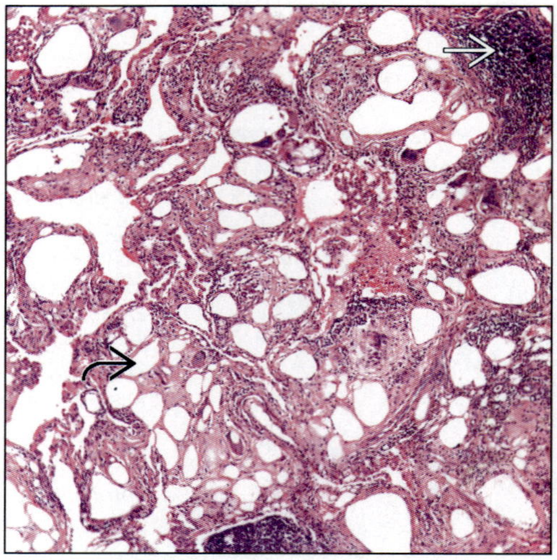

Low-power view of lipoid pneumonia shows the characteristic "Swiss cheese" appearance. Note the number of cystic spaces ➩ and focal areas of inflammation ➡.

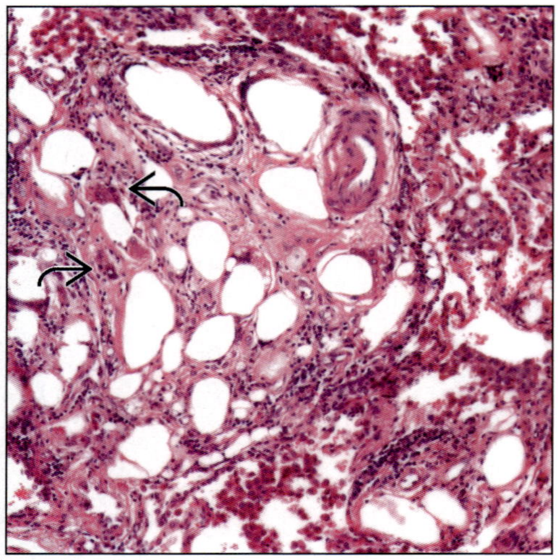

With this closer view of lipoid pneumonia, note the presence of several multinucleated giant cells ➩. The normal lung architecture is lost, and the inflammatory reaction is minimal.

TERMINOLOGY

Synonyms

- Cholesterol pneumonia, lipoid pneumonia, golden pneumonia, exogenous/endogenous lipoid pneumonia

Definitions

- Type of pneumonia secondary to aspiration; can be classified as
  - Endogenous
  - Exogenous

ETIOLOGY/PATHOGENESIS

Etiology

- Exogenous
  - Aspiration of oily substances
    - Mineral oil
    - Vegetable oil
    - Petroleum jelly
    - Oil mists
    - Some radiographic contrast media
- Endogenous
  - Result of pulmonary obstruction or gastroesophageal reflux
  - May result from breakdown of cell membrane or lipoprotein secretions

CLINICAL ISSUES

Epidemiology

- Incidence
  - Rare; may be seen in bedridden patients
- Age
  - Can occur in any age group, children or elderly
- Gender
  - No gender predilection

Presentation

- Cough
- Chest pain
- Dyspnea
- Fever

Treatment

- In cases of endogenous lipoid pneumonia, dealing with cause of obstruction may be beneficial
- In cases of exogenous lipoid pneumonia, identification and stopping of probable cause is crucial
- Antibiotics may be necessary

Prognosis

- Depends on origin, but in some cases, endogenous lipoid pneumonia can be fatal

IMAGE FINDINGS

Radiographic Findings

- May be a mixture of interstitial and alveolar pattern

MACROSCOPIC FEATURES

General Features

- Soft and yellowish consolidated areas

MICROSCOPIC PATHOLOGY

Histologic Features

- Proliferation of foamy histiocytes
  - Intraalveolar
  - Interstitial
- Cholesterol cleft granulomas
- Foreign body giant cell reaction
  - Around fat droplets in exogenous pneumonia
  - May be absent in cases of endogenous pneumonia
- Fat droplets in interstitium

PARAFFINOMA (LIPOID PNEUMONIA)

Key Facts

Terminology
- Synonyms
  - Cholesterol pneumonia, lipoid pneumonia, golden pneumonia
- Definition: Type of pneumonia that could be secondary to aspiration; can be classified as
  - Endogenous
  - Exogenous

Etiology/Pathogenesis
- Exogenous
  - Aspiration of oily substances
  - Mineral oil
  - Vegetable oil
  - Petroleum jelly
  - Oil mists
  - Some radiographic contrast media
- Endogenous
  - Result of pulmonary obstruction or gastroesophageal reflux
  - May result as a breakdown of cell membrane or lipoprotein secretions

Clinical Issues
- Rare; may be seen in bedridden patients
- Can occur in any age group, children or elderly

Microscopic Pathology
- Proliferation of foamy histiocytes
- Cholesterol cleft granulomas
- Foreign body giant cell reaction
- Fat droplets in interstitium
- Inflammatory reaction may be minimal

Histochemical Features of Lipoid Pneumonia

Stain	Result
PAS	Negative for intracellular glycogen
D-PAS	Negative for intracellular mucin
Mucicarmine	Negative for intracellular mucin
Oil red O	Positive in fat droplets

- Inflammatory reaction may be minimal

Cytologic Features
- Fat droplets in interstitium
- Positive staining in frozen tissue for oil red O

DIFFERENTIAL DIAGNOSIS

Mycobacterial Infection
- Shows organisms with acid-fast bacilli stain
- Unusual to have fat droplets

Rosai-Dorfman Disease (R-D Disease)
- Characteristically shows the presence of emperipolesis
- Infiltrate is predominantly composed of histiocytes
- Does not show presence of fat droplets
- Shows negative staining for oil red O

Juvenile Xanthogranuloma (JXG)
- Presents as pulmonary mass
- Histiocytic infiltrate destroys lung parenchyma
- Oil red O is negative
- Immunohistochemical studies for histiocytic markers show positive staining

Langerhans Cell Histiocytosis (LCH)
- Characteristically shows positive staining for S100 protein and CD1a
- Characteristically presents as multiple pulmonary nodules
- Presence of eosinophils favors diagnosis of LCH

DIAGNOSTIC CHECKLIST

Pathologic Interpretation Pearls
- Fat droplets
- Positive staining for oil red O
- Giant cell reaction

SELECTED REFERENCES

1. Marchiori E et al: Lipoid pneumonia in 53 patients after aspiration of mineral oil: comparison of high-resolution computed tomography findings in adults and children. J Comput Assist Tomogr. 34(1):9-12, 2010
2. Weinberg I et al: Exogenous lipoid pneumonia caused by paraffin in an amateur fire breather. Occup Med (Lond). 60(3):234-5, 2010
3. Armangil D et al: Lipoid pneumonia caused by intranasal butter application in a newborn infant. . J Paediatr Child Health. 45(7-8):475-6, 2009
4. Rollins CE et al: Disseminated lipogranulomas and sudden death from self-administered mineral oil injection. Am J Forensic Med Pathol. 18(1):100-3, 1997
5. Borrie J et al: Paraffinoma of lung: lipoid pneumonia. Report of two cases. Thorax. 28(2):214-21, 1973

PARAFFINOMA (LIPOID PNEUMONIA)

Microscopic Features

*(**Left**) Classic Swiss cheese-like appearance admixed with inflammatory reaction is shown. Note the presence of large ↪ and small → "empty" spaces typical of this process. The interstitium shows only mild inflammatory changes. (**Right**) Different view of a paraffinoma with widening of the interstitium ↪ gives the appearance of a fibrinous component with focal inflammatory reaction →. Still, one can identify large empty spaces ⇨.*

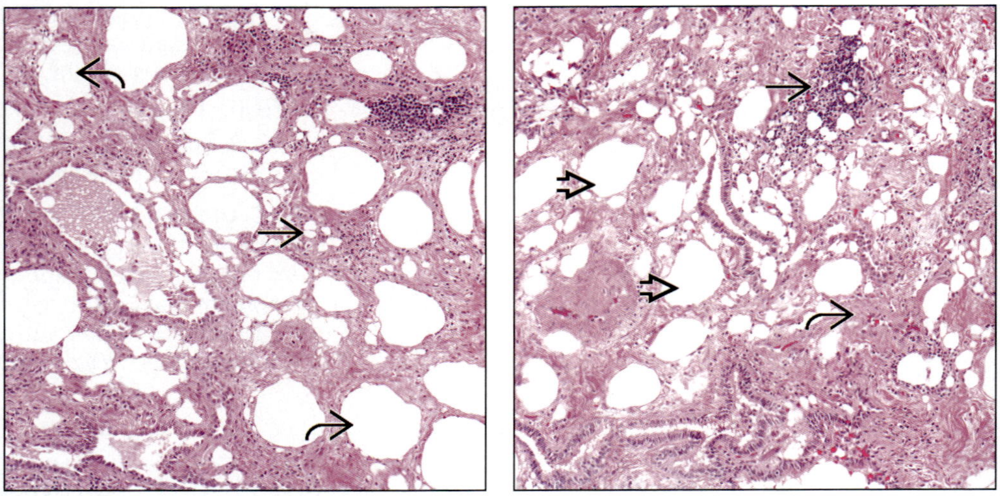

*(**Left**) Pulmonary paraffinoma shows some preservation of lung architecture in which the alveoli are filled with histiocytes ↪ with focal areas of inflammatory reaction composed of lymphocytes →. This pattern would suggest an infectious process. (**Right**) Higher magnification shows characteristic fat droplets ↪ with focal inflammation ⇨ and the presence of multinucleated giant cells forming an ill-defined granuloma →.*

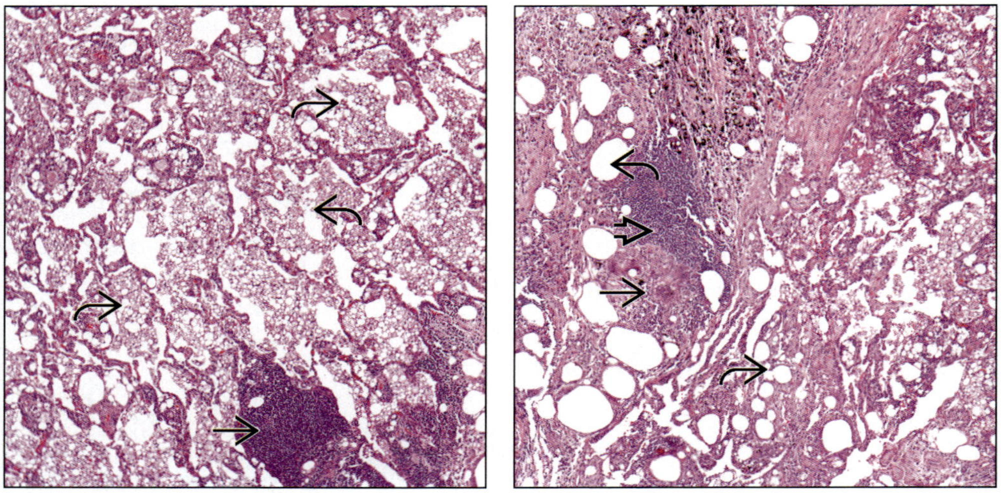

*(**Left**) Low-power view shows collections of intraalveolar foamy histiocytes ↪ giving the appearance of an infectious process. In addition, there are focal areas of inflammatory reaction ⇨. (**Right**) Closer view of a pulmonary paraffinoma shows some inflammatory changes and destruction of the normal pulmonary architecture. Note the presence of fat droplets of different sizes ↪.*

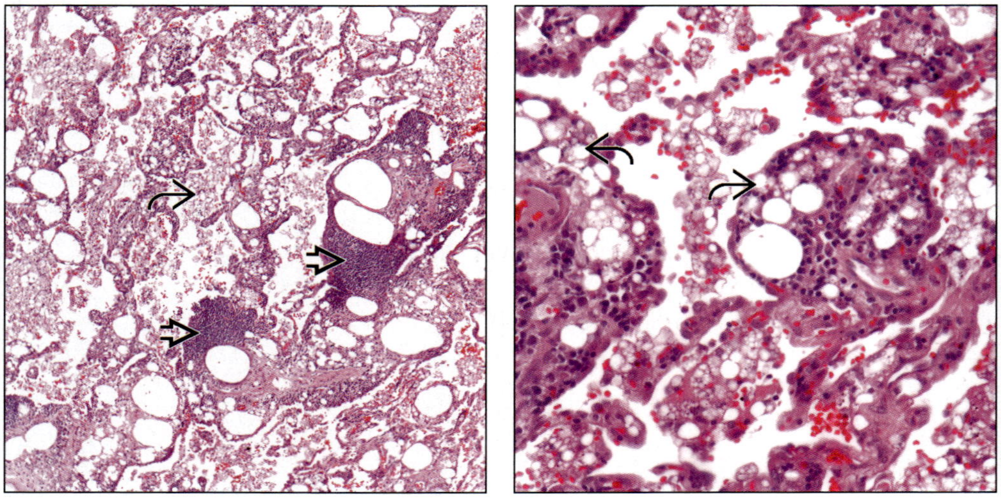

Microscopic Features

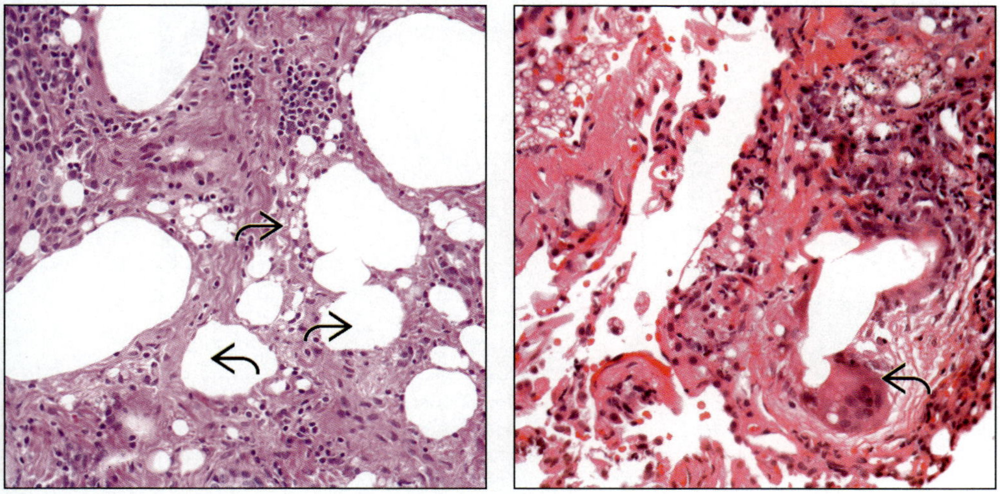

(Left) *Distorted pulmonary parenchyma shows the presence of fat droplets* ↪ *of different sizes. There is very little in terms of inflammatory reaction.* ***(Right)*** *Pulmonary paraffinoma shows a giant cell component* ↪ *around a pulmonary vessel. Such a finding is common, although in some cases the giant cell reaction is not necessarily attached to a pulmonary vessel.*

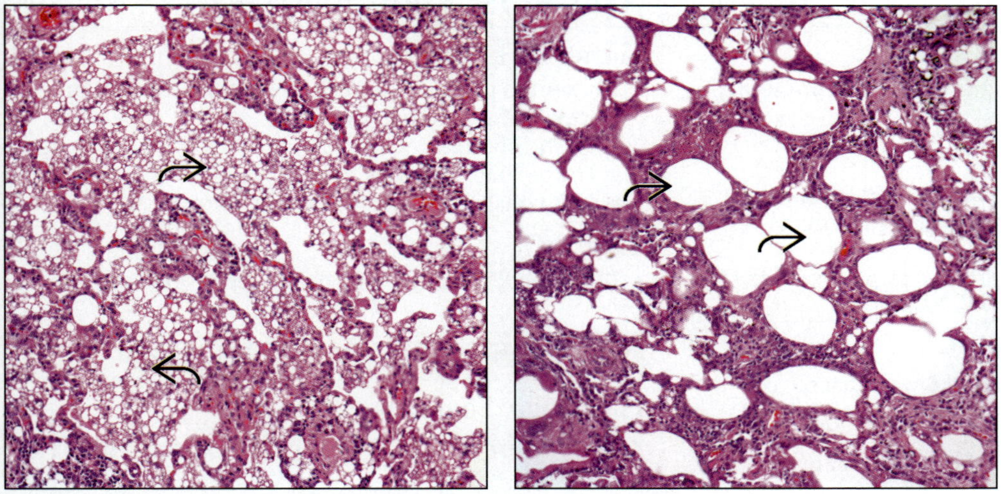

(Left) *Marked collection of intraalveolar macrophages admixed with more conventional areas of fat droplets* ↪ *is shown, with destruction of the normal lung architecture. These findings are typical of this process.* ***(Right)*** *In some cases, the process appears to be more homogeneous with large fat droplets, which mimic alveolar structures* ↪*. In addition, there is a subtle inflammatory reaction.*

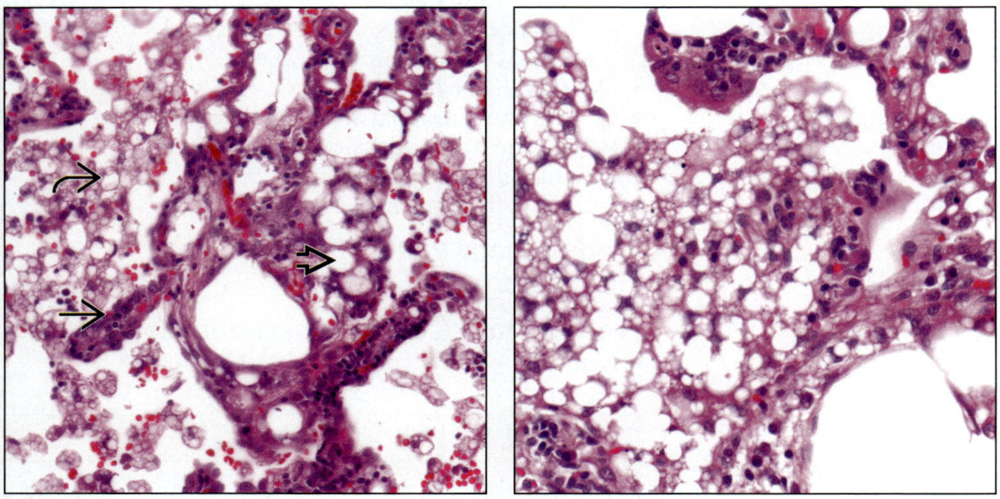

(Left) *Closer magnification reveals the presence of some intraalveolar macrophages* ↪*. Note the presence of remnants of alveolar lining* →*. In addition, numerous fat droplets are present, which are characteristic of paraffinoma* ⇨*.* ***(Right)*** *Higher magnification shows foamy histiocytes admixed with fat droplets and some remaining alveolar lining. These features are typical of pulmonary paraffinoma.*

PLACENTAL TRANSMOGRIFICATION

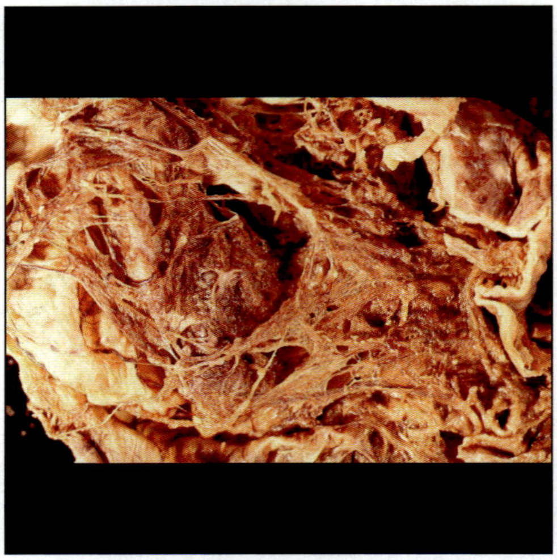

This portion of lung shows placental transmogrification. Note the grotesque appearance of the lung parenchyma.

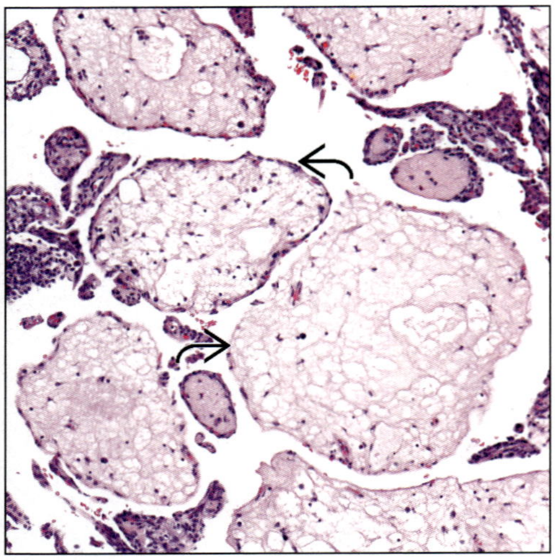

High-power view shows some of the "placentoid" structures ⮳ typical of placental transmogrification of the lung. Note the presence of the different sizes and the edematous internal composition.

TERMINOLOGY

Synonyms

- Placentoid bullous lesion, giant bullous emphysema, pulmonary lipomatosis

Definitions

- Benign unusual condition characterized by bizarre changes in shape of normal lung parenchyma

ETIOLOGY/PATHOGENESIS

Environmental Exposure

- Some cases have been associated with tobacco use

Infectious Agents

- Some cases have been associated with pneumonic process

CLINICAL ISSUES

Epidemiology

- Incidence
  - This process can be seen in the elderly or young adults

Presentation

- Cough
- Fever
- Pneumonia

Treatment

- Surgical approaches
  - Complete surgical resection

Prognosis

- Good

MACROSCOPIC FEATURES

General Features

- Ill-defined process with complete degeneration of normal lung parenchyma
  - Cystic changes
  - Grape-like structures
  - Soft consistency and yellowish color

Size

- Ill-defined; may involve entire lobe or lobe segment

MICROSCOPIC PATHOLOGY

Histologic Features

- Papillary features without cellular atypia or mitotic activity
- Papillary component may show
  - Myxoid changes
  - Lipomatous changes
  - Edematous changes
  - Minimal inflammatory changes
- Placental-like pattern
- In focal areas, residual alveolated tissue may be present
- In focal areas, residual airway may be seen
- Lack of pulmonary fibrosis
- Focal calcifications may be seen

Predominant Pattern/Injury Type

- Ill-defined

Predominant Cell/Compartment Type

- Foamy

DIFFERENTIAL DIAGNOSIS

Pneumonia

- Show areas of acute and chronic inflammation that are usually absent in placental transmogrification

PLACENTAL TRANSMOGRIFICATION

Key Facts

Terminology
- Synonyms: Placentoid bullous lesion, giant bullous emphysema, pulmonary lipomatosis
- Benign unusual condition characterized by bizarre changes in shape of normal lung parenchyma

Etiology/Pathogenesis
- Some cases have been associated with tobacco use, others with a pneumonic process

Clinical Issues
- Process can be seen in adult or young adults

Macroscopic Features
- Ill-defined process with complete degeneration of normal lung parenchyma
- Cystic changes
- Grape-like structures
- Soft consistency and yellowish color
- Ill-defined; may involve entire lobe or lobe segment

Top Differential Diagnoses
- Pneumonia
  - Shows areas of acute and chronic inflammatory cells, which are commonly absent in transmogrification
- Emphysema
  - There is very little residual alveoli in transmogrification
  - Extensive areas of papillary-like structures with adipose tissue
- Papillary carcinoma
  - Most likely would present as pulmonary mass

Immunohistochemistry

Antibody	Reactivity	Staining Pattern	Comment
CK-PAN	Positive	Cytoplasmic	In surface epithelium
S100	Positive	Cytoplasmic	Adipose tissue component
TTF-1	Positive	Nuclear	In entrapped pneumocytes
CD34	Negative		
Thyroglobulin	Negative		

- Macroscopic features of pneumonia do not resemble the bizarre features of transmogrification
- Highly unusual for pneumonic process to show presence of adipose tissue

Emphysema
- Presence of papillary structures with myxoid or lipomatous changes would be unusual for emphysema
- Entire lung parenchyma is destroyed in transmogrification
  - Leaves little residual alveoli

Papillary Carcinoma
- Lack of nuclear atypia or mitosis is feature of placental transmogrification
- Presence of myxoid or lipomatous changes would be unusual for carcinoma
- Macroscopic feature of transmogrification is diffuse
  - Carcinoma would be a localized tumor mass

DIAGNOSTIC CHECKLIST

Clinically Relevant Pathologic Features
- Gross appearance

Pathologic Interpretation Pearls
- Placental-like pattern with myxoid &/or lipomatous changes

SELECTED REFERENCES

1. Moran CA et al: Unusual non-neoplastic lesions of the lung. Semin Diagn Pathol. 24(3):199-208, 2007
2. Vogel-Claussen J et al: Placental transmogrification of the lung. J Thorac Imaging. 20(3):233-5, 2005
3. Cavazza A et al: Placental transmogrification of the lung: clinicopathologic, immunohistochemical and molecular study of two cases, with particular emphasis on the interstitial clear cells. Hum Pathol. 35(4):517-21, 2004
4. Brevetti GR et al: Pulmonary placental transmogrification: diagnosis and treatment. J Thorac Cardiovasc Surg. 118(5):966-7, 1999
5. Hochholzer L et al: Pulmonary lipomatosis: a variant of placental transmogrification. Mod Pathol. 10(8):846-9, 1997
6. Horsley WS et al: Unilateral giant bullous emphysema with placental transmogrification of the lung. Ann Thorac Surg. 64(1):226-8, 1997
7. Fidler ME et al: Placental transmogrification of the lung, a histologic variant of giant bullous emphysema. Clinicopathological study of three further cases. Am J Surg Pathol. 19(5):563-70, 1995
8. Mark EJ et al: Placentoid bullous lesion of the lung. Hum Pathol. 26(1):74-9, 1995
9. McChesny T et al: Placental transmogrification of the lung: a unique case with remarkable histopathologic features. Lab Invest. 40:245-6, 1979

PLACENTAL TRANSMOGRIFICATION

Microscopic Features

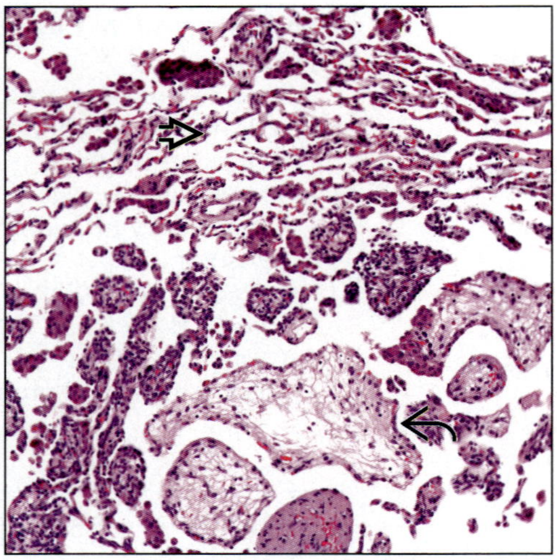
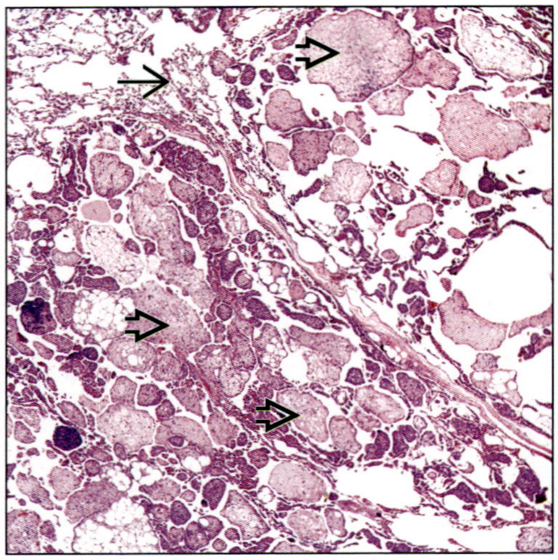

(Left) *Placental transmogrification shows the classical "placentoid" structures ; however, normal alveolar structures are also present . Most of the time normal lung parenchyma is only focally present.* ***(Right)*** *Placental transmogrification of the lung shows large and small placentoid structures destroying residual normal lung parenchyma . This growth pattern may be seen in some primary or metastatic carcinomas of the lung.*

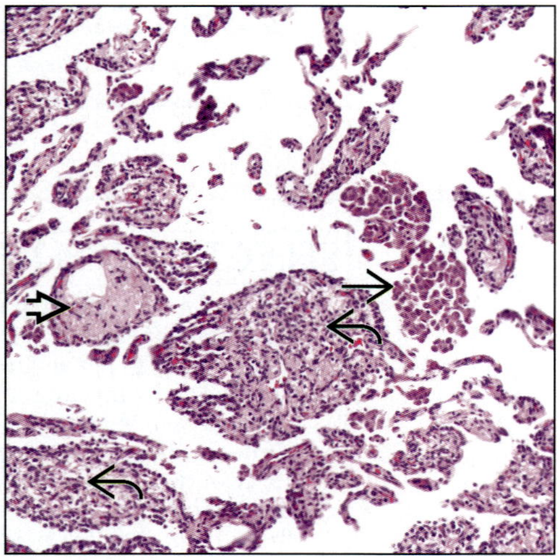
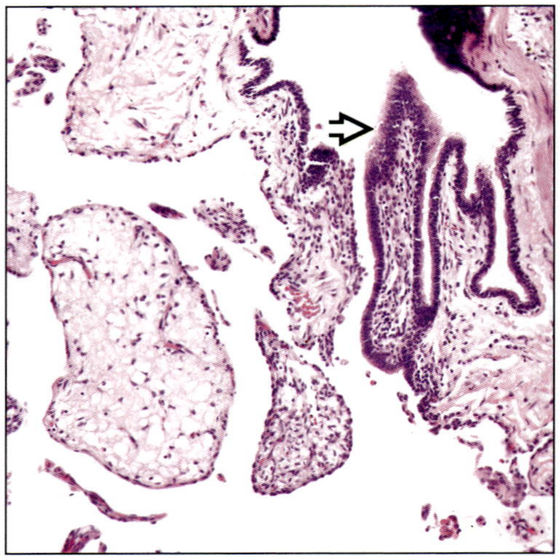

(Left) *Some of the "placentoid" structures composing placental transmogrification may show a more cellular component while others remain more edematous . Focal residual macrophages are also seen .* ***(Right)*** *Although placental transmogrification destroys the normal lung parenchyma, one is still able to recognize focal areas in which there is residual airway . It is important to note that placental transmogrification does not involve the airway.*

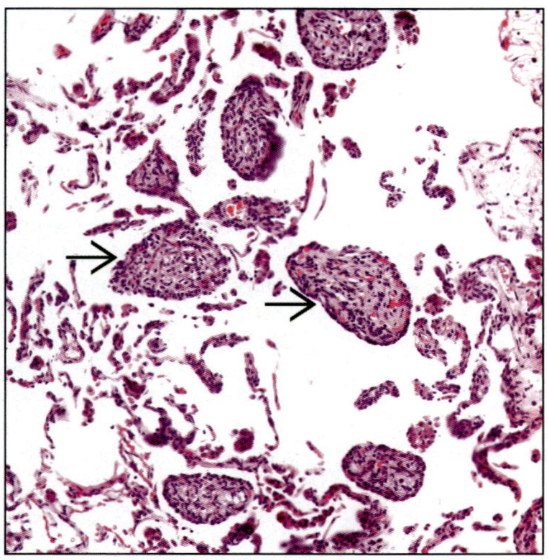
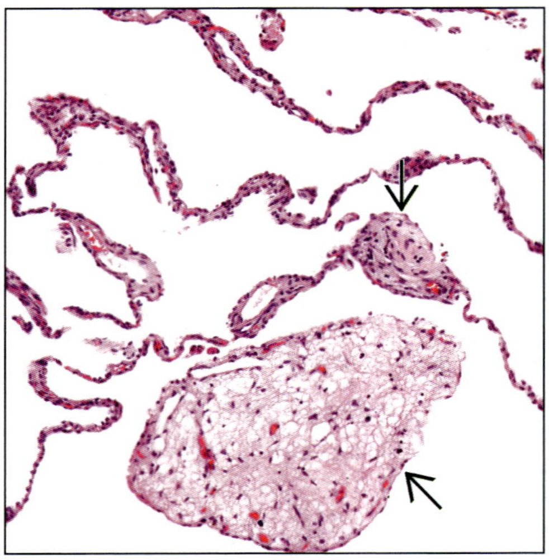

(Left) *Small, elongated, more cellular structures are present mixed with relatively normal alveolar structures in placental transmogrification. These structures resemble morular structures present in some adenocarcinomas.* ***(Right)*** *Predominantly normal-appearing alveolar structures and a couple of structures classical of placental transmogrification of the lung are present. The presence of these structures in small biopsies should raise the possibility of placental transmogrification.*

Microscopic Features

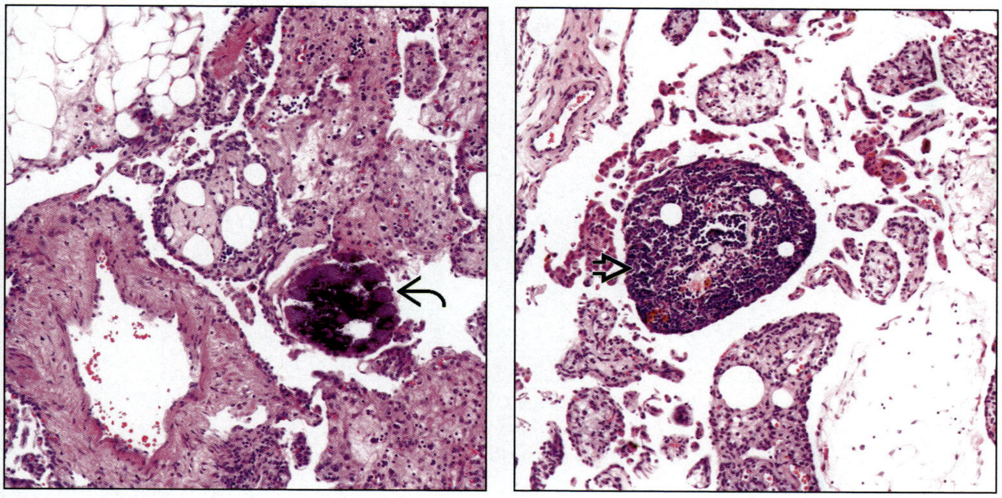

(Left) *Although an unusual feature, the presence of dystrophic calcifications ↶ may be seen in focal areas of placental transmogrification.* ***(Right)*** *Placental transmogrification of the lung shows one of the placentoid structures with marked inflammatory reaction ⇨. Inflammatory changes are also not a common feature of this process; most of these placentoid structures lack an inflammatory reaction.*

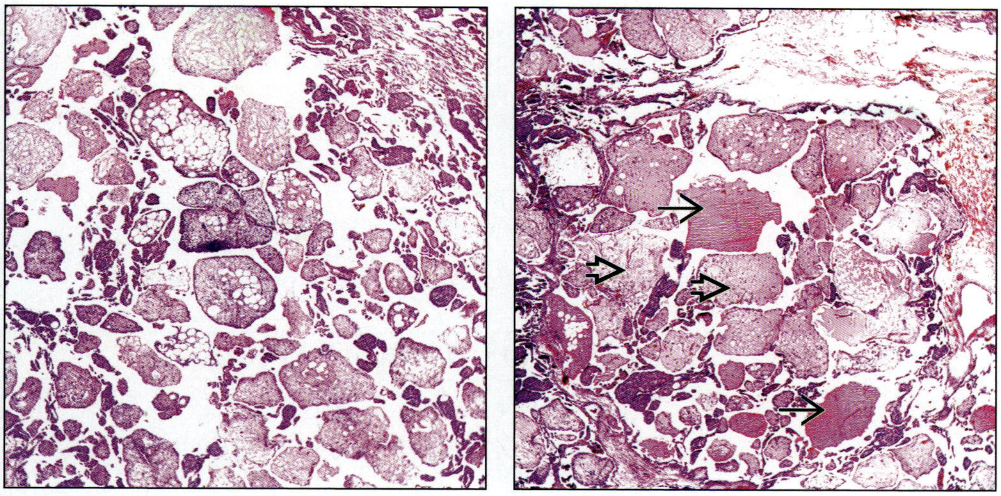

(Left) *Placental transmogrification of the lung shows structures of different sizes with almost total replacement of lung parenchyma. Note that in some of these placentoid structures, adipose tissue is present.* ***(Right)*** *Some of the placentoid structures show myxoid changes ⇨ while others show more edematous changes →. These changes are commonly seen in these cases and may represent aging changes.*

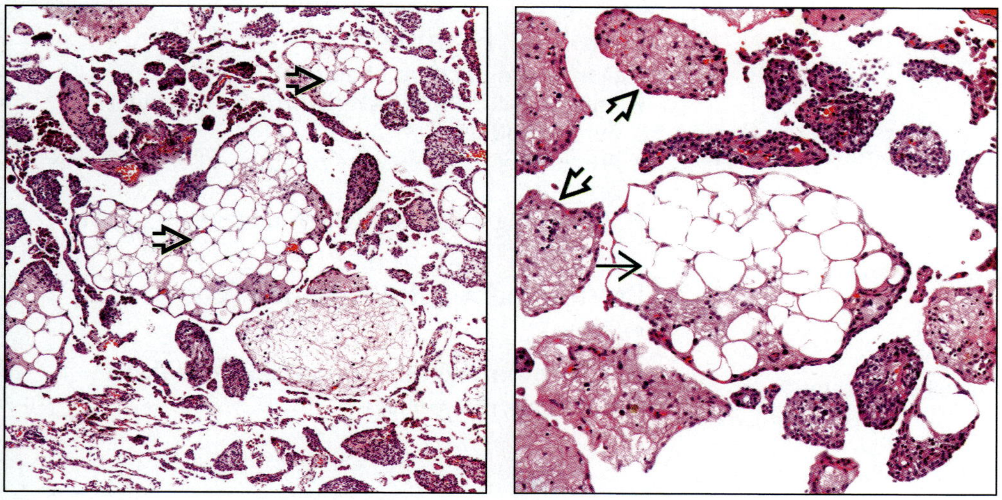

(Left) *Placentoid structures in placental transmogrification show prominent lipomatous changes ⇨. These histological features led some authors to coin the term lipomatosis.* ***(Right)*** *Higher magnification of placentoid structures in placental transmogrification of the lung shows prominent lipomatous changes →. Note adjacent structures with more myxoid change ⇨.*

ROSAI-DORFMAN DISEASE

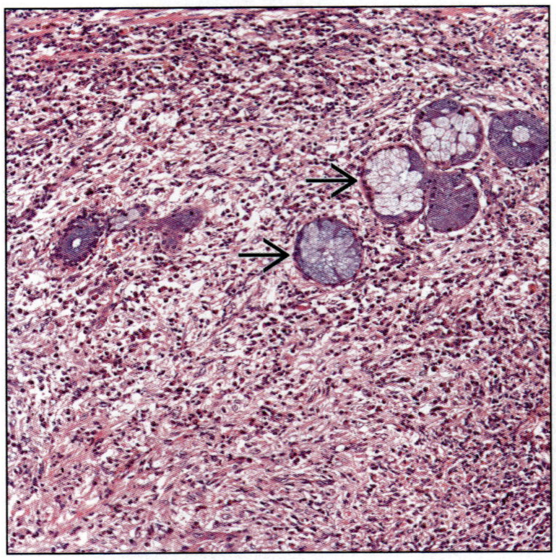

Primary Rosai-Dorfman disease of the lung shows residual endobronchial glands ⇒ and prominent histiocytic proliferation admixed with inflammatory cells.

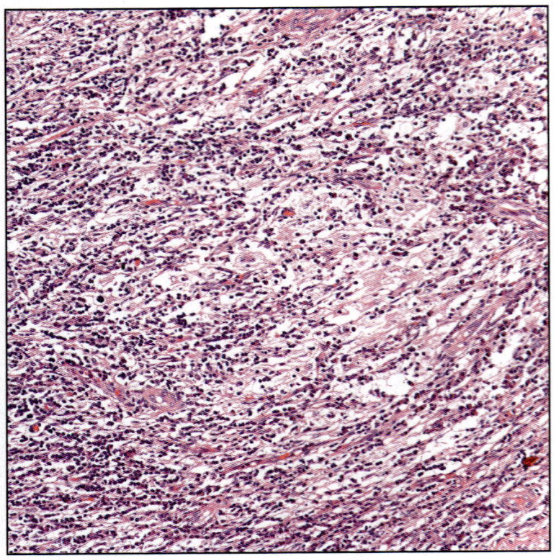

Primary Rosai-Dorfman disease of the lung shows prominent histiocytic proliferation admixed with inflammatory cells.

TERMINOLOGY

Abbreviations

- Rosai-Dorfman (R-D) disease

Synonyms

- Sinus histiocytosis with massive lymphadenopathy (SHML)

Definitions

- Histiocytic proliferation primarily affecting lymph nodes

ETIOLOGY/PATHOGENESIS

Etiology

- Unknown
- Possible infectious origin
- Possible immunologic response

CLINICAL ISSUES

Epidemiology

- Incidence
  - Unusual tumoral condition more commonly seen in lymph nodes
  - May appear in extranodal sites in approximately 20% of cases
  - Respiratory system is most unusual site of occurrence
- Age
  - May occur at any age
    - Cases described in lung have been in adults

Presentation

- Cough
- Shortness of breath
- Chest pain

Treatment

- Surgical resection is treatment of choice
- Chemotherapy can be used in more severe and extensive cases
  - However, its use has not shown meaningful results

Prognosis

- Generally good
- In a few cases, fatal course may be seen, but that is unusual
- Some patients may live with persistent disease

MACROSCOPIC FEATURES

General Features

- Pulmonary mass indistinguishable from bronchogenic carcinoma

MICROSCOPIC PATHOLOGY

Histologic Features

- Diffuse proliferation of large histiocytes
- Presence of histiocytes engulfing lymphocytes (emperipolesis)
- Presence of inflammatory reaction, namely plasma cells
- When lung is affected, lymph nodes may also be involved

Predominant Pattern/Injury Type

- Sheets

Predominant Cell/Compartment Type

- Histiocyte/macrophage

ROSAI-DORFMAN DISEASE

Key Facts

Terminology
- Synonym: Sinus histiocytosis with massive lymphadenopathy (SHML)

Etiology/Pathogenesis
- Unknown
- Possible infectious origin
- Possible immunologic response

Clinical Issues
- R-D disease is unusual tumoral condition more commonly seen in lymph nodes
- May appear in extranodal sites in ~ 20% of cases
- Respiratory system is most unusual site of occurrence
- Surgical resection is treatment of choice
- Chemotherapy can be used in more severe and extensive cases
  - However, its use has not shown meaningful results
- Prognosis
  - May follow nonaggressive course
  - In a few cases, fatal course may be observed, but that is unusual
  - Some patients may live with persistent disease
  - Number of cases involving lung is too small to make definitive conclusions

Top Differential Diagnoses
- Infectious process
  - Histochemical stains for fungi and acid-fast bacilli are negative
- Erdheim-Chester disease (E-C disease)
- Langerhans cell histiocytosis (LCH)
- Juvenile xanthogranuloma (JXG)

Immunohistochemistry

Antibody	Reactivity	Staining Pattern	Comment
S100	Positive	Cytoplasmic	In large histiocytes
CD68	Positive	Cytoplasmic	In histiocytes
CD163	Positive	Cytoplasmic	
CD15	Positive	Cytoplasmic	May stain other inflammatory cells
α-1-antichymotrypsin	Positive	Cytoplasmic	In histiocytes
CD1a	Negative		
FXIIIA	Negative		

DIFFERENTIAL DIAGNOSIS

Infectious Process
- Histochemical stains for fungi and acid-fast bacilli are negative

Erdheim-Chester (E-C) Disease
- May show similar immunophenotype
- Shows histiocytes of normal size, while R-D disease shows large histiocytes
- Absence of emperipolesis in E-C disease
- Different growth pattern, namely in septum and pleura

Langerhans Cell Histiocytosis (LCH)
- Shows positive staining for CD1a, while R-D disease is negative
- LCH in lung usually shows numerous nodules, while R-D presents as single mass
- Histiocytes in LCH are rather small with grooves, while those in R-D are large without grooves
- Ultrastructural studies in LCH usually show classic Birbeck granules

Juvenile Xanthogranuloma (JXG)
- Usually presents as multiple nodules in lung
- More common in young adults
- Usually also shows dermal involvement
- JXG and R-D disease may share similar immunophenotype

DIAGNOSTIC CHECKLIST

Clinically Relevant Pathologic Features
- Tissue distribution

Pathologic Interpretation Pearls
- Diffuse presence of large histiocytes
- Marked presence of plasma cells
- Histiocytes engulfing lymphocytes (emperipolesis)

SELECTED REFERENCES

1. Ohori NP et al: Rosai-Dorfman disease of the pleura: a rare extranodal presentation. Hum Pathol. 34(11):1210-1, 2003
2. Foucar E et al: Sinus histiocytosis with massive lymphadenopathy (Rosai-Dorfman disease): review of the entity. Semin Diagn Pathol. 7(1):19-73, 1990
3. Bonetti F et al: Immunohistological analysis of Rosai-Dorfman histiocytosis. A disease of S-100 + CD1-histiocytes. Virchows Arch A Pathol Anat Histopathol. 411(2):129-35, 1987
4. Wright DH et al: Sinus histiocytosis with massive lymphadenopathy (Rosai-Dorfman disease): report of a case with widespread nodal and extra nodal dissemination. Histopathology. 5(6):697-709, 1981

ROSAI-DORFMAN DISEASE

Microscopic Features

*(**Left**) Low-power view of R-D disease of the lung shows the presence of an airway → that is not involved by the process. Adjacent lung parenchyma is obliterated by a histiocytic proliferation →. (**Right**) R-D disease of the lung shows transitional areas between normal lung parenchyma → and the histocytic process → that is obliterating normal lung parenchyma.*

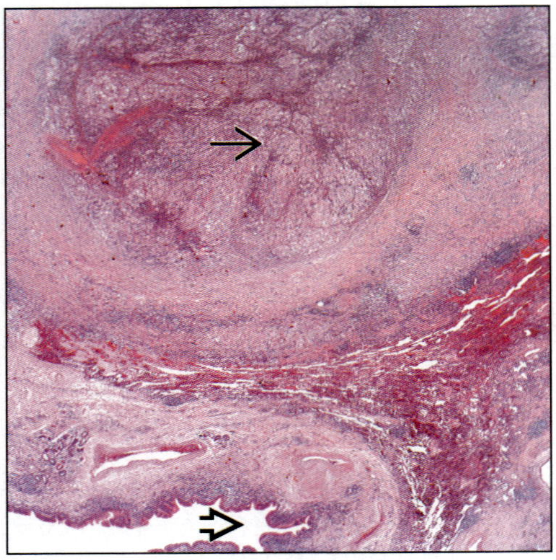

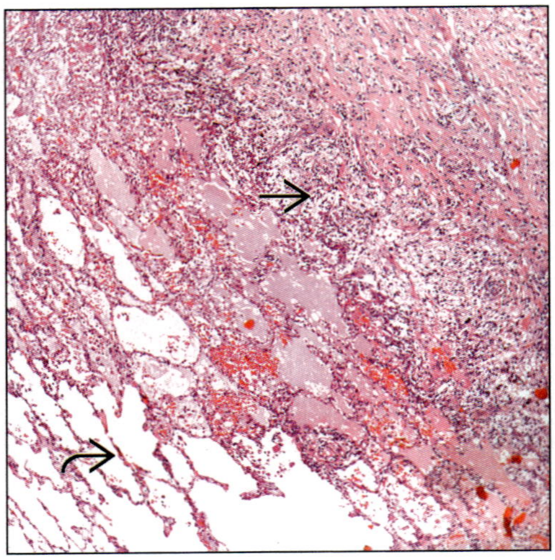

*(**Left**) R-D disease shows a prominent histiocytic cellular proliferation approaching the bronchial cartilage →. Although the bronchial cartilage is not involved, the process lingers in the cartilaginous surface. (**Right**) R-D disease shows residual bronchial glands → that are not involved by the process. R-D disease characteristically obliterates alveolated lung parenchyma.*

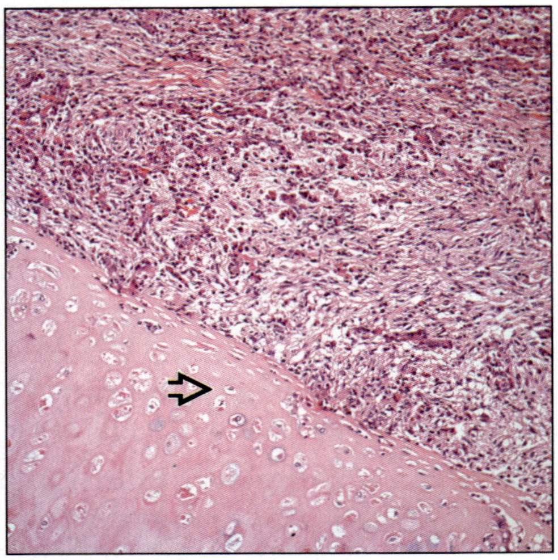

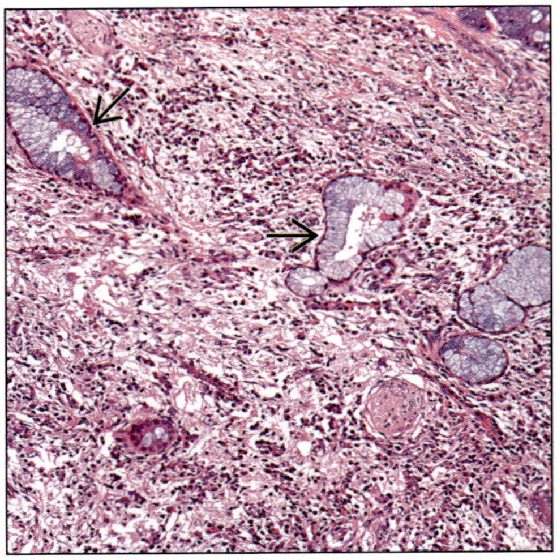

*(**Left**) Histiocytic proliferation is not easily identified in this case of R-D disease. The lung parenchyma appears to be congested by fresh blood →, and the adjacent lung appears to be heavily inflamed →. (**Right**) Histocytic proliferation is not easily identified in this case of R-D disease. The lung parenchyma has been replaced by dense collagen with only a discrete histiocytic infiltrate in between collagen fibers.*

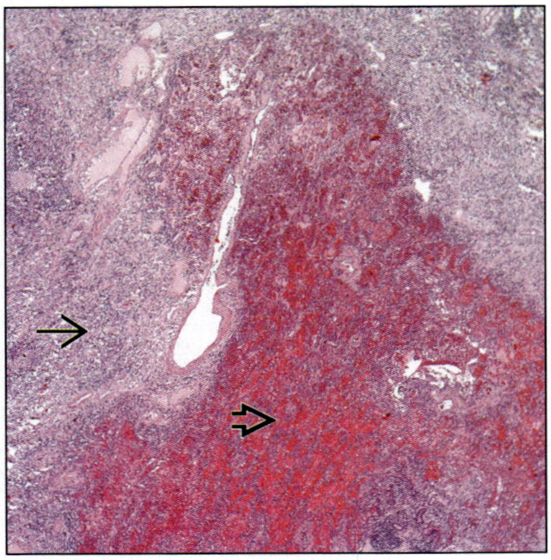

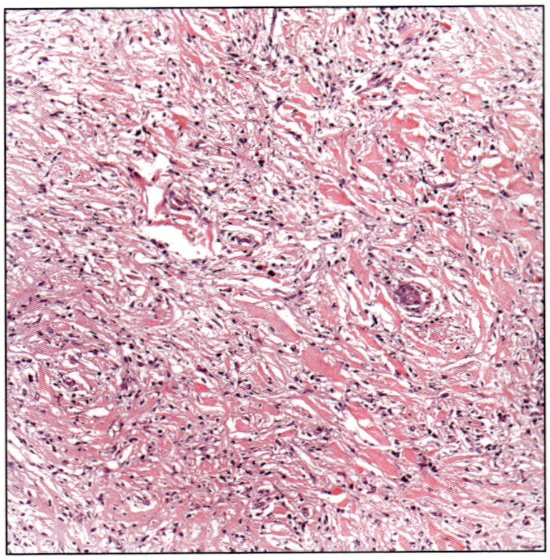

ROSAI-DORFMAN DISEASE

Microscopic Features

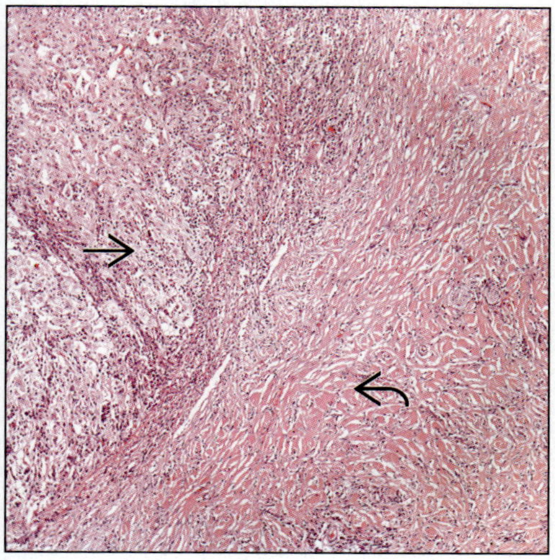

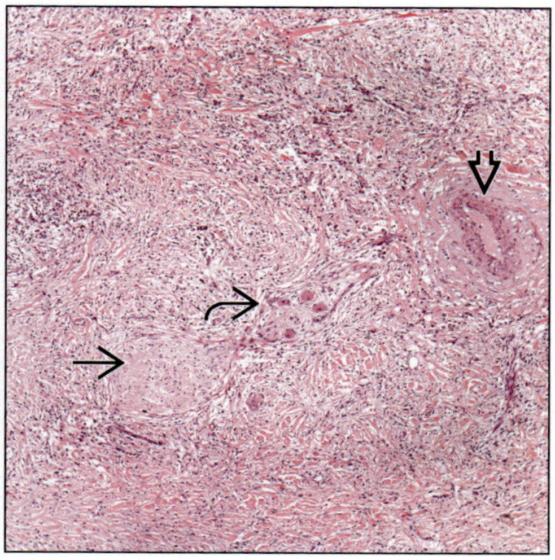

(Left) R-D disease shows transitional areas between dense collagenization of the lung parenchyma ↗ and a more prominent histiocytic proliferation →. The histological changes of R-D disease in the lung may vary in cellularity as is demonstrated in this image. **(Right)** R-D disease shows several normal structures entrapped by the histiocytic proliferation. A nerve →, pulmonary vessel ⇨, and ganglion cells ↗ are shown.

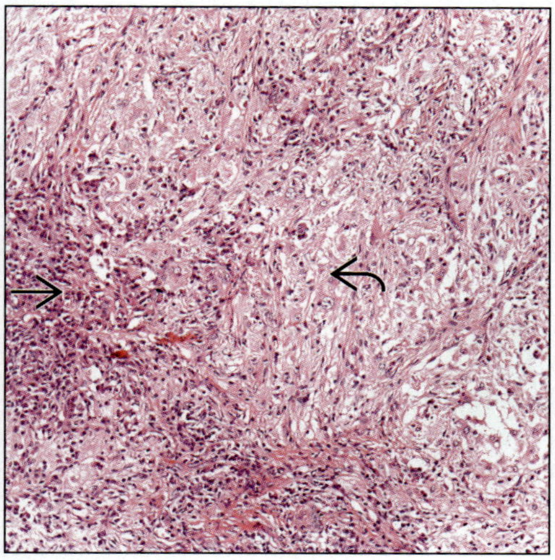

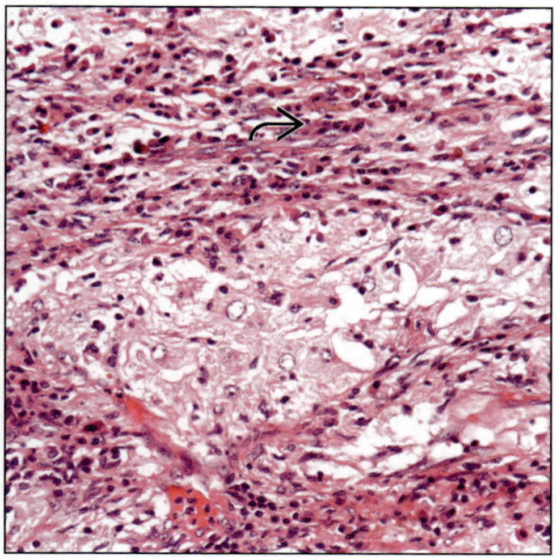

(Left) R-D disease shows a prominent histiocytic proliferation composed of large histiocytes with abundant eosinophilic cytoplasm ↗. In addition, note the presence of an inflammatory infiltrate composed almost exclusively of plasma cells →. Plasma cells are invariably present in all cases of R-D disease. **(Right)** R-D disease shows large histiocytes with round to oval nuclei and abundant eosinophilic cytoplasm. Note the presence of plasma cells ↗.

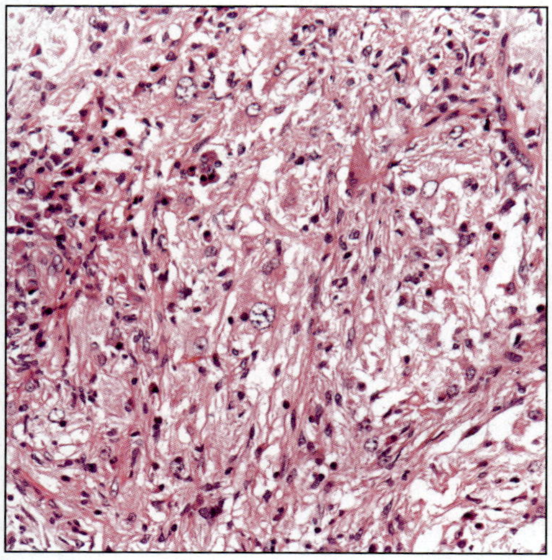

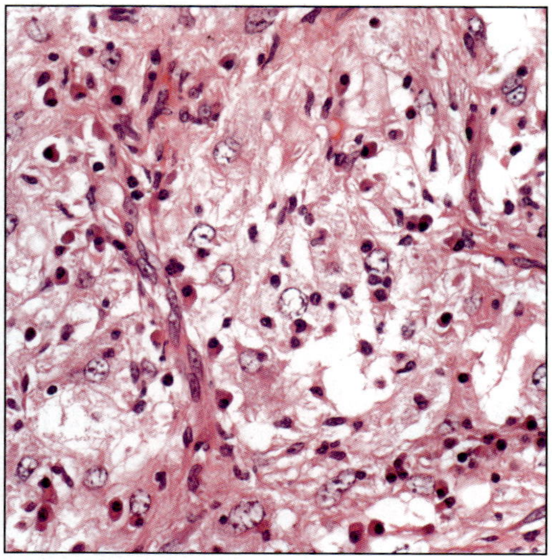

(Left) R-D disease shows the characteristic histiocytic proliferation composed of large histiocytes. However, in some areas, the inflammatory response is minimal. **(Right)** R-D disease shows large histiocytes, some of them engulfing lymphocytes. Emperipolesis is one of the most important characteristics of R-D disease, even though in some cases it may be difficult to identify.

ANGIOLYMPHOID HYPERPLASIA WITH EOSINOPHILIA

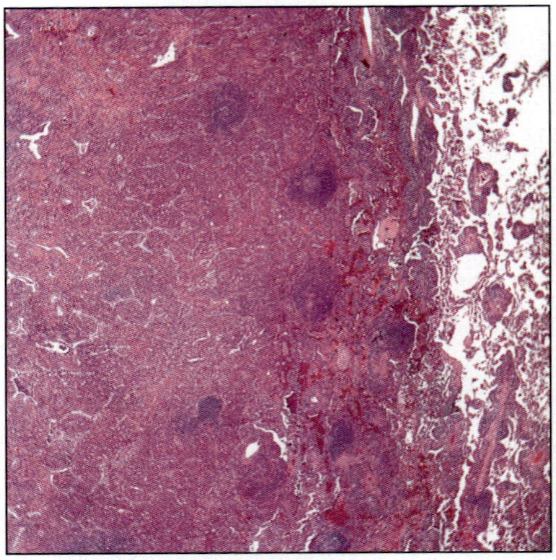

Low-power view shows angiolymphoid hyperplasia with eosinophilia presenting as a pulmonary mass. The lesion is fairly well circumscribed.

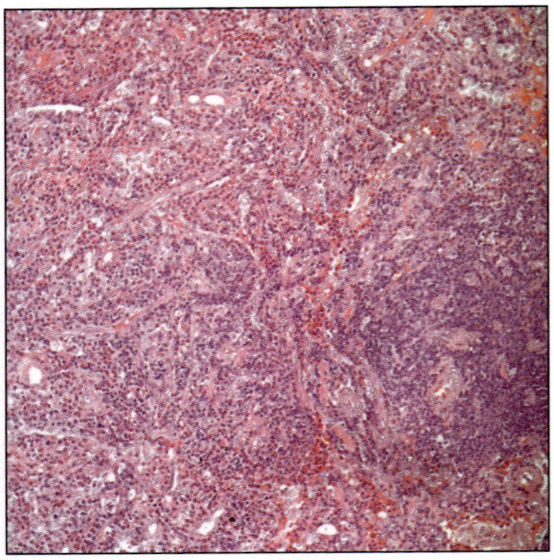

High-power view of ALHE shows the characteristic features of lymphoid aggregates, proliferation of small vessels, and prominent eosinophilic infiltrate.

TERMINOLOGY

Abbreviations

- Angiolymphoid hyperplasia with eosinophilia (ALHE)

Synonyms

- Epithelioid hemangioma

Definitions

- Benign vascular tumor characterized by vascular proliferation, lymphoid hyperplasia, and eosinophilia

CLINICAL ISSUES

Presentation

- Cough
- Dyspnea
- Asthma

Treatment

- Surgical approaches
  - Complete surgical resection
    - Lobectomy
    - Wedge resection

Prognosis

- Good when lesions are limited to the lung

MACROSCOPIC FEATURES

General Features

- Tumor nodule
  - Necrosis &/or hemorrhage are absent
  - Well circumscribed but not encapsulated

Size

- 2-3 cm in diameter

MICROSCOPIC PATHOLOGY

Histologic Features

- Eosinophilia and proliferation of epithelioid endothelial cells

Predominant Cell/Compartment Type

- Endothelial
- Lymphocyte

DIFFERENTIAL DIAGNOSIS

Hodgkin Lymphoma (HD)

- Absence of Reed-Sternberg cells in ALHE
- Negative staining for HD markers
- Often HD presents in lung with multiple pulmonary nodules

Eosinophilic Pneumonia

- ALHE characteristically shows presence of vascular proliferation and lymphoid hyperplasia, which are not present in eosinophilic pneumonia
- In eosinophilic pneumonia, alveoli are filled with eosinophils
- Eosinophilic pneumonia does not show endothelial or lymphoid hyperplasia

Parasitic Infection

- ALHE does not show acute inflammation
- Negative staining for infectious organisms
- No parasitic organisms are identified on conventional stains

Non-Hodgkin Lymphoma

- Presence of inflammatory infiltrate would be unusual for lymphoma
- Immunomarkers would show evidence of polyclonality in ALHE

ANGIOLYMPHOID HYPERPLASIA WITH EOSINOPHILIA

Key Facts

Terminology
- Angiolymphoid hyperplasia with eosinophilia (ALHE)
- Epithelioid hemangioma

Clinical Issues
- Presentation
  - Cough
  - Dyspnea
  - Asthma
- Treatment of choice: Complete surgical resection
  - Lobectomy
  - Wedge resection
- Prognosis: Good

Microscopic Pathology
- Lymphoid hyperplasia
- Endothelial hyperplasia
- Inflammatory reaction
- Eosinophilia

Top Differential Diagnoses
- Hodgkin lymphoma (HD)
  - Absence of Reed-Sternberg cells in ALHE
  - Negative staining for HD markers
- Eosinophilic pneumonia
  - ALHE characteristically shows presence of vascular proliferation and lymphoid hyperplasia
- Parasitic infection
  - ALHE does not show acute inflammation
  - Negative staining for infectious organisms

Diagnostic Checklist
- Endothelial and lymphoid hyperplasia
- Eosinophilia

Immunohistochemistry

Antibody	Reactivity	Staining Pattern	Comment
CD31	Positive	Cytoplasmic	Endothelial cells
CD34	Positive	Cytoplasmic	Endothelial cells
CD20	Positive		Lymphocytes
CD45	Positive		Lymphoid cells
CK-PAN	Positive	Cytoplasmic	Alveolar lining cells
CD15	Negative		
CD30	Negative		
ALK1	Negative		

DIAGNOSTIC CHECKLIST

Clinically Relevant Pathologic Features
- Tissue distribution

Pathologic Interpretation Pearls
- Endothelial and lymphoid hyperplasia are characteristic of ALHE
- Eosinophilia coupled with endothelial and lymphoid hyperplasia

SELECTED REFERENCES

1. Cham E et al: Epithelioid hemangioma (angiolymphoid hyperplasia with eosinophilia) arising on the extremities. J Cutan Pathol. 37(10):1045-52, 2010
2. Sotiriou E et al: Angiolymphoid hyperplasia with eosinophilia: good response to photodynamic therapy. Clin Exp Dermatol. 34(8):e629-31, 2009
3. Trindade F et al: Giant angiolymphoid hyperplasia with eosinophilia on the chest. J Cutan Pathol. 36(4):493-6, 2009
4. Dewan P et al: Angiolymphoid hyperplasia with eosinophilia affecting the penis. Br J Dermatol. 159(3):755-7, 2008
5. Koizumi H et al: Spontaneous regression of generalized angiolymphoid hyperplasia with eosinophilia in a 2-year-old boy. Acta Derm Venereol. 88(4):395-6, 2008
6. Thompson MJ et al: Angiolymphoid hyperplasia with eosinophilia affecting the eyelids. Arch Ophthalmol. 125(7):987, 2007
7. Macarenco RS et al: Angiolymphoid hyperplasia with eosinophilia showing prominent granulomatous and fibrotic reaction: a morphological and immunohistochemical study. Am J Dermatopathol. 28(6):514-7, 2006
8. Moran CA et al: Angiolymphoid hyperplasia with eosinophilia (epithelioid hemangioma) of the lung: a clinicopathologic and immunohistochemical study of two cases. Am J Clin Pathol. 123(5):762-5, 2005
9. Zarrin-Khameh N et al: Angiolymphoid hyperplasia with eosinophilia associated with pregnancy: a case report and review of the literature. Arch Pathol Lab Med. 129(9):1168-71, 2005
10. Fetsch JF et al: Observations concerning the pathogenesis of epithelioid hemangioma (angiolymphoid hyperplasia). Mod Pathol. 4(4):449-55, 1991
11. Chan JK et al: Epithelioid haemangioma (angiolymphoid hyperplasia with eosinophilia) and Kimura's disease in Chinese. Histopathology. 15(6):557-74, 1989
12. Suster S: Nodal angiolymphoid hyperplasia with eosinophilia. Am J Clin Pathol. 88(2):236-9, 1987
13. Olsen TG et al: Angiolymphoid hyperplasia with eosinophilia. A clinicopathologic study of 116 patients. J Am Acad Dermatol. 12(5 Pt 1):781-96, 1985
14. Rosai J et al: The histiocytoid hemangiomas. A unifying concept embracing several previously described entities of skin, soft tissue, large vessels, bone, and heart. Hum Pathol. 10(6):707-30, 1979

ANGIOLYMPHOID HYPERPLASIA WITH EOSINOPHILIA

Microscopic Features

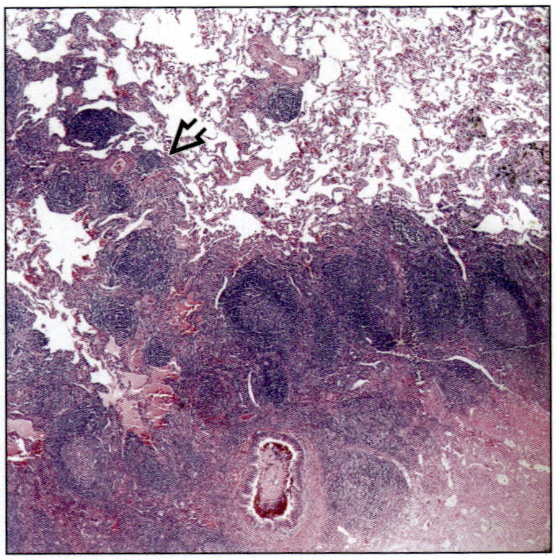

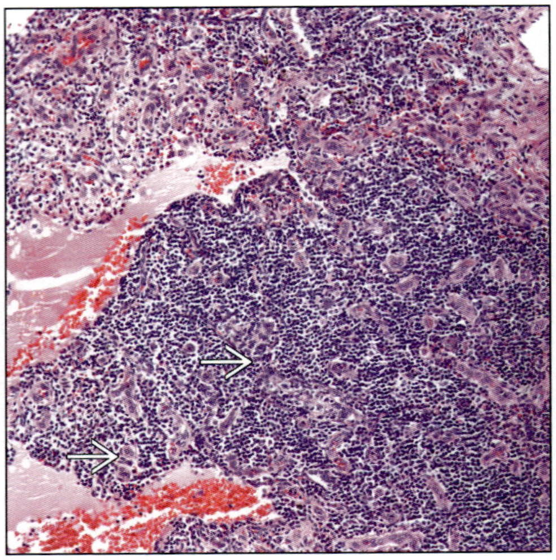

(Left) *Low-power view of ALHE shows a prominent lymphoid component with hyperplastic changes and an ill-defined tumor within the lung parenchyma. Note the spread of the tumor toward other areas of lung parenchyma ⇨.* ***(Right)*** *Prominent lymphoid component in ALHE of the lung obliterates numerous small blood vessels ➡. The eosinophilic component is not marked.*

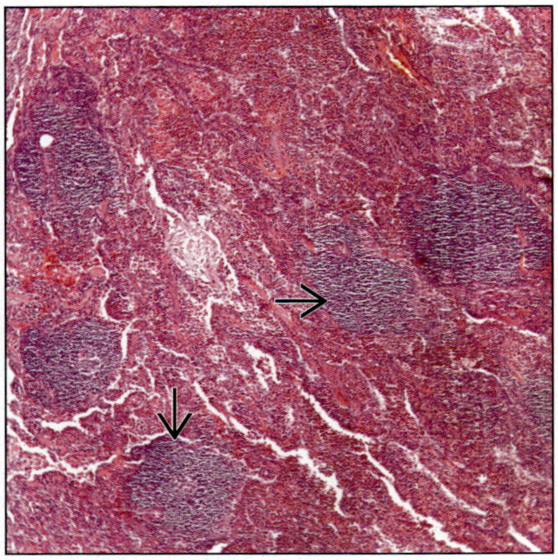

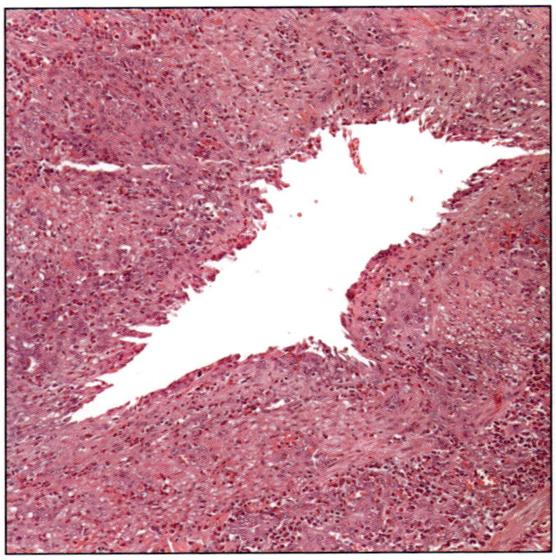

(Left) *ALHE shows more classical features with several germinal centers ⇨, blood vessel proliferation, and prominent infiltrate of eosinophils.* ***(Right)*** *ALHE in the lung shows a large pulmonary vessel with a prominent inflammatory infiltrate in the walls. The lumen is not obstructed; however, numerous eosinophils are easily identified in the walls of the vessels.*

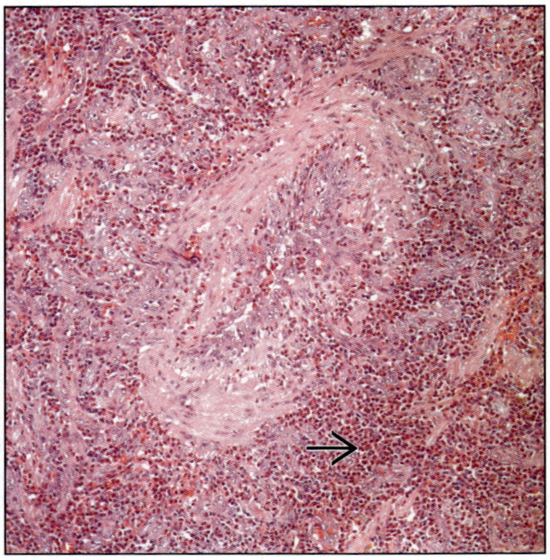

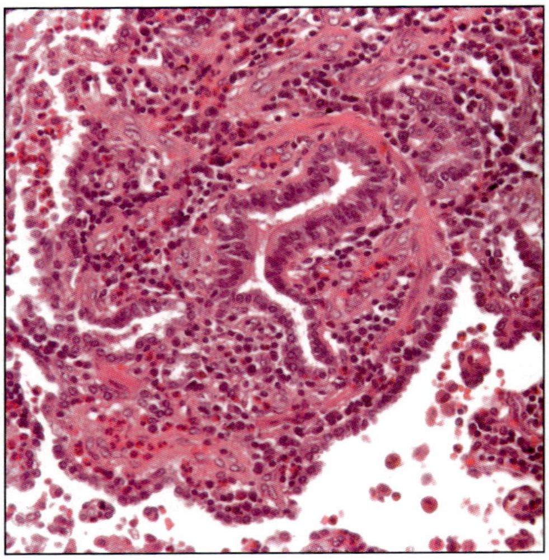

(Left) *Different view of a pulmonary vessel compressed by the inflammatory infiltrate. Even in the compressed lumen, it is still possible to identify inflammatory cells (eosinophils). Note the prominent eosinophilic component ⇨ in the adjacent lung parenchyma.* ***(Right)*** *ALHE in the lung involves the peribronchial soft tissue and adjacent alveolar structures. The presence of eosinophils is easily identified.*

Microscopic Features

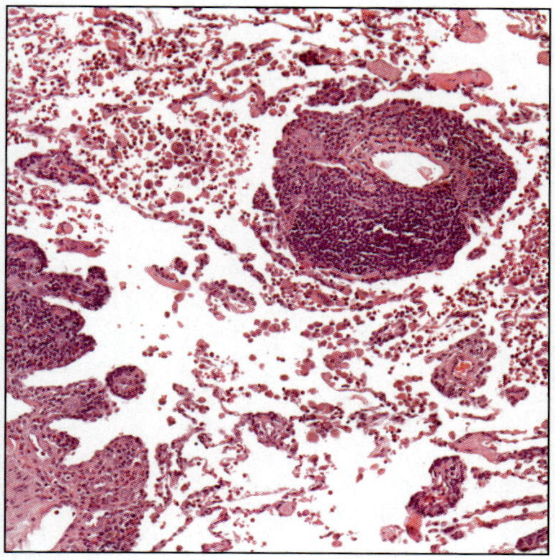
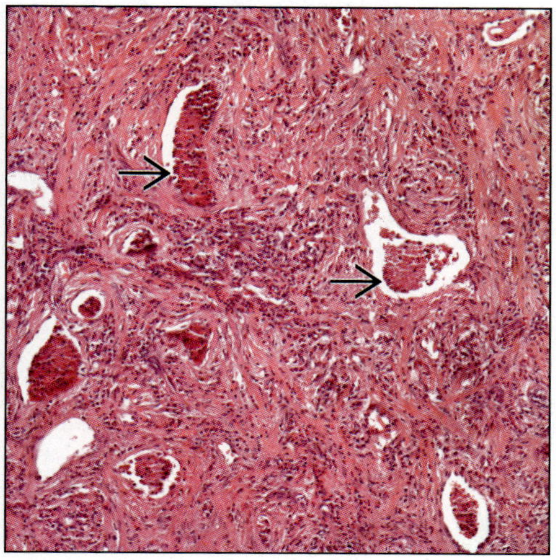

(Left) *Adjacent areas of lung parenchyma may also be affected by ALHE. In this case, small vessels away from the main tumor nodule show inflammatory changes with lymphoid aggregate.* ***(Right)*** *In other areas of the lung, ALHE demonstrates prominent eosinophilic infiltrate in areas of dense fibrosis. Note the dilated vascular structures ⇨ lined by hyperplastic endothelial cells with prominent epithelioid features.*

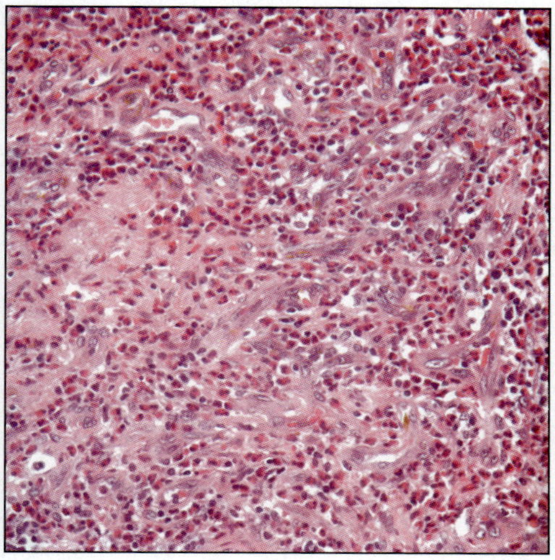
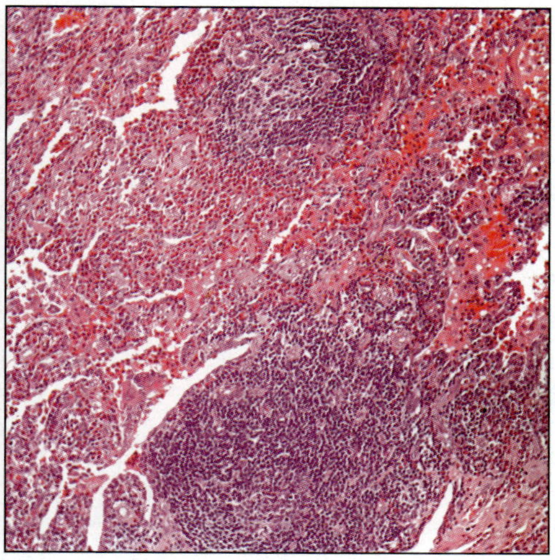

(Left) *High-power view of ALHE reveals numerous vascular channels showing hyperplastic changes. Also note the presence of marked eosinophilia.* ***(Right)*** *Different view of ALHE in the lung shows lymphoid hyperplasia, a proliferation of vessels, and prominent eosinophilic infiltrate. It is difficult to recognize normal lung parenchyma.*

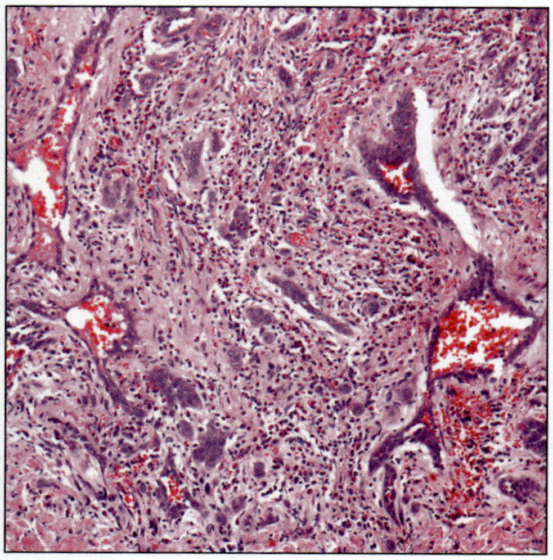
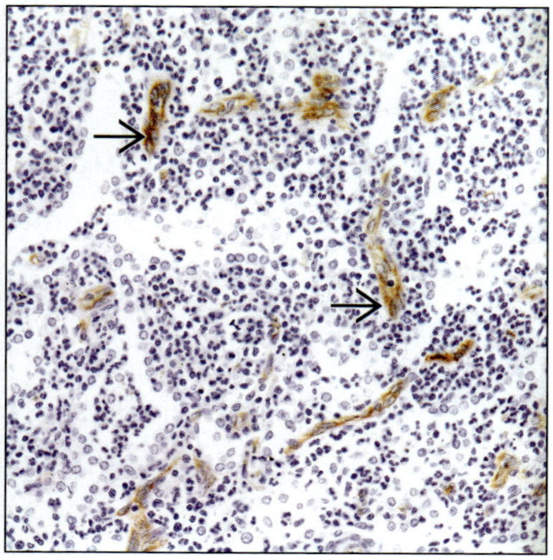

(Left) *ALHE in the lung shows a pattern in which the process is affecting predominantly small vessels, which appear compressed and surrounded by a prominent inflammatory infiltrate composed mainly of eosinophils.* ***(Right)*** *CD31 immunostain shows positive staining in the vascular structures ⇨ in ALHE of the lung. In some cases, immunostains are important to identify the vascular component.*

ATYPICAL ADENOMATOUS HYPERPLASIA

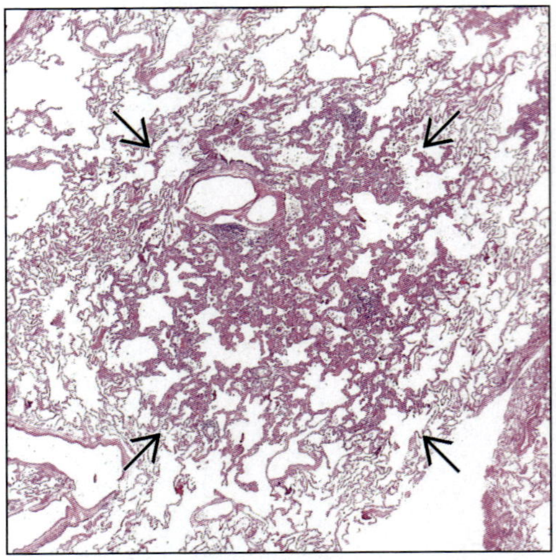

Scanning magnification of atypical adenomatous hyperplasia of the lung shows a well-delineated area ➔ of lung parenchyma that stands out from the surrounding tissue.

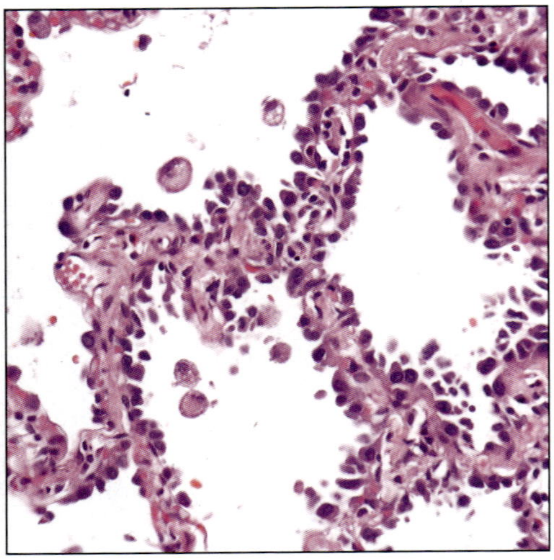

Higher magnification of atypical adenomatous hyperplasia shows alveolar septa lined by cells with enlarged, hyperchromatic nuclei with mild fibrosis of the underlying interstitium.

TERMINOLOGY

Abbreviations

- Atypical adenomatous hyperplasia (AAH)

Synonyms

- Bronchioloalveolar adenoma

Definitions

- Microscopic proliferation of atypical alveolar lining cells measuring < 5 mm in greatest diameter

ETIOLOGY/PATHOGENESIS

Pathogenesis

- Recent studies support that these lesions may be the earliest precursors of peripheral lung adenocarcinoma

CLINICAL ISSUES

Epidemiology

- Incidence
  - May be present in up to 50% of lung specimens surgically resected for lung adenocarcinoma
  - Most commonly associated with adenocarcinoma than with other histologic types of lung cancer
  - No data available on progression rate to bronchioloalveolar cell carcinoma
- Age
  - Adults and elderly patients
- Gender
  - Appears to be more common in female patients
- Ethnicity
  - Higher prevalence in Asians, where bronchioloalveolar adenocarcinoma is most common type of lung cancer

Presentation

- Asymptomatic
- Incidental finding in lung specimens resected for cancer or other conditions

Natural History

- Asymptomatic, incidental microscopic finding
- No known morbidity or mortality
- Lesions are believed to represent precursor lesions to well-differentiated adenocarcinoma
- No increased risk of subsequent development of cancer has been found in patients with these incidental lesions

Prognosis

- No studies to support that AAH worsens prognosis of patients with existing lung cancer

IMAGE FINDINGS

General Features

- Morphology
  - No characteristic radiologic features for AAH
  - Most lesions are completely invisible, even on high-resolution CT scans

MACROSCOPIC FEATURES

General Features

- Lesions are grossly very difficult to visualize and most often pass unnoticed

Size

- Usually < 5 mm in greatest diameter but may be as large as 1 cm in diameter
- Lesions with similar features > 0.5 cm in diameter are generally considered bronchioloalveolar cell carcinomas

ATYPICAL ADENOMATOUS HYPERPLASIA

Key Facts

Terminology
- Microscopic proliferation of atypical alveolar lining cells measuring < 5 mm in greatest diameter

Clinical Issues
- Incidental microscopic finding in lung tissues removed for other reasons

Microscopic Pathology
- Lining cells are round, cuboidal, or low columnar
- Hobnail cells or "peg" cells with apical snouts are often seen
- Nuclei are round and hyperchromatic with evenly dispersed chromatin
- Intranuclear inclusions may be present in some cells

Ancillary Tests
- Atypical cells are strongly positive for TTF-1
- MIB-1/Ki-67 proliferation index is very low (< 1%)

MICROSCOPIC PATHOLOGY

Histologic Features
- Focal lesion composed of mildly to moderately atypical cells lining alveoli and, sometimes, respiratory bronchioles
- Absence of background fibrosis or inflammation
- Lesions stand out against background lung because of increased size and hyperchromatism of lining cells

Cytologic Features
- Lining cells are round, cuboidal, or low columnar
- Hobnail cells or "peg" cells with apical snouts are often seen
- Occasional short tufts of cells may protrude into lumen, but papillary structures are not seen
- Nuclei are round and hyperchromatic with evenly dispersed chromatin
- Occasional large, moderately atypical cells may be seen
- Intranuclear inclusions may be present in some cells
- Mitoses or areas of necrosis are rare

ANCILLARY TESTS

Immunohistochemistry
- Atypical cells are strongly positive for TTF-1
- MIB-1/Ki-67 proliferation index is very low (< 1%)

Electron Microscopy
- Transmission
  - Ultrastructurally show admixtures of cells with features of Clara cells and of type II pneumocytes

DIFFERENTIAL DIAGNOSIS

Bronchioloalveolar Cell Carcinoma (BAC)
- May be indistinguishable morphologically from AAH
- Arbitrary size criterion has been proposed of 0.5 cm diameter for separating BAC from AAH
  - Size may not be a reliable criterion for making this distinction
  - Most cases < 0.5 cm are regarded as atypical adenomatous hyperplasia
  - Most cases > 0.5 cm in diameter are regarded as bronchioloalveolar cell carcinoma

Reactive Bronchioloalveolar Cell Hyperplasia (RBCH)
- RBCH is generally observed against background of pneumonitis whereas AAH is seen against background of normal lung

SELECTED REFERENCES

1. Seki M et al: Multiple lung adenocarcinomas and AAH treated by surgical resection. Lung Cancer. 55(2):237-40, 2007

IMAGE GALLERY

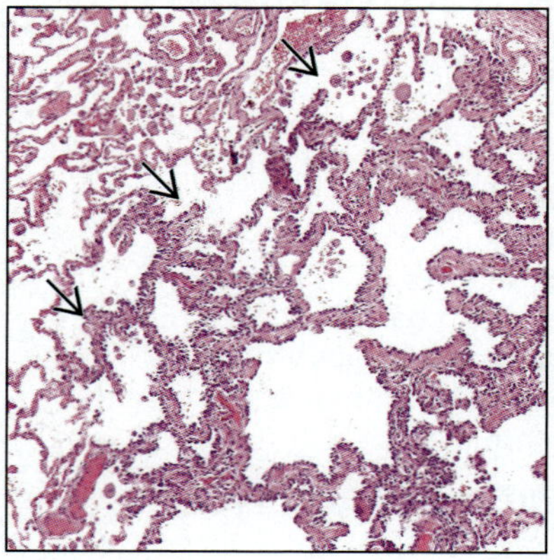
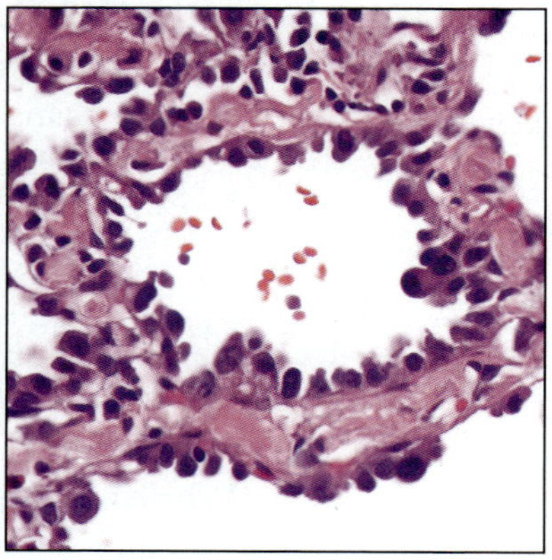
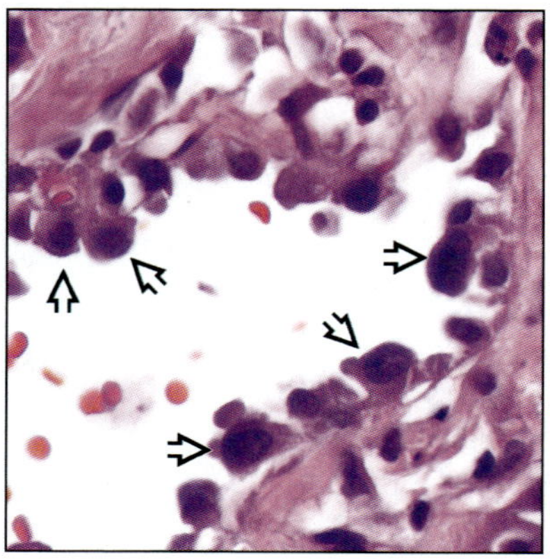

(Left) *Atypical adenomatous hyperplasia shows a well-defined area ⇒ in which the alveolar walls are lined by cells that are larger and more hyperchromatic than those in the surrounding lung parenchyma.* ***(Center)*** *Higher magnification of alveolar adenomatous hyperplasia shows large cells lining the walls of the alveoli.* ***(Right)*** *Higher magnification of alveolar adenomatous hyperplasia shows atypical alveolar lining cells with enlarged, hyperchromatic nuclei and a hobnail configuration ⇨.*

LYMPHANGIOLEIOMYOMATOSIS

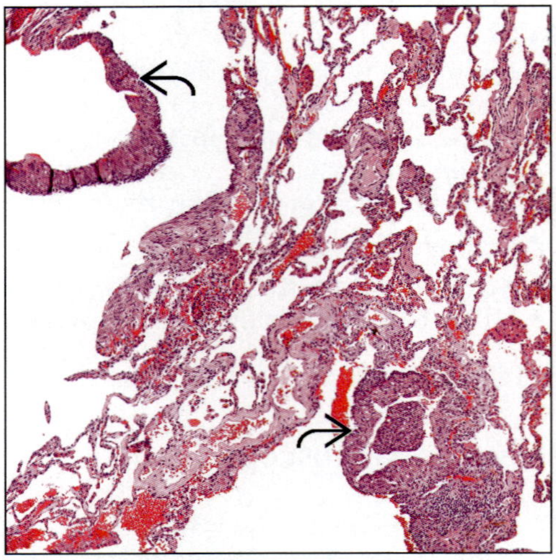

Low-power view of LAM shows 2 focal areas of muscle proliferation ➔. Note that the rest of the pulmonary parenchyma appears to be within normal limits.

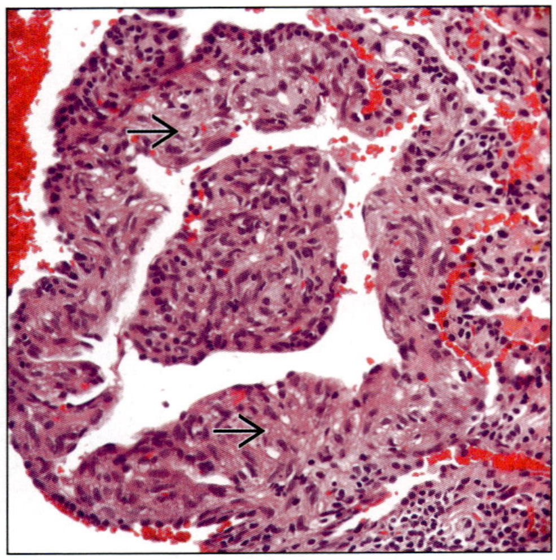

High-power magnification of LAM shows the classical presence of smooth muscle proliferation. The muscle proliferation is obvious and has obliterated the normal alveolar lining ➔.

TERMINOLOGY

Abbreviations

- Lymphangioleiomyomatosis (LAM)

Synonyms

- Lymphangiomyomatosis

Definitions

- Nonneoplastic lung condition characterized by presence of immature muscle proliferation

ETIOLOGY/PATHOGENESIS

Etiology

- Unknown etiology
- May share similar genetic relationship with tuberous sclerosis complex

CLINICAL ISSUES

Epidemiology

- Incidence
  - LAM occurs in approximately 2 cases per million patients
  - May be underreported
- Age
  - More common in premenopausal women
  - Rarely described in children
- Gender
  - Commonly affects women

Presentation

- Cough
- Shortness of breath
- Chylous effusion
- Pneumothorax
- Hemoptysis

Treatment

- No specific treatment
- Hormonal manipulation
- Oophorectomy
- Lung transplantation

Prognosis

- Predominantly cystic lesions may have poor prognosis
- 85% survival at 5 years
- 70% survival at 10 years

IMAGE FINDINGS

General Features

- Bilateral multiple nodular and cystic changes in lung parenchyma
- Unilateral involvement is also possible

MACROSCOPIC FEATURES

General Features

- Multiple cysts with honeycomb appearance

MICROSCOPIC PATHOLOGY

Histologic Features

- Cystic changes
- Hemorrhage
- Spindle cell proliferation
  - In alveolar walls
  - Lining cystic structures
  - With focal clear cell change
  - Lacking atypia or mitotic activity
- Adjacent lung parenchyma may show type II pneumocyte hyperplasia

Predominant Pattern/Injury Type

- Cystic

LYMPHANGIOLEIOMYOMATOSIS

Key Facts

Terminology
- Lymphangioleiomyomatosis (LAM)

Etiology/Pathogenesis
- Unknown etiology
- May share similar genetic relationship with tuberous sclerosis complex

Clinical Issues
- Incidence
  - More common in premenopausal women
  - Rarely described in children
- Symptoms
  - Cough
  - Shortness of breath
  - Chylous effusion
  - Pneumothorax
  - Hemoptysis

Microscopic Pathology
- Cystic changes
- Spindle cell proliferation lining cystic structures

Top Differential Diagnoses
- Leiomyoma
  - Usually forms a tumor mass
  - Unusual for leiomyoma to present with prominent cystic changes
- Leiomyosarcoma
  - LAM lacks atypia or mitotic activity
- Tuberous sclerosis
  - Such distinction may not be possible on histologic grounds alone
  - It is important to obtain a clinical history

Immunohistochemistry

Antibody	Reactivity	Staining Pattern	Comment
Actin-sm	Positive	Cytoplasmic	In muscle component
Desmin	Positive	Cytoplasmic	In muscle component
HMB-45	Positive	Cytoplasmic	More often in clear cells
IGF-1	Positive	Cytoplasmic	
MMP-1	Positive	Cytoplasmic	
ER	Positive	Nuclear	May be focal
PR	Positive	Nuclear	May be focal
S100	Negative		
CK-PAN	Negative		Positive in alveolar cell and entrapped lung

Predominant Cell/Compartment Type
- Smooth muscle

DIFFERENTIAL DIAGNOSIS

Leiomyoma
- Usually forms a tumor mass
- Unusual for leiomyoma to present with prominent cystic changes

Leiomyosarcoma
- LAM lacks atypia or mitotic activity

Tuberous Sclerosis
- Such distinction may not be possible on histologic grounds alone
- It is important to obtain a clinical history of tuberous sclerosis

DIAGNOSTIC CHECKLIST

Clinically Relevant Pathologic Features
- Gross appearance

Pathologic Interpretation Pearls
- Cystic changes with smooth muscle proliferation
- Spindle cells are positive for SMA and HMB-45
- Spindle cells are positive for ER/PR

SELECTED REFERENCES

1. Maruyama H et al: Multifocal micronodular pneumocyte hyperplasia and lymphangioleiomyomatosis in tuberous sclerosis with a TSC2 gene. Mod Pathol. 14(6):609-14, 2001
2. Beasly MB et al: Histologic predictors of survival in 101 cases of pulmonary lymphangioleiomyomatosis (LAM): prognostic significance of histologic score. Am J Respir Crit Care Med. 161: A15, 2000
3. Urban T et al: Pulmonary lymphangioleiomyomatosis. A study of 69 patients. Groupe d'Etudes et de Recherche sur les Maladies "Orphelines" Pulmonaires (GERM"O"P). Medicine (Baltimore). 78(5):321-37, 1999
4. Kitaichi M et al: Pulmonary lymphangioleiomyomatosis: a report of 46 patients including a clinicopathologic study of prognostic factors. Am J Respir Crit Care Med. 151(2 Pt 1):527-33, 1995
5. Capron F et al: Pulmonary lymphangioleiomyomatosis and Bourneville's tuberous sclerosis with pulmonary involvement: the same disease? Cancer. 52(5):851-5, 1983

Microscopic Features

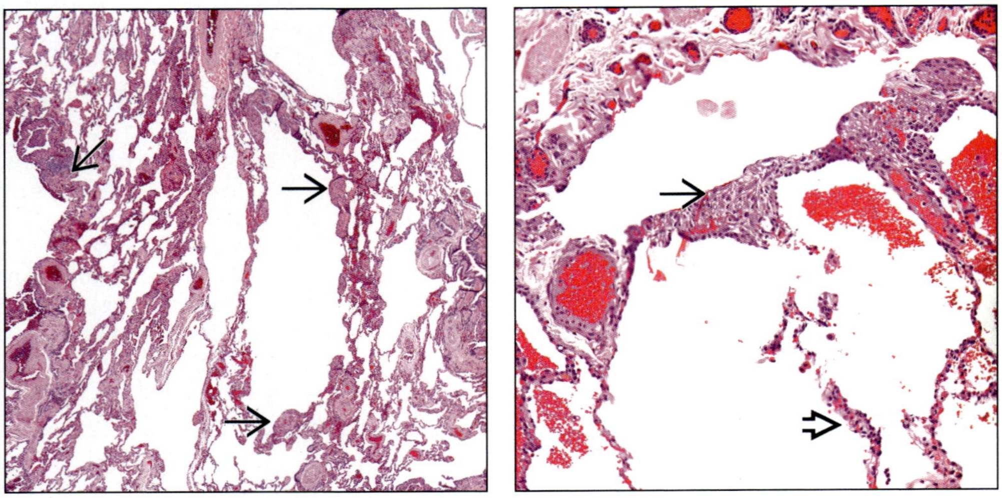

(Left) *Low-power view of lung parenchyma in LAM shows little change at this magnification. However, note the presence of cysts and the thickening of some of those cyst's walls →.* ***(Right)*** *Higher magnification shows alternating normal alveolar structures ⇨ and other cystic structures lined by smooth muscle proliferation → in pulmonary lymphangioleiomyomatosis.*

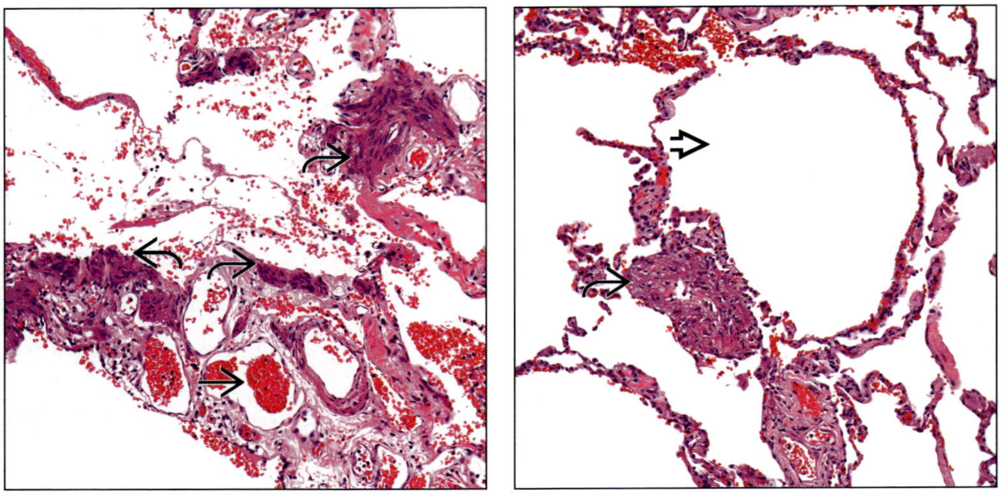

(Left) *LAM shows areas of nonneoplastic vascular proliferation →; some of the vessels contain fresh blood. Note the presence of muscle proliferation adjacent to the dilated vascular structures ↪.* ***(Right)*** *This LAM shows a very subtle area of muscle proliferation ↪ adjacent to an alveolar space ⇨. In some cases, the presence of muscle may be only focal and can easily be missed in a cursory review.*

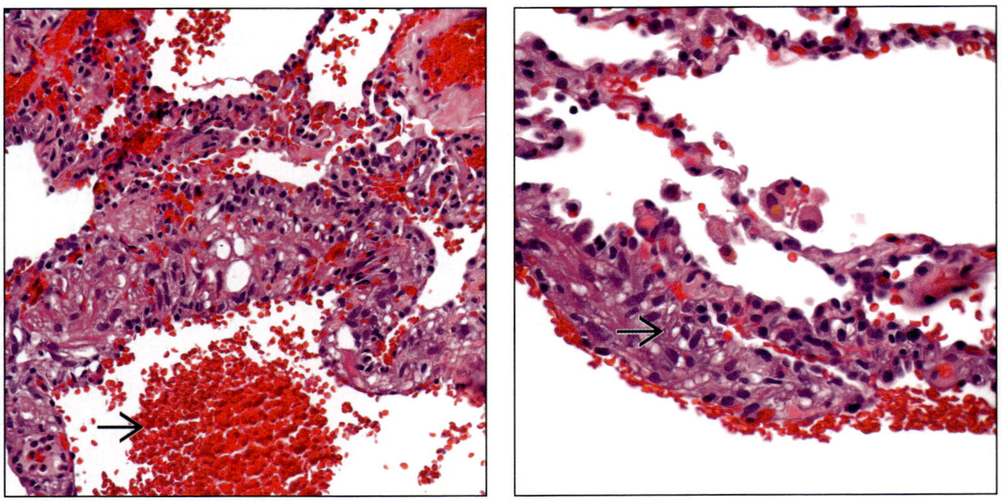

(Left) *This LAM shows areas of congestion and hemorrhage with the presence of fresh blood →. However, note that the alveolar wall has been replaced by a muscle proliferation, which also shows some clear cell changes. Due to the areas of hemorrhage and congestion, these areas can be missed.* ***(Right)*** *High-power view of the smooth muscle proliferation in LAM is shown. Note that in some areas, the cellular proliferation demonstrates focal clear cells →.*

Microscopic Features

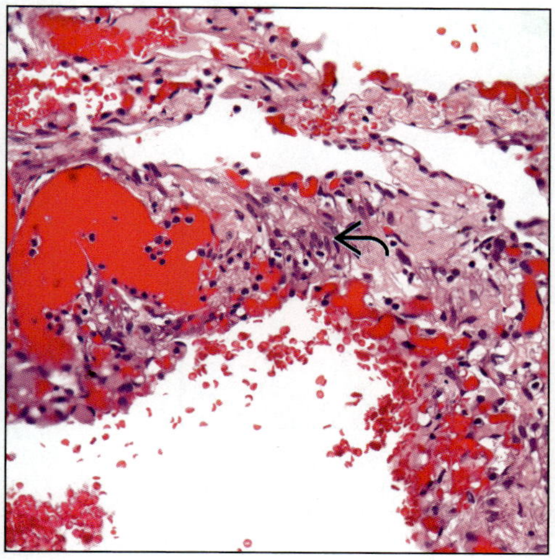

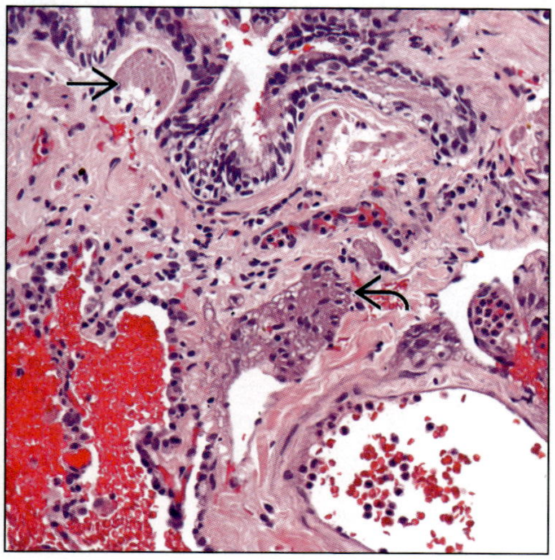

(Left) *The presence of hemorrhage and congestion in LAM can at times be very marked, and areas of muscle proliferation can be difficult to find. Note here that the muscle proliferation* ↪ *can be easily missed.* ***(Right)*** *The presence of muscle proliferation must be separated from the normal muscle layers that surround normal airway structures. Note the presence of the difference of the muscle of LAM* ↪ *in contrast to the normal muscular layer around the airway* →.

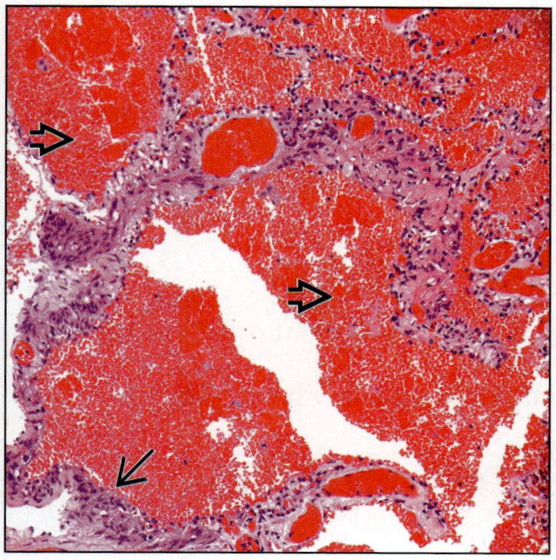

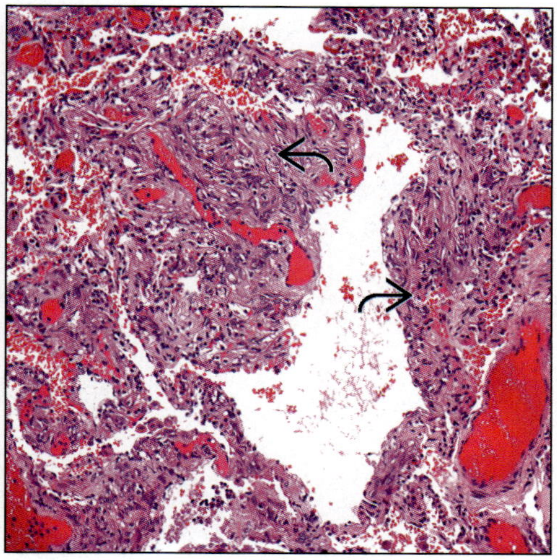

(Left) *Despite the presence of dilated alveolar spaces filled with fresh blood* ⇨*, one is still able to see smooth muscle proliferation* →*.* ***(Right)*** *In some cases of LAM, the muscle proliferation can be marked and can actually mimic a smooth muscle tumor. The muscle proliferation* ↪ *in this case is extensive, destroying normal lung architecture.*

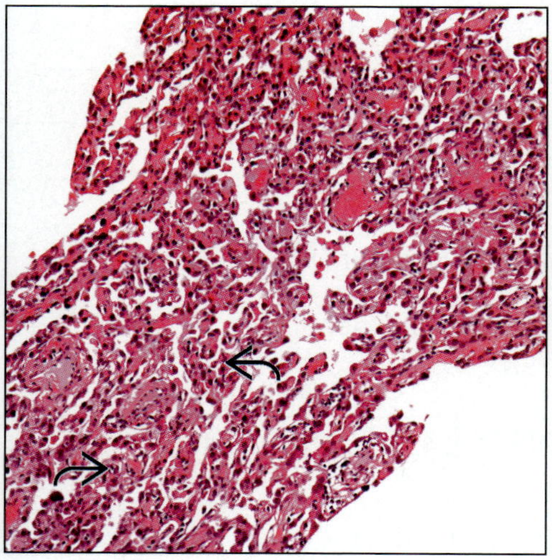

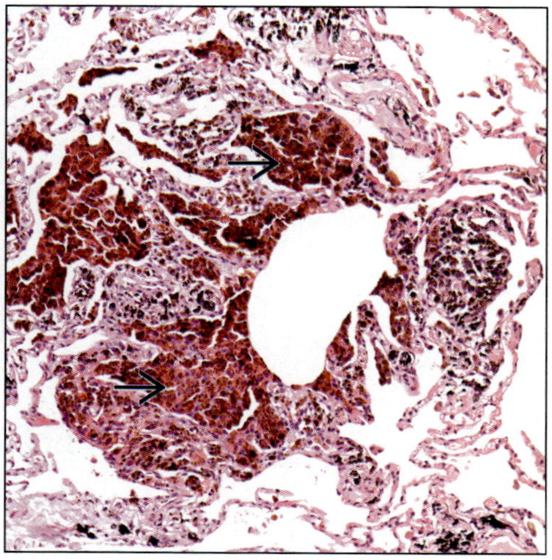

(Left) *An unusual feature that may be seen in some cases of LAM is the presence of pneumocyte hyperplasia* ↪*. Such change may be in the form of small nodules that can raise the possibility of a malignant epithelial neoplasm.* ***(Right)*** *One additional feature that may be seen in most of the cases of LAM is the presence of hemosiderin-laden macrophages* → *filling alveolar spaces, as shown here.*

CAPILLARY HEMANGIOMATOSIS

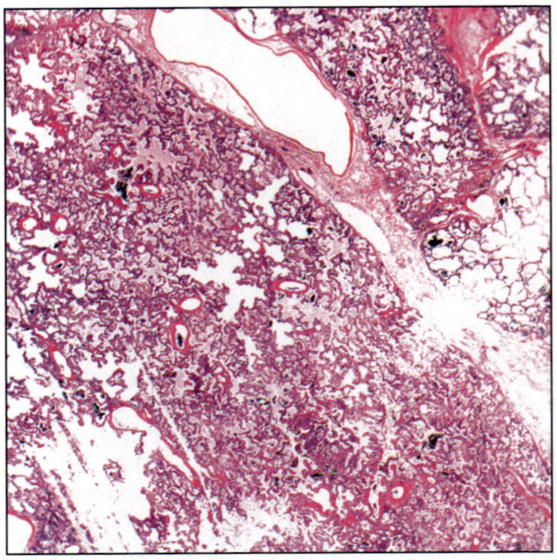

Low-power view shows a lung section with capillary hemangiomatosis. At this power, the lung may look within normal limits, and in a cursory review, the pathological process can be easily missed.

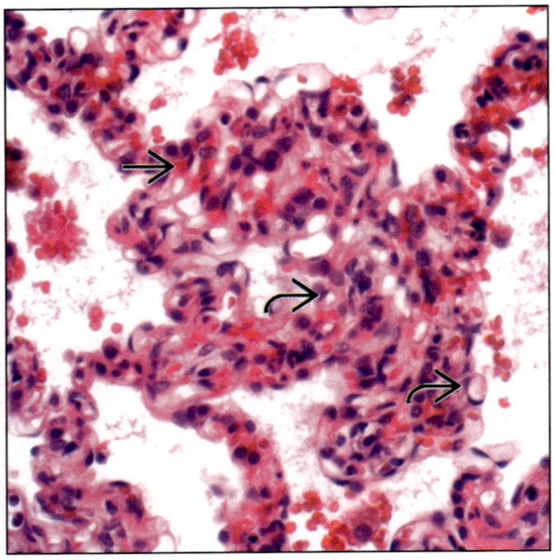

High-power view of capillary hemangiomatosis of the lung shows the classical proliferation of small capillaries ⮫ with numerous extravasated red cells →.

TERMINOLOGY

Abbreviations

- Capillary hemangiomatosis (CH)

Definitions

- Benign condition characterized by proliferation of small capillaries in pulmonary interstitium

ETIOLOGY/PATHOGENESIS

Etiology

- Possible autosomal recessive inheritance has been observed
- May also appear as an incidental finding

CLINICAL ISSUES

Epidemiology

- Incidence
  - Unusual occurrence
- Age
  - It may occur in any age group
    - Most cases appear to be more commonly diagnosed in 3rd or 4th decade of life
- Gender
  - No gender predilection
- Ethnicity
  - No ethnic predilection

Site

- Pulmonary interstitium

Presentation

- Cough
- Hemoptysis
- Respiratory distress
- Chest pain
- Pulmonary hypertension
- Interstitial lung disease

Treatment

- Surgical approaches
  - Due to extensive nature of process, radical approach may be necessary
  - Lobectomy or pneumonectomy
- Drugs
  - Interferon α-2a

Prognosis

- Good if diagnosed earlier and if the process is less diffuse
- Can be fatal due to pulmonary hemorrhage

MACROSCOPIC FEATURES

General Features

- Congested lung parenchyma
- Sponge-like appearance
- Multicystic changes in lung parenchyma

MICROSCOPIC PATHOLOGY

Histologic Features

- Interstitial congestion
- Proliferation of small capillaries
- Capillaries may infiltrate into bronchi and larger vessels
- Presence of double capillaries
- Lack of cytologic atypia

DIFFERENTIAL DIAGNOSIS

Capillaritis

- In cases of capillaritis, there is usually inflammatory reaction associated with the process
- May not be as diffuse as capillary hemangiomatosis

CAPILLARY HEMANGIOMATOSIS

Key Facts

Terminology
- Benign condition characterized by proliferation of small capillaries in pulmonary interstitium

Etiology/Pathogenesis
- Possible autosomal recessive inheritance has been mentioned
- May also appear as an incidental finding

Clinical Issues
- Unusual occurrence
- It may occur in any age group
- Most cases appear to be more commonly diagnosed in 3rd or 4th decade of life
- Symptoms
  - Cough
  - Hemoptysis
  - Respiratory distress
  - Chest pain
  - Pulmonary hypertension
  - Interstitial lung disease
- Prognosis
  - Good if diagnosed earlier
  - Can be fatal in advanced stages

Top Differential Diagnoses
- Capillaritis
- Cavernous hemangioma
- Capillary hemangioma
- Pulmonary hemorrhage
- Angiosarcoma
- Normal lung parenchyma

Histochemical Features

Stain	Result
Elastic van Gieson	May highlight some capillaries

Immunohistochemical Features

Stain	Result
SD-40	May decorate capillary proliferation
CD-31	May show positive staining in capillaries
CD-34	May decorate capillary proliferation
Factor VIII	May show positive staining in capillary proliferation
Ulex	May show positive staining in capillary proliferation

Cavernous Hemangioma
- Shows more circumscription
- Vascular proliferation is more obvious with larger vessels

Capillary Hemangioma
- Vascular proliferation in capillary hemangioma is larger than in capillary hemangiomatosis
- May be more circumscribed
- May present as pulmonary nodule or mass

Pulmonary Hemorrhage
- Blood lakes are formed in alveoli
- Does not show presence of capillary proliferation

Angiosarcoma
- Most likely will present as multiple pulmonary nodules rather than diffuse pattern
- Displays more cytologic atypia and mitotic activity

Normal Lung Parenchyma
- Does not show extensive capillary proliferation

DIAGNOSTIC CHECKLIST

Clinically Relevant Pathologic Features
- Diffuse capillary proliferation in pulmonary interstitium

Pathologic Interpretation Pearls
- Extensive capillary proliferation without atypia

SELECTED REFERENCES

1. McGuire F et al: Pulmonary capillary hemangiomatosis associated with CREST syndrome: a case report and review of the literature. Respiration. 80(5):435-8, 2010
2. Fugo K et al: Solitary capillary hemangioma of the lung: report of 2 resected cases detected by high-resolution CT. Am J Surg Pathol. 30(6):750-3, 2006
3. Lantuéjoul S et al: Pulmonary veno-occlusive disease and pulmonary capillary hemangiomatosis: a clinicopathologic study of 35 cases. Am J Surg Pathol. 30(7):850-7, 2006
4. Sullivan A et al: Pulmonary capillary hemangiomatosis: an immunohistochemical analysis of vascular remodeling. Eur J Med Res. 11(5):187-93, 2006
5. Sullivan A et al: Pulmonary capillary hemangiomatosis: an immunohistochemical analysis of vascular remodeling in a fatal case. Chest. 128(6 Suppl):576S, 2005

Microscopic Features

*(**Left**) Pulmonary capillary hemangiomatosis shows a dilated vascular structure ⇨ in the septum of the lung. In either side of this dilated vascular structure, there is lung parenchyma, which at this power looks only congested. (**Right**) Areas of fibroconnective tissue deposition may be encountered ⇨. However, note that the alveolar spaces are rather dilated, and the interstitium is widened by a proliferation of capillaries.*

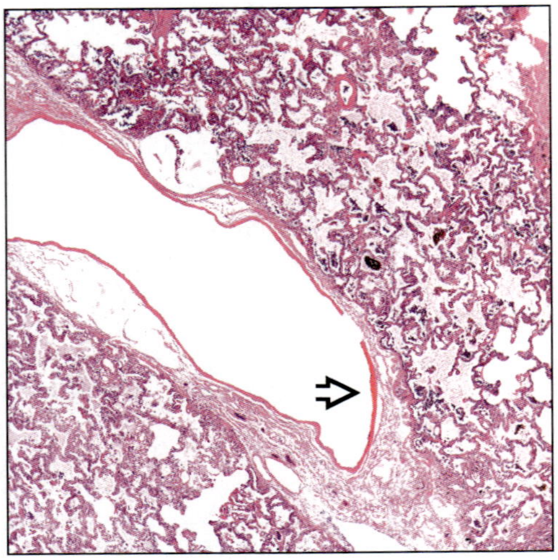

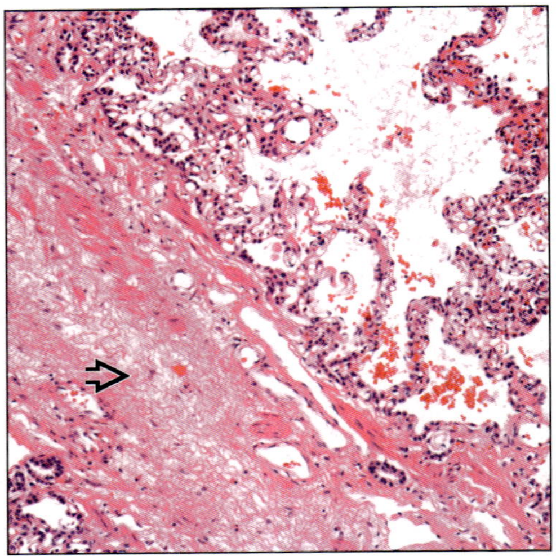

*(**Left**) In some areas, there may be pigmented macrophages within alveolar spaces →. This feature may be secondary to hemorrhage as there may be breakdown of capillaries within the pulmonary interstitium. (**Right**) High-power view shows a cluster of pigmented macrophages → within what may have been an alveolar space. Also note that the adjacent pulmonary parenchyma is almost replaced by a capillary proliferation ↗.*

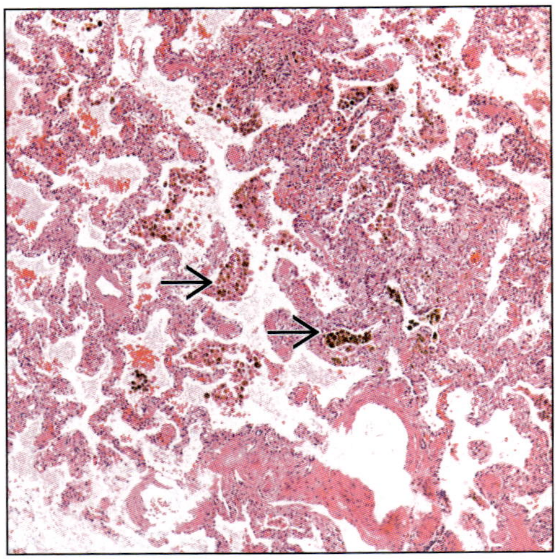

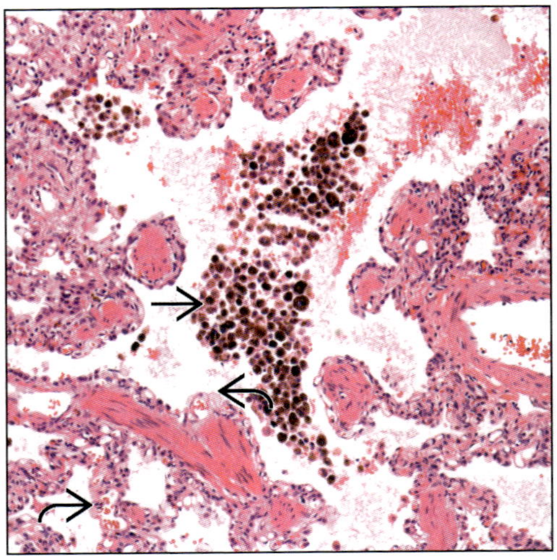

*(**Left**) Pulmonary capillary hemangiomatosis with areas of intraalveolar acellular edematous material ↗ gives a vague appearance of pulmonary edema. (**Right**) High-power view shows easily identifiable capillary proliferation ↗ lining not only the alveolar walls but also the interstitium. The edematous material within the alveolar spaces may be a secondary phenomenon that may be seen in some cases.*

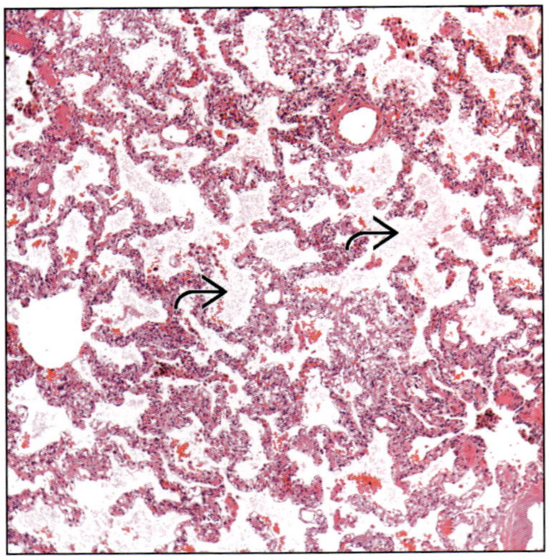

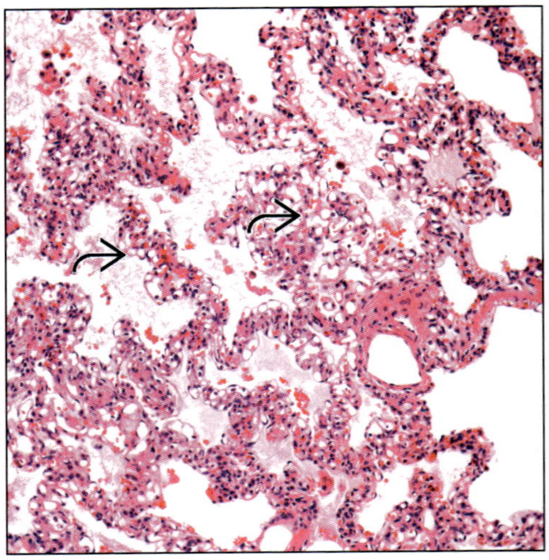

CAPILLARY HEMANGIOMATOSIS

Microscopic Features

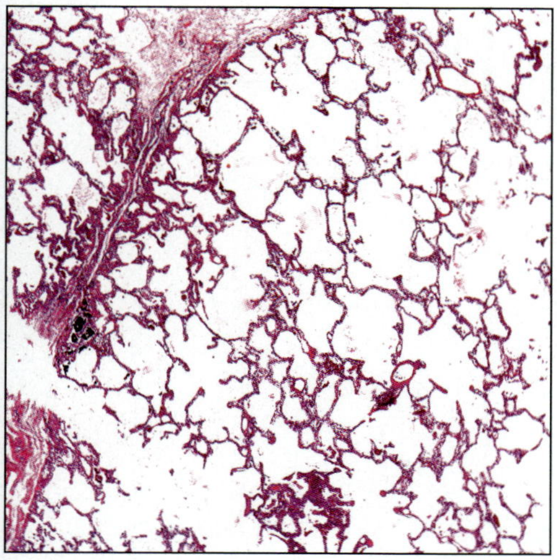

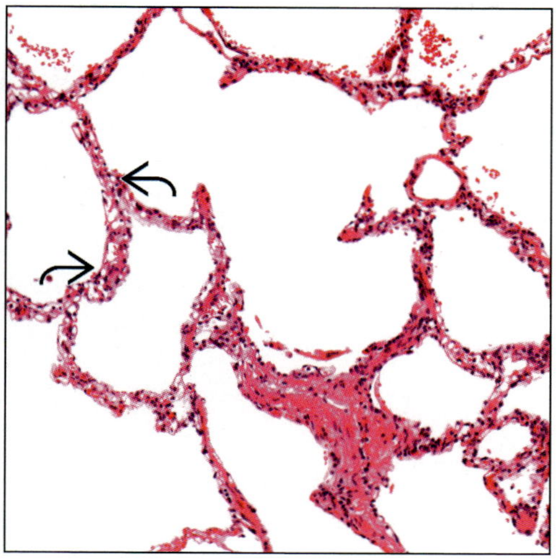

(Left) *Low-power view shows pulmonary hemangiomatosis with an appearance mimicking emphysematous changes. The true nature of this process may be easily missed if not properly examined at higher magnification.* ***(Right)*** *High-power view shows an emphysematous-like area in which there is some breakdown of alveolar walls. Note that the alveolar lining is being replaced by a capillary proliferation* ↷.

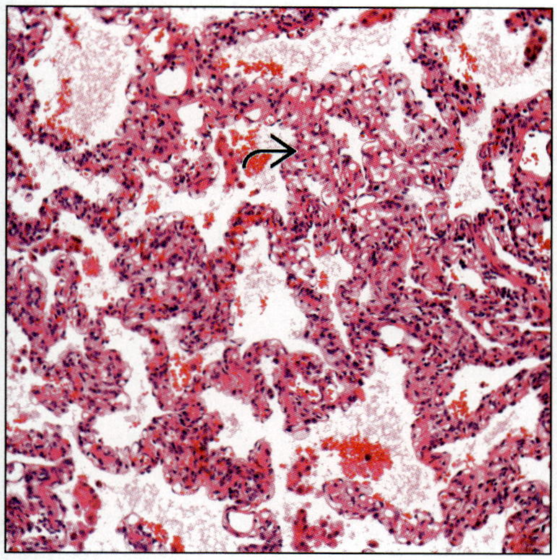

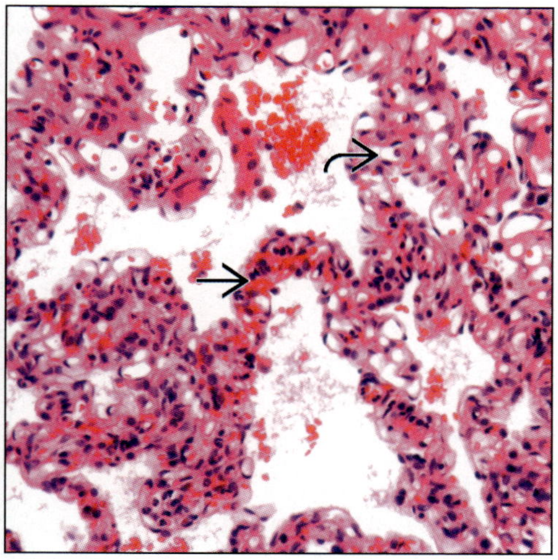

(Left) *Pulmonary capillary hemangiomatosis shows widening of the interstitium and easily identifiable capillary proliferation* ↷. *The lung parenchyma may in some cases preserve some of the normal lung architecture.* ***(Right)*** *The capillary proliferation is composed of small capillaries* ↷ *with extravasated red cells* →. *However, the capillary proliferation does not show any atypical features or mitotic activity.*

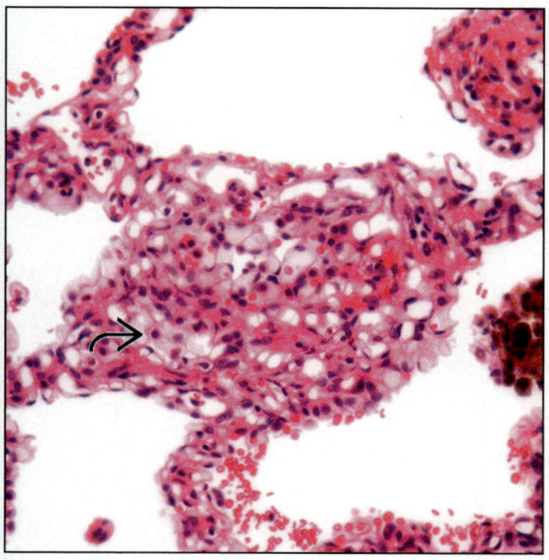

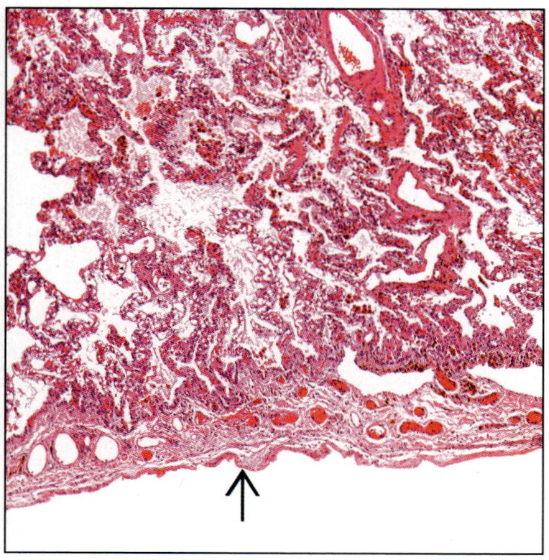

(Left) *Focal area of a more solid capillary proliferation* ↷ *in pulmonary hemangiomatosis is shown. These features are reminiscent of capillary hemangiomas of the subcutis.* ***(Right)*** *Although the process of capillary hemangiomatosis may be diffuse, involving extensive areas of the lung parenchyma, the process does not appear to involve the pleura, as is illustrated in this case with sparing of the pleural surface* →.

PROTOCOL FOR LUNG CANCER SPECIMEN EXAMINATION

Lung: Resection

Surgical Pathology Cancer Case Summary (Checklist)

Specimen

___ Lung
___ Lobe(s) of lung (specify): ____________________
___ Bronchus (specify): ____________________
___ Other (specify): ____________________
___ Not specified

Procedure

___ Major airway resection
___ Wedge resection
___ Segmentectomy
___ Lobectomy
___ Bilobectomy
___ Pneumonectomy
___ Other (specify): ____________________
___ Not specified

Specimen Integrity

___ Intact
___ Disrupted
___ Indeterminate

Specimen Laterality

___ Right
___ Left
___ Not specified

Tumor Site (select all that apply)

___ Upper lobe
___ Middle lobe
___ Lower lobe
___ Other(s) (specify): ____________________
___ Not specified

Tumor Size

Greatest dimension: ________ cm
*Additional dimensions: ________ x ________ cm
___ Cannot be determined

Histologic Type

___ Carcinoma, type cannot be determined
___ Non-small cell carcinoma, subtype cannot be determined
___Small cell carcinoma
___Combined small cell carcinoma (small cell carcinoma and non-small cell component)
Specify type of non-small cell carcinoma component: ____________________
___ Squamous cell carcinoma
___ Squamous cell carcinoma, papillary variant
___ Squamous cell carcinoma, clear cell variant
___ Squamous cell carcinoma, small cell variant
___ Squamous cell carcinoma, basaloid variant
___ Adenocarcinoma
___ Adenocarcinoma, mixed subtype
___ Acinar adenocarcinoma
___ Papillary adenocarcinoma
___ Bronchioalveolar carcinoma

___ Bronchioalveolar carcinoma, nonmucinous
___ Bronchioalveolar carcinoma, mucinous
___ Bronchioalveolar carcinoma, mixed nonmucinous and mucinous
___ Solid adenocarcinoma
___ Fetal adenocarcinoma
___ Mucinous (colloid) adenocarcinoma
___ Mucinous cystadenocarcinoma
___ Signet ring adenocarcinoma
___ Clear cell adenocarcinoma
___ Large cell carcinoma
___ Large cell neuroendocrine carcinoma
___ Combined large cell neuroendocrine carcinoma
Specify type of other non-small cell carcinoma component: ___
___ Basaloid carcinoma
___ Lymphoepithelioma-like carcinoma
___ Clear cell carcinoma
___ Large cell carcinoma with rhabdoid phenotype
___ Adenosquamous carcinoma
___ Sarcomatoid carcinoma
___ Pleomorphic adenoma
___ Spindle cell carcinoma
___ Giant cell carcinoma
___ Carcinosarcoma
___ Pulmonary blastoma
___ Typical carcinoid tumor
___ Atypical carcinoid tumor
___ Mucoepidermoid carcinoma
___ Adenoid cystic carcinoma
___ Epithelial-myoepithelial carcinoma
___ Other (specify): ___

Histologic Grade

___ Not applicable
___ GX: Cannot be assessed
___ G1: Well differentiated
___ G2: Moderately differentiated
___ G3: Poorly differentiated
___ G4: Undifferentiated
___ Other (specify): ___

Visceral Pleura Invasion

___ Not identified
___ Present
___ Indeterminate

Tumor Extension (select all that apply)

___ Not applicable
___ Not identified
___ Superficial spreading tumor with invasive component limited to bronchial wall
___ Tumor involves main bronchus 2 cm or more distal to the carina
___ Parietal pleura
___ Chest wall
*Specify involved structure(s): ___
___ Diaphragm
___ Mediastinal pleura
___ Phrenic nerve

PROTOCOL FOR LUNG CANCER SPECIMEN EXAMINATION

___ Parietal pericardium
___ Tumor in main bronchus < 2 cm distal to carina but does not involve carina
___ Mediastinum
*Specify involved structures: ___
___ Heart
___ Great vessels
___ Trachea
___ Esophagus
___ Vertebral body
___ Carina
___ Other (specify): ___

Margins (select all that apply)

Bronchial margin
___ Not applicable
___ Cannot be assessed
___ Uninvolved by invasive carcinoma
___ Involved by invasive carcinoma
___ Squamous cell carcinoma in situ (CIS) present at bronchial margin
___ Squamous cell carcinoma in situ (CIS) not identified at bronchial margin

Vascular margin
___ Not applicable
___ Cannot be assessed
___ Uninvolved by invasive carcinoma
___ Involved by invasive carcinoma

Parenchymal margin
___ Not applicable
___ Cannot be assessed
___ Uninvolved by invasive carcinoma
___ Involved by invasive carcinoma

Parietal pleural margin
___ Not applicable
___ Cannot be assessed
___ Uninvolved by invasive carcinoma
___ Involved by invasive carcinoma

Chest wall margin
___ Not applicable
___ Cannot be assessed
___ Uninvolved by invasive carcinoma
___ Involved by invasive carcinoma

Other attached tissue margin (specify): ___
___ Not applicable
___ Cannot be assessed
___ Uninvolved by invasive carcinoma
___ Involved by invasive carcinoma
If all margins uninvolved by invasive carcinoma: Distance of invasive carcinoma from closest margin: ___ mm
Specify margin: ___

Treatment Effect

___ Not applicable
___ Cannot be determined
___ > 10% residual viable tumor
___ < 10% residual viable tumor

**Tumor-associated Atelectasis or Obstructive Pneumonitis*

*___ Extends to hilar region but does not involve entire lung

*____ Involves entire lung

Lymph-Vascular Invasion

____ Not identified

____ Present

____ Indeterminate

**Lymph Nodes*

*Extranodal extension

*____ Not identified

*____ Present

Pathologic Staging (pTNM)

TNM descriptors (required only if applicable)

____ m (multiple primary tumors)

____ r (recurrent)

____ y (post-treatment)

Primary tumor (pT)

____ PTX: Cannot be assessed, or tumor proven by presence of malignant cells in sputum or bronchial washings but not visualized by imaging or bronchoscopy

____ pT0: No evidence of primary tumor

____ pTis: Carcinoma in situ

____ pT1a: Tumor ≤ 2 cm in greatest dimension, surrounded by lung or visceral pleura, without bronchoscopic evidence of invasion more proximal than the lobar bronchus (i.e., not in the main bronchus); or superficial spreading tumor of any size with its invasive component limited to the bronchial wall, which may extend proximally to the main bronchus

____ pT1b: Tumor > 2 cm but ≤ 3 cm in greatest dimension, surrounded by lung or visceral pleura, without bronchoscopic evidence of invasion more proximal than the lobar bronchus (i.e., not in the main bronchus)

____ PT2a: Tumor > 3 cm but ≤ 5 cm in greatest dimension surrounded by lung or visceral pleura, without bronchoscopic evidence of invasion more proximal than the lobar bronchus (i.e., not in the main bronchus); or tumor ≤ 5 cm in greatest dimension with any of the following features of extent: Involves main bronchus ≥ distal to the carina; invades the visceral pleura; associated with atelectasis or obstructive pneumonitis that extends to the hilar region but does not involve the entire lung

____ pT2b: Tumor > 5 cm but ≤ 7 cm in greatest dimension

____ pT3: Tumor > 7 cm in greatest dimension; or tumor of any size that directly invades any of the following: Parietal pleural chest wall (including superior sulcus tumors), diaphragm, phrenic nerve, mediastinal pleura, parietal pericardium; or tumor of any size in the main bronchus < 2 cm distal to the carina but without involvement of the carina; or tumor of any size associated with atelectasis or obstructive pneumonitis of the entire lung; or tumors of any size with separate tumor nodule(s) in same lobe

____ PT4: Tumor of any size that invades any of the following: Mediastinum, heart, great vessels, trachea, recurrent laryngeal nerve, esophagus, vertebral body, carina; or tumor of any size with separate tumor nodule(s) in a different lobe of ipsilateral lung

Regional lymph nodes (pN)

____ pNX: Cannot be assessed

____ pN0: No regional lymph node metastasis

____ pN1: Metastasis in ipsilateral peribronchial &/or ipsilateral hilar lymph nodes, and intrapulmonary nodes, including involvement by direct extension

____ pN2: Metastasis in ipsilateral mediastinal &/or subcarinal lymph node(s)

____ pN3: Metastasis in contralateral mediastinal, contralateral hilar, ipsilateral or contralateral scalene, or supraclavicular lymph node(s)

____ No nodes submitted or found

Number of lymph nodes examined

Specify: __________

____ Number cannot be determined (explain): ______________________________

Number of lymph nodes involved

Specify: __________

____ Number cannot be determined (explain): ______________________________

If lymph node(s) involved, specify involved nodal station(s): ______________________________

Distant Metastasis (pM)

____ Not applicable

____ pM1a: Separate tumor nodule(s) in contralateral lung; tumor with pleural nodules or malignant pleural (or pericardial) effusion

____ pM1b: Distant metastases (in extrathoracic organs)

*Specify site(s), if known: ______________________________

Additional Pathologic Findings (select all that apply)

*____ None identified

PROTOCOL FOR LUNG CANCER SPECIMEN EXAMINATION

*___ Atypical adenomatous hyperplasia
*___ Squamous dysplasia
*___ Metaplasia (specify type): ____________________
*___ Diffuse neuroendocrine hyperplasia
*___ Inflammation (specify type): ____________________
*___ Emphysema
*___ Other (specify): ____________________

Ancillary Studies (select all that apply)

*___ Epidermal growth factor receptor (EGFR) analysis results
(Specify method): ____________________
*___ *KRAS* mutational analysis
(Specify results): ____________________
*___ Other (specify): ____________________

**Data elements with asterisks are not required. However, these elements may be clinically important but are not yet validated or regularly used in patient management. Adapted with permission from College of American Pathologists, "Protocol for the Examination of Specimens from Patients with Primary Non-Small Cell carcinoma, Small Cell Carcinoma, or Carcinoid Tumor of the Lung." Web posting date: February, 2011, www.cap.org.*

Tumor Staging

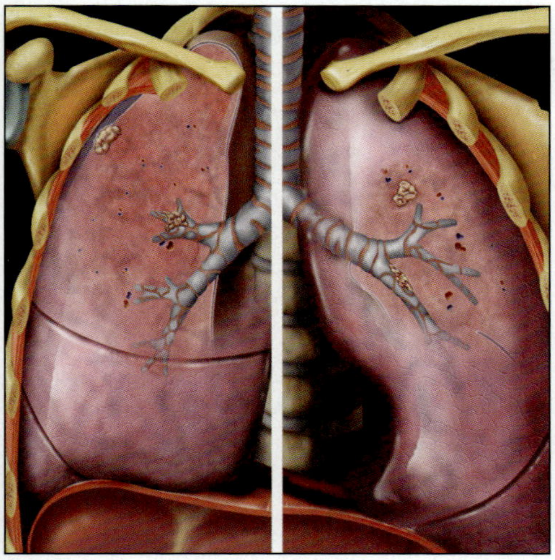

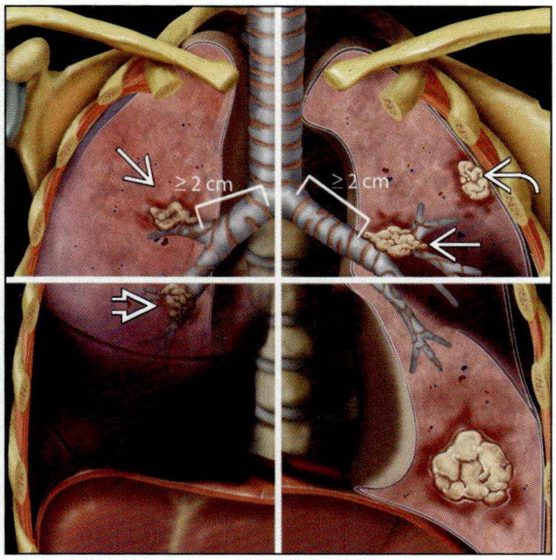

(Left) *Graphic depicts T1 tumors: ≤ 3 cm, surrounded by lung/visceral pleura, no invasion of main bronchus. T1a: Tumor ≤ 2 cm or superficial spreading tumor invading bronchial wall (may extend to main bronchus). T1b: Tumor > 2 cm but ≤ 3 cm.* ***(Right)*** *Graphic depicts T2 tumors involving main pulmonary bronchus, > 2 cm distal to carina, invading visceral pleura, and associated with atelectasis/pneumonitis of portion of lung. T2a: Tumor > 3 cm but ≤ 5 cm. T2b: Tumor > 5 cm but ≤ 7 cm.*

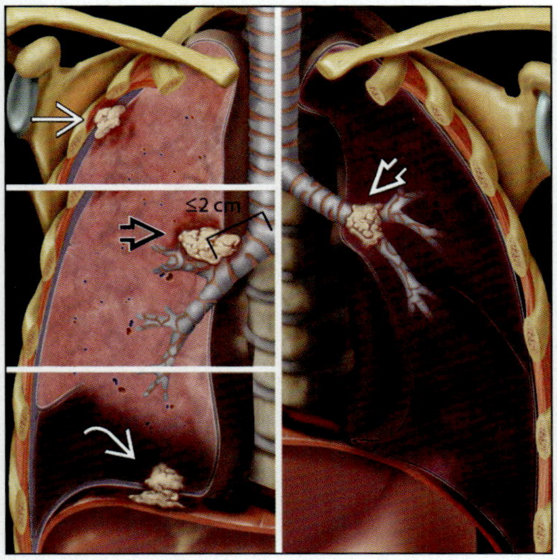

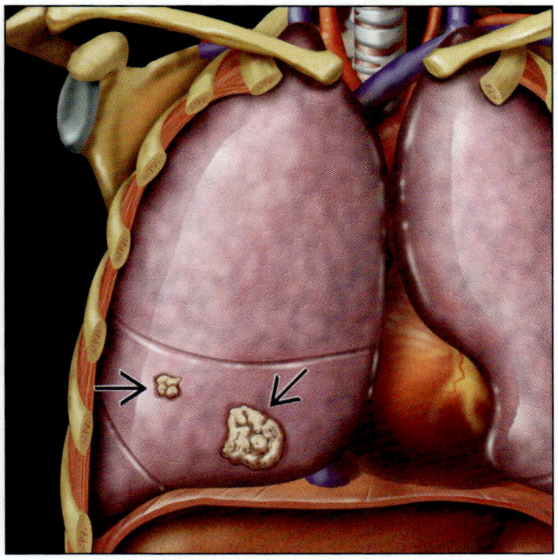

(Left) *Graphic depicts T3 tumors invading chest wall, tumor in main bronchus, < 2 cm distal to carina, invading diaphragm, and tumor with associated atelectasis/pneumonitis of entire left lung.* ***(Right)*** *Graphic depicts two separate tumor nodules in the same pulmonary lobe, designated T3.*

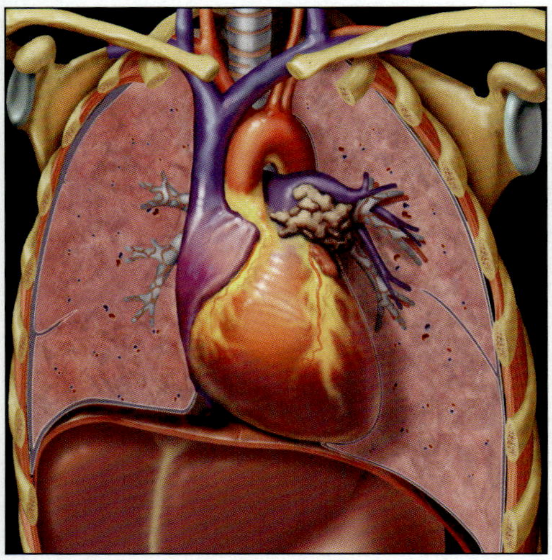

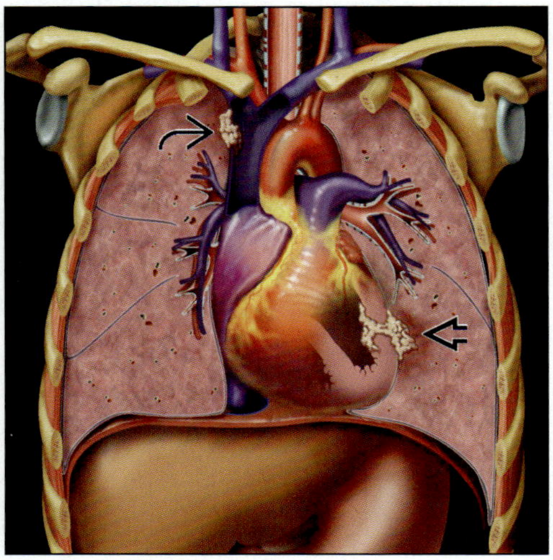

(Left) *Graphic depicts a T4 hilar tumor invading the great vessels. T4 tumors can be any size.* ***(Right)*** *Graphic depicts 2 T4 tumors: One invades the superior vena cava and another invades the myocardium.*

PROTOCOL FOR LUNG CANCER SPECIMEN EXAMINATION

Tumor Staging

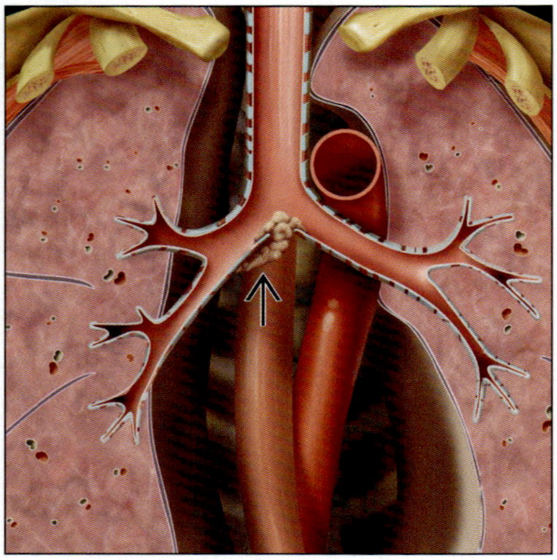
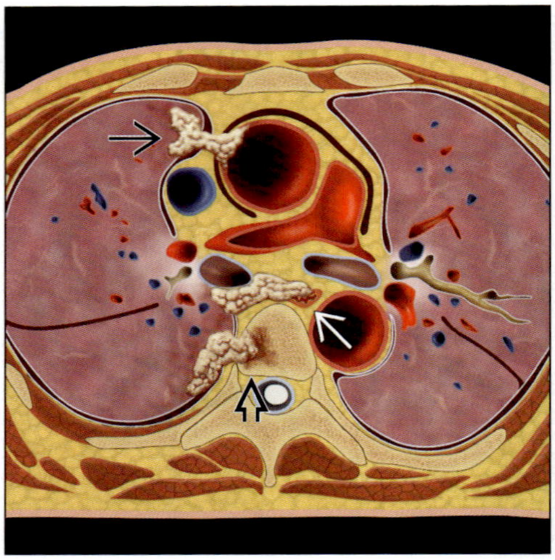

(Left) *Graphic depicts T4 tumor due to involvement of carina →.* ***(Right)*** *Graphic depicts axial view of T4 tumors invading the ascending aorta →, mediastinum and esophagus ➡, and a thoracic vertebral body ⇨.*

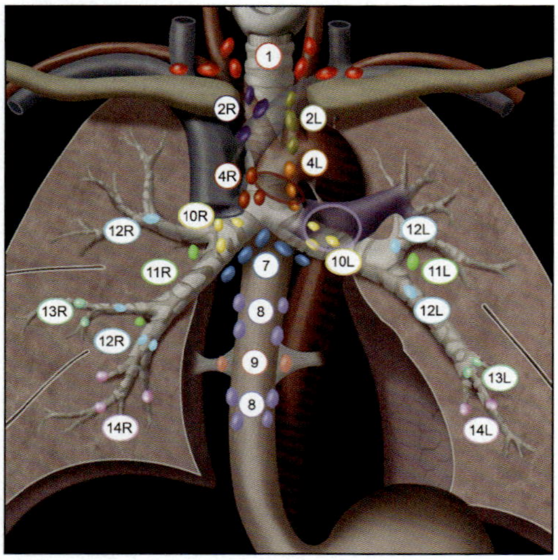

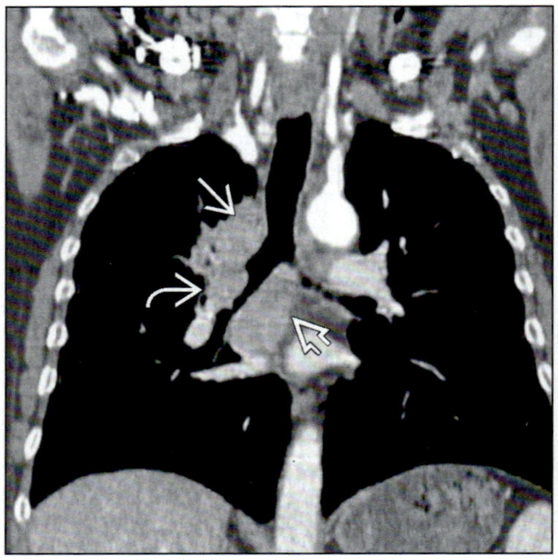

(Left) *IASLC lymph node map: Supraclavicular: 1 low cervical, supraclavicular, and sternal notch nodes; upper zone: 2R and 2L upper paratracheal, 3a prevascular, 3p retrotracheal, 4R and 4L lower paratracheal; AP zone: 5 subaortic, 6 paraaortic; subcarinal: 7 subcarinal; lower zone: 8 paraesophageal, 9 pulmonary ligament; hilar/interlobar zone: 10 hilar, 11 interlobar; peripheral zone: 12 lobar, 13 segmental, 14 subsegmental.* ***(Right)*** *Coronal CT shows subcarinal ⇨, paratracheal ➡, and hilar ↗ adenopathy.*

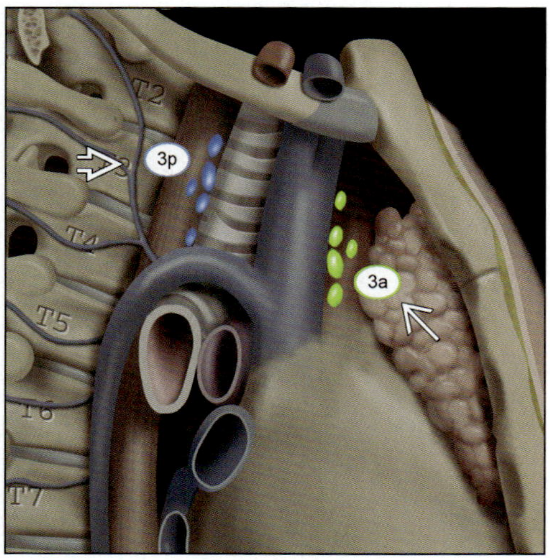

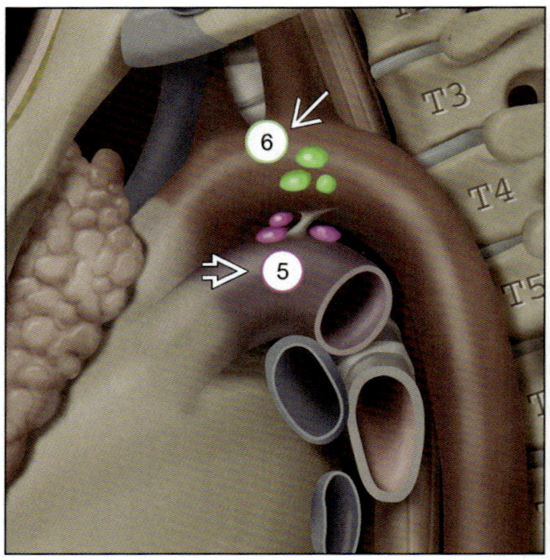

(Left) *Graphic depicts 3a prevascular ➡ and 3p retrotracheal ⇨ nodes.* ***(Right)*** *Graphic depicts AP zone lymph nodes: 5 subaortic ⇨ and 6 paraaortic (ascending aorta or phrenic) ➡.*

METASTATIC CARCINOMA

Metastatic Carcinoma of Colon

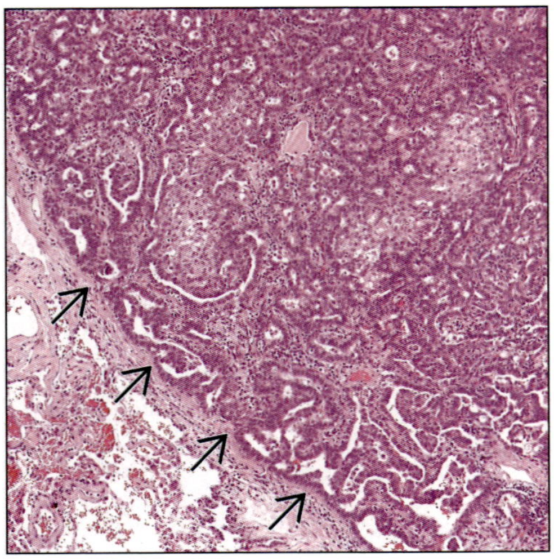

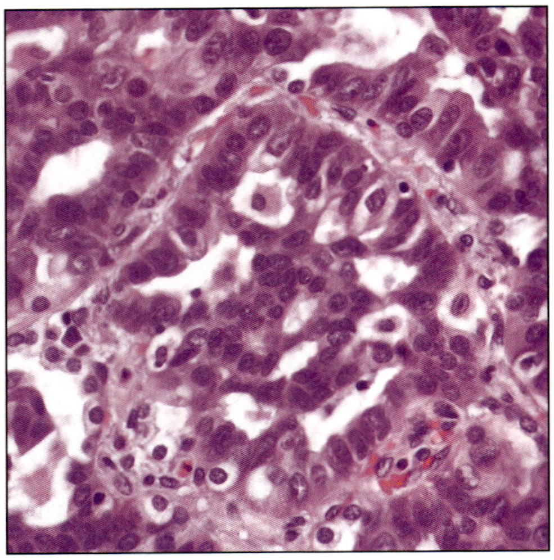

(Left) *Scanning magnification of lung nodule in metastatic carcinoma of the colon shows a well-circumscribed tumor mass with glandular, solid, and cribriform areas. Notice sharp circumscription from the surrounding lung parenchyma* ⇒. ***(Right)*** *Higher magnification of a lung metastasis from a colon adenocarcinoma shows prominent cribriform arrangement of glands, a feature that is often observed in carcinomas of colonic origin but is very unusual in primary lung cancer.*

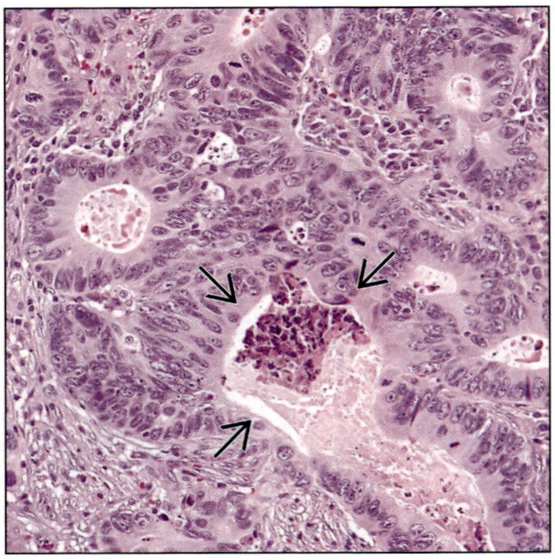

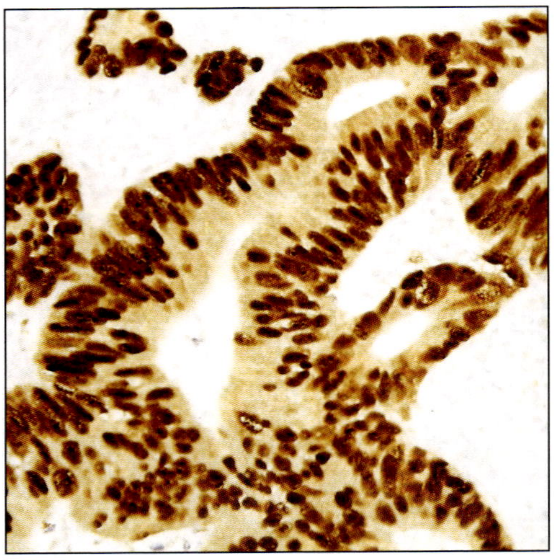

(Left) *Metastasis of colonic adenocarcinoma to the lung shows a focus of "dirty" necrosis in the center of a gland* ⇒. *The necrosis is composed of nuclear debris admixed with inflammatory cells and fibrinous exudate.* ***(Right)*** *Immunohistochemical staining for CDX-2 antibody in metastatic colonic adenocarcinoma shows strong nuclear staining of the tumor cells. CDX-2 is a transcription factor that is highly expressed in colon carcinoma but not in lung cancer.*

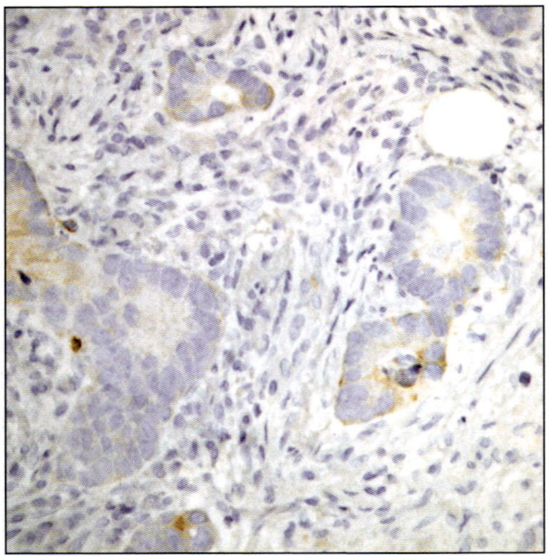

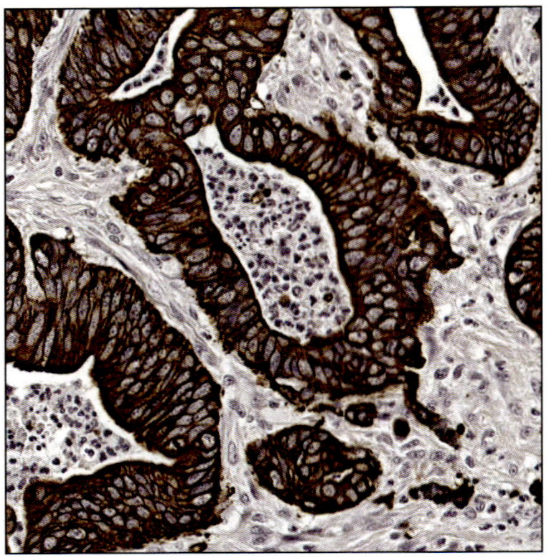

(Left) *Immunohistochemical staining of colon adenocarcinoma metastasis to the lung with TTF-1 antibody shows a negative reaction in the tumor cells. TTF-1 is highly specific and sensitive for primary lung adenocarcinoma.* ***(Right)*** *Immunohistochemical staining of metastatic adenocarcinoma of the colon to the lung with CK20 shows strong positivity in the tumor cells. CK20 is preferentially expressed in colonic adenocarcinoma. Stains for CK7 in the pictured tumor were negative.*

Neoplasms, Metastatic

BENIGN METASTASIZING LEIOMYOMA

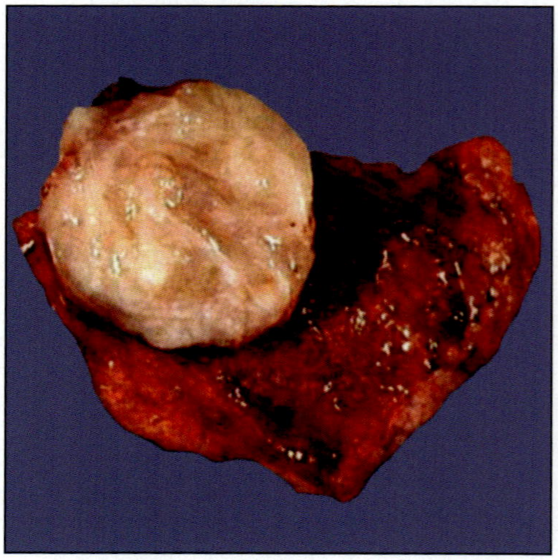

Gross appearance of benign metastasizing leiomyoma of the lung in a 50-year-old woman shows a well-circumscribed, fleshy nodule that bulges above the cut surface.

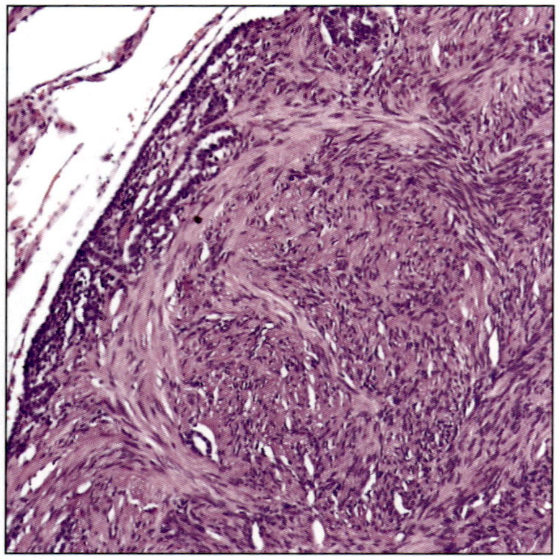

Histologic appearance of benign metastasizing leiomyoma to the lung shows a well-circumscribed nodule composed of fascicles of bland-appearing smooth muscle cells.

TERMINOLOGY

Abbreviations

- Benign metastasizing leiomyoma (BML)

Synonyms

- Adenomyomatous hamartoma

Definitions

- Benign smooth muscle proliferation of the lung arising in women with history of previously resected uterine leiomyoma

ETIOLOGY/PATHOGENESIS

Pathogenesis

- Remote implantation of benign cells released into circulation during surgery
- True metastases from very low-grade, well-differentiated leiomyosarcomas
- Recent studies have demonstrated a clonal origin by molecular-genetic analysis

CLINICAL ISSUES

Epidemiology

- Incidence
  - Very rare condition
- Age
  - 30-50 years of age
- Gender
  - Exclusively observed in women

Site

- No site predilection in the lungs
- Lesions are usually multiple and may be bilateral, suggesting metastatic disease

Presentation

- Mostly asymptomatic and discovered incidentally on chest x-rays

Natural History

- Lesions may regress spontaneously or following hormonal manipulation
- Growth of nodules typically ceases with onset of menopause
- Nodules may be discovered after removal of uterine leiomyomas or concurrent with them

Treatment

- Surgical approaches
  - Nodulectomy or lobectomy, depending on size of lesion
- Hormonal therapy

Prognosis

- Excellent prognosis following surgery

IMAGE FINDINGS

Radiographic Findings

- Lesions are often multiple and can be bilateral
- Lesions may be solitary and present as a "coin lesion"

MACROSCOPIC FEATURES

General Features

- Well-circumscribed, tan-white nodule
- Whorled, homogeneous rubbery tissue that bulges above the cut surface
- No evidence of hemorrhage or necrosis

Size

- Nodules range from small (3 mm diameter) to large (> 5 cm in greatest diameter)

BENIGN METASTASIZING LEIOMYOMA

Key Facts

Clinical Issues
- 30-50 years of age
- Exclusively observed in women
- Lesions are usually multiple and may be bilateral, suggesting metastatic disease

Macroscopic Features
- Well-circumscribed, tan-white nodule

Microscopic Pathology
- Fascicles of monotonous, bland-appearing spindle cells that are sharply separated from the surrounding lung parenchyma
- Lesions may entrap normal respiratory mucosa and airspaces in the vicinity of the lesions (adenomyomatous hamartoma)
- Spindle cells have blunt-ended nuclei showing dispersed chromatin pattern and small or inconspicuous nucleoli
- Spindle cells are surrounded by a scant rim of fibrillary eosinophilic cytoplasm
- No evidence of nuclear pleomorphism, mitoses, or tumor cell necrosis

Ancillary Tests
- Spindle cells are positive for smooth muscle actin (SMA), desmin, calponin, and H-caldesmon
  - Stain positive with Bcl-2 (a feature shared with müllerian-derived smooth muscle)
  - May show expression of estrogen and progesterone receptors

MICROSCOPIC PATHOLOGY

Histologic Features
- Fascicles of monotonous, bland-appearing spindle cells that are sharply separated from the surrounding uninvolved lung parenchyma
- Spindle cell fascicles may appear cut at right angles
- Lesions may entrap normal respiratory mucosa and airspaces at the periphery of the lesions (adenomyomatous hamartoma)

Cytologic Features
- Spindle cells have blunt-ended nuclei showing dispersed chromatin pattern and small or inconspicuous nucleoli
- Spindle cells are surrounded by a scant rim of fibrillary eosinophilic cytoplasm
- No evidence of nuclear pleomorphism, mitoses, or tumor cell necrosis
- Some cases may show prominent areas of stromal fibrosis

ANCILLARY TESTS

Immunohistochemistry
- Spindle cells are positive for smooth muscle actin (SMA), desmin, calponin, and H-caldesmon
  - Negative for other differentiation markers, including cytokeratins, EMA, and S100 protein
  - Stain positive with Bcl-2 (a feature shared with müllerian-derived smooth muscle)
  - Show expression of estrogen and progesterone receptors

Electron Microscopy
- Transmission
  - Spindle cells show basal lamina material, pinocytotic vesicles, and intracytoplasmic microfilaments with focal densities

DIFFERENTIAL DIAGNOSIS

Solitary Fibrous Tumor
- Bland spindle cell proliferation characterized by rope-like linear deposition of stromal collagen within the tumor
- Prominent hemangiopericytic, herringbone, and storiform patterns
- Tumor cells are positive for CD34, CD99, and Bcl-2 and are negative for SMA, desmin, and calponin

Schwannoma
- Bland spindle cell proliferation with focal palisading of nuclei (Verocay bodies) and degenerative stromal changes
- Prominent perivascular hyalinization and cystic/myxoid changes
- Tumor cells are strongly positive for S100 protein and negative for smooth muscle markers

Metastatic Low-Grade Leiomyosarcoma
- Spindle cell proliferation shows mild to moderate cytologic atypia and nuclear pleomorphism
- Low mitotic activity (2-3 mitoses per 10 high-power fields)
- History of leiomyosarcoma of soft tissue or other location is indispensable for definitive diagnosis

SELECTED REFERENCES

1. Nuovo GJ et al: Benign metastasizing leiomyoma of the lung: clinicopathologic, immunohistochemical, and micro-RNA analyses. Diagn Mol Pathol. 17(3):145-50, 2008
2. Rao AV et al: Pulmonary benign metastasizing leiomyoma following hysterectomy: a clinicopathologic correlation. J Thorac Oncol. 3(6):674-6, 2008
3. Nucci MR et al: Distinctive cytogenetic profile in benign metastasizing leiomyoma: pathogenetic implications. Am J Surg Pathol. 31(5):737-43, 2007
4. Patton KT et al: Benign metastasizing leiomyoma: clonality, telomere length and clinicopathologic analysis. Mod Pathol. 19(1):130-40, 2006

BENIGN METASTASIZING LEIOMYOMA

Histologic Features

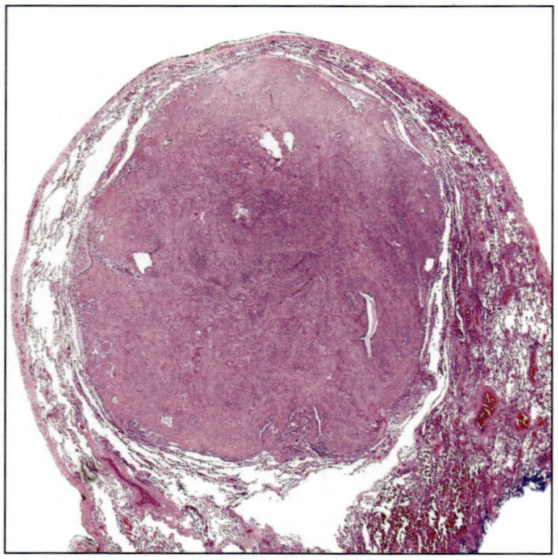

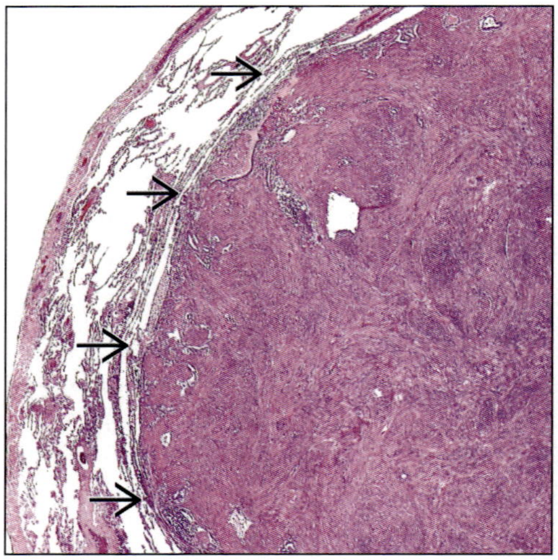

(Left) *Scanning magnification of a small lung nodule with benign metastasizing leiomyoma shows a well-circumscribed intraparenchymatous nodule that is completely surrounded by normal pulmonary parenchyma.* ***(Right)*** *Higher magnification of benign metastasizing leiomyoma of the lung shows a well-circumscribed but unencapsulated tumor nodule → sharply demarcated from the surrounding lung parenchyma. No evidence of hemorrhage or necrosis is identified.*

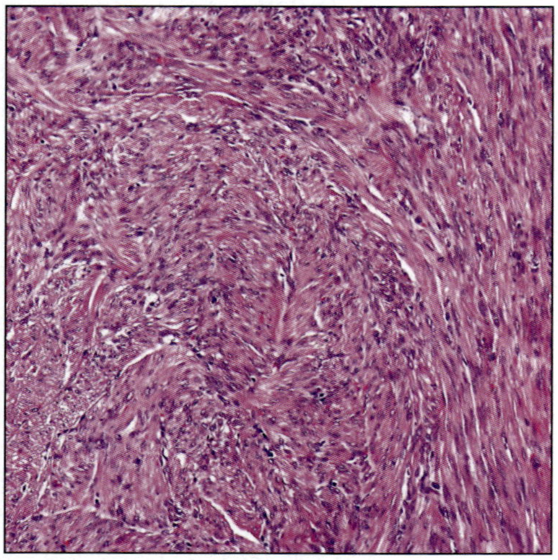

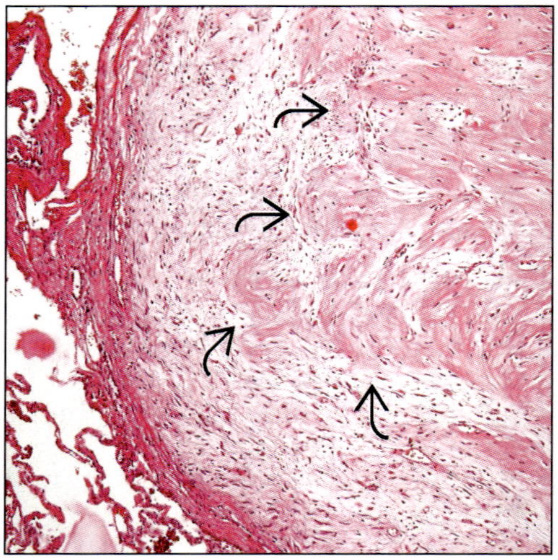

(Left) *Higher magnification of benign metastasizing leiomyoma of the lung shows a bland-appearing spindle cell proliferation displaying a fascicular architecture with fascicles that intersect at right angles.* ***(Right)*** *Benign metastasizing leiomyoma of the lung shows focal myxoid stromal changes and areas of stromal hyalinization →. Occasional cases of benign metastasizing leiomyoma can display such changes, simulating a benign peripheral nerve sheath tumor.*

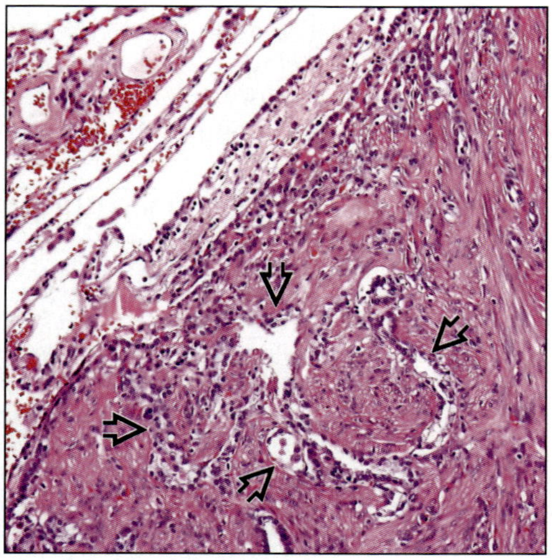

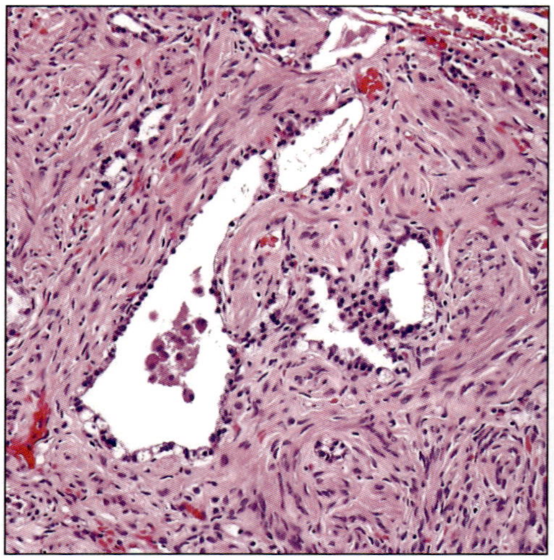

(Left) *Entrapment of glands → is seen at the periphery of this benign metastasizing leiomyoma to the lung. Cases showing these features have been designated as benign metastasizing adenomyoma or adenomyomatous hamartoma.* ***(Right)*** *Higher magnification from benign metastasizing adenomyoma shows entrapped glandular structures. The entrapped glandular epithelial structures are usually distributed along the periphery but may also be located deeper within the lesion.*

Cytologic and Immunohistochemical Features

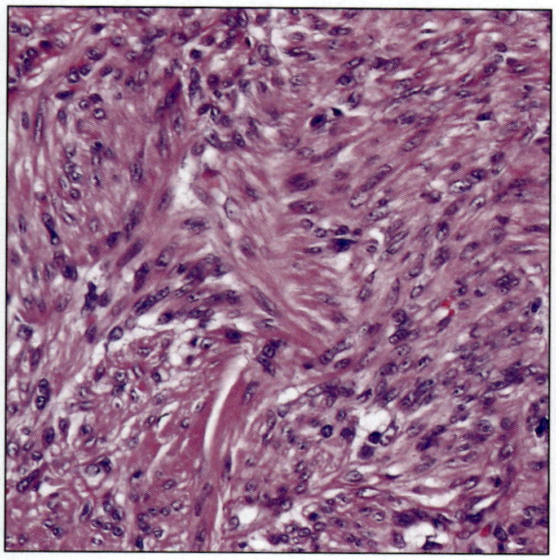

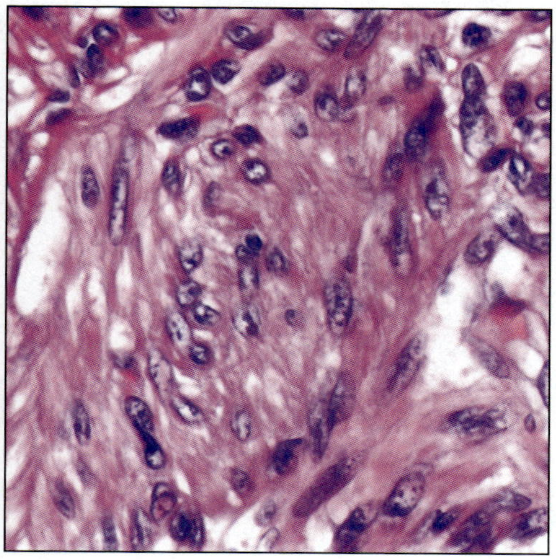

(Left) *Higher magnification of benign metastasizing leiomyoma of the lung shows a fascicular proliferation of bland-appearing spindle cells. The cells are devoid of nuclear pleomorphism, cytologic atypia, or mitotic activity. Presence of any of the above features should prompt consideration of a leiomyosarcoma.* ***(Right)*** *Higher magnification of a benign metastasizing leiomyoma to the lung shows bland-appearing spindle cells with oval to spindle nuclei and fibrillary cytoplasm.*

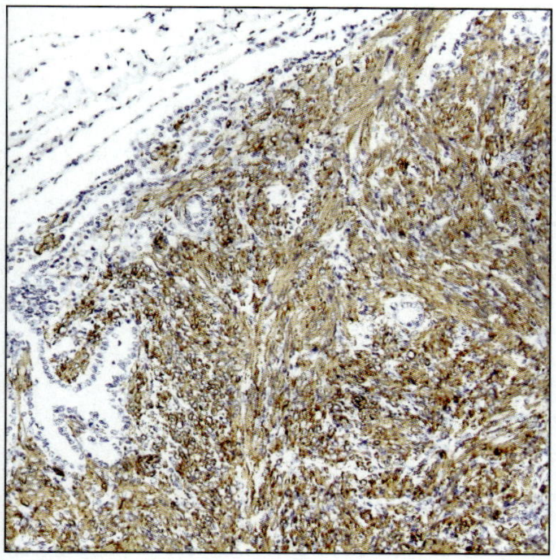

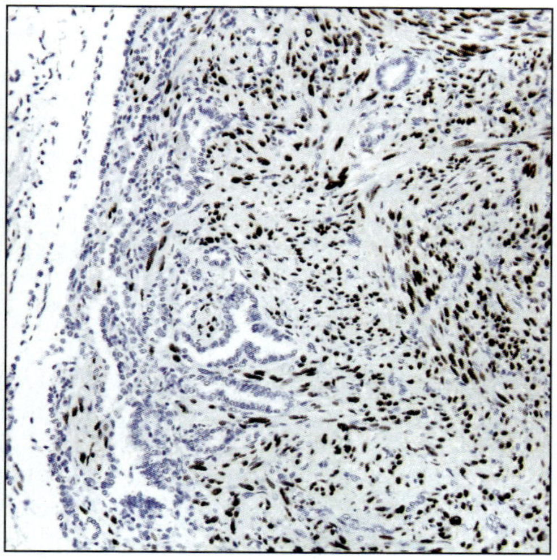

(Left) *Immunohistochemical staining for smooth muscle-specific antigen (SMA) shows strong positivity of the spindle tumor cells in this example of benign metastasizing leiomyoma to the lung.* ***(Right)*** *Immunohistochemical staining for progesterone receptors (PR) in benign metastasizing leiomyoma of the lung shows strong nuclear positivity in the majority of spindle cells. Staining for estrogen and progesterone receptors is a characteristic feature of these tumors.*

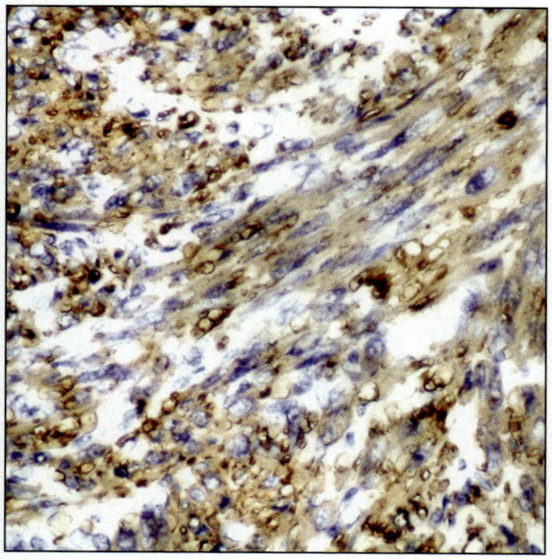

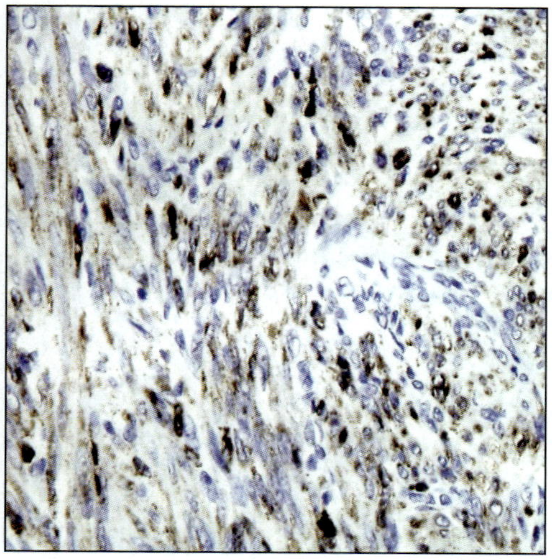

(Left) *Immunohistochemical staining for calponin shows strong cytoplasmic positivity for this antigen in benign metastasizing leiomyoma of the lung.* ***(Right)*** *Immunohistochemical staining for Bcl-2 oncogene shows positive staining for this antigen in many of the spindle tumor cells. Bcl-2 positivity is a feature of müllerian-derived (female genital) smooth muscle neoplasms that is not shared with other types of smooth muscle tumors in which Bcl-2 positivity is quite limited or absent.*

METASTATIC CARCINOMA

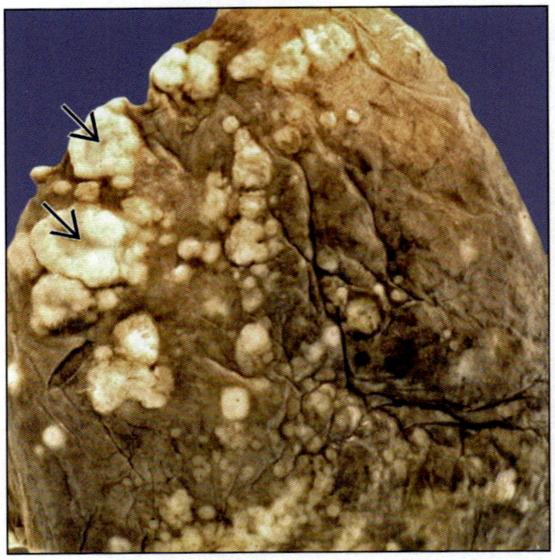

Gross appearance of metastatic adenocarcinoma to the lung shows the pleural surface studded by multiple nodules of varying sizes. Notice central umbilication in some of the tumor nodules ➔.

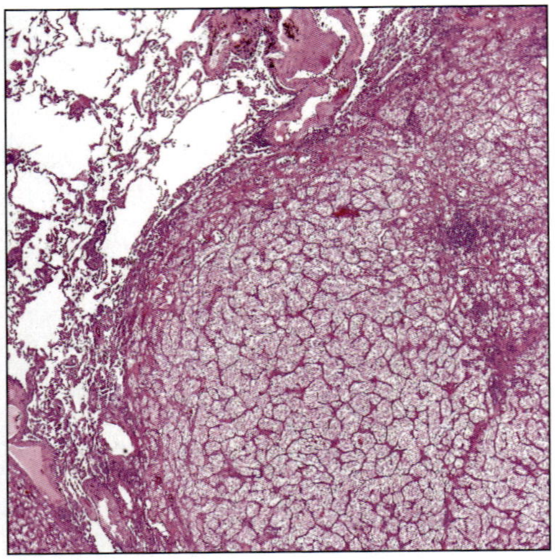

Histologic appearance of a metastasis from a renal cell carcinoma to the lungs shows a well-demarcated nodule composed of nests of large cells with abundant clear cytoplasm.

TERMINOLOGY

Definitions

- Tumor nodules appearing in the lung as a result of spread from another primary site

ETIOLOGY/PATHOGENESIS

Metastatic Models

- Majority of lung metastases occur via hematogenous route by spread through general circulation
- Malignant tumors may also reach the lung through lymphatic dissemination
- Less common mechanism of spread to the lung involves large vessel tumor emboli, especially via the pulmonary artery (liver and renal cancer)

CLINICAL ISSUES

Presentation

- Cough
- Chest pain
- Dyspnea
- Hemoptysis
- Pleural effusion
- Cor pulmonale and pulmonary hypertension
- Most common primary sites: Genital, gastrointestinal and genitourinary tracts, pancreatohepatobiliary tract, head and neck

Treatment

- Surgical approaches
  - Solitary metastatic nodules may respond well to surgical excision
- Adjuvant therapy
  - Chemotherapy and radiation therapy are used for palliation of symptoms in advanced cases

Prognosis

- Generally poor but may vary based on type of tumor, grade, and presence of other metastatic lesions
- Patients with late metastases from low-grade indolent tumors (such as adenoid cystic carcinoma of salivary gland) may have good survival

IMAGE FINDINGS

General Features

- Location
  - Most common locations are lower lobes in subpleural distribution
- Size
  - May vary from microscopic nodules to large nodules > 5 cm in diameter
- Morphology
  - Lesions are most commonly multiple and of varying sizes
  - Solitary "coin" lesion can be present in up to 9% of cases
  - Rounded contour is most likely to be associated with metastasis, as opposed to the "spiculated" appearance of primary lung cancer

CT Findings

- CT is best imaging tool to characterize pattern and spread of disease

MACROSCOPIC FEATURES

General Features

- Multiple bilateral nodules of various sizes, most commonly in peripheral, subpleural areas in lower lobes
- Endobronchial metastases may be polypoid and fill the lumen of the affected bronchus

METASTATIC CARCINOMA

Key Facts

Clinical Issues
- Cough, chest pain, dyspnea, hemoptysis, and pleural effusion are most common presenting symptoms
- Most common primary sites: Genital, gastrointestinal and genitourinary tracts, pancreatohepatobiliary tract, head and neck

Image Findings
- Most common locations are lower lobes in subpleural distribution
- May vary from microscopic nodules to large nodules > 5 cm in diameter
- Lesions are most commonly multiple and of varying sizes
- Solitary "coin" lesion can be present in up to 9% of cases

Macroscopic Features
- Multiple bilateral nodules most commonly in peripheral, subpleural areas of lower lobes

Microscopic Pathology
- Tumor nodule formation composed of glandular or papillary structures, squamous islands, or poorly differentiated sheets of cells
- Bronchioloalveolar (lepidic) pattern of growth with neoplastic cells lining alveolar spaces
- Endobronchial pattern of growth with polypoid tumor mass filling the bronchial lumen
- Miliary pattern of growth with diffuse small (< 0.5 cm) nodules diffusely studding the lung parenchyma
- Lymphangitis carcinomatosa pattern characterized by plugging of peribronchial lymphatics by tumor cells

- Miliary pattern of metastases may resemble miliary tuberculosis
- Pleural nodules show characteristic central umbilication

MICROSCOPIC PATHOLOGY

Histologic Features
- Histologic patterns of growth
  - Tumor nodule formation composed of glandular or papillary structures, squamous islands, or poorly differentiated sheets of cells
  - Bronchioloalveolar (lepidic) pattern of growth with neoplastic cells lining alveolar spaces
  - Endobronchial pattern of growth with polypoid tumor mass filling bronchial lumen
  - Miliary pattern of growth with diffuse small (< 0.5 cm) nodules diffusely studding lung parenchyma
  - Lymphangitis carcinomatosa pattern characterized by microscopic plugging of peribronchial lymphatics by tumor cells

Cytologic Features
- May vary depending on type of tumor and degree of differentiation
  - Cells may be mucinous, clear, oncocytic, granular, signet ring, hobnailed, pleomorphic, or spindled

ANCILLARY TESTS

Immunohistochemistry
- Primary lung carcinomas are usually TTF-1 positive, CK7 positive, and CK20 negative
  - TTF-1 may be negative in up to 40% of pulmonary primary tumors
  - Other tumors can also express CK7, including GI primary tumors, renal cell carcinomas, gynecologic neoplasms, and bladder carcinoma
- Certain specific antibodies can be of value in identifying source of a primary lesion, including
  - PSA and PSAP for prostate cancer
  - CDX-2 for gastrointestinal tract primary cancers (colon, rectum, pancreas, biliary tract, etc.)
  - Hepar-1 (hepatocyte antigen) for hepatocellular carcinoma
  - Thyroglobulin for thyroid carcinoma
  - Renal cell carcinoma (RCC) antigen for renal cell carcinoma
  - Villin surface protein for colorectal cancer
  - WT1 for serous papillary carcinoma of ovary
  - Mammoglobin and estrogen and progesterone receptors for breast cancer

DIFFERENTIAL DIAGNOSIS

Colorectal Carcinoma
- Immunohistochemistry for CDX-2 and CD20 are positive
- Dirty necrosis, mucinous features, and cribriform growth pattern are commonly seen
- Stains for TTF-1 are always negative

Renal Cell Carcinoma
- Sheets and islands of clear cells with abundant cytoplasm
- "Blood lakes" (pools of red blood cells) are commonly present in center of tumor cell islands
- Usually show low-grade nuclear features but may exhibit sarcomatoid features

Pancreatic or Biliary Adenocarcinoma
- Commonly associated with stromal desmoplasia and mucinous features
- Immunohistochemistry is helpful because tumors are negative for TTF-1 and positive for CDX2

Endometrial Adenocarcinoma
- Subnuclear vacuolization, cribriform pattern, and squamoid "morules" are often present
- Tumor cells are positive for ER/PR and negative for TTF-1

METASTATIC CARCINOMA

Immunohistochemistry

Antibody	Reactivity	Staining Pattern	Comment
Primary Lung Carcinoma			
TTF-1	Positive	Nuclear	Positive in > 75% of cases, mostly in adenocarcinoma
CK7	Positive	Cytoplasmic	Positive in 97% of cases
p63	Positive	Nuclear	Positive in squamous cell carcinomas
CK20	Negative	Cytoplasmic	Positive in rare mucinous primaries only
Colorectal Carcinoma			
CK20	Positive	Cytoplasmic	Positive in 89% of cases
CDX-2	Positive	Nuclear	Positive in 91% of cases
TTF-1	Negative	Nuclear	May be positive in 2% of cases
CK7	Negative	Cytoplasmic	May be positive in 13% of cases
Breast Carcinoma			
CK7	Positive	Cytoplasmic	Positive in 93% of cases
TTF-1	Negative	Nuclear	Positive in no cases
ERP	Positive	Nuclear	Positive in 70% of cases; non small cell lung cancer can be positive if 6F11 clone used
CK20	Negative	Cytoplasmic	May be positive in 4% of cases
Thyroid Carcinoma			
TTF-1	Positive	Nuclear	Positive in 98% of cases
CK7	Positive	Cytoplasmic	Positive in 100% of cases
Thyroglobulin	Positive	Cytoplasmic	Positive in 89% of cases
CK20	Negative	Cytoplasmic	Positive in no cases
Renal Cell Carcinoma			
RCC	Positive	Cytoplasmic	Positive in 78% of cases, but very inconsistent antibody
TTF-1	Negative	Nuclear	Positive in no cases
CK7	Negative	Cytoplasmic	May be positive in 15% of cases
CK20	Negative	Cytoplasmic	May be positive in 2% of cases
Prostatic Carcinoma			
PSA	Positive	Cytoplasmic	Positive in 89% of cases
TTF-1	Negative	Nuclear	May be positive in 16% of cases
CK7	Negative	Cytoplasmic	Positive in no cases
CK20	Negative	Cytoplasmic	May be positive in 22% of cases

DIAGNOSTIC CHECKLIST

Clinically Relevant Pathologic Features

- Clinical history of previous tumor elsewhere is indispensable for proper diagnosis
- Comparison of lung lesion with histology of previous tumors is also of critical importance for definitive diagnosis
- Correlation with endoscopic and imaging studies is critical to rule out occult malignancy

Pathologic Interpretation Pearls

- Multiple and bilateral nodules in lower lobes
- Immunohistochemistry is most useful ancillary technique
    - Clinicopathologic correlation should always be carried out regardless of results of immunohistochemical stains

SELECTED REFERENCES

1. Jagirdar J: Application of immunohistochemistry to the diagnosis of primary and metastatic carcinoma to the lung. Arch Pathol Lab Med. 132(3):384-96, 2008
2. Sica G et al: Immunohistochemical expression of estrogen and progesterone receptors in primary pulmonary neuroendocrine tumors. Arch Pathol Lab Med. 132(12):1889-95, 2008
3. Lin X et al: Diagnostic value of CDX-2 and TTF-1 expressions in separating metastatic neuroendocrine neoplasms of unknown origin. Appl Immunohistochem Mol Morphol. 15(4):407-14, 2007
4. Compérat E et al: Variable sensitivity and specificity of TTF-1 antibodies in lung metastatic adenocarcinoma of colorectal origin. Mod Pathol. 18(10):1371-6, 2005
5. Li MK et al: CDX-2, a new marker for adenocarcinoma of gastrointestinal origin. Adv Anat Pathol. 11(2):101-5, 2004
6. Suster S et al: Unusual manifestations of metastatic tumors to the lungs. Semin Diagn Pathol. 12(2):193-206, 1995

Growth Patterns in Lung Metastases

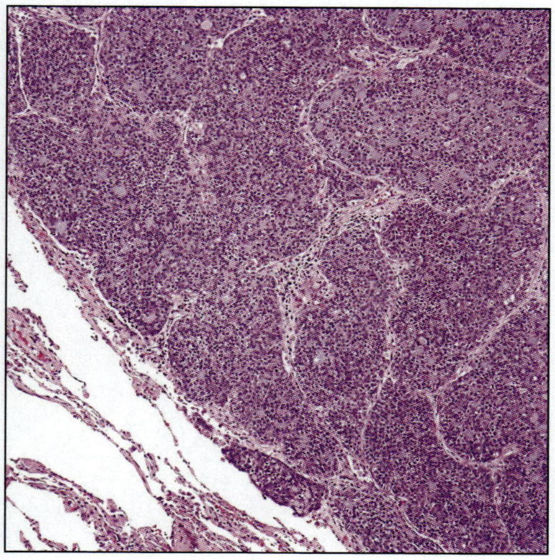

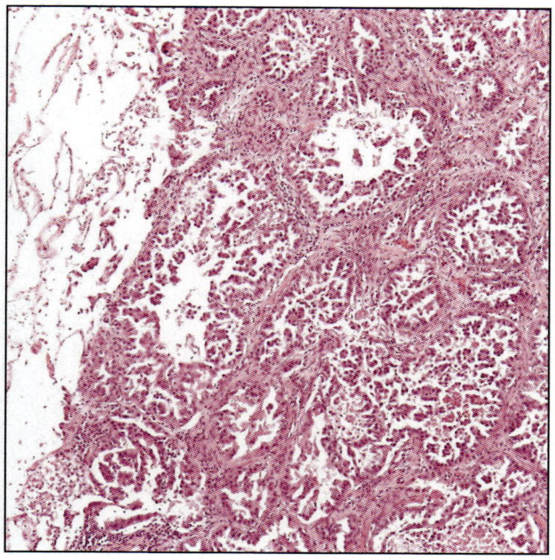

(Left) *Solid pattern of growth in a lung metastasis from a poorly differentiated carcinoma of breast shows irregular islands composed of a compact population of poorly differentiated tumor cells without glandular or other type of differentiation.* ***(Right)*** *Solid pattern of metastasis to the lung from an adenocarcinoma of the ovary shows a papillary pattern of growth. The tumor is sharply demarcated from the surrounding lung parenchyma and contains numerous papillary and micropapillary structures.*

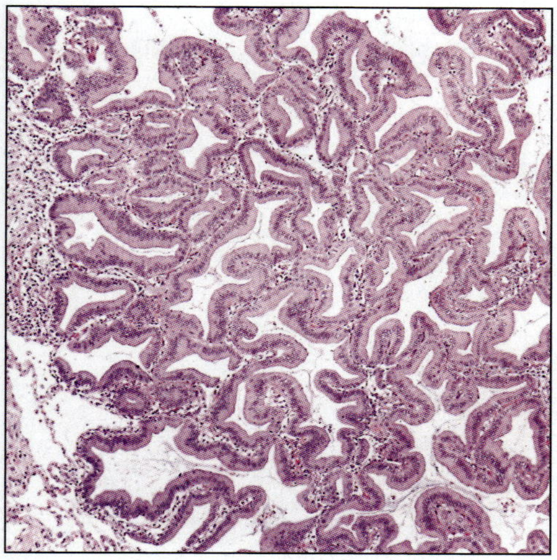

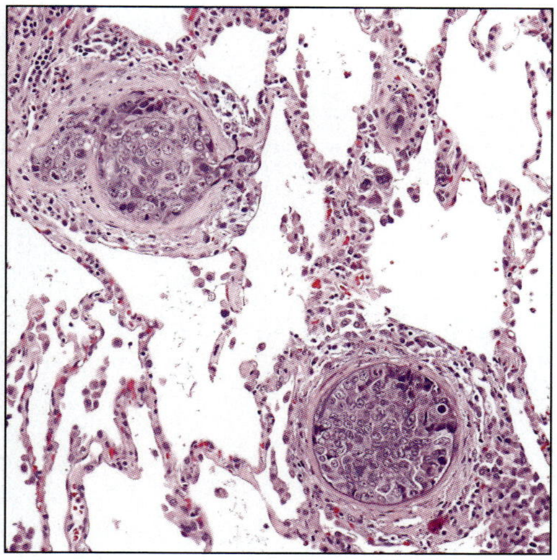

(Left) *Lepidic pattern of growth in metastatic carcinoma of the pancreas to the lung shows mucinous cells extending along the alveolar walls. Tumors with these features can be confused for the mucinous variant of bronchioloalveolar cell carcinoma.* ***(Right)*** *Metastatic carcinoma of breast to the lung with miliary pattern shows microscopic tumor nests scattered throughout lung parenchyma. The clinical and radiologic presentation in these cases resembles that of interstitial lung disease.*

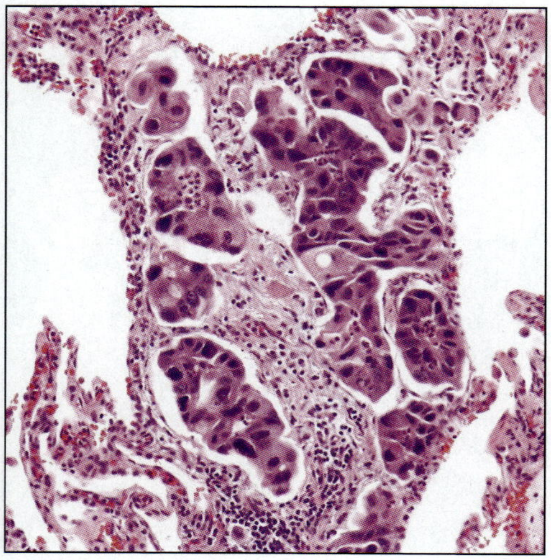

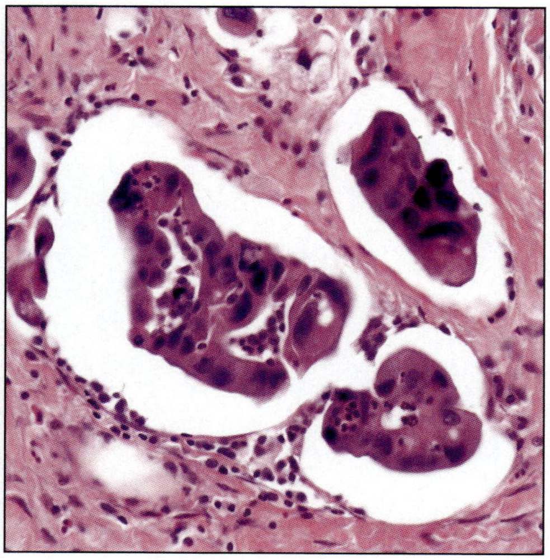

(Left) *Scanning magnification in lymphangitis carcinomatosa shows emboli of tumor cells from ovarian carcinoma distributed along lymphatic routes in the lung. The clinical and radiographic presentation in these cases simulate an interstitial lung process.* ***(Right)*** *High magnification of lymphangitic pattern of spread in metastatic ovarian carcinoma to the lung shows clusters of atypical tumor cells lying free within the lumen of dilated lymphatics.*

Metastatic Carcinoma of Colon

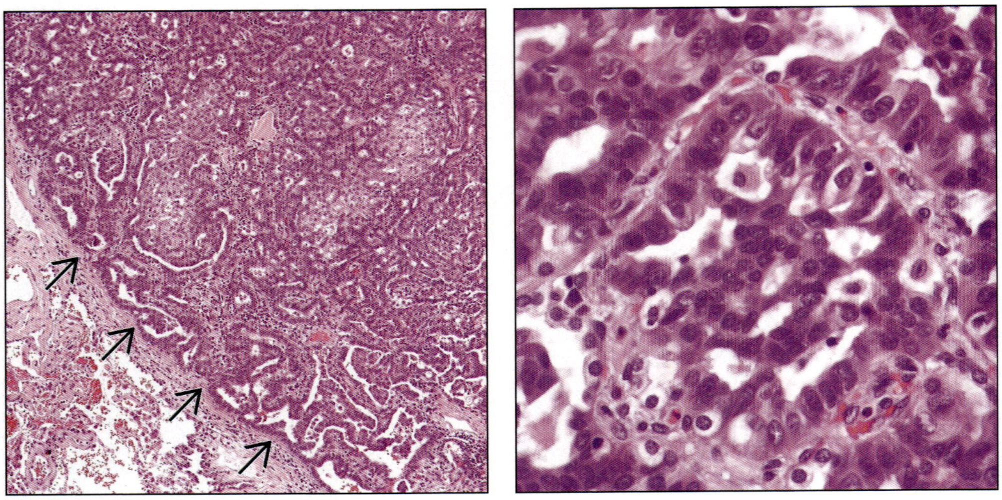

(Left) *Scanning magnification of lung nodule in metastatic carcinoma of the colon shows a well-circumscribed tumor mass with glandular, solid, and cribriform areas. Notice sharp circumscription from the surrounding lung parenchyma* ➔. ***(Right)*** *Higher magnification of a lung metastasis from a colon adenocarcinoma shows prominent cribriform arrangement of glands, a feature that is often observed in carcinomas of colonic origin but is very unusual in primary lung cancer.*

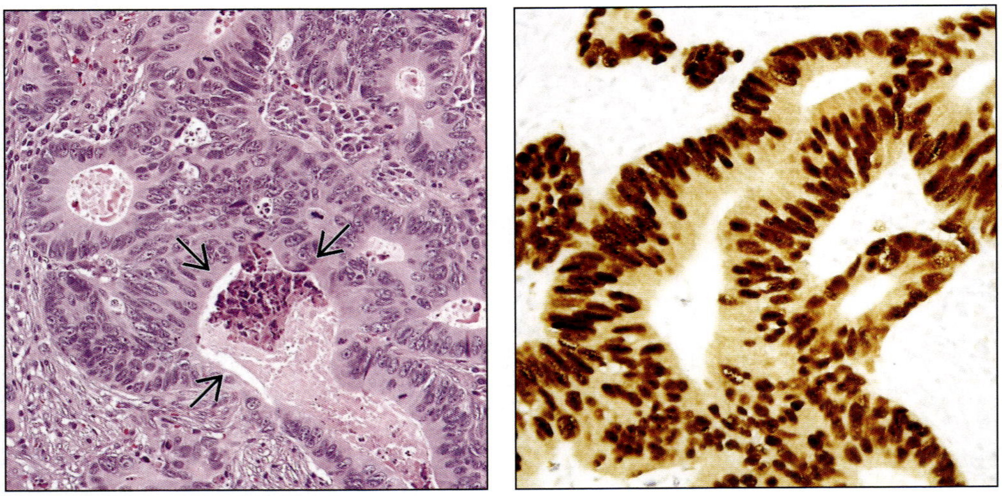

(Left) *Metastasis of colonic adenocarcinoma to the lung shows a focus of "dirty" necrosis in the center of a gland* ➔. *The necrosis is composed of nuclear debris admixed with inflammatory cells and fibrinous exudate.* ***(Right)*** *Immunohistochemical staining for CDX-2 antibody in metastatic colonic adenocarcinoma shows strong nuclear staining of the tumor cells. CDX-2 is a transcription factor that is highly expressed in colon carcinoma but not in lung cancer.*

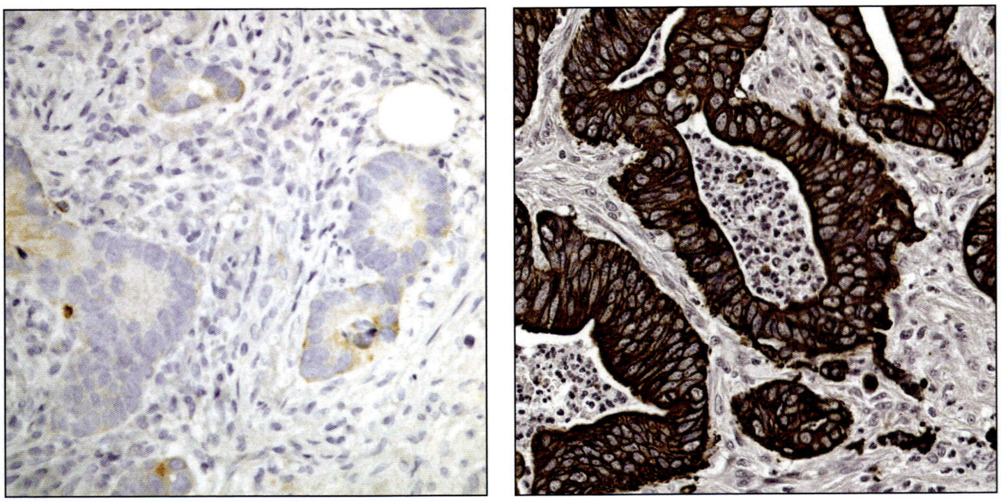

(Left) *Immunohistochemical staining of colon adenocarcinoma metastasis to the lung with TTF-1 antibody shows a negative reaction in the tumor cells. TTF-1 is highly specific and sensitive for primary lung adenocarcinoma.* ***(Right)*** *Immunohistochemical staining of metastatic adenocarcinoma of the colon to the lung with CK20 shows strong positivity in the tumor cells. CK20 is preferentially expressed in colonic adenocarcinoma. Stains for CK7 in the pictured tumor were negative.*

Metastatic Breast Carcinoma

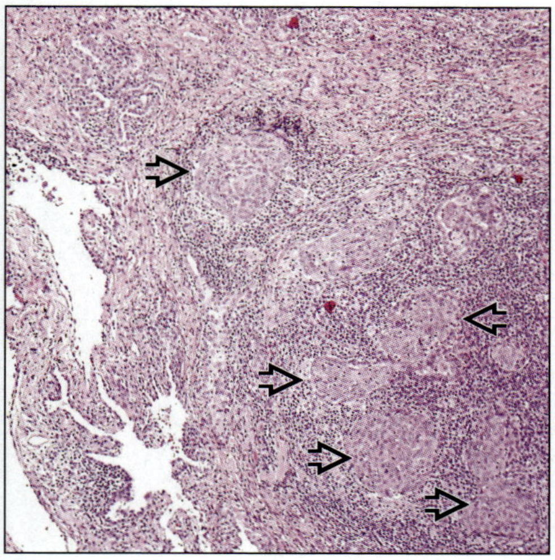

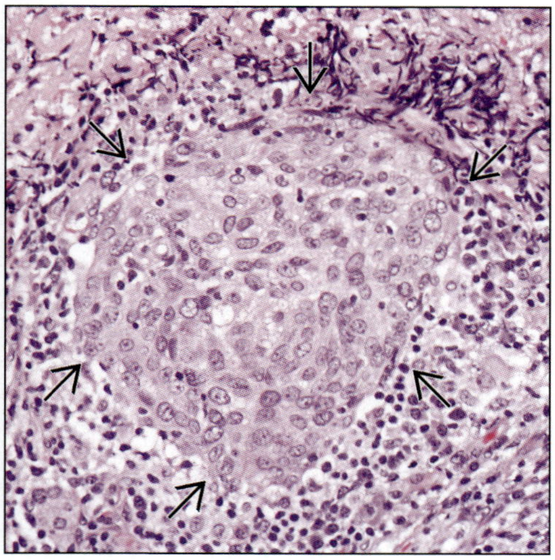

(Left) *Scanning magnification of a lung metastasis from a breast carcinoma shows ill-defined nodules ⇨ adjacent to dilated bronchial spaces that are surrounded by heavy lymphocytic infiltrates.* ***(Right)*** *Higher magnification of a small nodule of a metastatic breast carcinoma to the lung shows a compact population of epithelioid cells → surrounded by dense lymphoid stroma. Evaluation of such cases in the absence of a pertinent history can be extremely difficult.*

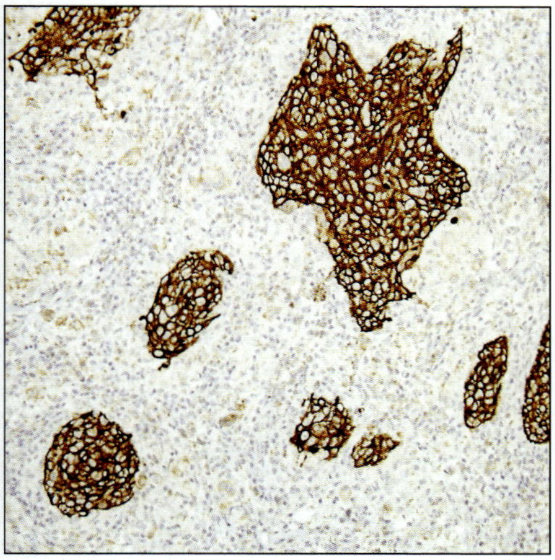

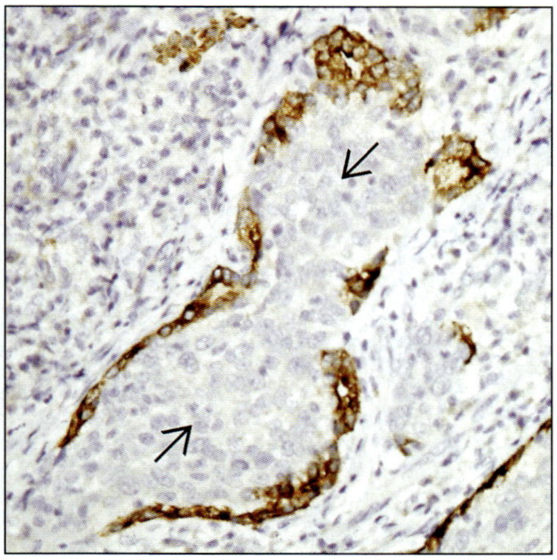

(Left) *Immunohistochemical staining of a metastatic carcinoma of the breast to the lungs with CK5/6 shows strong positivity in the islands of tumor cells. This marker is strongly positive in > 85% of breast cancers.* ***(Right)*** *Immunohistochemical staining for CK7 in a metastatic carcinoma of breast to the lung shows strong positivity of residual entrapped respiratory epithelium surrounding the tumor cell island →. CK20 was also negative in the tumor cells in this case.*

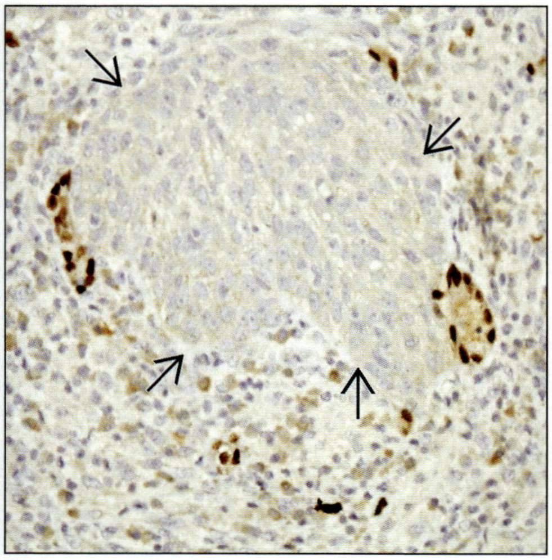

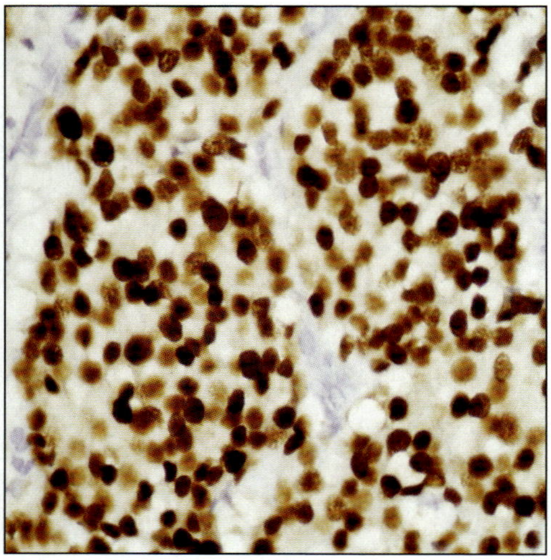

(Left) *Immunohistochemical staining for TTF-1 in metastatic breast cancer to the lung shows strong nuclear positivity in a few small residual airspaces entrapped at the periphery of a metastatic tumor cell island →. TTF-1 is a transcription factor expressed in lung epithelial cells but not in breast cancer.* ***(Right)*** *Immunohistochemical staining of metastatic breast cancer to the lung for estrogen receptors shows strong nuclear positivity for this antibody. The primary tumor was also positive.*

METASTATIC CARCINOMA

Metastatic Renal Cell Carcinoma

(Left) Scanning magnification of lung nodule due to metastatic clear cell renal cell carcinoma shows a sharply demarcated tumor → composed of nests of cells with abundant clear cytoplasm. *(Right)* Higher magnification of metastatic renal cell carcinoma to the lung shows nests of large tumor cells with abundant clear cytoplasm and small hyperchromatic nuclei. Notice "pools" of blood in the center of the tumor cell nests. Intratumoral hemorrhage is a common feature of these tumors.

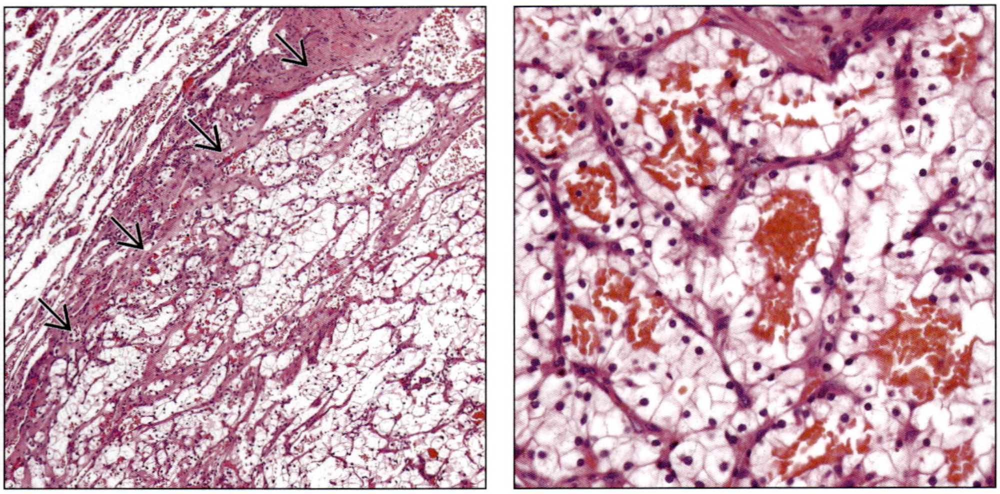

(Left) Immunohistochemical staining of metastatic clear cell renal cell carcinoma to the lung shows strong cytoplasmic positivity for broad-spectrum cytokeratin AE1/AE3. These tumors react with low-molecular weight cytokeratins but are usually negative for CK7 and CK20. *(Right)* Lung metastasis of a renal cell carcinoma shows consistent positivity of the tumor cells for epithelial membrane antigen (EMA). The tumors also react with vimentin, CD10, Pax-2, and Pax-8 antibodies.

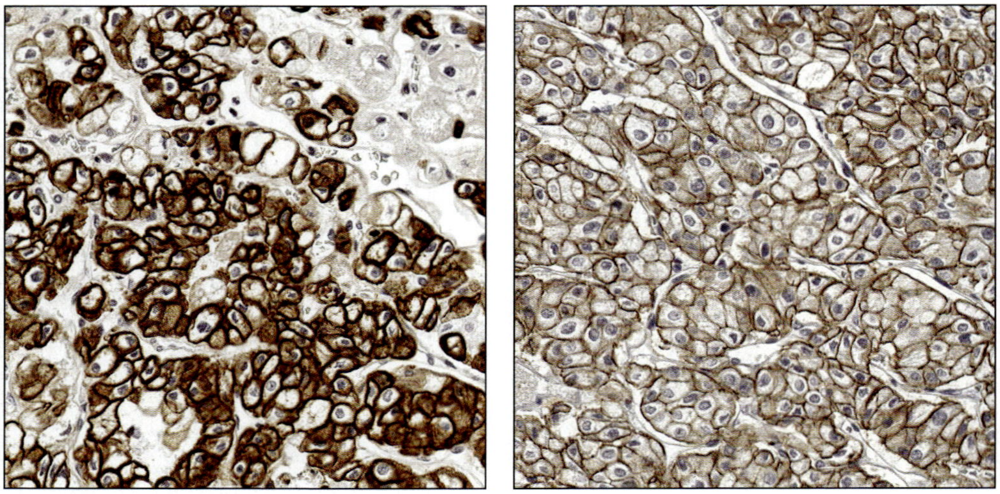

(Left) Metastatic renal cell carcinoma to the lung with sarcomatoid features shows entrapment of residual bronchial cartilage ➢ by pleomorphic and spindle tumor cells. These tumors can be very difficult to distinguish from a spindle cell sarcoma. Identification of cytoplasmic positivity for cytokeratins and a history of previous kidney tumor are indispensable for diagnosis. *(Right)* Pleomorphic and spindle cells are seen in this lung metastasis of sarcomatoid renal cell carcinoma.

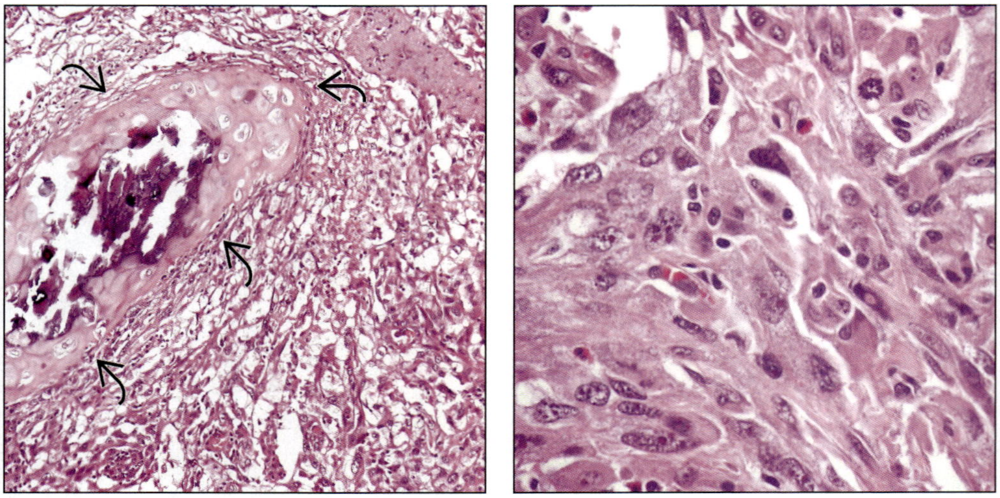

METASTATIC CARCINOMA

Metastatic Papillary Thyroid Carcinoma

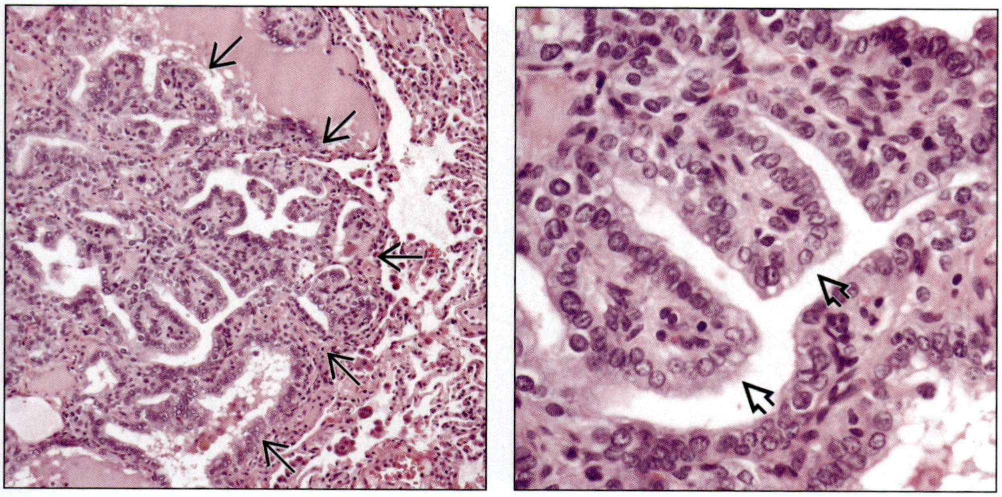

(Left) *Scanning magnification of metastatic papillary thyroid carcinoma to the lung shows proliferation of epithelial cells forming papillary structures* → *separated from the surrounding lung parenchyma.* ***(Right)*** *Higher magnification of a metastasis to the lung of a papillary thyroid carcinoma shows small finger-like papillary structures* ⇨*. The papillae are lined by a single layer of cells with oval to round nuclei with clearing of the nuclear chromatin.*

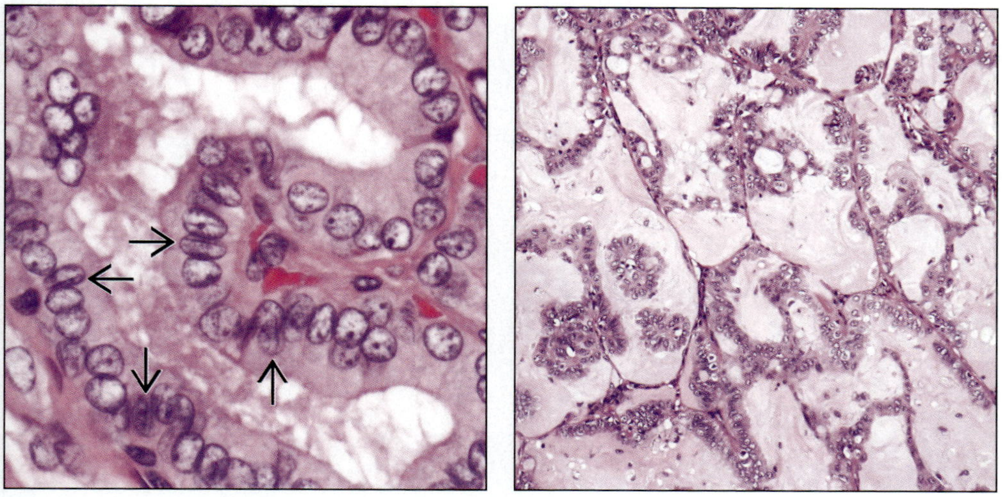

(Left) *Higher magnification of pulmonary metastasis from a papillary thyroid carcinoma shows characteristic nuclear features, including enlargement of nuclei, prominent clearing of the nuclear chromatin with margination to the periphery, and occasional longitudinal nuclear grooves* →*.* ***(Right)*** *Striking lepidic pattern of growth is seen in this pulmonary metastasis of papillary thyroid carcinoma resembling a bronchioloalveolar cell carcinoma.*

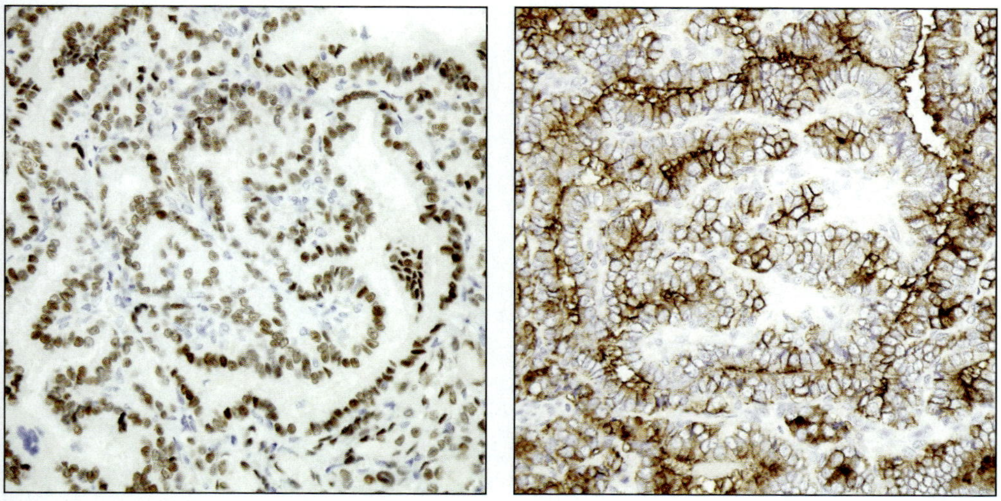

(Left) *Immunohistochemical staining for TTF-1 in a pulmonary metastasis of a papillary thyroid carcinoma shows strong nuclear positivity. This antibody is of limited utility in this diagnostic setting since it will also strongly stain the nuclei of primary pulmonary adenocarcinoma.* ***(Right)*** *Immunohistochemical staining of metastatic papillary thyroid carcinoma (PTC) to the lung with thyroglobulin antibodies shows cytoplasmic positivity in the tumor cells, supporting the diagnosis of PTC.*

METASTATIC CARCINOMA

Metastases from Urogenital Tract

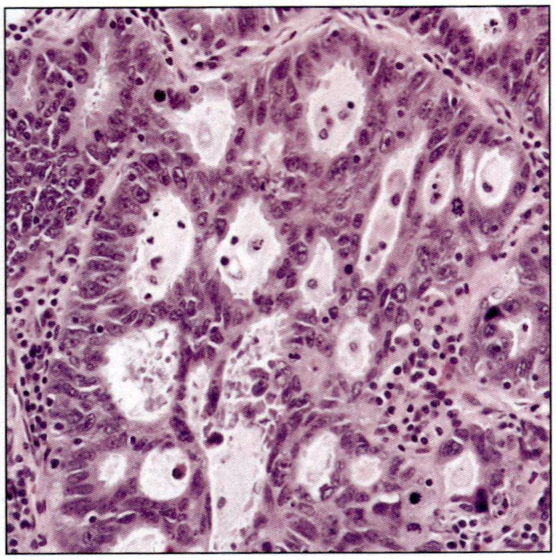

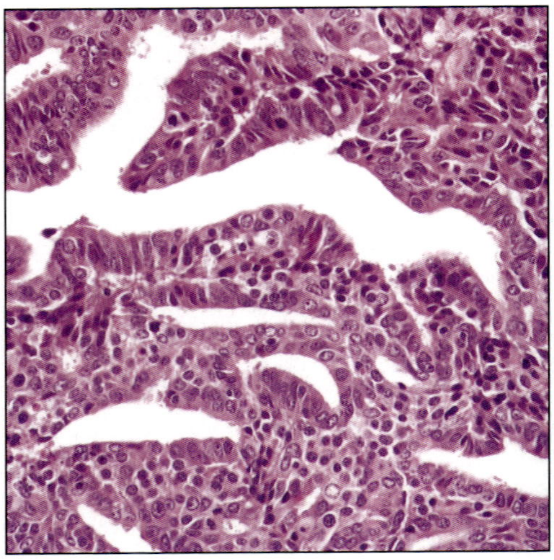

(Left) *Metastatic adenocarcinoma of the endocervix to the lung shows a cribriform pattern of glandular growth. Tumors with these features can resemble primary lung adenocarcinoma; however, they are negative for TTF-1 and show strong nuclear positivity for p16 and monoclonal CEA.* ***(Right)*** *Metastasis of endometrial adenocarcinoma to the lung shows atypical glandular structures separated by inflammatory stroma. These tumors express CK7, ER/PR, and vimentin but are negative for TTF-1.*

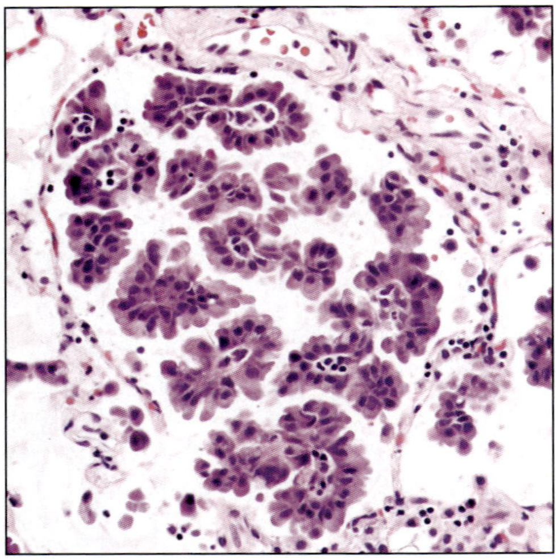

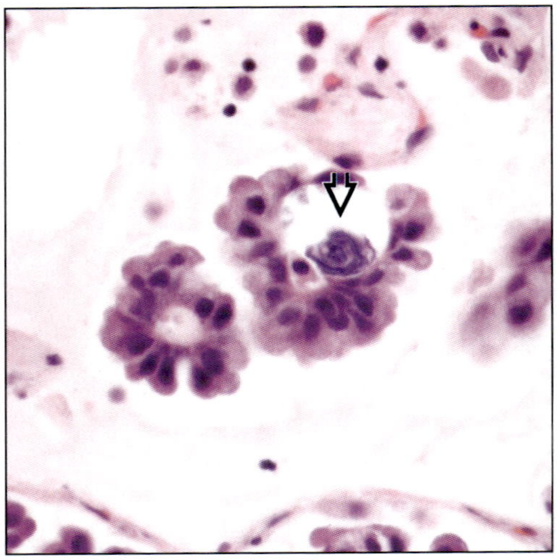

(Left) *Metastasis of serous papillary carcinoma of the ovary to the lung shows papillary structures lying within the lumen of a distended alveolus and lined by atypical cells with hyperchromatic nuclei. These tumors are usually strongly positive for WT1 and also stain for ER/PR antibodies.* ***(Right)*** *Higher magnification in a lung metastasis from a serous papillary carcinoma of the ovary shows micropapillary structures. Notice the psammoma body at the base of the papilla ⇨.*

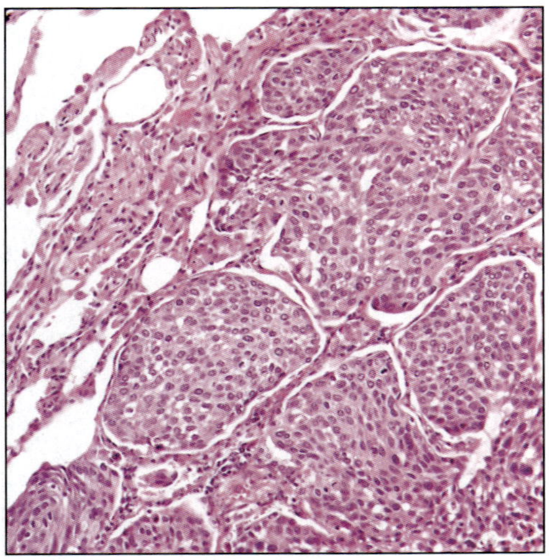

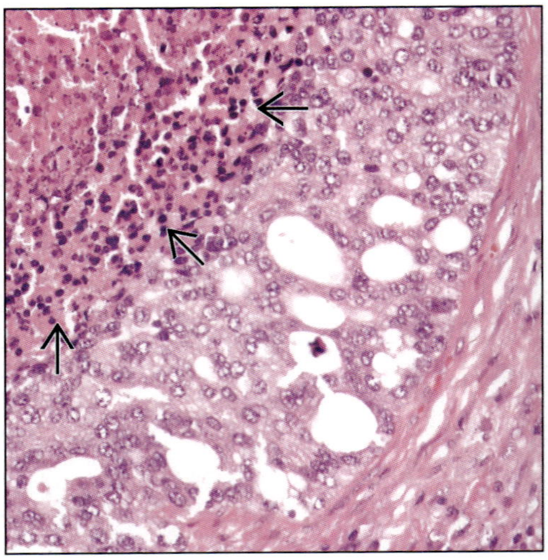

(Left) *Metastases to the lung from a transitional cell carcinoma of the urinary bladder show nests of uniform oval to spindle cells separated from the surrounding pulmonary parenchyma. Most cases of urothelial carcinoma are positive for both CK7 and CK20 and, in about 66% of cases, for uroplakin.* ***(Right)*** *Metastasis of prostate adenocarcinoma to the lung shows a cribriform pattern of growth and central necrosis →. Prostate cancer reacts strongly with PSA, PSAP, and AMACR (P504S) antibodies.*

Other Metastases to the Lung

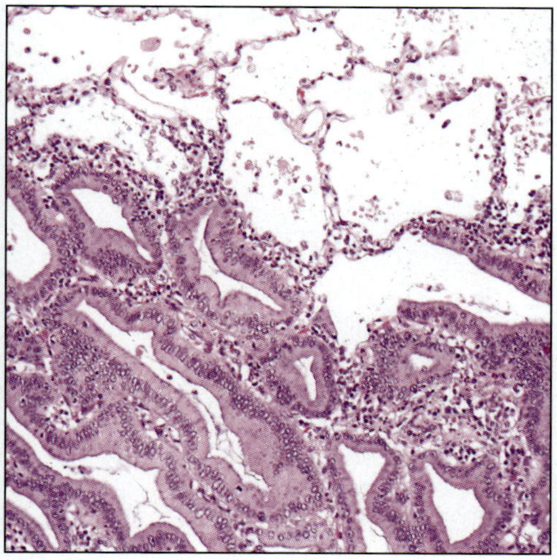

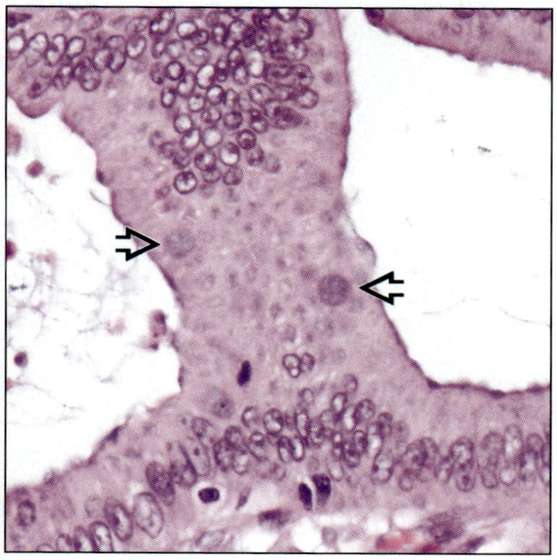

(Left) *Metastatic adenocarcinoma of the pancreas to the lung shows well-differentiated glandular proliferation with tall columnar cells that contain abundant cytoplasm. These tumors can closely resemble well-differentiated lung adenocarcinoma; they are strongly positive for CK7 but lack nuclear expression of TTF-1.* ***(Right)*** *Higher magnification of ductal adenocarcinoma of the pancreas metastatic to the lung shows mucin-secreting cells ⇨ scattered throughout.*

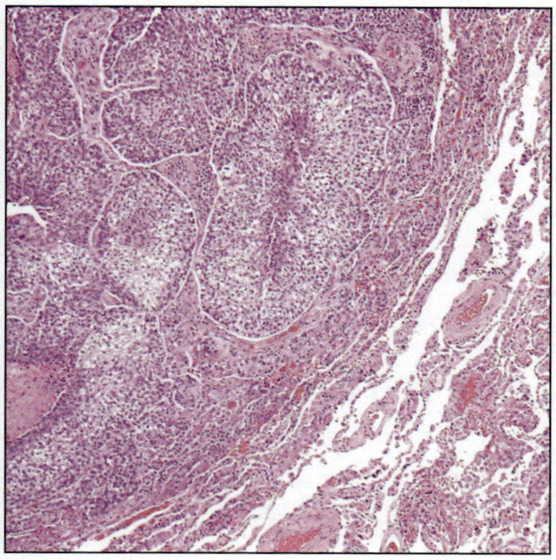

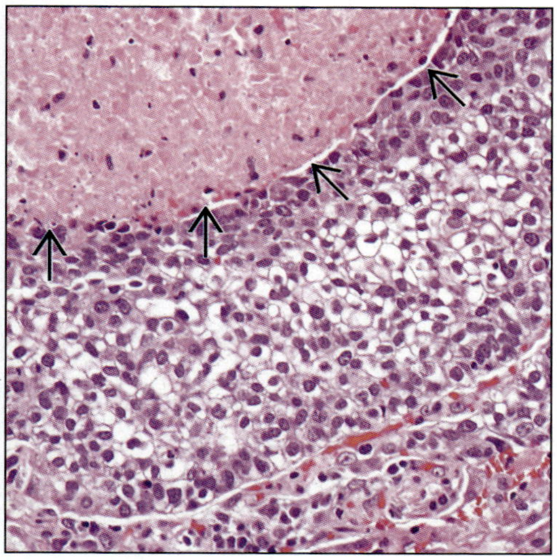

(Left) *Metastasis of squamous cell carcinoma of the larynx to the lung shows islands of large tumor cells with prominent clearing of the cytoplasm. In the absence of a clinical history, it may be impossible to distinguish a solitary metastasis from a primary squamous cell carcinoma of the lung.* ***(Right)*** *Higher magnification of a metastatic squamous cell carcinoma of the larynx to the lung shows poorly differentiated squamous cell islands circumscribing an area of necrosis →.*

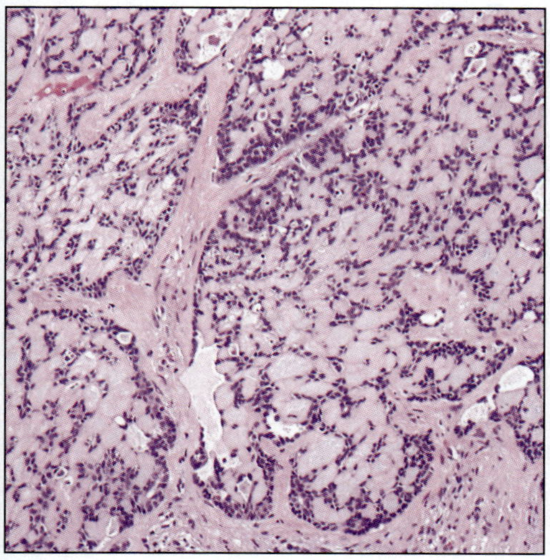

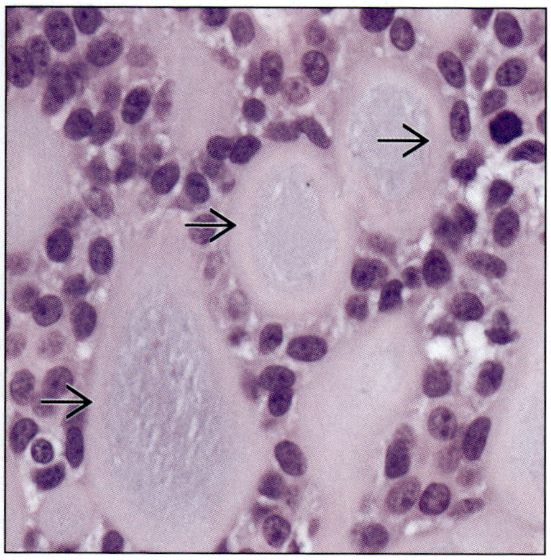

(Left) *Metastatic adenoid cystic carcinoma of the salivary gland to the lung shows strands of epithelial cells with cylindromatous growth pattern. The tumors can metastasize up to 15 years after removal of the primary and may be impossible to separate from a primary salivary gland-type lung tumor. Clinical history is indispensable for diagnosis.* ***(Right)*** *Higher magnification of metastatic adenoid cystic carcinoma shows "cylinders" lined by an eosinophilic rim of basal lamina material →.*

METASTATIC SARCOMA

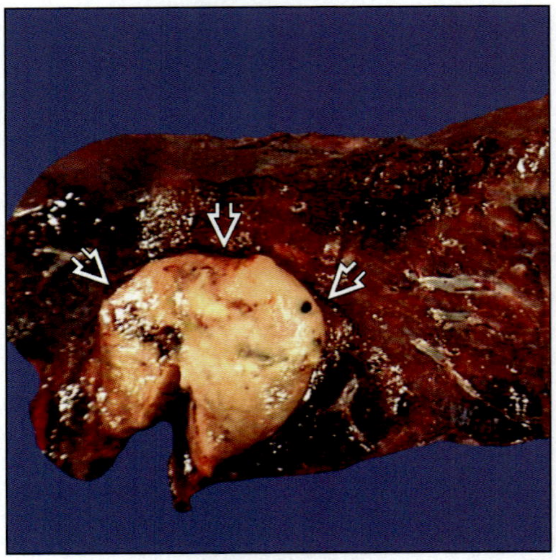

Gross appearance of a metastatic leiomyosarcoma from soft tissue to the lung shows a well-circumscribed, round mass that is sharply separated from the surrounding lung parenchyma ⇨.

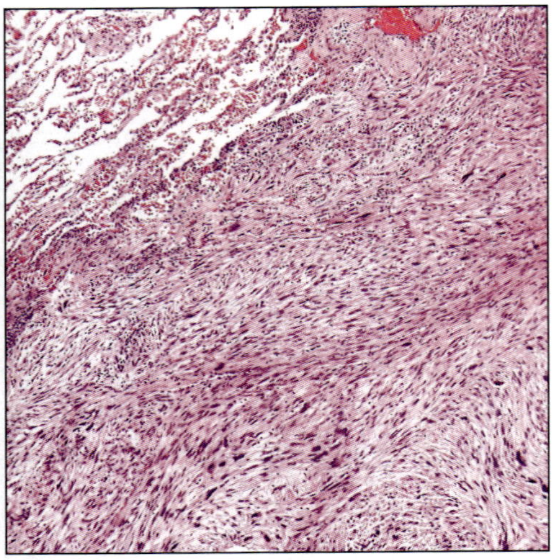

Histologic appearance of metastatic leiomyosarcoma to the lung shows a well-demarcated tumor nodule with fascicles of atypical spindle cells showing marked nuclear pleomorphism.

TERMINOLOGY

Definitions

- Formation of sarcomatous nodules in the lung as a result of hematogenous spread from distant sites

CLINICAL ISSUES

Presentation

- Multiple nodules on chest x-ray
- Cough
- Dyspnea
- Hemoptysis

Natural History

- Lung is most common site of metastases for soft tissue sarcomas from trunk and extremities
- Most common primary source of lung metastasis from soft tissue sarcomas is from lower extremities
- Most common types of metastatic sarcomas to the lung are
  - Leiomyosarcoma (21%)
  - Pleomorphic high-grade sarcoma (malignant fibrous histiocytoma) (18%)
  - Synovial sarcoma (14%)
  - Liposarcoma (12%)

Treatment

- Surgical approaches
  - Surgical excision for solitary or peripheral lesions
  - Adjuvant chemotherapy for multiple and bilateral lesions

Prognosis

- Good prognosis in patients with resectable tumors and in patients with metastases from uterine leiomyosarcoma
- Metastasectomy can double median survival and 3-year survival for patients with metastatic soft tissue sarcoma
- Patient age > 50 years old is adverse prognostic factor

IMAGE FINDINGS

General Features

- Location
  - Usually distributed in lower lobes, bilaterally
- Size
  - Variable size, from microscopic to large masses (> 5 cm in diameter)

CT Findings

- Best imaging tool to characterize the number of tumor nodules, location, and resectability

MACROSCOPIC FEATURES

General Features

- Bilateral nodules, mostly small and interstitial, most commonly in lower lobes
- Gray-white, whorled rubbery tissue that bulges from cut surface
- Can show extensive hemorrhage and necrosis
- May show prominent cystic changes
- Can have myxoid or mucinous cut surface or may be rubbery, like cartilage
- Metastases of osteosarcoma may be gritty and hard

MICROSCOPIC PATHOLOGY

Histologic Features

- May vary depending on type of sarcoma
  - **Spindle cell sarcomas**
    - Fascicles of atypical spindle cells with variable cellularity, pleomorphism, and mitotic activity
    - Most common types: Leiomyosarcoma, myxofibrosarcoma, synovial sarcoma, malignant peripheral nerve sheath tumor, and osteosarcoma

Key Facts

Clinical Issues
- Multiple nodules on chest x-ray
- Cough
- Dyspnea
- Lung is most common site of metastases for soft tissue sarcomas from trunk and extremities
- Good prognosis in patients with resectable tumors and in patients with metastases from uterine leiomyosarcoma

Microscopic Pathology
- **Spindle cell sarcomas**
  - Most common types are leiomyosarcoma, myxofibrosarcoma, synovial sarcoma, osteosarcoma, malignant schwannoma
- **Epithelioid cell sarcomas**
  - Most common types include epithelioid sarcoma, angiosarcoma, alveolar soft parts sarcoma
- **Pleomorphic cell sarcomas**
  - Most common type is pleomorphic high-grade sarcoma (so-called malignant fibrous histiocytoma)
- **Small round blue cell sarcomas**
  - Most common types include rhabdomyosarcoma, Ewing sarcoma/PNET, round cell liposarcoma, small desmoplastic round cell tumor

Ancillary Tests
- Immunohistochemistry is very helpful tool for differential diagnosis
- Most important distinction is between sarcomatoid carcinoma (keratin positive) and true spindle cell sarcoma

- **Epithelioid cell sarcomas**
  - Sheets of large round to polygonal atypical cells with abundant cytoplasm resembling a carcinoma
  - Most common types include epithelioid sarcoma, angiosarcoma, and alveolar soft part sarcoma
- **Pleomorphic cell sarcomas**
  - Sheets of large pleomorphic or anaplastic tumor cells with atypical nuclei and abnormal mitoses
  - Most common type is pleomorphic high-grade sarcoma (so-called malignant fibrous histiocytoma)
- **Small round blue cell sarcomas**
  - Sheets of atypical, undifferentiated small round blue cells
  - Most common types include rhabdomyosarcoma, Ewing sarcoma/PNET, small desmoplastic round cell tumor, and round cell liposarcoma

ANCILLARY TESTS

Immunohistochemistry
- Very helpful tool for differential diagnosis
- Most important distinction is between sarcomatoid carcinoma (keratin positive) and a true spindle cell sarcoma
- Specific antibodies may be of value for further subtyping of tumor and defining cell lineage

Cytogenetics
- Chromosomal translocations can be associated with specific types of sarcomas, i.e., t(x;18) in synovial sarcoma

Molecular Genetics
- Specific chimeric fusion products resulting from genetic translocations can be detected using molecular techniques
  - FISH and PCR can be used to detect the *EWSR-1* fusion product in Ewing sarcoma or the *SYT-SXX* fusion product in synovial sarcoma

DIFFERENTIAL DIAGNOSIS

Metastatic Malignant Melanoma
- Can resemble a sarcoma due to mixed spindle and epithelioid cell morphology
- Prominent "nesting" pattern, intracellular melanin pigment, and large eosinophilic nucleoli are characteristic
- Tumor cells react strongly with S100 protein and melanocytic-associated markers (HMB-45, Melan-A, tyrosinase, and MiTF)

Primary Lung Sarcoma
- Any type of soft tissue sarcoma can arise as a primary in lung; however, this is an extremely rare event
- Thorough clinical history to rule out possibility of late or occult metastasis from soft tissue site is indispensable for diagnosis

Sarcomatoid (Spindle Cell) Carcinoma of Lung
- Sheets of pleomorphic and atypical spindle cells, usually in association with preexisting adenocarcinoma or squamous cell carcinoma
- Extensive sampling is recommended to identify well-differentiated adenocarcinoma or squamous cell carcinoma component
- Spindle cells are strongly positive for epithelial markers (cytokeratins, EMA, MOC31, etc.)

Pulmonary Carcinosarcoma
- Biphasic malignant neoplasm composed of a true malignant epithelial component (squamous or adenocarcinoma) and true sarcoma component
- Epithelial component must stain with epithelial markers or show ultrastructural features of epithelial differentiation
- Sarcomatous component must resemble well-defined types of sarcomas or be devoid of reactivity for epithelial markers

METASTATIC SARCOMA

Immunohistochemistry

Antibody	Reactivity	Staining Pattern	Comment
Metastatic Leiomyosarcoma			
SMAD4	Positive	Cytoplasmic	Should stain strongly and diffusely
Desmin	Positive	Cytoplasmic	May be present in only 50-60% of cases
CK-PAN	Negative	Cytoplasmic	May be positive focally in a small percentage of cases
EMA	Negative	Cell membrane & cytoplasm	May be positive in a small percentage of cases
Metastatic Synovial Sarcoma			
CK-PAN	Positive	Cytoplasmic	Usually only focal, weak positivity in scattered cells
EMA	Positive	Cell membrane & cytoplasm	Usually only focal positivity
Bcl-2	Positive	Cytoplasmic	Usually strong and diffuse positivity in majority of tumor cells
CD99	Positive	Cytoplasmic	Present at least focally in > 75% of cases
Metastatic Epithelioid Sarcoma			
CK-PAN	Positive	Cytoplasmic	Strongly positive in all cases
Vimentin	Positive	Cytoplasmic	Strongly positive in all cases
CD34	Positive	Cytoplasmic	Positive in about 50% of cases
Ewing Sarcoma/PNET			
CD99	Positive	Cell membrane	Diffusely positive in all cases
FLI-1	Positive	Nuclear	Positive in about 70% of cases
CK-PAN	Negative	Not applicable	May be present focally in a small number of cases
Metastatic Epithelioid Angiosarcoma			
CD31	Positive	Cell membrane & cytoplasm	Most specific and sensitive marker for angiosarcoma
CD34	Positive	Cytoplasmic	Sensitive but relatively nonspecific marker
CK-PAN	Positive	Cytoplasmic	Cytokeratins may be positive in a high percentage of epithelioid vascular neoplasms
TTF-1	Negative	Not applicable	
Metastatic Endometrial Stromal Sarcoma			
CD10	Positive	Cytoplasmic	Diffuse CD10 positivity in absence of reactivity for H-caldesmon or desmin is characteristic
ERP	Positive	Nuclear	ER/PR positivity is seen in all cases
PRP	Positive	Nuclear	
CK-PAN	Negative	Not applicable	Focal keratin positivity may be seen in rare cases

Pulmonary Blastoma

- Biphasic malignant neoplasm with epithelial component resembling fetal lung and spindle cell sarcomatous component
- Epithelial component is positive for cytokeratin and TTF-1
- Sarcomatous component stains as specific subtype of sarcoma or is composed of primitive spindle cell sarcoma, NOS

DIAGNOSTIC CHECKLIST

Clinically Relevant Pathologic Features

- Metastatic sarcomas to the lung are much more frequent than primary lung sarcomas
- Obtaining prior history of soft tissue sarcoma elsewhere is most important step for establishing diagnosis of metastasis

Pathologic Interpretation Pearls

- Metastases of soft tissue sarcomas to the lungs can change their morphology at the metastatic site
- Clinicopathologic correlation is most important step for establishing correct diagnosis

SELECTED REFERENCES

1. Kaifi JT et al: Indications and approach to surgical resection of lung metastases. J Surg Oncol. 102(2):187-95, 2010
2. Nishiyama N et al: Lung metastases from various malignancies combined with primary lung cancer. Gen Thorac Cardiovasc Surg. 58(10):538-41, 2010
3. García Franco CE et al: Long-term results after resection for soft tissue sarcoma pulmonary metastases. Interact Cardiovasc Thorac Surg. 9(2):223-6, 2009
4. Absalon MJ et al: Pulmonary nodules discovered during the initial evaluation of pediatric patients with bone and soft-tissue sarcoma. Pediatr Blood Cancer. 50(6):1147-53, 2008
5. Pfannschmidt J et al: Pulmonary metastasectomy in patients with soft tissue sarcomas: experiences in 50 patients. Thorac Cardiovasc Surg. 54(7):489-92, 2006

METASTATIC SARCOMA

Spindle Cell Sarcomas

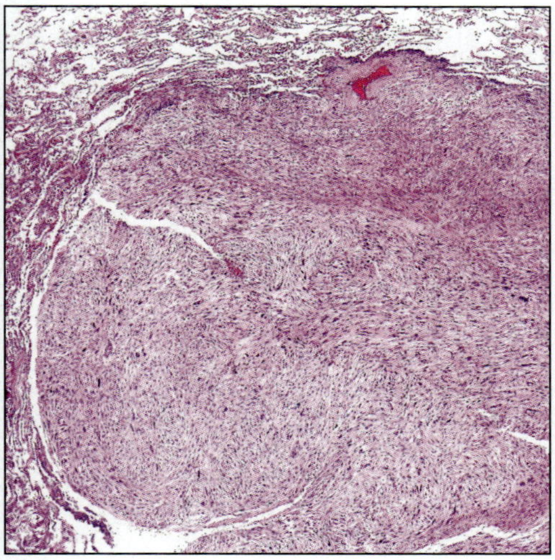

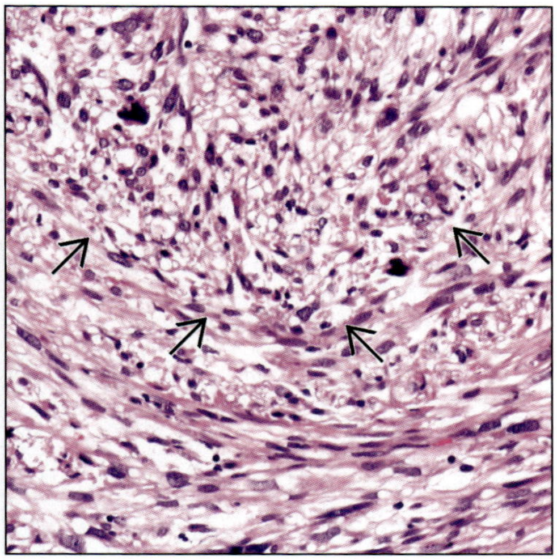

***(Left)** Scanning magnification of metastasis of uterine leiomyosarcoma to the lung shows a well-circumscribed nodule composed of atypical spindle cell proliferation that is sharply separated from the surrounding pulmonary parenchyma.* ***(Right)** Higher magnification of pulmonary metastasis of uterine leiomyosarcoma shows fascicles of atypical cells that are cut at right angles resulting in some of the cells appearing round → while others (below) appear spindled.*

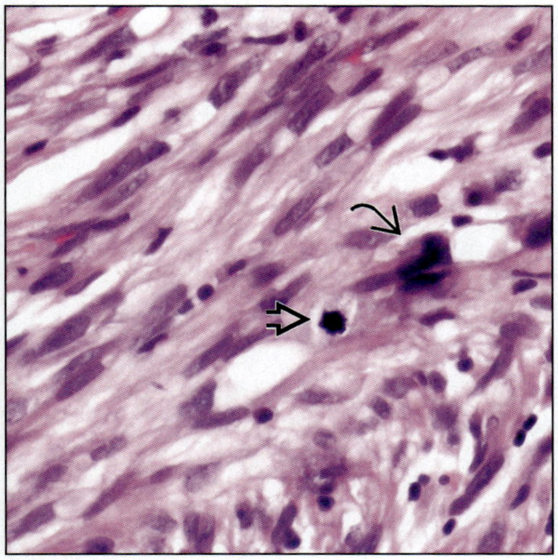

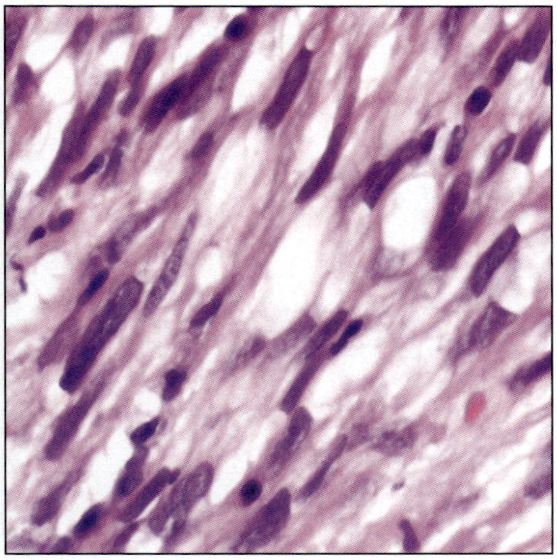

***(Left)** Higher magnification of pulmonary metastasis of uterine leiomyosarcoma shows a bizarre tumor cell → and mitotic figure →. The tumor cells reacted strongly with antibodies for smooth muscle actin, smooth muscle myosin, and desmin.* ***(Right)** Higher magnification of metastatic uterine leiomyosarcoma to the lung shows another characteristic feature of these tumors: The nuclei are cigar-shaped and display blunted ends rather than the tapered ends seen in other types of sarcomas.*

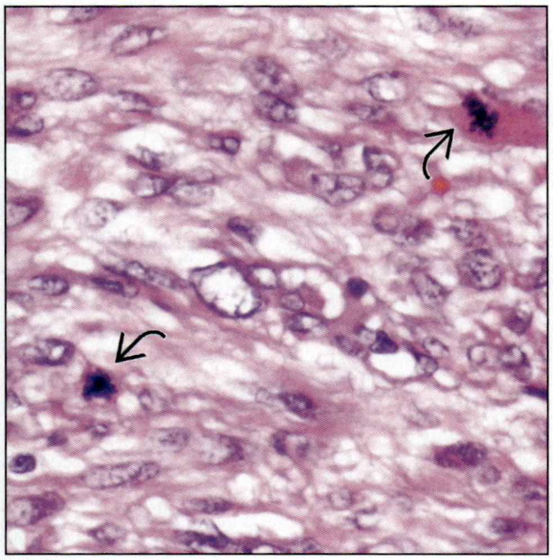

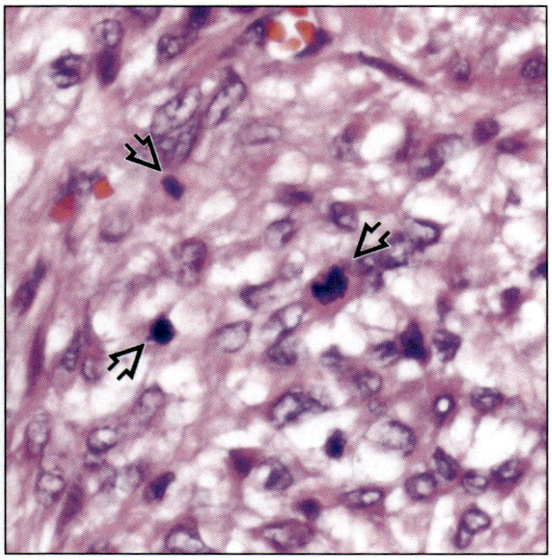

***(Left)** Metastasis to the lung from leiomyosarcoma of soft tissue (thigh) shows a population of atypical tumor cells with pleomorphic and vesicular nuclei and scattered mitotic figures →.* ***(Right)** Metastasis of leiomyosarcoma of soft tissue to the lung shows high mitotic activity admixed with a population of atypical spindle cells. This high-power field contains 3 mitotic figures →. The tumor also showed extensive areas of tumor necrosis and areas with nuclear pleomorphism.*

METASTATIC SARCOMA

Metastatic Osteosarcoma

(Left) *Scanning magnification of intrapulmonary metastasis from osteosarcoma of the femur shows a well-circumscribed nodule* → *surrounded by normal lung parenchyma and containing abundant osteoid matrix.* ***(Right)*** *High magnification of metastasis of osteosarcoma to the lung shows abundant osteoid matrix circumscribing a focus of stromal spindle cell proliferation* →*. Not all metastases from osteosarcoma are well-differentiated and show obvious osteoid matrix as this one does.*

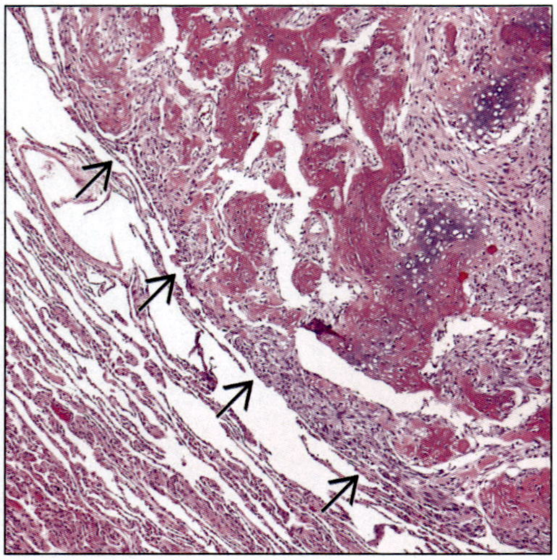

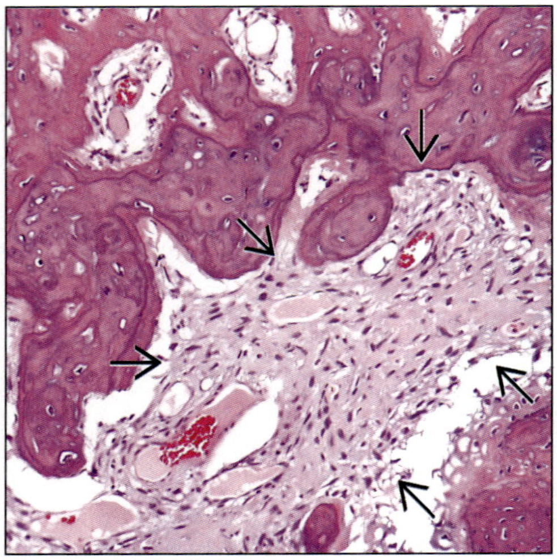

(Left) *Endobronchial metastasis from osteosarcoma of the tibia shows a polypoid tumor mass protruding into the lumen of the bronchus* →*.* ***(Right)*** *Scanning magnification from the wall of the bronchus shows atypical spindle cell proliferation containing thin, irregular strands of immature osteoid matrix* ↗*. Benign osseous metaplasia can occasionally occur in a variety of other sarcomas and must be distinguished from osteoid matrix in osteosarcoma.*

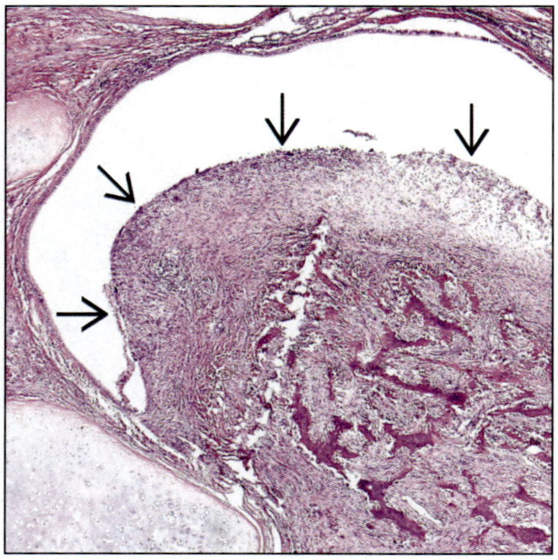

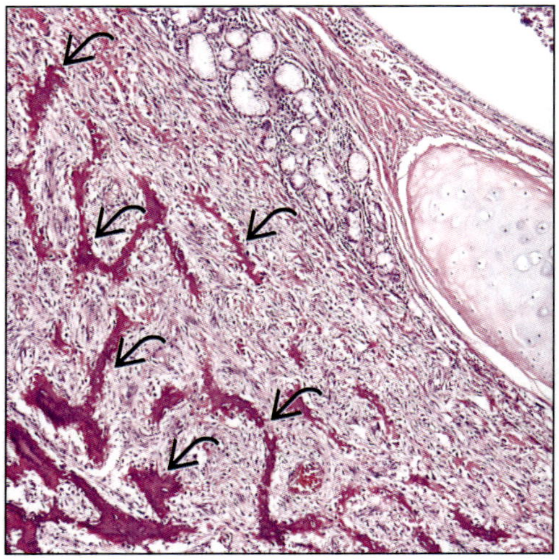

(Left) *Higher magnification from a metastasis of osteosarcoma to the lung shows an immature osteoid matrix surrounded by atypical spindle cell population embedded in abundant collagenous stroma.* ***(Right)*** *High magnification from metastatic osteosarcoma to the lung shows a small focus of osteoid* ⇨*. The surrounding connective tissue stroma shows a sparse spindle cell population with cytologic atypia. Scattered mitoses were noted in other areas of the tumor.*

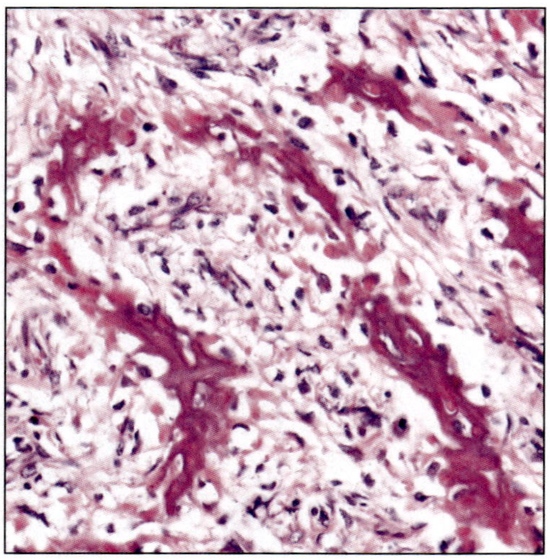

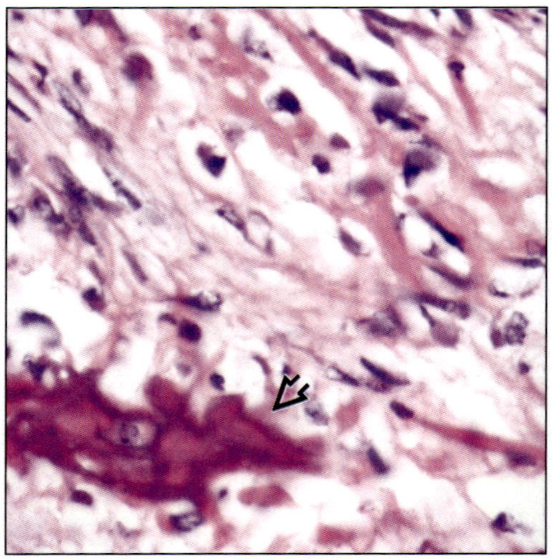

Metastases of Epithelioid Sarcomas

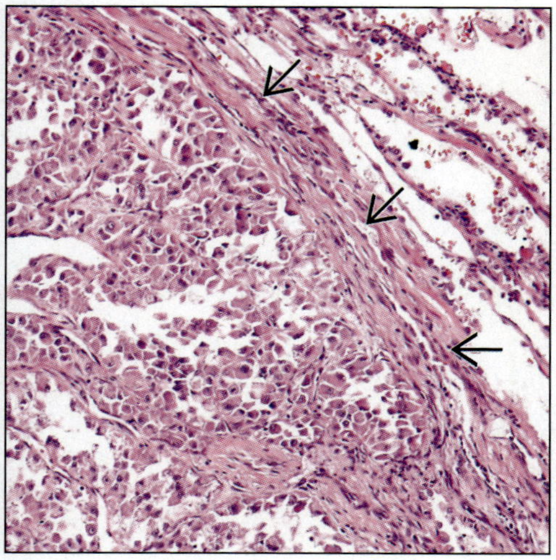

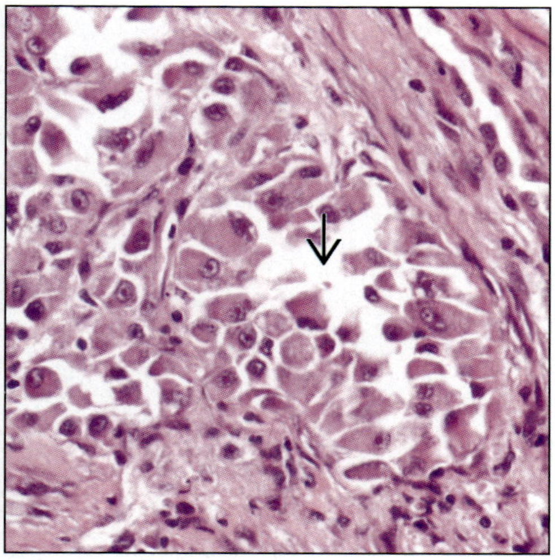

(Left) *Metastasis to the lung of alveolar soft part sarcoma of the thigh shows the proliferation of large epithelioid cells with abundant cytoplasm* → *that are sharply separated from the surrounding pulmonary parenchyma.* ***(Right)*** *Higher magnification from metastasis of an alveolar soft part sarcoma to the lung shows a vague alveolar pattern with large epithelioid cells aggregating around a central lumen* →*. The lung is a favored site of metastasis for this tumor.*

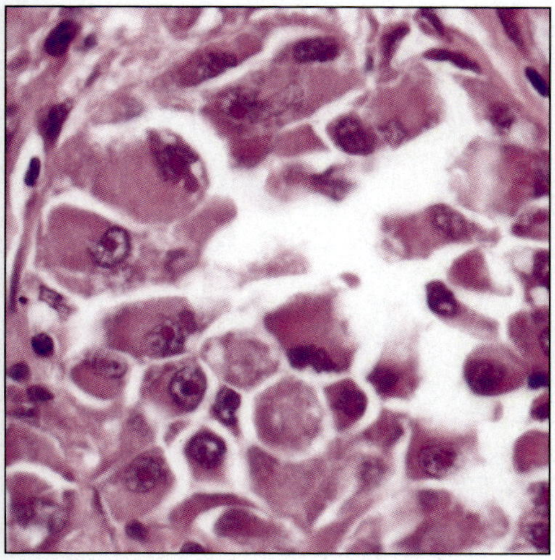

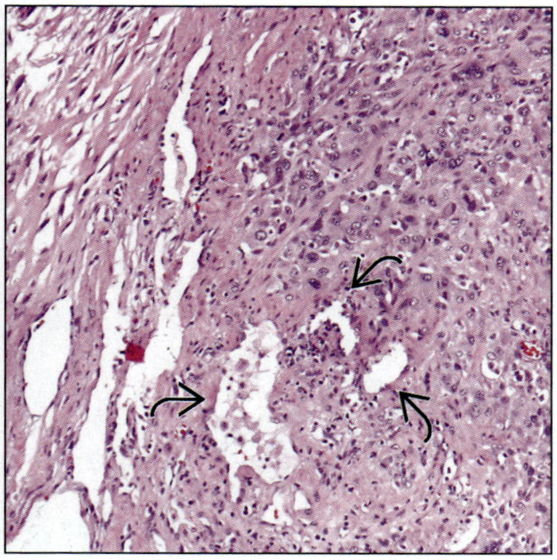

(Left) *High magnification of a metastasis to the lung from an alveolar soft part sarcoma of soft tissue shows a discohesive population of large, epithelioid cells with abundant granular cytoplasm. The cells display large round nuclei with prominent eosinophilic nucleoli.* ***(Right)*** *Lung metastasis of epithelioid sarcoma from the arm in a 32-year-old man shows sheets of large epithelioid cells with abundant cytoplasm surrounding entrapped residual alveolar spaces* ↪*.*

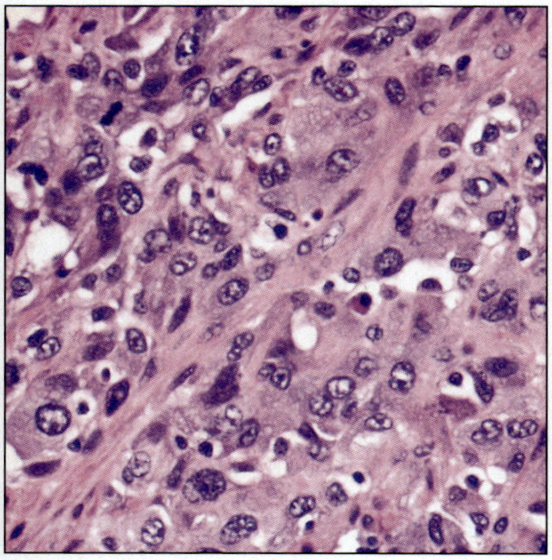

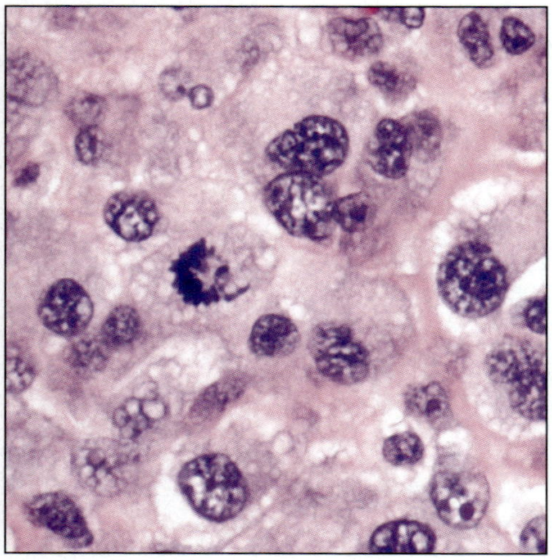

(Left) *High magnification of lung metastases in epithelioid sarcoma shows sheets of large cells with enlarged nuclei and an abundant rim of cytoplasm. These tumor cells were positive for cytokeratin, vimentin, and CD34. The tumors can be easily confused for large cell carcinoma of the lung. Clinical history is indispensable for diagnosis.* ***(Right)*** *Higher magnification of lung metastasis from epithelioid sarcoma shows large cells with abundant cytoplasm & mitotic activity.*

METASTATIC SARCOMA

Metastatic Epithelioid Angiosarcoma

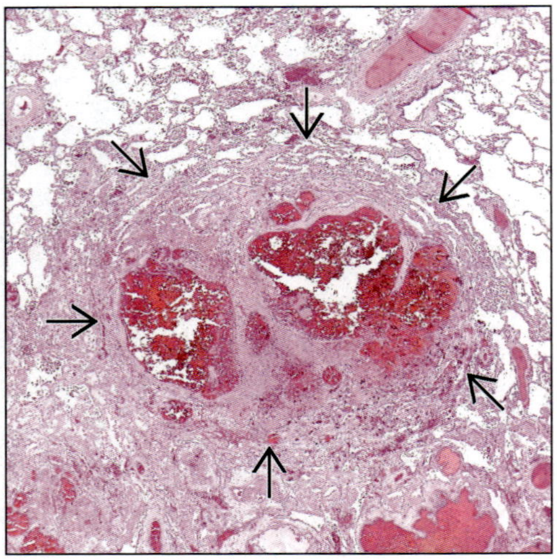

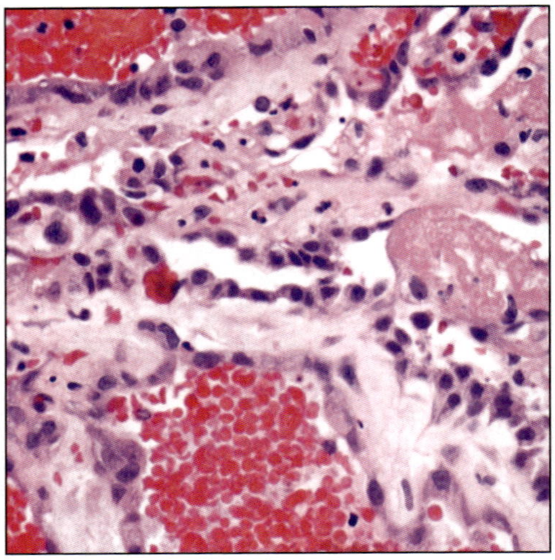

(Left) *Multiple hemorrhagic tumor nodules ➔ are seen studding the lung parenchyma in this metastasis from an epithelioid angiosarcoma from the heart.* ***(Right)*** *Higher magnification from a hemorrhagic tumor nodule in lung parenchyma from metastasis of an angiosarcoma of the heart shows poorly formed, anastomosing vascular channels lined by atypical, hyperchromatic endothelial cells. The vascular channels merged with solid areas containing similar cells in the stroma.*

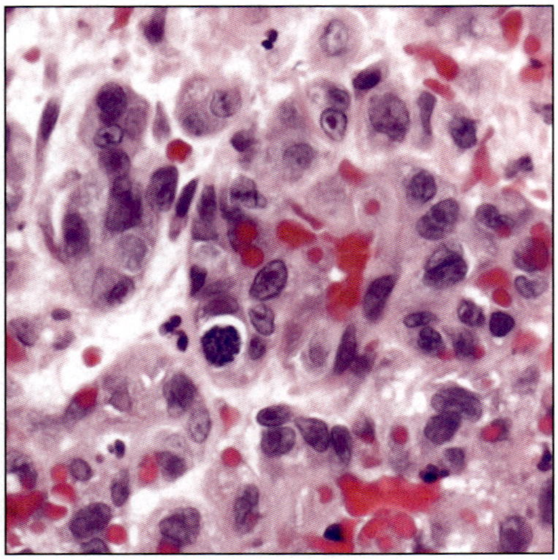

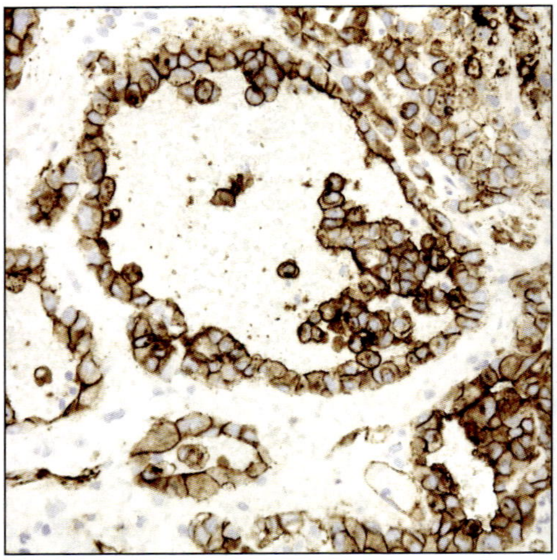

(Left) *A solid focus containing sheets of apparently cohesive epithelioid cells in the stroma is seen in this metastasis to the lung from angiosarcoma of the heart. The tumor cells are round with large nuclei and occasional mitoses, and the cells contain prominent nucleoli and a rim of ample to eosinophilic cytoplasm.* ***(Right)*** *Immunohistochemical staining of a metastatic angiosarcoma to the lung with CD31 shows strong membrane and cytoplasmic staining for this antibody.*

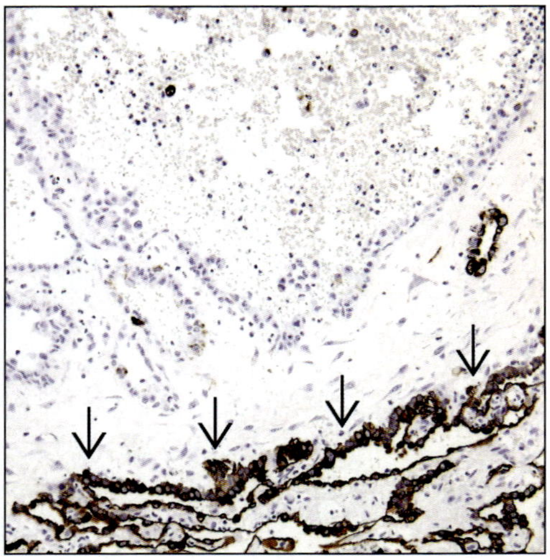

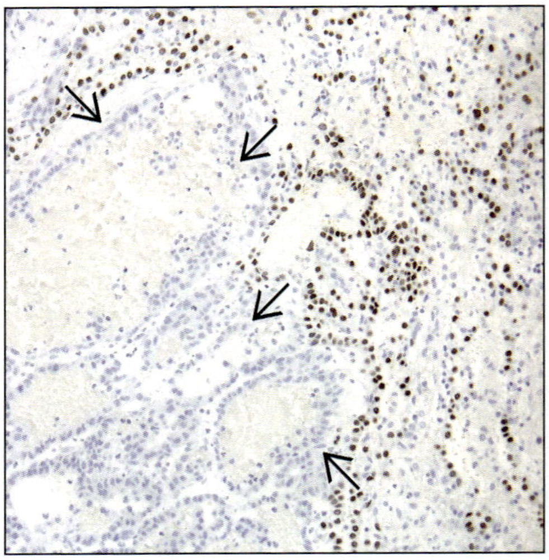

(Left) *Immunohistochemical staining of a metastasis from an angiosarcoma of the heart to the lung with CK7 shows strong positivity of the normal lung respiratory mucosa for this marker ➔ but negative staining of the tumor cells (above).* ***(Right)*** *Immunohistochemical staining of metastatic epithelioid angiosarcoma to the lung with the lung-specific marker, TTF-1, shows nuclear positivity in the respiratory epithelium surrounding the tumor but not in the tumor cells ➔.*

Metastatic Pleomorphic Sarcomas

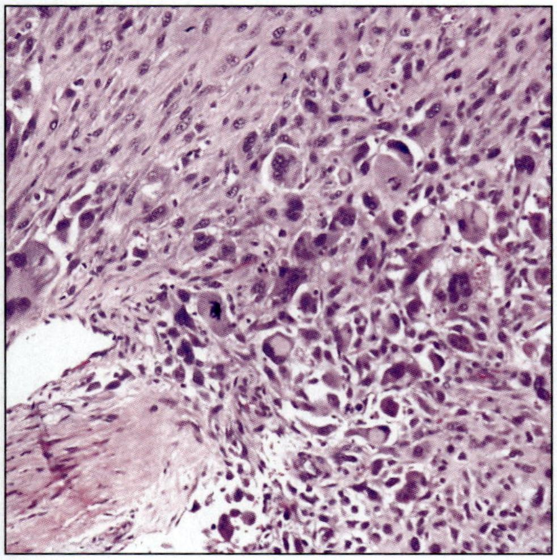
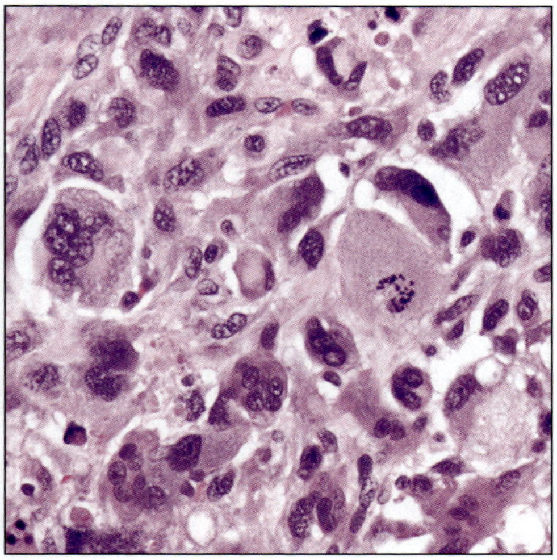

(Left) *Metastasis to the lung from a pleomorphic high-grade sarcoma of the thigh ("malignant fibrous histiocytoma") shows a highly pleomorphic tumor cell population destroying the lung parenchyma.* ***(Right)*** *High magnification of a malignant fibrous histiocytoma-type of metastasis is characterized by the extreme pleomorphism of the tumor cells. This morphologic appearance can be observed in metastases coming from a variety of well-differentiated sarcomas from other sites.*

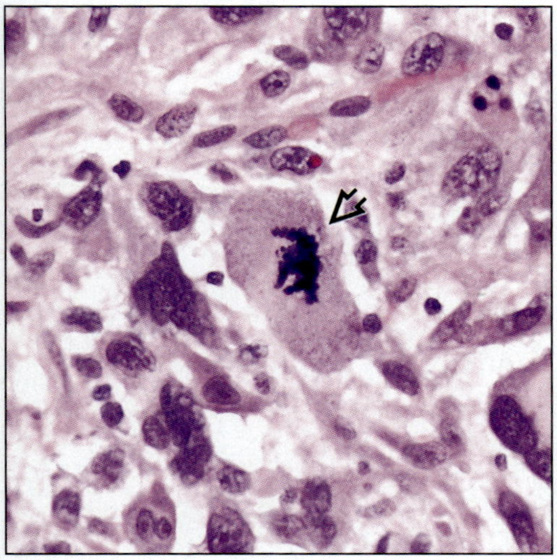
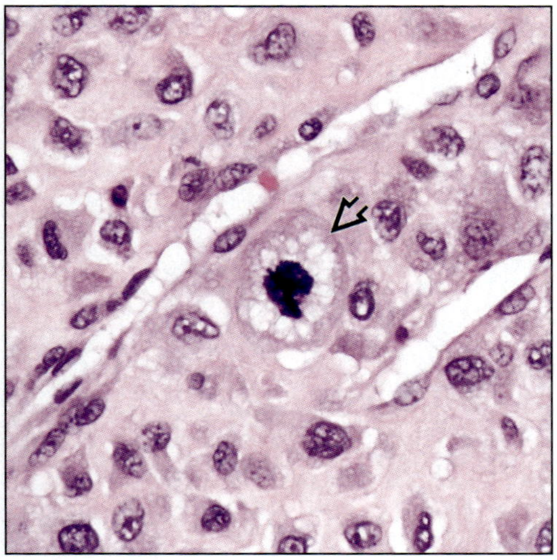

(Left) *Higher magnification of a metastatic pleomorphic high-grade sarcoma to the lung shows highly atypical tumor cells surrounding an abnormal mitotic figure ⇨.* ***(Right)*** *High-power view of a metastasis from a pleomorphic high-grade sarcoma to the lung shows a large atypical cell with abundant, finely vacuolated cytoplasm, resembling a lipoblast ⇨. Lipoblast-like atypical cells can be seen in a variety of sarcomas other than liposarcomas and may not be an indication of a liposarcoma metastasis.*

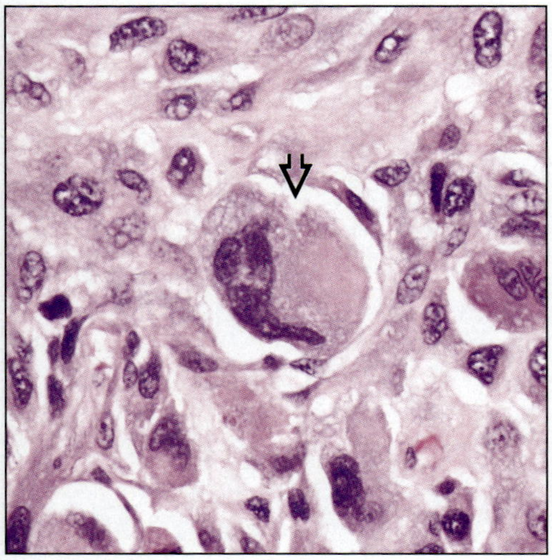
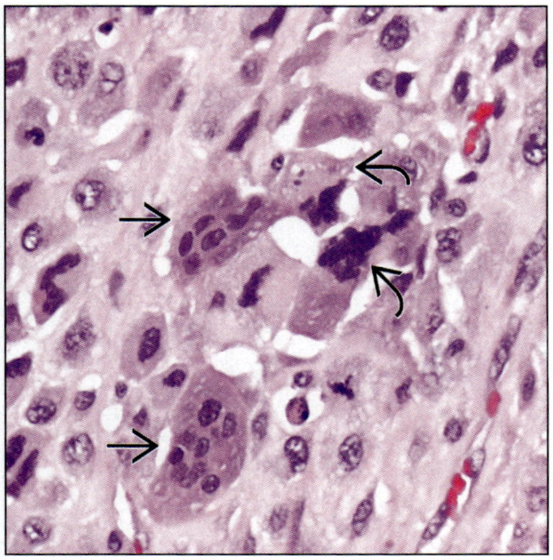

(Left) *High magnification of a lung metastasis from a pleomorphic high-grade sarcoma of soft tissue shows a large, atypical multinucleated cell ⇨ with abundant eosinophilic cytoplasm, reminiscent of a malignant histiocytic cell.* ***(Right)*** *High magnification of a pulmonary metastasis from a pleomorphic high-grade sarcoma of soft tissue (MFH) shows benign osteoclast-type multinucleated giant cells → alongside malignant, pleomorphic multinucleated giant cells ↷.*

METASTATIC SARCOMA

Metastatic Small Round Blue Cell Sarcomas

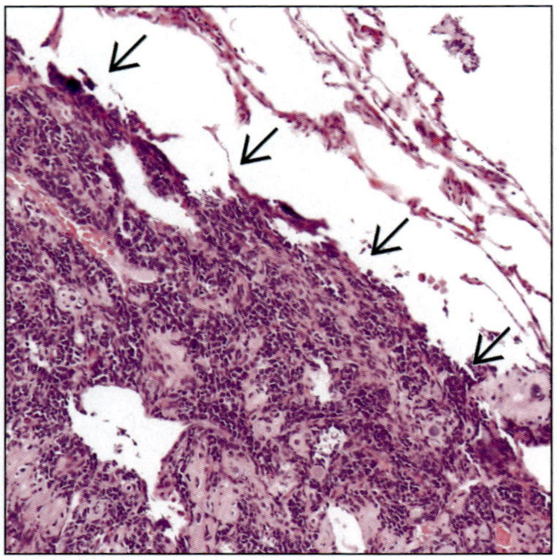

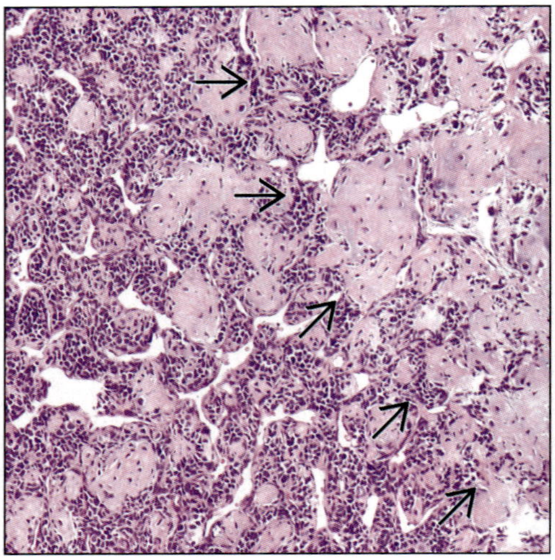

(Left) *Scanning magnification of a lung metastasis from an extraskeletal mesenchymal chondrosarcoma shows a well-circumscribed tumor nodule* → *surrounded by normal lung parenchyma.* ***(Right)*** *Lung metastasis from an extraskeletal mesenchymal chondrosarcoma shows areas of immature chondroid matrix* → *imperceptibly merging with an atypical small round blue cell neoplastic population (left). Numerous ectatic and branching hemangiopericytic vascular spaces are noted throughout.*

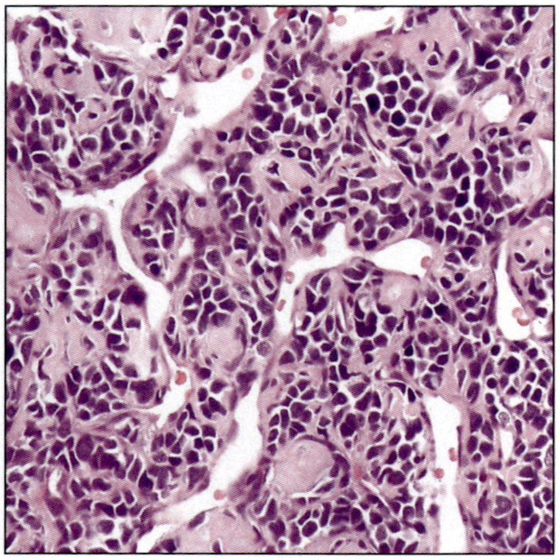

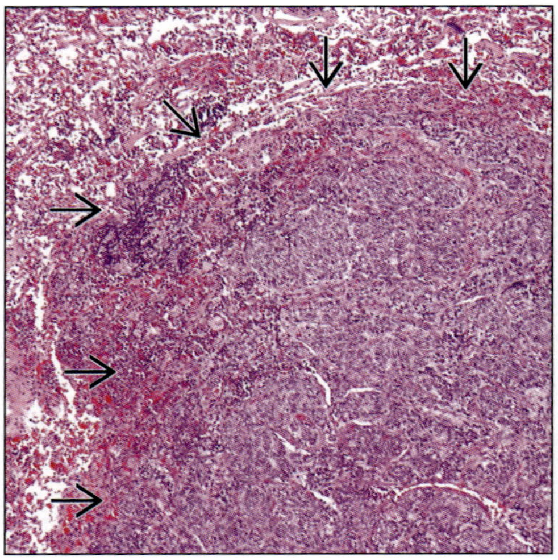

(Left) *High magnification of a pulmonary metastasis from an extraskeletal mesenchymal chondrosarcoma shows a small round blue cell population flanking a proliferation of branching dilated vascular spaces. The "hemangiopericytic" appearance is quite characteristic for this tumor.* ***(Right)*** *Scanning magnification shows a pulmonary metastasis from a Ewing sarcoma of pelvis* →*. Tumors with similar morphologic features can arise in the soft tissues, in a variety of somatic organs, and in the pleura.*

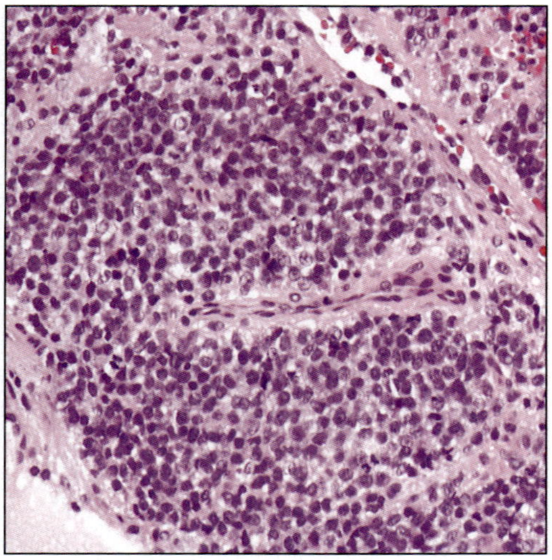

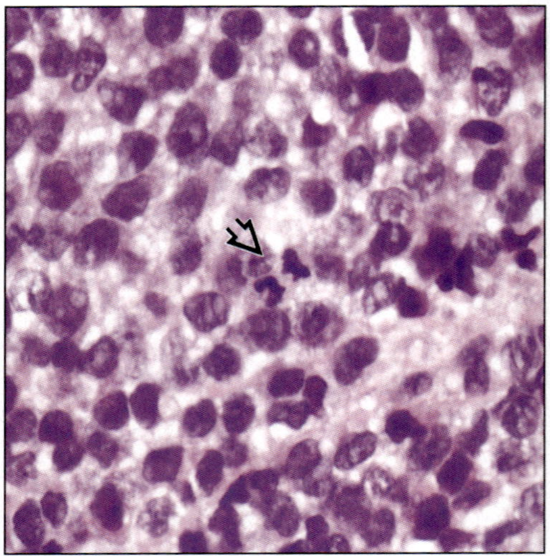

(Left) *Pulmonary metastasis from Ewing sarcoma/PNET shows a dense population of sheets of primitive-appearing small round blue cells. A wide variety of tumors can adopt this morphology. Immunohistochemical and molecular studies are indispensable to determine the exact type of tumor.* ***(Right)*** *High magnification of a metastasis from a Ewing/PNET to the lung shows sheets of primitive small round blue cells with dense nuclear chromatin and small nucleoli. Notice the mitotic figure* ⇨*.*

Metastatic Small Round Blue Cell Sarcomas

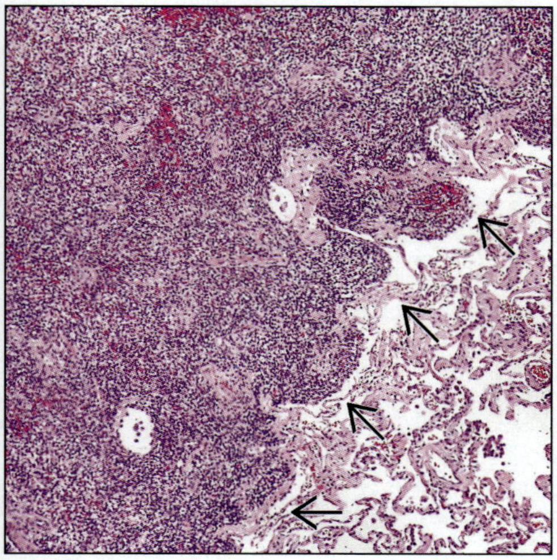

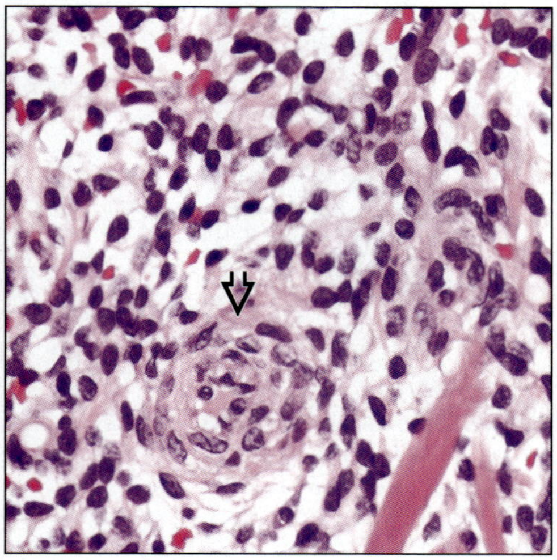

(Left) *Scanning magnification of a pulmonary metastasis from an endometrial stromal sarcoma of the uterus shows a well-demarcated nodule* → *showing sheets of small round blue cells without any specific architecture.* ***(Right)*** *High magnification of pulmonary metastases from endometrial stromal sarcoma of the uterus shows monotonous small round blue cell population surrounding a small vessel* ⊳*. The presence of these scattered small vessels with thickened walls is a characteristic of this tumor.*

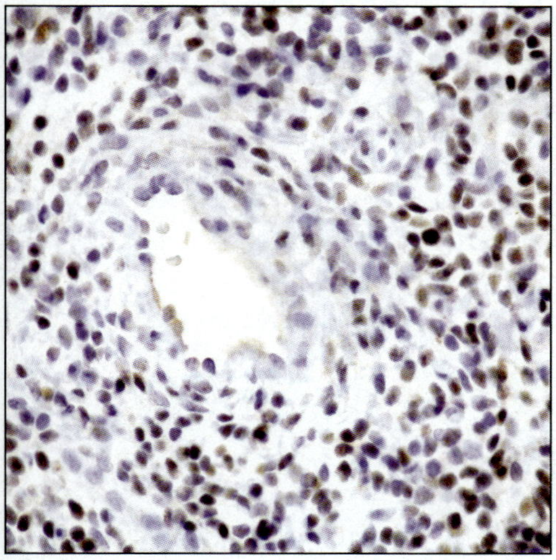

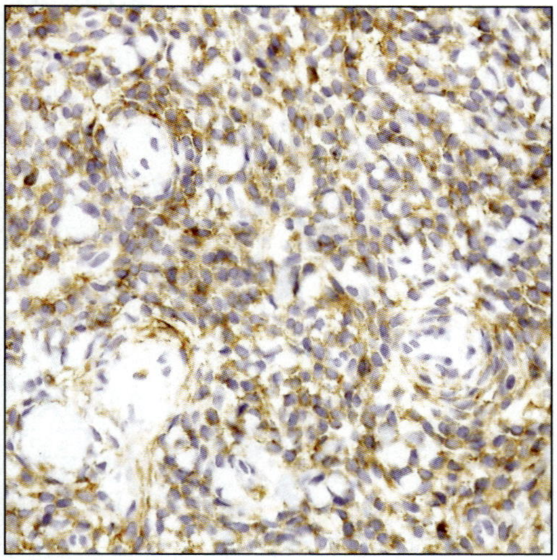

(Left) *Immunohistochemical staining of a pulmonary metastasis from endometrial stromal sarcoma of the uterus for estrogen receptors (ER) shows strong nuclear positivity for this antibody in the majority of the small round blue tumor cells. ER/PR positivity is a distinctive feature of these tumors.* ***(Right)*** *Immunohistochemical staining of a pulmonary metastasis from endometrial stromal sarcoma from the uterus for CD10 shows cytoplasmic positivity in the majority of the tumor cells.*

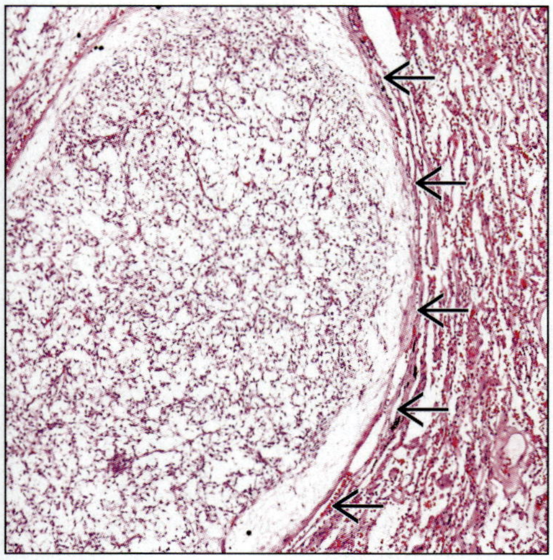

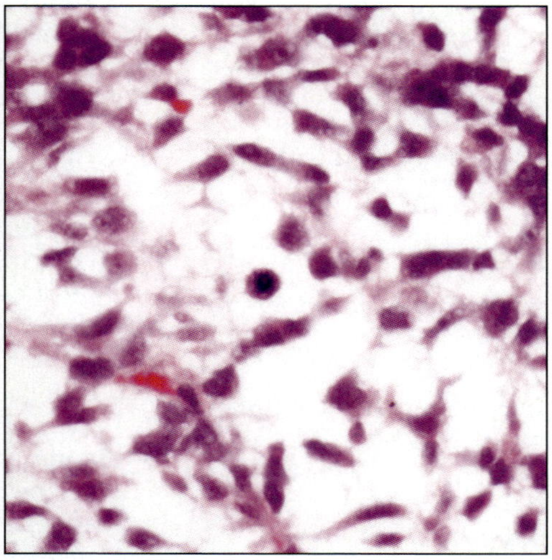

(Left) *Scanning magnification of a pulmonary metastasis from a round cell/myxoid liposarcoma of soft tissue shows a well-circumscribed nodule* → *sharply separated from the surrounding lung parenchyma.* ***(Right)*** *High magnification of a lung metastasis from a round cell/ myxoid liposarcoma shows a primitive population of small round blue cells without any distinguishing features of differentiation. Cytogenetic or molecular studies for the demonstration of the CHOP translocation are indicated.*

METASTATIC MALIGNANT MELANOMA

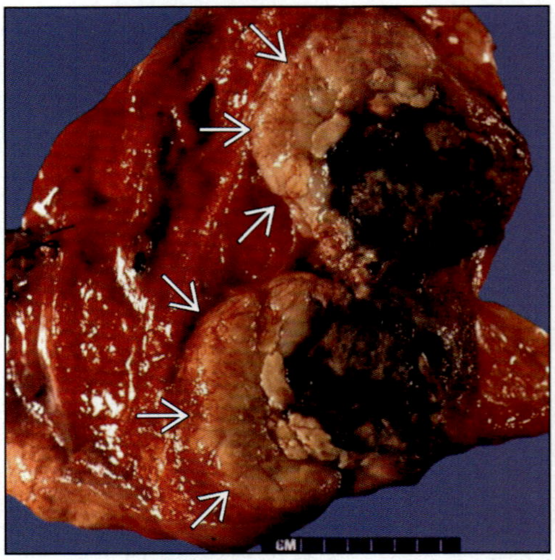

Gross appearance of a bisected nodule ➔ containing a lung metastasis of malignant melanoma shows a well-circumscribed tan nodule with an area of black discoloration due to melanin pigment deposition.

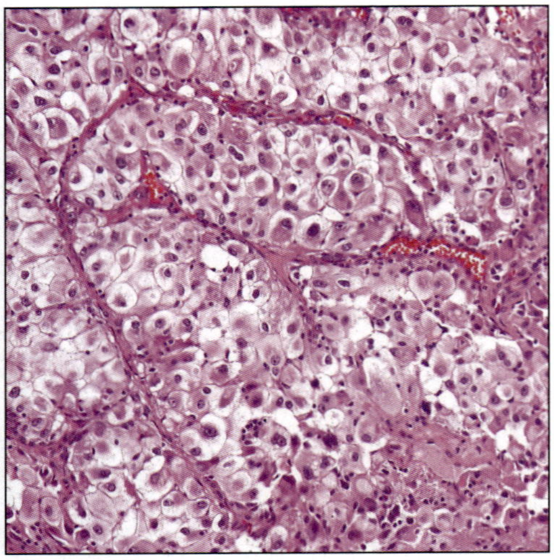

Histologic appearance of metastatic malignant melanoma in the lung shows nests of large, epithelioid tumor cells with enlarged nuclei, prominent nucleoli, and abundant eosinophilic cytoplasm.

CLINICAL ISSUES

Epidemiology

- Incidence
  - Lung is frequent site of metastasis for malignant melanoma
- Age
  - Middle-aged to elderly patients

Presentation

- Cough
- Hemoptysis
- Dyspnea
- Atelectasis
- Pleural effusion

Treatment

- Surgical approaches
  - Surgical excision for solitary lesions may improve median survival
- Adjuvant therapy
  - Chemotherapy may be used for multiple and bilateral tumors

Prognosis

- Melanoma metastases to lungs are associated with advanced stage and poor prognosis

IMAGE FINDINGS

General Features

- Location
  - Multiple, well-defined nodules in periphery of lungs
  - Endobronchial metastases
- Morphology
  - Round, well-defined nodules
  - Can show cavitation and necrosis

MACROSCOPIC FEATURES

General Features

- Usually well circumscribed but unencapsulated
- Tan or white, homogeneous cut surface with areas of hemorrhage and necrosis
- Tumors may be deeply pigmented due to heavy melanin deposition

Size

- Several millimeters to > 5 cm in greatest diameter

MICROSCOPIC PATHOLOGY

Histologic Features

- **Epithelioid melanoma**
  - Nests or islands of large epithelioid cells with abundant eosinophilic cytoplasm that may resemble carcinoma
  - Tumor cells contain enlarged nuclei with prominent nucleoli
- **Spindle cell melanoma**
  - Nests or short fascicles of atypical spindle cells resembling sarcoma
  - Differential diagnosis includes sarcomatoid lung carcinoma, metastatic sarcomatoid renal cell carcinoma, and spindle cell sarcoma
- **Mixed spindle and epithelioid cell melanoma**
  - Most common form of metastatic melanoma, showing admixture of both spindle and epithelioid cells
  - Can be confused for a variety of other primary and metastatic sarcomas in the lung
- **Pleomorphic melanoma**
  - Characterized by sheets of pleomorphic and anaplastic tumor cells with bizarre nuclei and frequent abnormal mitoses

METASTATIC MALIGNANT MELANOMA

Key Facts

Clinical Issues
- Lung is frequent site of metastasis for malignant melanoma
- Middle-aged to elderly patients

Image Findings
- Multiple, well-defined nodules in periphery of lungs
- Endobronchial metastases

Microscopic Pathology
- Can show large variety of morphologic appearances, including epithelioid, spindle, signet ring cell, rhabdoid, and small cell melanoma
- Hallmark of malignant melanoma is presence of cells with marked cytologic atypia
- Majority of tumor cells are large, pleomorphic, with enlarged nuclei and prominent eosinophilic nucleoli
- Cells may also be small and relatively bland-appearing with minimal cytologic atypia

Ancillary Tests
- S100 protein is positive in nearly 100% of cases (nuclear and cytoplasmic stain)
- In most cases, melanocytic-associated markers are positive: HMB-45, Melan-A, tyrosinase, microphthalmia transcription factor (MiTF)
- Aberrant expression of epithelial markers (keratins, CEA, EMA) can be seen in small percentage of cases
- Other markers can also be expressed, including CD10, CD56, CD68, CD99, CD117, calretinin, NSE, vimentin, and Bcl-2, but are nonspecific

  - Tumors may resemble pleomorphic high-grade sarcoma (MFH) or pleomorphic/anaplastic carcinoma of lung
- **"Rhabdoid" melanoma**
  - Composed of sheets of large tumor cells with eccentric, densely eosinophilic cytoplasmic inclusions
  - Tumor cells can resemble rhabdomyoblastic cells in rhabdomyosarcoma or in "malignant rhabdoid tumor"
- **Signet ring cell melanoma**
  - Sheets of tumor cells characterized by signet ring cell morphology
  - Cells will show enlarged, hyperchromatic nuclei displaced to periphery by abundant cytoplasm
- **Small cell melanoma**
  - Dense sheets of monotonous small round tumor cells with hyperchromatic nuclei and scant cytoplasm
  - Tumors can resemble malignant lymphoma, carcinoid tumors, and other small round blue cell tumors

Cytologic Features
- Hallmark of malignant melanoma is presence of cells with marked cytologic atypia
- Majority of tumor cells are large, pleomorphic, with enlarged nuclei and prominent eosinophilic nucleoli
- Frequent mitotic figures; abnormal mitoses are often encountered
- Cells may also be small and relatively bland-appearing with minimal cytologic atypia

ANCILLARY TESTS

Immunohistochemistry
- S100 protein is positive in nearly 100% of cases (nuclear and cytoplasmic stain)
- In most cases, melanocytic-associated markers are positive: HMB-45, Melan-A, tyrosinase, microphthalmia transcription factor (MiTF)
- Aberrant expression of epithelial markers (keratins, CEA, EMA) can be seen in small percentage of cases
- Other markers can also be expressed, including CD10, CD56, CD68, CD99, CD117, calretinin, NSE, vimentin, and Bcl-2, but are nonspecific

DIFFERENTIAL DIAGNOSIS

Sarcomatoid Carcinoma
- Tumor cells are positive for epithelial markers (cytokeratin, EMA, MOC31) and negative for S100 and melanocytic markers

Metastatic Renal Cell Carcinoma
- Can show similar morphology with nests of tumor cells with abundant eosinophilic or granular cytoplasm
- Tumor cells are positive for cytokeratin, EMA, and RCC marker, and negative for melanoma-associated markers and S100

Spindle and Epithelioid Cell Sarcomas
- Tumors such as leiomyosarcoma, epithelioid sarcoma, and synovial sarcoma may resemble melanoma morphologically
- Absence of melanocytic-associated markers and reactivity for other specific lineage-associated markers are helpful adjuncts for diagnosis

Pleomorphic High-Grade Sarcoma (MFH)
- Usually vimentin positive only and does not express melanocytic-associated markers

SELECTED REFERENCES

1. Kobayashi S et al: Pulmonary metastasis with endobronchial spread from sinonasal melanoma during a 9-year follow-up. Intern Med. 49(8):777-9, 2010
2. Oliaro A et al: Pulmonary metastasectomy for melanoma. J Thorac Oncol. 5(6 Suppl 2):S187-91, 2010
3. Lee JH et al: Biological factors, tumor growth kinetics, and survival after metastasectomy for pulmonary melanoma. Ann Surg Oncol. 16(10):2834-9, 2009

METASTATIC MALIGNANT MELANOMA

Epithelioid Melanoma

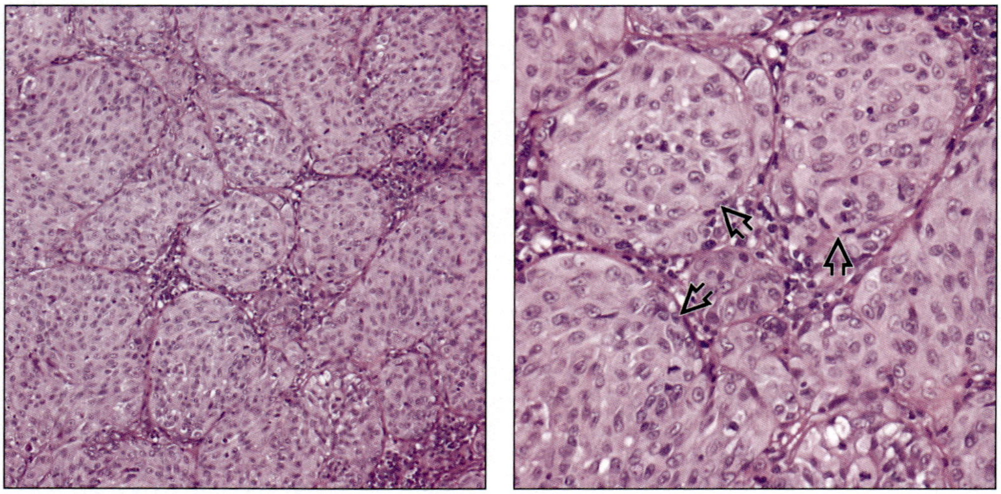

(Left) *Pulmonary metastasis from epithelioid melanoma shows classical morphology of metastatic melanoma characterized by discrete, well-formed nests or thèques of large, epithelioid cells with enlarged nuclei surrounded by abundant cytoplasm.* ***(Right)*** *Higher magnification of a metastasis to the lung from an epithelioid malignant melanoma of the skin shows discrete nests ➪ of tumor cells with large, round to oval nuclei surrounded by abundant eosinophilic cytoplasm.*

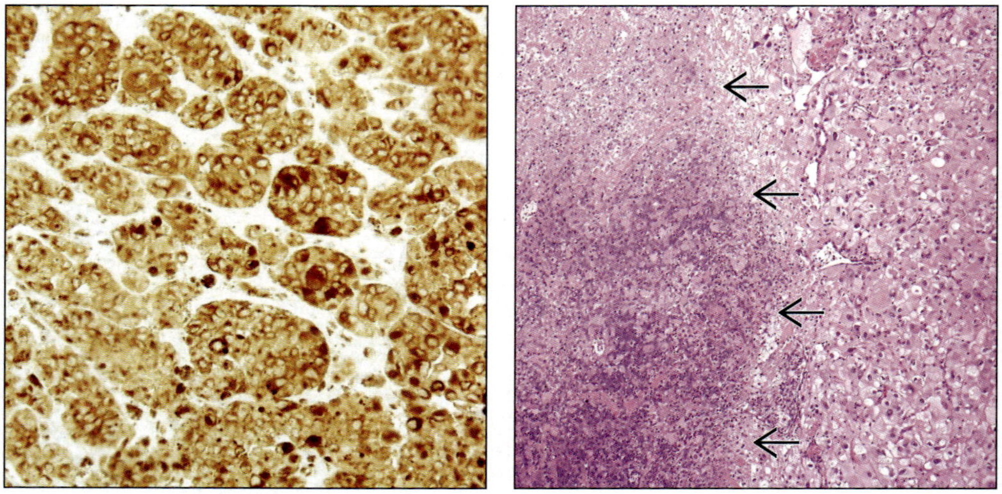

(Left) *Immunohistochemical staining of metastatic malignant melanoma to the lung with S100 protein shows strong cytoplasmic and nuclear positivity in the vast majority of the tumor cells. Notice the nested configuration of the tumor cells highlighted by the stain.* ***(Right)*** *Metastatic epithelioid malignant melanoma to the lung shows sheets of large, atypical tumor cells flanking an extensive area of necrosis →. Necrosis is a frequent finding in these tumors.*

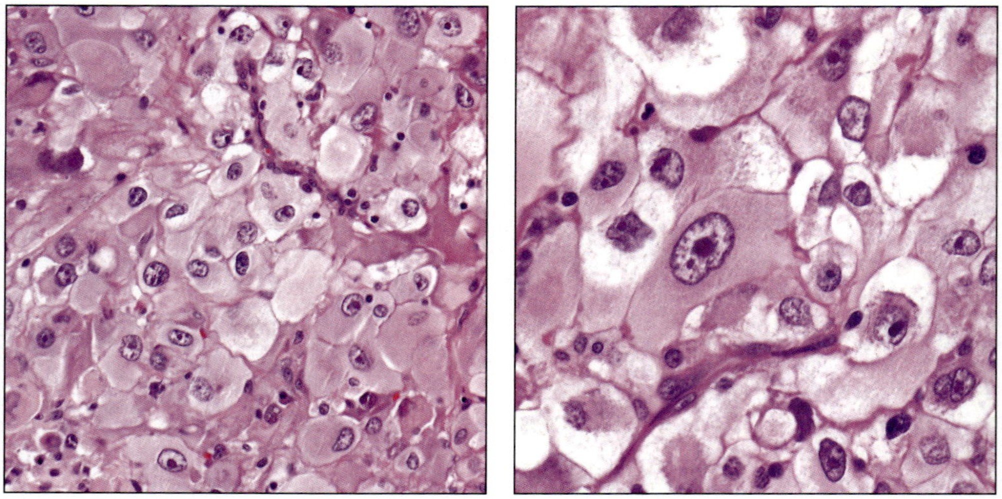

(Left) *Higher magnification of metastasis of epithelioid malignant melanoma to the lung shows characteristic appearance with large cells displaying sharp cell borders, giving the appearance of cohesiveness and raising the diagnostic possibility of an epithelial neoplasm (i.e., large cell carcinoma) in the differential diagnosis.* ***(Right)*** *Higher magnification of metastatic melanoma shows cells with enlarged nuclei, prominent nucleoli, and abundant cytoplasm.*

METASTATIC MALIGNANT MELANOMA

Spindle Cell Melanoma

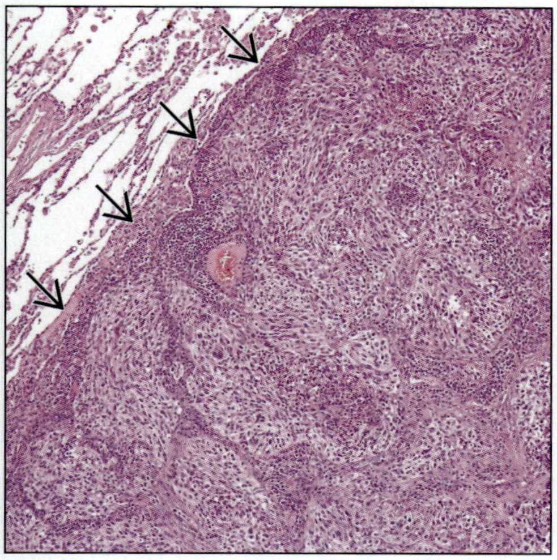

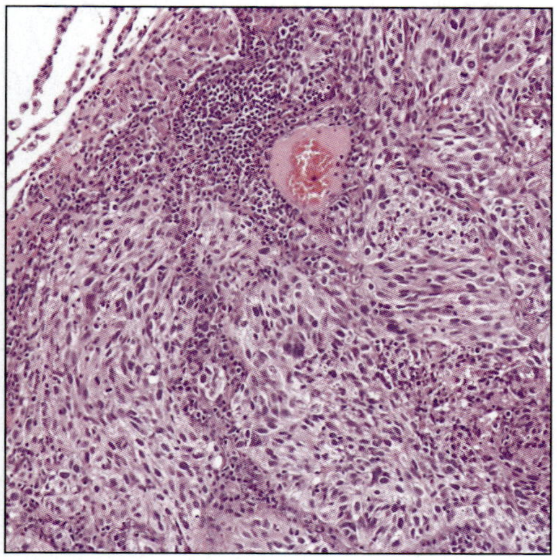

(Left) *Metastasis to the lung from spindle cell melanoma of the forearm shows nests of spindle cells* ⇒ *that are sharply demarcated from the surrounding lung parenchyma.* ***(Right)*** *Higher magnification of metastasis from a spindle cell melanoma shows well-defined nests of tumor cells. The tumor cells are characterized by their spindle appearance, with elongated, tapered nuclei surrounded by a rim of eosinophilic cytoplasm. The nesting patterns are a clue to the diagnosis.*

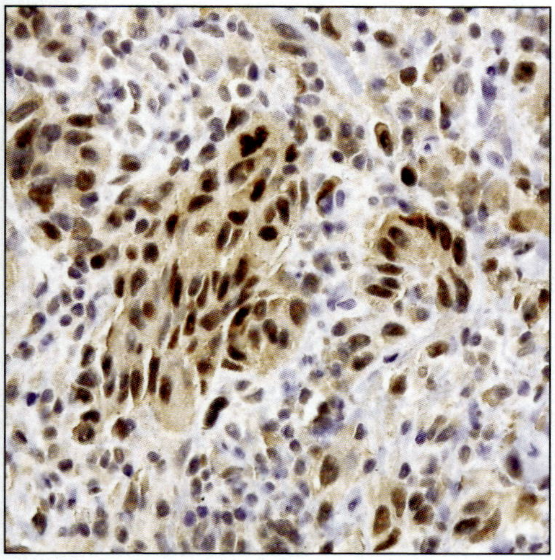

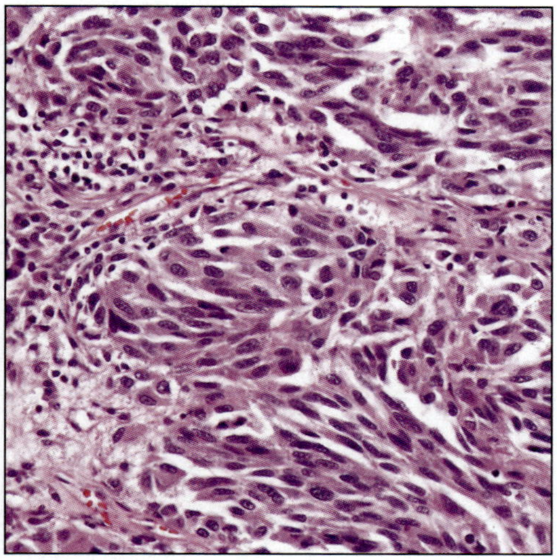

(Left) *Immunohistochemical staining of metastasis to the lung from spindle cell melanoma with S100 shows strong cytoplasmic and nuclear positivity of the spindle tumor cells for this antigen.* ***(Right)*** *Metastasis to the lung from a spindle cell ocular melanoma shows poorly formed nests of tumor cells with a spindle morphology. Spindle cell melanomas may lose their nested pattern and show a fascicular appearance that may be confused for a sarcoma or sarcomatoid carcinoma.*

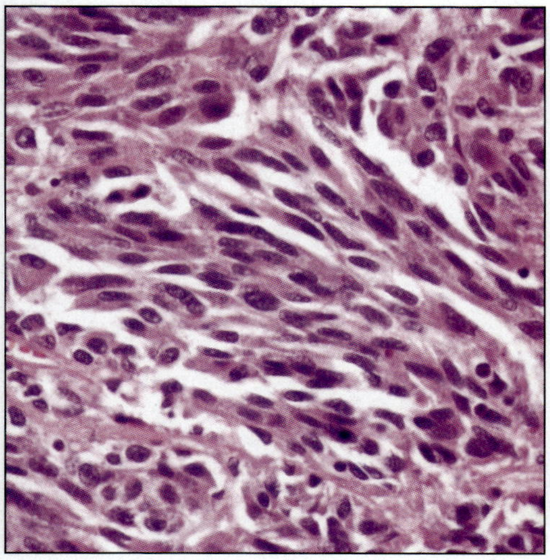

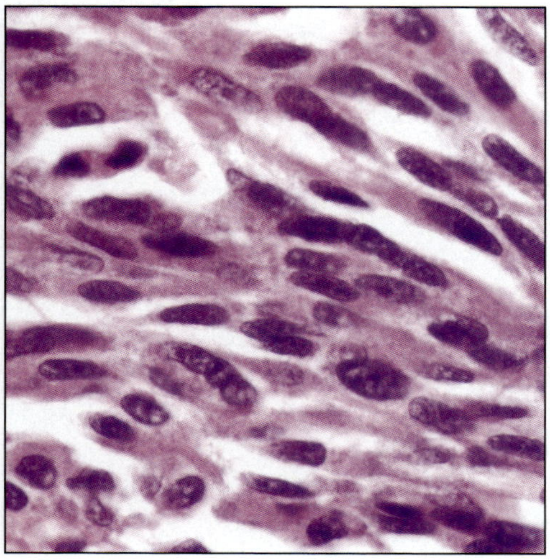

(Left) *Higher magnification of metastatic ocular spindle cell melanoma shows fascicles of tumor cells composed of atypical cells with hyperchromatic nuclei and scant rim of eosinophilic cytoplasm. Tumors like this may resemble leiomyosarcoma or spindle cell carcinomas.* ***(Right)*** *Higher magnification of metastasis to the lung from ocular spindle cell melanoma shows spindle cells with hyperchromatic nuclei and occasional nucleoli surrounded by a rim of eosinophilic cytoplasm.*

Endobronchial Metastasis of Melanoma

(Left) *Endobronchial metastasis of malignant melanoma shows a polypoid tumor mass growing into the lumen of the bronchus. Notice distended bronchial lumen lined by a single layer of bronchial epithelium* →*. Endobronchial metastases of melanoma need to be distinguished from primary lung neoplasms that can show this same growth pattern.* ***(Right)*** *Endobronchial metastasis of malignant melanoma shows transition between the normal bronchial mucosa and the malignant melanoma* ⇨*.*

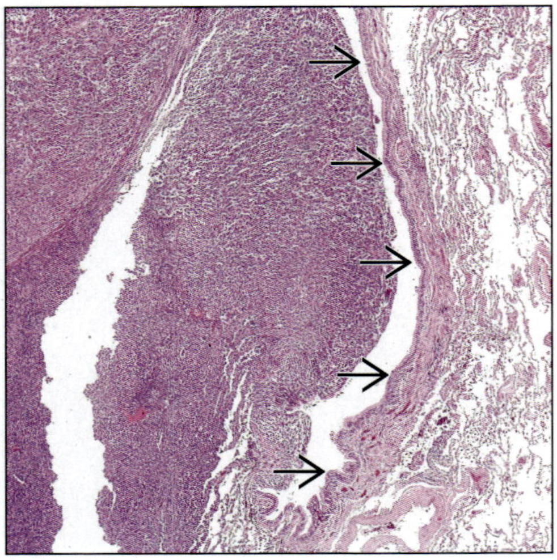

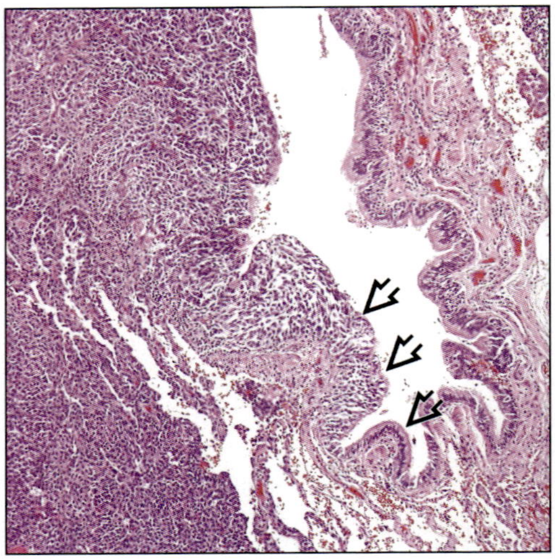

(Left) *Higher magnification of endobronchial metastasis from malignant melanoma shows gradual replacement of the bronchial epithelium by the melanoma cells* →*. At times it may be impossible to separate cases like this from a primary malignant melanoma of the bronchus in the absence of a clinical history.* ***(Right)*** *Higher magnification illustrates transition between normal bronchial epithelium with tall columnar ciliated cells and endobronchial metastatic malignant melanoma.*

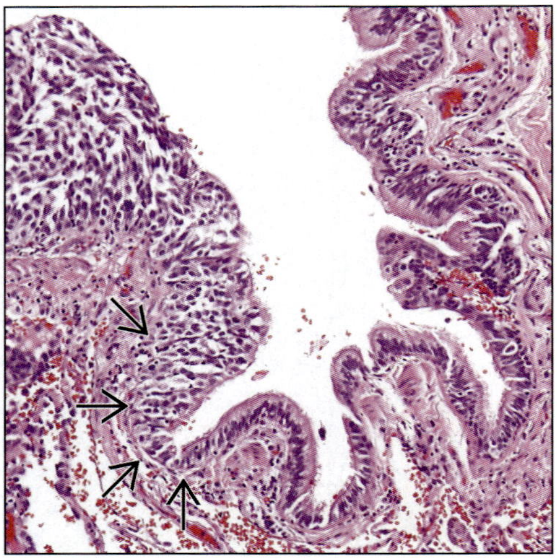

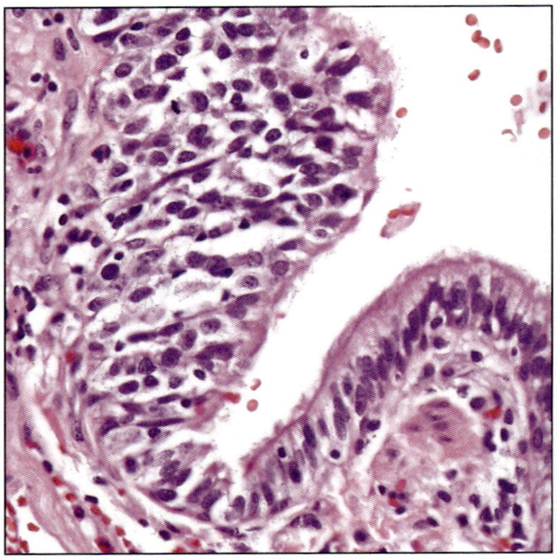

(Left) *Solid area of the tumor in endobronchial metastasis of malignant melanoma shows heavy deposition of dark melanin pigment. The presence of melanin pigment serves to facilitate the diagnosis in pigmented metastases of malignant melanoma.* ***(Right)*** *Higher magnification of endobronchial metastasis of pigmented malignant melanoma shows heavy deposition of dark brown pigment in the cytoplasm of the tumor cells. A hint of nesting pattern of the tumor cells can be appreciated.*

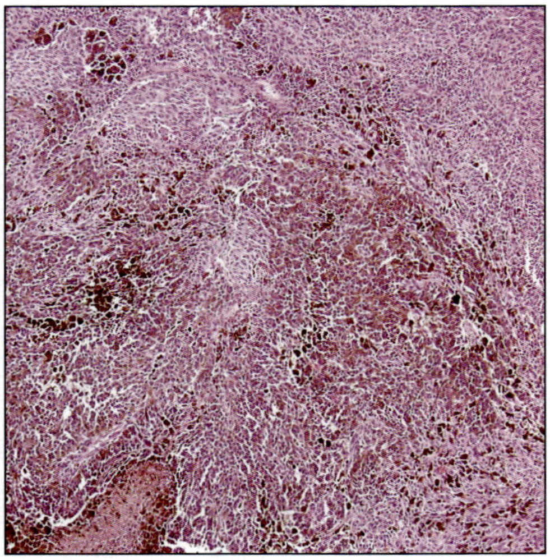

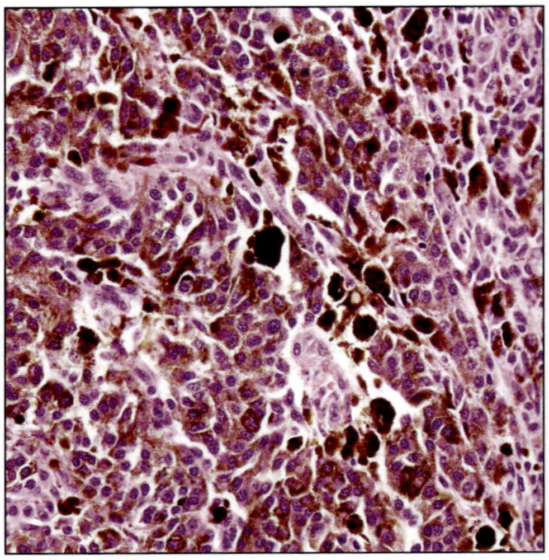

Unusual Variants of Melanoma

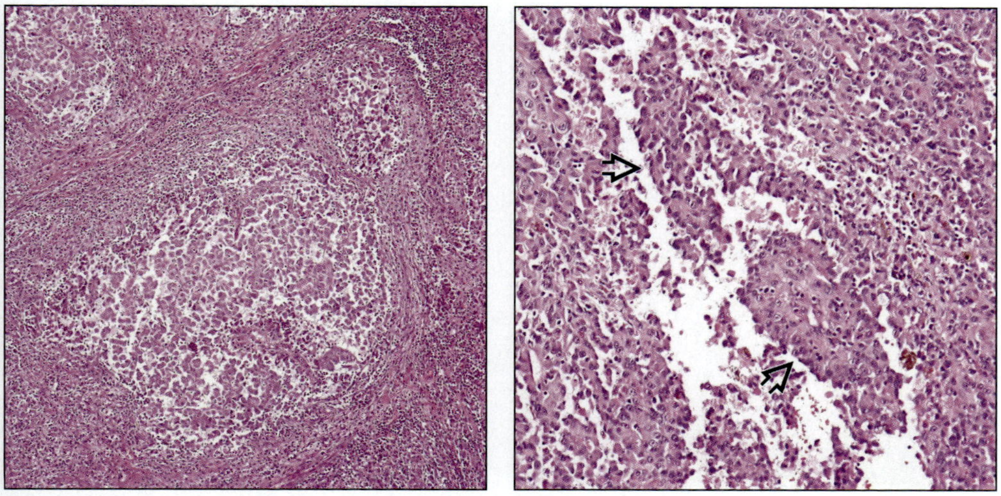

*(**Left**) Metastatic malignant melanoma to the lung shows a vague pseudopapillary pattern of growth resulting from dehiscence of tumor cells. (**Right**) Higher magnification of metastatic malignant melanoma to the lung shows irregular pseudopapillary structures resulting from artifactual breakdown of the tumor cells ➩. Tumors with these features can often be confused for a variety of primary and metastatic papillary carcinomas of the lung.*

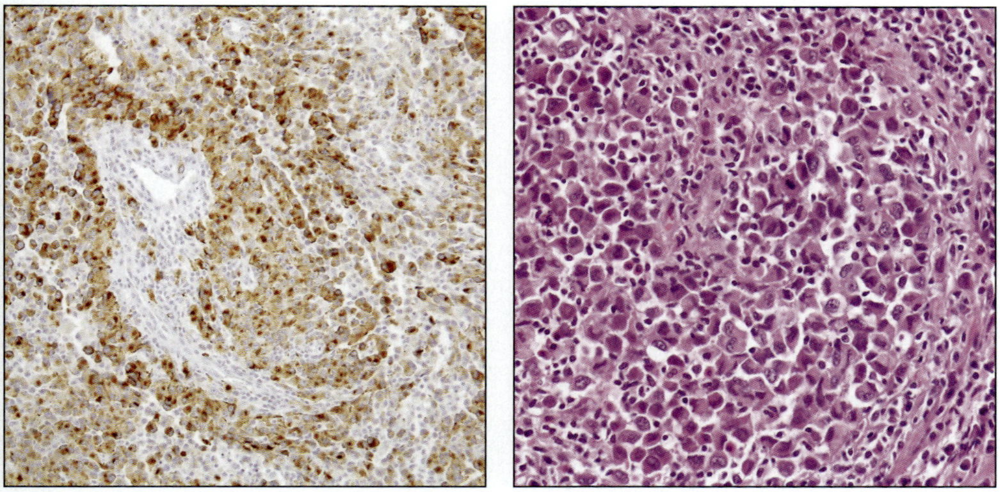

*(**Left**) Immunohistochemical staining with S100 in pulmonary metastasis of malignant melanoma with pseudopapillary pattern of growth shows strong nuclear and cytoplasmic positivity in the tumor cells. (**Right**) Metastasis to the lung from malignant melanoma shows a discohesive population of cells with large nuclei and abundant eccentric cytoplasm imparting the cells a "rhabdoid" appearance. The differential diagnosis includes rhabdomyosarcoma and malignant rhabdoid tumor.*

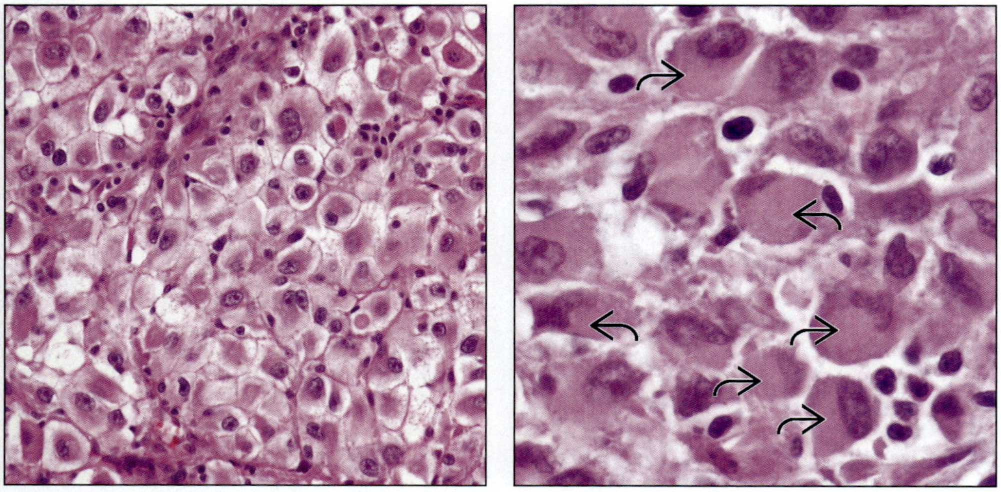

*(**Left**) Higher magnification of metastasis to the lung from "rhabdoid" malignant melanoma shows sheets of large tumor cells with abundant cytoplasm and dense eosinophilic cytoplasmic inclusions. These features are nonspecific and can be observed in a wide variety of malignant neoplasms, including neuroendocrine malignancies, sarcomas, and carcinomas. (**Right**) Higher magnification of "rhabdoid" cells in metastatic melanoma of lung shows characteristic cytoplasmic inclusions ↪.*

METASTATIC MALIGNANT MELANOMA

Small Cell Variant of Malignant Melanoma

*(**Left**) Scanning magnification of lung metastasis of malignant melanoma, small cell variant, shows a well-defined tumor nodule → separated from the surrounding normal lung parenchyma. (**Right**) Higher magnification of pulmonary metastasis from malignant melanoma, small cell variant, shows sheets of uniform small tumor cells with no discernible growth pattern. Tumors like this can be confused for malignant lymphoma or small cell neuroendocrine carcinoma.*

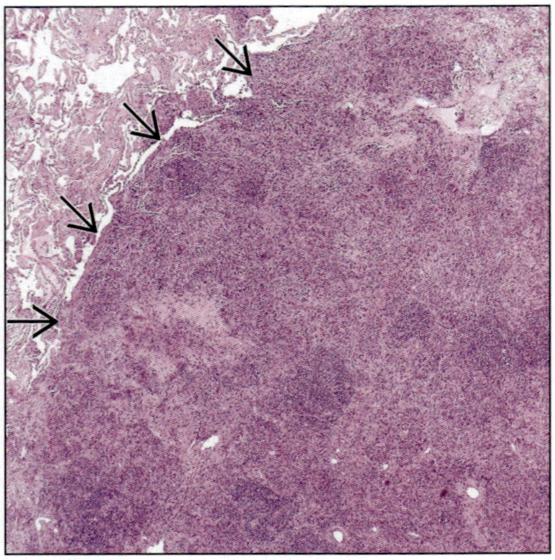

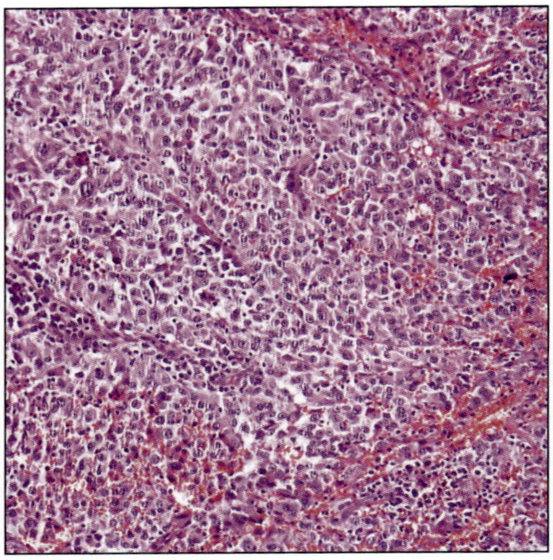

*(**Left**) Infiltration and destruction of the wall of a bronchiole → is seen in this example of pulmonary metastasis of malignant melanoma of small cell type. Epitheliotropism is commonly encountered in malignant melanoma at metastatic sites. (**Right**) Metastasis to the lung from malignant melanoma of small cell type shows a monotonous population of small tumor cells simulating a malignant lymphoma, a highly unusual morphologic appearance that can be very difficult to diagnose.*

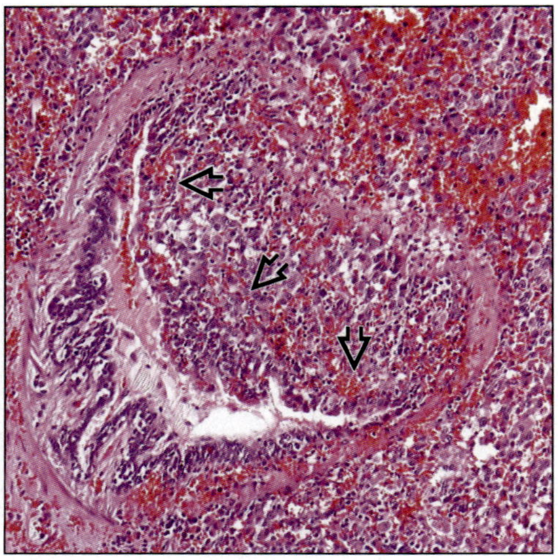

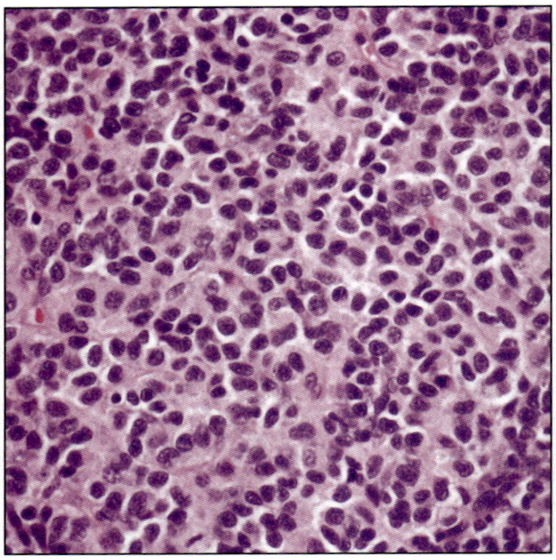

*(**Left**) Higher magnification of pulmonary metastasis of small cell melanoma shows sheets of small, round tumor cells with hyperchromatic nuclei, absent or very inconspicuous nucleoli, paucity of mitotic figures, and indistinct rim of cytoplasm surrounding the tumor cells. (**Right**) Higher magnification from pulmonary metastasis of malignant melanoma, small cell variant, shows a few scattered cells displaying cytoplasmic melanin pigment →, a helpful clue for the diagnosis.*

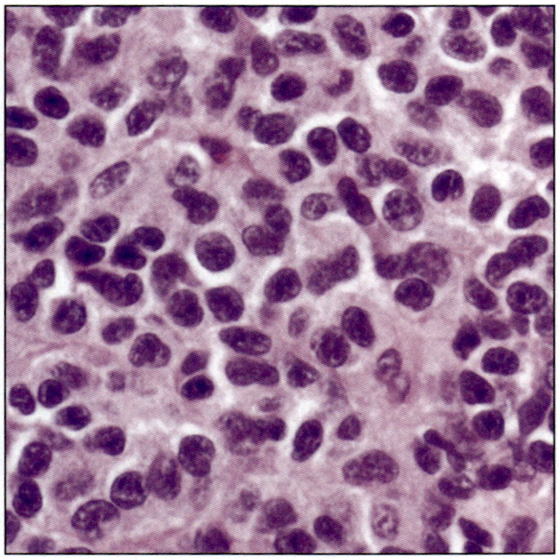

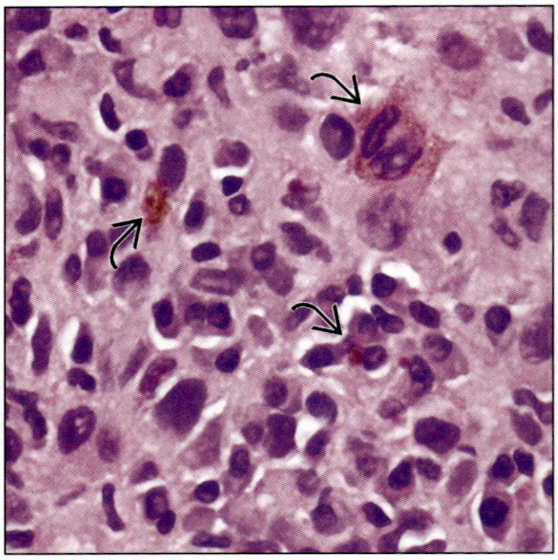

Immunohistochemical Features of Melanoma

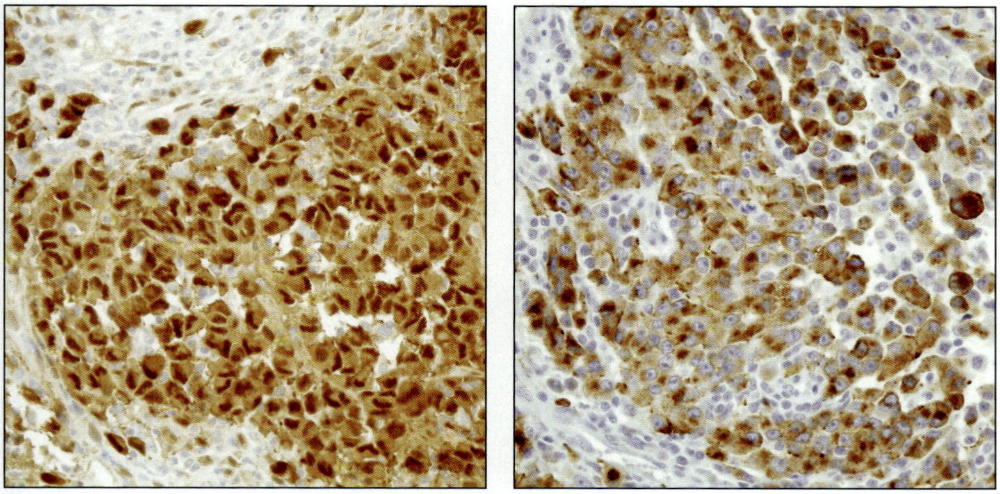

(Left) *Immunohistochemical staining of metastatic malignant melanoma for S100 protein shows strong nuclear and cytoplasmic staining of the tumor cells. This antigen is very sensitive but not very specific for malignant melanoma.* ***(Right)*** *Immunohistochemical staining of metastatic malignant melanoma to lung with HMB-45 melanoma-associated marker shows strong positivity in the tumor cells. This marker may not always be expressed at metastatic sites and is less sensitive than S100.*

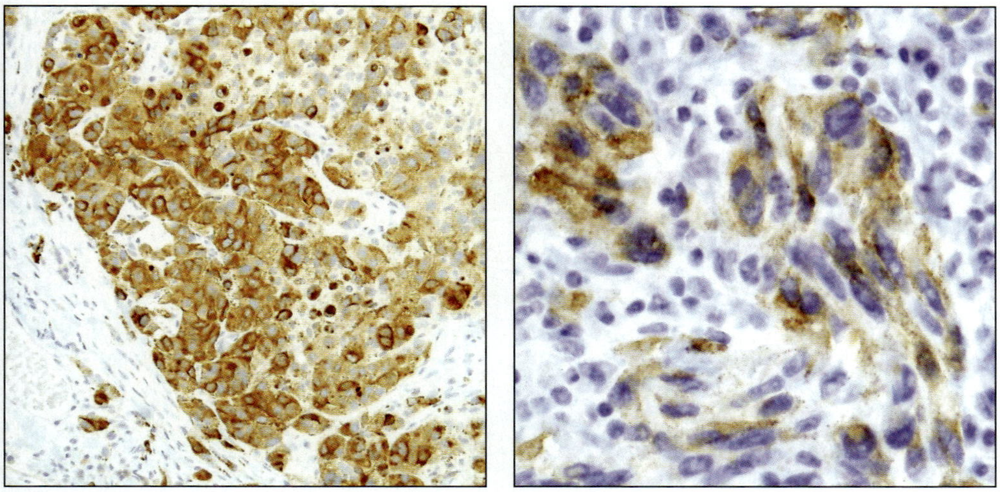

(Left) *Immunohistochemical staining of metastatic melanoma to the lung with Melan-A shows the strong positivity of tumor cells for this marker. Melan-A is a good alternative for a melanocyte-specific marker in the diagnosis of malignant melanoma at metastatic sites.* ***(Right)*** *Immunohistochemical staining of metastatic spindle cell melanoma with Melan-A (clone A103) shows cytoplasmic positivity in the spindle tumor cells. Use of this antibody can be helpful in HMB-45 negative cases.*

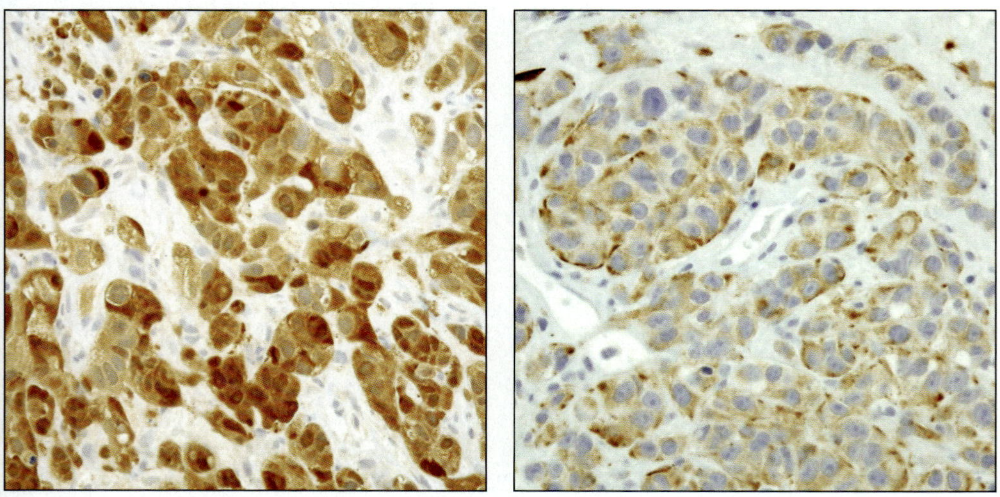

(Left) *Immunohistochemical staining of metastatic malignant melanoma to the lung with CEA polyclonal antibody shows cytoplasmic positivity in the tumor cells. CEA positivity can occur in a subset of malignant melanomas causing diagnostic difficulties that most likely result from cross-reactivity with nonspecific antigens.* ***(Right)*** *Faint cytoplasmic staining is seen in metastatic melanoma with EMA antibodies. Occasional cases of metastatic melanoma may react with EMA antibodies.*

Nonneoplastic and Systemic Conditions

DIFFUSE ALVEOLAR DAMAGE

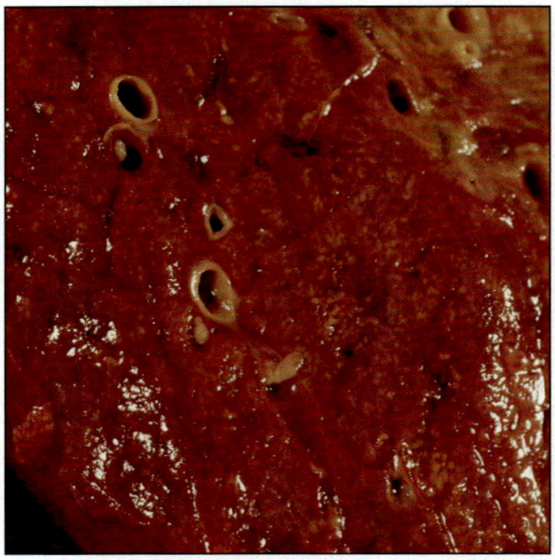

Gross appearance of the lung on cut surface in a patient with diffuse alveolar damage shows beefy red, congested, and edematous parenchyma.

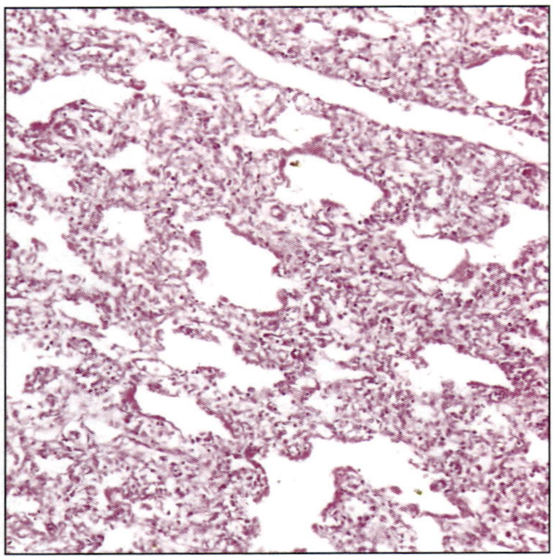

Histologic appearance of diffuse alveolar damage shows airspaces lined by hyaline membranes and thickened alveolar septa containing inflammatory exudate.

TERMINOLOGY

Abbreviations

- Diffuse alveolar damage (DAD)

Synonyms

- Acute respiratory distress syndrome, shock lung, post-perfusion lung, hyaline membrane disease

Definitions

- Acute inflammatory reaction involving endothelial and epithelial cells of alveolus

ETIOLOGY/PATHOGENESIS

Etiology

- Can result from variety of lung injuries
  - Bacterial and viral infection
  - Drugs and inhaled toxins
  - Shock, trauma, burns
  - Sepsis
  - Allograft rejection
  - Radiation
  - Collagen vascular disease
  - Idiopathic

CLINICAL ISSUES

Epidemiology

- Incidence
  - 18-50 persons per 100,000 population per year
- Age
  - Children to adults

Presentation

- Tachypnea and rapidly progressive dyspnea
- Hypoxemia (PaO_2/FiO_2 ratio < 200)
- Respiratory failure with noncardiogenic pulmonary edema

Natural History

- Nonspecific histologic pattern of acute lung injury that may occur in wide variety of clinical settings
- Idiopathic cases are designated acute interstitial pneumonia (AIP) or Hamman-Rich syndrome
- Clinical syndrome associated with DAD is known as acute respiratory distress syndrome (ARDS)
- Rapid clinical onset, usually within 24-48 hours of precipitating event
- About 50% of patients may undergo spontaneous resolution with supportive therapy
- Oxygen therapy and mechanical ventilation may play significant role in causing development of tissue injury

Treatment

- Supportive therapy using mechanical ventilation with low tidal volumes
- Treatment of underlying precipitating condition (e.g., infection, shock, etc.)

Prognosis

- High overall mortality (~ 50% of patients)
- Death occurs after 1st 72 hours due to secondary infection, sepsis, or multisystem organ failure
- Surviving patients may recover normal lung function or go on to develop interstitial fibrosis

IMAGE FINDINGS

Radiographic Findings

- Bilateral basilar opacities are most common finding

CT Findings

- Intense parenchymal opacification due to lung consolidation or compressive atelectasis in dependent lung
- Ground-glass opacities with inhomogeneous distribution

DIFFUSE ALVEOLAR DAMAGE

Key Facts

Terminology
- Acute inflammatory reaction involving endothelial and epithelial cells of the alveolus

Clinical Issues
- Nonspecific histologic pattern of acute lung injury that may occur in wide variety of clinical settings
- Idiopathic cases are designated acute interstitial pneumonia (AIP) or Hamman-Rich syndrome
- Clinical syndrome associated with DAD is known as acute respiratory distress syndrome (ARDS)
- About 50% of patients may undergo spontaneous resolution with supportive therapy
- High overall mortality (~ 50% of patients)
- Surviving patients may recover normal lung function or go on to develop interstitial fibrosis

Microscopic Pathology
- Early, acute phase characterized by capillary congestion, edema, and intraalveolar hemorrhage
- Formation of hyaline membranes (pink fibrinous material lining alveolar walls) is hallmark of acute phase
- Interstitial inflammatory exudates (lymphocytes, plasma cells, and histiocytes)
- Organizing phase shows proliferation of type II pneumocytes with cytologic atypia
- Fibroblastic proliferation forms fibrinous intraalveolar plugs of granulation tissue reminiscent of organizing pneumonia
- Dense interstitial fibrosis with widening of alveolar septa is seen in late stages

MACROSCOPIC FEATURES

General Features
- Markedly enlarged and heavy lungs (3-4x normal weight)
- Dark, red to blue cut surface with marked congestion and edema in early stages
- Red-brown or gray, rubbery, and firm cut surface in later stages

MICROSCOPIC PATHOLOGY

Histologic Features
- Process is progressive and moves through 3 phases
  - **Exudative (acute) phase**
    - Early, acute phase characterized by capillary congestion, edema, and intraalveolar hemorrhage
    - Formation of hyaline membranes (pink fibrinous material lining alveolar walls) is hallmark of acute phase
    - Injury of type I pneumocytes and endothelial cells resulting in exudation of proteins and fluid into interstitium
    - Necrosis of type I pneumocytes with sloughing into alveolar lumens
    - Interstitial inflammatory exudates (lymphocytes, plasma cells, and histiocytes)
    - Microvascular thromboemboli (fibrin thrombi in capillaries or fibrin clots in medium-sized arterioles)
  - **Proliferative (organizing) phase**
    - Organization of exudate with proliferation of type II pneumocytes and fibroblasts
    - Proliferating pneumocytes can display large nuclei with prominent nucleoli and marked cytologic atypia
    - Fibroblastic proliferation forms fibrinous intraalveolar plugs of granulation tissue reminiscent of organizing pneumonia
    - Fibroblastic proliferation distends the alveolar walls forming loose organizing connective tissue
    - Vascular thromboemboli are present and may lead to peripheral infarcts
  - **Fibrotic (chronic) phase**
    - Seen in patients who survive on a ventilator > 3-4 weeks
    - Dense interstitial fibrosis with widening of alveolar septa
    - Squamous metaplasia of bronchiolar epithelium
    - Extensive honeycombing of lung parenchyma in very late stages

DIAGNOSTIC CHECKLIST

Pathologic Interpretation Pearls
- Morphologic findings are nonspecific and need to be correlated with clinical picture for definitive diagnosis
- Similar histologic findings can be observed secondarily in other processes unrelated to the respiratory distress syndrome
- Histologic phases of DAD may show considerable overlap
- Special stains for organisms or viruses may be of value in cases suspected of infection

SELECTED REFERENCES

1. Chung JH et al: CT predictors of mortality in pathology confirmed ARDS. Eur Radiol. 21(4):730-7, 2011
2. Beasley MB: The pathologist's approach to acute lung injury. Arch Pathol Lab Med. 134(5):719-27, 2010
3. de Hemptinne Q et al: ARDS: a clinicopathological confrontation. Chest. 135(4):944-9, 2009
4. Kang D et al: Two forms of diffuse alveolar damage in the lungs of patients with acute respiratory distress syndrome. Hum Pathol. 40(11):1618-27, 2009

DIFFUSE ALVEOLAR DAMAGE

Acute Exudative Phase

*(**Left**) Early stage of diffuse alveolar damage of the lung shows capillary congestion, edema, and intraalveolar hemorrhage. Microvascular thromboemboli ⇨ composed of fibrin thrombi in capillaries or in medium-sized arterioles can also be observed. (**Right**) Interstitial edema is seen in the early stages of diffuse alveolar damage, admixed with interstitial inflammatory exudates, including small lymphocytes, plasma cells, and histiocytes.*

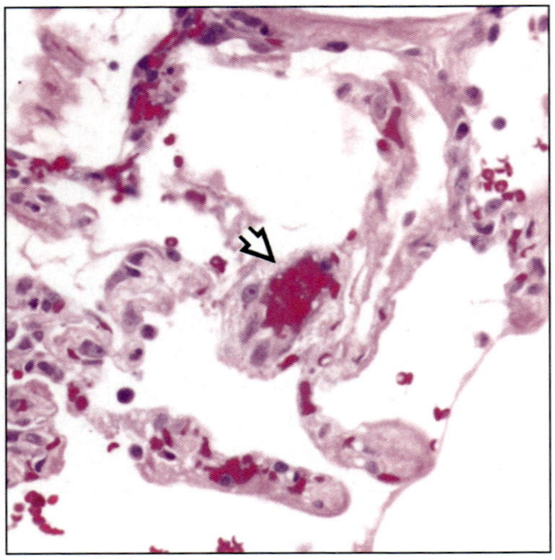

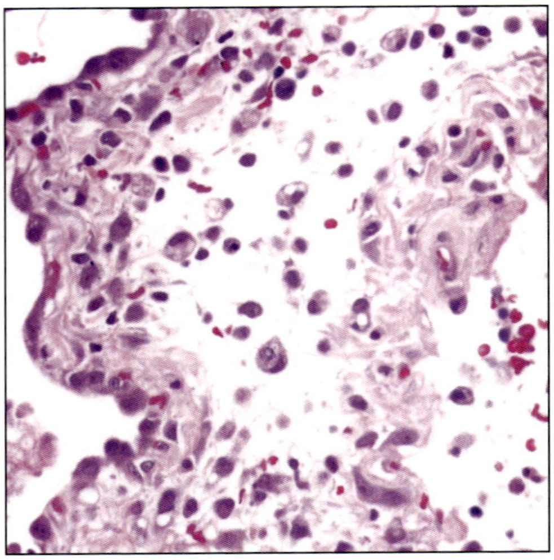

*(**Left**) Acute exudative stage of diffuse alveolar damage shows injury of type II pneumocytes with necrosis of epithelial lining cells and sloughing into the lumen, accompanied by exudation of protein and fluid into the interstitium. (**Right**) Hyaline membrane formation is also an early event in the exudative phase of diffuse alveolar damage. The hyaline membranes appear as a layer of pink, amorphous, and homogeneous material → lining the alveolar lumens.*

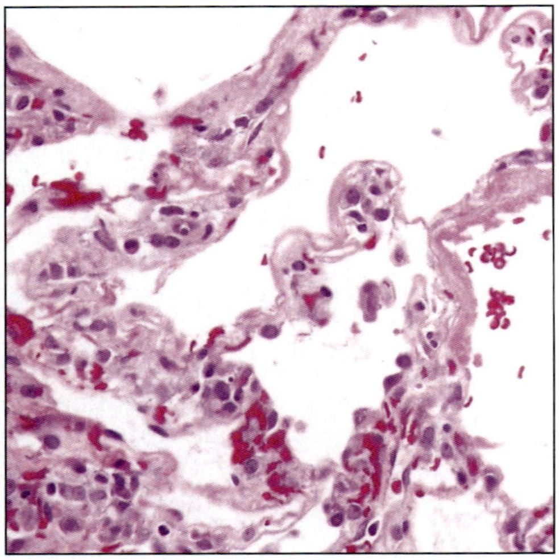

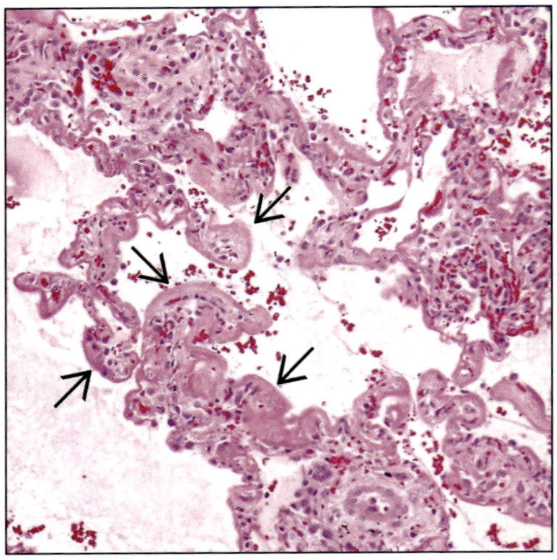

*(**Left**) Hyaline membrane formation is seen in the early stages of diffuse alveolar damage. The hyaline membrane in this case of acute lung injury is characterized by a thick band of homogeneous eosinophilic material → that lines the alveolar surface and replaces the native respiratory epithelium. (**Right**) Higher magnification of hyaline membrane in diffuse alveolar damage shows a thick band of dense, eosinophilic material covering the surface of the alveolar wall.*

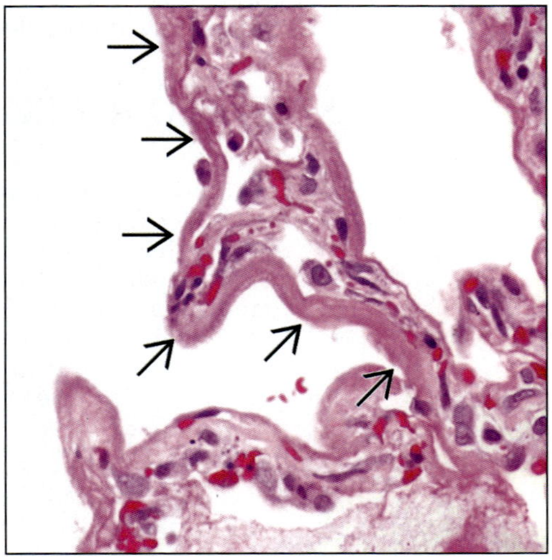

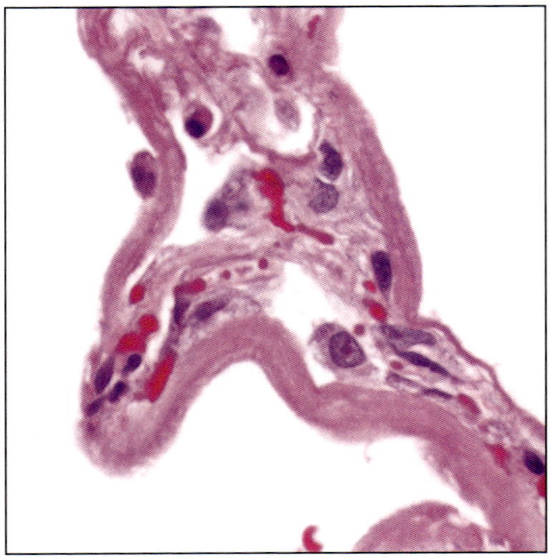

Organizing Proliferative Phase

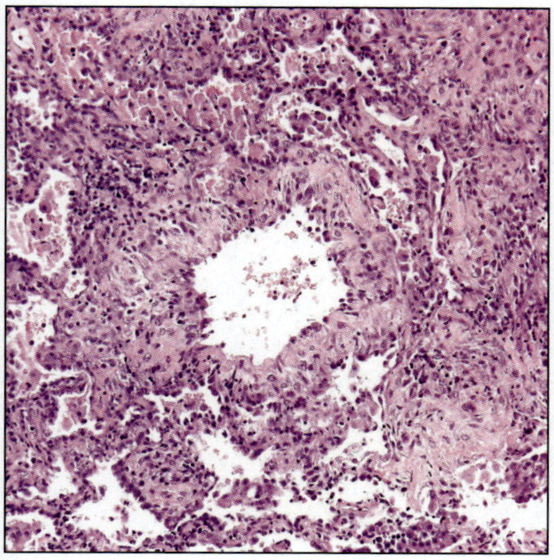
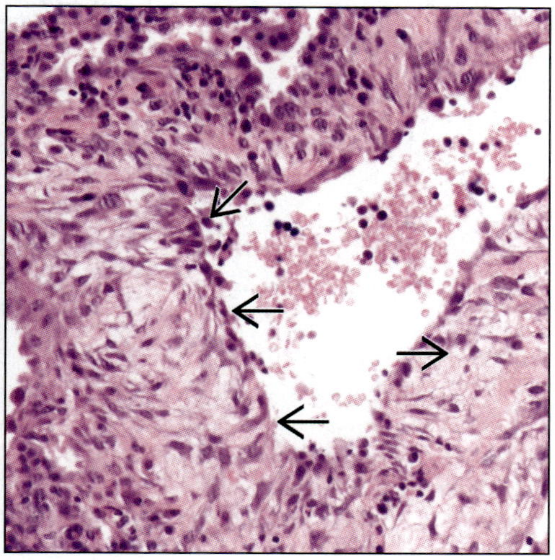

(Left) *Proliferative (organizing) phase of diffuse alveolar damage shows organization of the interstitial exudate with proliferation of type II pneumocytes and fibroblasts.* ***(Right)*** *Higher magnification of proliferative phase of diffuse alveolar damage shows fibroblastic proliferation in the wall of the alveoli with residual inflammation and granulation tissue-like changes of the interstitium* ➔*. The appearance is reminiscent of fibroblastic foci in UIP, but the process is more diffuse.*

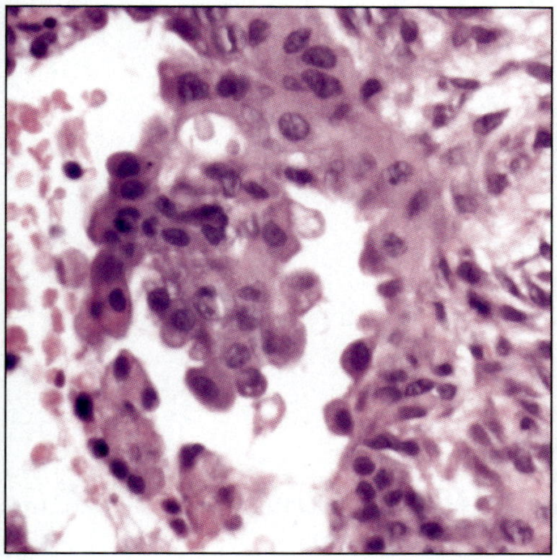
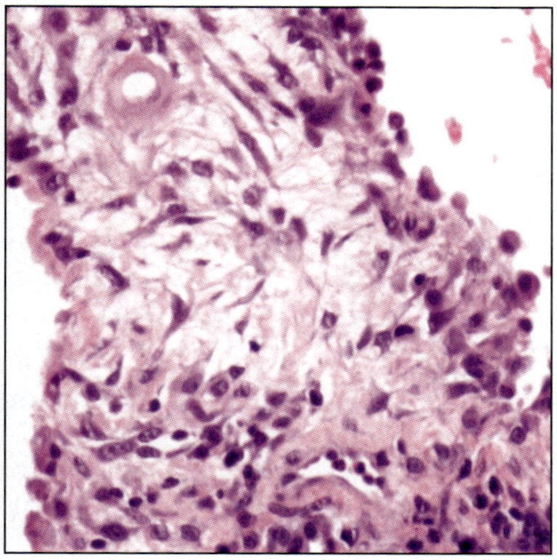

(Left) *Proliferative (organizing) phase of diffuse alveolar damage shows reactive proliferation of type II pneumocytes displaying large nuclei with prominent nucleoli, an ample rim of eosinophilic cytoplasm, and marked cytologic atypia.* ***(Right)*** *Proliferative phase of diffuse alveolar damage shows young fibroblastic proliferation in the interstitium of the alveolar walls with spindled fibroblasts embedded in lightly staining myxoid stroma admixed with scattered inflammatory cells.*

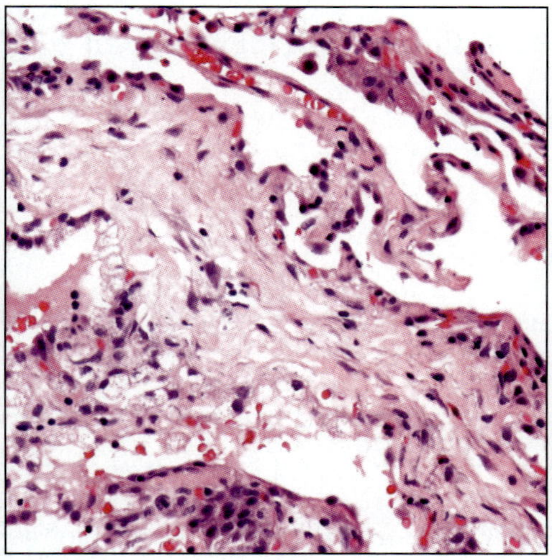
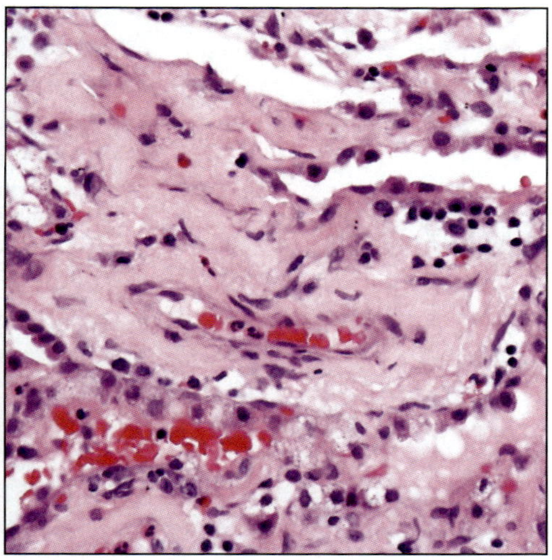

(Left) *Late, chronic phase of diffuse alveolar damage may show dense interstitial fibrosis, particularly in patients who have been on a respirator for more than 3-4 weeks. There is widening of the alveolar septa by dense collagenous fibrosis with minimal inflammatory infiltrates and complete disappearance of the hyaline membranes.* ***(Right)*** *Higher magnification of the chronic phase of diffuse alveolar damage shows thickening of alveolar septa by dense fibrosis.*

BRONCHIOLITIS OBLITERANS WITH ORGANIZING PNEUMONIA

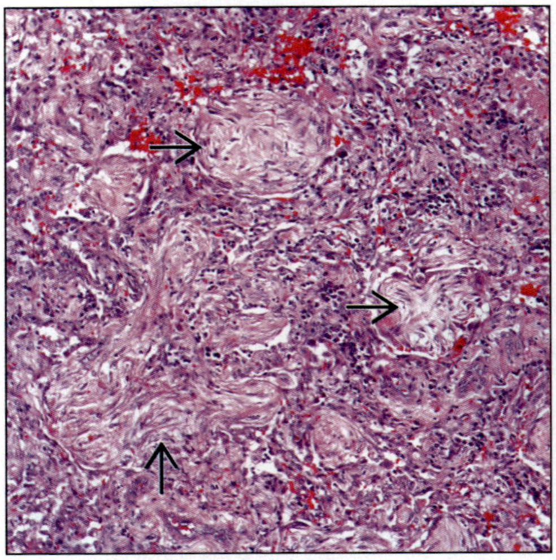

BOOP is shown with areas of young fibrous plugs in alveolar spaces ⇒. These features are characteristic of organizing pneumonia. Note the presence of an inflammatory component.

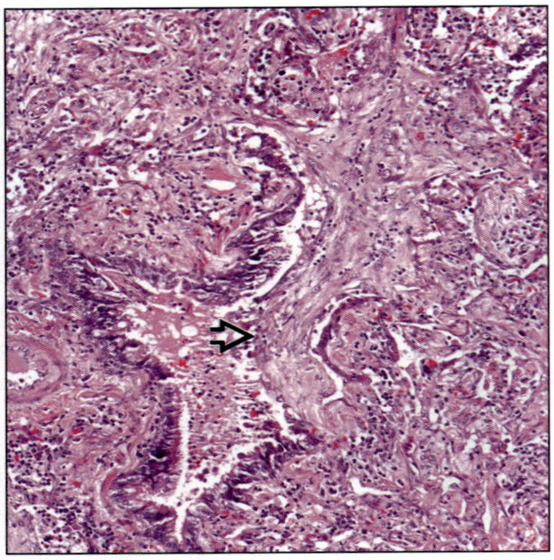

Young fibrous tissue ⇒ partially obstructs and destroys bronchial lumen and epithelium, respectively. This particular feature is also important in the diagnosis of BOOP.

TERMINOLOGY

Abbreviations

- Bronchiolitis obliterans with organizing pneumonia (BOOP)

Synonyms

- Cryptogenic organizing pneumonia (COP), bronchiolitis obliterans

Definitions

- Idiopathic interstitial and airway process with features of pneumonia

ETIOLOGY/PATHOGENESIS

Etiology

- No definitive etiology has been specified for BOOP
- Histopathologic features of BOOP may be seen secondary to diverse conditions

CLINICAL ISSUES

Epidemiology

- Incidence
  - Definitive incidence of BOOP is not known
  - It has been stated at < 10 per 100,000 patient admissions
- Age
  - Usually in adults
- Gender
  - No gender predilection
- Ethnicity
  - No ethnic predilection

Site

- Process may appear in any lung or lung segment

Presentation

- Cough
- Dyspnea
- Fever
- Malaise
- Flu-like symptoms
- Headache

Laboratory Tests

- Leukocytosis
- Elevation of erythrocyte sedimentation rate
- C-reactive protein is positive

Treatment

- Drugs
  - Corticosteroids
  - Azathioprine or cyclophosphamide in some patients who do not respond to steroids

Prognosis

- Most patients respond to corticosteroid therapy

Associated Conditions with Histology of BOOP

- Infectious conditions
  - Viral
  - Bacterial
  - Fungal
- Collagen vascular disease
- Radiation
- Hypersensitivity
- Autoimmune process

MACROSCOPIC FEATURES

General Features

- Diagnosis of BOOP is essentially done on open biopsy specimens
  - Thus, no specific macroscopic features have been associated with BOOP

BRONCHIOLITIS OBLITERANS WITH ORGANIZING PNEUMONIA

Key Facts

Terminology
- Synonyms: Cryptogenic organizing pneumonia (COP), bronchiolitis obliterans
- Definition
  - Idiopathic interstitial and airway disease process with features of pneumonia

Etiology/Pathogenesis
- No definitive etiology has been specified
- Histopathologic features of BOOP may be seen secondary to diverse conditions

Clinical Issues
- Symptoms
  - Cough
  - Dyspnea
  - Fever
  - Flu-like symptoms
- Treatment
  - Corticosteroids

Top Differential Diagnoses
- Usual interstitial pneumonitis (UIP)
- Diffuse alveolar damage (DAD)
- Organizing diffuse alveolar damage (O-DAD)
- Inflammatory pseudotumor (IPT)

Diagnostic Checklist
- Loose young fibrocollagenous polypoid plugs in alveoli and airway
- Mild inflammatory changes
- Loose organizing fibrosis

MICROSCOPIC PATHOLOGY

Histologic Features
- Loose organizing fibrosis
- Intraluminal fibrocollagenous polypoid plugs
  - Bronchioles
  - Alveoli
  - Alveolar ducts
- Mild inflammatory changes

DIFFERENTIAL DIAGNOSIS

Usual Interstitial Pneumonitis (UIP)
- Shows relatively normal areas of lung parenchyma intermixed with areas of interstitial fibrosis
- Usually bilateral and diffuse
- Honeycombing-like changes in lung parenchyma are characteristic of UIP

Diffuse Alveolar Damage (DAD)
- Generally shows presence of hyaline membranes
- Shows hyperplasia of type II pneumocytes

Infectious Pneumonia
- Generally shows areas of acute and chronic inflammation
- Use of special histochemical stains for microorganisms or tissue cultures will lead to correct interpretation

Organizing Diffuse Alveolar Damage (O-DAD)
- May show areas of intraluminal fibrosis similar to BOOP
- Shows hyaline membranes and type II pneumocyte hyperplasia
- O-DAD is diffuse process

Inflammatory Pseudotumor (IPT)
- Shows predominantly plasma cell or fibrohistiocytic component
- Will not show presence of intraalveolar fibrocollagenous plugs

DIAGNOSTIC CHECKLIST

Clinically Relevant Pathologic Features
- Tissue distribution

Pathologic Interpretation Pearls
- Loose young fibrocollagenous polypoid plugs in alveoli and airway
- Mild inflammatory changes
- Loose organizing fibrosis

SELECTED REFERENCES

1. Drakopanagiotakis F et al: Organizing pneumonia. Am J Med Sci. 335(1):34-9, 2008
2. Sara AG et al: Bronchiolitis obliterans organizing pneumonia: Pathogenesis, clinical features, imaging and therapy review. Ann Thorac Med. 3(2):67-75, 2008
3. Lazor R: [Cryptogenic and secondary organizing pneumonia.] Rev Prat. 57(20):2243-8, 2007
4. Yoshihara S et al: Bronchiolitis obliterans syndrome (BOS), bronchiolitis obliterans organizing pneumonia (BOOP), and other late-onset noninfectious pulmonary complications following allogeneic hematopoietic stem cell transplantation. Biol Blood Marrow Transplant. 13(7):749-59, 2007
5. Cordier JF: Cryptogenic organising pneumonia. Eur Respir J. 28(2):422-46, 2006
6. Schlesinger C et al: The organizing pneumonias : a critical review of current concepts and treatment. Treat Respir Med. 5(3):193-206, 2006
7. Angel L et al: Bronchiolitis obliterans. Semin Respir Crit Care Med. 21(2):123-34, 2000

BRONCHIOLITIS OBLITERANS WITH ORGANIZING PNEUMONIA

Microscopic Features

*(**Left**) Low-power view of BOOP shows a well-demarcated area of organization ➡ giving the appearance of a nodule within the lung parenchyma. Still, areas of uninvolved lung parenchyma ↪ are present. (**Right**) BOOP may present as a well-demarcated nodule that partially obliterates the normal lung parenchyma. Note here the presence of a well-demarcated nodule ➡ in contrast to normal lung parenchyma ↪.*

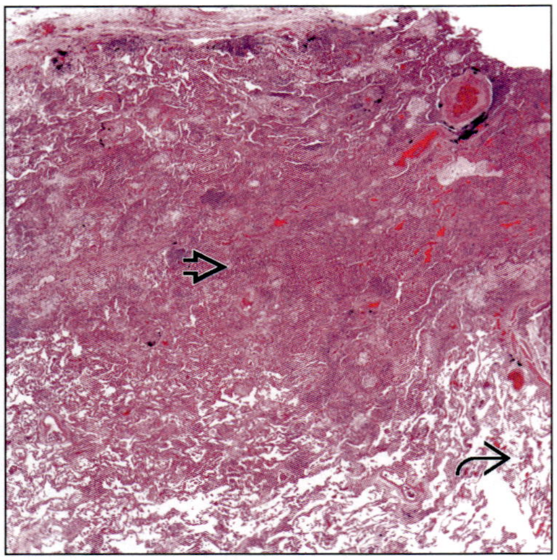

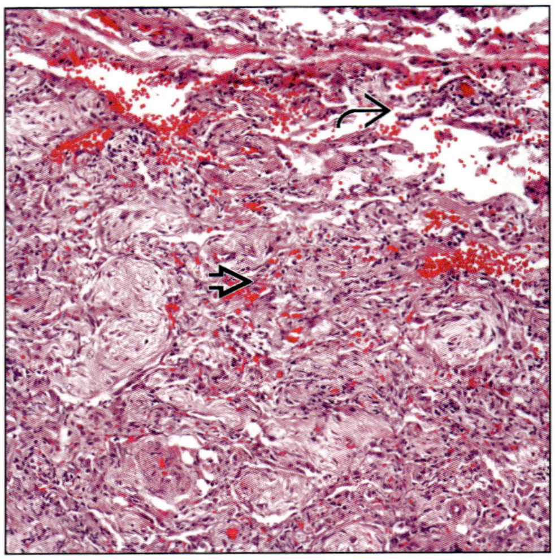

*(**Left**) This closer view shows fibroblastic plugs ➡ made of young fibroconnective tissue. These structures are destroying the normal alveolated lung parenchyma. This image may mimic cases of organizing diffuse alveolar damage. (**Right**) High-power magnification of a fibroblastic plug shows some spindle cellular proliferation admixed with fibroconnective tissue. Cellular atypia may be seen in some cases.*

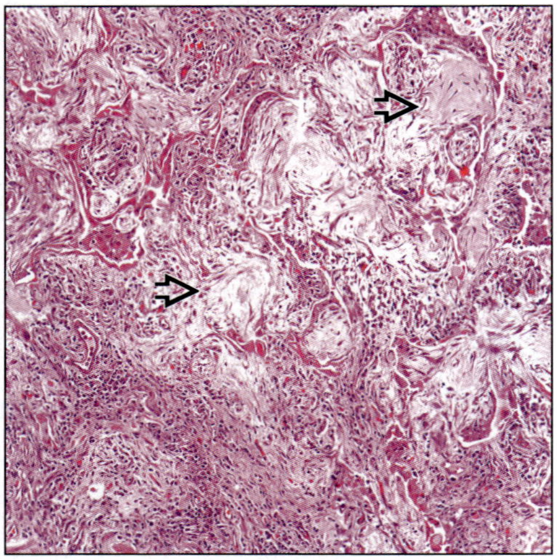

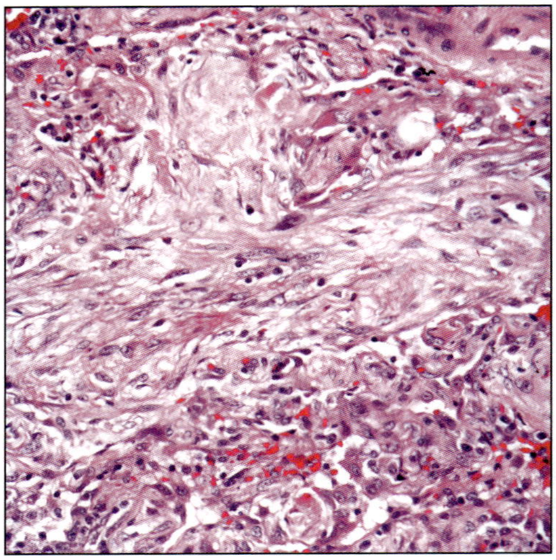

*(**Left**) Fibroblastic plugs ↪ are shown involving alveolar spaces and dispersed haphazardly in the lung parenchyma. In addition, there is hyperplasia of type II pneumocytes. (**Right**) One important component in the diagnosis of BOOP is the presence of similar fibroblastic plugs in the the airways. Note the presence of polypoid structures filling the airway.*

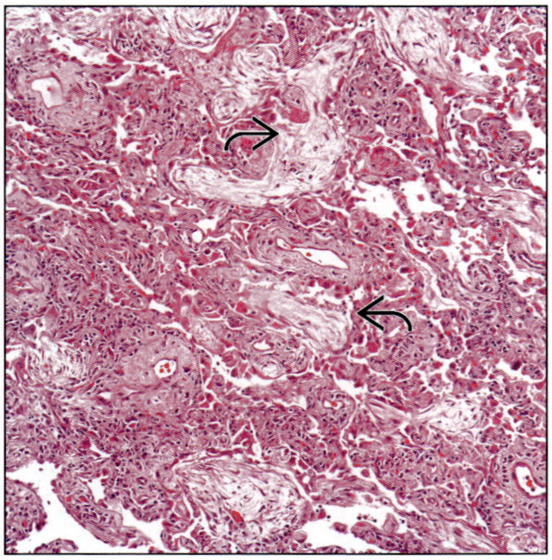

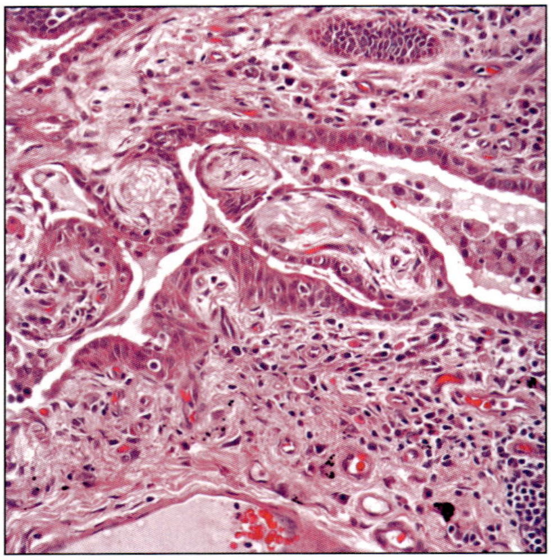

BRONCHIOLITIS OBLITERANS WITH ORGANIZING PNEUMONIA

Microscopic Features

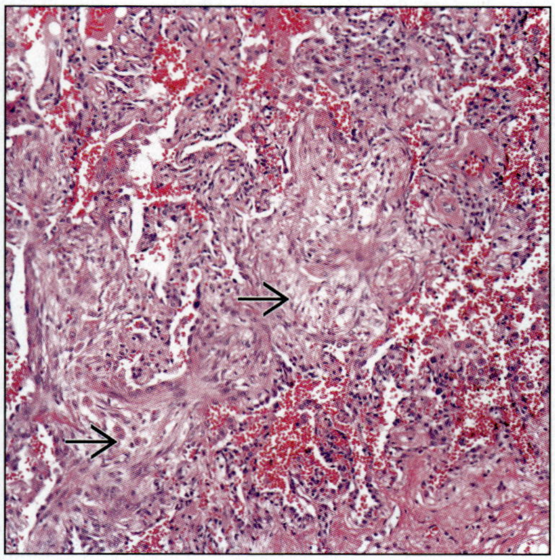

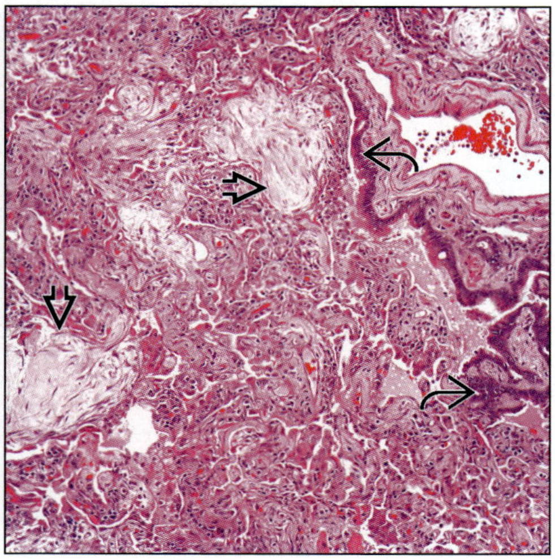

(Left) *BOOP shows the presence of young fibrous → tissue penetrating alveolar spaces. The tissue appears to be dissecting interstitium. Still areas of uninvolved lung parenchyma are present.* ***(Right)*** *In some cases of BOOP, the presence of airway obstruction can be difficult to appreciate. In this case, the airway ↪ appears to be partially destroyed, and the presence of fibrous plugs ⇨ appears to be more in the alveolated areas than in the airway.*

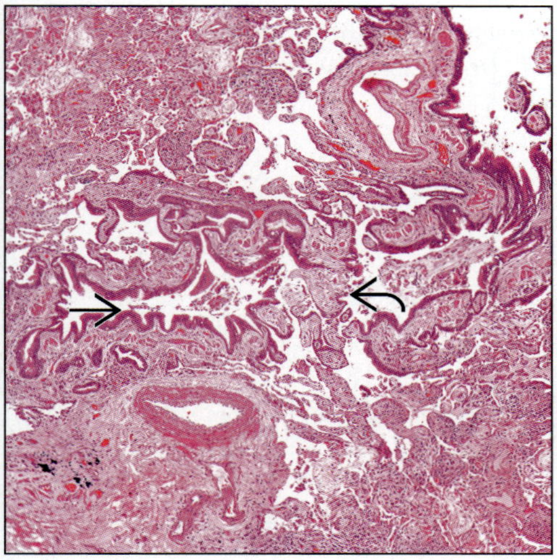

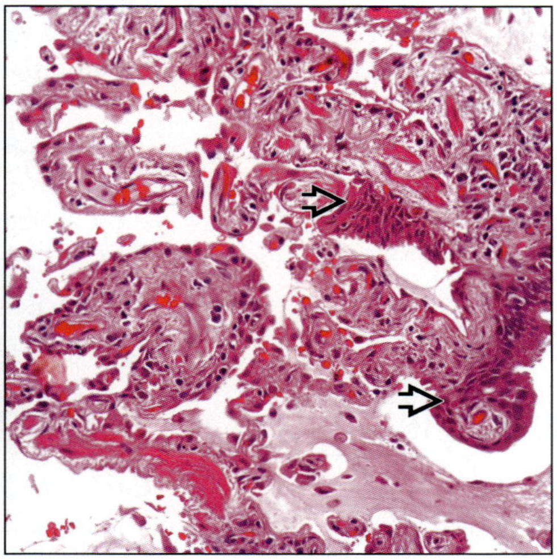

(Left) *In other areas of BOOP, strips of bronchial epithelium → are present as well as identifiable airway. In addition, polypoid structures ↪ composed of young fibrous tissue are apparent in the lumen of the airway.* ***(Right)*** *Closer view shows some of those polypoid structures are composed of fibroconnective tissue and some of them are lined by low cuboidal type of epithelium. In addition, note the presence of residual normal bronchial epithelium ⇨.*

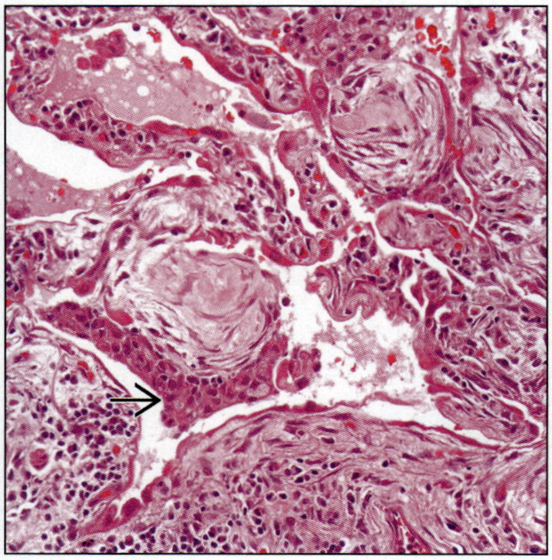

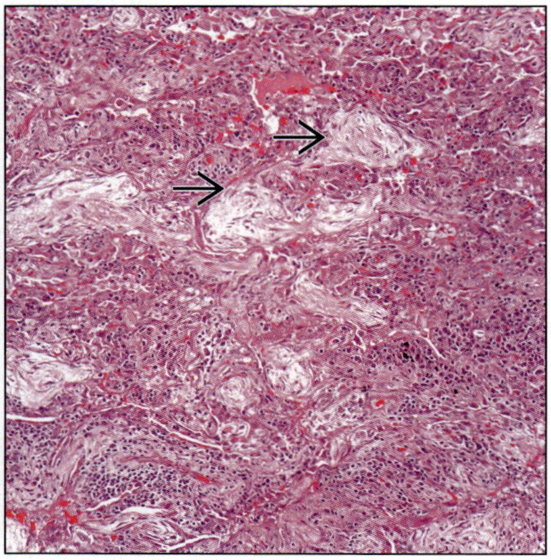

(Left) *Remaining bronchial structure is shown with squamous metaplasia → and some polypoid fibrous plugs in this lumen. These features are characteristic of BOOP.* ***(Right)*** *Areas of BOOP are shown with more conventional areas of organizing pneumonia. Note the presence of the so-called Masson bodies →, young fibrocollagenous tissue, and inflammatory infiltrate.*

RESPIRATORY BRONCHIOLITIS

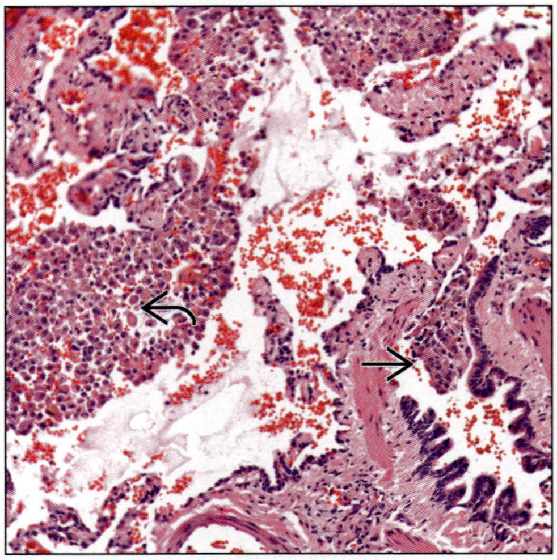

Respiratory bronchiolitis shows collections of pigmented macrophages within the airway ➔ and in adjacent alveolar spaces ➔.

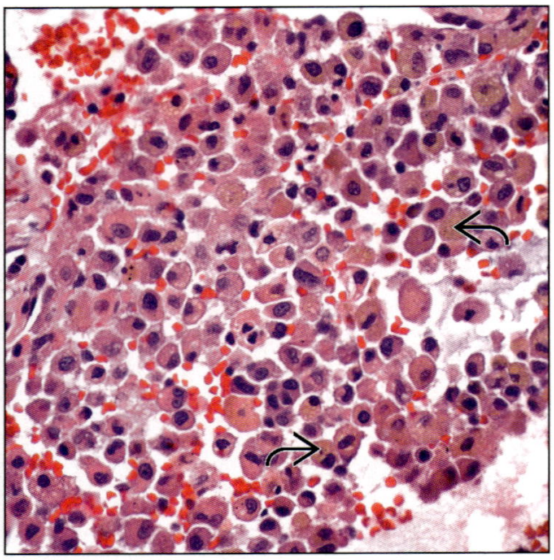

High-power magnification shows a collection of macrophages in respiratory bronchiolitis. Note that some of the macrophages show pigment ➔.

TERMINOLOGY

Abbreviations

- Respiratory bronchiolitis-interstitial lung disease (RB-ILD)

Synonyms

- Smoker's bronchiolitis
- Small airway disease

Definitions

- Mild form of interstitial lung disease

ETIOLOGY/PATHOGENESIS

Environmental Exposure

- Closely associated with smoking history
- Occupational exposure to fumes

CLINICAL ISSUES

Epidemiology

- Incidence
  - No hard data on incidence
- Age
  - Generally in adults
- Gender
  - No gender predilection
- Ethnicity
  - No ethnic preference

Site

- Small airways of lung parenchyma

Presentation

- Cough
- Dyspnea
- Wheezing
- Flu-like symptoms

Laboratory Tests

- There are no specific laboratory findings for RB
- Pulmonary function tests may be normal or show only minimal changes

Treatment

- Drugs
  - Corticosteroids
- Cessation of smoking

Prognosis

- Very good prognosis

MACROSCOPIC FEATURES

General Features

- Most of the time, diagnosis of RB-ILD is made during open lung biopsy

MICROSCOPIC PATHOLOGY

Histologic Features

- Pigmented macrophages in lumens of airway
- Collections of intraalveolar pigmented macrophages around airways
- Goblet cell metaplasia may be present in bronchial epithelium
- Mild interstitial fibrosis may be present
- Most of alveolated lung parenchyma appears normal
- Absence of marked interstitial fibrosis
- Absence of marked inflammatory changes

DIFFERENTIAL DIAGNOSIS

Desquamative Interstitial Pneumonitis (DIP)

- Shows more diffuse process
- Prominent collections of intraalveolar macrophages

Key Facts

Terminology
- Respiratory bronchiolitis-interstitial lung disease (RB-ILD)
- Synonym: Smoker's bronchiolitis
- Mild form of interstitial lung disease

Etiology/Pathogenesis
- Closely associated with smoking history
- Occupational exposure to fumes

Clinical Issues
- Symptoms
  - Cough
  - Dyspnea
  - Wheezing
  - Flue-like symptoms
- Laboratory findings
  - There are no specific laboratory findings for RB
  - Pulmonary function tests may be normal
- Treatment
  - Cessation of smoking
  - Corticosteroids

Top Differential Diagnoses
- Desquamative interstitial pneumonitis (DIP)
- Langerhans cell histiocytosis (LCH)
- Usual interstitial pneumonitis (UIP)

Diagnostic Checklist
- Collections of pigmented macrophages in lumens of airways
- Collections of intraalveolar macrophages around small airways
- Absence of marked interstitial fibrosis

Langerhans Cell Histiocytosis (LCH)
- Shows presence of histiocytic cellular proliferation
- May show prominent eosinophilic component
- Not limited to small airways
- Immunohistochemical study for CD1a will show positive staining in histiocytes of LCH

Usual Interstitial Pneumonitis (UIP)
- Shows areas of remodeling lung parenchyma
- Shows honeycombing changes of lung parenchyma
- Shows extensive areas of interstitial fibrosis

Eosinophilic Pneumonia
- Shows prominent intraalveolar collections of eosinophils
- Is a diffuse process
- Presence of collections of intraalveolar macrophages in airway is not a feature of eosinophilic pneumonia

Pneumonia
- Shows prominent acute and chronic inflammatory changes
- Is a more diffuse process
- Histochemical stains for organisms or tissue cultures will lead to correct interpretation

DIAGNOSTIC CHECKLIST

Clinically Relevant Pathologic Features
- Tissue distribution

Pathologic Interpretation Pearls
- Collections of pigmented macrophages in lumens of airways
- Collections of intraalveolar macrophages around small airways
- Absence of marked interstitial fibrosis
- Subtle changes in small airways
- Absence of marked inflammatory changes

SELECTED REFERENCES

1. Argiriadi PA et al: High resolution computed tomography in idiopathic interstitial pneumonias. Mt Sinai J Med. 76(1):37-52, 2009
2. Attili AK et al: Smoking-related interstitial lung disease: radiologic-clinical-pathologic correlation. Radiographics. 28(5):1383-96; discussion 1396-8, 2008
3. Kawabata Y et al: Smoking-related changes in the background lung of specimens resected for lung cancer: a semiquantitative study with correlation to postoperative course. Histopathology. 53(6):707-14, 2008
4. Patel RR et al: Cigarette smoking and diffuse lung disease. Drugs. 68(11):1511-27, 2008
5. Prezant DJ et al: Upper and lower respiratory diseases after occupational and environmental disasters. Mt Sinai J Med. 75(2):89-100, 2008
6. Rao RN et al: Smoking-related interstitial lung disease. Ann Diagn Pathol. 12(6):445-57, 2008
7. Vassallo R et al: Tobacco smoke-related diffuse lung diseases. Semin Respir Crit Care Med. 29(6):643-50, 2008
8. Portnoy J et al: Respiratory bronchiolitis-interstitial lung disease: long-term outcome. Chest. 131(3):664-71, 2007
9. Woo OH et al: Respiratory bronchiolitis-associated interstitial lung disease in a nonsmoker: radiologic and pathologic findings. AJR Am J Roentgenol. 188(5):W412-4, 2007
10. Franquet T et al: Disorders of the small airways: high-resolution computed tomographic features. Semin Respir Crit Care Med. 24(4):437-44, 2003
11. Wells AU et al: Respiratory bronchiolitis-associated interstitial lung disease. Semin Respir Crit Care Med. 24(5):585-94, 2003
12. Elkin SL et al: Desquamative interstitial pneumonia and respiratory bronchiolitis-associated interstitial lung disease. Semin Respir Crit Care Med. 22(4):387-98, 2001

RESPIRATORY BRONCHIOLITIS

Microscopic Features

*(**Left**) Low-power view of a section from lung parenchyma shows extensive congestion. At this power, the diagnostic features of respiratory bronchiolitis are not easily recognized. (**Right**) Lung parenchyma is shown with an intraalveolar collection of red cells. The lung parenchyma is congested, probably as a result of the surgical procedure and not necessarily as a feature of respiratory bronchiolitis.*

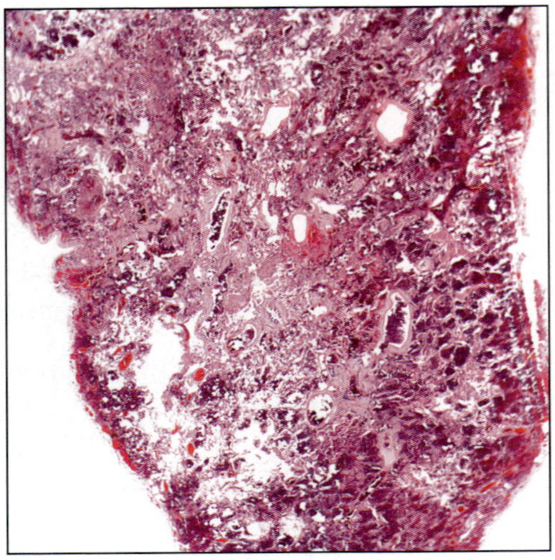

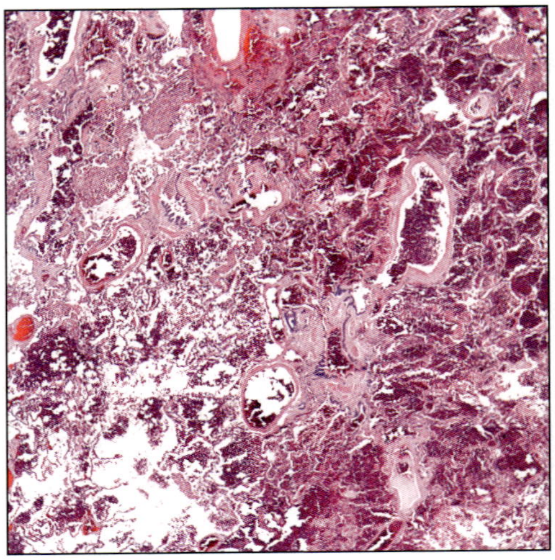

*(**Left**) Other areas of respiratory bronchiolitis in which collections of red cells are admixed with collections of macrophages are shown. Note the presence of an airway structure ↶. (**Right**) In some cases, discrete areas of interstitial fibrosis may be apparent; however, note the presence of intraalveolar red cells with the absence of pigmented macrophages.*

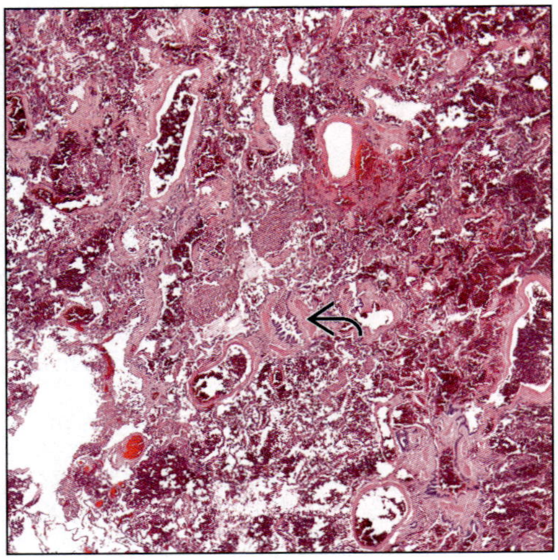

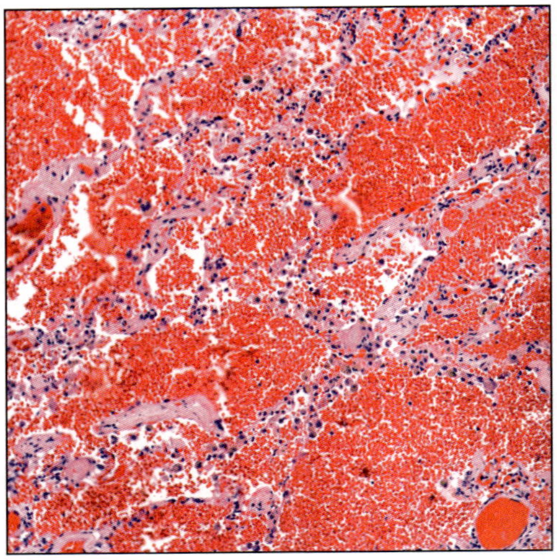

*(**Left**) Other areas of respiratory bronchiolitis show combined intraalveolar collections of red cells → and macrophages ↶. Note that the basic architecture of the lung parenchyma is preserved. (**Right**) Closer view shows a collection of macrophages, some of them with pigment in their cytoplasm ↶. Although this is an important feature of respiratory bronchiolitis, by itself, it is not diagnostic.*

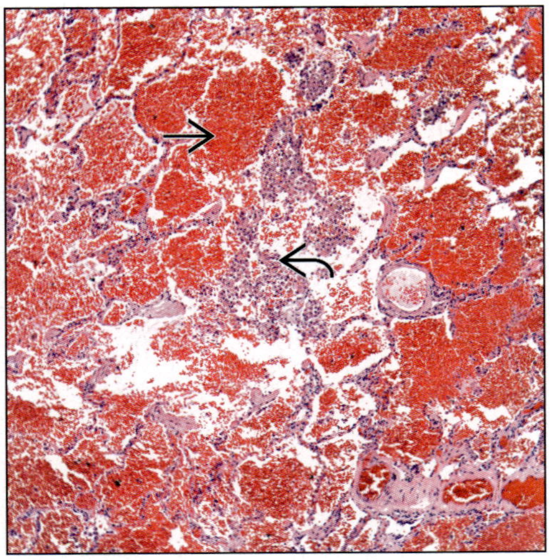

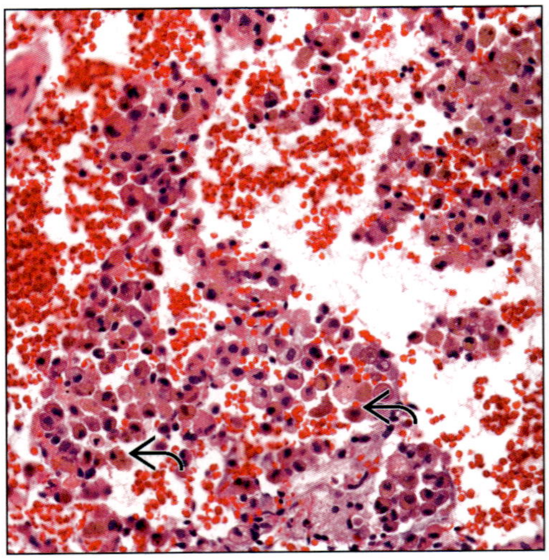

RESPIRATORY BRONCHIOLITIS

Microscopic Features

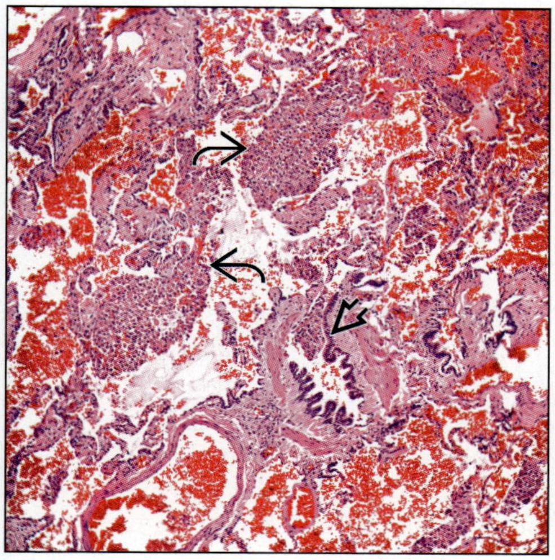

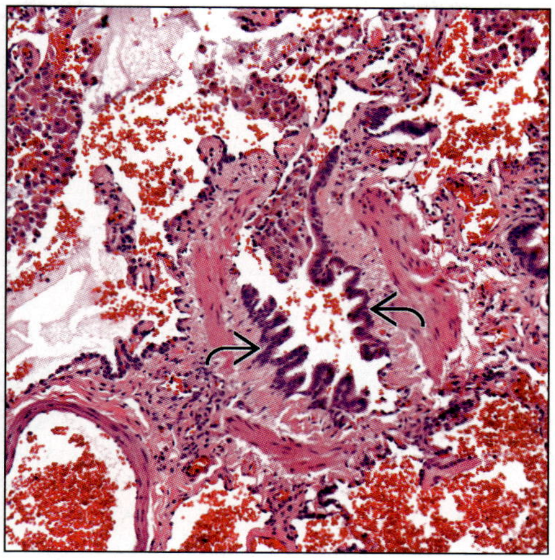

(Left) *Respiratory bronchiolitis shows the most important and characteristic histological features, mainly the presence of pigmented macrophages in the bronchial lumen* → *and collections of pigmented macrophages in the adjacent peribronchial areas* →. ***(Right)*** *Closer view of an airway shows collections of pigmented macrophages. Note that the bronchial epithelium is still within normal limits* →.

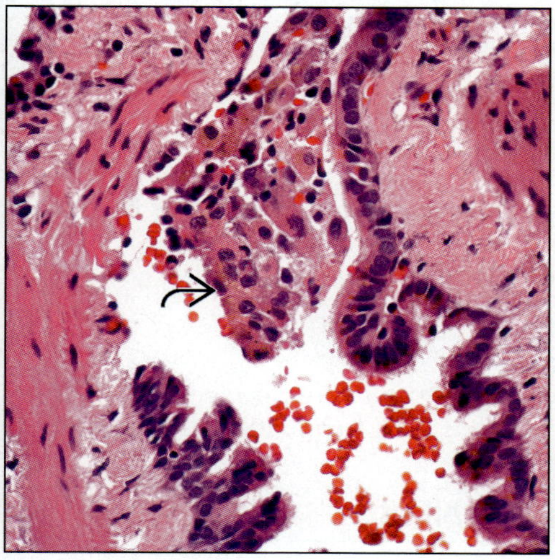

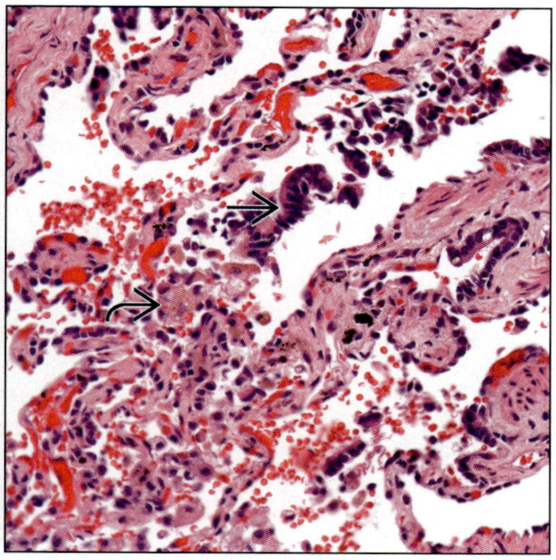

(Left) *High-power view shows the airway containing pigmented macrophages* →. *The bronchial epithelium is still showing ciliated epithelium. This histological feature is important in the diagnosis of respiratory bronchiolitis.* ***(Right)*** *In some areas of respiratory bronchiolitis, the airway may not show the usual concentric luminal space; rather, the airway is partially distorted* → *yet contains numerous pigmented macrophages* →.

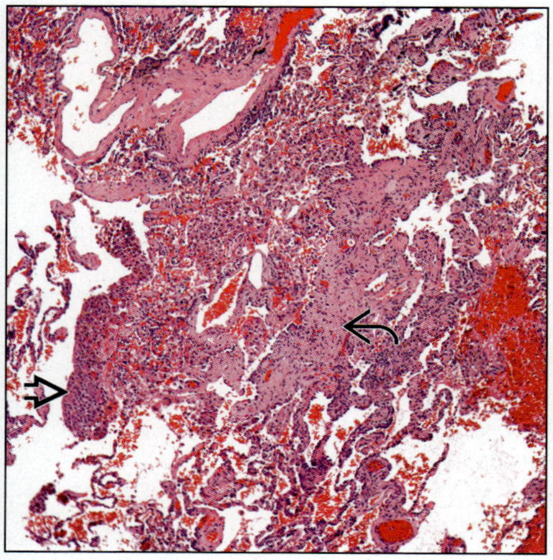

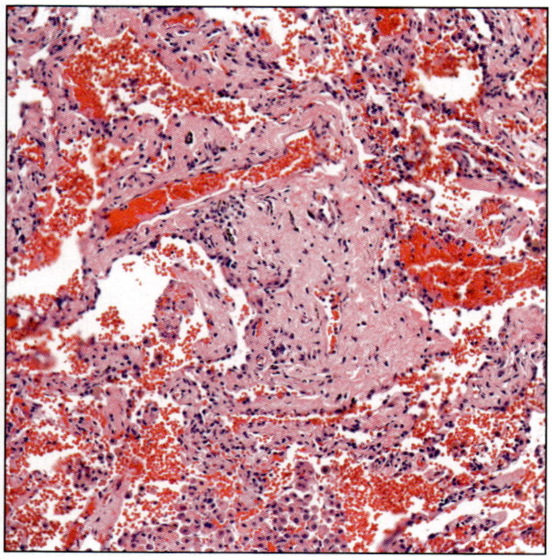

(Left) *Low-power view of respiratory bronchiolitis shows areas with collections of pigmented macrophages* → *and focal scarring* → *with mild inflammatory reaction.* ***(Right)*** *The presence of areas of scarring may be only focal in cases of respiratory bronchiolitis. Extensive areas of fibrosis or scarring are not features of respiratory bronchiolitis.*

USUAL INTERSTITIAL PNEUMONIA

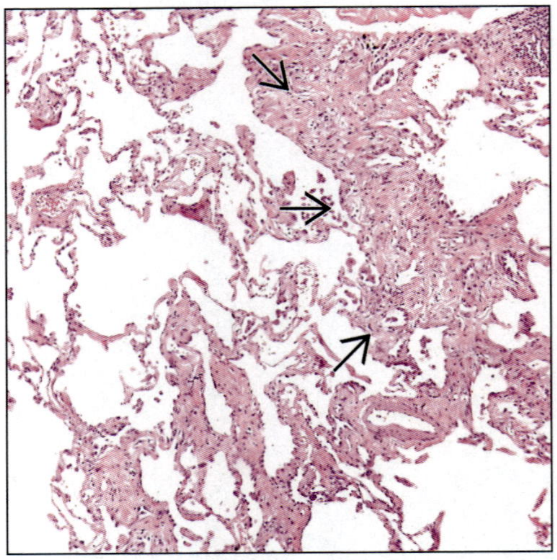

Scanning magnification in usual interstitial pneumonia shows areas of lung parenchyma with thickened alveolar walls ⇒ surrounded by areas of normal lung parenchyma.

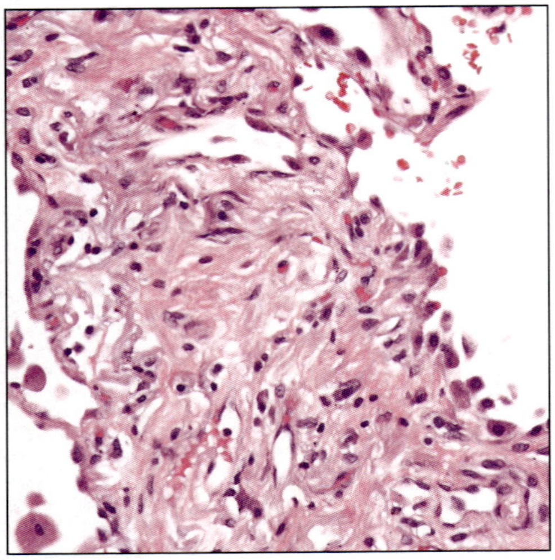

Higher magnification of thickened alveolar wall in usual interstitial pneumonia shows heavy deposition of collagen fibers admixed with sparse inflammatory infiltrate.

TERMINOLOGY

Abbreviations

- Usual interstitial pneumonia (UIP)

Synonyms

- Idiopathic interstitial fibrosis, idiopathic pulmonary fibrosis, cryptogenic fibrosing alveolitis

Definitions

- Pattern of lung damage characterized by bilateral, diffuse, interstitial inflammation and fibrosis

ETIOLOGY/PATHOGENESIS

Pathogenesis

- Unknown (idiopathic)
- May be associated with a variety of clinical conditions, including
  - Collagen-vascular disease
  - Drug toxicity
  - Pneumoconiosis and other environmental exposures

CLINICAL ISSUES

Epidemiology

- Incidence
  - Approximately 10 cases per 100,000 people per year
- Age
  - 50-70 years of age
- Gender
  - More common in men

Presentation

- Insidious onset of dyspnea and nonproductive cough
- Tachypnea
- Bibasilar, late inspiratory crackles
- Clubbing of fingers in > 40% of patients
- Pulmonary hypertension (in late stages)
- Restriction and impairment of gas exchange on pulmonary function tests

Treatment

- Surgical approaches
  - Lung transplantation
- Drugs
  - Immunosuppressive and cytotoxic agents have not been very effective
  - Gamma interferon

Prognosis

- Poor prognosis
- Mean survival ranges from 3.5-5 years
- Respiratory failure is most frequent cause of death

IMAGE FINDINGS

Radiographic Findings

- Bilateral, symmetrical, linear opacities showing reticular pattern
- Ground-glass opacities
- Honeycombing and decreased lung volume
- Abnormalities involve mainly lower lobes of lung
- Normal chest x-rays may be seen in ~ 10% of patients

CT Findings

- HRCT shows reticular pattern with honeycombing involving mainly subpleural lung regions
- Intralobular linear opacities with irregular thickening of interlobular septa
- Irregular pleural, vascular, and bronchial interfaces with the lung parenchyma
- In more advanced stages there is traction bronchiectasis and honeycombing
- Typical findings may be seen on HRCT even when chest x-rays appear normal
- Bilateral process with basilar and peripheral predominance

USUAL INTERSTITIAL PNEUMONIA

Key Facts

Terminology
- Pattern of lung damage characterized by bilateral, diffuse, interstitial inflammation and fibrosis

Clinical Issues
- Insidious onset of dyspnea and nonproductive cough
- Poor prognosis
- Mean survival ranges from 3.5-5 years

Image Findings
- HRCT shows reticular pattern with honeycombing involving mainly subpleural lung regions
- In more advanced stages there is traction bronchiectasis and honeycombing

Macroscopic Features
- Peripheral subpleural areas of fibrosis of lung parenchyma predominantly in lower lobes
- Peripheral honeycomb cystic changes in more advanced lesions

Microscopic Pathology
- Areas of lung parenchyma showing interstitial inflammation and fibrosis adjacent to areas of normal parenchyma
- Areas of diseased lung are seen in various stages of evolution ("temporal heterogeneity")
- Interstitial fibrosis causes widening of alveolar septa due to collagen deposition admixed with inflammatory cells
- "Fibroblastic foci" are present, composed of loose connective tissue admixed with fibroblastic cells
- Areas of fibrosis with cystic spaces result in "honeycombing" effect

MACROSCOPIC FEATURES

General Features
- Peripheral subpleural areas of fibrosis of lung parenchyma, predominantly in lower lobes
- Peripheral honeycomb cystic changes in more advanced lesions

MICROSCOPIC PATHOLOGY

Histologic Features
- Areas of lung parenchyma showing interstitial inflammation and fibrosis adjacent to areas of normal parenchyma
- Areas of diseased lung are seen in various stages of evolution ("temporal heterogeneity")
- Interstitial fibrosis causes widening of alveolar septa due to collagen deposition admixed with inflammatory cells
- Interstitial inflammatory infiltrate includes small lymphocytes, plasma cells, and histiocytes with occasional lymphoid follicles
- "Fibroblastic foci" are present, composed of loose connective tissue admixed with fibroblastic cells
- Focal accumulation of alveolar macrophages ("DIP-like" appearance)
- Bronchiolization of alveolar lining ("Lambertosis") may be observed
- Squamous metaplasia in areas of scarring can be seen in late stages
- Smooth muscle stromal proliferation may accompany stromal scarring
- Areas of fibrosis with cystic spaces result in "honeycombing" effect
- Episodes of acute exacerbation may result in foci of diffuse alveolar damage superimposed on UIP

DIAGNOSTIC CHECKLIST

Clinically Relevant Pathologic Features
- Transbronchial biopsies are not useful for evaluation of interstitial fibrosis
- Multiple open lung biopsies are indicated for definitive diagnosis
- Biopsies must be obtained from multiple lobes, avoiding the lung apices
- About 50% of patients can be diagnosed on clinical and radiologic grounds alone without a biopsy

Pathologic Interpretation Pearls
- "Temporal heterogeneity" (lesions at various stages of evolution) serve to distinguish UIP from NSIP
- Clinical history is indispensable for cases associated with underlying collagen-vascular disorders
- Scanning magnification showing variegation and admixture of abnormal foci with normal lung parenchyma is diagnostic
- Advanced stages with extensive fibrosis and honeycombing may be impossible to diagnose in absence of a history

SELECTED REFERENCES

1. Borchers AT et al: Idiopathic Pulmonary Fibrosis-an Epidemiological and Pathological Review. Clin Rev Allergy Immunol. 40(2):117-34, 2011
2. Chan AL et al: Therapeutic Update in Idiopathic Pulmonary Fibrosis. Clin Rev Allergy Immunol. Epub ahead of print, 2011
3. Force SD et al: Bilateral lung transplantation offers better long-term survival, compared with single-lung transplantation, for younger patients with idiopathic pulmonary fibrosis. Ann Thorac Surg. 91(1):244-9, 2011
4. Cavazza A et al: The role of histology in idiopathic pulmonary fibrosis: an update. Respir Med. 104 Suppl 1:S11-22, 2010
5. Coward WR et al: The pathogenesis of idiopathic pulmonary fibrosis. Ther Adv Respir Dis. 4(6):367-88, 2010

USUAL INTERSTITIAL PNEUMONIA

Histologic Features

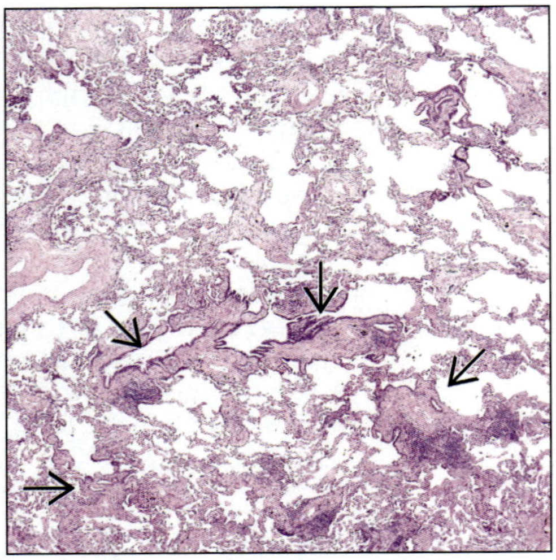
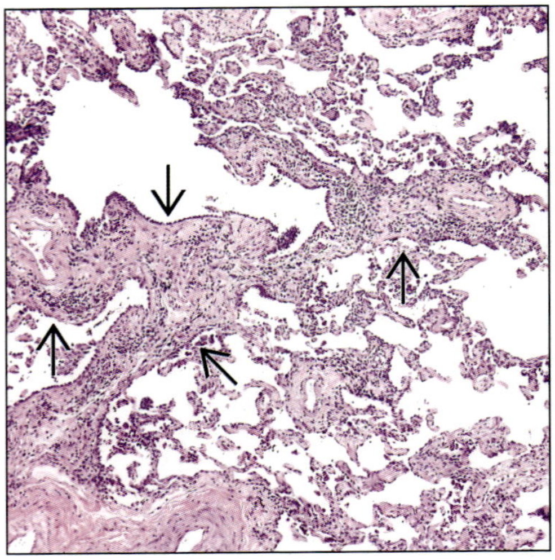

(Left) *Scanning magnification in a patient with usual interstitial pneumonia shows focal areas of interstitial fibrosis* → *surrounded by areas of spared, normal lung parenchyma. This variegation in histology, with lesions present in different stages of organization, is described as "temporal heterogeneity."* ***(Right)*** *Higher magnification in a patient with usual interstitial pneumonia shows interstitial fibrosis with widened alveolar septa* → *circumscribing normal lung parenchyma.*

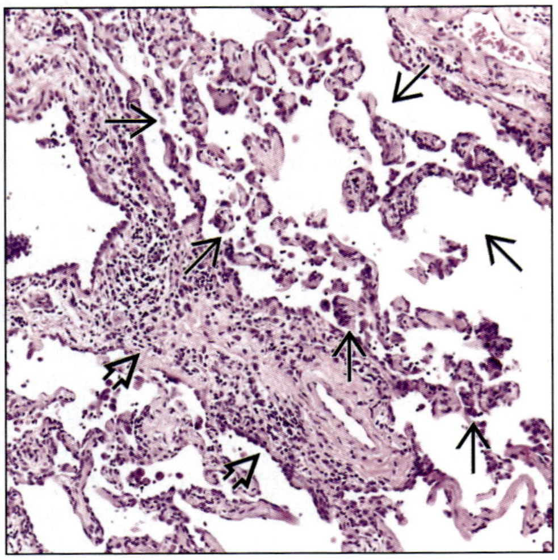
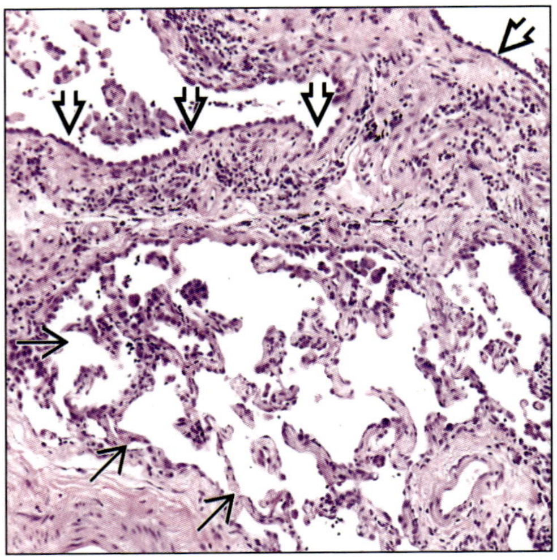

(Left) *Higher magnification of lung involved with usual interstitial pneumonia shows thickened alveolar septa* ⇨ *containing a dense lymphoid cell infiltration admixed with fibrous tissue deposition. Notice the normal intervening lung parenchyma* →. ***(Right)*** *Higher magnification in usual interstitial pneumonia shows thickened alveolar septa* ⇨ *with scattered inflammatory cells admixed with fibrous tissue. The thickened alveolar septa circumscribe normal lung parenchyma* →.

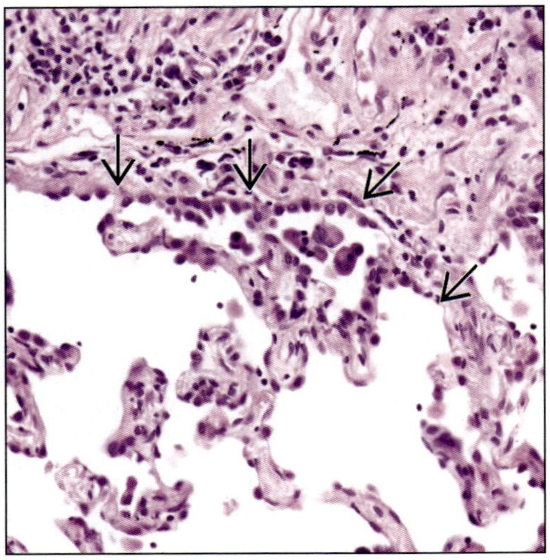
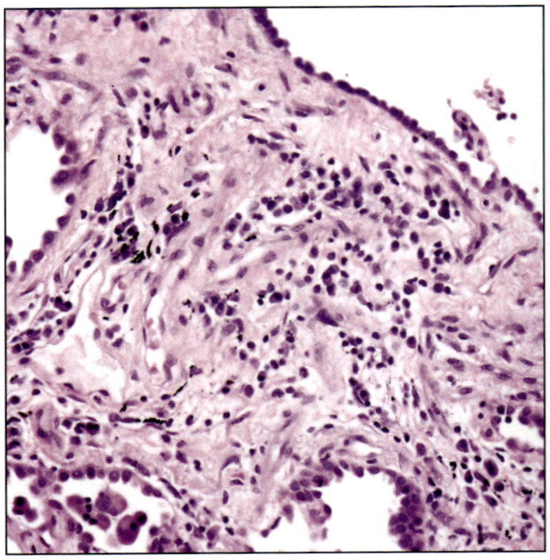

(Left) *Higher magnification in usual interstitial pneumonia shows thickened alveolar septa with chronic inflammation and fibrosis (top). The underlying entrapped lung parenchyma shows alveolar septa of normal thickness without inflammation or fibrosis* →. ***(Right)*** *Higher magnification of thickened alveolar septa in usual interstitial pneumonia shows numerous scattered small lymphocytes and plasma cells embedded in abundant collagenous stroma.*

Special Features

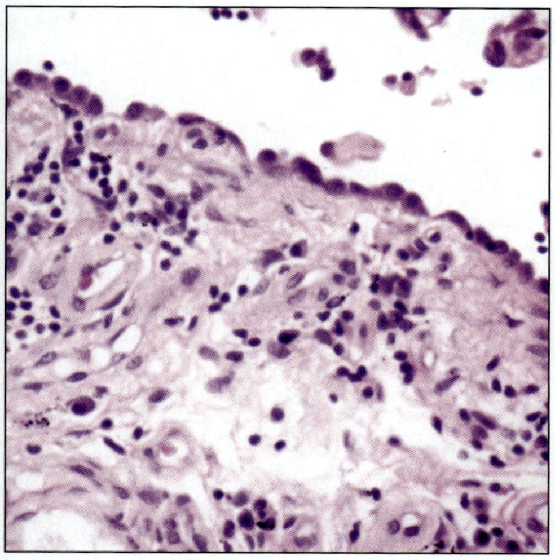
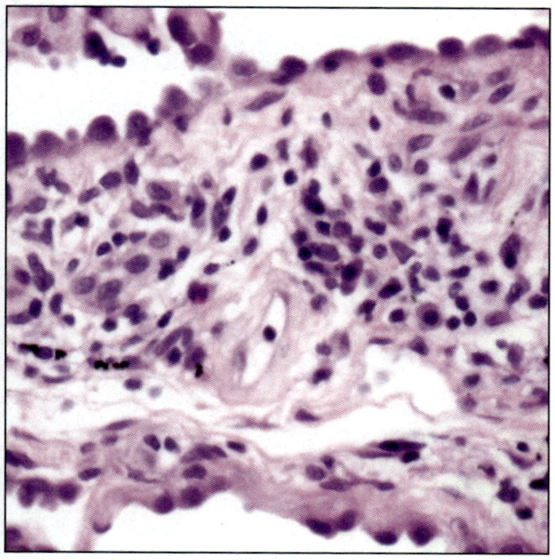

(Left) *Higher magnification in usual interstitial pneumonia illustrates an area of interstitial fibrosis with scattered inflammatory infiltrate and deposition of early, young collagenous tissue in the interstitium.* ***(Right)*** *Higher magnification from thickened alveolar septa in a patient with usual interstitial fibrosis shows mixed inflammatory infiltrate chiefly composed of small lymphocytes and scattered plasma cells and histiocytes deposited around small vessels.*

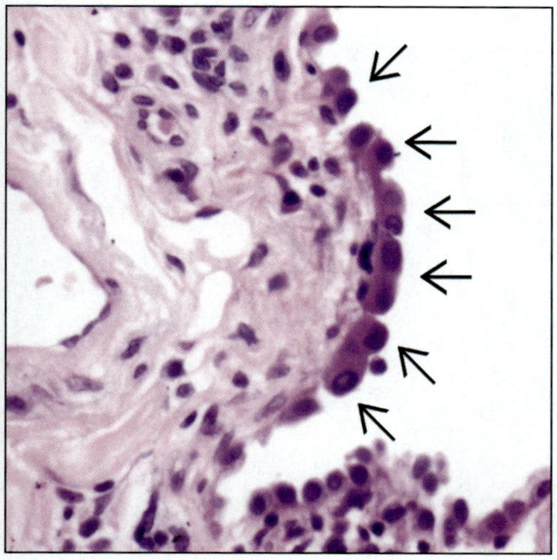
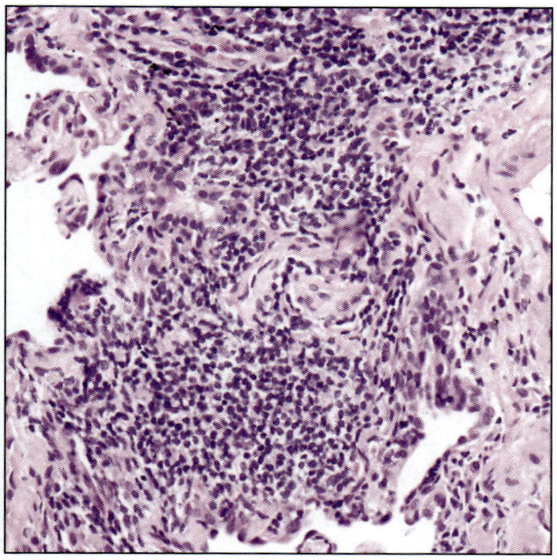

(Left) *Higher magnification of thickened alveolar septa in a patient with usual interstitial pneumonia shows mixed inflammatory infiltrate with lymphocytes and plasma cells, and hyperplasia of type II pneumocytes* → *in the alveolar lining cells.* ***(Right)*** *Lymphoid aggregate is seen in a case of usual interstitial pneumonia showing widening of alveolar septa with numerous small lymphoid cells. Lymphoid follicle formation with germinal centers should raise the possibility of lymphoid interstitial pneumonia.*

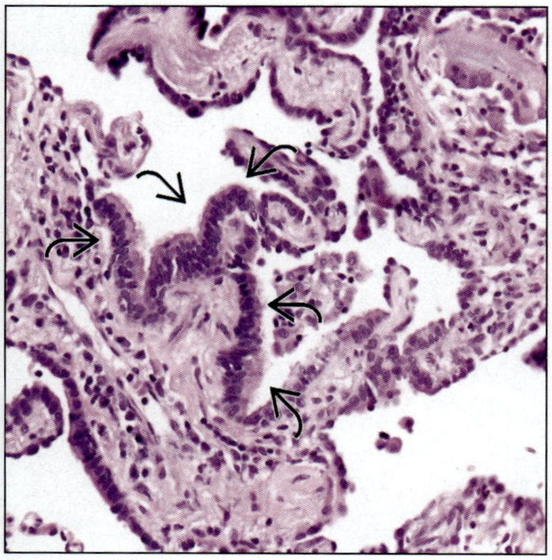
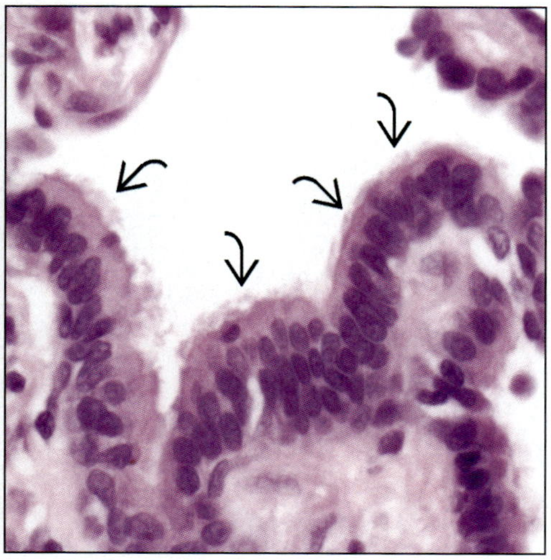

(Left) *Scanning magnification of usual interstitial pneumonia shows a focus of bronchiolization of alveolar lining (Lambertosis)* ↷*, a metaplastic phenomenon in which the alveolar lining cells are transformed into tall columnar ciliated epithelium.* ***(Right)*** *Higher magnification from a focus of bronchiolar metaplasia (Lambertosis) in a patient with usual interstitial pneumonia shows tall columnar cells with parallel elongated nuclei and abundant cytoplasm. Notice the surface cilia* ↷*.*

USUAL INTERSTITIAL PNEUMONIA

Histologic Features

(Left) *Scanning magnification in usual interstitial pneumonia shows extensive areas of interstitial fibrosis* → *blending imperceptibly with normal, uninvolved lung parenchyma at the bottom of the figure. The focal, patchy character of the fibrosing changes is quite typical of usual interstitial fibrosis.* ***(Right)*** *Higher magnification of usual interstitial pneumonia shows an area affected by interstitial fibrosis with widening of the alveolar septa and chronic inflammatory infiltrates.*

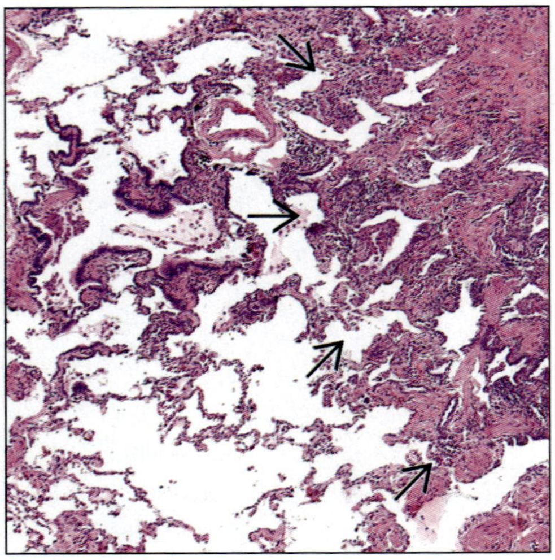

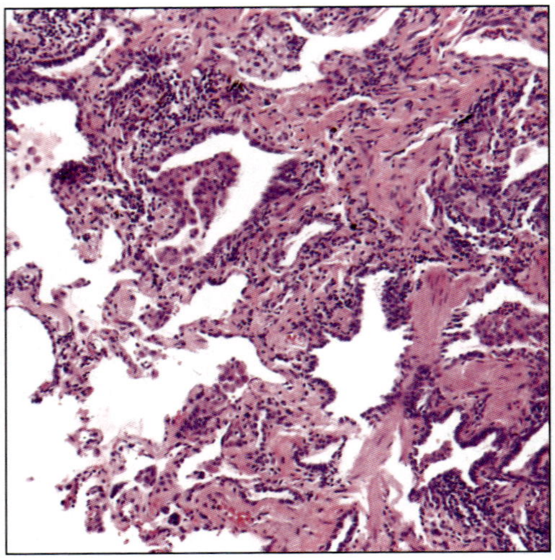

(Left) *Higher magnification from the wall of an alveolus in usual interstitial pneumonia shows abundant deposition of fibrocollagenous tissue in the interstitium admixed with a mixed inflammatory infiltrate. The thick collagen bundles are arranged in a haphazard fashion.* ***(Right)*** *Microscopic focus of bronchiolization is seen in a case of usual interstitial pneumonia. The change is quite subtle and consists of gradual metaplasia of alveolar lining cells into tall columnar ciliated epithelium* →.

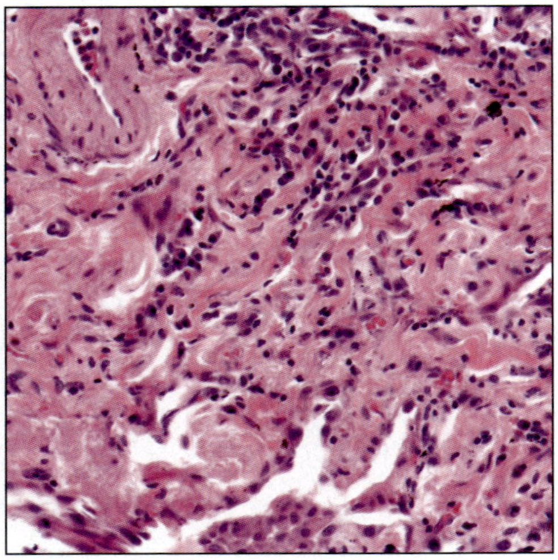

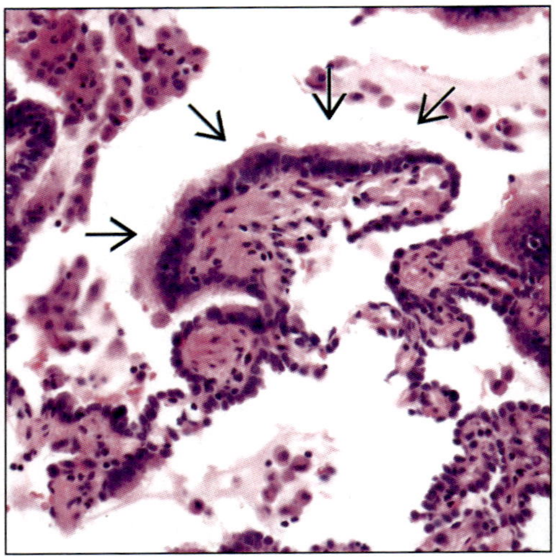

(Left) *Scanning magnification of usual interstitial pneumonia shows widening of alveolar septa by fibrosis and inflammation, and multiple foci of eosinophilic intraalveolar macrophages resulting in a DIP-like appearance.* ***(Right)*** *Usual interstitial pneumonia with DIP-like effect shows clusters of alveolar macrophages with abundant eosinophilic cytoplasm within a dilated alveolar lumen. This may be observed focally in UIP and should not be confused with desquamative interstitial pneumonia.*

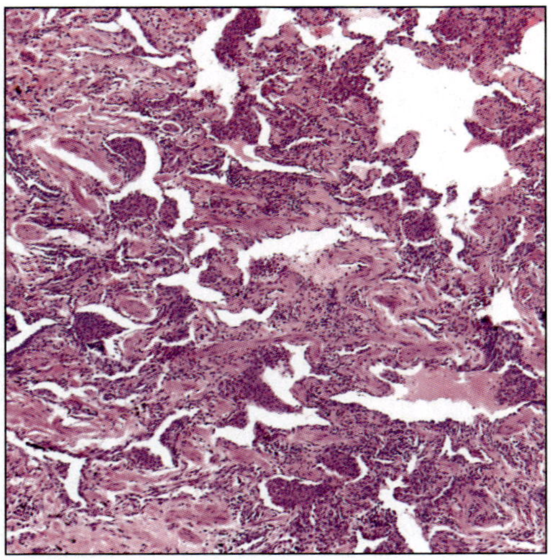

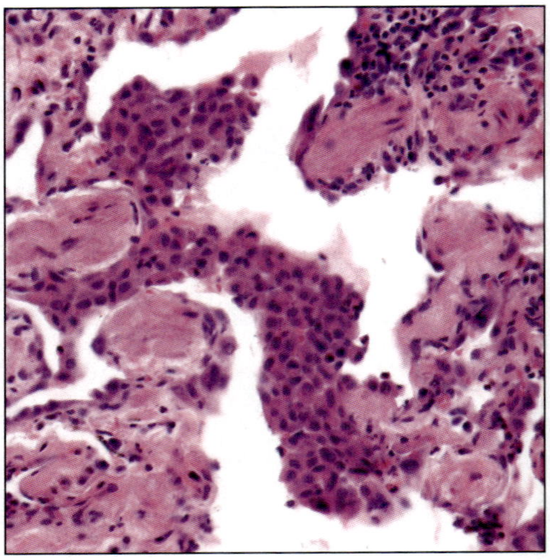

Histologic Features

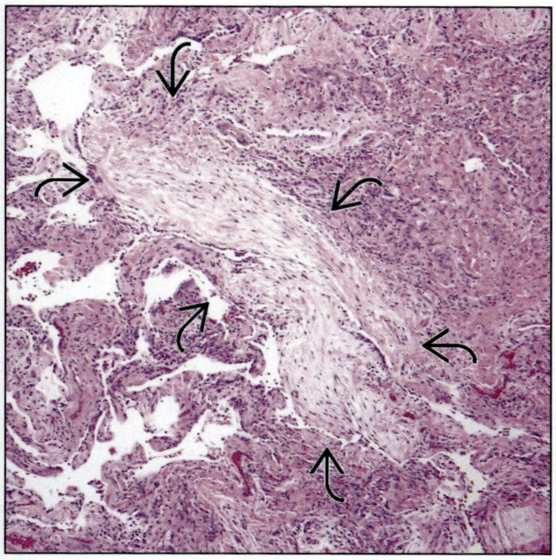

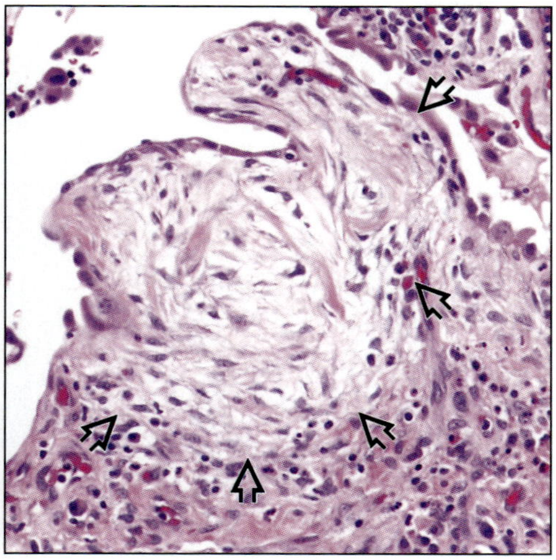

(Left) *Scanning magnification in a case of usual interstitial pneumonia shows a large fibroblastic focus →. This area is composed of loose connective tissue admixed with fibroblastic cells against a faintly myxoid matrix. Fibroblastic foci are a distinctive feature of usual interstitial pneumonia.* ***(Right)*** *Fibroblastic focus → in an usual interstitial pneumonia shows young collagen admixed with spindled fibroblasts in the interstitium displaying a faintly myxoid background.*

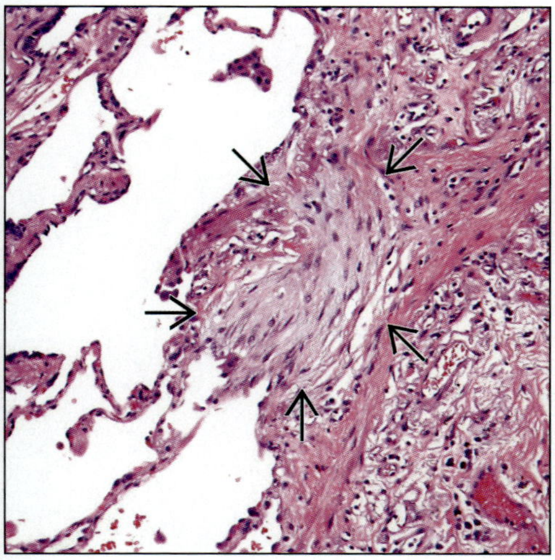

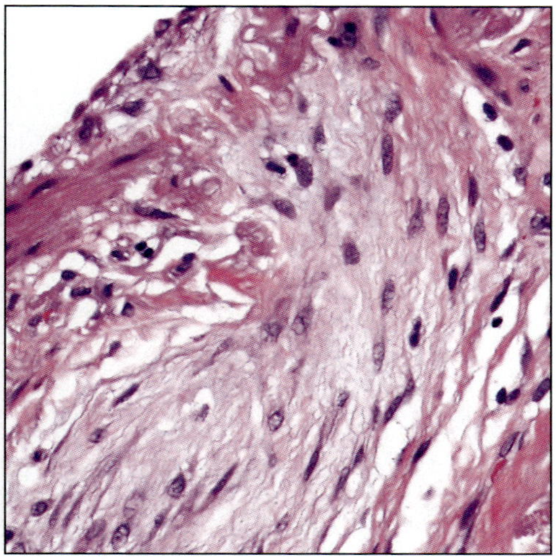

(Left) *Scanning magnification in usual interstitial pneumonia shows a fibroblastic focus in the wall of the alveolus adjacent to normal pulmonary parenchyma →. Notice the parallel, linear disposition of the spindle fibroblastic cells admixed with the young collagen.* ***(Right)*** *Higher magnification of the fibroblastic focus in usual interstitial pneumonia shows bland-appearing spindled fibroblasts embedded in a slightly myxoid young collagenous matrix.*

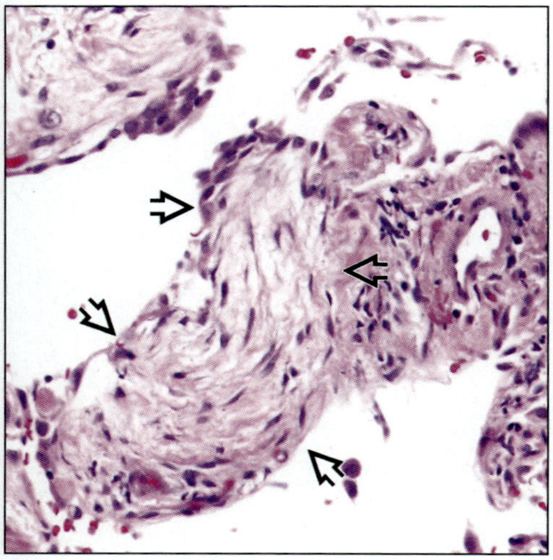

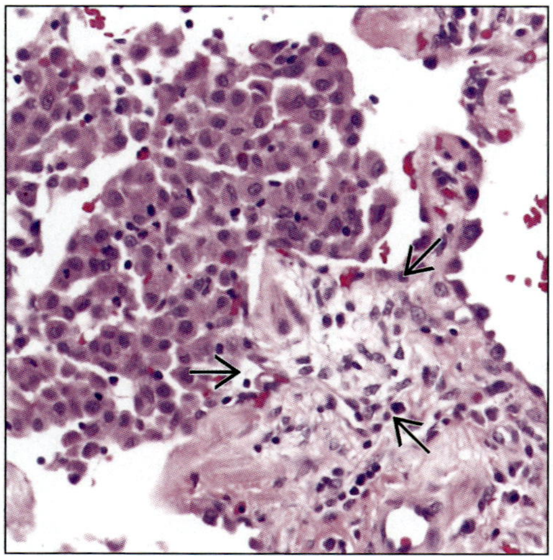

(Left) *Fibroblastic focus located within the wall of an alveolus → in usual interstitial pneumonia shows spindled fibroblasts embedded in collagenous matrix. The interstitial location is distinctive as opposed to the intraalveolar location in organizing pneumonia.* ***(Right)*** *Early fibroblastic focus formation → in usual interstitial pneumonia is seen alongside clusters of intraalveolar macrophages with abundant eosinophilic cytoplasm (DIP-like appearance) within the alveolar lumen.*

USUAL INTERSTITIAL PNEUMONIA

End-stage Changes

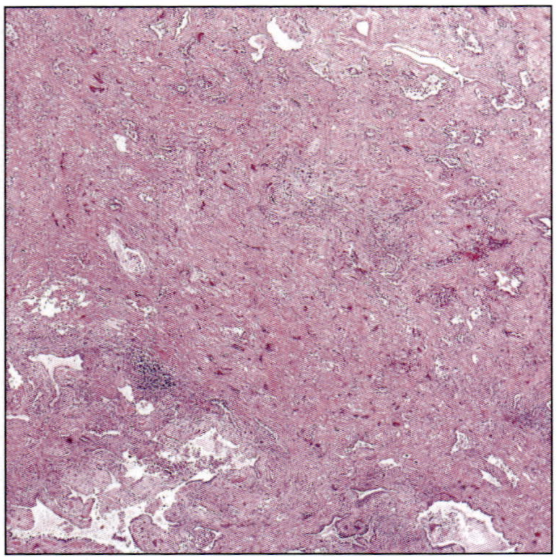

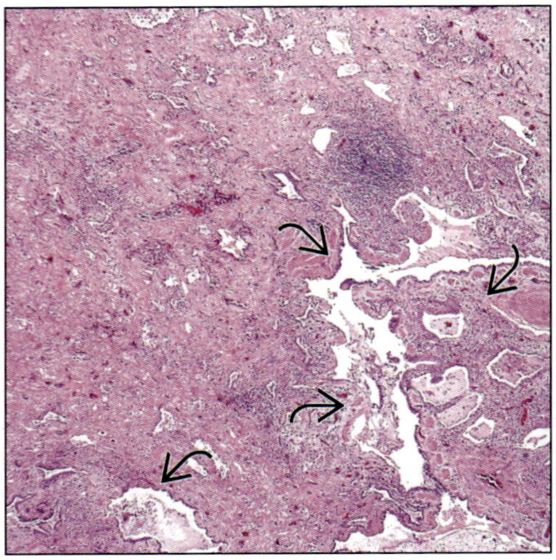

(Left) *End-stage fibrosis in patient with usual interstitial pneumonia shows almost total remodeling of lung parenchyma with almost complete obliteration of the underlying architecture and replacement by dense connective tissue.* ***(Right)*** *Scanning magnification in end-stage idiopathic interstitial fibrosis (usual interstitial pneumonia) shows almost total obliteration of lung parenchyma by fibrous tissue with only a few small residual foci of lung parenchyma* ↷.

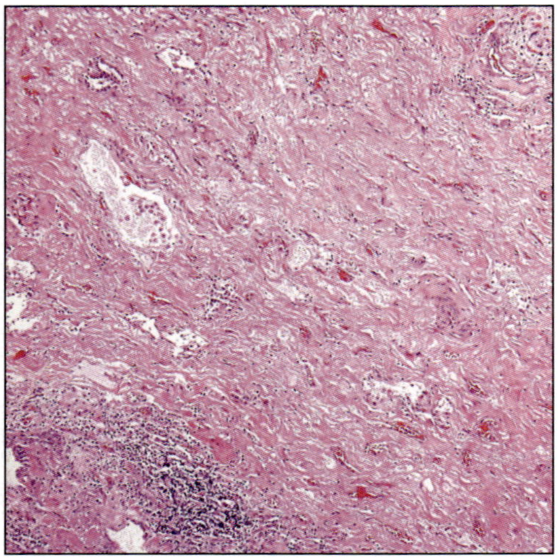

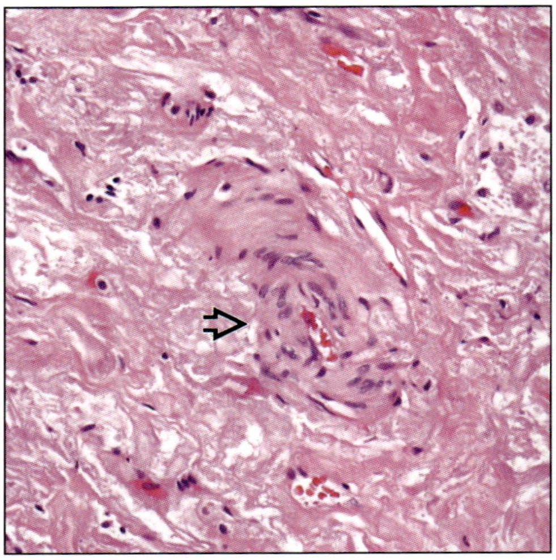

(Left) *Higher magnification from an area of dense fibrosis in end-stage idiopathic pulmonary fibrosis (usual interstitial pneumonia) shows almost total replacement of the lung parenchyma by paucicellular collagenous tissue.* ***(Right)*** *Higher magnification of collagenized area in end-stage idiopathic pulmonary fibrosis (usual interstitial pneumonia) shows deposition of mature, paucicellular collagen with a few scattered inflammatory cells in the background. Notice the entrapped small vessel* ⇨.

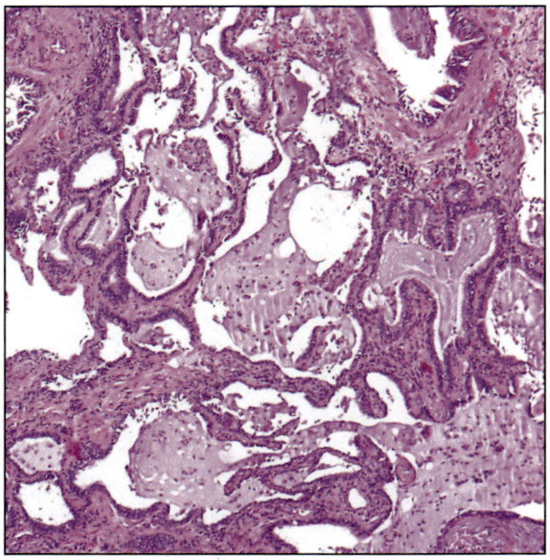

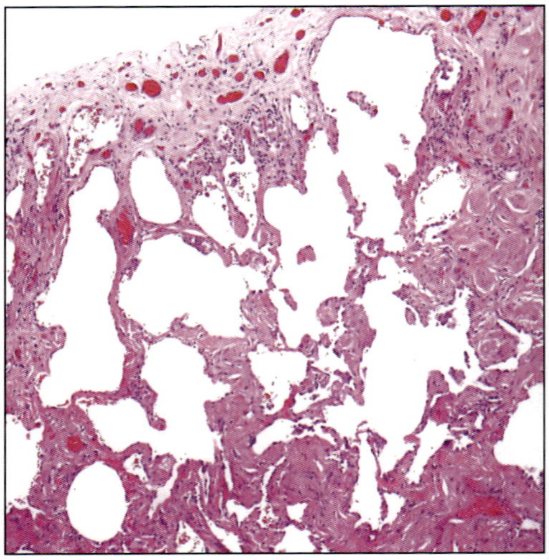

(Left) *Honeycombing of lung parenchyma is seen in advanced stages of idiopathic pulmonary fibrosis (usual interstitial pneumonia) and is characterized by massive dilatation of air spaces, which become filled with mucin.* ***(Right)*** *Scanning magnification in end-stage idiopathic pulmonary fibrosis shows honeycombing of lung parenchyma with dilated airspaces surrounded by fibrotic alveolar septa. It may be difficult to determine the correct diagnosis in such cases without comparison with previous films.*

End-stage Changes

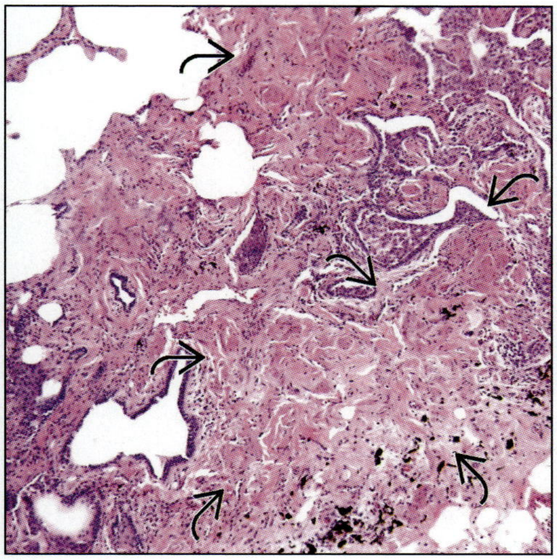

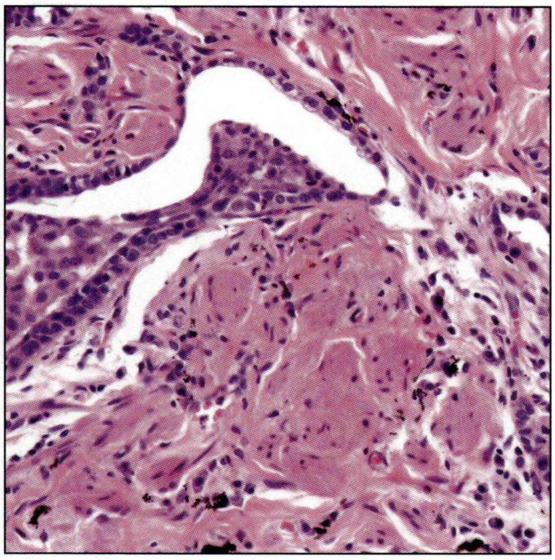

(Left) *Advanced, end-stage changes in idiopathic pulmonary fibrosis (usual interstitial pneumonia) show a few residual airspaces surrounded by collagenous stroma with smooth muscle metaplasia* ⇨. ***(Right)*** *Higher magnification in advanced stages of usual interstitial fibrosis shows a residual compressed airspace with multiple small foci of smooth muscle proliferation in the interstitium. Smooth muscle metaplasia is usually a late event in usual interstitial pneumonia.*

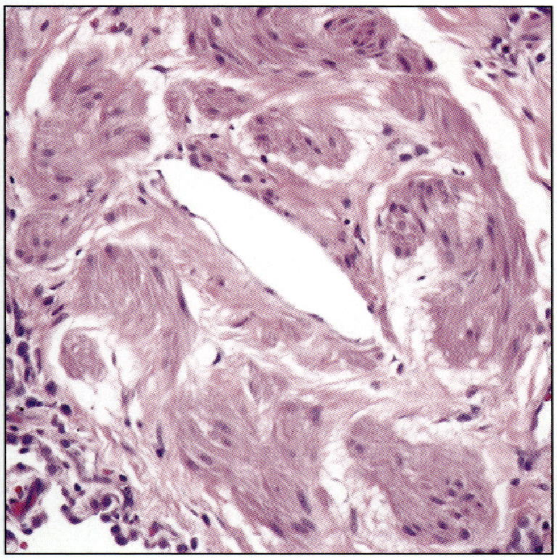

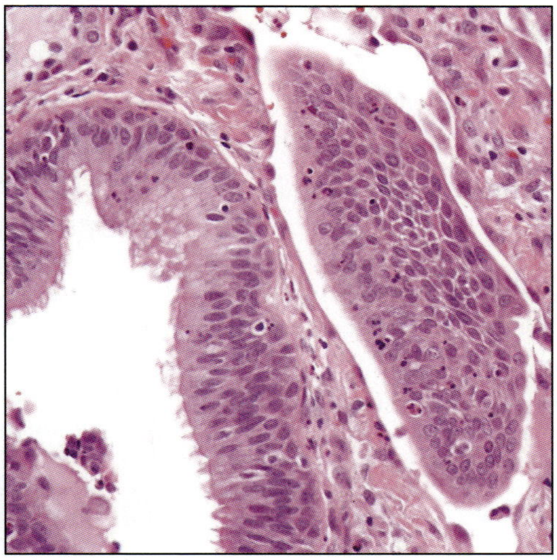

(Left) *Focus of smooth muscle is seen in the pulmonary interstitium of a patient with advanced usual interstitial pneumonia. The smooth muscle metaplasia can result in a cobblestone gross appearance and has been termed, by some, "pulmonary cirrhosis."* ***(Right)*** *Metaplastic phenomena are rather common in end-stage idiopathic pulmonary fibrosis. This image depicts a focus of bronchial metaplasia (left) side-by-side with a focus of squamous metaplasia (right).*

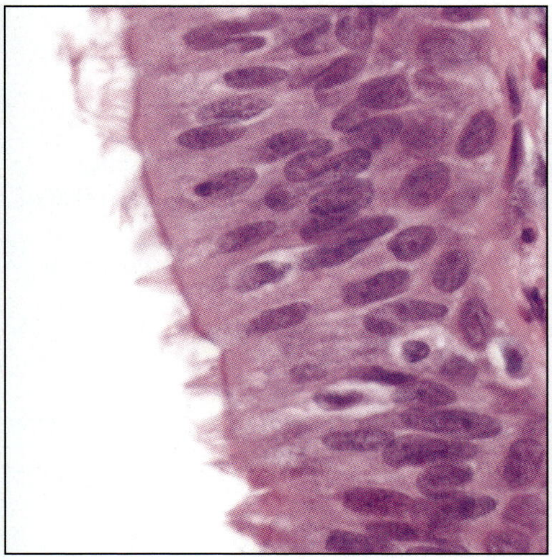

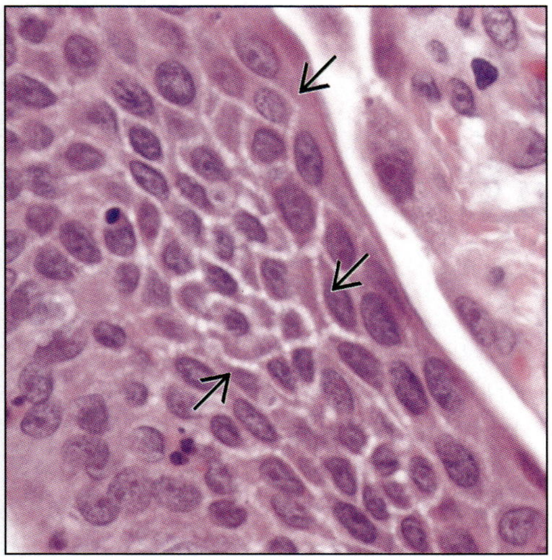

(Left) *Higher magnification from a focus of bronchial metaplasia in end-stage idiopathic pulmonary fibrosis (usual interstitial pneumonia) shows columnar cell metaplasia with prominent cilia on the luminal surface.* ***(Right)*** *Higher magnification in focus of squamous metaplasia in end-stage idiopathic pulmonary fibrosis (usual interstitial pneumonia) shows polygonal cells with large nuclei and pavement-like architecture displaying intercellular bridges* →.

DESQUAMATIVE INTERSTITIAL PNEUMONIA

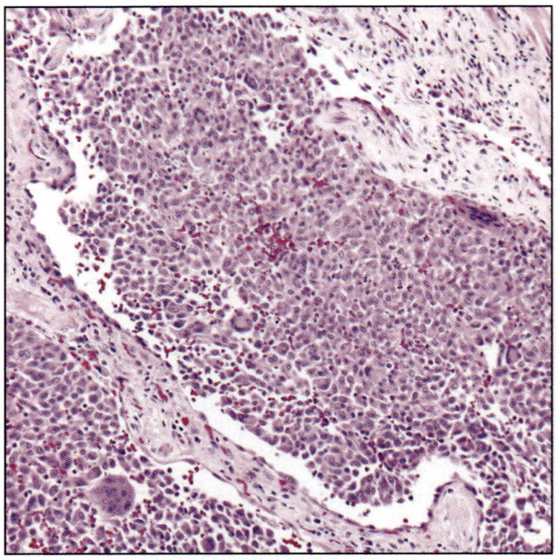

Desquamative interstitial pneumonia shows plugging and distention of airspaces by monotonous infiltrate of alveolar macrophages filling the lumen.

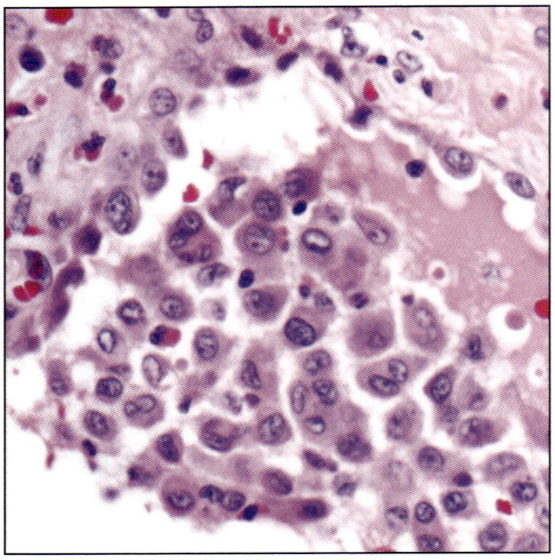

Higher magnification of desquamative interstitial pneumonia shows collection of alveolar macrophages with vesicular nuclei and abundant eosinophilic cytoplasm within the alveolar lumen.

TERMINOLOGY

Abbreviations

- Desquamative interstitial pneumonia (DIP)

Definitions

- A distinctive histologic reaction pattern to lung injury related to cigarette smoking

ETIOLOGY/PATHOGENESIS

Environmental Exposure

- Strong epidemiologic link to cigarette smoking

CLINICAL ISSUES

Epidemiology

- Incidence
  - Unknown
- Age
  - 40-50 years
- Gender
  - More common in males (2:1)

Presentation

- Dyspnea
- Cough
- Crackles on auscultation
- Clubbing in 40% of patients

Laboratory Tests

- Lung function tests show a restrictive pattern with decreased diffusion capacity

Natural History

- Subacute onset (weeks to months) of symptoms
- Cessation of smoking generally leads to regression of symptoms and radiologic changes
- Patients with moderate to severe disease respond well to administration of corticosteroids
- Recurrences occur when patients resume smoking

Treatment

- Steroids
- Smoking cessation

Prognosis

- Much better survival than UIP and other interstitial pneumonias
- Approximately 95% 5-year survival and 70% 10-year survival
- Very small number of patients may progress to diffuse interstitial fibrosis requiring transplantation

IMAGE FINDINGS

Radiographic Findings

- Bilateral symmetric areas of ground-glass opacification in lower lung zones
- Reticular pattern observed in 50% of cases due to localized areas of fibrosis

CT Findings

- Bilateral and symmetric, panlobular ground-glass pattern seen in lower lung zones on HRCT in 100% of cases
- Round, small thin-walled cysts within ground-glass opacities
- Irregular linear opacities (reticular pattern) in periphery of lower lung zones

MICROSCOPIC PATHOLOGY

Histologic Features

- Histologic hallmark is diffuse and extensive intraalveolar deposition of alveolar macrophages

DESQUAMATIVE INTERSTITIAL PNEUMONIA

Key Facts

Terminology
- A distinctive histologic reaction pattern to lung injury related to cigarette smoking

Clinical Issues
- Dyspnea
- Cough
- Cessation of smoking generally leads to regression of symptoms and radiologic changes
- Patients with moderate to severe disease respond well to administration of corticosteroids
- Much better survival than UIP and other interstitial pneumonias

Image Findings
- Bilateral symmetric areas of ground-glass opacification in lower lung zones
- Reticular pattern observed in 50% of cases due to localized areas of fibrosis

Microscopic Pathology
- Histologic hallmark is diffuse and extensive intraalveolar deposition of alveolar macrophages
- Minimal fibrosis with only mild thickening of alveolar septa and mild chronic inflammatory infiltrate
- Absence of organizing fibroblastic foci
- All lesions in same stage of evolution (absence of "temporal heterogeneity")

Ancillary Tests
- Cells filling alveoli are positive for CD68 macrophage-associated antigen and negative for cytokeratin

- Minimal fibrosis with only mild thickening of alveolar septa and mild chronic inflammatory infiltrate
- Absence of organizing fibroblastic foci
- All lesions in same stage of evolution (absence of "temporal heterogeneity")

Cytologic Features
- Intraalveolar macrophages may contain finely granular brown pigment (hemosiderin)
- Intraalveolar laminated basophilic concretions ("blue bodies") may be present

ANCILLARY TESTS

Immunohistochemistry
- Cells filling alveoli are positive for CD68 macrophage-associated antigen and negative for cytokeratin

Histochemistry
- Cells filling alveoli stain strongly positive with iron stains, such as Prussian blue

DIFFERENTIAL DIAGNOSIS

Usual Interstitial Pneumonia (UIP)
- UIP may show DIP-like effect with focal areas containing abundant intraalveolar macrophages
- Interstitial fibrosis and inflammation are prominent with active remodeling of lung architecture
- Alternating areas of interstitial fibrosis alongside normal lung parenchyma are characteristic
- Fibroblastic foci are commonly seen
- Smooth muscle proliferation, squamous metaplasia, and honeycombing are common findings in advanced stages

Nonspecific DIP-like Reaction
- Areas resembling DIP can occur as a nonspecific reaction adjacent to a variety of unrelated lesions, such as tumors, scars, etc.
- Focalized process found incidentally in the vicinity of lesions resected for other causes
- Radiologic correlation will not show bilateral symmetric ground-glass opacities

Histiocyte-rich Infections
- Certain infections such as *Mycobacterium avium intracellulare* (MAI), *Cryptococcus*, and *Rhodococcus equi* may show DIP-like areas
- Special stains for organisms (AFB, GMS, PAS, etc.) will serve to highlight causative agent

Chronic Eosinophilic Pneumonia (CEP)
- CEP patients treated with corticosteroids may resemble DIP due to disappearance of eosinophils secondary to steroids
- Prominent peripheral eosinophilia is distinctive for CEP but is not a feature of DIP

DIAGNOSTIC CHECKLIST

Pathologic Interpretation Pearls
- Term "desquamative" is a misnomer; cells filling alveoli are histiocytes, not desquamated epithelial cells
- Process is closely related to "respiratory bronchiolitis interstitial lung disease" (RB-ILD), a condition also related to smoking
- DIP and RB-ILD may be different stages within same spectrum in response pattern of lung to smoking

SELECTED REFERENCES

1. Tazelaar HD et al: Desquamative interstitial pneumonia. Histopathology. 58(4):509-16, 2011
2. Rao RN et al: Smoking-related interstitial lung disease. Ann Diagn Pathol. 12(6):445-57, 2008
3. Vassallo R et al: Tobacco smoke-related diffuse lung diseases. Semin Respir Crit Care Med. 29(6):643-50, 2008
4. Hidalgo A et al: Smoking-related interstitial lung diseases: radiologic-pathologic correlation. Eur Radiol. 16(11):2463-70, 2006

DESQUAMATIVE INTERSTITIAL PNEUMONIA

Histologic Features

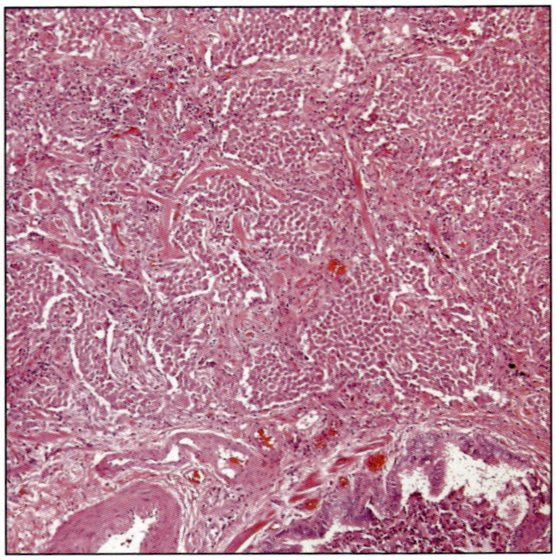
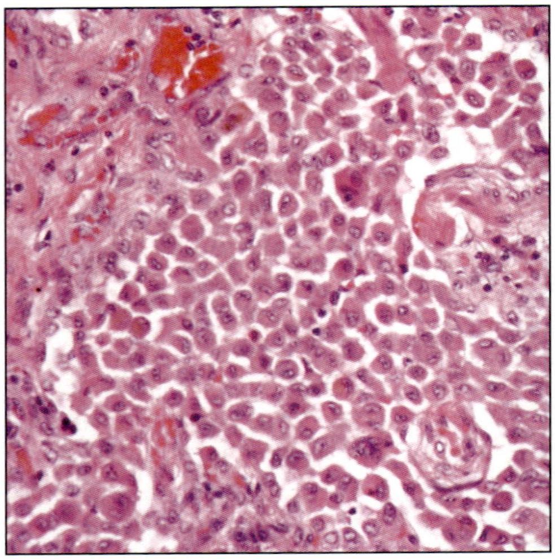

(Left) *Scanning magnification of desquamative interstitial pneumonia shows massive expansion of alveolar spaces by dense, monotonous population of alveolar macrophages completely filling the lumens.* ***(Right)*** *Higher magnification of desquamative interstitial pneumonia shows a monotonous discohesive population of histiocytic cells that are completely filling the alveolar lumen. Notice absence of lymphocytes, neutrophils, or other types of inflammatory cells admixed with the histiocytes.*

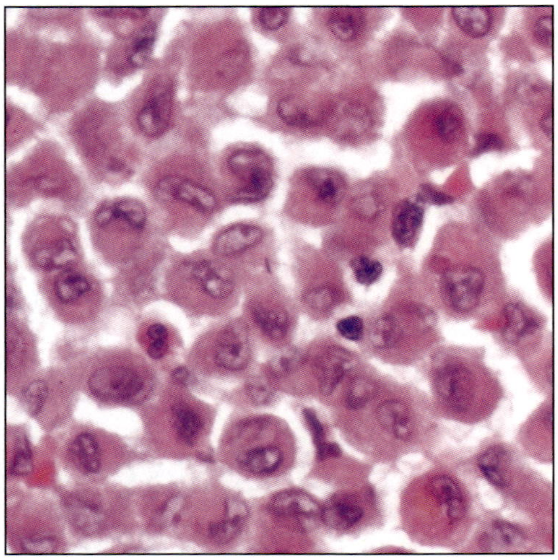
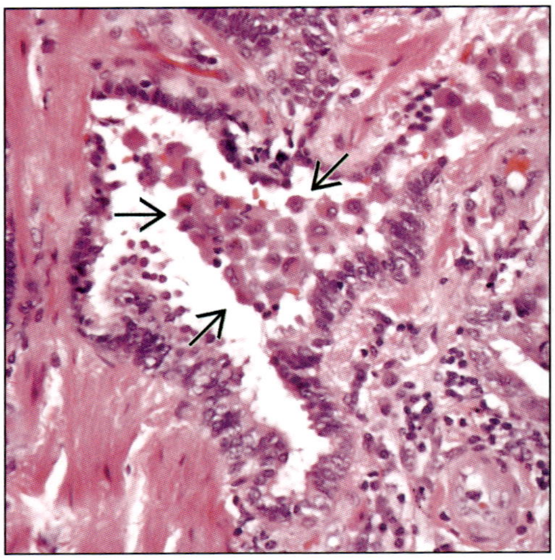

(Left) *Higher magnification of desquamative interstitial pneumonia (DIP) shows monotonous sheets of histiocytes with irregular nuclei and an abundant rim of eosinophilic cytoplasm. Some of the histiocytes contain finely granular hemosiderin pigment in their cytoplasm.* ***(Right)*** *Areas adjacent to the infiltrates may show evidence of respiratory bronchiolitis with pigmented macrophages lying within the lumen of small bronchioles →. DIP is closely related to cigarette smoking.*

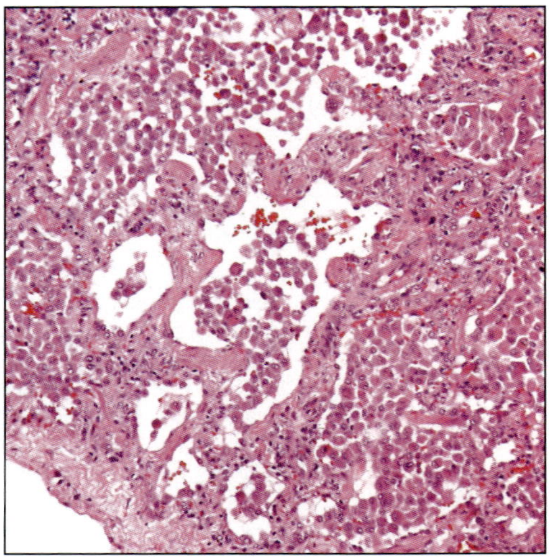
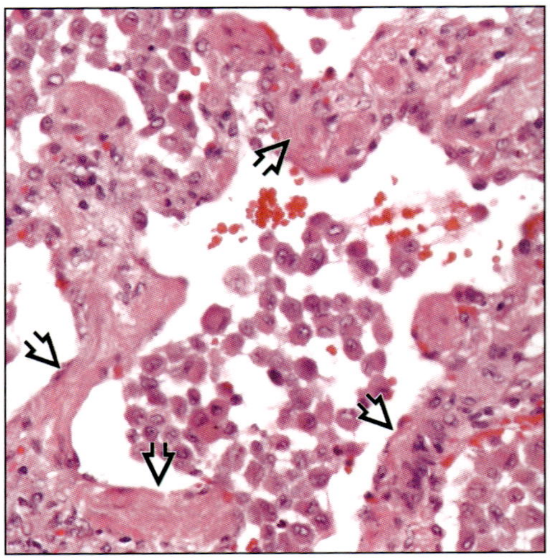

(Left) *Desquamative interstitial pneumonia shows monotonous deposition of alveolar macrophages showing temporal uniformity; i.e., all the lesions are in the same stage of evolution and do not show variability from field to field.* ***(Right)*** *Higher magnification of desquamative interstitial pneumonia shows minimal fibrosis with only mild thickening of alveolar septa ⇨ and mild chronic inflammatory infiltrates. Notice the absence of organizing fibroblastic foci.*

Histologic and Immunohistochemical Features

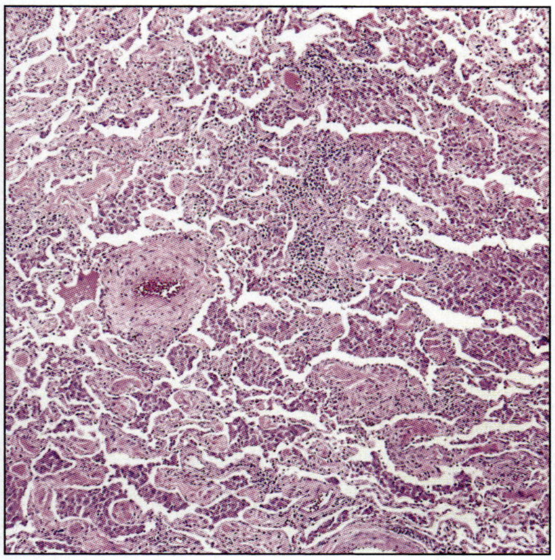

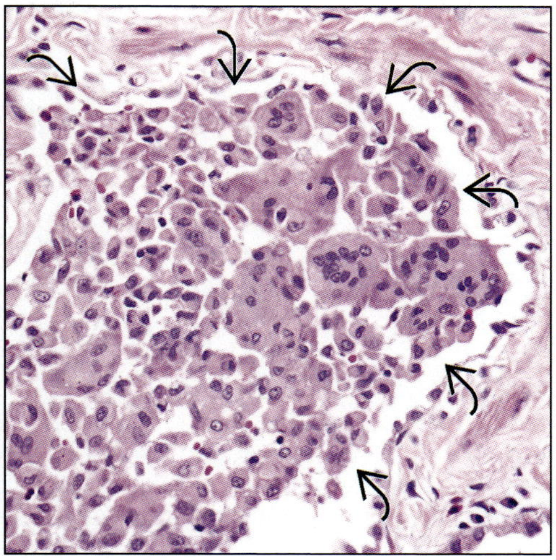

(Left) *Desquamative interstitial pneumonia is characterized by a monotonous deposition of alveolar macrophages filling the alveolar lumina. The process is characterized by minimal interstitial fibrosis and inflammation and displays a uniform histologic appearance ("temporal uniformity").* ***(Right)*** *Higher magnification of desquamative interstitial pneumonia shows a monotonous population of macrophages occupying the alveolar lumen ⮫.*

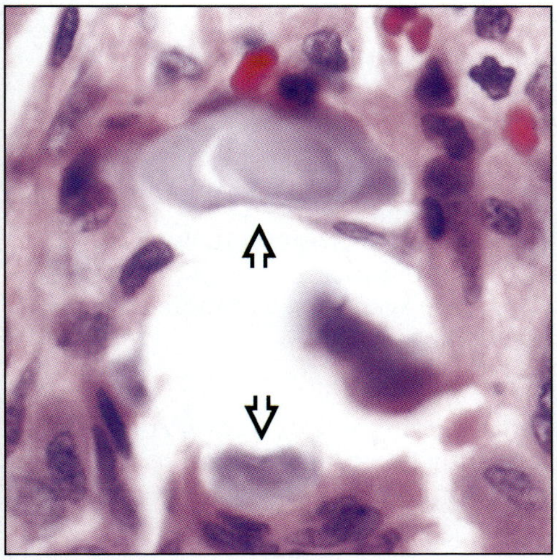

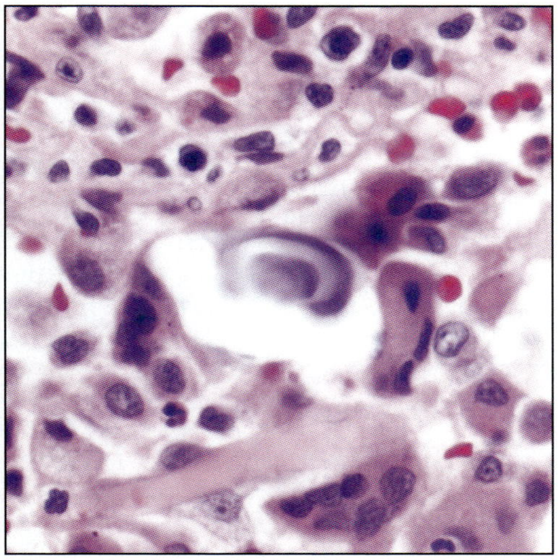

(Left) *Intraalveolar laminated basophilic concretions ⇨ (so-called blue bodies) can occasionally be identified admixed with the histiocytic infiltrate in desquamative interstitial pneumonia. These are nonspecific inclusions composed mostly of calcium carbonate admixed with mucopolysaccharide matrix and iron.* ***(Right)*** *Higher magnification shows laminated structure corresponding to basophilic concretion (so-called blue bodies) in desquamative interstitial pneumonia.*

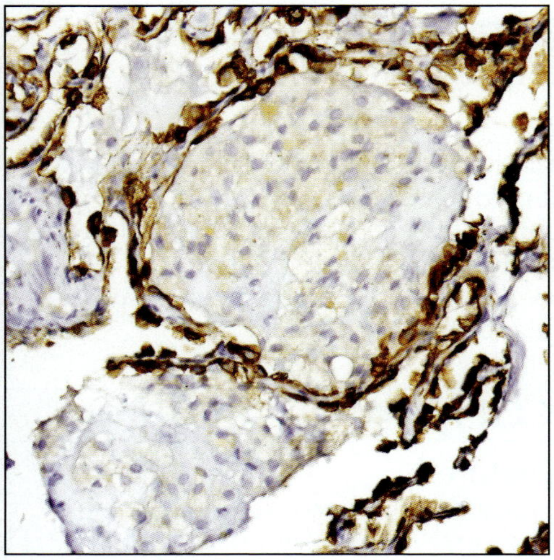

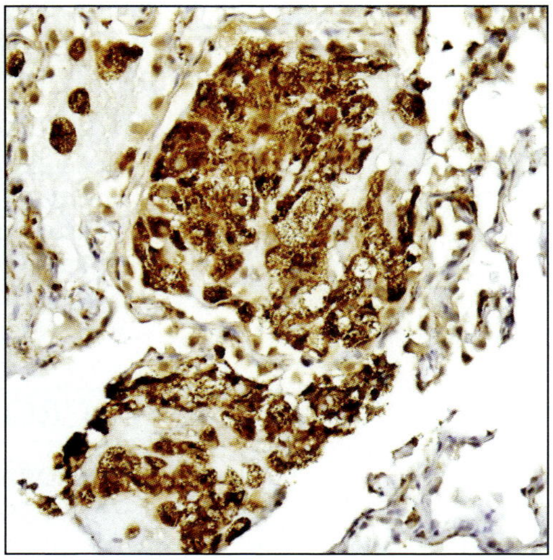

(Left) *Immunohistochemical staining of desquamative interstitial pneumonia for cytokeratin AE1/AE3 shows positivity in the alveolar epithelial cells but is negative in the intraalveolar macrophages. "Desquamative" is a misnomer since the infiltrate is composed of histiocytes and not desquamated epithelial cells.* ***(Right)*** *Immunohistochemical staining of desquamative interstitial pneumonia with CD68 shows strong positivity in the intraalveolar macrophages.*

NONSPECIFIC INTERSTITIAL PNEUMONIA

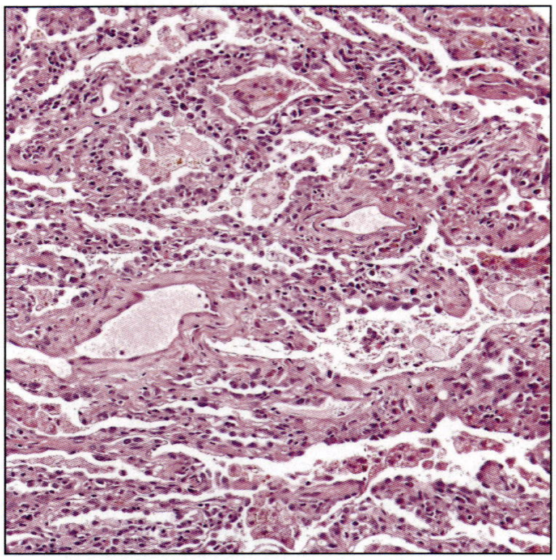

Nonspecific interstitial pneumonia pattern in the lungs shows uniform thickening of the alveolar septa with a monotonous population of inflammatory cells showing temporal uniformity.

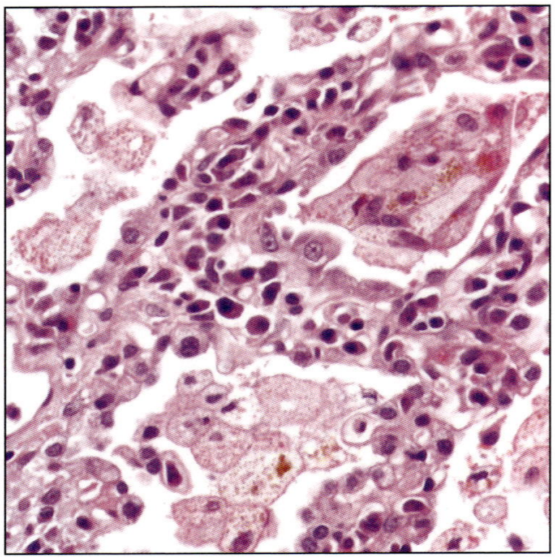

Higher magnification of nonspecific interstitial pneumonia shows uniform thickening of the alveolar septa by inflammatory elements, including lymphocytes and plasma cells.

TERMINOLOGY

Abbreviations

- Nonspecific interstitial pneumonia (NSIP)

Definitions

- Special pattern of fibrosing idiopathic interstitial pneumonia with much better prognosis than usual interstitial pneumonia

ETIOLOGY/PATHOGENESIS

Etiology

- Unknown
- Substantial number of cases are related to underlying collagen-vascular disease

CLINICAL ISSUES

Epidemiology

- Age
    - 25-60 years (average: 50 years)
- Gender
    - Slightly more common in women

Site

- Diffuse, bilateral process, predominantly distributed in lower lobes

Presentation

- Dyspnea
- Cough
- Fever
- Clubbing of fingers (up to 40% of patients)

Natural History

- Disease has insidious onset with slowly progressive exertional dyspnea over 8-18 months
- Dramatic response to corticosteroids during early stages
- Fibrosing histologic variant of NSIP has worse prognosis than nonfibrosing ("cellular") variant
- Average 5-year survival > 80%

Treatment

- Drugs
    - Dramatic response to corticosteroids, especially during early phases of process
    - Immunosuppressive agents used in more advanced or refractory cases

Prognosis

- > 75% of patients will improve or recover completely following treatment with corticosteroids
- Patients with fibrosing variant of NSIP may progress to UIP

IMAGE FINDINGS

Radiographic Findings

- Diffuse ground-glass opacities in lower lobes

CT Findings

- Reticular opacities in 80% of patients, often admixed with ground-glass opacities
- Traction bronchiectasis out of proportion to degree of reticular opacities
- Ground-glass opacities in 75% of patients, may often exceed reticular opacities

MICROSCOPIC PATHOLOGY

Histologic Features

- Process is characterized by interstitial fibrosis and inflammation in varying proportions

Key Facts

Clinical Issues

- 25-60 years (average: 50 years)
- Diffuse, bilateral process, predominantly distributed in lower lobes
- Dyspnea
- Cough
- Fever
- Disease has insidious onset with slowly progressive exertional dyspnea over 8-18 months
- Dramatic response to corticosteroids during early stages
- > 75% of patients will improve or recover completely following treatment with corticosteroids

Microscopic Pathology

- Process is characterized by interstitial fibrosis and inflammation in varying proportions
- Findings are characterized by absence of temporal heterogeneity (i.e., all lesions in same stage of evolution)
- Underlying lung architecture is often preserved
- 2 major patterns are recognized
  - Cellular pattern is characterized by dense lymphoid infiltration of alveolar septa with preservation of underlying lung architecture
  - Fibrosing pattern is characterized by uniform expansion of alveolar septa by collagen deposition, without fibroblastic foci

Diagnostic Checklist

- Not a specific pathologic entity but a reaction pattern to unknown underlying stimulus
- Diagnosis of exclusion (i.e., absence of features of UIP, DIP, LIP, BOOP, etc.)

- Findings are characterized by absence of temporal heterogeneity (i.e., all lesions in same stage of evolution)
- Underlying lung architecture is often preserved
- 2 major patterns are recognized
  - NSIP with cellular pattern
    - Characterized by mild to moderate interstitial chronic inflammation
    - Inflammatory infiltrate is composed of small lymphocytes and plasma cells
    - Lymphoid aggregates may also be present
  - NSIP with fibrosing pattern
    - Characterized primarily by interstitial deposition of loose or dense fibrous tissue
    - Distribution of fibrous tissue is uniform and monotonous, without variation from field to field
    - Absence of fibroblastic foci
    - Pattern of fibrosis may be patchy and discontinuous throughout lung
    - May be combinations of cellular and fibrosing pattern in same biopsy

DIFFERENTIAL DIAGNOSIS

Hypersensitivity Pneumonitis

- Contains scattered, small, poorly formed epithelioid granulomas
- Clinical history of exposure to allergens is important for differential diagnosis
- Usually more severe in mid and upper lung zones, rather than in lower zones

Lymphoid Interstitial Pneumonia (Diffuse BALT Hyperplasia)

- Interstitial infiltration by lymphoid infiltrate is dense and distorts underlying lung architecture
- Lymphoid infiltrate involves interlobular septa, perivascular and peribronchiolar spaces, and pleura
  - Lymphoid infiltrate in cellular NSIP involves mainly alveolar septa with preservation of underlying architecture

Usual Interstitial Pneumonia (UIP)

- Inflammatory and fibrotic changes are characterized by temporal heterogeneity (i.e., lesions are at varying stages of evolution)
- UIP shows prominent fibroblastic foci, a feature not seen in NSIP
- Honeycombing of lung parenchyma is a common feature of UIP that should not be seen in NSIP
- Imaging features in HRCT are quite distinctive and may serve to separate equivocal cases

Collagen-Vascular Diseases

- Clinical history and laboratory tests are important for establishing correct diagnosis

DIAGNOSTIC CHECKLIST

Clinically Relevant Pathologic Features

- Not a specific pathologic entity but a reaction pattern to an unknown underlying stimulus
- Diagnosis of exclusion (i.e., absence of features of UIP, DIP, LIP, BOOP, or other specific process)
- Histologic features may overlap with several other conditions, including LIP, hypersensitivity pneumonitis, and collagen vascular diseases
- Clinical and radiographic correlation is indispensable for diagnosis

SELECTED REFERENCES

1. Akira M et al: Long-term follow-up high-resolution CT findings in non-specific interstitial pneumonia. Thorax. 66(1):61-5, 2011
2. Sato T et al: Non-specific interstitial pneumonia; as the first clinical presentation of various collagen vascular disorders. Rheumatol Int. 26(6):551-5, 2006
3. Nicholson AG: Classification of idiopathic interstitial pneumonias: making sense of the alphabet soup. Histopathology. 41(5):381-91, 2002

NONSPECIFIC INTERSTITIAL PNEUMONIA

Cellular Pattern

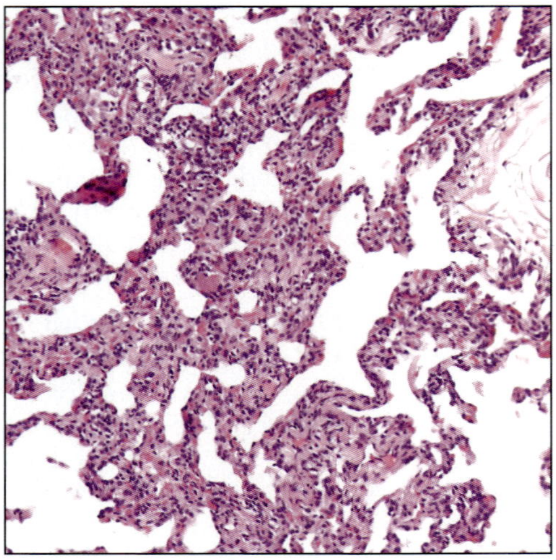

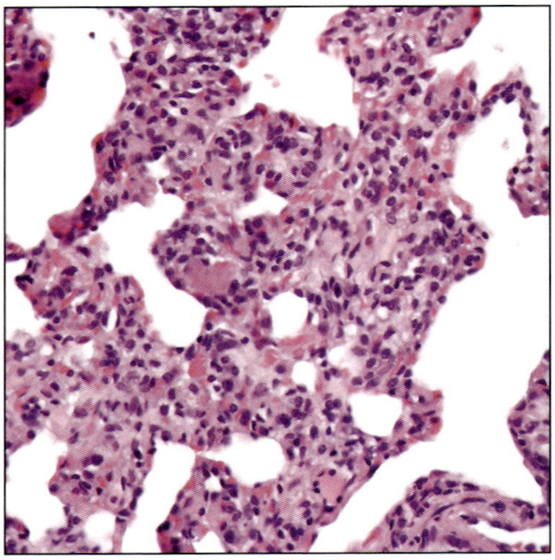

(Left) *Scanning magnification in nonspecific interstitial pneumonia shows moderate thickening of the alveolar septa with interstitial chronic inflammation. The lesions are uniform throughout and show temporal uniformity (i.e., all are at the same stage of evolution), which imparts them with a monotonous appearance.* ***(Right)*** *Higher magnification in nonspecific interstitial pneumonia shows uniform thickening of the alveolar septa by a monotonous population of lymphoid cells.*

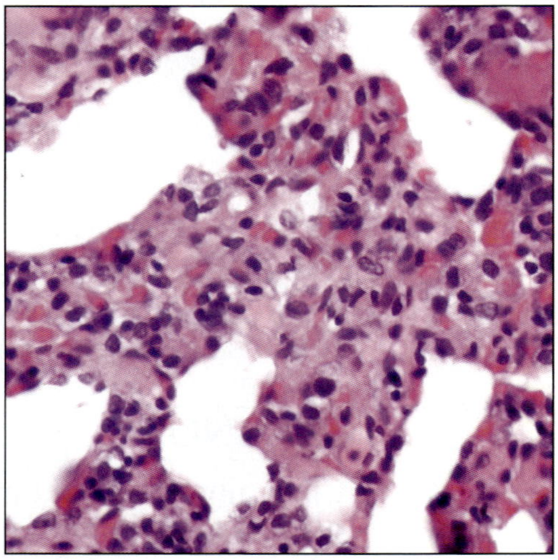

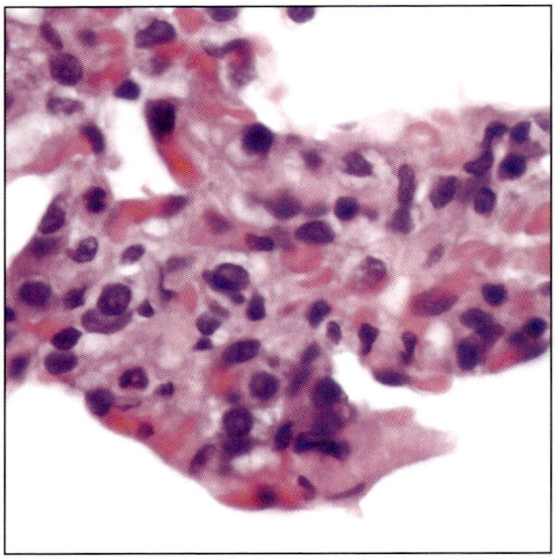

(Left) *Higher magnification of nonspecific interstitial pneumonia shows distended alveolar walls with early collagen deposition and dense lymphoid cell infiltrates. Cases like this need to be distinguished from lymphoid interstitial pneumonia and extrinsic allergic alveolitis.* ***(Right)*** *Higher magnification from nonspecific interstitial pneumonia with cellular pattern shows a thickened alveolar wall containing dense inflammatory cell infiltrate.*

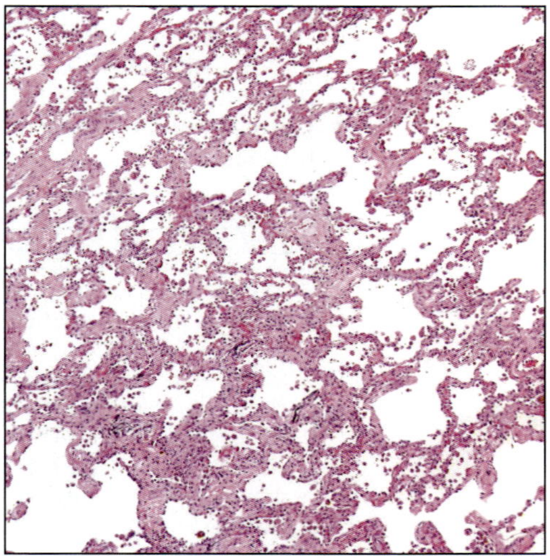

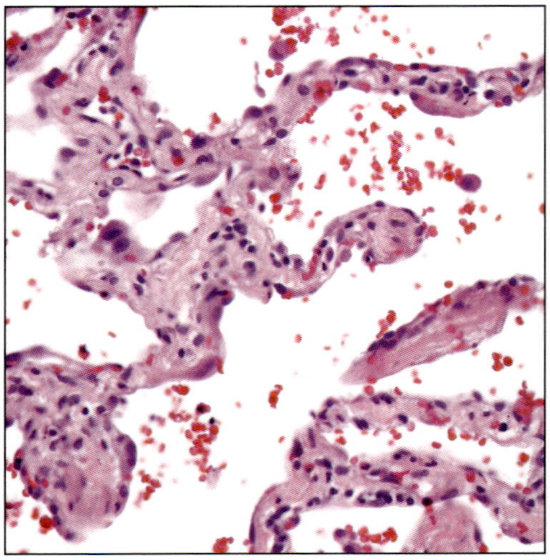

(Left) *Scanning magnification of nonspecific interstitial pneumonia, late cellular phase, shows fibrotic, uniformly distended alveolar walls with a few residual inflammatory elements. The lesions are strikingly similar from area to area and do not show the entrapment of normal lung parenchyma characteristic of UIP.* ***(Right)*** *Higher magnification of the late cellular phase of nonspecific interstitial pneumonia shows fibrotic alveolar septa with some residual lymphocytes.*

Fibrosing Pattern

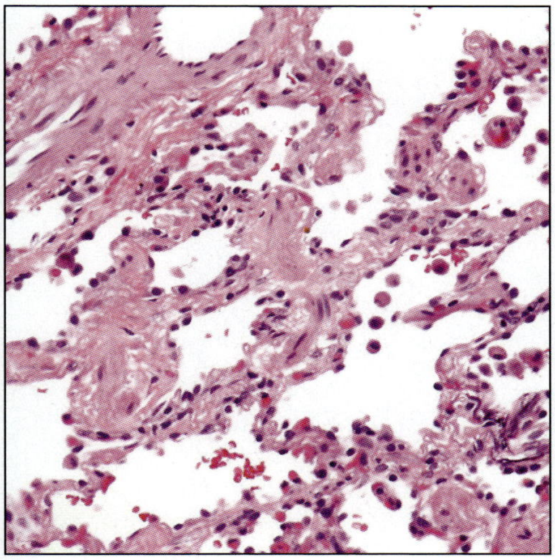
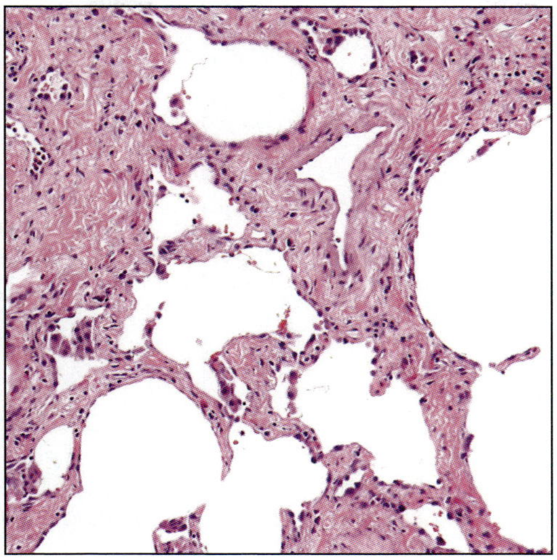

(Left) *Fibrosing pattern of nonspecific interstitial pneumonia shows thickened alveolar septa that are primarily distended by abundant fibrocollagenous tissue. Notice the uniformity of the process, which looks the same throughout, unlike the heterogeneous appearance of UIP, which shows lesions in varying stages of evolution.* ***(Right)*** *Nonspecific interstitial pneumonia, fibrosing pattern, shows thickened alveolar septa with a paucity of inflammatory elements.*

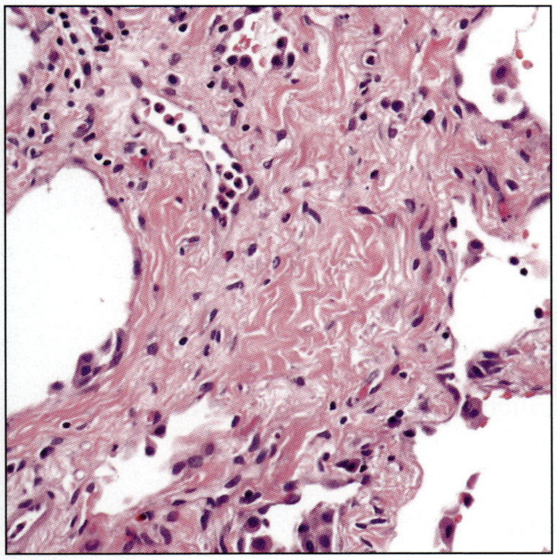
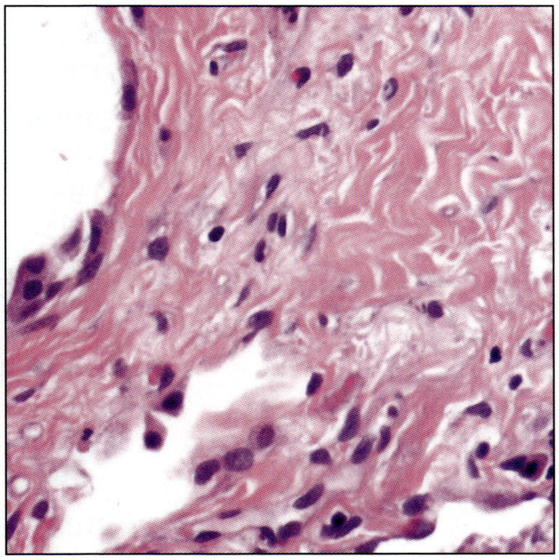

(Left) *Higher magnification of the fibrosing pattern in nonspecific interstitial pneumonia shows thickening of the alveolar septum due to dense collagen deposition. There are still a few small lymphocytes noted, but the damage is predominantly at the expense of collagen deposition.* ***(Right)*** *Higher magnification of an alveolar wall in the fibrosing pattern of nonspecific interstitial pneumonia shows thick collagen bundles with only a few scattered inflammatory cells.*

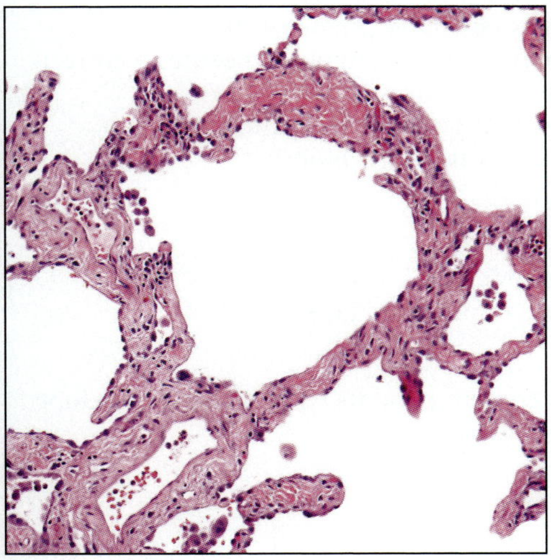
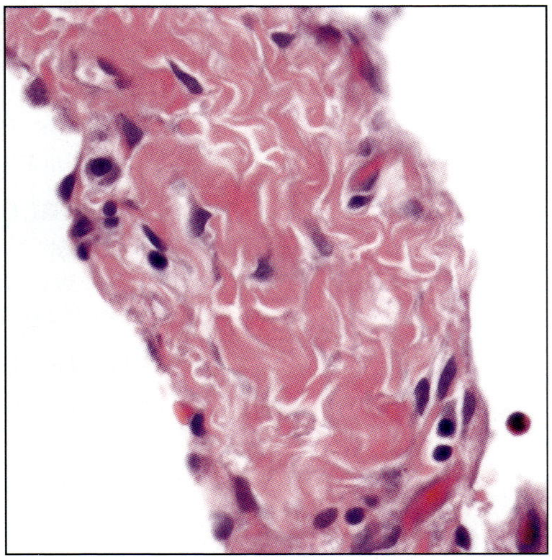

(Left) *Fibrosing pattern of nonspecific interstitial pneumonia shows mildly thickened alveolar walls with few lymphocytes and heavy interstitial collagen deposition. Cases with these features are associated with a poorer prognosis and may lead to honeycombing of the lung.* ***(Right)*** *Higher magnification of the sclerosing pattern of nonspecific interstitial pneumonia shows heavy interstitial collagen deposition with a few spindled fibroblasts.*

EXTRINSIC ALLERGIC ALVEOLITIS

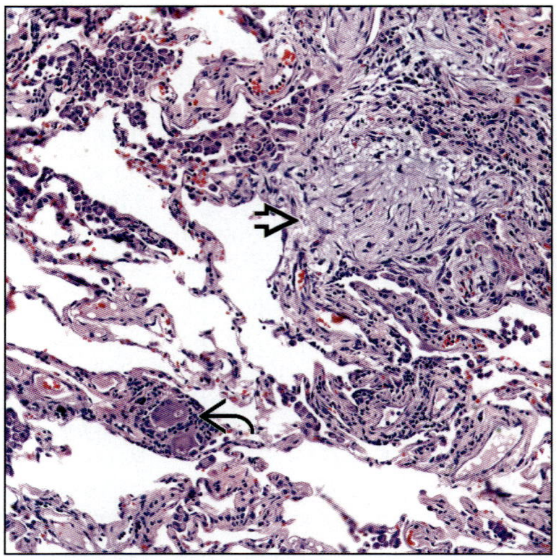

Hypersensitivity pneumonitis shows the 2 most important features for its diagnosis: Areas of bronchiolitis obliterans ⇒ and the presence of ill-defined granulomas ↷.

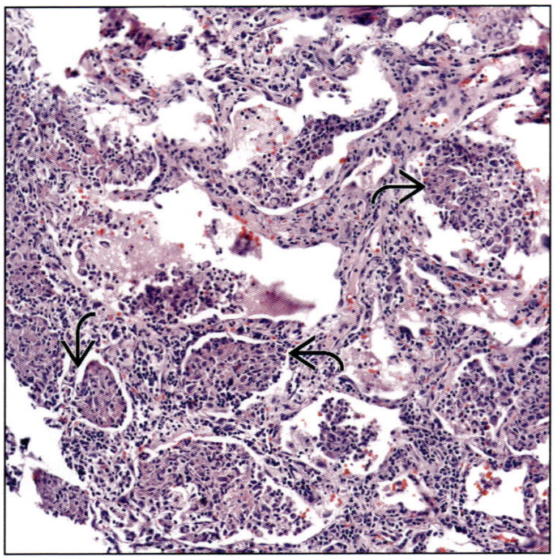

In other areas of lung parenchyma, there is a discrete presence of numerous noncaseating granulomas ↷. The presence of ill-defined granulomas is characteristic of HP.

TERMINOLOGY

Synonyms
- Hypersensitivity pneumonitis (HP)

Definitions
- Granulomatous lung disease secondary to inhalation of organic antigens or chemicals

ETIOLOGY/PATHOGENESIS

Environmental Exposure
- History of exposure to organic antigens
  - *Saccharopolyspora rectivirgula* in "farmer's lung" (moldy hay)
  - *Thermoactinomyces sacchari* in bagassosis (sugar cane workers)
  - Animal protein from bird feathers and feces from birds

Pathogenesis
- HP represents immune complex-mediated (type III) T-cell and delayed (type IV) hypersensitivity reaction

CLINICAL ISSUES

Epidemiology
- Incidence
  - Exact incidence of HP is unknown
    - However, HP may be more prevalent in people exposed to birds
- Age
  - Usually in adults
- Gender
  - No predilection for any particular gender
- Ethnicity
  - No predilection for any particular ethnic group

Site
- Lung without predilection for specific side or lung segment

Presentation
- Cough
- Dyspnea
- Fever
- Chills
- Wheezing
- Malaise

Laboratory Tests
- Pulmonary function tests may be abnormal
- Erythrosedimentation may be elevated
- C-protein may be elevated

Natural History
- Acute hypersensitivity pneumonitis
  - 4-6 hours after exposure to antigen
  - Episode may last 12-18 hours
- Chronic hypersensitivity pneumonitis
  - Patients may have continuous exposure to antigen over months or years
  - Patients may not experience acute episode
  - This type eventually gets biopsied

Treatment
- Drugs
  - Corticosteroids
- Stop exposure to potential antigen

Prognosis
- Prognosis is good in patients who have not developed pulmonary fibrosis

EXTRINSIC ALLERGIC ALVEOLITIS

Key Facts

Terminology
- Hypersensitivity pneumonitis (HP)
- Granulomatous lung disease secondary to inhalation of organic antigens or chemicals

Etiology/Pathogenesis
- History of exposure to organic antigens
- *Saccharopolyspora tectivirgula* in "farmer's lung" (moldy hay)
- *Thermoactinomyces sacchari* in bagassosis (sugar cane workers)
- Animal protein from bird feathers and feces from birds

Clinical Issues
- Acute hypersensitivity pneumonitis
  - 4-6 hours after exposure to antigen
  - Episode may last 12-18 hours
- Chronic hypersensitivity pneumonitis
  - Patients may have continuous exposure to antigen over longer periods of time
  - Patients may not experience acute episode
  - This type of HP eventually gets biopsied
- Treatment
  - Corticosteroids

Top Differential Diagnoses
- Sarcoidosis
- Usual interstitial pneumonitis (UIP)
- BOOP

Diagnostic Checklist
- Areas of BOOP
- Noncaseous granulomatous inflammation

MACROSCOPIC FEATURES

General Features
- Diagnosis of HP is generally performed by open lung biopsy

MICROSCOPIC PATHOLOGY

Histologic Features
- Areas of organizing pneumonia
- Intrabronchial budding of fibrocollagenous tissue
- Noncaseating granulomatous inflammation
- Patchy appearance in lung parenchyma
- Mild inflammatory peribronchial and interstitial changes

DIFFERENTIAL DIAGNOSIS

Sarcoidosis
- Rarely shows combined features of BOOP and noncaseous granulomatous reaction
- Granulomatous component in HP is rather ill-defined in contrast with the one seen in sarcoidosis

Usual Interstitial Pneumonitis (UIP)
- Rarely shows presence of noncaseous granulomatous inflammation
- Shows more extensive areas of pulmonary fibrosis

Bronchiolitis Obliterans and Organizing Pneumonia (BOOP)
- HP shows areas of BOOP
- Combination of BOOP and noncaseous granulomatous inflammation is hallmark of HP

Infectious Process
- Use of histochemical stains (AFB, PAS, and GMS) and tissue cultures are helpful in ruling out such possibility

DIAGNOSTIC CHECKLIST

Clinically Relevant Pathologic Features
- Tissue distribution

Pathologic Interpretation Pearls
- Areas of BOOP
- Noncaseous granulomatous inflammation
- Ill-defined granulomas

SELECTED REFERENCES

1. Akashi T et al: Histopathologic analysis of sixteen autopsy cases of chronic hypersensitivity pneumonitis and comparison with idiopathic pulmonary fibrosis/usual interstitial pneumonia. Am J Clin Pathol. 131(3):405-15, 2009
2. Churg A et al: Pathologic patterns and survival in chronic hypersensitivity pneumonitis. Am J Surg Pathol. 33(12):1765-70, 2009
3. Girard M et al: Hypersensitivity pneumonitis. Allergy. 64(3):322-34, 2009
4. Hirschmann JV et al: Hypersensitivity pneumonitis: a historical, clinical, and radiologic review. Radiographics. 29(7):1921-38, 2009
5. Koschel D et al: Hypersensitivity pneumonitis associated with the use of temozolomide. Eur Respir J. 33(4):931-4, 2009
6. Lima MS et al: Subacute and chronic hypersensitivity pneumonitis: histopathological patterns and survival. Respir Med. 103(4):508-15, 2009
7. van Heemst RC et al: Hypersensitivity pneumonitis caused by occupational exposure to phytase. Eur Respir J. 33(6):1507-9, 2009
8. Lacasse Y et al: Myths and controversies in hypersensitivity pneumonitis. Semin Respir Crit Care Med. 29(6):631-42, 2008

EXTRINSIC ALLERGIC ALVEOLITIS

Microscopic Features

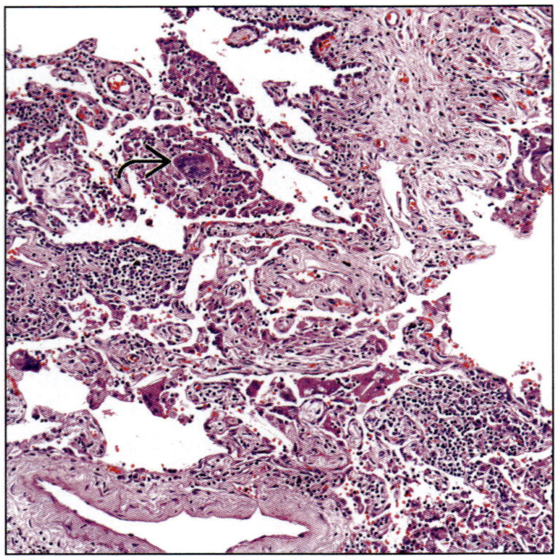
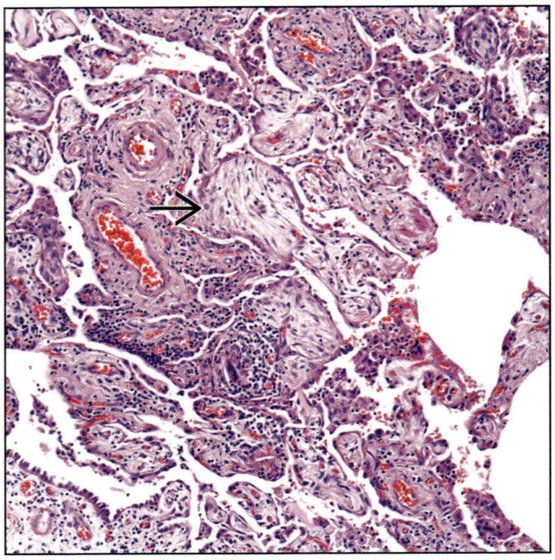

(Left) *HP shows an ill-defined granulomatous reaction, noncaseous type. Adjacent lung parenchyma shows widening of the interstitium with focal areas of fibrosis.* ***(Right)*** *HP shows areas similar to those seen in organizing pneumonia, namely the presence of fibroblastic polypoid plugs, so-called Masson bodies. There is mild inflammatory infiltrate.*

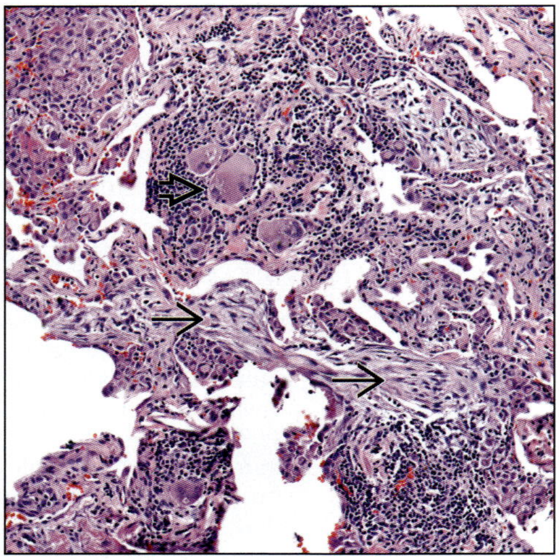
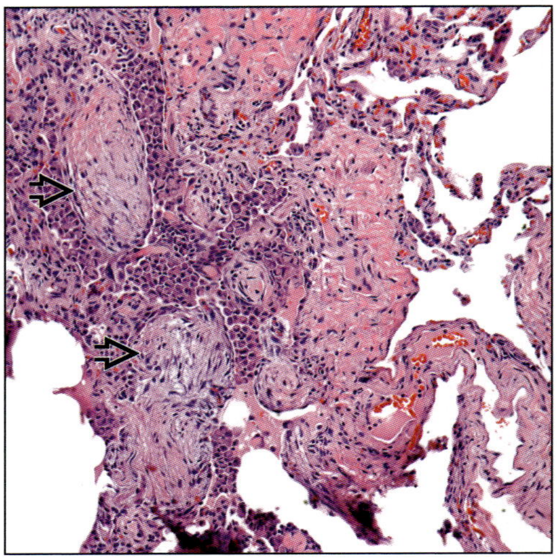

(Left) *The classical features of HP, namely the presence organizing pneumonia and the presence of an ill-defined granulomatous component, are present. These features are diagnostic of HP.* ***(Right)*** *The presence of young fibroblastic plugs may be the most obvious features in cases of HP. Thus, careful attention should be given to the finding of the granulomatous component in order to diagnose HP.*

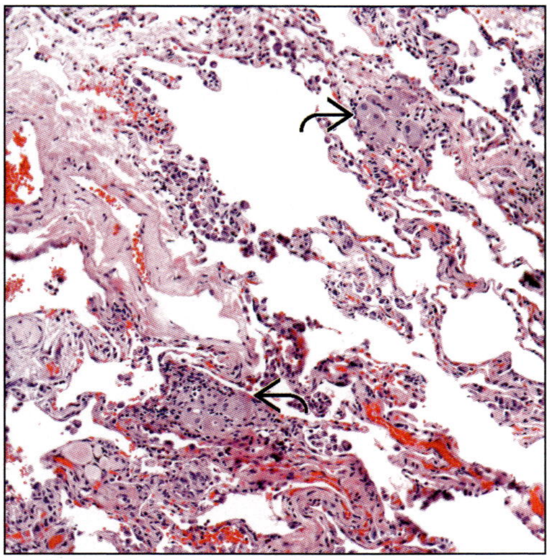
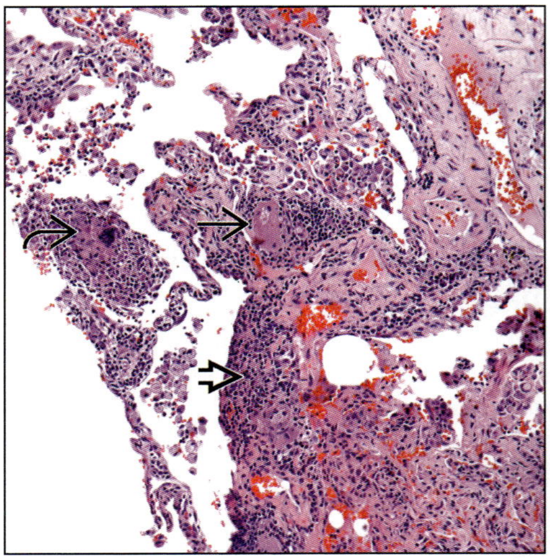

(Left) *Low-power view shows an HP in which the lung appears to be within normal limits; however, note the presence of discrete granulomas. This component can be easily ignored in cases of HP.* ***(Right)*** *HP shows more inflammatory components, including lymphocytes. There is also the presence of a small granuloma and giant cells embedded in the inflammatory component.*

EXTRINSIC ALLERGIC ALVEOLITIS

Microscopic Features

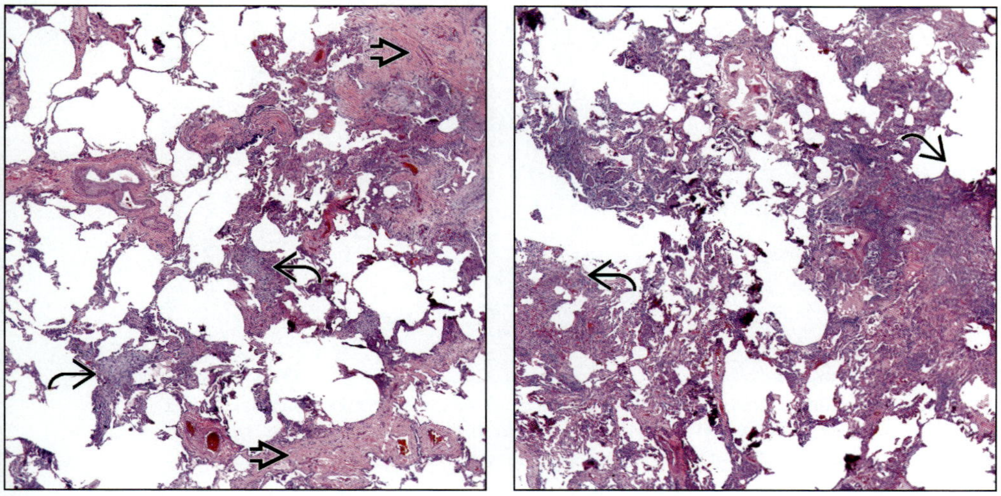

(Left) *Low-power view of HP shows the presence of fibroblastic plugs ➔ admixed with areas of relatively uninvolved lung parenchyma. In focal areas, there is mild interstitial scarring ⇨.* ***(Right)*** *Two distinct nodules ➔ are present within the lung parenchyma giving the appearance of organizing pneumonia. Although this is an important histological feature, equally important is the presence of granulomas.*

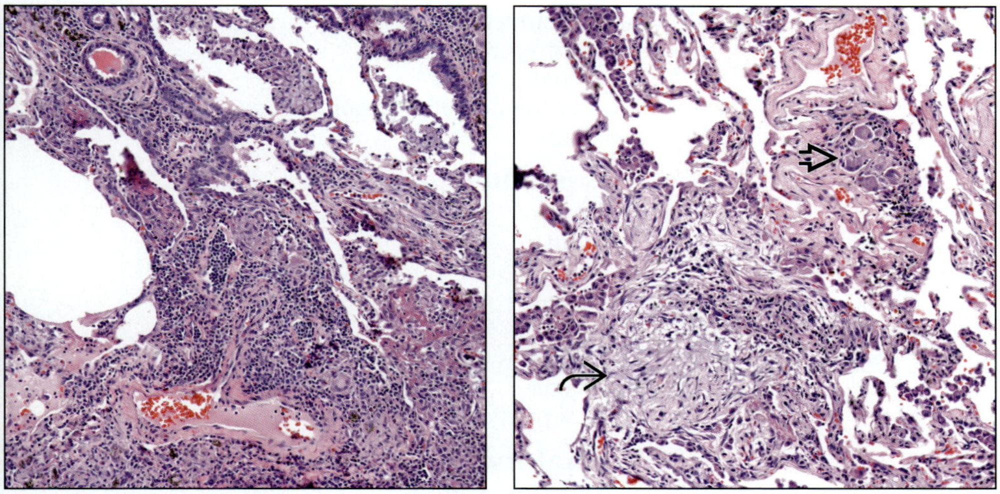

(Left) *HP shows areas with a more inflammatory component, namely lymphocytes. This feature may suggest an infectious or reactive process.* ***(Right)*** *Closer view at a fibroblastic plug shows the spindle fibroblastic proliferation ➔. In addition, note the presence of a granulomatous component ⇨. Adjacent lung parenchyma appears uninvolved.*

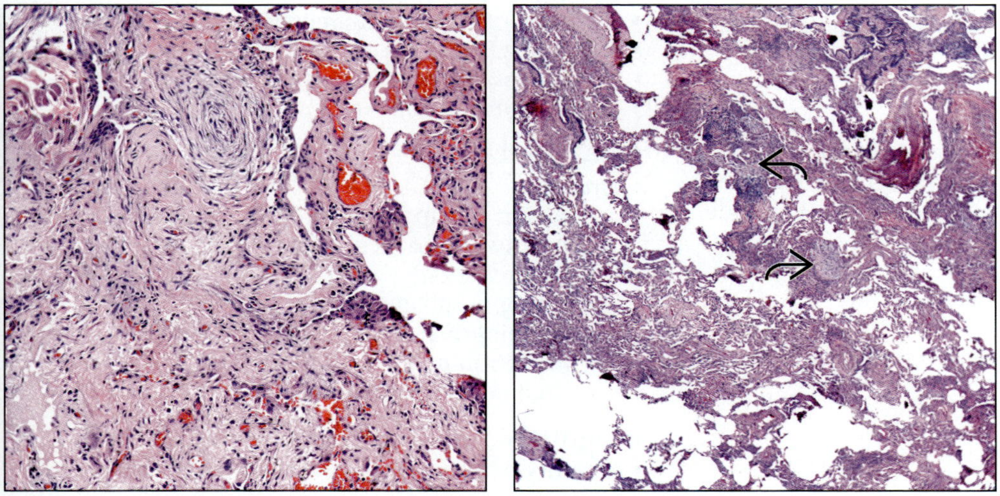

(Left) *In some cases of HP, areas of scarring or fibrosis may be present, suggesting the possibility of developing an interstitial fibrotic lung disease.* ***(Right)*** *A section of lung parenchyma shows areas of what appear to be "normal" lung parenchyma alternating with areas of focal organizing pneumonia ➔. The presence of areas of organizing pneumonia and a granulomatous component are characteristic of HP.*

ALLERGIC ANGIITIS AND GRANULOMATOSIS (CHURG-STRAUSS)

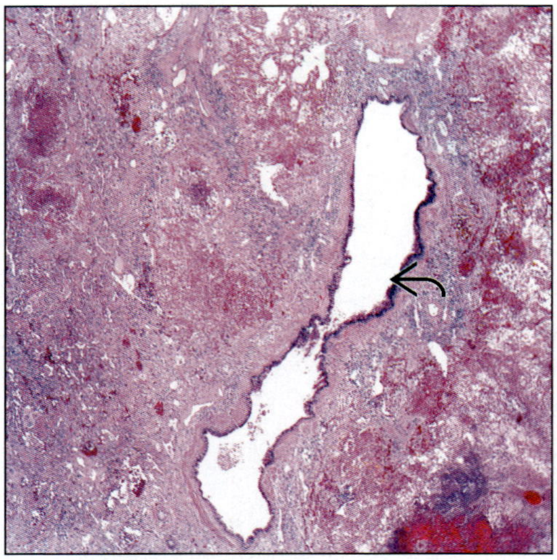

Lung parenchyma is shown partially destroyed by a fibrinous infiltrate composed of mixed inflammatory infiltrate. Note the presence of an airway structure that is still identifiable →.

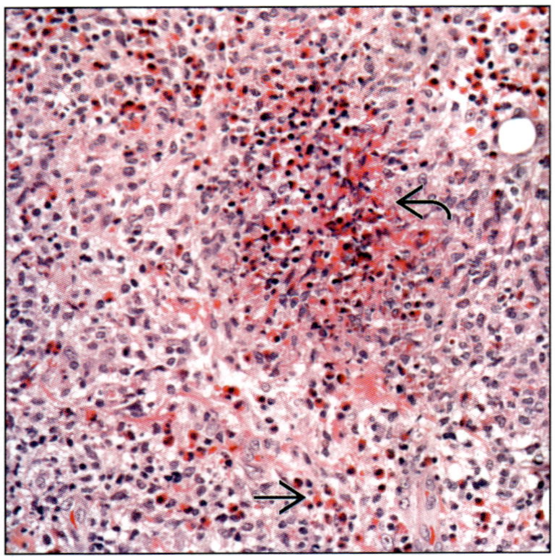

The presence of eosinophilic microabscess → is a common feature in cases of Churg-Strauss syndrome. Note also the presence of tissue eosinophilia →.

TERMINOLOGY

Abbreviations

- Allergic angiitis and granulomatosis (AAG)

Synonyms

- Churg-Strauss syndrome

Definitions

- Systemic process characterized by presence of vasculitis, blood eosinophilia, and asthma

ETIOLOGY/PATHOGENESIS

Etiology

- No definitive etiology has been defined for Churg-Strauss syndrome
- Probably an autoimmune process

CLINICAL ISSUES

Epidemiology

- Incidence
  - No clear population study has been performed to evaluate exact incidence of this syndrome
  - It is believed that 10% of patients with well-defined vasculitides may belong to Churg-Strauss syndrome
- Age
  - More common in adults
  - May vary from 3rd to 6th decade of life
- Gender
  - No apparent gender predilection for Churg-Strauss syndrome
- Ethnicity
  - No apparent predilection

Site

- Since this process is systemic, it may involve different systems, including
  - Respiratory system
  - Cardiovascular
  - Gastrointestinal
  - Renal
  - Central nervous system
  - Skin

Presentation

- Rhinitis
- Asthma
- Cough
- Dyspnea
- Erythema
- Arthralgias
- Myalgia
- Neuropathy

Laboratory Tests

- Blood eosinophilia
- p-ANCA commonly positive although c-ANCA may also be positive in some cases
- Elevation of erythrosedimentation rate
- Elevated IgE levels
- Leukocytosis
- Hypergammaglobulinemia

Treatment

- Drugs
  - Different therapeutic approaches have been tried, depending on particular case
    - Corticosteroids
    - Cyclophosphamide
    - Azathioprine
    - Interefron-α
    - High doses of immunoglobulin

Prognosis

- Majority of patients respond to steroid treatment
- Churg-Strauss syndrome may follow rapid and severe course unresponsive to treatment

ALLERGIC ANGIITIS AND GRANULOMATOSIS (CHURG-STRAUSS)

Key Facts

Terminology
- Systemic process characterized by presence of vasculitis, blood eosinophilia, and asthma

Etiology/Pathogenesis
- No definitive etiology has been defined for Churg-Strauss syndrome
- Probably an autoimmune process

Clinical Issues
- Incidence
  - More common in adults
- Since this process is systemic, it may involve different systems, including
  - Respiratory
  - Cardiovascular
  - Gastrointestinal
  - Renal
  - Central nervous
  - Skin
- Laboratory findings
  - Blood eosinophilia
  - p-ANCA commonly positive although c-ANCA may also be positive in some cases
- Treatment
  - Different therapeutic approaches have been tried depending on particular case
- Prognosis
  - Majority of patients respond to treatment with steroids
  - Churg-Strauss syndrome may follow rapid and severe course unresponsive to treatment

MACROSCOPIC FEATURES

General Features
- No pathognomonic gross findings for Churg-Strauss syndrome
  - May depend on severity and the tissues involved

MICROSCOPIC PATHOLOGY

Histologic Features
- Vasculitis
  - This process may affect capillaries, veins, and arteries
- Granulomatous reaction
  - Necrotizing
  - Non-necrotizing
- Tissue eosinophilia
- Bronchitis
- Fibrinoid pneumonia

DIFFERENTIAL DIAGNOSIS

Wegener Granulomatosis (WG)
- WG commonly involves kidneys
  - Churg-Strauss commonly involves cardiovascular system
- WG commonly has positive c-ANCA
  - Churg-Strauss more commonly has positive p-ANCA

Eosinophilic Pneumonia (EP)
- Eosinophilic abscess is more commonly seen in intraalveolar spaces
- Does not show extensive areas of necrosis and granulomatous reaction
- Does not involve other systems, such as cardiovascular system
- Most likely negative for p-ANCA or c-ANCA

Infectious Conditions
- Fungal
  - Special histochemical stains, including PAS and GMS, should be performed; tissue cultures are highly recommended
- Parasitic
  - *Strongyloides stercoralis* and *Toxocara canis*
    - Both of these parasites can be identified on light microscopic examination

DIAGNOSTIC CHECKLIST

Clinically Relevant Pathologic Features
- Organ distribution

Pathologic Interpretation Pearls
- Vasculitis
- Granulomatous inflammation
- Asthma

SELECTED REFERENCES

1. Kane GC et al: Involvement of the heart by small and medium vessel vasculitis. Curr Opin Rheumatol. 21(1):29-34, 2009
2. Sinico RA et al: Churg-Strauss angiitis. Best Pract Res Clin Rheumatol. 23(3):355-66, 2009
3. Grau RG: Churg-Strauss syndrome: 2005-2008 update. Curr Rheumatol Rep. 10(6):453-8, 2008
4. Jennette JC et al: New insight into the pathogenesis of vasculitis associated with antineutrophil cytoplasmic autoantibodies. Curr Opin Rheumatol. 20(1):55-60, 2008
5. Nathani N et al: Churg-Strauss syndrome and leukotriene antagonist use: a respiratory perspective. Thorax. 63(10):883-8, 2008
6. Alberts WM: Pulmonary manifestations of the Churg-Strauss syndrome and related idiopathic small vessel vasculitis syndromes. Curr Opin Pulm Med. 13(5):445-50, 2007

ALLERGIC ANGIITIS AND GRANULOMATOSIS (CHURG-STRAUSS)

Microscopic Features

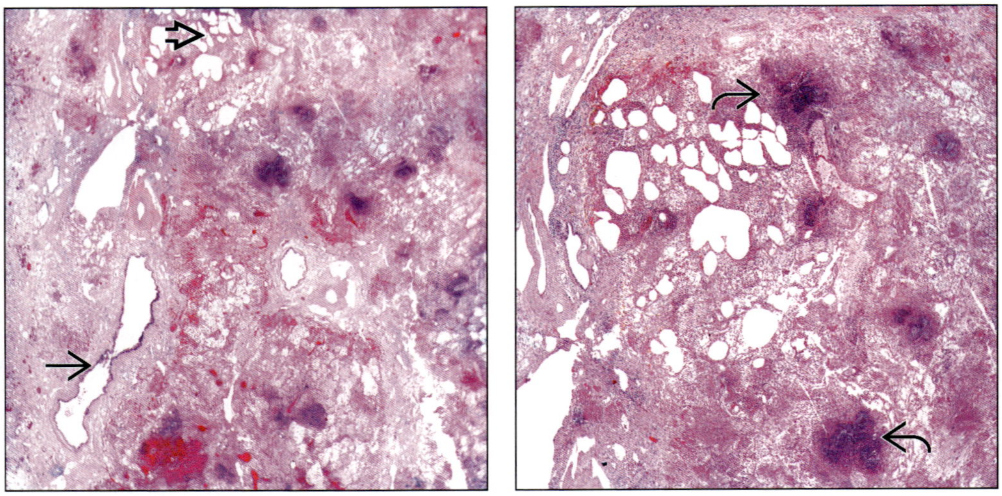

(Left) *Low-power view of Churg-Strauss syndrome shows areas of still recognizable airway structures → and alveolated tissue ⇨. Most of the lung parenchyma is destroyed by a fibrinous inflammatory infiltrate.* ***(Right)*** *Churg-Strauss syndrome shows the presence of numerous microabscesses ↷. This feature may be seen in infectious cases as well as in Wegener granulomatosis.*

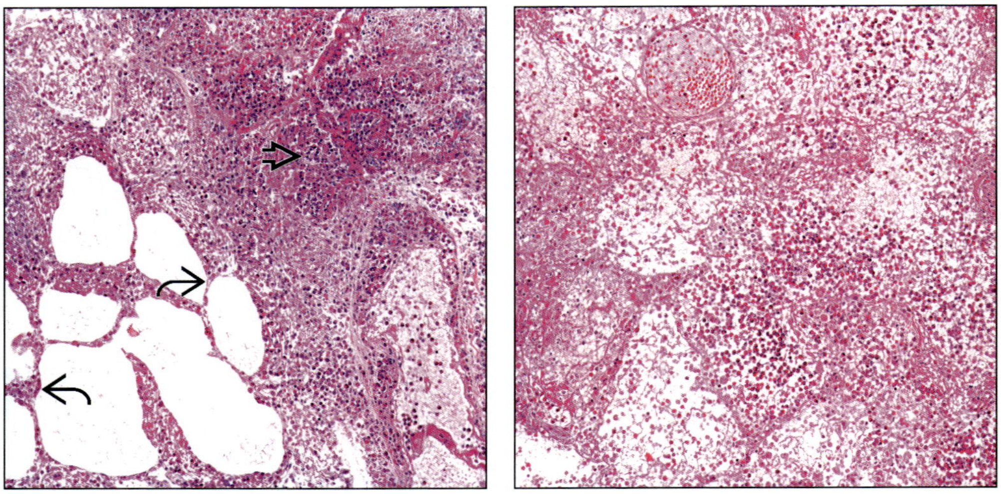

(Left) *Extensive areas of necrosis with eosinophils ⇨. However, in some areas one is still able to identify the outline of alveoli ↷.* ***(Right)*** *Higher magnification of the fibrinopurulent infiltrate in the lung parenchyma in Churg-Strauss. At this power, it is difficult to recognize either lung parenchyma or vascular structures.*

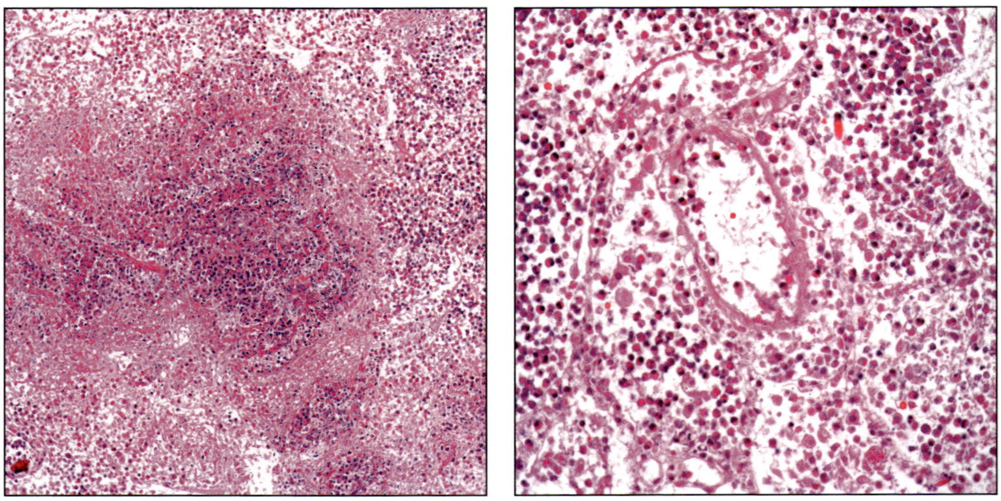

(Left) *Necrosis and microabscesses are commonly seen in cases of Churg-Strauss as they may also be seen in cases of Wegener granulomatosis.* ***(Right)*** *High-power magnification shows that the inflammatory infiltrate is composed predominantly of eosinophils. This type of infiltrate should raise the suspicion of Churg-Strauss syndrome in the proper clinical setting.*

Microscopic Features

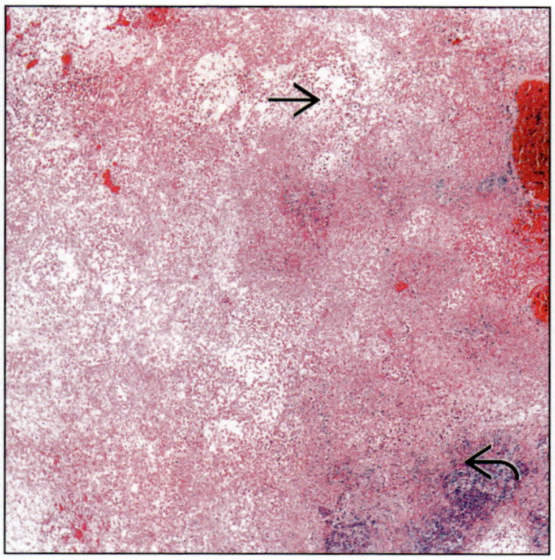

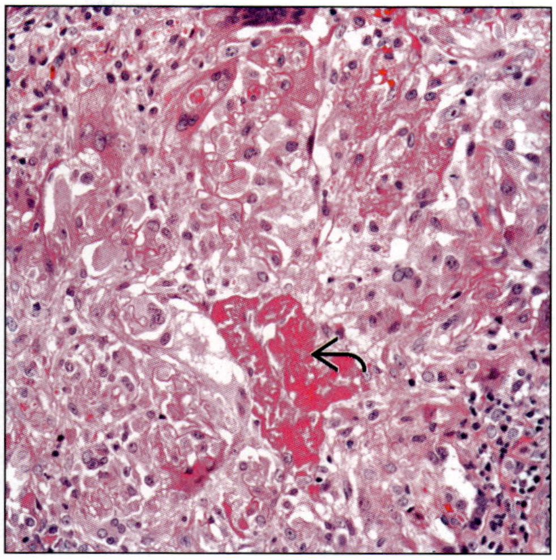

(Left) *Low-power view shows areas of necrosis ↩ and fibrinoid exudate → destroying lung parenchyma. Similar features may be seen in Wegener granulomatosis.* ***(Right)*** *High-power view of areas showing focal fibrinoid exudate ↩ are surrounded by the remains of lung parenchyma with marked inflammatory changes.*

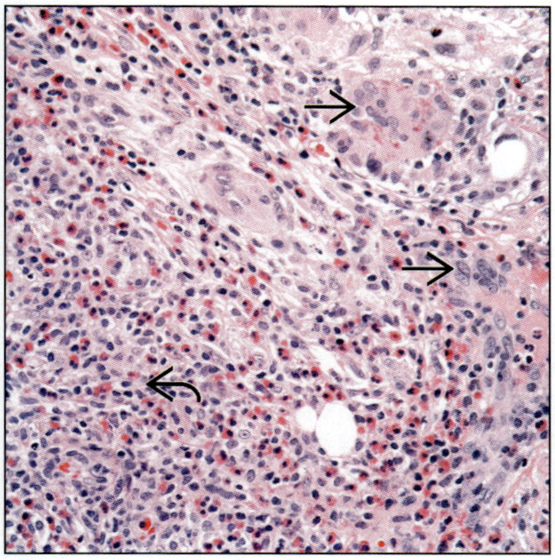

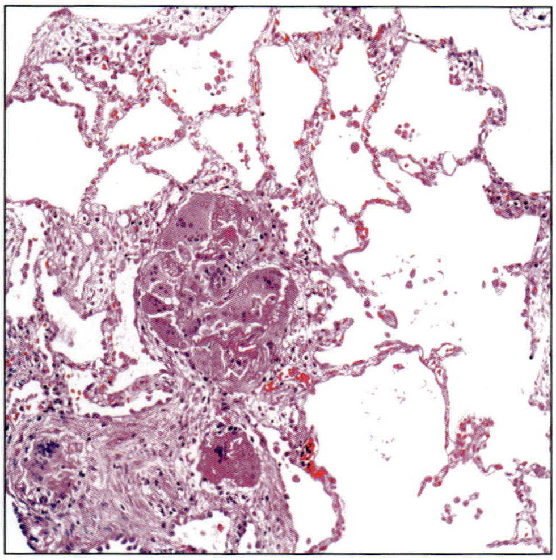

(Left) *Prominent tissue eosinophilia ↩ admixed with scattered multinucleated giant cells → is a common feature of Churg-Strauss syndrome.* ***(Right)*** *In areas away from the acute inflammatory reaction and eosinophilia, the presence of granulomas in otherwise uninvolved lung parenchyma is common. Special stains are important to rule out infection.*

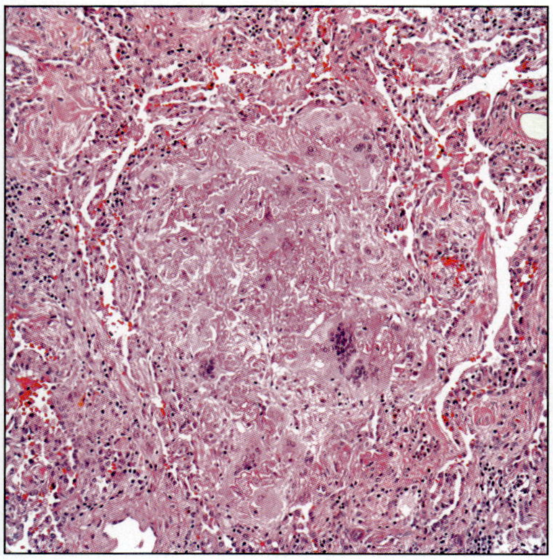

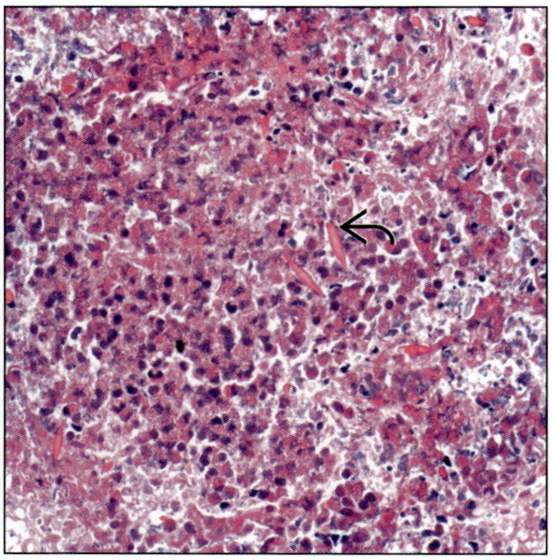

(Left) *High-power view shows a focal granulomatous reaction in Churg-Strauss syndrome. This feature may be seen in cases of infectious origin.* ***(Right)*** *Areas of tissue necrosis and prominent inflammatory changes are admixed with crystalloid material ↩. These features should also raise suspicion for underlying asthma.*

BRONCHOCENTRIC GRANULOMATOSIS

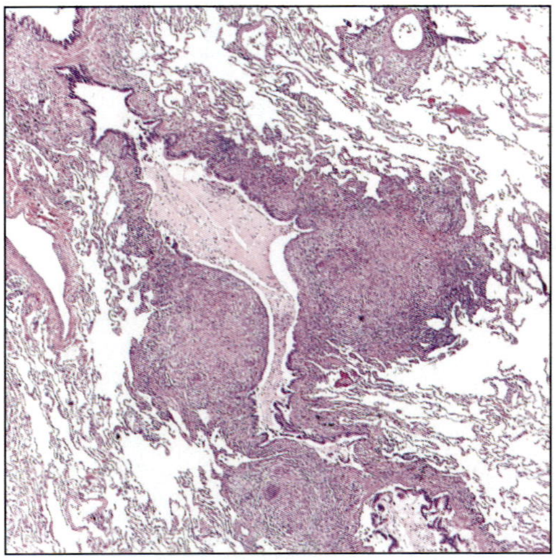

Bronchocentric granulomatosis shows multiple epithelioid granulomas composed of epithelioid histiocytes circumscribing a bronchus.

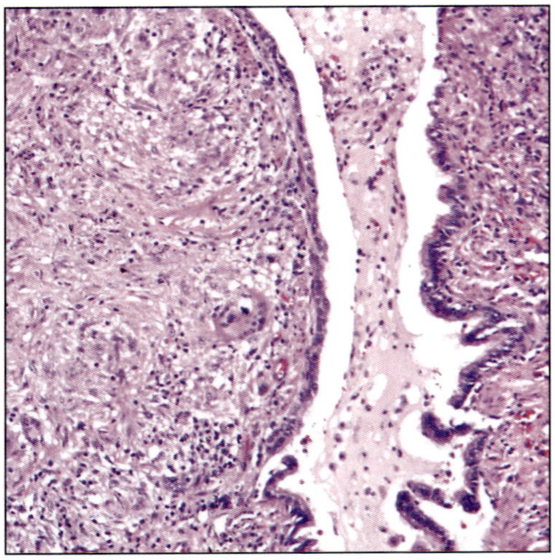

Higher magnification of bronchocentric granulomatosis shows epithelioid granulomas with multinucleated giant cells.

TERMINOLOGY

Abbreviations

- Bronchocentric granulomatosis (BCG)

Definitions

- Reaction pattern of lung parenchyma characterized by broncho- and bronchiolocentric necrotizing granulomatous inflammation

ETIOLOGY/PATHOGENESIS

Environmental Exposure

- Process can be related to infectious and noninfectious causes
  - Infections associated with BCG include mycobacteria, fungi (*Aspergillus*, *Histoplasma*, etc.), and parasites (*Echinococcus*)
  - Noninfectious causes of BCG include Wegener granulomatosis and rheumatoid arthritis
  - Allergic causes of BCG include allergic aspergillosis in association with mucoid impaction

CLINICAL ISSUES

Epidemiology

- Incidence
  - Most cases of BCG are allergic and associated with allergic bronchopulmonary aspergillosis
  - About 50% of patients have history of chronic asthma
- Age
  - No particular age distribution

Site

- BCG affects mostly larger bronchi but may also involve more distant bronchioles

Presentation

- Fever
- Cough
- Wheezing
- Peripheral eosinophilia
- Mucoid impaction

Endoscopic Findings

- Frequent finding is mucoid impaction with "allergic" mucin

Laboratory Tests

- Elevated IgE levels and serum precipitins to *Aspergillus* are important clues in allergic cases
- Antinuclear antibody testing is helpful to rule out Wegener granulomatosis
- Cultures are important to rule out specific infectious agents

Natural History

- Noninfectious cases occur mainly in asthmatic patients with mucus impaction
- Infectious cases show more variable findings, ranging from localized consolidation to nodular parenchymal lesions
- Cavitation is most often encountered in cases associated with infectious etiology

Treatment

- Steroids are treatment of choice for both infectious and noninfectious BCG

IMAGE FINDINGS

Radiographic Findings

- Mucoid impaction shows band-like or branching opacities in bronchial distribution
- Nonasthmatic individuals may show spiculated nodules or masses that can undergo cavitation

Key Facts

Terminology
- Reaction pattern of lung parenchyma characterized by broncho- and bronchiolocentric necrotizing granulomatous inflammation

Clinical Issues
- Most cases of BCG are allergic and associated with allergic bronchopulmonary aspergillosis
- About 50% of patients have history of chronic asthma
- Frequent finding is mucoid impaction with "allergic" mucin
- Noninfectious cases occur mainly in asthmatic patients with mucus impaction
- Infectious cases show more variable findings, ranging from localized consolidation to nodular parenchymal lesions

Microscopic Pathology
- Destruction of walls of small bronchi and bronchioles by necrotizing granulomatous inflammation
- Bronchial walls are replaced by palisading histiocytic reaction
- Abundant necrotic debris seen in lumens of bronchioles with numerous neutrophils and eosinophils
- Impaction of proximal airways by allergic mucin
- Eosinophils are particularly prominent in cases associated with allergic bronchopulmonary aspergillosis
- Multinucleated giant cells may be present, particularly around necrotic debris

MICROSCOPIC PATHOLOGY

Histologic Features
- Destruction of walls of small bronchi and bronchioles by necrotizing granulomatous inflammation
- Bronchial walls are replaced by palisading histiocytic reaction
- Abundant necrotic debris seen in lumen of bronchioles with numerous neutrophils and eosinophils
- Impaction of proximal airways by allergic mucin
- Early lesions may show only chronic bronchitis with intact bronchial wall
- More advanced lesions will show chronic and acute bronchitis with destruction of normal elastic lamina of bronchioles

Cytologic Features
- Eosinophils are particularly prominent in cases associated with allergic bronchopulmonary aspergillosis
- Multinucleated giant cells may be present, particularly around necrotic debris

DIFFERENTIAL DIAGNOSIS

Wegener Granulomatosis
- May also show prominent bronchocentric distribution with destruction of bronchial walls
  - In addition to bronchocentric granulomas, there will also be evidence of vasculitis and microabscesses
  - Extensive areas of parenchymal necrosis with abundant neutrophilic debris
  - Positive c-ANCA in serum favors Wegener granulomatosis

Sarcoidosis
- Abundant epithelioid granulomas that can occasionally undergo necrotizing changes
- Distribution of granulomas is not restricted to bronchiolar walls and follows lymphangitic distribution
- Absence of allergic mucin, eosinophilia, or organisms on special stains
- Characteristic clinical and radiographic presentation often associated with lymphadenopathy

Foreign Body Granulomas
- Secondary to aspiration
- Can cause necrotizing granulomatous reaction surrounding foreign material
- Complete destruction of bronchial wall is unusual
- Foreign material is usually recognizable under polarized light

DIAGNOSTIC CHECKLIST

Clinically Relevant Pathologic Features
- Most important consideration is to rule out infection or Wegener granulomatosis when encountering bronchocentric granulomas
- History of asthma is most important clue for allergic cases

Pathologic Interpretation Pearls
- BCG resembles any necrotizing granuloma of infectious etiology except that it is bronchiolocentric in distribution
- Chronic bronchitis and scattered non-necrotizing granulomas are not sufficient for diagnosis in the absence of palisaded necrotizing inflammation

SELECTED REFERENCES

1. Yousem SA: Bronchocentric injury in Wegener's granulomatosis: a report of five cases. Hum Pathol. 22(6):535-40, 1991
2. Myers JL: Bronchocentric granulomatosis. Disease or diagnosis? Chest. 96(1):3-4, 1989
3. Clee MD et al: Bronchocentric granulomatosis: a review and thoughts on pathogenesis. Br J Dis Chest. 77(3):227-34, 1983

BRONCHOCENTRIC GRANULOMATOSIS

Histologic Features

*(**Left**) Bronchocentric granulomatosis of the lung shows multiple large, epithelioid granulomas coalescing around a bronchiole →. The lumen of the bronchiole is collapsed and distorted by the surrounding granulomas. (**Right**) Higher magnification of bronchocentric granulomatosis shows dense epithelioid granulomas surrounding a bronchial lumen. Early lesions do not show necrotizing changes, but there is evidence of bronchitis with inflammatory infiltrate in the bronchial lumen.*

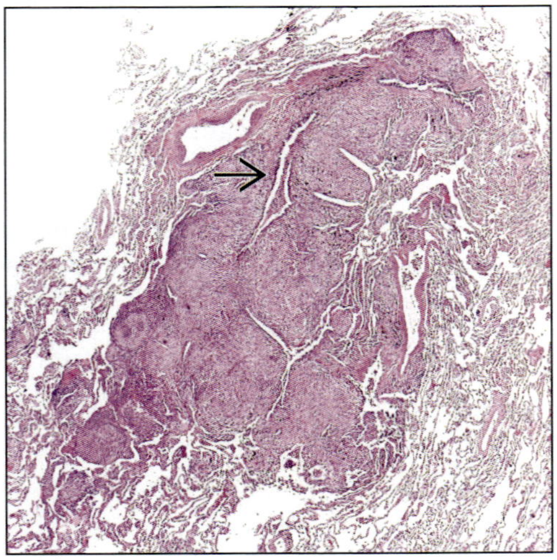

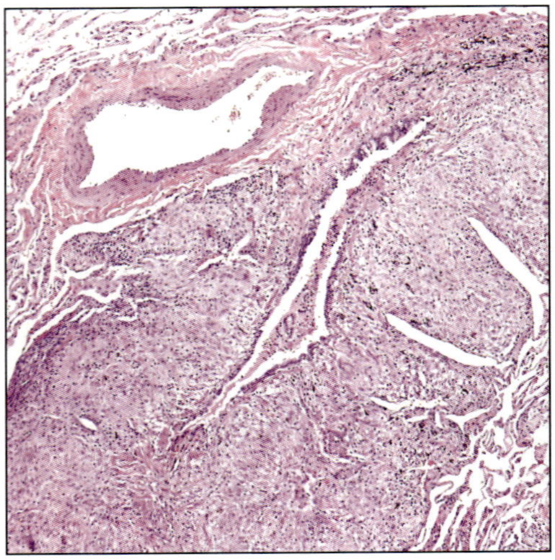

*(**Left**) Higher magnification of bronchocentric granulomatosis shows a bronchial lumen surrounded by epithelioid histiocytes and a few multinucleated giant cells. The lumen of the bronchus contains scant inflammatory infiltrate admixed with fibrin. (**Right**) Bronchocentric granulomatosis shows partial destruction of the wall of a bronchus by granulomatous inflammation. An ill-defined palisading granuloma can be observed → adjacent to the bronchial wall.*

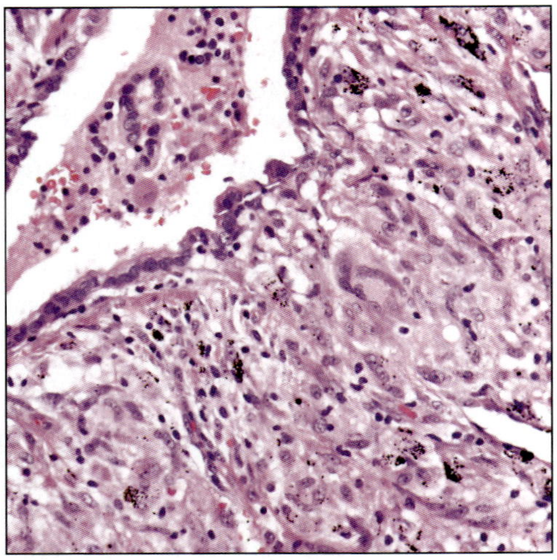

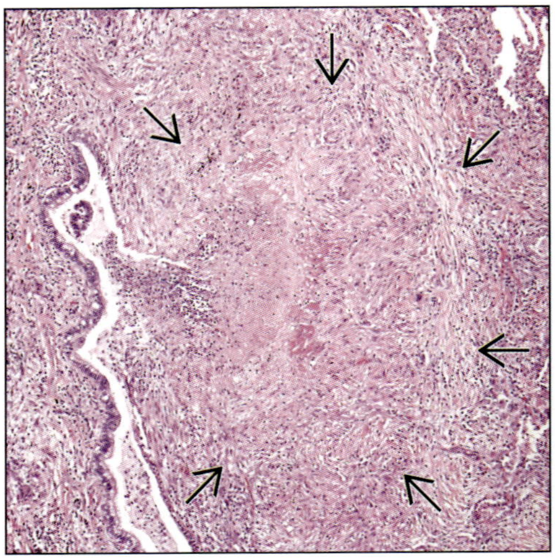

*(**Left**) Higher magnification of the bronchial wall in bronchocentric granulomatosis shows partial destruction of the wall of the bronchus by severe acute and chronic inflammation with abundant necrotic debris and neutrophilic infiltrate ↷. (**Right**) Higher magnification of a bronchial wall in bronchocentric granulomatosis shows acute inflammation with abundant neutrophils, karyorrhexis, and necrotic debris surrounded by a rim of epithelioid histiocytes.*

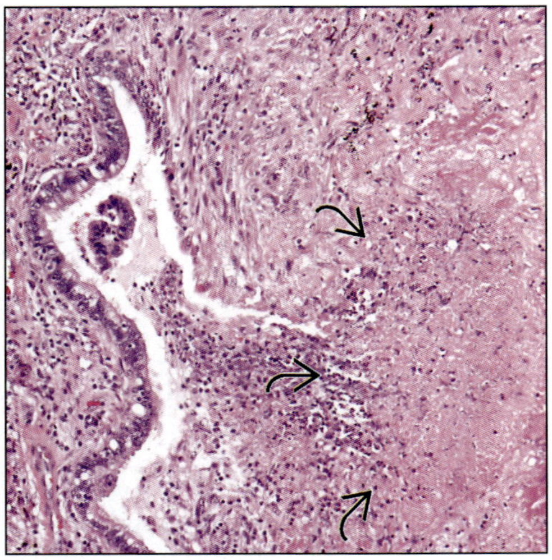

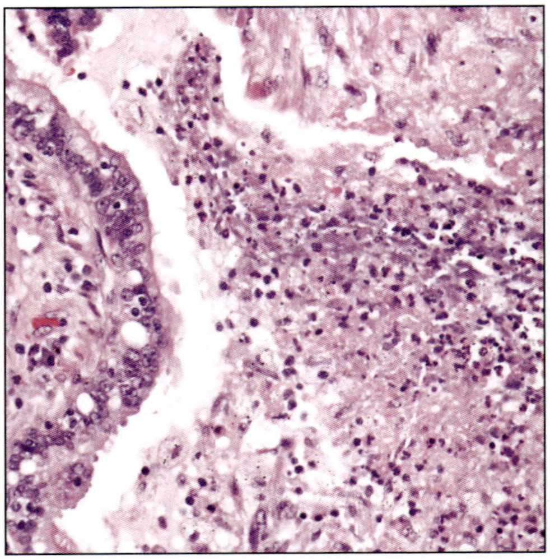

BRONCHOCENTRIC GRANULOMATOSIS

Histologic Features

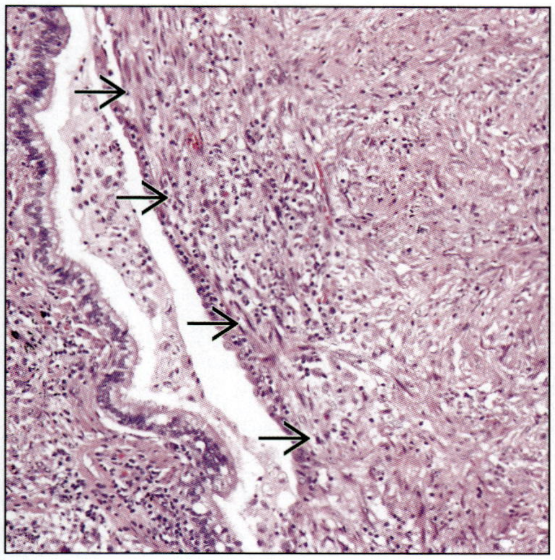

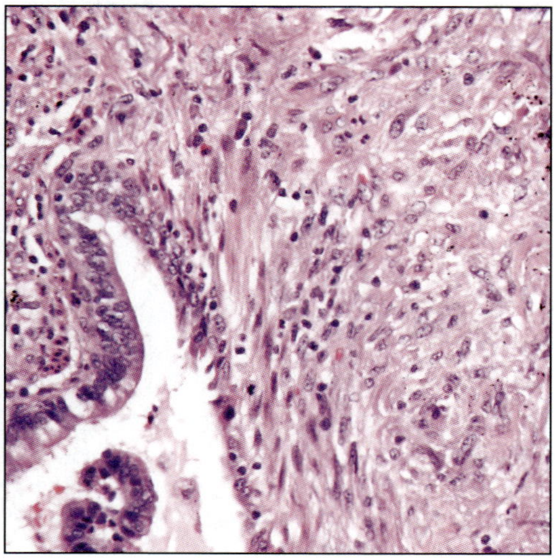

(Left) *Bronchocentric granulomatosis shows partial destruction of the wall of a bronchus by chronic inflammation. The involved wall of the bronchus contains a large epithelioid granuloma* → *composed of sheets of large epithelioid histiocytes admixed with scant lymphoid cells.* ***(Right)*** *Higher magnification of an affected bronchial wall in bronchocentric granulomatosis shows partial destruction and thinning of the wall by adjacent sheets of epithelioid histiocytes.*

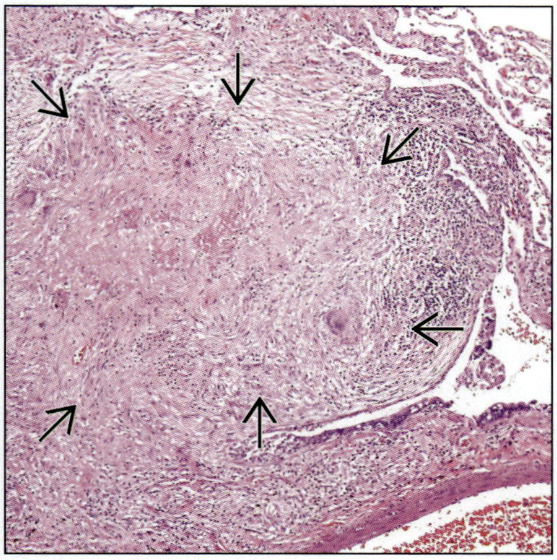

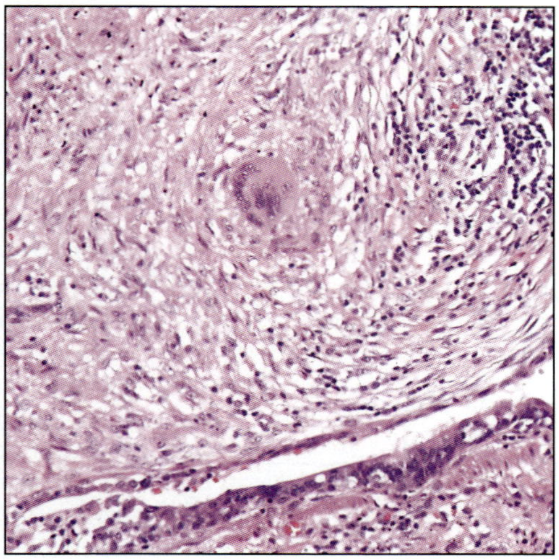

(Left) *Bronchocentric granulomatosis shows compression and distortion of a bronchial lumen by a large epithelioid granuloma* → *involving lung parenchyma around the bronchioles.* ***(Right)*** *Higher magnification of a small bronchiole in bronchocentric granulomatosis shows a large epithelioid granuloma with a multinucleated giant cell and few scattered small lymphocytes. Absence of vasculitis is a helpful clue to distinguish this from Wegener granulomatosis.*

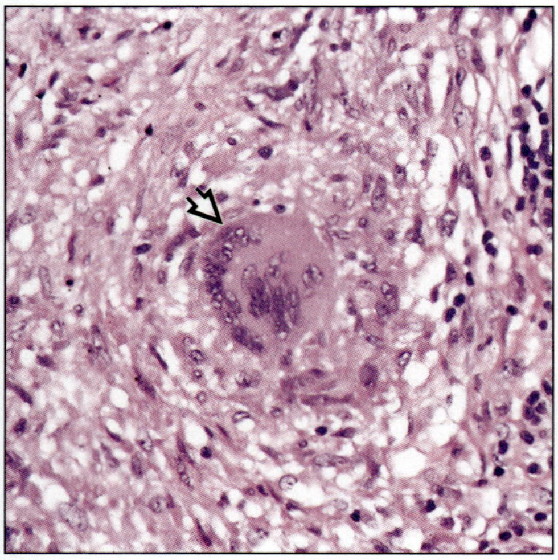

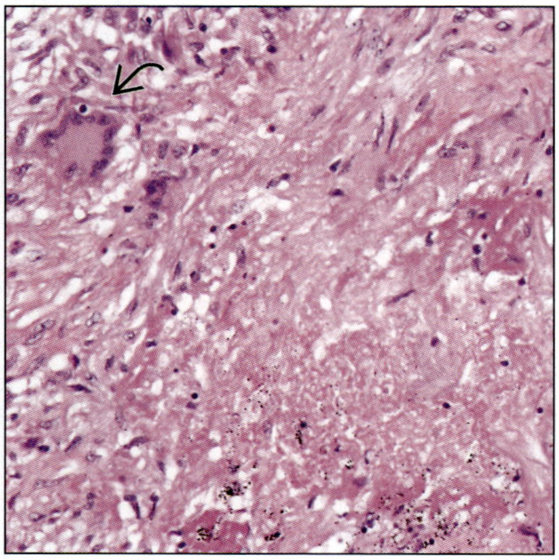

(Left) *Higher magnification of epithelioid granuloma in bronchocentric granulomatosis shows sheets of epithelioid histiocytes with a single multinucleated giant cell in the center* ⇒*.* ***(Right)*** *Granulomatous inflammation in the wall of a bronchus in patient with bronchocentric granulomatosis shows abundant necrotic debris surrounded by palisading histiocytes. Notice the single residual multinucleated giant cell* ↗ *at the edges of the necrotic field.*

WEGENER GRANULOMATOSIS

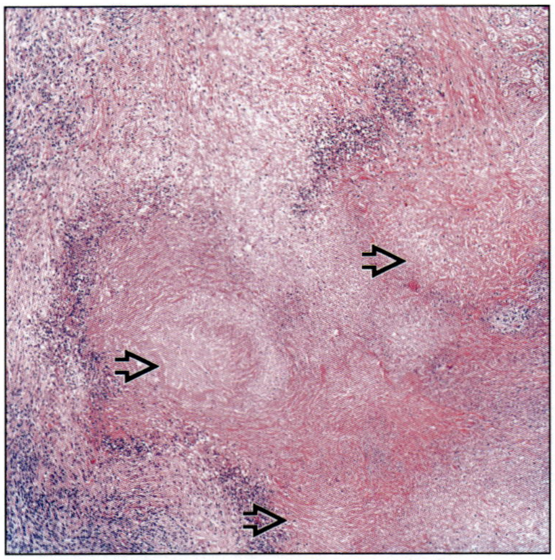

Low-power view of Wegener granulomatosis displays extensive areas of necrosis ➪, so-called geographic necrosis with total destruction of the normal lung parenchyma.

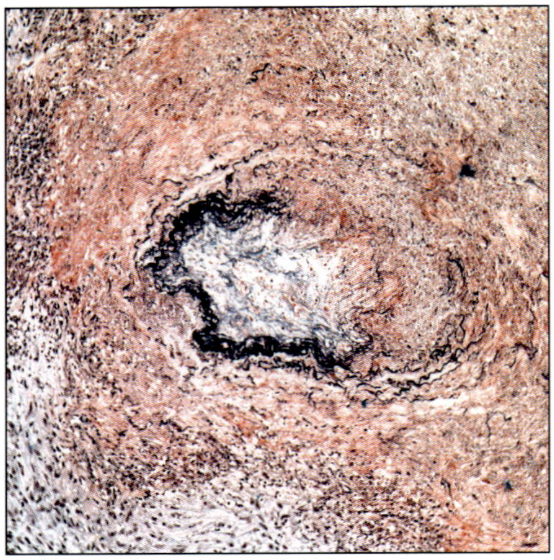

High-power view of a vessel stained with elastic van Gieson in Wegener granulomatosis shows partial destruction of the vascular wall.

TERMINOLOGY

Abbreviations

- Wegener granulomatosis (WG)

Definitions

- Systemic inflammatory process characterized by vasculitis and granulomatous reaction

ETIOLOGY/PATHOGENESIS

Etiology

- No definitive etiology is known for WG

CLINICAL ISSUES

Epidemiology

- Incidence
  - Incidence of this condition varies and can be up to 8 per 1,000,000 people
- Age
  - More common in adults, usually in 5th decade of life
  - Rarely occurs in young people or children
- Gender
  - No apparent predilection
- Ethnicity
  - No ethnic predilection

Site

- Since WG process is systemic, it can affect any particular system
  - Sites may include
    - Upper and lower respiratory system
    - Genitourinary system, mainly kidney
    - Ocular system
    - Breast

Presentation

- Rhinorrea
- Oral and nasal ulcers
- Cough
- Dyspnea
- Pleuritic pain
- Hemoptysis

Laboratory Tests

- Antineutrophil cytoplasmic antibodies
  - Cytoplasmic antineutrophilic antibody (c-ANCA) is positive in nearly all cases of WG
  - Perinuclear antineutrophilic antibody (p-ANCA) not as specific as c-ANCA, as it may be seen positive in other conditions
- Erythrocyte sedimentation rate is usually elevated
- Leukocytosis
- Thrombocytopenia
- Anemia (normochromic-normocytic)

Treatment

- Drugs
  - Cyclophosphamide and prednisone
  - Trimethoprim and sulfamethoxazole

Prognosis

- Untreated WG is fatal
- Treated patients do relatively well, and remissions are common
- Younger patients appear to fare better than older patients

MACROSCOPIC FEATURES

General Features

- Multiple bilateral cavitary and solid pulmonary nodules
- Areas of necrosis are usually present

WEGENER GRANULOMATOSIS

Key Facts

Etiology/Pathogenesis

- No definitive etiology is known for WG

Clinical Issues

- Incidence
  - More common in adults, usually in 5th decade of life
- Since WG is systemic and can affect any particular system; these sites may include
  - Upper and lower respiratory system
  - Genitourinary system, mainly kidney
  - Ocular system
  - Breast
- Laboratory findings
  - c-ANCA is positive in nearly all cases of WG
  - p-ANCA is not as specific as c-ANCA, as it may be positive in other conditions
  - Leukocytosis
  - Erythrocyte sedimentation rate is usually elevated
- Treatment
  - Cyclophosphamide and prednisone
  - Trimethoprim and sulfamethoxazole
- Prognosis
  - Untreated WG is fatal
  - Treated patients do relatively well, but remissions are common

Top Differential Diagnoses

- Lymphomatoid granulomatosis
  - Usually shows atypical lymphoid proliferation
- Churg-Strauss syndrome
  - Commonly associated with asthma
- Infectious process

MICROSCOPIC PATHOLOGY

Histologic Features

- Geographic necrosis
  - Extensive areas of necrosis
  - Microabscesses
- Vasculitis
  - Arteries, veins, &/or capillaries
- Prominent inflammatory response composed of lymphocytes, neutrophils, macrophages, and giant cells
- Granulomatous reaction
  - All types of giant cells may be present

DIFFERENTIAL DIAGNOSIS

Lymphomatoid Granulomatosis

- There is vasculitis, but usually, infiltrate is more monotonous and atypical
- Extensive areas of geographic necrosis are uncommon
- Immunohistochemical studies are helpful in this diagnosis

Churg-Strauss Syndrome

- Both conditions show evidence of vasculitis
- Most commonly will show positive p-ANCA and negative c-ANCA
- Commonly associated with asthma

Infectious Process

- WG shows necrosis and granulomatous inflammation that may mimic any infectious process
- Infectious process needs to be ruled out with histochemical stains
  - Includes PAS, GMS, and AFB
  - In addition, tissue cultures are highly recommended

DIAGNOSTIC CHECKLIST

Clinically Relevant Pathologic Features

- Organ distribution

Pathologic Interpretation Pearls

- Geographic necrosis
- Vasculitis
- Granulomatous inflammation

SELECTED REFERENCES

1. Allende DS et al: Wegener's granulomatosis of the breast: a rare entity with daily clinical relevance. Ann Diagn Pathol. 13(5):351-7, 2009
2. Ananthakrishnan L et al: Wegener's granulomatosis in the chest: high-resolution CT findings. AJR Am J Roentgenol. 192(3):676-82, 2009
3. Gómez-Puerta JA et al: Antineutrophil cytoplasmic antibody-associated vasculitides and respiratory disease. Chest. 136(4):1101-11, 2009
4. Csernok E et al: Proteinase 3, protease-activated receptor-2 and interleukin-32: linking innate and autoimmunity in Wegener's granulomatosis. Clin Exp Rheumatol. 26(3 Suppl 49):S112-7, 2008
5. Moosig F et al: Wegener's granulomatosis: the current view. Clin Rev Allergy Immunol. 35(1-2):19-21, 2008
6. Renaudineau Y et al: Renal involvement in Wegener's granulomatosis. Clin Rev Allergy Immunol. 35(1-2):22-9, 2008
7. Seo P: Wegener's granulomatosis: managing more than inflammation. Curr Opin Rheumatol. 20(1):10-6, 2008
8. Weeda LW Jr et al: Wegener's granulomatosis. Oral Maxillofac Surg Clin North Am. 20(4):643-9, 2008

WEGENER GRANULOMATOSIS

Imaging and Microscopic Features

(Left) *Chest x-ray shows bilateral pulmonary involvement. This radiologic image is not diagnostic of Wegener granulomatosis as it may be seen in other conditions.* ***(Right)*** *Low power of Wegener granulomatosis shows extensive areas of necrosis destroying most of the lung parenchyma. There is very little inflammatory component.*

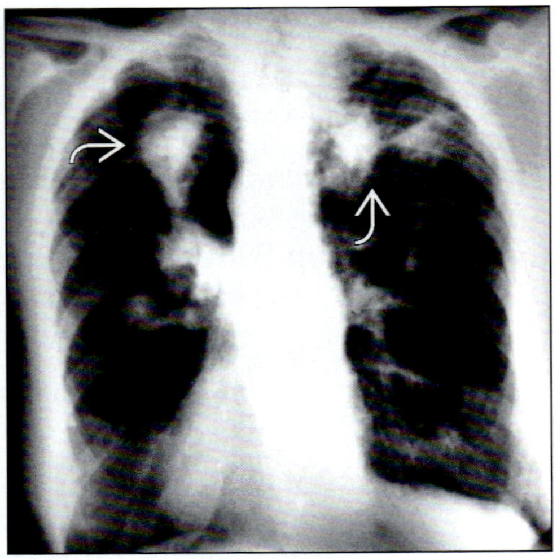

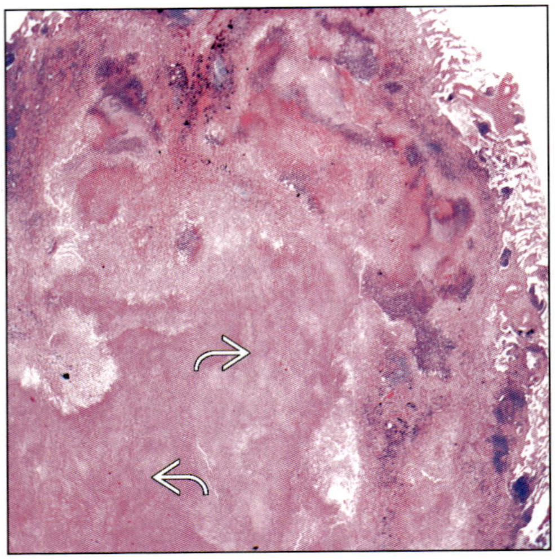

(Left) *Small microabscesses are a common feature in cases of Wegener granulomatosis, and their presence should not dissuade from the diagnosis of WG.* ***(Right)*** *In other parts of the lung, the necrosis merges with areas of fibrosis and prominent acute inflammatory changes. These features may also be seen in cases of infectious origin.*

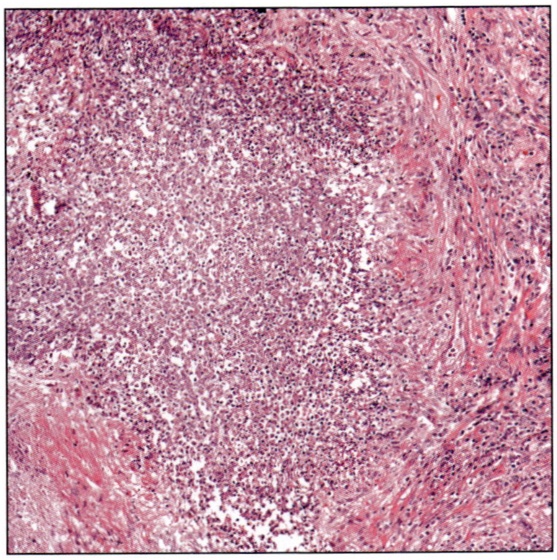

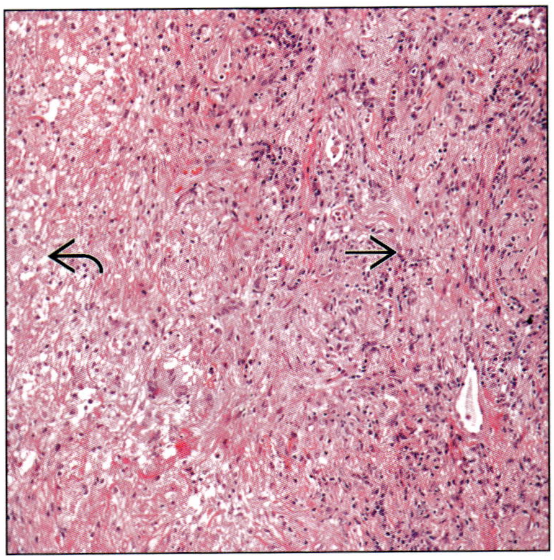

(Left) *Wegener granulomatosis shows areas of acute inflammation admixed with numerous multinucleated giant cells. This feature may not be present in all the cases of WG.* ***(Right)*** *Wegener granulomatosis shows a pulmonary vessel that is markedly involved by vasculitis. Adjacent tissue shows prominent acute inflammatory changes.*

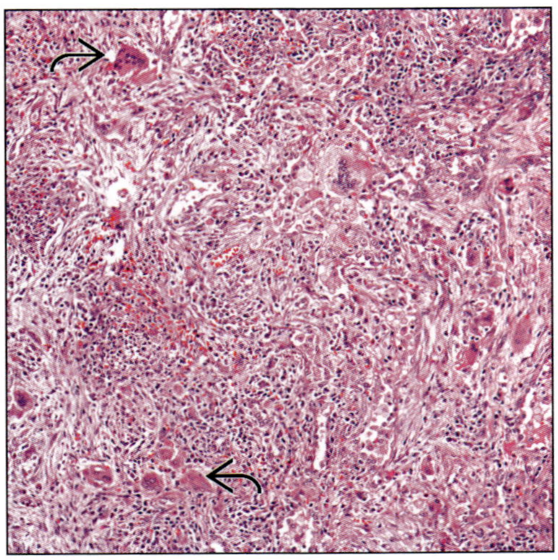

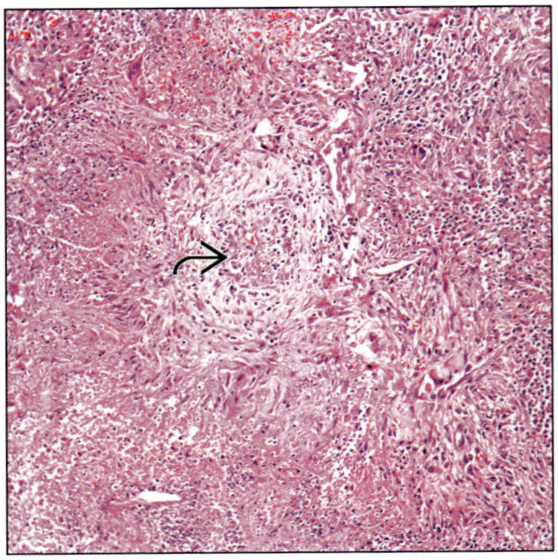

WEGENER GRANULOMATOSIS

Microscopic Features

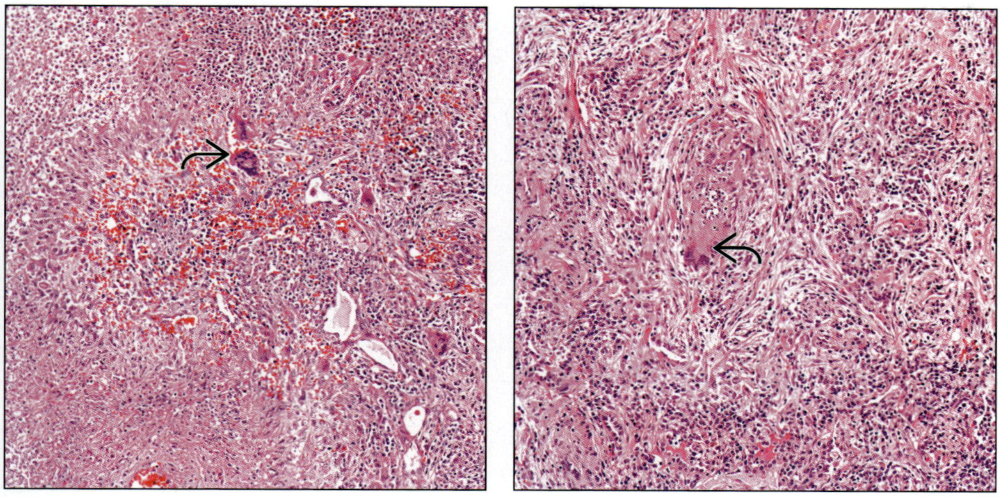

(Left) *Pulmonary parenchyma totally destroyed by acute inflammation shows granulomatous inflammation and the presence of multinucleated giant cells →. These features are commonly seen in Wegener granulomatosis.* ***(Right)*** *Multinucleated giant cells → can be seen singly and without forming a conventional granulomatous reaction embedded in otherwise fibrotic tissue with acute inflammation.*

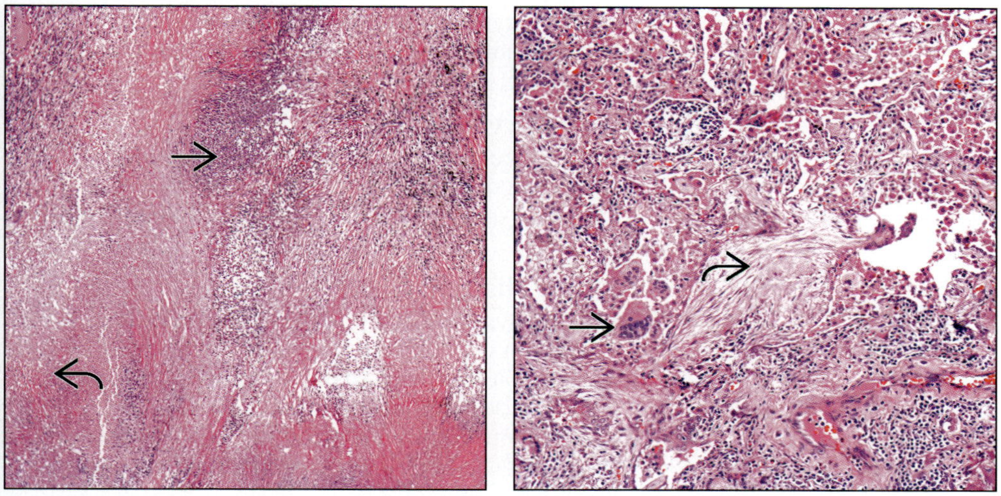

(Left) *Extensive areas of necrosis → are admixed with focal areas of acute inflammation →. Because these features may be seen in infectious cases, the use of histochemical stains for organisms is required.* ***(Right)*** *Wegener granulomatosis shows areas of organizing pneumonia with the presence of "Masson bodies" →. In addition, note the presence of numerous multinucleated giant cells →.*

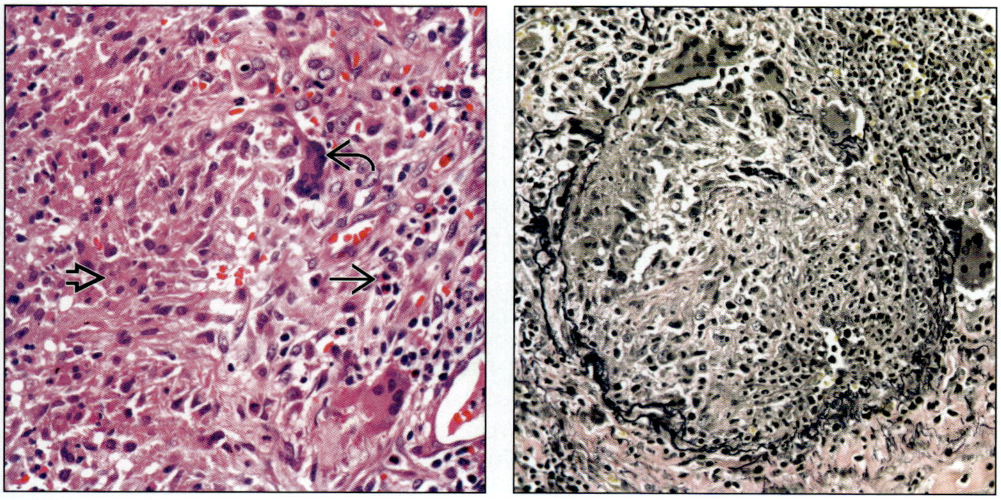

(Left) *High-power view of the inflammatory infiltrate in Wegener granulomatosis shows multinucleated giant cells →, histiocytes →, and eosinophils →.* ***(Right)*** *High-power view (elastic van Gieson stain) shows a vessel with destruction of the vascular wall and prominent inflammatory changes (vasculitis). This is an important diagnostic feature of Wegener granulomatosis.*

SARCOIDOSIS

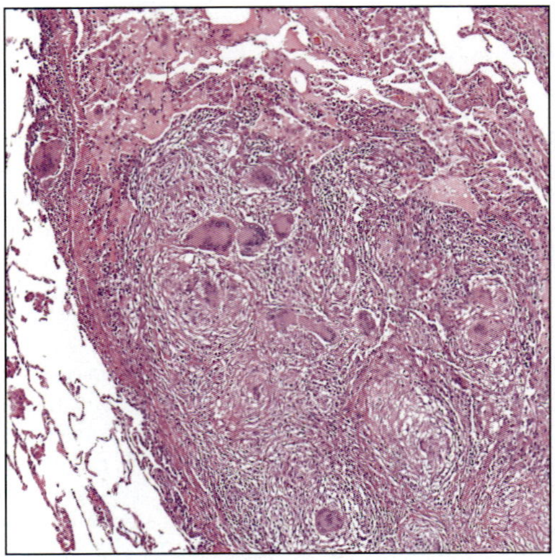

Pulmonary sarcoidosis shows well-circumscribed collections of histiocytes without evidence of necrosis and abundant multinucleated giant cells.

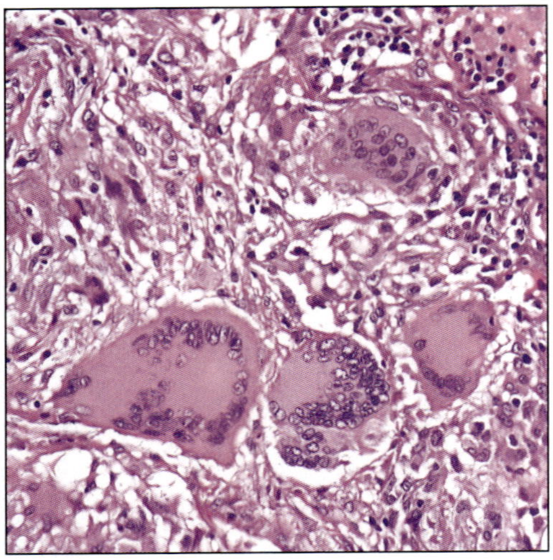

Higher magnification from sarcoid granuloma of the lung shows numerous histiocytes and large, multinucleated giant cells.

TERMINOLOGY

Definitions

- Multiorgan disease characterized by nonnecrotizing epithelioid granulomas

ETIOLOGY/PATHOGENESIS

Environmental Exposure

- Etiology is unknown, but evidence suggests it may represent exaggerated cellular immune response to an unidentified antigen

Genetic Predisposition

- Marked familial clustering of cases

CLINICAL ISSUES

Epidemiology

- Incidence
  - About 10 per 100,000 people per year
- Age
  - Young adults (from 20-40 years of age)
- Gender
  - Slight female predominance
- Ethnicity
  - Increased incidence in African Americans

Site

- Most commonly affected sites include lungs (95% of patients) and lymphatic organs
- Other organs involved include liver, spleen, skin, heart, and eyes; central nervous system (CNS) may also be involved

Presentation

- Fatigue
- Anorexia
- Weight loss
- Fever
- Triad of erythema nodosum, bilateral hilar lymphadenopathy, and polyarthralgia (Löfgren syndrome) seen in 20-50% of patients

Laboratory Tests

- Hyperglobulinemia due to nonspecific polyclonal activation of B cells by helper T cells
- Elevation of serum levels of angiotensin-converting enzyme

Natural History

- May be asymptomatic and discovered incidentally on chest x-rays
- Symptomatic patients may present with insidious chronic disease or an acute presentation
- Spontaneous resolution is commonly the rule
- Progressive and disabling organ failure may occur in up to 10% of patients

Treatment

- Drugs
  - Corticosteroids (prednisone)
  - Immunosuppressive or cytotoxic drugs

Prognosis

- Most cases involute spontaneously
- Mortality may occur in a small percentage of patients (1-5%) due to progressive lung, heart, or CNS involvement

IMAGE FINDINGS

Radiographic Findings

- Symmetric bilateral hilar and mediastinal lymph node enlargement, ± associated interstitial lung abnormalities
- Symmetrical, bilateral reticulonodular or nodular opacifications mainly involving middle and upper lung zones

SARCOIDOSIS

Key Facts

Etiology/Pathogenesis
- Etiology unknown, but evidence suggests it may represent exaggerated cellular immune response to an unidentified antigen

Clinical Issues
- Most commonly affected sites include lungs (95% of patients) and lymphatic organs
- May be asymptomatic and discovered incidentally on chest x-rays
- Symptomatic patients may present with insidious chronic disease or an acute presentation

Microscopic Pathology
- Multiple small, nonnecrotizing interstitial epithelioid granulomas distributed along bronchovascular bundles and interlobular septa
- Nodular sarcoidosis shows confluence of granulomas with large tumor nodule formation
- Granulomas are frequently distributed along bronchial submucosa, accounting for high yield in bronchoscopic biopsies
- Interstitial inflammation is absent or inconspicuous
- Vasculitis and foci of necrosis may sometimes accompany the granulomas
- Granulomas are composed of aggregates of epithelioid histiocytes ± multinucleated giant cells

Diagnostic Checklist
- Sarcoidosis is a diagnosis of exclusion made by clinician rather than pathologist
- Special stains for organisms (AFB, PAS, GMS) should always be done to rule out infection

CT Findings
- HRCT shows small nodules 2-5 mm in diameter with irregular margins and perilymphatic distribution
- Nodules are distributed along the bronchi and pulmonary vessels and along the interlobar fissures and interlobular septa

MACROSCOPIC FEATURES

General Features
- Cut surface shows multiple minute white nodules distributed along bronchovascular bundles
- Confluence of lesions can lead to formation of large nodules measuring several centimeters in diameter ("nodular sarcoidosis")

MICROSCOPIC PATHOLOGY

Histologic Features
- Multiple small, nonnecrotizing interstitial epithelioid granulomas distributed along bronchovascular bundles and interlobular septa
- Nodular sarcoidosis shows confluence of granulomas with large tumor nodule formation
- Granulomas are frequently distributed along bronchial submucosa, accounting for high yield in bronchoscopic biopsies
- Interstitial inflammation is absent or inconspicuous
- Vasculitis and foci of necrosis may sometimes accompany the granulomas
- Interstitial fibrosis may develop in a small percentage of advanced cases that may lead to end-stage honeycomb lung

Cytologic Features
- Granulomas are composed of aggregates of epithelioid histiocytes ± multinucleated giant cells
- Concentric fibrosis may surround the outer layer of the epithelioid granulomas in advanced cases
- Granulomas may contain asteroid bodies (star-shaped crystals)
- Schaumann bodies (small lamellar calcifications) are seen in up to 70% of patients
- Rounded, birefringent basophilic calcifications can also be encountered in fibrotic granulomas

DIFFERENTIAL DIAGNOSIS

Fungal Infections
- Majority of deep fungal infections are characterized by necrotizing granulomas
- Clinical history and fungal stain (GMS, PAS) will help identify the specific organisms

Mycobacterial Infections
- Tuberculosis usually shows caseating granulomas and organisms on acid-fast stains (AFB, Ziehl-Neelsen)
- *Mycobacterium avium intracellulare* (MAI) may have punctate areas of necrosis and stain positive for modified Fite-Farraco stains

Berylliosis
- History of exposure to beryllium

DIAGNOSTIC CHECKLIST

Pathologic Interpretation Pearls
- Sarcoidosis is a diagnosis of exclusion made by clinician rather than pathologist
- Battery of special stains for organisms (AFB, PAS, GMS) should always be done in cases suspected of sarcoidosis to rule out infection

SELECTED REFERENCES

1. Iannuzzi MC et al: Sarcoidosis: clinical presentation, immunopathogenesis, and therapeutics. JAMA. 305(4):391-9, 2011
2. Morgenthau AS et al: Recent advances in sarcoidosis. Chest. 139(1):174-82, 2011
3. Hsu RM et al: Histologic, microbiologic, and clinical correlates of the diagnosis of sarcoidosis by transbronchial biopsy. Arch Pathol Lab Med. 120(4):364-8, 1996

SARCOIDOSIS

Histologic Features

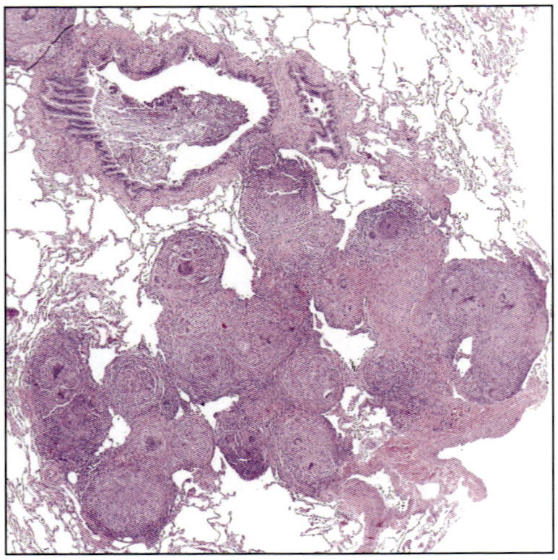
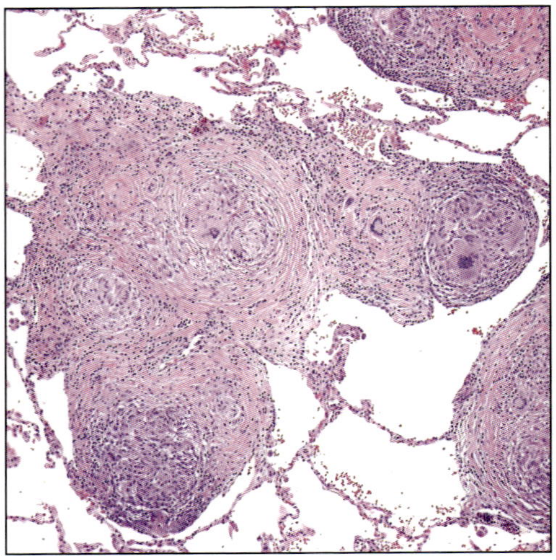

(Left) *Pulmonary sarcoidosis shows multiple small, nonnecrotizing interstitial epithelioid granulomas distributed along bronchovascular bundles. Notice some of the granulomas are in close proximity to the bronchial submucosa, which accounts for the high diagnostic yield on bronchoscopic biopsies.* ***(Right)*** *Higher magnification of interstitial granulomas in a patient with sarcoidosis shows focal accumulations of epithelioid histiocytes admixed with scattered multinucleated giant cells.*

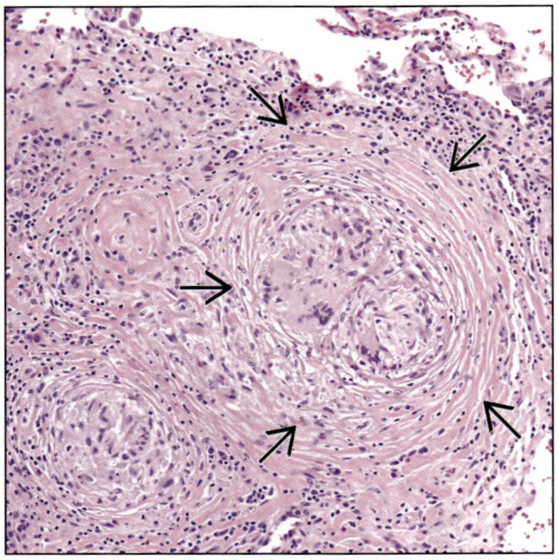
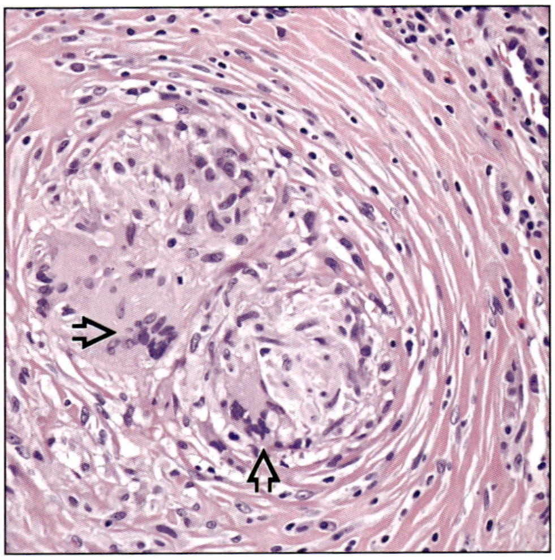

(Left) *Higher magnification of epithelioid granulomas in pulmonary sarcoidosis shows a concentric rim of fibrosis surrounding one of the granulomas →. Notice the sparse inflammatory cells scattered in the interstitium outside of the granulomas.* ***(Right)*** *Higher magnification of a sclerotic granuloma in pulmonary sarcoidosis shows concentric layers of collagenous tissue circumscribing clusters of epithelioid histiocytes with a few multinucleated giant cells ⇨.*

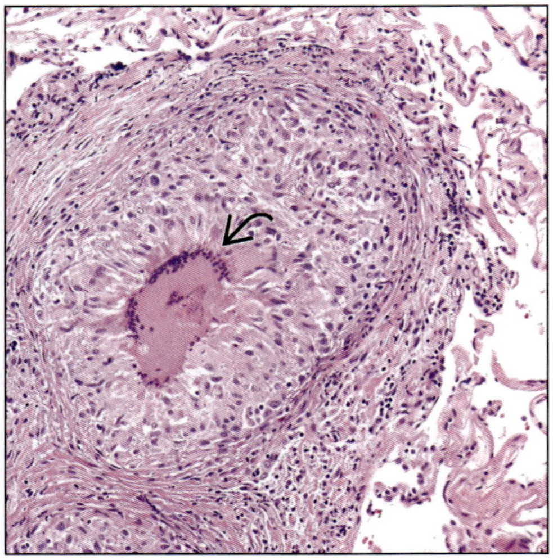
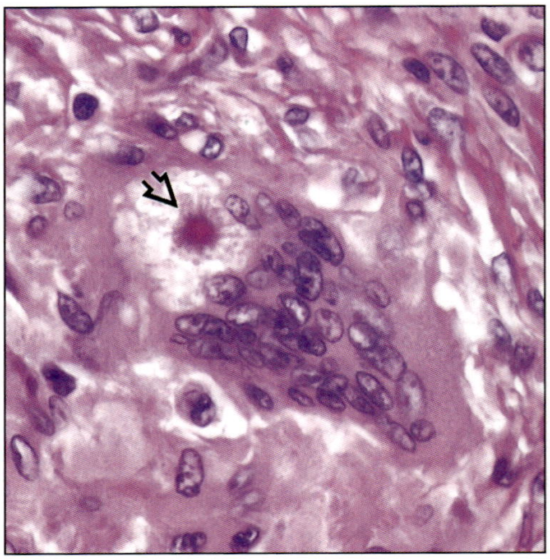

(Left) *Higher magnification of an epithelioid granuloma in pulmonary sarcoidosis shows a concentric arrangement of epithelioid histiocytes around a large multinucleated giant cell with abundant eosinophilic cytoplasm ↷.* ***(Right)*** *Sarcoid granuloma of the lung shows a multinucleated giant cell containing a star-shaped asteroid body ⇨. The asteroid bodies are made up of crystals located within the cytoplasm of the giant cells. These structures are very distinctive but nonspecific.*

SARCOIDOSIS

Histologic Features

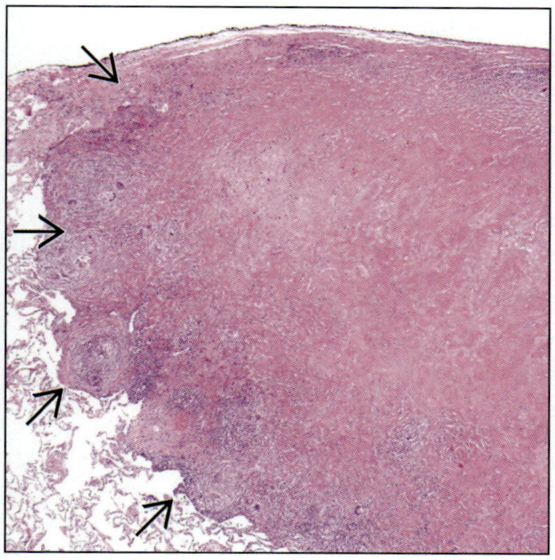

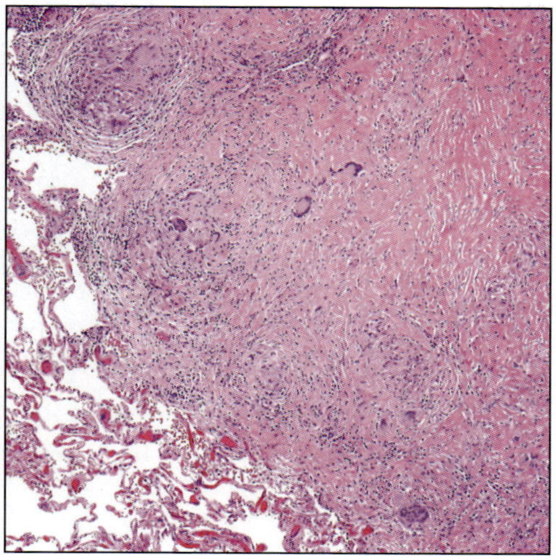

(Left) *Confluence of granulomas in pulmonary sarcoidosis may lead to the formation of a large nodular mass* → *that can be confused radiologically for malignancy. Such cases have been termed nodular sarcoidosis.* ***(Right)*** *Nodular sarcoidosis usually displays extensive stromal hyalinization with only a few scattered multinucleated giant cells remaining, admixed with collagenous matrix. The granulomas in such instances may be small and very subtle.*

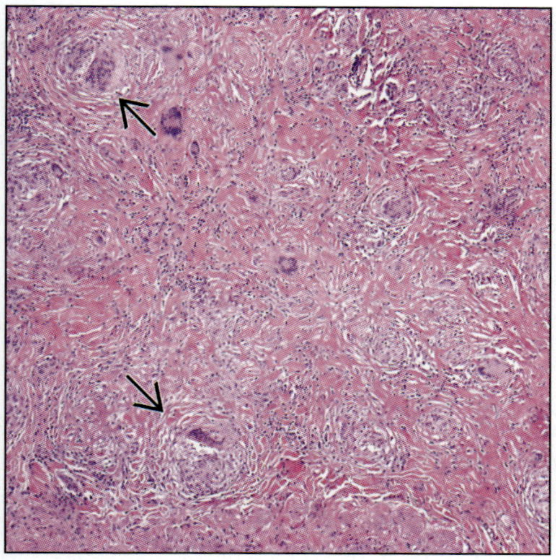

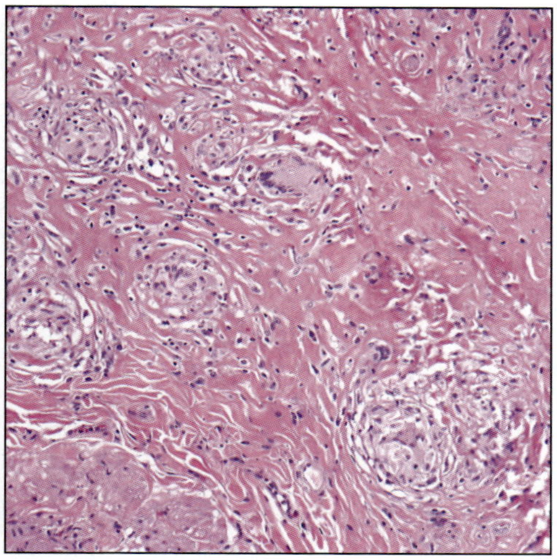

(Left) *Higher magnification of nodular sarcoidosis of the lung shows extensive sclerosis and hyalinization of the stroma with scattered multinucleated giant cells. Discrete, small epithelioid granuloma formation is also noted* →. ***(Right)*** *Higher magnification of the sclerotic area within a nodular sarcoidosis of the lung shows massive stromal sclerosis due to the deposition of acellular collagen. The small scattered epithelioid granulomas are better appreciated at this magnification.*

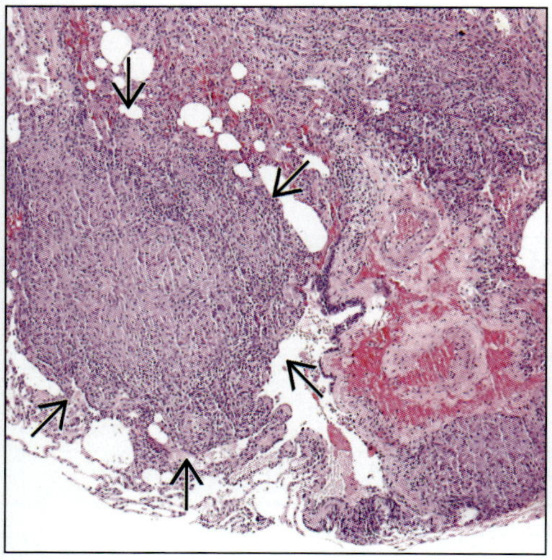

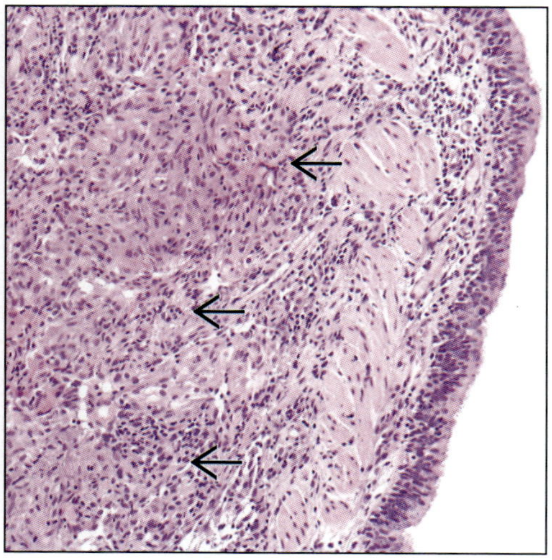

(Left) *Endoscopic biopsy in a patient with scattered interstitial infiltrates on a CT scan suspicious for interstitial fibrosis shows a sarcoid granuloma* → *adjacent to the wall of the bronchus. The peribronchial location makes it very easy to identify the granulomas on endoscopic biopsies.* ***(Right)*** *Sometimes the granulomas are not well-formed, and endoscopic biopsies may yield only ill-defined clusters of epithelioid histiocytes* → *without multinucleated giant cells.*

HARD METAL PNEUMOCONIOSIS PNEUMONITIS

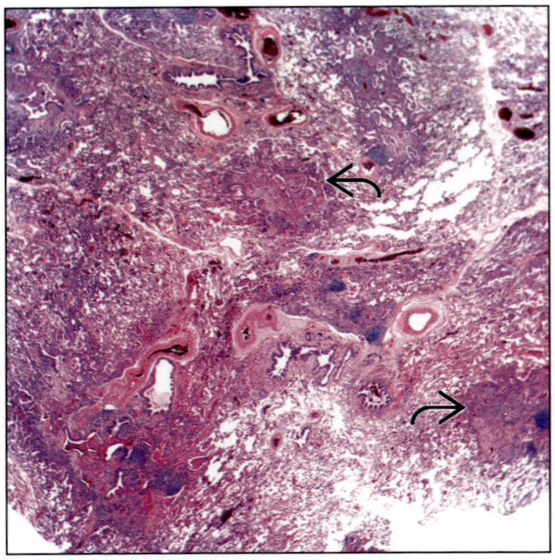

Low-power view of hard metal pneumonitis shows a patchy and subtle nodular growth pattern. There are at least 2 nodule-like ⮫ areas within the lung parenchyma.

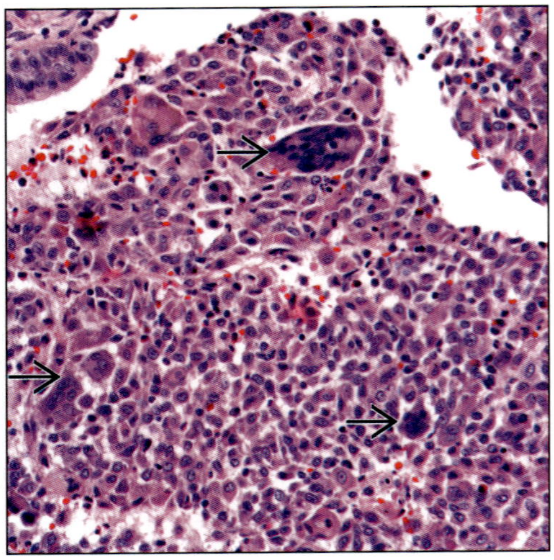

High-power view of hard metal pneumonitis shows a collection of intraalveolar macrophages admixed with multinucleated giant cells →.

TERMINOLOGY

Synonyms

- Hard metal lung disease, cobalt lung disease

Definitions

- Type of pneumonitis caused by exposure to hard metal (cobalt and others)

ETIOLOGY/PATHOGENESIS

Environmental Exposure

- Exposure to hard metal
  - Hard metal is combination of tungsten with cobalt

Pathogenesis

- Possibly immunologically mediated disease

CLINICAL ISSUES

Epidemiology

- Incidence
  - No hard data documenting true incidence of hard metal lung disease
- Age
  - Adults are more commonly affected
- Gender
  - No apparent gender predilection
- Ethnicity
  - No apparent ethnic predilection

Site

- Lung without predilection for any side or segment

Presentation

- Cough
- Dyspnea
- Chest pain
- Wheezing
- Rhinitis
- Conjunctivitis
- Dermatitis
- Asthma
- Malaise

Laboratory Tests

- Radiographic features are nonspecific
- Increased cobalt in urine
- Increased cobalt in blood
- IgE antibodies to cobalt may be present in serum

Treatment

- Drugs
  - Corticosteroids
  - In cases not responding to corticosteroids
    - Cyclophosphamide
    - Azathioprine
    - Lung transplantation
  - Most important aspect is to avoid contact with cobalt

Prognosis

- If patients are kept away form further exposure to cobalt and treated with corticosteroids, their prognosis may be good
- Fatal cases have been reported

MACROSCOPIC FEATURES

General Features

- Diagnosis of this process is performed with open lung biopsy

MICROSCOPIC PATHOLOGY

Histologic Features

- Subtle nodular or patchy appearance
- Intraalveolar macrophages

Key Facts

Terminology
- Type of pneumonitis caused by exposure to hard metal (cobalt)

Etiology/Pathogenesis
- Exposure to hard metal
- Hard metal is combination of tungsten with cobalt

Clinical Issues
- Symptoms
  - Cough
  - Dyspnea
  - Rhinitis
  - Dermatitis
  - Asthma
- Laboratory findings
  - Increased cobalt in urine
  - Increased cobalt in blood
- Treatment
  - Corticosteroids

Top Differential Diagnoses
- Usual interstitial pneumonitis
- Desquamative interstitial pneumonitis
- Infectious pneumonia
- Langerhans cell histiocytosis

Diagnostic Checklist
- Presence of giant cells
- Patchy and subtle nodular appearance
- Inflammatory reaction
- Lymphoid aggregates
- History of exposure to hard metal

- Easily identifiable multinucleated giant cells
- Lymphoid aggregates
- Discrete interstitial fibrosis may be present

DIFFERENTIAL DIAGNOSIS

Usual Interstitial Pneumonitis
- Shows presence of extensive areas of interstitial fibrosis alternating with areas of relatively normal alveolated lung parenchyma
- Does not show multinucleated giant cells

Desquamative Interstitial Pneumonitis
- Generally displays collections of intraalveolar macrophages
- Shows only mild and subtle interstitial fibrosis
- Does not show multinucleated giant cells

Infectious Pneumonia
- Use of special histochemical stains (GMS, PAS, and AFB) and tissue cultures are important to rule out infectious origin
- History of exposure to hard metal will be relevant to point to right interpretation

Langerhans Cell Histiocytosis (LCH)
- Shows nodular and cystic growth pattern
- Shows giant cells but also displays other inflammatory component in which eosinophils may be prominent
- Immunohistochemical stain for CD1a is helpful in diagnosis of LCH
- History of hard metal exposure will be unusual for LCH

DIAGNOSTIC CHECKLIST

Clinically Relevant Pathologic Features
- Symptom complex

Pathologic Interpretation Pearls
- Presence of giant cells
- Patchy and subtle nodular appearance
- Inflammatory reaction
- Lymphoid aggregates
- History of exposure to hard metal

SELECTED REFERENCES

1. Enriquez LS et al: Hard metal pneumoconiosis: a case of giant-cell interstitial pneumonitis in a machinist. Respir Care. 52(2):196-9, 2007
2. Kinoshita M et al: Giant cell interstitial pneumonia in two hard metal workers: the role of bronchoalveolar lavage in diagnosis. Respirology. 4(3):263-6, 1999
3. Schwarz Y et al: Evaluation of workers exposed to dust containing hard metals and aluminum oxide. Am J Ind Med. 34(2):177-82, 1998
4. Figueroa S et al: Hard metal interstitial pulmonary disease associated with a form of welding in a metal parts coating plant. Am J Ind Med. 21(3):363-73, 1992
5. Sahle W: Possible role of tungsten oxide whiskers in hard-metal pneumoconiosis. Chest. 102(4):1310, 1992
6. Cugell DW et al: The respiratory effects of cobalt. Arch Intern Med. 150(1):177-83, 1990
7. Knape H: [Hard metal-induced lung changes. Hard metal asthma--interstitial hard metal pneumopathy.] Pneumologie. 44(7):862-5, 1990
8. Ohori NP et al: Giant-cell interstitial pneumonia and hard-metal pneumoconiosis. A clinicopathologic study of four cases and review of the literature. Am J Surg Pathol. 13(7):581-7, 1989

HARD METAL PNEUMOCONIOSIS PNEUMONITIS

Microscopic Features

*(**Left**) Low-power view shows a small nodule , which at this power may suggest the possibility of organizing pneumonia. The remaining lung parenchyma appears within normal limits. (**Right**) Hard metal pneumonitis shows areas of organization admixed with areas that show lymphoid aggregates . These features by themselves are not specific and may be seen in other types of pneumonitis.*

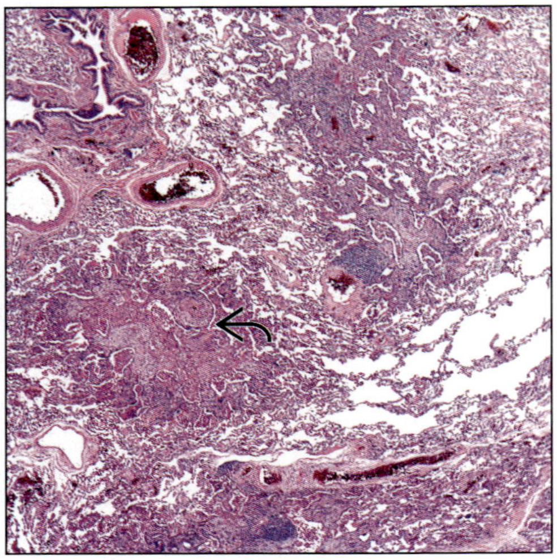

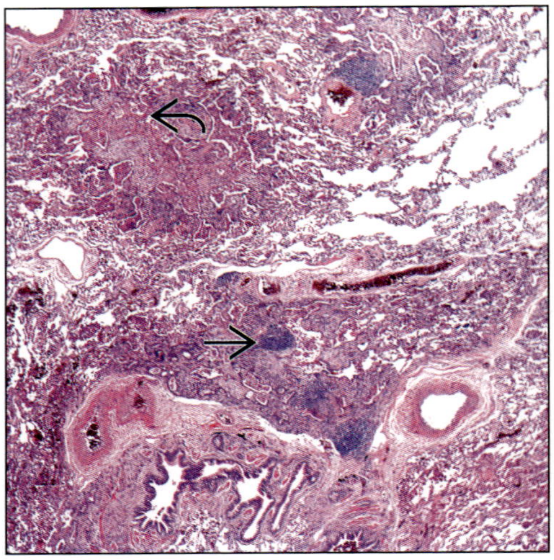

*(**Left**) Areas of discrete interstitial fibrosis are present. Also note the scattered multinucleated giant cells as well as a small lymphoid aggregate . (**Right**) Hard metal pneumonitis shows collections of intraalveolar macrophages, inflammatory changes, and a lymphoid aggregate. Note that in the collections of macrophages, it is possible to identify giant cells .*

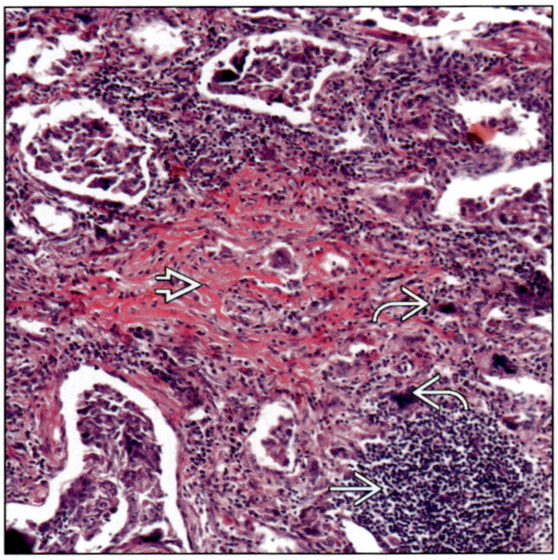

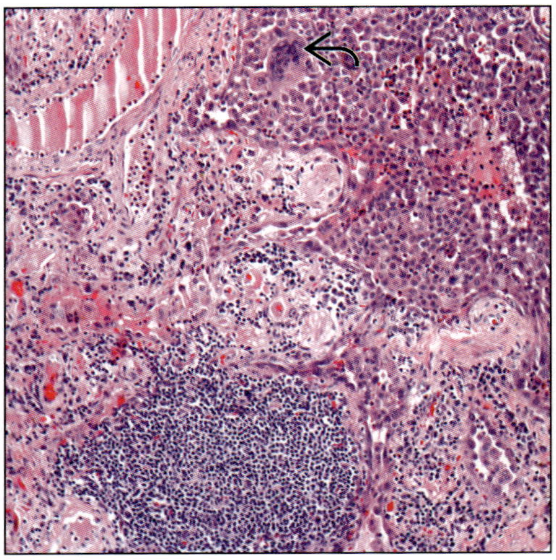

*(**Left**) Areas with more discrete fibrosis and collections of intraalveolar macrophages can be identified. The presence of scattered giant cells may also be seen. (**Right**) High-power view of an airway shows peribronchial fibrosis and intraluminal presence of macrophages and giant cells. Surrounding areas appear to show inflammatory changes.*

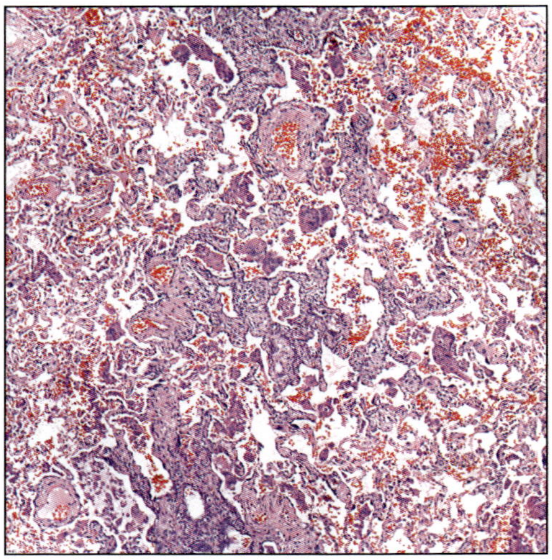

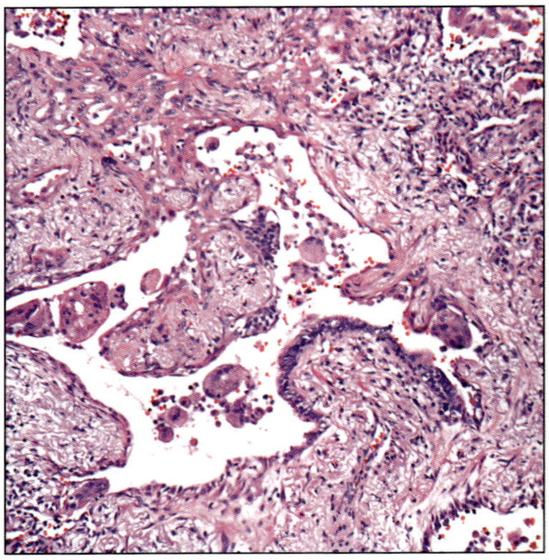

Microscopic Features

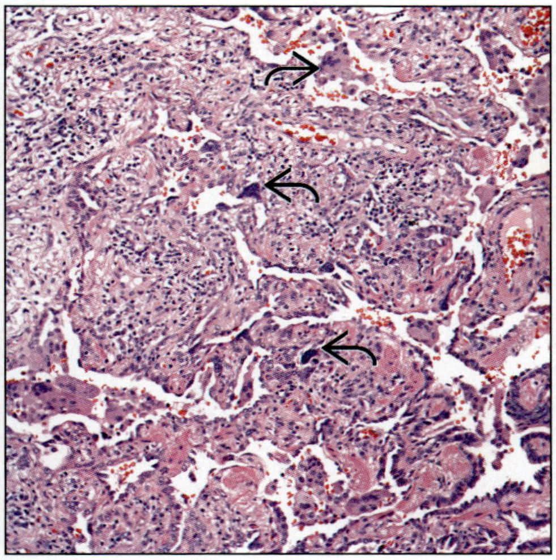

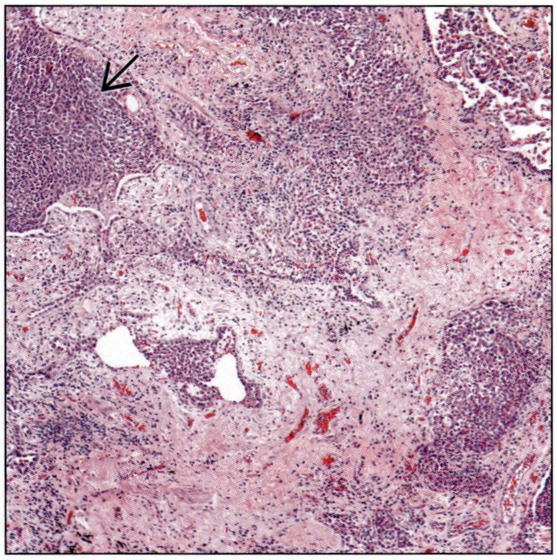

(Left) *Hard metal pneumonitis shows lung parenchyma with marked inflammatory changes and hyperplastic changes of the bronchial and alveolar lining, as well as accumulation of macrophages and giant cells →.* ***(Right)*** *Areas of prominent scarring can be seen in hard metal pneumonitis. Note the adjacent accumulation of macrophages →.*

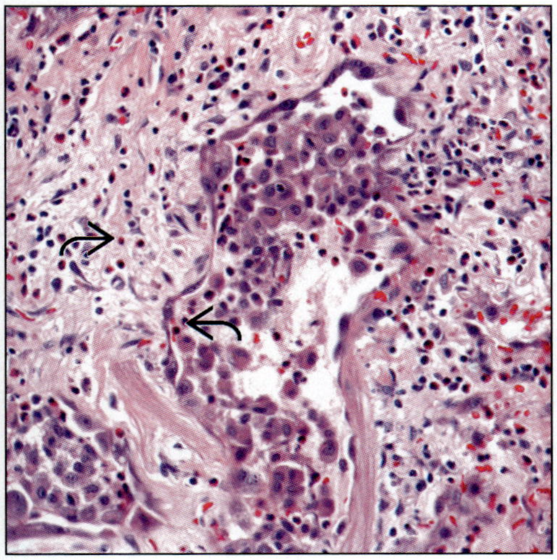

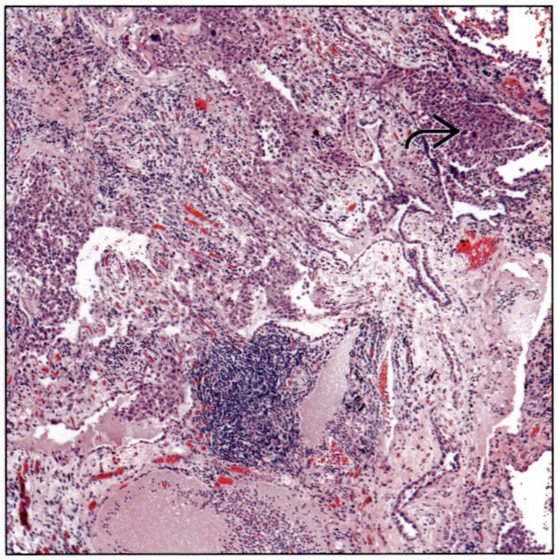

(Left) *Collections of macrophages and eosinophils may also be seen in vascular spaces. Note the presence of eosinophils not only inside the vessels but also in adjacent tissue →.* ***(Right)*** *Hard metal pneumonitis shows a combination of collections of macrophages admixed with giant cells →, inflammatory changes, and lymphoid aggregates.*

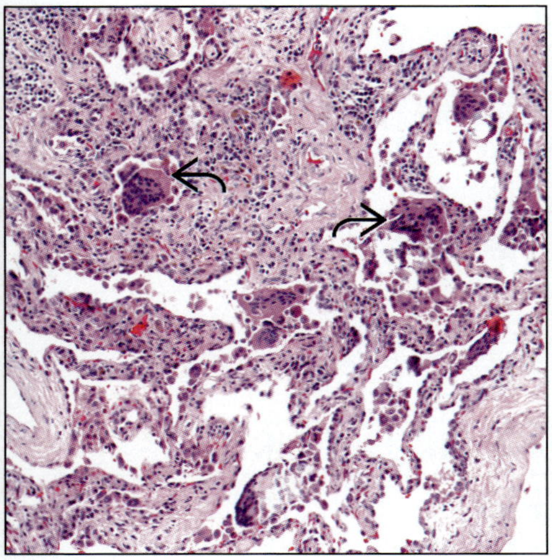

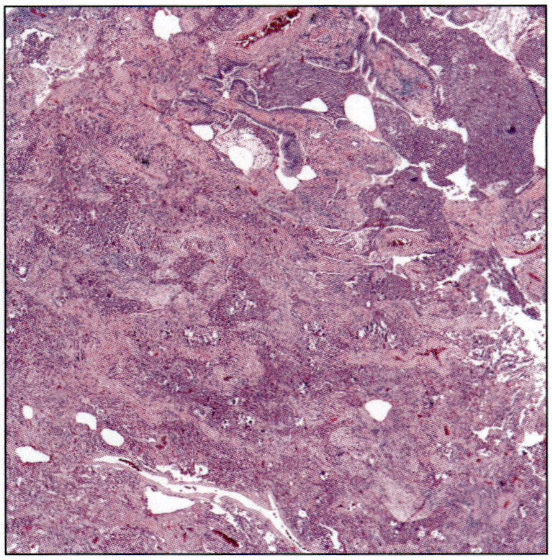

(Left) *This higher magnification shows the collections of macrophages and the obvious presence of multinucleated giant cells →. This is one of the most important histopathological features of hard metal pneumonitis.* ***(Right)*** *Low-power view of hard metal pneumonitis shows discrete interstitial fibrosis and collections of macrophages. These features may be seen in other types of pneumonitis.*

ASBESTOS-RELATED INTERSTITIAL FIBROSIS

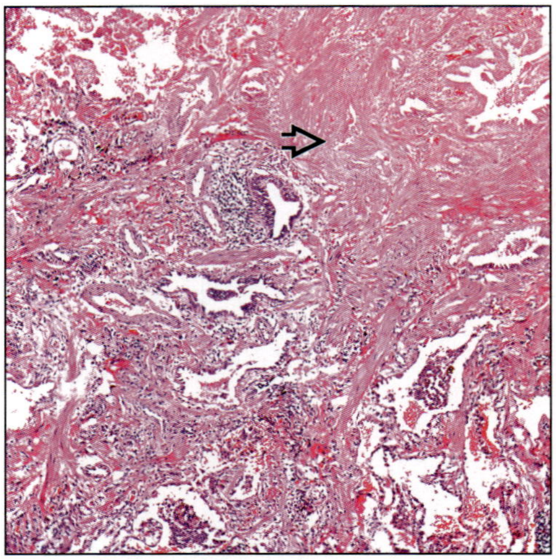

Low-power magnification of lung shows extensive areas of interstitial fibrosis. The normal lung architecture has been replaced by fibrocollagenous tissue.

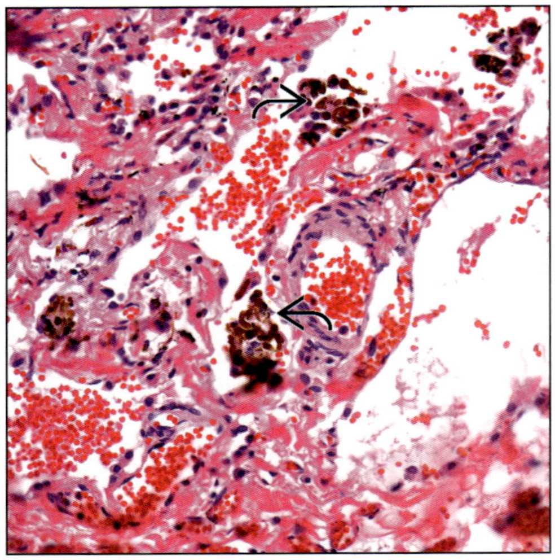

Closer magnification of lung tissue shows numerous asbestos bodies floating in airspaces. There is discrete interstitial fibrosis and minimal inflammatory reaction.

TERMINOLOGY

Synonyms

- Asbestosis

Definitions

- Interstitial pulmonary fibrosis secondary to inhalation of asbestos dust

ETIOLOGY/PATHOGENESIS

Environmental Exposure

- Combination of hydrated silicates
  - Silica
  - Iron
  - Magnesium
- 2 types of asbestos fibers have been identified
  - Serpentine
    - Chrysotile (more common in industry)
    - Somewhat soluble in lung fluids
  - Amphibole
    - Amosite
    - Crocidolite

CLINICAL ISSUES

Epidemiology

- Age
  - Usually occurs in adults
- Gender
  - More common in males
  - Females may also be affected
- Ethnicity
  - No ethnic predilection

Site

- Lung
- Pleura

Presentation

- Shortness of breath
- Cough
- Dyspnea
- Clubbing of fingers
- Pleural effusion

Laboratory Tests

- Pulmonary function test
  - Restrictive disease

Natural History

- Latent period
  - Varies from 15-20 years
  - Disease may occur earlier depending on exposure
- Occupational exposure
  - Direct
  - Indirect

Treatment

- No specific treatment for asbestosis
- Stop exposure

Prognosis

- Pulmonary fibrosis may progress
  - May be fatal in patients with severe pulmonary fibrosis

IMAGE FINDINGS

Radiographic Findings

- Bilateral interstitial opacities

MACROSCOPIC FEATURES

General Features

- Extensive areas of scarring
- Spongy appearance

ASBESTOS-RELATED INTERSTITIAL FIBROSIS

Key Facts

Terminology
- Asbestosis
  - Interstitial pulmonary fibrosis secondary to inhalation of asbestos dust

Etiology/Pathogenesis
- 2 types of asbestos fibers have been identified
- Serpentine
  - Chrysotile (more common in industry)
  - Somewhat soluble in lung fluids
- Amphibole
  - Amosite
  - Crocidolite

Clinical Issues
- Latent period
  - Varies from 15-20 years
  - Disease may occur earlier depending on exposure
- Occupational exposure
  - Direct
  - Indirect
- Symptoms
  - Shortness of breath
  - Cough
  - Dyspnea
  - Clubbing of finger
  - Pleural effusion
- Laboratory tests
  - Pulmonary functions tests
  - Restrictive disease

MICROSCOPIC PATHOLOGY

Histologic Features
- Interstitial fibrosis
  - Nonuniform interstitial fibrosis
  - Honeycombing of lung parenchyma
  - Residual areas of uninvolved lung parenchyma
  - Intraalveolar collection of pigmented macrophages
- Peribronchiolar fibrosis
- Round atelectasis
- Identification of asbestos bodies or fibers in lung parenchyma

ANCILLARY TESTS

Identification of Asbestos Bodies
- X-ray diffraction analysis should show asbestos bodies
- Mass spectrometry may also identify asbestos bodies
- Histochemical stains for iron in tissue sections will disclose asbestos bodies

DIFFERENTIAL DIAGNOSIS

Usual Interstitial Pneumonitis
- Both conditions may share similar histological features
- Does not show asbestos bodies
- Negative staining for asbestos bodies using iron stains

Desquamative Interstitial Pneumonitis (DIP)
- Shows a more homogeneous pattern of intraalveolar macrophages and fibrosis
- Shows more subtle interstitial fibrosis
- Negative results for asbestos bodies using iron stains

DIAGNOSTIC CHECKLIST

Clinically Relevant Pathologic Features
- Age distribution
- Gross appearance

Pathologic Interpretation Pearls
- UIP type of interstitial fibrosis
- Identification of asbestos bodies in tissue
  - Histochemical stains for iron
  - X-ray diffraction analysis
  - Mass spectrometry

SELECTED REFERENCES

1. Antonescu-Turcu AL et al: Parenchymal and airway diseases caused by asbestos. Curr Opin Pulm Med. 16(2):155-61, 2010
2. Brody AR: Asbestos and lung disease. Am J Respir Cell Mol Biol. 42(2):131-2, 2010
3. Roggli VL et al: Pathology of asbestosis- An update of the diagnostic criteria: Report of the asbestosis committee of the college of american pathologists and pulmonary pathology society. Arch Pathol Lab Med. 134(3):462-80, 2010
4. Schneider F et al: Asbestos fiber content of lungs with diffuse interstitial fibrosis: An analytical scanning electron microscopic analysis of 249 cases. Arch Pathol Lab Med. 134(3):457-61, 2010
5. Harding AH et al: Mortality among British asbestos workers undergoing regular medical examinations (1971-2005). Occup Environ Med. 66(7):487-95, 2009
6. Kamp DW: Asbestos-induced lung diseases: an update. Transl Res. 153(4):143-52, 2009
7. Mizell KN et al: Antemortem diagnosis of asbestosis by screening chest radiograph correlated with postmortem histologic features of asbestosis: a study of 273 cases. J Occup Med Toxicol. 4:14, 2009
8. Wick MR et al: Asbestosis: demonstration of distinctive interstitial fibroelastosis: a pilot study. Ann Diagn Pathol. 13(5):297-302, 2009

ASBESTOS-RELATED INTERSTITIAL FIBROSIS

Microscopic Features

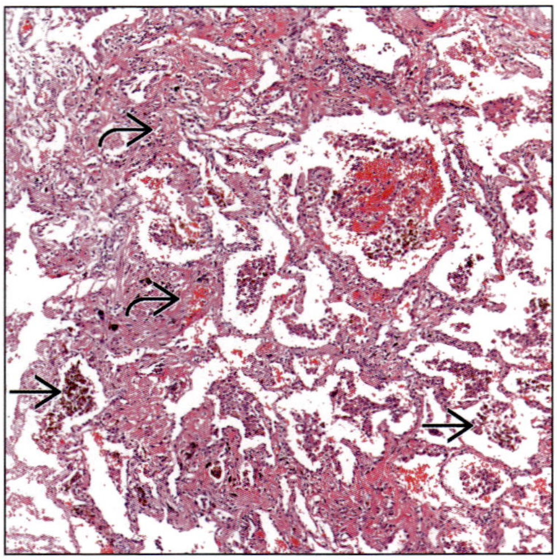

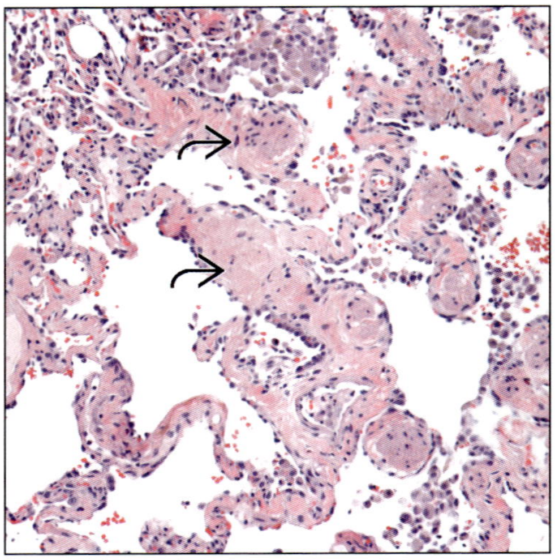

(Left) *Low-power magnification of lung shows the presence of marked interstitial fibrosis with collections of pigmented macrophages within some alveolar spaces.* ***(Right)*** *Interstitial pulmonary fibrosis can be prominent, mimicking the histological features of usual interstitial pneumonitis. However, the identification of asbestos bodies is essential for the diagnosis.*

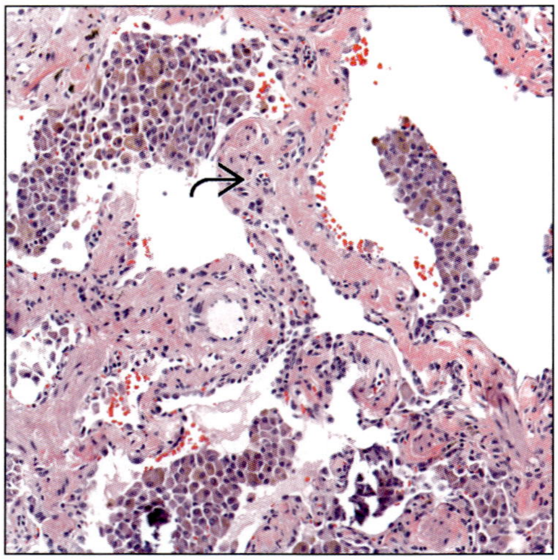

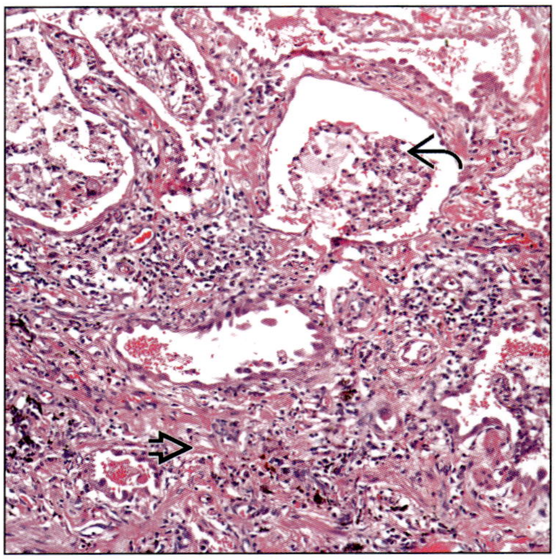

(Left) *This lung biopsy specimen shows extensive areas of fibrosis with collections of pigmented macrophages within airspaces. These changes are similar to those seen in usual interstitial pneumonitis.* ***(Right)*** *Extensive areas of fibrosis replace lung parenchyma with only focal areas of residual airspaces containing collections of macrophages.*

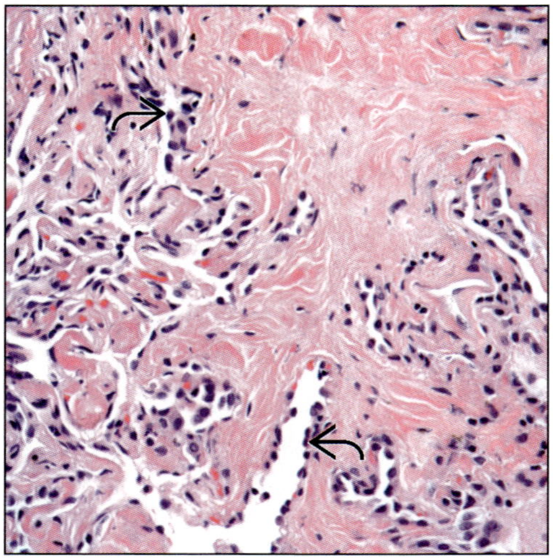

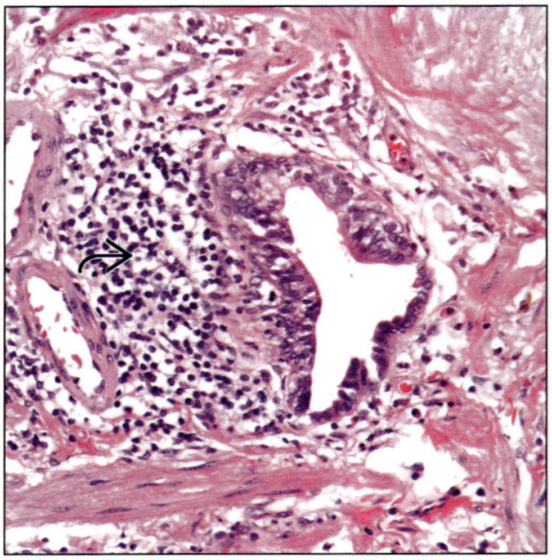

(Left) *Closer view shows marked interstitial fibrosis with entrapment of residual alveolar lining. These features are indistinguishable from other interstitial fibrotic lung diseases.* ***(Right)*** *Residual airway shows peribronchiolar inflammation composed mainly of lymphocytes. This feature is commonly seen in cases of asbestosis.*

Microscopic Features

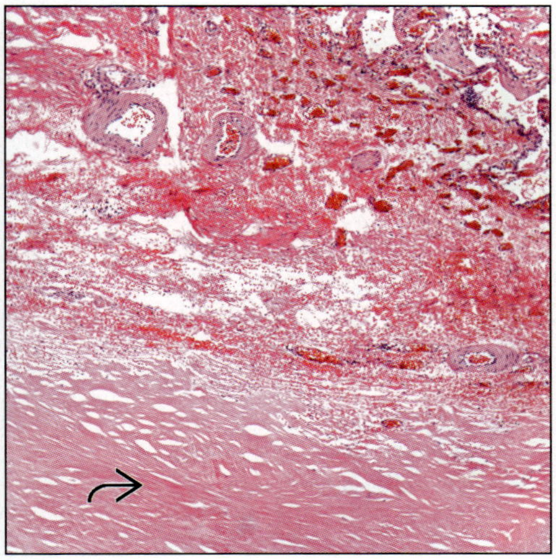

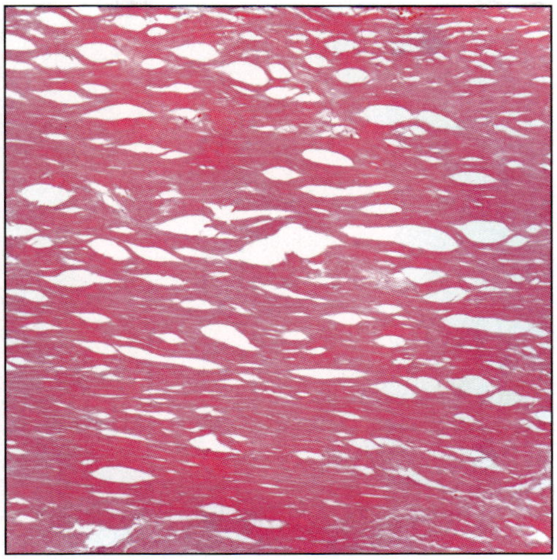

(Left) *Asbestosis in the lung is not limited to lung parenchyma, as the process may also involve pleura. Note the presence of a pleural plaque, which is composed essentially of dense hyaline matrix.* ***(Right)*** *Closer view of a pleural plaque shows dense hyalinization with minimal cellular reaction. This is a common finding in cases of asbestos exposure.*

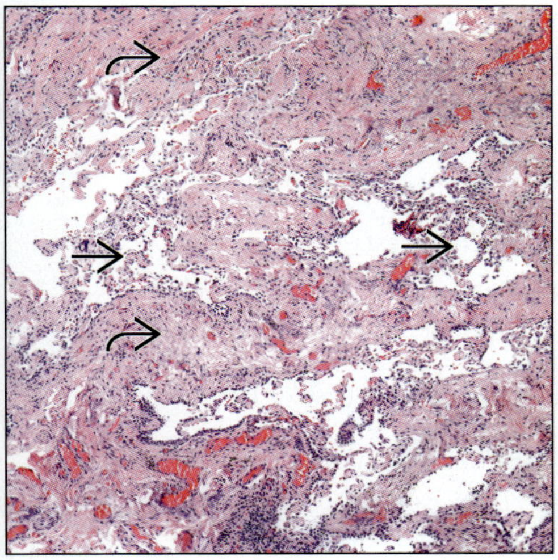

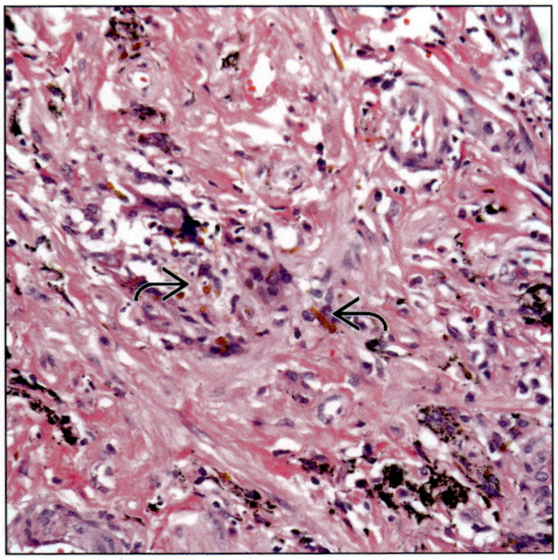

(Left) *In some cases of pulmonary asbestosis, the lung parenchyma is replaced with fibroconnective tissue, leaving only focal areas of of uninvolved lung parenchyma.* ***(Right)*** *Extensive areas of fibrosis with anthracotic pigment and numerous asbestos bodies are shown. Asbestos bodies are generally found in areas containing viable lung parenchyma.*

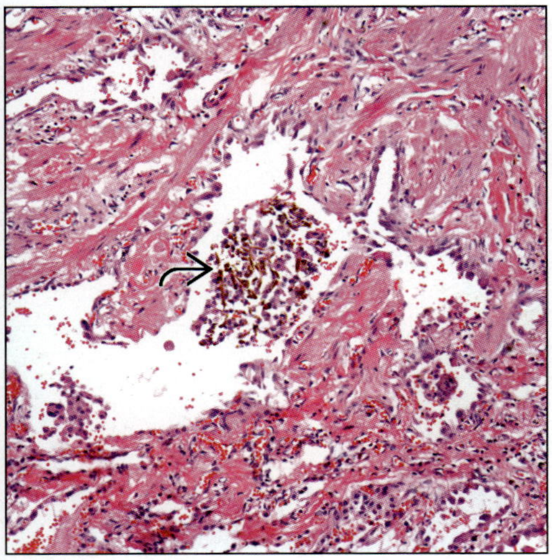

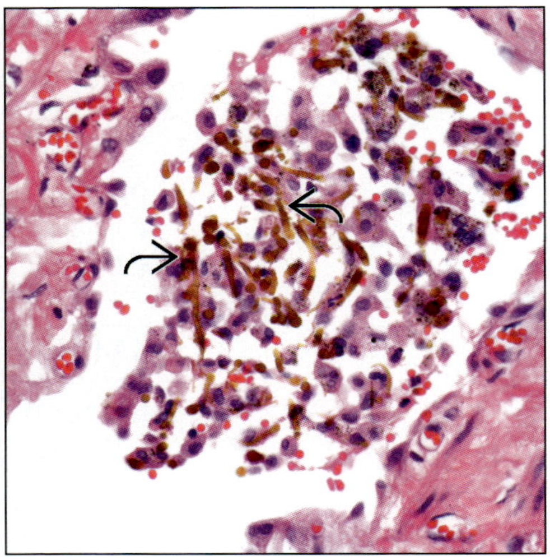

(Left) *Numerous asbestos bodies are floating within airspaces. The finding of asbestos bodies is essential for the diagnosis of asbestosis.* ***(Right)*** *Closer magnification demonstrates numerous asbestos bodies admixed with macrophages. This is the most important finding in cases of asbestosis.*

IDIOPATHIC PULMONARY HEMOSIDEROSIS

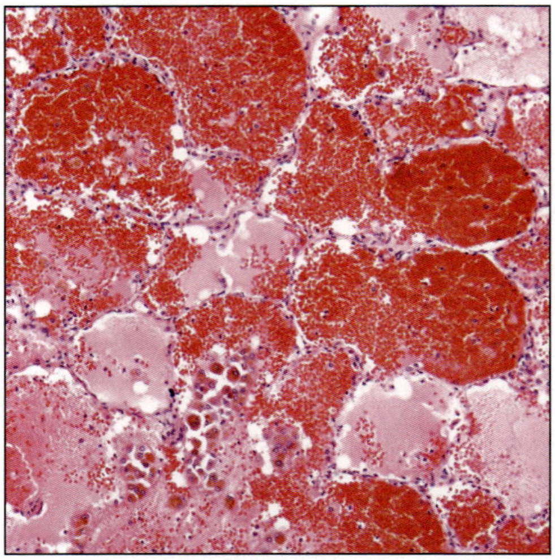

Histologic appearance of the lung in idiopathic pulmonary hemosiderosis shows massive fresh intraalveolar hemorrhage.

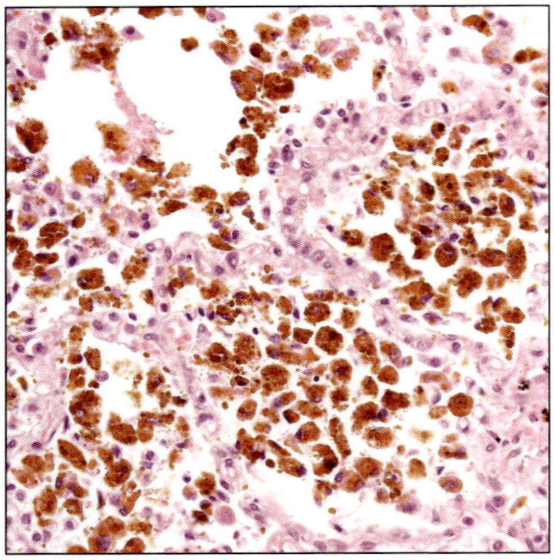

Idiopathic pulmonary hemosiderosis shows abundance of intraluminal hemosiderin-laden macrophages in alveolar lumens.

TERMINOLOGY

Abbreviations

- Idiopathic pulmonary hemosiderosis (IPH)

Synonyms

- Idiopathic pulmonary hemorrhage

Definitions

- Intrapulmonary hemorrhage of unknown etiology that is unassociated with other systemic manifestations

ETIOLOGY/PATHOGENESIS

Etiology

- Unknown
- No immunologic mechanism has been identified
- Familial clustering has been reported, supporting genetic susceptibility

CLINICAL ISSUES

Epidemiology

- Age
  - Affects children more commonly than adults
  - About 20% of patients are adults, usually < 30 years old
- Gender
  - Male predominance (M:F = 2:1) in adults
  - Equal gender distribution in children

Site

- Localized to lungs; no systemic involvement

Presentation

- Hemoptysis
- Iron deficiency anemia
- Cough
- Dyspnea
- Acute phase may lead to fulminant hemoptysis with respiratory failure
- Chronic phase may lead to pulmonary fibrosis

Laboratory Tests

- ANCA and ABMA tests are negative
- Absence of immune complexes
- Normal renal function tests

Natural History

- Sudden onset of cough and hemoptysis in child or young adult
- No evidence of systemic disease or laboratory test abnormalities
- Episodes of pulmonary hemorrhage are recurrent and intermittent
- 25% of patients die rapidly due to massive hemorrhage
- 50% of patients develop chronic disease with persistent anemia and eventual interstitial fibrosis
- 25% of patients recover completely without recurrence

Treatment

- Drugs
  - Corticosteroids

Prognosis

- Patients can show variable response to steroid therapy
- Median survival: 3-5 years

IMAGE FINDINGS

General Features

- Diffuse bilateral consolidation

Radiographic Findings

- Acute phase: Diffuse ground-glass infiltrates predominantly in lower lobes
- Chronic phase: Parenchymal reticulonodular infiltrates with fibrosis

IDIOPATHIC PULMONARY HEMOSIDEROSIS

Key Facts

Terminology
- Intrapulmonary hemorrhage of unknown etiology that is unassociated with other systemic manifestations

Clinical Issues
- Affects children more commonly than adults
- About 20% of patients are adults > 30 years old
- Hemoptysis
- Iron deficiency anemia
- Cough
- Dyspnea

Microscopic Pathology
- Hemorrhage diffusely involving alveolar spaces
- Abundance of intraluminal hemosiderin-laden macrophages within bronchial lumens
- Iron stains are strongly positive in alveolar macrophages

MACROSCOPIC FEATURES

General Features
- Cut section of lung shows dark brown, homogeneous, indurated parenchyma

MICROSCOPIC PATHOLOGY

Histologic Features
- Hemorrhage diffusely involving alveolar spaces
- Abundance of intraluminal hemosiderin-laden macrophages within bronchial lumens
- Interstitial thickening seen in more advanced stages, with type II pneumocyte hyperplasia and interstitial fibrosis
- Minimal interstitial inflammation

ANCILLARY TESTS

Electron Microscopy
- Transmission
  - No evidence of immunoglobulin deposits by ultrastructure

Histochemistry
- Iron stains are strongly positive in alveolar macrophages

DIFFERENTIAL DIAGNOSIS

Goodpasture Syndrome
- Has both lung and kidney involvement
- Due to circulating antibasement membrane antibodies (ABMA)
- Serologic studies demonstrate antiglomerular basement membrane (anti-GBM) antibodies
- Linear deposition of IgG and complement can be demonstrated in basement membrane of alveoli by immunofluorescence

DIAGNOSTIC CHECKLIST

Pathologic Interpretation Pearls
- IPH cannot be distinguished on routine histology from Goodpasture syndrome
- Serologic studies to demonstrate circulating ABMA or immunofluorescence detection of anti-GBM antibodies is required for diagnosis

SELECTED REFERENCES

1. Le Clainche L et al: Long-term outcome of idiopathic pulmonary hemosiderosis in children. Medicine (Baltimore). 79(5):318-26, 2000
2. Cohen S: Idiopathic pulmonary hemosiderosis. Am J Med Sci. 317(1):67-74, 1999

IMAGE GALLERY

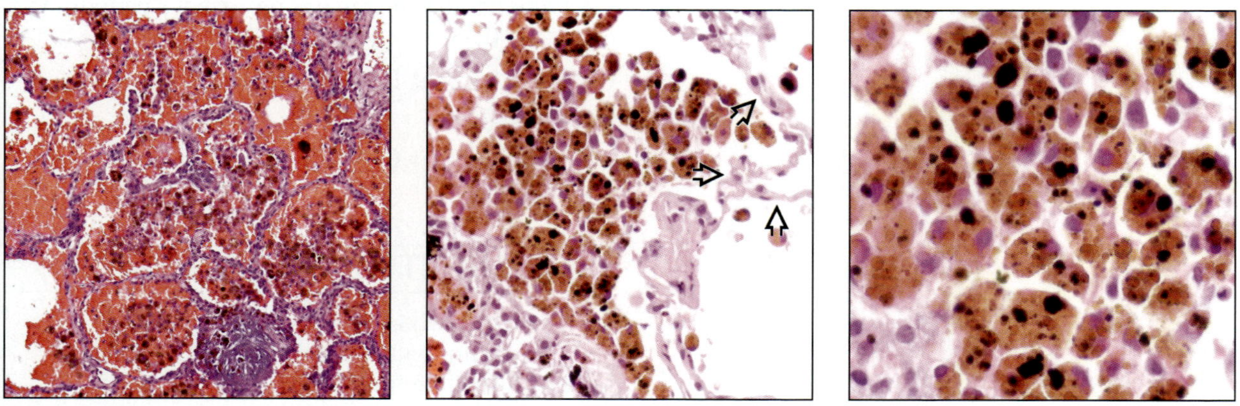

(Left) *Scanning magnification in a patient with idiopathic pulmonary hemosiderosis shows distended alveolar spaces filled with blood and hemosiderin-laden macrophages.* ***(Center)*** *Higher magnification of an airspace in idiopathic pulmonary hemosiderosis shows normal alveolar walls ⇨ devoid of interstitial fibrosis or inflammation.* ***(Right)*** *Higher magnification in idiopathic pulmonary hemosiderosis shows abundant hemosiderin-laden macrophages.*

ALVEOLAR PROTEINOSIS

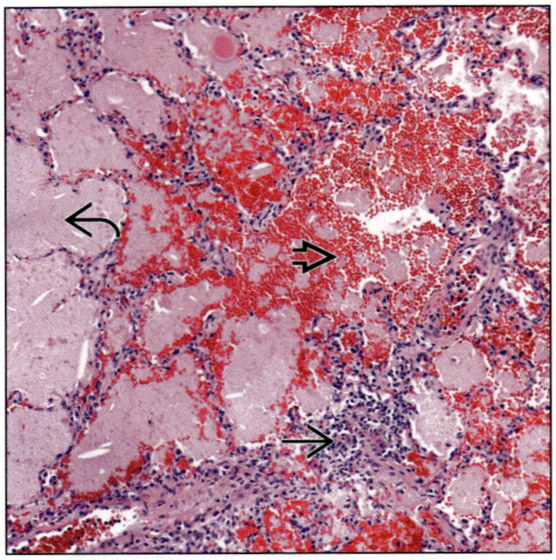

Pulmonary alveolar proteinosis shows alveolar filling by a proteinaceous material ⇒ as well as fresh blood ⇒. In addition, a mild inflammatory infiltrate is also present →.

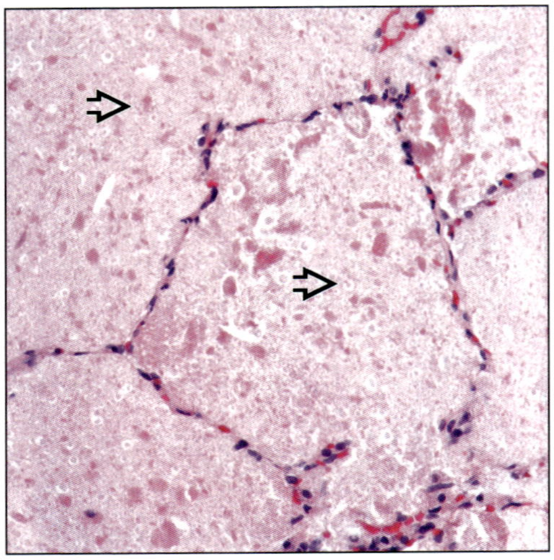

High-power view of alveolar proteinosis shows complete filling of the alveolar spaces by granular acellular proteinaceous material ⇒.

TERMINOLOGY

Abbreviations

- Pulmonary alveolar proteinosis (PAP)

Definitions

- Nonneoplastic condition in which alveoli are filled with proteinaceous material

ETIOLOGY/PATHOGENESIS

Etiology

- Pulmonary alveolar proteinosis has been seen in association with the following
  - Infectious conditions
  - Immunosuppression
  - Hematologic malignancies

CLINICAL ISSUES

Epidemiology

- Incidence
  - Condition of unusual occurrence
- Age
  - Condition has been reported to occur in any age group
- Gender
  - No gender predilection

Presentation

- Cough
- Dyspnea
- Chest pain
- Fever

Treatment

- Spontaneous remission in some cases
- Pulmonary lavage

Prognosis

- Generally good prognosis
- Depends on associated condition
- Some patients may not respond to treatment

IMAGE FINDINGS

General Features

- Reticulonodular pattern
- Small acinar pattern
- Focal consolidation

MACROSCOPIC FEATURES

General Features

- Congested lung parenchyma

MICROSCOPIC PATHOLOGY

Histologic Features

- Alveolar filling by proteinaceous material
- Preservation of normal alveolar architecture
- No evidence of interstitial fibrosis
- Proteinaceous material is positive for periodic acid-Schiff (PAS)

Predominant Pattern/Injury Type

- Diffuse

Predominant Cell/Compartment Type

- Granular

DIFFERENTIAL DIAGNOSIS

Pneumocystis Pneumonia

- Silver stains will show presence of organisms
- PAS histochemical stain is negative

ALVEOLAR PROTEINOSIS

Key Facts

Terminology
- Nonneoplastic condition in which alveoli are filled with proteinaceous material

Clinical Issues
- Presentation
  - Cough
  - Dyspnea
  - Chest pain
  - Fever
- Treatment
  - Pulmonary lavage
  - Spontaneous remission in some cases

Image Findings
- Reticulonodular pattern
- Small acinar pattern
- Focal consolidation

Microscopic Pathology
- Alveolar filling by proteinaceous material
- Preservation of normal alveolar architecture
- Proteinaceous material is positive for periodic acid-Schiff (PAS)

Top Differential Diagnoses
- *Pneumocystis* pneumonia
  - Silver stains will show presence of organisms
  - PAS histochemical stain is negative
- Pulmonary edema
  - Pulmonary edema fluid is negative for PAS histochemical stain

Immunohistochemistry

Antibody	Reactivity	Staining Pattern	Comment
CD68	Negative		May be positive in alveolar macrophages
S100	Negative		May be positive in alveolar macrophages
AE1/AE3	Negative		
CD45	Negative		

Histochemical Features of Alveolar Proteinosis

Histochemical Stain	Result
Periodic acid-Schiff (PAS)	Positive in proteinaceous material
Periodic acid-Schiff with diastase digestion (D-PAS)	Negative in proteinaceous material
Mucicarmine	Negative
Silver stains for organisms (GMS)	Negative

- PCP and PAP may be associated with immunosuppression
- In both conditions, there is filling of alveolar spaces by acellular material

Pulmonary Edema
- In pulmonary edema, fluid filling the spaces is rather bright and not granular
- Pulmonary edema fluid is negative for PAS histochemical stain

DIAGNOSTIC CHECKLIST

Clinically Relevant Pathologic Features
- Tissue distribution
- Prominent intraalveolar pattern

Pathologic Interpretation Pearls
- Granular proteinaceous material filling alveolar spaces
- Intraalveolar proteinaceous material is positive for PAS histochemical stain

SELECTED REFERENCES

1. Huizar I et al: Alveolar proteinosis syndrome: pathogenesis, diagnosis, and management. Curr Opin Pulm Med. 15(5):491-8, 2009
2. Luisetti M et al: Plasmapheresis for treatment of pulmonary alveolar proteinosis. Eur Respir J. 33(5):1220-2, 2009
3. Frazier AA et al: From the archives of the AFIP: pulmonary alveolar proteinosis. Radiographics. 28(3):883-99; quiz 915, 2008
4. Sauni R et al: Pulmonary alveolar proteinosis induced by silica dust? Occup Med (Lond). 57(3):221-4, 2007
5. Prakash UB et al: Pulmonary alveolar phospholipoproteinosis: experience with 34 cases and a review. Mayo Clin Proc. 62(6):499-518, 1987
6. Kariman K et al: Pulmonary alveolar proteinosis: prospective clinical experience in 23 patients for 15 years. Lung. 162(4):223-31, 1984
7. McCook TA et al: Pulmonary alveolar proteinosis in children. AJR Am J Roentgenol. 137(5):1023-7, 1981
8. Bedrossian CW et al: Alveolar proteinosis as a consequence of immunosuppression. A hypothesis based on clinical and pathologic observations. Hum Pathol. 11(5 Suppl):527-35, 1980
9. Rosen SH et al: Pulmonary alveolar proteinosis. N Engl J Med. 258(23):1123-42, 1958

ALVEOLAR PROTEINOSIS

Microscopic Features

*(**Left**) In some cases of alveolar proteinosis, the lumen of the airway may also be involved →. Adjacent structures are within normal limits; a lymphoid aggregate is also present →. (**Right**) In areas, the airway may appear to be involved and partially destroyed → in alveolar proteinosis. The adjacent alveolar spaces show the typical alveolar filling →.*

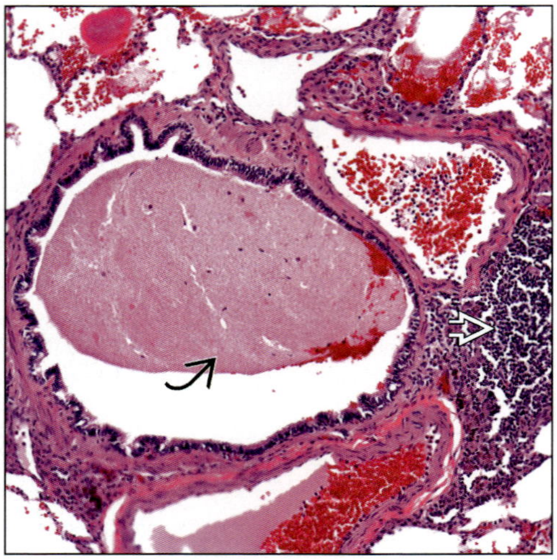

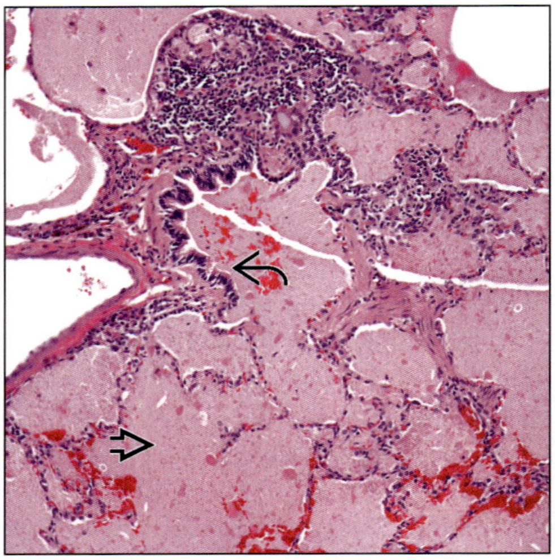

*(**Left**) Alveolar proteinosis shows extensive areas of hemorrhage almost obscuring the process. In a few areas, it is still possible to identify diagnostic areas →. These findings may pose a problem in making a definitive diagnosis. (**Right**) In some cases, the areas of hemorrhage → and alveolar proteinosis have a clear demarcation →, thus making the interpretation of alveolar proteinosis easier.*

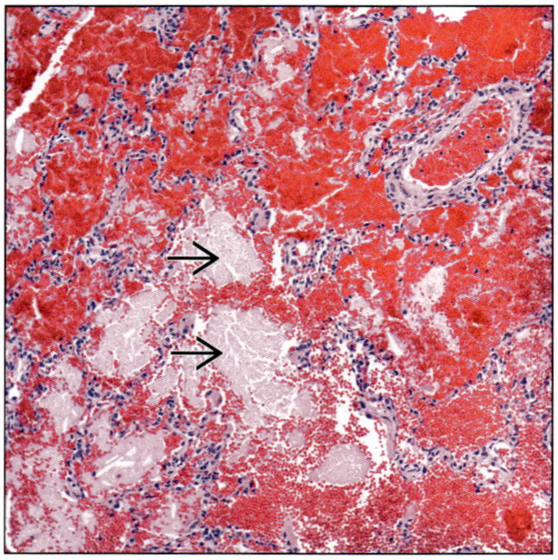

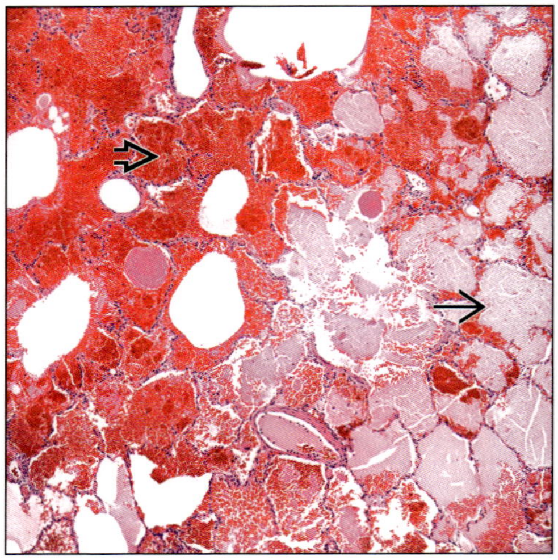

*(**Left**) Alveolar proteinosis shows areas containing cholesterol cleft granuloma →. This feature is also rather unusual since, in the majority of cases of PAP, no reactive changes are associated with it. (**Right**) Adjacent lung parenchyma in alveolar proteinosis may show areas of pneumonitis with the accumulation of alveolar macrophages →.*

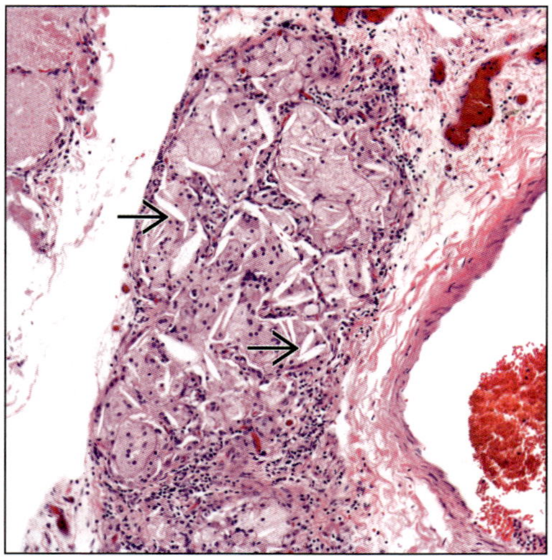

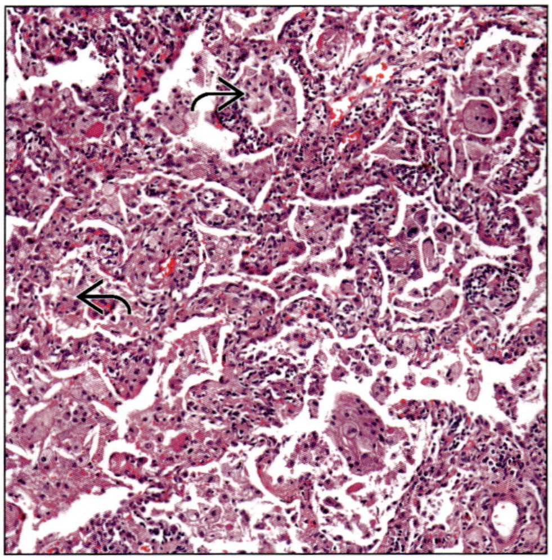

ALVEOLAR PROTEINOSIS

Microscopic Features

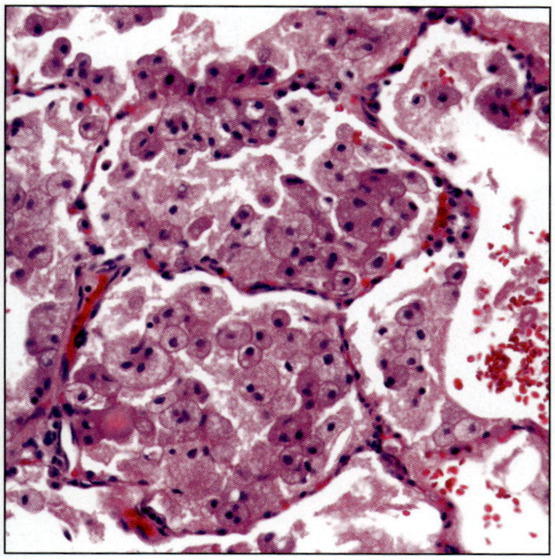
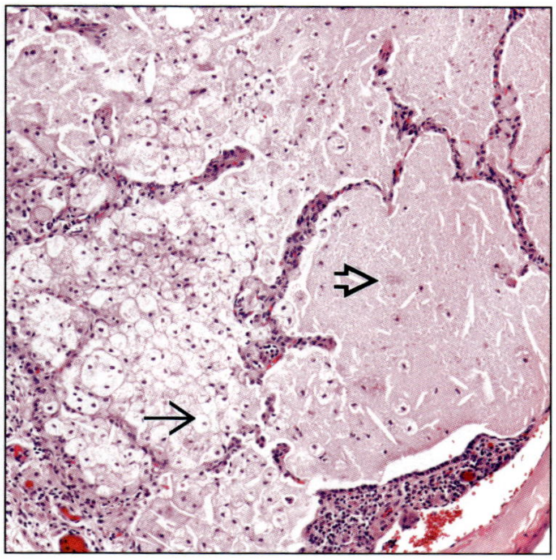

(Left) *Alveolar proteinosis shows an area in which the alveoli are filled with foamy macrophages. No proteinaceous material is present within the alveoli.* ***(Right)*** *In some cases, the classic features of alveolar proteinosis are present and admixed with numerous macrophages. These findings may suggest the possibility of obstructive pneumonia with edematous changes.*

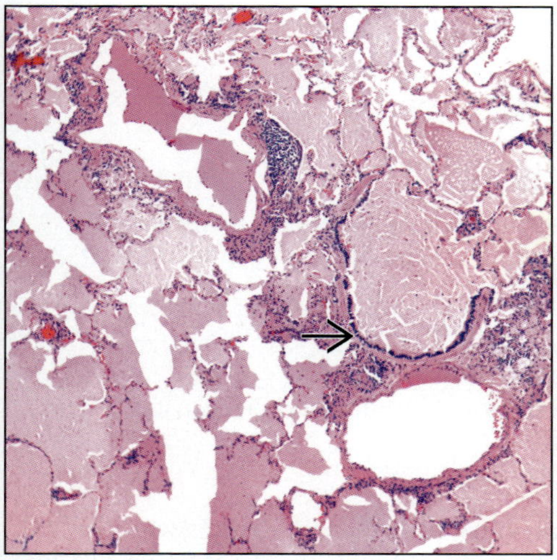
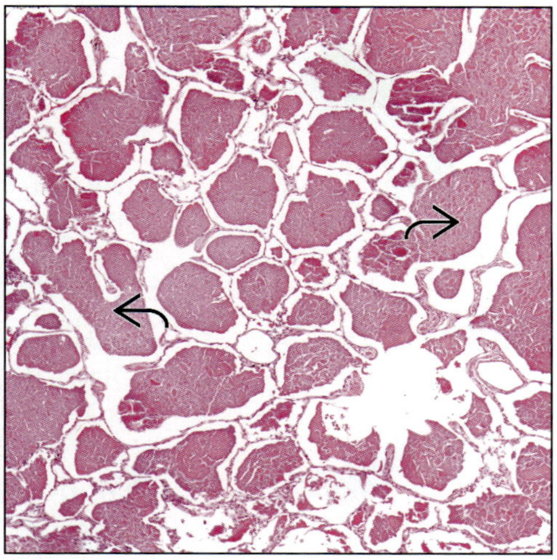

(Left) *Alveolar proteinosis is shown partially destroying an airway, which is also filled with the proteinaceous material. Although the name alveolar proteinosis implies alveolar disease, the process may also involve airway structures.* ***(Right)*** *Conventional feature of alveolar proteinosis in which the normal lung architecture is preserved. However, the alveoli are filled with proteinaceous material.*

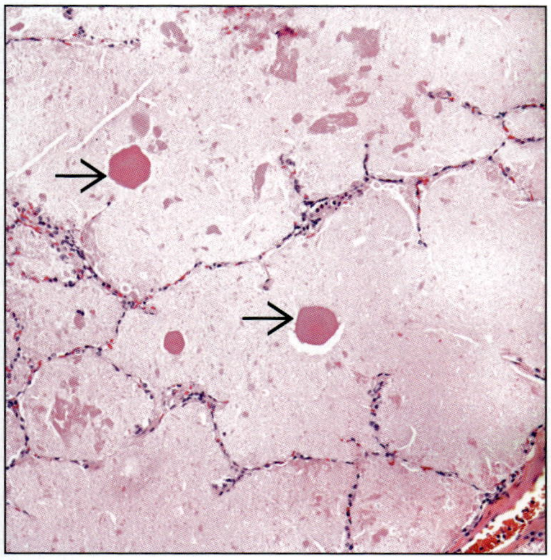
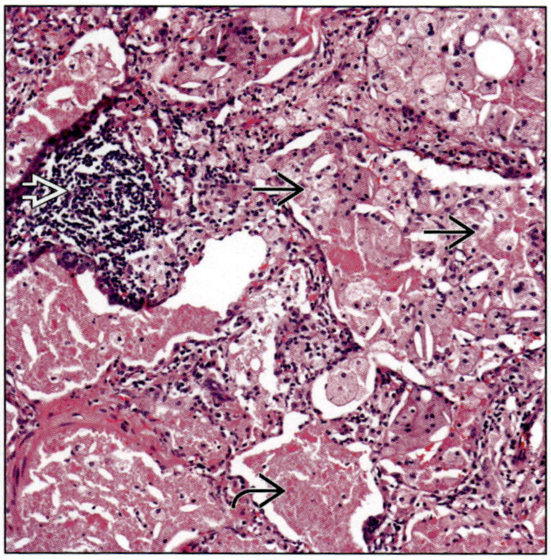

(Left) *Higher magnification of alveolar proteinosis shows the classical granular proteinaceous material with small clumps of bright eosinophilic material. There is no cellularity, including macrophages.* ***(Right)*** *Alveolar proteinosis shows areas of focal lymphoid aggregate, intraalveolar foamy macrophages, and classic proteinaceous material.*

PULMONARY AMYLOIDOSIS

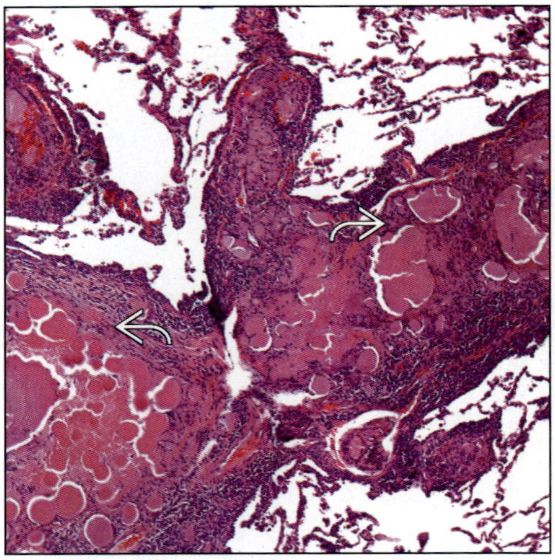

Low-power view demonstrates lung parenchyma with nodules ➔ of different sizes composed of an amorphous acellular material replacing lung parenchyma.

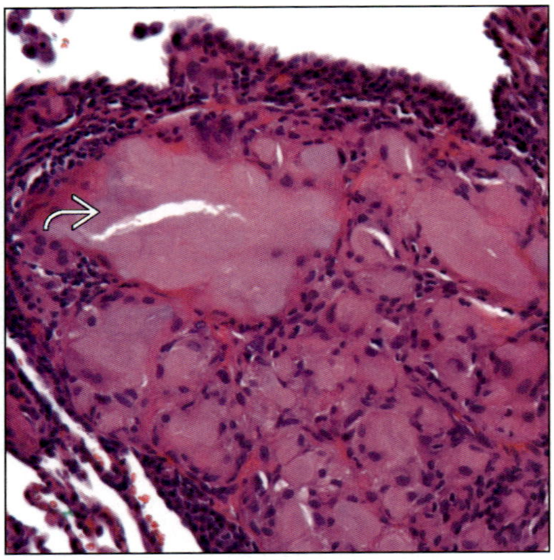

Closer view of the amorphous material replacing normal lung parenchyma is shown. The material is acellular ➔ with a haphazard distribution.

TERMINOLOGY

Synonyms

- Amyloidoma

Definitions

- Nonneoplastic process characterized by deposition of amorphous proteinaceous material that may involve lung either primarily or secondarily

ETIOLOGY/PATHOGENESIS

May Develop Secondary to

- Systemic amyloidosis
- Light chain disease
- Multiple myeloma
- Waldenström macroglobulinemia
- Familial neuropathy
- Niemann-Pick disease
- Gaucher disease
- Sjögren syndrome
- MALT lymphoma of lung

CLINICAL ISSUES

Epidemiology

- Incidence
  - Rare condition in lung
- Age
  - Generally affects adults
- Gender
  - No apparent gender predilection
- Ethnicity
  - No apparent ethnic predilection

Site

- Lung

Presentation

- Dyspnea
- Cough
- Chest pain
- Asymptomatic

Laboratory Tests

- Potassium permanganate oxidation technique
  - Separates amyloid type AA from other forms of amyloid

Treatment

- Surgical approaches
  - Surgical resection of tumor nodules is usually performed

Prognosis

- Depends on clinical background, such as whether patient has systemic amyloidosis or any other disease associated with amyloid deposition

MACROSCOPIC FEATURES

General Features

- Lung parenchyma can have 1 or more pulmonary nodules

Size

- Varies; between 1 and > 10 cm

MICROSCOPIC PATHOLOGY

Histologic Features

- Several distinct patterns of amyloid deposition in lung
  - Nodular
  - Interstitial
  - Diffuse
  - Plaque-like

PULMONARY AMYLOIDOSIS

Key Facts

Terminology
- Nonneoplastic process characterized by deposition of amorphous proteinaceous material that may involve lung either primarily or secondarily

Etiology/Pathogenesis
- Secondary to
  - Systemic amyloidosis
  - Light chain disease
  - Multiple myeloma
  - MALT lymphoma of lung
  - Sjögren syndrome
  - Familial neuropathy
  - Gaucher disease

Microscopic Pathology
- Several distinct patterns of amyloid deposition
  - Nodular
  - Interstitial
  - Diffuse
  - Plaque-like
- Cytologic features
  - Amorphous acellular material
  - Presence of giant cells toward periphery of lesion
  - Ossification may be present
  - Inflammatory reaction

Top Differential Diagnoses
- Hyalinizing granuloma of lung
- Alveolar proteinosis
- Intrapulmonary solitary fibrous tumor (I-SFT)
- Pneumocystis pneumonia
- Pneumonia

Cytologic Features
- Amorphous acellular material
- Presence of giant cells toward periphery of lesion
- Ossification may be present
- Inflammatory reaction, namely plasma cells

ANCILLARY TESTS

Histochemistry
- Congo red: Positive
  - Characteristic apple-green birefringence under polarized light
- Crystal violet: Positive, metachromatic
- PAS: Negative
- GMS: Negative

Immunohistochemistry
- Kappa: Polyclonal
- Lambda: Polyclonal
- CD34: Negative

DIFFERENTIAL DIAGNOSIS

Hyalinizing Granuloma of Lung
- Shows negative staining for Congo red
- Composed of thick collagen
- More fibrosing process than pulmonary amyloidosis

Alveolar Proteinosis
- Negative for Congo red
- Classically has proteinaceous material within alveolar spaces only
- Positive staining for PAS while amyloid is negative
- Neither giant cells nor interstitial involvement

Intrapulmonary Solitary Fibrous Tumor (I-SFT)
- More collagen deposition
- Negative staining for Congo red
- Positive staining for CD34 and Bcl-2

Pneumocystis Pneumonia
- Shows preservation of alveolar parenchyma
- Intraalveolar foamy exudate
- Minimal inflammatory reaction
- GMS positive for organisms
- Congo red negative for amyloid

Pneumonia
- Preservation of alveolar parenchyma
- Presence of inflammatory infiltrate; predominantly polymorphonuclear cells
- Gram stain shows presence of bacteria

DIAGNOSTIC CHECKLIST

Pathologic Interpretation Pearls
- Amorphous material
  - Congo red histochemical stain positive
- Giant cells
  - Usually in periphery
- Plasma cells

SELECTED REFERENCES

1. Cottin V et al: Interstitial pulmonary amyloidosis. Respiration. 75(2):210, 2008
2. Seith A et al: Isolated nodular pulmonary amyloidosis. Intern Med J. 38(4):293-4, 2008
3. Biewend ML et al: The spectrum of localized amyloidosis: a case series of 20 patients and review of the literature. Amyloid. 13(3):135-42, 2006
4. Lachmann HJ et al: Amyloidosis and the lung. Chron Respir Dis. 3(4):203-14, 2006
5. Berk JL et al: Pulmonary and tracheobronchial amyloidosis. Semin Respir Crit Care Med. 23(2):155-65, 2002
6. Hui AN et al: Amyloidosis presenting in the lower respiratory tract. Clinicopathologic, radiologic, immunohistochemical, and histochemical studies on 48 cases. Arch Pathol Lab Med. 110(3):212-8, 1986

PULMONARY AMYLOIDOSIS

Microscopic Features

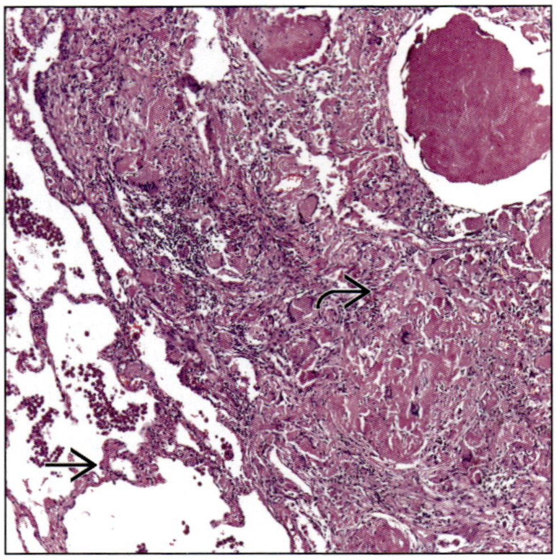

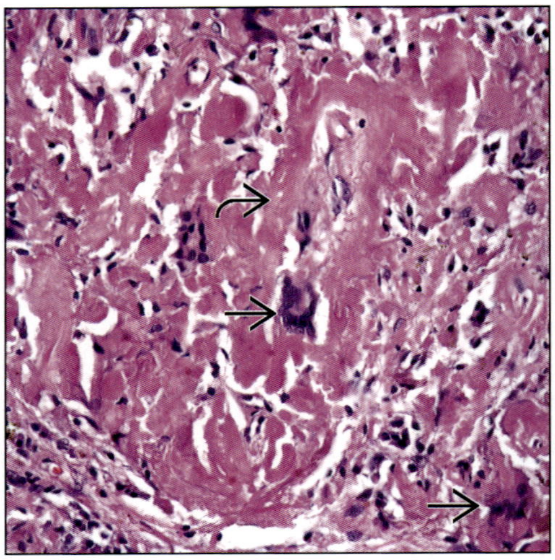

*(**Left**) Low magnification of amyloid deposition in the lung shows both uninvolved lung parenchyma → and extensive areas of lung parenchyma replaced by amyloid ↪. (**Right**) Closer view of amyloid deposition in the lung shows areas composed of an acellular material ↪; however, note the presence of multinucleated giant cells → admixed with the amorphous material.*

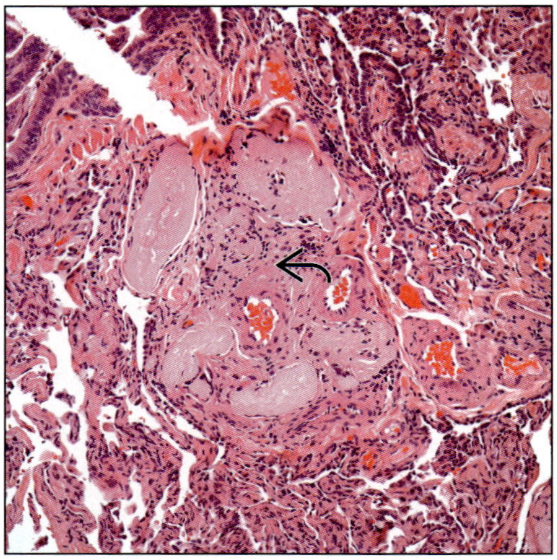

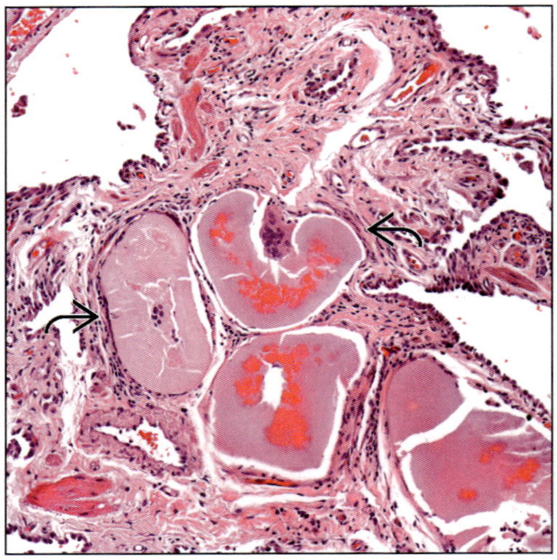

*(**Left**) In some cases the presence of amyloid may not be so obvious, and the amorphous material may be deposited in a more interstitial distribution ↪. In such cases, the diagnosis of pulmonary amyloidosis can be easily missed. (**Right**) Amyloid deposition ↪ in a pattern involving predominantly the interstitium is shown. Note that the adjacent lung parenchyma seems to be within normal limits.*

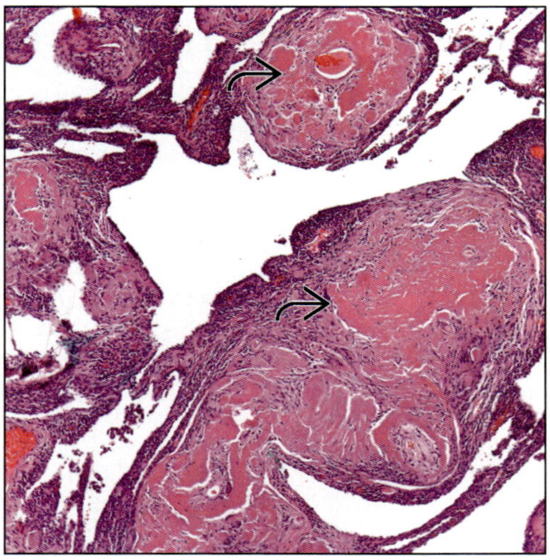

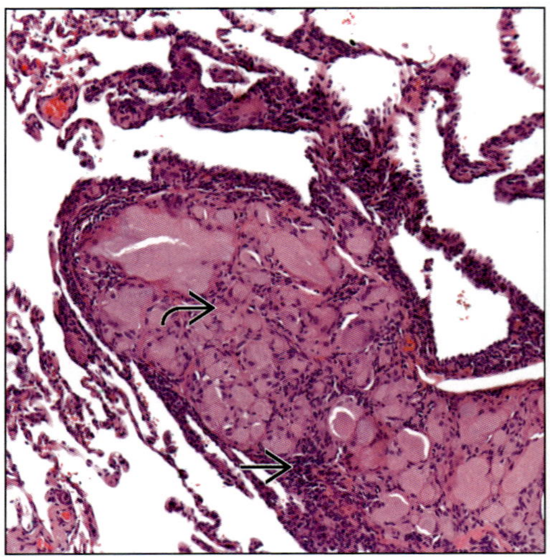

*(**Left**) In some cases of amyloid deposition ↪, the normal architecture of the lung parenchyma is distorted, which can give the impression of a fibrotic interstitial lung disease. (**Right**) Lung parenchyma with amyloid deposition ↪ and a rim of inflammatory reaction is shown. Also note the presence of a mild inflammatory reaction within the amyloid →.*

PULMONARY AMYLOIDOSIS

Microscopic Features

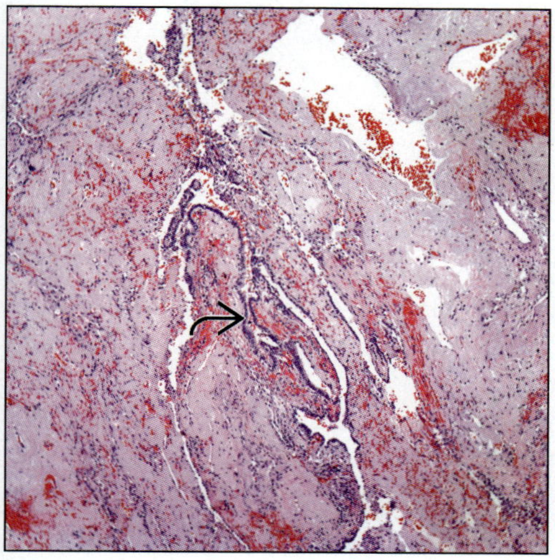
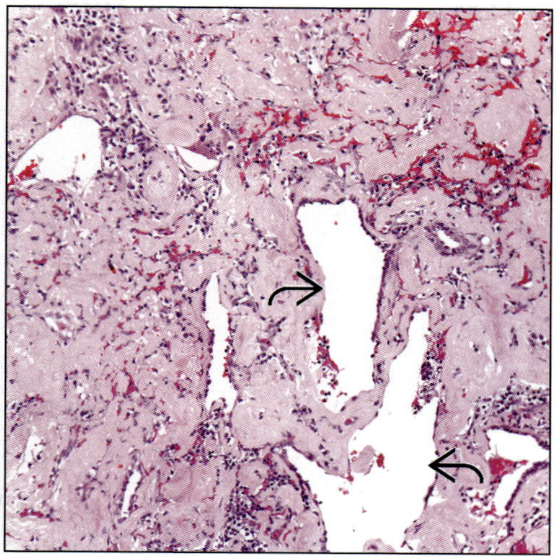

(Left) *In some cases of amyloid deposition, there are only focal residual areas of normal lung tissue, as in this case with focal areas of respiratory epithelium* ↪ *within the amyloid.* ***(Right)*** *In some cases, amyloid deposition may show ectatic spaces* ↪ *that can mimic dilated vascular structures, which could be easily mistaken for a vascular neoplasm.*

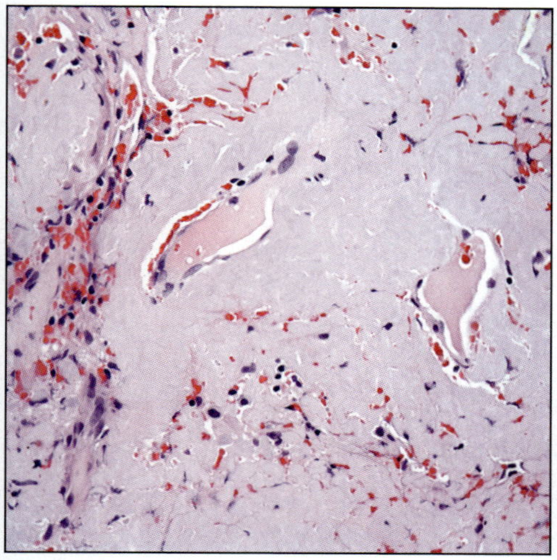
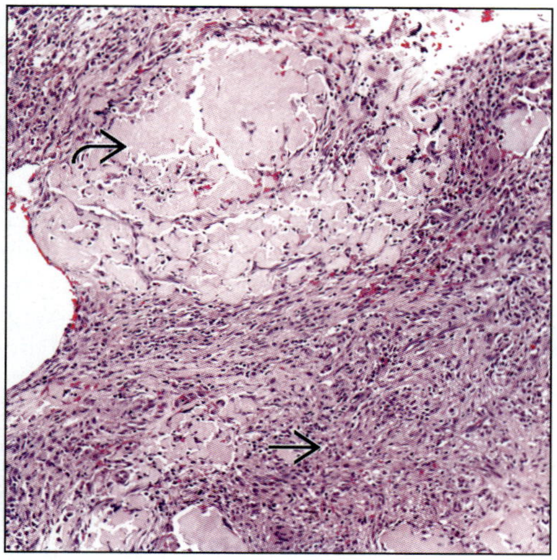

(Left) *Higher magnification of amyloid displays an amorphous material with minimal inflammatory reaction. This histologic feature is characteristic, and a Congo red stain must be requested for further evaluation.* ***(Right)*** *Focal areas of lung parenchyma are obliterated by amyloid deposition* ↪*. However, note the presence of a spindle cell proliferation* →*, which by itself could be mistaken for a spindle cell neoplasm.*

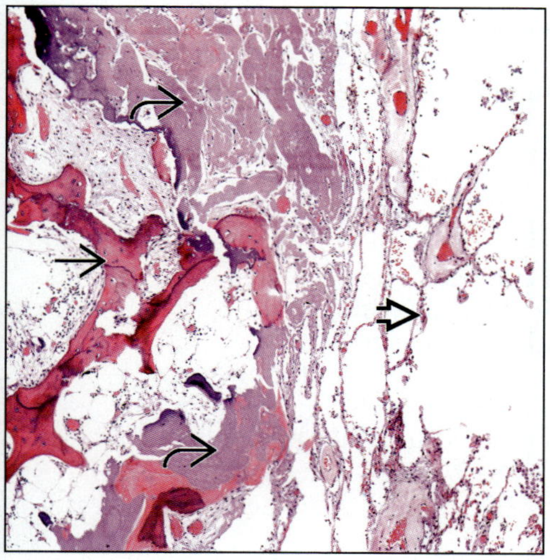
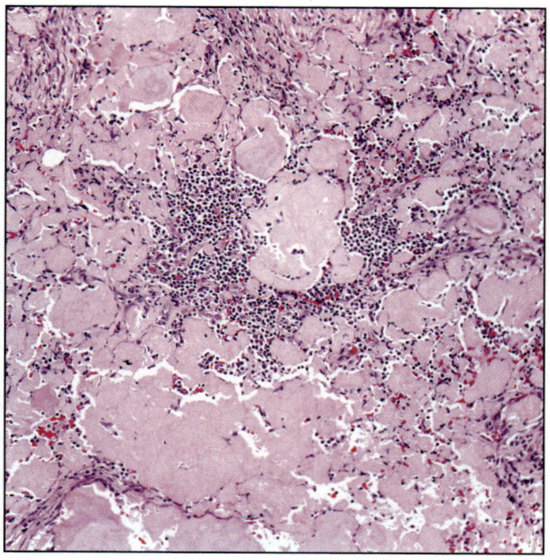

(Left) *Another rather unusual histological feature of amyloid in the lung is the presence of metaplastic bone. Note the presence of normal lung parenchyma* ⇨*, metaplastic bone* →*, and amyloid* ↪*.* ***(Right)*** *Extensive areas of amyloid admixed with an inflammatory reaction composed predominantly of lymphocytes are seen. Because in some cases amyloid may be associated with lymphoma or plasma cell malignancy, it is very important to carefully rule out these possibilities.*

EOSINOPHILIC PNEUMONIA

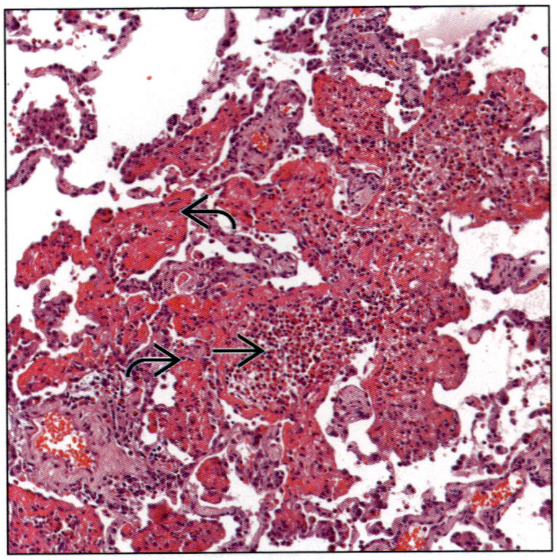

Eosinophilic pneumonia shows pulmonary parenchyma with a fibrinous intraalveolar exudate ➢. Note the presence of numerous inflammatory cells in the center of the exudate ➔.

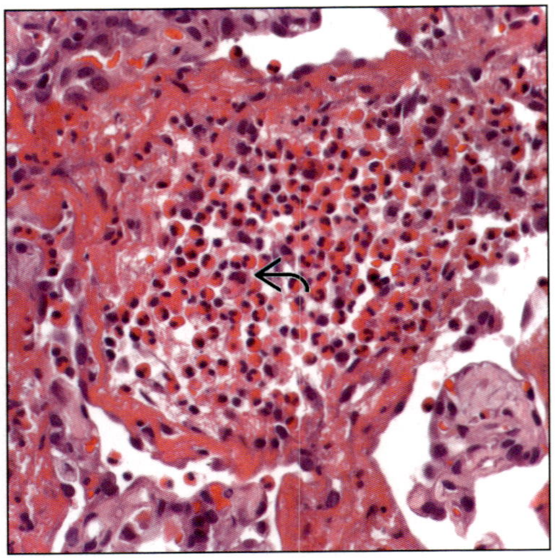

Higher magnification shows numerous eosinophils ➢ admixed with macrophages. This finding is essential for the diagnosis of eosinophilic pneumonia.

TERMINOLOGY

Synonyms

- Loeffler syndrome

Definitions

- Patchy pulmonary infiltrates characterized by the presence of eosinophils as the main inflammatory component

ETIOLOGY/PATHOGENESIS

Causes

- Parasites
  - *Ascaris*
  - Filariasis
  - *Strongyloides*
  - *Toxocara*
- Ingestants and inhalants
  - L-tryptophan
  - Cocaine
- Fungal infections
  - *Aspergillus*
  - *Candida*
  - *Curvularia*
- Drug toxicity
  - Antibiotics
- Unknown etiology

CLINICAL ISSUES

Epidemiology

- Gender
  - Females are more commonly affected in chronic phase

Presentation

- Symptomatology will depend on type of process
  - Simple (Loeffler syndrome)
    - Self-limited
    - Fleeting pulmonary infiltrates
  - Tropical
    - Fever
    - Cough
    - Dyspnea
  - Chronic
    - Fever
    - Chills
    - Dyspnea
    - Weight loss
    - History of asthma
  - Acute
    - Fever
    - Marked respiratory difficulty

Laboratory Tests

- Peripheral eosinophilia in chronic phase
- Elevated IgE in serum in chronic phase

Natural History

- Eosinophilic pneumonia can present in 4 different forms
  - Simple (Loeffler syndrome)
  - Tropical
  - Chronic
  - Acute

Treatment

- Depends on etiology of process
  - Avoidance of possible drug
  - Identification of parasite
  - In cases of chronic eosinophilic pneumonia
    - Steroids may be useful
- In cases of simple eosinophilic pneumonia, process is self-limited

Prognosis

- Will depend on etiology of process
- Most patients follow a recovery process

EOSINOPHILIC PNEUMONIA

Key Facts

Terminology
- Synonyms
  - Loeffler syndrome
- Definition
  - Patchy pulmonary infiltrates characterized by presence of eosinophils as main inflammatory component

Etiology/Pathogenesis
- Parasites
- Ingestants and inhalants
- Fungal infections
- Drug toxicity
- Unknown etiology

Clinical Issues
- Presentation
  - Simple (Loeffler syndrome)
  - Tropical
  - Chronic
  - Acute
- Treatment
  - Depends on etiology of process
- Prognosis
  - Most patients follow a recovery process

Microscopic Pathology
- Histological Features
  - Filling of alveolar spaces by eosinophils and macrophages
  - Intraalveolar acellular exudate
  - Eosinophilic intraalveolar necrosis may be present

IMAGE FINDINGS

Radiographic Findings
- Fleeting pulmonary infiltrates

MICROSCOPIC PATHOLOGY

Histologic Features
- Filling of alveolar spaces by eosinophils and macrophages
- Charcot-Leyden crystal may be present
- Intraalveolar acellular exudate
- Eosinophilic intraalveolar necrosis may be present
- Bronchiolitis obliterans and organizing pneumonia (BOOP) areas may be present
- Areas of diffuse alveolar damage may be present

DIFFERENTIAL DIAGNOSIS

Churg-Strauss Syndrome
- Infiltrates in eosinophilic pneumonia are intraalveolar
- Eosinophilic pneumonia does not show vasculitis
- Eosinophilic pneumonia does not show positive p-ANCA in serum

Langerhans Cell Histiocytosis (LCH)
- Eosinophilic pneumonia shows fleeting infiltrates while LCH shows multiple pulmonary nodules
- Shows the typical nodules (so-called Medusa's head)
- Shows positive staining for S100 protein and CD1a

Dirofilariasis
- Dirofilariasis usually presents with necrotizing intrapulmonary nodule
- Identification of parasite within necrotizing nodule is diagnostic of dirofilariasis
- Eosinophilic infiltrate may be seen in periphery of necrotizing nodule

Fibrinous Pneumonitis
- Lacks presence of eosinophils
- Fleeting pulmonary infiltrates would be unusual finding
- Clinical background of fibrinous pneumonitis is different

DIAGNOSTIC CHECKLIST

Clinically Relevant Pathologic Features
- Symptom complex
- Tissue distribution

Pathologic Interpretation Pearls
- Intraalveolar presence of eosinophilic infiltrate

SELECTED REFERENCES

1. Swartz J et al: Acute eosinophilic pneumonia complicating Coccidioides immitis pneumonia: a case report and literature review. Respiration. 77(1):102-6, 2009
2. Katz U et al: Pulmonary eosinophilia. Clin Rev Allergy Immunol. 34(3):367-71, 2008
3. Jeong YJ et al: Eosinophilic lung diseases: a clinical, radiologic, and pathologic overview. Radiographics. 27(3):617-37; discussion 637-9, 2007
4. Vijayan VK: Tropical pulmonary eosinophilia: pathogenesis, diagnosis and management. Curr Opin Pulm Med. 13(5):428-33, 2007
5. Wechsler ME: Pulmonary eosinophilic syndromes. Immunol Allergy Clin North Am. 27(3):477-92, 2007
6. Allen J: Acute eosinophilic pneumonia. Semin Respir Crit Care Med. 27(2):142-7, 2006
7. Chitkara RK et al: Parasitic pulmonary eosinophilia. Semin Respir Crit Care Med. 27(2):171-84, 2006
8. Marchand E et al: Idiopathic chronic eosinophilic pneumonia. Semin Respir Crit Care Med. 27(2):134-41, 2006
9. Cottin V et al: Eosinophilic pneumonias. Allergy. 60(7):841-57, 2005

EOSINOPHILIC PNEUMONIA

Microscopic Features

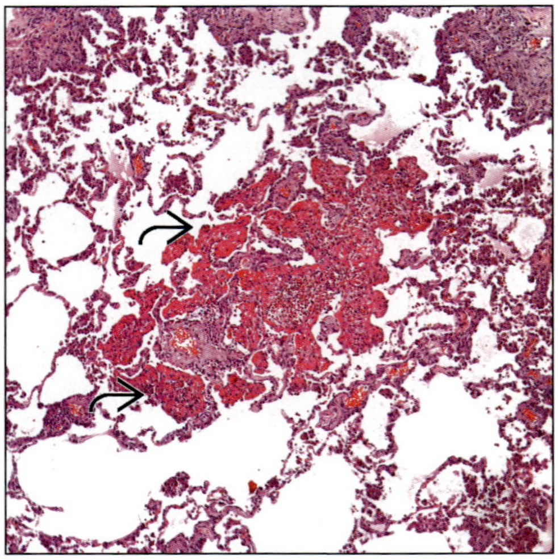

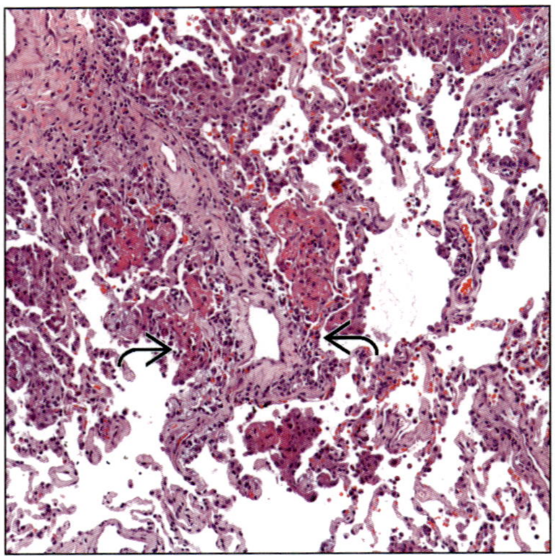

(Left) *Low-power magnification of eosinophilic pneumonia shows a fibrinous inflammatory exudate predominantly in intraalveolar location ↷. This feature may be seen in some cases of acute fibrinous pneumonia.* ***(Right)*** *In other areas, the fibrinous exudate is also found around perivascular structures ↷, giving the impression of an inflammatory vascular process.*

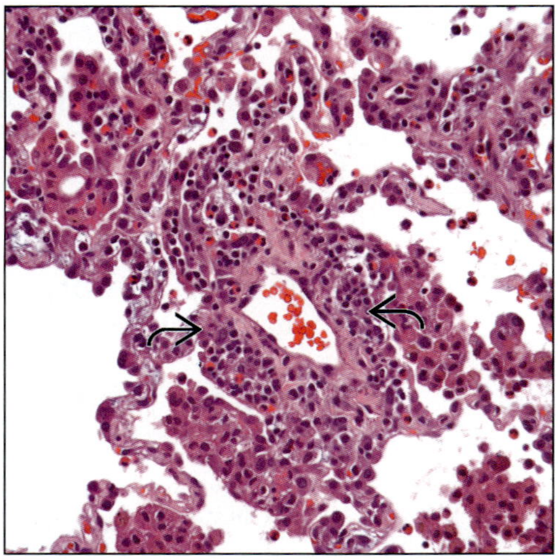

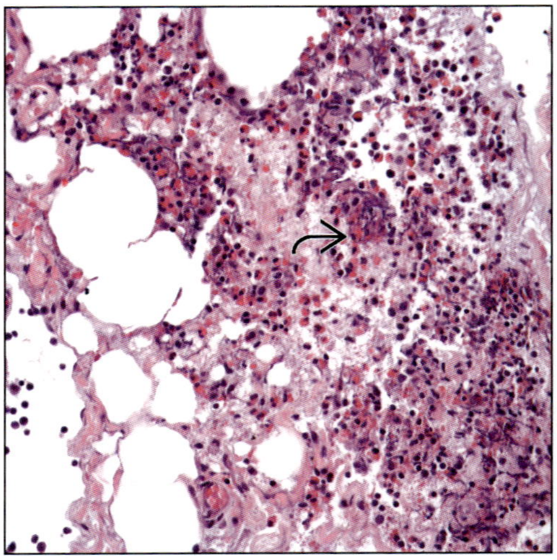

(Left) *In some cases of eosinophilic pneumonia away from the eosinophilic abscesses that are commonly seen, the inflammatory response may be more subtle, showing a perivascular inflammatory reaction ↷ without the fibrinous exudate.* ***(Right)*** *In addition to the commonly seen intraalveolar eosinophilic abscess, an eosinophilic reaction ↷ is also seen toward the periphery of the lung into the visceral pleura.*

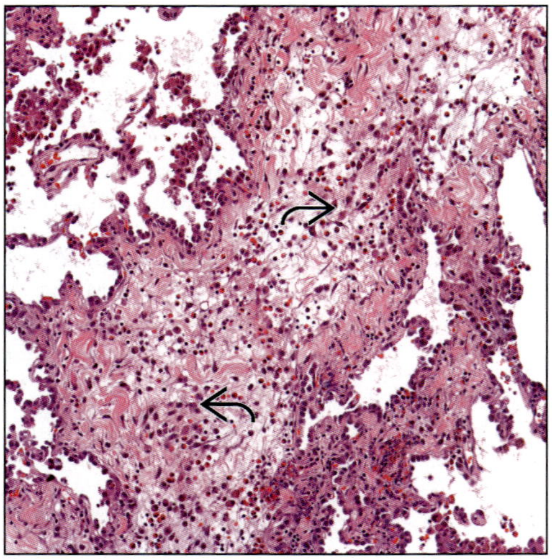

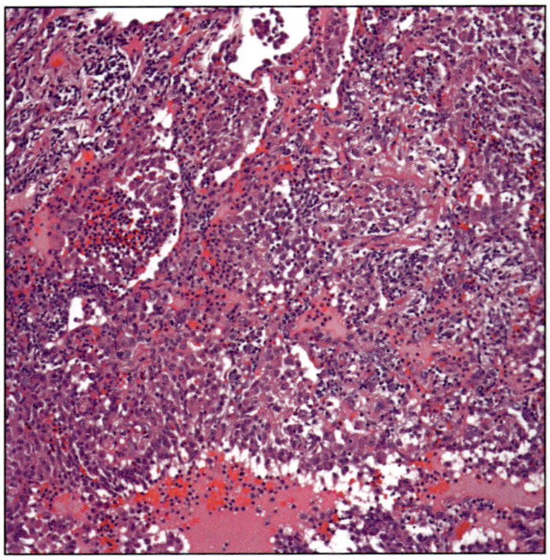

(Left) *Eosinophilic pneumonia shows extensive deposition of inflammatory cells, predominantly composed of eosinophils. The eosinophilic infiltrate ↷ involves the pulmonary septum.* ***(Right)*** *Eosinophilic pneumonia shows areas of organization. The eosinophilic infiltrate is mixed with other inflammatory cells and macrophages, obscuring the diagnosis.*

EOSINOPHILIC PNEUMONIA

Microscopic Features

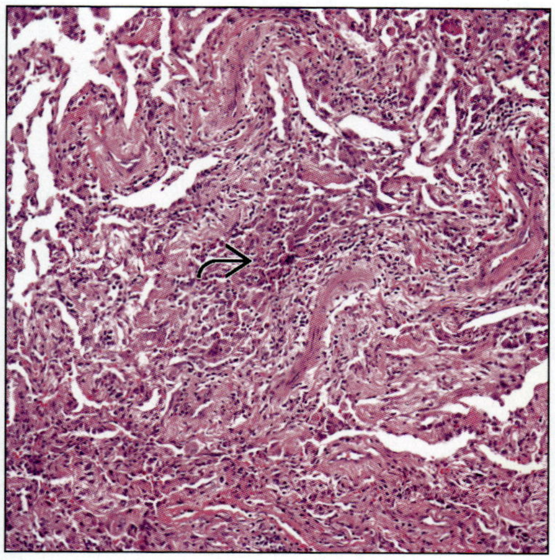

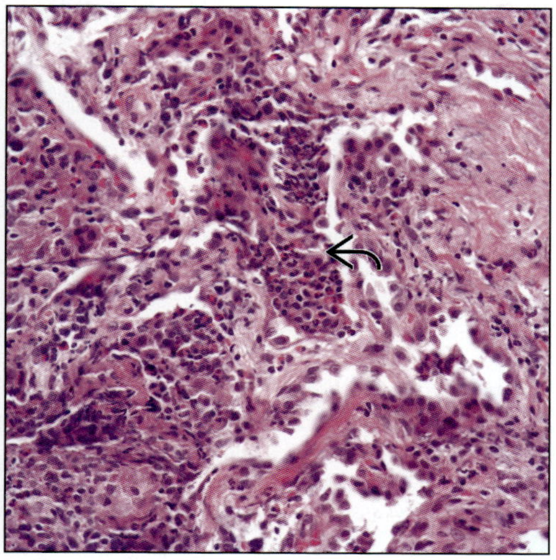

(Left) *In some cases of eosinophilic pneumonia, the lung parenchyma is collapsed, and the presence of the eosinophilic abscess ⮫ is not readily observed, making the diagnosis more challenging.* ***(Right)*** *Eosinophilic pneumonia shows an eosinophilic abscess ⮫ in the background of collapsed alveolar structures.*

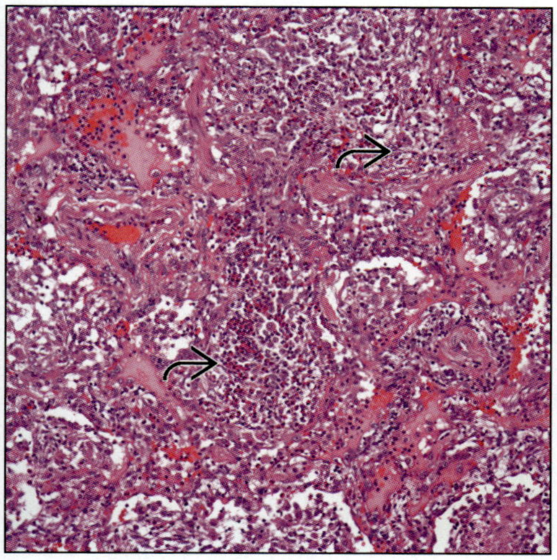

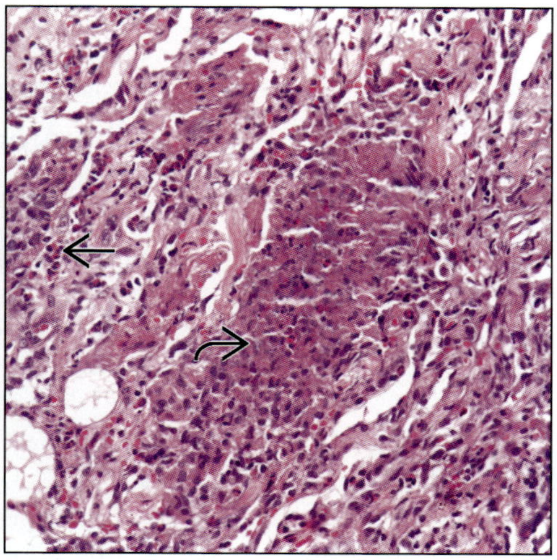

(Left) *Eosinophilic pneumonia shows alveolar filling ⮫ of inflammatory cells predominantly composed of eosinophils. At this magnification, this process can easily be mistaken for a conventional pneumonia.* ***(Right)*** *Classic eosinophilic abscess ⮫ in an eosinophilic pneumonia is shown. Adjacent to the abscess are numerous interstitial eosinophils →.*

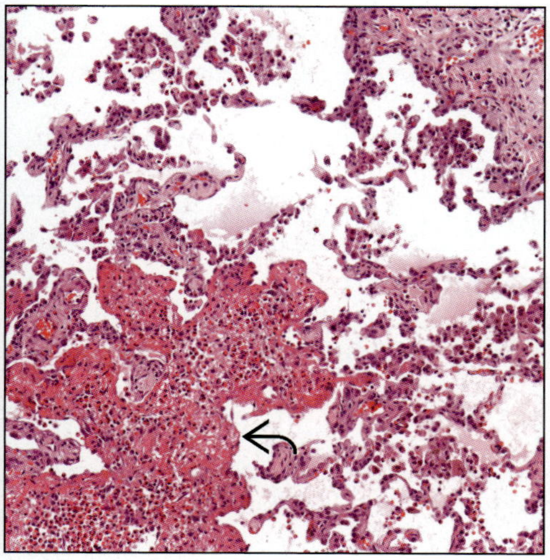

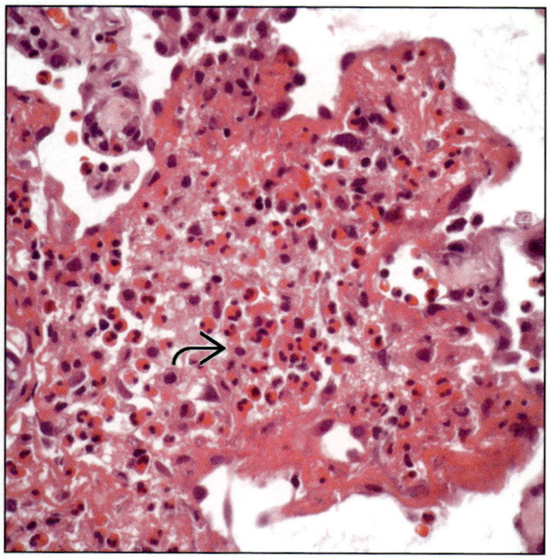

(Left) *Eosinophilic pneumonia shows conventional features of intraalveolar fibrinous exudate ⮫. The cellular proliferation within the fibrinous exudate is composed predominantly of eosinophils.* ***(Right)*** *Higher magnification demonstrates that the fibrinous exudates contain numerous eosinophils ⮫, which are essential for the diagnosis of eosinophilic pneumonia.*

LANGERHANS CELL HISTIOCYTOSIS

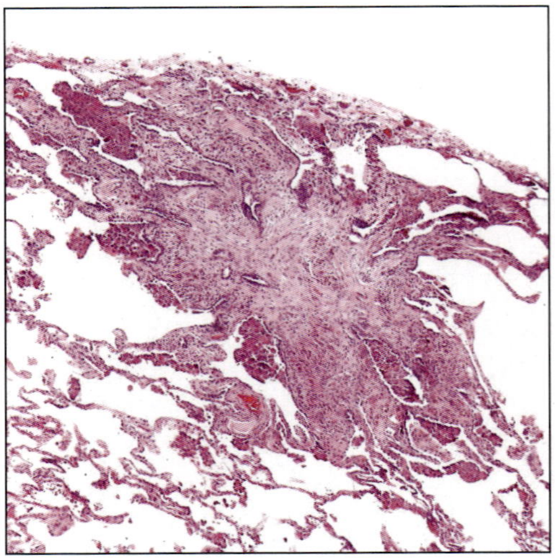

Histologic appearance of a focus of Langerhans cell histiocytosis shows a stellate-shaped area in the periphery of the lung with sparse cellular proliferation.

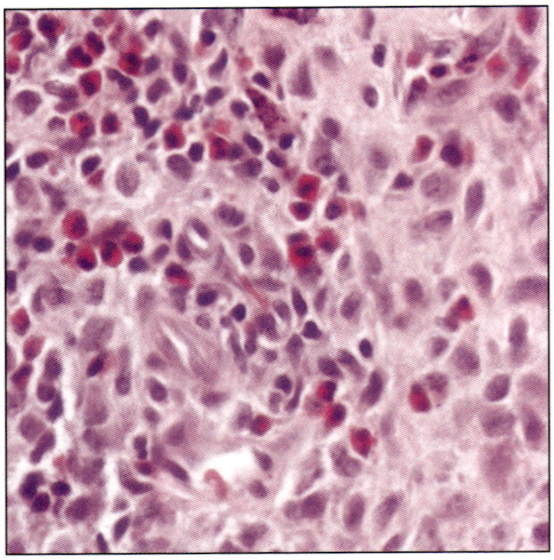

Higher magnification of a pulmonary focus of Langerhans cell histiocytosis shows proliferation of small spindled Langerhans cells admixed with abundant eosinophils.

TERMINOLOGY

Abbreviations

- Langerhans cell histiocytosis (LCH)

Synonyms

- Eosinophilic granuloma, Langerhans cell granulomatosis, histiocytosis-X

Definitions

- Proliferation of Langerhans cells that form multiple interstitial, bilateral, peribronchiolar pulmonary nodules

ETIOLOGY/PATHOGENESIS

Pathogenesis

- Clonality studies in the lung have suggested both reactive and neoplastic process
- 95% of patients are cigarette smokers, suggesting link with cigarette smoking

CLINICAL ISSUES

Epidemiology

- Incidence
  - Highest incidence is in cigarette smokers (95% of patients)
- Age
  - 18-40 years
- Gender
  - Slight male predominance

Site

- Predominantly affects upper and mid-zones of lungs

Presentation

- Cough
- Dyspnea
- Chest pain
- Systemic symptoms (malaise, fever, weight loss)
- Extrapulmonary involvement seen in 15% of patients
- Asymptomatic in approximately 15% of patients

Laboratory Tests

- Pulmonary function tests show restrictive disease with decreased diffusing capacity

Natural History

- Some patients may experience spontaneous remissions while others may progress to end-stage pulmonary fibrosis
- Disease often regresses with cessation of smoking

Treatment

- Steroids
- Cessation of smoking
- Immunosuppressive therapy in refractory cases
- Spontaneous resolution in some cases

Prognosis

- Usually reversible with cessation of smoking
- 15% of patients show progressive disease that may be fatal
  - Progressive cases may require lung transplantation

IMAGE FINDINGS

Radiographic Findings

- Interstitial process with predilection for the mid and upper lobes of lung with sparing of costophrenic angles

CT Findings

- HRCT shows small nodules and cystic spaces showing upper and mid lung patchy distribution

LANGERHANS CELL HISTIOCYTOSIS

Key Facts

Terminology

- Proliferation of Langerhans cells that form multiple interstitial, bilateral, peribronchiolar pulmonary nodules

Clinical Issues

- Highest incidence is in cigarette smokers (95% of patients)
- 18-40 years
- Predominantly affects upper and mid zones of the lungs
- Asymptomatic in approximately 15% of patients

Microscopic Pathology

- Interstitial proliferation of Langerhans cells distributed along small airways (bronchioles and alveolar ducts)
- Larger lesions produce stellate-shaped or round nodules around bronchioles
- Lesions may be paucicellular or contain abundant Langerhans cells
- Nodular lesions may show cystic changes and cavitation
- Langerhans cells show round to oval nuclei with frequent nuclear irregularities and nuclear infolding (grooves)
- Langerhans cells are accompanied by abundant eosinophils

Ancillary Tests

- Langerhans cells are positive for S100 protein and CD1a
- Zipper-like structures (Birbeck granules) are pathognomonic on electron microscopy

MACROSCOPIC FEATURES

General Features

- Usually seen as small (2 mm diameter) nodules
- Advanced stages may show extensive interstitial fibrosis

MICROSCOPIC PATHOLOGY

Histologic Features

- Interstitial proliferation of Langerhans cells distributed along small airways (bronchioles and alveolar ducts)
- Larger lesions produce stellate-shaped or round nodules around bronchioles
- Lesions may be paucicellular or contain abundant Langerhans cells
- Nodular lesions may show cystic changes and cavitation
- Lesions are often accompanied by evidence of respiratory bronchiolitis

Cytologic Features

- Langerhans cells show round to oval nuclei with frequent nuclear irregularities and nuclear infolding (grooves)
- Langerhans cells are accompanied by abundant eosinophils
- Multinucleated histiocytes may accompany the cellular infiltrate
- Late or more advanced lesions may be almost totally devoid of Langerhans cells and replaced by stromal fibrosis

ANCILLARY TESTS

Immunohistochemistry

- Langerhans cells are positive for S100 protein, Langerin, and CD1a

Electron Microscopy

- Transmission
    - Zipper-like structures (Birbeck granules) are pathognomonic

DIFFERENTIAL DIAGNOSIS

Eosinophilic Pneumonia

- Intraalveolar infiltrate of eosinophils without Langerhans cells

Usual Interstitial Pneumonia

- Alternating areas of normal and fibrotic parenchyma with "temporal heterogeneity"
- Diffuse interstitial pattern of fibrosis, unlike nodular and stellate pattern of fibrosis in LCH

DIAGNOSTIC CHECKLIST

Clinically Relevant Pathologic Features

- In healed cases, diagnosis is based on presence of stellate peribronchiolar scarring in the setting of typical HRCT changes

Pathologic Interpretation Pearls

- Stellate peribronchiolar lesions with cystic changes in upper lobes of lung are characteristic
- Admixture of eosinophils with mononuclear cells displaying prominent nuclear infolding is also characteristic

SELECTED REFERENCES

1. Nagarjun Rao R et al: Histiocytic disorders of the lung. Adv Anat Pathol. 17(1):12-22, 2010
2. Allen TC: Pulmonary Langerhans cell histiocytosis and other pulmonary histiocytic diseases: a review. Arch Pathol Lab Med. 132(7):1171-81, 2008
3. Attili AK et al: Smoking-related interstitial lung disease: radiologic-clinical-pathologic correlation. Radiographics. 28(5):1383-96; discussion 1396-8, 2008
4. Rao RN et al: Smoking-related interstitial lung disease. Ann Diagn Pathol. 12(6):445-57, 2008

LANGERHANS CELL HISTIOCYTOSIS

Histologic and Immunohistochemical Features

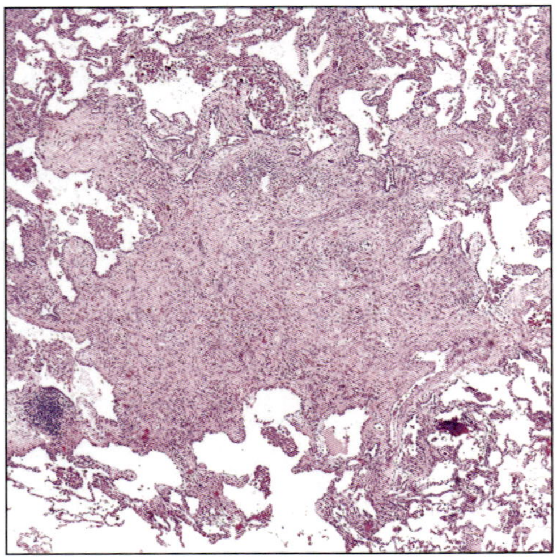
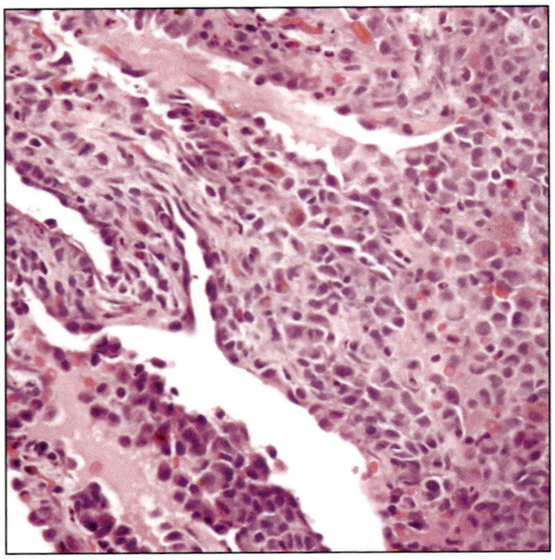

*(**Left**) Scanning magnification of a pulmonary lesion in Langerhans cell histiocytosis shows a characteristic stellate-shaped area of consolidation of lung parenchyma composed of a monotonous population of small round to oval cells. The lesions show a tendency to follow the distribution of bronchioles and vascular bundles. (**Right**) Higher magnification of a pulmonary lesion in Langerhans cell histiocytosis shows a dense population of Langerhans cells admixed with eosinophils and hemosiderin-laden macrophages.*

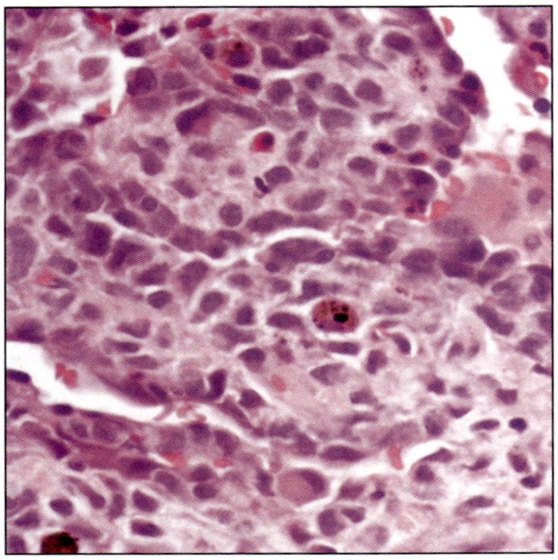
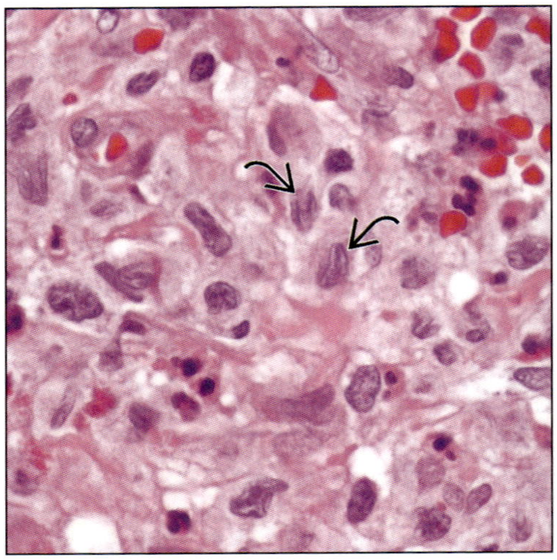

*(**Left**) High magnification of a pulmonary lesion of Langerhans cell histiocytosis shows interstitial infiltration by Langerhans cell proliferation. Interstitial spread of the process may lead to symptoms. (**Right**) Higher magnification of pulmonary Langerhans cell histiocytosis shows histiocytic cells with elongated nuclei surrounded by an ample rim of eosinophilic cytoplasm. The nuclei show a cerebriform appearance with occasional faint longitudinal nuclear grooves →.*

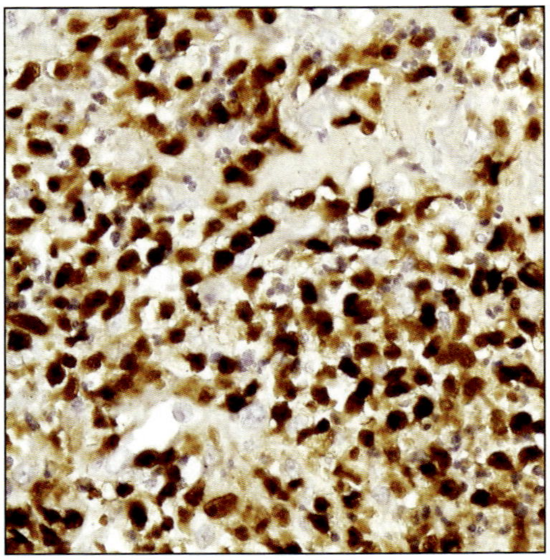
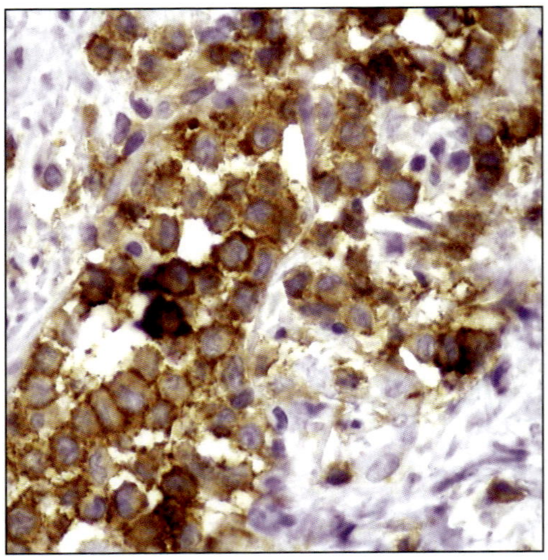

*(**Left**) Immunohistochemical staining for S100 protein in pulmonary Langerhans cell histiocytosis shows nuclear positivity in the Langerhans cells scattered throughout the lesion. (**Right**) Immunohistochemical staining for CD1a in pulmonary Langerhans cell histiocytosis shows strong membrane positivity in the Langerhans cells. The combination of S100 protein positivity with CD1a positivity in the same cells, in the appropriate setting, is diagnostic of this condition.*

LANGERHANS CELL HISTIOCYTOSIS

Histologic Features

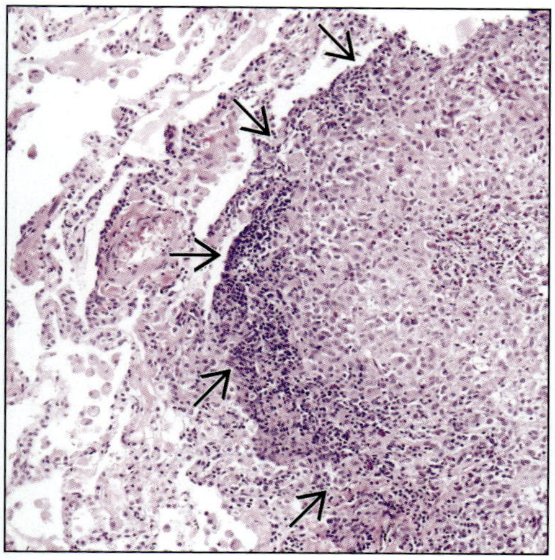

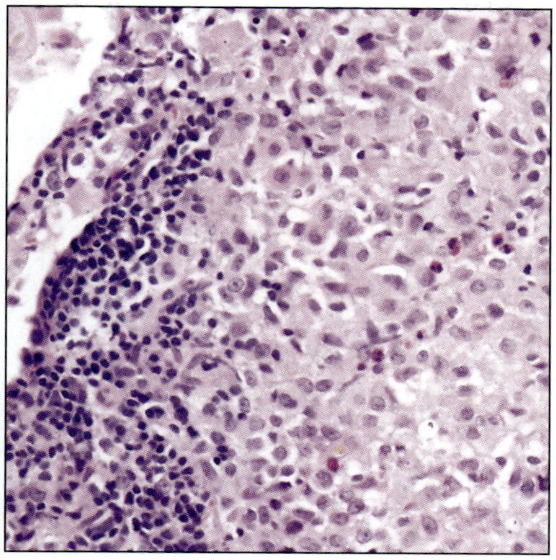

(Left) *Scanning magnification of a nodular lesion ⇒ in pulmonary Langerhans cell histiocytosis shows a well-demarcated nodule composed of sheets of epithelioid cells that are sharply demarcated from the surrounding pulmonary parenchyma.* ***(Right)*** *Higher magnification of a nodular lesion in a patient with pulmonary Langerhans cell histiocytosis shows sheets of monotonous tumor cells with round to oval nuclei and abundant lightly eosinophilic cytoplasm.*

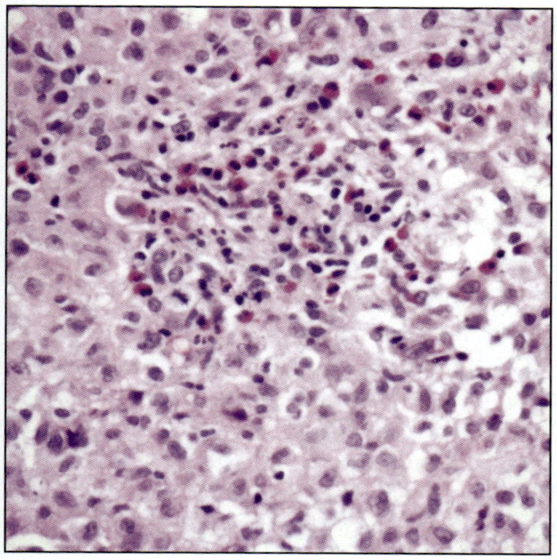

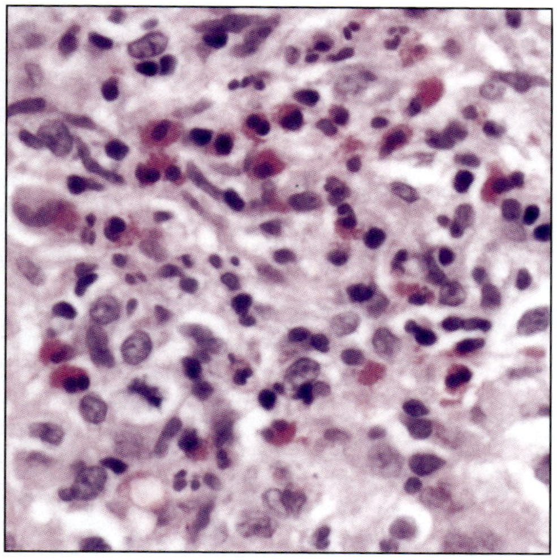

(Left) *Higher magnification of pulmonary Langerhans cell histiocytosis shows sheets of round to oval cells with abundant lightly eosinophilic cytoplasm admixed with scattered eosinophils.* ***(Right)*** *Higher magnification of a pulmonary lesion in Langerhans cell histiocytosis shows sheets of Langerhans cells with round to oval nuclei surrounded by an ample rim of lightly eosinophilic cytoplasm. There are numerous mature eosinophils scattered in the background.*

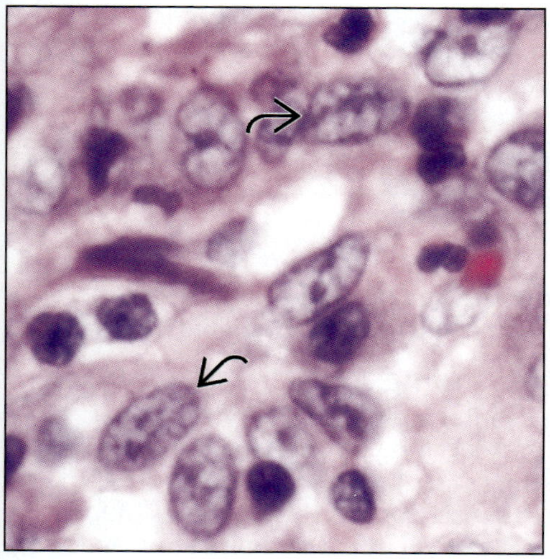

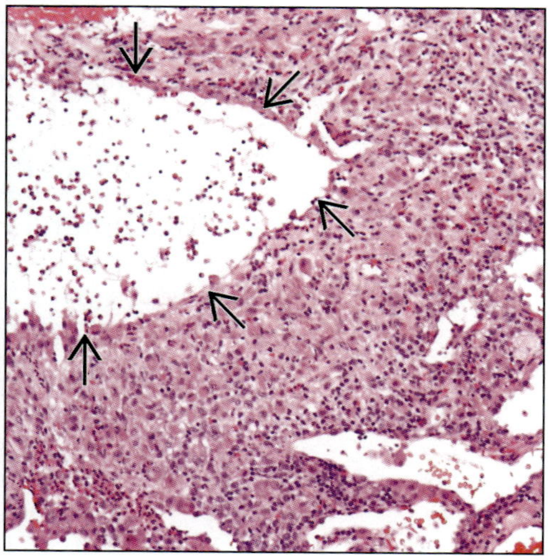

(Left) *Higher magnification of pulmonary Langerhans cell histiocytosis shows oval to spindle cells with vesicular nuclei that display nuclear convolutions and occasional longitudinal nuclear grooves ⇒. Nuclear convolutions and longitudinal nuclear grooves are 2 of the distinguishing features of Langerhans cells at the microscopic level.* ***(Right)*** *Pulmonary Langerhans cell histiocytosis shows a focus of central cavitation ⇒ (a characteristic feature of this process) frequently observed on CT scans.*

ERDHEIM-CHESTER DISEASE

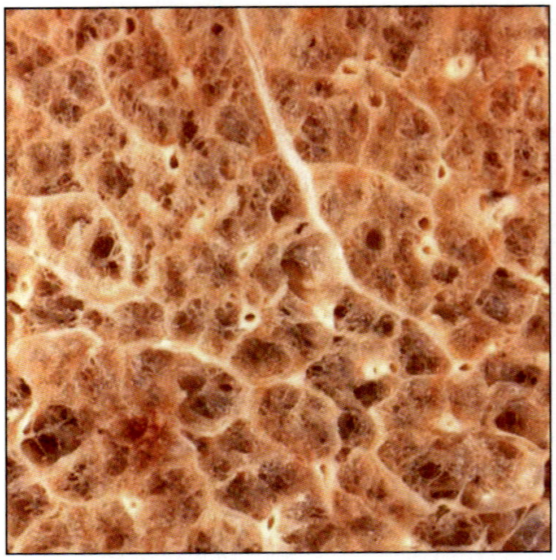

Gross appearance of the lung in Erdheim-Chester disease shows thickened interlobular septa with dilatation of airspaces.

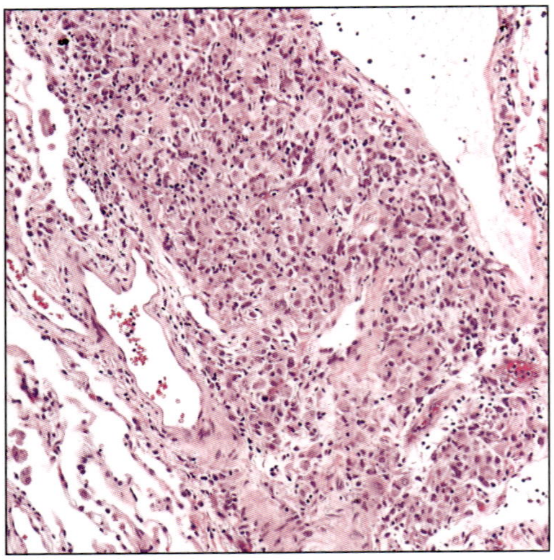

Erdheim-Chester disease of the lung shows characteristic widening of the interlobular septa by diffuse infiltration of foamy histiocytes.

TERMINOLOGY

Abbreviations

- Erdheim-Chester disease (ECD)

Synonyms

- Chester-Erdheim disease, lipoid granulomatosis

Definitions

- Rare histiocytic infiltrative disorder that most commonly affects bones but may affect other organs, including lung

ETIOLOGY/PATHOGENESIS

Etiology

- Unknown
- Has been proposed to be "macrophage counterpart" of Langerhans cell histiocytosis
- Study using HUMARA assay has demonstrated monoclonality in histiocytic cells in some cases

CLINICAL ISSUES

Epidemiology

- Incidence
  - Extremely rare condition
- Age
  - 25-70 years of age
- Gender
  - Slight male predominance

Site

- Bone involvement is most common site
- Extraskeletal involvement is seen in 50% of patients, including
  - Lung and pleura
  - Central nervous system
  - Kidney and retroperitoneum
  - Breast and skin
  - Heart and pericardium

Presentation

- Dyspnea
- Fever
- Weight loss
- Bone pain

Natural History

- Pulmonary involvement may precede skeletal manifestations in some cases
- Eventually, all patients develop skeletal manifestations
- Development of clearly delimited bilateral and symmetrical metaphyseal and diaphyseal areas of cortical sclerosis of long bones is classical
- Progressive disorder; morbidity and mortality depend on the presence or absence of extraskeletal involvement

Prognosis

- About 60% of patients die due to respiratory failure
- Patients with central nervous system involvement may die due to brain deterioration

IMAGE FINDINGS

General Features

- Location
  - Diffuse interstitial bilateral infiltrates with thickening of the pleura and interlobular septa

Radiographic Findings

- Characteristic radiographic finding is interstitial opacities with thickening of interlobular fissures and septa in the lung
- Symmetrical osteosclerosis of the diaphyses of long bones is the classical finding that helps confirm the diagnosis

ERDHEIM-CHESTER DISEASE

Key Facts

Terminology
- Rare histiocytic infiltrative disorder that most commonly affects bones but may affect other organs, including lung

Clinical Issues
- Bone involvement is most common site
- 50% of patients have extraskeletal involvement, including lungs
- Progressive disorder; morbidity and mortality depend on the presence or absence of extraskeletal involvement

Image Findings
- Diffuse interstitial bilateral infiltrates with thickening of the pleura and interlobular septa
- Characteristic radiographic finding is interstitial opacities with thickening of interlobular fissures and septae in the lung
- Symmetrical osteosclerosis of the diaphyses of long bones

Microscopic Pathology
- Diffuse infiltration of histiocytes along lymphatic routes, including the pleura, septa, and perivascular and peribronchiolar interstitium
- Characteristic thickening of the pleura that tracks into lung parenchyma along the interlobular septa

Ancillary Tests
- Histiocytes are positive for CD68 and factor XIIIa
- Scattered S100 positive cells may be identified

CT Findings
- Interlobular septal thickening with areas of ground-glass attenuation and centrilobular, nodular opacities
- Bullous or cystic lesions may also be seen
- Pleural thickening and pleural or pericardial effusion

MICROSCOPIC PATHOLOGY

Histologic Features
- Diffuse infiltration of histiocytes along lymphatic routes, including the pleura, septa, and perivascular and peribronchiolar interstitium
- Characteristic thickening of the pleura that tracks into lung parenchyma along the interlobular septa
- Histiocytic cell infiltrate is admixed with stromal fibrosis in varying degrees

Cytologic Features
- Histiocytes are generally small with round or oval nuclei and a scant rim of cytoplasm
- Histiocytes may be accompanied by small lymphocytes, plasma cells, and eosinophils
- Absence of nuclear atypia, mitotic figures, or anaplasia
- Absence of osteoclastic giant cells or grooved, convoluted nuclei

ANCILLARY TESTS

Immunohistochemistry
- Histiocytes are positive for CD68 and factor XIIIa
- Scattered S100 positive cells may be identified
  - Stains for CD1a, CD45RB, and CD21 are negative
  - Stains for cytokeratins are negative

Electron Microscopy
- Transmission
  - Cells show cytoplasmic phagolysosomes containing lipid
  - No Birbeck granules are identified

DIFFERENTIAL DIAGNOSIS

Langerhans Cell Histiocytosis
- Histiocytic cells have oval nuclei with longitudinal grooves and nuclear convolutions
- Prominent eosinophilic infiltration is present admixed with the histiocytic cells
- Osteoclastic giant cells are often present admixed with the infiltrate
- Histiocytic cells are positive for CD1a and S100 protein
- Histiocytic cells contain distinctive organelles (Birbeck granules) on electron microscopy

Sinus Histiocytosis with Massive Lymphadenopathy (Rosai-Dorfman Disease)
- Histiocytic disorder of unknown etiology that can also involve the lung
- Usually forms well-circumscribed lesions without pleural involvement or septal distribution
- Histiocytes are large with enlarged, vesicular nuclei and abundant cytoplasm
- Histiocytic cells
  - Display prominent emperipolesis
  - Are accompanied by abundant plasma cells
  - Strongly positive for S100 protein

SELECTED REFERENCES

1. Bisceglia M et al: Erdheim-Chester disease: clinical and pathologic spectrum of four cases from the Arkadi M. Rywlin slide seminars. Adv Anat Pathol. 10(3):160-71, 2003
2. Wittenberg KH et al: Pulmonary involvement with Erdheim-Chester disease: radiographic and CT findings. AJR Am J Roentgenol. 174(5):1327-31, 2000
3. Chetritt J et al: Chester-Erdheim disease: a neoplastic disorder. Hum Pathol. 30(9):1093-6, 1999
4. Egan AJ et al: Erdheim-Chester disease: clinical, radiologic, and histopathologic findings in five patients with interstitial lung disease. Am J Surg Pathol. 23(1):17-26, 1999

ERDHEIM-CHESTER DISEASE

Histologic Features

(Left) *Characteristic appearance of Erdheim-Chester disease of the lung shows a thickened pleura in continuity with a widened interlobular septa → containing a proliferation of histiocytes.* ***(Right)*** *Higher magnification of the pleura in pulmonary involvement by Erdheim-Chester disease shows dramatic widening ⇨ by a proliferation of small histiocytes. A few admixed small lymphocytes are also present against a mildly fibrotic stroma.*

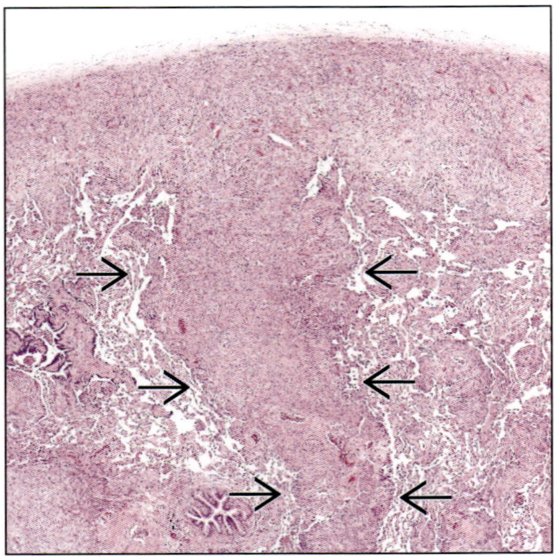

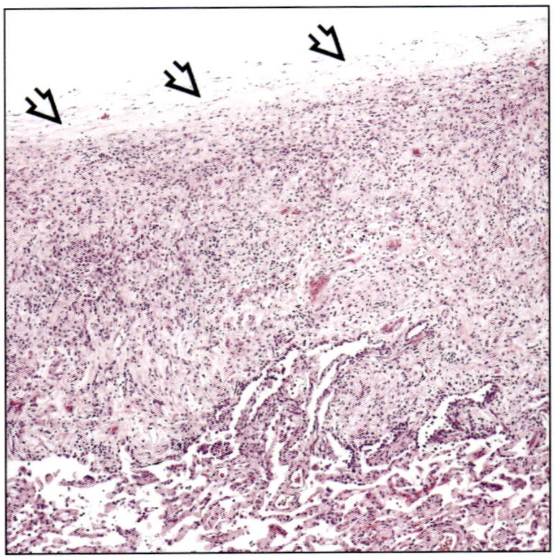

(Left) *Erdheim-Chester disease of the lung shows widening of the perivascular interstitium by the proliferation of small histiocytes admixed with variable degrees of stromal sclerosis.* ***(Right)*** *Higher magnification of lung infiltrate in a patient with Erdheim-Chester disease shows a mononuclear cell population primarily composed of histiocytes admixed with scattered small lymphocytes, plasma cells, and occasional eosinophils. The histiocytic infiltrate is accompanied by stromal fibrosis.*

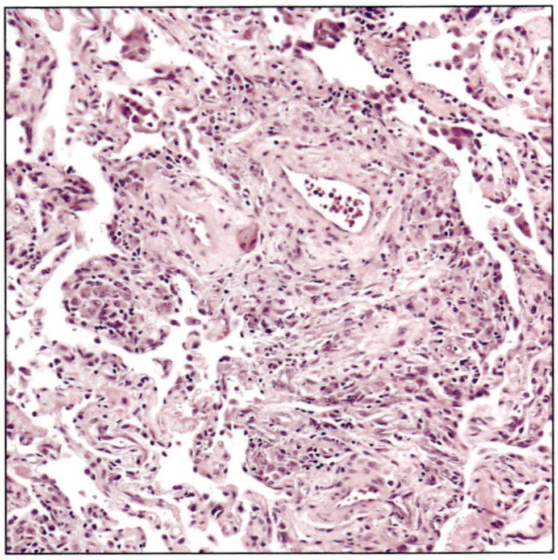

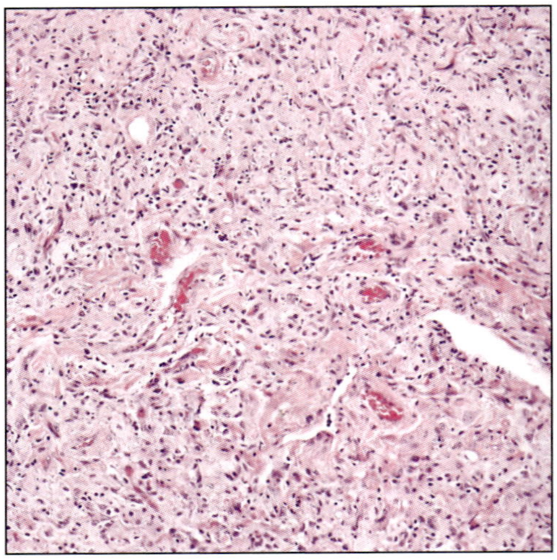

(Left) *Higher magnification of lung involvement in a patient with Erdheim-Chester disease shows a sparse population of small lymphocytes scattered between small histiocytes.* ***(Right)*** *Higher magnification of lung involved with Erdheim-Chester disease shows histiocytic proliferation characterized by round to oval nuclei surrounded by a scant rim of amphophilic to eosinophilic cytoplasm. A few rare cells can show multinucleation, but nuclear atypia and mitoses are not encountered.*

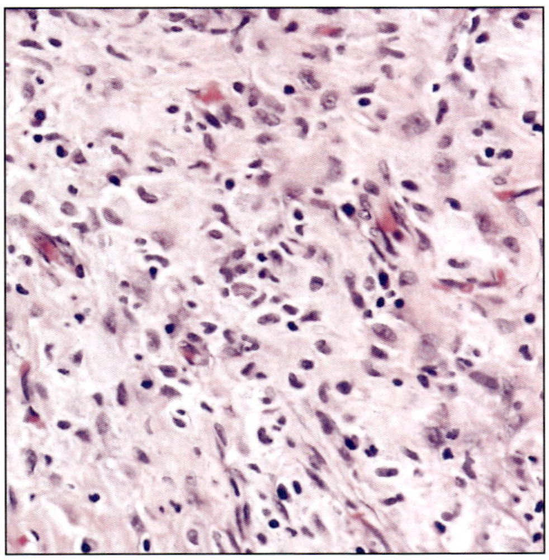

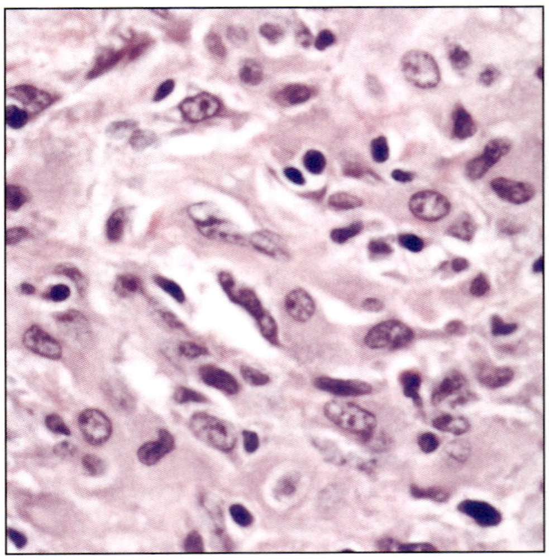

Other Features

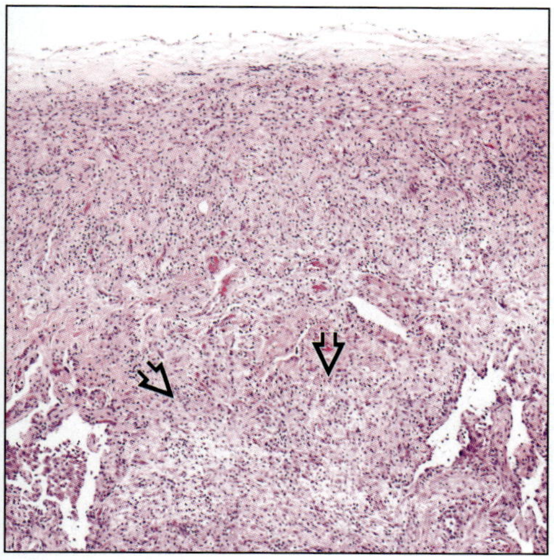

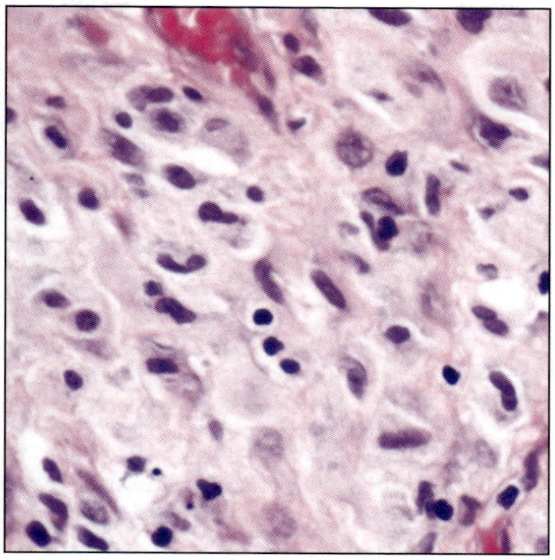

(Left) *Histologic appearance of Erdheim-Chester disease of the lung shows massive widening of the pleura by the proliferation of small, bland-appearing histiocytes that extend along the interlobular septa into the lung parenchyma ⇨.* ***(Right)*** *Higher magnification of Erdheim-Chester disease involving the lung shows a bland-appearing population of histiocytes admixed with a few scattered small lymphocytes. The histiocytes are singly scattered in a dense collagenous matrix.*

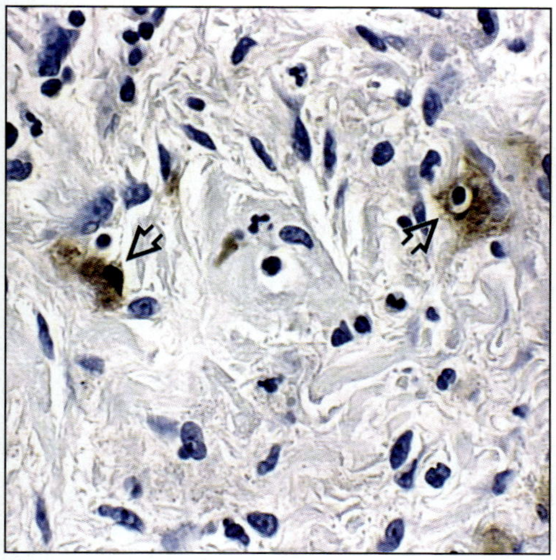

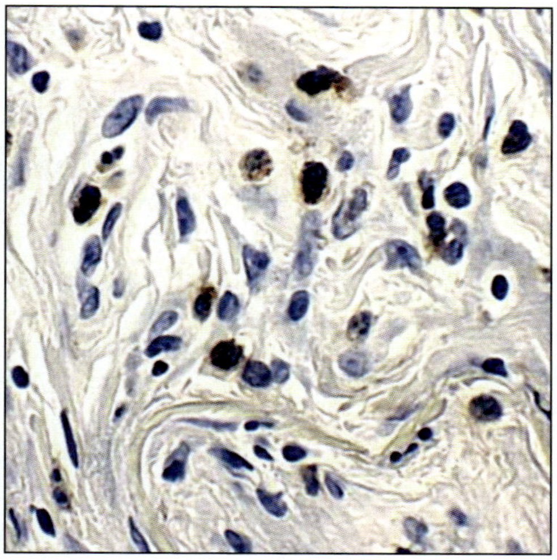

(Left) *Immunohistochemical staining of Erdheim-Chester disease with S100 protein shows a few cells ⇨ displaying nuclear and cytoplasmic positivity for this antigen.* ***(Right)*** *Immunohistochemical staining of Erdheim-Chester disease involving the lung for CD68 shows scattered small histiocytes that stain positive for this antibody. The cells are negative for CD1a antibodies and do not otherwise display the cytological or ultrastructural features of Langerhans cells.*

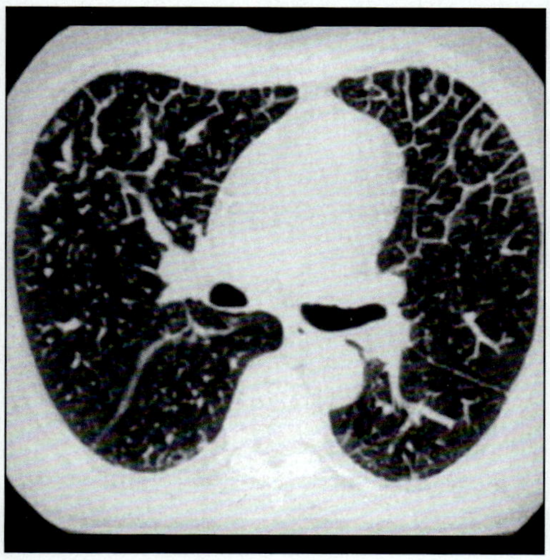

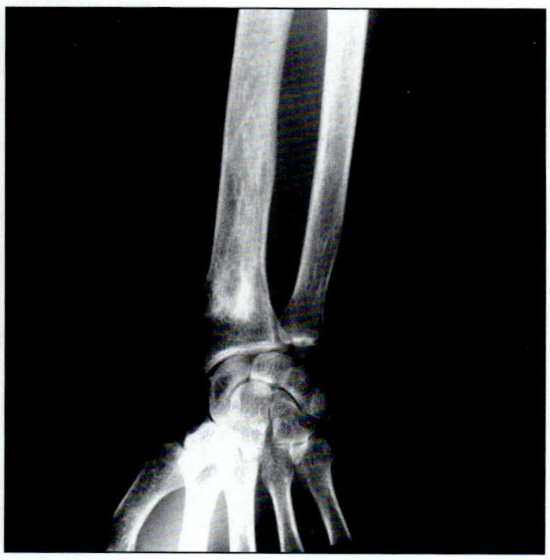

(Left) *CT scan of the chest in a patient with Erdheim-Chester disease shows a typical radiographic image characterized by interlobular septal thickening with areas of ground-glass attenuation.* ***(Right)*** *Radiograph of the hand and forearm shows characteristic symmetrical osteosclerosis of the long bones. This radiographic appearance is typical for Erdheim-Chester disease and permits confirmation of the histologic diagnosis.*

ALVEOLAR MICROLITHIASIS

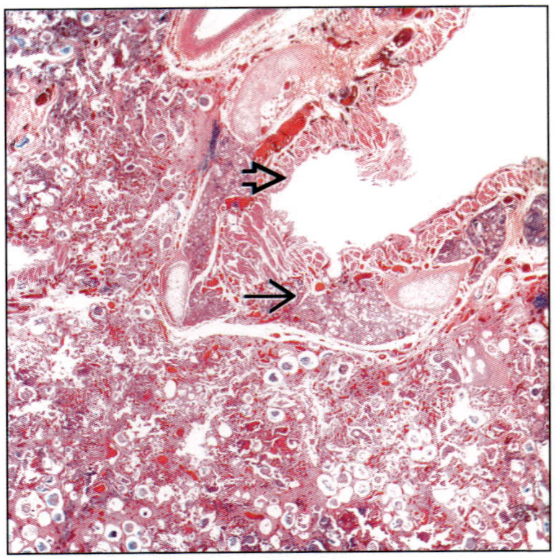

Low-power view of alveolar microlithiasis shows the main bronchus ⇨ and adjacent bronchial glands not involved by the process →.

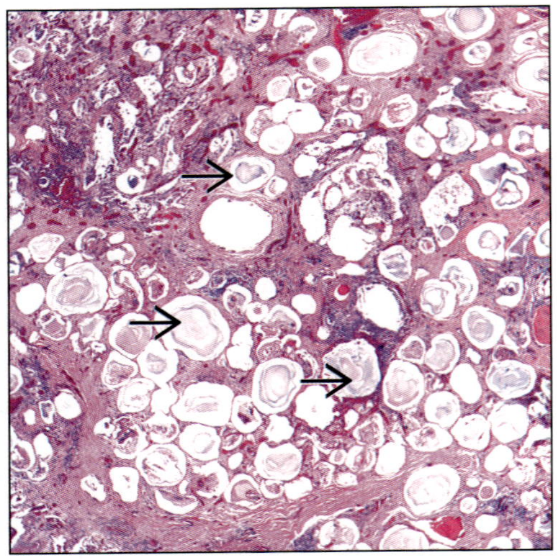

Pulmonary microlithiasis shows numerous calcospherites → in an intraalveolar location. This pattern is classical of pulmonary alveolar microlithiasis.

TERMINOLOGY

Synonyms

- Pulmonary microlithiasis

Definitions

- Extensive deposition of microliths in alveolar spaces

ETIOLOGY/PATHOGENESIS

Etiology

- Rare condition of unknown etiology
- Familial pattern has been observed in some cases

CLINICAL ISSUES

Presentation

- Cough
- Shortness of breath
- Malaise
- Fatigue
- Decrease in respiratory performance
- No metabolic abnormalities

Laboratory Tests

- Normal calcium and phosphates in serum
- No signs of hyperparathyroidism
- Decreased pulmonary function tests

Natural History

- This condition may become apparent at any age and may follow a rapid fatal course
- May become apparent in younger patients with variable course
  - Protracted course
  - Rapid course with respiratory failure and death

Treatment

- No specific treatment

Prognosis

- Variable

IMAGE FINDINGS

General Features

- "Sandstorm" pattern

MACROSCOPIC FEATURES

General Features

- Honeycomb changes in lung parenchyma

MICROSCOPIC PATHOLOGY

Histologic Features

- Intraalveolar deposition of spherical calcifications
- Each calcospherite measures about 250-750 μm
- Laminated bodies with "onion skin" features
- Interstitial fibrosis may be seen
- Areas of ossification may be present
- Minimal inflammatory reaction
- Chemical analysis shows calcospherites to be made of phosphorus and calcium

Predominant Pattern/Injury Type

- Calcification

DIFFERENTIAL DIAGNOSIS

Metastatic Calcification (Dendritic Calcification)

- Calcification follows alveolar wall and interstitium
- Absence of calcospherites in intraalveolar spaces
- Generally, there is history of underlying condition, which is not the case with microlithiasis

Key Facts

Terminology
- Extensive deposition of microliths in alveolar spaces

Etiology/Pathogenesis
- Rare condition of unknown etiology
- Familial pattern has been observed in some cases
- Can occur at any age

Clinical Issues
- Decrease in respiratory performance
- No metabolic abnormalities
- No specific treatment
- Variable
- Protracted course
- Rapid course with respiratory failure and death

Image Findings
- "Sandstorm" pattern

Microscopic Pathology
- Intraalveolar deposition of spherical calcifications
- Each calcospherite measures about 250-750 μm
- Laminated bodies with "onion skin" features
- Chemical analysis shows calcospherites to be made of phosphorus and calcium

Top Differential Diagnoses
- Metastatic calcification (dendritic calcification)
  - Absence of calcospherites in intraalveolar spaces
- Corpora amylacea
  - "Onion skin" features of microlithiasis are not present in corpora amylacea
  - Corpora is usually not intraalveolar location

Histochemical Features of Alveolar Microlithiasis

Stain	Result
Von Kossa	Positive in microliths
Iron	May show positive staining in some microliths
Mucicarmine	Negative
PAS	Negative
D-PAS	Negative
*Chemical Analysis**	
Calcium	High in chemical analysis
Phosphorus	High in chemical analysis

Chemical analysis is the best procedure to determine the composition of the microliths.

- Chemical analysis of metastatic calcification and that of microlithiasis is different

Corpora Amylacea
- Less extensive distribution than microlithiasis
- "Onion skin" features of microlithiasis are not present in corpora amylacea
- Overall, presence of corpora amylacea is haphazard and commonly involves interstitium
- Presence of corpora amylacea may be seen in otherwise normal lung
- Chemical analysis of corpora amylacea is different

Blue Bodies
- These bodies are present only focally in areas of lung parenchyma and are much smaller than microliths
- Will not have distribution of microlithiasis
- Sporadic
- Blue bodies are commonly seen in inflammatory conditions of lung
- Chemical analysis is also different

DIAGNOSTIC CHECKLIST

Pathologic Interpretation Pearls
- Intraalveolar calcospherites with "onion skin" features

SELECTED REFERENCES

1. Dahabreh M et al: Pulmonary alveolar microlithiasis in an 8-month-old infant. Ann Trop Paediatr. 29(1):55-9, 2009
2. Horvatić Herceg G et al: "Sandstorm" image: bone scintigraphy in pulmonary alveolar microlithiasis. Eur J Nucl Med Mol Imaging. 36(8):1353, 2009
3. Moran CA et al: Unusual non-neoplastic lesions of the lung. Semin Diagn Pathol. 24(3):199-208, 2007
4. Eggert CH et al: Metastatic pulmonary calcification in a dialysis patient: case report and a review. Hemodial Int. 10 Suppl 2:S51-5, 2006
5. Wang HY et al: Pulmonary alveolar microlithiasis: report of four familial cases. Chin Med J (Engl). 2004 Jun;117(6):950-2. Erratum in: Chin Med J (Engl). 119(10):870, 2006
6. Burke LM et al: Pulmonary alveolar microlithiasis. Critical Care Int. 8:6-7, 1998
7. Moran CA et al: Pulmonary alveolar microlithiasis. A clinicopathologic and chemical analysis of seven cases. Arch Pathol Lab Med. 121(6):607-11, 1997
8. Prakash UB et al: Pulmonary alveolar microlithiasis. A review including ultrastructural and pulmonary function studies. Mayo Clin Proc. 58(5):290-300, 1983
9. Koss MN et al: Pulmonary blue bodies. Hum Pathol. 12(3):258-66, 1981

ALVEOLAR MICROLITHIASIS

Gross and Microscopic Features

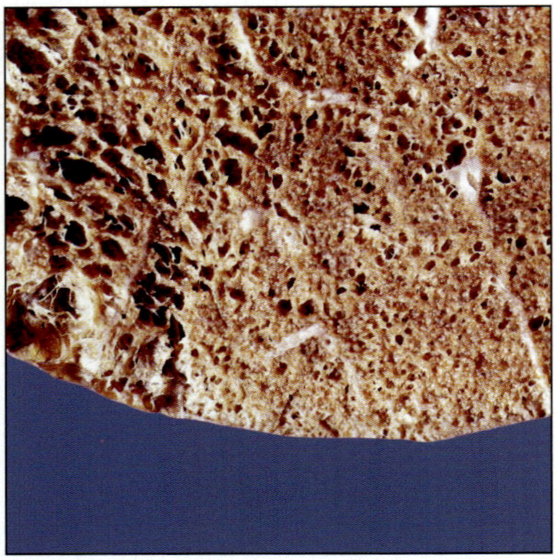

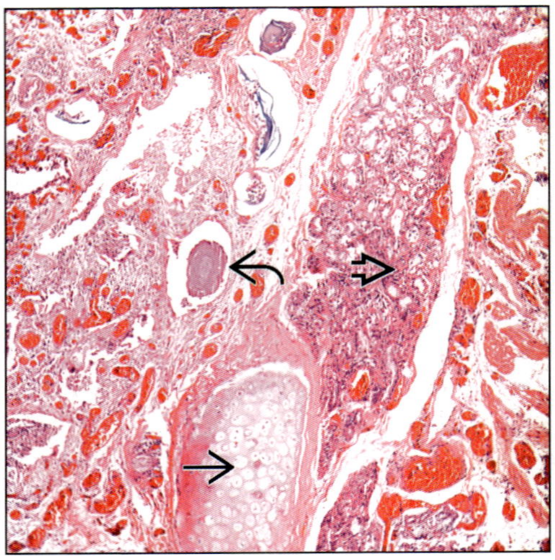

(Left) *Portion of lung shows a honeycomb appearance. This pattern, although not classical of alveolar microlithiasis, may be seen in some advanced cases. Similar features may be seen in cases of pulmonary fibrosis.* ***(Right)*** *Low-power view of the bronchial wall shows the bronchial cartilage → and endobronchial glands ⇨ not involved by the process, which is essentially an intraalveolar process ↷. Thus, bronchial biopsies will rarely be diagnostic of this process.*

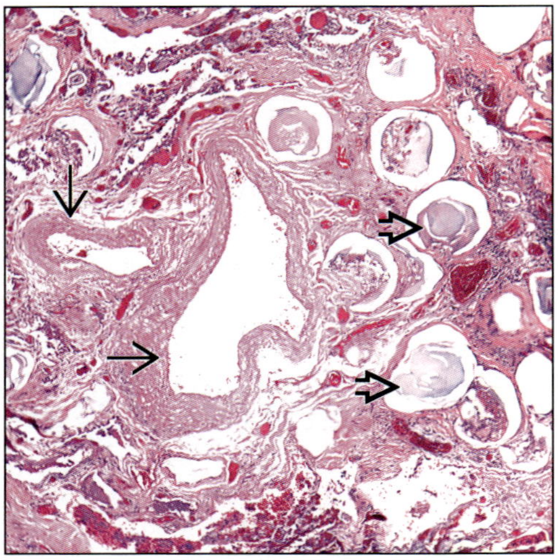

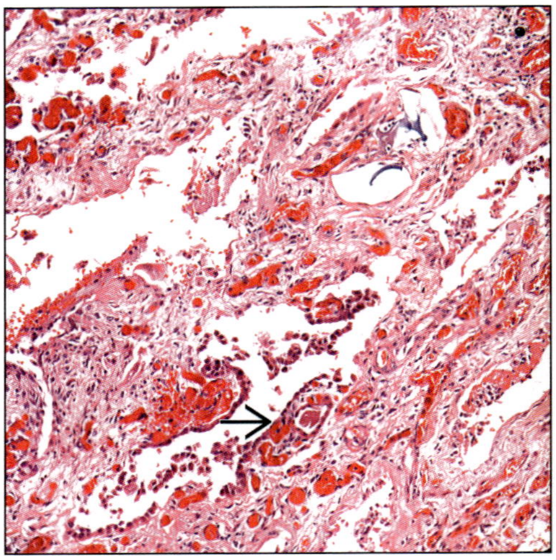

(Left) *Lung parenchyma shows prominent dilated vascular structures not involved by the process →. Adjacent alveolar structures are filled with microliths ⇨. This is the classical pattern of distribution of this unusual process.* ***(Right)*** *Uninvolved lung parenchyma shows areas of fibrosis with only remnants of epithelial lining →. No microliths are present. Even in resected material, skip areas of uninvolved lung parenchyma will be present.*

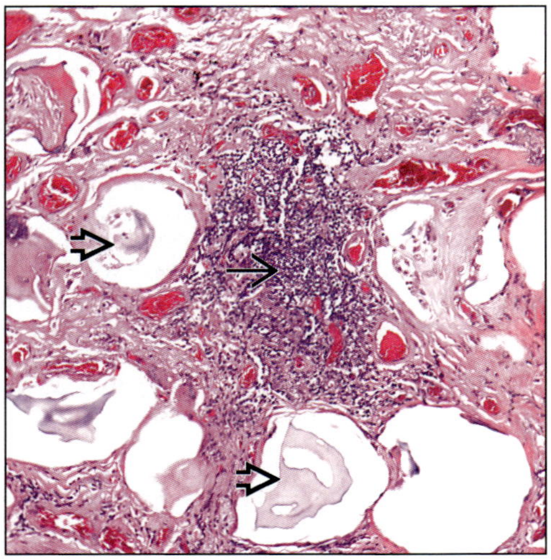

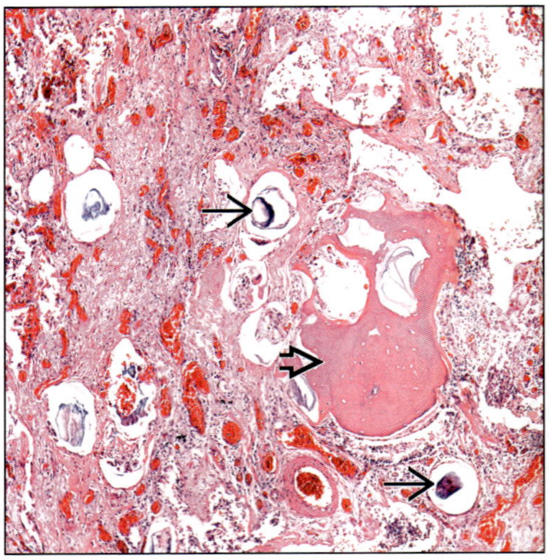

(Left) *Alveolar microlithiasis shows areas of fibrosis with chronic inflammation →. Adjacent alveolar structures are filled with microliths ⇨. The microliths do not show the classical structural features and may be confused with foreign material.* ***(Right)*** *A common finding in alveolar microlithiasis → is the presence of ossification ⇨. Note the difference between the 2 processes. In the ossified component, one can still see bone rims.*

Microscopic Features

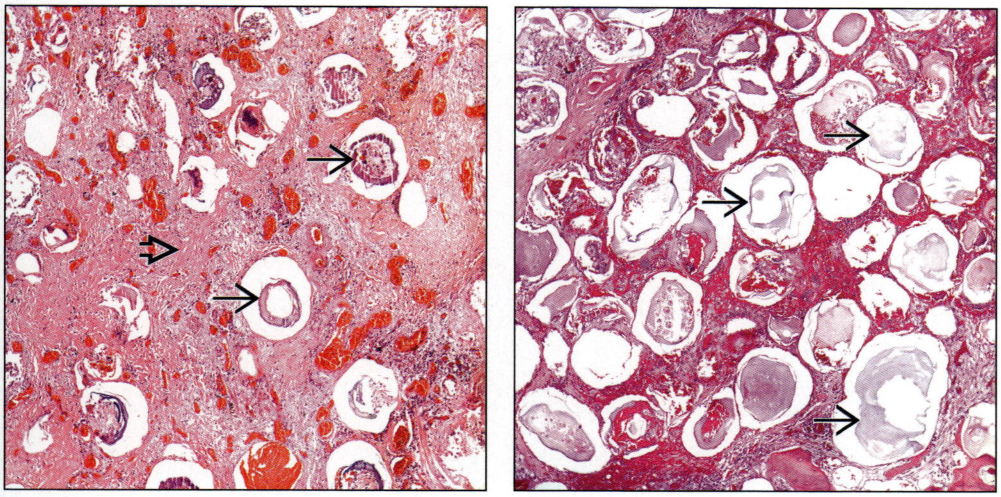

(Left) *Alveolar microlithiasis shows degenerated microliths* →*. Extensive fibrosis of the lung parenchyma is also present* ⇒*. This pattern may suggest a fibrotic lung disease with foreign material.* ***(Right)*** *Alveolar microlithiasis shows numerous microliths with a more cartilaginous appearance* →*. The morphological features of the microliths are different from the classical ones showing the "onion skin" features.*

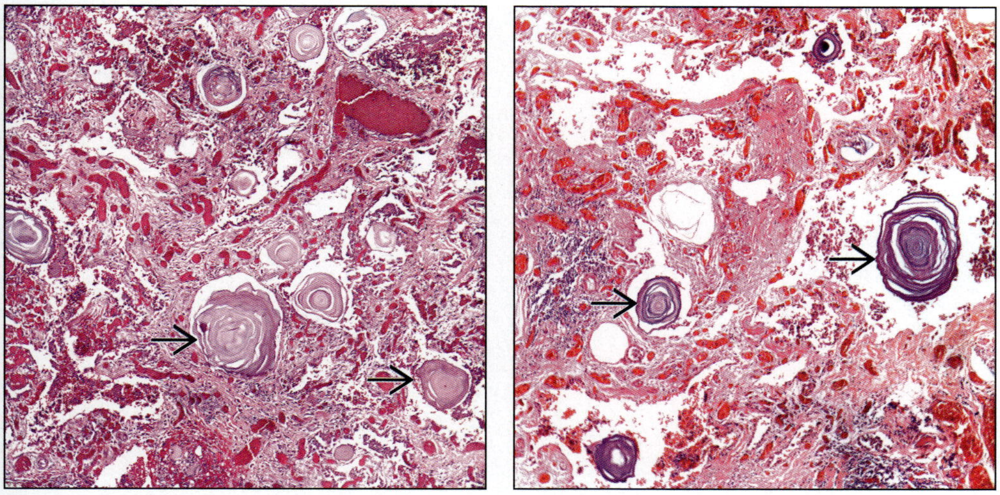

(Left) *Low-power view of alveolar microlithiasis shows only a few microliths* → *embedded in a predominantly fibrotic lung parenchyma. Although the number of microliths is not prominent, their morphology is classical and diagnostic of alveolar microlithiasis.* ***(Right)*** *Typical appearance of microliths in alveolar microlithiasis shows the classical "onion skin" changes* →*. Even though they are not numerous, they are diagnostic.*

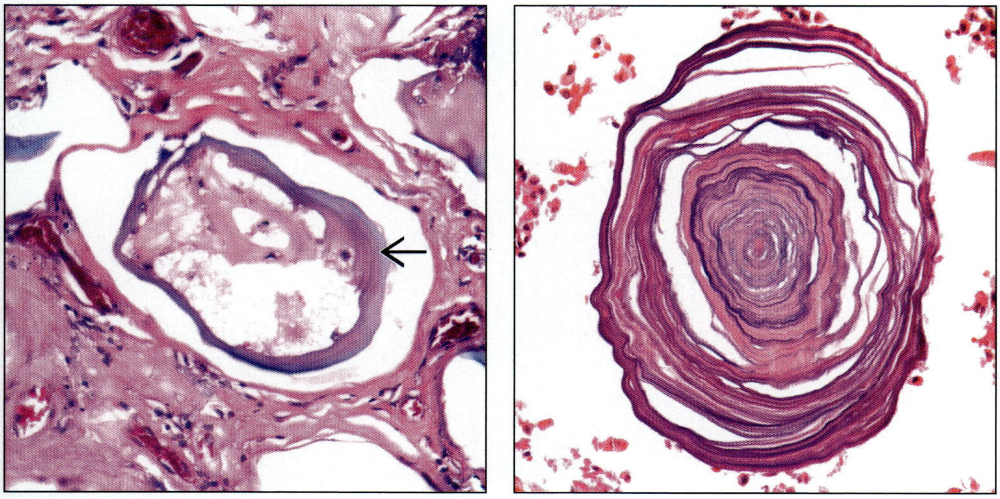

(Left) *High-power view of a microlith shows degenerative changes in which the structure has only a thin rim of calcification* →*. The "onion skin" pattern is not present. These degenerative changes in the microliths may be related to the long course of the process.* ***(Right)*** *High-power view of a microlith in alveolar microlithiasis shows the "onion skin" changes of this structure. This morphological appearance is classical and diagnostic of alveolar microlithiasis.*

Parasitic Disorders

STRONGYLOIDIASIS

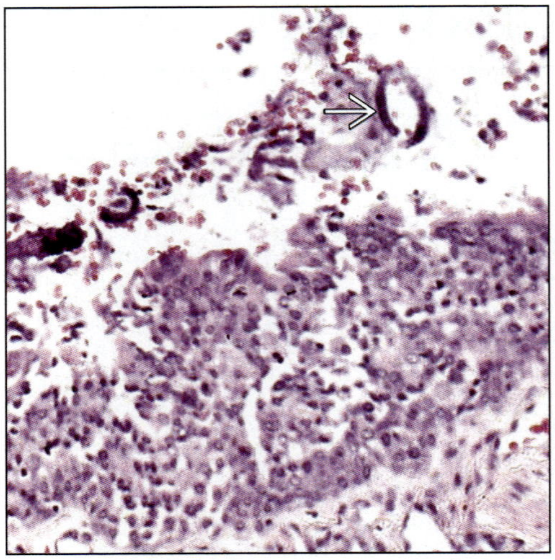

Low-power view of a pulmonary airway shows respiratory epithelium with inflammatory changes and focal necrosis. Even at this power, it is possible to identify some filariform larvae ➡.

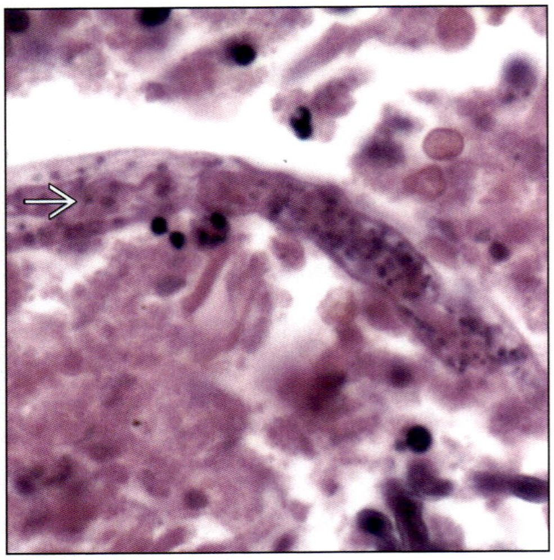

High-power view shows rhabditiform larvae of Strongyloides ➡ admixed with necrosis. The rhabditiform larva is most commonly encountered on histological examinations.

TERMINOLOGY

Synonyms

- Cochin China diarrhea, thread worm infection

Definitions

- Parasitic infection caused by a nematode

ETIOLOGY/PATHOGENESIS

Infectious Agents

- *Strongyloides stercoralis*

3 Cycles of Infection

- Direct
  - Filariform larvae penetrate the skin
    - Cutaneous phase may last a few days
- Indirect
  - Rhabditiform larvae mature into free-living males and females in the soil
- Autoinfection
  - Rhabditiform larvae become infective filariform larvae in intestine or skin of the host

CLINICAL ISSUES

Epidemiology

- Incidence
  - Worldwide distribution
  - More common in tropical countries
  - High in conditions that promote fecal contamination
- Age
  - Affects any age group
- Gender
  - Infection may be more common in males
- Ethnicity
  - No ethnic predisposition

Presentation

- Skin itching
- Skin edema
- Urticaria
- Low-grade fever
- Cough
- Dyspnea
- Hemoptysis
- Bronchopneumonia
- Intermittent diarrhea
- Cramping
- Constipation
- Anemia
- Asymptomatic

Laboratory Tests

- Eosinophilia
- Leukocytosis
- Feces study is important in diagnosis
- Enzyme-linked immunosorbent assays (ELISA) for IgG antibodies to antigens of larvae of *Strongyloides*

Treatment

- Drugs
  - Thiabendazole
  - Albendazole

Prognosis

- Depends on immune status of patient
  - In immunocompromised patients, disseminated hyperinfection can take place
  - In nonimmunocompromised patients, prognosis is good after treatment

MICROSCOPIC PATHOLOGY

Histologic Features

- Inflammatory reaction with prominent eosinophils
- Suppurative exudate
- Presence of larvae

STRONGYLOIDIASIS

Key Facts

Terminology
- Synonyms
  - Cochin China diarrhea, thread worm infection
- Definition
  - Parasitic infection caused by nematode

Clinical Issues
- Epidemiology
  - Worldwide distribution
  - More common in tropical countries
  - High in conditions that promote fecal contamination
- Symptoms
  - Urticaria
  - Cough
  - Dyspnea
  - Hemoptysis
  - Bronchopneumonia
  - Intermittent diarrhea
- Laboratory tests
  - Eosinophilia
  - Leukocytosis
  - Feces study is important in diagnosis
  - Enzyme-linked immunosorbent assays (ELISA) for IgG antibodies to antigens of larvae of *Strongyloides*

Microscopic Pathology
- Inflammatory reaction with prominent eosinophils
- Suppurative exudate
- Presence of larvae
- Presence of adult worm

Diagnostic Methods for Identification of Strongyloidiasis

Method	Result
Fresh stools	Identification of larvae or adult worm
Tissue biopsy	Identification of larvae or adult worm
Aspirates	Identification of larvae
ELISA for IgG antibodies	May be elevated

Histochemical Features

Stain	Result
Hematoxylin-eosin	Identifies larvae and adult worm
Movat	Accentuates outlines of adult worm
Giemsa	Identifies larvae
Papanicolaou stain	Identifies larvae

- Presence of adult worm

DIFFERENTIAL DIAGNOSIS

Parasitic Infections
- Hookworm
- Ascariasis
  - Morphology and size of those parasites are different from *Strongyloides*

Bronchopneumonia
- Even though there may be inflammatory component, bacterial pneumonia will lack presence of larvae

Dirofilaria immitis
- *Dirofilaria* is larger parasite
- Dirofilaria generally form necrotic tumor nodules
- Presence of larvae would be more in keeping with *Strongyloides*

DIAGNOSTIC CHECKLIST

Pathologic Interpretation Pearls
- Prominent inflammatory reaction with increased eosinophils
- Presence of larvae
- Presence of adult worm

SELECTED REFERENCES

1. Apewokin S et al: Strongyloides hyperinfection diagnosed by bronchoalveolar lavage in an immunocompromized host. Cytopathology. 21(5):345-7, 2010
2. Basile A et al: Disseminated Strongyloides stercoralis: hyperinfection during medical immunosuppression. J Am Acad Dermatol. 63(5):896-902, 2010
3. Bon B et al: Evaluation of a rapid enzyme-linked immunosorbent assay for diagnosis of strongyloidiasis. J Clin Microbiol. 48(5):1716-9, 2010
4. Feely NM et al: Strongyloides stercoralis hyperinfection: difficulties in diagnosis and treatment. Anaesthesia. 65(3):298-301, 2010

STRONGYLOIDIASIS

Microscopic Features

*(**Left**) Pulmonary parenchyma shows focal areas of an ill-defined granulomatous reaction. Such a finding is unusual in cases of strongyloidiasis. (**Right**) Pulmonary parenchyma shows a rhabditiform larva of Strongyloides ➔. Note the absence of reactive changes in the adjacent lung parenchyma. In some cases, the parasites are not numerous and are difficult to identify.*

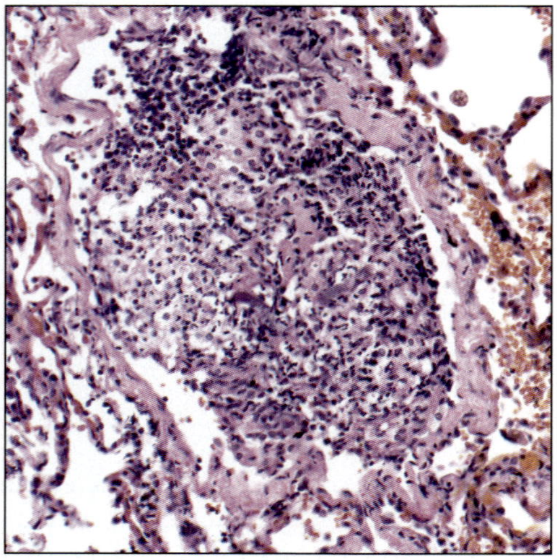

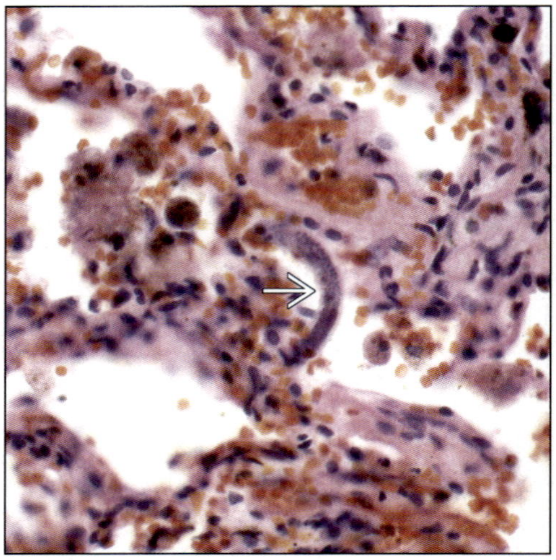

*(**Left**) High power shows Strongyloides eggs ➔ admixed with epithelial cells most likely exfoliated from the bronchial respiratory epithelium. Once again, the reaction is not marked. (**Right**) A single rhabditiform larva of Strongyloides ➔ is present. In this particular case, there is an associated inflammatory reaction with some destruction of the normal lung architecture.*

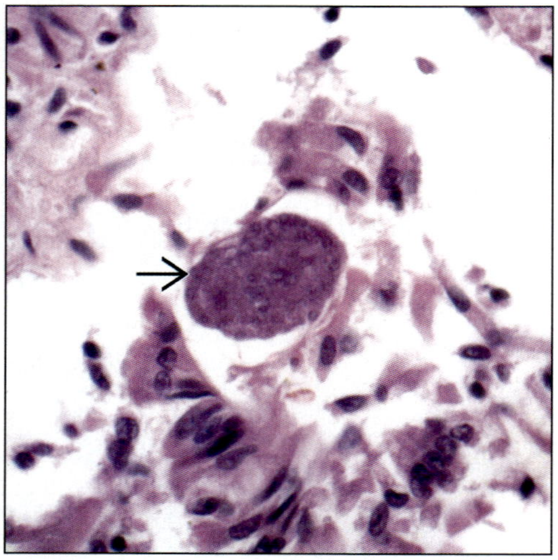

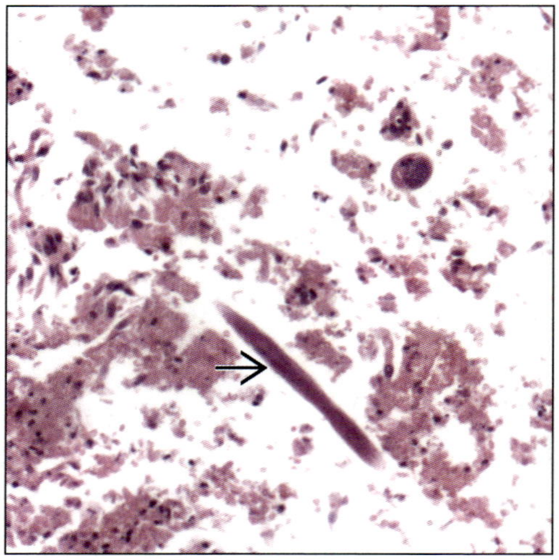

*(**Left**) The diagnosis of pulmonary strongyloidiasis can also be accomplished by aspiration cytology. This aspiration depicts the presence of inflammatory cells and numerous Strongyloides forms, difficult to visualize at this power. (**Right**) On higher magnification, the presence of filariform larvae of Strongyloides ➔ is easily detected, and they are admixed with epithelial and inflammatory cells.*

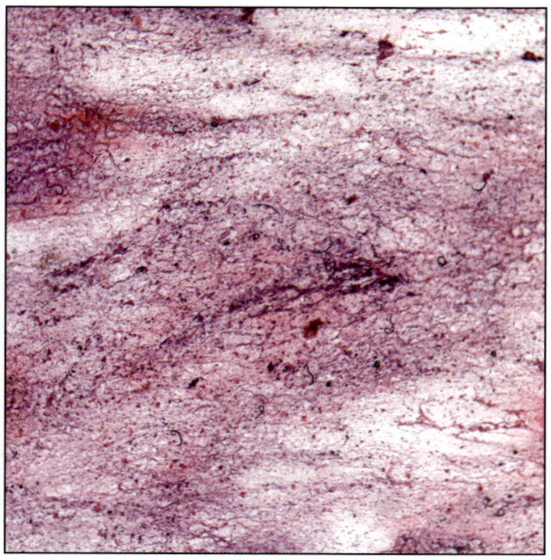

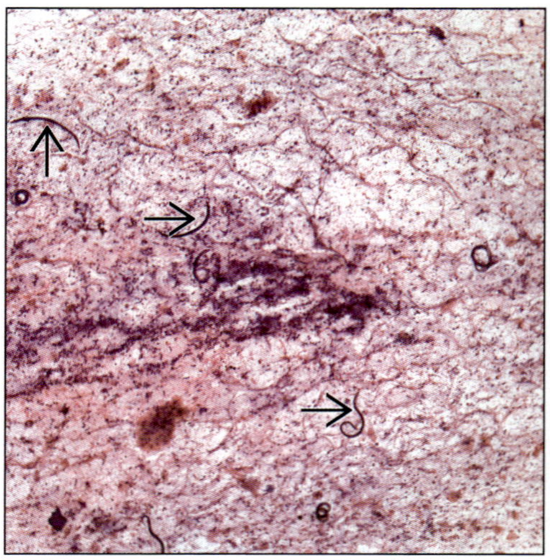

STRONGYLOIDIASIS

Microscopic Features

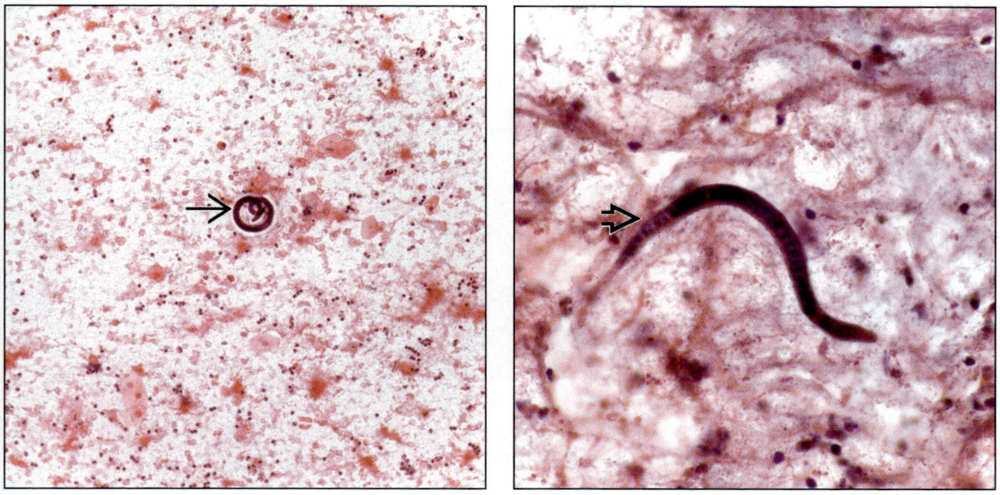

(Left) *Pulmonary aspirate shows numerous cellular debris admixed with blood and a single rhabditiform larva of Strongyloides →, which is enough to establish a diagnosis of pulmonary infection.* ***(Right)*** *High-power magnification shows a filariform larva of Strongyloides ⇨. Similar features may be seen in filarial diseases. Note the absence of a prominent inflammatory reaction in this lung aspirate.*

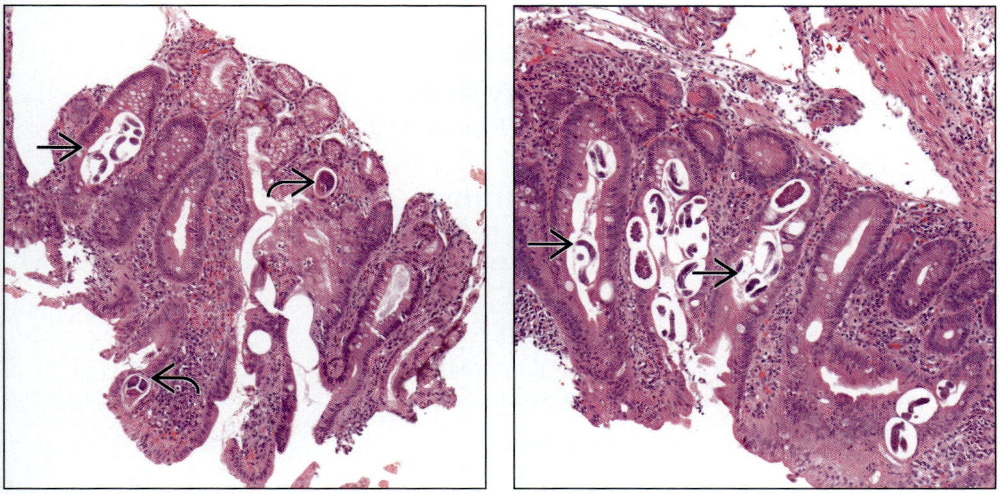

(Left) *Low-power magnification shows a duodenal biopsy in which the glands are filled with numerous filariform larvae of Strongyloides →. Also note the presence of adult parasites ↗.* ***(Right)*** *In this high magnification, the glandular component of the duodenum is filled with numerous filariform larvae of Strongyloides →, similar to those encountered in the lung parenchyma.*

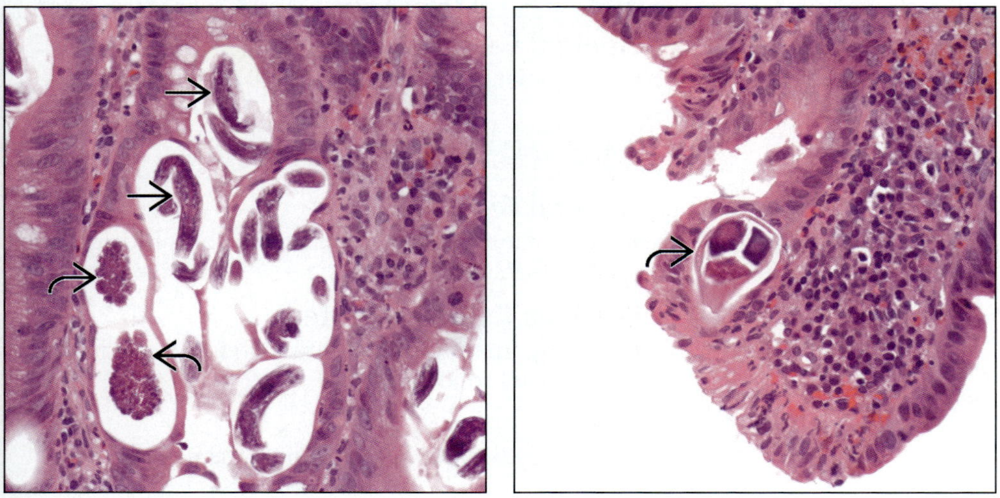

(Left) *High-power view shows numerous rhabditiform larvae of Strongyloides →. Also note the presence of eggs of Strongyloides ↗.* ***(Right)*** *High-power view shows an adult Strongyloides ↗. This finding appears to be more commonly seen in intestinal biopsies than in pulmonary infection.*

DIROFILARIASIS

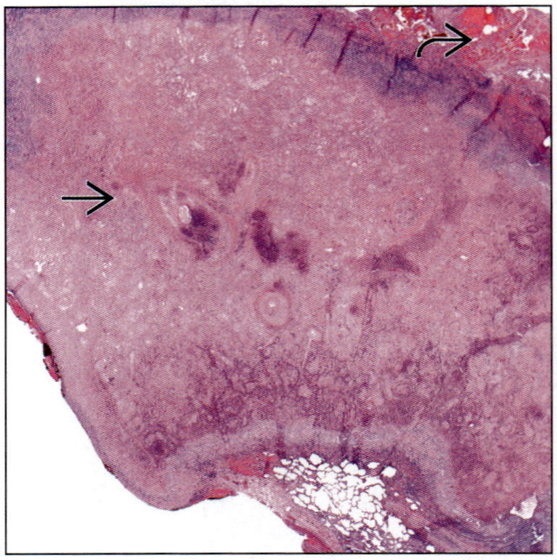

Low-power view of a necrotic pulmonary nodule → shows that the nodule is well demarcated and destroys normal lung parenchyma. A little rim of normal lung parenchyma is still present ↷.

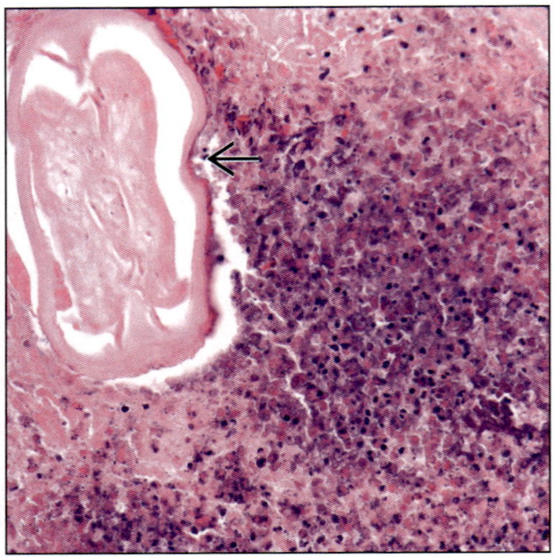

High-power view of a nonviable worm typical of dirofilariasis is present →. The worm is embedded in necrotic material, which makes it difficult to identify.

TERMINOLOGY

Definitions

- Infectious condition caused by helminth

ETIOLOGY/PATHOGENESIS

Etiology

- Caused by *Dirofilaria immitis*
  - Dirofilariasis is more common in dogs
  - Humans are accidental hosts

CLINICAL ISSUES

Epidemiology

- Incidence
  - Uncommon infectious condition
- Age
  - Can occur at any age, and infection has been described in children and adults
  - More common in adults
- Gender
  - May be more common in males than in females
- Ethnicity
  - No ethnic predilection

Site

- Worms lodge in the heart but die before reaching maturity
- Worms pass into pulmonary arteries
- Right lung appears to be more commonly involved
- Peripheral lung lesions are by far more common
- Central lung lesions are unusual

Presentation

- Symptoms
  - Cough
  - Dyspnea
  - Wheezing
  - Chest pain
  - Fever
    - Some patients may be asymptomatic

Laboratory Tests

- Eosinophilia may be present in about 10-15% of patients

Natural History

- Not associated with immunosuppression
- In some cases, it is associated with history of previous malignancy

Treatment

- Surgical approaches
  - Complete surgical resection is curative

Prognosis

- Excellent

IMAGE FINDINGS

General Features

- May present as single or multiple lung nodules

MACROSCOPIC FEATURES

General Features

- Well-circumscribed necrotic nodule of soft consistency ± hemorrhage

Sections to Be Submitted

- It is important to submit entire nodule as worms may be difficult to identify

Size

- May vary from 1 cm to > 5 cm in diameter

DIROFILARIASIS

Key Facts

Etiology/Pathogenesis
- Caused by *Dirofilaria immitis*
- Dirofilariasis is more common in dogs
- Humans are accidental hosts

Clinical Issues
- Uncommon infectious condition
- Can occur at any age, and infection has been described in children and adults
  - More common in adults
- May be more common in males than in females
- As it occurs in dogs, worms lodge in the heart but die before reaching maturity
- Worms pass into pulmonary arteries
- Peripheral lung lesions are by far more common
- Clinical presentation
  - Cough
  - Dyspnea
  - Wheezing
  - Chest pain
  - Fever
- Laboratory findings
  - Eosinophilia may be present in 10-15% of patients
- Treatment
  - Complete surgical resection is curative

Microscopic Pathology
- Histological features
  - Well-demarcated necrotic nodule
  - Intravascular presence of nonviable worms
  - Worms may be present in necrotic tissue and not in vessels
  - Prominent inflammatory reaction
  - Nonnecrotizing granulomas may be present

Commonly Used Histochemical Stains in Pulmonary Dirofilariasis

Special Stain	Result
PAS	Highlights presence of worms
Movat	Highlights cuticle of worms
Trichrome	Highlights presence of worms
Elastic van Gieson	Highlights pulmonary vessels containing worms

MICROSCOPIC PATHOLOGY

Histologic Features
- Well-demarcated necrotic nodule
- Prominent inflammatory reaction
- Dilated pulmonary vessels
- Intravascular presence of nonviable worms
- Worms may be present within necrotic tissue and not in vessels
- Charcot-Leyden crystals may be present in about 25% of cases
- Nonnecrotizing granulomas may also be present
  - In adjacent lung parenchyma, other changes may take place, including
    - Desquamative interstitial pneumonitis-like (DIP-like) reaction
    - Follicular bronchiolitis
    - Organizing pneumonia
    - Microcalcifications
    - Cholesterol cleft granulomas
    - Fibrinous pleuritis

DIFFERENTIAL DIAGNOSIS

Other Infectious Conditions
- Fungal
  - Use of silver stains will help in identifying fungal organisms
- Mycobacterial
  - Use of Ziehl-Nielsen or Fite-Faraco stains will help in identification of acid fast-bacilli
- *Strongyloides*
  - Rarely presents as necrotic pulmonary nodule
  - Shows filariform organisms, which does not occur with dirofilariasis

Wegener Granulomatosis (WG)
- May show necrotic areas but will not show presence of worms
- Laboratory test for c-ANCA may show positive results in WG and negative results in dirofilariasis

Churg-Strauss Syndrome
- May also show necrosis and eosinophilia
- Negative for presence of worms

Carcinoma
- It is essential to identify presence of malignant component

DIAGNOSTIC CHECKLIST

Pathologic Interpretation Pearls
- Necrotic nodule
- Intravascular presence of worms

SELECTED REFERENCES

1. Mulanovich EA et al: A case of Dirofilaria pulmonary infection coexisting with lung cancer. J Infect. 56(4):241-3, 2008
2. Flieder DB et al: Pulmonary dirofilariasis: a clinicopathologic study of 41 lesions in 39 patients. Hum Pathol. 30(3):251-6, 1999

DIROFILARIASIS

Microscopic Features

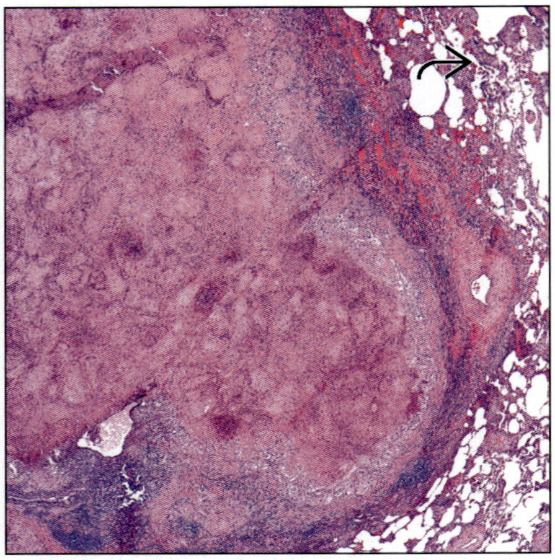
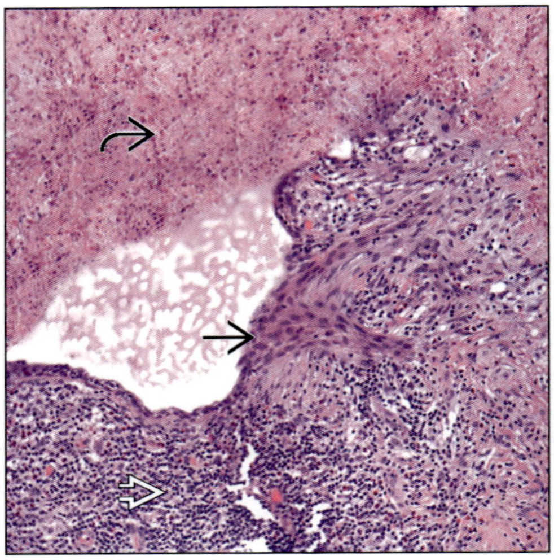

(Left) *Low-power view of a well-demarcated pulmonary nodule shows destruction of normal lung parenchyma. The nodule shows extensive necrosis with a rim of normal lung parenchyma.* ***(Right)*** *Necrotic pulmonary nodule replacing lung parenchyma also shows focal areas of squamous metaplastic changes accompanied by an inflammatory reaction.*

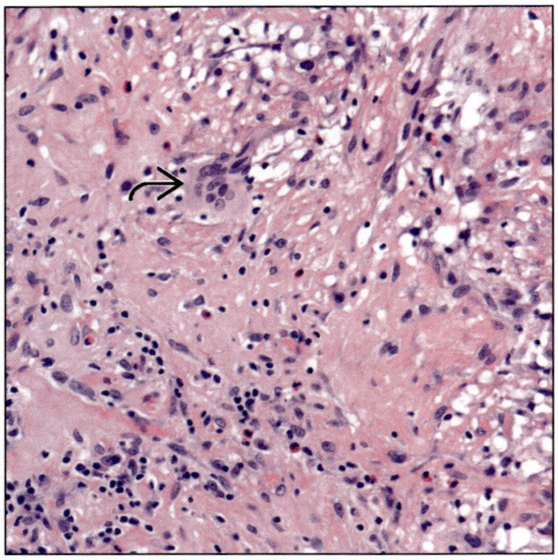
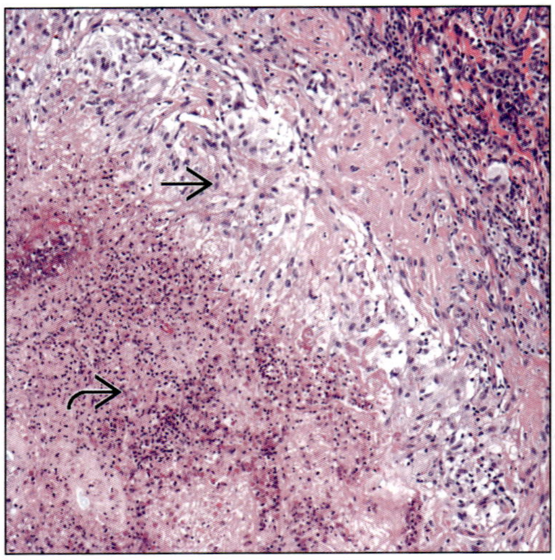

(Left) *High-power view of the peripheral aspect of the necrotic pulmonary nodule shows histiocytic reaction and the presence of multinucleated giant cells. Such features may be seen in other infectious conditions.* ***(Right)*** *Intermediate-power view shows the interface between areas of necrosis with prominent eosinophilic inflammatory reaction and areas of a histiocytic reaction. These features also suggest the possibility of another pulmonary infection.*

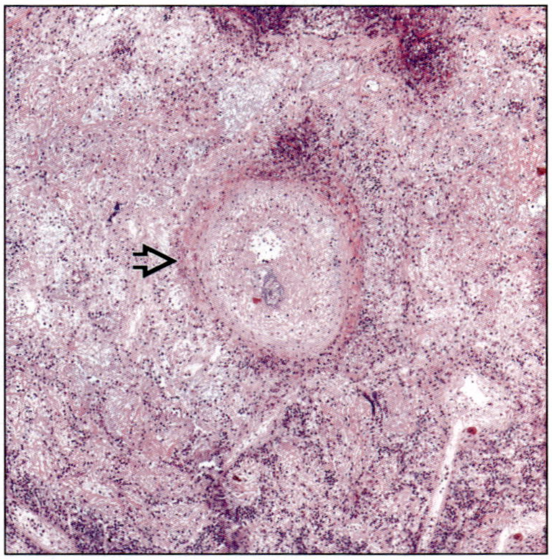
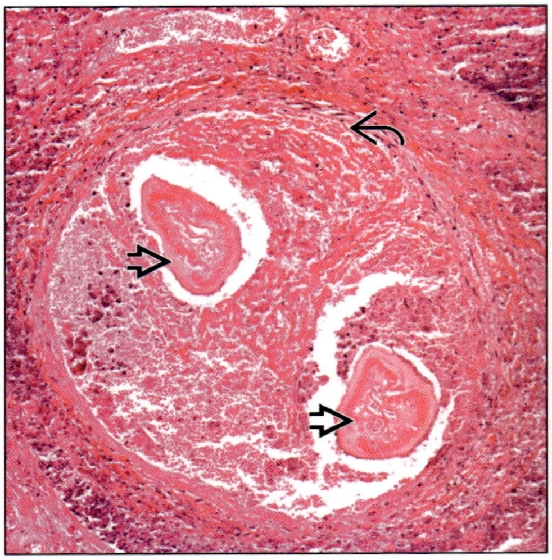

(Left) *Pulmonary dirofilariasis shows a nodule with extensive necrosis and inflammatory reaction. Note the presence, even with the conventional stain, of an obstructed pulmonary vessel.* ***(Right)*** *Two worms of Dirofilaria are present embedded in a necrotic background. Still, the outlines of a pulmonary vessel can be recognized. This is a typical presentation of Dirofilaria.*

DIROFILARIASIS

Microscopic Features

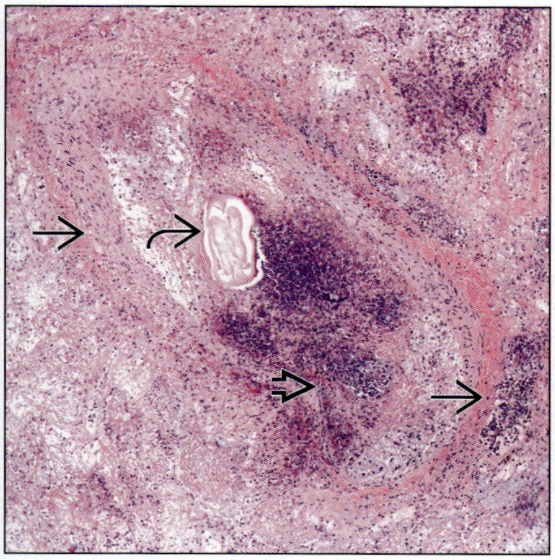
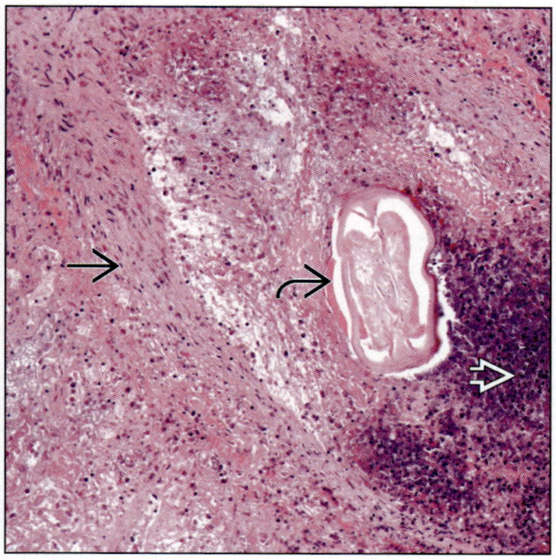

(Left) *Pulmonary dirofilariasis shows the classical pulmonary nodule with extensive necrosis. Note the outline of the pulmonary vessel →, which is filled with necrotic material ⇨, and in the center, the presence of Dirofilaria immitis ↪.* ***(Right)*** *High-power magnification shows the parasite of Dirofilaria immitis ↪ embedded in necrotic material ⇨ and within a large pulmonary vessel →. The salient feature of Dirofilaria immitis here is the presence of a thick cuticle.*

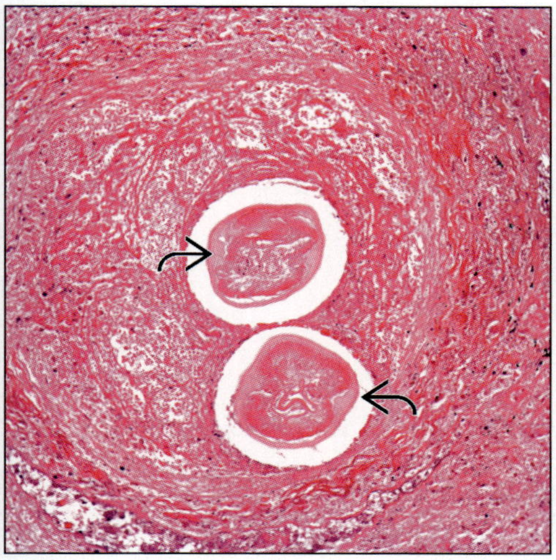
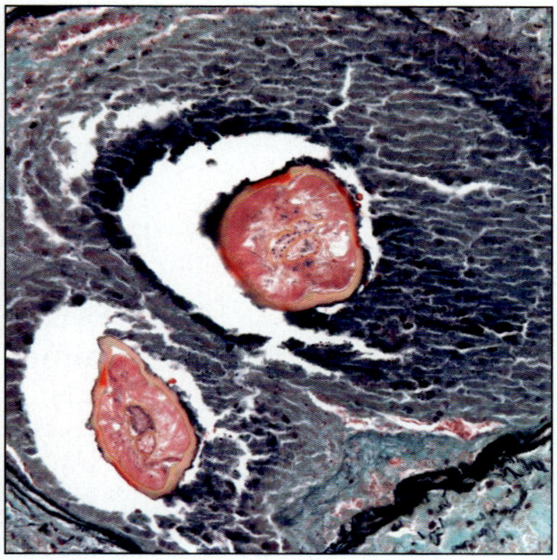

(Left) *In some cases, the presence of Dirofilaria is more obvious as in this low-power view of 2 worms ↪ that have a targetoid appearance.* ***(Right)*** *In some cases, the use of other histochemical stains, such as Movat, are important in highlighting the worms and distinguishing their internal organs.*

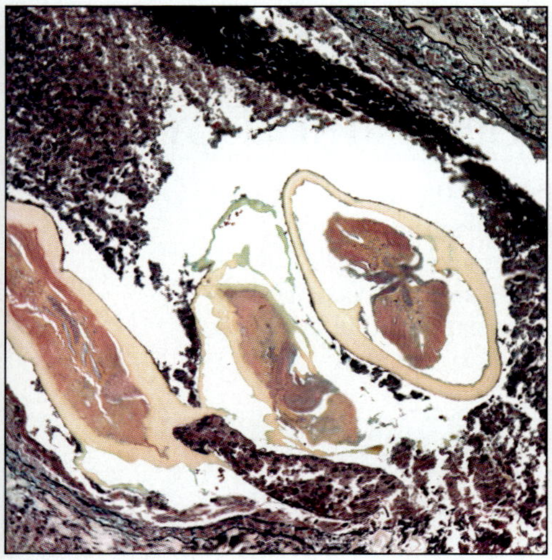
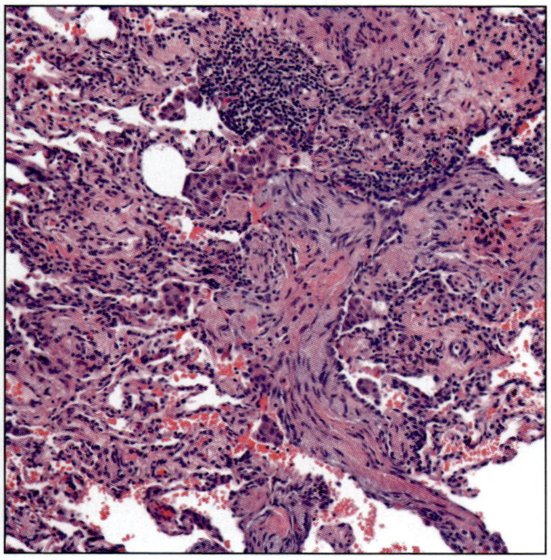

(Left) *Another histochemical stain that may be useful in the identification of the parasites, mainly when there is a lot of necrotic material, is an Elastic stain, which not only highlights the parasite but also the remains of the affected vessel.* ***(Right)*** *Adjacent lung parenchyma in cases of dirofilariasis may show different features, including organizing pneumonia as it is depicted in this case. Other features may also include nonnecrotizing lung nodules.*

SCHISTOSOMIASIS

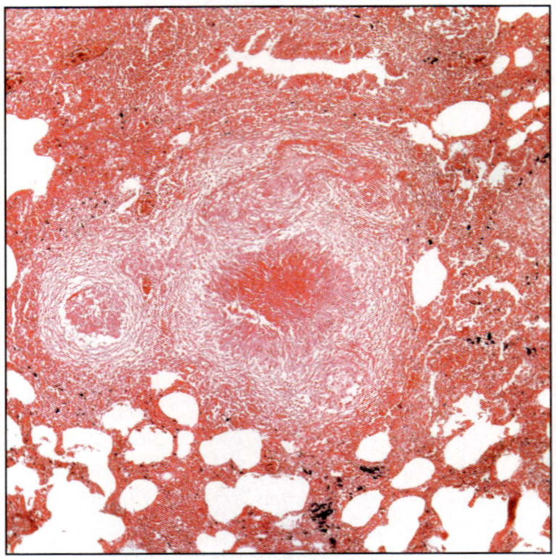

Lung parenchyma with an easily identifiable granulomatous reaction shows that the center of the granulomas contain necrosis and hemorrhage. These changes can be seen in other infections as well.

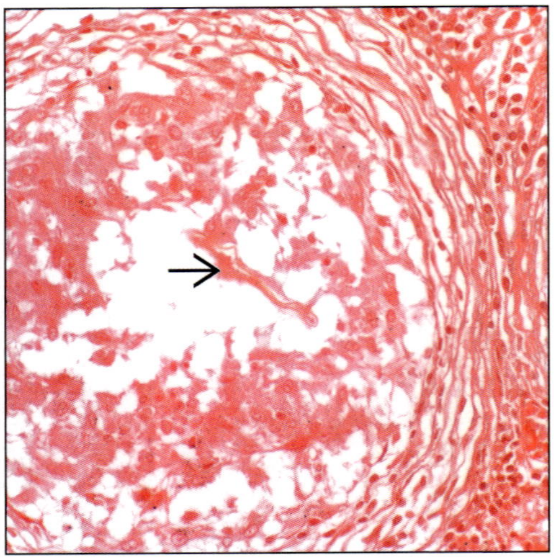

High-power view of the central necrosis of the granulomatous reaction shows the outlines of Schistosoma →. This organism can be easily missed in a cursory review.

TERMINOLOGY

Synonyms

- Bilharziasis

Definitions

- Infection caused by Trematoda (flukes)

ETIOLOGY/PATHOGENESIS

Infectious Agents

- 3 most common types affecting humans are
  - *Schistosoma haematobium* (urinary tract)
  - *Schistosoma mansoni* (intestinal tract)
  - *Schistosoma japonicum* (intestinal tract)
    - Snails are intermediate host

Pathogenesis in Pulmonary Schistosomiasis

- *Schistosoma* eggs travel via the portal-systemic collateral veins to the lung

CLINICAL ISSUES

Epidemiology

- Incidence
  - Approximately 10% worldwide
- Age
  - Any age group can potentially be affected
- Gender
  - No gender predilection
- Ethnicity
  - No ethnic predilection

Presentation

- Acute phase
  - Fever
  - Cough
  - Asthma-like symptoms
  - Urticaria
  - Diarrhea
  - Hepatomegaly
  - Splenomegaly
  - Lymphadenopathy
- Chronic phase
  - Acute symptoms subside over a period of weeks
  - Patients may be asymptomatic

Laboratory Tests

- Eosinophilia
- Possible false-positive HIV test

Treatment

- Drugs
  - Praziquantel (all types of *Schistosoma*)
  - Oxamniquine (*S. mansoni*)
  - Metrifonate (*S. haematobium*)

Prognosis

- Good if treated early and patients not immunocompromised
- Can follow aggressive course in immunocompromised individuals

MICROSCOPIC PATHOLOGY

Histologic Features

- Granulomatous reaction
- Granulomatous endarteritis
- Thickening of pulmonary vasculature
- *Schistosoma* eggs deposited in arterioles
- Acute inflammatory reaction

DIFFERENTIAL DIAGNOSIS

Fungal Granulomatous Infection

- Presence of fungal organisms demonstrated by fungal stains

SCHISTOSOMIASIS

Key Facts

Terminology
- Synonym
  - Bilharziasis
- Definition
  - Infection caused by Trematoda (flukes)

Etiology/Pathogenesis
- 3 most common types that affect humans are
  - *Schistosoma haematobium* (urinary tract)
  - *Schistosoma mansoni* (intestinal tract)
  - *Schistosoma japonicum* (intestinal tract)
- Pathogenesis
  - Snails are intermediate host
  - *Schistosoma* eggs travel via the portal-systemic collateral veins to the lung

Clinical Issues
- Acute phase
- Chronic phase
- Laboratory findings
  - Eosinophilia
  - Possible false-positive HIV test
- Treatment
  - Good if treated early and patient not immunocompromised
  - Can be fatal in some cases

Top Differential Diagnoses
- Fungal granulomatous infection
- Pulmonary tuberculosis
- Pulmonary hypertension
- Bacterial bronchopneumonia

Diagnostic Aids

Study	Description	Result
Stool examination	Fresh stools	Identification of *Schistosoma* eggs
Urine test	Fresh urine	Identification of *Schistosoma* eggs
Kato method	Quantification of eggs in fresh stools	Identification of *Schistosoma* eggs
Tissue biopsy	Tissue of the gastrointestinal, genitourinary, or pulmonary tract	Identification of *Schistosoma* eggs
Hematoxylin-eosin stain	From any tissue	Identification of *Schistosoma* eggs
Ziehl-Neelsen stain	Shells and spines of *Schistosoma* eggs are acid fast	Helps highlight *Schistosoma* eggs

- Fungal organisms present within the granulomatous reaction
- Unusual for a fungal infection to show organisms only within vessels

Pulmonary Tuberculosis
- Histochemical stains for acid-fast bacilli aid the identification of bacilli
- Thickening of pulmonary vasculature is unusual
- Acid-fast bacilli are distributed haphazardly rather than in pulmonary vessels

Pulmonary Hypertension
- As in schistosomiasis, thickening of pulmonary vasculature is a feature of pulmonary hypertension
- However, *Schistosoma* eggs are absent

Bacterial Bronchopneumonia
- As in schistosomiasis, acute inflammatory reaction may be seen in bronchopneumonia
- Thickening of pulmonary vasculature is unusual
- Gram stain may show presence of bacteria
- Absence of parasites

DIAGNOSTIC CHECKLIST

Clinically Relevant Pathologic Features
- Symptom complex
  - Pulmonary hypertension
  - Hepatosplenomegaly

Pathologic Interpretation Pearls
- Granulomatous endarteritis
- Presence of Schistosoma eggs in vessels is of utmost importance

SELECTED REFERENCES

1. Dawson-Hahn EE et al: Eosinophilia and the seroprevalence of schistosomiasis and strongyloidiasis in newly arrived pediatric refugees: an examination of Centers for Disease Control and Prevention screening guidelines. J Pediatr. 156(6):1016-8, 1018, 2010
2. Everett DB et al: Association of schistosomiasis with false-positive HIV test results in an African adolescent population. J Clin Microbiol. 48(5):1570-7, 2010
3. Graham BB et al: Schistosomiasis-associated pulmonary hypertension: pulmonary vascular disease: the global perspective. Chest. 137(6 Suppl):20S-29S, 2010
4. Keiser J et al: Efficacy and safety of mefloquine, artesunate, mefloquine-artesunate, and praziquantel against Schistosoma haematobium: randomized, exploratory open-label trial. Clin Infect Dis. 50(9):1205-13, 2010
5. Kouriba B et al: [Immunity in human schistosomiasis: hope for a vaccine.] Med Trop (Mars). 70(2):189-97, 2010
6. Osada Y et al: Parasitic helminths: new weapons against immunological disorders. J Biomed Biotechnol. 2010:743758, 2010

SCHISTOSOMIASIS

Microscopic Features

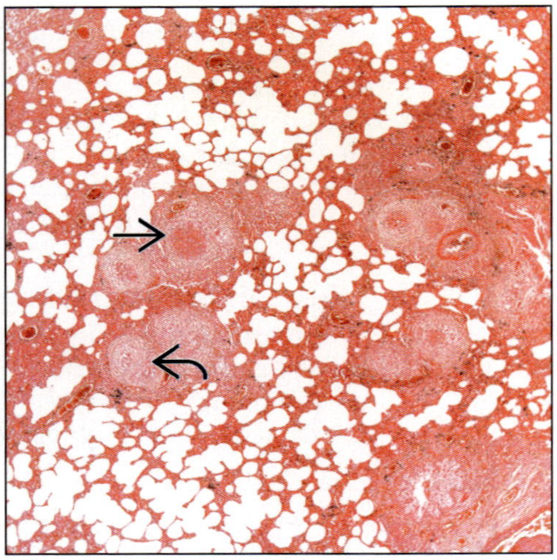

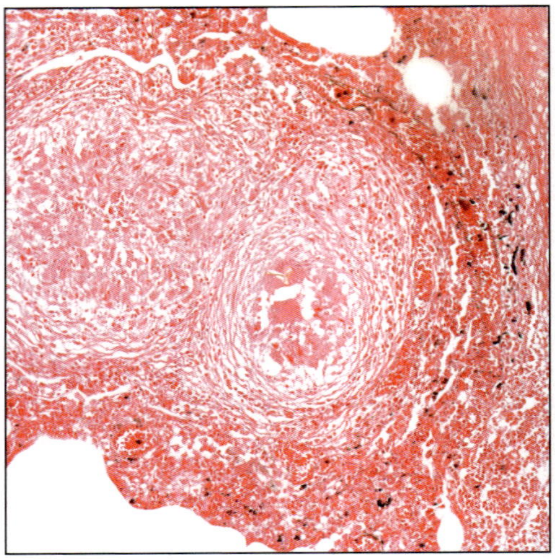

(Left) *Low-power view of a section of lung shows a florid granulomatous reaction. Note that part of the granulomatous area has central necrosis → while other areas do not contain caseous material ↷. Remaining portions of lung are within normal limits.* ***(Right)*** *Higher magnification of the granulomatous reactions shows central necrosis, and it is in these areas that the parasite will most likely be identifiable. However, similar features may also be seen in other infections.*

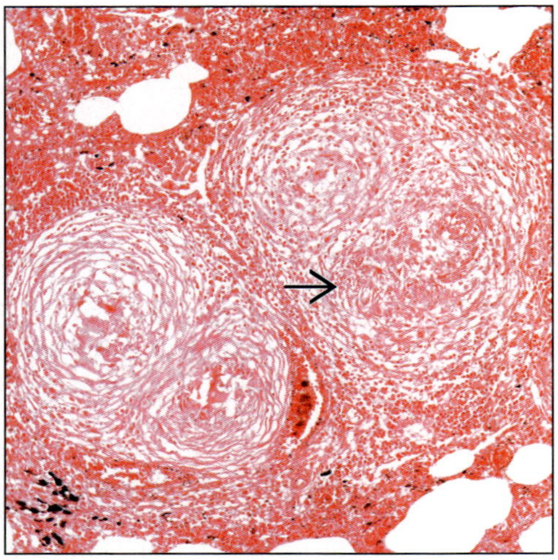

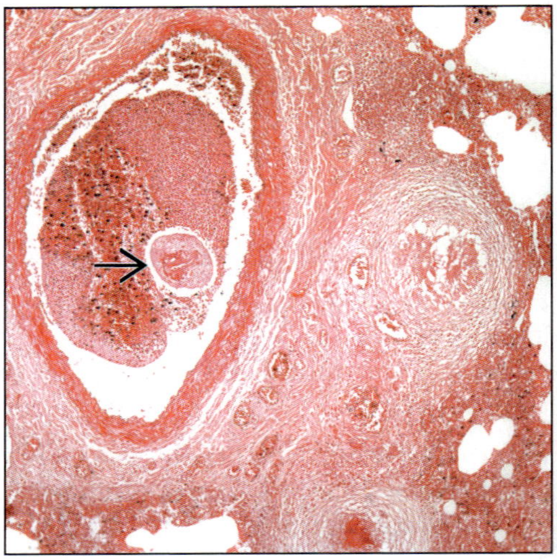

(Left) *In some areas, the granulomas are tightly packed, almost mimicking the granulomas seen in sarcoidosis. Note, however, the presence of central necrosis and acute inflammation →. These features would be unusual for sarcoid granulomas.* ***(Right)*** *In other portions of the lung parenchyma, the vessels are dilated, containing blood and, in some cases, schistosomes, as in this case where the parasite → is admixed with blood within the vessel.*

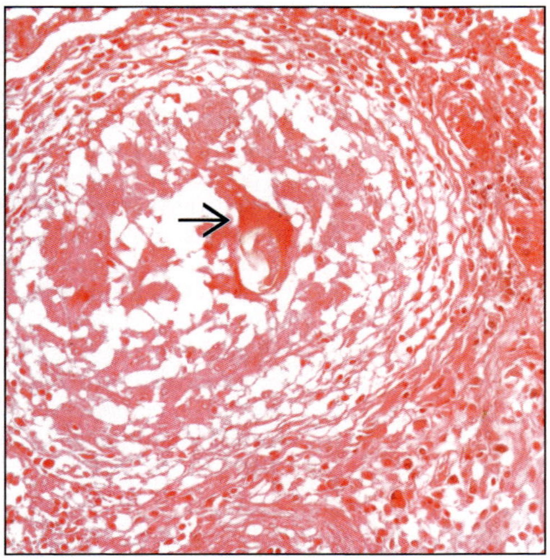

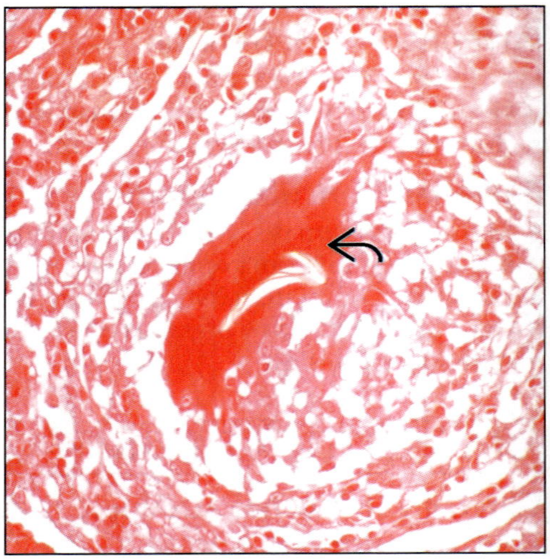

(Left) *Usually schistosomes are encountered in areas of central necrosis within the granulomatous reaction. In this case, the parasite → is admixed with necrosis. However, the parasite is not well preserved and can be easily missed.* ***(Right)*** *Higher magnification shows a not so well-preserved Schistosoma ↷ embedded in a central area of necrosis. Schistosoma is not well preserved in the lungs, in contrast to other organs, which can make identification difficult.*

Microscopic Features

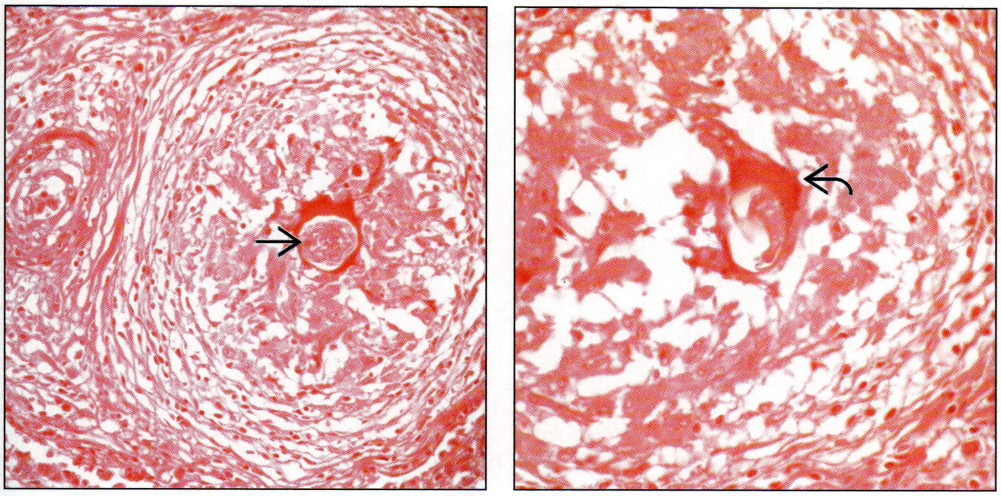

(Left) In some granulomas, the parasite → is more easily identifiable. In this granuloma with concentric fibrosis and central necrosis, for example, the organism is easily diagnosed. **(Right)** In other granulomas, one can see only the outlines of the organism ↪, making the diagnosis more difficult since the remnants can be easily dismissed as foreign material or artifact.

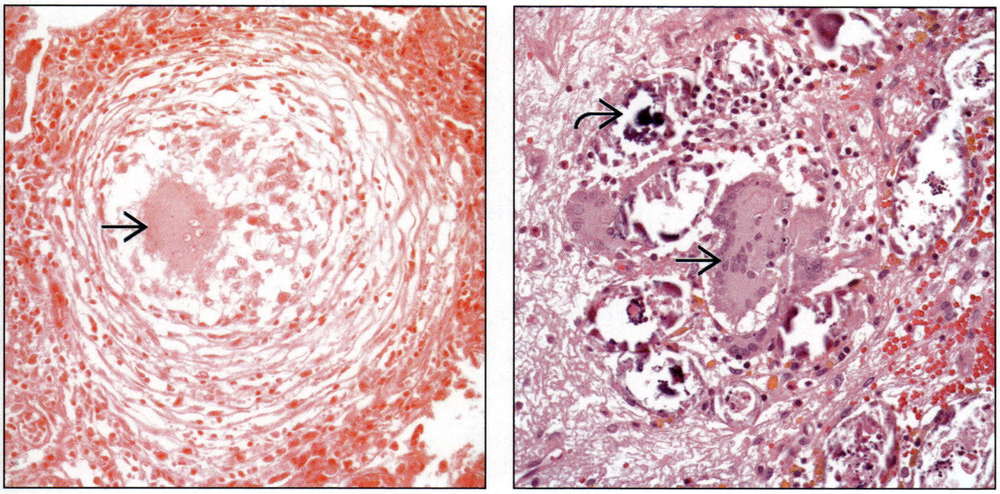

(Left) Unlike granulomas containing fragments of the parasite, some granulomas do not show evidence of parasitic infection. Essentially, such granulomas show central necrosis with the presence of multinucleated giant cells →. **(Right)** Other areas of the lung parenchyma may show numerous multinucleated giant cells → with calcifications ↪. In these areas, it is also possible to identify the presence of Schistosoma.

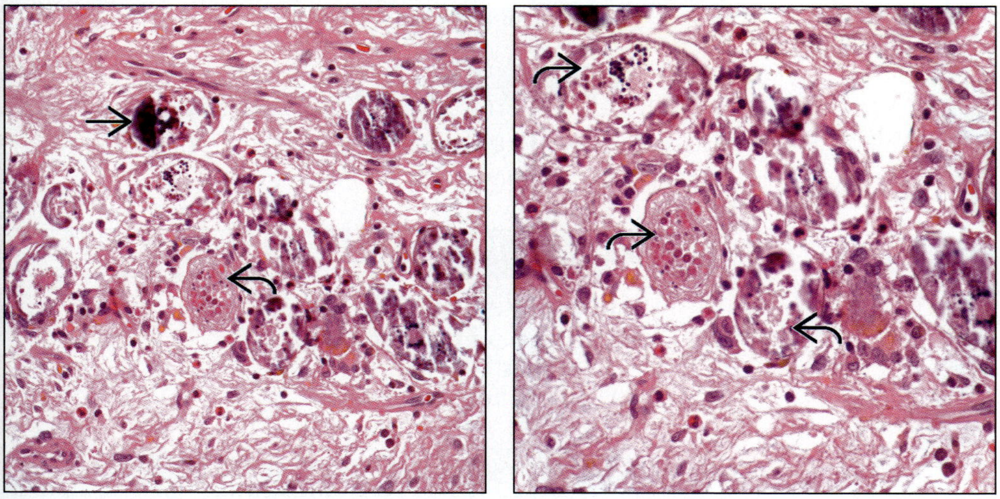

(Left) In some unusual cases, parasites ↪ are easily identifiable admixed with mild inflammatory changes and the presence of calcifications →. **(Right)** High-power view of Schistosoma ↪ demonstrates classic organisms. Unfortunately, such cases are few since in most cases the intact parasite is hard to identify. In many cases, the presence of granulomas and marked inflammatory changes may obscure the parasites.

ECHINOCOCCOSIS (HYDATID CYST)

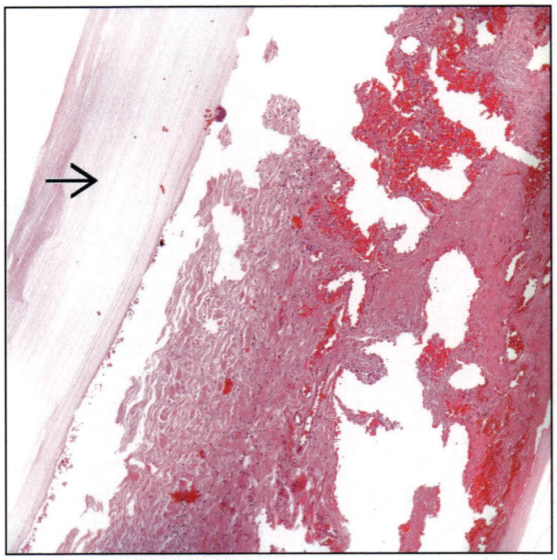

Lung parenchyma shows on 1 side a laminated structure ⇒ of hyaline material characteristic of an echinococcal cyst.

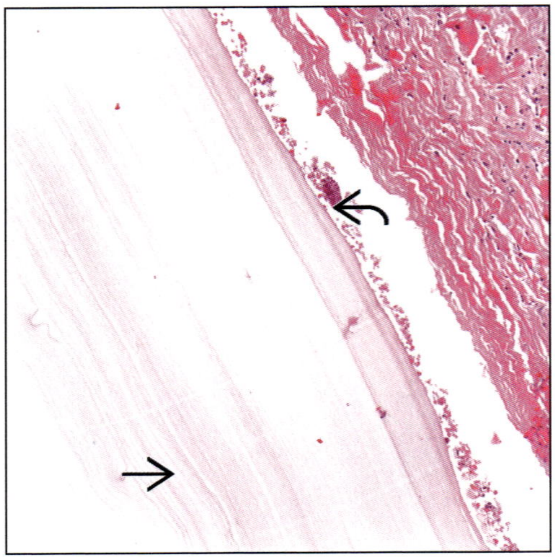

Closer view shows that the cystic lesion is rimmed by a very thin germinal layer ↶. Still, the laminated nature of the cystic structure ⇒ can be identified.

TERMINOLOGY

Synonyms

- Hydatidosis, echinococcosis

Definitions

- Infectious condition caused by tapeworms

ETIOLOGY/PATHOGENESIS

Infectious Agents

- *Echinococcus*
  - 4 types
    - *E. granulosus*
    - *E. multilocularis*
    - *E. vogeli*
    - *E. oligarthrus*

CLINICAL ISSUES

Epidemiology

- Incidence
  - Worldwide distribution
    - Predominantly in sheep- and cattle-raising regions
- Age
  - Can occur in any age group
- Gender
  - Appears to be more common in females
- Ethnicity
  - No ethnic predilection

Presentation

- Symptoms
  - Cough
  - Chest pain
  - Dyspnea
  - Hemoptysis
  - Pneumothorax
- Infection can involve
  - Lung
  - Liver
  - Brain
  - Spleen
  - Kidney
  - Bone
- Patients may be asymptomatic

Natural History

- Eggs can contaminate fruits, vegetables, water, or hands

Treatment

- Surgical approaches
  - Complete surgical resection of the cyst
- Drugs
  - Albendazole
  - Combined mebendazole with praziquantel

Prognosis

- Good after treatment
- Can develop serious morbidity

IMAGE FINDINGS

General Features

- Cystic lesion

MACROSCOPIC FEATURES

General Features

- Unilocular or multilocular cysts
- Thin walls
- Light tan fluid contents

MICROSCOPIC PATHOLOGY

Histologic Features

- Bronchopneumonia

ECHINOCOCCOSIS (HYDATID CYST)

Key Facts

Terminology
- Synonyms
  - Hydatidosis, echinococcosis
- Definition
  - Infectious condition caused by tapeworms

Etiology/Pathogenesis
- 4 types of *Echinococcus*
  - *E. granulosus*
  - *E. multilocularis*
  - *E. vogeli*
  - *E. oligarthrus*

Clinical Issues
- Epidemiology
  - Worldwide distribution
  - Predominantly in sheep- and cattle-raising regions
- Symptoms
  - Cough
  - Dyspnea
  - Hemoptysis
  - Pneumothorax
- Infection can also involve
  - Liver
  - Brain
  - Spleen
  - Kidney
  - Bone
- Natural history
  - Eggs can contaminate fruits, vegetables, water, or hands

Histochemical Stains in the Diagnosis of Echinococcus

Stain	Comment
Hematoxylin and eosin	Clearly identifies the parasite
GMS (silver stain)	Highlights hooklets and lamination of cyst wall
Ziehl-Neelsen	Highlights internal components of parasite
Periodic acid-Schiff (PAS)	May accentuate laminations of cyst wall

- Abscess formation
- Identification of the parasite
  - Cystic structures
  - Laminations of the cyst wall
  - Outer laminated membrane
  - Thin germinal membrane
  - Calcareous corpuscles

DIFFERENTIAL DIAGNOSIS

Other Parasitic Infections
- Strongyloidiasis
  - Commonly shows presence of larvae
- Dirofilariasis (*Dirofilaria immitis)*
  - Does not present as cystic lesion
  - Usually necrotic granuloma
- Schistosomiasis
  - Does not present as unilocular or multilocular cyst
  - Morphology of *Schistosoma* differs from *Echinococcus*

Bacterial Bronchopneumonia
- Abscess formation and acute inflammation may be seen in both bacterial bronchopneumonia and echinococcosis
- Identification of bacterial organisms
- Absence of hydatid cyst

DIAGNOSTIC CHECKLIST

Pathologic Interpretation Pearls
- Unilocular or multilocular cyst
- Identification of the parasite
- Cystic structures
- Laminations of the wall of the cyst
- Identification of a thin germinal membrane and a laminated outer membrane

SELECTED REFERENCES

1. Erbey F et al: Coexistence of non-Hodgkin's lymphoma and cyst hydatid disease and successful medical treatment. J Pediatr Hematol Oncol. 32(6):524, 2010
2. Matsumoto J et al: Primary alveolar echinococcosis: course of larval development and antibody responses in intermediate host rodents with different genetic backgrounds after oral infection with eggs of Echinococcus multilocularis. Parasitol Int. 59(3):435-44, 2010
3. Mehta KD et al: Comparative evaluation of thoracoscopy versus thoracotomy in the management of lung hydatid disease. World J Surg. 34(8):1828-31, 2010
4. Rangarajan V et al: Pulmonary hydatid cyst detected on FDG PET-CT. Clin Nucl Med. 35(4):298-9, 2010
5. Tennert U et al: Pitfall alveolar echinococcosis in non-endemic areas. Alveolar echinococcosis migrating northward. Ann Hepatol. 9(1):99-103, 2010

ECHINOCOCCOSIS (HYDATID CYST)

Microscopic Features

*(**Left**) Low-power view of a pulmonary cystic lesion shows pulmonary parenchyma surrounding the cyst ⇨. Even at this power, it is possible to identify the presence of a well-formed outer layer of the cyst ↗. (**Right**) Different view shows a pulmonary hydatid cyst in which the classical laminated wall is not that easily identifiable. The cyst appears to be surrounded just by alveolated lung parenchyma ⇨.*

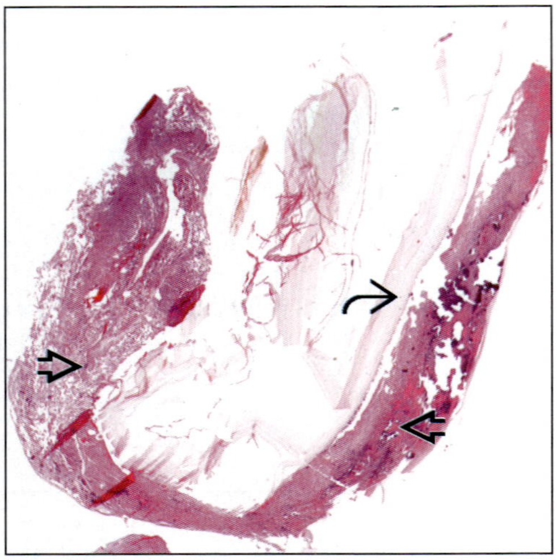

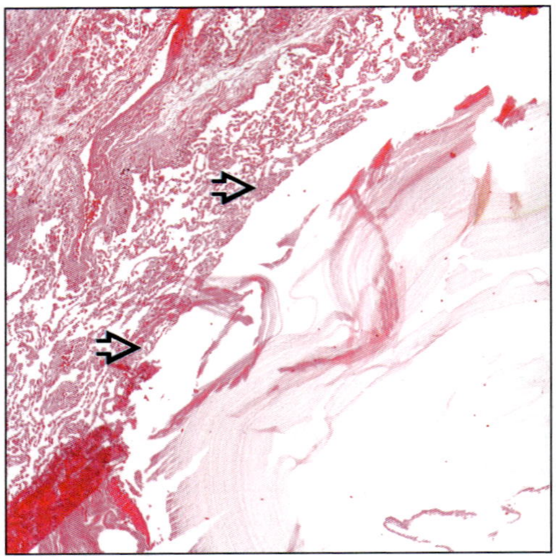

*(**Left**) In some cases of hydatid cyst, the cystic wall also appears to be surrounded by dense fibrous connective tissue ⇨ forming a capsule around the cystic structure. Even at this magnification, the classical laminations ↗ of the cystic wall can be identified. (**Right**) Hydatid cyst composed of a laminated cystic structure ⇨ with a very thin germinal layer ↗ is shown. Note that the cystic structure here is not surrounded by dense fibrous connective tissue.*

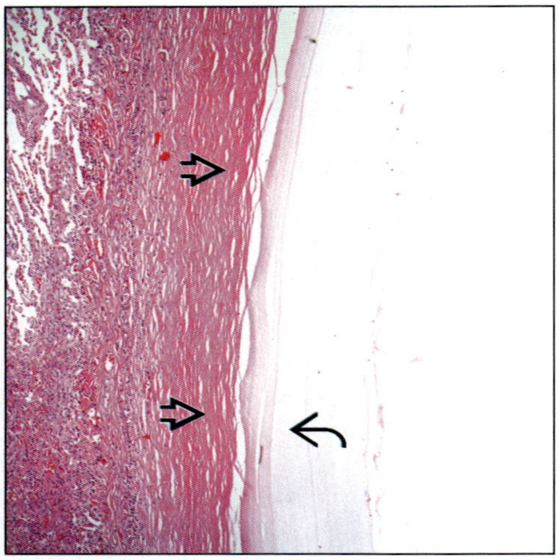

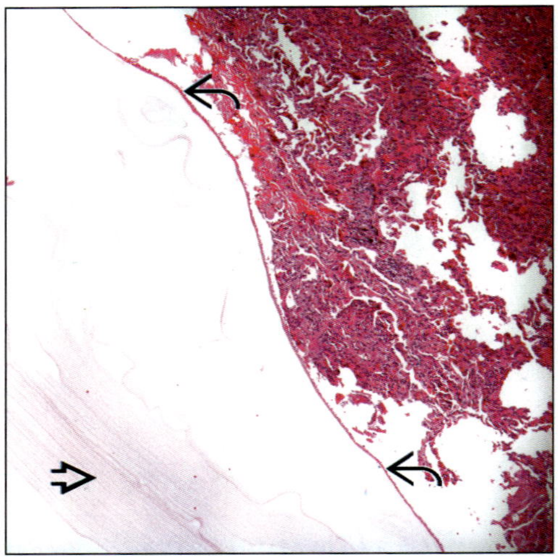

*(**Left**) Low-power view shows a hydatid cyst in which the surrounding lung parenchyma appears congested with dilated vascular spaces ↗. Note that the hydatid cyst is easily identifiable →. (**Right**) Closer view shows that the hydatid cyst contains a laminated wall → and a thin germinal layer ↗. Note the absence of any inflammatory changes within the wall of the cyst. The features are characteristic of echinococcosis.*

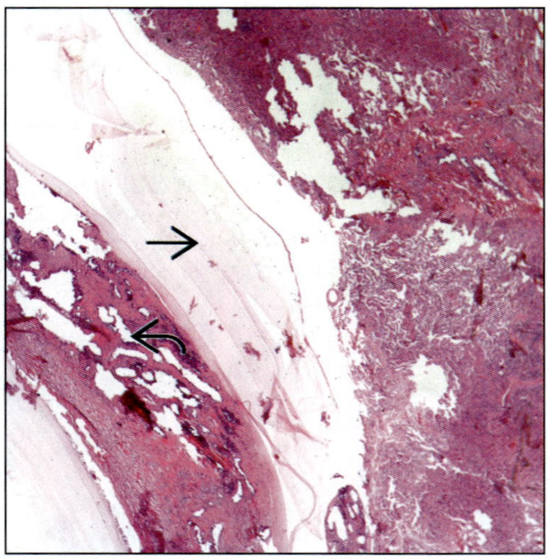

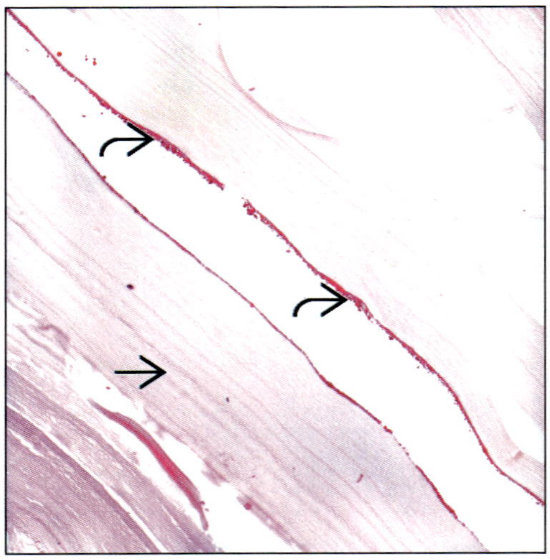

ECHINOCOCCOSIS (HYDATID CYST)

Microscopic Features

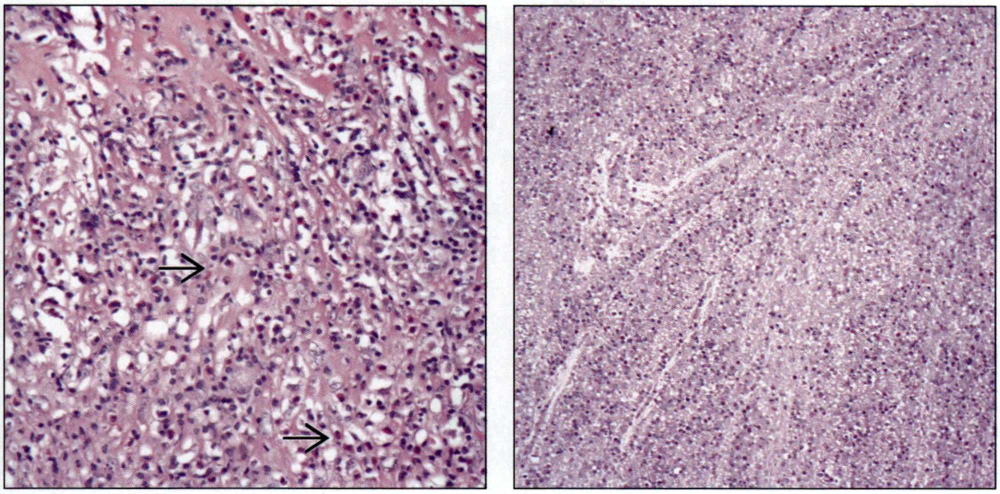

(Left) *Areas adjacent to the hydatid cyst may show inflammation with marked eosinophils, as are present in this particular case.* ***(Right)*** *In other areas, the presence of viable cystic structures may not be readily identifiable, and prominent areas of necrosis can obscure the diagnosis.*

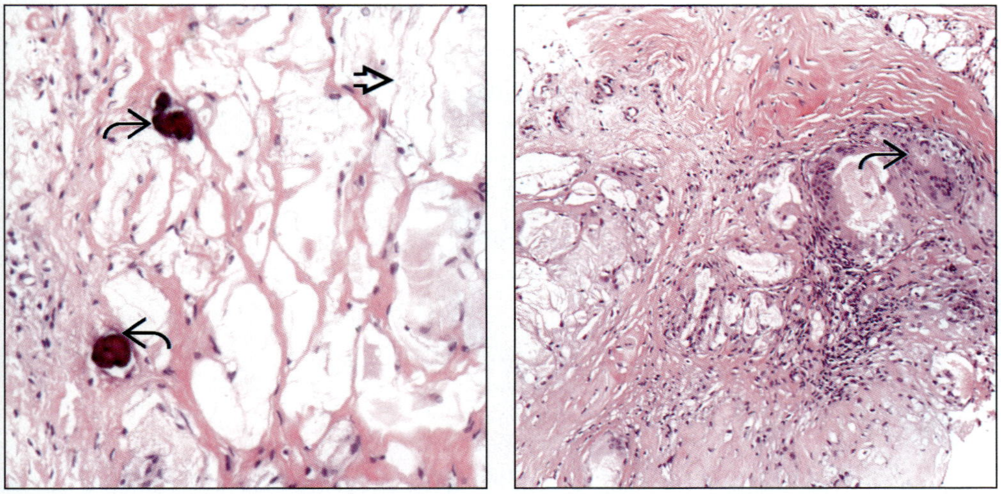

(Left) *The presence of calcifications and areas of myxoid change is not common but may occur in some cases in areas adjacent to the cyst. These features are not specific for the diagnosis of echinococcosis.* ***(Right)*** *The presence of a granulomatous reaction in the form of multinucleated giant cells, although not common, may be seen in some cases. Note how the multinucleated giant cells are admixed with myxoid changes and inflammatory reaction.*

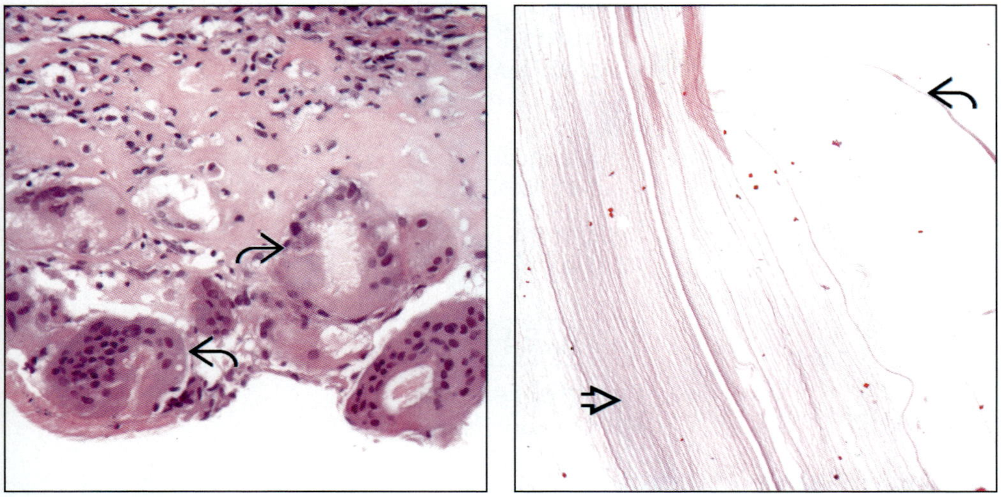

(Left) *In some cases, the presence of multinucleated giant cells is easily recognizable and may be misleading for another infectious condition. Proper identification of the cyst is necessary for diagnosis.* ***(Right)*** *Classic features of the echinococcal cyst include a laminated wall and a thin germinal layer. Note the absence of any inflammatory changes within the wall of the cyst.*

PARAGONIMIASIS

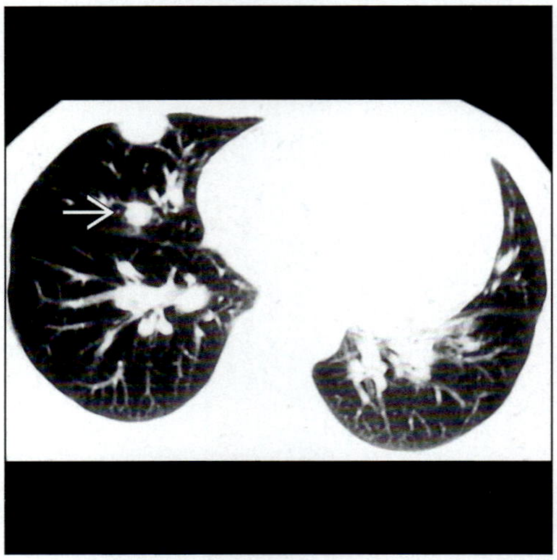

CT scan of the thorax shows intrapulmonary nodules ➡. This presentation may be confused with other conditions, including neoplastic processes.

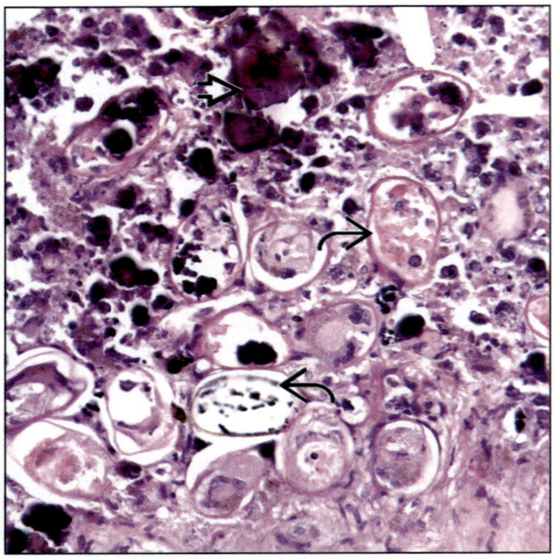

Numerous paracytic structures are present ↗ admixed with calcifications ⇨ and minimal inflammatory reaction. These features are in keeping with paragonimiasis.

TERMINOLOGY

Synonyms

- Pulmonary distomiasis, lung fluke disease, parasitic hemoptysis, tojil (earth-borne disease), and gregarinosis

Definitions

- Infectious condition caused by trematode

ETIOLOGY/PATHOGENESIS

Environmental Exposure

- Raw or partially cooked crab or crayfish
- Contaminated drinking water

Infectious Agents

- Although there are numerous species of *Paragonimus*, most common in humans is
  - *Paragonimus westermani* (Asia)
  - *Paragonimus mexicanus* (Latin America)
    - Requires 7 different phases in life cycle
    - Requires 3 hosts to complete life cycle
    - Incubation period is ~ 70 days

CLINICAL ISSUES

Epidemiology

- Incidence
  - Worldwide distribution
- Age
  - More common in younger patients
- Gender
  - Males appear to be more commonly infected
- Ethnicity
  - No ethnic predilection

Site

- Infection can involve
  - Lung
  - Brain
  - Skin/subcutis

Presentation

- Symptoms
  - Abdominal pain
  - Diarrhea
  - Nausea
  - Vomiting
  - Fatigue
  - Fever
  - Cough
  - Night sweats
  - Chest pain
  - Hemoptysis
  - Hydropneumothorax
- Asymptomatic

Laboratory Tests

- Eosinophilia

Treatment

- Surgical approaches
  - Surgical resection
- Drugs
  - Praziquantel
  - Bithionol

Prognosis

- Good

IMAGE FINDINGS

General Features

- Pulmonary mass

PARAGONIMIASIS

Key Facts

Terminology
- Synonyms: Pulmonary distomiasis, lung fluke disease, parasitic hemoptysis, tojil (earth-borne disease), and gregarinosis
- Infectious condition caused by trematode

Etiology/Pathogenesis
- Raw or partially cooked crab or crayfish
- Contaminated drinking water
- Infectious agent; most common in humans are
  - *Paragonimus westermani* (Asia)
  - *Paragonimus mexicanus* (Latin America)

Clinical Issues
- Infection can involve
  - Lung
  - Brain
  - Skin/subcutis
- Laboratory results
  - Eosinophilia
- Treatment
  - Surgical resection
- Alternative treatment
  - Praziquantel
  - Bithionol

Image Findings
- Pulmonary mass

Microscopic Pathology
- Identification of parasite or eggs
- Granulomatous reaction
- Necrosis

Diagnostic Aids

Study	Finding
Sputum	Eggs of parasite
Feces	Eggs of parasite
Fluid from pleura or abdomen	Eggs of parasite
Skin biopsy	Identification of parasite or eggs
Pulmonary resection or biopsy	Identification of parasite or eggs
Brain biopsy or resection	Identification of parasite or eggs
Omental biopsy	Identification of parasite or eggs

MACROSCOPIC FEATURES

General Features
- Necrotic mass
- Well circumscribed but not encapsulated
- Soft and light tan in color

Size
- May vary from 1 cm to > 5 cm

MICROSCOPIC PATHOLOGY

Histologic Features
- Abscess formation
- Tissue eosinophilia
- Necrosis
- Hemorrhage
- Granulomatous reaction
- Identification of parasite or eggs

DIFFERENTIAL DIAGNOSIS

Other Parasites
- *Clonorchis sinensis*
- *Fasciola hepatica*
- *Schistosoma*
  - Size of eggs and morphology of *Paragonimus* are different

DIAGNOSTIC CHECKLIST

Pathologic Interpretation Pearls
- Identification of parasite
  - Sputum
  - Feces
  - Tissue

SELECTED REFERENCES

1. Lane MA et al: Human paragonimiasis in North America following ingestion of raw crayfish. Clin Infect Dis. 49(6):e55-61, 2009
2. Osaki T et al: Pulmonary Paragonimus westermani with false-positive fluorodeoxyglucose positron emission tomography mimicking primary lung cancer. Gen Thorac Cardiovasc Surg. 55(11):470-2, 2007
3. Yoo IeR et al: Two cases of pulmonary paragonimiasis on FDG-PET CT imaging. Ann Nucl Med. 20(4):311-5, 2006
4. Choo JD et al: Chronic cerebral paragonimiasis combined with aneurysmal subarachnoid hemorrhage. Am J Trop Med Hyg. 69(5):466-9, 2003
5. Dainichi T et al: A case of cutaneous paragonimiasis with pleural effusion. Int J Dermatol. 42(9):699-702, 2003
6. Meehan AM et al: Severe pleuropulmonary paragonimiasis 8 years after emigration from a region of endemicity. Clin Infect Dis. 35(1):87-90, 2002

PARAGONIMIASIS

Imaging, Gross, and Microscopic Features

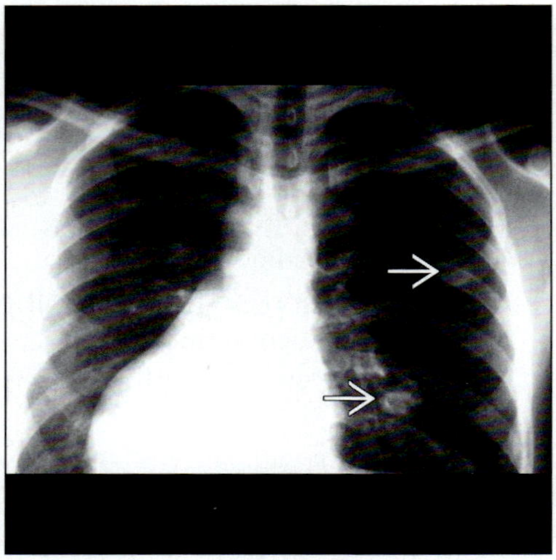

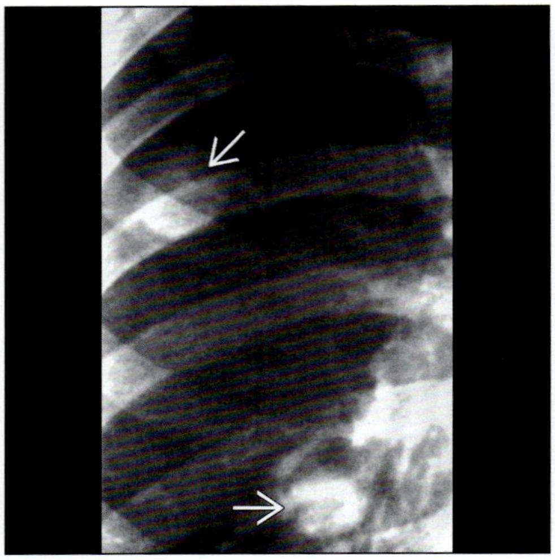

(Left) *Chest x-ray shows intrapulmonary nodules →. This appearance may be confused with metastatic tumors of the lung.* ***(Right)*** *Closer view of chest x-ray of the lung fields demonstrates the presence of intrapulmonary nodules →, raising the possibility of a malignant neoplasm involving lung parenchyma.*

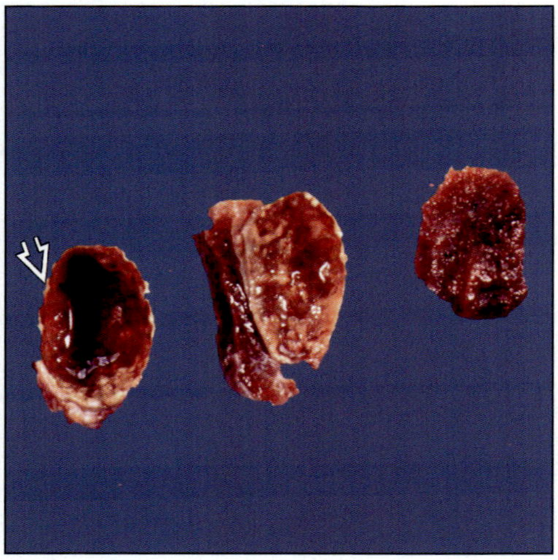

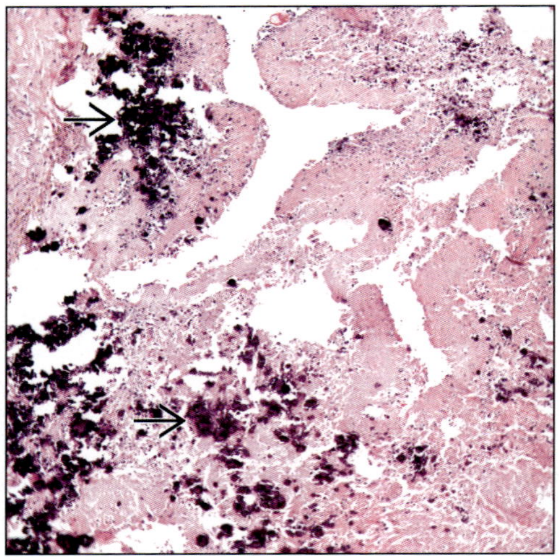

(Left) *Wedge resection of a pulmonary nodule of paragonimiasis shows a cystic structure with a thick capsule ⇨. The cyst appears to be hemorrhagic and somewhat yellowish. Adjacent lung parenchyma is congested.* ***(Right)*** *Low-power view of pulmonary paragonimiasis shows extensive areas of fibrinous exudate accompanied by areas of calcification →. At this power, it is difficult to identify the presence of the organisms.*

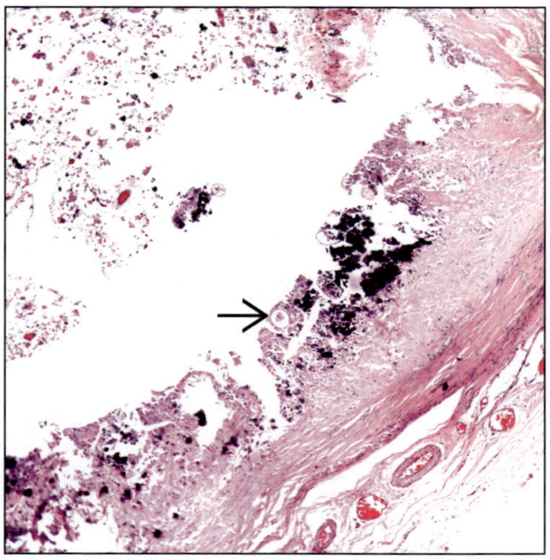

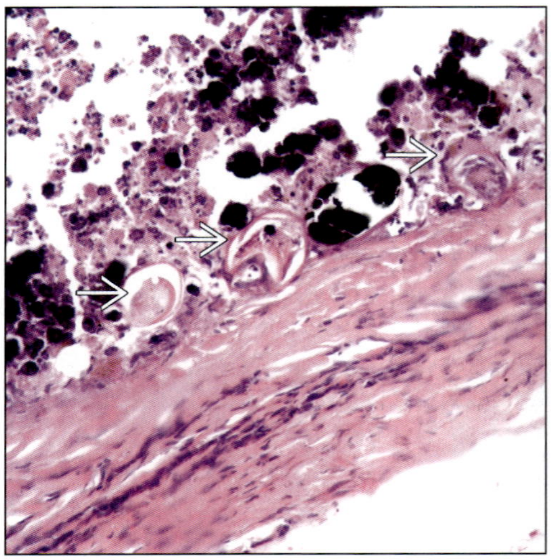

(Left) *Cystic structure shows a thick capsule and extensive fibrinous material admixed with calcifications and eggs or Paragonimus →. In some cases, the presence of calcifications may make the identification of the parasite much more difficult.* ***(Right)*** *High-power magnification shows collapsed eggs of Paragonimus → admixed with calcifications. Note that there is minimal associated inflammatory change.*

PARAGONIMIASIS

Microscopic Features

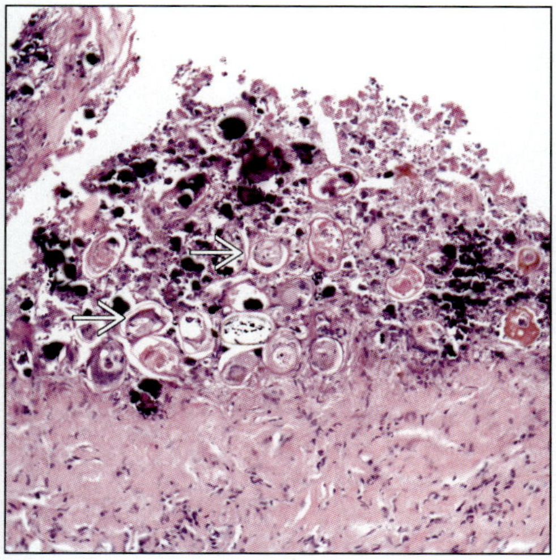

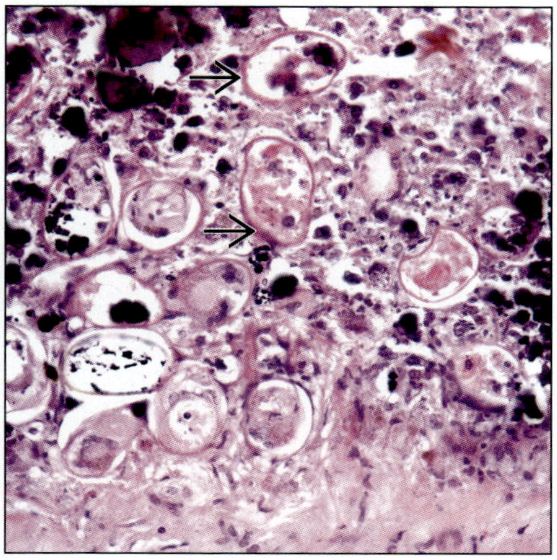

(Left) *Different view of a cystic structure demonstrates numerous eggs of Paragonimus* → *admixed with calcifications.* ***(Right)*** *High-power view of eggs of Paragonimus shows a thickened shell and operculum* →*. These characteristics are important in order to differentiate Paragonimus from other parasites.*

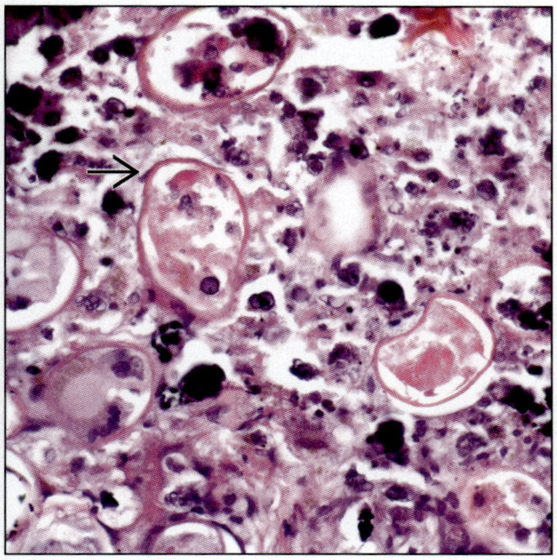

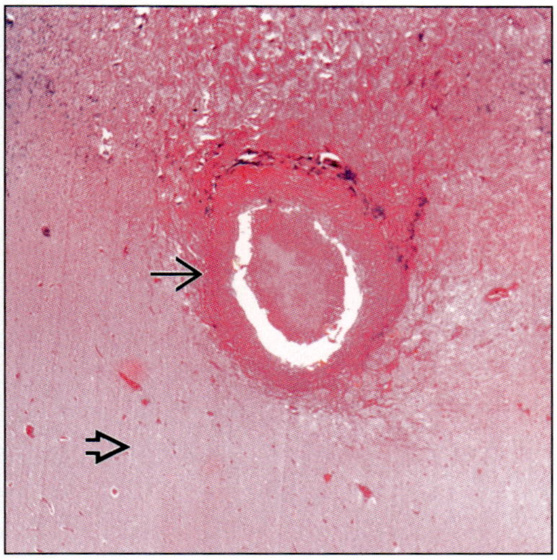

(Left) *Eggs of Paragonimus admixed with calcifications and mild inflammatory reaction are shown. The features of a thickened shell and operculum* → *are characteristics of Paragonimus.* ***(Right)*** *Paragonimus in the brain shows a cystic lesion* → *with central necrosis and mild inflammatory reaction. Note the rest of the glial tissue does not show marked inflammatory changes* ⇨*.*

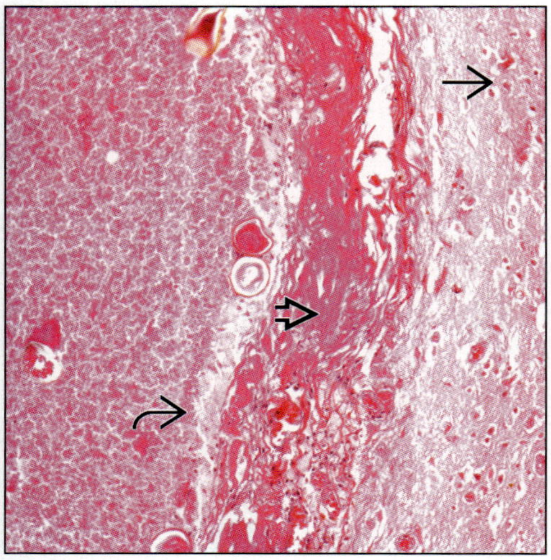

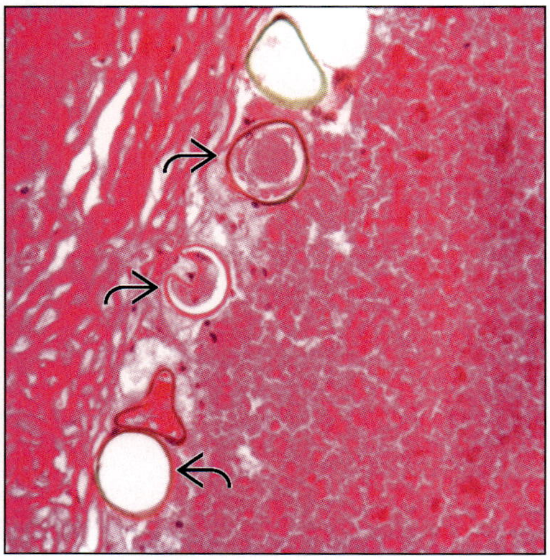

(Left) *Higher magnification of Paragonimus in the brain shows a distinct interphase between the cystic lesion* ↷ *and the normal glial tissue* →*. Note the presence of a thickened capsule* ⇨*.* ***(Right)*** *Higher magnification of Paragonimus in the brain shows the presence of numerous collapsed eggs of Paragonimus* ↷*. Note the presence of a thickened shell, which is a characteristic of the eggs of Paragonimus.*

Infectious Diseases

CRYPTOCOCCOSIS

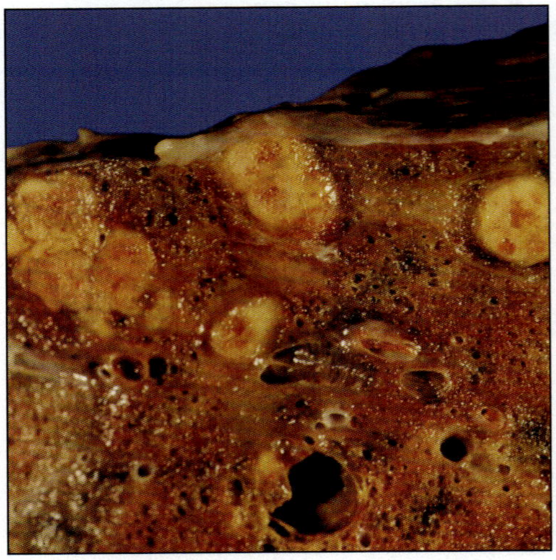

Gross appearance of cryptococcal infection in the lung shows multiple cryptococcomas distributed in the periphery of the upper lobe.

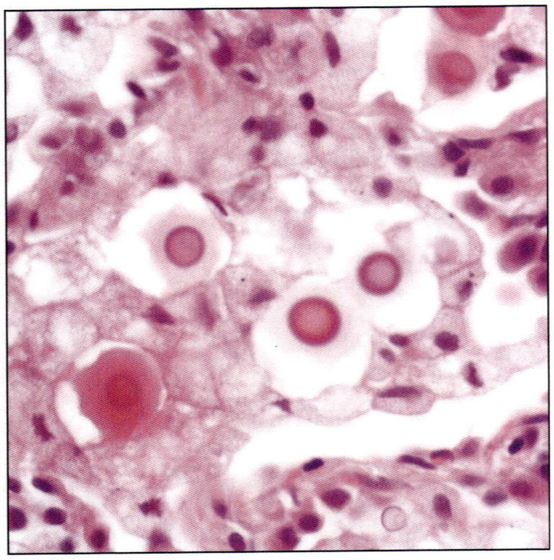

Histologic appearance of cryptococcal pneumonia shows round to oval yeast with thick mucinous capsule creating a "halo" effect.

TERMINOLOGY

Definitions

- Lung infection caused by inhalation of *Cryptococcus neoformans* spores

ETIOLOGY/PATHOGENESIS

Environmental Exposure

- Organisms are found in soil, especially soil contaminated with pigeon droppings

CLINICAL ISSUES

Epidemiology

- Incidence
  - Worldwide distribution; unknown incidence

Presentation

- Acute pulmonary infection is most often asymptomatic
- Progressive infection is associated with the following symptoms
  - Cough
  - Low-grade fever
  - Pleuritic pain
  - Weight loss

Natural History

- Acute pulmonary infection can be asymptomatic or self-limited
- Progressive infection is seen in immunocompromised hosts and involves lungs and meninges
- Sequel of self-limited infection is formation of small subpleural fibrocaseous nodules without calcifications
- Disease is most severe in immunocompromised patients

Treatment

- Surgical approaches
  - Surgical excision of pulmonary nodules may be helpful to reduce mortality
- Drugs
  - Amphotericin B
  - Fluconazole

Prognosis

- Good response to antifungal agents
- Infection with *C. gattii* in immunocompetent patients is associated with significant mortality despite therapy

IMAGE FINDINGS

General Features

- Morphology
  - Focal pulmonary nodule or masses
  - Multifocal peripheral pulmonary nodules predominantly in upper lobes
  - Unilateral or bilateral parenchymal consolidation
  - Immunocompromised patients may show diffuse, bilateral, reticular, or nodular interstitial opacities or miliary nodules
  - Fibrosis and calcification are not associated with cryptococcosis

MACROSCOPIC FEATURES

General Features

- Well-defined nodules (cryptococcomas) show central necrosis and cavitation but absence of calcifications
- Nodules may be minute, resembling miliary tuberculosis
- Areas of patchy consolidation can be seen that display a mucoid cut surface
- Immunocompromised patients can present with cystic lesions

CRYPTOCOCCOSIS

Key Facts

Terminology
- Lung infection caused by inhalation of *Cryptococcus neoformans* spores

Clinical Issues
- Acute pulmonary infection can be asymptomatic or self-limited
- Progressive infection is seen in immunocompromised hosts and involves lungs and meninges

Microscopic Pathology
- Nodular granulomatous lesions with multinucleated giant cells containing intracellular organisms
- Nodular lesions may progress to form necrotizing granulomas with palisading histiocytes
- Multiple organisms can be seen lying free within alveolar spaces with no inflammation in alveolar walls
- *C. neoformans* yeast are small (4-6 µm in diameter), eosinophilic, round to oval, and occasionally appear refractile with single budding
- Cells appear to be surrounded by a halo that actually represents a mucinous capsule
- Capsule-deficient variant of *C. neoformans* is found in immunocompromised patients

Ancillary Tests
- Organisms stain with silver stains (GMS) and PAS
- Capsule of organisms stains strongly with mucicarmine and Alcian blue stains
- Capsule-deficient variant of *C. neoformans* stains with Fontana-Masson stain

MICROSCOPIC PATHOLOGY

Histologic Features
- Reaction pattern of lung to organisms depends on immune status of patient
  - Immunocompetent patients generally develop granulomatous reaction to organisms
    - Nodular granulomatous lesions with multinucleated giant cells containing intracellular organisms
    - Nodular lesions may progress to form necrotizing granulomas with palisading histiocytes
    - Granulomatous lesions may exhibit prominent stromal fibrosis
  - Immunocompromised patients will not exhibit a granulomatous response to organisms
    - Multiple organisms can be seen lying free within alveolar spaces with no inflammation in alveolar walls
    - Organisms may be accompanied by abundant histiocytes within alveolar lumens, mimicking lipoid pneumonia

Cytologic Features
- *C. neoformans* yeast are small (4-6 µm in diameter), eosinophilic, round to oval, occasionally appear refractile, and are easily seen on H&E stains
  - Characterized by single budding attached by narrow base to parent cell
- Cells appear to be surrounded by a halo that actually represents a mucinous capsule
- Capsule-deficient variant of *C. neoformans* is found in immunocompromised patients

ANCILLARY TESTS

Histochemistry
- Organisms stain with silver stains (GMS) and PAS
- Capsule of organisms stains strongly with mucicarmine and Alcian blue stains
- Capsule-deficient variant of *C. neoformans* stains with Fontana-Masson stain

DIFFERENTIAL DIAGNOSIS

Other Fungal Infections
- *C. neoformans* can be mistaken for any yeast-forming fungus but is the only one with true mucinous capsule
- Capsule-deficient variant of *C. neoformans* can be confused for *Histoplasma*, *Blastomyces*, *Coccidioides*, and *Candida*
  - Fontana-Masson stain is useful to identify wall of organism and separate it from other fungi
- Blastomycosis can be distinguished from cryptococcosis due to its broad-based budding yeast

DIAGNOSTIC CHECKLIST

Clinically Relevant Pathologic Features
- Capsule-deficient organisms can be confused for other fungi due to absence of mucicarmine positivity

Pathologic Interpretation Pearls
- Only fungus that stains positive with mucicarmine stain

SELECTED REFERENCES

1. Bavishi AV et al: A case of pulmonary cryptococcosis caused by capsule-deficient cryptococcus neoformans in an immunocompetent patient. Respir Care. 55(7):937-41, 2010
2. Goldman JD et al: Cryptococcosis in the immunocompetent patient. Respir Care. 55(11):1499-503, 2010
3. Pappas PG et al: Invasive fungal infections among organ transplant recipients: results of the Transplant-Associated Infection Surveillance Network (TRANSNET). Clin Infect Dis. 50(8):1101-11, 2010

CRYPTOCOCCOSIS

Histologic Features

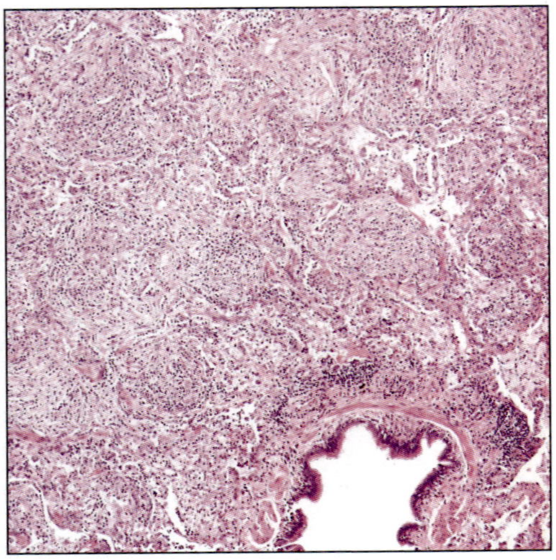

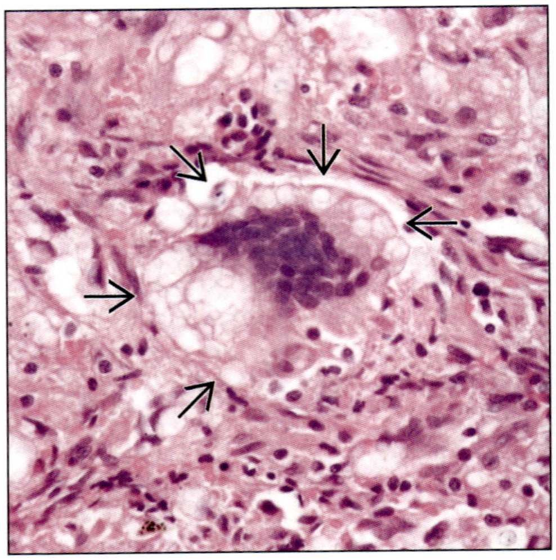

(Left) *Nodular granulomatous lesion in the lung of an immunocompetent patient with cryptococcosis shows sheets of epithelioid histiocytes surrounding a bronchus. Advanced lesions will undergo central necrosis and cavitation with peripheral palisading of histiocytes.* ***(Right)*** *Higher magnification of a granulomatous lesion in immunocompetent patient with cryptococcosis shows numerous organisms located within the cytoplasm of a multinucleated giant cell →.*

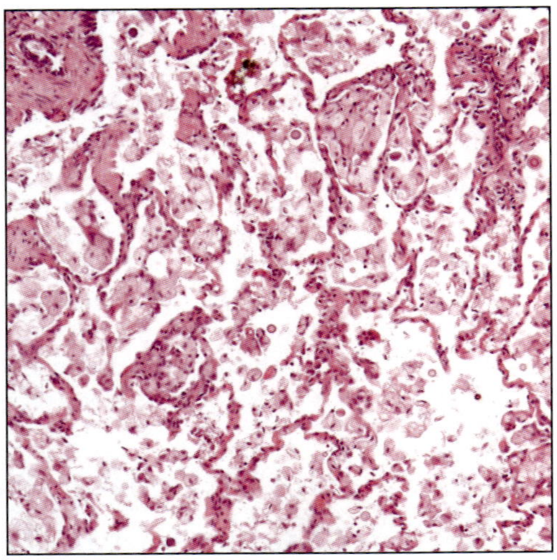

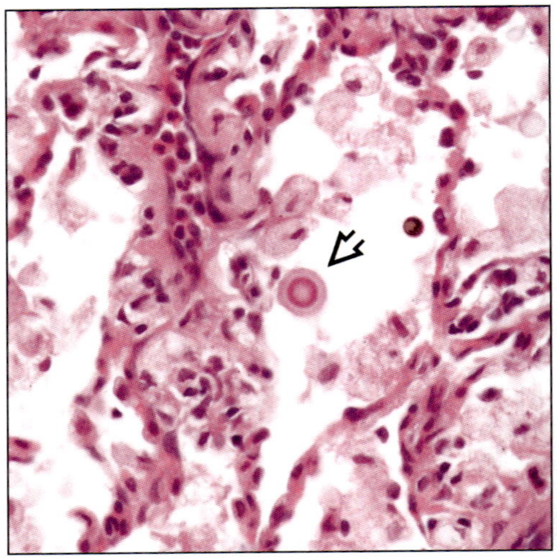

(Left) *Scanning magnification of cryptococcal pneumonia in an immunocompromised patient shows minimal reaction of lung parenchyma with no inflammatory response and abundant organisms lying free within the alveolar lumens.* ***(Right)*** *Higher magnification of cryptococcal pneumonia in an immunocompromised patient shows minimal inflammatory reaction and organisms lying free within the alveolar lumens ⇨. The organisms can be easily visualized on H&E without the need for special stains.*

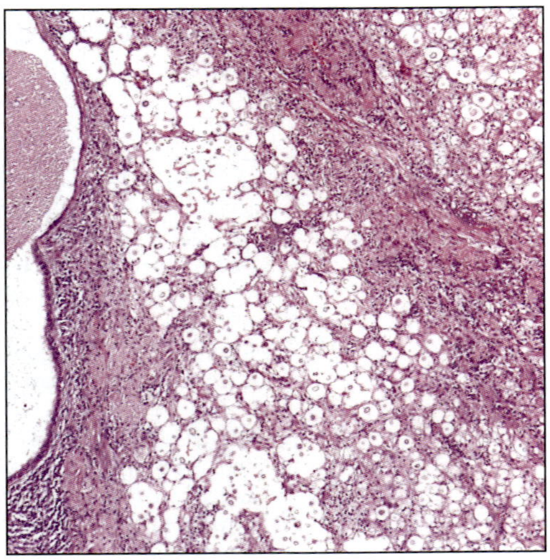

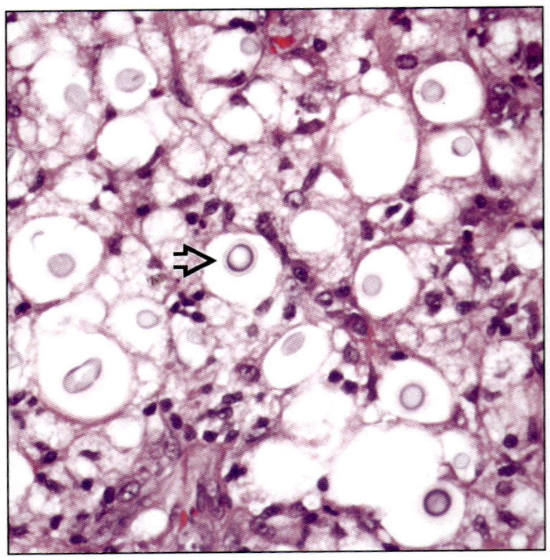

(Left) *Cryptococcal pneumonia in an AIDS patient shows multiple organisms lying free within the alveolar lumens.* ***(Right)*** *Higher magnification of cryptococcal pneumonia in an immunocompromised patient with AIDS shows numerous round to oval yeast with refractile cell walls and "halo" effect ⇨ caused by the presence of a thick mucinous capsule. There are numerous foamy macrophages seen admixed with the organisms. Cases like this can be confused for lipoid pneumonia.*

CRYPTOCOCCOSIS

Cytology and Special Stains

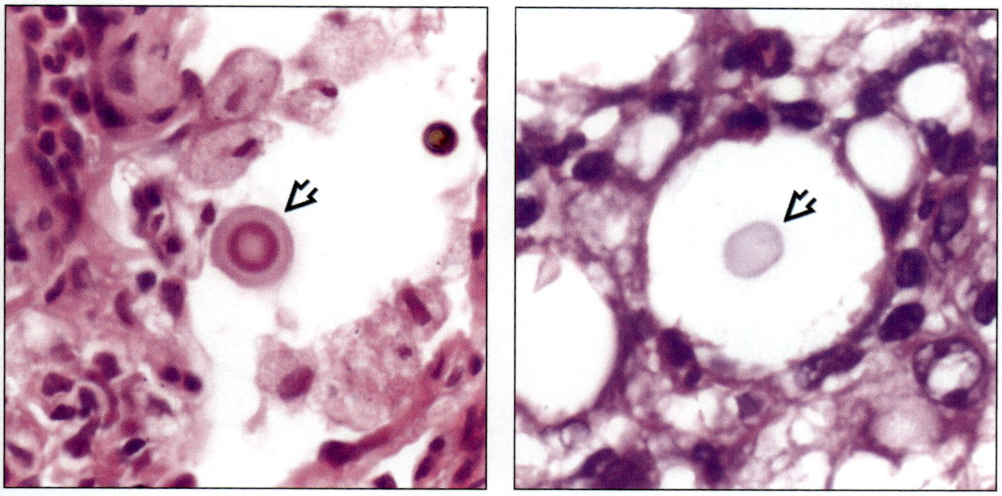

(Left) *High magnification in cryptococcal pneumonia shows classical appearance of cryptococcus, displaying round yeast ⇨ with a halo around the nucleus caused by the presence of a thick mucinous capsule. The capsule can be highlighted with mucicarmine.* ***(Right)*** *Higher magnification shows a capsule-deficient variant of Cryptococcus ⇨ in the lung. The absence of a thick capsule allows these forms to be easily mistaken for other types of yeast, including histoplasmosis, blastomycosis, etc.*

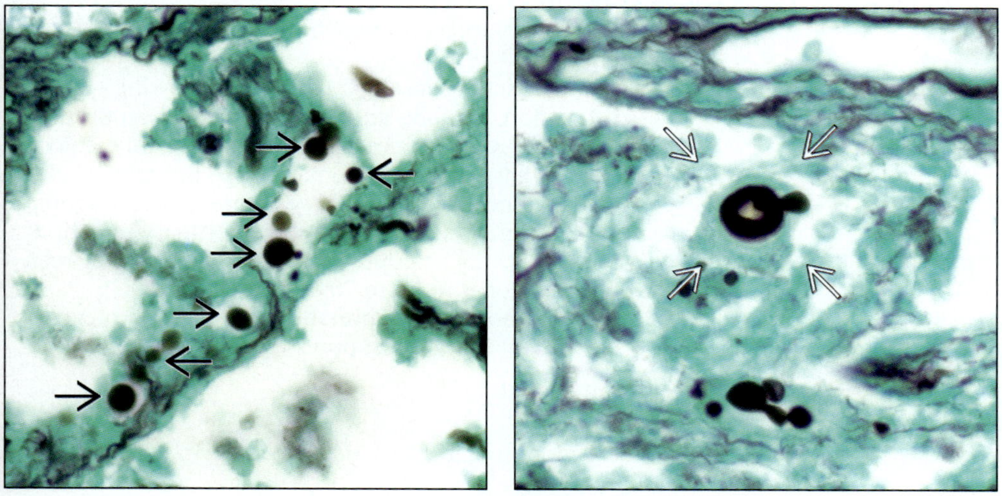

(Left) *Histochemical staining with Grocott methenamine silver (GMS) stain in a patient with pulmonary cryptococcosis shows numerous small yeast lying free within the airspaces →.* ***(Right)*** *Higher magnification of cryptococcal pneumonia in an immunocompromised patient with AIDS, stained with Gomori methenamine silver (GMS), shows a budding yeast ➡. The budding yeasts in cryptococcosis are characterized by single buds attached to the parent cell by a narrow base.*

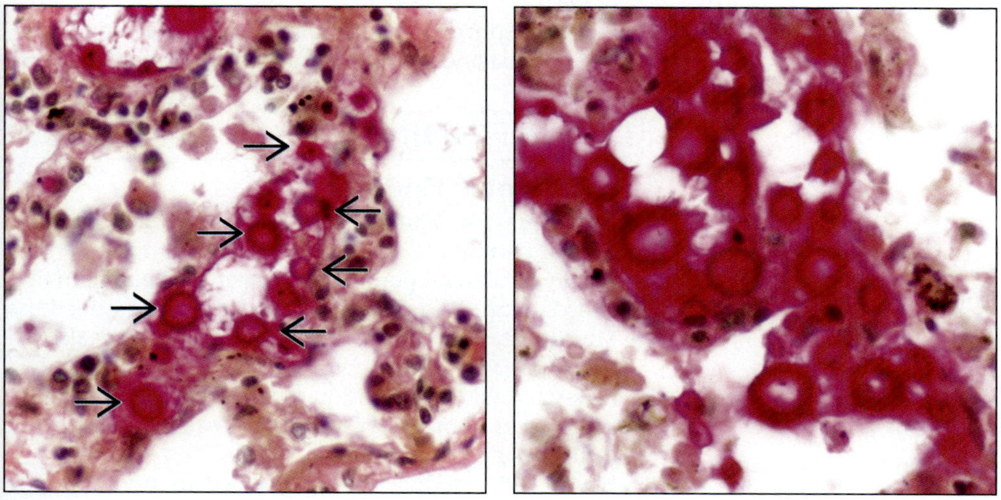

(Left) *Cryptococcal pneumonia stained with mucicarmine displays multiple organisms that show strong positivity →. Mucicarmine may be very useful in the context of differentiating Cryptococcus from other fungal organisms, as this is the only fungus that contains a mucicarmine positive capsule.* ***(Right)*** *Higher magnification of cryptococcal pneumonia stained with mucicarmine histochemical reaction shows accentuation of the capsule by the stain.*

COCCIDIOIDOMYCOSIS

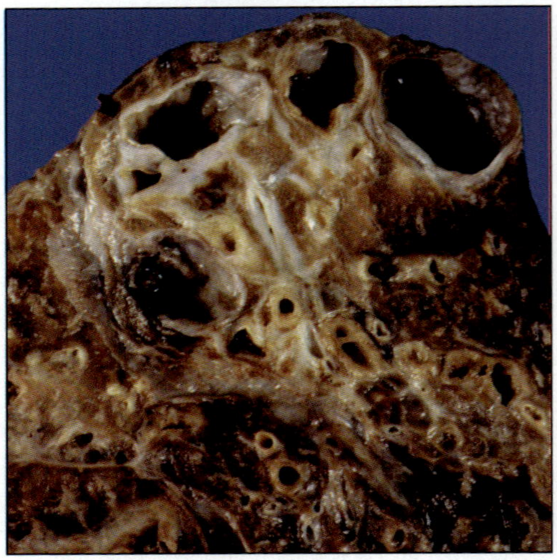

Cut surface of the lung in a patient with cavitary lesions due to coccidioidomycosis shows large, thin-walled subpleural cavities lined by fibrous tissue with necrotic debris.

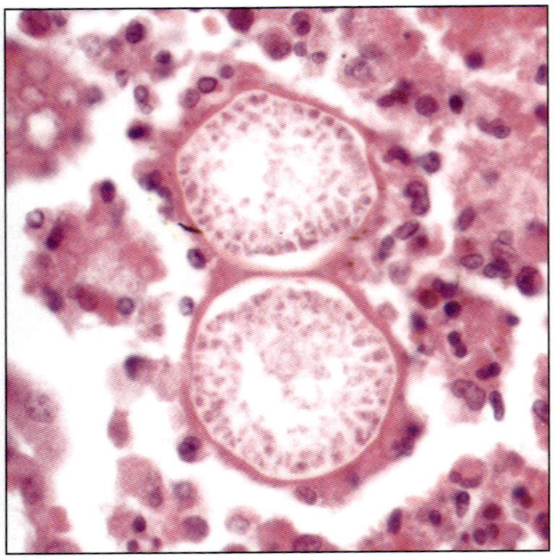

Histologic appearance of coccidioidomycosis in the lung shows 2 large round spherules surrounded by a thin capsule and containing numerous endospores.

TERMINOLOGY

Synonyms

- San Joaquin Valley fever

Definitions

- Pulmonary infection caused by inhalation of fungal spores of *Coccidioides immitis*

ETIOLOGY/PATHOGENESIS

Environmental Exposure

- Organisms preferentially grow in hot, dry, or semi-arid climates (e.g., desert)

CLINICAL ISSUES

Epidemiology

- Incidence
  - Organism is endemic in Southwestern United States, Mexico, and Central and South America

Presentation

- Majority of patients are asymptomatic
- Symptomatic patients present with
  - Fever with influenza-like illness
  - Cough
  - Myalgias and arthralgias
  - Pleuritic pain
  - Erythema nodosum or erythema multiforme (in 20% of patients)

Laboratory Tests

- Serum IgM antibodies to *C. immitis* can be detected 2-3 weeks after onset of infection in 75% of patients
- Serum IgG antibodies are detected in later stages in up to 90% of patients

Natural History

- Pulmonary infection may be acute, persistent, or chronic
- Acute infection develops 1-4 weeks following inhalation of spores and leads to fungal pneumonia
- Chronic progressive infection can mimic tuberculosis with miliary dissemination and high mortality
- Residual localized pulmonary nodule (coccidioidoma) can be seen as a sequel of resolved primary infection
- Solitary cavitary nodules with thin walls may be seen in upper lobes in up to 70% of cases
- Extrapulmonary dissemination can occur in pregnant women and immunosuppressed patients

Treatment

- Drugs
  - Amphotericin B

Prognosis

- Most patients recover spontaneously without evidence of persistent disease
- Persistent pneumonia in immunosuppressed patients can be fatal and requires antifungal treatment

IMAGE FINDINGS

Radiographic Findings

- Chest x-rays in acute infection can be normal in up to 20% of patients
- Patchy, unilateral perihilar, or lower lobe parenchymal consolidation is seen in primary pulmonary infection
- Multifocal, peripheral, subpleural nodules may also occur
- Parenchymal consolidation may resolve in some areas and appear in others, resulting in so-called phantom infiltrates
- Healing will produce solitary pulmonary nodules or thin-walled cavities

COCCIDIOIDOMYCOSIS

Key Facts

Terminology
- Pulmonary infection caused by inhalation of fungal spores of *Coccidioides immitis*

Clinical Issues
- Organism is endemic in Southwestern United States, Mexico, and Central and South America
- Pulmonary infection may be acute, persistent, or chronic
- Chronic progressive infection can mimic tuberculosis with miliary dissemination and high mortality
- Solitary cavitary nodules with thin walls may be seen in upper lobes in up to 70% of cases
- Extrapulmonary dissemination can occur in pregnant women and immunosuppressed patients

Microscopic Pathology
- Primary pulmonary infection is characterized by an acute suppurative pneumonia with neutrophilic infiltrates
- Granulomatous lesions are characterized by solid epithelioid granulomas that can cavitate and undergo central necrosis
- Organism is characterized by a large, round to oval spherule (30-100 μm) containing multiple endospores
- Immature spherules lack endospores

Ancillary Tests
- GMS stains both mature spherules and endospores
- Immature spherules are PAS positive

- Pulmonary nodules are typically single, peripheral, spherical, and well-defined without calcifications
- Thin-walled (so-called grape skin) cavities that may change in size over time are characteristic
- Cavitary lesion may rupture into pleural space and produce pneumothorax or bronchopleural fistula
- Disseminated disease shows miliary nodules or diffuse reticular and nodular interstitial pulmonary opacities

MACROSCOPIC FEATURES

General Features
- Chronic progressive coccidioidal pneumonia is characterized by consolidation and cavitary lesions
- Fibrous-walled cavities may contain gray-brown, friable fungus balls
- Coccidioidoma is characterized by a discrete, well-demarcated lesion without calcifications
- Rarely, endobronchial nodules may cause bronchial obstruction

MICROSCOPIC PATHOLOGY

Histologic Features
- Primary pulmonary infection is characterized by an acute suppurative pneumonia with neutrophilic infiltrates
- Granulomatous lesions are characterized by solid epithelioid granulomas that can cavitate and undergo central necrosis
- Some cases may develop an eosinophilic pneumonia in which eosinophilic infiltrate is admixed with numerous organisms
- Necrotizing granulomas may be multiple or solitary and have a fibrotic rim surrounding a central necrotic zone
- Necrotizing granulomas show peripheral palisading of histiocytes admixed with multinucleated giant cells
- Mature spherules may be difficult to identify in necrotizing granulomas and they may only contain a few immature spherules
- Immature spherules may become lined with eosinophilic radiating material resulting in Splendore-Hoeppli phenomenon

Cytologic Features
- Organism is characterized by a large, round to oval spherule (30-100 μm) containing multiple endospores
- Mature spherules have a 1-2 μm thick refractile wall
- Immature spherules lack endospores
- Endospores are 2-5 μm in diameter and have punctate cytoplasmic inclusions that are PAS(+) and GMS(-)
- Under certain conditions, endospores can germinate within the host tissue, resulting in vegetative forms
- Vegetative forms consist of 2-4 μm thick septate branching hyphae and 2-5 μm barrel-shaped arthroconidia

ANCILLARY TESTS

Histochemistry
- GMS stains both mature spherules and endospores
- Immature spherules are PAS positive

DIFFERENTIAL DIAGNOSIS

Histoplasmosis
- Yeast form of *H. capsulatum* may resemble the endospores in *C. immitis* but are characterized by the presence of buds

Blastomycosis
- Yeast forms of *B. dermatidis* may resemble the endospores of *C. immitis* but are characterized by broad-based budding forms

SELECTED REFERENCES

1. Ampel NM: New perspectives on coccidioidomycosis. Proc Am Thorac Soc. 7(3):181-5, 2010
2. Spinello IM et al: Pulmonary coccidioidomycosis. Semin Respir Crit Care Med. 29(2):166-73, 2008

COCCIDIOIDOMYCOSIS

Histologic Findings

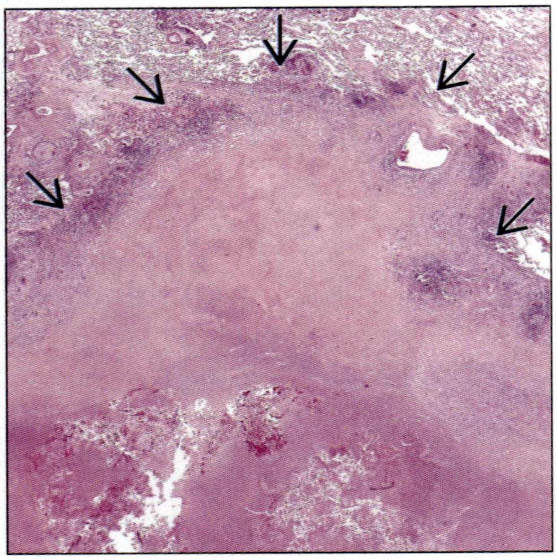

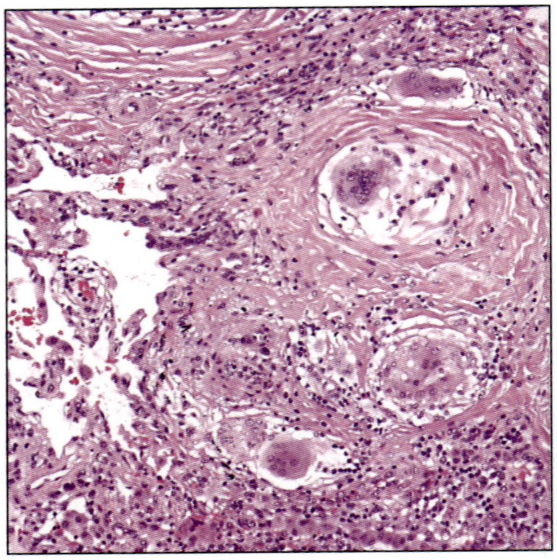

(Left) *Granulomatous lesion in pulmonary coccidioidomycosis shows a well-circumscribed nodule (coccidioidoma) → with extensive central necrosis and peripheral palisading of histiocytes.* ***(Right)*** *Scattered small epithelioid granulomas with multinucleated giant cells are seen in pulmonary coccidioidomycosis. Organisms are not numerous in granulomatous lesions and are often found within the areas of necrosis. They can be easily visualized with H&E without the need for special stains.*

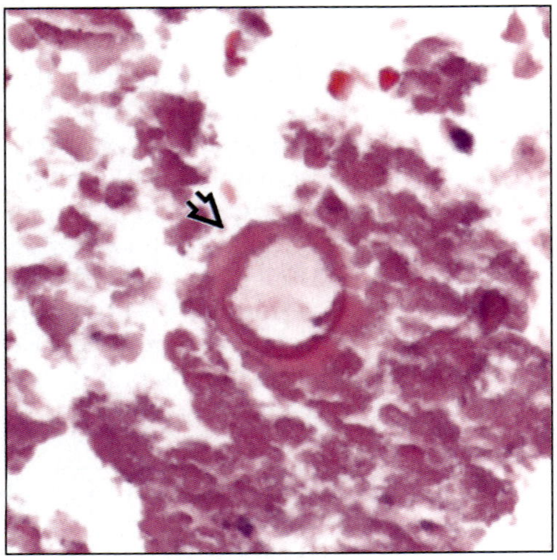

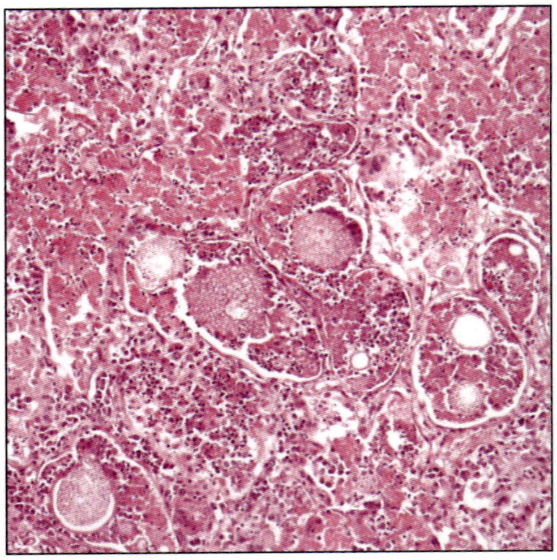

(Left) *Higher magnification of the organism in pulmonary coccidioidomycosis with localized granulomatous reaction (coccidioidoma) shows a single degenerating spherule ⇨ devoid of endospores. The extensive necrosis often makes it difficult to identify viable organisms in these cases.* ***(Right)*** *Typical reaction in primary pulmonary infection with coccidioides shows acute suppurative pneumonia with neutrophilic infiltrates and abundant organisms lying within alveolar lumens.*

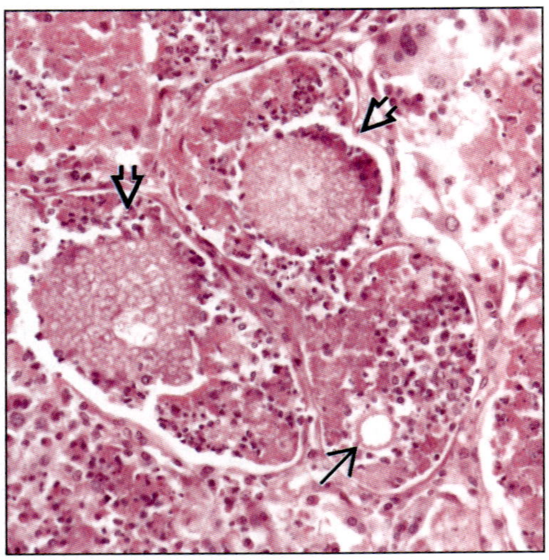

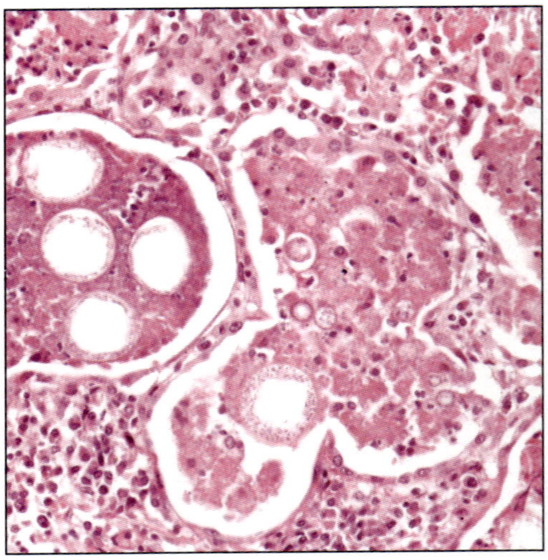

(Left) *Higher magnification of acute infection by coccidioidomycosis in the lung shows 2 large spherules ⇨ filled with numerous endospores and surrounded by abundant neutrophilic infiltrates. Notice also a smaller empty spherule → corresponding to an immature organism.* ***(Right)*** *Acute suppurative pneumonia in a patient with acute coccidioidomycosis shows multiple large spherules within distended alveolar lumens. Notice the intense neutrophilic infiltration in the interstitium.*

Cytology and Special Stains

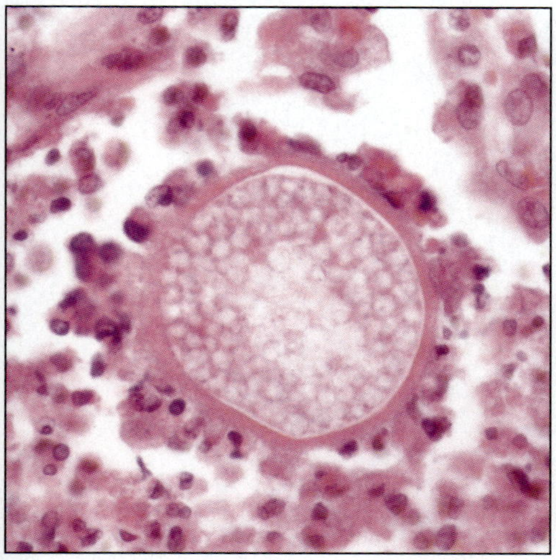
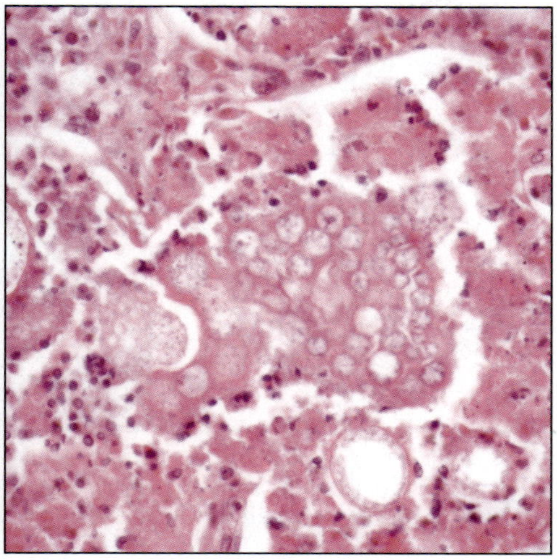

(Left) *Pulmonary coccidioidomycosis shows a large round spherule filled with endospores. Notice Splendore-Hoeppli phenomenon characterized by radiating clusters of neutrophils admixed with fibrinous exudate along the outer surface of the structure.* ***(Right)*** *Pulmonary coccidioidomycosis shows destruction of alveolar walls by acute fibrinopurulent exudate admixed with mature and immature spherules. Some spherules have ruptured, releasing their endospores.*

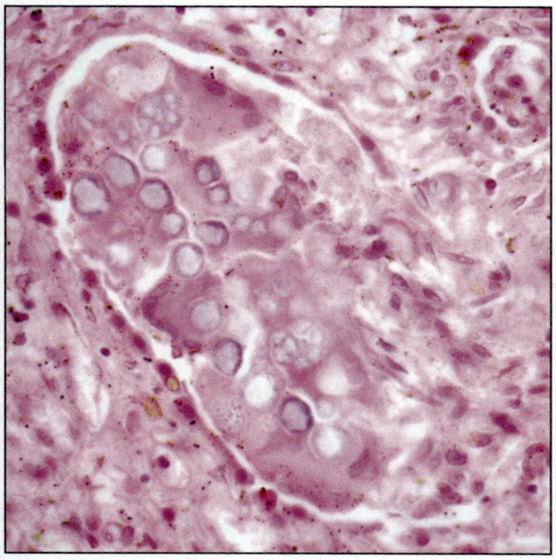
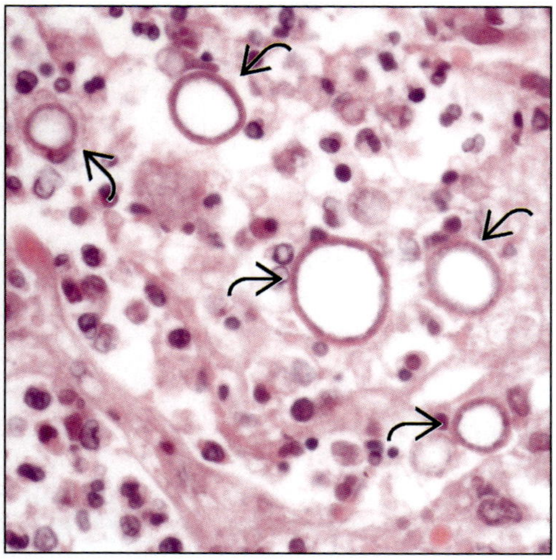

(Left) *Pulmonary coccidioidomycosis shows infiltration and dilatation of alveolar lumen by clusters of immature spherules. There is little inflammatory infiltration in this immunocompromised patient with AIDS.* ***(Right)*** *Primary pulmonary infection by coccidioidomycosis shows scattered immature spherules of C. immitis admixed with suppurative neutrophilic exudate. Notice the thin wall of the spherules* ➔*, which are empty and devoid of endospores.*

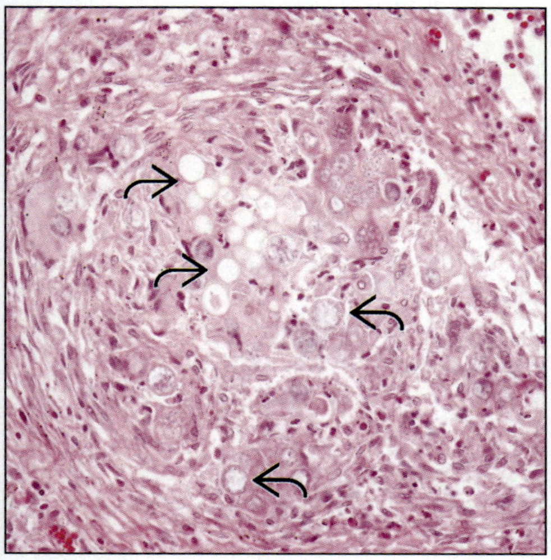
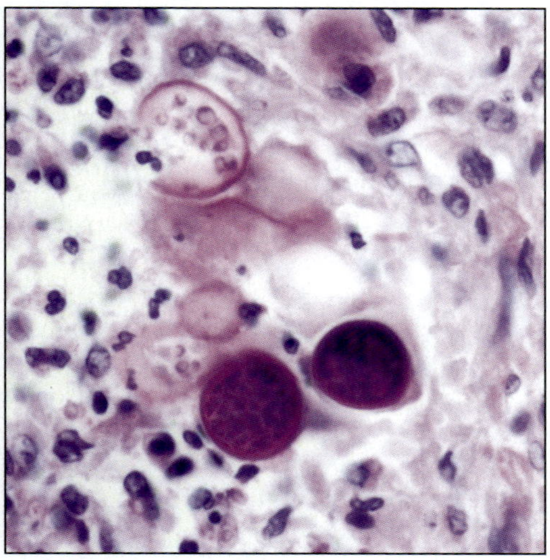

(Left) *Chronic infection with coccidioidomycosis in the lung shows small epithelioid granuloma containing multiple immature spherules* ➔ *devoid of endospores. The organisms are admixed with multinucleated giant cells.* ***(Right)*** *A histochemical stain for PAS in chronic pulmonary coccidioidomycosis highlights the organisms. Notice the stain is strongly positive in the endospores as well as in the large spherules. Immature spherules also stain with the PAS stain.*

PNEUMOCYSTOSIS

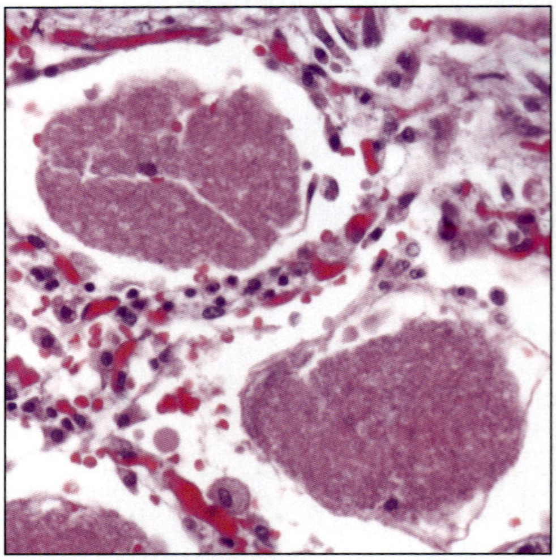

Histologic appearance of pulmonary pneumocystosis is characterized by abundant frothy intraalveolar eosinophilic exudates that contain multiple organisms.

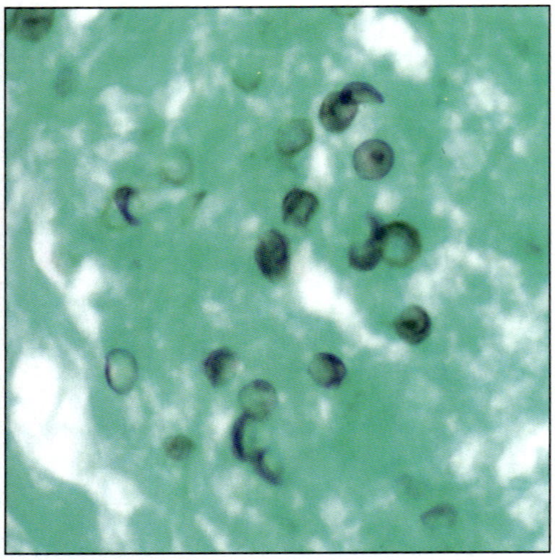

Histochemical stain for GMS in pulmonary pneumocystosis shows the typical organisms with crescentic forms as well as some cysts with dark-staining central dots.

TERMINOLOGY

Abbreviations

- Pneumocystosis pneumonia (PCP)

Definitions

- Lung infection caused by fungus *Pneumocystis jiroveci* (formerly *P. carinii*)

CLINICAL ISSUES

Epidemiology

- Incidence
  - Organisms are globally distributed

Presentation

- Clinical presentation of Pneumocystis pneumonia can be quite variable
  - Some patients may be completely asymptomatic or show only minimal symptoms, including
    - Nonproductive cough, dyspnea, fever
  - Some patients may follow a rapidly fatal course with progressive respiratory failure
    - Insidious onset with respiratory and generalized symptoms of fever, dyspnea, tachypnea, cough, weight loss, and fatigue
- Favorable prognosis when appropriately treated; relapses are common in AIDS patients

Laboratory Tests

- HIV-infected patients with CD4 counts < 200 cell/μL are 5x more likely to develop PCP

Natural History

- Infection is acquired by inhalation, with primary infection occurring early in life and remaining latent in host
- Reinfection occurs when host becomes immunocompromised
- 2 major clinical forms
  - Infantile form ("plasma cell interstitial pneumonia") affects premature and malnourished infants
  - Adult (sporadic) form occurs in AIDS patients and other immunocompromised patients with impaired CD4(+) lymphoid cells

Treatment

- Drugs
  - Trimethoprim-sulfamethoxazole
  - Pentamidine isethionate
  - Early adjunctive treatment with corticosteroids can reduce morbidity and mortality

Prognosis

- Survival rates of 50-90% with appropriate treatment

IMAGE FINDINGS

Radiographic Findings

- Early stages show a fine pattern of ground-glass opacities involving perihilar regions
- Untreated cases progress to perihilar or diffuse bilateral airspace consolidation involving mainly lower lobes

CT Findings

- HRCT shows characteristic symmetrical, bilateral ground-glass opacities with geographic distribution
- AIDS patients show tendency to develop bilateral thin-walled cysts in 30% of cases showing subpleural distribution
- Atypical cases may show nodules, thick-walled cavities, and focal or asymmetric areas of consolidation

MACROSCOPIC FEATURES

General Features

- Consolidation of pulmonary parenchyma with pale-gray or tan granular cut surface

PNEUMOCYSTOSIS

Key Facts

Terminology

- Lung infection caused by fungus *Pneumocystis jiroveci* (formerly *P. carinii*)

Clinical Issues

- Infantile form ("plasma cell interstitial pneumonia") affects premature and malnourished infants
- Adult (sporadic) form occurs in AIDS patients and other immunocompromised patients with impaired CD4(+) lymphoid cells
- Insidious onset with respiratory and generalized symptoms of fever, dyspnea, tachypnea, cough, weight loss, and fatigue
- Favorable prognosis when appropriately treated; relapses are common in AIDS patients

Microscopic Pathology

- Typical pattern is characterized by foamy, granular eosinophilic intraalveolar exudates containing organisms
- Alveolar exudate is composed of fibrin admixed with abundant trophozoites and cysts, surfactant, and cellular debris
- Cysts are oval (4-7 μm) with collapsed or crescentic forms and exhibit grooves, folds, and dark-staining central dots

Ancillary Tests

- Cysts are best stained in tissues with GMS
- Antibodies against Pneumocystis can be used to highlight organisms in tissue sections by immunoperoxidase technique

- Nodules or cavities may occasionally be identified
- Small subpleural blebs and cysts are often noted in upper lobes

MICROSCOPIC PATHOLOGY

Histologic Features

- Histologic reaction patterns can be quite variable
  - Typical pattern is characterized by foamy, granular eosinophilic intraalveolar exudates containing organisms
    - Alveolar exudate is composed of fibrin admixed with abundant trophozoites and cysts, surfactant, and cellular debris
    - Alveolar exudate may be focal or diffuse and can be accompanied by mild interstitial inflammation and type II pneumocyte hyperplasia
  - Atypical patterns
    - Dense interstitial lymphoid infiltrates (LIP-like pattern), which may obscure alveolar exudates
    - Interstitial fibrosis and organizing pneumonia may be seen in resolving phase of process
    - Diffuse alveolar damage pattern with hyaline membranes
    - Absence of characteristic foamy alveolar exudate can be seen in up to 50% of non-HIV patients
    - Miliary pattern of involvement with multiple small, scattered foci of PCP
    - Cavitary lesions (including subpleural blebs), intraparenchymatous cysts, or necrotizing granulomas may be seen
    - Granulomatous pattern with clusters of epithelioid histiocytes and multinucleated giant cells lining alveolar walls
    - Interstitial microcalcifications can be seen in small percentage of patients and should raise possibility of PCP
    - Vacular invasion by exudate containing organisms and vasculitis can be seen in small percentage of patients

Cytologic Features

- Organisms have 3 life stages: Sporozoites, trophozoites, and cysts
- Cysts are the most commonly encountered and are oval (4-7 μm) with collapsed or crescentic forms
- Cysts may display prominent grooves or folds and small, darkly staining, dot-like structures at their centers

ANCILLARY TESTS

Histochemistry

- Cysts are best stained in tissues with GMS
- Trophozoites are seen only in smears stained with Giemsa (Diff-Quik)

Immunohistochemistry

- Antibodies against Pneumocystis can be used to highlight organisms in tissue sections by immunoperoxidase technique

DIFFERENTIAL DIAGNOSIS

Histoplasmosis

- *H. capsulatum* may show similar morphology to Pneumocystis, including central dark dots
  - Pneumocystis lacks budding forms unlike *H. capsulatum*, which is characterized by budding yeast

SELECTED REFERENCES

1. Matsumura Y et al: Clinical characteristics of Pneumocystis pneumonia in non-HIV patients and prognostic factors including microbiological genotypes. BMC Infect Dis. 11(1):76, 2011

PNEUMOCYSTOSIS

Histologic Features

*(**Left**) Typical histologic appearance of pulmonary pneumocystosis is characterized by foamy, granular eosinophilic intraalveolar exudates → containing abundant organisms. The organisms cannot be easily visualized on routine microscopy and usually require the use of special stains. (**Right**) Typical appearance of pulmonary pneumocystosis shows frothy intraalveolar eosinophilic exudates. Notice the lack of damage or inflammation in the alveolar walls.*

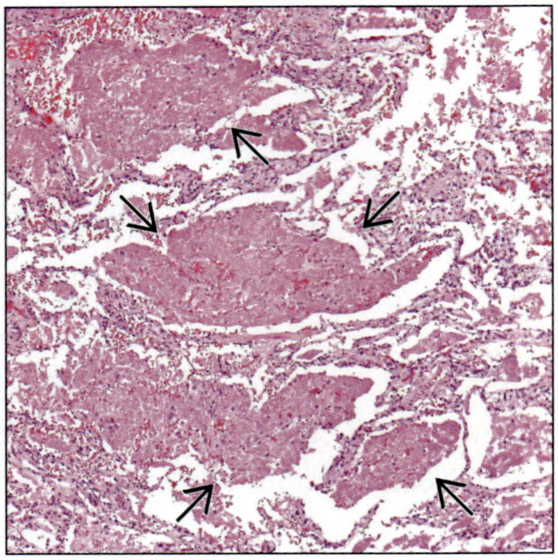

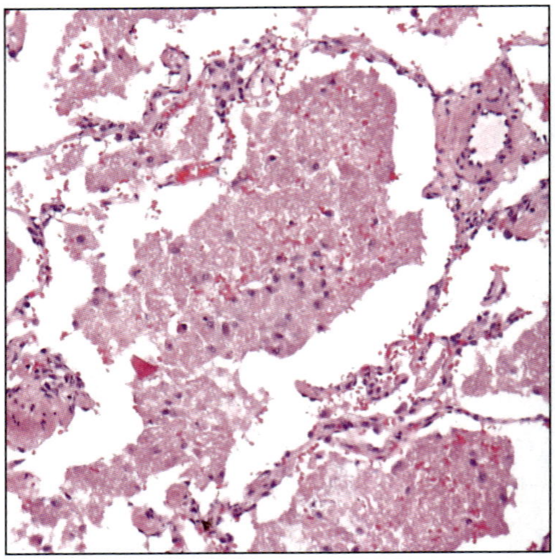

*(**Left**) Higher magnification of the frothy intraalveolar exudate shows mostly fibrin admixed with a few scattered inflammatory cells. Numerous small round "ghosts" of cells are seen in the background, which correspond to the unstained organisms. (**Right**) Acute pulmonary pneumocystosis is characterized by diffuse alveolar damage associated with intraalveolar exudates. Notice the frothy alveolar exudates ⇨ and the hyaline membranes lining the alveoli →.*

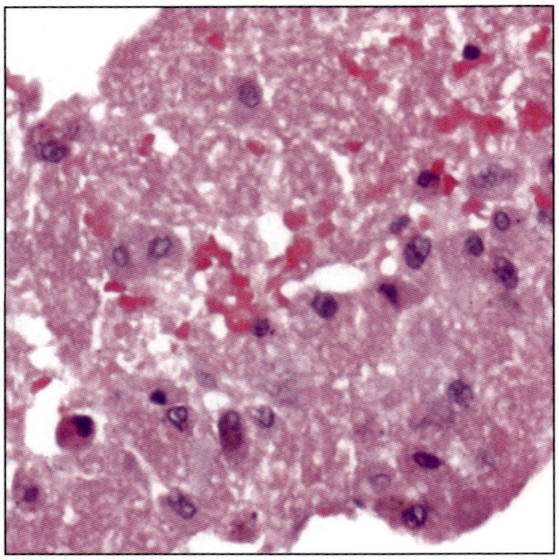

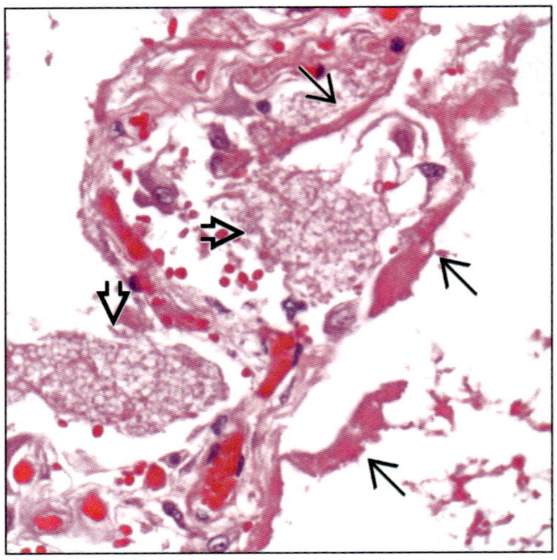

*(**Left**) Acute pulmonary pneumocystosis shows abundant frothy intraalveolar exudate and hyperplasia of type II pneumocytes in the lining of the airspace →. (**Right**) Pulmonary pneumocystosis simulating lymphoid interstitial pneumonia (LIP) shows frothy intraalveolar exudate within the alveolar lumen ⇨ surrounded by a dense lymphoid infiltrate that is distending and replacing the alveolar walls. Cases like this may be confused for LIP if the exudate is overlooked.*

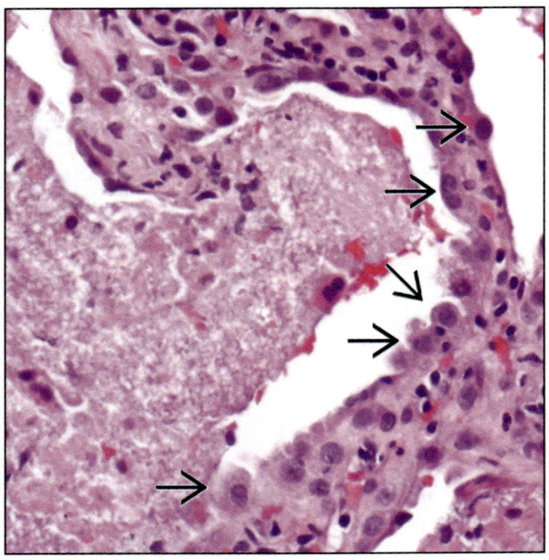

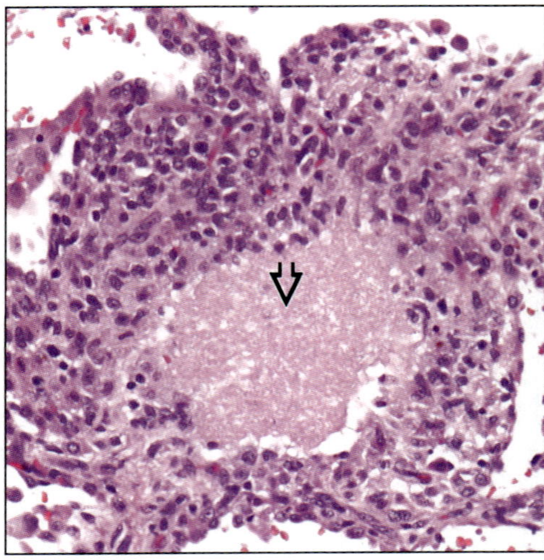

PNEUMOCYSTOSIS

Histology and Special Stains

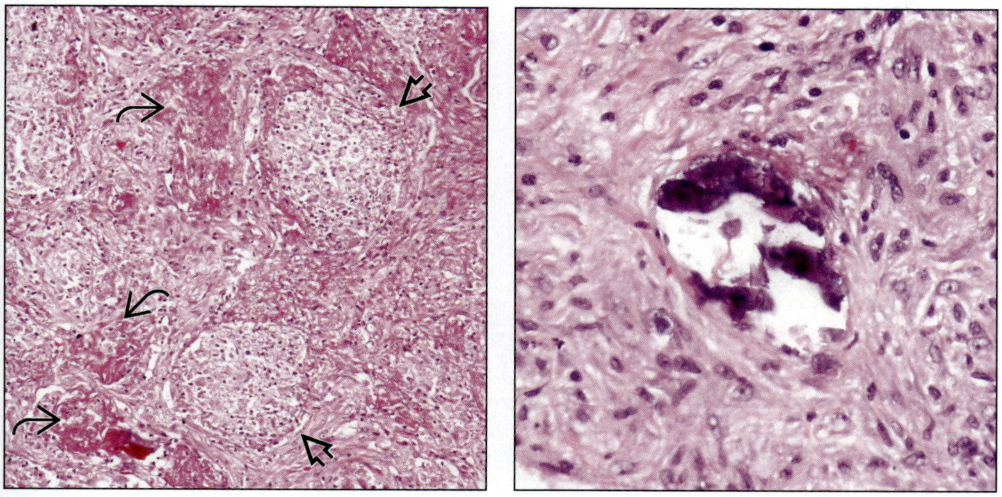

(Left) *Pulmonary pneumocystosis with granulomatous reaction shows well-formed epithelioid granulomas* ⇨ *adjacent to discrete foci containing frothy eosinophilic exudates* ↪. *The granulomas can sometimes obscure the diagnosis when the exudates are minimal.* ***(Right)*** *Stromal calcification is seen in a case of granulomatous pulmonary pneumocystosis. Interstitial calcifications can be seen in a small proportion of patients with pneumocystosis and are a helpful clue for diagnosis.*

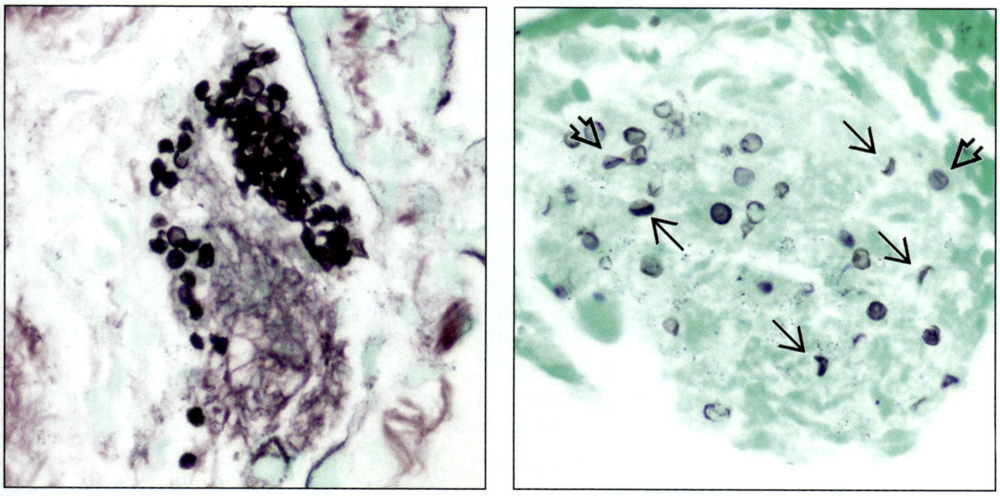

(Left) *Pulmonary pneumocystosis stained with Gomori methenamine silver (GMS) shows numerous small round organisms lying within the alveolar exudate.* ***(Right)*** *Pulmonary pneumocystosis stained with Gomori methenamine silver (GMS) shows small oval cysts. The cysts can display collapsed or crescentic forms* → *and have been described as disc or boat-shaped. They can also display distinctive longitudinal grooves or folds* ⇨.

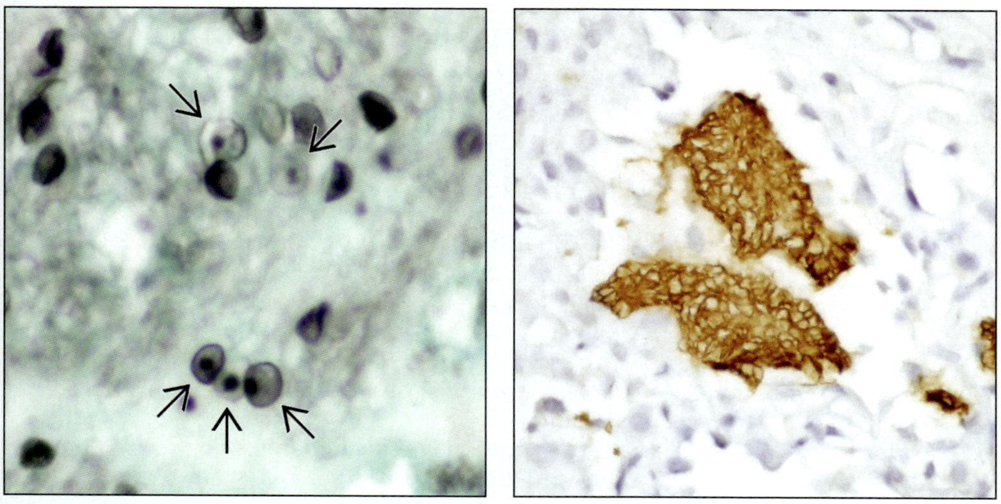

(Left) *Pulmonary pneumocystosis stained with Gomori methenamine silver (GMS) stain shows another characteristic feature of the cysts, which is the presence of dark-staining central "dots"* →. ***(Right)*** *Immunohistochemical staining in pulmonary pneumocystosis with antibodies against Pneumocystis shows multiple organisms lying within the alveolar lumens. The organisms show a dark brown reaction with this antibody.*

BLASTOMYCOSIS

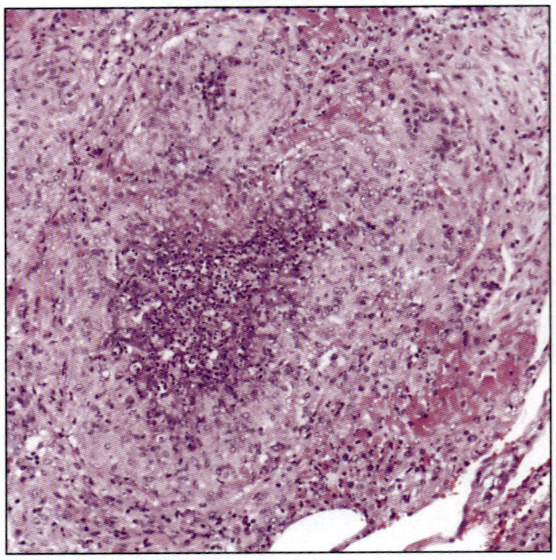

Scanning magnification of a suppurative, epithelioid granuloma in pulmonary blastomycosis shows a dense collection of epithelioid histiocytes with central necrosis and neutrophilic infiltrates.

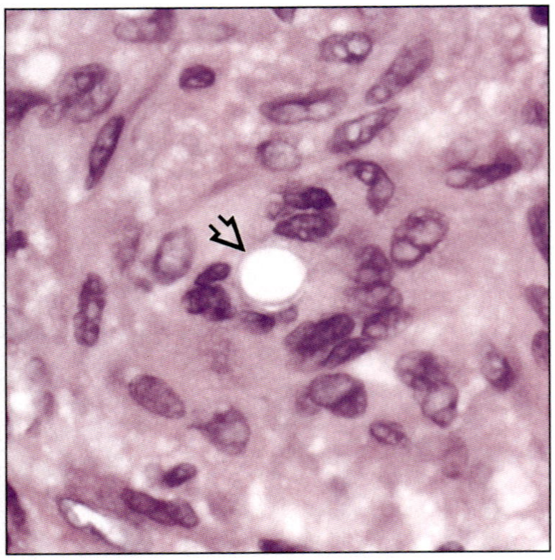

Higher magnification from an epithelioid granuloma in pulmonary blastomycosis shows abundant epithelioid histiocytes surrounding a large (~ 10 μm), oval yeast form ⇨ with a thin refractile capsule.

TERMINOLOGY

Synonyms

- North American blastomycosis

Definitions

- Pulmonary infection caused by inhalation of the fungus *Blastomyces dermatidis*

ETIOLOGY/PATHOGENESIS

Environmental Exposure

- Natural habitat for the fungus is most likely wood

CLINICAL ISSUES

Epidemiology

- Incidence
  - Geographic distribution in the USA: Mississippi, Missouri, and Ohio River valleys
  - Mostly restricted to North America although cases have been described in other countries in South America, Asia, and the Middle East
- Age
  - Young adults
- Gender
  - Male predilection

Presentation

- Acute infection is usually self-limited and may simulate a bacterial pneumonia
  - Cough
  - Sudden onset of fever and chills
  - Myalgias and arthralgias
- Chronic infection presents with gradual onset of cough, low-grade fever, hemoptysis, weight loss, and pleuritic pain

Laboratory Tests

- Culture is most definitive way to establish the diagnosis but may take up to 3 weeks to be positive

Natural History

- Infection may be acute or chronic; most often self-limited and accompanied by flu-like symptoms
- Some cases in acute phase may lead to respiratory distress syndrome and cavitary lesions
- Extrapulmonary hematogenous spread may occur to a variety of organs, in particular skin and bone
- Not a common infection in immunocompromised patients, but the disease is more aggressive in HIV(+) patients
- Advanced chronic cases may lead to development of sclerosing mediastinitis

Treatment

- Drugs
  - Amphotericin B used in severe life-threatening infections
  - Ketoconazole used in mild or moderate infections

Prognosis

- Acute primary blastomycosis usually self-limited

IMAGE FINDINGS

Radiographic Findings

- Focal or diffuse parenchymal consolidation affecting upper lobes
- Solitary or multiple nodules can occur in about 30% of patients
- Single or multiple cavities can be seen in 15-20% of patients
- Pleural effusion and pleural thickening seen in up to 15% of patients

CT Findings

- Localized mass with air bronchograms

Key Facts

Terminology
- Pulmonary infection caused by inhalation of the fungus *Blastomyces dermatidis*

Clinical Issues
- Geographic distribution in the USA: Mississippi, Missouri, and Ohio River valleys
- Acute infection is usually self-limited and may simulate bacterial pneumonia

Microscopic Pathology
- Typical reaction of lung parenchyma to *B. dermatidis* is suppuration with abscess formation
- Advanced stages show necrotizing palisading granulomas
- Organisms are round to oval budding yeasts measuring 8-15 μm with thick, refractile cell walls
- Organisms stain positive with GMS and may also stain positive for PAS

- Hilar &/or mediastinal lymphadenopathy

MACROSCOPIC FEATURES

General Features
- Lesions may be nodular and localized or diffuse with a miliary pattern of spread
- Chronic lesions show fibrosis and hyalinization of the nodules, with cavitation similar to other fungal processes

MICROSCOPIC PATHOLOGY

Histologic Features
- Typical reaction of lung parenchyma to *B. dermatidis* is suppuration with abscess formation
- Advanced stages show necrotizing palisaded granulomas
- Granulomas may become fibrotic and cavitary, but calcification is very uncommon

Cytologic Features
- Organisms are round to oval yeasts measuring 8-15 μm with thick, refractile cell walls
- Yeasts frequently show budding, with a broad base attached to the parent cell
- Organisms are more numerous in suppurative than in granulomatous lesions

ANCILLARY TESTS

Immunofluorescence
- Direct immunofluorescence or immunohistochemistry in deparaffinized tissue sections is a sensitive way to make the diagnosis

Histochemistry
- Organisms stain positive with GMS and may also stain positive for PAS

DIFFERENTIAL DIAGNOSIS

Cryptococcosis
- Does not show broad-based budding yeast, and the capsule-deficient variant is negative for mucicarmine stains
- Capsule-deficient *Cryptococcus* is positive with Fontana-Masson stain (unlike blastomycosis, which is negative)

SELECTED REFERENCES

1. Mukhopadhyay S: Role of histology in the diagnosis of infectious causes of granulomatous lung disease. Curr Opin Pulm Med. 17(3):189-96, 2011
2. Patel AJ et al: Diagnosis of blastomycosis in surgical pathology and cytopathology: correlation with microbiologic culture. Am J Surg Pathol. 34(2):256-61, 2010

IMAGE GALLERY

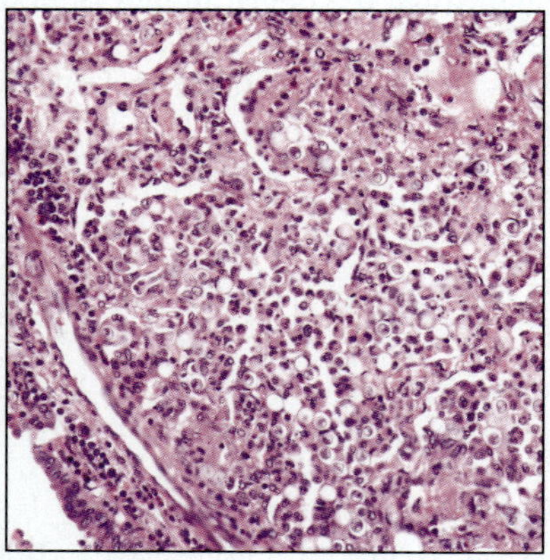

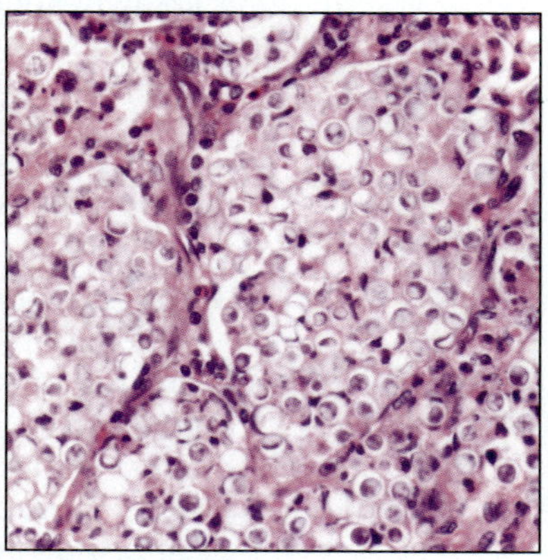

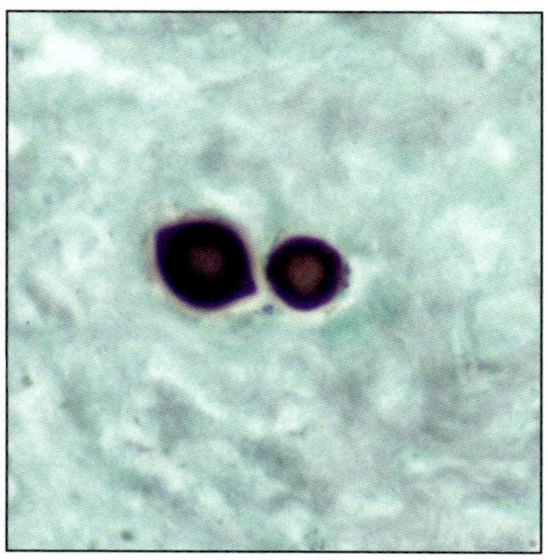

(Left) *Acute bronchopneumonia with suppurative inflammation and numerous organisms is seen in acute pulmonary blastomycosis.* ***(Center)*** *Higher magnification from an acute lesion of pulmonary blastomycosis shows numerous yeast forms stuffing the alveolar lumens. The organisms are easily recognized on routine histology due to their thick, refractile cell walls.* ***(Right)*** *Pulmonary blastomycosis stained with Gomori methenamine silver (GMS) shows round to oval yeast with thick walls.*

HISTOPLASMOSIS

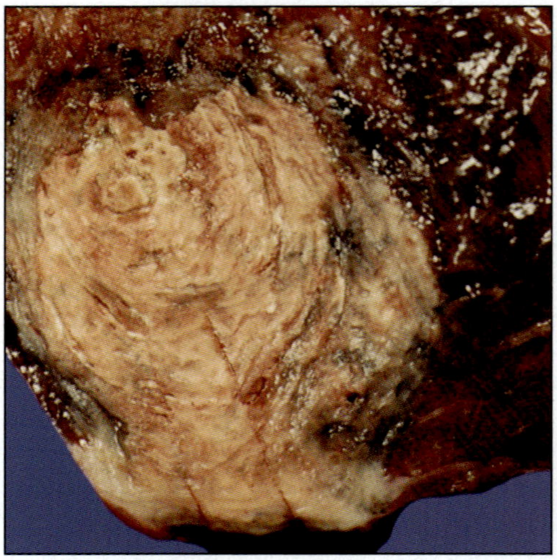

Gross appearance of a pulmonary histoplasma granuloma shows a distinctive lamellar pattern of concentric fibrosis with progressive stages of calcification.

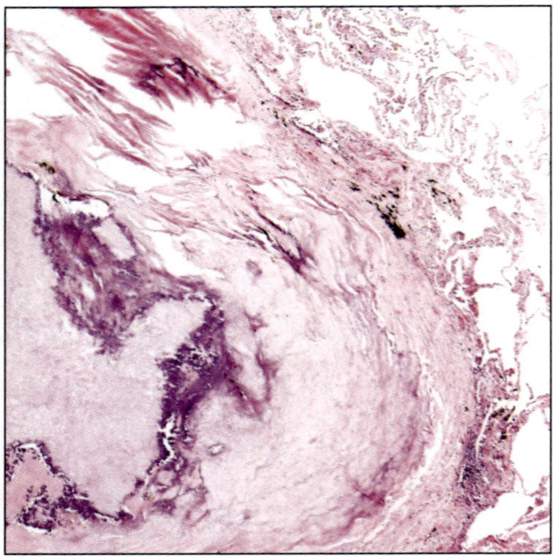

Histologic appearance of an old hyalinized histoplasma granuloma of the lung shows concentric layers of fibrotic and calcified material surrounding a hyalinized central core.

TERMINOLOGY

Definitions

- Disease caused by inhalation of the fungus *Histoplasma capsulatum*

ETIOLOGY/PATHOGENESIS

Environmental Exposure

- The fungus lives in soil and is endemic to the south-central United States, especially the Mississippi and Ohio valleys
- Infection caused by inhalation of infected dust, most commonly from bird droppings

CLINICAL ISSUES

Epidemiology

- Incidence
  - Approximately 500,000 new cases occur annually

Presentation

- Clinical forms of histoplasmosis include benign self-limited, acute, chronic, progressive disseminated, and with mediastinal involvement
- Most patients with primary pulmonary infection are asymptomatic (75% of patients)
- Patients with acute pulmonary histoplasmosis present with a self-limited disease in the upper lobes that resolves spontaneously
- Patients exposed to a large inoculum may develop life-threatening infection with acute respiratory distress syndrome
- Symptoms usually develop 2 weeks after exposure and include fever, chills, cough, and muscle pain
- Complications of the infection include calcified pulmonary nodules, chronic cavitary lesions, or mediastinal fibrosis
- Immunosuppressed patients generally develop progressive disseminated disease involving other organs

Treatment

- Drugs
  - Progressive disseminated disease requires treatment with antifungal agents such as amphotericin B, ketoconazole, etc.

Prognosis

- Acute primary infection is self-limited and resolves spontaneously without treatment
- Progressive disseminated disease in immunocompromised patients is associated with 80% mortality without treatment

IMAGE FINDINGS

Radiographic Findings

- Majority of patients with primary infection have normal chest x-rays
- Acute infection shows focal or multifocal parenchymal consolidation associated with ipsilateral hilar lymphadenopathy
- Resolving phase will show the development of nodular opacities (histoplasmoma)
- Pulmonary nodules and hilar adenopathy often show central calcification
- Mediastinal involvement presents with focal densities or with diffuse fibrosing mediastinitis

MACROSCOPIC FEATURES

General Features

- In acute histoplasmosis, cut section shows patchy pneumonia
- Disseminated histoplasmosis characterized by congestion and scattered granulomas on cut section

Key Facts

Terminology
- Disease caused by inhalation of the fungus *Histoplasma capsulatum*

Clinical Issues
- Clinical forms of histoplasmosis include benign self-limited, acute, chronic, progressive disseminated, and with mediastinal involvement
- Immunosuppressed patients generally develop progressive disseminated disease involving other organs

Microscopic Pathology
- Acute infection characterized by acute fibrinous pneumonia with abundant organisms within macrophages in alveolar spaces
- Disseminated infection characterized by granulomatous inflammation that may show central areas of necrosis
- Granulomas may show characteristic lamellar patten of concentric fibrosis with progressive stages of calcification
- Organisms are round or oval, small (2-4 μm), uninucleated, and devoid of a capsule, with single narrow-based buds
- Organisms can also show a small, dark-staining central "dot" similar to those seen in Pneumocystis
- Cytoplasm of the yeast can be retracted from the cell wall, forming a "halo" that resembles a capsule
- Organisms are highlighted in tissue sections with GMS stains
- PAS also stains *Histoplasma* but more weakly

- Chronic histoplasmosis shows diffuse, bilateral infiltrates associated with cavitary lesions resembling tuberculosis
- Solitary lesions (histoplasmoma) are round, subpleural, and show a pattern of laminated, concentric calcification

MICROSCOPIC PATHOLOGY

Histologic Features
- Acute infection characterized by acute fibrinous pneumonia with abundant organisms within macrophages in alveolar spaces
- Disseminated infection characterized by granulomatous inflammation that may show central areas of necrosis
- Occasionally small, solid, non-necrotizing epithelioid granulomas may develop that can mimic sarcoidosis
- Chronic infection characterized by formation of necrotizing granulomas
- Granulomas may show characteristic lamellar patten of concentric fibrosis with progressive stages of calcification
- Necrotizing granulomas can sometimes involve bronchi and bronchioles resembling bronchocentric granulomatosis
- Histoplasmomas consist of large necrotizing granulomas surrounded by a fibrous capsule with large central zones of necrosis that may become calcified
- Disseminated form in immunosuppressed patients shows extensive tissue infiltration with abundant organisms and no tissue reaction

Cytologic Features
- *Histoplasma* is seen in tissues in yeast form and are usually multiple and clustered
- Organisms are round or oval, small (2-4 μm), uninucleated, and devoid of a capsule, with single narrow-based buds
- Organisms can also show a small, dark-staining central "dot" similar to those seen in Pneumocystis
- Cytoplasm of the yeast can be retracted from the cell wall, forming a "halo" that resembles a capsule
- Organisms are extremely rare in tissue sections and require use of special stains to visualize
- Organisms are usually present in the centers of necrotizing granulomas or within macrophages

ANCILLARY TESTS

Histochemistry
- Organisms are best stained with GMS
- PAS stains will also identify the organisms, particularly in acute infection when they are numerous

Immunofluorescence
- Direct immunofluorescence on histologic sections can help establish diagnosis

DIFFERENTIAL DIAGNOSIS

Pneumocystosis
- *P. jiroveci* may show identical morphology to histoplasma (including central "dots") but is not found within large necrotizing granulomas

Blastomycosis
- *B. dermatidis* may show identical morphology to histoplasma but is characterized by broad-based budding yeast and thicker walls

Capsule-deficient Cryptococcus
- Cell walls are strongly positive for Fontana-Masson and may also be weakly positive for mucicarmine

SELECTED REFERENCES

1. Mukhopadhyay S: Role of histology in the diagnosis of infectious causes of granulomatous lung disease. Curr Opin Pulm Med. 17(3):189-96, 2011
2. Hage CA et al: Pulmonary histoplasmosis. Semin Respir Crit Care Med. 29(2):151-65, 2008

HISTOPLASMOSIS

Histologic Features

*(**Left**) Necrotizing palisading granuloma in pulmonary histoplasmosis shows a well-defined collection of epithelioid histiocytes surrounding a centrally necrotic area ⇨. The organisms cannot be visualized on routine histology and require the use of special stains for identification. (**Right**) Higher magnification of a palisaded necrotizing granuloma in a patient with pulmonary histoplasmosis shows a necrotic center bordered by a rim of palisaded histiocytes →.*

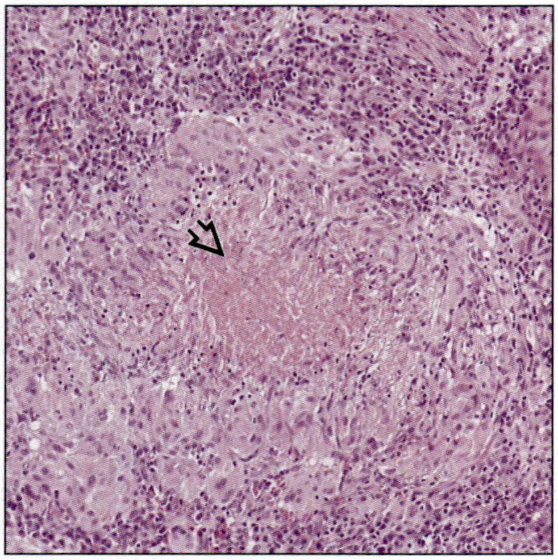

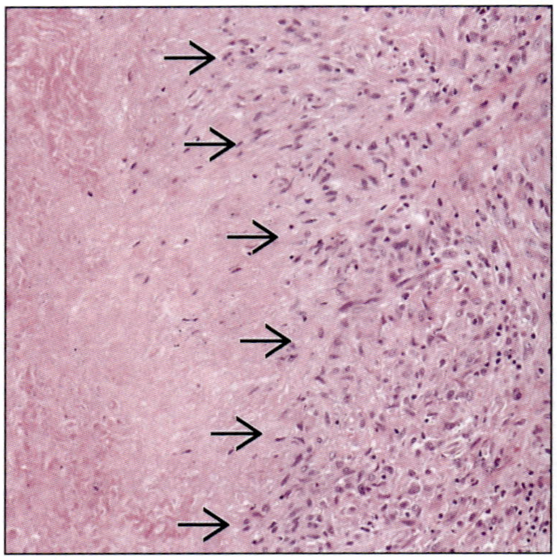

*(**Left**) Suppurative granuloma in pulmonary histoplasmosis shows a well-defined rim of epithelioid histiocytes → circumscribing a dense zone of suppuration containing abundant neutrophilic infiltrates ⇨. (**Right**) Higher magnification of a suppurative granuloma in pulmonary histoplasmosis shows a rim of epithelioid histiocytes ↷ showing a sharp transition with a central area of suppuration. Sheets of neutrophils are seen, but organisms could not be visualized on routine stains.*

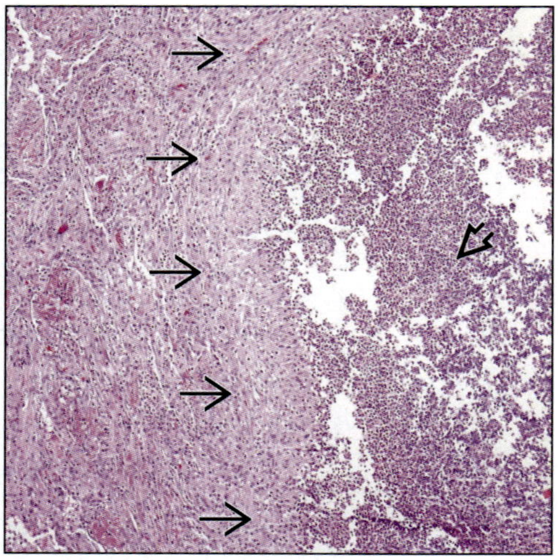

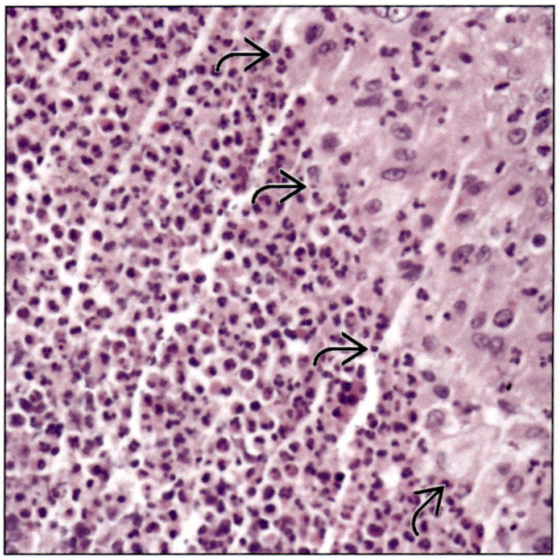

*(**Left**) Non-necrotizing epithelioid granuloma (so-called productive granuloma) in a patient with pulmonary histoplasmosis shows focalized accumulation of epithelioid histiocytes devoid of central areas of necrosis. Cases like this can mimic sarcoidosis, but special stains will reveal evidence of the characteristic organisms. (**Right**) Higher magnification of non-necrotizing epithelioid granuloma in a patient with pulmonary histoplasmosis shows multinucleated giant cells.*

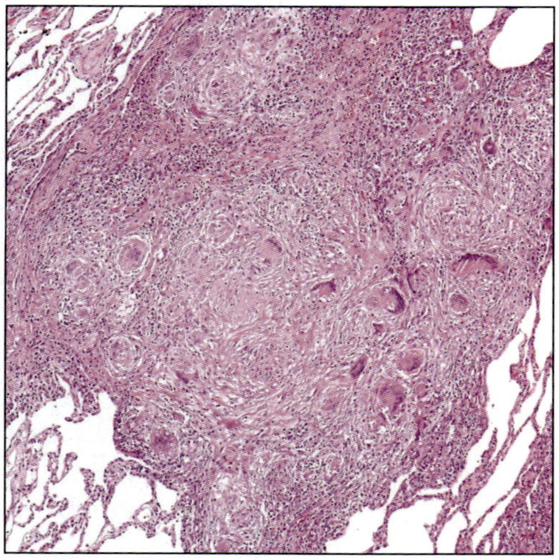

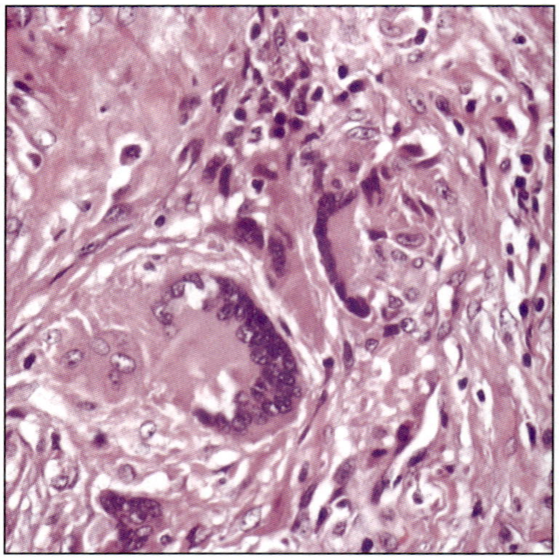

Histology and Special Stains

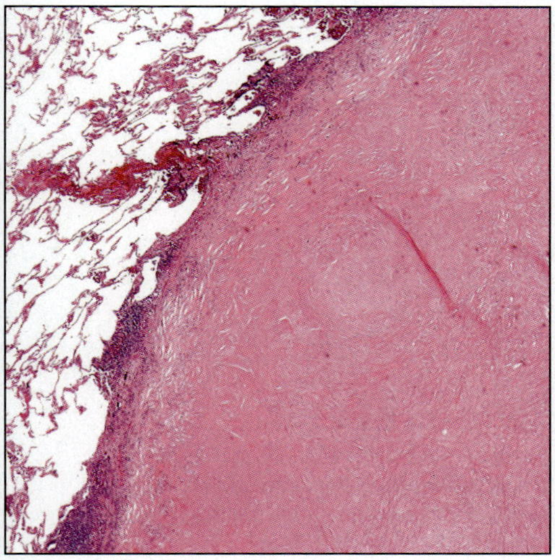

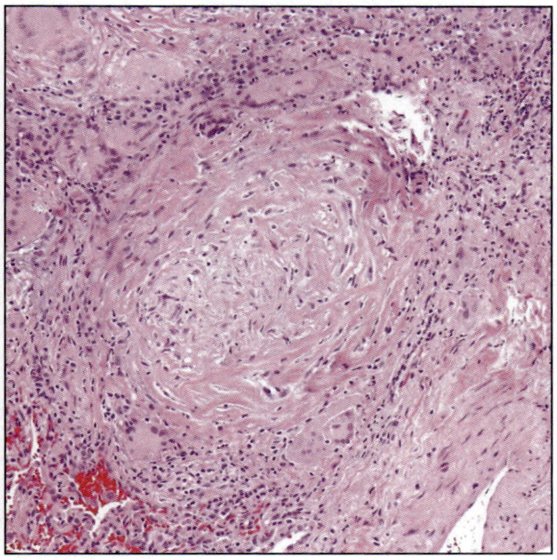

(Left) *Solitary histoplasmoma in pulmonary histoplasmosis shows a characteristic well-circumscribed nodule that is sharply separated from the surrounding lung parenchyma with extensive central areas of necrosis.* ***(Right)*** *Hyalinizing granuloma in a patient with pulmonary histoplasmosis shows a well-circumscribed collection of epithelioid histiocytes with concentric layers of hyalinized collagen. Progression of the process leads to formation of a fibrous capsule and calcification.*

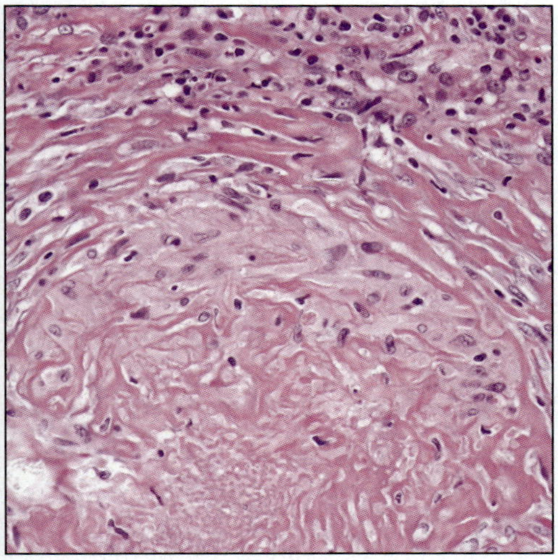

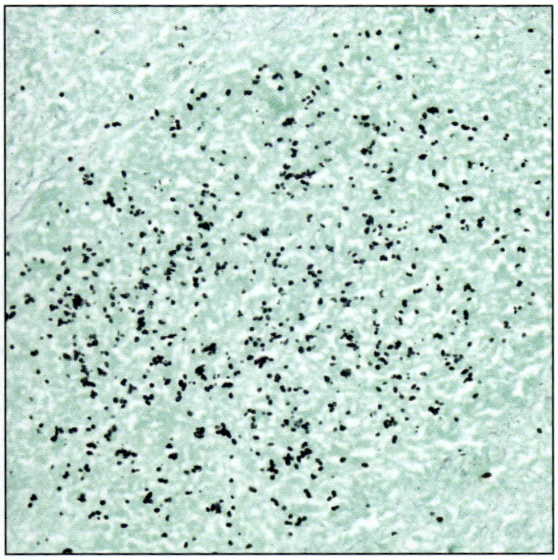

(Left) *Higher magnification of a fibrosing granuloma in pulmonary histoplasmosis shows dense deposits of hyalinized collagen arranged in layers around the periphery of the granuloma.* ***(Right)*** *Gomori methenamine silver (GMS) stain in a necrotizing granuloma of a patient with pulmonary histoplasmosis shows numerous organisms forming clusters in the central portion of the granuloma. The number of organisms can vary and decreases with the age of the lesions.*

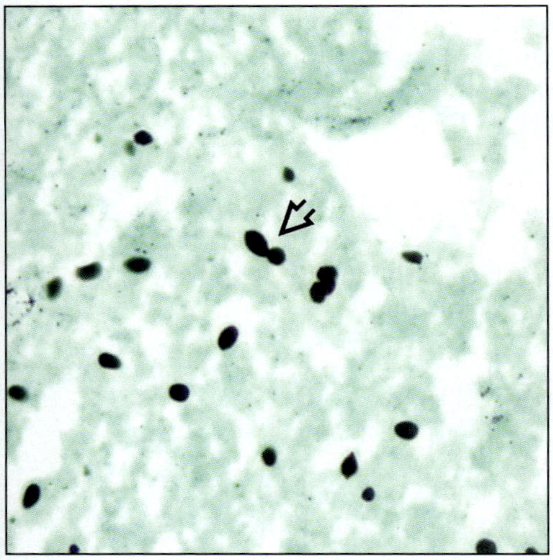

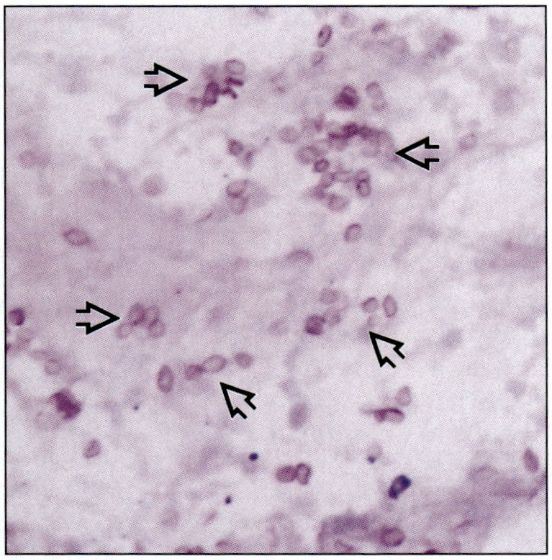

(Left) *Higher magnification of pulmonary histoplasmosis stained with Gomori methenamine silver (GMS) shows small round to oval yeast devoid of a capsule. One of the organisms shows budding, with a single narrow-based bud ⇨.* ***(Right)*** *High magnification of pulmonary histoplasmosis stained with periodic acid-Schiff (PAS) stain shows numerous clusters of scattered small yeasts ⇨. Notice that the organisms stain much less intensely than with the GMS stain.*

TUBERCULOSIS

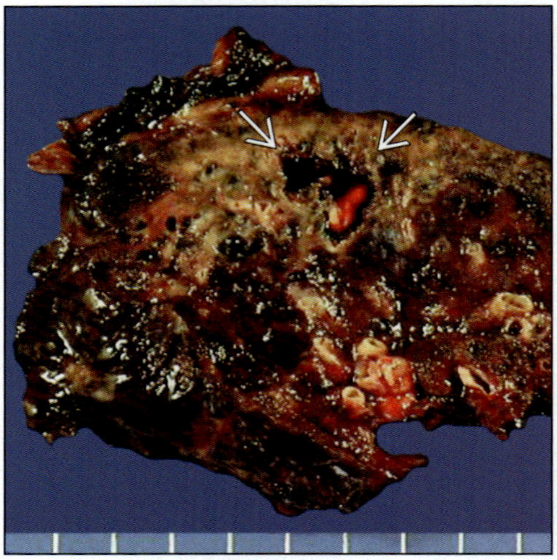

Gross appearance of the lung in active pulmonary tuberculosis shows subpleural areas of consolidation with cavitary lesions containing caseous material in the lumen ➔.

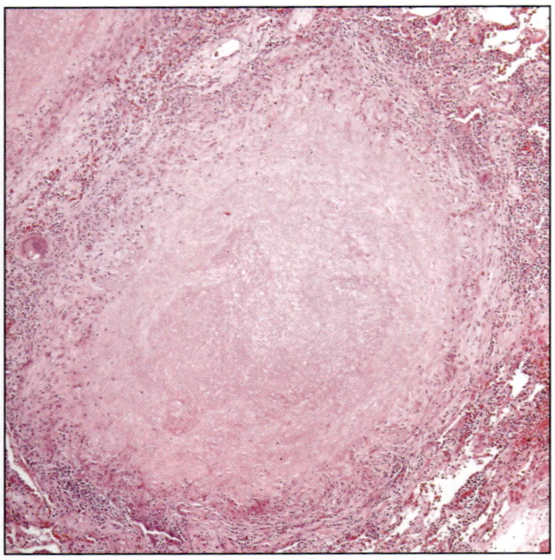

Typical histologic appearance of pulmonary tuberculosis characterized by necrotizing caseating granuloma shows peripheral palisading of histiocytes surrounding a necrotic center.

TERMINOLOGY

Abbreviations

- Tuberculosis (TB)

Definitions

- Lung infection caused by inhalation of *Mycobacterium tuberculosis*

ETIOLOGY/PATHOGENESIS

Infectious Agents

- Tuberculosis transmitted through inhalation of airborne droplets contaminated with the bacillus

CLINICAL ISSUES

Epidemiology

- Incidence
  - About 1/3 of the world's population is infected with tuberculosis; more prevalent in underdeveloped countries
  - About 10% of HIV-infected patients will develop active disease annually

Presentation

- Primary TB is defined as an infection occurring in a previously uninfected host
  - Primary infection is usually asymptomatic and leads to formation of the Ghon complex (apical nodule with calcification) and hilar lymphadenopathy
  - Progressive primary TB occurs when the primary foci do not involute and progress to disseminated, cavitary lesions
  - Fulminant infection with dissemination via the bloodstream can lead to miliary tuberculosis
- Secondary or chronic TB is defined as active disease developing in a previously sensitized host
  - Most common mechanism of secondary TB is reactivation of a latent focus of infection
  - May also be the result of massive reinfection from external source
  - Symptoms include cough, weight loss, fatigue, and fever with cavitary lesions in the upper lobes
  - Often associated with chronic, debilitating diseases or immunosuppressive states (AIDS, transplant, cancer, diabetes, alcoholism)

Natural History

- Symptomatic TB is a disease mainly of debilitated and immunosuppressed patients
- TB is a major cause of death in individuals infected with HIV

Treatment

- Drugs
  - Successful treatment of TB requires multidrug therapy for prolonged period of time
  - Most traditional drugs include isoniazid, para-aminosalicylic acid, streptomycin, rifampin, ethambutol, and pyrazinamide
  - Drug-resistant strains of TB require use of novel compounds

Prognosis

- Mortality rate for active tuberculosis is ~ 50% if left untreated
- Poor prognosis is seen in patients with drug-resistant strains and in AIDS patients

IMAGE FINDINGS

Radiographic Findings

- Most common manifestation of primary TB is focal apical airspace consolidation with hilar lymphadenopathy (Ranke complex)

TUBERCULOSIS

Key Facts

Terminology

- Lung infection caused by inhalation of *Mycobacterium tuberculosis*

Clinical Issues

- Primary infection usually asymptomatic and leads to formation of the Ghon complex (apical nodule with calcification) and hilar lymphadenopathy
- Progressive primary TB occurs when the primary foci do not involute and progress to disseminated, cavitary lesions
- Most common mechanism of secondary TB is reactivation of a latent focus of infection
- Often associated with chronic, debilitating diseases or immunosuppressive states (AIDS, transplant, cancer, diabetes, alcoholism)

Microscopic Pathology

- Basic pathologic manifestation of TB is granulomatous inflammation, with necrotizing, palisading epithelioid granulomas
- Palisading granulomas can progress to complete fibrosis and calcification
- Necrotizing granulomas may enlarge to form cavities with central liquefaction that may range from 3-10 cm in diameter
- Mycobacteria are slender rods measuring 4 μm in length; they cannot be visualized on routine histology and require special stains

Ancillary Tests

- Best stain for *M. tuberculosis* is the Ziehl-Neelsen stain, which stains acid-fast bacilli (AFB)

- Postprimary tuberculosis shows lobular and peribronchial consolidation, cavitation, and intraparenchymatous nodules

CT Findings

- Mediastinal lymph nodes characteristically display low-density centers with peripheral rim enhancement
- Consolidation with variably sized cavities with thick walls
- Small nodular opacities with centrilobular distribution associated with branching opacities ("tree-in-bud" appearance)
- Centrilobular distribution of nodular opacities reflects a bronchiolocentric process and is highly suggestive of intrabronchial spread
- Miliary tuberculosis shows randomly distributed small nodules, usually too numerous to count

MACROSCOPIC FEATURES

General Features

- Cut section often displays consolidation resembling bacterial pneumonia with areas of caseous (i.e., cheese-like) necrosis
- Advanced lesions are characterized by cavitation that may often lead to erosion into a bronchus with intrabronchial spread
- Cavitation is often distributed in the upper lobes; cavities have thick walls and measure from 3-10 cm in diameter
- TB can also present as a mass or circumscribed nodule (tuberculoma) with central necrosis, calcification, or fibrosis
- Miliary TB is characterized by numerous small (1-2 mm) nodules diffusely distributed throughout the lungs
- Pleural involvement is characterized by a thick, shaggy pleura studded by discrete granulomas and associated with pleural effusion

MICROSCOPIC PATHOLOGY

Histologic Features

- Basic pathologic manifestation of TB is granulomatous inflammation, with necrotizing, palisading epithelioid granulomas
- Palisading granulomas can progress to complete fibrosis and calcification
- Necrotizing granulomas may enlarge to form cavities with central liquefaction that may range from 3-10 cm in diameter

Cytologic Features

- Granulomas can be necrotizing or non-necrotizing and contain abundant epithelioid macrophages and Langhans-type giant cells
- Mycobacteria are slender rods measuring 4 μm in length; they cannot be visualized on routine histology and require special stains

ANCILLARY TESTS

Histochemistry

- Best stain for *M. tuberculosis* is the Ziehl-Neelsen stain, which stains acid-fast bacilli (AFB)
- Other useful stains include the Fite stain and the auramine-rhodamine fluorescent stain

PCR

- PCR detects mycobacterial DNA, but a positive reaction is not accepted as valid unless at least 1 organism can be visualized in tissue

SELECTED REFERENCES

1. Alsumrain M et al: Intracavitary and endobronchial tuberculosis. ScientificWorldJournal. 11:130-2, 2011
2. Sia IG et al: Current concepts in the management of tuberculosis. Mayo Clin Proc. 86(4):348-61, 2011
3. WHO global tuberculosis control report 2010: Summary. Cent Eur J Public Health. 18(4):237, 2010

TUBERCULOSIS

Histologic Features and Special Stains

(Left) *Scanning magnification of area of consolidation of the lung in postprimary tuberculosis shows extensive, confluent areas of necrosis of lung parenchyma with liquefaction and intervening areas of granulomatous inflammation.* ***(Right)*** *Higher magnification of an area of liquefactive necrosis in pulmonary tuberculosis shows abundant pink fibrinopurulent exudate surrounding an epithelioid granuloma ⮫. There is complete loss of the underlying pulmonary architecture in the area of necrosis.*

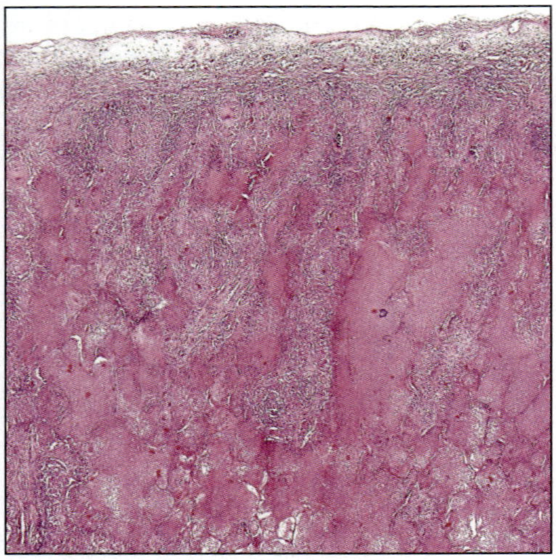

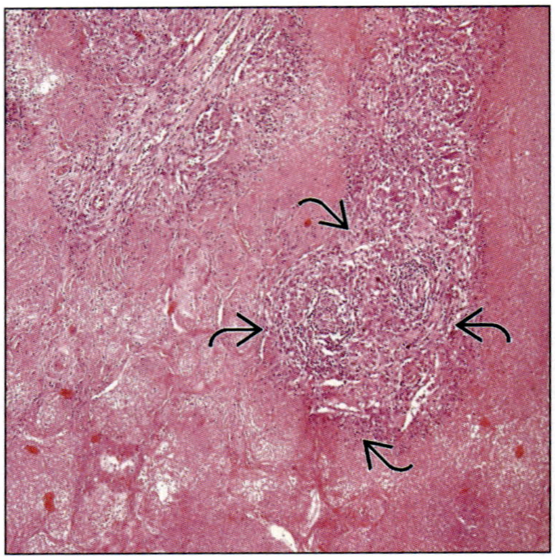

(Left) *Higher magnification from an area of liquefactive necrosis in postprimary pulmonary tuberculosis shows necrotic fibrinopurulent exudate focally admixed with a residual epithelioid histiocytic granuloma ➡.* ***(Right)*** *A necrotizing palisaded granuloma with central focus of caseous necrosis is seen in this patient with an advanced lesion of postprimary tuberculosis. Notice the epithelioid histiocytes at the periphery of the granuloma and scattered multinucleated giant cells ⇨.*

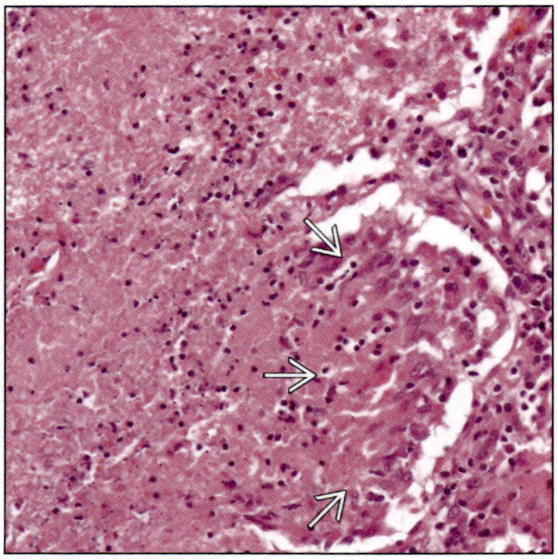

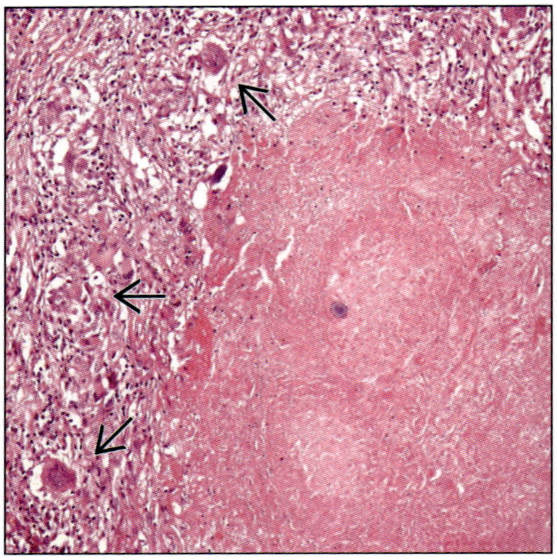

(Left) *Higher magnification from the edges of a large necrotizing palisaded granuloma in postprimary pulmonary tuberculosis shows several Langhans-type multinucleated giant cells.* ***(Right)*** *Higher magnification of the center of a granuloma in cavitating pulmonary tuberculosis shows a few slender acid-fast organisms (stained in red). The mycobacteria are slender rods that cannot be visualized on routine microscopy and are usually quite scanty.*

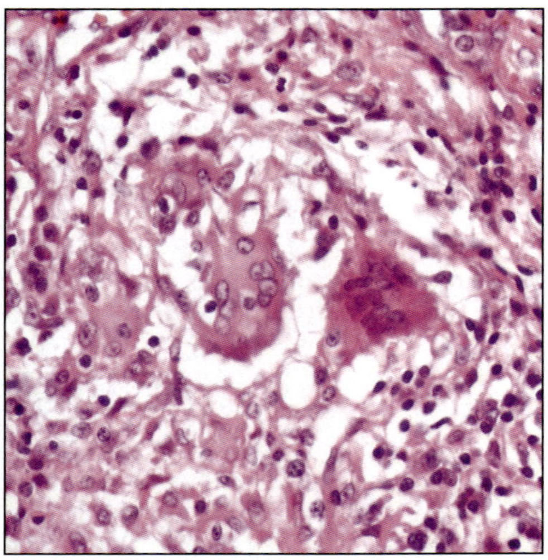

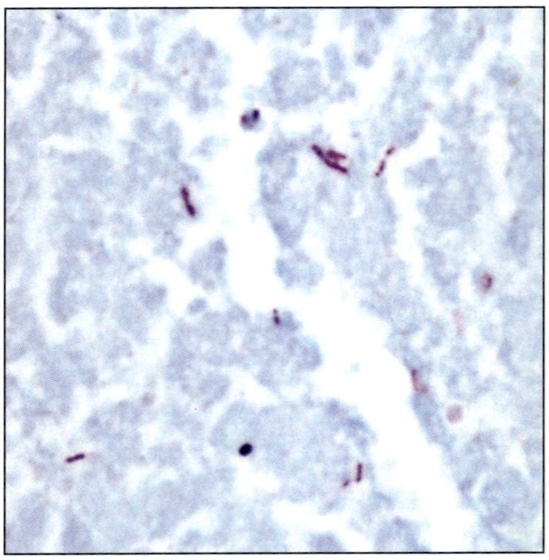

Other Histologic Features

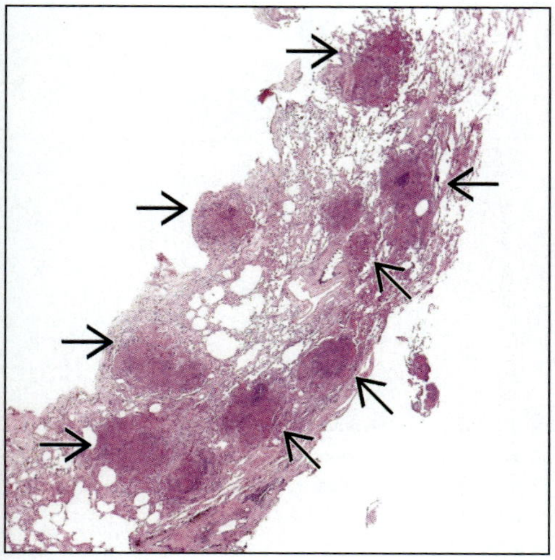
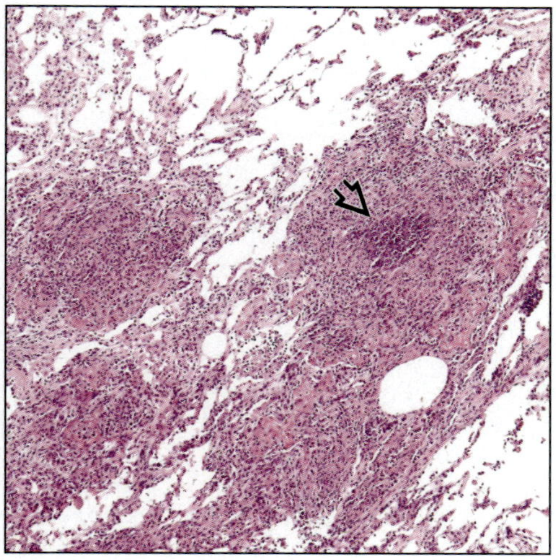

*(**Left**) Scanning magnification shows miliary pattern of spread in pulmonary tuberculosis, with multiple microscopic nodules ➔ scattered throughout the lung parenchyma. (**Right**) Higher magnification of lung parenchyma involved with miliary tuberculosis shows multiple small nodules containing epithelioid granulomas admixed with inflammatory infiltrates in the surrounding lung parenchyma. Notice one of the granulomas ➲ has a focus of necrosis and suppuration.*

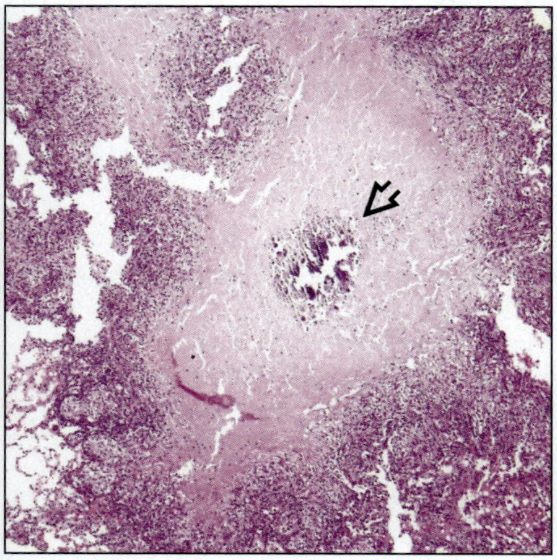
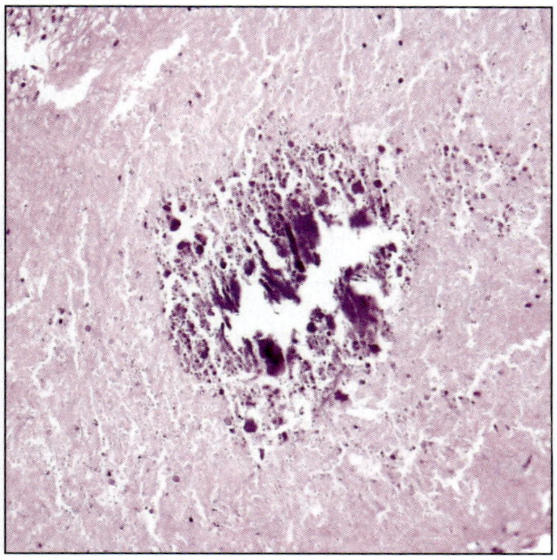

*(**Left**) Necrotizing palisaded granuloma in a patient with postprimary pulmonary tuberculosis shows a central area of extensive necrosis with a central focus of calcification ➲. Foci of fibrosis and calcification are a common occurrence in old necrotizing palisaded granulomas in pulmonary tuberculosis. (**Right**) Higher magnification from the center of a necrotizing palisaded granuloma in pulmonary tuberculosis shows irregular areas of dystrophic calcification.*

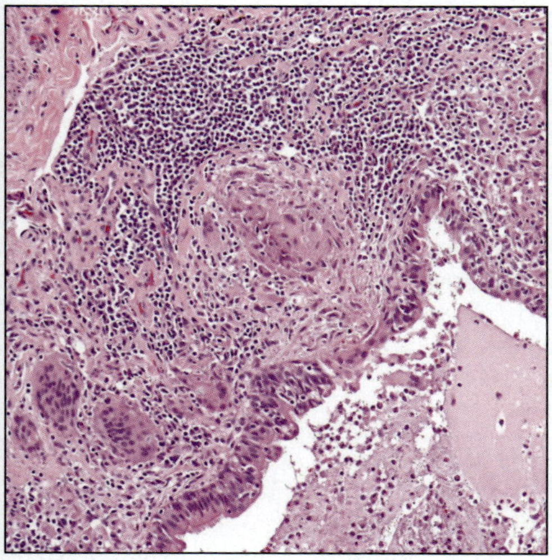
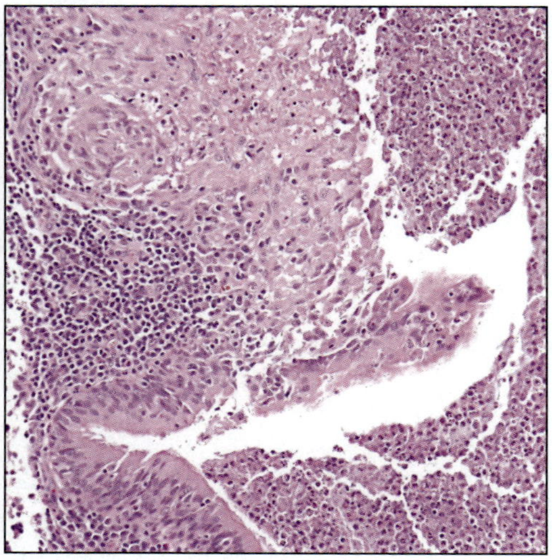

*(**Left**) Scanning magnification shows a bronchus with multiple small epithelioid granulomas surrounding the bronchial wall in a patient with postprimary pulmonary tuberculosis. Notice that there is early involvement of the mucosa of the bronchus by the inflammation resembling a pattern of bronchocentric granulomatosis. (**Right**) Higher magnification of bronchocentric granulomatosis-like pattern of involvement of the bronchial wall in a patient with pulmonary tuberculosis.*

HERPES SIMPLEX VIRUS

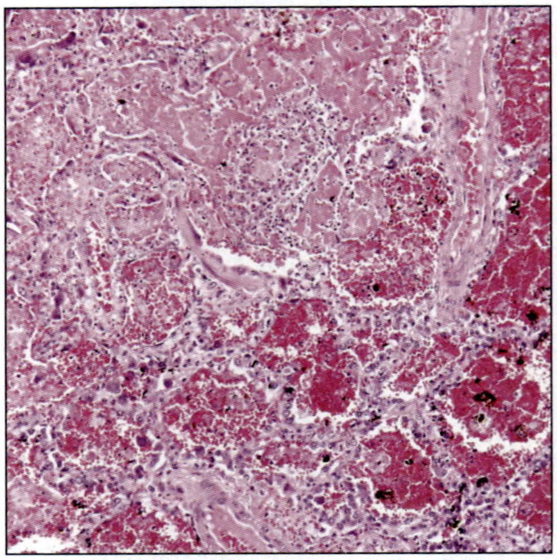

Histologic appearance of hemorrhagic necrotizing pneumonia in a patient with herpes simplex virus (HSV) infection shows extensive destruction of lung parenchyma with fibrinous intraalveolar exudates.

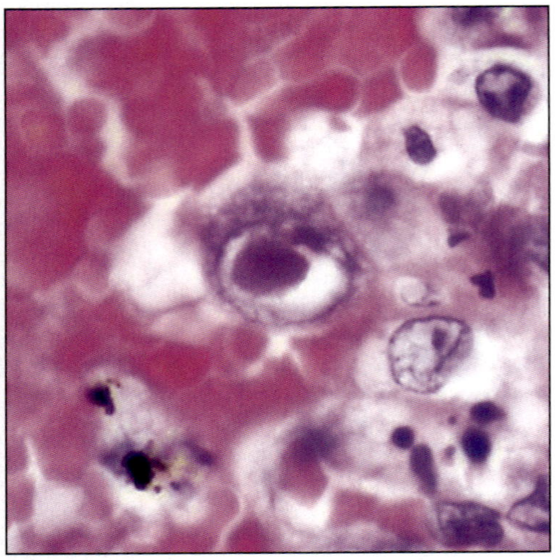

Higher magnification of acute necrotizing and hemorrhagic HSV pneumonia shows a characteristic viral inclusion composed of dense eosinophilic intranuclear mass surrounded by a clear halo.

TERMINOLOGY

Abbreviations

- Herpes simplex virus (HSV)

Definitions

- Lung infection caused by double-stranded DNA herpes simplex virus-1

ETIOLOGY/PATHOGENESIS

Infectious Agents

- Most cases of neonatal disease are acquired from infected mothers during labor
- Adult HSV pneumonia is most often caused by inhalation of viral particles from mucocutaneous lesions in oropharynx

CLINICAL ISSUES

Epidemiology

- Incidence
  - HSV pneumonia is seen in neonates as well as in immunosuppressed patients
  - Incidence of neonatal HSV infection is approximately 1 in every 3,000 deliveries
  - Disseminated HSV infection develops in approximately 25% of infected neonates
- Age
  - Wide age range, from neonates to elderly patients

Presentation

- HSV pneumonia is most often preceded by mucocutaneous infection
- Newborn infants, severely immunosuppressed or burned patients, and patients with trauma are at highest risk for infection
- Infants with disseminated neonatal infection show signs and symptoms about 1 week after birth
- Clinical picture in neonatal infection resembles bacterial sepsis with pneumonia, shock, and disseminated intravascular coagulation
- In adults, disseminated infection produces acute hemorrhagic bronchopneumonia
- Ulcerative necrotizing tracheobronchitis can also accompany pneumonia in adults

Natural History

- HSV has worldwide distribution with no recognizable gender or racial predilection
- In infants, disease is transmitted by mother during passage of fetus through infected birth canal
- In adults, infection may be due to contamination from mucocutaneous sources or reactivation of latent infection
- Disease is associated with high mortality if left untreated

Treatment

- Drugs
  - Antiviral therapy (acyclovir, valacyclovir, famciclovir, etc.)
  - Foscarnet is treatment of choice in acyclovir-resistant patients

Prognosis

- Primary HSV infection of upper respiratory tract usually resolves spontaneously without treatment
- Infection in immunosuppressed patients requires treatment with antiviral drugs
- Disseminated disease in neonates carries 30% mortality rate

IMAGE FINDINGS

Radiographic Findings

- Multifocal, bilateral nodular densities between 5-10 mm in greatest diameter

HERPES SIMPLEX VIRUS

Key Facts

Terminology
- Lung infection caused by double-stranded DNA herpes simplex virus-1

Clinical Issues
- In infants, disease is transmitted by mother during passage of fetus through infected birth canal
- In adults, infection may be due to contamination from mucocutaneous sources or reactivation of latent infection

Microscopic Pathology
- Pattern of involvement in lung may present as necrotizing pneumonia or as diffuse interstitial pneumonitis
- HSV diffuse interstitial pneumonitis closely resembles diffuse alveolar damage (DAD)
- Infected cells are characterized by presence of intranuclear inclusions
  - Cowdry type A inclusions: Eosinophilic intranuclear inclusion separated from nuclear membrane by a halo
  - Cowdry type B inclusions: Homogeneous, amphophilic, and glassy intranuclear inclusions
- Multinucleated epithelial cells with multiple eosinophilic intranuclear inclusions may also be present

Ancillary Tests
- Antibodies to HSV using formalin-fixed paraffin-embedded tissue sections are quite sensitive
- Virus particles are encapsulated and targetoid and measure 100-110 nm by electron microscopy

- Nodular opacities may coalesce to form more extensive areas of consolidation

CT Findings
- Patchy ground-glass opacities and consolidation
- Findings are typically diffuse and bilateral
- Pleural effusions

MACROSCOPIC FEATURES

General Features
- Cut section shows heavy, congested, and firm lungs with multiple necrotic and hemorrhagic nodules
- Hematogenous dissemination will produce a miliary pattern of distribution of lesions

MICROSCOPIC PATHOLOGY

Histologic Features
- Pattern of involvement in lung may present as necrotizing pneumonia or as diffuse interstitial pneumonitis
- HSV diffuse interstitial pneumonitis closely resembles diffuse alveolar damage (DAD)
- Miliary pattern of spread can be seen in cases of hematogenous dissemination of HSV to lungs
- Herpetic foci show extensive necrosis and karyorrhectic debris with hemorrhage and neutrophilic infiltration
- Cells with intranuclear inclusions are best appreciated at edges of necrotic foci

Cytologic Features
- Infected cells are characterized by presence of intranuclear inclusions
  - Cowdry type A inclusions
    - Eosinophilic intranuclear inclusion separated from nuclear membrane by a halo
  - Cowdry type B inclusions
    - Homogeneous, amphophilic, and glassy intranuclear inclusions
- Multinucleated epithelial cells with multiple eosinophilic intranuclear inclusions may also be present

ANCILLARY TESTS

Immunohistochemistry
- Antibodies to HSV using formalin-fixed paraffin-embedded tissue sections are quite sensitive

Electron Microscopy
- Transmission
  - Virus particles are encapsulated and measure approximately 100-110 nm in diameter
  - Virus particles have targetoid appearance and are arranged in a lattice-like pattern

DIFFERENTIAL DIAGNOSIS

Adenovirus
- Has intranuclear inclusions identical to HSV but also contains "smudge" cells not seen in HSV

Measles
- Similar inclusions to HSV but inclusions are both intranuclear and cytoplasmic, unlike HSV, in which they are exclusively intranuclear

Varicella-Zoster
- Produce identical inclusions to HSV; can only be distinguished by immunohistochemistry or molecular methods

SELECTED REFERENCES

1. Chong S et al: Herpes simplex virus pneumonia: high-resolution CT findings. Br J Radiol. 83(991):585-9, 2010
2. Witt MN et al: Occurrence of HSV-1-induced pneumonitis in patients under standard immunosuppressive therapy for rheumatic, vasculitic, and connective tissue disease. BMC Pulm Med. 9:22, 2009

HERPES SIMPLEX VIRUS

Necrotizing Pneumonia Pattern

*(**Left**) Scanning magnification of hemorrhagic necrotizing pneumonia in a patient with herpes simplex virus infection shows complete destruction of the airways with irregular areas of hemorrhage and necrosis ➚. (**Right**) Higher magnification of hemorrhagic necrotizing pneumonia in a patient with herpes simplex virus infection shows complete destruction of lung parenchyma with loss of the normal alveolar architecture and sparse inflammatory infiltrates.*

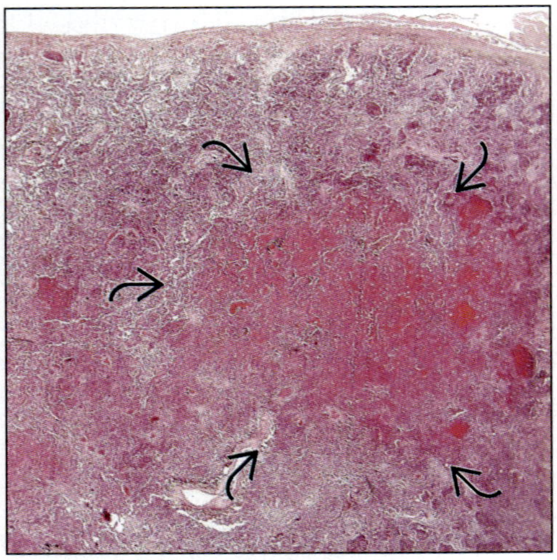

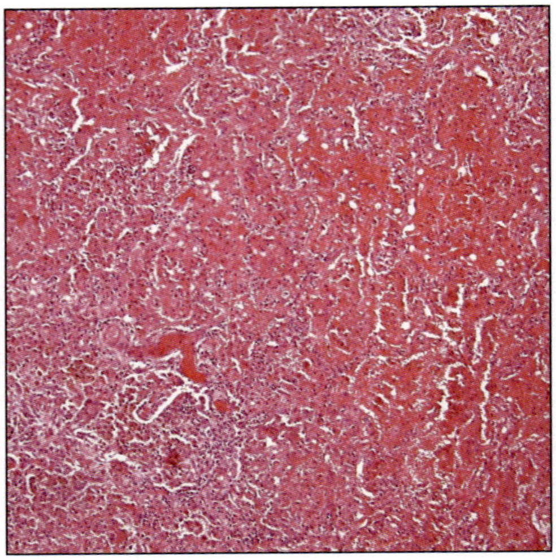

*(**Left**) Scanning magnification of the lung in a patient with necrotizing herpes simplex virus pneumonia shows well-defined nodular areas of necrosis ➚ separated by a residual cartilaginous plate ➪. Necrotizing HSV pneumonia is usually airway centered and involves bronchi and bronchioles. (**Right**) Higher magnification from the edge of an area of necrosis in necrotizing HSV pneumonia shows a characteristic intranuclear inclusion ➪ with peripherally marginated nuclear chromatin.*

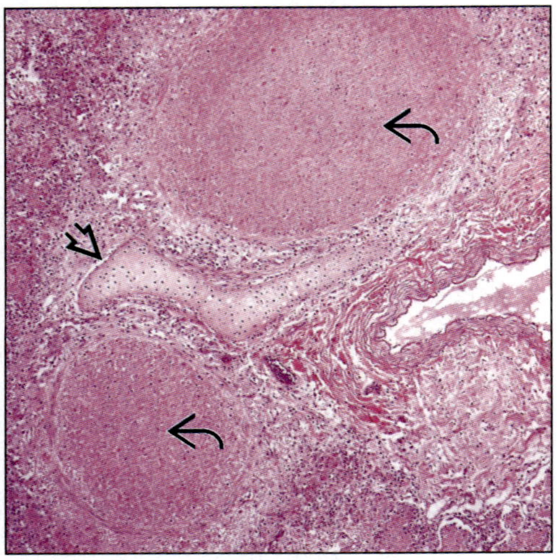

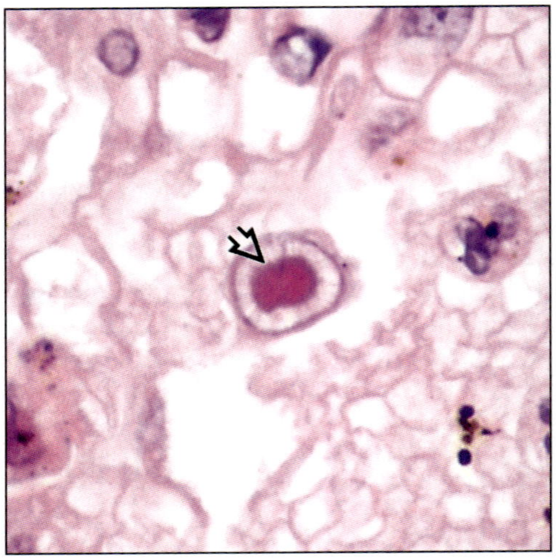

*(**Left**) Scanning magnification of lung involved with necrotizing herpes simplex virus pneumonia shows complete destruction of the bronchial lining mucosa by dense inflammatory infiltrates with filling of the bronchial lumen by abundant fibrinopurulent exudate. (**Right**) Necrotizing tracheobronchitis and bronchiolitis in a patient with herpes simplex virus pneumonia shows extensive destruction of the wall of the bronchus by inflammatory exudate ➚.*

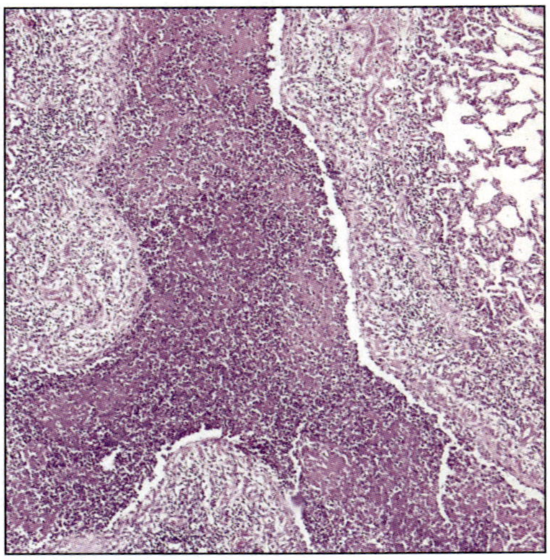

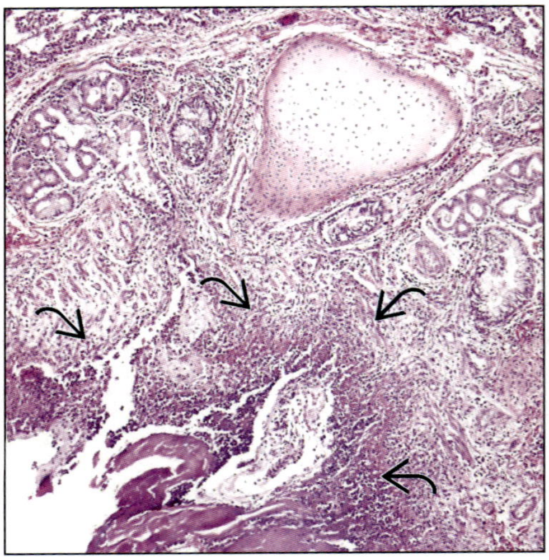

Interstitial Pneumonia Pattern

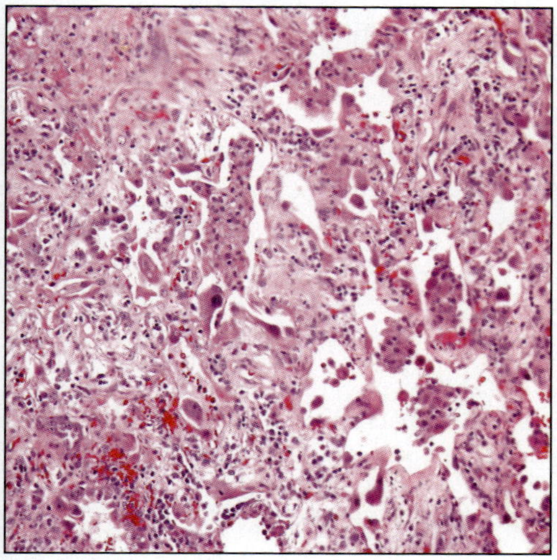

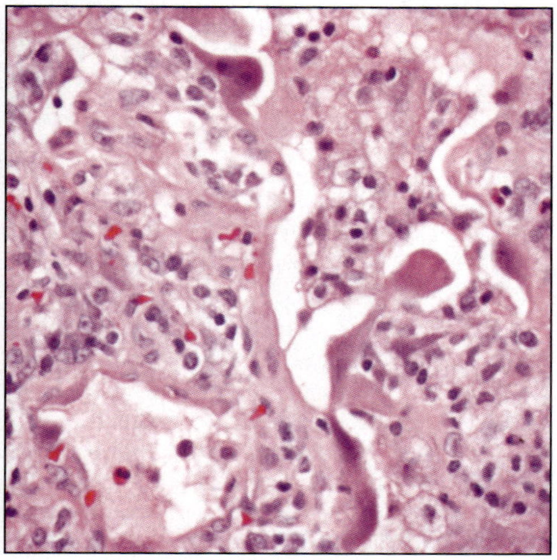

(Left) *Diffuse interstitial pneumonia pattern in lung infection with herpes simplex virus shows preservation of lung alveolar architecture with thickening of alveolar septa by chronic inflammatory cell infiltrates.* ***(Right)*** *Higher magnification of herpes simplex virus pneumonia with diffuse interstitial pattern shows hyaline membrane formation, interstitial edema, and pneumocyte hyperplasia, all features seen in diffuse alveolar damage.*

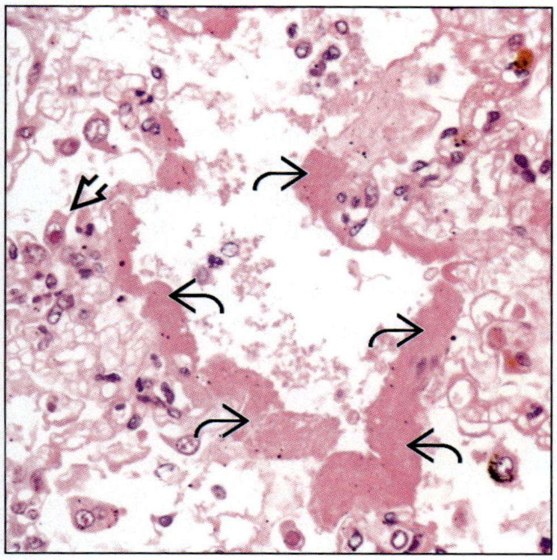

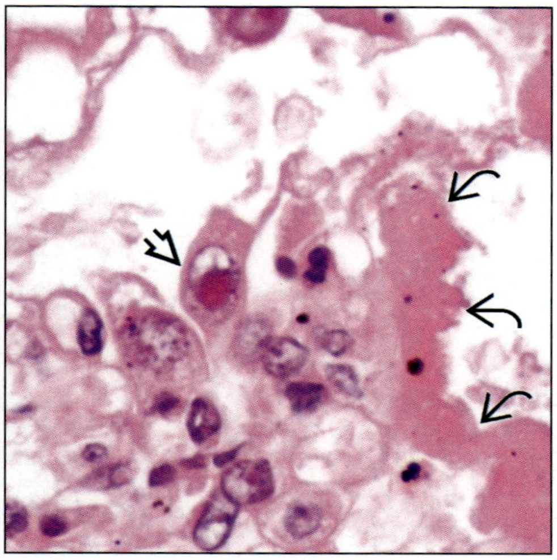

(Left) *Interstitial pattern of involvement in herpes simplex virus pneumonia shows thick eosinophilic hyaline membranes lining the wall of an alveolus ↷. Notice an infected cell containing a large, bright eosinophilic inclusion ⇨.* ***(Right)*** *Higher magnification of herpes simplex virus pneumonia with interstitial pattern of involvement shows large intranuclear inclusion surrounded by a clear halo ⇨ adjacent to a hyaline membrane ↷.*

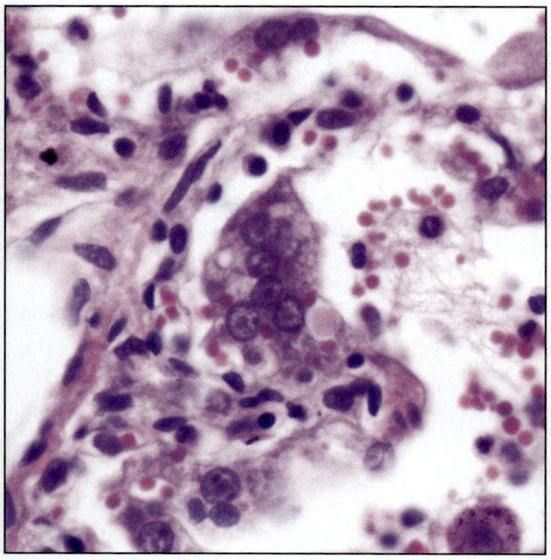

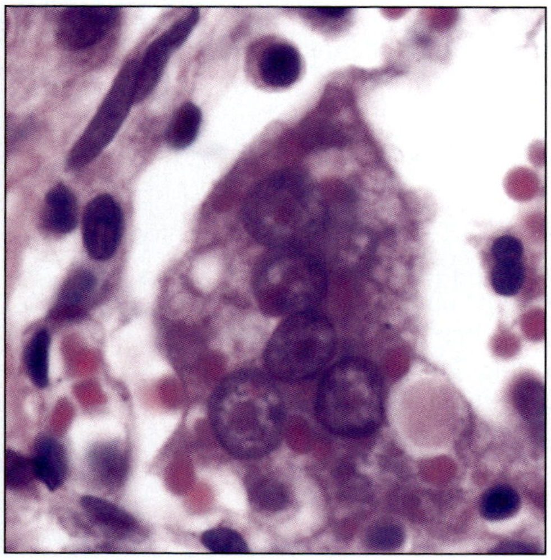

(Left) *Infected epithelial multinucleated giant cell in the lung of a patient infected with herpes simplex virus shows multiple small uniform nuclei containing round eosinophilic inclusions. Similar cells can also be seen in varicella-zoster and measles infection.* ***(Right)*** *Higher magnification of multinucleated giant cell in the lung of a patient with herpes simplex virus infection shows uniform small nuclei containing small intranuclear inclusions.*

CYTOMEGALOVIRUS

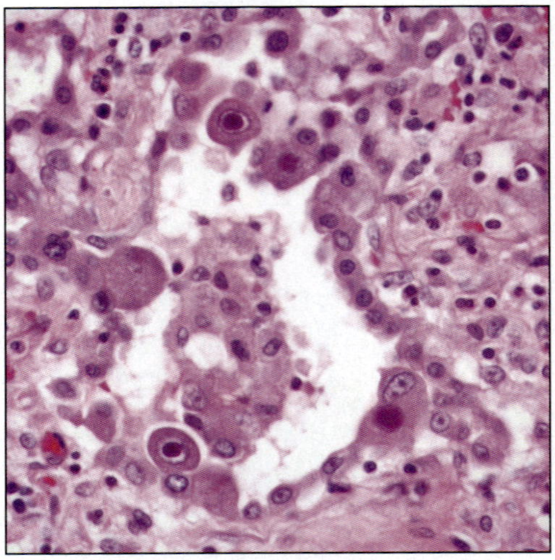

Histologic appearance of CMV pneumonitis in an immunosuppressed patient shows interstitial inflammation with a few alveolar lining cells containing the characteristic viral intranuclear inclusions.

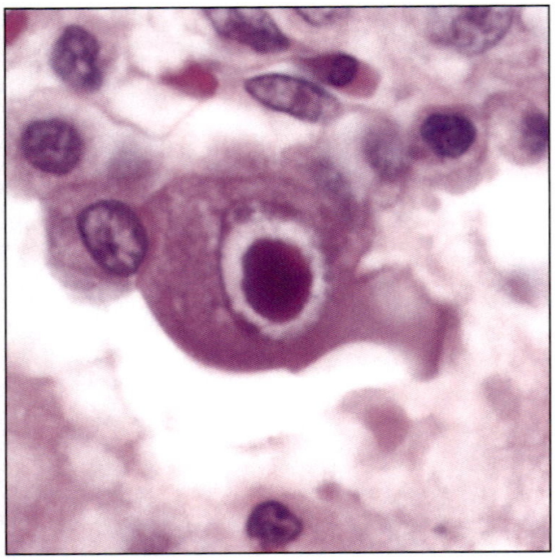

Higher magnification of cytopathic effect in CMV pneumonia shows a cell displaying cytomegaly with a large, single intranuclear inclusion surrounded by a clear halo in the periphery.

TERMINOLOGY

Abbreviations

- Cytomegalovirus (CMV)

Definitions

- Infection of the lung caused by cytomegalovirus

ETIOLOGY/PATHOGENESIS

Infectious Agents

- CMV is a double-stranded DNA herpesvirus with an icosahedral capsid that contains 120 capsomeres
- Measures 120 to 200 nm and has an envelope derived from the nuclear membrane

CLINICAL ISSUES

Epidemiology

- Incidence
  - One of the most common opportunistic infections in AIDS and organ transplant patients
- Age
  - Seen in congenital, perinatal, childhood and adult age groups

Presentation

- CMV pneumonitis causes fever, nonproductive cough, and shortness of breath with hypoxemia
- Diagnosis of CMV pneumonia is based on evaluation of lung biopsy or bronchoalveolar lavage specimens
  - Presence of CMV in blood, urine, or sputum is not evidence of CMV pneumonia; tissue confirmation is required for diagnosis
  - Serologic demonstration of CMV infection is not sufficient for diagnosis of CMV pneumonia; tissue confirmation is required

Natural History

- Primary infection can occur in utero or shortly after birth and is generally asymptomatic, leading to latent status
- Immune deficiency or immunosuppression causes CMV to reactivate and disseminate
- Reactivation may lead to minimal disease or be symptomatic to fulminant depending on degree of immunodeficiency
- CMV can cause a variety of infections that affect multiple organs, including liver, lung, CNS, lymph nodes, etc.
- Disseminated CMV infection can cause pneumonitis, hepatitis, adrenalitis, encephalitis, leukopenia, and other systemic manifestations

Treatment

- Drugs
  - Ganciclovir, foscarnet, and intravenous immunoglobulin

Prognosis

- CMV pneumonia can be fatal in immunosuppressed patients

IMAGE FINDINGS

Radiographic Findings

- Bilateral nodular or reticular interstitial opacities
- Bilateral ground-glass opacities are less commonly seen
- Pleural effusions may be seen in about 1/3 of patients
- Patients with mixed infections may have additional features that will complicate radiologic interpretation

CT Findings

- HRCT studies show consolidation with micronodules, ground-glass opacities, and irregular reticular opacities

CYTOMEGALOVIRUS

Key Facts

Clinical Issues

- One of the most common opportunistic infections in AIDS and organ transplant patients
- Diagnosis of CMV pneumonia is based on evaluation of lung biopsy or bronchoalveolar lavage specimens
- Disseminated CMV infection can cause pneumonitis, hepatitis, adrenalitis, encephalitis, leukopenia, and other systemic manifestations

Microscopic Pathology

- Cytopathic effects of CMV involve both nucleus and cytoplasm of infected cells and lead to cytomegaly
- Can infect a large variety of cell types in lung, including pneumocytes, endothelial cells, fibroblasts, and macrophages
- Intranuclear inclusions in CMV are larger than cytoplasmic inclusions and may measure up to 20 µm in diameter
- Nuclear inclusions are usually basophilic, round to oval, and show a peripheral halo with accentuation of nuclear membrane
- Cytoplasmic inclusions are basophilic to eosinophilic and smaller than intranuclear inclusions (1-3 µm in diameter)

Ancillary Tests

- Anti-CMV antibodies by immunoperoxidase technique are sensitive and specific for the organisms
- DNA in situ hybridization for CMV is another sensitive and reliable method for identification of the organisms

MICROSCOPIC PATHOLOGY

Histologic Features

- Patterns of lung involvement in CMV
  - Minimal disease characterized by scattered or isolated CMV inclusions without significant changes in lung parenchyma
  - Miliary disease characterized by miliary pattern of distribution with microscopic nodules containing chronic inflammation and viral inclusions
  - Diffuse interstitial pneumonitis characterized by interstitial inflammation that may progress to diffuse alveolar damage

Cytologic Features

- Cytopathic effects of CMV involve both nucleus and cytoplasm of infected cells and lead to cytomegaly
- Can infect a large variety of cell types in lung, including pneumocytes, endothelial cells, fibroblasts, and macrophages
- Intranuclear inclusions are larger than cytoplasmic inclusions and may measure up to 20 µm in diameter
- Nuclear inclusions are usually basophilic, round to oval, and show a peripheral halo with accentuation of nuclear membrane
- Cytoplasmic inclusions are basophilic to eosinophilic and smaller than intranuclear inclusions (1-3 µm in diameter)

ANCILLARY TESTS

Histochemistry

- Intranuclear inclusions are positive with Feulgen stain
- Cytoplasmic inclusions are positive for PAS and GMS stains

Immunohistochemistry

- Anti-CMV antibodies by immunoperoxidase technique are sensitive and specific for the organisms

In Situ Hybridization

- DNA in situ hybridization for CMV is another sensitive and reliable method for identification of the organisms

DIFFERENTIAL DIAGNOSIS

Other Viral Pneumonias

- Other viral pneumonias with cytopathic inclusions lack the cytomegaly and distinct large basophilic intranuclear inclusions of CMV

DIAGNOSTIC CHECKLIST

Pathologic Interpretation Pearls

- CMV inclusions may be very scant and difficult to recognize; immunohistochemical staining should be done routinely for identification in suspected cases
- Mixed infections are often encountered in immunosuppressed patients; attention must be paid for other signs of pathogens in patients with CMV
- CMV and pneumocystosis are a common and frequent combination in AIDS patients

SELECTED REFERENCES

1. Torres HA et al: Fatal cytomegalovirus pneumonia in patients with haematological malignancies: an autopsy-based case-control study. Clin Microbiol Infect. 14(12):1160-6, 2008
2. Drew WL: Laboratory diagnosis of cytomegalovirus infection and disease in immunocompromised patients. Curr Opin Infect Dis. 20(4):408-11, 2007
3. Tang HJ et al: Opportunistic infections in adults with acquired immunodeficiency syndrome: a comparison of clinical and autopsy findings. J Microbiol Immunol Infect. 39(4):310-5, 2006

CYTOMEGALOVIRUS

Histologic Features

(Left) Scanning magnification of miliary form of CMV infection in the lung shows a small cellular nodule ➙ that is well delimited from the surrounding pulmonary parenchyma and contains dense inflammatory infiltrates. **(Right)** Higher magnification from the center of the nodule in miliary form of CMV pulmonary infection shows dense inflammatory cell infiltrates with a few scattered cells displaying cytomegaly and large, densely basophilic intranuclear inclusions ➙.

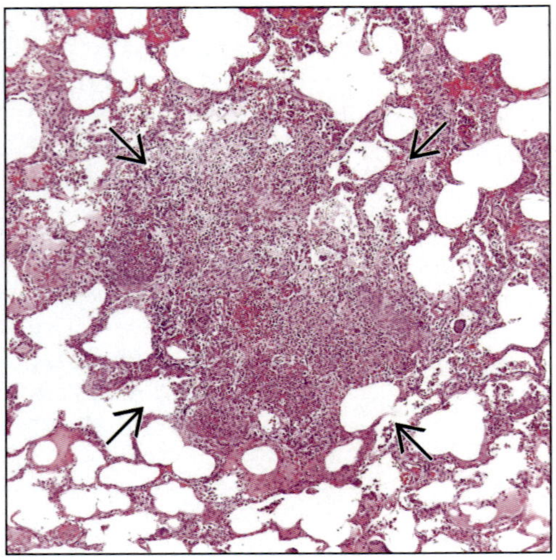

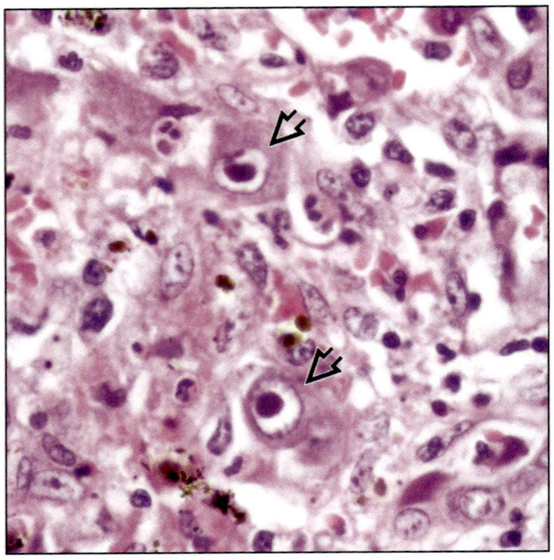

(Left) Scanning magnification in CMV lung infection with a diffuse interstitial pneumonic pattern shows thickening and expansion of alveolar septa by dense inflammatory cell infiltrates and filling of the alveolar lumina by eosinophilic fibrinous material. **(Right)** Higher magnification of diffuse interstitial CMV pneumonitis shows hyaline membrane formation lining the walls of an alveolar space ➙. Notice that the contiguous alveolar space contains 2 cells with prominent basophilic intranuclear inclusions ➙.

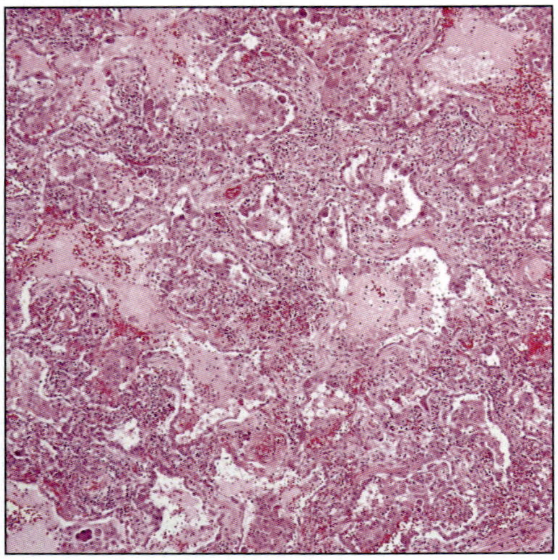

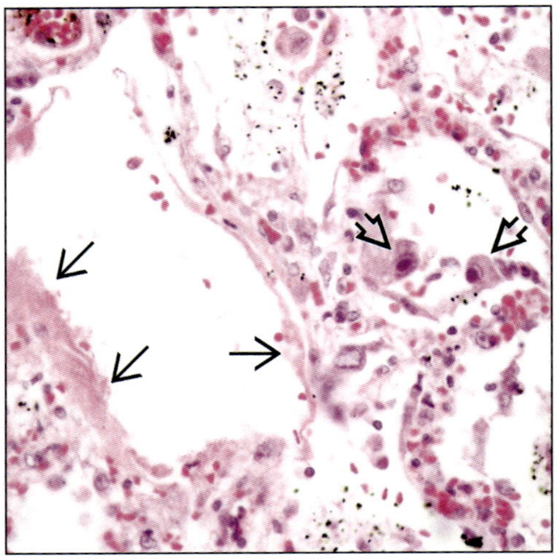

(Left) Massive superinfection by CMV in an infant with AIDS shows a massive accumulation of cells with marked viral cytopathic effect. The infected cells are forming sheets and show characteristic cytomegaly with large viral inclusions. On cursory examination, the sheets of cells can be confused for a malignant process. **(Right)** Higher magnification of massive CMV pneumonitis in a child with AIDS shows sheets of large cells with viral cytopathic effect and large basophilic intranuclear inclusions.

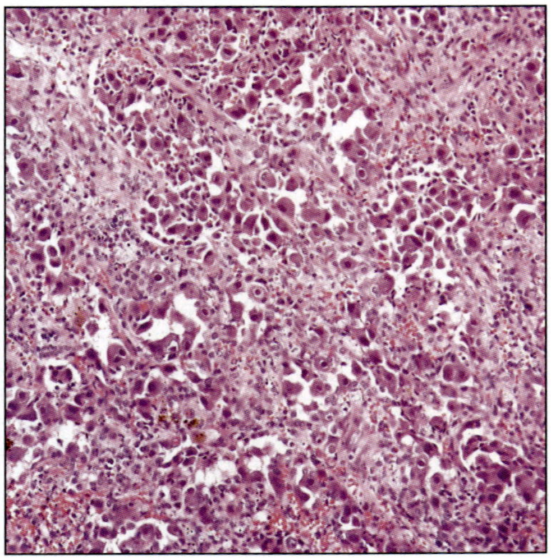

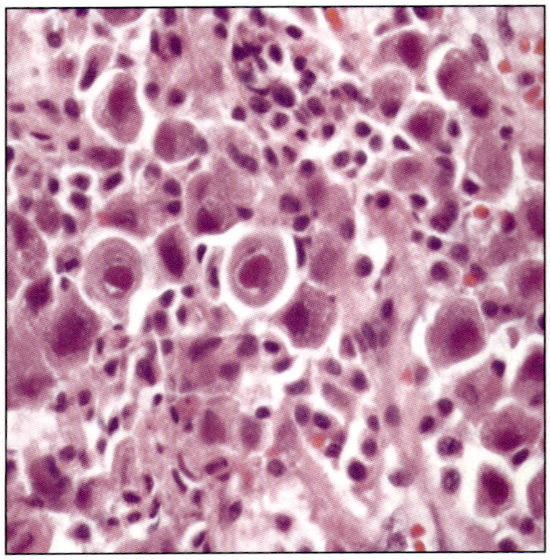

Cytology and Special Stains

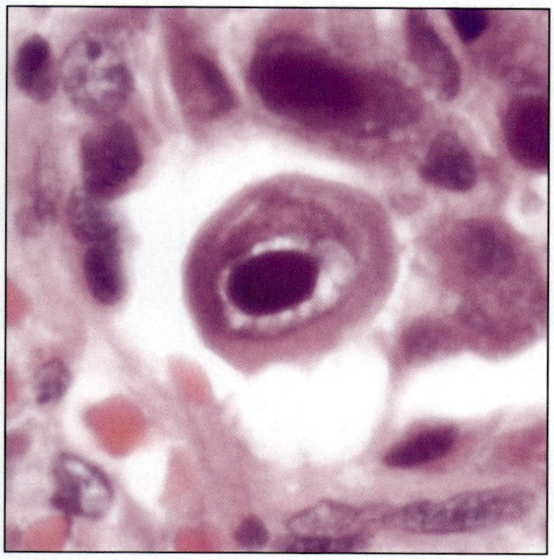

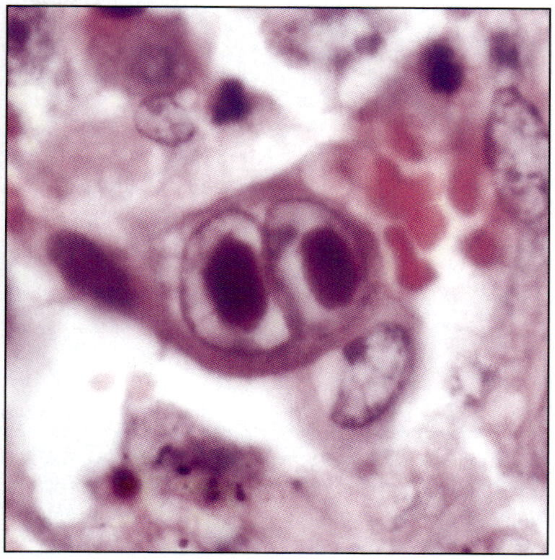

(Left) *Viral cytopathic effect in CMV pneumonia is characterized by a single, large basophilic intranuclear inclusion that is surrounded by a clear halo. There is usually accentuation of the nuclear membrane. The inclusions can be round or oval.* ***(Right)*** *Cytopathic effect in CMV pneumonitis shows 2 cells side-by-side displaying characteristic "owl-eyed" double nuclear inclusions surrounded by a clear halo. The appearance of these cells is reminiscent of the Reed-Sternberg cell.*

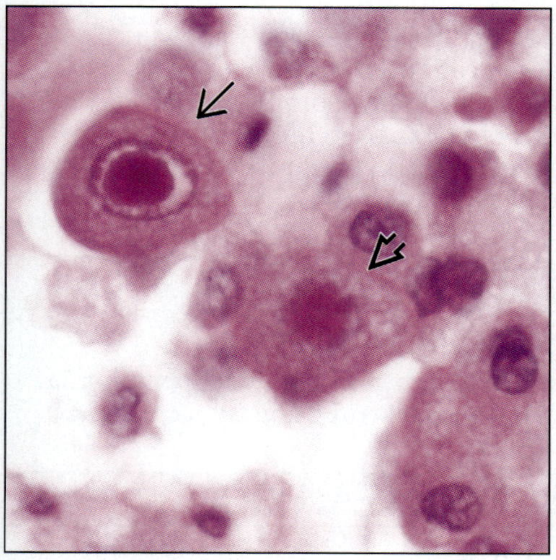

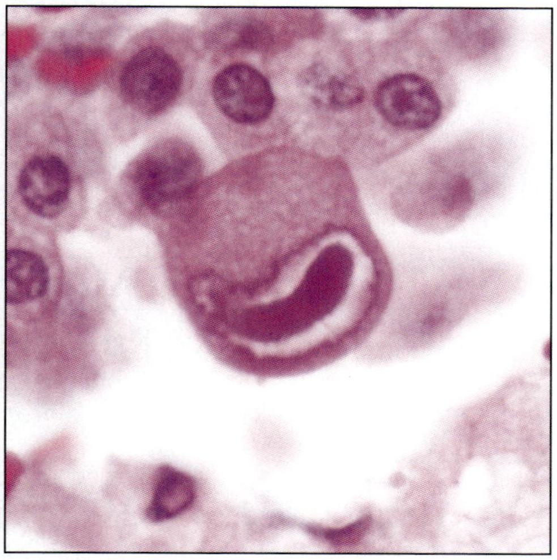

(Left) *Cytopathic effect in CMV pneumonitis shows 1 cell with classical basophilic intranuclear inclusion* → *lying next to another cell lacking a basophilic intranuclear inclusion but containing a smaller, eosinophilic cytoplasmic inclusion* ⇨. ***(Right)*** *Cytopathic effect in CMV pneumonitis shows an infected cell containing a boat-shaped, crescentic intranuclear inclusion. Notice the clear halo surrounding the inclusion and the accentuation of the nuclear membrane.*

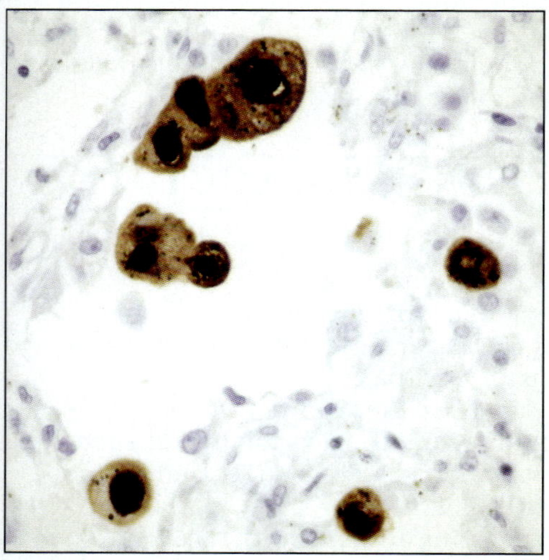

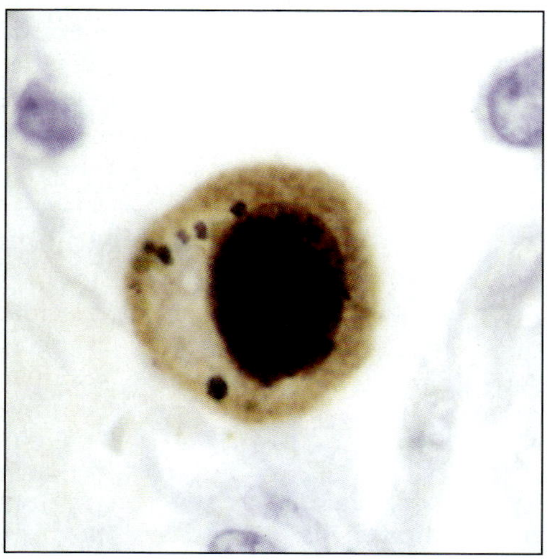

(Left) *IHC staining for CMV in a patient with CMV pneumonitis shows strong positivity in several scattered infected cells. Infected cells may be few in some cases of CMV pneumonitis and can be easily missed on histopathologic examination; routine use of immunohistochemistry is therefore recommended for proper identification in suspected cases.* ***(Right)*** *Higher magnification shows positive staining for CMV antibody by immunohistochemistry in CMV pneumonitis.*

ADENOVIRUS

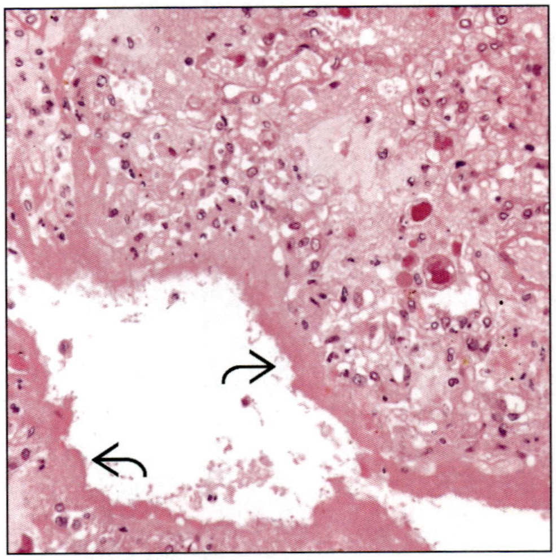

Histologic appearance of acute necrotizing alveolitis in a patient with adenovirus pneumonia shows interstitial edema with inflammatory exudates and hyaline membrane formation ➔ similar to DAD.

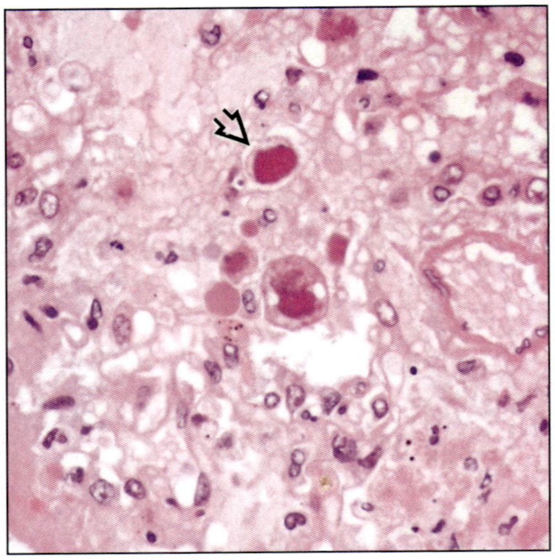

Higher magnification of adenovirus pneumonia shows several intranuclear eosinophilic inclusions. The presence of "smudge cells" ➔ (eosinophilic inclusions filling the nucleus) is distinctive for adenovirus.

TERMINOLOGY

Definitions

- Pulmonary infection caused by adenovirus

ETIOLOGY/PATHOGENESIS

Infectious Agents

- > 50 known serotypes
  - Serotypes 3, 7, and 21 are most common in children
  - Serotypes 3, 4, and 7 are most common in adults

CLINICAL ISSUES

Epidemiology

- Incidence
  - Accounts for about 10% of all pneumonias in children and infants
  - Epidemics have been reported in military personnel
  - Common in immunocompromised patients

Presentation

- Acute respiratory disease
  - Fever
  - Chills
  - Myalgias
  - Pharyngitis and tracheobronchitis
- Adenovirus pneumonia
  - Similar symptoms to other types of pneumonia
  - May be fatal in immunosuppressed patients, particularly transplant and AIDS patients

Treatment

- Drugs
  - Medical support and management of symptoms
  - Severe cases may be treated with intravenous ribavirin
  - Vaccines for serotypes 4 and 7 have been used with success in military personnel

Prognosis

- Can resolve spontaneously, leaving some sequelae, or may progress to death over 2-3 weeks
  - Sequelae of disease include bronchiectasis, bronchiolitis obliterans, or chronic lung disease
- Adenovirus pneumonia in immunocompromised patients is almost always fatal

IMAGE FINDINGS

Radiographic Findings

- Bilateral, multifocal, lobar or segmental pneumonia with bronchial wall thickening and hyperaeration

MACROSCOPIC FEATURES

General Features

- Lungs are heavy and edematous
- Mucosa in main bronchi is generally congested and hemorrhagic
- Cut surface of lung may show yellow friable nodules corresponding to necrotic foci

MICROSCOPIC PATHOLOGY

Histologic Features

- 2 major patterns of lung injury
  - Necrotizing bronchitis/bronchiolitis
    - Necrosis of walls of airways due to severe acute inflammatory infiltrate
    - Airway lumens are filled with necrotic eosinophilic debris and fibrinopurulent exudate
    - Mucosa of bronchioles is denuded and necrotic
  - Necrotizing alveolitis
    - Acute necrotizing alveolitis with hyaline membranes and fibrinous alveolar exudates resembling diffuse alveolar damage (DAD)

ADENOVIRUS

Key Facts

Clinical Issues
- Accounts for about 10% of all pneumonias in children and infants
- Epidemics have been reported in military personnel

Microscopic Pathology
- 2 major patterns of lung injury
  - Necrotizing bronchitis/bronchiolitis with necrosis of walls of airways due to severe acute inflammatory infiltrate
  - Acute necrotizing alveolitis with hyaline membranes and fibrinous alveolar exudates resembling diffuse alveolar damage (DAD)
- "Smudge cell"
  - Basophilic inclusion that obscures nuclear membrane and fills entire nucleus
- Intranuclear eosinophilic inclusions
  - Surrounded by a halo separating them from nuclear membrane (similar to those seen in HSV)

- Walls of alveoli show interstitial edema and neutrophilic and mononuclear inflammatory infiltrates

Cytologic Features
- 2 types of intranuclear inclusions
  - Cowdry type A intranuclear eosinophilic inclusions
    - Surrounded by a halo separating them from nuclear membrane
  - "Smudge cells"
    - Dark eosinophilic to basophilic inclusion that obscures nuclear membrane and fills entire nucleus

ANCILLARY TESTS

Immunohistochemistry
- Immunohistochemistry and DNA in situ can be used in formalin-fixed paraffin-embedded tissue for specific diagnosis

Electron Microscopy
- Characteristic paracrystalline arrays of virions that measure 70-90 nm in diameter

PCR
- Molecular assays with gene amplification or DNA in situ hybridization can be used for identification

Culture
- Optimal way to establish the diagnosis
  - Provides added advantage of serotyping

Serologic Testing
- Requires demonstration of IgM antibody or 4x increase in IgG antibody

DIAGNOSTIC CHECKLIST

Pathologic Interpretation Pearls
- Eosinophilic intranuclear inclusions are identical to those seen in herpes simplex virus or Cytomegalovirus
- Identification of "smudge cells" is helpful for distinguishing adenovirus from other viral infections

SELECTED REFERENCES

1. Pavia AT: Viral infections of the lower respiratory tract: old viruses, new viruses, and the role of diagnosis. Clin Infect Dis. 52 Suppl 4:S284-9, 2011
2. Trei JS et al: Spread of adenovirus to geographically dispersed military installations, May-October 2007. Emerg Infect Dis. 16(5):769-75, 2010
3. Chong DC et al: Respiratory viruses in pediatric necropsies: an immunohistochemical study. Pediatr Dev Pathol. 12(3):211-6, 2009

IMAGE GALLERY

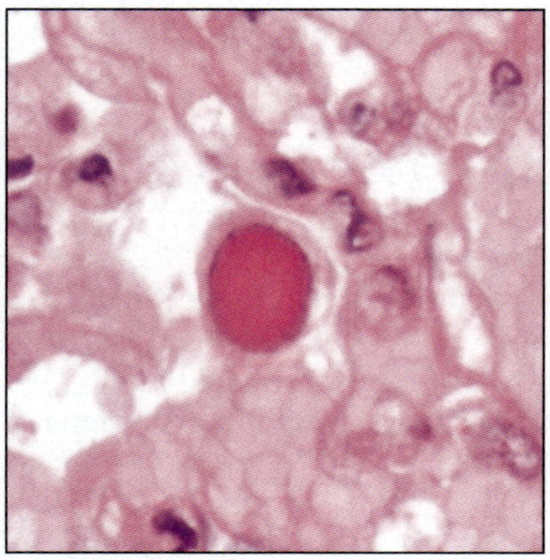

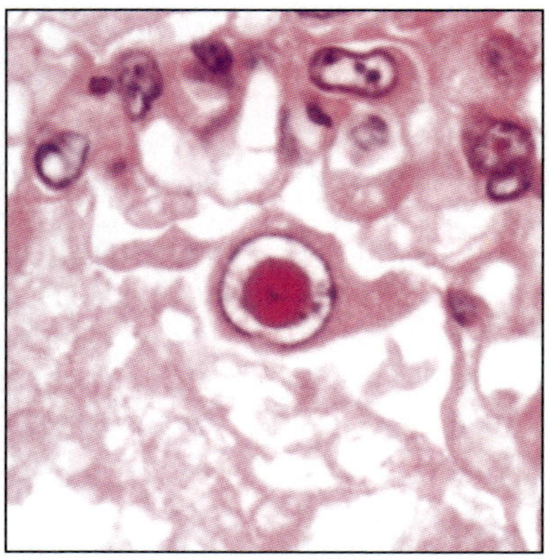

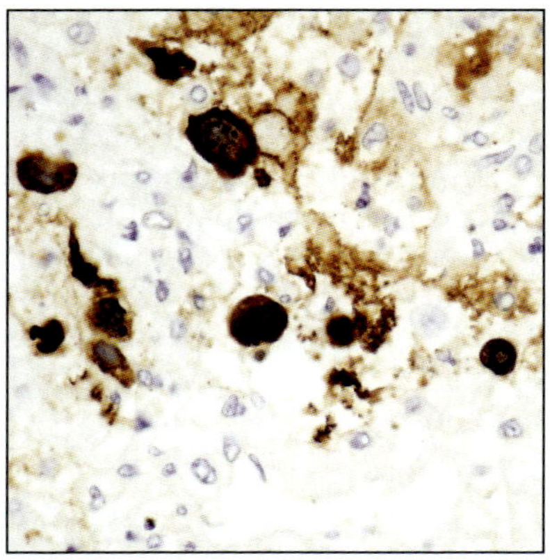

(Left) "Smudge" cells are distinctive for adenovirus pneumonia and are characterized by large eosinophilic inclusions that completely fill the nucleus and obliterate the nuclear membrane. ***(Center)*** Cowdry type A intranuclear eosinophilic inclusion in adenovirus pneumonia shows characteristic clear halo separating it from the nuclear envelope. Identical inclusions can be seen in HSV pneumonia. ***(Right)*** Immunohistochemical staining with antibodies to adenovirus shows strong positivity in the intranuclear inclusions.

MEASLES PNEUMONIA

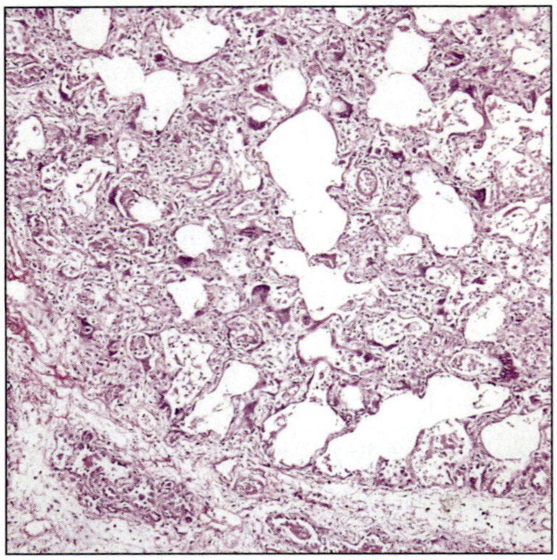

Histological appearance on scanning magnification of giant cell interstitial pneumonia in a patient with measles infection shows expansion of alveolar walls by mononuclear cell infiltrate admixed with giant cells.

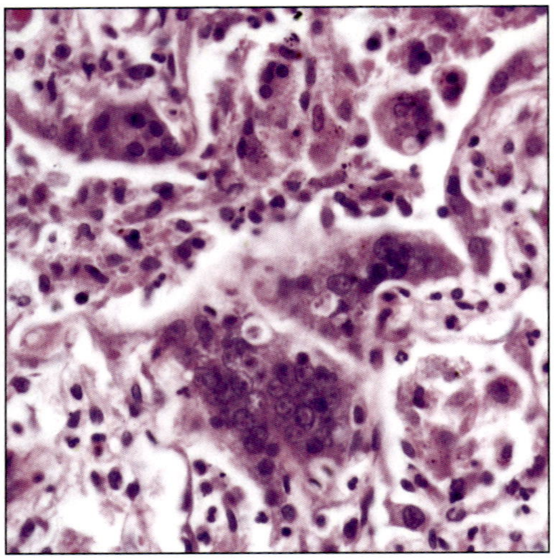

Higher magnification of the infiltrate in giant cell interstitial pneumonia due to measles shows multinucleated giant cells containing abundant small, uniform nuclei surrounded by inflammatory cell infiltrate.

TERMINOLOGY

Definitions

- Highly contagious pulmonary infection caused by measles virus (rubeola)

ETIOLOGY/PATHOGENESIS

Infectious Agents

- Causative agent is a single-stranded, enveloped virus of the family Paramyxoviridae, genus *Morbillivirus*
- Virus is spread by aerosols and droplets from respiratory secretions of acute cases

CLINICAL ISSUES

Epidemiology

- Incidence
  - Worldwide infection, particularly prevalent in underdeveloped countries
  - Recrudescence has occurred in some urban areas of USA due to diminished use of vaccine
  - Mortality is 1 in 1,000 patients
- Age
  - Children and young adults

Presentation

- Prodromal period consists of fever, cough, rhinorrhea, and conjunctivitis, with Koplik spots in buccal mucosa
- Erythematous maculopapular rash develops 3 days after onset and involves the face, trunk, and extremities
- Pulmonary complications include secondary pneumonia, giant cell pneumonia, and atypical pneumonia

Natural History

- Exposure in children < 6 years of age usually results in lifelong immunity
- Most adults have lifelong immunity either due to vaccination or previous exposure
- Clinical infection has incubation period of 1-2 weeks followed by prodromal period and skin rash
- Symptoms usually resolve spontaneously over period of days with complete resolution
- Pulmonary complications usually occur in immunocompromised or debilitated patients and may progress to fatal pneumonia

Treatment

- Drugs
  - Immune globulin may be helpful if administered within 1st week of exposure

Prognosis

- Measles pneumonia can be fatal in immunocompromised patients

IMAGE FINDINGS

Radiographic Findings

- Bilateral fine reticular opacities and patchy consolidation throughout the lungs

CT Findings

- Ground-glass opacities, small nodules, and consolidation

MACROSCOPIC FEATURES

General Features

- Cut surface shows features of patchy or lobar bronchopneumonia
- Advanced cases usually show congested and hemorrhagic cut surface with pulmonary edema

MEASLES PNEUMONIA

Key Facts

Etiology/Pathogenesis

- Causative agent is a single-stranded, enveloped virus of the family Paramyxoviridae, genus *Morbillivirus*

Clinical Issues

- Exposure in children < 6 years of age usually results in lifelong immunity
- Pulmonary complications usually occur in immunocompromised or debilitated patients and may progress to fatal pneumonia

Microscopic Pathology

- Necrotizing bronchiolitis with extensive destruction of epithelial lining of bronchioles
- Squamous metaplasia of bronchial and bronchiolar lining epithelium
- Giant cell interstitial pneumonia with numerous multinucleated epithelial giant cells
- Interstitial mononuclear inflammatory cell infiltrate
- Abundant intraalveolar exudate with hyaline membrane formation indistinguishable from DAD
- Giant cells can show up to 60 nuclei and are prominently enlarged (up to 100 μm in diameter)
- Multinucleated giant cells contain homogeneous, small eosinophilic intranuclear and cytoplasmic inclusions

Ancillary Tests

- Presence of virus can be confirmed by immunohistochemistry using specific measles antibodies
- Viral particles can be identified in cells by using specific probes by DNA in situ hybridization

MICROSCOPIC PATHOLOGY

Histologic Features

- Necrotizing bronchiolitis with extensive destruction of epithelial lining of bronchioles
- Squamous metaplasia of bronchial and bronchiolar lining epithelium
- Giant cell interstitial pneumonia with numerous multinucleated epithelial giant cells
- Interstitial mononuclear inflammatory cell infiltrate
- Proliferation of alveolar type II pneumocytes
- Abundant intraalveolar exudate with hyaline membrane formation indistinguishable from DAD
- Secondary bacterial pneumonia can superimpose as complication of measles pneumonia

Cytologic Features

- Viral cytopathic changes involving tracheal and bronchial mucosal epithelial cells
- Giant cells can show up to 60 nuclei and are prominently enlarged (up to 100 μm in diameter)
- Multinucleated giant cells contain homogeneous, small eosinophilic intranuclear and cytoplasmic inclusions

ANCILLARY TESTS

Immunohistochemistry

- Presence of virus can be confirmed by immunohistochemistry using specific measles antibodies

In Situ Hybridization

- Viral particles can be identified in cells by using specific probes by DNA in situ hybridization

Serologic Testing

- Detection of viral antigens can be accomplished by hemagglutination inhibition, neutralization, or enzyme immunoassay
- Presence of specific IgM antibodies can be used to diagnose recent infection

Electron Microscopy

- Nuclear inclusions resemble tubular or rod-shaped particles with blunt tips

DIFFERENTIAL DIAGNOSIS

Parainfluenza and Respiratory Syncytial Virus (RSV) Infection

- Also produces a giant cell interstitial pneumonia similar to that of measles
  - Viral inclusions in parainfluenza virus and RSV pneumonia are only cytoplasmic, not intranuclear
  - Definitive diagnosis requires viral isolation, demonstration of viral antigen, serologic testing, or ultrastructural examination

Varicella-Zoster Virus Infection

- Also characterized by giant cell interstitial pneumonia similar to that of measles
  - Inclusions in varicella-zoster pneumonia are similar to the intranuclear inclusions in measles, but cytoplasmic inclusions are not seen

Hard Metal Pneumoconiosis

- Produces a giant cell interstitial pneumonia secondary to inhalation of heavy metal particles (tungsten, carbide, titanium, etc.)
  - Giant cells in hard metal pneumoconiosis are multinucleated histiocytes rather than virally infected epithelial cells
  - Histiocytic giant cells in hard metal pneumoconiosis do not contain viral inclusions

SELECTED REFERENCES

1. Piastra M et al: Measles-induced respiratory distress, air-leak and ARDS. Eur J Clin Microbiol Infect Dis. 29(2):181-5, 2010
2. Moussallem TM et al: Lung involvement in childhood measles: severe immune dysfunction revealed by quantitative immunohistochemistry. Hum Pathol. 38(8):1239-47, 2007

MEASLES PNEUMONIA

Giant Cell Interstitial Pneumonia

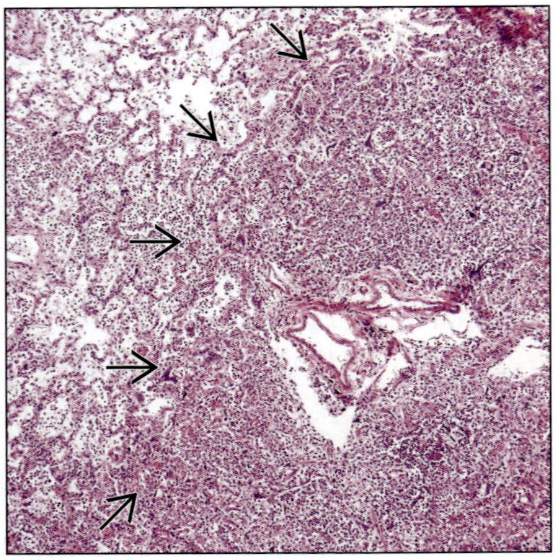

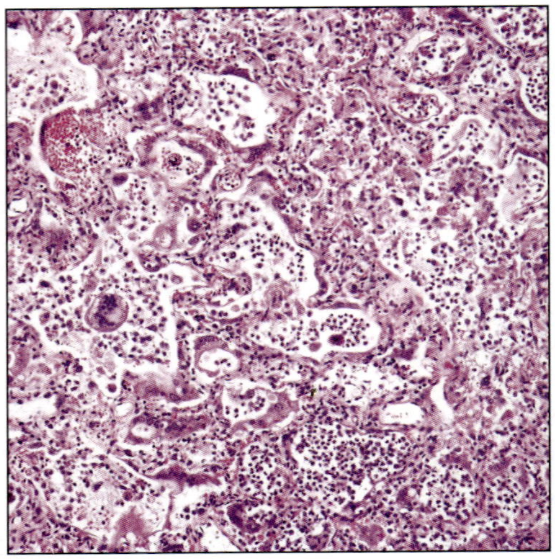

(Left) *Scanning magnification of lung parenchyma in a patient with measles infection shows a well-circumscribed area of consolidation → merging with the adjacent lung parenchyma. The area of consolidation contains heavy inflammatory cell infiltrates.* ***(Right)*** *Higher magnification of lung with giant cell interstitial pneumonia in a patient with measles shows intraalveolar inflammatory infiltrates and thickening of the walls of the alveoli secondary to inflammation and giant cells.*

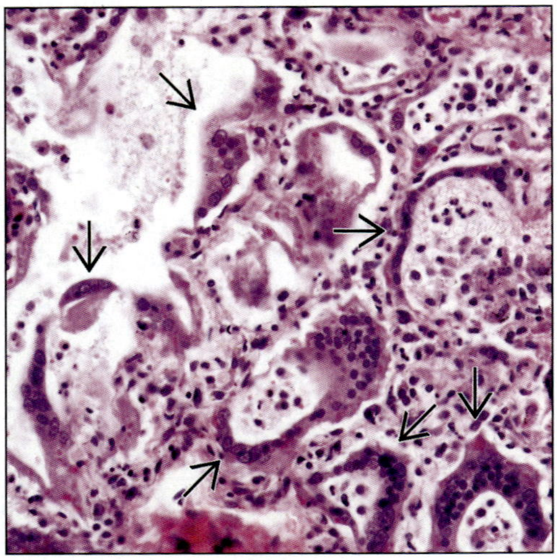

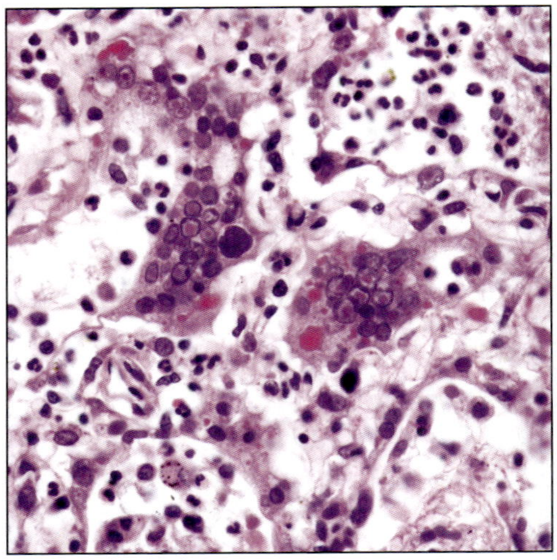

(Left) *Higher magnification of giant cell interstitial pneumonia in a patient with measles shows numerous giant cells with multiple nuclei. The nuclei of the giant cells → characteristically wrap around the alveolar walls and surround the inflammatory cells in the lumen.* ***(Right)*** *Giant cells in measles giant cell interstitial pneumonia show a large number of small, round uniform nuclei, most of which contain small eosinophilic intranuclear inclusions.*

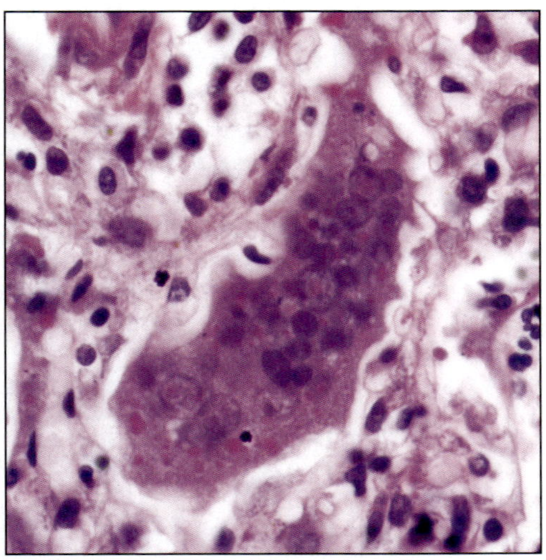

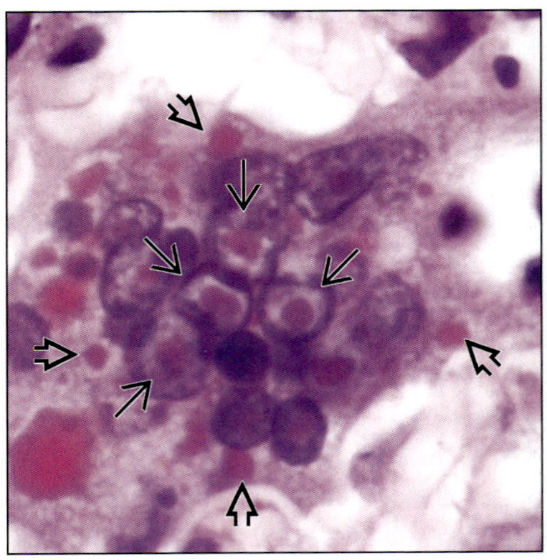

(Left) *Higher magnification of a giant cell in measles interstitial pneumonia shows multiple small nuclei and scattered intracytoplasmic and intranuclear inclusions. The giant cells are not histiocytic in origin but rather are modified epithelial cells.* ***(Right)*** *Higher magnification of a multinucleated epithelial giant cell in measles giant cell interstitial pneumonia shows small eosinophilic intranuclear inclusions with a targetoid appearance →. Notice similar inclusions within the cytoplasm ⇨.*

Additional Histologic Features

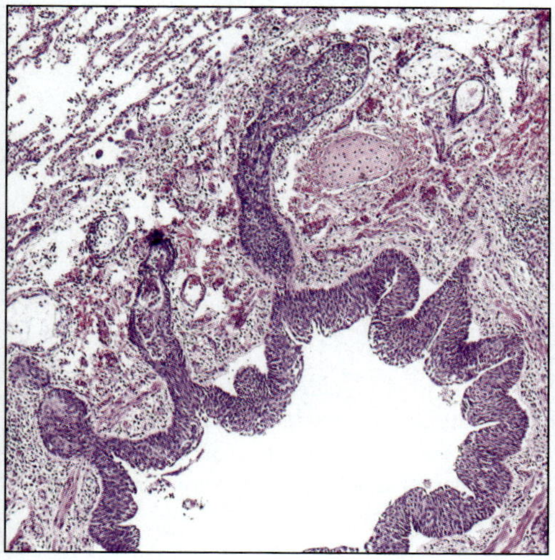

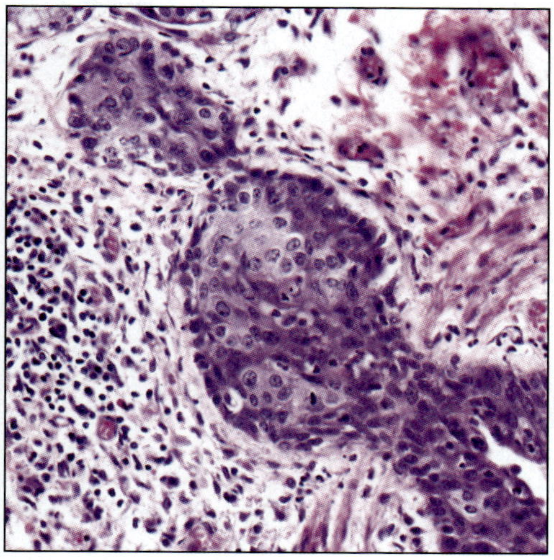

(Left) *Scanning magnification of the lung in a patient with measles pneumonia shows severe acute and chronic inflammation of a bronchus with extensive squamous metaplasia of the bronchial lining mucosa.* ***(Right)*** *Higher magnification of the wall of a secondary bronchus in a patient with measles pneumonia shows squamous metaplasia of the lining epithelium. The islands of squamous metaplasia are surrounded by chronic inflammation mainly composed of a mononuclear cell infiltrate.*

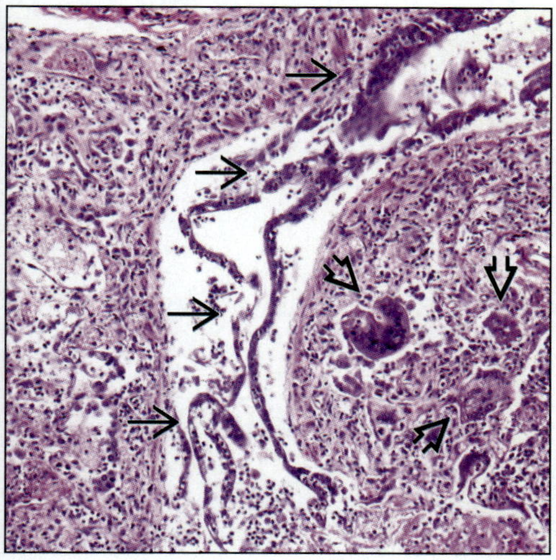

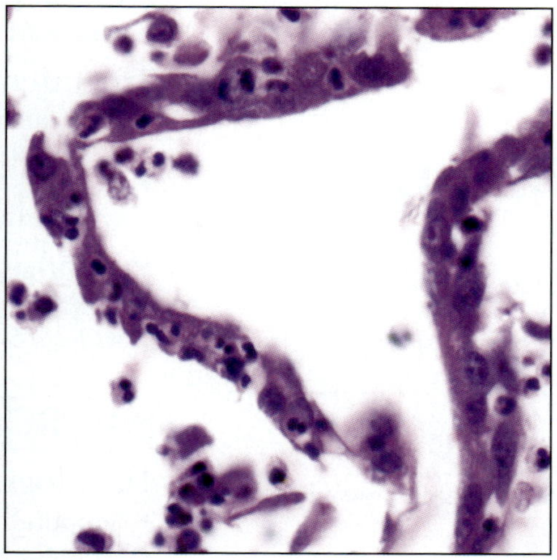

(Left) *Section of lung in a patient with pulmonary involvement by measles pneumonia shows necrotizing bronchiolitis with extensive destruction of the bronchiolar mucosa* →*. Notice a few scattered multinucleated giant cells distributed throughout the adjacent parenchyma* ⇨*.* ***(Right)*** *Higher magnification from focus of necrotizing bronchiolitis in patient with measles pneumonia shows infiltration of mucosa by mononuclear cell inflammatory infiltrate.*

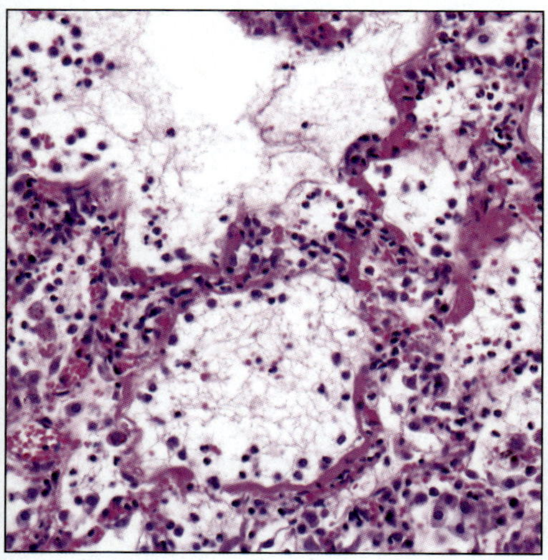

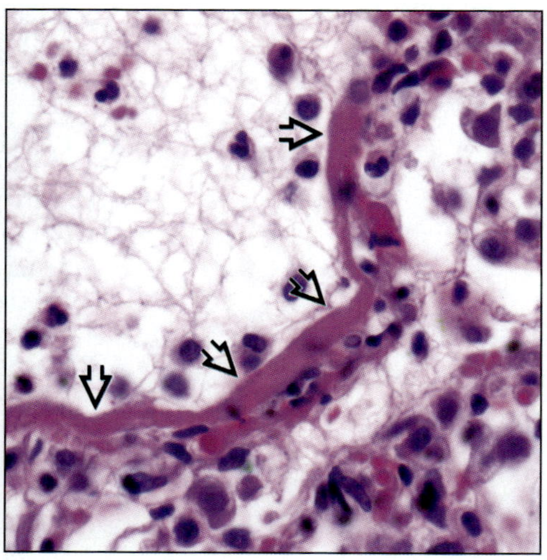

(Left) *Acute lung injury in a patient with measles pneumonia shows edema and congestion of alveolar septa with dense mononuclear cell inflammatory infiltrates. The alveolar lumens contain edema fluid and scattered inflammatory cells and are lined by a thin layer of dense eosinophilic material similar to that seen in diffuse alveolar damage.* ***(Right)*** *Higher magnification from measles pneumonia displays dense eosinophilic hyaline membrane lining the wall of an alveolar space* ⇨*.*

SPOROTRICHOSIS

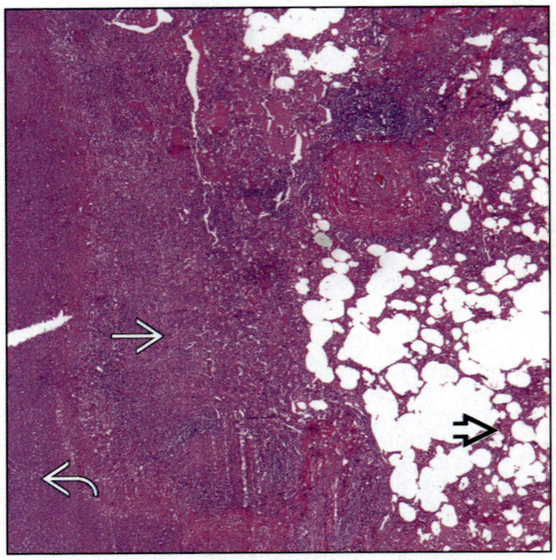

Low-power view of pulmonary sporotrichosis shows areas of necrosis with a rim of fibrosis with acute and chronic inflammation. Note the presence of uninvolved lung parenchyma.

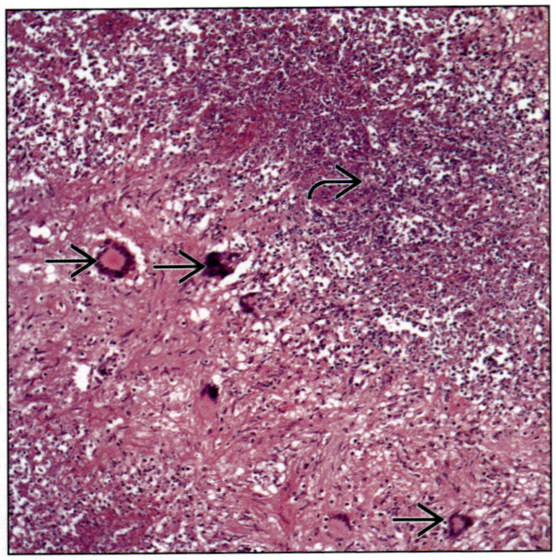

Higher magnification of pulmonary sporotrichosis shows areas of abscess formation and granulomatous reaction with presence of multinucleated giant cells.

TERMINOLOGY

Definitions

- Chronic mycotic infection

ETIOLOGY/PATHOGENESIS

Infectious Agents

- *Sporothrix schenckii* (*Sporotrichum schenckii*)

CLINICAL ISSUES

Epidemiology

- Incidence
  - Worldwide distribution with variable prevalence
- Age
  - Any age group may be affected

Site

- Infection predominantly affects
  - Skin
  - Lymph nodes
- Infection may also involve
  - Lung
  - Bone
  - Mucosal membranes
    - Nose
    - Mouth
    - Pharynx

Presentation

- Fever
- Dyspnea
- Chest pain

Laboratory Tests

- Blood and tissue cultures

Natural History

- May start as a penetrating wound

Treatment

- Surgical approaches
  - In some cases, wedge resection or even lobectomy
- Drugs
  - Antifungal treatment

Prognosis

- May be fatal in immunocompromised patients with widespread infection

MICROSCOPIC PATHOLOGY

Histologic Features

- Suppurative pneumonia
- Granulomatous inflammation
- Abscess formation
  - Presence of fungal organisms
  - Asteroid bodies
  - Splendore-Hoeppli phenomenon

DIFFERENTIAL DIAGNOSIS

Other Infectious Diseases

- Histoplasmosis
  - Splendore-Hoeppli and asteroid bodies unusual in histoplasmosis
  - Cultures reveal the correct fungal organisms
- Cryptococcus
  - Mucicarmine stain positive in cryptococcal infections but negative in sporotrichosis
  - Tissue cultures reveal the correct organism
- Coccidioidomycosis
  - Coccidioides is a larger fungal organism
  - Coccidioides shows the presence of endospores, which are not present in sporotrichosis
- Bacterial pneumonia

SPOROTRICHOSIS

Key Facts

Terminology
- Chronic mycotic infection

Etiology/Pathogenesis
- *Sporothrix schenckii* (*Sporotrichum schenckii*)

Clinical Issues
- Infection predominantly affects
  - Skin
  - Lymph nodes
- Infections may also involve
  - Lung
  - Bone
  - Mucosal membranes
- Process may start as a penetrating wound

Microscopic Pathology
- Suppurative pneumonia
- Granulomatous inflammation
- Abscess formation

Histochemical Stains

Stain	Result
Silver stain (GMS)	Positive staining of fungal organisms
Periodic acid-Schiff (PAS)	Highlights fungal organisms
Mucicarmine	Negative staining of fungal organisms
Acid-fast bacilli	Negative
Fite-Faraco	Negative

Tissue culture is the most important study to define the type of fungal organism.

  - Suppurative pneumonia may be seen in both bacterial pneumonia and sporotrichosis
  - GMS and PAS histochemical stains negative
- Atypical mycobacterial disease
  - Suppurative pneumonia may be seen in both atypical mycobacterial disease and sporotrichosis
  - Acid-fast histochemical stains positive for presence of acid-fast bacilli
  - GMS and PAS histochemical stains negative

DIAGNOSTIC CHECKLIST

Pathologic Interpretation Pearls
- Fungal organisms
- Asteroid bodies
- Splendore-Hoeppli phenomenon
- Numerous yeasts
- Budding yeasts

SELECTED REFERENCES

1. Hussein MR: Mucocutaneous Splendore-Hoeppli phenomenon. J Cutan Pathol. 35(11):979-88, 2008
2. Schubach A et al: Epidemic sporotrichosis. Curr Opin Infect Dis. 21(2):129-33, 2008
3. Zeegelaar JE et al: Imported tropical infectious ulcers in travelers. Am J Clin Dermatol. 9(4):219-32, 2008
4. Scheinfeld N: A review of the new antifungals: posaconazole, micafungin, and anidulafungin. J Drugs Dermatol. 6(12):1249-51, 2007
5. Kauffman CA: Endemic mycoses: blastomycosis, histoplasmosis, and sporotrichosis. Infect Dis Clin North Am. 20(3):645-62, vii, 2006
6. Yelverton CB et al: Fatal sporotrichosis. Cutis. 78(4):253-6, 2006

IMAGE GALLERY

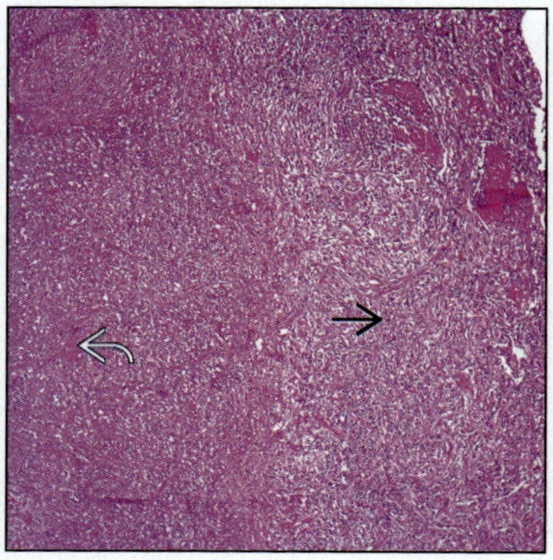

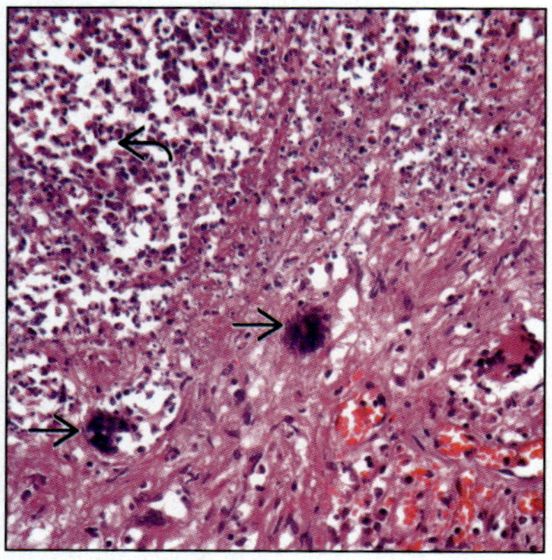

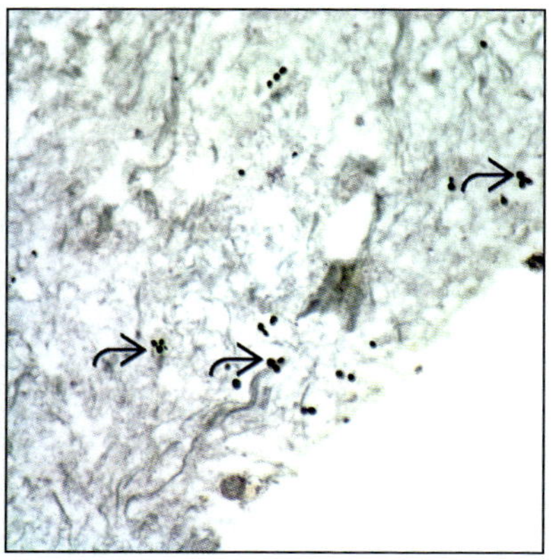

(Left) *Pulmonary sporotrichosis shows extensive areas of necrosis and fibrosis. Note that the presence of multinucleated giant cells is not prominent.* ***(Center)*** *Pulmonary sporotrichosis shows acute inflammatory changes and granulomatous inflammation with numerous multinucleated giant cells.* ***(Right)*** *Silver stain shows the presence of numerous budding yeast forms. There is narrow budding, which is characteristic of sporotrichosis.*

KLEBSIELLA PNEUMONIA

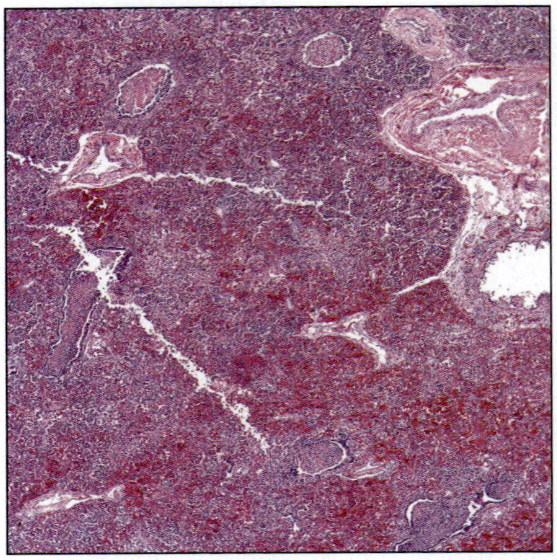

Low-power view of a section of lung parenchyma shows extensive areas of congestion and inflammation. Note the absence of alveolated tissue.

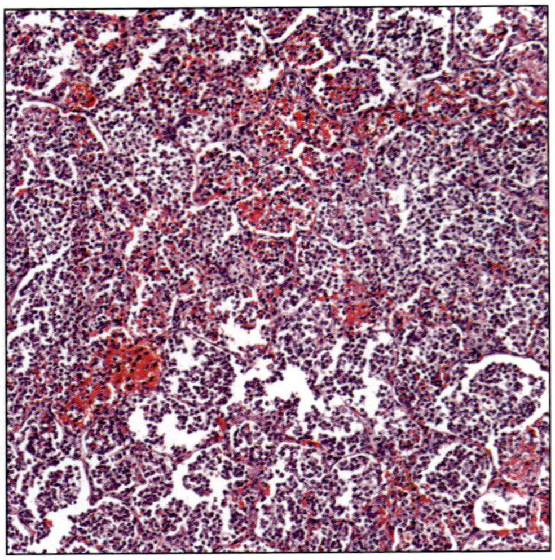

Higher magnification shows areas of abscess formation with prominent acute inflammation and fibrinous exudate. These features, although not pathognomonic of Klebsiella pneumonia, are suggestive.

TERMINOLOGY

Synonyms

- Friedlander pneumonia

Definitions

- Infectious condition caused by Gram-negative bacteria

ETIOLOGY/PATHOGENESIS

Infectious Agents

- *Klebsiella pneumoniae*
  - Nonmotile, usually encapsulated bacillus
  - > 80 different types

CLINICAL ISSUES

Epidemiology

- Incidence
  - Klebsiella pneumonia appears to be more common in
    - Hospitalized patients
    - Nursing homes
    - Alcoholics
    - Diabetic patients
    - Individuals with poor oral hygiene
- Age
  - More common in adults
- Gender
  - No gender predilection
- Ethnicity
  - No ethnic predisposition

Site

- Posterior segment of the right upper lobe is more commonly affected

Presentation

- Fever
- Cough
- Hemoptysis
- Chest pain
- Malaise
- Weight loss

Laboratory Tests

- Leukocytosis
- Increased erythrocyte sedimentation rate
- Cultures positive for Gram-negative bacilli

Treatment

- Drugs
  - Antibiotics

Prognosis

- Depends on setting in which illness occurs
- May be fatal in 20-60% of patients

IMAGE FINDINGS

Radiographic Findings

- Bilateral multifocal consolidations or cavitations

MACROSCOPIC FEATURES

General Features

- Necrosis
- Hemorrhage
- Abscess formation

MICROSCOPIC PATHOLOGY

Histologic Features

- Alveolar destruction
- Prominent polymorphonuclear leukocyte reaction
- Edematous fluid mixed with mononuclear cells
- Mucicarminophilic exudate
- Abscess formation

Key Facts

Terminology
- Synonym
  - Friedlander pneumonia
- Definition
  - Infectious condition caused by Gram-negative bacteria

Etiology/Pathogenesis
- *Klebsiella pneumoniae*
  - Nonmotile, usually encapsulated bacillus
  - > 80 different types

Clinical Issues
- Klebsiella pneumonia appears to be more common in
  - Hospitalized patients
  - Nursing homes
  - Alcoholics
  - Diabetics
  - Individuals with poor hygiene
- Presentation
  - Fever
  - Cough
  - Hemoptysis
  - Chest pain
  - Malaise
  - Weight loss
- Prognosis
  - Depends on setting in which illness occurs
  - May be fatal in 20-60% of patients
- Treatment
  - Antibiotics

Histochemical Features of Klebsiella Pneumonia

Stains	Result
Gram	Identification of Gram-negative bacilli
Brown-Hopps	Identification of Gram-negative bacilli
Mucicarmine	Negative in organisms; positive in exudate

- Pulmonary gangrene

Cytologic Features
- Consolidation with acute inflammation
- Cavitation
- Abscess formation

DIFFERENTIAL DIAGNOSIS

Bacterial Pneumonia
- Gram stain distinguishes Gram-positive from Gram-negative pneumonia
- Bacterial cultures help in identifying Klebsiella
- Mucicarminophilic exudate appears to be more common in Klebsiella pneumonia

Pulmonary Tuberculosis
- Although tuberculosis may show areas of cavitation, Gram stain is negative
- Tuberculosis stains positive for acid-fast bacilli
- Tuberculosis shows specific culture results

Carcinoma
- In some cases, cavitation may occur in cases of non-small cell carcinoma
- Identification of malignant cells is of utmost importance

DIAGNOSTIC CHECKLIST

Pathologic Interpretation Pearls
- Mucicarminophilic exudate
- Cavitation
- Abscess formation
- Gram-negative bacilli
- Positive cultures

SELECTED REFERENCES

1. Antoniadou A et al: Colistin-resistant isolates of Klebsiella pneumoniae emerging in intensive care unit patients: first report of a multiclonal cluster. J Antimicrob Chemother. 59(4):786-90, 2007
2. Couto RC et al: A 10-year prospective surveillance of nosocomial infections in neonatal intensive care units. Am J Infect Control. 35(3):183-9, 2007
3. Wu CL et al: Early evolution of arterial oxygenation in severe community-acquired pneumonia: a prospective observational study. J Crit Care. 22(2):129-36, 2007
4. Labombardi VJ et al: Use of cefepime for the treatment of infections caused by extended spectrum beta-lactamase-producing Klebsiella pneumoniae and Escherichia coli. Diagn Microbiol Infect Dis. 56(3):313-5, 2006
5. Lomaestro BM et al: The spread of Klebsiella pneumoniae carbapenemase-producing K. pneumoniae to upstate New York. Clin Infect Dis. 43(3):e26-8, 2006
6. Omwandho CO et al: Early pregnancy loss and neonatal deaths associated with Klebsiella pneumonia infection: a mini review of possible occupational health risk. Arch Gynecol Obstet. 273(5):258-60, 2006

KLEBSIELLA PNEUMONIA

Microscopic Features

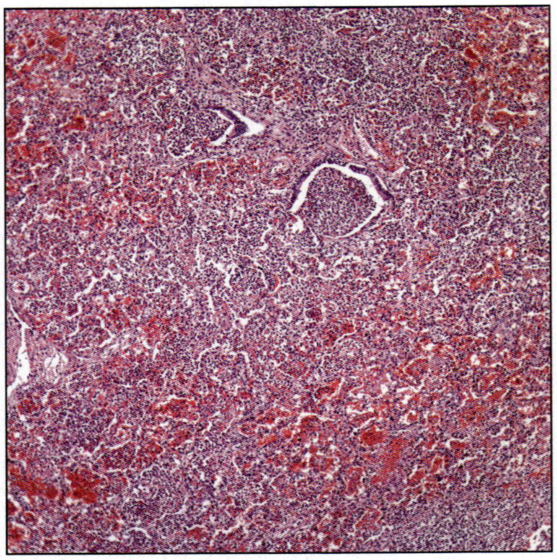
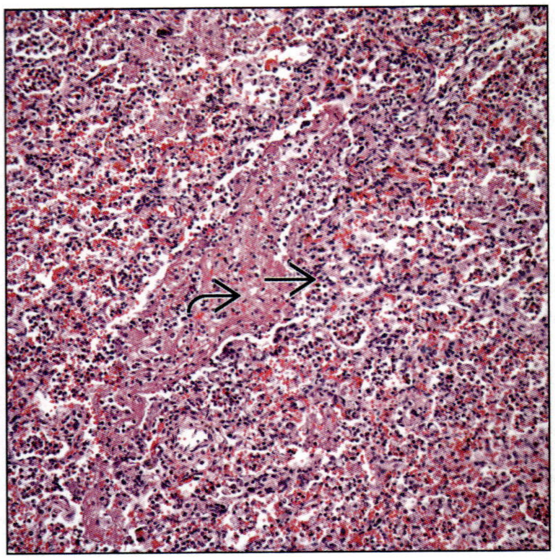

*(**Left**) Low-power view of Klebsiella pneumonia shows extensive congestion and fibrinous exudate admixed with inflammatory reaction. These features, although not specific for Klebsiella pneumonia, should prompt the use of cultures and special stains. (**Right**) High-power view of lung parenchyma shows areas of fibrinous exudate ↗ and a prominent inflammatory component → with abscess formation. The use of special histochemical stains for bacteria is warranted in such cases.*

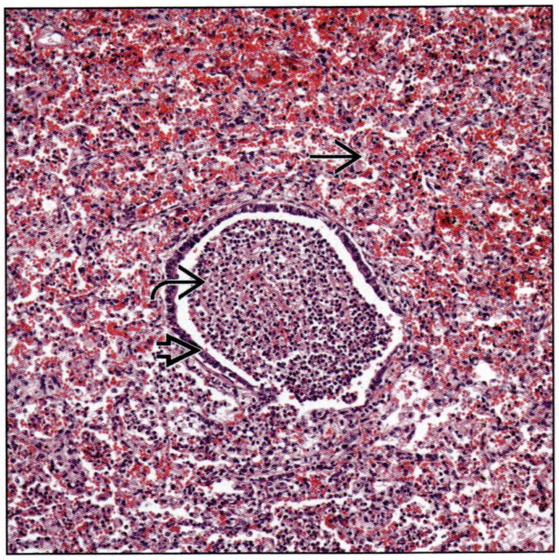
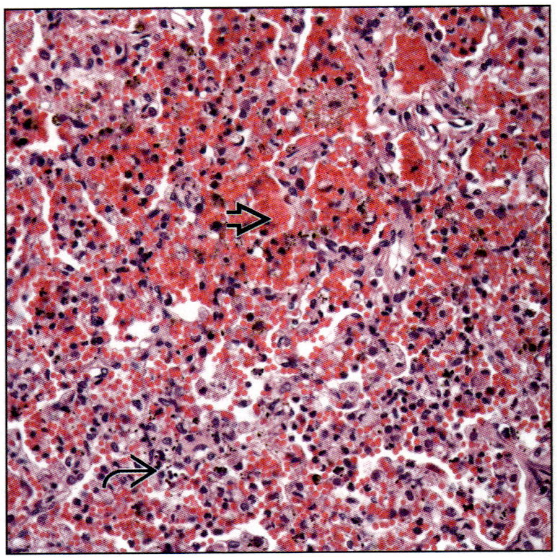

*(**Left**) Klebsiella pneumonia shows abscess formation ↗ within the airway ⇨ while the adjacent lung parenchyma → shows congestion and inflammatory changes. (**Right**) Closer view of the inflammatory component shows that it consists of acute inflammatory cells ↗ admixed with red cells ⇨. Once again, even though these changes are not specific for Klebsiella pneumonia, they should raise the possibility of this diagnosis in the right setting.*

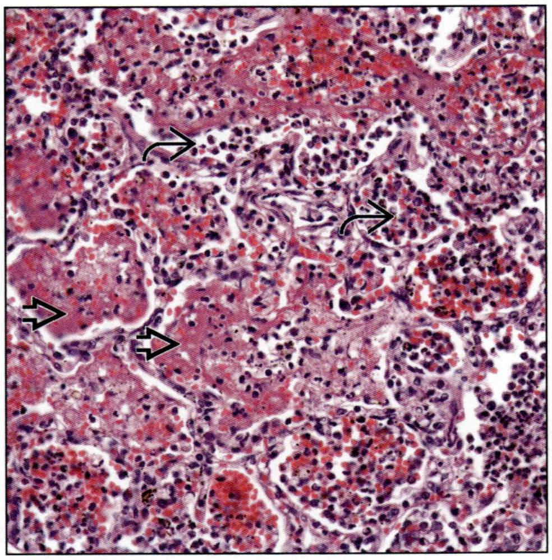
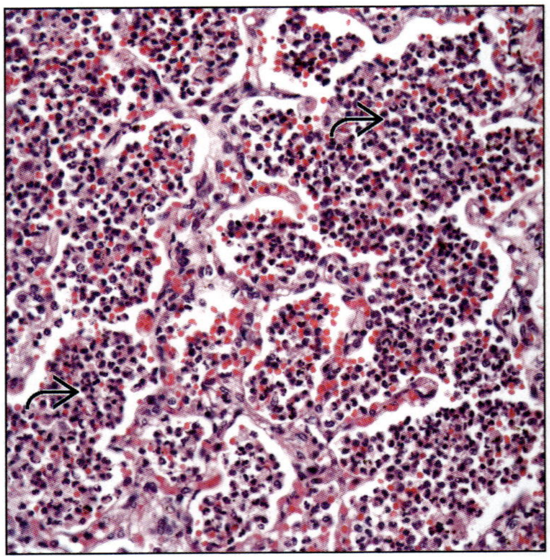

*(**Left**) Klebsiella pneumonia shows extensive areas of fibrinous component ⇨ admixed with acute inflammatory cells ↗. The process is clearly infectious and requires the use of cultures and special histochemical stains for identification of the organism. (**Right**) High-power magnification shows that alveoli are filled with acute inflammatory cells ↗. Basically, the normal lung parenchyma is destroyed by the infectious process.*

Microscopic Features

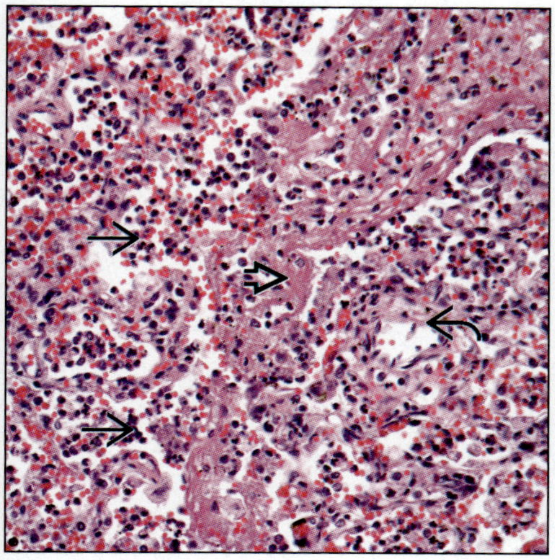
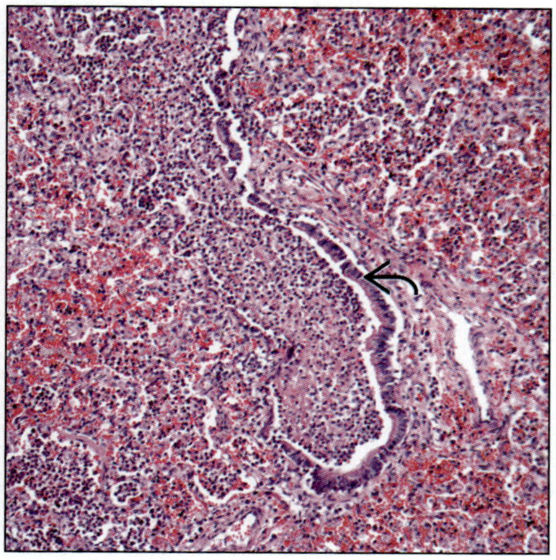

(Left) *In some cases of Klebsiella pneumonia, the basic alveolar outline is not recognizable due to the inflammatory process. In this case, the acute inflammatory cells are admixed with fibrin leaving only a few recognizable structures, such as pulmonary vessels.* ***(Right)*** *Klebsiella pneumonia shows partial destruction of the airway. Note the presence of abscess formation and the destruction of the adjacent normal lung parenchyma.*

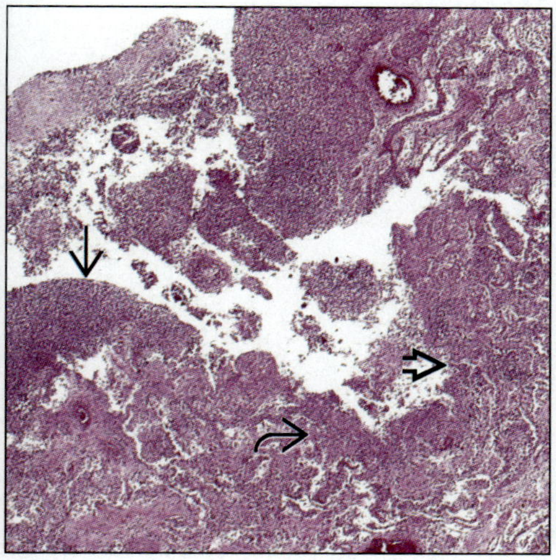
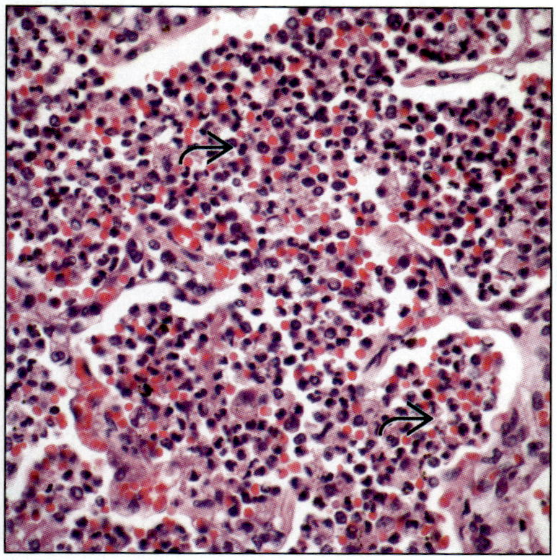

(Left) *Klebsiella pneumonia involving main bronchi shows erosion and destruction of the normal mucosa and the presence of abscess formation. These changes may be seen in small biopsy specimens.* ***(Right)*** *The involvement of the lung parenchyma characterized by alveoli filled with acute inflammatory cells is the most common pattern in cases of Klebsiella pneumonia.*

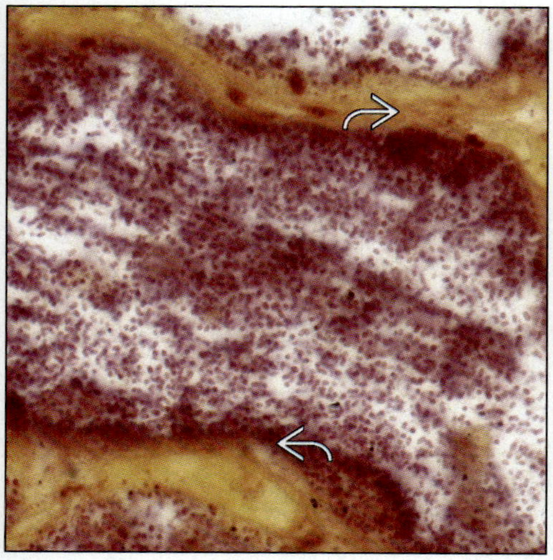
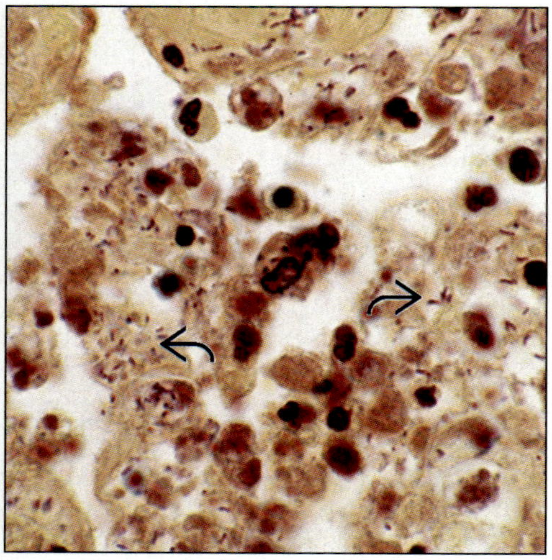

(Left) *Mucin histochemical stain shows the classical mucicarminophilic exudate that is commonly seen in cases of Klebsiella pneumonia. Such a finding is helpful in making the diagnosis.* ***(Right)*** *Brown-Hopps histochemical stain is useful in the diagnosis of Klebsiella pneumonia as it may demonstrate the presence of bacterial forms, which may not be readily identifiable in the conventional H&E. Note the presence of numerous organisms compatible with Klebsiella.*

SARS PNEUMONIA

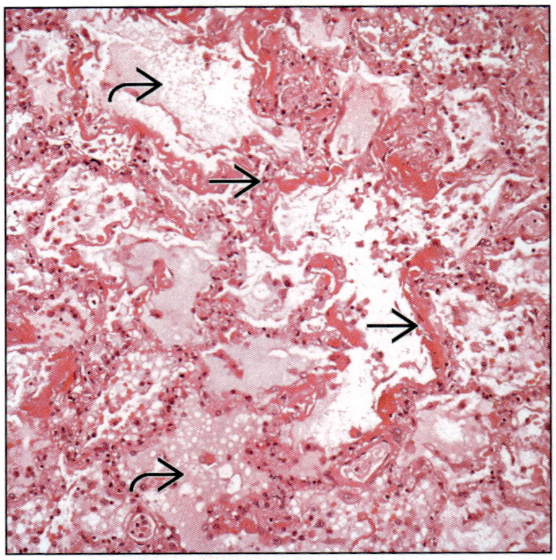

SARS infection shows extensive areas of congestion, edema ↪, and hyaline membranes →. All these features are compatible with diffuse alveolar damage caused by SARS-CoV.

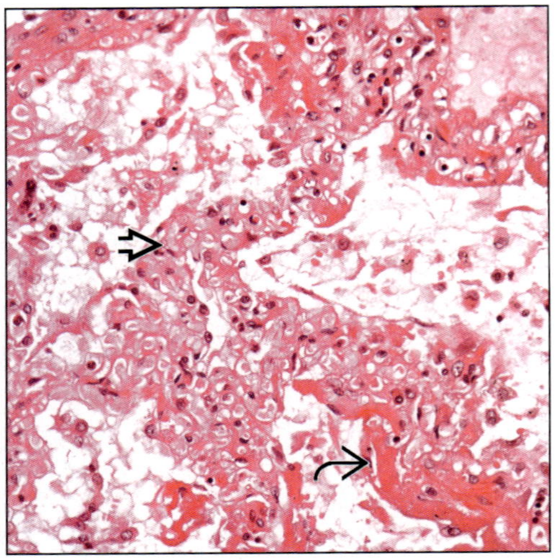

SARS shows the classic features of hyaline membranes ↪ and pneumocyte type II hyperplasia ⇨, which are compatible with DAD.

TERMINOLOGY

Abbreviations

- Severe acute respiratory syndrome (SARS)

Definitions

- Infectious viral disease

ETIOLOGY/PATHOGENESIS

Infectious Agents

- SARS coronavirus (SARS-CoV)
- Single-stranded RNA virus
- Virus has also been isolated from
  - Urine
  - Feces

Pathogenesis

- Highly complex
- It may involve
  - Immune system
  - Hyperinduction of chemokines and cytokines
  - Insufficient interferon reaction
  - Compromised cellular immune response
  - Metallopeptidase (ACE2) identified as functional receptor for SARS-CoV
- SARS can be transmitted by
  - Direct contact
  - Droplet
  - Airborne route

CLINICAL ISSUES

Epidemiology

- Incidence
  - Difficult to establish but at the end of the initial epidemic of 2003, > 8,000 probable cases had been reported
- Age
  - Affects any age group
- Gender
  - No gender predilection
- Ethnicity
  - Probably more common in China

Presentation

- Flu-like symptoms
- Fever
- Cough
- Chills
- Malaise
- Shortness of breath

Treatment

- No specific treatment
- Some patients treated with steroids
- Antiviral therapy

Prognosis

- Mortality is ~ 10%
- Elderly patients (> 60 years of age) may account for 50% of fatal cases
- In younger patients, mortality has been estimated to be < 10%
- Mortality appears to be higher in males than females

MACROSCOPIC FEATURES

General Features

- Congested lungs

MICROSCOPIC PATHOLOGY

Histologic Features

- Diffuse alveolar damage (DAD)
  - Pneumocyte type II hyperplasia
  - Hyaline membranes
- Organizing phase of DAD

SARS PNEUMONIA

Key Facts

Terminology
- Severe acute respiratory syndrome (SARS)

Etiology/Pathogenesis
- Etiological agent
  - SARS coronavirus (SARS-CoV)
- SARS can be transmitted by
  - Direct contact
  - Droplet
  - Airborne route

Clinical Issues
- Symptomatology
  - Flu-like symptoms
- Prognosis
  - Mortality is ~ 10%
  - More fatal cases in elderly patients > 60 years of age
  - Mortality in younger individuals is < 10%

  - Hyaline membranes
  - Fibroblastic plugs in alveolar spaces
  - Pneumocyte type II hyperplasia
- Bronchiolitis obliterans and organizing pneumonia
- Multinucleated giant cells
- Other organs may also be affected, including
  - Gastrointestinal tract
  - Hematopoietic
  - Central nervous system
  - Skeletal muscle
  - Heart
  - Thyroid
  - Testes

ANCILLARY TESTS

In Situ Hybridization
- Identification of viral particles

PCR
- Identification of viral particles

Electron Microscopy
- Identification of viral particles

DIFFERENTIAL DIAGNOSIS

Avian Influenza A (H5N1)
- Although it also shows DAD, avian influenza follows a more aggressive course with marked necrosis and hemorrhage in the lungs
- Multinucleated giant cells present in SARS are not present in avian influenza

DIAGNOSTIC CHECKLIST

Pathologic Interpretation Pearls
- Diffuse alveolar damage
- Organizing phase of DAD
- Multinucleated giant cells

SELECTED REFERENCES

1. Cleri DJ et al: Severe acute respiratory syndrome (SARS). Infect Dis Clin North Am. 24(1):175-202, 2010
2. Hui DS et al: Severe acute respiratory syndrome and coronavirus. Infect Dis Clin North Am. 24(3):619-38, 2010
3. Guo Y et al: Pathogenetic mechanisms of severe acute respiratory syndrome. Virus Res. 133(1):4-12, 2008
4. Wong SS et al: The management of coronavirus infections with particular reference to SARS. J Antimicrob Chemother. 62(3):437-41, 2008
5. Cheng VC et al: Severe acute respiratory syndrome coronavirus as an agent of emerging and reemerging infection. Clin Microbiol Rev. 20(4):660-94, 2007

IMAGE GALLERY

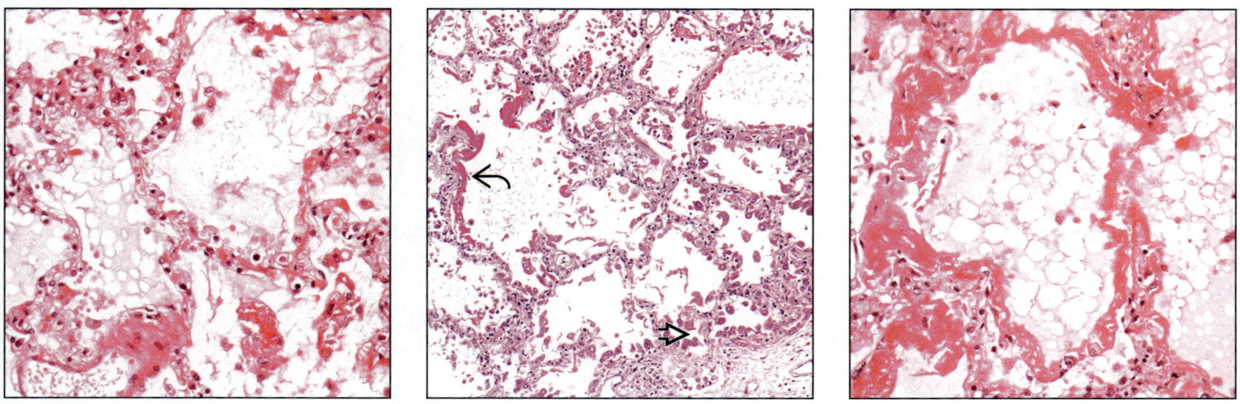

(Left) *In some areas, the presence of hyaline membranes may not be as apparent; however, the presence of type II pneumocyte hyperplasia can still be identified. Note the presence of intraalveolar edema.* ***(Center)*** *In other areas, features of DAD are more apparent. Note the presence of type II pneumocyte hyperplasia ⇨ and hyaline membranes ⇨.* ***(Right)*** *Alveolar walls entirely lined by a hyaline membrane are commonly seen in fulminant cases of DAD as shown here.*

NOCARDIOSIS

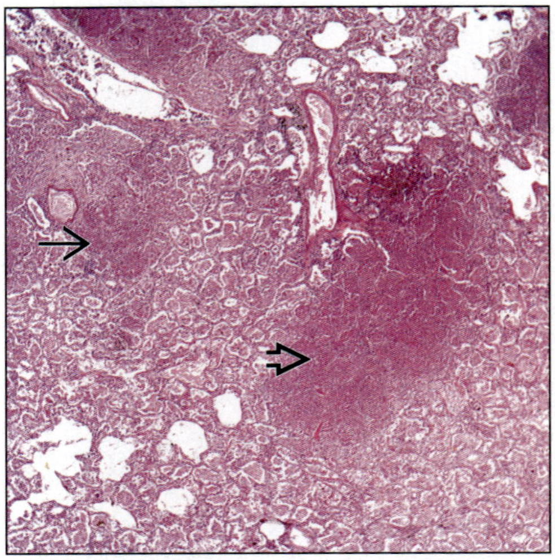

Low-power view of a suppurative pneumonia shows abscess formation ⇨. The remaining portions of the lung show acute inflammatory changes and a small developing abscess →.

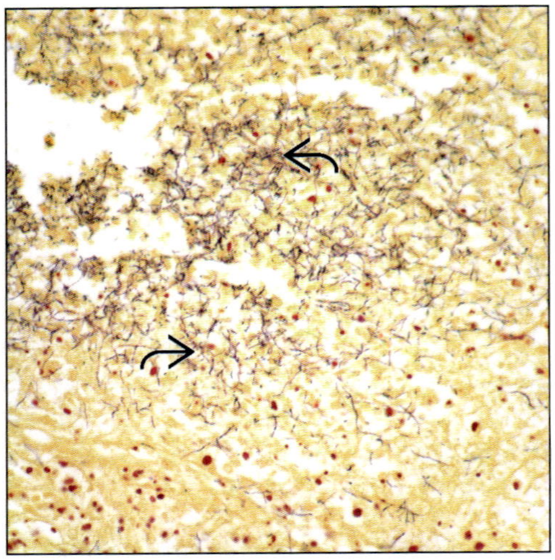

Gram histochemical stains show numerous filamentous bacterial organisms ↪ embedded in a pulmonary abscess. Gram stain is important in demonstrating nocardiosis.

TERMINOLOGY

Definitions

- Infectious condition

ETIOLOGY/PATHOGENESIS

Infectious Agents

- *Nocardia asteroides*
  - Aerobic, partially acid-fast branching actinomycete
  - Rarely measures > 1 μm in diameter
- Other types of *Nocardia* may also be the pathogenic agent

CLINICAL ISSUES

Epidemiology

- Incidence
  - Worldwide distribution
- Age
  - More common in adults
- Gender
  - No gender predilection
- Ethnicity
  - No ethnic predilection

Site

- Nocardiosis predominantly affects
  - Lungs
  - Brain
  - Meninges

Presentation

- Fever
- Dyspnea
- Chest pain
- Weight loss
- Anorexia
- General malaise

Laboratory Tests

- Blood cultures
- Tissue cultures

Treatment

- Drugs
  - Antibiotics
    - Penicillin
    - Sulfonamides

Prognosis

- If treated early, prognosis may be good
- If spreads to brain and meninges, may be fatal

MICROSCOPIC PATHOLOGY

Histologic Features

- Acute suppurative pneumonia
- Abscess formation

DIFFERENTIAL DIAGNOSIS

Other Infectious Conditions

- Bacterial pneumonia
  - Both infections may share similar histopathological features
  - Presence of acid-fast organisms with special stains is more typical of *Nocardia*
  - Tissue cultures would reveal the correct organism
- Atypical mycobacterial disease
  - Both infections may share similar histopathological features
  - Bacilli of mycobacterial infection are short
  - Bacilli of mycobacterial disease are negative for Gram stains
  - Tissue cultures would reveal the correct organism
- Actinomycosis

NOCARDIOSIS

Key Facts

Etiology/Pathogenesis
- *Nocardia asteroides*
  - Aerobic, partially acid-fast branching actinomycete
  - Rarely measures > 1 µm in diameter
- Other types of *Nocardia* may also be the pathogenic agent

Clinical Issues
- Nocardiosis predominantly affects
  - Lungs
  - Brain
  - Meninges

Microscopic Pathology
- Acute suppurative pneumonia
- Abscess formation

Diagnostic Checklist
- Positive staining for
  - Gram
  - Ziehl-Neelsen

Histochemical Stains

Stain	Result
Gram	Positive staining of organism
GMS	Positive staining of organism
Ziehl-Neelsen/Fite-Faraco	Positive staining of organism
PAS	Negative
Gridley	Negative

Tissue cultures are the best method to identify the organisms.

  - Presence of granules may aid in separating *Nocardia* from other actinomyces as *Nocardia* would not show granules
- Other fungal infections
  - GMS positivity may be shared by other fungal organisms
  - Acid-fast histochemical stains are negative in other fungal infections
  - Gram stain may also be negative in other common fungal infections

DIAGNOSTIC CHECKLIST

Pathologic Interpretation Pearls
- Suppurative pneumonia
- Abscess formation
- Delicate filamentous organisms
- Branching at right angles
- Absence of granules
- Positive staining for
  - Gram
  - GMS
  - Ziehl-Neelsen
  - Fite-Faraco

SELECTED REFERENCES

1. Ambrosioni J et al: Nocardiosis: updated clinical review and experience at a tertiary center. Infection. 38(2):89-97, 2010
2. Sullivan DC et al: Bacteria that masquerade as fungi: actinomycosis/nocardia. Proc Am Thorac Soc. 7(3):216-21, 2010
3. Rodrigues C et al: [Thoracic nocardiosis.] Rev Port Pneumol. 15(6):1199-204, 2009

IMAGE GALLERY

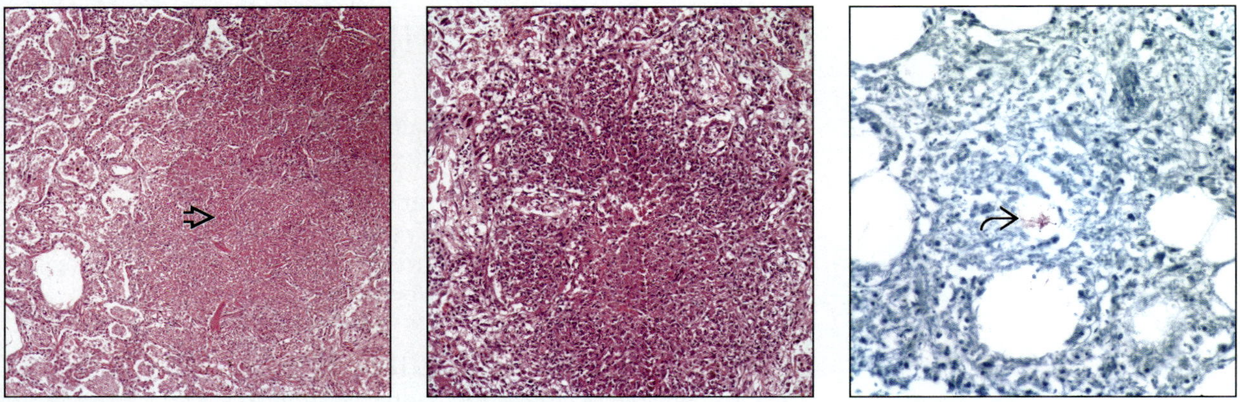

(Left) *Low-power view of an acute pneumonic process shows severe acute inflammation with abscess formation ⇨. The remaining portion of the lung shows changes similar to those seen in diffuse alveolar damage.* ***(Center)*** *Closer view at a pulmonary abscess caused by nocardiosis shows the presence of severe acute inflammation. The presence of organisms is not apparent in conventional H&E stains.* ***(Right)*** *A cluster of organisms ➚ is present with the Ziehl-Neelsen stain.*

ACTINOMYCOSIS

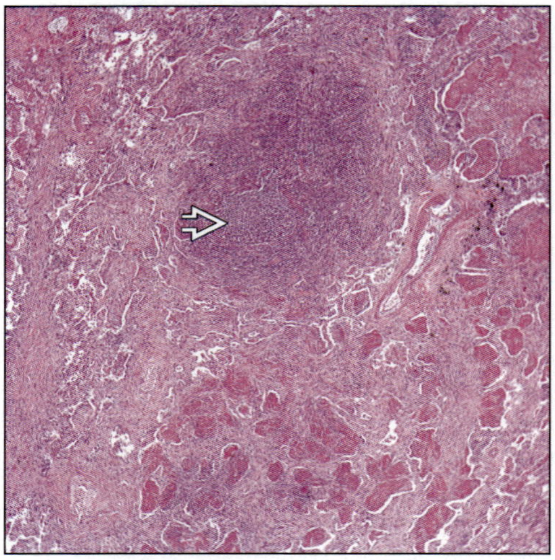

Low-power view shows suppurative pneumonia with abscess formation ➡. The rest of the lung parenchyma shows acute fibrinous pneumonia.

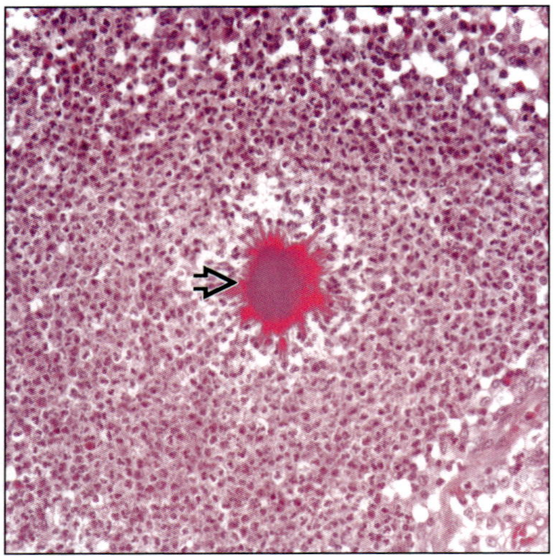

High-power view of the abscess shows the presence of acute inflammatory cells. Actinomycosis ➡ with the characteristic grains is present in the center.

TERMINOLOGY

Definitions

- Chronic suppurative infectious condition

ETIOLOGY/PATHOGENESIS

Infectious Agents

- *Actinomyces israelii*
  - Common saprophyte of the mouth and tonsils
- Other types isolated from infections include
  - *A. naeslundii*
  - *A. propionicus*
  - *A. eriksonii*

CLINICAL ISSUES

Epidemiology

- Incidence
  - Worldwide distribution
- Age
  - Affects any age group but may be more common in adults
- Gender
  - No gender predilection
- Ethnicity
  - No ethnic predilection

Site

- May involve
  - Cervicofacial area
  - Lungs
  - Abdomen

Presentation

- Fever
- Dyspnea
- Cough
- Chest pain
- Suppurative skin lesion in cervicofacial area

Laboratory Tests

- Tissue cultures
- Anaerobic cultures

Treatment

- Drugs
  - Broad-spectrum antibiotics

Prognosis

- Good if treated early
- May be difficult to control in immunocompromised patients

MICROSCOPIC PATHOLOGY

Histologic Features

- Suppurative pneumonia
- Abscess formation
- Presence of "sulfur" granules in the abscess
  - Deep purple granules
  - Round to oval granules
  - 100-300 μm in diameter
- Identification of Gram-positive filamentous organisms

DIFFERENTIAL DIAGNOSIS

Nocardiosis

- Absence of "sulfur" granules
- Tissue cultures would reveal the correct organism

Candida Infection

- Absence of granules
- In unusual circumstances, *Candida* may be weakly positive for Gram stain
- Tissue cultures would reveal the correct organism

Aspergillosis Infection

- Absence of "sulfur" granules

ACTINOMYCOSIS

Key Facts

Etiology/Pathogenesis

- *Actinomyces israelii*
  - Common saprophyte of the mouth and tonsils
- Other types isolated from infections include
  - *A. naeslundii*
  - *A. propionicus*
  - *A. eriksonii*

Clinical Issues

- May involve the following areas
  - Cervicofacial area
  - Lungs
  - Abdomen

Microscopic Pathology

- Suppurative pneumonia
- Abscess formation
- Presence of "sulfur" granules in the abscess

Histochemical Stains

Stain	Result
Gram	Positive staining of the filamentous organism
GMS	Positive staining of the organism
PAS	Negative
Gridley	Negative
Ziehl-Neelsen	Negative
Mucicarmine	Negative

Tissue cultures are the best method to separate the organisms from other infectious agents.

- Unusual for *Aspergillus* to be positive for Gram stain
- Tissue cultures would reveal the correct organism

Histoplasmosis

- Unusual for *Histoplasma* to show acute suppurative pneumonia
- Negative for Gram stain
- Absence of "sulfur" granules
- More commonly shows a granulomatous reaction
- Tissue cultures would reveal the correct organism

DIAGNOSTIC CHECKLIST

Pathologic Interpretation Pearls

- Suppurative pneumonia
- Abscess formation
- Presence of "sulfur" granules
- Filamentous bacteria

SELECTED REFERENCES

1. Song JU et al: Treatment of thoracic actinomycosis: A retrospective analysis of 40 patients. Ann Thorac Med. 5(2):80-5, 2010
2. Sullivan DC et al: Bacteria that masquerade as fungi: actinomycosis/nocardia. Proc Am Thorac Soc. 7(3):216-21, 2010
3. Bastian A et al: [Thoracic actinomycosis: diagnostic pitfalls and therapeutic considerations.] Pneumologie. 63(2):86-92, 2009

IMAGE GALLERY

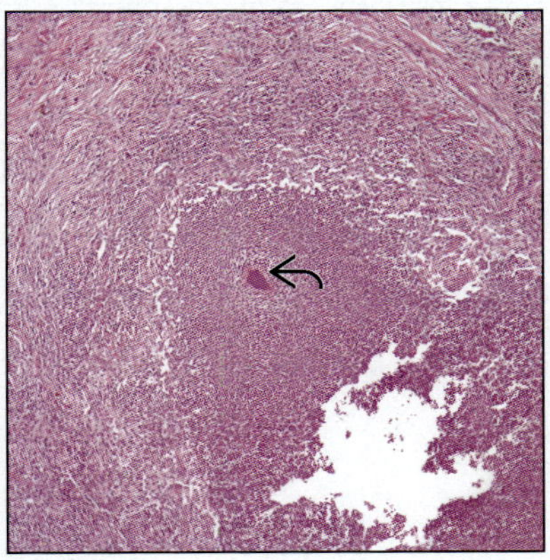

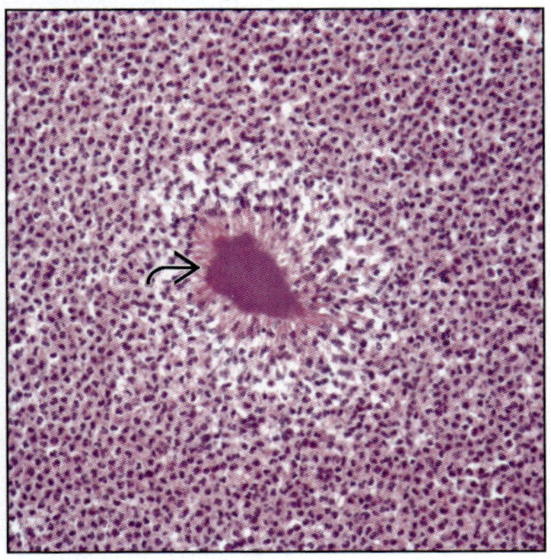

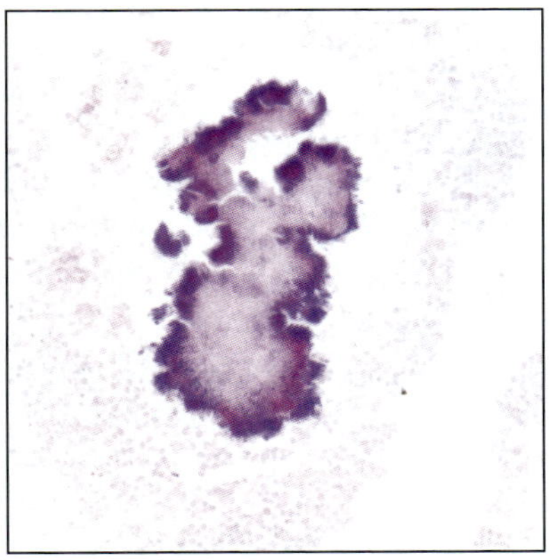

(Left) *Low-power view of an acute suppurative pneumonia shows the presence of an abscess formation. The presence of actinomycosis ⇨ can still be observed toward the periphery.* ***(Center)*** *High-power view of actinomycosis ⇨ embedded in an abscess shows the presence of the purple color of the organism and the characteristic granular appearance.* ***(Right)*** *Actinomycosis in a Gram stain shows a purple color. It is possible to observe the presence of filamentous organisms.*

ASPERGILLOSIS

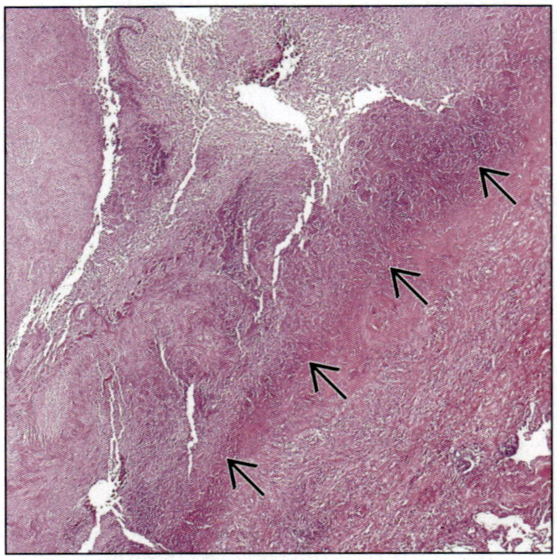

Fungus ball in pulmonary aspergilloma shows a cavity containing abundant necrotic material ⇒ admixed with numerous layers of hyphal forms of aspergillus.

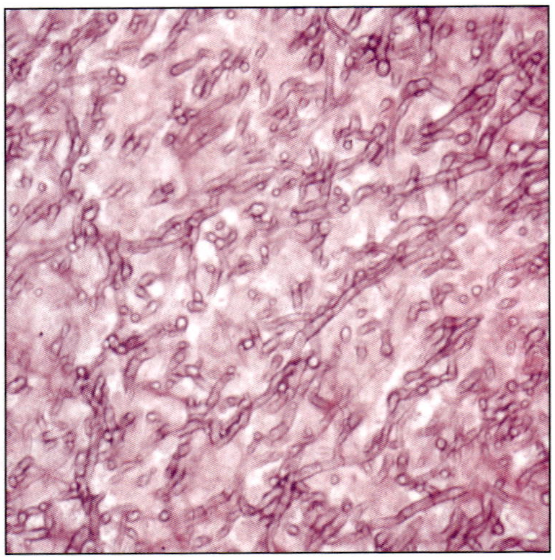

Higher magnification from the necrotic center of a fungus ball (aspergilloma) shows numerous slender and septate hyphae that branch at acute angles.

TERMINOLOGY

Definitions

- Infection caused by fungus of the species *Aspergillus*

ETIOLOGY/PATHOGENESIS

Infectious Agents

- Most common species that cause infection are *A. fumigatus*, *A. flavus*, and *A. niger*

CLINICAL ISSUES

Presentation

- Several clinical forms of aspergillosis
  - Colonizing (saprophytic) form in which preexisting cavities are secondarily colonized by the organisms, which form a fungus ball
  - Allergic bronchopulmonary aspergillosis seen in patients with asthma or cystic fibrosis
  - Acute invasive aspergillosis tends to occur preferentially in immunocompromised patients
  - Chronic necrotizing aspergillosis seen in patients with chronic underlying lung disease such as COPD or collagen vascular disorders
- Fungus balls may be asymptomatic and discovered incidentally or can present with massive, life-threatening hemoptysis
- Immunosuppressed patients with acute invasive aspergillosis present with cough, fever, and pleuritic pain; simulates bacterial bronchopneumonia

Laboratory Tests

- Serum precipitins against *Aspergillus* can be found in > 95% of patients with fungus balls
- Sputum cultures can help identify the organisms in patients with fungus balls but may not be helpful in invasive aspergillosis

Treatment

- Drugs
  - Amphotericin B is the drug of choice for acute invasive aspergillosis and chronic necrotizing aspergillosis

IMAGE FINDINGS

Radiographic Findings

- Aspergilloma (fungus ball) shows a soft tissue nodule within a preexistent pulmonary cavity or bronchiectatic airway
  - Fungus ball is usually outlined by a crescent of air along its nondependent surface ("air crescent" sign)
- Invasive aspergillosis shows multifocal opacities with ill-defined borders that may progress to large foci of consolidation

CT Findings

- Invasive aspergillosis shows focal or multifocal nodular opacities surrounded by ground-glass attenuation ("halo" sign)

MACROSCOPIC FEATURES

General Features

- Fungus balls appear as friable greenish to brown soft material lying within a distended cavity
- Necrotizing tracheobronchitis is characterized by the formation of a shaggy pseudomembrane growing along mucosa of the trachea
- Acute invasive aspergillosis is characterized by a target lesion corresponding to an area of infarction surrounded by a hemorrhagic rim

ASPERGILLOSIS

Key Facts

Terminology
- Infection caused by fungus of the species *Aspergillus*

Clinical Issues
- Fungus balls may be asymptomatic and discovered incidentally or can present with massive, life-threatening hemoptysis
- Immunosuppressed patients with acute invasive aspergillosis present with cough, fever, and pleuritic pain; infection simulates bacterial bronchopneumonia

Microscopic Pathology
- Acute invasive aspergillosis shows foci of necrotic and hemorrhagic parenchyma associated with occlusion of vessel lumens by fungal hyphae
- Wedge-shaped infarcts can also occur when large arteries are occluded by fungus
- Chronic necrotizing aspergillosis shows large areas of parenchymal consolidation by necrotizing granulomas containing fungal hyphae
- Bronchocentric granulomatosis pattern characterized by necrotizing granulomas surrounding bronchiolar walls
- Conidial or fruiting heads occur in lesions exposed to air and consist of a vesicle with sterigmata surrounded by chains of conidia
- Organisms consist of septate hyphae 3-6 µm in width that branch at acute angles (45°)

Ancillary Tests
- Organisms can be seen on H&E stains but are best highlighted with PAS and GMS stains

MICROSCOPIC PATHOLOGY

Histologic Features
- **Fungus ball (aspergilloma)**
  - Masses of mycelia that grow in layers within a cavity
- **Necrotizing pseudomembranous tracheobronchitis**
  - Pseudomembrane lining the mucosa contains a mixture of mucus, inflammatory cells, necrotic tissue, and fungal hyphae with conidial heads
- **Acute invasive aspergillosis**
  - Foci of necrotic, infarcted, and hemorrhagic parenchyma associated with occlusion of vessel lumens by fungal hyphae
  - Wedge-shaped infarcts can also occur when large arteries are occluded by fungus
  - Infarcts lead to progressive cavitation in which fungus balls later develop
- **Chronic necrotizing aspergillosis**
  - Large areas of parenchymal consolidation by necrotizing granulomas containing fungal hyphae
  - Bronchocentric granulomatosis pattern characterized by necrotizing granulomas surrounding bronchiolar walls

Cytologic Features
- Organisms consist of septate hyphae 3-6 µm in width that branch at acute angles (45°)
- Hyphae may undergo degenerative changes, such as swollen hyphal segments, that may make it difficult to distinguish them from other fungi
- Conidial or fruiting heads occur in lesions exposed to air and consist of a vesicle with sterigmata surrounded by chains of conidia
- In chronic granulomatous lesions, hyphae may be surrounded by proteinaceous debris with the Splendore-Hoeppli phenomenon
- Birefringent calcium oxalate crystals may be encountered admixed with the hyphal elements

ANCILLARY TESTS

Histochemistry
- Organisms can be seen on H&E stains but are best highlighted with PAS and GMS stains

DIFFERENTIAL DIAGNOSIS

Fusarium Infection
- *Fusarium* has wider hyphae (3-8 µm) that branch at 90° angles and show constrictions at branching points
- Some branches in *Fusarium* hyphae can show small ovoid conidia at their tips or located laterally on short conidiophores
- Morphologic overlap between *Fusarium* and *Aspergillus* can be significant; definitive diagnosis may require cultures or other methods

Pseudoallescheria boydii Infection
- *Pseudoallescheria* has slightly thinner hyphae (2-5 µm) than *Aspergillus* and a more haphazard branching pattern
- *P. boydii* may show vesicles and oval conidia measuring 5-10 µm that grow on short conidiophores
- Morphologic overlap with *Aspergillus* can be significant; definitive diagnosis requires culture, immunohistochemistry, or direct immunofluorescence

Zygomycetes Infection
- *Zygomycetes* have broad hyphae that range from 5-25 µm and appear twisted, folded, or swollen with an irregular branching pattern

SELECTED REFERENCES

1. Chai LY et al: Recent advances in invasive pulmonary aspergillosis. Curr Opin Pulm Med. 17(3):160-6, 2011
2. Ader F: Invasive pulmonary aspergillosis in patients with chronic obstructive pulmonary disease: an emerging fungal disease. Curr Infect Dis Rep. 12(6):409-16, 2010

ASPERGILLOSIS

Histologic Features

*(**Left**) Acute invasive pulmonary aspergillosis shows an occluded vessel ➔ surrounded by an extensive area of ischemic infarction due to plugging of the lumen with fungal organisms. (**Right**) Higher magnification from the center of the vessel shows branching septate hyphae ➪ admixed with necrotic debris and scattered red blood cells. The areas of infarction caused by the occlusion of vessels may eventually lead to cavitation followed by the development of fungus balls.*

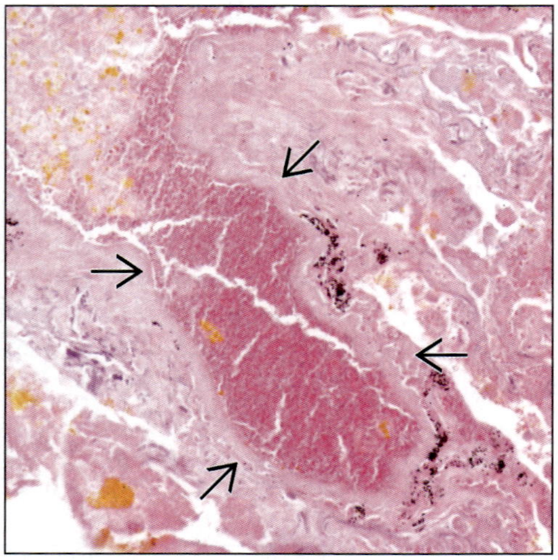

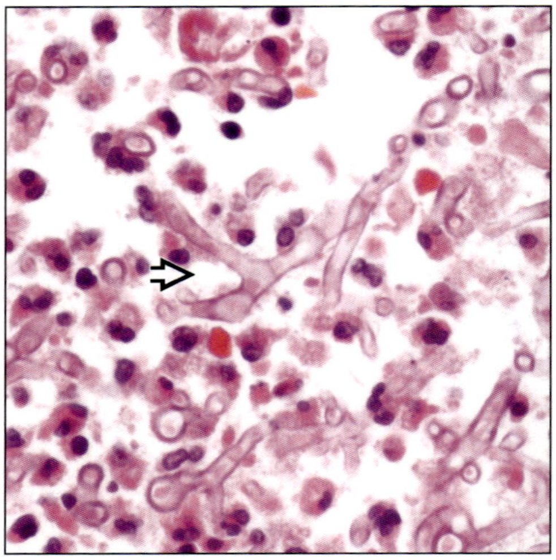

*(**Left**) Necrotizing palisaded granuloma ➔ circumscribing an area of necrosis is seen admixed with abundant hyphal organisms in chronic necrotizing pulmonary aspergillosis. The granulomas can sometimes involve the bronchiolar walls, resulting in a pattern of bronchocentric granulomatosis. (**Right**) Higher magnification from the edge of a necrotizing granuloma in chronic necrotizing aspergillosis shows abundant epithelioid histiocytes circumscribing a mass of tangled hyphal organisms ➔.*

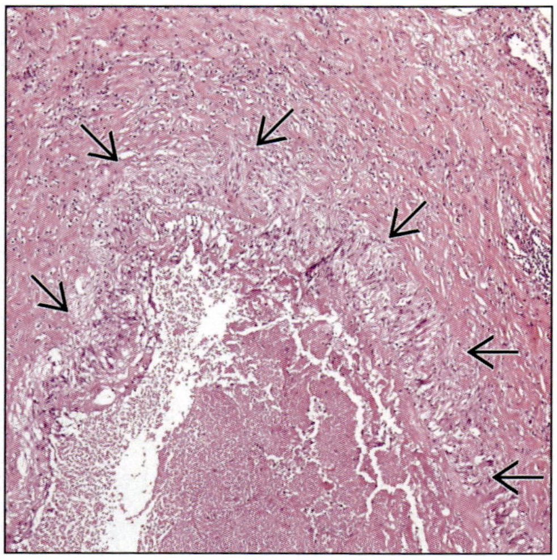

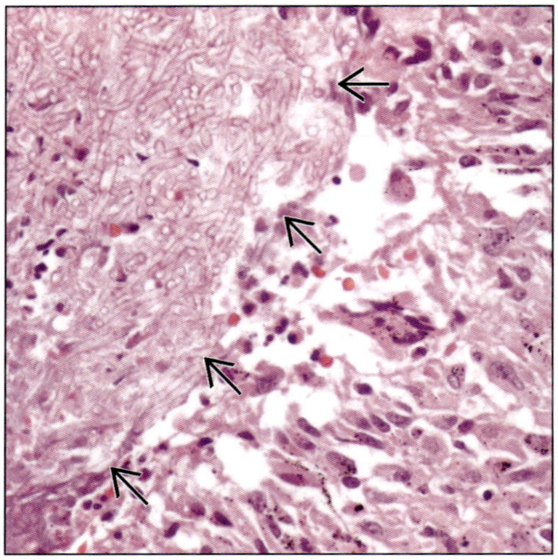

*(**Left**) A dilated bronchiole with extensive squamous metaplasia of the lining epithelium shows masses of hyphal forms plugging the lumen in a case of chronic necrotizing pulmonary aspergillosis. (**Right**) Higher magnification of the wall of a dilated bronchiole in a patient with chronic necrotizing pulmonary aspergillosis shows extensive squamous metaplasia of the lining bronchiolar epithelium. Notice the masses of hyphal organisms plugging the lumen ↷.*

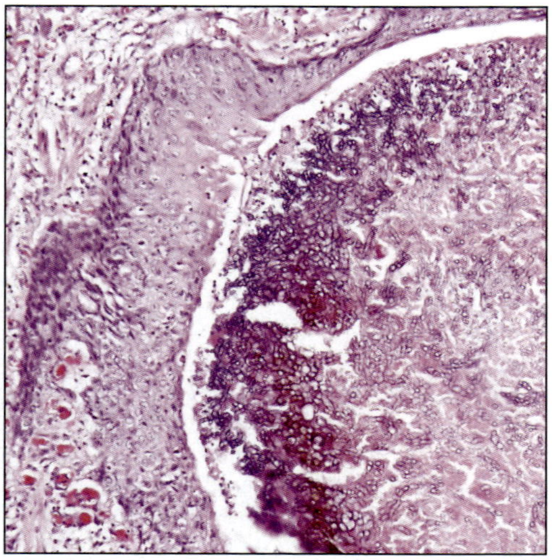

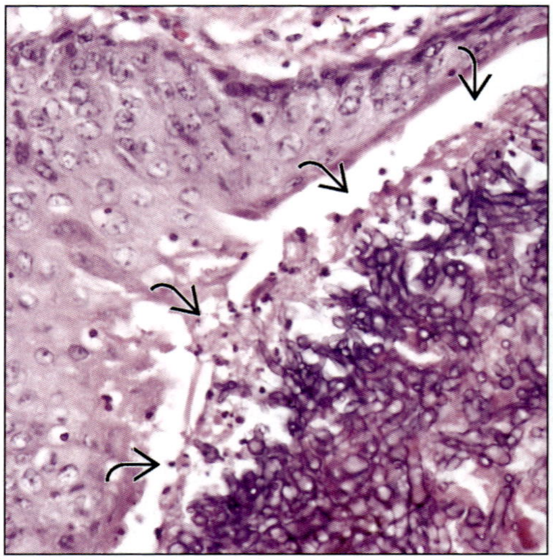

ASPERGILLOSIS

Organisms and Special Stains

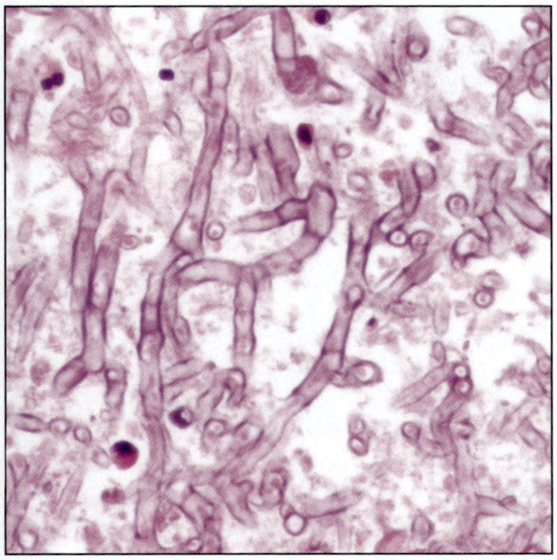

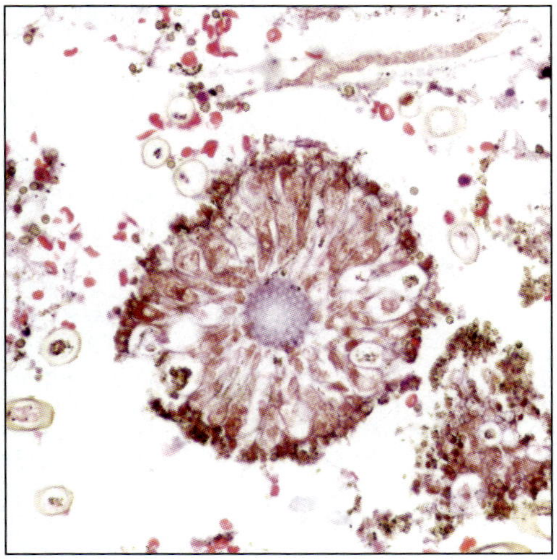

(Left) *Pulmonary aspergillosis shows clusters of hyphal organisms that are easy to identify on routine staining with hematoxylin and eosin (H&E). The organisms consist of septate hyphae that show branching in acute angles.* ***(Right)*** *A conidial head ("fruiting body") consists of a round vesicle with sterigmata that are surrounded by chains of conidia. Conidial heads are frequently encountered in cavitary lesions that are exposed to air.*

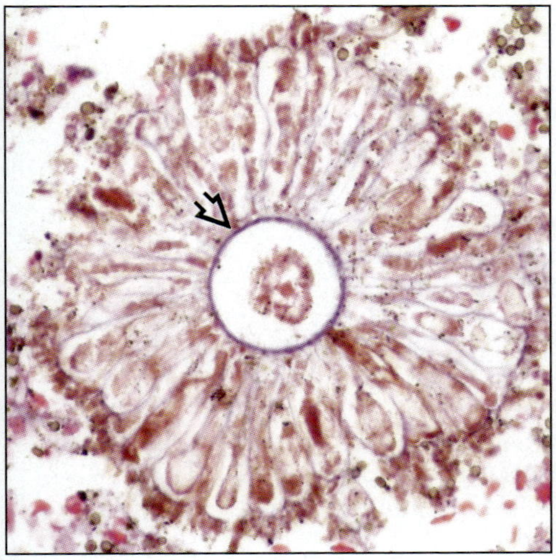

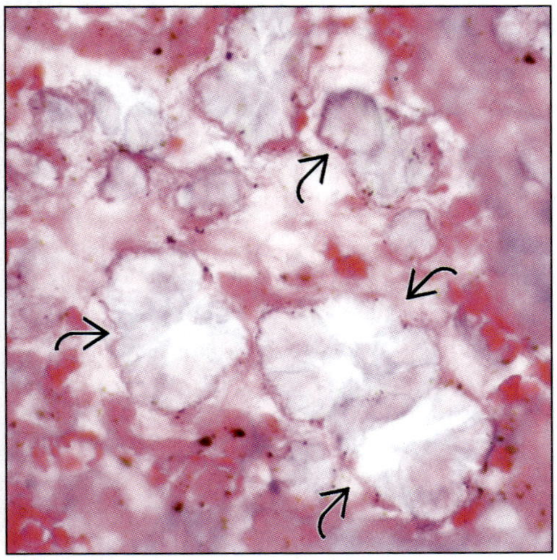

(Left) *A conidial head is seen in a case of an aspergilloma in a lung abscess from an elderly patient that shows a central vesicle ⇨ with radiating sterigmata and conidia. Notice the proteinaceous material admixed with necrotic debris surrounding the conidial head (so-called Splendore-Hoeppli phenomenon).* ***(Right)*** *Birefringent calcium oxalate crystals are seen ⮫ in the center of an aspergilloma. They can be best appreciated under polarized light.*

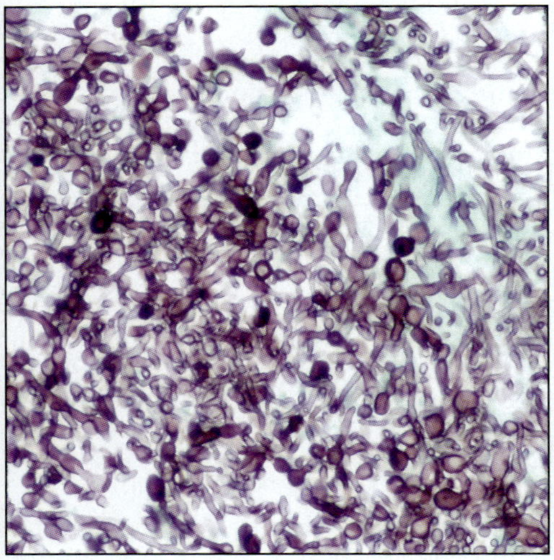

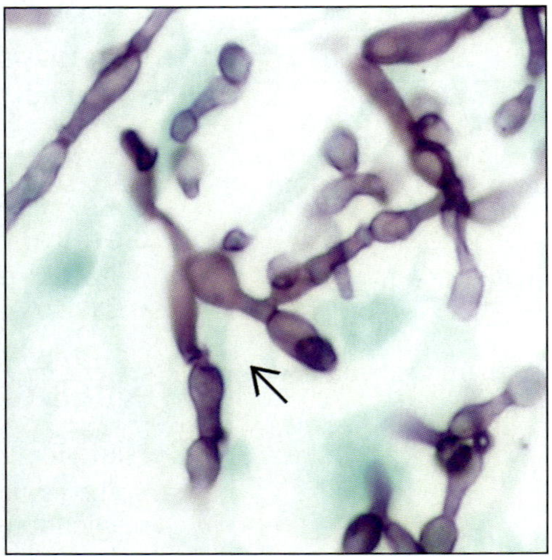

(Left) *The mass of hyphal structures in the center of an aspergilloma are strongly positive for Gomori methenamine silver (GMS) stain. The organisms can also be stained with the PAS stain.* ***(Right)*** *Higher magnification of Aspergillus stained with Gomori methenamine silver (GMS) shows septate hyphae branching at acute angles →. Sometimes degenerative changes such as swelling of hyphal segments can make it difficult to distinguish them from other fungi.*

BOTRYOMYCOSIS

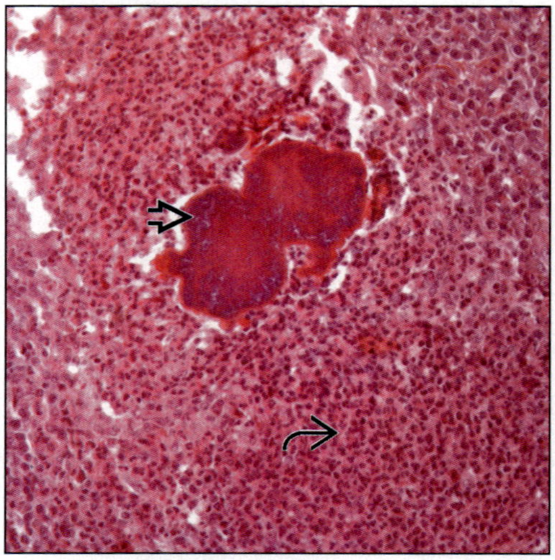

Pulmonary botryomycosis shows abscess formation ➔, and in the center of the abscess there is an eosinophilic clump of bacterial organisms ➔.

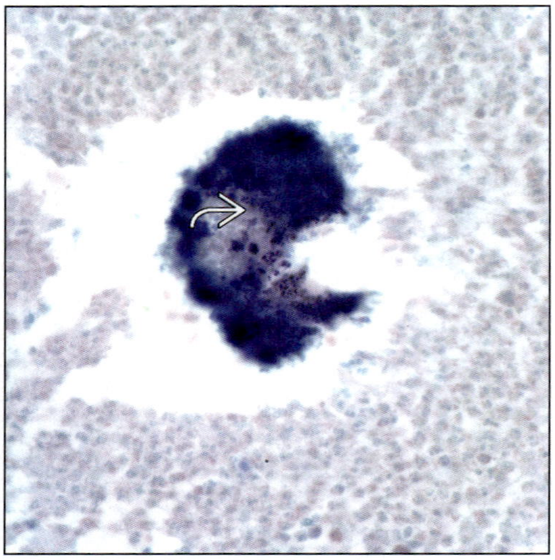

Higher magnification shows the presence of the characteristic grains ➔, a feature of botryomycosis.

TERMINOLOGY

Definitions

- Chronic, purulent, granulomatous bacterial infection

ETIOLOGY/PATHOGENESIS

Infectious Agents

- Can be caused by different bacterial organisms
  - *Staphylococcus aureus*
  - *Pseudomonas aeruginosa*
  - *Escherichia coli*
  - *Proteus vulgaris*

Pathogenesis

- Not well understood; possibilities include
  - Decreased T and B lymphocyte function
  - Unusual tissue response
  - Foreign body

CLINICAL ISSUES

Epidemiology

- Age
  - Can affect any age group from small children to elderly individuals
- Gender
  - May be more common in males than females

Site

- Ordinarily more common in skin and subcutaneous tissue
- Can involve different anatomic areas
  - Lung
  - Upper respiratory tract
  - Liver
  - Kidney
  - Brain
  - Lymph node

Presentation

- Ulcers
- Draining sinuses
- Fever
- Chest pain
- Hemoptysis

Natural History

- More common in patients with
  - Immunodeficiency
  - Diabetes
  - Alcoholism
  - Poor hygiene

Treatment

- Surgical approaches
  - Surgical excision of affected tissue
- Drugs
  - Antibiotics
- Best results may be obtained with combination of surgical resection and long-term antibiotic therapy

Prognosis

- Depends on setting in which infection occurs

IMAGE FINDINGS

General Features

- Discrete pulmonary mass
- Cavitary pulmonary lesion

MICROSCOPIC PATHOLOGY

Histologic Features

- Abscess formation
- Splendore-Hoeppli phenomenon
- Purulent inflammatory reaction
- Granules within abscess
- Nonfilamentous bacteria

BOTRYOMYCOSIS

Key Facts

Terminology
- Chronic, purulent, granulomatous bacterial infection

Etiology/Pathogenesis
- Can be caused by different bacterial organisms

Clinical Issues
- Symptoms
  - Ulcers
  - Draining sinuses
  - Fever
  - Chest pain
  - Hemoptysis
- More common in patients with
  - Immunodeficiency
  - Diabetes
  - Alcoholism
  - Poor hygiene

Histochemical Stains Commonly Used in the Diagnosis of Botryomycosis

Histochemical Stain	Result
Giemsa	Shows presence of granules and enhances Splendore-Hoeppli phenomenon
Brown-Hopps	Shows presence of granules
Luxol fast	Enhances Splendore-Hoeppli phenomenon
Ziehl-Neelsen	Enhances Splendore-Hoeppli phenomenon; negative for acid-fast bacilli or filamentous bacteria
GMS	Negative for fungal organisms
PAS	Enhances Splendore-Hoeppli phenomenon, but negative for fungal organisms
Gridley	Negative for fungal organisms
Tissue cultures	Most important study to isolate the specific type of organism

DIFFERENTIAL DIAGNOSIS

Actinomycosis
- True fungi shown on silver stains
- May show granules
- May show Splendore-Hoeppli phenomenon

Nocardiosis
- Granules and nonfilamentous bacteria will be unusual in *Nocardia* infections
- Fite stains will show presence of filamentous bacteria

SELECTED REFERENCES

1. Vera-Alvarez J et al: Primary pulmonary botryomycosis diagnosed by fine needle aspiration cytology: a case report. Acta Cytol. 50(3):331-4, 2006
2. Hodgson R et al: Pulmonary botryomycosis: a difficult diagnosis in the preoperative patient. J Thorac Cardiovasc Surg. 130(3):924-5, 2005
3. Kathir K et al: Primary pulmonary botryomycosis: an important differential diagnosis for lung cancer. Respirology. 6(4):347-50, 2001
4. Tuggey JM et al: Primary pulmonary botryomycosis: a late complication of foreign body aspiration. Thorax. 55(12):1068-9, 2000
5. Neafie RC et al: Unusual infections in humans. Clin Microbiol Rev. 6(1):34-56, 1993
6. Paz HL et al: Primary pulmonary botryomycosis. A manifestation of chronic granulomatous disease. Chest. 101(4):1160-2, 1992
7. Brunken RC et al: Immunologic abnormalities in botryomycosis. A case report with review of the literature. J Am Acad Dermatol. 9(3):428-34, 1983
8. Speir WA Jr et al: Primary pulmonary botryomycosis. Chest. 60(1):92-3, 1971

IMAGE GALLERY

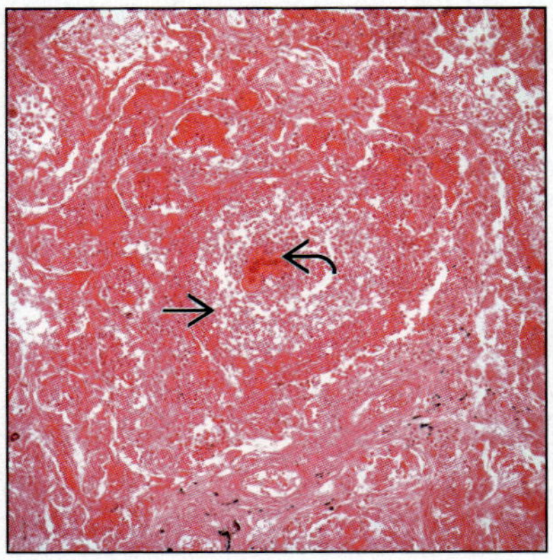
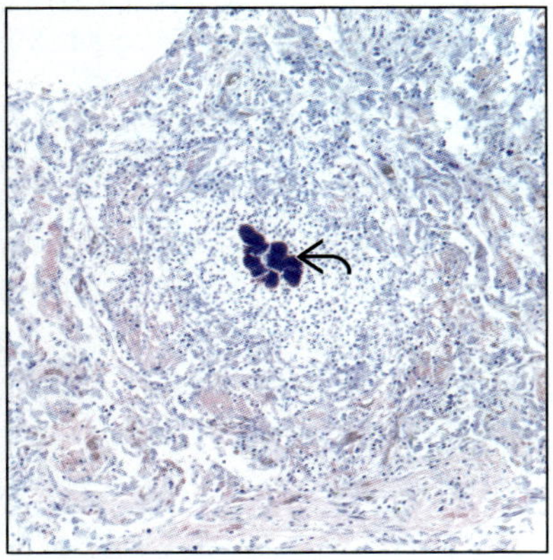
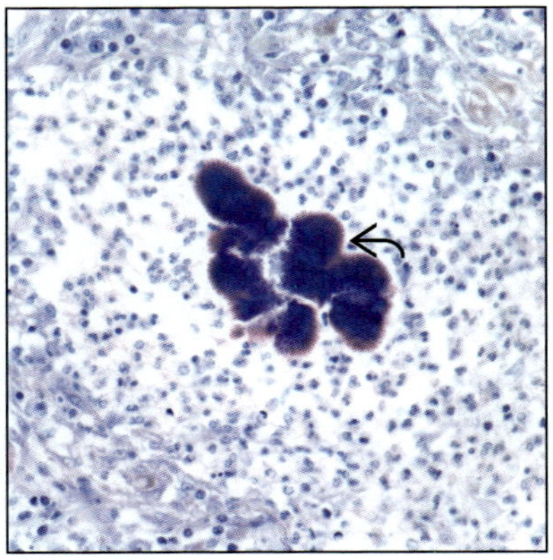

(Left) *Pulmonary botryomycosis shows abscess formation ⇒ filling the alveolar space. At the center, there is bacterial infection ⇒, typical of botryomycosis.* ***(Center)*** *Low-power view highlights the organisms ⇒. The use of special stains in many cases is useful to highlight the presence of grains.* ***(Right)*** *Higher magnification shows botryomycosis ⇒ embedded in an abscess formation.*

MALAKOPLAKIA

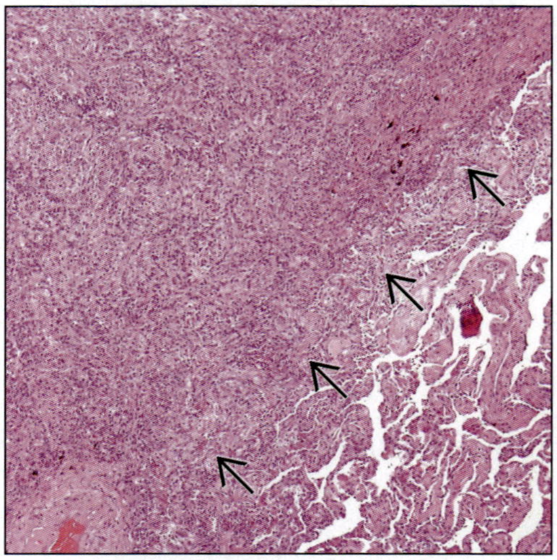

Histologic appearance of pulmonary malakoplakia due to Rhodococcus equi infection shows normal pulmonary parenchyma flanked by an area of consolidation ➔ that contains a dense histiocytic reaction.

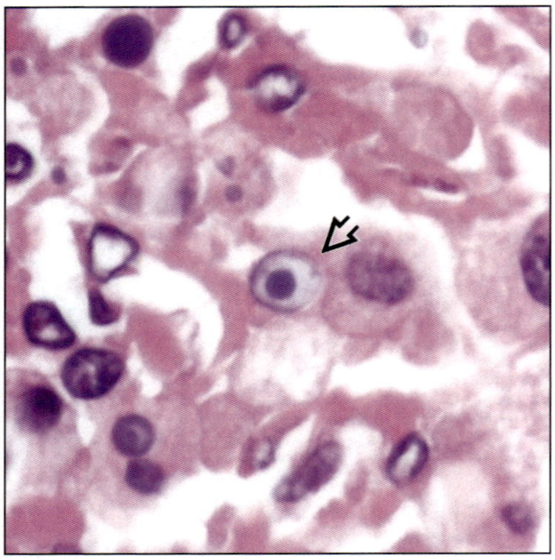

Higher magnification of lung infection by malakoplakia shows sheets of histiocytes with occasional small, concentric, and targetoid calcific bodies with a central core ➪ (Michaelis-Gutmann bodies).

TERMINOLOGY

Definitions

- Distinctive chronic inflammatory process characterized by histiocytic proliferation admixed with microcalcifications (Michaelis-Gutmann bodies)

ETIOLOGY/PATHOGENESIS

Infectious Agents

- Response to infection with *Rhodococcus equi*, *E. coli*, and *Acinetobacter*
- *R. equi* is aerobic, usually Gram-positive coccobacillus of worldwide distribution found in soil and feces of animals, especially horses
- Human infection is acquired through inhalation of contaminated soil

CLINICAL ISSUES

Epidemiology

- Incidence
  - Most cases reported are associated with *R. equi* infection in AIDS patients or immunocompromised hosts
- Age
  - Adults between 30-60 years of age

Presentation

- Cough
- Fever
- Dyspnea
- Chest pain

IMAGE FINDINGS

Radiographic Findings

- Dense single focus of parenchymal consolidation
- Predilection for upper lobes of lung
- Cavitation with thick walls simulating post-primary tuberculosis
- Bilateral and multifocal pulmonary involvement may also occur

CT Findings

- Large cavitary mass with thick fibrous capsule in upper lobes

MACROSCOPIC FEATURES

General Features

- Lesions are more often solitary, although multifocal and bilateral lesions can sometimes be encountered
- Cut section shows well-circumscribed yellow-cream area of consolidation that can simulate a neoplasm
- Lesions can show cavitation lined by thick capsule and forming abscess

MICROSCOPIC PATHOLOGY

Histologic Features

- Sheets of histiocytes admixed with inflammatory cells, particularly plasma cells
- Abscess formation with abundant fibrinopurulent exudate
- Organizing pneumonia may be present at periphery of lesion with hyperplasia of type II pneumocytes
- Histiocytic infiltrate may adopt slightly spindled appearance reminiscent of inflammatory pseudotumor, plasma cell type

Cytologic Features

- Histiocytes have large round to oval nuclei with vesicular chromatin and abundant eosinophilic cytoplasm

Key Facts

Clinical Issues

- Most cases reported are associated with *R. equi* infection in AIDS patients or immunocompromised hosts
- Presentation
  - Cough, fever, dyspnea

Microscopic Pathology

- Sheets of histiocytes admixed with inflammatory cells, particularly plasma cells
- Abscess formation with abundant fibrinopurulent exudate
- Histiocytes have large round to oval nuclei with vesicular chromatin and abundant eosinophilic cytoplasm
- Scattered small calcific structures (Michaelis-Gutmann bodies) can be seen within histiocytes or in interstitium
  - Round to oval structures with concentric targetoid appearance
  - Small round to oval structures with glassy homogeneous appearance

Ancillary Tests

- Michaelis-Gutmann bodies can be readily identified with alizarin red or von Kossa calcium stains
- In case of *R. equi* infection, organisms can be stained with tissue Gram stains (Brown and Brenn stain; Brown and Hopps stain)
- Michaelis-Gutmann bodies consist of large phagolysosomes that contain fragments of bacterial organisms on electron microscopy

- Scattered small calcific structures (Michaelis-Gutmann bodies) can be seen within histiocytes or in interstitium
  - Michaelis-Gutmann bodies consist of concentric, laminated foci of calcifications, 2-10 μm in diameter
    - Round to oval structures with targetoid appearance, showing dark peripheral rim surrounding clear halo and containing dark central zone
    - Small gray-blue round or oval structures with glassy homogeneous appearance

ANCILLARY TESTS

Histochemistry

- Michaelis-Gutmann bodies can be readily identified with alizarin red or von Kossa calcium stains
- Michaelis-Gutmann bodies can also be stained with PAS (pink-red), GMS (dark brown), Giemsa (dark blue), and iron (dark blue) stains
- In case of *R. equi* infection, organisms can be stained with tissue Gram stains (Brown and Brenn stain; Brown and Hopps stain)
  - Organisms appear as small Gram-positive bacilli that may be pleomorphic in shape
- Organisms are also weakly acid-fast positive and can be seen on modified Fite-Faraco stain but do not stain with Ziehl-Neelsen stain

Electron Microscopy

- Transmission
  - Michaelis-Gutmann bodies consist of large phagolysosomes that contain fragments of bacterial organisms

DIFFERENTIAL DIAGNOSIS

Mycobacterial Pneumonia

- *Mycobacterium avium intracellulare* (MAI) infection can present with sheets of foamy histiocytes admixed with inflammatory infiltrates
  - MAI infection shows abundant foamy cytoplasm in macrophages rather than dense eosinophilic cytoplasm of malakoplakia
  - Organisms in MAI are strongly positive with AFB and modified AFB (Fite-Faraco) stains
  - MAI infection lacks Michaelis-Gutmann bodies

Lipid Storage Disorders

- Gaucher disease or Niemann-Pick disease can show prominent histiocytic infiltrates in lung parenchyma, similar to malakoplakia
  - Infiltrates in storage diseases are usually diffuse rather than localized and form discrete mass as in malakoplakia
  - PAS stains will highlight intracytoplasmic inclusions (Michaelis-Gutmann bodies) in malakoplakia but not in storage disease
  - Histiocytes in Gaucher disease show characteristic "wrinkled-paper" appearance
  - Clinical history and specialized testing are necessary for specific diagnosis of storage disease

Rosai-Dorfman Disease

- Will also form discrete localized tumor masses composed of sheets of histiocytes admixed with plasma cells
  - Histiocytes may show enlarged atypical nuclei with emperipolesis
  - Prominent cuffing of vessel walls by sheets of plasma cells
  - Not associated with Michaelis-Gutmann bodies
  - Histiocytes stain strongly positive for S100 protein
    - Histiocytes in malakoplakia are uniformly negative for S100 protein

SELECTED REFERENCES

1. Guerrero MF et al: Pulmonary malacoplakia associated with Rhodococcus equi infection in patients with AIDS: case report and review. Clin Infect Dis. 28(6):1334-6, 1999

MALAKOPLAKIA

Histologic Features

*(**Left**) Scanning magnification of a focus of pulmonary malakoplakia shows a well-circumscribed area composed of sheets of large histiocytic cells → separated from the normal lung parenchyma by a fibrotic band of connective tissue. (**Right**) Higher magnification of pulmonary malakoplakia shows sheets of histiocytes with abundant eosinophilic cytoplasm. Notice a few scattered Michaelis-Gutmann bodies ↷ in the background; they can sometimes be hard to find without the aid of special stains.*

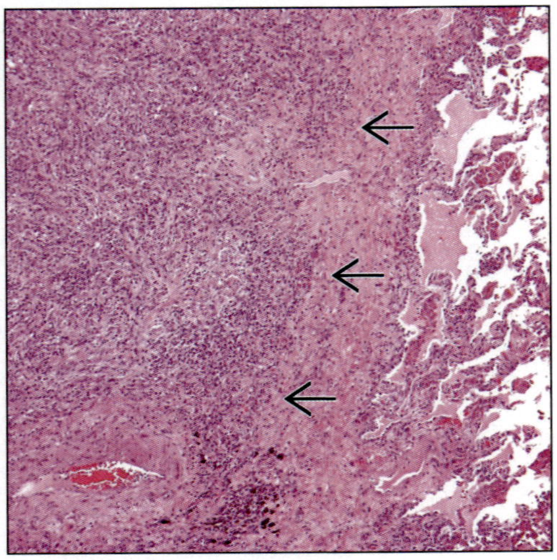
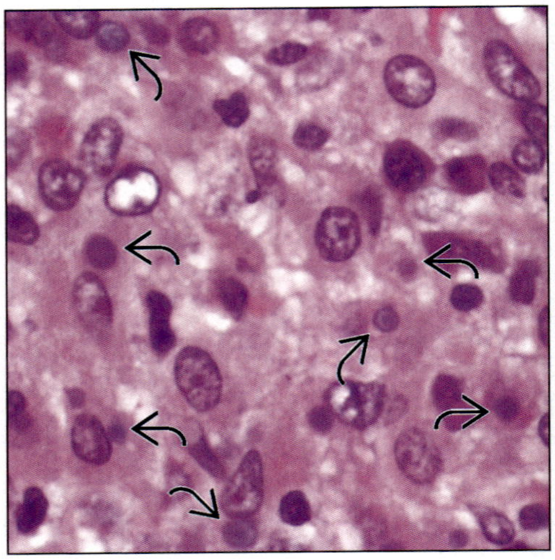

*(**Left**) Heavy plasma cell infiltrates ↷ can often be seen in pulmonary malakoplakia. Such cases can be confused for extranodal Rosai-Dorfman disease involving the lung. Absence of reactivity of the surrounding histiocytes for S100 protein will help rule out that diagnostic possibility. (**Right**) Periphery of the lesion in a case of pulmonary malakoplakia shows organizing pneumonia with hyperplasia of type II pneumocytes and intraalveolar fibrin plugs with fibroblastic proliferation.*

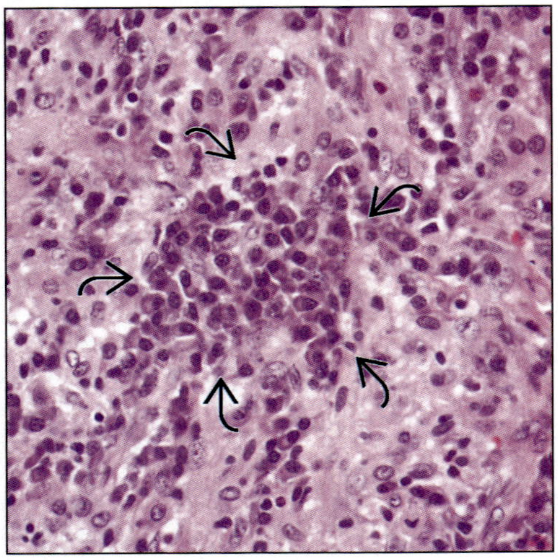
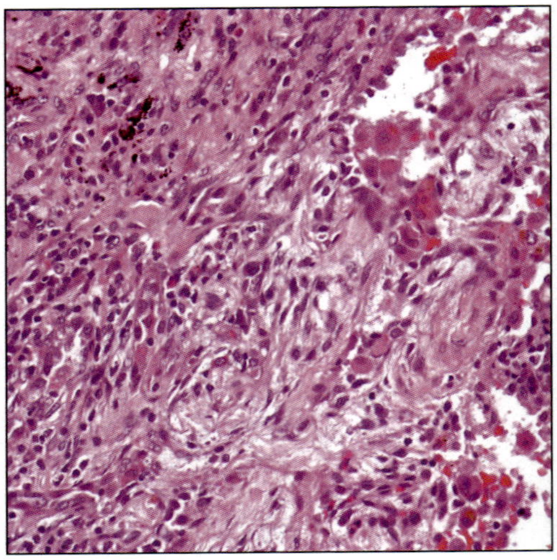

*(**Left**) Spindling of the histiocytes showing a vague storiform pattern is seen in this example of pulmonary malakoplakia. Cases such as this can be confused for inflammatory pseudotumor of the plasma cell type. Careful attention and identification of Michaelis-Gutmann bodies is indispensable for correct diagnosis. (**Right**) Higher magnification of pulmonary malakoplakia shows scattered histiocytes with oval to spindle-shaped nuclei admixed with abundant mature plasma cells.*

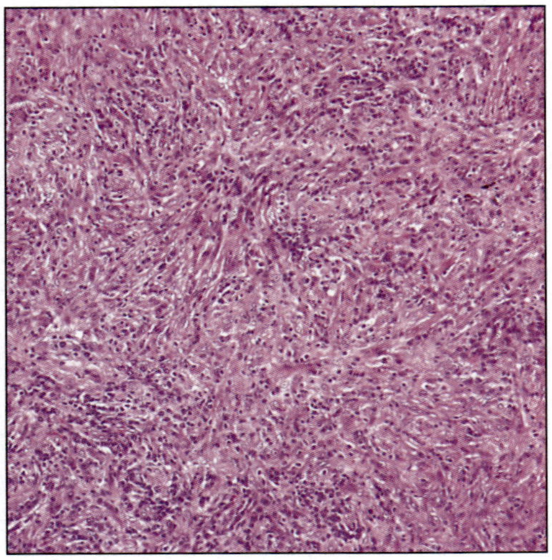
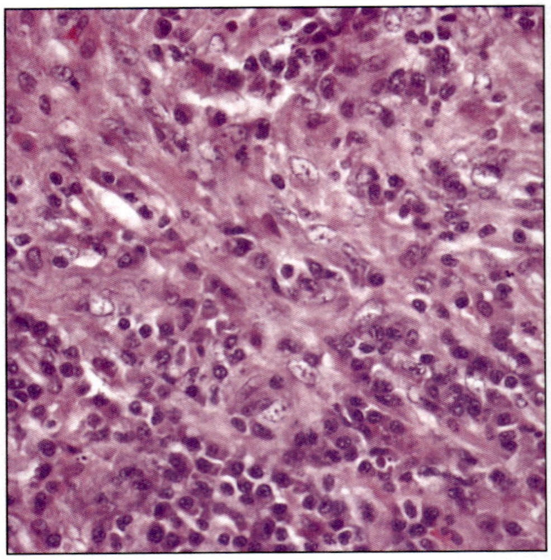

Cytology and Special Stains

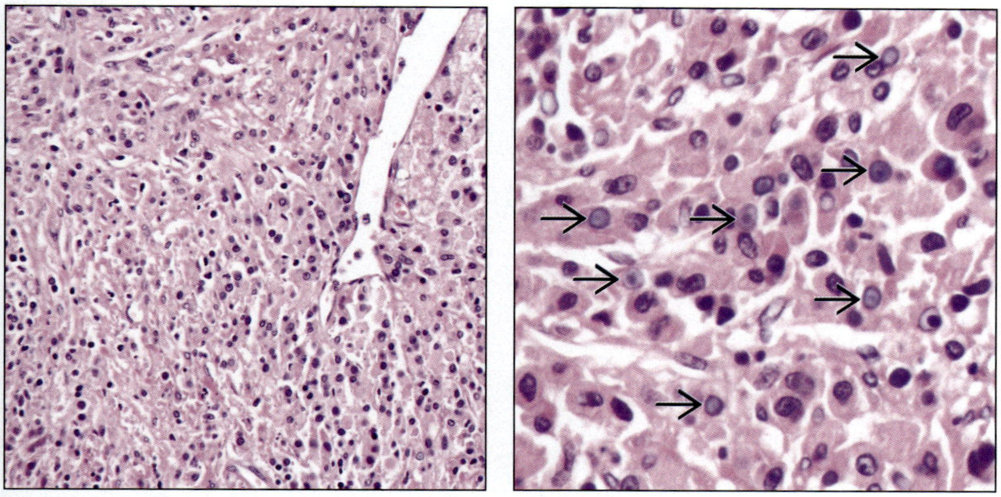

(Left) *Typical appearance of histiocytic reaction in pulmonary malakoplakia shows sheets of histiocytes admixed with other chronic inflammatory cells. The process resembles a xanthogranulomatous inflammation, inflammatory pseudotumor, or Rosai-Dorfman disease.* ***(Right)*** *Higher magnification of pulmonary malakoplakia shows sheets of histiocytic cells admixed with other inflammatory cell elements. There are multiple small round gray-blue structures scattered throughout* ➔.

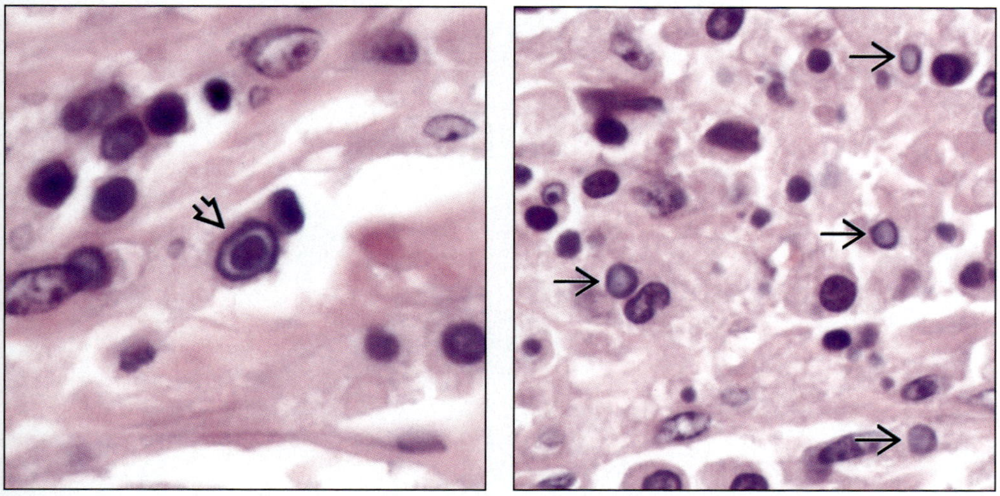

(Left) *Characteristic histologic appearance of a Michaelis-Gutmann body* ⇨ *shows target-shaped structure composed of concentric laminations containing a dark central core surrounded by a halo. Such bodies may be found within macrophages or lying free in the interstitium.* ***(Right)*** *Michaelis-Gutmann bodies are not always laminated or with target-like appearance but may be homogeneous with a light glassy center* ➔. *They may be quite difficult to find, requiring special stains.*

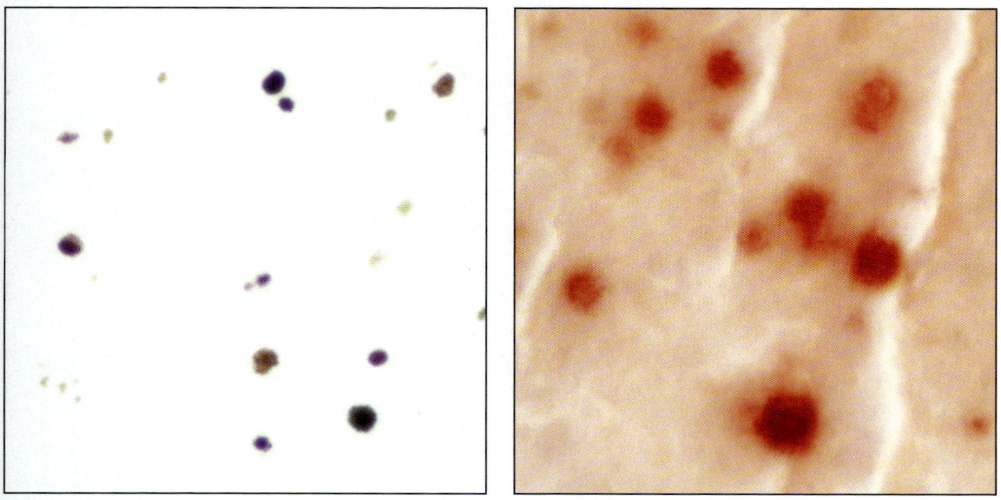

(Left) *Michaelis-Gutmann bodies can be readily identified with the use of histochemical stains. One of the most useful stains is the von Kossa calcium stain, which stains the small, dot-like structures dark brown or black.* ***(Right)*** *Another useful stain for identifying Michaelis-Gutmann bodies in pulmonary malakoplakia is alizarin red, which stains these structures bright red-orange. Other stains that may be used include PAS, GMS, and Giemsa.*

Neoplasms, Benign

MESOTHELIAL HYPERPLASIA

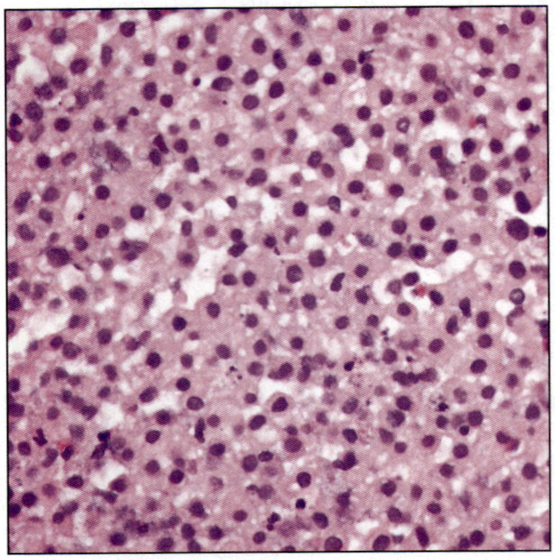

Mesothelial hyperplasia shows sheets of monotonous mesothelial cells with mild cytologic atypia and abundant pale eosinophilic cytoplasm. The cells are quite monotonous.

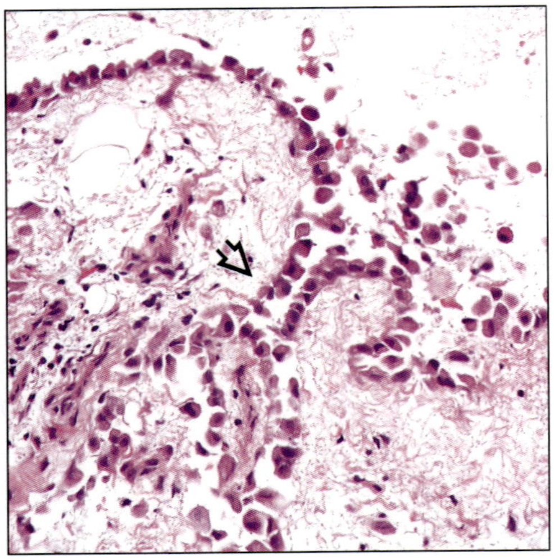

Pleural biopsy specimen shows benign mesothelial hyperplasia. Notice the single layer of epithelioid cells with mild cytologic atypia tracking into an invagination of the pleura ➯.

TERMINOLOGY

Abbreviations

- Mesothelial hyperplasia (MH)

Definitions

- Proliferation of benign reactive mesothelial cells lining pleural surface

ETIOLOGY/PATHOGENESIS

Pathogenesis

- Reaction to injury, such as recurrent effusions, inflammation, or neoplasia
- As a result of surgical procedures, such as in cardiac MICE (monocytic incidental cardiac excrescences)

CLINICAL ISSUES

Presentation

- Asymptomatic
- Incidental finding in pleural biopsies done for other causes
- Finding in pleural fluid cytology for assessment of pleural effusion
- May arise in pericardium forming small excrescences (cardiac MICE)

Prognosis

- Benign
- Usually regresses spontaneously when stimulus is removed

MICROSCOPIC PATHOLOGY

Histologic Features

- Focal thickening of pleural surface by sheets of mesothelial cells
- Formation of small papillary excrescences that project into free pleural space
- May harbor psammoma bodies
- Process is confined to surface of pleura and does not invade underlying structures
- When in pericardium (cardiac MICE), lesions are composed of reactive mesothelial cells admixed with epithelioid histiocytes

Cytologic Features

- Variable nuclear enlargement with mild increase in chromatin pattern
- Nucleolar prominence
- Variable mitotic activity
- Process may vary in cytological composition
  - Simple mesothelial hyperplasia composed of bland-appearing cuboidal mesothelial cells
  - Atypical mesothelial hyperplasia composed of atypical mesothelial cells with complex architecture
  - May be admixed with histiocytes, such as in cardiac MICE

DIFFERENTIAL DIAGNOSIS

Malignant Mesothelioma, Early Stage

- Differs from hyperplasia by showing infiltration of underlying fat, muscle, or adjacent tissues
- Definite stromal invasion with fibroblastic response favors malignant mesothelioma
- Presence of tumor cell necrosis favors mesothelioma

Metastatic Papillary Carcinoma

- May resemble metastasis from papillary carcinoma of thyroid, lung, ovary, uterus, or breast
- Thorough clinical history is essential to rule out tumor at another location
- Multiple and bilateral lesions are more likely to be metastatic
- Symptomatic lesions are more likely to be metastatic

MESOTHELIAL HYPERPLASIA

Key Facts

Clinical Issues
- Incidental finding in pleural biopsy specimens done for other causes
- Finding in pleural fluid cytology for assessment of pleural effusion
- Usually regresses spontaneously when stimulus is removed

Microscopic Pathology
- Focal thickening of pleural surface by sheets of mesothelial cells
- Formation of small papillary excrescences that project into free pleural space
- Process is confined to surface of pleura and does not invade underlying structures
- Variable nuclear enlargement with mild increase in chromatin pattern
- Nucleolar prominence
- Variable mitotic activity

Diagnostic Checklist
- Small and focal process; generally seen as incidental finding
- Demonstration of absence of invasion is most important feature for distinguishing from early malignant mesothelioma
- Role of immunohistochemistry is very limited for separating mesothelial hyperplasia from malignant mesothelioma
- Reactive, hyperplastic mesothelial cells share the same markers with malignant mesothelioma
  - No molecular or cytogenetic markers are available for distinguishing between them

- Immunohistochemical stains may help in differential diagnosis
  - TTF-1 positivity favors carcinoma metastatic from lung or thyroid
  - ERP/PRP positivity favors uterine, ovarian, or breast carcinoma

Müllerian Rests and Proliferations
- Pleural endometriosis
  - Rare condition, usually in young women of child-bearing age
  - Well-formed glandular structures are predominantly seen in endometriosis
  - Cells lining glands are devoid of cytologic atypia or mitotic activity in endometriosis
  - Glandular structures are surrounded by dense spindle cell stroma in endometriosis
  - Presence of scattered hemosiderin-laden macrophages in stroma and glandular lumens in endometriosis

DIAGNOSTIC CHECKLIST

Clinically Relevant Pathologic Features
- Gross appearance
  - Usually constitutes microscopic finding
- Mitotic rate
  - Low, usually with no abnormal mitoses
- Nuclear features
  - Mild to moderate nuclear atypia
  - Moderate increase in chromatin pattern
  - Prominent nucleoli
- Cytoplasmic features
  - Abundant eosinophilic cytoplasm
- Tissue distribution
  - Focal, usually forms skip lesions
- Invasive pattern
  - Usually confined to surface of pleura
  - Invasion or infiltration of fat, muscle, or lung parenchyma signifies malignancy

Pathologic Interpretation Pearls
- Small and focal process; generally seen as incidental finding
- Demonstration of absence of invasion is most important feature for distinguishing from early malignant mesothelioma
- Role of immunohistochemistry is very limited for separating mesothelial hyperplasia from malignant mesothelioma
  - Reactive, hyperplastic mesothelial cells mostly share the same markers with malignant mesothelioma
  - Strong EMA/MUC1 positivity has been observed to be more common in malignant mesothelioma than in mesothelial hyperplasia
  - Strong desmin positivity has been observed more commonly in mesothelial hyperplasia than in malignant mesothelioma
  - Strong Ki-67 labeling (> 9%) favors malignant mesothelioma over mesothelial hyperplasia

SELECTED REFERENCES

1. Taheri ZM et al: The diagnostic value of Ki-67 and repp86 in distinguishing between benign and malignant mesothelial proliferations. Arch Pathol Lab Med. 132(4):694-7, 2008
2. Cagle PT et al: Differential diagnosis of benign and malignant mesothelial proliferations on pleural biopsies. Arch Pathol Lab Med. 129(11):1421-7, 2005
3. Attanoos RL et al: The use of immunohistochemistry in distinguishing reactive from neoplastic mesothelium. A novel use for desmin and comparative evaluation with epithelial membrane antigen, p53, platelet-derived growth factor-receptor, P-glycoprotein and Bcl-2. Histopathology. 43(3):231-8, 2003
4. Cury PM et al: The use of histological and immunohistochemical markers to distinguish pleural malignant mesothelioma and in situ mesothelioma from reactive mesothelial hyperplasia and reactive pleural fibrosis. J Pathol. 189(2):251-7, 1999
5. Henderson DW et al: Reactive mesothelial hyperplasia vs mesothelioma, including mesothelioma in situ: a brief review. Am J Clin Pathol. 110(3):397-404, 1998

MESOTHELIAL HYPERPLASIA

Microscopic Features

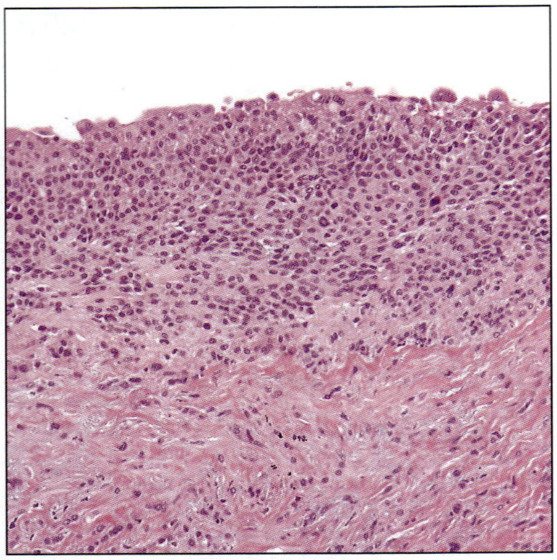
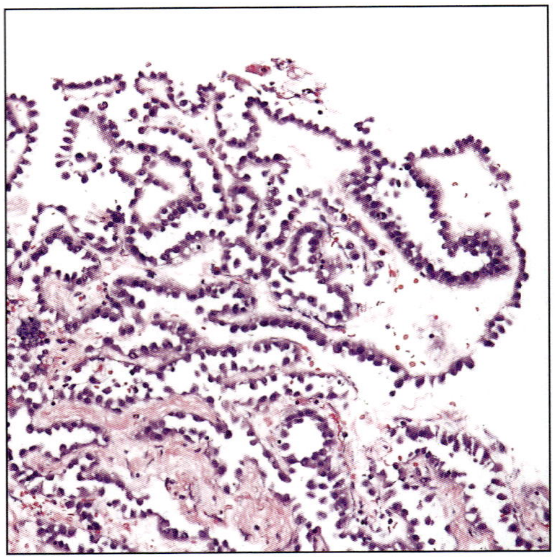

(Left) *Mesothelial hyperplasia, diffuse type, is seen with thickening of the pleural surface caused by sheets of epithelioid cells in a diffuse, solid pattern. Notice the sharp demarcation from the underlying pleural connective tissue.* ***(Right)*** *In mesothelial hyperplasia, papillary type, hyperplastic mesothelial cells are forming small papillary fronds lined by a single layer of cells.The process may be confused for malignant mesothelioma or a metastasis from papillary carcinoma.*

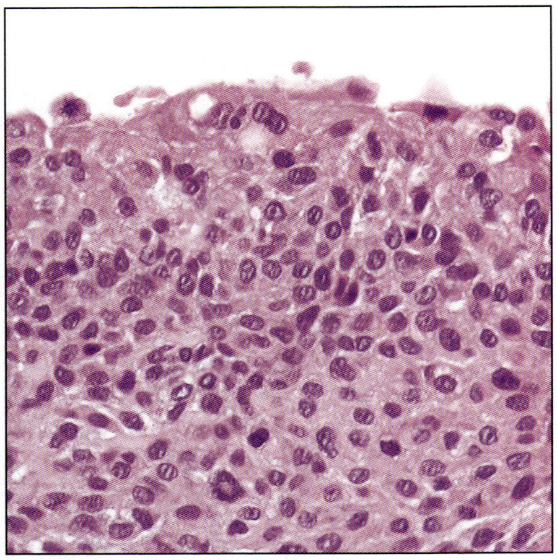
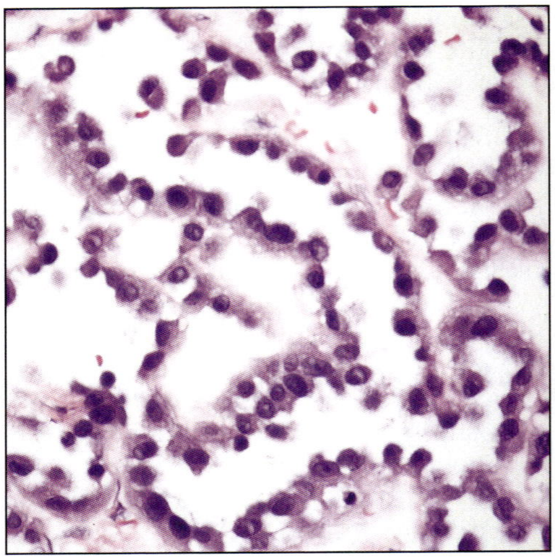

(Left) *In this mesothelial hyperplasia, diffuse type, high magnification shows solid mesothelial hyperplasia with sheets of round to polygonal cells with moderate atypia. No papillary structures are seen.* ***(Right)*** *In mesothelial hyperplasia, papillary type, high magnification of papillary fronds shows a single layer of hyperchromatic cells lining the papillae. The cells contain enlarged nuclei with a dense chromatin pattern and often display a "hobnail" configuration.*

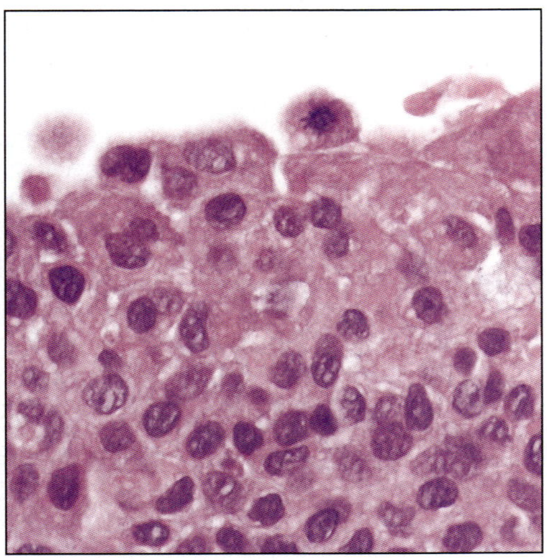
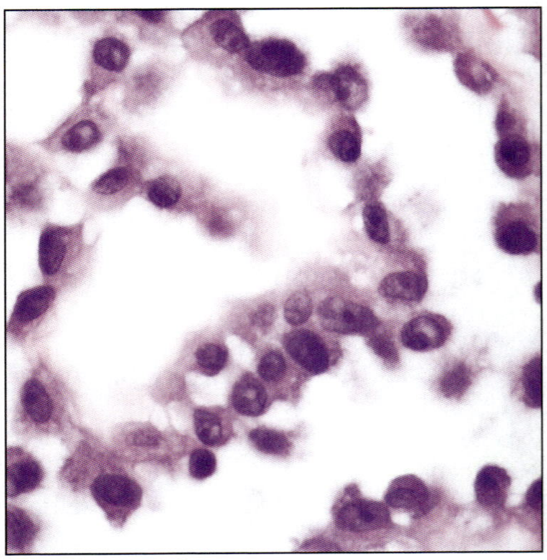

(Left) *Higher magnification of solid mesothelial hyperplasia shows cells with enlarged nuclei, prominent nucleoli, and a dense chromatin pattern in this mesothelial hyperplasia, diffuse type. Some of the cells contain a single small nucleolus.* ***(Right)*** *Higher magnification of papillary mesothelial hyperplasia shows cells with enlarged, atypical nuclei and small nucleoli in this mesothelial hyperplasia, papillary type. Some of the cells can show prominent eosinophilic nucleoli.*

Atypical Mesothelial Hyperplasia

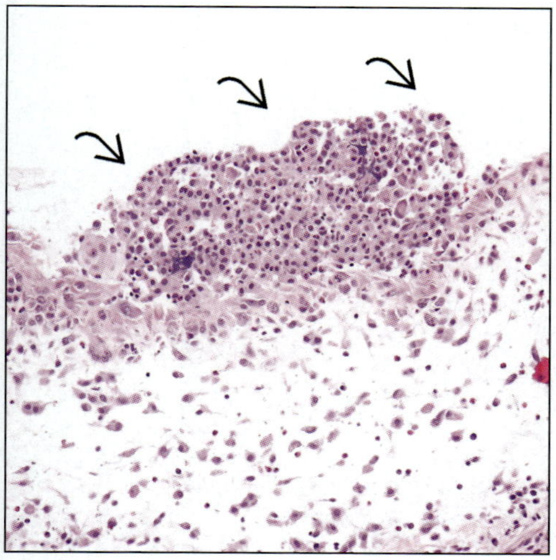

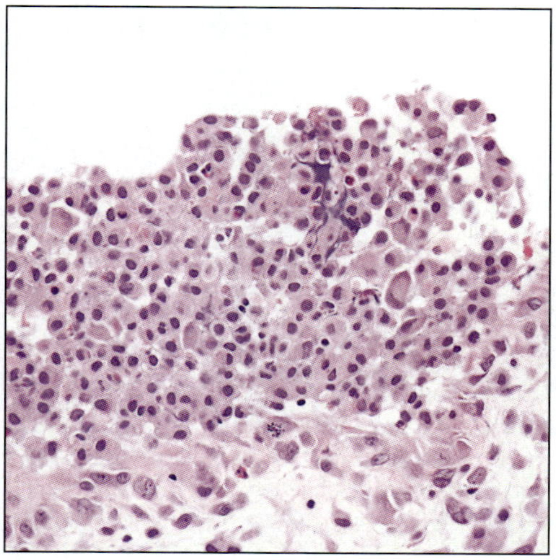

(Left) *Focus of pleural atypical mesothelial hyperplasia ⮫ is characterized by focal thickening of the pleural surface by proliferation of atypical round epithelioid cells. Small foci like this can be mistaken for metastatic carcinoma.* ***(Right)*** *High magnification shows densely packed epithelioid cells with abundant eosinophilic cytoplasm. There is some degree of nuclear pleomorphism and cytologic atypia noted.*

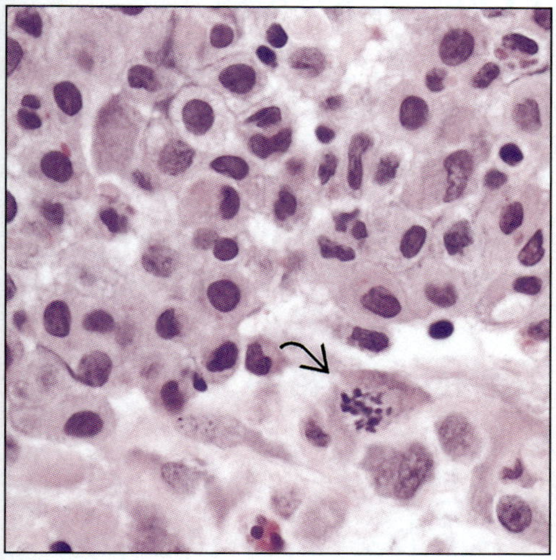

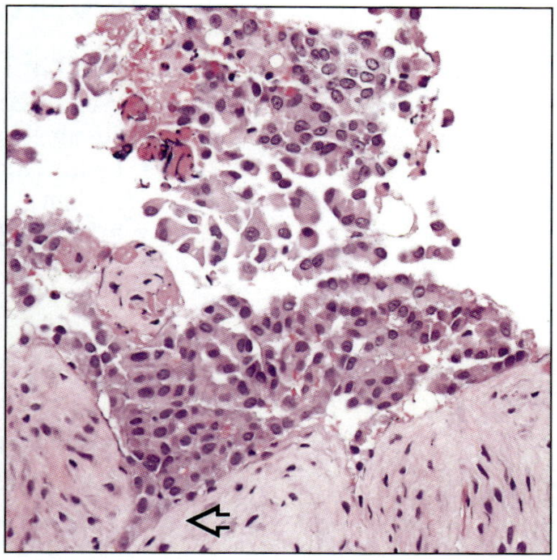

(Left) *Higher magnification shows significant cytologic atypia with enlarged, hyperchromatic nuclei and an abnormal mitosis ⮫. The cells show some degree of nuclear pleomorphism with variation in size and shape of the mesothelial cells.* ***(Right)*** *Atypical mesothelial hyperplasia of the pleura shows densely packed proliferation of epithelioid cells along the pleural surface. The area toward the base ⇨ is suggestive of a focus of invasion.*

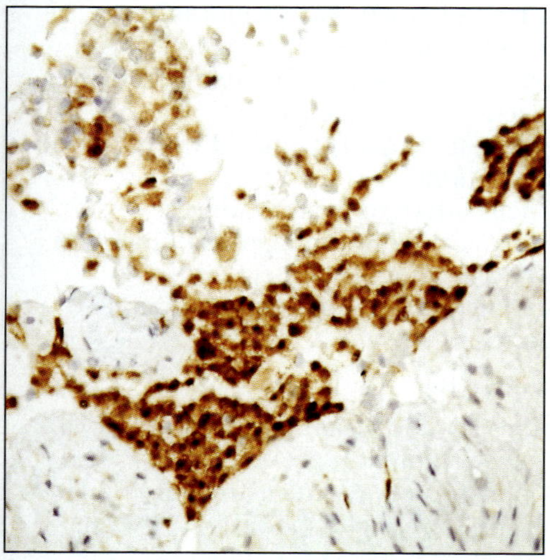

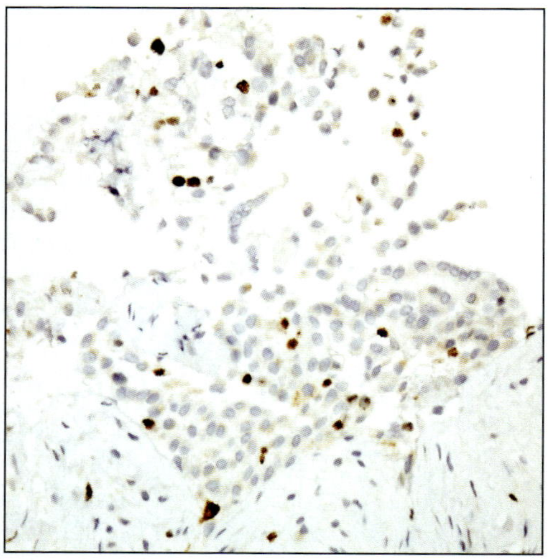

(Left) *Immunohistochemical staining shows positive nuclear and cytoplasmic staining of the epithelioid cells for calretinin antibodies.* ***(Right)*** *Immunoperoxidase staining shows scattered nuclear positivity in a few of the epithelioid cells (< 10%) for the proliferation marker, Ki-67.*

SOLITARY FIBROUS TUMOR

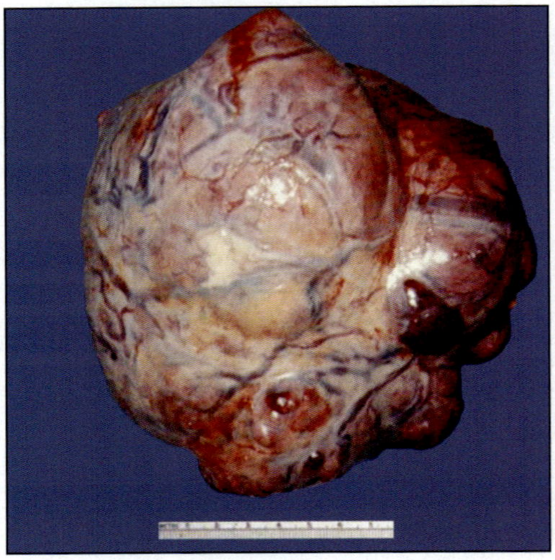

Typical gross appearance of solitary fibrous tumor of the pleura shows a lobulated and well-circumscribed firm mass covered by a thin, shiny capsule with striking vascular markings.

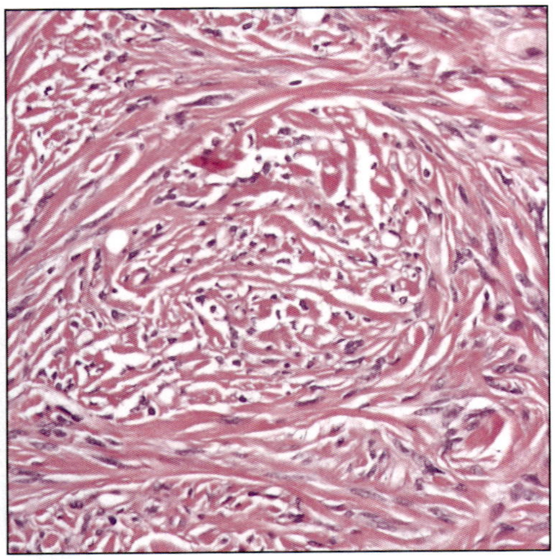

Typical histologic appearance of solitary fibrous tumor of the pleura shows rope-like strands of keloidal collagen flanked by small hyperchromatic spindle cells.

TERMINOLOGY

Abbreviations

- Solitary fibrous tumor (SFT)

Synonyms

- Submesothelial fibroma
- Fibrous mesothelioma
- Localized fibrous tumor
- Pleural fibroma

Definitions

- Benign neoplastic proliferation of submesothelial fibroblastic cells

ETIOLOGY/PATHOGENESIS

Pathogenesis

- Arises from submesothelial fibroblasts
- No relationship with asbestos exposure

CLINICAL ISSUES

Presentation

- Asymptomatic; incidental finding on routine chest x-ray
- Cough
- Pleuritic pain
- Dyspnea
- Hypoglycemia (5% of patients)
- Pulmonary osteoarthropathy with clubbing of fingers
- Most frequent in adults; no sex predilection

Treatment

- Surgical excision

Prognosis

- Excellent prognosis following complete excision with clear margins

MACROSCOPIC FEATURES

General Features

- Well circumscribed and encapsulated
- Sessile, broad-based pleural mass
- Pedunculated mass attached to pleural surface by short pedicle
- Rubbery, homogeneous, and whorled cut surface
- Size: 5-20 cm in greatest diameter
- Smooth, shiny outer surface

MICROSCOPIC PATHOLOGY

Histologic Features

- Bland-appearing spindle cell proliferation
- Variegation in growth patterns
- May incorporate entrapped air spaces at interphase with lung parenchyma
- May show prominent myxoid stromal changes
- May contain metaplastic bone or abnormal "amianthoid" collagen fibers
- Stroma is highly vascularized with angiofibromatous or hemangiopericytic vascular pattern
- Spindle cell areas are variably admixed with areas of stromal hyalinization
- Most distinctive pattern of hyalinization is characterized by parallel linear deposits of rope-like collagen separating tumor cells
- Areas with degeneration of collagen may simulate tumor cell necrosis

Cytologic Features

- Oval to spindle cells with scant cytoplasm and oval nuclei with dense chromatin pattern
- Spindle cells may show wavy nuclei resembling schwannian cells
- Multinucleated giant cells may be present
- Very low mitotic activity (1-3 per 10 high-power fields)

SOLITARY FIBROUS TUMOR

Key Facts

Clinical Issues
- Asymptomatic; incidental finding on routine chest x-ray
- Cough
- Pleuritic pain
- Dyspnea
- Hypoglycemia (5% of patients)
- Pulmonary osteoarthropathy with clubbing of fingers

Microscopic Pathology
- Bland-appearing spindle cell proliferation
- Variegation in growth patterns within same tumor
- May show prominent myxoid stromal changes
- Stroma is highly vascularized with angiofibromatous or hemangiopericytic vascular pattern
- Spindle cell areas are variably admixed with areas of stromal hyalinization
- Most distinctive pattern of hyalinization is characterized by parallel linear deposits of rope-like collagen separating tumor cells
- Oval to spindle cells with scant cytoplasm and oval nuclei with dense chromatin pattern
- Very low mitotic activity (1-3 per 10 high-power fields)
- Cells are positive for vimentin, CD34, Bcl-2, and CD99

Diagnostic Checklist
- Circumscription and encapsulation
- Bland-appearing spindle cell proliferation with prominent vascular pattern and variable degrees of stromal sclerosis
- Fascicular, short storiform, hemangiopericytic, neural palisading, and synovial sarcoma-like growth patterns

ANCILLARY TESTS

Immunohistochemistry
- Cells are positive for vimentin, CD34, Bcl-2, and CD99
- Focal positivity has been reported in some cases for cytokeratin and SMA; otherwise negative for all other markers
- Diagnosis of exclusion; CD34 positivity is not exclusive for this tumor and may be seen in a variety of other spindle cell tumors

Ultrastructure
- Features of fibroblastic cells
- May display immature cell junctions at tips of slender cytoplasmic processes

DIFFERENTIAL DIAGNOSIS

Sarcomatoid Mesothelioma
- More pronounced cytologic atypia, nuclear pleomorphism, and mitotic activity are seen in sarcomatoid mesothelioma
- Diffuse, as opposed to localized, growth pattern in sarcomatoid mesothelioma
- Strong cytokeratin and calretinin positivity favors sarcomatoid mesothelioma
- Strong CD34, Bcl-2, and CD99 positivity favors solitary fibrous tumor

Pleural Monophasic Synovial Sarcoma
- More pronounced cytologic atypia and mitotic activity are seen in synovial sarcoma
- Invasive features favor synovial sarcoma over solitary fibrous tumor
- Cytokeratin and EMA positivity is typically seen in synovial sarcoma but not in solitary fibrous tumor
- Most synovial sarcomas are negative for CD34, but Bcl-2 and CD99 are positive in both tumors
- Cytogenetic translocation (x;18) is characteristic of synovial sarcoma and is absent in solitary fibrous tumor

Peripheral Nerve Sheath Tumors
- Palisading of tumor cells with Anthony type A foci are more common in schwannian tumors
- S100 protein positivity is distinctive for peripheral nerve sheath tumors and is negative in solitary fibrous tumors
- Both can express Bcl-2 and CD34, but CD34 is more strongly expressed in solitary fibrous tumors
- Ultrastructural finding of complex, interdigitating cytoplasmic cell processes is characteristic of schwannian tumors

DIAGNOSTIC CHECKLIST

Clinically Relevant Pathologic Features
- Circumscription and encapsulation
- Pulmonary osteoarthropathy with clubbing of fingers
- Hypoglycemia
- Often found incidentally on routine chest x-rays

Pathologic Interpretation Pearls
- Bland-appearing spindle cell proliferation with prominent vascular pattern and variable degrees of stromal sclerosis
- Fascicular, short storiform, hemangiopericytic, neural palisading, and synovial sarcoma-like growth patterns
- Variegation of histologic growth patterns within same lesion
- Immunohistochemical positivity for CD34, Bcl-2, and CD99
- No distinctive or pathognomonic markers available; diagnosis is by exclusion of other spindle cell tumors
- So far, no known molecular or cytogenetic abnormalities
- Distinction from synovial sarcoma in cellular examples of solitary fibrous tumors may require molecular studies to demonstrate t(x;18)

SOLITARY FIBROUS TUMOR

Immunohistochemistry

Antibody	Reactivity	Staining Pattern	Comment
Vimentin	Positive	Cytoplasmic	Diffuse, strong staining in all cells
CD34	Positive	Cytoplasmic	Positive in 60-90% of cases
Bcl-2	Positive	Cytoplasmic	Strongly positive in 80-100% of cases
CD99	Positive	Cytoplasmic	Positive in 60-80% of cases
AE1/AE3	Negative		May be rarely positive in some cases
Actin-sm	Negative		May be rarely positive in some cases
S100	Negative		
Caldesmon	Negative		

Histologic Growth Patterns in Solitary Fibrous Tumors

Solid Spindle Cell Component	Diffuse Sclerosing Component
Fascicular spindle cell growth pattern	Fine linear pattern of intercellular sclerosis
Short storiform pattern of growth	Coarse linear pattern of sclerosis (rope-like collagen)
Hemangiopericytic growth pattern	Diffuse, confluent areas of sclerosis
Herringbone growth pattern	Angiofibromatous growth pattern
Wavy neural growth pattern	Myxoid stromal changes
Synovial sarcoma-like cellular growth pattern	Metaplastic bone and "amianthoid" fibers
Neural-type palisaded growth pattern	Degeneration of collagen resembling necrosis

SELECTED REFERENCES

1. Cardillo G et al: Solitary fibrous tumors of the pleura: an analysis of 110 patients treated in a single institution. Ann Thorac Surg. 88(5):1632-7, 2009
2. Harrison-Phipps KM et al: Solitary fibrous tumors of the pleura: results of surgical treatment and long-term prognosis. J Thorac Cardiovasc Surg. 138(1):19-25, 2009
3. Kalebi AY et al: Surgically cured hypoglycemia secondary to pleural solitary fibrous tumour: case report and update review on the Doege-Potter syndrome. J Cardiothorac Surg. 4:45, 2009
4. Liu CC et al: Solitary fibrous tumors of the pleura: clinicopathological characteristics, immunohistochemical profiles, and surgical outcomes with long-term follow-up. Thorac Cardiovasc Surg. 56(5):291-7, 2008
5. Lu C et al: Solitary fibrous tumor of the pleura: an analysis of 13 cases. World J Surg. 32(8):1663-8, 2008
6. Perna V et al: Localized (solitary) fibrous tumors of the pleura: an analysis of 15 patients. Int J Surg. 6(4):298-301, 2008
7. Schirosi L et al: Pleuro-pulmonary solitary fibrous tumors: a clinicopathologic, immunohistochemical, and molecular study of 88 cases confirming the prognostic value of de Perrot staging system and p53 expression, and evaluating the role of c-kit, BRAF, PDGFRs (alpha/beta), c-met, and EGFR. Am J Surg Pathol. 32(11):1627-42, 2008
8. Chang JC et al: Hypoglycemia in a patient with a huge malignant solitary fibrous tumor of the pleura. Pathol Int. 57(12):791-3, 2007
9. Sung SH et al: Solitary fibrous tumors of the pleura: surgical outcome and clinical course. Ann Thorac Surg. 79(1):303-7, 2005
10. Bini A et al: Solitary fibrous tumor of the pleura. A single institution's experience. J Cardiovasc Surg (Torino). 45(2):167-8, 2004
11. de Perrot M et al: Solitary fibrous tumors of the pleura. Ann Thorac Surg. 74(1):285-93, 2002
12. Magdeleinat P et al: Solitary fibrous tumors of the pleura: clinical characteristics, surgical treatment and outcome. Eur J Cardiothorac Surg. 21(6):1087-93, 2002
13. Tateishi U et al: Solitary fibrous tumor of the pleura: MR appearance and enhancement pattern. J Comput Assist Tomogr. 26(2):174-9, 2002
14. Cardillo G et al: Localized (solitary) fibrous tumors of the pleura: an analysis of 55 patients. Ann Thorac Surg. 70(6):1808-12, 2000
15. de Perrot M et al: Clinical behavior of solitary fibrous tumors of the pleura. Ann Thorac Surg. 67(5):1456-9, 1999
16. de Saint Aubain Somerhausen N et al: Myxoid solitary fibrous tumor: a study of seven cases with emphasis on differential diagnosis. Mod Pathol. 12(5):463-71, 1999
17. Fukasawa Y et al: Solitary fibrous tumor of the pleura causing recurrent hypoglycemia by secretion of insulin-like growth factor II. Pathol Int. 48(1):47-52, 1998
18. Suster S et al: Expression of bcl-2 oncoprotein in benign and malignant spindle cell tumors of soft tissue, skin, serosal surfaces, and gastrointestinal tract. Am J Surg Pathol. 22(7):863-72, 1998
19. Nascimento AG: Solitary fibrous tumor: a ubiquitous neoplasm of mesenchymal differentiation. Adv Anat Pathol. 3:388-95, 1996
20. Flint A et al: CD-34 and keratin expression distinguishes solitary fibrous tumor (fibrous mesothelioma) of pleura from desmoplastic mesothelioma. Hum Pathol. 26(4):428-31, 1995
21. Moran CA et al: The spectrum of histologic growth patterns in benign and malignant fibrous tumors of the pleura. Semin Diagn Pathol. 9(2):169-80, 1992
22. England DM et al: Localized benign and malignant fibrous tumors of the pleura. A clinicopathologic review of 223 cases. Am J Surg Pathol. 13(8):640-58, 1989
23. Said JW et al: Localized fibrous mesothelioma: an immunohistochemical and electron microscopic study. Hum Pathol. 15(5):440-3, 1984

Classical Sclerosing Pattern

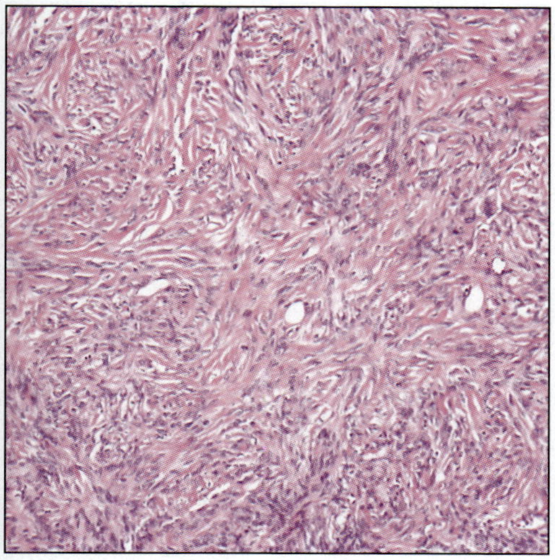
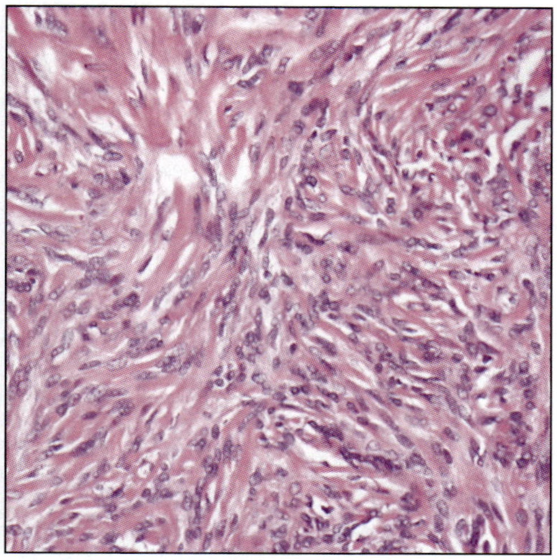

(Left) *Solitary fibrous tumor of the pleura shows cellular proliferation with a storiform pattern of growth. Tumors with this growth pattern can be easily confused with fibrohistiocytic neoplasms.* ***(Right)*** *High magnification of solitary fibrous tumor of the pleura shows a storiform pattern of growth. Short fascicles of small spindle cells are seen radiating from the center in a pinwheel fashion along with the surrounding stromal collagen fibers.*

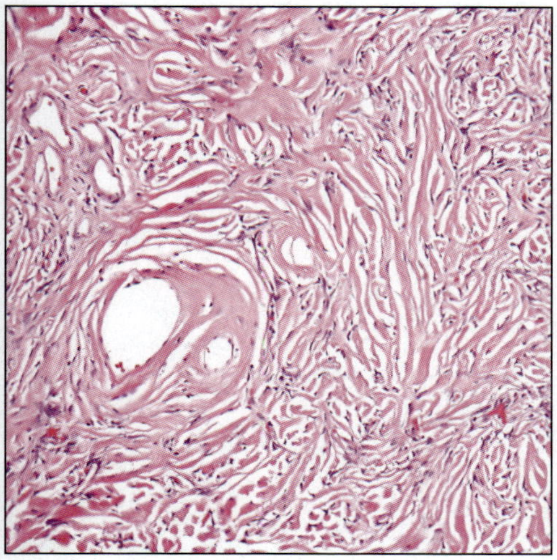
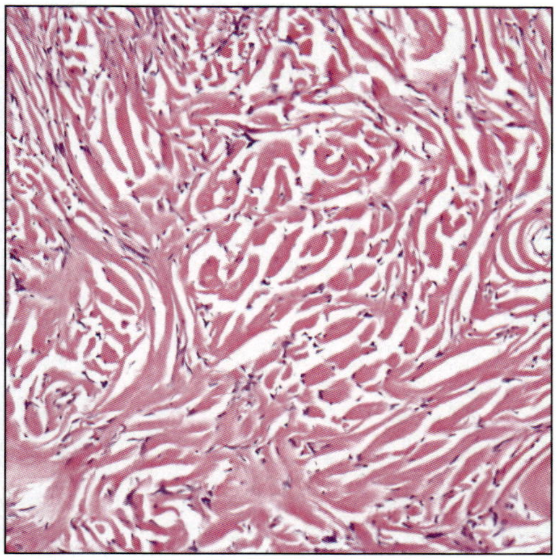

(Left) *Typical appearance of solitary fibrous tumor of the pleura is characterized by rope-like strands of acellular, hyalinized collagen flanked by small hyperchromatic spindle cells. The parallel arrangement of the strands of collagen is quite characteristic for this tumor.* ***(Right)*** *High magnification of typical sclerosing pattern in solitary fibrous tumor of the pleura shows parallel strands of rope-like keloidal collagen flanked by small spindle cells.*

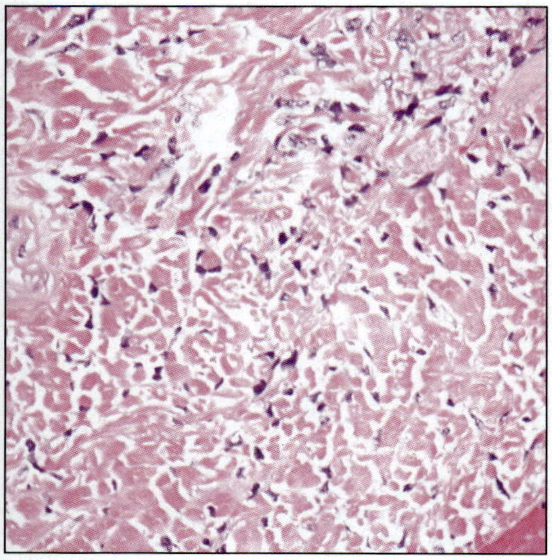
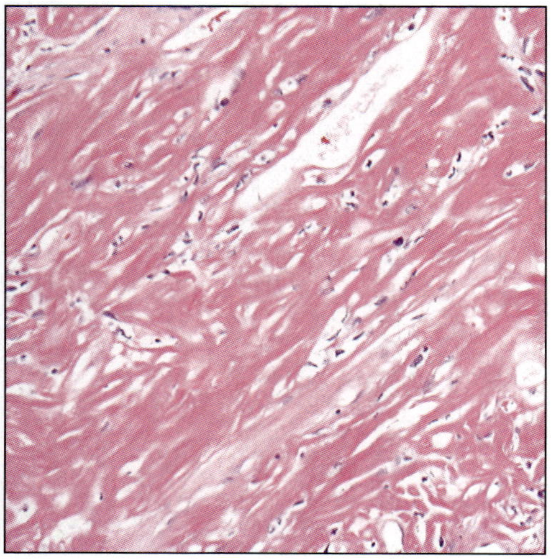

(Left) *A more advanced stage of stromal sclerosis is seen in solitary fibrous tumor of the pleura showing abundant collagen deposition with few scattered residual round to oval nuclei compressed by the stromal collagen.* ***(Right)*** *Advanced stage of stromal collagen deposition in solitary fibrous tumor of the pleura shows acellular bands of hyalinized intercellular collagen with very few scattered small spindle cells in the background.*

SOLITARY FIBROUS TUMOR

Unusual Growth Patterns

(Left) *This neural-like appearance of solitary fibrous tumor of the pleura is characterized by longitudinal fascicles of spindle cells with wavy nuclei. Tumors with this appearance can closely resemble peripheral nerve sheath tumors.* ***(Right)*** *Higher magnification of solitary fibrous tumor of the pleura with a neural-like appearance shows elongated spindle cells with wavy nuclei and tapering cell processes simulating a schwannian neoplasm.*

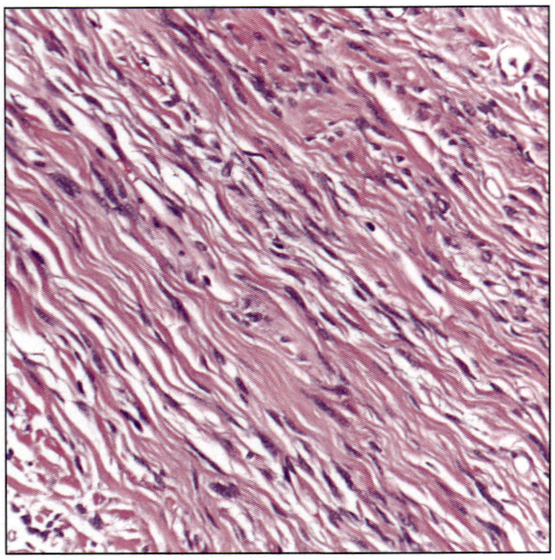

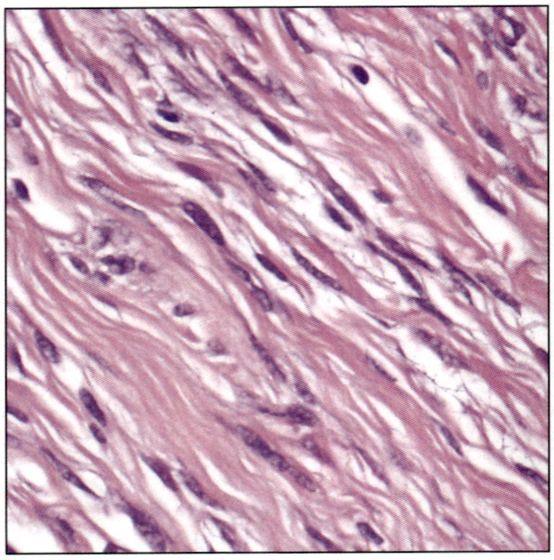

(Left) *Solitary fibrous tumor of the pleura shows prominent myxoid stroma surrounding the tumor cell population. The tumor cells are composed of small, spindle to stellate cells with dark nuclei and an inconspicuous rim of cytoplasm.* ***(Right)*** *High magnification of solitary fibrous tumor of the pleura with prominent myxoid stroma shows a bland-appearing proliferation of small, stellate to spindle cells with hyperchromatic nuclei and a scant, indistinct rim of cytoplasm.*

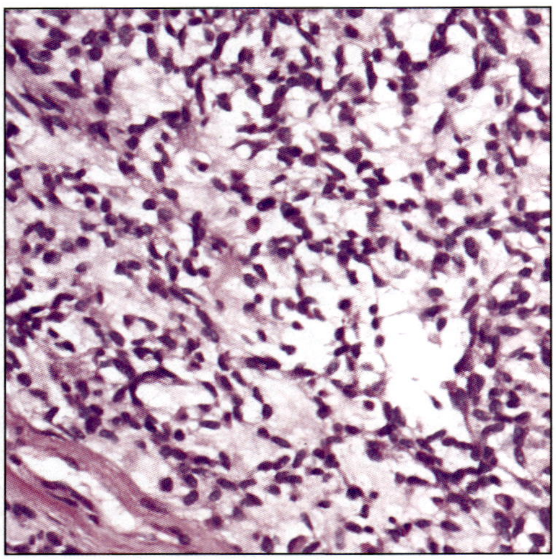

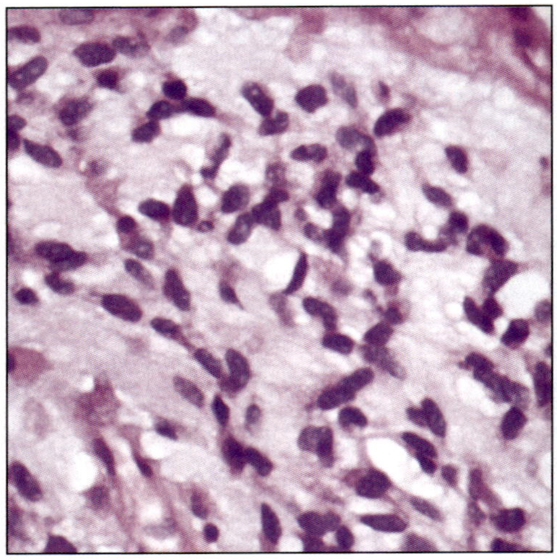

(Left) *Solitary fibrous tumor of the pleura with epithelioid cell morphology shows peritheliomatous distribution of round epithelioid tumor cells. Notice the entrapment of small dilated vascular spaces in the center of the cellular nodule* ➔*.* ***(Right)*** *Higher magnification of solitary fibrous tumor of the pleura with epithelioid features shows a monotonous population of round epithelioid cells with an abundant rim of eosinophilic cytoplasm.*

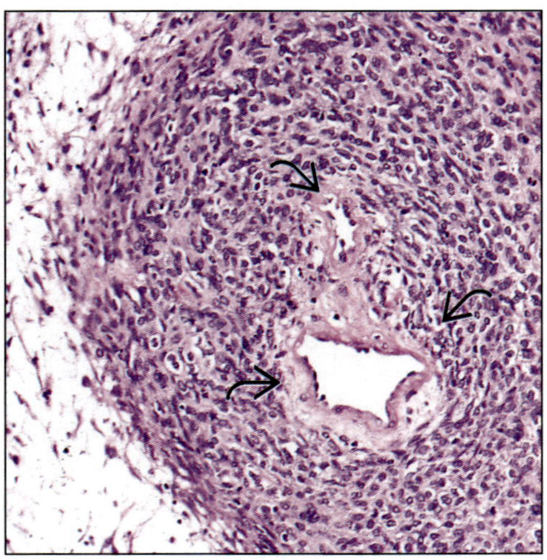

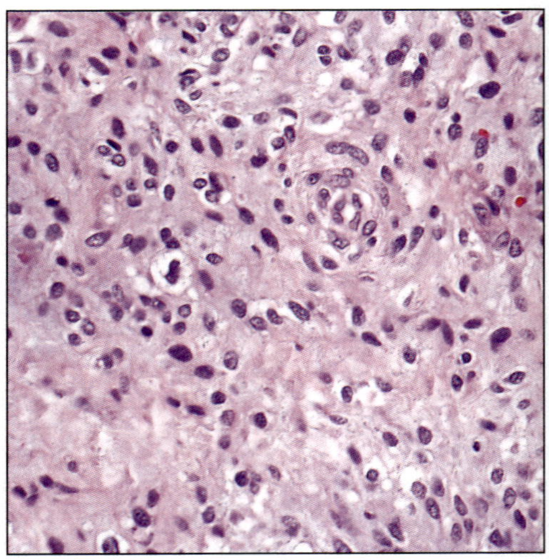

Vascular Growth Patterns

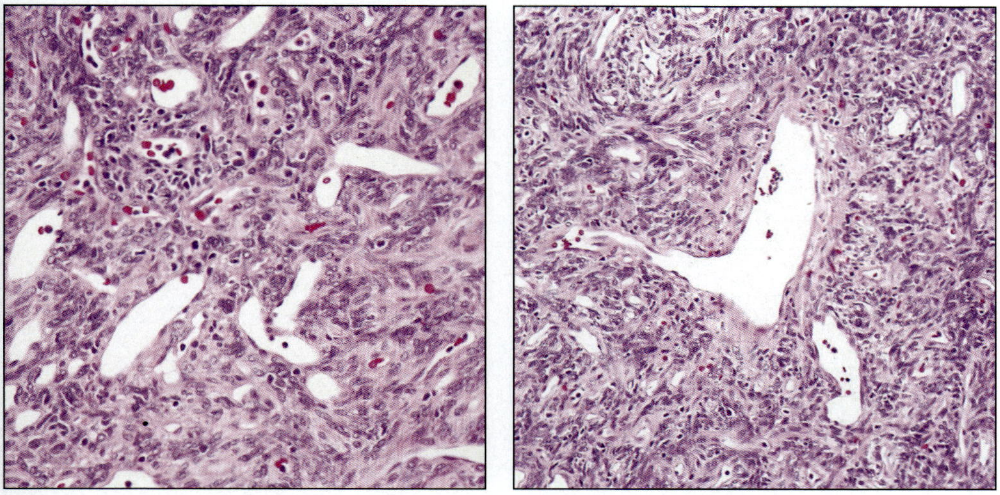

(Left) *Solitary fibrous tumor of the pleura shows abundant branching small vessels with patent lumens resulting in a striking hemangiopericytoma-like appearance. The hemangiopericytoma variant of SFT is another typical morphologic manifestation of these tumors.* ***(Right)*** *Higher magnification of solitary fibrous tumor of the pleura with hemangiopericytoma-like growth pattern shows a dilated small vessel branching at right angles, resulting in a "staghorn" appearance.*

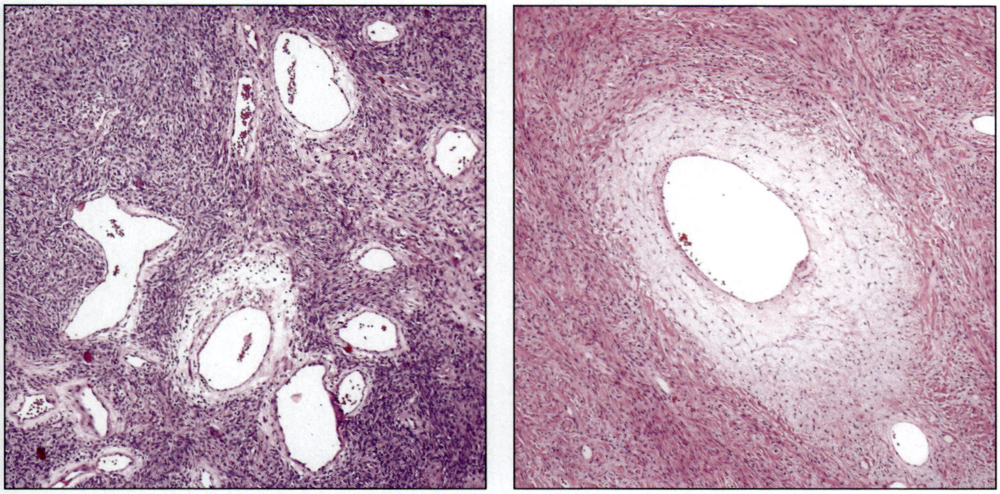

(Left) *Solitary fibrous tumor of the pleura shows multiple dilated small vessels with wide patent lumens and perivascular stromal sclerosis resulting in an angiofibromatous growth pattern.* ***(Right)*** *Solitary fibrous tumor of the pleura with angiofibromatous pattern of growth shows a dilated vessel in the center with perivascular sclerosis and edema and solid spindle cell proliferation circumferentially surrounding the dilated vascular space.*

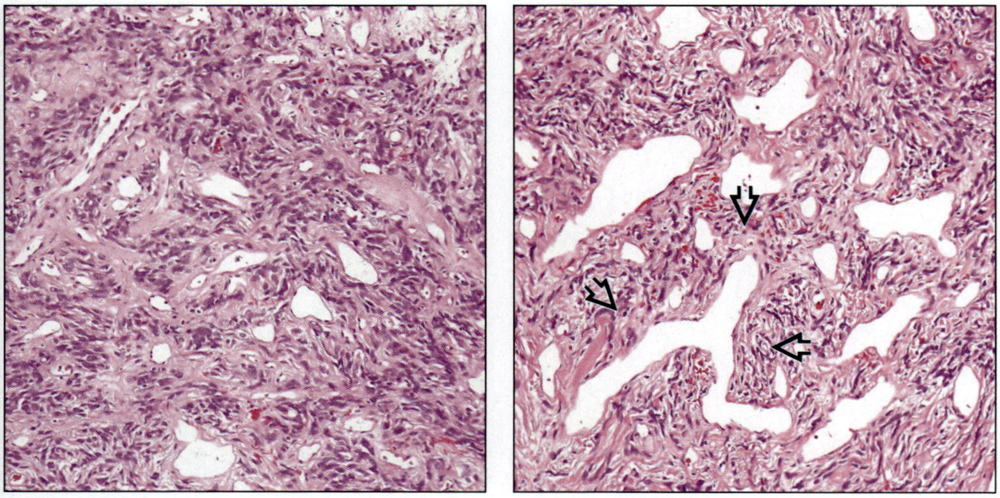

(Left) *Solitary fibrous tumor of the pleura shows a dense population of plump epithelioid cells surrounding small dilated vascular spaces with patent lumens.* ***(Right)*** *Solitary fibrous tumor of the pleura with prominent hemangiopericytic growth pattern shows a dense population of spindle cells in the stroma surrounding irregular, branching, and dilated vascular spaces with open lumens displaying an occasional "staghorn" configuration* ⇨.

SOLITARY FIBROUS TUMOR

Entrapment of Airspaces

(Left) *Solitary fibrous tumor of the pleura shows entrapment of airspaces within the tumor ⇨ near the interface between the lung and the tumor. The entrapped airspaces can simulate a biphasic malignant neoplasm.* ***(Right)*** *Solitary fibrous tumor of the pleura shows entrapped airspaces deep within the tumor and away from the adjacent lung parenchyma ⇨. The distribution of these epithelial-lined structures primarily at the periphery of the lesion is quite characteristic.*

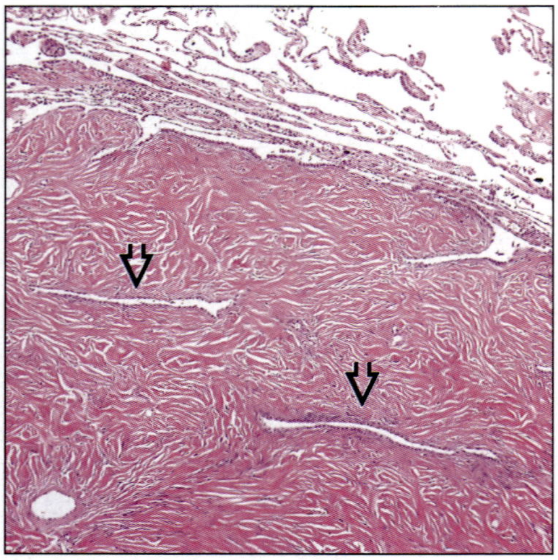

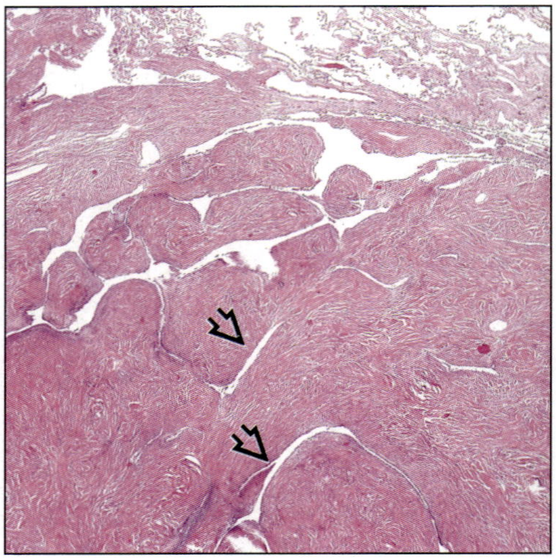

(Left) *Higher magnification of entrapped airspaces in solitary fibrous tumor of the pleura shows luminal spaces lined by columnar epithelium and surrounding fibrous tissue cores containing dense hyalinized collagen.* ***(Right)*** *Solitary fibrous tumor of the pleura shows a more advanced stage of entrapment of airspaces within the substance of the tumor. In this example, the stroma surrounding the entrapped airspaces is completely sclerotic.*

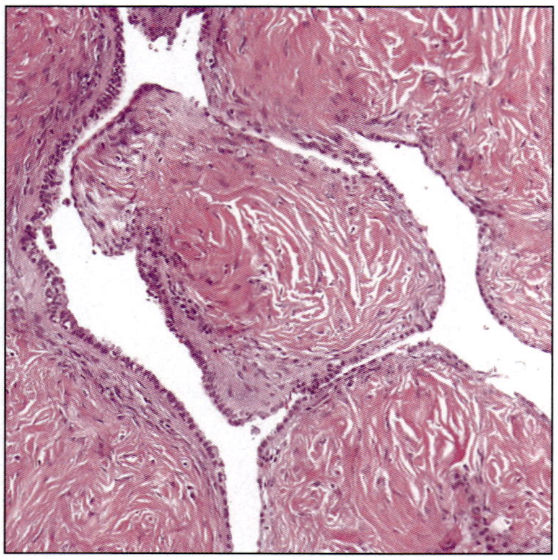

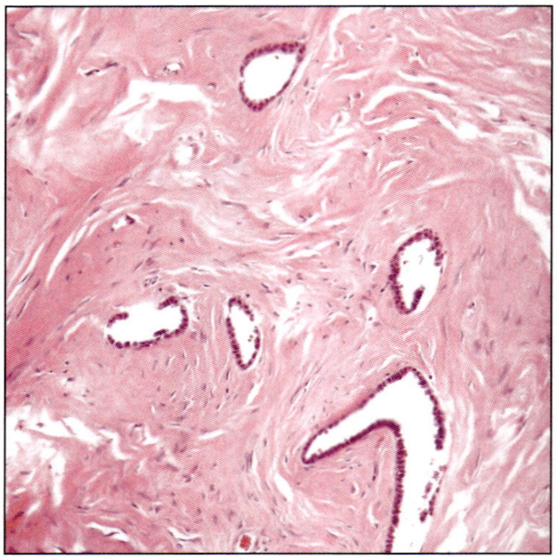

(Left) *Higher magnification of residual entrapped airspace in solitary fibrous tumor of the pleura shows atrophy of the epithelial lining in the luminal side of the structure, which is lined primarily by a single layer of small, cuboidal epithelial cells.* ***(Right)*** *Entrapped airspace in solitary fibrous tumor of the pleura shows irregularly dilated luminal space lined by variable epithelium ranging from flat to cuboidal to tall columnar epithelium.*

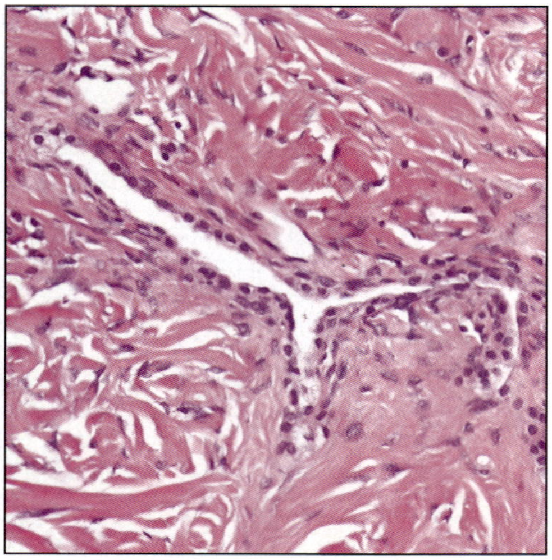

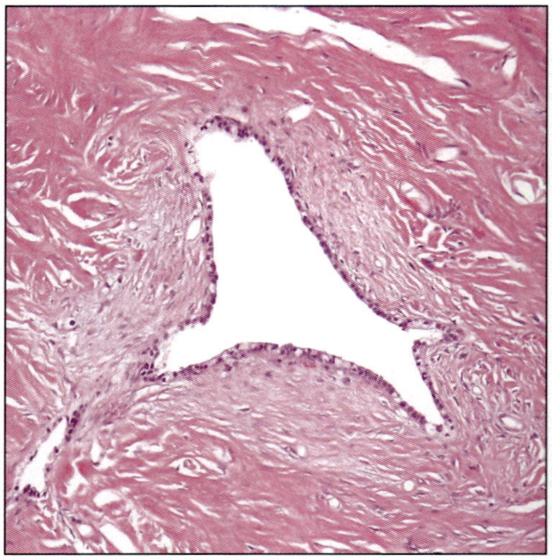

Cellular Growth Pattern

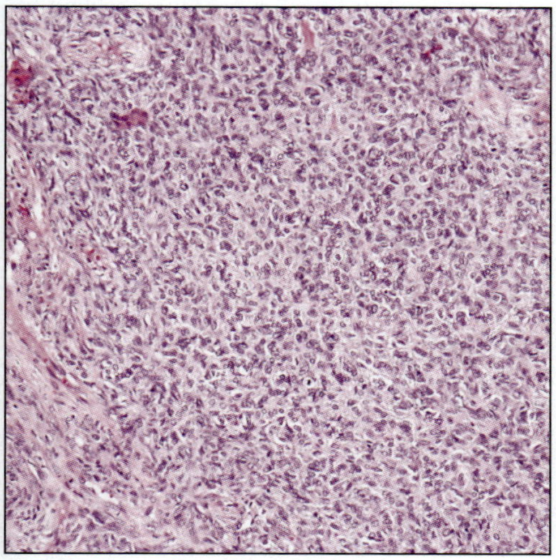

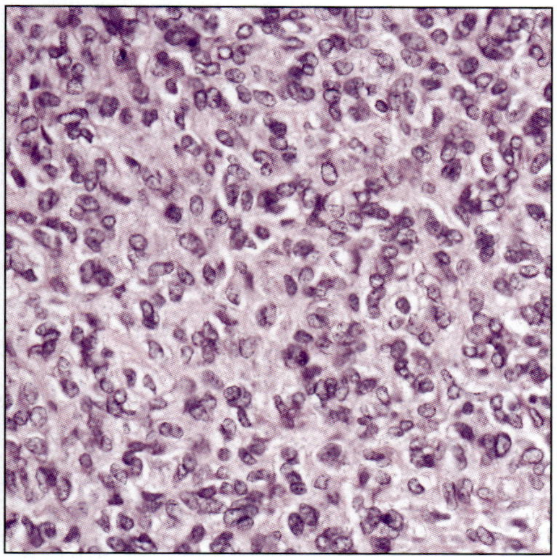

(Left) *Solitary fibrous tumor of the pleura growing as diffuse sheets of cells shows dense cellularity. The tumor cells are small and mostly round epithelioid rather than the conventional spindle cells commonly observed in these tumors.* ***(Right)*** *Higher magnification of solitary fibrous tumor of the pleura characterized by a predominantly round cell population shows densely packed round to oval cells with vesicular nuclei and surrounded by a scant rim of amphophilic cytoplasm.*

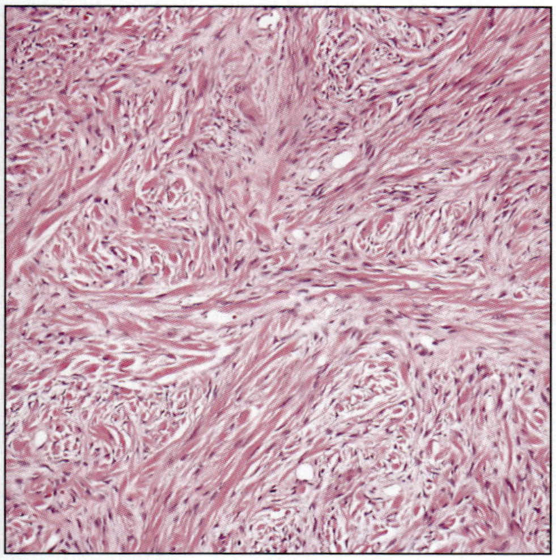

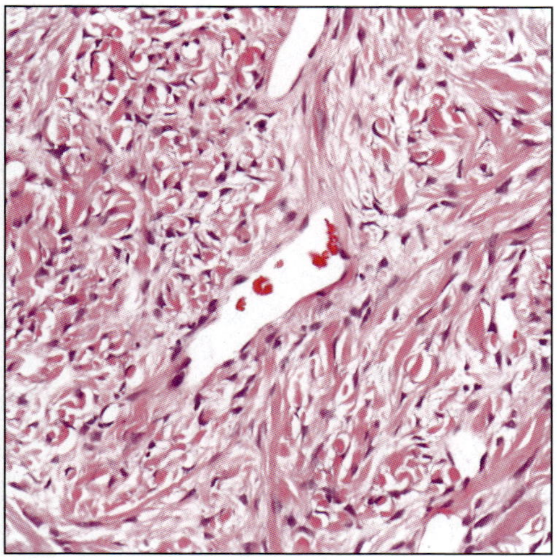

(Left) *Solitary fibrous tumor of pleura shows a proliferation of small spindle cells set against a background of hyalinized stromal collagen. The lesion is quite cellular and uniform with even distribution of the short spindle cells among the collagen fibers.* ***(Right)*** *High magnification of solitary fibrous tumor of the pleura shows a uniform population of small, dark spindle cells set against a heavily collagenized stroma. Despite the heavy collagenization, the lesion is quite cellular.*

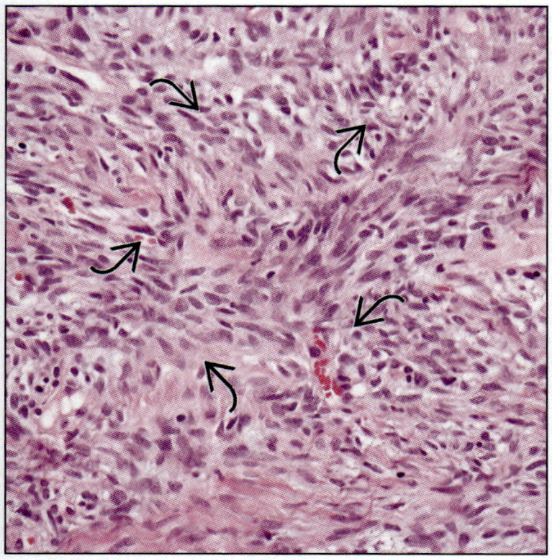

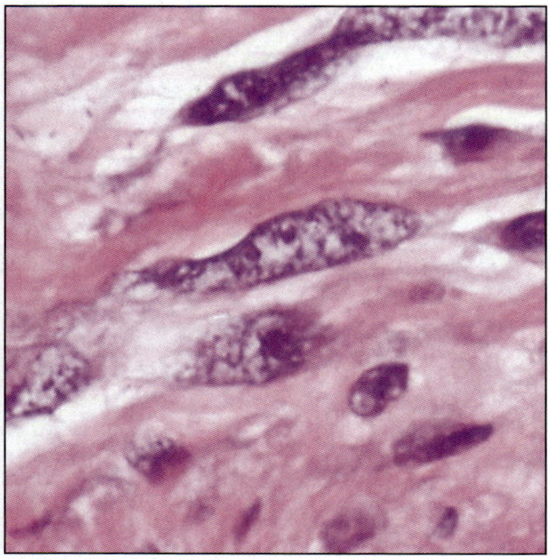

(Left) *Solitary fibrous tumor of the pleura shows a cellular spindle cell proliferation with a discrete storiform growth pattern. The spindle cells seem to be radiating from the central portion of the spindle cell fascicles like the spokes of a wheel* ➢*.* ***(Right)*** *High magnification of solitary fibrous tumor of the pleura shows spindle cells with elongated nuclei, a dispersed chromatin pattern, and multiple small nucleoli surrounded by a scant rim of amphophilic cytoplasm.*

SOLITARY FIBROUS TUMOR

Dense Spindle Cell Growth Pattern

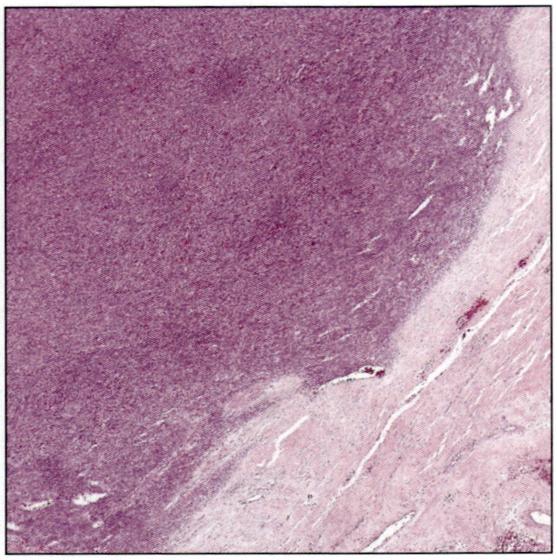

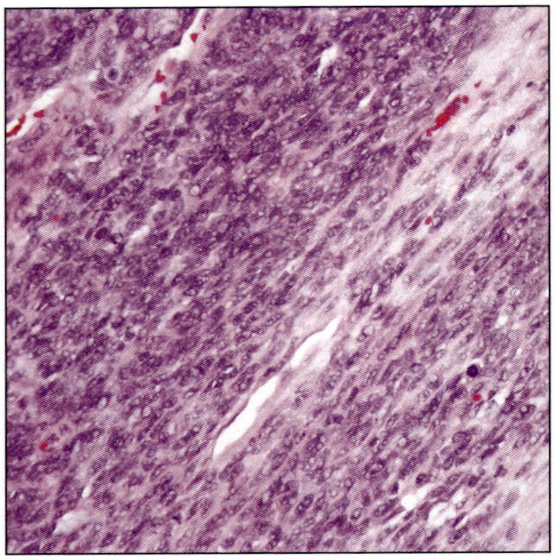

(Left) *Densely cellular, synovial sarcoma-like variant of solitary fibrous tumor of the pleura shows solid proliferation of tightly packed spindle cells on scanning magnification.* ***(Right)*** *Higher magnification of cellular spindle cell variant of solitary fibrous tumor of the pleura shows sheets of hyperchromatic spindle cells with very little intervening stroma. Scattered mitotic figures can also be seen in these tumors, highlighting the similarity with synovial sarcoma.*

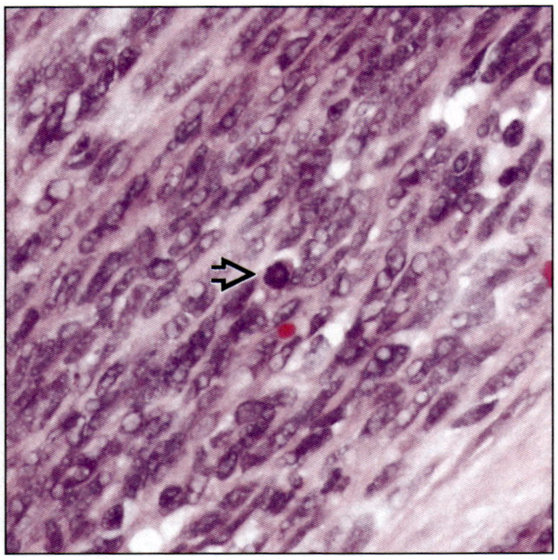

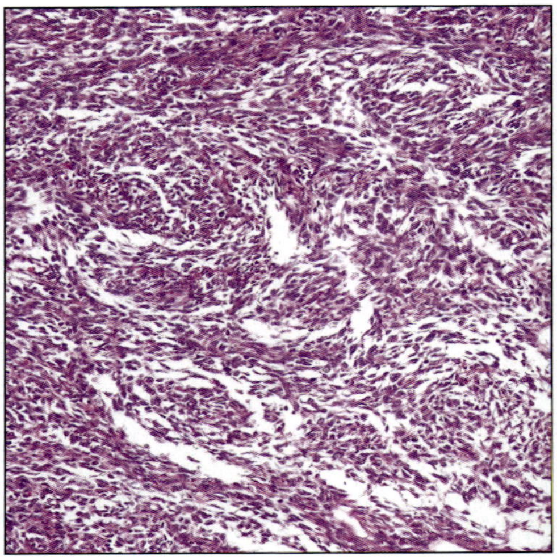

(Left) *Higher magnification of cellular variant of solitary fibrous tumor of the pleura shows a monotonous population of spindle cells with vesicular nuclei and occasional mitotic figures ⇨. Tumors with these features can be easily mistaken for examples of synovial sarcoma of the pleura.* ***(Right)*** *Solitary fibrous tumor of the pleura shows solid spindle cell proliferation with little intervening stroma that may closely resemble monophasic synovial sarcoma.*

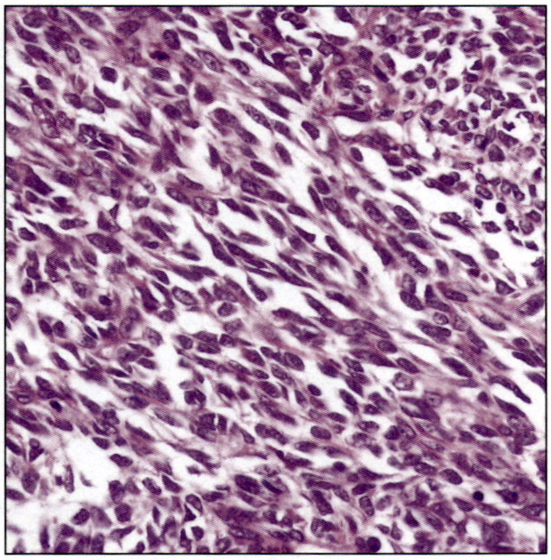

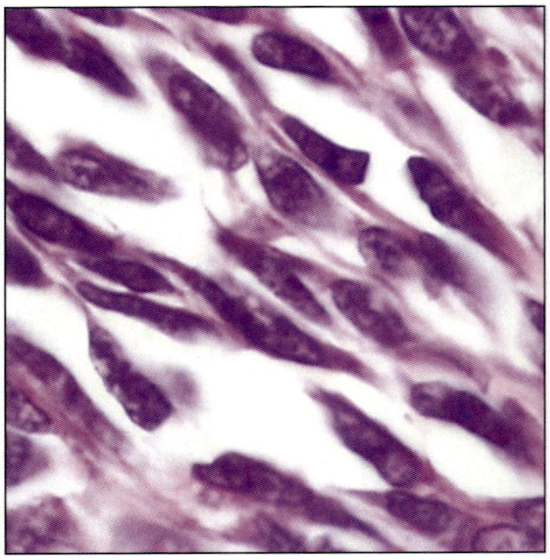

(Left) *Higher magnification of solitary fibrous tumor of the pleura composed of a monotonous proliferation of spindle cells with little intervening stroma closely resembles monophasic synovial sarcoma.* ***(Right)*** *Detail of the spindle cells in cellular variant of solitary fibrous tumor of the pleura resembling monophasic synovial sarcoma shows hyperchromatic spindle cells with a dense chromatin pattern, inconspicuous nucleoli, and tapered cytoplasmic processes.*

Immunohistochemical Features

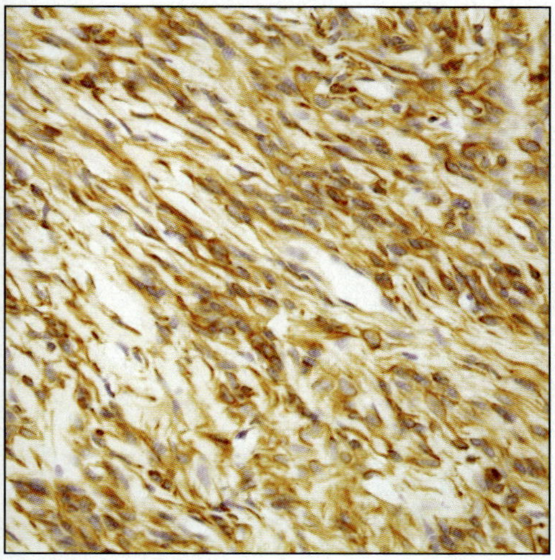
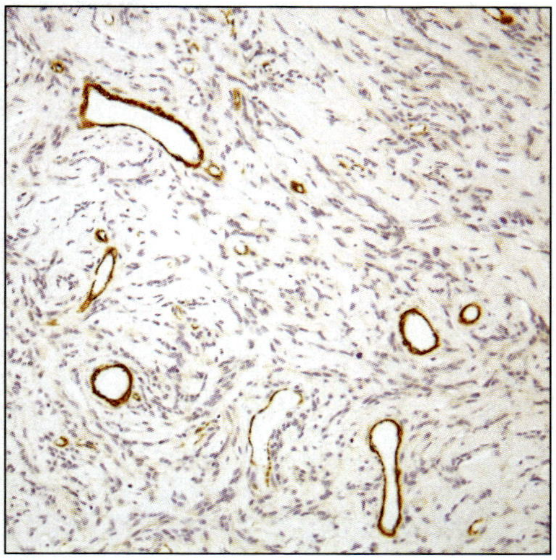

(Left) *Immunohistochemical stain for vimentin in solitary fibrous tumor of the pleura shows strong positivity in all of the spindle cells. This marker is positive in 100% of cases of solitary fibrous tumors in all locations.* ***(Right)*** *Immunohistochemical staining for smooth muscle actin (SMA) in solitary fibrous tumor of the pleura highlights the positive staining of the muscle layer of small vessels but shows negative staining in the tumor cells.*

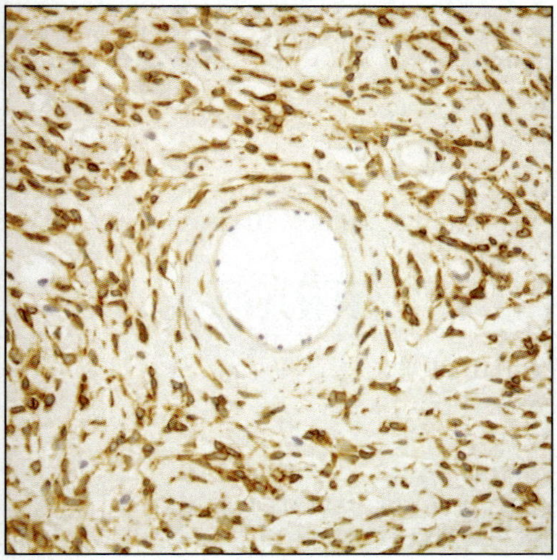
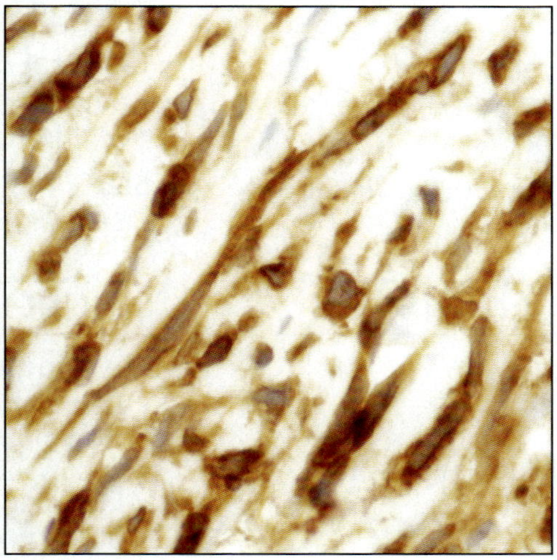

(Left) *Immunohistochemical staining of solitary fibrous tumor of the pleura with antibodies to Bcl-2 shows strong positivity of the tumor cells for this marker. Notice the concentric arrangement of the positive tumor cells surrounding the vessel wall (center).* ***(Right)*** *Immunohistochemical staining for Bcl-2 in solitary fibrous tumor of the pleura shows strong cytoplasmic positivity of the spindle cells for this marker. Nearly 100% of cases of SFT are positive for this marker.*

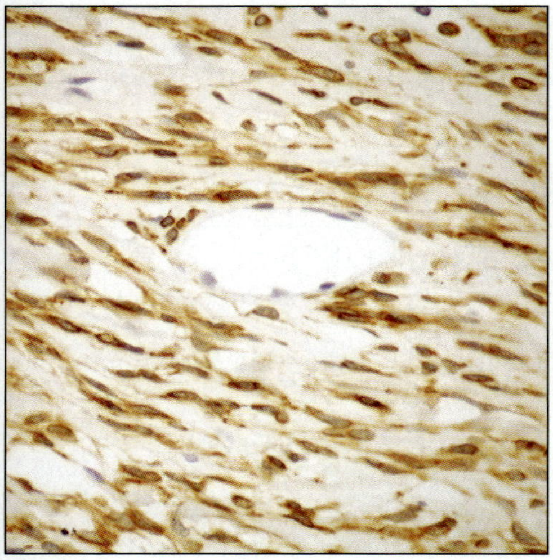
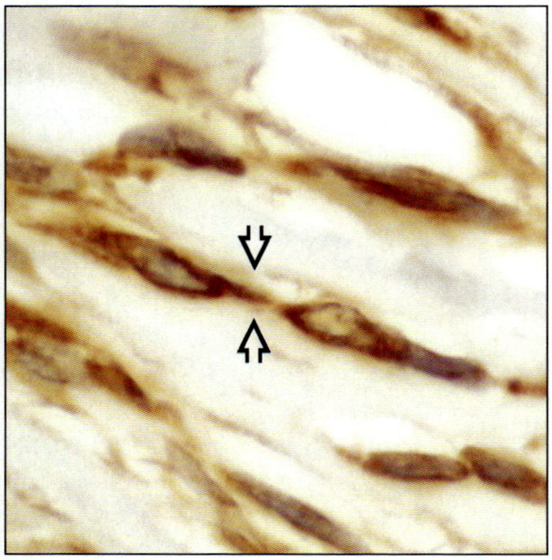

(Left) *Immunohistochemical staining of solitary fibrous tumor of the pleura for CD34 shows positive staining in the majority of the tumor cells. CD34 stains positively in approximately 60-80% of the cases of solitary fibrous tumors.* ***(Right)*** *Immunohistochemical staining for CD34 in solitary fibrous tumor of the pleura shows a positive cytoplasmic rim in 2 adjacent tumor cells that appear to be touching each other via slender cytoplasmic prolongations* ⇨.

CALCIFIED FIBROUS PSEUDOTUMOR

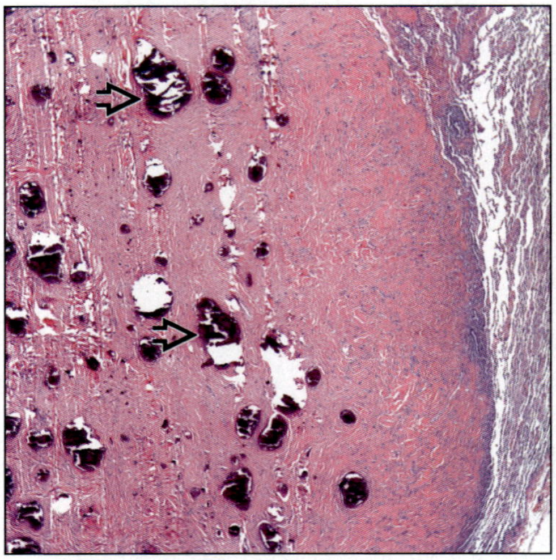

Low-power view shows a calcifying fibrous pseudotumor of the pleura. Note the presence of numerous calcifications ➡ embedded in a fibrous stroma with mild inflammatory changes.

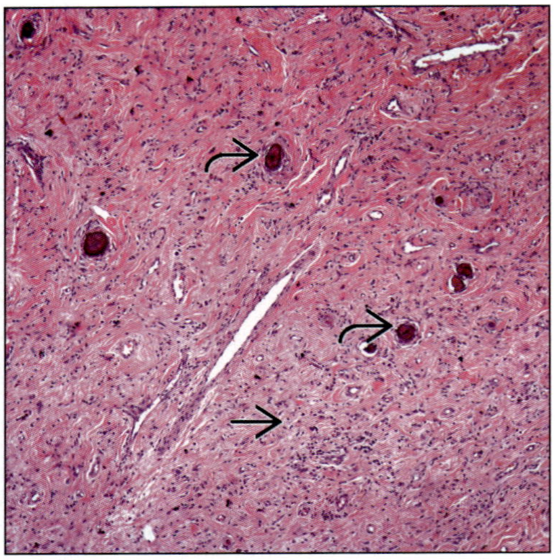

The tumor is composed of a bland spindle cell proliferation ➡ with scattered inflammatory cells and the presence of psammomatous calcifications ➡.

TERMINOLOGY

Abbreviations

- Calcified fibrous pseudotumor (CFPT)

Definitions

- Benign fibrocollagenous tumor with dystrophic or psammomatous calcifications

ETIOLOGY/PATHOGENESIS

Possible Etiologies

- Fibroinflammatory in nature
- Reactive process
- Late sclerosing stage of myofibroblastic tumor

CLINICAL ISSUES

Epidemiology

- Incidence
  - Very uncommon tumor in thoracic cavity
- Age
  - Usually occurs in adults from 20-55 years old
- Gender
  - No gender predilection

Presentation

- Cough
- Chest pain
- Shortness of breath
- Asymptomatic

Treatment

- Surgical approaches
  - Complete surgical resection

Prognosis

- Good
- Recurrences may occur

MACROSCOPIC FEATURES

General Features

- Single pleural mass
- Multiple pleural nodules

Size

- Tumors may vary from 1 cm to > 10 cm in diameter

MICROSCOPIC PATHOLOGY

Histologic Features

- Dense fibrocollagenous tissue
- Psammoma bodies
- Dystrophic calcifications
- Lymphoplasmacytic inflammatory reaction
- Absence of nuclear atypia or mitotic activity
- Absence of necrosis &/or hemorrhage

Predominant Pattern/Injury Type

- Fibrous

Predominant Cell/Compartment Type

- Fibroblast

DIFFERENTIAL DIAGNOSIS

Solitary Fibrous Tumor (SFT)

- Shows different growth pattern in same tumor
- Positive staining for Bcl-2
- Rarely shows dystrophic calcification &/or psammoma bodies

Sarcomatoid Mesothelioma (SM)

- Shows diffuse pleural involvement
- Shows nuclear atypia and mitotic activity
- Positive for CK-PAN

CALCIFIED FIBROUS PSEUDOTUMOR

Key Facts

Terminology
- Calcified fibrous pseudotumor (CFPT)

Clinical Issues
- Cough
- Chest pain
- Shortness of breath
- Asymptomatic

Macroscopic Features
- Single pleural mass
- Multiple pleural nodules

Microscopic Pathology
- Dense fibrocollagenous tissue
- Psammoma bodies
- Dystrophic calcifications
- Lymphoplasmacytic inflammatory reaction
- Absence of nuclear atypia or mitotic activity
- Absence of necrosis &/or hemorrhage

Top Differential Diagnoses
- Solitary fibrous tumor
  - Shows different growth pattern in same tumor
  - Positive staining for Bcl-2
  - Rarely shows dystrophic calcification &/or psammoma bodies
- Sarcomatoid mesothelioma
  - Shows diffuse pleural involvement
  - Shows nuclear atypia and mitotic activity
  - Positive for CK-PAN
- Fibrous plaque
  - CFPT generally shows psammoma bodies &/or dystrophic calcification

Immunohistochemistry

Antibody	Reactivity	Staining Pattern	Comment
CD34	Positive	Cytoplasmic	In some cases
Vimentin	Positive	Cytoplasmic	
Bcl-2	Negative		
Actin-sm	Negative		May be positive in some fibroblasts
Desmin	Negative		
CK-PAN	Negative		Some fibroblasts may stain with keratin
S100	Negative		Macrophages may stain for S100
EMA	Negative		
Calretinin	Negative		If there are residual mesothelial cells, they may be positive
CK5/6	Negative		
SOX9	Negative		

Fibrous Plaque
- CFPT generally shows psammoma bodies &/or dystrophic calcification
- Fibrous plaque generally consists of dense fibrocollagenous tissue ± inflammatory changes

Inflammatory Pseudotumor (IPT)
- Shows presence of marked inflammatory reaction composed mainly of plasma cells
- Shows presence of pulmonary parenchymal involvement
- May also show presence of fibroblastic spindle cell component
- Rarely shows presence of calcifications

DIAGNOSTIC CHECKLIST

Clinically Relevant Pathologic Features
- Tissue distribution

Pathologic Interpretation Pearls
- Fibrocollagenous tissue
- Psammoma bodies
- Dystrophic calcifications
- Lymphoplasmacytic inflammatory reaction, focal

SELECTED REFERENCES

1. Shibata K et al: Multiple calcifying fibrous pseudotumors disseminated in the pleura. Ann Thorac Surg. 85(2):e3-5, 2008
2. Suh JH et al: Multiple calcifying fibrous pseudotumor of the pleura. J Thorac Oncol. 3(11):1356-8, 2008
3. Mito K et al: Multiple calcifying fibrous tumors of the pleura. Virchows Arch. 446(1):78-81, 2005
4. Jang KS et al: Calcifying fibrous pseudotumor of the pleura. Ann Thorac Surg. 78(6):e87-8, 2004
5. Soyer T et al: Calcifying fibrous pseudotumor of lung: a previously unreported entity. J Pediatr Surg. 39(11):1729-30, 2004
6. Ammar A et al: Calcifying fibrous pseudotumor of the pleura: a rare location. Ann Thorac Surg. 76(6):2081-2, 2003
7. Cavazza A et al: [Calcified pseudotumor of the pleura: description of a case.] Pathologica. 94(4):201-5, 2002
8. Pinkard NB et al: Calcifying fibrous pseudotumor of pleura. A report of three cases of a newly described entity involving the pleura. Am J Clin Pathol. 105(2):189-94, 1996

CALCIFIED FIBROUS PSEUDOTUMOR

Microscopic Features

*(**Left**) Calcifying pseudotumor of the pleura shows good circumscription from the lung parenchyma ⮫. The tumor is not encapsulated and has a rim of inflammatory infiltrate →. (**Right**) The presence of calcifications ⮫ may be very subtle. In some areas, there may only be a few, while in other areas there may be multiple.*

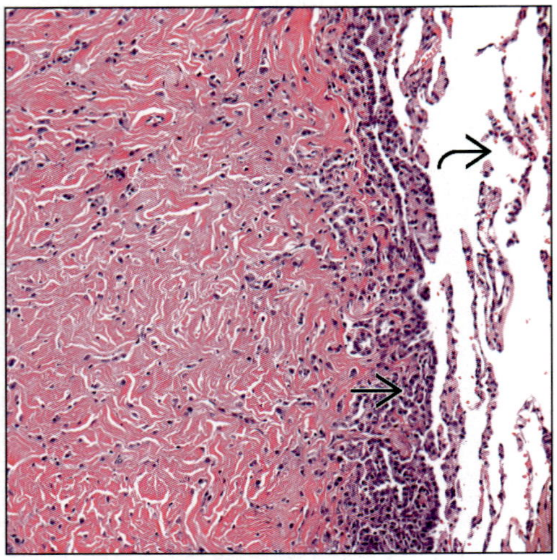

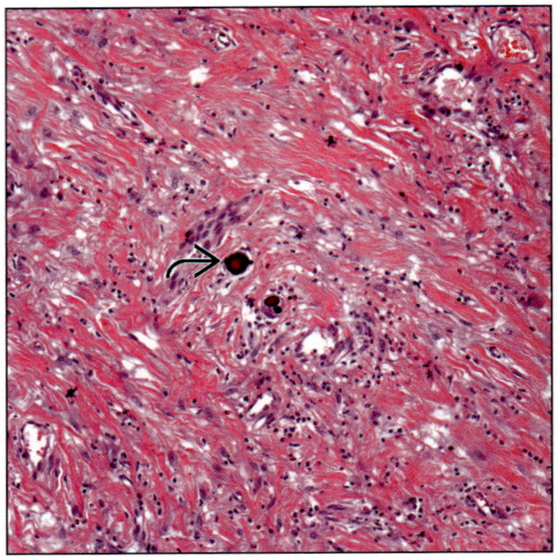

*(**Left**) Calcified fibrous pseudotumor shows extensive areas of hyalinization ⇨ with only focal areas of inflammatory reaction. This pattern could easily be confused with solitary fibrous tumor of the pleura. The presence of calcifications are important in arriving at a correct interpretation. (**Right**) High-power view of CFPT shows extensive hyalinization with a cluster of inflammatory cells, namely plasma cells →. Note the absence of calcifications in these areas.*

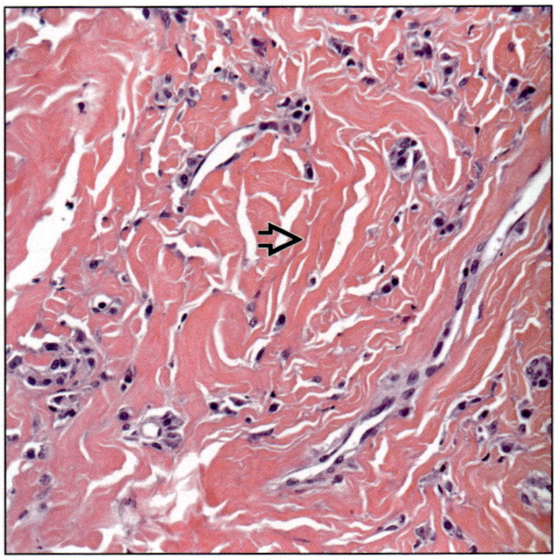

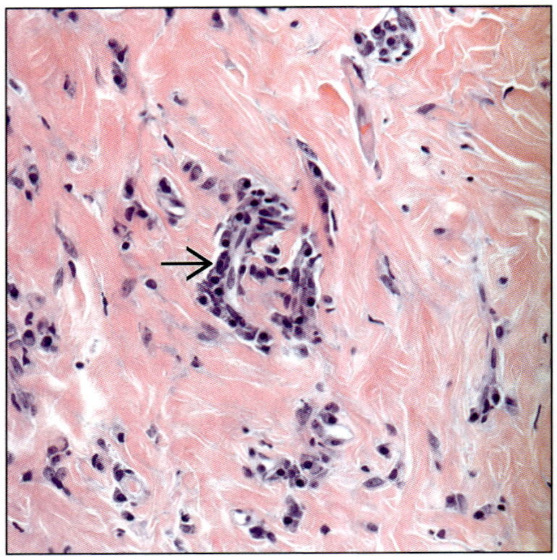

*(**Left**) Calcified fibrous pseudotumor shows collagenization with proliferation of small capillaries →. Very minimal inflammatory reaction is seen. This growth pattern may also be seen in cases of solitary fibrous tumors of the pleura. (**Right**) Extensive collagenization with little cellularity. Note the presence of a small calcification ⮫ and also the presence of dilated blood vessels.*

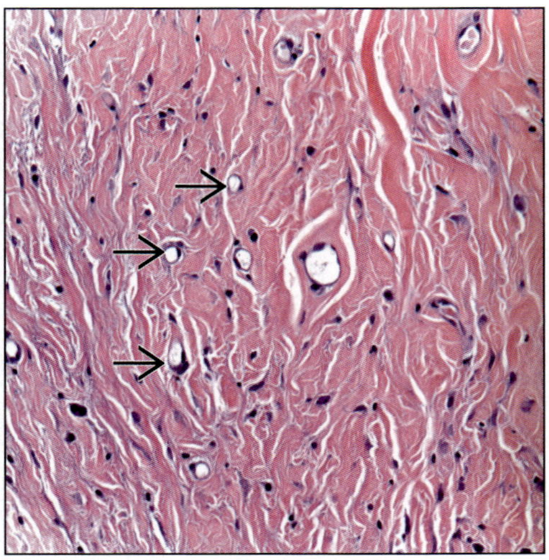

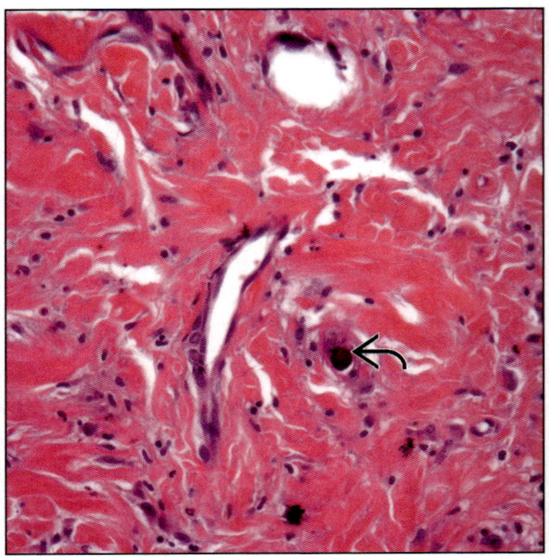

Microscopic Features

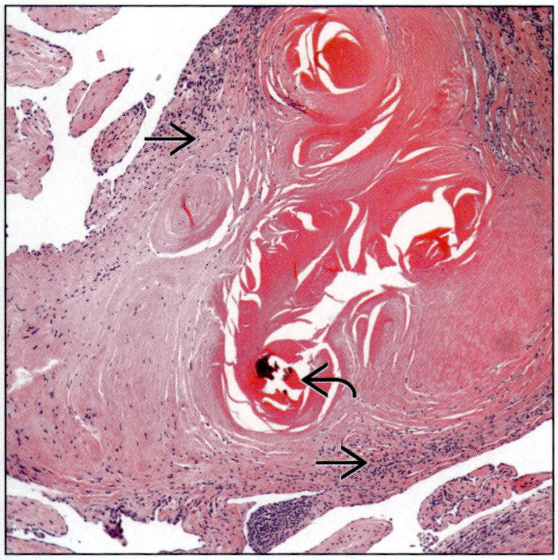

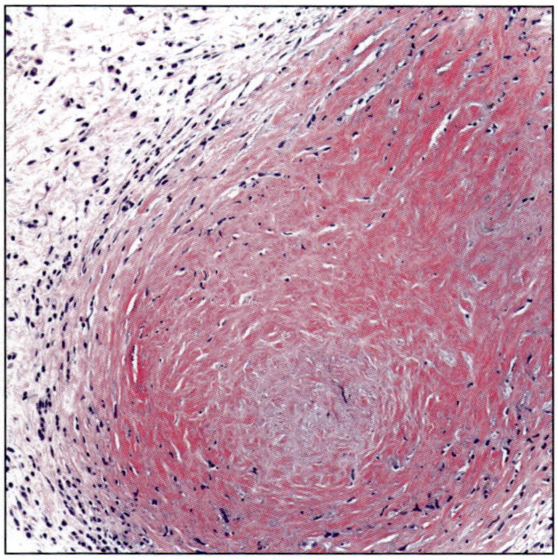

(Left) *Some cases may show extensive areas of collagenization with only focal calcifications ↪. Note the presence of a spindle cell proliferation →.* ***(Right)*** *In some other areas, there is only dense collagen deposition with no calcifications. The presence of calcifications is important for the diagnosis.*

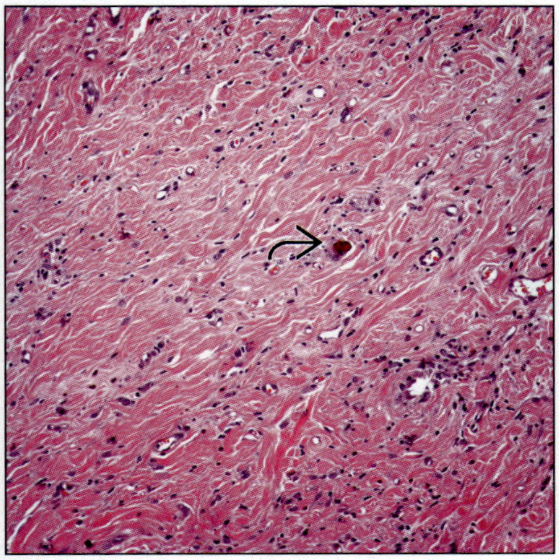

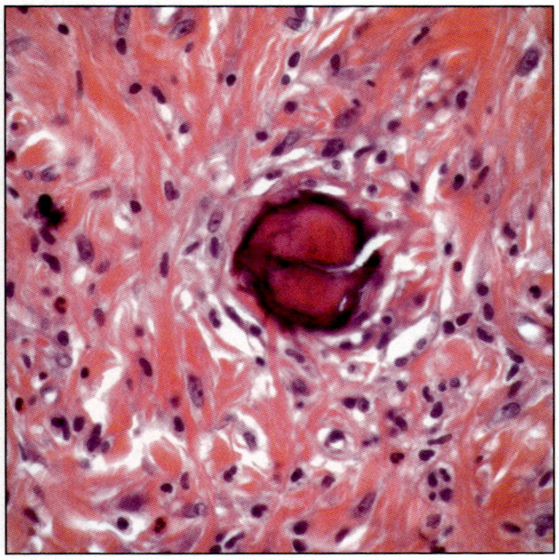

(Left) *Only a small calcification ↪ is present in this tumor. Otherwise, these features may be seen in other mesenchymal neoplasms, mainly solitary fibrous tumor.* ***(Right)*** *In this high-power view of a calcification in a calcified fibrous pseudotumor, the calcification is similar to those described as psammoma bodies, which can be seen in neoplastic and nonneoplastic conditions. However, in this setting it is diagnostic of CFPT.*

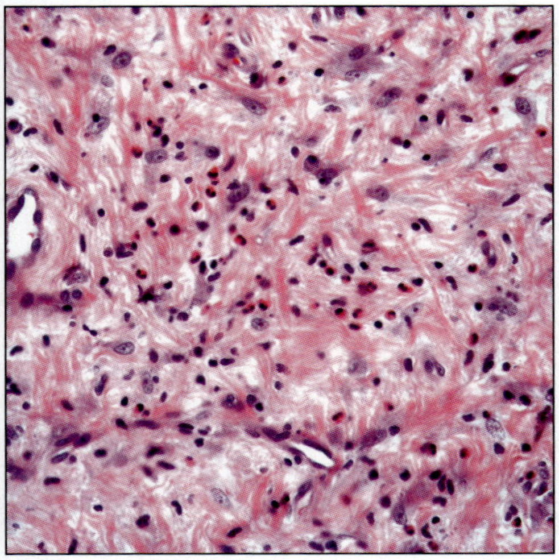

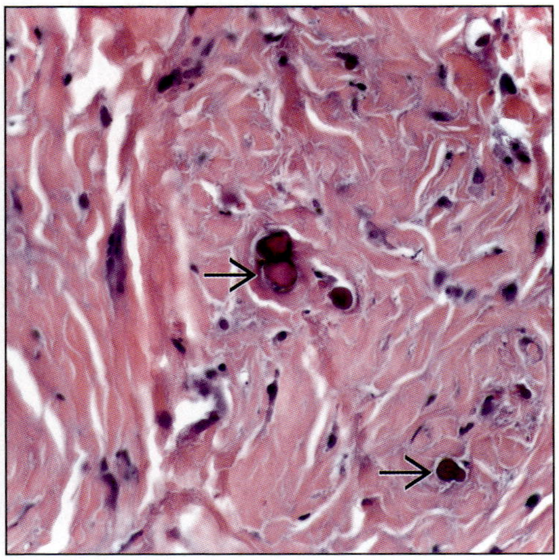

(Left) *Inflammatory reaction with presence of numerous eosinophils is commonly encountered in these tumors.* ***(Right)*** *In some cases of calcified fibrous pseudotumor of the pleura, the calcification may not be so obvious and large. In this case, the calcifications are rather small → and embedded in a collagenous stroma. These features are common in CFPT of the pleura.*

Neoplasms, Malignant, Primary

Epithelial Neoplasms

Pleural Mesothelioma Protocols

OVERVIEW OF MALIGNANT PLEURAL NEOPLASMS

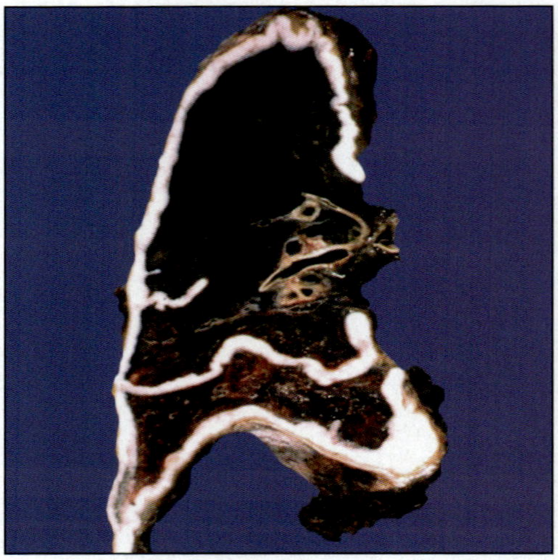

Cut section of the lung in a patient with malignant pleural mesothelioma shows a thick rind of whitish tumor tissue surrounding the outer surface of the lung and extending along the interlobar fissures.

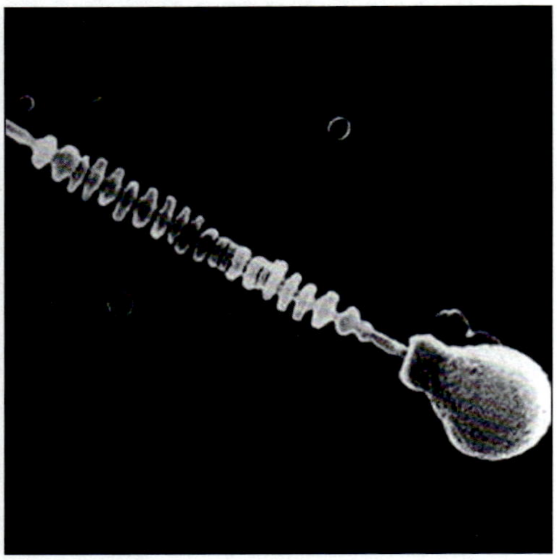

Scanning electron micrograph of an asbestos fiber measuring approximately 35 μm in length shows a bulb-shaped end attached to a longitudinal core with a beaded appearance.

TERMINOLOGY

Definitions

- Malignant pleural neoplasms may be primary or secondary
  - Primary malignant pleural neoplasms
    - Malignant mesothelioma (most common primary malignant pleural neoplasm)
    - Malignant lymphoma of pleura (primary effusion lymphoma and pyothorax-associated lymphoma)
    - Primary mesenchymal tumors of pleura
  - Secondary pleural neoplasms
    - Metastases to pleura are most common type of malignancy involving pleura
    - Metastases from lung carcinoma are most common type of secondary tumor of pleura
    - Other common types of pleural metastases include breast, kidney, gastrointestinal, and female genital tract cancer

ETIOLOGY/PATHOGENESIS

Etiology

- Occupational exposure to asbestos has been established as most important cause for development of malignant mesothelioma
  - Asbestos-related mesotheliomas are associated with long latency period (30-40 years)
  - Asbestos fiber types are associated with varying degrees of carcinogenicity
    - Amphiboles (amosite and crocidolite) are most potent ones; crocidolite is more dangerous of the 2
    - Chrysotile is the least potent carcinogen among asbestos fibers and associated with the lowest risk
- Syrian monkey virus (SV40) has been associated with development of mesothelioma in exposed individuals
  - SV40 induces breaks in human DNA strands in human mesothelial cells inactivating tumor suppressor *TP53* and *RB* genes
  - SV40 was found in contaminated polio vaccines during the 1950s and 1960s, spreading to millions of people
  - Role of latent infection with SV40 for causing malignant mesothelioma still remains to be established
- Other causes of mesothelioma include the non-asbestos fiber, erionite (found only in Cappadocia, Turkey), and ionizing radiation

EPIDEMIOLOGY

Age Range

- Malignant mesothelioma can occur in any age group, from children to adults
- Most prevalent in adults over 60 years of age

Gender

- Marked male predilection (in USA, male:female ratio is 9:1)

Incidence

- Incidence in men in USA is about 20 per 1,000,000 persons per year
- Incidence in women in USA is about 2-3 per 1,000,000 persons per year
- Incidence in other countries is higher; e.g., in Australia and UK it is about 50-60 per 1,000,000 persons per year

CLINICAL IMPLICATIONS

Clinical Presentation

- Most common presenting symptoms are recurrent pleural effusions, progressive dyspnea, and chest pain

- Constitutional symptoms include malaise, weight loss, weakness, and fatigue

Clinical Risk Factors

- Certain occupations are associated with higher risk of exposure to asbestos
  - Workers in shipyard industry
  - Workers in insulation and heating trades and construction workers
  - Workers in mining and milling industry of asbestos
- Marked increase in incidence is observed when risk factors are combined with cigarette smoking

Staging

- AJCC (7th edition) pathologic staging
  - Primary tumor (T)
    - TX: Primary tumor cannot be assessed
    - T0: No evidence of primary tumor
    - T1: Tumor limited to ipsilateral parietal pleura ± mediastinal or diaphragmatic pleural involvement
    - T1a: No involvement of visceral pleura
    - T1b: Tumor also involving visceral pleura
    - T2: Tumor involving each of the ipsilateral pleural surfaces with at least involvement of diaphragm or of underlying lung parenchyma
    - T3: Locally advanced but potentially resectable tumor involving all ipsilateral pleural surfaces and extension into fat, fascia, chest wall, or pericardium
    - T4: Locally advanced and technically unresectable tumor with extension through chest wall, diaphragm, mediastinum, spine, pericardium
  - Regional lymph nodes (N)
    - NX: Regional lymph nodes cannot be assessed
    - N0: No regional lymph node metastases
    - N1: Metastases in ipsilateral bronchopulmonary or hilar lymph nodes
    - N2: Metastases in subcarinal or ipsilateral mediastinal lymph nodes (including internal mammary and peridiaphragmatic nodes)
    - N3: Metastases in contralateral mediastinal or internal mammary nodes and ipsilateral or contralateral supraclavicular lymph nodes
  - Metastases (M)
    - M0: No distant metastases
    - M1: Distant metastases

Prognostic Factors

- Histologic type
  - Pure epithelioid mesothelioma is associated with slightly better outcome
  - Sarcomatoid and biphasic mesotheliomas are associated with more aggressive course
- Presenting symptoms (chest pain, dyspnea, and weight loss) are associated with worse prognosis
- Younger age at presentation, low stage, and good performance status are associated with better prognosis

MACROSCOPIC FINDINGS

General Features

- Pleural mesothelioma shows a tendency to spread along pleural surface
  - Initial manifestation may be as multiple tiny nodules studding visceral or parietal pleura
  - Over time, nodules enlarge and become confluent, forming plaques and larger nodules
  - In more advanced stages, entire pleural surface is covered by a rind of tumor that may vary in thickness
  - Tumor tends to invade pleural fissures and infiltrate surface of lung parenchyma
  - Tumor eventually spreads to regional and intrathoracic lymph nodes
  - Invasion of chest wall fat and muscle is characteristic
  - Spread through diaphragm can occasionally occur, leading to seeding of peritoneal cavity, and ascites
- Rarely, mesothelioma may grow as a localized, sharply circumscribed mass, termed localized malignant mesothelioma
  - Such tumors are generally associated with better prognosis

MICROSCOPIC FINDINGS

General Features

- Malignant mesothelioma is divided histopathologically into epithelioid, sarcomatoid, and mixed (biphasic) types
- Special histologic variants of mesothelioma include desmoplastic, lymphohistiocytic, and deciduoid types
- Well-differentiated papillary mesothelioma is distinct variant with papillary architecture and absence of invasion and indolent behavior

Molecular Genetic Alterations

- Inactivation of *CDKN2A/ARF* locus at 9p21 leading to loss of p16 expression is a frequent finding
- Deletions at 3p21 is common in epithelioid mesothelioma but rare in sarcomatoid and biphasic tumors

SELECTED REFERENCES

1. Campbell NP et al: Update on malignant pleural mesothelioma. Semin Respir Crit Care Med. 32(1):102-10, 2011
2. Kao SC et al: Molecular biomarkers in malignant mesothelioma: state of the art. Pathology. 43(3):201-12, 2011
3. Suster S et al: Malignant mesothelioma: current status of histopathologic diagnosis and molecular profile. Expert Rev Mol Diagn. 5(5):715-23, 2005

MALIGNANT MESOTHELIOMA

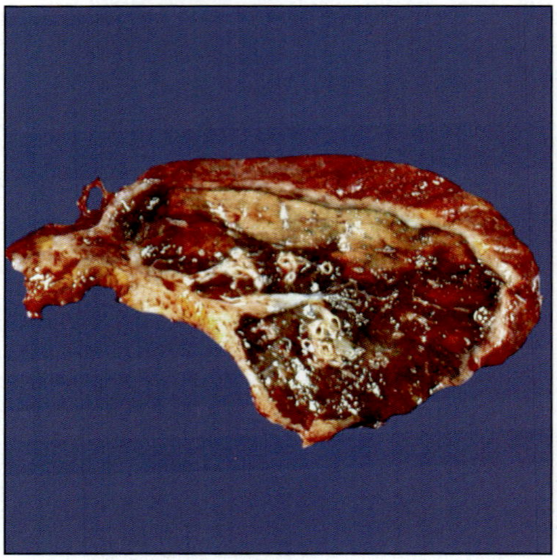

Extrapulmonary pneumonectomy consisting of both visceral and parietal pleuras, lung, and portions of diaphragm and pericardium is shown. Note the marked pleural thickening.

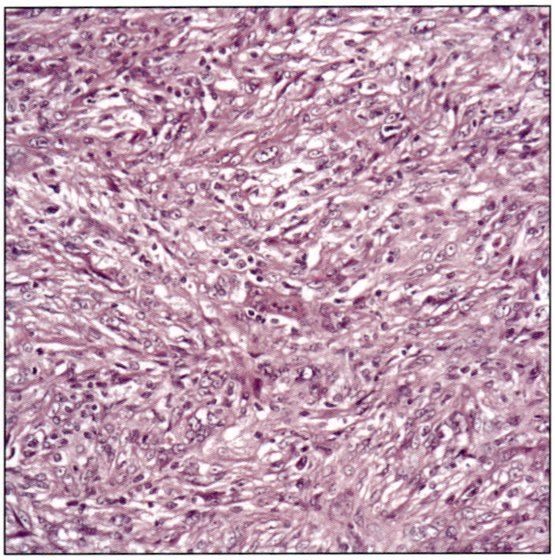

Sarcomatoid malignant mesothelioma shows a spindle cell proliferation closely mimicking the features of a mesenchymal neoplasm.

TERMINOLOGY

Synonyms

- Epithelioma
  - Term used in older literature

Definitions

- Malignant neoplasm arising in serosal surfaces

ETIOLOGY/PATHOGENESIS

Environmental Exposure

- Mesotheliomas have been linked closely to asbestos exposure

Other Possible Etiologies

- Viral infection SV40
- De novo

CLINICAL ISSUES

Epidemiology

- Incidence
  - Rare tumor that accounts for approximately 4-7 cases per 1,000,000 individuals
- Age
  - More common in 5th and 6th decades of life
- Gender
  - More common in men

Presentation

- Weight loss
- Chest pain
- Cough
- Shortness of breath
- Pleural effusion

Treatment

- Surgical approaches
  - Extrapulmonary pneumonectomy
  - Decortication
  - Pleural peeling
- Adjuvant therapy
  - Chemotherapy

Prognosis

- Poor
  - 12-18 month average survival

MACROSCOPIC FEATURES

General Features

- Diffuse thickening of pleura
- In rare cases, tumor will present as localized pleural-based tumor

MICROSCOPIC PATHOLOGY

Histologic Features

- Homogeneous cellular proliferation without much mitotic activity or cellular pleomorphism

Predominant Pattern/Injury Type

- Tubulo-papillary
- Sarcomatoid
- Biphasic

Predominant Cell/Compartment Type

- Epithelial
- Spindle

Other Growth Patterns

- Clear cell
  - This pattern is characterized by presence of cellular proliferation in which cells show clear cytoplasm
  - Low mitotic count
  - Most of these tumors do not show extensive areas of necrosis
- Deciduoid

Key Facts

Etiology/Pathogenesis

- Mesotheliomas have been linked closely to asbestos exposure

Clinical Issues

- Rare tumor that accounts for approximately 4-7 cases per 1,000,000 individuals
- Tumor is more common in 5th & 6th decades of life
- Weight loss
- Chest pain
- General malaise
- Extrapulmonary pneumonectomy
- Decortication
- More common in men

Microscopic Pathology

- Tubulo-papillary
- Sarcomatoid
- Biphasic
- Clear cell
- Deciduoid
- Adenomatoid
- Glandular
- Mucohyaline
- Cartilaginous and osseous metaplasia
- Desmoplastic
- Lymphohistiocytic

Top Differential Diagnoses

- Adenocarcinoma
- Sarcoma
- Synovial sarcoma

    - This pattern is composed of medium-sized cells with excentric nuclei and inconspicuous nucleoli
    - Low mitotic count
    - Necrosis and prominent nuclear atypia are not common
- Adenomatoid
    - Cords of neoplastic cells forming cystic spaces
    - Signet ring cell-like
    - Low mitotic count
    - Areas of necrosis or hemorrhage are not common
- Glandular
    - Prominent glandular component
    - Glands of different sizes
    - Most closely mimics adenocarcinoma
- Mucohyaline
    - Extensive pools of mucoid material
    - Neoplastic cells embedded or floating in pools of mucoid material
- Cartilaginous and osseous metaplasia
    - Very unusual growth pattern
    - Tumor shows extensive areas of cartilaginous or osseous differentiation
    - Numerous osteoclast giant cells
- Desmoplastic
    - Low cellularity
    - Easily mistaken for a benign tumor
    - Neoplastic cells, either spindle or oval, dissecting fibrocollagen
    - Areas of necrosis are not readily apparent
- Lymphohistiocytic
    - Mixture of epithelioid cells, lymphocytes, and histiocytes
    - May mimic thymoma or lymphoma

ANCILLARY TESTS

Electron Microscopy

- Transmission
    - Elongated microvilli
    - Well-developed cell junctions

DIFFERENTIAL DIAGNOSIS

Metastatic Adenocarcinoma

- Shows positive staining for carcinomatous epitopes, including CEA, MOC31, and BER-EP4
- History of primary tumor elsewhere is important

Sarcoma

- Sarcomas encasing lung parenchyma are rather unusual
- It would be unusual for mesothelioma to stain with mesenchymal markers other than vimentin
- Clinical history is important to rule out a metastasis

Synovial Sarcoma

- Either mono- or biphasic tumors may mimic mesothelioma
- Monophasic tumors will show positive staining for Bcl-2, which would be unusual in mesothelioma
- Synovial sarcoma shows characteristic X;18 translocation

Thymoma

- In cases of lymphohistiocytic mesothelioma
    - Use of immunohistochemical studies show strong p63(+) in thymoma
- Although thymomas may occur as pleural tumors, they are more common in anterior mediastinum

Metastatic Clear Cell Carcinoma

- In cases of clear cell mesothelioma
    - Use of immunohistochemical studies will lead to correct interpretation

Metastatic Osteogenic Sarcoma

- In cases of mesothelioma with osseous and cartilaginous components
    - Clinical history of previous osteosarcoma will be necessary for correct diagnosis

MALIGNANT MESOTHELIOMA

Immunohistochemistry

Antibody	Reactivity	Staining Pattern	Comment
CK-PAN	Positive	Cytoplasmic	
CK5/6	Positive	Cytoplasmic	In epithelioid neoplasms; also positive in squamous cell carcinomas
Calretinin	Positive	Nuclear & cytoplasmic	In epithelioid neoplasms/focally in sarcomatoid
HBME-1	Positive	Cytoplasmic	Also positive in carcinomas
WT1	Positive	Nuclear	Also positive in carcinomas
Thrombomodulin	Positive	Cytoplasmic	Also positive in carcinomas
Mesothelin	Positive	Cell membrane	Also positive in carcinomas
CEA-M	Negative		
CD15	Negative		
EpCAM/BER-EP4/ CD326	Negative		In 27% of mesotheliomas, it may be positive
MOC-31	Negative		May be seen focally positive in some mesotheliomas
TTF-1	Negative		

Histochemical Features of Mesothelioma

Stain	Reactivity
Periodic acid-Schiff (PAS)	Positive
Periodic acid-Schiff after diastase (D-PAS)	Negative
Mucicarmine	Negative
Iron	Identifies ferruginous bodies in lung parenchyma

DIAGNOSTIC CHECKLIST

Clinically Relevant Pathologic Features

- Invasive pattern
  - Penetration of tumor cells into fat

SELECTED REFERENCES

1. Arrossi AV et al: Histologic assessment and prognostic factors of malignant pleural mesothelioma treated with extrapleural pneumonectomy. Am J Clin Pathol. 130(5):754-64, 2008
2. Borasio P et al: Malignant pleural mesothelioma: clinicopathologic and survival characteristics in a consecutive series of 394 patients. Eur J Cardiothorac Surg. 33(2):307-13, 2008
3. Flores RM et al: Extrapleural pneumonectomy versus pleurectomy/decortication in the surgical management of malignant pleural mesothelioma: results in 663 patients. J Thorac Cardiovasc Surg. 135(3):620-6, 626, 2008
4. Klebe S et al: Malignant mesothelioma with heterologous elements: clinicopathological correlation of 27 cases and literature review. Mod Pathol. 21(9):1084-94, 2008
5. Miles SE et al: Clinical consequences of asbestos-related diffuse pleural thickening: A review. J Occup Med Toxicol. 3:20, 2008
6. Schipper PH et al: Malignant pleural mesothelioma: surgical management in 285 patients. Ann Thorac Surg. 85(1):257-64; discussion 264, 2008
7. Suster S et al: Applications and limitations of immunohistochemistry in the diagnosis of malignant mesothelioma. Adv Anat Pathol. 13(6):316-29, 2006
8. Wick MR et al: Immunohistochemical differential diagnosis of pleural effusions, with emphasis on malignant mesothelioma. Curr Opin Pulm Med. 7(4):187-92, 2001
9. Moran CA et al: The role of immunohistochemistry in the diagnosis of malignant mesothelioma. Semin Diagn Pathol. 17(3):178-83, 2000
10. Ordóñez NG: Epithelial mesothelioma with deciduoid features: report of four cases. Am J Surg Pathol. 24(6):816-23, 2000
11. Ordóñez NG: In search of a positive immunohistochemical marker for mesothelioma: an update. Adv Anat Pathol. 5(1):53-60, 1998
12. Ordóñez NG: Value of cytokeratin 5/6 immunostaining in distinguishing epithelial mesothelioma of the pleura from lung adenocarcinoma. Am J Surg Pathol. 22(10):1215-21, 1998
13. Ordóñez NG et al: Clear cell mesothelioma. Ultrastruct Pathol. 20(4):331-6, 1996
14. Henderson DW et al: Lymphohistiocytoid mesothelioma: a rare lymphomatoid variant of predominantly sarcomatoid mesothelioma. Ultrastruct Pathol. 12(4):367-84, 1988
15. Yousem SA et al: Malignant mesotheliomas with osseous and cartilaginous differentiation. Arch Pathol Lab Med. 111(1):62-6, 1987

Sarcomatoid (Spindle Cell) Mesothelioma

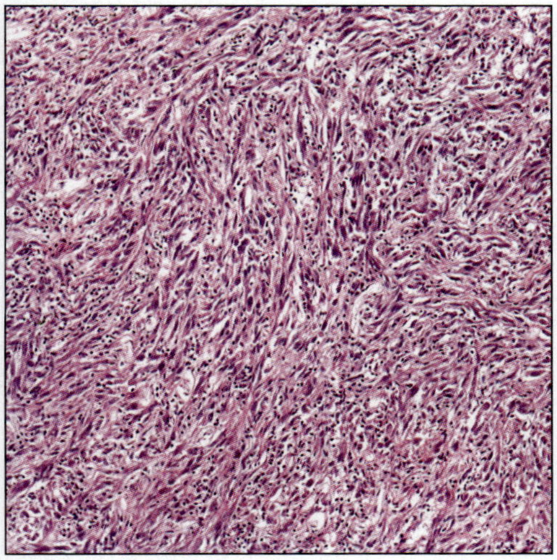
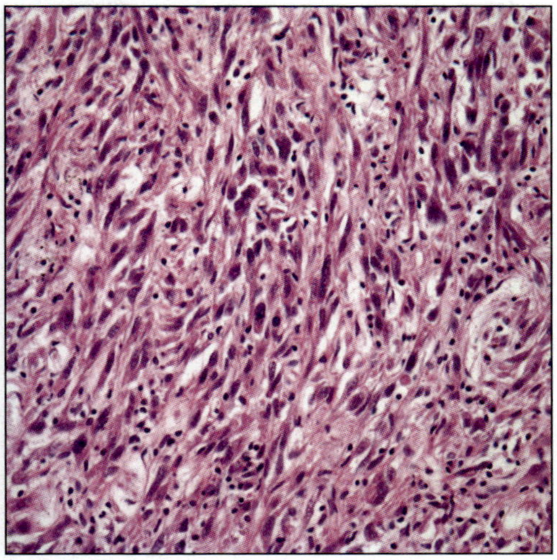

*(**Left**) Intermediate-power view shows the spindle cellular proliferation with a vague storiform pattern, admixed with inflammatory cells. This pattern is indistinguishable from any other high-grade sarcoma. (**Right**) Higher magnification shows spindle cells with marked cellular atypia and scattered mitotic figures. This pattern closely mimics any pleomorphic sarcoma or malignant fibrous histiocytoma.*

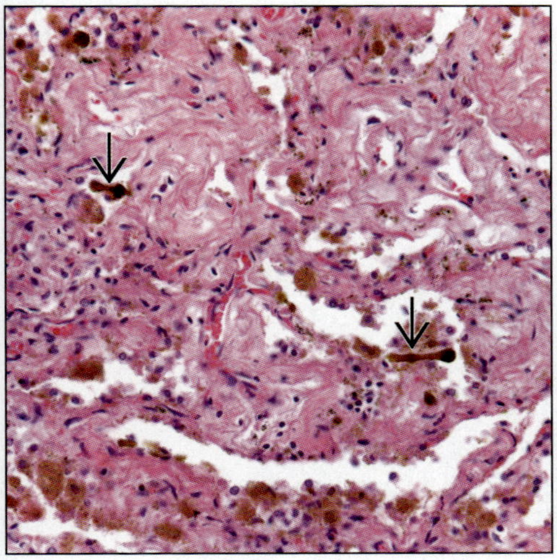
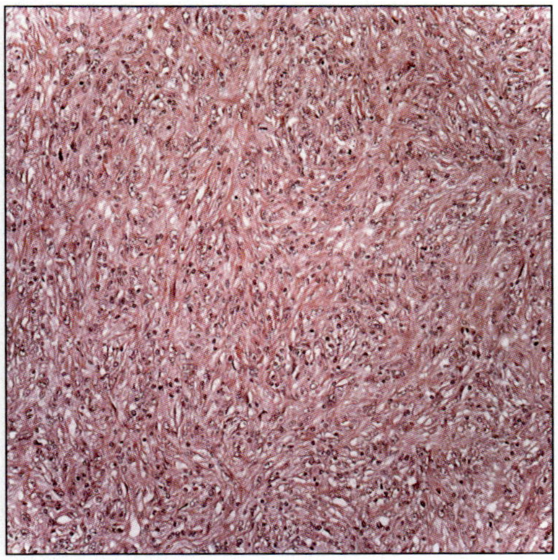

*(**Left**) Adjacent lung parenchyma shows numerous ferruginous bodies →. In many cases, these structures can be easily identified with conventional H&E stains. However, in cases in which these structures are not readily recognizable, the use of iron histochemical stains is recommended. (**Right**) Sarcomatoid mesothelioma shows more bland spindle cell proliferation admixed with inflammatory cells. This growth pattern is reminiscent of fibrosarcoma.*

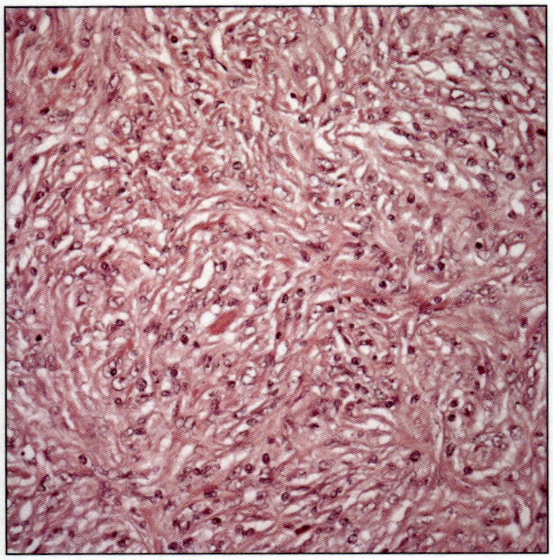
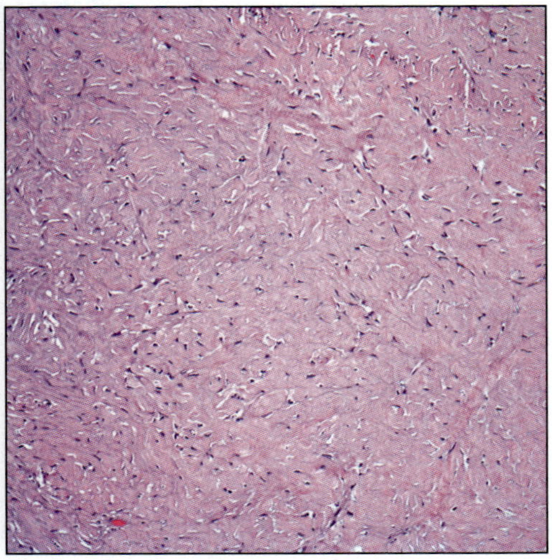

*(**Left**) Sarcomatoid mesothelioma is shown with desmoplastic features. In a cursory evaluation, this tumor can be easily confused for a benign fibrous pleurisy. Careful review of the histology usually leads to a correct interpretation. However, in some cases the cellularity may be scant. (**Right**) Desmoplastic mesothelioma shows prominent hyalinized stroma with only minimal cellular proliferation. On cursory review, this type of mesothelioma can be easily misdiagnosed.*

MALIGNANT MESOTHELIOMA

Microscopic Features

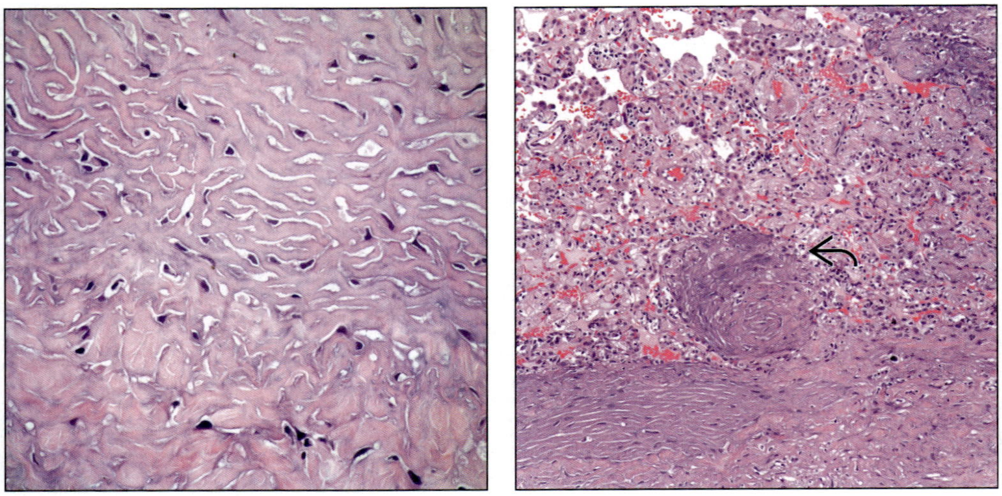

(Left) *Closer magnification of a desmoplastic mesothelioma shows abundant collagen deposition with a subtle spindle cell component. However, there is no evidence of nuclear atypia or mitotic activity.* ***(Right)*** *One additional feature that may be helpful in the diagnosis of desmoplastic mesothelioma is the penetration of the tumor into adipose tissue or into lung parenchyma as is illustrated here ↶.*

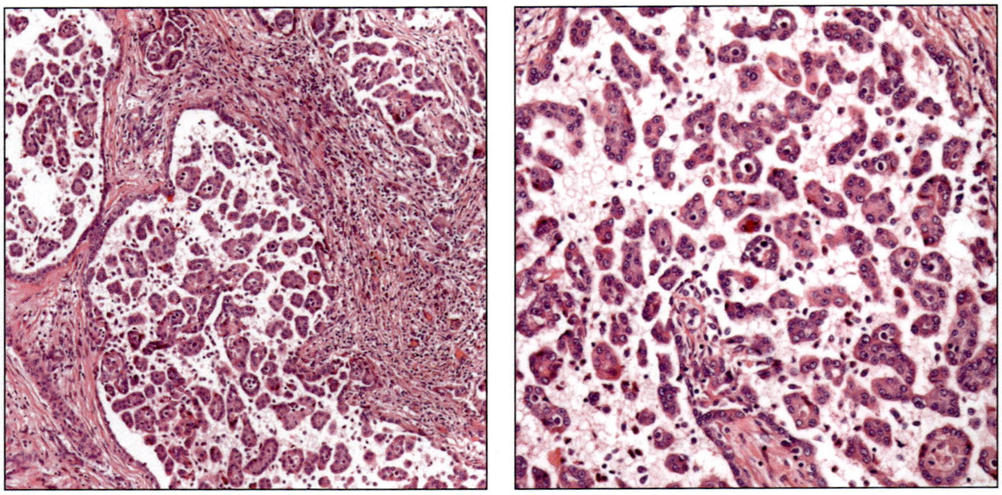

(Left) *Epithelioid malignant mesothelioma on intermediate-power view shows the presence of a papillary tumor dissecting areas of fibroconnective tissue. This histological growth pattern should raise the suspicion of malignant mesothelioma.* ***(Right)*** *Higher magnification shows tumor cells arranged in small papillary projections. Note the presence of a homogeneous cellular proliferation without much nuclear atypia or mitotic figures.*

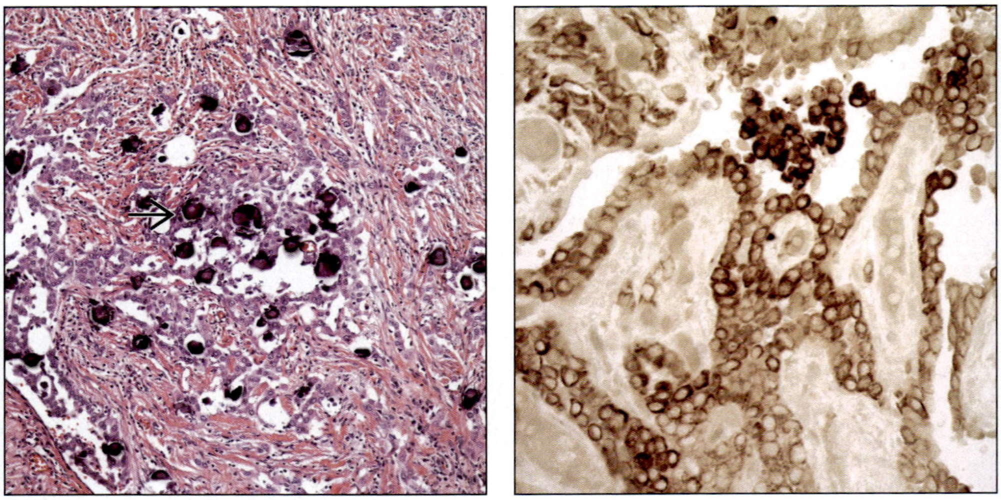

(Left) *Higher magnification shows psammoma bodies closely admixed with neoplastic cells. In the tubulo-papillary growth pattern, it is common to identify psammoma bodies →. However, these calcifications may be seen in calcifying fibrous pseudotumor of the pleura.* ***(Right)*** *Immunohistochemical study for CK5/6 shows strong positive staining in tumor cells.*

Microscopic Features

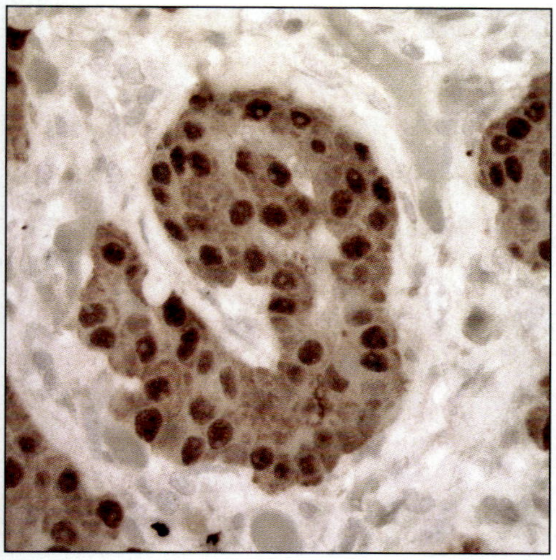

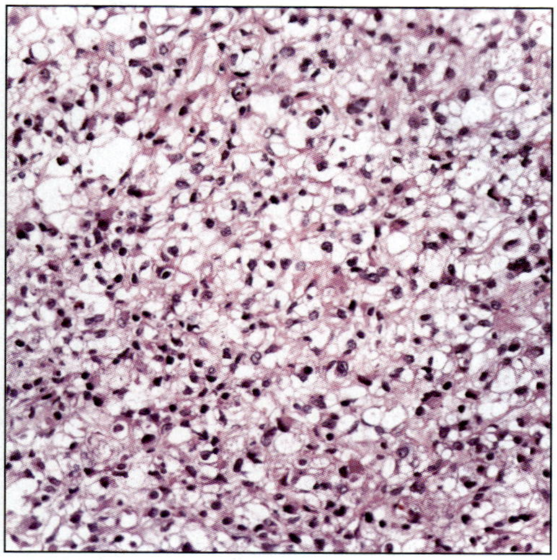

(Left) Calretinin and keratin 5/6 are commonly used in the work-up of mesothelioma, and their interpretation should be performed taking into account the results of other carcinomatous epitopes. *(Right)* High magnification of a malignant mesothelioma shows prominent clear cells with round to oval nuclei and clear cytoplasm. This pattern can mimic metastatic renal cell carcinoma.

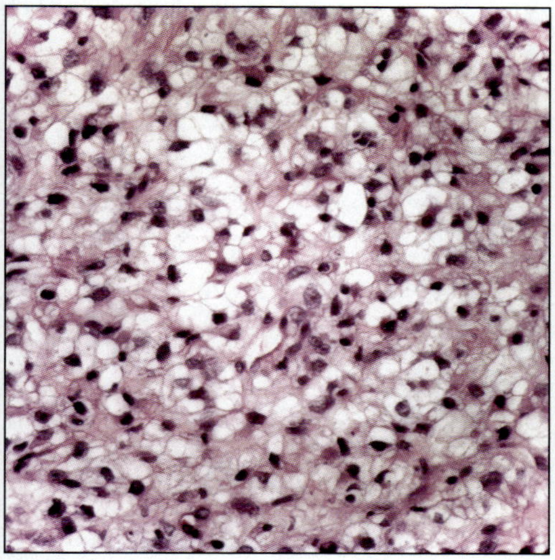

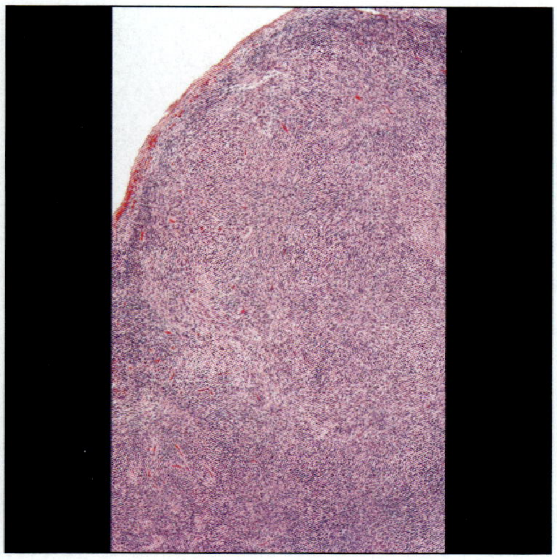

(Left) A closer view shows malignant cells with clear cytoplasm and round nuclei. Note the absence of cellular pleomorphism and mitotic activity. Similar features may be seen in metastatic carcinomas of renal or thyroid origin. *(Right)* Low-power view of a lymphohistiocytoid mesothelioma shows a dense atypical cellular proliferation, which at this power mimics a benign lesion.

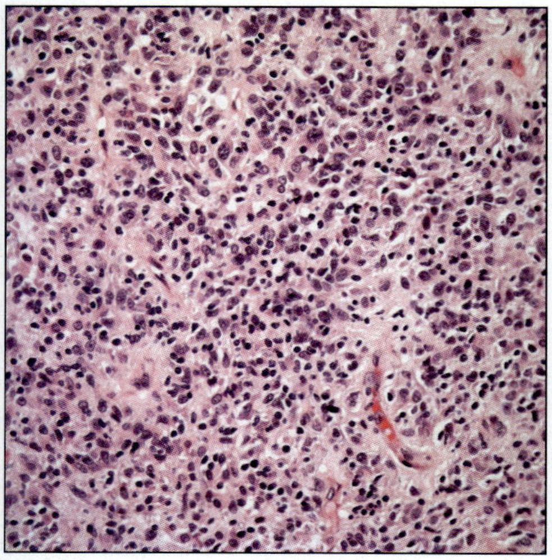

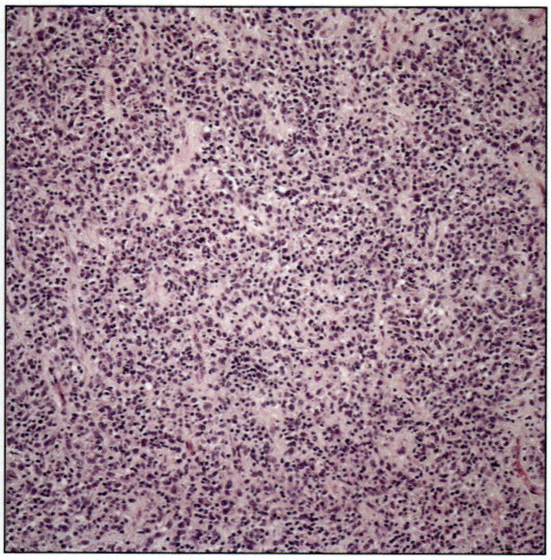

(Left) High-power view clearly shows the presence of epithelioid cells admixed with lymphocytes, giving the impression of a lymphohistiocytic type of proliferation. Similar features may be seen in pleural thymomas. *(Right)* Intermediate-power view shows a mixture of epithelioid cells and lymphocytes distributed in a diffuse pattern. At this power, this is indistinguishable from cases of thymoma; therefore, close analysis of the histology and IHC is recommended.

MALIGNANT MESOTHELIOMA

Microscopic Features

*(**Left**) Intermediate magnification shows a tumor composed of spindle cells, osteoid →, and cartilage ↷. This is the so-called mesothelioma with osseous and cartilaginous differentiation. (**Right**) Higher magnification shows the presence of osteoid ↷ and cartilage → admixed with spindle cells. This variant of mesothelioma can be easily confused with metastasis from skeletal osteosarcoma.*

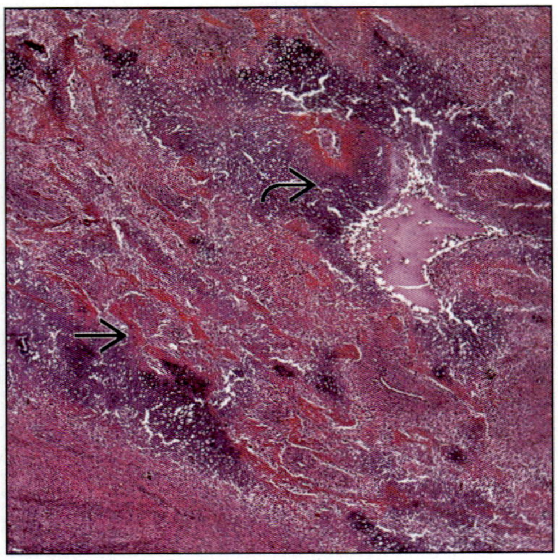

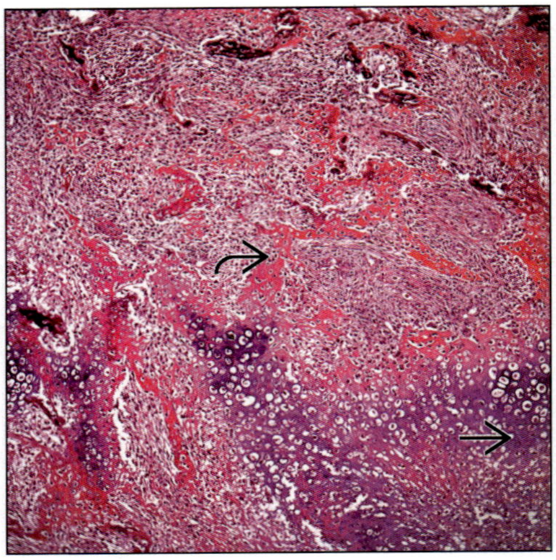

*(**Left**) Intermediate-power view of a malignant mesothelioma shows neoplastic cells with areas of necrosis. These morphologic features have also been referred to as "transitional mesothelioma." (**Right**) High-power view shows pleomorphic cells with marked nuclear atypia and scattered mitotic figures. Although the features are of an epithelioid mesothelioma, often these tumors are difficult to classify.*

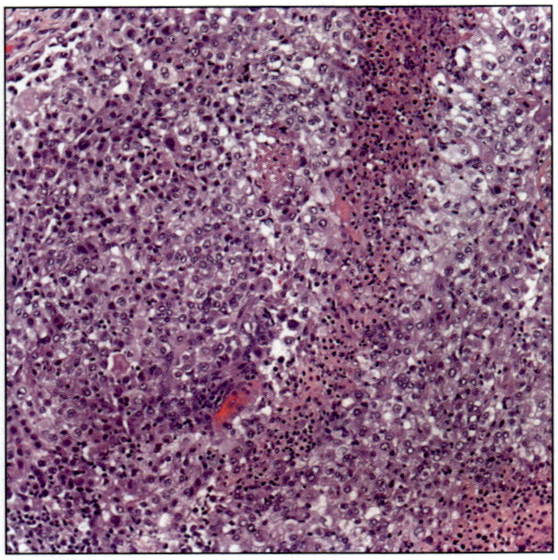

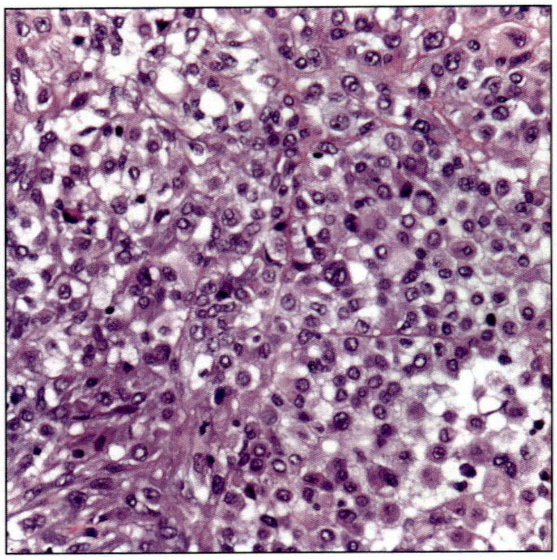

*(**Left**) Intermediate-power view shows a malignant mesothelioma with prominent mucinous component and neoplastic cells floating in pools of mucin →. Because of the presence of extensive areas of mucoid deposition, this tumor may be confused with adenocarcinomas. (**Right**) High-power view shows a mesothelioma with extensive extracellular deposition of mucoid material. Note the presence of clusters of neoplastic cells of mesothelial origin → floating in the pools of mucin.*

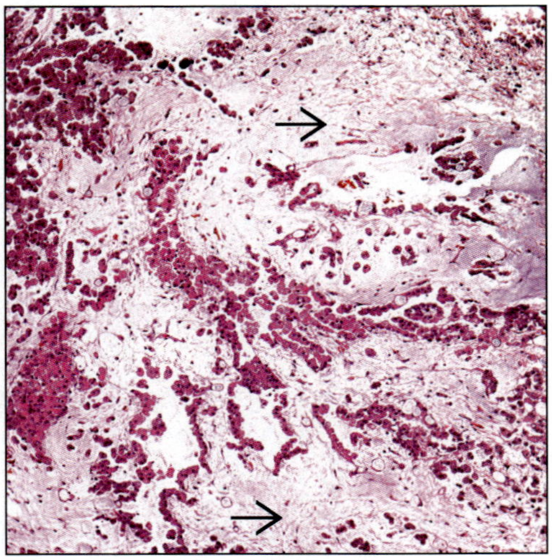

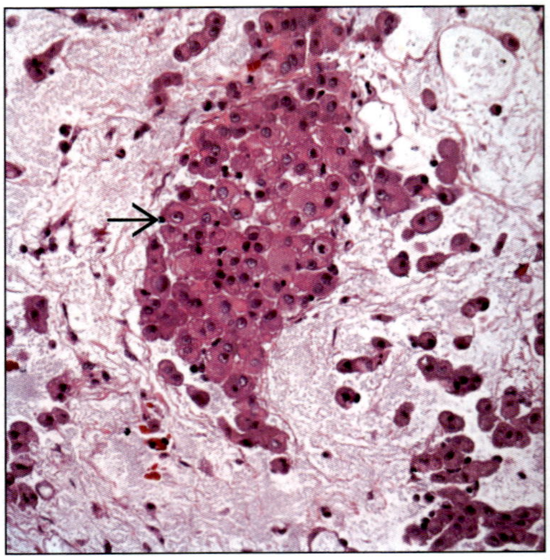

Microscopic Features

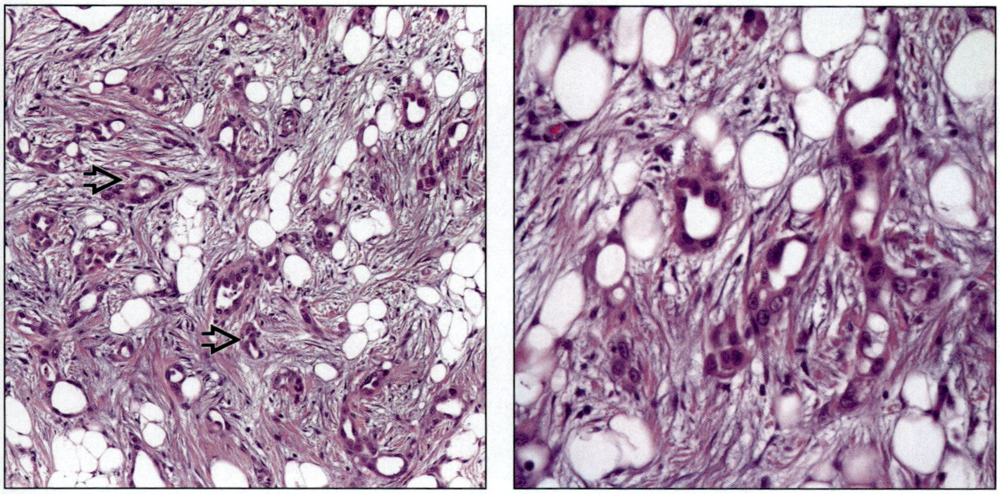

(Left) Higher magnification of glandular proliferation ⇨ involving fibroconnective and adipose tissue in a malignant mesothelioma is shown. **(Right)** Higher magnification shows malignant glands with minimal cytological atypia and virtual absence of mitotic activity. This pattern mimics an adenomatoid tumor, and care must be used in not confusing this pattern with a benign adenomatoid tumor.

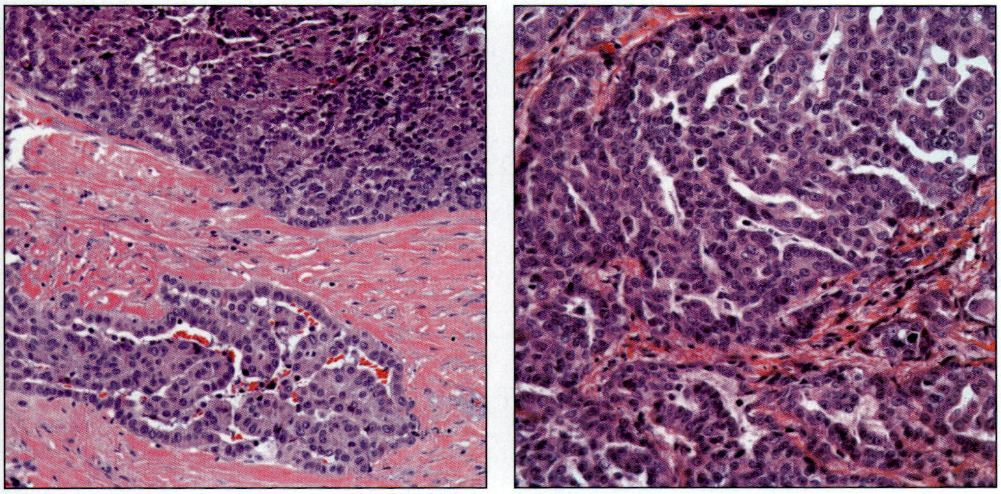

(Left) High-power view of a malignant mesothelioma shows a homogeneous cellular proliferation with absence of mitotic activity and nuclear pleomorphism. This is one of the most common histological growth patterns of malignant mesothelioma. **(Right)** Low-power view shows a neoplastic cellular proliferation arranged in short papillary projections and tubules. Note the absence of marked nuclear atypia or mitotic activity.

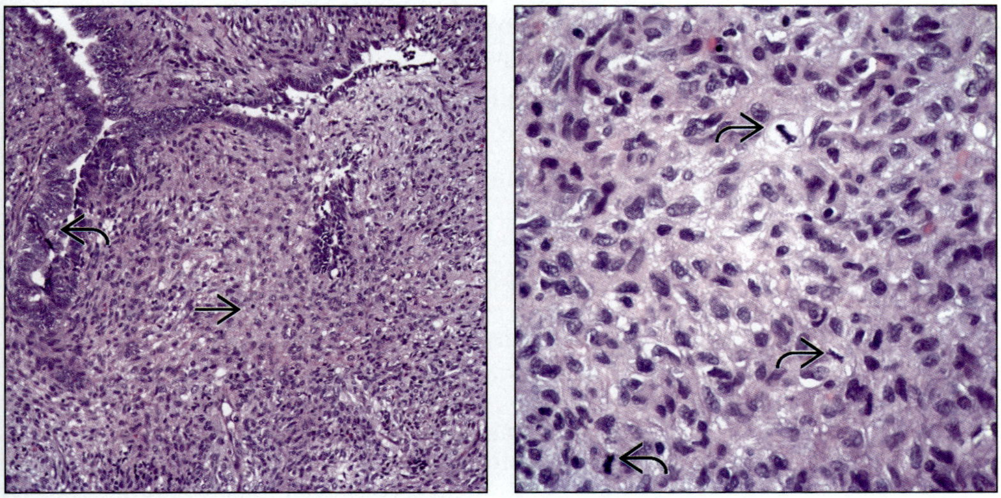

(Left) Biphasic malignant mesothelioma shows 2 distinct components: Epithelioid ↪ and sarcomatoid →. In some cases, the epithelioid component may be minimal, and the tumor may have a predominant sarcomatoid component. **(Right)** Closer magnification of the sarcomatoid component in a biphasic mesothelioma. Note the presence of prominent cellular and nuclear atypia. Mitotic figures are easily identified ↪.

PSEUDOMESOTHELIOMATOUS ADENOCARCINOMA

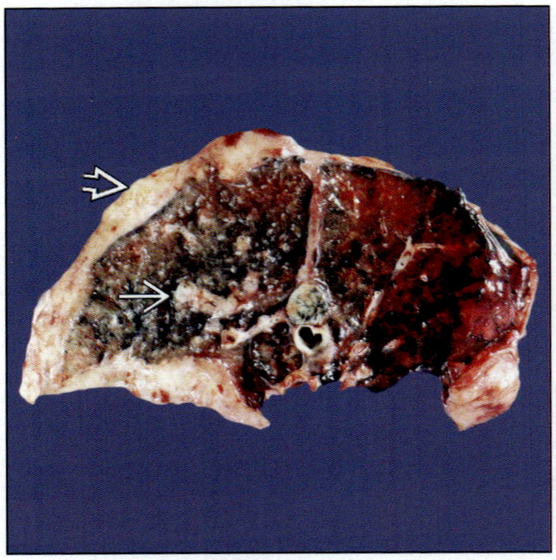

In this pseudomesotheliomatous adenocarcinoma, note the presence of diffuse pleural thickening ➡, as well as the presence of distinct intrapulmonary nodules ➡.

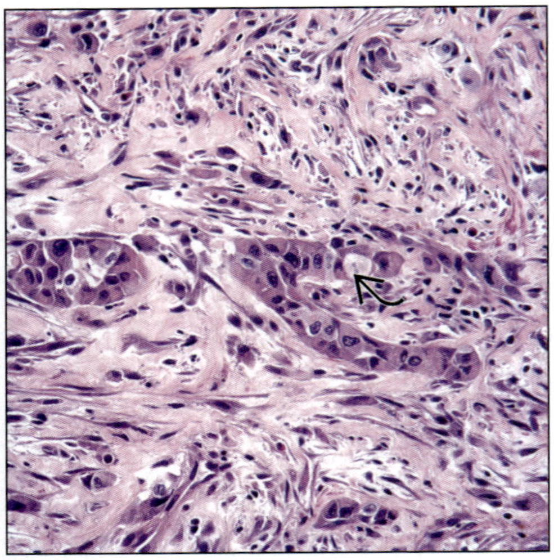

Malignant glands are invading fibroconnective tissue of the pleura. Note the presence of malignant cells, some of them showing intracytoplasmic mucin ➡.

TERMINOLOGY

Definitions

- Malignant epithelial neoplasm of lung origin growing along pleural surface

ETIOLOGY/PATHOGENESIS

Environmental Exposure

- Has been linked to the following
  - Tobacco smoke
  - Asbestos exposure
  - Iron exposure
  - Stone dust exposure

CLINICAL ISSUES

Epidemiology

- Incidence
  - Tumor of rare occurrence
- Age
  - Majority of patients are > 50 years old
- Gender
  - Tumor may be more common in men

Presentation

- Cough
- Shortness of breath
- Chest pain
- Weight loss
- Pleural effusion

Treatment

- Adjuvant therapy
  - Chemotherapy

Prognosis

- Poor with survival of < 18 months

IMAGE FINDINGS

General Features

- Tumor mimics radiographic findings of mesothelioma

MACROSCOPIC FEATURES

General Features

- Thickening of pleura
- Encasement of lung parenchyma
- Tumor growth along pulmonary septum
- Discrete peripheral intrapulmonary tumor

MICROSCOPIC PATHOLOGY

Histologic Features

- Glandular formation
- Desmoplastic reaction
- Papillary pattern in some cases
- Cellular atypia
- Mitotic figures

Predominant Pattern/Injury Type

- Infiltrative

Predominant Cell/Compartment Type

- Epithelial

DIFFERENTIAL DIAGNOSIS

Mesothelioma, Epithelioid Type

- Both tumors may shows similar histopathological features
- Histochemical studies are important (DPAS and mucicarmine)
- Immunohistochemistry: Carcinomatous epitopes positive (CEA-M, TAG72, MOC-31, CD15, TTF-1)

PSEUDOMESOTHELIOMATOUS ADENOCARCINOMA

Key Facts

Terminology

- Malignant epithelial neoplasm of lung origin growing along pleural surface

Etiology/Pathogenesis

- Has been linked to the following
  - Tobacco use
  - Asbestos exposure
  - Iron exposure
  - Stone dust exposure

Clinical Issues

- Cough
- Shortness of breath
- Chest pain
- Weight loss
- Pleural effusion

Macroscopic Features

- Thickening of pleura
- Encasement of lung parenchyma
- Tumor growth along pulmonary septum
- Discrete peripheral intrapulmonary tumor

Microscopic Pathology

- Glandular formation
- Desmoplastic reaction
- Papillary pattern in some cases

Top Differential Diagnoses

- Mesothelioma, epithelioid type
  - Immunohistochemistry: Carcinomatous epitopes positive (CEA-M, TAG72, MOC-31, CD15, TTF-1)

Immunohistochemistry

Antibody	Reactivity	Staining Pattern	Comment
CEA-M	Positive	Cytoplasmic	
CD15	Positive	Cytoplasmic	
MOC-31	Positive	Cytoplasmic	
EpCAM/BER-EP4/ CD326	Positive	Cell membrane & cytoplasm	May be positive in ~ 25% of mesotheliomas
TTF-1	Positive	Nuclear	If of lung origin
CK-PAN	Positive	Cytoplasmic	
TAG72	Positive	Cell membrane & cytoplasm	
Calretinin	Negative		May be positive in some carcinomas
CK5/6	Negative		
p63	Negative		

Histochemical Features

Stain	Result
Mucicarmine	Positive for intracellular mucin
D-PAS	Positive for intracellular mucin
PAS	May show positive staining for intracellular glycogen

DIAGNOSTIC CHECKLIST

Clinically Relevant Pathologic Features

- Gross appearance

Pathologic Interpretation Pearls

- Glandular proliferation
- Glands with cellular atypia and mitotic figures
- Positive CEA-M, TAG72, CD15, MOC-31, TTF-1

SELECTED REFERENCES

1. Pardo J et al: Pseudomesotheliomatous carcinoma of the lung with a distinct morphology, immunohistochemistry, and comparative genomic hybridization profile. Ann Diagn Pathol. 11(4):241-51, 2007
2. Attanoos RL et al: 'Pseudomesotheliomatous' carcinomas of the pleura: a 10-year analysis of cases from the Environmental Lung Disease Research Group, Cardiff. Histopathology. 43(5):444-52, 2003
3. Attems JH et al: Pseudomesotheliomatous adenocarcinoma of the lung with rhabdoid features. Pathol Res Pract. 197(12):841-6, 2001
4. Shah IA et al: Pseudomesotheliomatous carcinoma involving pleura and peritoneum: A clinicopathologic and immunohistochemical study of three cases. Ann Diagn Pathol. 3(3):148-59, 1999
5. Koss MN et al: Adenocarcinoma simulating mesothelioma: a clinicopathologic and immunohistochemical study of 29 cases. Ann Diagn Pathol. 2(2):93-102, 1998
6. Koss M et al: Pseudomesotheliomatous adenocarcinoma: a reappraisal. Semin Diagn Pathol. 9(2):117-23, 1992
7. Harwood TR et al: Pseudomesotheliomatous carcinoma of the lung. A variant of peripheral lung cancer. Am J Clin Pathol. 65(2):159-67, 1976

PSEUDOMESOTHELIOMATOUS ADENOCARCINOMA

Microscopic Features

(Left) *This case of pseudomesotheliomatous adenocarcinoma of the lung shows areas of fibrinous pleuritis ⇨, and adjacent fibrocollagen is infiltrated by neoplastic cells forming small glands →. Note the fibrocollagenous stroma with mild inflammatory infiltrate ↗.* ***(Right)*** *Neoplastic cellular proliferation arranged in cords are invading fibroconnective tissue of the pleura. This pattern may be seen in some cases of mesothelioma.*

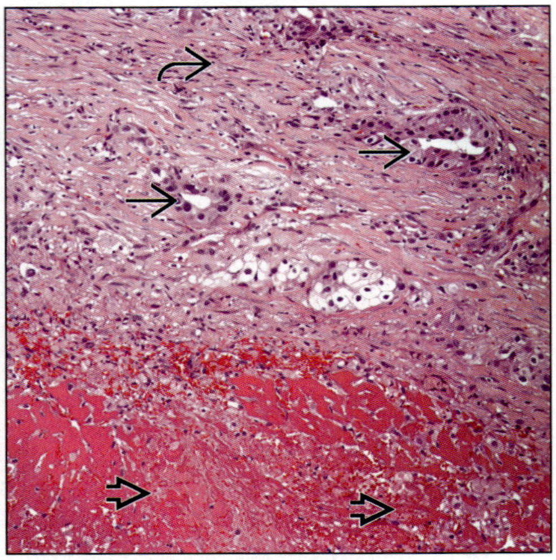

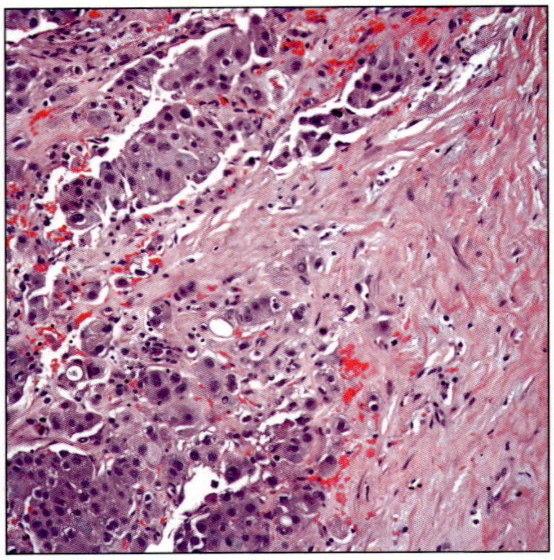

(Left) *Pleural tissue with adipose tissue is invaded by a glandular proliferation →. This feature may also be seen in cases of mesothelioma, thus the need for immunohistochemical stains.* ***(Right)*** *Solid neoplastic cellular proliferation is composed of medium-sized cells with ample eosinophilic cytoplasm. The growth pattern closely mimics mesothelioma.*

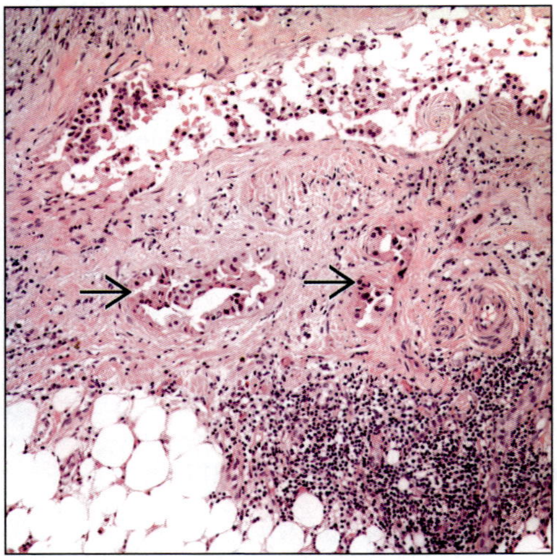

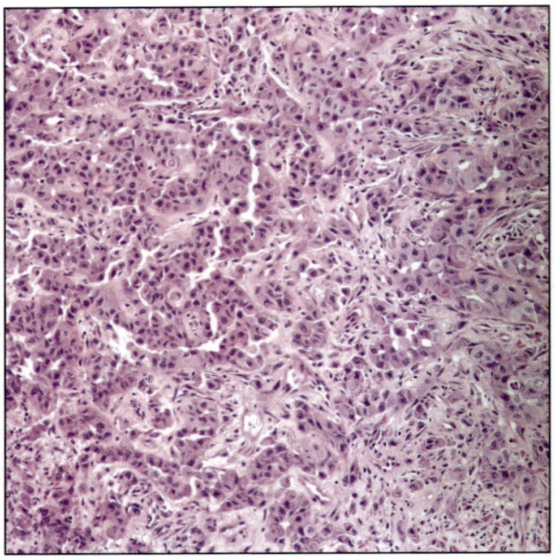

(Left) *More pleomorphic malignant component admixed with areas of fibrinoid pleuritis ⇨. This features is more common in adenocarcinomas than in mesotheliomas.* ***(Right)*** *Clusters of malignant cells ⇨ embedded in a fibrous stroma → giving the appearance of a biphasic mesothelioma. It is important to keep this feature in mind to avoid an incorrect diagnosis.*

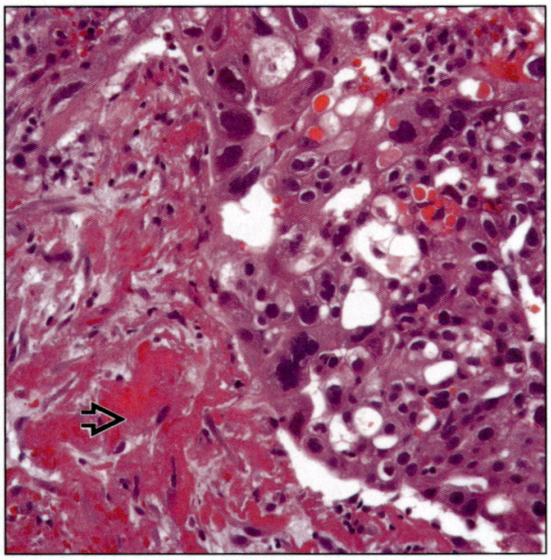

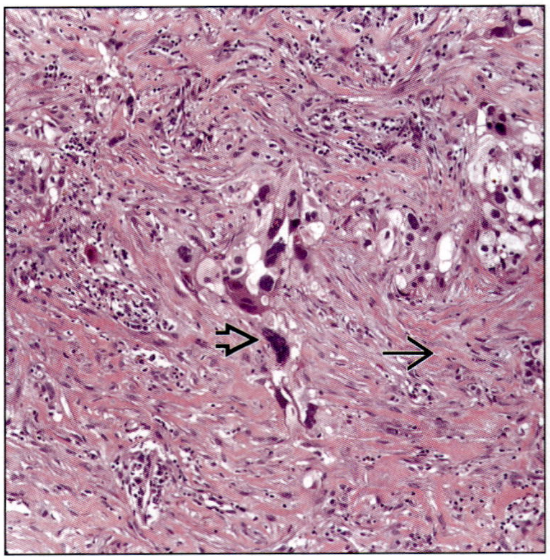

Microscopic Features

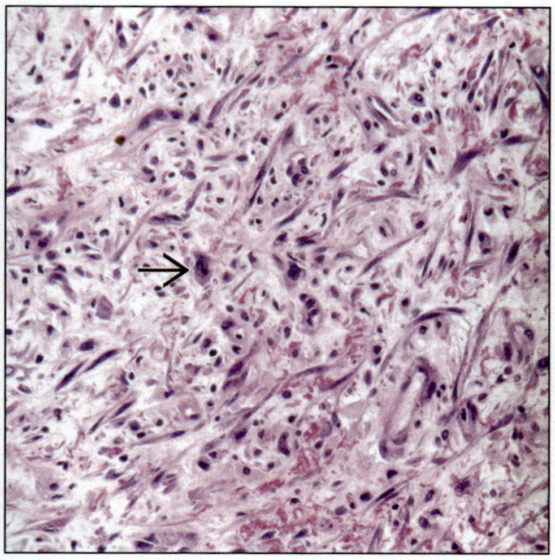
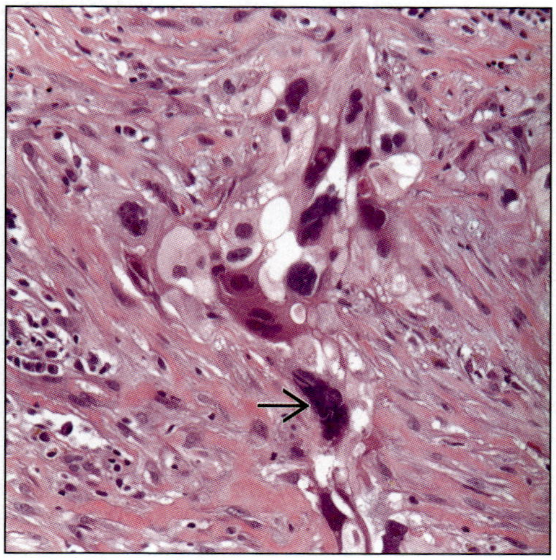

(Left) *Prominent reactive changes are shown in the pleura mixed with neoplastic cells, some of them with atypical mitotic figures* →. *This pattern could be misinterpreted as biphasic cellular proliferation and diagnosed as mesothelioma.* ***(Right)*** *Pseudomesotheliomatous adenocarcinoma shows prominent cellular atypia, namely cells with prominent nucleoli and multinucleated malignant cells* →. *These features are unusual for mesotheliomas.*

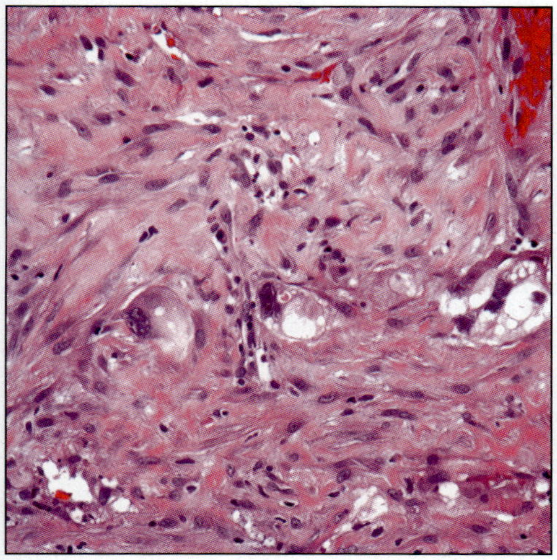
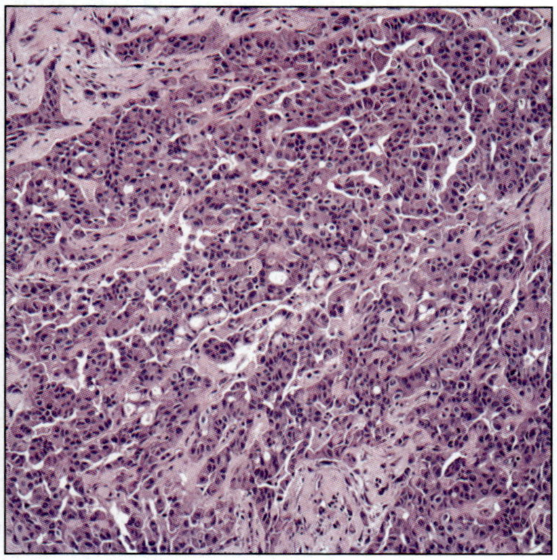

(Left) *In cases of limited tissue for analysis, the presence of single malignant cells embedded in a fibrous stroma would prompt the use of immunohistochemical stains.* ***(Right)*** *More conventional features of adenocarcinoma. The tumor is showing cords and glandular formation.*

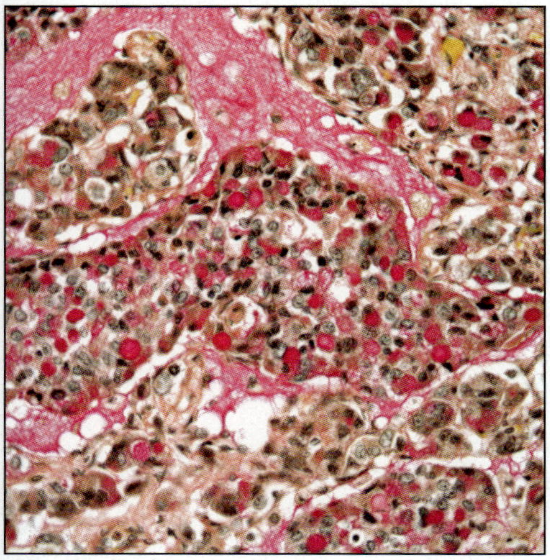
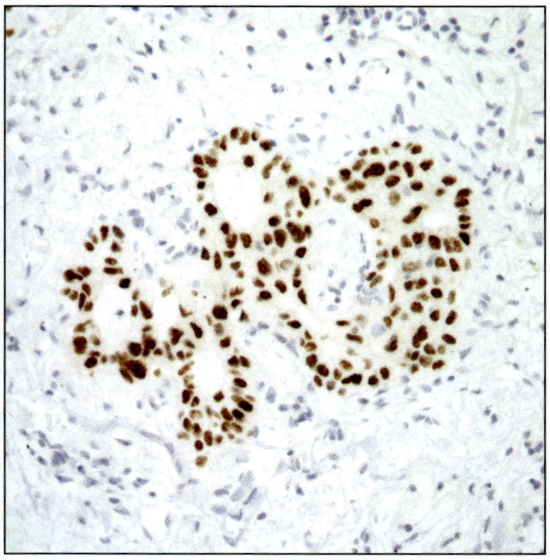

(Left) *The presence of intracellular mucin is one important feature in favor of the diagnosis of adenocarcinoma as it is illustrated in this case.* ***(Right)*** *Positive nuclear staining for TTF-1 is strong evidence in favor of adenocarcinoma of lung origin.*

MUCOEPIDERMOID CARCINOMA OF THE PLEURA

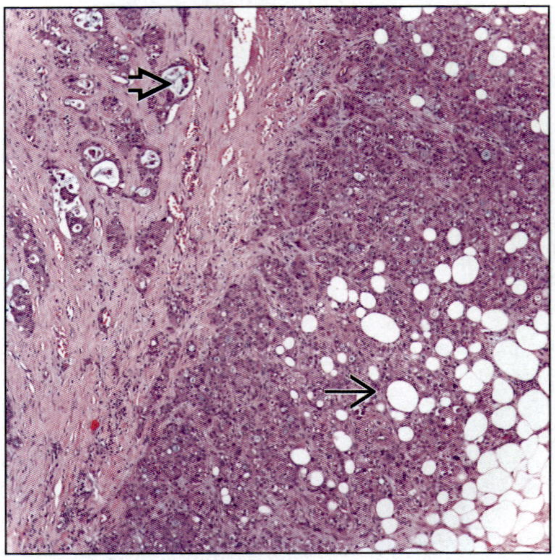

Pleural MEC shows invasion of the tumor into the adipose tissue ➔. Similar features may also be seen in mesotheliomas. However, note the presence of cystic structures containing mucin ➲.

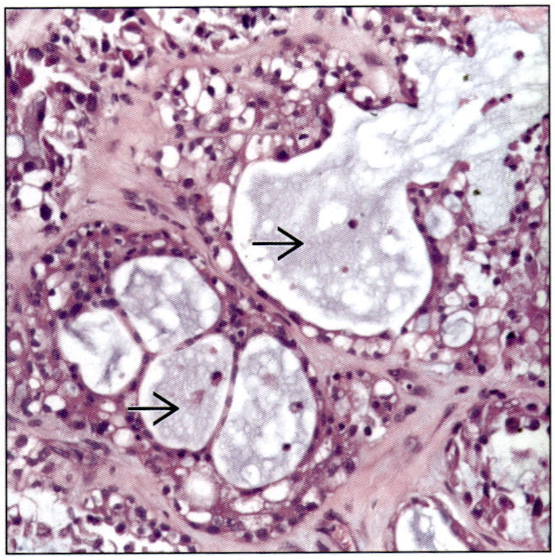

MEC shows gland-like structures of different sizes with mucoid material ➔. The neoplastic cellular proliferation is rather homogeneous.

TERMINOLOGY

Abbreviations

- Pleural mucoepidermoid carcinoma (MEC)

Definitions

- Primary salivary gland-type tumor of pleura

ETIOLOGY/PATHOGENESIS

Etiology

- Although etiology of this tumor in pleura is unknown, it is possible that it may arise from entrapped glands in pleura

CLINICAL ISSUES

Epidemiology

- Incidence
  - Exceedingly rare tumor in pleura
- Age
  - Has been described only in adults
- Gender
  - No gender predilection

Presentation

- Chest pain
- Shortness of breath

Treatment

- Surgical approaches
  - Complete resection of tumor
    - Lobectomy
    - Decortication
    - Simple resection of pleural tumor
- Adjuvant therapy
  - Possible chemotherapy

Prognosis

- May be good depending on histological grade of tumor
- Difficult to assess due to the few cases reported

IMAGE FINDINGS

General Features

- Pleural-based mass
- Diffuse involvement of pleura has not been recorded for these tumors

MACROSCOPIC FEATURES

General Features

- Tumor mass well circumscribed and attached to pleura

Size

- May vary from 2 cm to > 5 cm

MICROSCOPIC PATHOLOGY

Histologic Features

- Epidermoid component without keratinization
- Mucus-secreting cells admixed with epidermoid component
- Mild cellular atypia
- Low mitotic activity
- Possible sclerotic stroma

Predominant Pattern/Injury Type

- Squamoid

Predominant Cell/Compartment Type

- Epithelial, squamous

MUCOEPIDERMOID CARCINOMA OF THE PLEURA

Key Facts

Terminology
- MEC

Clinical Issues
- Symptoms
  - Chest pain
  - Shortness of breath

Image Findings
- Pleural-based mass
- Diffuse involvement of pleura has not been recorded for these tumors

Microscopic Pathology
- Epidermoid component without keratinization
- Mucus-secreting cells admixed with epidermoid component
- Mild cellular atypia
- Low mitotic activity
- Possible sclerotic stroma

Top Differential Diagnoses
- Adenocarcinoma
  - MEC lacks the presence of malignant glandular component
- Squamous cell carcinoma
  - Presence of keratinization unusual in MEC
  - Mucus-producing cells (mucocytes) admixed with epidermoid component in MEC
- Synovial sarcoma
  - Spindle cell component in synovial sarcoma is malignant
  - Sclerotic component in MEC is fibroblastic benign

Immunohistochemistry

Antibody	Reactivity	Staining Pattern	Comment
CK-PAN	Positive	Cytoplasmic	Also positive in other carcinomas
p63	Positive	Nuclear	Also positive in squamous cell carcinomas
EMA	Positive	Cell membrane	Also positive in other carcinomas
CK5/6	Positive	Cytoplasmic	Also positive in mesotheliomas and squamous cell carcinomas
CEA-M	Positive	Cytoplasmic	
Vimentin	Positive	Cytoplasmic	In spindle cell component of sclerotic areas
Androgen receptor	Positive	Nuclear	In some cases
S100	Negative		
Actin-HHF-35	Negative		
Desmin	Negative		

Histochemical Features

Stain	Comment
Mucicarmine	Positive for intracellular mucin in mucinophages
D-PAS	Positive for intracellular mucin in mucinophages
PAS	Positive in some cell for glycogen content

DIFFERENTIAL DIAGNOSIS

Adenocarcinoma
- Peripheral adenocarcinoma shows presence of intrapulmonary mass
- Shows presence of neoplastic glandular proliferation
- Does not show presence of intermediate cells

Squamous Cell Carcinoma
- Presence of keratinization is unusual and favors squamous cell carcinoma over MEC
- Mucus-producing cells (mucocytes) admixed with epidermoid component in MEC

Synovial Sarcoma
- Spindle cell component in synovial sarcoma is malignant
- Sclerotic component in MEC is fibroblastic benign

DIAGNOSTIC CHECKLIST

Clinically Relevant Pathologic Features
- Gross appearance

Pathologic Interpretation Pearls
- Epidermoid component without keratinization
- Mucus-secreting cells (mucocytes) admixed with epidermoid component
- Focal oncocytic features may be seen
- In sclerosing variant, spindle cell stroma is benign

SELECTED REFERENCES

1. Moran CA et al: Primary mucoepidermoid carcinoma of the pleura. A clinicopathologic study of two cases. Am J Clin Pathol. 120(3):381-5, 2003

MUCOEPIDERMOID CARCINOMA OF THE PLEURA

Microscopic Features

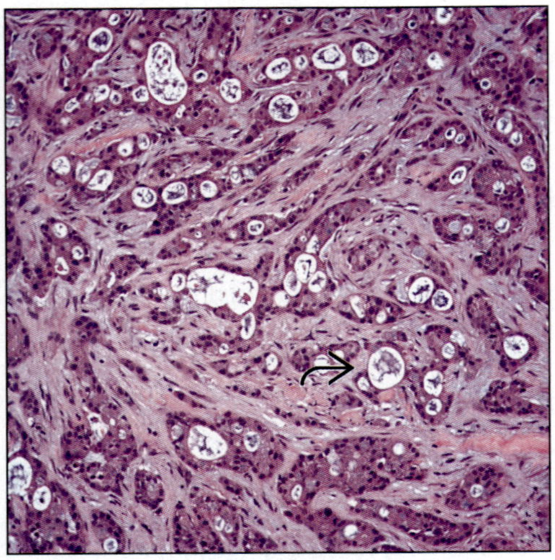
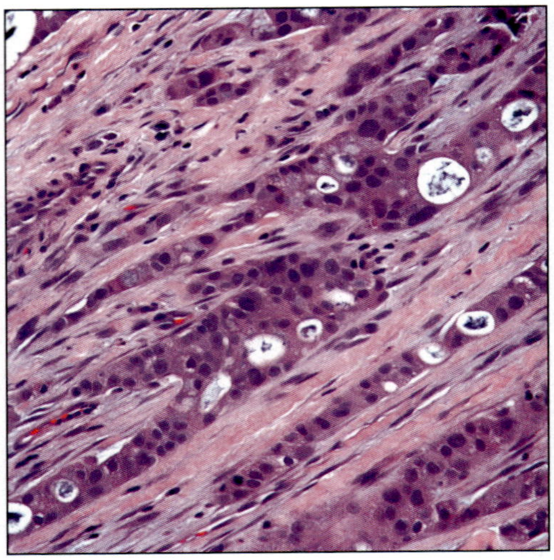

(Left) *MEC of the pleura shows more conventional areas of epidermoid component with the presence of mucinous cells →. Even at this power, one can see the oncocytic features present in this tumor.* ***(Right)*** *In some areas, the pattern of growth is that of cords of neoplastic cells embedded in a collagenous stroma. The tumor does not show evidence of increased mitotic activity or necrosis.*

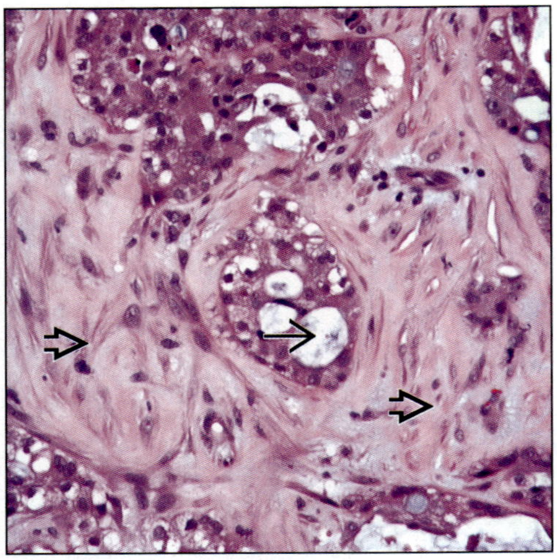
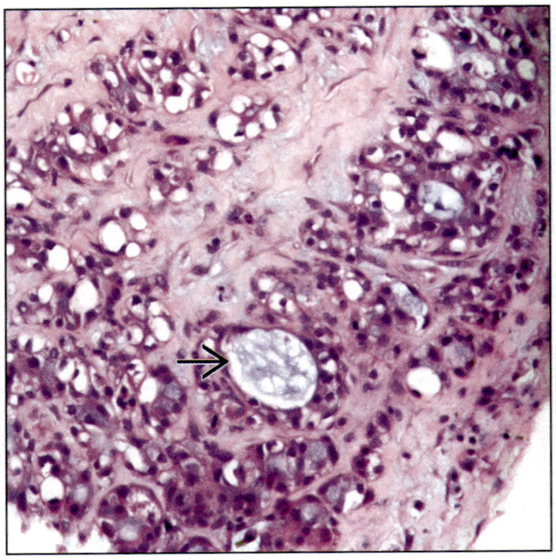

(Left) *Closer view shows the neoplastic cells arranged in a pseudoglandular pattern with intraluminal mucin →. Note the desmoplastic reaction around the tumor cells ⇨.* ***(Right)*** *MEC with a more nested pattern and 1 obvious dilated gland-like structure →. The cellular proliferation has rather oncocytic and clear cell features. This growth pattern is unusual for conventional mesotheliomas or adenocarcinomas.*

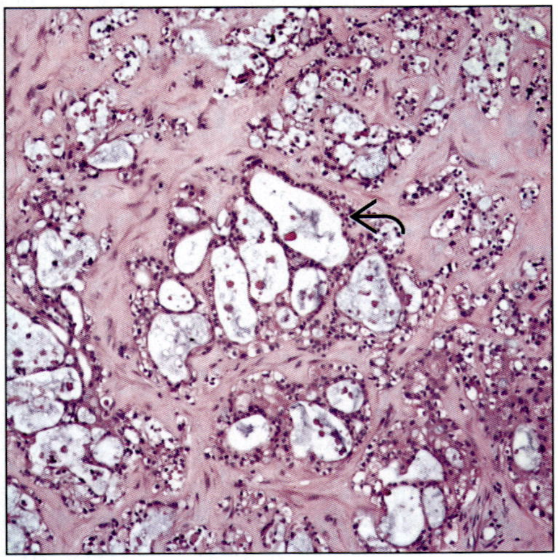
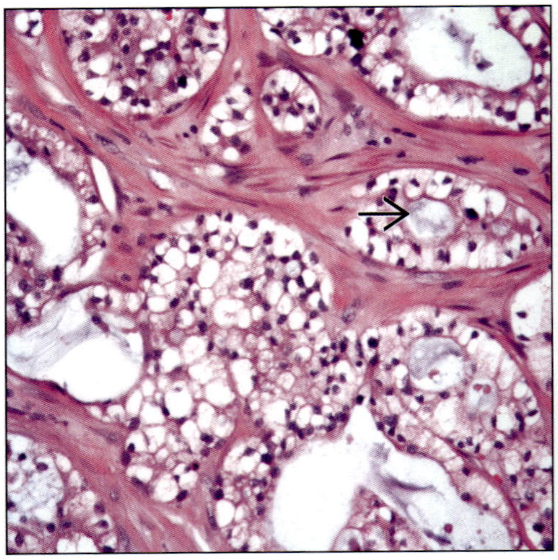

(Left) *In some areas, the neoplastic cells are seen in association with cystic areas, which contain flattened epithelium →.* ***(Right)*** *Pleural MEC with prominent clear cell features. This feature may be only focal in these tumors. Note the presence of intraluminal mucin →.*

MUCOEPIDERMOID CARCINOMA OF THE PLEURA

Microscopic Features

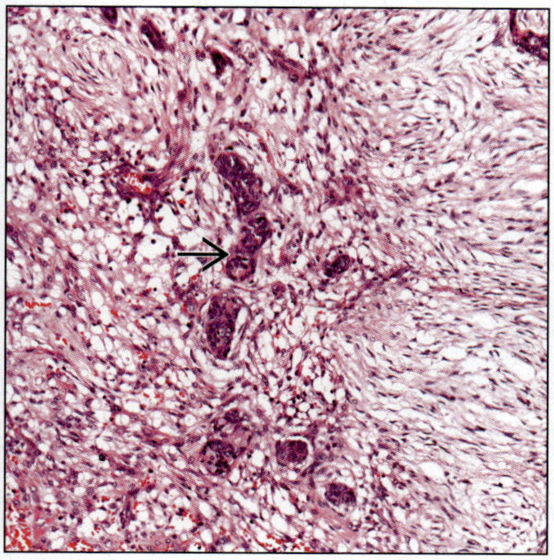

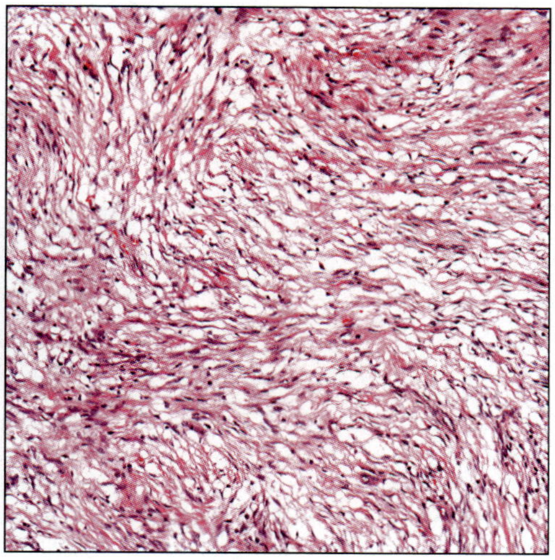

(Left) *Sclerosing MEC with extensive areas of spindle fibroblastic proliferation. In some areas, the presence of an epidermoid component → may be only minimal.* ***(Right)*** *Closer view of the sclerosing areas shows fibroconnective tissue with fibroblastic proliferation. Note the absence of cellular atypia or mitotic activity.*

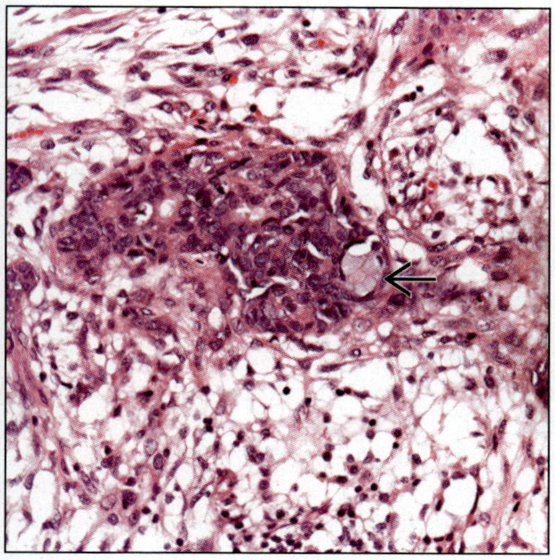

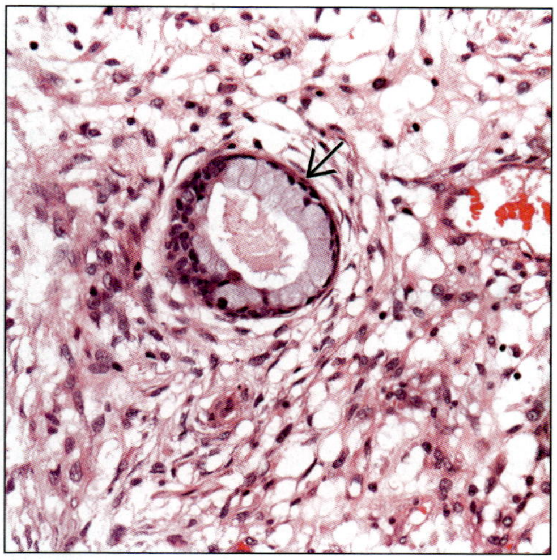

(Left) *Closer view of the epithelial component of a sclerosing variant of MEC shows the neoplastic cells with vague epidermoid features and only focal mucus-producing cells →.* ***(Right)*** *Different view of the epithelial component of a sclerosing variant of MEC shows a classical area of epidermoid cells and mucus-producing → cells embedded in a collagenous stroma. The use of histochemical stain for mucin, such as mucicarmine, shows positive staining in these areas.*

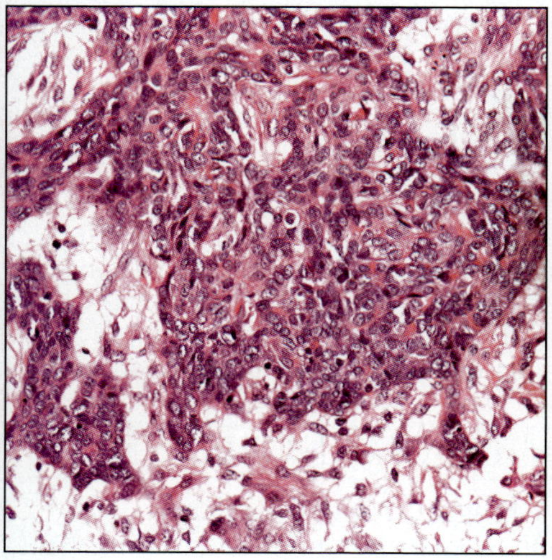

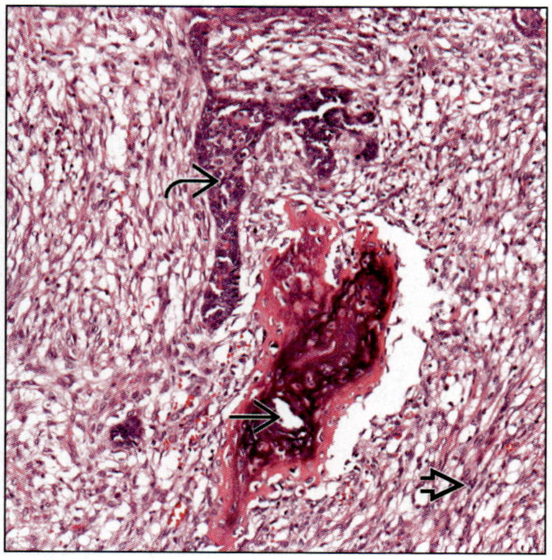

(Left) *Closer view at the epithelial component of a MEC sclerosing variant shows the epidermoid component with mild to moderate nuclear atypia and scattered mitotic figures. These features may also be seen in cases of metastatic squamous cell carcinomas to the pleura.* ***(Right)*** *Sclerosing MEC shows the classical sclerosed areas ⇨ with islands of epidermoid carcinoma ↷ and metaplastic bone formation →.*

ANGIOSARCOMA

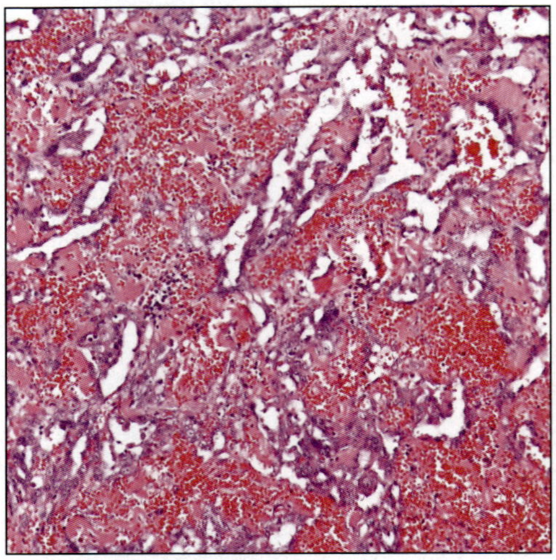

The pleura in pleural angiosarcoma is replaced by an extensively hemorrhagic cellular proliferation composed of anastomosing vessel-like channels that are lined by large, atypical endothelial cells.

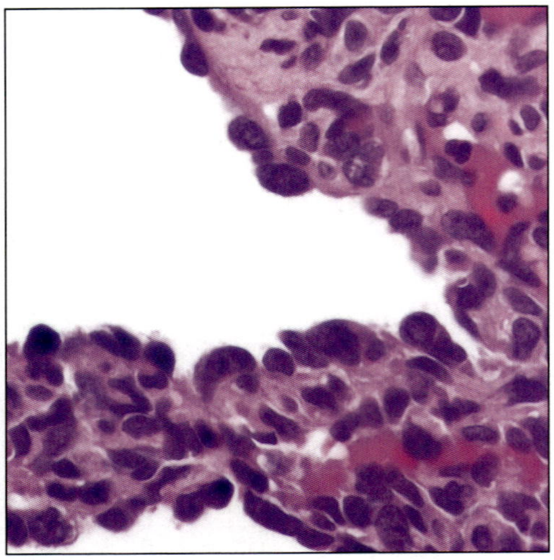

A dilated vascular space is seen in pleural angiosarcoma that is lined by large, hyperchromatic cells with round to oval nuclei with inconspicuous nucleoli and scant cytoplasm with "hobnail" features.

TERMINOLOGY

Abbreviations

- Angiosarcoma (AS)

Definitions

- Malignant pleural neoplasm showing evidence of vascular endothelial differentiation

ETIOLOGY/PATHOGENESIS

Unknown

- No association with occupational exposure to asbestos

CLINICAL ISSUES

Presentation

- Chest pain
- Dyspnea
- Recurrent hemorrhagic pleural effusions
- Age range: 22-79 years (average: 57 years)
- History of prior chronic pyothorax reported in Japan

Treatment

- Surgical excision
- Radiation therapy
- Chemotherapy

Prognosis

- Poor prognosis
- Highly aggressive behavior
- Median survival approximately 12 months

MACROSCOPIC FEATURES

General Features

- Diffuse, plaque-like thickening encasing pleura
- Abundant hemorrhage and necrosis
- Infiltration of adjacent structures

MICROSCOPIC PATHOLOGY

Histologic Features

- Solid atypical epithelioid or spindle cell proliferation
- Anastomosing vessel-like channels lined by atypical cells
- Extensive hemorrhage and necrosis
- Infiltration of adjacent structures

Cytologic Features

- Enlarged nuclei with dense chromatin pattern
- Prominent nucleoli
- Frequent mitoses, including atypical (abnormal) mitoses
- Cells may be predominantly epithelioid (epithelioid variant of angiosarcoma) and resemble an epithelial neoplasm
- Conventional type is composed of spindle and pleomorphic tumor cells resembling a spindle cell sarcoma

ANCILLARY TESTS

Immunohistochemistry

- CD31, CD34, and FVIIIRAg positive in tumor cells
- Cytokeratin may be (+) in cells of epithelioid variant
- Tumor cells are negative for most conventional mesothelioma markers
- Tumors cells are strongly positive for vimentin

DIFFERENTIAL DIAGNOSIS

Epithelioid Malignant Mesothelioma

- Typical tubulo-papillary growth pattern of epithelioid mesothelioma is absent in angiosarcoma

ANGIOSARCOMA

Key Facts

Macroscopic Features
- Diffuse, plaque-like growth encasing pleura
- Abundant hemorrhage and necrosis
- Infiltration of adjacent structures

Microscopic Pathology
- Solid atypical epithelioid or spindle cell proliferation
- Anastomosing vessel-like channels lined by atypical cells
- Extensive hemorrhage and necrosis
- Enlarged nuclei with dense chromatin pattern
- Prominent nucleoli
- Frequent mitoses, including atypical (abnormal) mitoses
- Cells may be predominantly epithelioid (epithelioid variant of angiosarcoma) and resemble an epithelial neoplasm
- Conventional type is composed of spindle and pleomorphic tumor cells resembling spindle cell sarcoma
- CD31 and CD34 positive in tumor cells
- Cytokeratin may be positive in cells of epithelioid variant
- Tumor cells are negative for most conventional mesothelioma markers

Diagnostic Checklist
- May simulate malignant mesothelioma radiologically and histologically
- Characterized by recurrent hemorrhagic pleural effusion
- Prognosis is similar to that of malignant mesothelioma
- Not associated with asbestos exposure

- Angiosarcoma tends to be more hemorrhagic than mesothelioma
- Presence of vessel-like spaces lined by atypical cells is rare in mesothelioma and typical of angiosarcoma
- CD31 and CD34 are negative in mesothelioma
- Tumor cells of epithelioid angiosarcoma may be positive for cytokeratin, similar to mesothelioma
- Tumor cells in mesothelioma are positive for calretinin, CK5/6, WT1, HBME-1, and other mesothelioma markers

Metastatic Adenocarcinoma
- Solid growth pattern and epithelioid cell features in angiosarcoma may simulate metastasis of carcinoma
- Epithelioid angiosarcoma may be positive for cytokeratin
- Anastomosing vessel-like channels favor angiosarcoma
- Tumor cells will be positive for a variety of epithelial markers in metastatic carcinoma, such as EMA/MUC1, CEA-M, MOC31, TTF-1, etc.
  - Tumor cells will be positive for CD31 and CD34 in angiosarcoma
- Clinical history or evidence of carcinoma elsewhere favors a metastatic carcinoma

Metastatic Amelanotic Melanoma
- Prominent nesting of tumor cells is typical of melanoma
- Intranuclear inclusions, binucleation, and pleomorphic cells with prominent nucleoli are more frequent in melanoma
- Presence of intracytoplasmic melanin pigment favors melanoma
- Melanoma (+) for S100, HMB45, and mart-1
  - Angiosarcoma will be positive for CD31 and CD34, and negative for melanocytic markers

DIAGNOSTIC CHECKLIST

Clinically Relevant Pathologic Features
- May simulate radiologically and histologically malignant mesothelioma
- Characterized by recurrent hemorrhagic pleural effusion
- May be of epithelioid or conventional (spindle cell) type
- Prognosis is similar to that of malignant mesothelioma
- Not associated with asbestos exposure

Pathologic Interpretation Pearls
- Look for extensive areas of hemorrhage and necrosis
- Look for anastomosing vessel-like channels lined by atypical endothelial cells
- CD31 and CD34 positivity in tumor cells is diagnostic
  - Think of this possibility when other tumor markers are equivocal or incomplete for malignant mesothelioma

SELECTED REFERENCES

1. Dainese E et al: Primary pleural epithelioid angiosarcoma. A case report and review of the literature. Pathol Res Pract. 206(6):415-9, 2010
2. Kurtz JE et al: Diffuse primary angiosarcoma of the pleura: a case report and review of the literature. Sarcoma. 8(4):103-6, 2004
3. Del Frate C et al: Pseudomesotheliomatous angiosarcoma of the chest wall and pleura. J Thorac Imaging. 18(3):200-3, 2003
4. Gladish GW et al: Primary thoracic sarcomas. Radiographics. 22(3):621-37, 2002
5. Zhang PJ et al: Malignant epithelioid vascular tumors of the pleura: report of a series and literature review. Hum Pathol. 31(1):29-34, 2000
6. Alexiou C et al: Primary angiosarcomas of the chest wall and pleura. Eur J Cardiothorac Surg. 14(5):523-6, 1998
7. Falconieri G et al: Pseudomesotheliomatous angiosarcoma: a pleuropulmonary lesion simulating malignant pleural mesothelioma. Histopathology. 30(5):419-24, 1997
8. Lin BT et al: Malignant vascular tumors of the serous membranes mimicking mesothelioma. A report of 14 cases. Am J Surg Pathol. 20(12):1431-9, 1996
9. McCaughey WT et al: Angiosarcoma of serous membranes. Arch Pathol Lab Med. 107(6):304-7, 1983

ANGIOSARCOMA

Pleural Angiosarcoma, Conventional Type

***(Left)** The pleura in conventional pleural angiosarcoma is replaced by an extensively hemorrhagic process. A sparsely cellular proliferation is seen in the center, containing scattered large cells admixed with abundant red blood cells. **(Right)** High-power view of pleural angiosarcoma shows scattered atypical cells with large, hyperchromatic nuclei and prominent basophilic nucleoli. Notice blood lakes containing abundant red blood cells interspersed with the atypical tumor cells.*

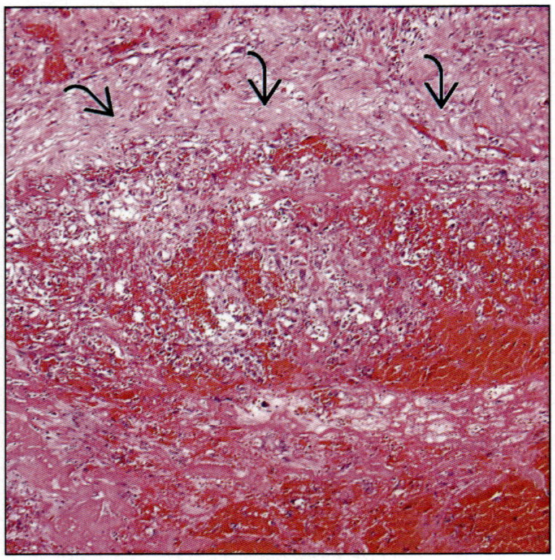

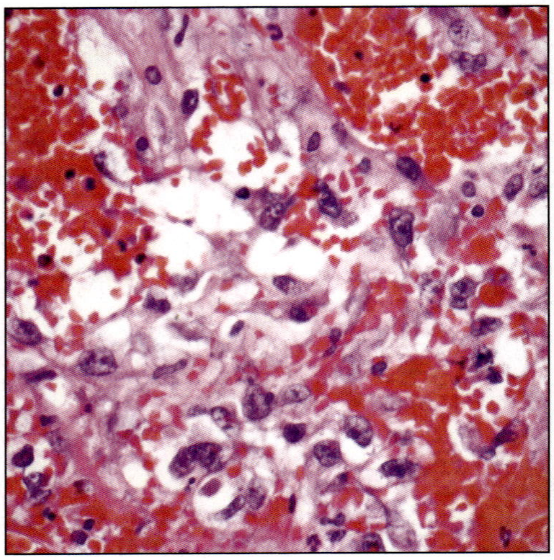

***(Left)** Multiple anastomosing vessel-like channels separated by abundant extravasated red blood cells are seen in conventional pleural angiosarcoma. Some of the atypical cells in the stroma are spindle-shaped. **(Right)** A malformed blood vessel is seen in the center of the field lined by large, hyperchromatic and atypical vascular endothelial cells in conventional pleural angiosarcoma. Note cells protruding into the vessel lumen in "hobnail" fashion.*

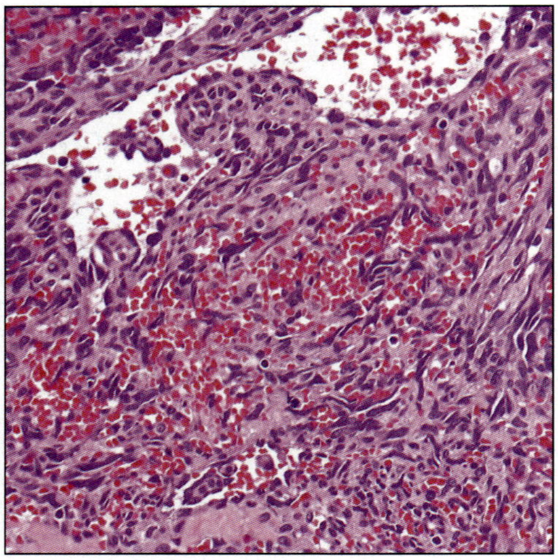

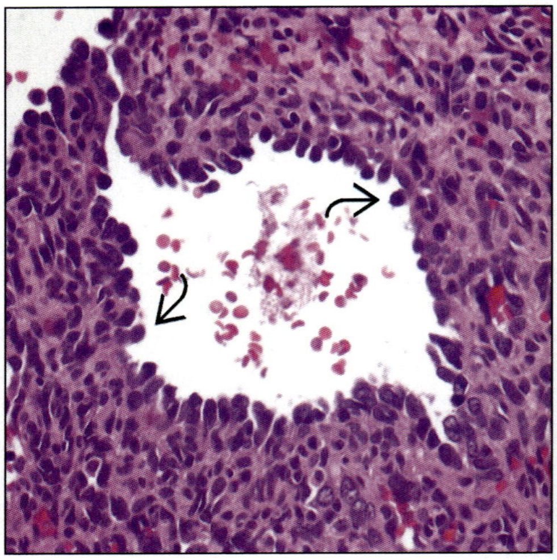

***(Left)** Solid areas (left) in conventional pleural angiosarcoma merge imperceptibly with vessel-like spaces. Note the dilated vessel at the bottom, which appears to be originating from the solid proliferation on the left. **(Right)** A large dilated and abnormal vessel is seen in the center of the field lined by atypical endothelial cells characterized by large, round to oval, hyperchromatic nuclei with scant cytoplasm in conventional pleural angiosarcoma.*

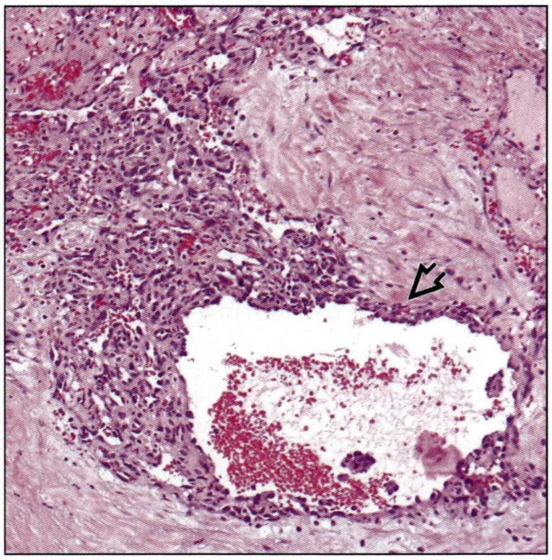

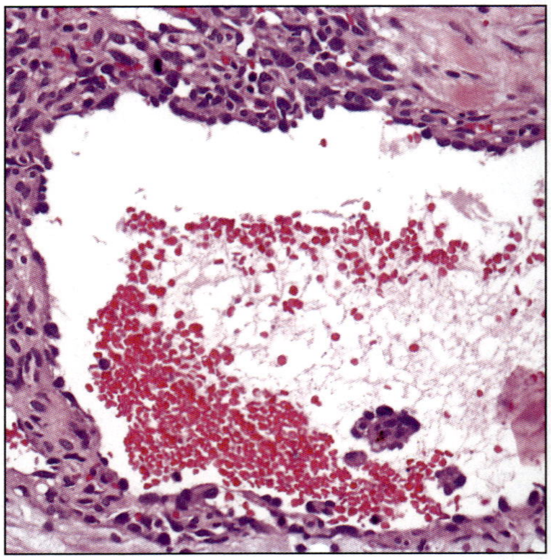

ANGIOSARCOMA

Pleural Angiosarcoma, Epithelioid Type

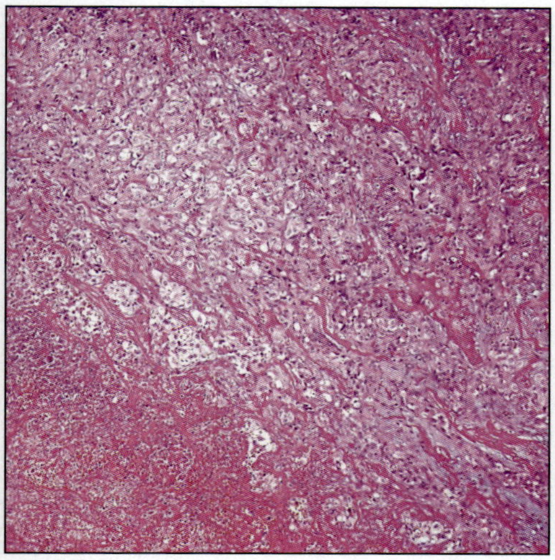
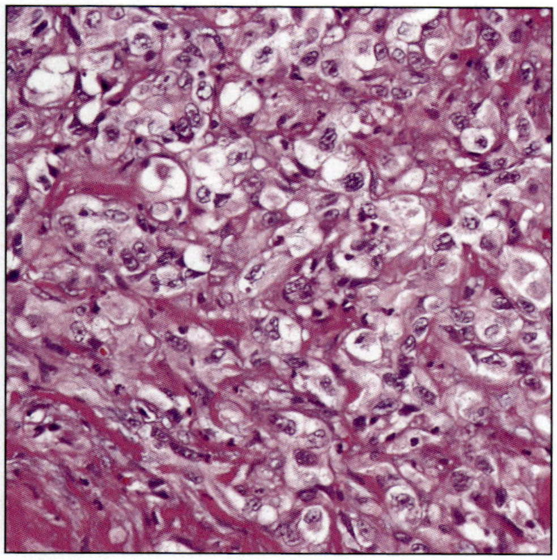

(Left) *The pleura is replaced by sheets of large, solid epithelioid cells devoid of recognizable vascular spaces in pleural angiosarcoma of the epithelioid type.* ***(Right)*** *High power shows solid sheets of large, epithelioid cells with abundant clear to lightly eosinophilic cytoplasm containing large, atypical nucleoli in epithelioid pleural angiosarcoma. Notice the absence of well-formed anastomosing vascular spaces lined by atypical endothelial cells.*

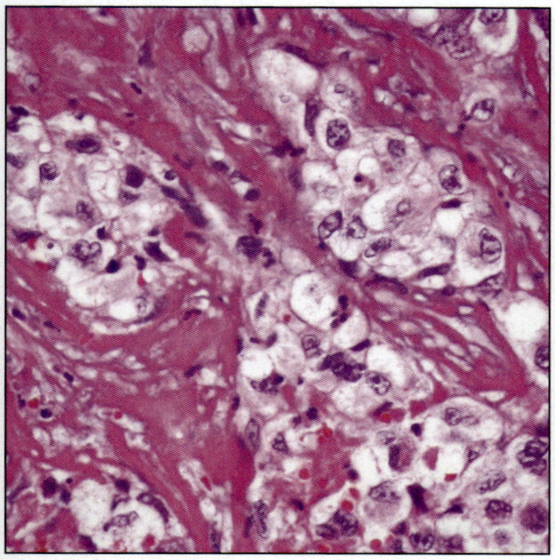
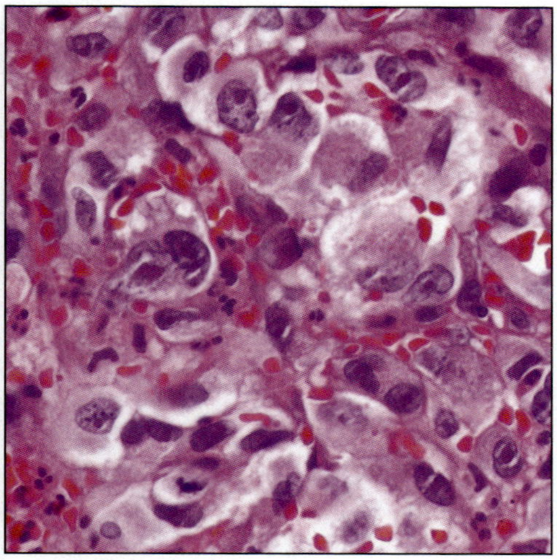

(Left) *Small solid nests of large epithelioid cells are seen, separated by bands of fibroconnective tissue in the stroma of a pleural angiosarcoma, epithelioid type. The cohesive and well-demarcated nature of these cell islands is reminiscent of a metastatic carcinoma.* ***(Right)*** *Nests of large, atypical epithelioid cells are seen in epithelioid pleural angiosarcoma. The cells contain abundant eosinophilic cytoplasm. The cell nuclei are large and hyperchromatic with prominent nucleoli.*

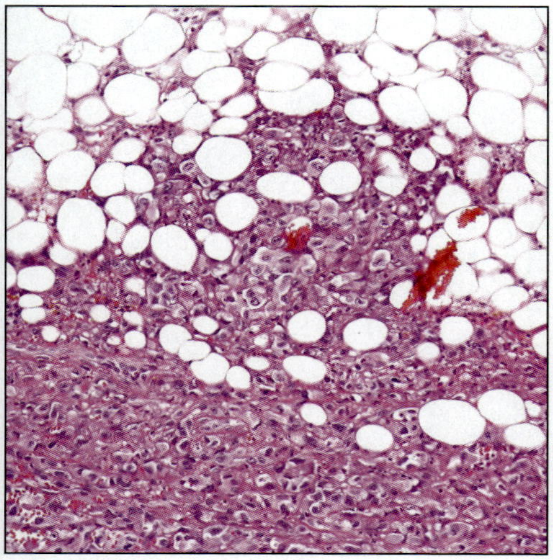
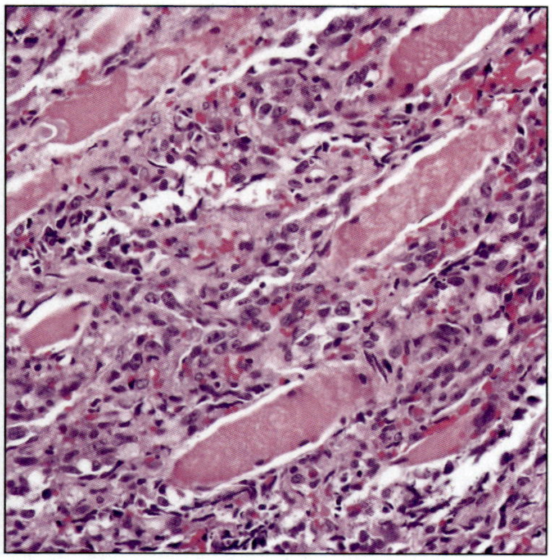

(Left) *Tumor is seen to infiltrate the subpleural adipose tissue in pleural angiosarcoma of epithelioid type. Notice how the adipocytes are spared by the infiltrating tumor cells.* ***(Right)*** *Extensive infiltration of skeletal muscle of the diaphragm is seen in a pleural epithelioid angiosarcoma. The skeletal muscle shows degeneration of the cytoplasm with loss of cross striations; however, it is not destroyed by the infiltrating epithelioid angiosarcoma tumor cells.*

Pleural Angiosarcoma, Epithelioid Type

*(**Left**) The pleura is replaced by a dense, solid cellular proliferation composed of sheets of large, epithelioid cells with abundant cytoplasm and large hyperchromatic nuclei in a pleural angiosarcoma of epithelioid type. (**Right**) High magnification shows sheets of large, epithelioid cells with abundant cytoplasm and large cell nuclei with prominent nucleoli in pleural epithelioid angiosarcoma. Notice the absence of angioformative elements and the cohesive aspect of the cell population.*

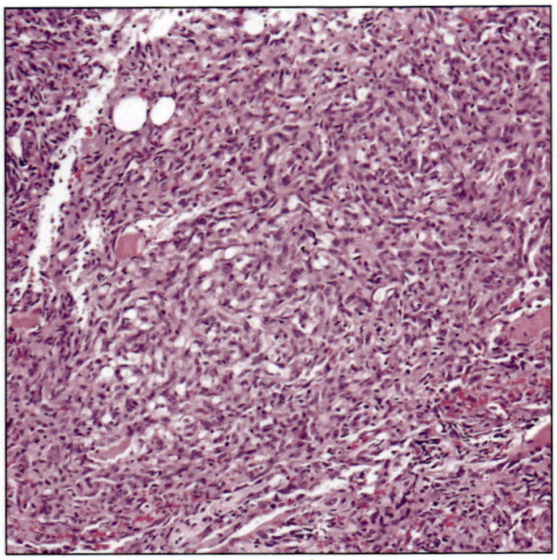

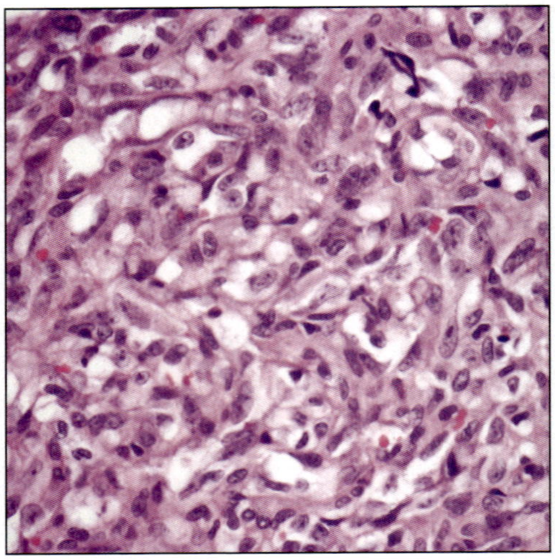

*(**Left**) This tumor shows an interesting feature, the presence of multiple large, epithelioid cells with prominent clear cytoplasmic vacuoles ⮫ simulating fat cells in epithelioid pleural angiosarcoma. (**Right**) Prominent cytoplasmic vacuolization is seen in this example of pleural angiosarcoma, epithelioid type. In some areas, the vacuoles displace the nuclei of the tumor cells toward the periphery of the cell, imparting them with a signet ring cell appearance ⇨.*

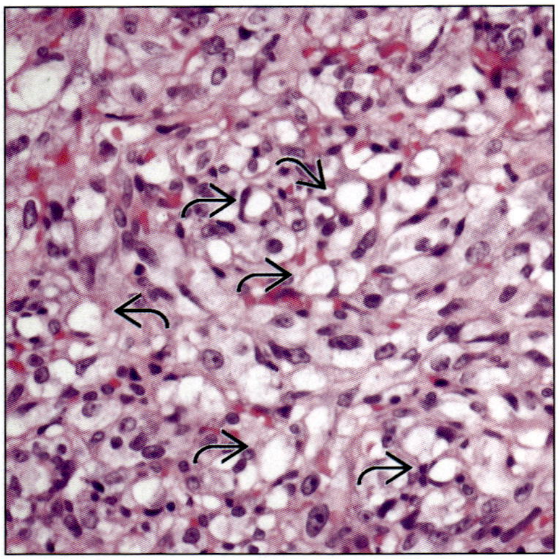

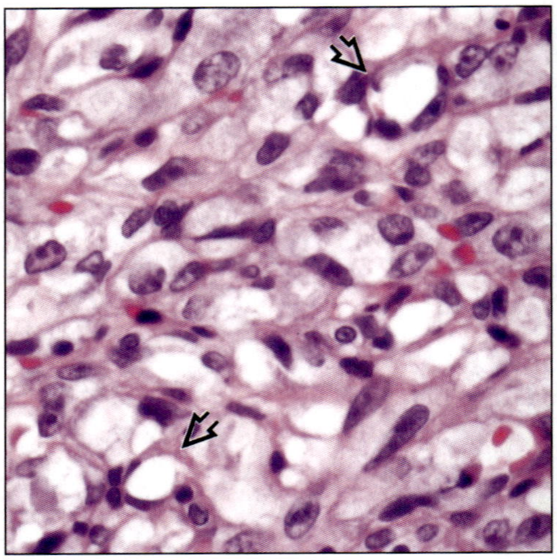

*(**Left**) Immunoperoxidase stain for CD31 shows positive cytoplasmic staining of the tumor cells for this antigen in a pleural angiosarcoma of epithelioid type. (**Right**) Immunoperoxidase stain for FVIIIRAg shows strong cytoplasmic staining of the epithelioid tumor cells in epithelioid pleural angiosarcoma. FVIIRAg shows a tendency to stain the circumference of the cytoplasmic vacuoles, highlighting the boundaries of these structures.*

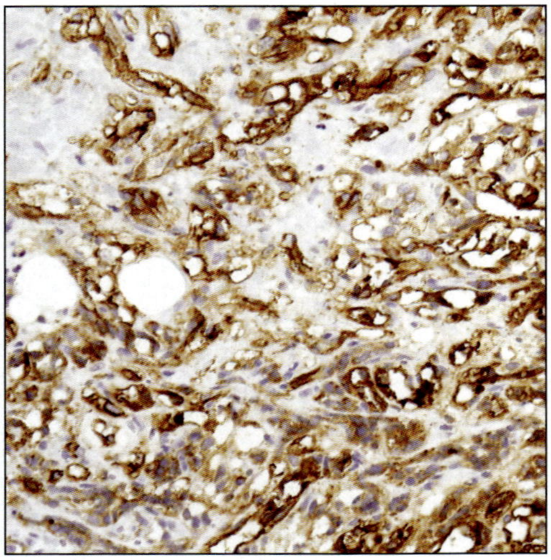

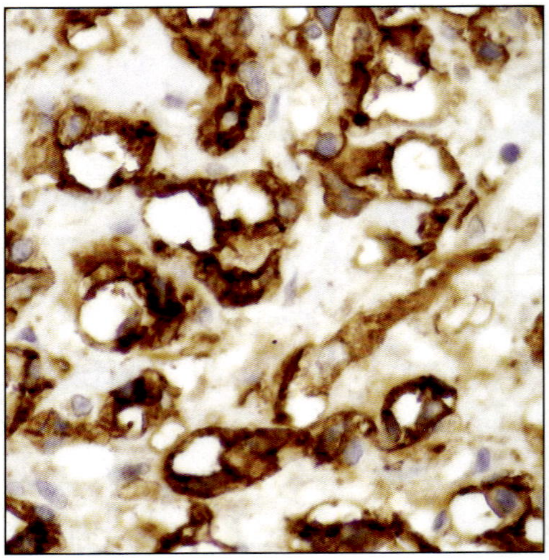

Pleural Angiosarcoma, Conventional Type

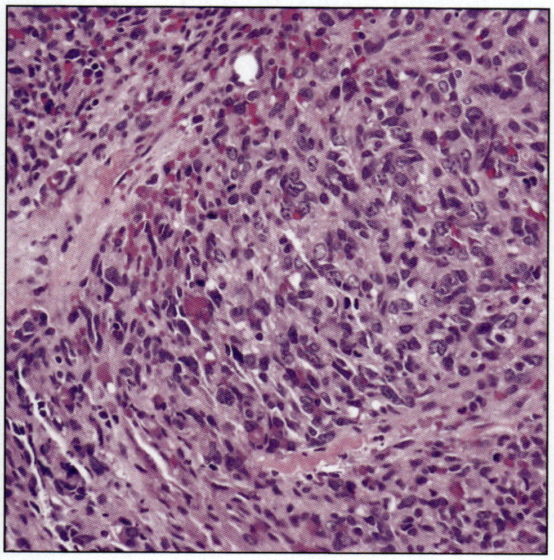

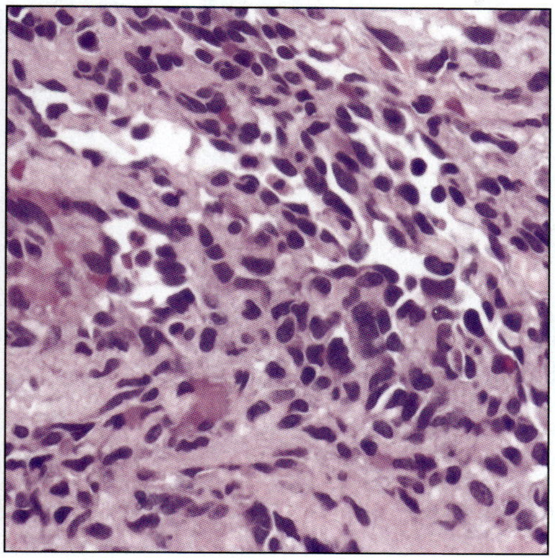

(Left) *The pleura is replaced by a solid proliferation of large atypical cells showing nuclear pleomorphism and focal spindling of the tumor cells in this example of pleural angiosarcoma, conventional type.* ***(Right)*** *This focus shows primitive, abortive and anastomosing vessel-like spaces lined by large, atypical endothelial cells with oval to spindle nuclei in pleural angiosarcoma. Notice that similar cells are also seen infiltrating the stroma and outside of the vessel-like lumens.*

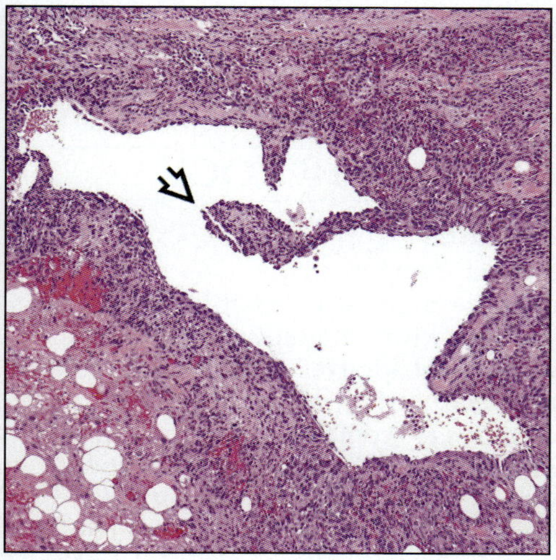

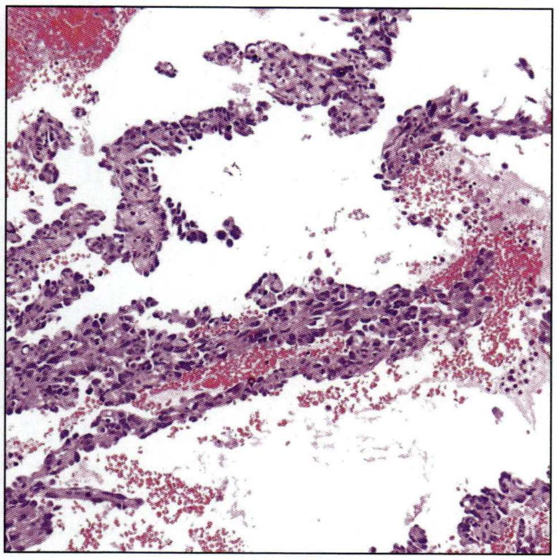

(Left) *There is a large, dilated space in the center of the field representing an abnormal, neoplastic vessel lined by atypical vascular endothelial cells in pleural angiosarcoma, conventional type. A focal projection into the lumen with pseudopapillary appearance is noted ⇨.* ***(Right)*** *Strands of tumor cells adopting a pseudopapillary appearance are seen projecting into an empty lumen in pleural angiosarcoma, conventional type. The structures are lined by atypical endothelial cells.*

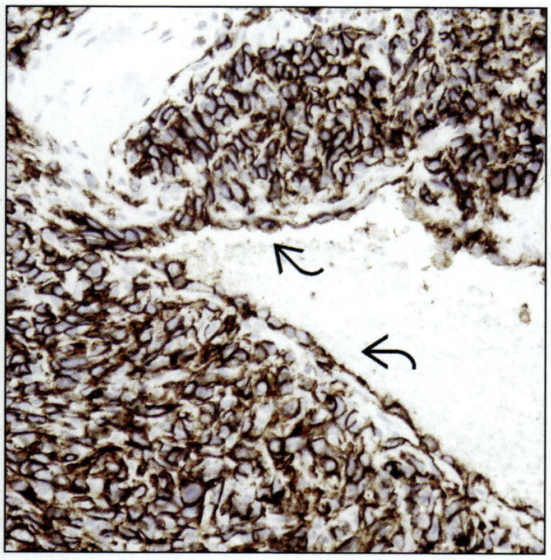

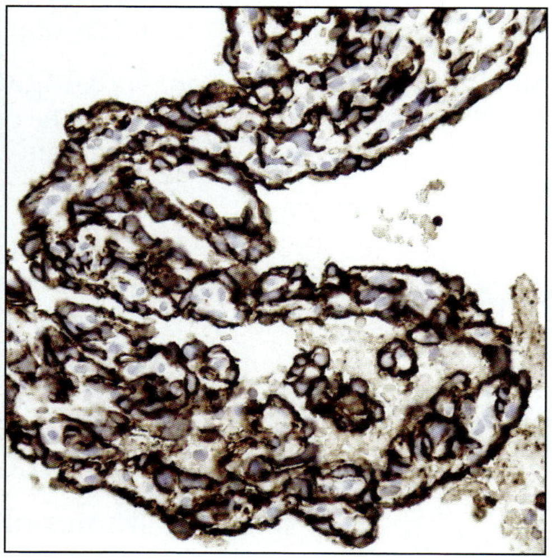

(Left) *Immunoperoxidase stain for CD31 shows strong cytoplasmic positivity of the tumor cells for this marker in a pleural angiosarcoma, conventional type. Notice that the cells lining the dilated vascular spaces are also strikingly positive ↗.* ***(Right)*** *Immunoperoxidase stain for CD34 shows strong cytoplasmic positivity of the tumor cells lining pseudopapillary structures and vascular spaces in this example of pleural angiosarcoma of conventional type.*

SYNOVIAL SARCOMA

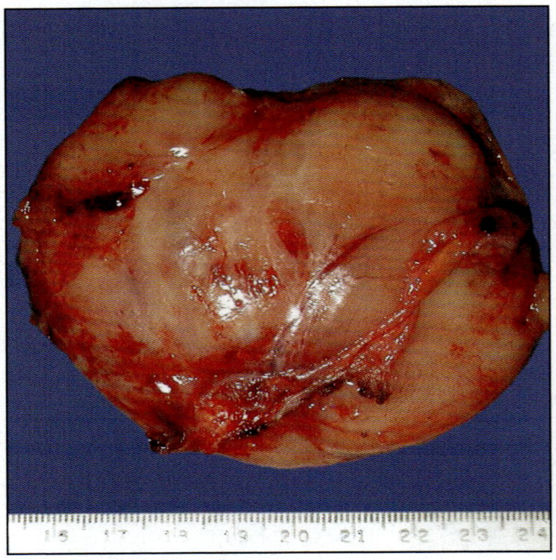

Gross appearance of primary synovial sarcoma of the pleura shows a well-circumscribed mass with a fleshy and soft appearance and a lobulated external surface.

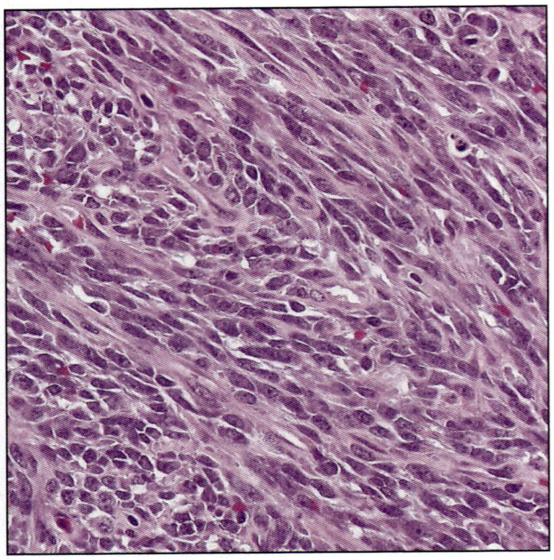

Typical histologic appearance of monophasic synovial sarcoma of the pleura shows monotonous fascicles of spindle cells almost completely devoid of connective tissue stroma.

TERMINOLOGY

Abbreviations

- Synovial sarcoma (SS)

Definitions

- Pleural malignant neoplasm composed of nonmesothelial cells showing epithelial differentiation with distinctive spindle cell pattern of growth and chromosomal translocation

ETIOLOGY/PATHOGENESIS

Pathogenesis

- Unknown

CLINICAL ISSUES

Presentation

- Chest pain
- Pleural effusion
- Pleural-based mass on CT scan
- Age range: 10-50 years (average: 25 years)

Treatment

- Surgical excision, radiation therapy, chemotherapy

Prognosis

- Similar prognosis to soft tissue counterpart
- Aggressive behavior with local recurrence and metastases

MACROSCOPIC FEATURES

General Features

- Large, well-circumscribed, pleural-based mass
- May extend along pleural surface mimicking malignant mesothelioma
- May infiltrate underlying structures
- May show cystic and hemorrhagic changes
- May attain large sizes (up to 16 cm in greatest dimension)

MICROSCOPIC PATHOLOGY

Histologic Features

- May be biphasic or monophasic
- Biphasic tumors are composed of cleft-like and glandular structures with intraluminal eosinophilic proteinaceous material admixed with population of atypical spindle cells
- Monophasic tumors are composed of monotonous atypical spindle cell proliferation with herringbone, storiform, or hemangiopericytic growth patterns
- Poorly differentiated variants are characterized by round epithelioid cells rather than spindle cells
- Variable mitotic activity (range: 2-10 mitoses per 10 high-power fields)
- May display hemorrhage and necrosis

Cytologic Features

- Spindle cell population is very monotonous and uniform
- Absence of nuclear pleomorphism or prominent nucleoli
- Glands lined by tall columnar cells with abundant cytoplasm in biphasic type
- Absence of fibrous stroma
- Absence of marked anaplasia or multinucleated tumor cells

ANCILLARY TESTS

Immunohistochemistry

- Focal (patchy) positivity for epithelial markers (cytokeratin and EMA)
- Strong positivity for Bcl-2 and CD99

Key Facts

Macroscopic Features

- Large, well-circumscribed, pleural-based mass
- May extend along pleural surface mimicking malignant mesothelioma
- May show cystic and hemorrhagic changes

Microscopic Pathology

- May be biphasic or monophasic
- Biphasic tumors are composed of cleft-like and glandular structures with intraluminal eosinophilic proteinaceous material admixed with population of atypical spindle cells
- Monophasic tumors are composed of monotonous atypical spindle cell proliferation with herringbone, storiform, or hemangiopericytic growth patterns
- Variable mitotic activity (range: 2-10 mitoses per 10 high-power fields)
- Spindle cell population is very monotonous and uniform
- Absence of nuclear pleomorphism or prominent nucleoli
- Glands lined by tall columnar cells with abundant cytoplasm in biphasic type
- Focal (patchy) positivity for epithelial markers (cytokeratin and EMA)
- Strong positivity for Bcl-2 and CD99
- Shares many markers with malignant mesothelioma, including calretinin and HBME-1
- Some cases may be positive for CD34
- Characteristic chromosomal translocation, t(X;18) (SYT-SSX) seen in > 80% of cases
- Distinctive translocation may be assayed by FISH, PCR, or DNA in situ hybridization

- Shares many markers with malignant mesothelioma, including calretinin and HBME-1
- May also stain with calponin and CD117

Cytogenetics

- Characteristic chromosomal translocation, t(X;18) (SYT-SSX) seen in > 80% of cases
- Distinctive translocation may be demonstrated by FISH, PCR, or DNA in situ hybridization
- Distinctive translocation has not been recognized in other similar tumors

DIFFERENTIAL DIAGNOSIS

Biphasic Malignant Mesothelioma

- More intimate admixture between glandular structures and spindle cell component seen in synovial sarcoma
- Extensive overlap in results of immunohistochemical staining
- Both tumors share cytokeratin, EMA, calretinin, and HMBE-1 positivity
- WT1 is positive in mesothelioma but consistently negative in synovial sarcoma
- Cytogenetic studies demonstrate t(X;18) in all synovial sarcomas; translocation is negative in mesothelioma

Sarcomatoid Malignant Mesothelioma

- Can be confused for monophasic spindle cell variant of synovial sarcoma
- Cell population more uniform in synovial sarcoma than in sarcomatoid mesothelioma
- Spindle cells in sarcomatoid mesothelioma show marked nuclear pleomorphism
- Both can be negative for epithelial (keratin, EMA) and mesothelial (calretinin, WT1, HBME-1) markers
- Demonstration of t(X;18) is most reliable way for separating the two

Solitary Fibrous Tumor/Malignant SFT

- Both can show very similar morphologic features
- Bcl-2, CD99, and CD34 reactivity can be shared by both synovial sarcoma and sarcomatoid mesothelioma
- Focal keratin or EMA positivity favors synovial sarcoma
- Demonstration of t(X;18) can help make definitive diagnosis of synovial sarcoma in equivocal cases

DIAGNOSTIC CHECKLIST

Clinically Relevant Pathologic Features

- More frequent in young adults than in mature or elderly patients
- Aggressive behavior with frequent recurrences and metastases

Pathologic Interpretation Pearls

- Uniformity of spindle cell population is important key for diagnosis of synovial sarcoma
- Demonstration of t(X;18) by molecular techniques is of value in equivocal cases

SELECTED REFERENCES

1. Bégueret H et al: Primary intrathoracic synovial sarcoma: a clinicopathologic study of 40 t(X;18)-positive cases from the French Sarcoma Group and the Mesopath Group. Am J Surg Pathol. 29(3):339-46, 2005
2. Essary LR et al: Primary pleuropulmonary synovial sarcoma: reappraisal of a recently described anatomic subset. Cancer. 94(2):459-69, 2002
3. Aubry MC et al: Primary monophasic synovial sarcoma of the pleura: five cases confirmed by the presence of SYT-SSX fusion transcript. Am J Surg Pathol. 25(6):776-81, 2001
4. Miettinen M et al: Calretinin and other mesothelioma markers in synovial sarcoma: analysis of antigenic similarities and differences with malignant mesothelioma. Am J Surg Pathol. 25(5):610-7, 2001
5. Nicholson AG et al: Synovial sarcoma of the pleura and its differentiation from other primary pleural tumours: a clinicopathological and immunohistochemical review of three cases. Histopathology. 33(6):508-13, 1998
6. Gaertner E et al: Biphasic synovial sarcomas arising in the pleural cavity. A clinicopathologic study of five cases. Am J Surg Pathol. 20(1):36-45, 1996

Microscopic Features

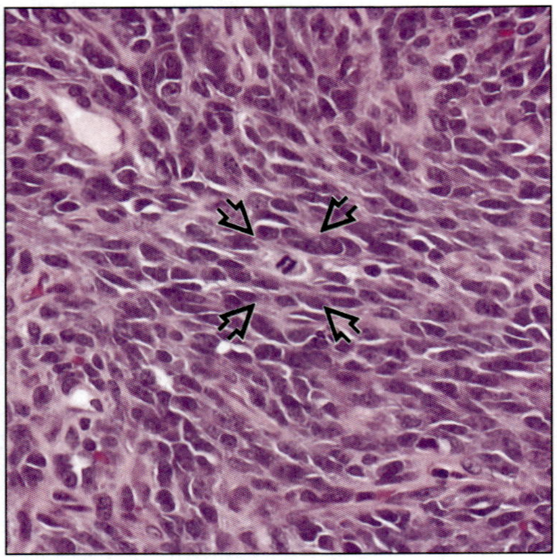
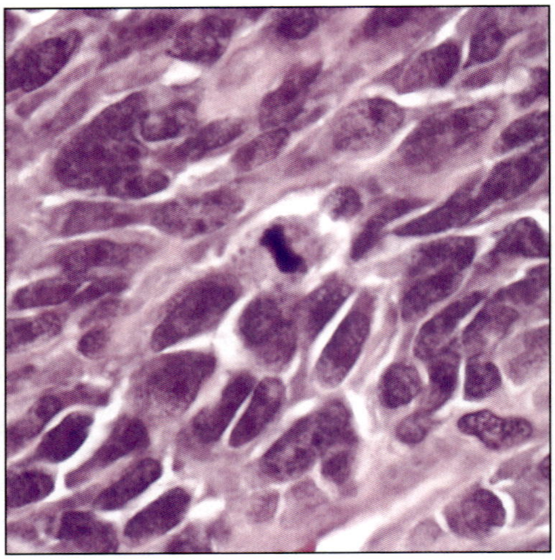

(Left) *Low magnification of monophasic synovial sarcoma of the pleura shows a monotonous population of spindle cells. A mitotic figure is seen in the center of the field ⊳.* *(Right)* *High magnification of monophasic synovial sarcoma of the pleura shows a monotonous population of atypical spindle cells. Notice the mitotic figure in the center. Mitotic activity can vary considerably in these tumors, from very scanty to more than 10 mitoses per 10 high-power fields.*

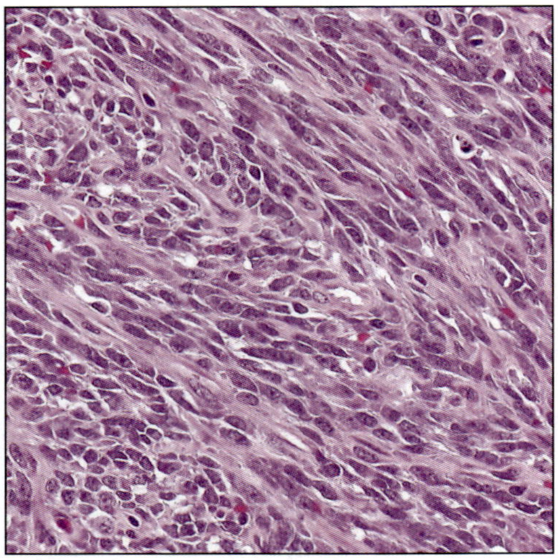
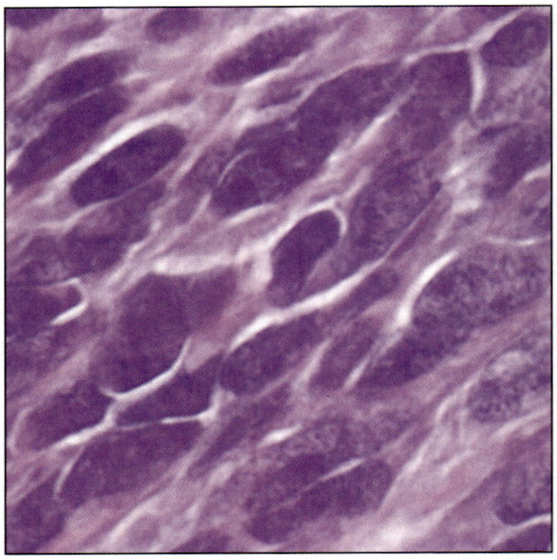

(Left) *Monophasic synovial sarcoma of the pleura shows fascicles of monotonous spindle cells without significant vascular markings and exhibiting a herringbone pattern of growth. This appearance can closely resemble that of sarcomatoid malignant mesothelioma.* *(Right)* *High magnification of monophasic synovial sarcoma of the pleura shows the monotonous character of the atypical spindle cells, with uniform nuclei showing a dispersed chromatic pattern and inconspicuous nucleoli.*

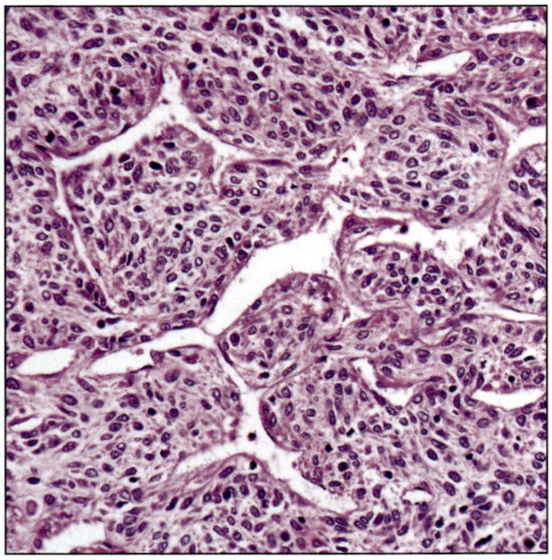
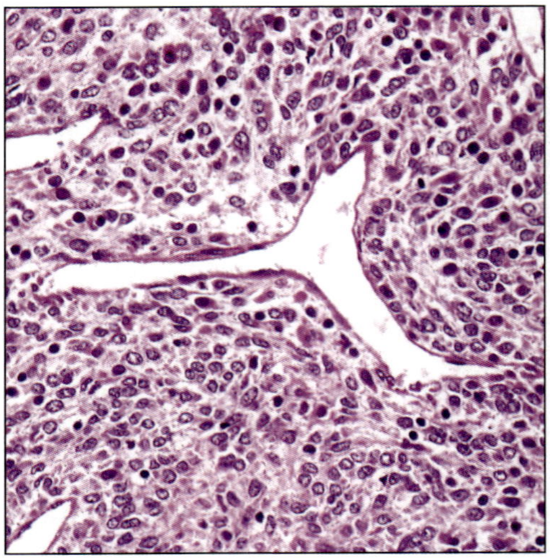

(Left) *Monophasic synovial sarcoma of the pleura shows a prominent hemangiopericytoma-like growth pattern. Multiple branching vessels with patent lumens are noted surrounded by the atypical spindle cells.* *(Right)* *High magnification of monophasic synovial sarcoma of the pleura with hemangiopericytoma-like growth patterns shows a small branching vessel with patent lumen surrounded by a dense population of monotonous spindle cells.*

Variants of Synovial Sarcoma

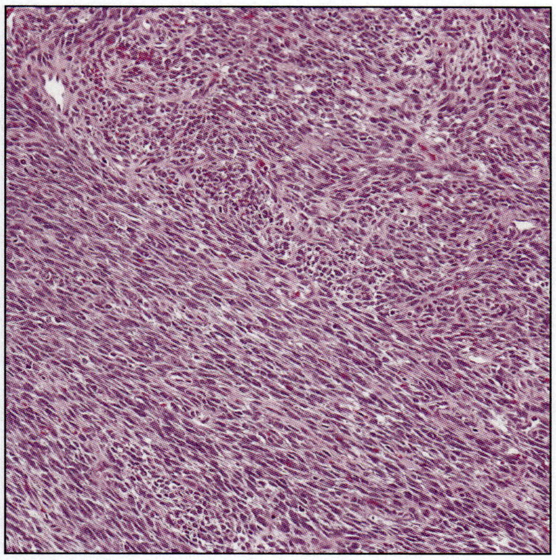

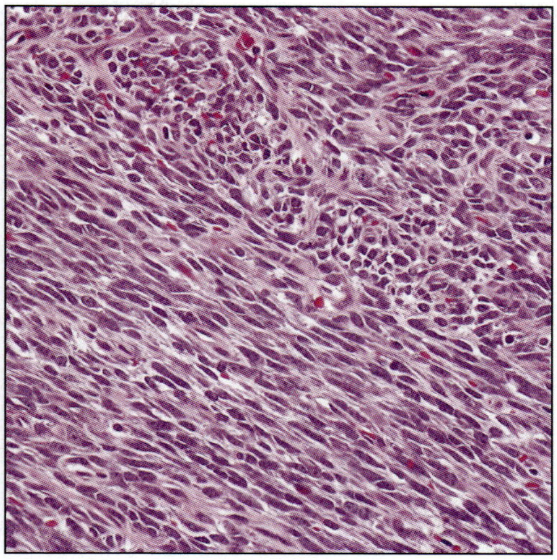

(Left) Scanning magnification of monophasic synovial sarcoma of the pleura shows fascicles of monotonous atypical spindle cells arranged in a herringbone pattern. The dense and monotonous atypical spindle cell proliferation is characteristic for this tumor. **(Right)** Scanning magnification of monophasic synovial sarcoma of the pleura shows fascicles of parallel tumor cells with a very monotonous appearance and scant intercellular stroma.

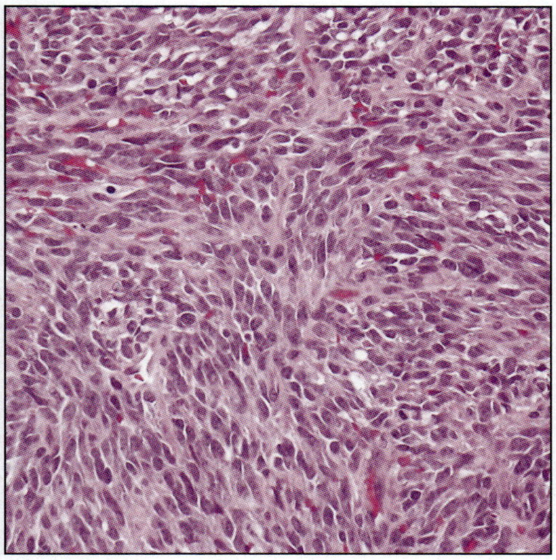

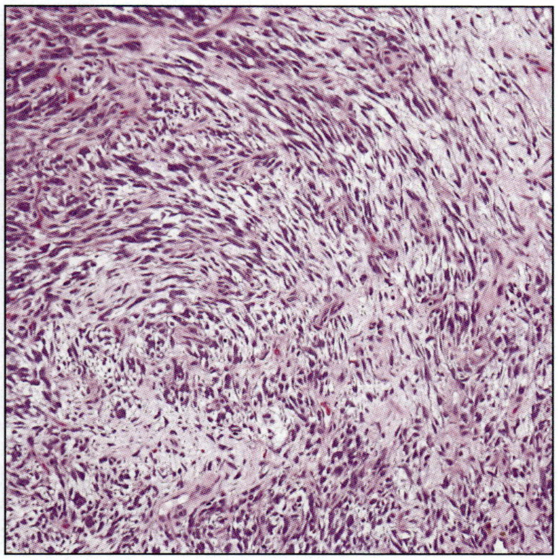

(Left) Monophasic synovial sarcoma of the pleura shows intersecting fascicles of monotonous tumor cells with a vague storiform pattern and a few scattered mitotic figures. This histologic appearance can closely resemble a "fibrohistiocytic" tumor. **(Right)** Monophasic synovial sarcoma of the pleura shows prominent myxoid intercellular matrix. This type of change is often seen in treated tumors that have been radiated prior to surgery or as a result of adjuvant chemotherapy.

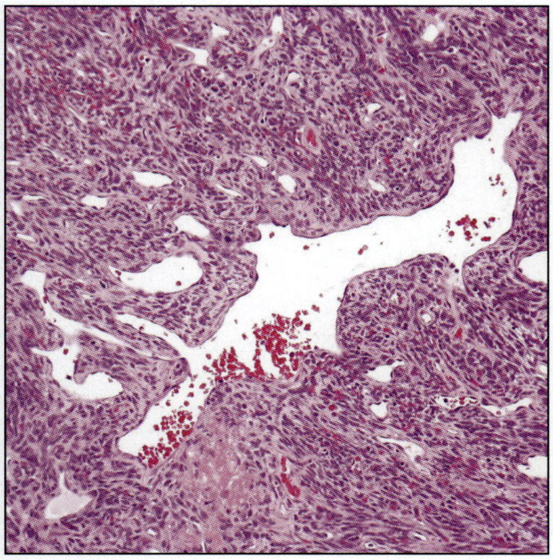

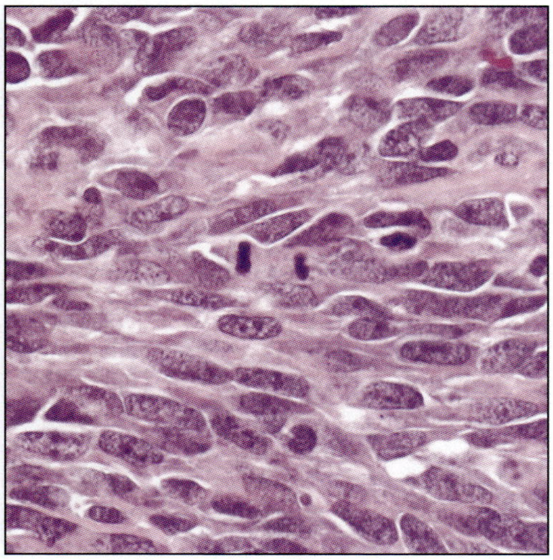

(Left) Monophasic synovial sarcoma of the pleura shows a focal hemangiopericytic growth pattern with branching vessels adopting a "staghorn" configuration. Tumors with these features were previously diagnosed as hemangiopericytoma. **(Right)** High magnification in monophasic synovial sarcoma of the pleura shows a monotonous population of tumor cells with tapered nuclei showing a dense chromatin pattern with inconspicuous nucleoli and scattered mitotic figures.

Monophasic Synovial Sarcoma of the Pleura

*(**Left**) Synovial sarcoma of the pleura shows alternating hypercellular and paucicellular areas. Notice a dense cuff of tumor cells surrounding a small vessel ➚. (**Right**) High magnification of a cellular area in monophasic synovial sarcoma of the pleura shows a monotonous population of hyperchromatic spindle cells. Notice the monotonous appearance of the spindle cells, which are devoid of significant nuclear pleomorphism. Scattered mitoses are present throughout the tumor ⇨.*

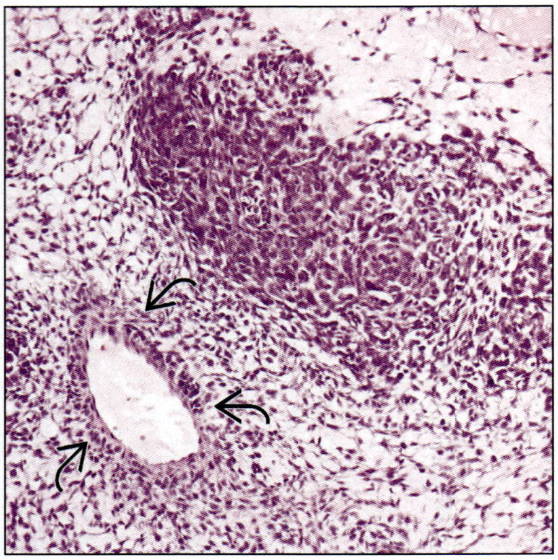

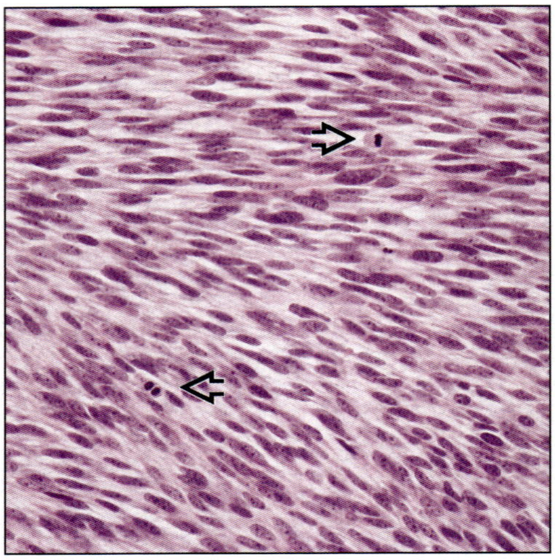

*(**Left**) Synovial sarcoma of the pleura shows a focus of coagulative tumor cell necrosis ➚. Notice the monotonous spindle tumor cells surrounding the area of necrosis. (**Right**) Synovial sarcoma of the pleura shows an area displaying striking stromal sclerosis with a sparse spindle cell population embedded in abundant collagenized stroma. Striking stromal hyalinization is rare in monophasic synovial sarcoma and is most often seen in cases after radiation or chemotherapy.*

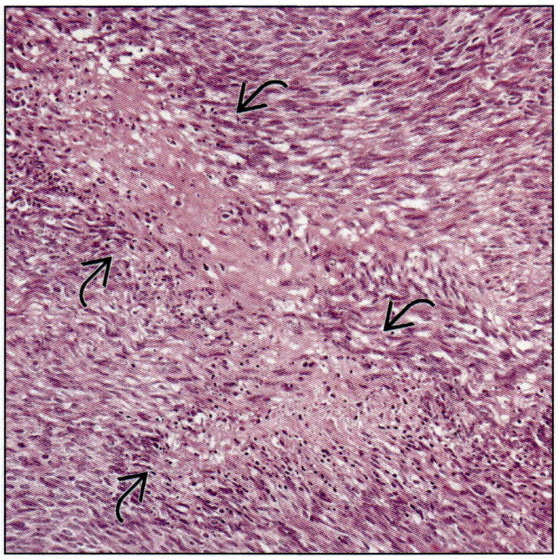

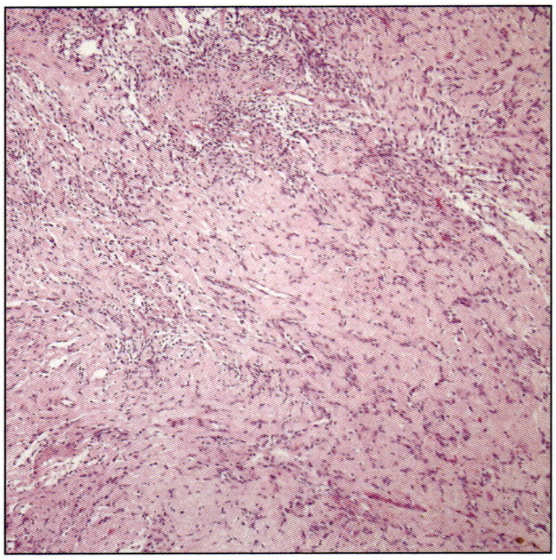

*(**Left**) Synovial sarcoma of the pleura with stromal sclerosis shows hyperchromatic spindle cells separated by abundant hyalinized stroma. Tumors with these features can be mistaken for solitary fibrous tumor, fibrosarcoma, and other types of spindle cell sarcomas. (**Right**) Synovial sarcoma of the pleura with stromal hyalinization shows a sparse population of hyperchromatic spindle cells embedded in abundant hyalinized connective tissue stroma.*

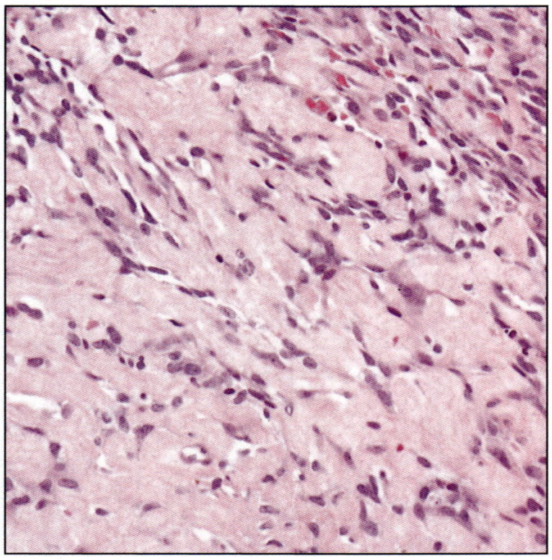

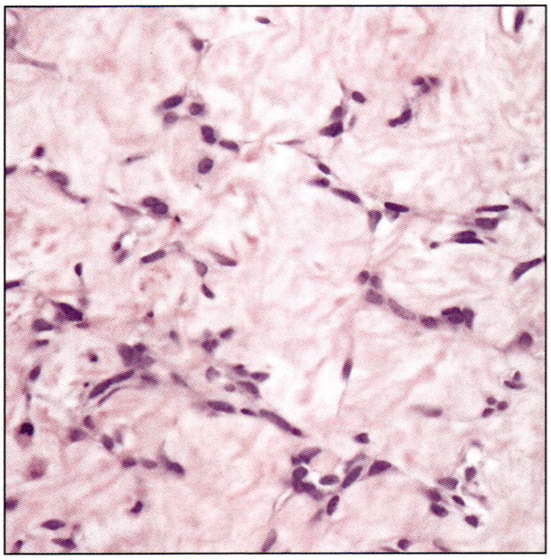

Immunohistochemical Features

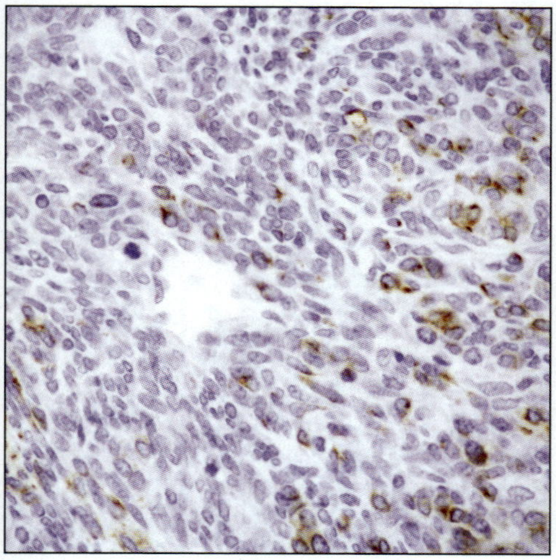

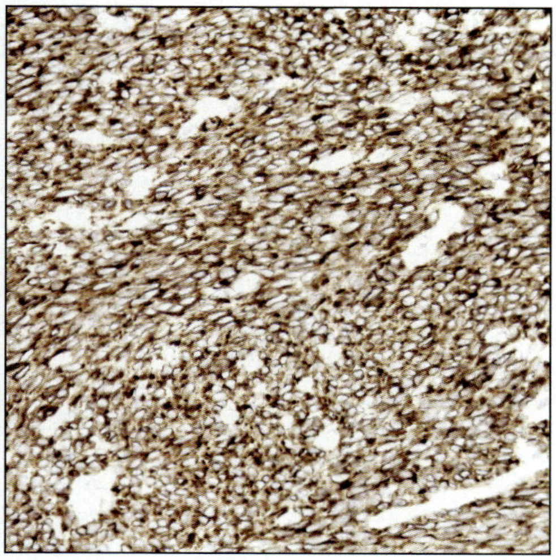

(Left) *Immunohistochemical stain for cytokeratin in monophasic synovial sarcoma of the pleura shows focal cytoplasmic positivity in scattered tumor cells. This is the typical staining pattern for cytokeratin in synovial sarcoma.* ***(Right)*** *Immunohistochemical staining of monophasic synovial sarcoma of the mediastinum for BCL2 oncogene shows strong positivity of the tumor cells. This marker is strongly expressed in practically all cases of monophasic synovial sarcoma.*

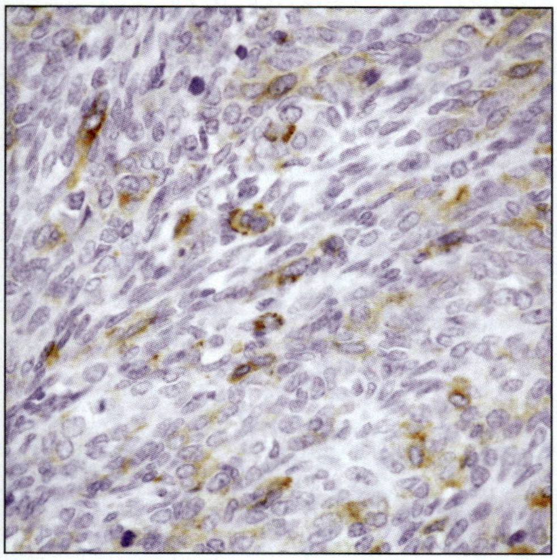

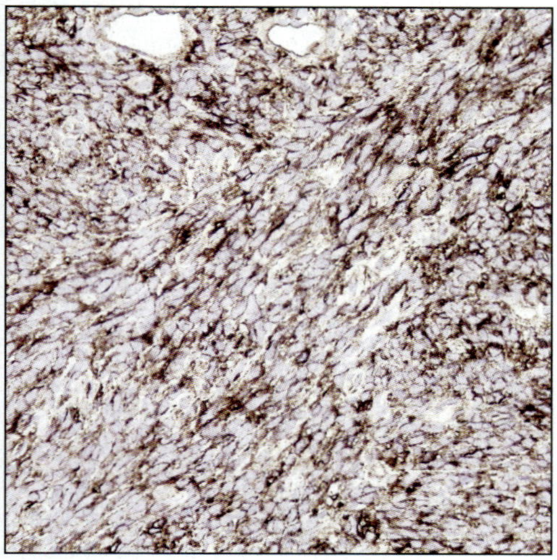

(Left) *Immunohistochemical stain for epithelial membrane antigen (EMA) is shown in monophasic synovial sarcoma of the pleura. The staining is patchy and often weak. EMA, however, may be a more sensitive marker for synovial sarcoma in cases that are keratin-negative.* ***(Right)*** *Immunohistochemical staining of monophasic synovial sarcoma of the mediastinum shows positive staining of the tumor cells for calponin.*

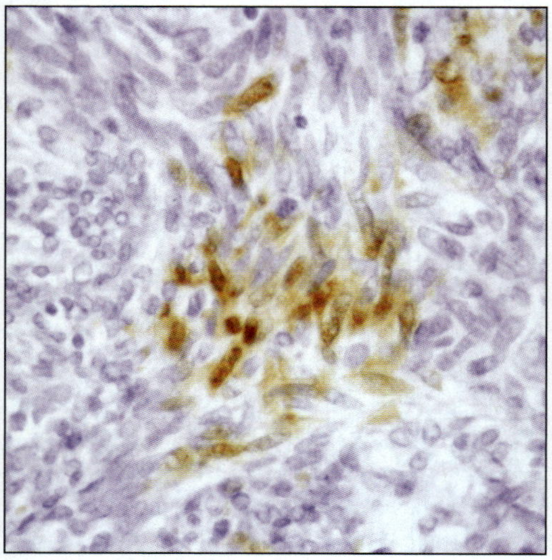

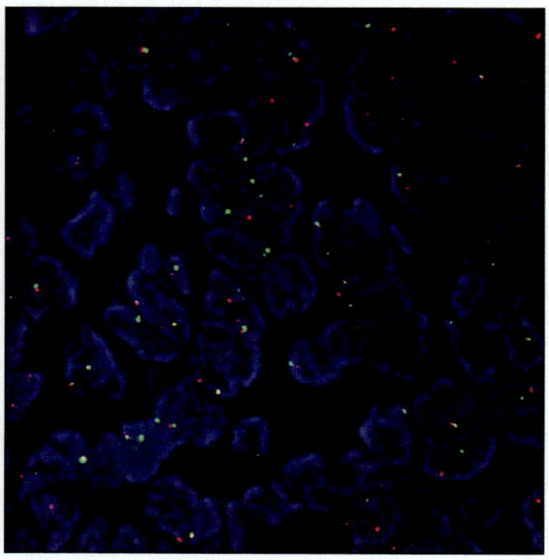

(Left) *Immunohistochemical stain for S100 protein shows monophasic synovial sarcoma. Notice focal nuclear positivity in a cluster of tumor cells. Up to 30% of monophasic synovial sarcoma has been reported to stain positive for this marker in 1 study.* ***(Right)*** *Fluorescence in situ hybridization (FISH) assay in a case of monophasic synovial sarcoma of the pleura demonstrates t(X;18) translocation by detecting the SYT-SSX fusion transcripts.*

MALIGNANT SOLITARY FIBROUS TUMOR (FIBROSARCOMA)

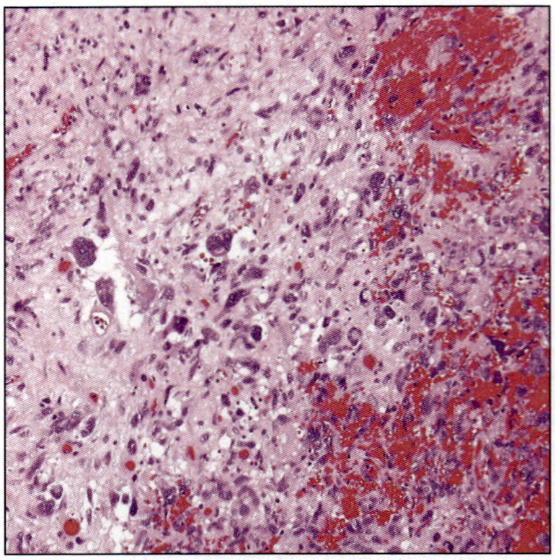

Malignant solitary fibrous tumor (pleural fibrosarcoma) shows scattered, discohesive atypical spindle cells admixed with pleomorphic large tumor cells and areas of hemorrhage.

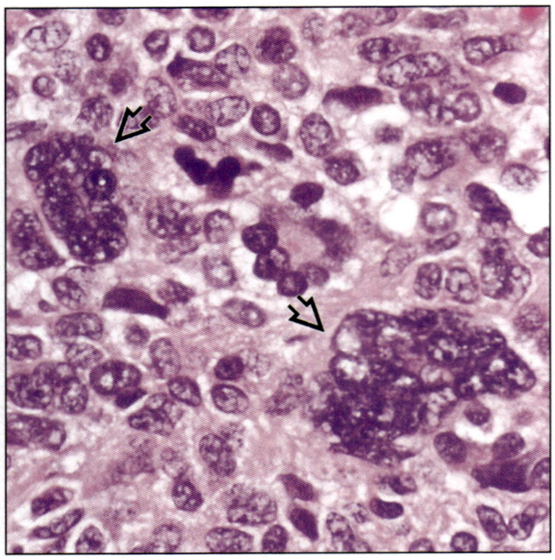

High power of malignant solitary fibrous tumor of the pleura shows highly atypical, pleomorphic, multinucleated tumor cells ⮚. Notice the more bland-appearing mononuclear cells in the background.

TERMINOLOGY

Abbreviations

- Malignant solitary fibrous tumor (MSFT)

Synonyms

- Pleural fibrosarcoma

Definitions

- Malignant neoplastic proliferation of submesothelial fibroblasts

CLINICAL ISSUES

Presentation

- Cough
- Pleuritic pain
- Dyspnea

Treatment

- Surgical excision
- Radiation
- Chemotherapy

Prognosis

- Based on staging and grade
- Usually aggressive behavior similar to high-grade sarcomas

MACROSCOPIC FEATURES

General Features

- Diffuse growth
- Poorly circumscribed
- Invasion of adjacent structures
- Areas of necrosis
- Hemorrhage
- May spread along pleural surface in a fashion reminiscent of malignant mesothelioma

MICROSCOPIC PATHOLOGY

Histologic Features

- Dense atypical spindle cell proliferation
- Fascicular, herringbone, storiform, and hemangiopericytic growth patterns
- May contain foci of "dedifferentiation"
- Areas of typical, low-grade solitary fibrous tumor must be identified to make diagnosis
- Infiltration of fat and surrounding tissues
- High mitotic activity (> 3 mitoses per 10 high-power fields)

Cytologic Features

- Atypical spindle cells with enlarged, hyperchromatic nuclei
- Marked nuclear pleomorphism
- Prominent nucleoli
- Tumor cell necrosis
- Bizarre giant cells and multinucleated cells

ANCILLARY TESTS

Immunohistochemistry

- Immunohistochemical stains are of limited value because markers associated with SFT may lose their expression in poorly differentiated variants
- Better differentiated areas stain positive for CD34, Bcl-2, CD99, and vimentin
- p53 and Ki-67 may show increased positivity in poorly differentiated areas

DIFFERENTIAL DIAGNOSIS

Sarcomatoid Mesothelioma

- May have similar clinical and radiological features
- Most sarcomatoid mesotheliomas are positive for cytokeratin

MALIGNANT SOLITARY FIBROUS TUMOR (FIBROSARCOMA)

Key Facts

Macroscopic Features

- Diffuse growth
- Poorly circumscribed
- Invasion of adjacent structures
- Areas of necrosis
- Hemorrhage

Microscopic Pathology

- Dense atypical spindle cell proliferation
- Fascicular, herringbone, storiform, and hemangiopericytic growth patterns
- May contain foci of "dedifferentiation"
- Areas of typical, low-grade solitary fibrous tumor must be identified to make diagnosis
- Atypical spindle cells with enlarged, hyperchromatic nuclei
- Marked nuclear pleomorphism
- Prominent nucleoli
- Tumor cell necrosis
- Bizarre giant cells and multinucleated cells
- Immunohistochemical stains are of limited value for diagnosis because markers associated with SFT may lose their expression in poorly differentiated variants
- Better differentiated areas stain positive for CD34, Bcl-2, CD99, and vimentin
- p53 and Ki-67 may show increased positivity in poorly differentiated areas

Diagnostic Checklist

- MSFT is largely a diagnosis of exclusion
- Other types of malignant spindle cell tumors of pleura must be ruled out 1st (e.g., sarcomatoid mesothelioma, synovial sarcoma, etc.)

- Need to identify areas typical for solitary fibrous tumor to diagnose malignant SFT

Pleural Synovial Sarcoma

- Spindle cell population is much more monotonous and uniform in synovial sarcoma
- No nuclear pleomorphism or giant cells seen in synovial sarcoma
- Synovial sarcoma is positive for cytokeratin and EMA
- Identification of t(x;18) by molecular techniques is diagnostic of synovial sarcoma and is absent in MSFT

Malignant Peripheral Nerve Sheath Tumor (MPNST)

- Histologic features may be very similar for both in high-grade tumors
- Electron microscopy of MPNST is distinctive and characterized by interdigitating cytoplasmic processes with basal lamina material

Metastatic Malignant Melanoma

- Histologic features may be very similar to MSFT
- Clinical history of malignant melanoma favors a metastasis
- Immunohistochemical positivity for S100 protein, HMB-45, and Melan-A is seen in melanoma

Metastatic Spindle Cell Sarcoma of Soft Tissue

- Variety of soft tissue spindle cell sarcomas can metastasize to pleura
- History of previous tumor elsewhere and bilateral lesions will favor a metastasis
  - Multiple local recurrences will favor primary tumor over a metastasis of sarcoma

Metastatic Sarcomatoid Renal Cell Carcinoma

- Histologic features may be very similar to MSFT
- Renal cell carcinoma will show positivity for cytokeratin, EMA, and CD10
- Clinical history of previous kidney tumor will favor a metastasis of renal cell carcinoma

DIAGNOSTIC CHECKLIST

Clinically Relevant Pathologic Features

- Gross appearance
  - Diffuse, infiltrative growth
  - Areas of hemorrhage and necrosis
  - Absence of a capsule
- Mitotic rate
  - > 3 mitoses per 10 high-power fields
  - Presence of atypical (abnormal) mitoses
- Nuclear features
  - Enlarged, hyperchromatic nuclei
  - Prominent nucleoli
  - Multinucleated cells

Pathologic Interpretation Pearls

- MSFT is largely a diagnosis of exclusion
- Other types of malignant spindle cell tumors of pleura must be ruled out 1st
- Immunohistochemical stains are not very specific in this setting and may be of limited value
- Most important feature for histologic diagnosis is identifying areas showing typical features of benign solitary fibrous tumor

SELECTED REFERENCES

1. Mosquera JM et al: Expanding the spectrum of malignant progression in solitary fibrous tumors: a study of 8 cases with a discrete anaplastic component--is this dedifferentiated SFT? Am J Surg Pathol. 33(9):1314-21, 2009
2. Hanau CA et al: Solitary fibrous tumor: histological and immunohistochemical spectrum of benign and malignant variants presenting at different sites. Hum Pathol. 26(4):440-9, 1995
3. Moran CA et al: The spectrum of histologic growth patterns in benign and malignant fibrous tumors of the pleura. Semin Diagn Pathol. 9(2):169-80, 1992

MALIGNANT SOLITARY FIBROUS TUMOR (FIBROSARCOMA)

Microscopic Features

*(**Left**) Malignant solitary fibrous tumor of the pleura shows a biphasic appearance with an area resembling conventional, benign solitary fibrous tumor (left) merging with hypercellular areas containing malignant elements (right). (**Right**) Preexisting benign solitary fibrous tumor component in malignant solitary fibrous tumor of pleura shows bland-appearing spindle cell proliferation devoid of cytologic atypia, nuclear pleomorphism, or any significant mitotic activity.*

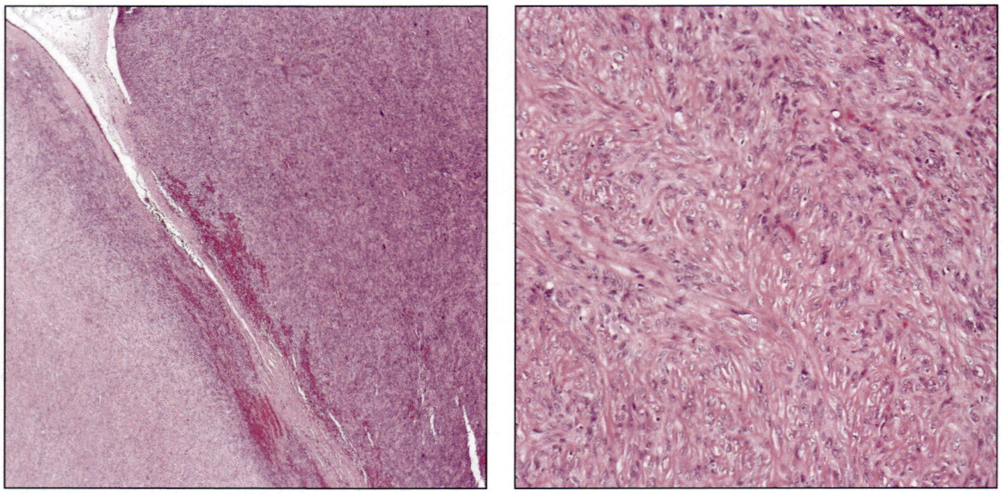

*(**Left**) Hypercellular, malignant component in malignant solitary fibrous tumor of pleura shows increased cellularity with significant nuclear pleomorphism. Notice scattered large pleomorphic and multinucleated tumor cells ↪. (**Right**) High-power view of a malignant solitary fibrous tumor of the pleura shows atypical spindle cell proliferation characterized by spindle cells with a dense chromatin pattern and occasional mitotic figures. Notice the large tumor cells with multiple nuclei →.*

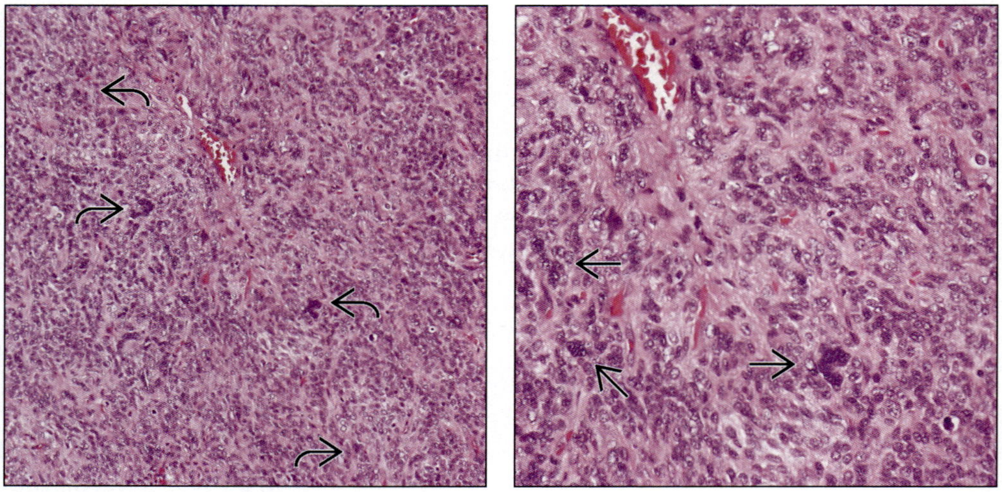

*(**Left**) High-power view of a malignant solitary fibrous tumor shows numerous bizarre multinucleated tumor cells with multiple enlarged nuclei. The nuclei in these cells show a dense chromatin pattern and vesiculation and contain scanty cytoplasm. (**Right**) High-power view of a malignant solitary fibrous tumor of the pleura shows a large multinucleated tumor cell. The giant tumor cell contains more than 20 nuclei and resembles a polykaryosome of Whartin-Finkeldey giant cell.*

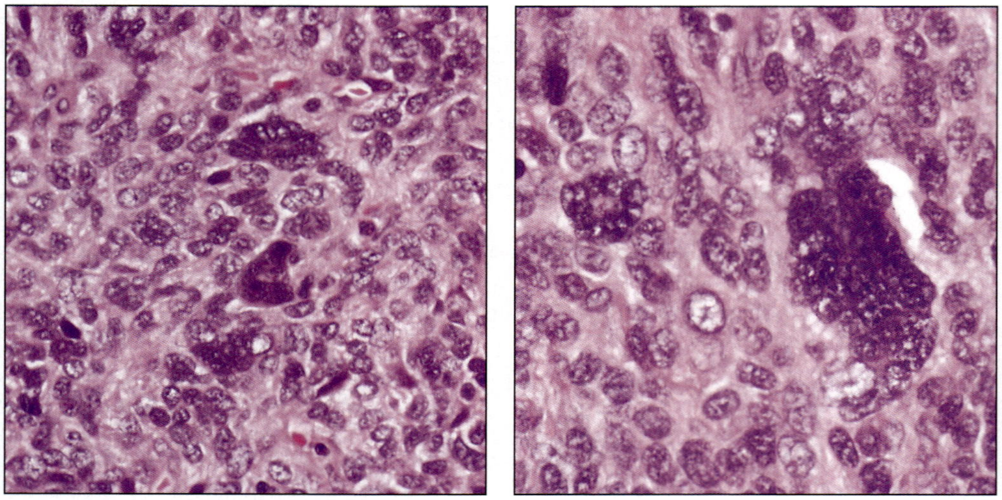

MALIGNANT SOLITARY FIBROUS TUMOR (FIBROSARCOMA)

Microscopic Features

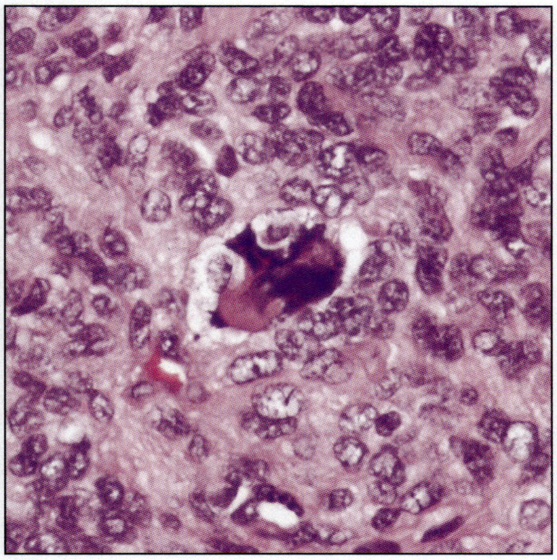
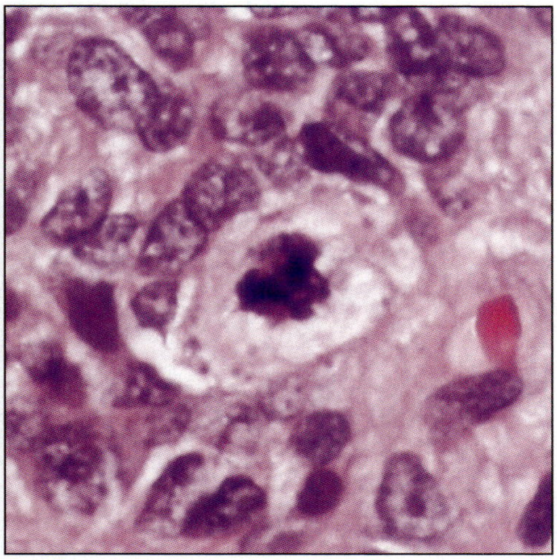

(Left) *Malignant solitary fibrous tumor of the pleura shows a bizarre, pleomorphic tumor cell with huge smudged nucleoli and retraction artifact surrounding the nucleus. Notice the monotonous population of mononuclear atypical cells surrounding the pleomorphic tumor cell.* ***(Right)*** *High magnification of malignant solitary fibrous tumor of the pleura (pleural fibrosarcoma) shows an abnormal mitotic figure within the mononuclear cell component of the tumor (center).*

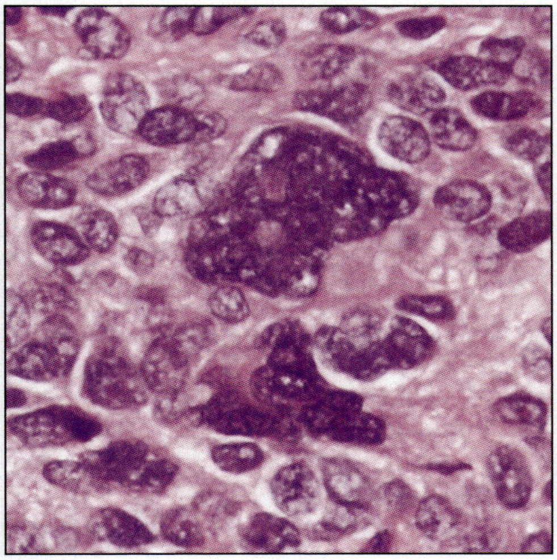
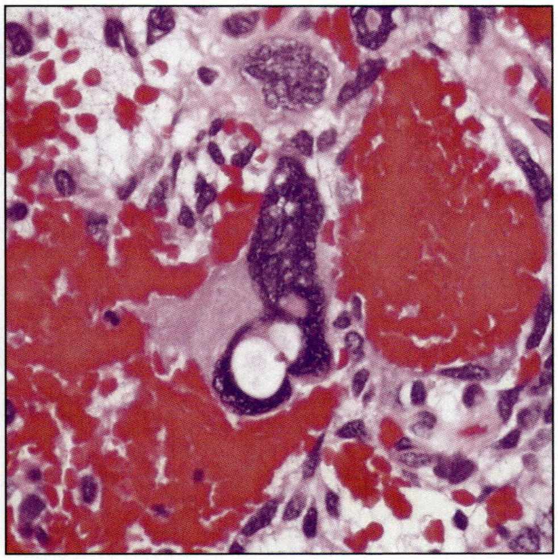

(Left) *High magnification of a malignant solitary fibrous tumor of the pleura shows several bizarre, hyperchromatic, and multinucleated tumor cells similar to the ones commonly observed in malignant fibrous histiocytoma.* ***(Right)*** *High magnification of a malignant solitary fibrous tumor of the pleura shows a bizarre tumor cell with intranuclear cytoplasmic inclusions. The appearance of the tumor cells and the abundant hemorrhage can closely simulate choriocarcinoma.*

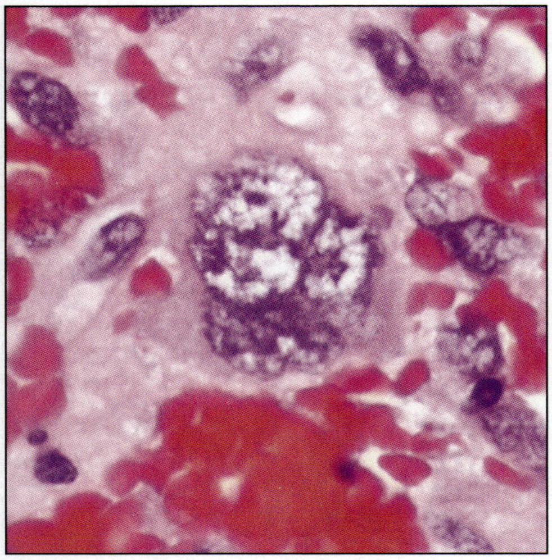
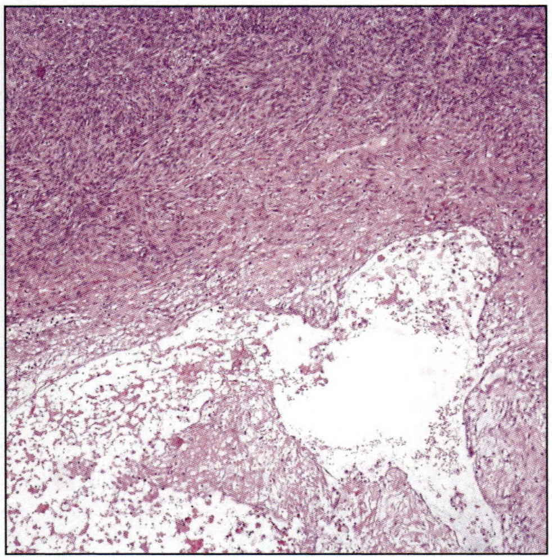

(Left) *High magnification of a malignant solitary fibrous tumor of the pleura shows a multinucleated tumor cell with vesicular nuclei and large eosinophilic nucleoli. These tumor cells can closely resemble the Reed-Sternberg cells seen in Hodgkin lymphoma.* ***(Right)*** *Malignant solitary fibrous tumor of the pleura shows an area of tumor cell necrosis adjacent to solid proliferation of atypical tumor cells.*

MALIGNANT SOLITARY FIBROUS TUMOR (FIBROSARCOMA)

Fibrosarcoma-like Malignant Solitary Fibrous Tumor

*(**Left**) Malignant solitary fibrous tumor of pleura shows a fibrosarcomatous appearance with fascicles of atypical spindle cells circumscribing an area of tumor cell necrosis →. (**Right**) Fibrosarcomatous variant of malignant solitary fibrous tumor of the pleura shows a large pleomorphic tumor cell ⇨. The surrounding cell population is composed of mildly atypical spindle cells with hyperchromatic nuclei surrounded by a scant rim of amphophilic cytoplasm.*

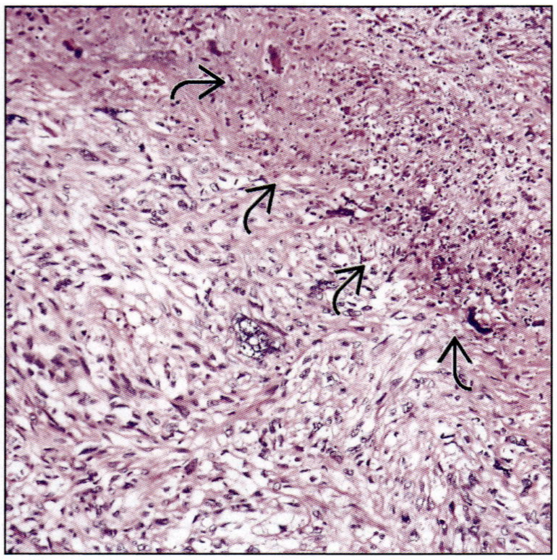

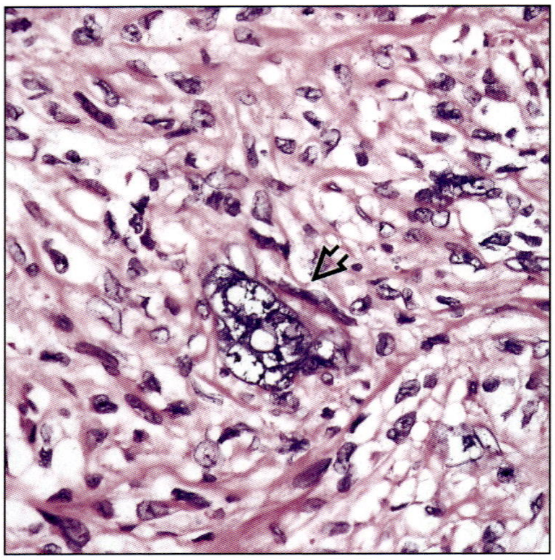

*(**Left**) Malignant solitary fibrous tumor of the pleura shows atypical spindle cell proliferation with collagenized stroma. Notice the scattered large, atypical, and often multinucleated tumor cells interspersed with the fibroblast-like spindle cells. (**Right**) Malignant solitary fibrous tumor of the pleura shows proliferation of atypical spindle cells with early features of tumor cell necrosis, apoptosis, and karrhyorrhexis.*

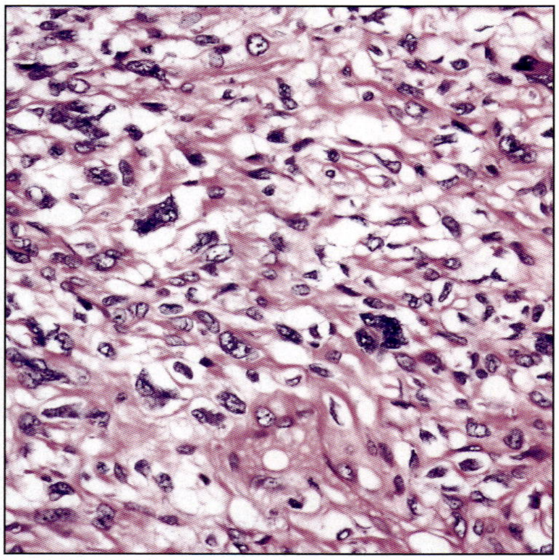

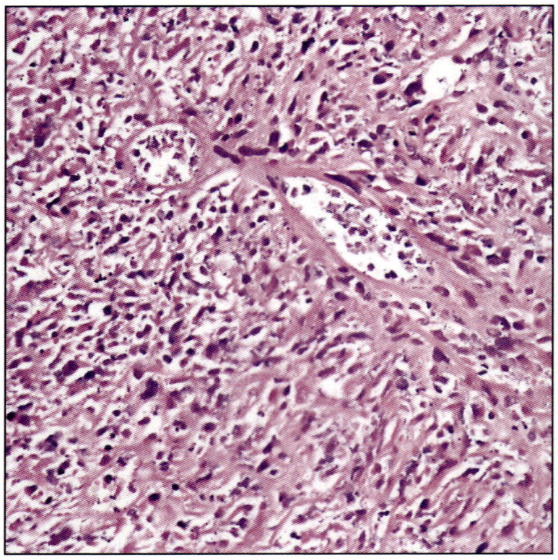

*(**Left**) Malignant solitary fibrous tumor of the pleura shows spindle cell proliferation with scattered mitotic figures and areas of necrosis embedded within abundant fibrous stroma. The tumor essentially resembles fibrosarcoma. (**Right**) High magnification of malignant solitary fibrous tumor of the pleura shows necrotic and dying spindle tumor cells and abundant scattered apoptotic bodies. Very few viable spindle tumor cells are seen in this field.*

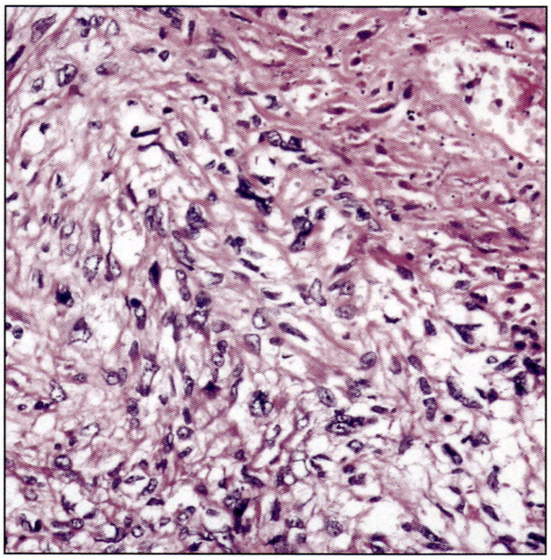

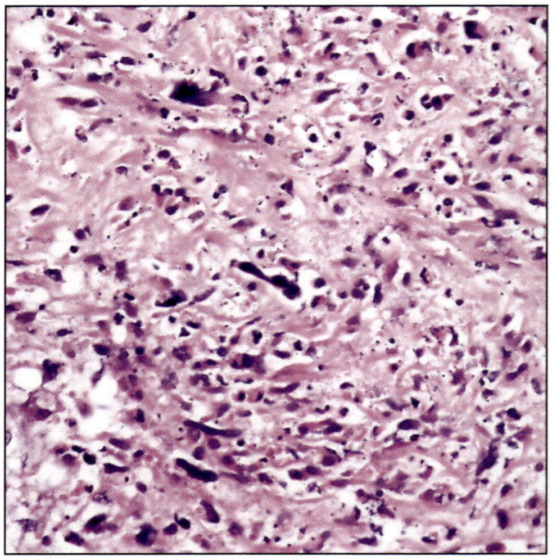

Fibrosarcoma-like Malignant Solitary Fibrous Tumor

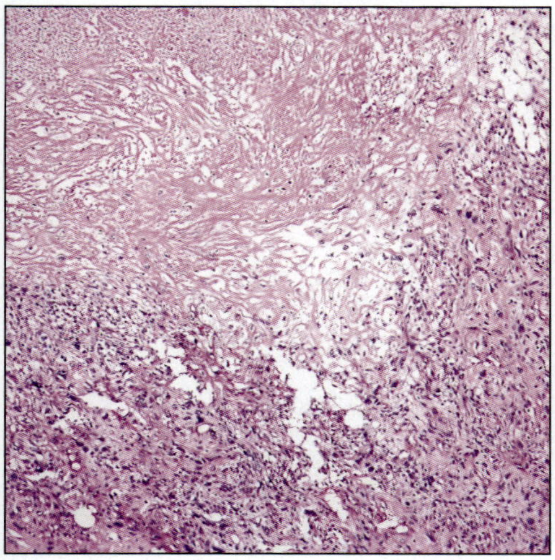
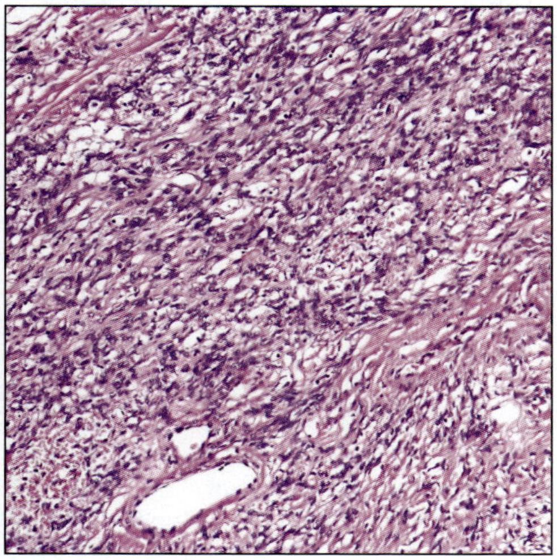

*(**Left**) Malignant solitary fibrous tumor of the pleura shows extensive areas of tumor cell necrosis (top). The viable portions of the tumor (bottom) are composed of an atypical spindle cell proliferation with collagenized stroma. (**Right**) Area of malignant solitary fibrous tumor shows a spindle cell population with preservation of the features of conventional solitary fibrous tumor and only early evidence of cytologic atypia.*

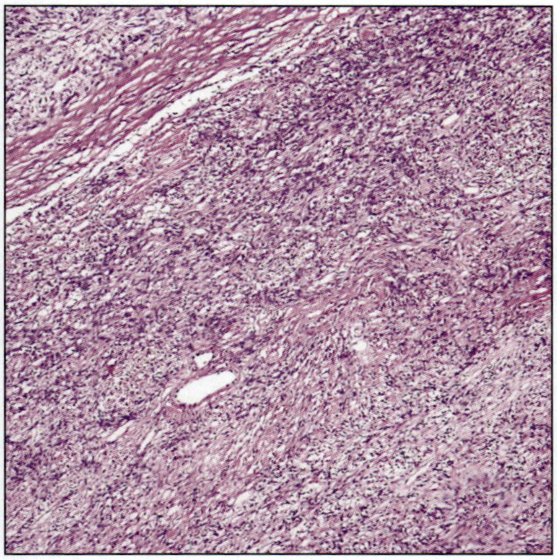
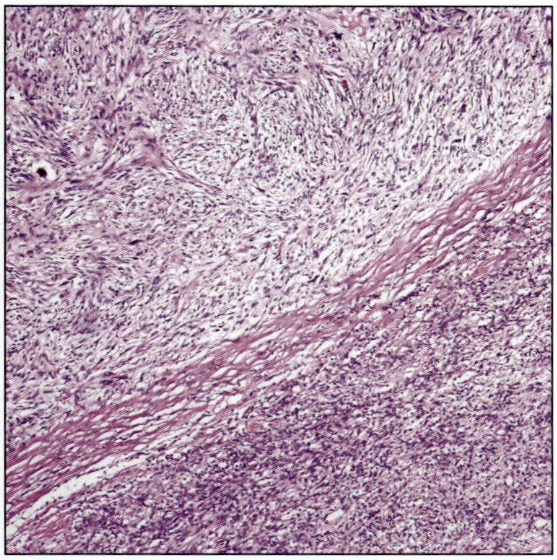

*(**Left**) Malignant solitary fibrous tumor of pleura shows fascicles of atypical spindle cells reminiscent of fibrosarcoma. Some of the original architecture of solitary fibrous tumor is still preserved in this area. (**Right**) Malignant solitary fibrous tumor of the pleura shows 2 distinct areas; a portion of the tumor (top) shows some myxoid stromal features and contains scattered large, atypical tumor cells, while a portion of the tumor (bottom) shows increased cellularity and atypia.*

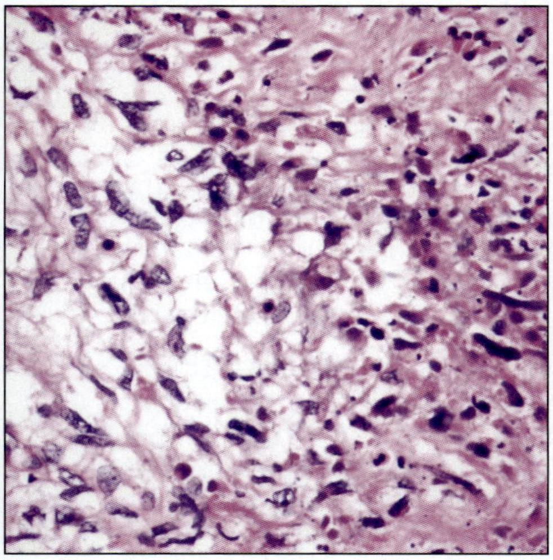
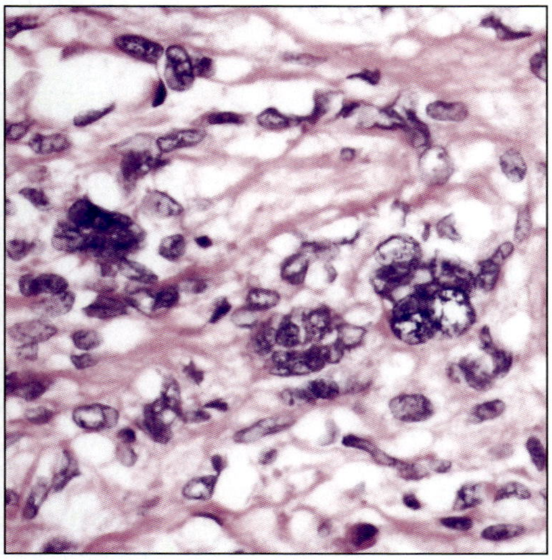

*(**Left**) Area of malignant solitary fibrous tumor shows viable tumor surrounded by extensive area of tumor cell necrosis. The viable tumor cells (left) show a dispersed chromatin pattern with prominent eosinophilic nucleoli. (**Right**) Malignant solitary fibrous tumor shows marked cytologic atypia, with large, multinucleated tumor cells with vesicular and hyperchromatic nuclei surrounded by mononuclear oval to spindle atypical cells embedded in collagenous stroma.*

SMOOTH MUSCLE TUMORS OF THE PLEURA

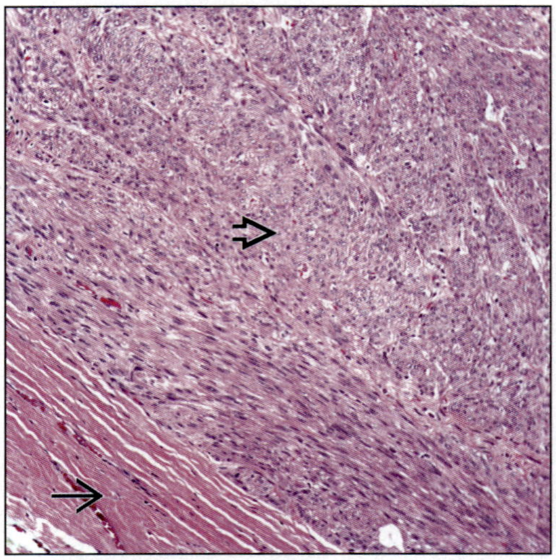

Pleural leiomyosarcoma shows the classical fascicular growth pattern composed of spindle cells ⇨. One is still able to recognize some residual pleural tissue →.

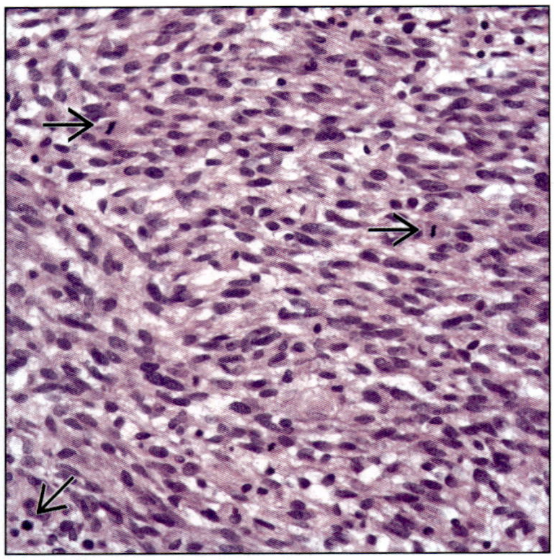

Higher magnification of a pleural leiomyosarcoma shows a spindle cell proliferation with nuclear atypia and scattered mitotic figures →.

TERMINOLOGY

Synonyms

- Leiomyoma, leiomyosarcoma

Definitions

- Spindle cell tumor with muscle differentiation

CLINICAL ISSUES

Epidemiology

- Incidence
  - Exceedingly rare tumors in pleura
- Age
  - Tumor affects individuals in wide range of ages (20-70 years)
- Gender
  - No apparent gender predilection

Presentation

- Chest pain
- Empyema
- Asymptomatic

Treatment

- Surgical approaches
  - Complete surgical resection
- Adjuvant therapy
  - In high-grade tumors, chemotherapy may be considered

Prognosis

- Depends on grade of tumor
  - Higher grade tumors have poor prognosis

MACROSCOPIC FEATURES

General Features

- Pleural-based tumors
- Diffuse involvement of pleura can occur
- Firm, white, and homogeneous surface
- Areas of hemorrhage &/or necrosis may be present

Size

- Between 10-18 cm

MICROSCOPIC PATHOLOGY

Histologic Features

- Spindle cell proliferation
- Fascicular pattern
- Variable mitotic activity
- Variable nuclear atypia
- Necrosis
- Hemorrhage

Predominant Pattern/Injury Type

- Sarcomatoid

Predominant Cell/Compartment Type

- Myoid

DIFFERENTIAL DIAGNOSIS

Solitary Fibrous Tumor (SFT)

- Shows positive staining for CD34 and Bcl-2
- Shows different growth patterns in the same tumor
- Would be unusual for SFT to show strong positive reaction for desmin and smooth muscle actin

Peripheral Nerve Sheath Tumor (PNST)

- May show positive staining for S100 protein
- Would be most unusual for PNST to show positive staining for desmin &/or smooth muscle actin

Desmoid Tumor

- Spindle cell proliferation of desmoid tumor is fibroblastic

SMOOTH MUSCLE TUMORS OF THE PLEURA

Key Facts

Clinical Issues

- Incidence
  - Exceedingly rare tumors in pleura
  - Tumor affects individuals in wide range of ages (20-70 years)
- Symptoms
  - Chest pain
  - Empyema
  - Asymptomatic

Macroscopic Features

- Pleural-based tumors
- Diffuse involvement of pleura can occur

Microscopic Pathology

- Spindle cell proliferation
- Fascicular pattern
- Variable mitotic activity
- Necrosis

Top Differential Diagnoses

- Solitary fibrous tumor (SFT)
  - Shows positive staining for CD34 and Bcl-2
  - Shows different growth patterns in the same tumor
- Peripheral nerve sheath tumor (PNST)
  - May show positive staining for S100 protein
  - Would be most unusual for PNST to show positive staining for desmin &/or smooth muscle actin
- Desmoid tumor
  - Spindle cell proliferation of desmoid tumor is fibroblastic
  - Would be unusual to show strong positive staining for desmin or smooth muscle actin

Immunohistochemistry

Antibody	Reactivity	Staining Pattern	Comment
Desmin	Positive	Cytoplasmic	Staining will vary depending on grade of tumor
Actin-sm	Positive	Cytoplasmic	Variable staining; can also be positive in some carcinomas
Caldesmon	Positive	Cytoplasmic	Stronger staining in lower grade tumors
CD34	Negative		
Bcl-2	Negative		
S100	Negative		
CK-PAN	Negative		May be positive in low-grade tumors

- Desmoid tumors would be unusual to show strong positive staining for desmin or smooth muscle actin

DIAGNOSTIC CHECKLIST

Clinically Relevant Pathologic Features

- Mitotic rate

Pathologic Interpretation Pearls

- Fascicular growth pattern
- Interlacing fascicles of elongated cells intersecting at right angles
- Mitotic count

GRADING

Uncertain Malignant Potential to Low Grade

- Spindle cells
- Fascicular growth pattern
- Mild nuclear atypia
- Scattered mitotic figures
- Absent necrosis &/or hemorrhage

Intermediate Grade

- Spindle cells
- Fascicular growth pattern
- Moderate nuclear atypia
- Necrosis &/or hemorrhage are present
- Mitotic activity easily identified (< 10 per 10 HPF)

High Grade

- Disorganized spindle cell proliferation
- Prominent nuclear atypia
- Atypical mitosis easily identified and numerous
- Necrosis &/or hemorrhage easily identified

SELECTED REFERENCES

1. Andino L et al: Pleuropulmonary desmoid tumors: immunohistochemical comparison with solitary fibrous tumors and assessment of beta-catenin and cyclin D1 expression. Arch Pathol Lab Med. 130(10):1503-9, 2006
2. Al-Daraji WI et al: Primary smooth muscle tumor of the pleura: a clinicopathological case report with ultrastructural observations and a review of the literature. Ultrastruct Pathol. 29(5):389-98, 2005
3. Takeshima Y et al: Extra-abdominal desmoid tumor presenting as an intrathoracic tumor: case report and literature review. Pathol Int. 51(10):824-8, 2001
4. Kubota Y et al: Myofibroblastic sarcoma of the pleura in a pig. J Vet Med Sci. 62(8):913-6, 2000
5. Proca DM et al: Smooth muscle tumor of the pleura. A case report and review of the literature. Arch Pathol Lab Med. 124(11):1688-92, 2000
6. Wilson RW et al: Desmoid tumors of the pleura: a clinicopathologic mimic of localized fibrous tumor. Mod Pathol. 12(1):9-14, 1999
7. Moran CA et al: Smooth muscle tumours of the pleura. Histopathology. 30(1):97-8, 1997

SMOOTH MUSCLE TUMORS OF THE PLEURA

Microscopic Features

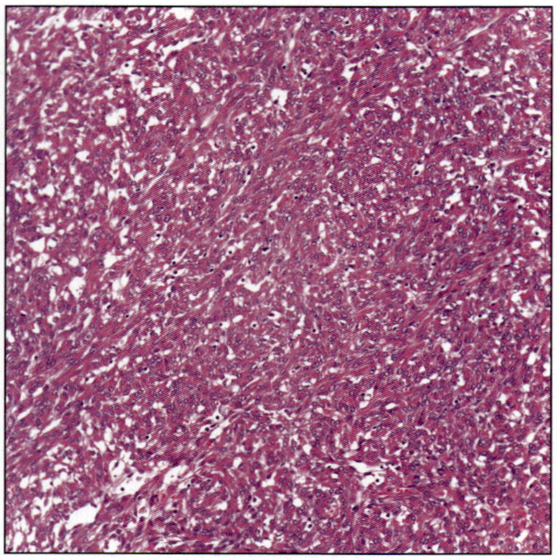

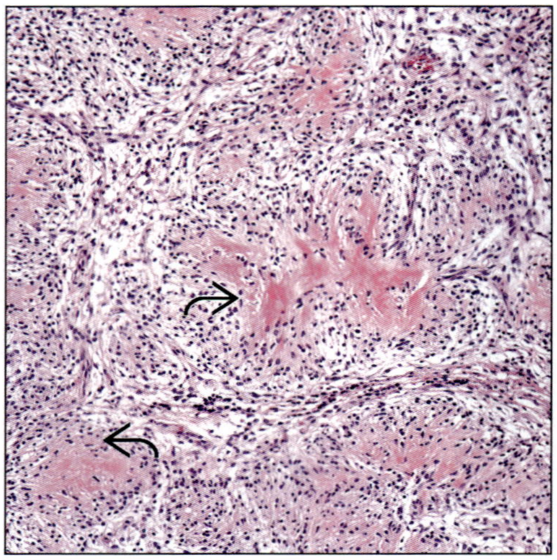

(Left) *Low-power view of a low-grade leiomyosarcoma of the pleura shows a spindle cellular proliferation with striking muscle appearance. Note the absence of hemorrhage or necrosis.* ***(Right)*** *Low-grade leiomyosarcoma shows a bland spindle cell proliferation with areas resembling the so-called amianthoid fibers ↪.*

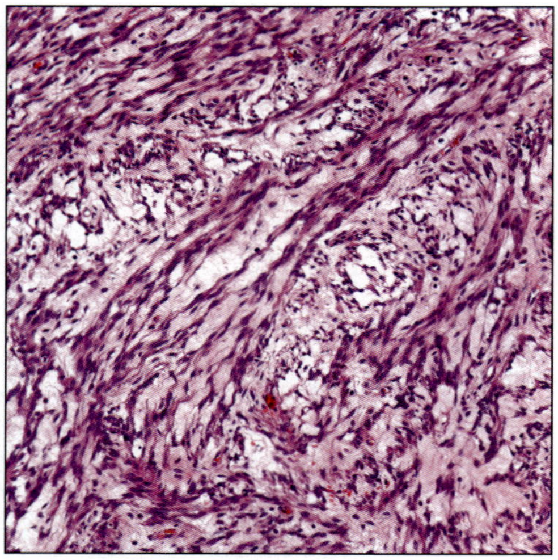

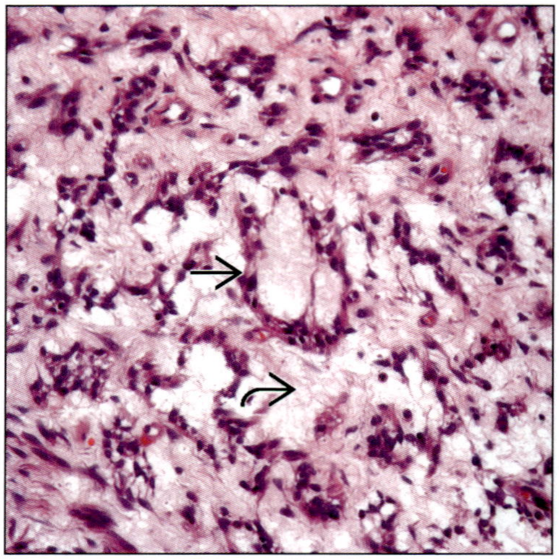

(Left) *Low-grade leiomyosarcoma of the pleura shows a spindle cell proliferation closely mimicking a neural tumor. Necrosis and hemorrhage are absent.* ***(Right)*** *Low-grade leiomyosarcoma with areas mimicking a glandular space → is seen with some myxoid changes ↪.*

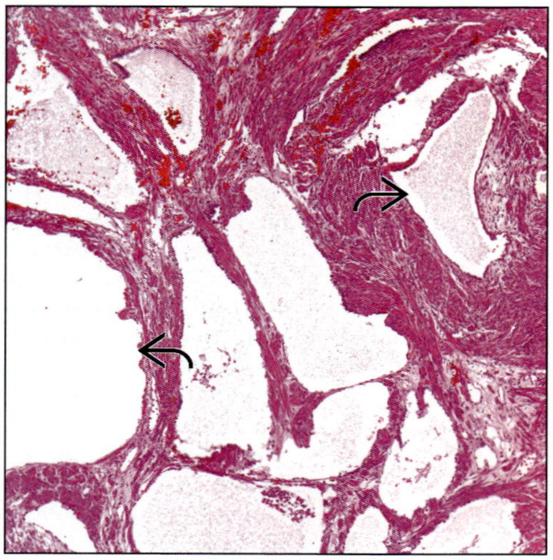

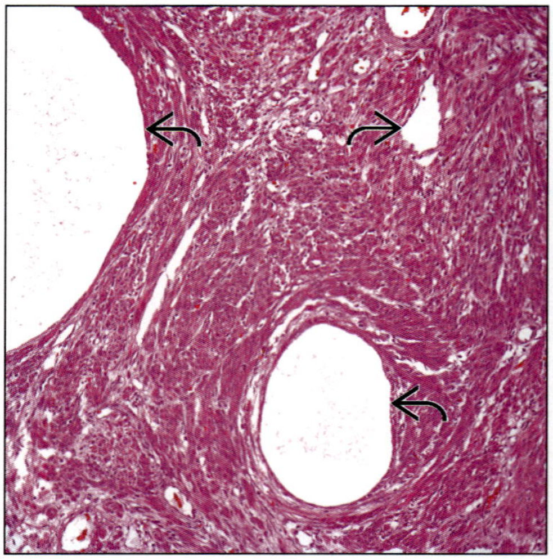

(Left) *Low-grade leiomyosarcoma shows prominent cystic changes ↪. Some of these cystic structures may be lined by flattened epithelium.* ***(Right)*** *Low-grade leiomyosarcoma is seen with more solid component and only focal small cystic structures ↪. In these areas, the nuclear atypia and mitotic activity may not be prominent.*

SMOOTH MUSCLE TUMORS OF THE PLEURA

Microscopic and Immunohistochemical Features

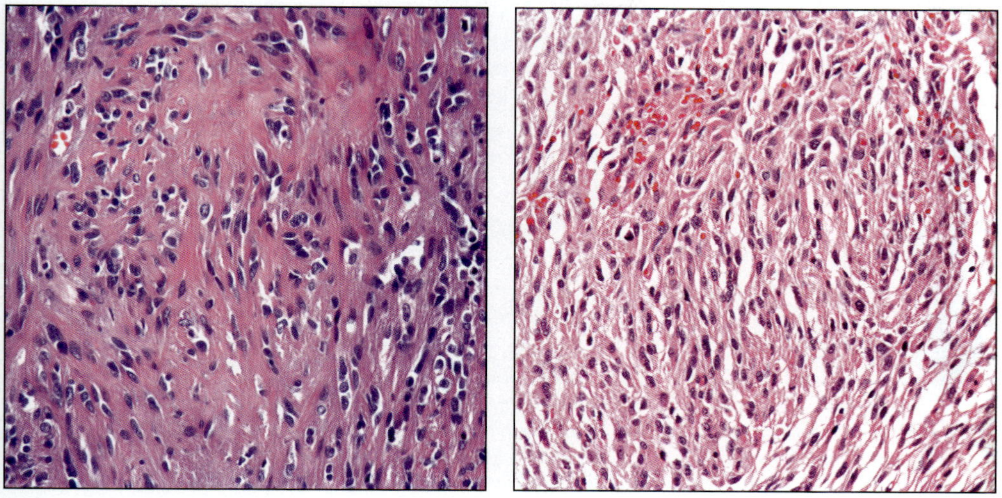

(Left) *Intermediate-grade leiomyosarcoma shows moderate nuclear atypia and spindle cells dissecting into collagenous tissue.* ***(Right)*** *Higher magnification shows mitotic activity and nuclear atypia. Note that the tumor still preserves a good fascicular arrangement, but the presence of nuclear pleomorphism and mitotic activity is a clue for a higher grade tumor.*

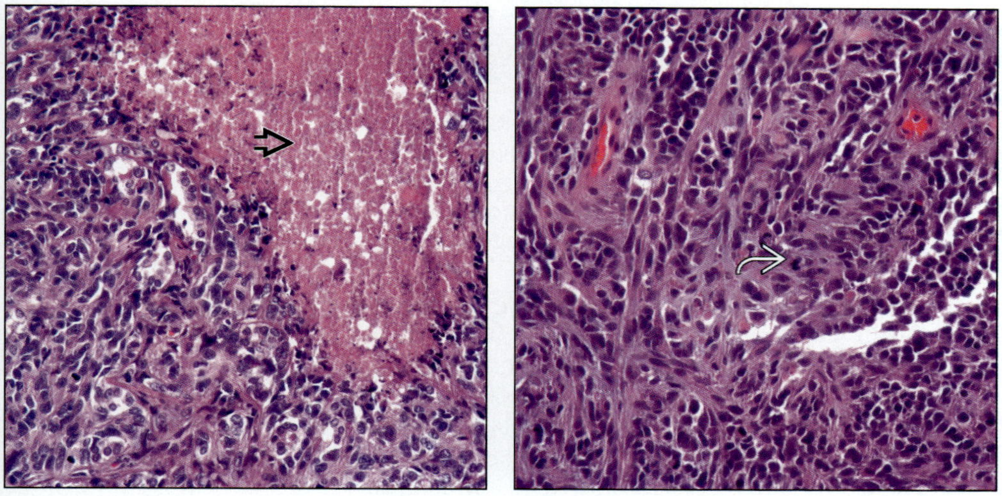

(Left) *High-grade leiomyosarcoma of the pleura shows areas of necrosis ⇨. Note the marked nuclear atypia, cellular pleomorphism, and mitotic activity.* ***(Right)*** *Higher magnification of a high-grade leiomyosarcoma shows prominent cellular and nuclear atypia as well as increased mitotic activity ↷.*

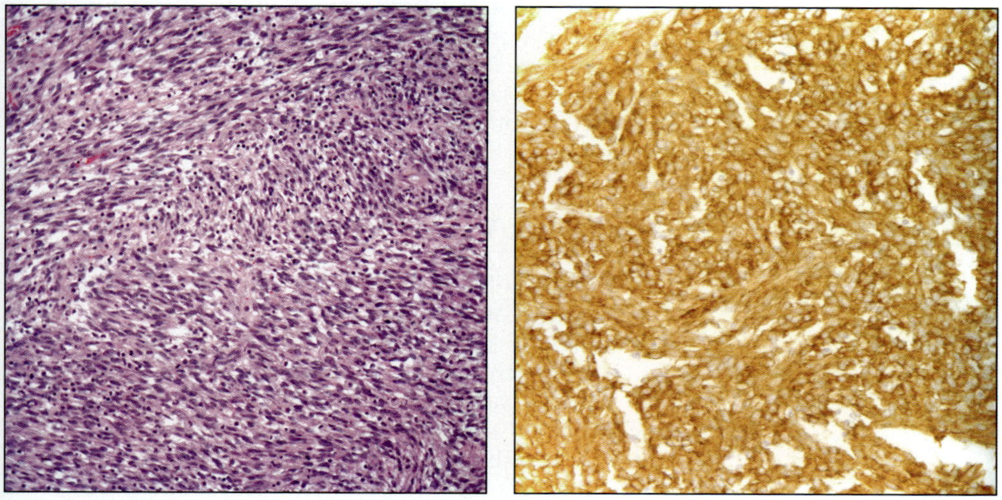

(Left) *More conventional features of leiomyosarcoma of the pleura show intersecting fascicles of tumor cells, which are typical for leiomyosarcomas.* ***(Right)*** *Desmin immunohistochemical stain shows strong positive reaction in tumor cells.*

DESMOPLASTIC SMALL ROUND CELL TUMOR

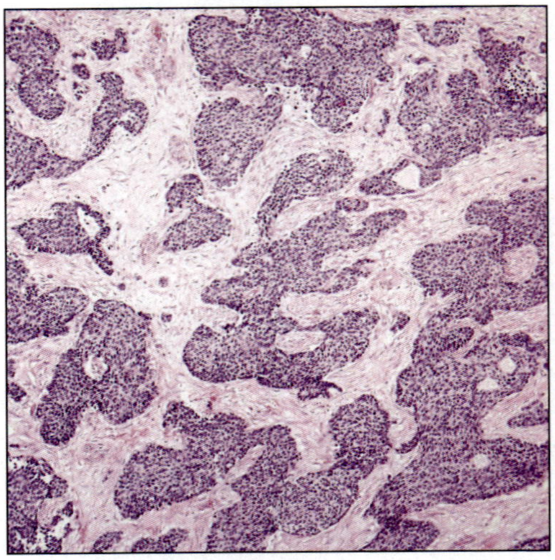

Desmoplastic small round cell tumor of the pleura shows islands of small round blue tumor cells surrounded by abundant, paucicellular, and desmoplastic connective tissue stroma.

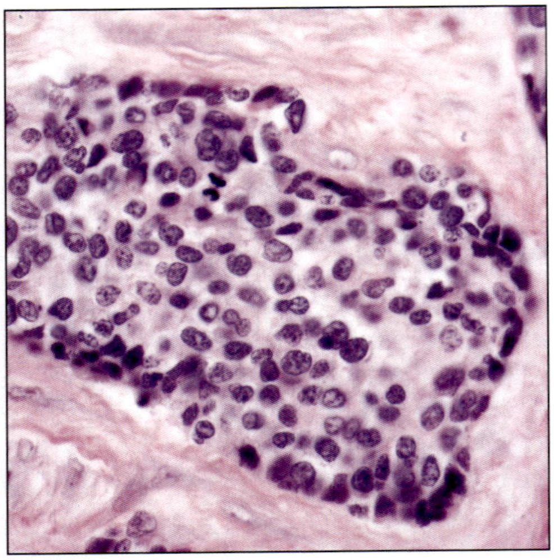

Small island of tumor cells in small desmoplastic round cell tumor shows primitive small blue cells with dispersed nuclear chromatin, small inconspicuous nucleoli, and occasional mitoses.

TERMINOLOGY

Abbreviations

- Desmoplastic small round cell tumor (DSRCT)

Synonyms

- Desmoplastic small cell tumor with divergent differentiation
- Polyphenotypic small round cell tumor
- Desmoplastic primitive neuroectodermal tumor

Definitions

- Primitive malignant neoplasm arising in serosal surfaces with distinctive histology composed of primitive small round blue cells embedded in abundant desmoplastic stroma

ETIOLOGY/PATHOGENESIS

Unknown

- May represent primitive mesothelial neoplasm (i.e., "mesoblastoma")

CLINICAL ISSUES

Presentation

- Male predilection
- Pain and weight loss
- Large pleural-based mass on chest x-rays and CT scans
- Most common in children and young adults (median age: 20 years)

Treatment

- Surgical excision
- Chemotherapy

Prognosis

- Poor prognosis
- Frequent local recurrence; rarely metastasizes
- Median survival is 24 months

MACROSCOPIC FEATURES

General Features

- Large, bulky tumors (> 10 cm in greatest dimension)
- May also grow in multinodular fashion
- Firm, homogeneous cut surface
- Hemorrhage and necrosis

MICROSCOPIC PATHOLOGY

Histologic Features

- Nests, trabeculae, or sheets of small round blue cells embedded in abundant desmoplastic fibrous stroma
- Nests may display peripheral palisading of tumor cells
- Rosette-like structures

Cytologic Features

- Small to intermediate-sized round to oval cells with scant cytoplasm
- Round to oval, hyperchromatic nuclei
- Small nucleoli
- High mitotic rate, often with atypical (abnormal) mitoses

ANCILLARY TESTS

Immunohistochemistry

- Staining pattern is polyphenotypic
- Vimentin, keratin, desmin, EMA, and WT1 consistently stain tumor cells in ~ 90% of cases
- Staining pattern for desmin and vimentin is characteristically dot-like and paranuclear
- May also show focal positivity for CD56, NSE, chromogranin, synaptophysin, and S100 protein

DESMOPLASTIC SMALL ROUND CELL TUMOR

Key Facts

Clinical Issues
- Most common in children and young adults (median age: 20 years)
- Male predilection
- Large pleural-based mass on chest x-rays and CT scans
- Poor prognosis
- Median survival is 24 months

Macroscopic Features
- Large, bulky tumors (> 10 cm in greatest dimension)

Microscopic Pathology
- Nests, trabeculae, or sheets of small round blue cells embedded in abundant desmoplastic fibrous stroma
- Rosette-like structures
- Small to intermediate-sized round to oval cells with scant cytoplasm
- High mitotic rate, often with atypical (abnormal) mitoses
- Staining pattern is polyphenotypic
- Vimentin, keratin, desmin, EMA, and WT1 consistently stain tumor cells in ~ 90% of cases
- Staining pattern for desmin and vimentin is characteristically dot-like and paranuclear
- May also show focal positivity for CD56, NSE, chromogranin, synaptophysin, and S100 protein
- Shows t(11:22)(p13;q12), similar to Ewing sarcoma/ PNET
- Unlike Ewing sarcoma, site on chromosome 11 is *WT-1* gene rather than *FLI-1* gene

Cytogenetics
- Unlike Ewing sarcoma, site on chromosome 11 is *WT-1* gene rather than *FLI-1* gene
- Shows t(11:22)(p13;q12), similar to Ewing sarcoma/ PNET

DIFFERENTIAL DIAGNOSIS

Peripheral Neuroectodermal Tumor (PNET)/ Ewing Sarcoma
- Similar cell population in both, but prominent desmoplastic stroma is not seen in PNET
- PNET does not show strong expression of polyphenotypic markers, such as desmin, keratin, and WT1
- PNET is strongly positive for CD99 in almost 100% of cases; CD99 is only seen in 20% of cases of DSRCT
- Translocation in PNET is t(11:22)(p24;q12); translocation in DSRCT is t(11:22)(p13;q12)

Metastatic Neuroendocrine Carcinoma
- Does not show prominent desmoplastic stroma separating tumor cell nests
- Has distinctive "smudged" or "salt & pepper" chromatin pattern
- Neuroendocrine carcinoma stains positive for neuroendocrine markers, such as chromogranin, CD56, and synaptophysin
- Neuroendocrine carcinomas do not express EMA, desmin, or WT1

Malignant Lymphoma
- Lymphomas show discohesive pattern of growth without striking desmoplasia
- Expresses CD45 and variety of other lymphoid markers, such as CD3, CD20, CD30, CD43, etc.
- Does not express keratin, desmin, WT1, and EMA
- Lymphoblastic lymphoma in children and adolescents shows nuclear positivity for TdT and lack of expression for CD99

DIAGNOSTIC CHECKLIST

Clinically Relevant Pathologic Features
- Preferentially affects children and young adults, although it can affect older patients

Pathologic Interpretation Pearls
- Distinctive combination of nests of small round blue cells surrounded by abundant desmoplastic fibrous stroma
- Primitive appearance of tumor cells
- High mitotic activity and areas of tumor cell necrosis
- Distinctive pattern of immunohistochemical staining: Keratin, EMA, vimentin, desmin, and WT1 positive
- Distinctive pattern of dot-like, paranuclear (Golgi zone) staining for vimentin and desmin
- Distinctive cytogenetic translocation, t(11:22)(p13;q12)

SELECTED REFERENCES

1. Jeong YJ et al: Neoplastic and nonneoplastic conditions of serosal membrane origin: CT findings. Radiographics. 28(3):801-17; discussion 817-8; quiz 912, 2008
2. Karavitakis EM et al: Desmoplastic small round cell tumor of the pleura. Pediatr Blood Cancer. 49(3):335-8, 2007
3. Lae ME et al: Desmoplastic small round cell tumor: a clinicopathologic, immunohistochemical, and molecular study of 32 tumors. Am J Surg Pathol. 26(7):823-35, 2002
4. Sápi Z et al: Desmoplastic small round cell tumour of the pleura: a case report with further cytogenetic and ultrastructural evidence of 'mesothelioblastemic' origin. Eur J Surg Oncol. 25(6):633-4, 1999
5. Ordóñez NG: Desmoplastic small round cell tumor: I: a histopathologic study of 39 cases with emphasis on unusual histological patterns. Am J Surg Pathol. 22(11):1303-13, 1998
6. Parkash V et al: Desmoplastic small round cell tumor of the pleura. Am J Surg Pathol. 19(6):659-65, 1995
7. Ladanyi M et al: Fusion of the EWS and WT1 genes in the desmoplastic small round cell tumor. Cancer Res. 54(11):2837-40, 1994

DESMOPLASTIC SMALL ROUND CELL TUMOR

Microscopic Features

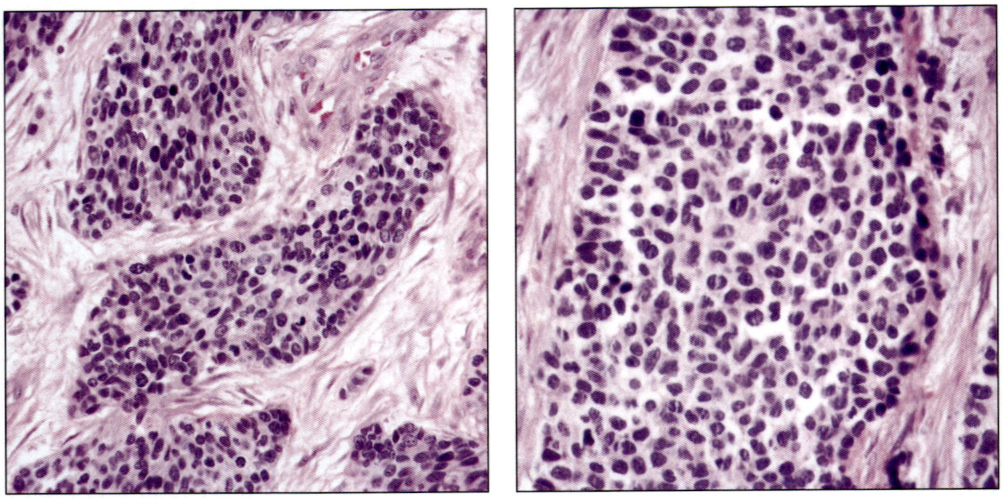

*(**Left**) Desmoplastic small round cell tumor shows irregular islands of tumor cells surrounded by dense fibroconnective tissue stroma. There is a hint of peripheral palisading in the tumor cell islands. (**Right**) High magnification of desmoplastic small round cell tumor of pleura shows a primitive cell population of small round blue cells with scant cytoplasm and scattered mitotic figures. The tumor lobules are sharply demarcated from the surrounding connective tissue stroma.*

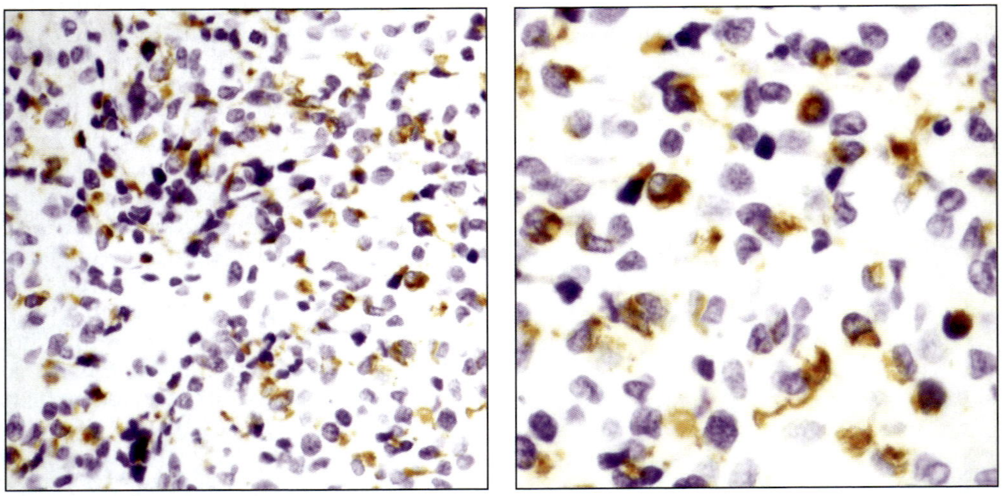

*(**Left**) Immunohistochemical staining of desmoplastic small blue cell tumor of the pleura for cytokeratin stain shows cytoplasmic positivity in the majority of the tumor cells for this marker. (**Right**) Immunohistochemical staining of desmoplastic small round blue cell tumor of the pleura for desmin shows cytoplasmic positivity in the majority of the tumor cells. The staining pattern is dot-like and paranuclear (Golgi zone) and very distinctive for this tumor.*

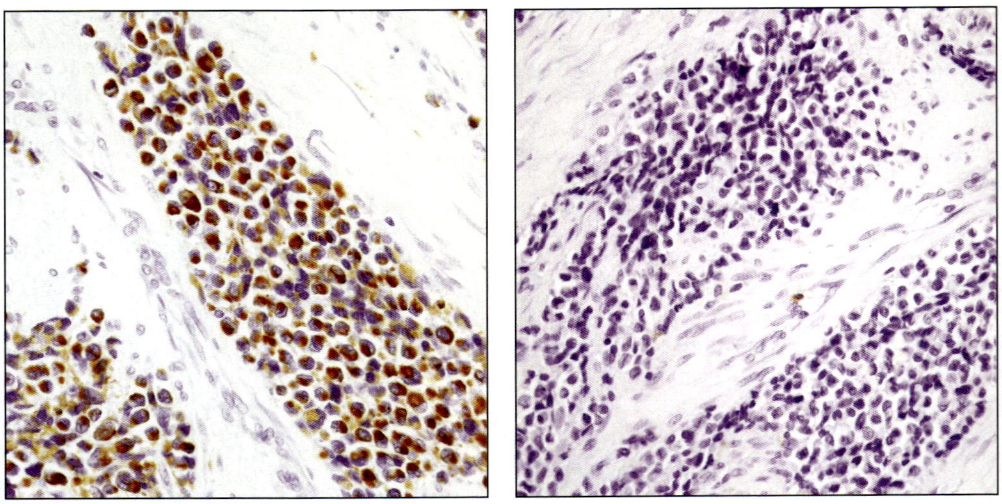

*(**Left**) Immunohistochemical staining of desmoplastic small round blue cell tumor of the pleura for vimentin shows the majority of the tumor cells are positive for this marker and display a distinctive dot-like, paranuclear (Golgi zone) staining pattern. (**Right**) Immunohistochemical staining of desmoplastic small round blue cell tumor for CD99 shows a negative reaction in the tumor cells. This serves to distinguish this tumor from PNET/Ewing sarcoma and lymphoblastic lymphoma.*

DESMOPLASTIC SMALL ROUND CELL TUMOR

Unusual Features

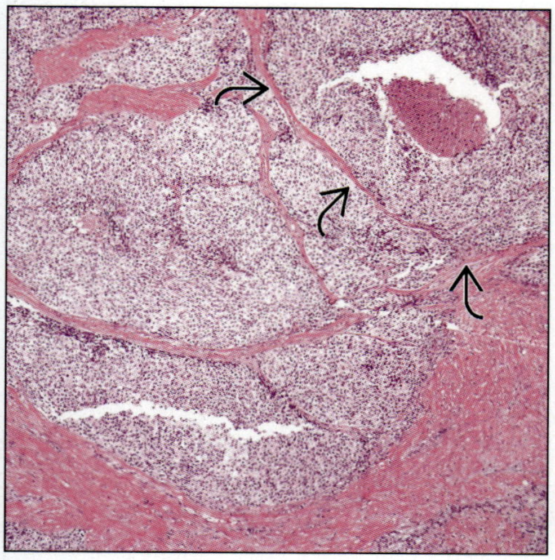

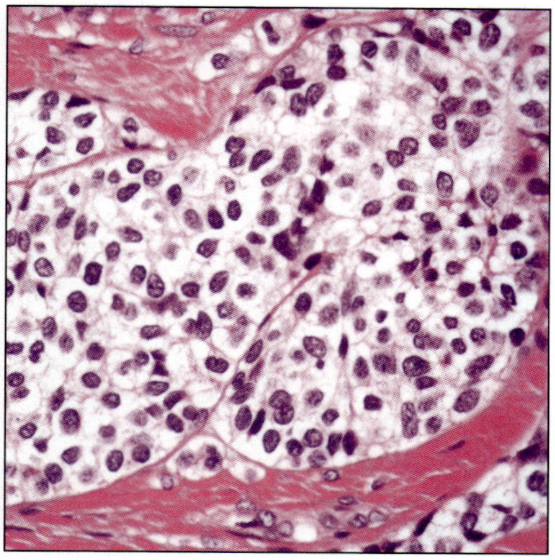

(Left) *Desmoplastic small round blue cell tumor of the pleura shows lobular architecture with foci of comedonecrosis* ➔*. The lobules are separated by broad bands of dense fibroconnective tissue.* ***(Right)*** *High magnification of desmoplastic small round blue cell tumor of the pleura shows islands of primitive small blue cells surrounded by a clear cytoplasmic halo. Tumors with this feature can be confused for a metastasis from clear cell carcinoma.*

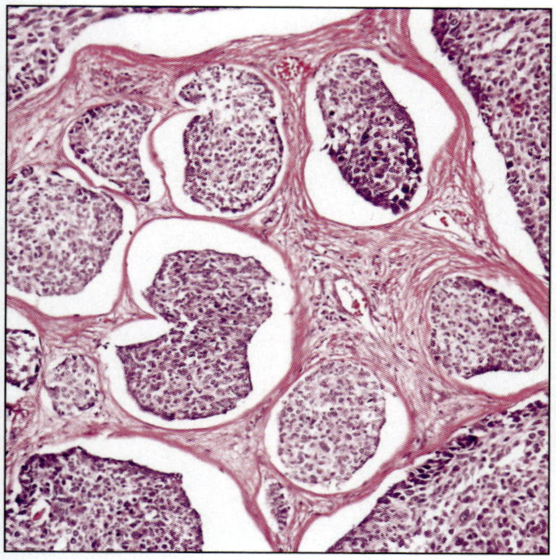

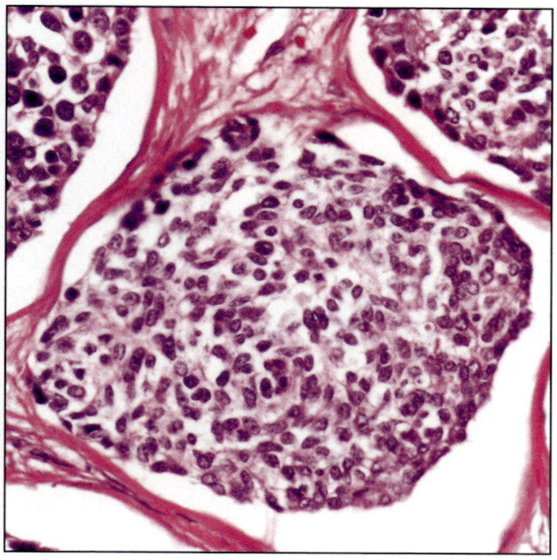

(Left) *Desmoplastic small round blue cell tumor shows islands of small blue cells with prominent stromal retraction artifact. The nesting appearance in this tumor is reminiscent of the "zellballen" or neuroendocrine growth pattern observed in neuroendocrine neoplasms.* ***(Right)*** *High magnification of desmoplastic small round blue cell tumor shows a nest of small round blue tumor cells surrounded by bands of collagenous stroma. This image can be confused for a neuroendocrine tumor.*

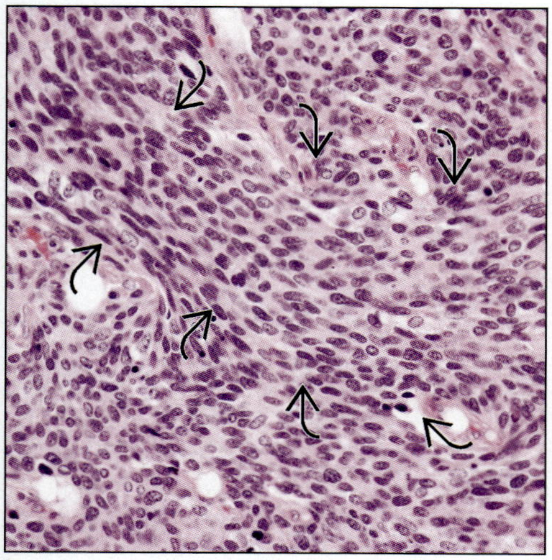

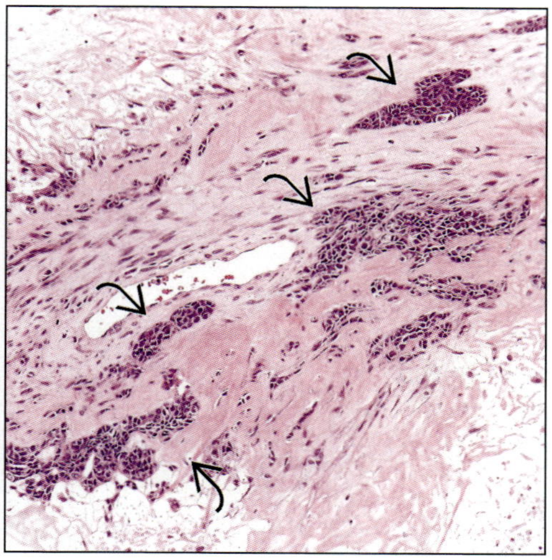

(Left) *Desmoplastic small round blue cell tumor shows spindling of the tumor cells* ➔*. Tumors with these features can be mistaken for other types of spindle cell tumors involving the pleura, including sarcomatoid malignant mesothelioma.* ***(Right)*** *Desmoplastic small round blue cell tumor shows extensive stromal hyalinization with only small, residual islands of tumor cells present in the stroma* ➔*. Such tumors can be mistaken for metastases of poorly differentiated carcinoma.*

PROTOCOL FOR MALIGNANT PLEURAL MESOTHELIOMA SPECIMEN EXAMINATION

Pleura: Resection

Surgical Pathology Cancer Case Summary (Checklist)

Specimen

___ Pleura
___ Other (specify): ___________________________
___ Not specified

Procedure

___ Pleural decortication
___ Pleurectomy
___ Extrapleural pneumonectomy
___ Other (specify): ___________________________
___ Not specified

Specimen Integrity

___ Intact
___ Disrupted
___ Indeterminate

Specimen Laterality

___ Right
___ Left
___ Not specified

Tumor Site (select all that apply)

___ Parietal pleura
___ Visceral pleura
___ Diaphragm
___ Other (specify): ___________________________
___ Not specified

****Tumor Size (for localized tumors only)***

*Greatest dimension: _________ cm
*Additional dimensions: _________ x _________ cm
*___ Cannot be determined

Tumor Focality

___ Localized
___ Diffuse
___ Cannot be determined

Histologic Type

___ Epithelioid mesothelioma
___ Sarcomatoid mesothelioma
___ Biphasic mesothelioma
___ Desmoplastic mesothelioma
___ Other (specify): ___________________________

Tumor Extension (select all that apply)

___ Parietal pleura without involvement of ipsilateral visceral pleura
___ Parietal pleura with focal involvement of ipsilateral visceral pleura
___ Confluent visceral pleural tumor (including fissure)
___ Into but not through diaphragm
___ Lung parenchyma
___ Endothoracic fascia
___ Into mediastinal fat
___ Solitary focus invading soft tissue of chest wall
___ Diffuse or multiple foci invading soft tissue of chest wall
___ Into but not through pericardium

____ Rib(s)

____ Mediastinal organ(s) (specify): ____________________________

____ Other (specify): ____________________________

Margins

____ Not applicable

____ Cannot be assessed

____ Margins negative for mesothelioma

____ Margin(s) involved by mesothelioma

Specify margin(s): ____________________________

Treatment Effect

____ Not applicable

____ Cannot be determined

____ > 50% residual viable tumor

____ < 50% residual viable tumor

Pathologic Staging (pTNM)

TNM descriptors (required only if applicable) (select all that apply)

____ m (multiple primary tumors)

____ r (recurrent)

____ y (post-treatment)

Primary tumor (pT)

____ pTX: Primary tumor cannot be assessed

____ pT0: No evidence of primary tumor

____ pT1a: Tumor limited to ipsilateral parietal pleura ± mediastinal or diaphragmatic pleural involvement; no involvement of visceral pleura

____ pT1b: Tumor involves ipsilateral parietal pleura ± mediastinal or diaphragmatic pleural involvement; tumor also involving visceral pleura

____ pT2: Tumor involves each of the ipsilateral pleural surfaces (parietal, mediastinal, diaphragmatic, and visceral pleura) with at least 1 of the following features:

Involvement of diaphragmatic muscle

Extension of tumor from visceral pleura into underlying pulmonary parenchyma

____ pT3: Locally advanced but potentially resectable tumor that involves all ipsilateral pleural surfaces (parietal, mediastinal, diaphragmatic, and visceral pleura), with at least 1 of the following features:

Involvement of the endothoracic fascia

Extension into mediastinal fat

Solitary completely resectable focus of tumor extending into soft tissues of chest wall

Nontransmural involvement of pericardium

____ pT4: Locally advanced technically unresectable tumor involving all ipsilateral pleural surfaces (parietal, mediastinal, diaphragmatic, and visceral pleura), with at least 1 of the following features:

Diffuse extension or multifocal masses of tumor in chest wall ± associated rib destruction

Direct transdiaphragmatic extension to peritoneum

Direct extension to contralateral pleura

Direct extension to mediastinal organs

Direct extension into spine

Extension through internal surface of pericardium ± a pericardial effusion

Tumor involving myocardium

Regional lymph nodes (pN)

____ pNX: Regional lymph nodes cannot be assessed

____ pN0: No regional lymph node metastases

____ pN1: Metastases in ipsilateral bronchopulmonary or hilar lymph nodes

____ pN2: Metastases in subcarinal or ipsilateral mediastinal lymph nodes including ipsilateral internal mammary and peridiaphragmatic nodes

____ pN3: Metastases in contralateral mediastinal, contralateral internal mammary, ipsilateral, or contralateral supraclavicular lymph nodes

____ No nodes submitted or found

Number of lymph nodes examined

Specify: ________

Number cannot be determined (explain): ____________________________

Number of lymph nodes involved

PROTOCOL FOR MALIGNANT PLEURAL MESOTHELIOMA SPECIMEN EXAMINATION

Specify: ________

____ Number cannot be determined (explain): ________________________

Distant metastasis (pM)

____ Not applicable

____ pM1: Distant metastasis

*Specify site(s), if known: ________________________

*Additional Pathologic Findings (select all that apply)

*____ None identified

*____ Asbestos bodies

*____ Pleural plaque

*____ Pulmonary interstitial fibrosis

*____ Inflammation (type): ________________________

*____ Other (specify): ________________________

*Ancillary Studies (select all that apply)

*____ Immunohistochemical stain(s) result(s) (specify stains): ________________________

*____ Histochemical stain(s) result(s) (specify stains): ________________________

*____ Electron microscopy results: ________________________

*____ Other (specify): ________________________

*Clinical History (select all that apply)

*____ Neoadjuvant therapy

*____ Other (specify): ________________________

*Data elements with asterisks are not required. However, these elements may be clinically important but are not yet validated or regularly used in patient management. Adapted with permission from College of American Pathologists, "Protocol for the Examination of Specimens from Patients with Malignant Pleural Mesothelioma." Web posting date: February, 2011, www.cap.org.

Other Lesions of the Pleura

PLEURAL ENDOMETRIOSIS

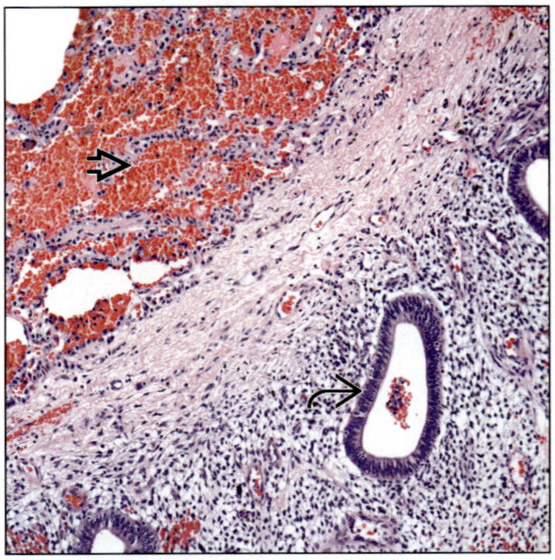

Pleuropulmonary endometriosis shows the classic features of endometrial glands ➚ embedded in a cellular stroma. Note the presence of adjacent lung parenchyma ➪ with congestion.

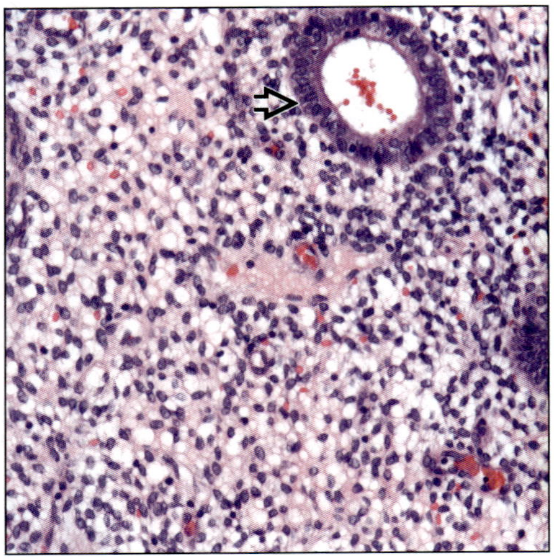

Higher magnification of pulmonary endometriosis shows a glandular structure ➪ with the appearance of an endometrial gland in the proliferative phase embedded in a cellular stroma.

TERMINOLOGY

Synonyms

- Endometrioma, deciduosis

Definitions

- Benign glandular proliferation of ectopic endometrial tissue in pleura

CLINICAL ISSUES

Epidemiology

- Incidence
  - Unusual occurrence in thoracic cavity
- Age
  - Predominantly in women of reproductive age
  - May be see in older postmenopausal women

Presentation

- Cough
- Pleuritic pain
- Shortness of breath
- Hemoptysis

Treatment

- Surgical approaches
  - Complete surgical resection

Prognosis

- Excellent

MICROSCOPIC PATHOLOGY

Histologic Features

- Glandular proliferation
- Glands in proliferative endometrial phase
- Glands with mitotic figures
- Mesenchymal-like stromal component
- Plasma cells in stromal component
- Medium-sized dilated vessels in stromal component
- Myxoid or edematous changes in stroma
- Cystic changes

Predominant Pattern/Injury Type

- Biphasic

Predominant Cell/Compartment Type

- Epithelial

DIFFERENTIAL DIAGNOSIS

Pleuropulmonary Blastoma (PPB)

- More common in younger individuals (< 20 years old)
- Commonly an intrapulmonary cystic neoplasm
- Epithelial component in both endometriosis and PPB is benign
- Spindle cell component in PPB is mesenchymal and commonly shows muscle differentiation
- Presence of scattered plasma cells is commonly seen in endometriosis
- Estrogen and progesterone receptors are positive in endometriosis and negative in PPB

Adenocarcinoma

- Glandular proliferation in endometriosis is embedded in cellular stroma
- Glands in endometriosis have appearance of proliferative phase of endometrial cycle
- Glandular component of endometriosis is benign

Biphasic Pulmonary Blastoma

- Both components in biphasic blastoma are malignant
- Mesenchymal component in blastoma is that of sarcoma
- Pulmonary blastoma generally is not cystic tumor

Biphasic Mesothelioma

- Both components of mesothelioma (epithelioid and sarcomatoid) are malignant

PLEURAL ENDOMETRIOSIS

Key Facts

Terminology
- Endometrioma, deciduosis

Clinical Issues
- Incidence
  - Unusual occurrence in thoracic cavity
  - Predominantly in women of reproductive age
  - May be seen in older postmenopausal women
- Symptoms
  - Cough
  - Pleuritic pain
  - Shortness of breath
  - Hemoptysis

Microscopic Pathology
- Glands in proliferative endometrial phase
- Plasma cells in stromal component
- Medium-sized dilated vessels in stromal component
- Myxoid or edematous changes in stroma
- Cystic changes

Top Differential Diagnoses
- Pleuropulmonary blastoma
  - More common in younger individuals (< 20 years old)
  - Commonly a cystic neoplasm
- Adenocarcinoma
  - Glandular proliferation in endometriosis is embedded in cellular stroma
  - Glands in endometriosis have appearance of proliferative phase of endometrial cycle
- Biphasic pulmonary blastoma
  - Both components in biphasic blastoma are malignant

Immunohistochemistry

Antibody	Reactivity	Staining Pattern	Comment
ER	Positive	Nuclear	Stromal component
PR	Positive	Nuclear	Stromal component
WT1	Positive	Nuclear	Stromal component
CK-PAN	Positive	Cytoplasmic	
CEA-M	Positive	Cytoplasmic	Glandular component
HER2	Positive	Cytoplasmic	Glandular component
CD15	Positive	Cytoplasmic	Glandular component
EMA	Positive	Cell membrane	
Vimentin	Positive	Cytoplasmic	In stromal tissue
S100	Negative		
Desmin	Negative		
Actin-HHF-35	Negative		
CD34	Negative		
Chromogranin-A	Negative		

- Sarcomatoid component in mesothelioma would be more atypical and may show pleomorphic features
- Immunohistochemical studies will lead to correct interpretation

DIAGNOSTIC CHECKLIST

Clinically Relevant Pathologic Features
- Gross appearance

Pathologic Interpretation Pearls
- Glands with appearance of proliferative phase of endometrial cycle
- Cellular stromal component
- Myxoid changes of stroma
- Prominent dilated vessels in stroma
- Scattered plasma cells in stroma

SELECTED REFERENCES

1. Augoulea A et al: Thoracic endometriosis syndrome. Respiration. 75(1):113-9, 2008
2. Costa F et al: [Thoracic endometriosis.] Rev Port Pneumol. 14(3):427-35, 2008
3. Kervancioglu S et al: Bronchial artery embolization in the management of pulmonary parenchymal endometriosis with hemoptysis. Cardiovasc Intervent Radiol. 31(4):824-7, 2008
4. Derman AY et al: Endometrioma presenting as a cavitary lung mass with intense 18F-FDG uptake on PET-CT. J Thorac Imaging. 22(2):172-5, 2007
5. Flieder DB et al: Pleuro-pulmonary endometriosis and pulmonary ectopic deciduosis: a clinicopathologic and immunohistochemical study of 10 cases with emphasis on diagnostic pitfalls. Hum Pathol. 29(12):1495-503, 1998
6. Karpel JP et al: Pulmonary endometriosis. Lung. 163(3):151-9, 1985
7. Foster DC et al: Pleural and parenchymal pulmonary endometriosis. Obstet Gynecol. 58(5):552-6, 1981

PLEURAL ENDOMETRIOSIS

Imaging, Gross, and Microscopic Features

*(**Left**) Lateral view of a chest x-ray shows a pulmonary lesion of pulmonary endometriosis →. However, there are not specific features for the diagnosis of endometriosis of the thoracopulmonary region. (**Right**) Gross photograph of pulmonary endometriosis. Note the cystic hemorrhagic lesion → attached to the lung parenchyma →. Although cystic hemorrhagic changes raise the suspicion of endometriosis, histopathologic examination is required.*

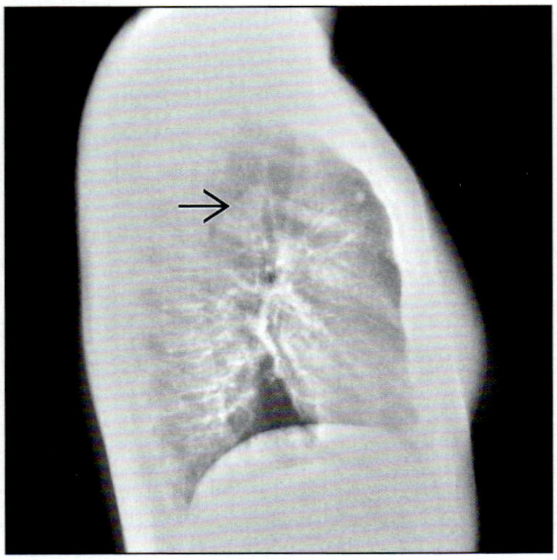

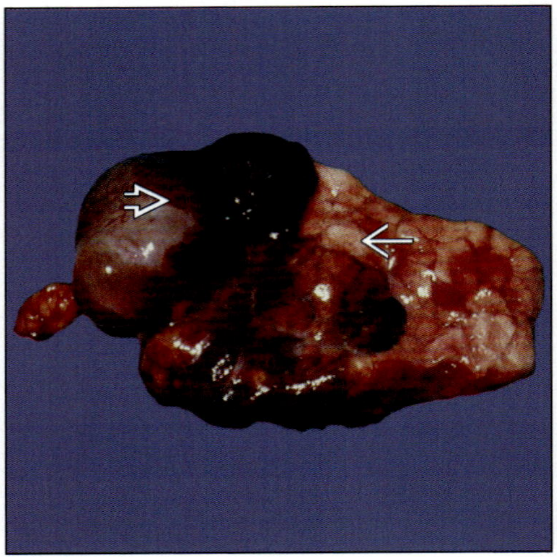

*(**Left**) Pulmonary endometriosis shows a biphasic cellular population, one composed of endometrial glands → and the other composed of stromal elements with dilated blood vessels →. (**Right**) Pleuropulmonary endometriosis shows typical features of endometrial gland embedded in a cellular stroma. Note the presence of numerous stromal vessels →.*

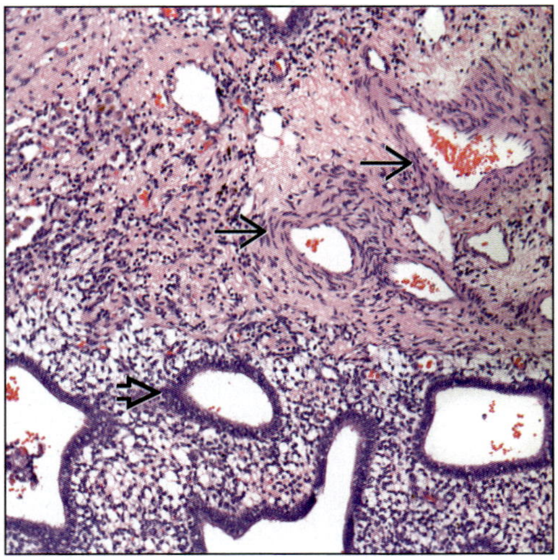

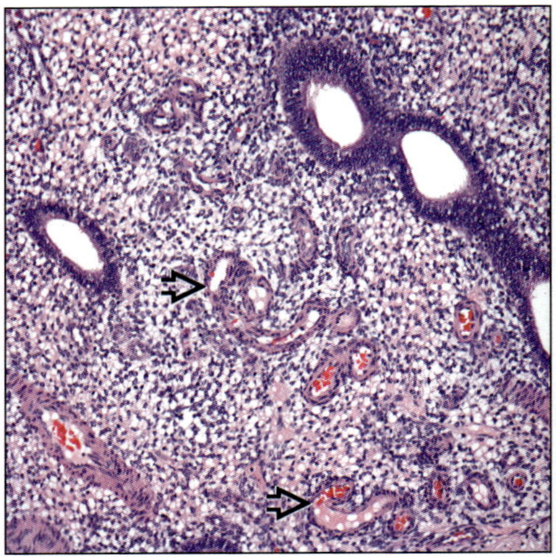

*(**Left**) In some cases of pleuropulmonary endometriosis, the stromal tissue may be extensive with only scattered glands →. In these cases, extensive search for the endometrial glands is warranted. (**Right**) Pleuropulmonary endometriosis shows extensive edematous reaction with stromal cells. No endometrial glands are present.*

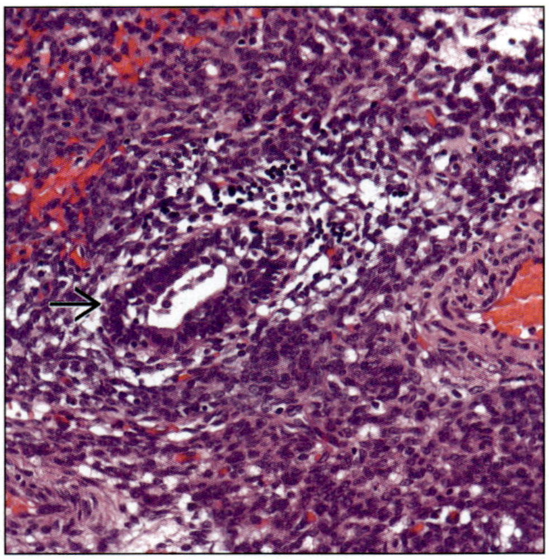

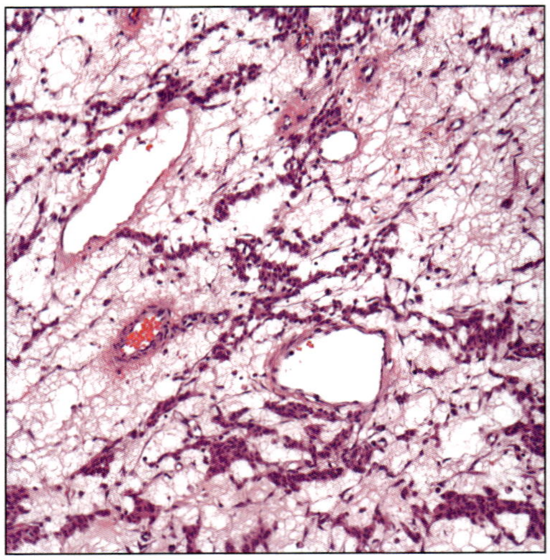

Microscopic Features

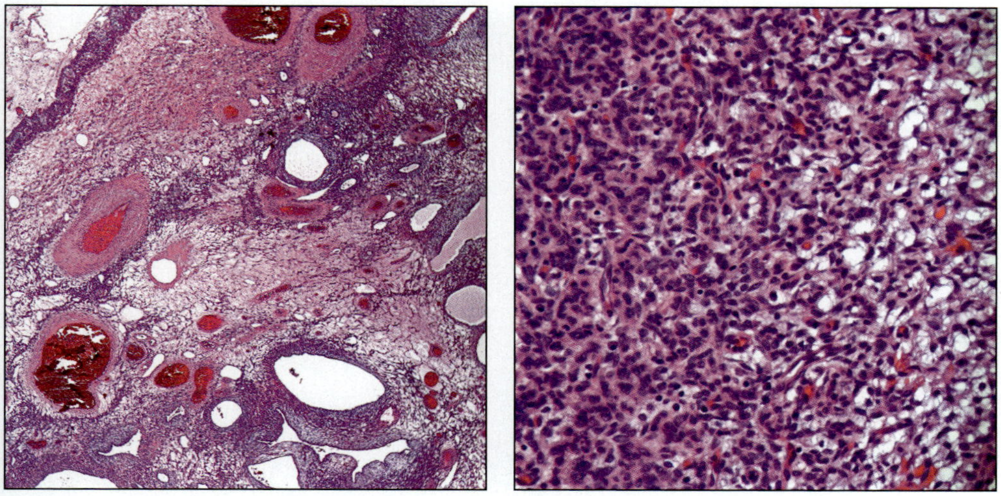

(Left) *Pulmonary endometriosis shows predominantly edematous changes in the stroma with dilated and congested blood vessels.* ***(Right)*** *The stromal component of pulmonary endometriosis shows spindle cells admixed with histiocytes and scattered plasma cells. The presence of plasma cells is not marked, and their findings are an important histological feature for the diagnosis of endometriosis.*

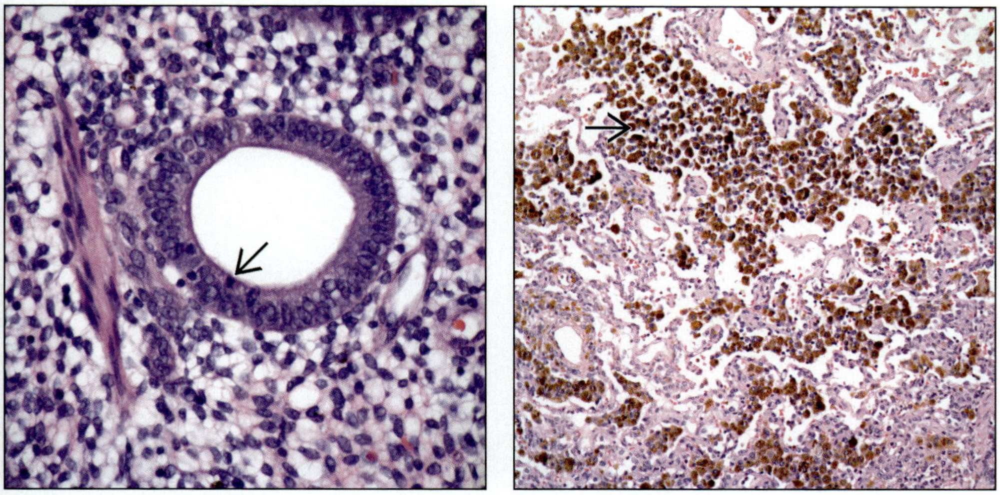

(Left) *High-power view of a gland in pulmonary endometriosis shows mitotic activity →. The appearance of this gland is reminiscent of the proliferative phase of the endometrial cycle.* ***(Right)*** *Lung parenchyma shows numerous hemosiderin-laden macrophages →. This feature may represent hemorrhagic changes due to the endometriotic process.*

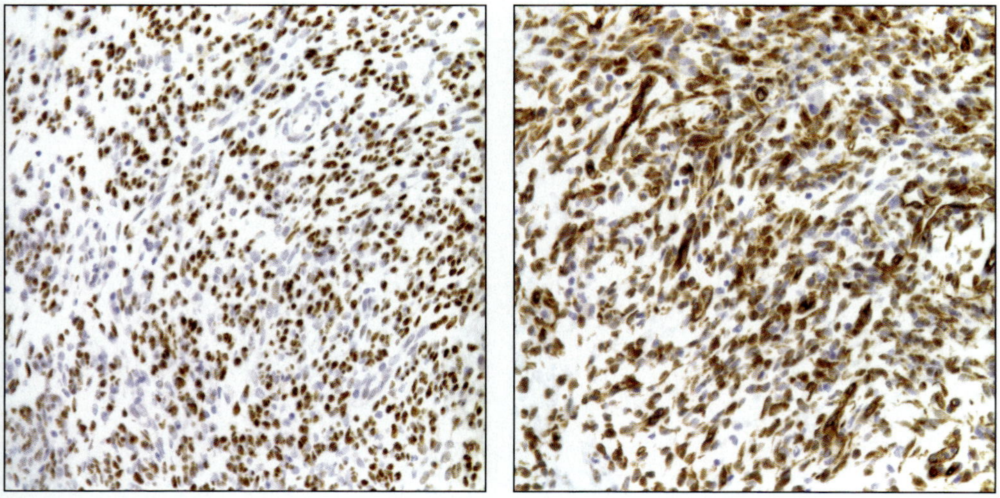

(Left) *Estrogen receptors (ER) immunohistochemical stain shows strong positive nuclear staining in endometriosis.* ***(Right)*** *WT1 immunohistochemical stain shows strong positive staining in endometriosis. These stains coupled with the negative staining for other specific markers are compatible with the diagnosis of endometriosis.*

Neoplasms, Benign

LYMPHANGIOMA

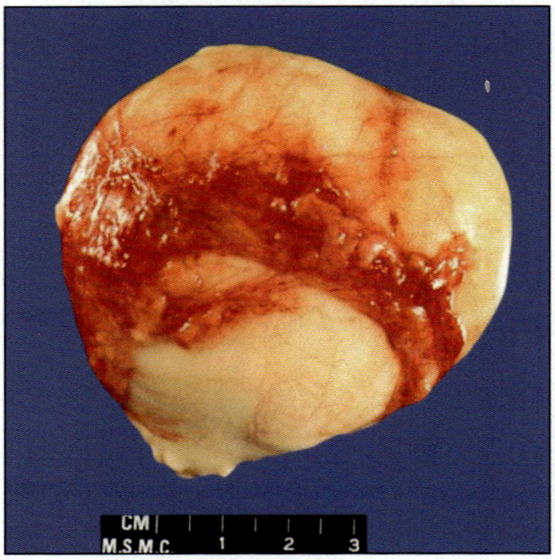

Gross appearance of cystic lymphangioma (cystic hygroma) in the anterior mediastinum of a child shows a well-circumscribed, distended cystic structure with a smooth and shiny outer surface.

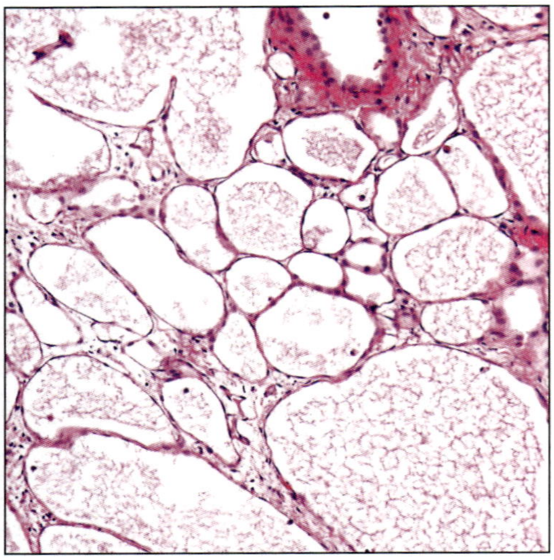

Histologic appearance of lymphangioma of anterior mediastinum shows dilated cystic spaces lined by a layer of flattened endothelial cells and containing proteinaceous fluid in their lumens.

TERMINOLOGY

Synonyms

- Cystic lymphangioma, cavernous lymphangioma, cystic hygroma, capillary lymphangioma

Definitions

- Benign, tumor-like proliferation of lymphatic vessels

ETIOLOGY/PATHOGENESIS

Developmental Anomaly

- Most likely represents hamartomatous process arising from sequestration of lymphatic tissue without connection to lymphatic system
- May occur as congenital malformation of lymphatic vascular channels

CLINICAL ISSUES

Site

- Neck mass with extension into mediastinum (75% of patients)
- Anterior mediastinal mass (15% of patients); can also arise in posterior and middle mediastinum
- May present as diffuse or multifocal process (lymphangiomatosis)

Presentation

- Cough
- Dyspnea
- May be asymptomatic and discovered incidentally on routine chest x-ray
- Rare tumor in mediastinum
- Majority of patients are pediatric, < 2 years of age
- Up to 50% of cases may be present at birth
- Congenital cases can be associated with hydrops fetalis and Turner syndrome
- Mass may enlarge, remain the same, or fluctuate in size over clinical evolution
- Rapid enlargement of mass can be observed following upper respiratory tract infection that blocks lymphatic drainage

Treatment

- Surgical excision
- Some cases may respond to sclerotherapy with sclerosing agents

Prognosis

- Surgery is usually curative
- May show repeated recurrences after surgery and require multiple surgical interventions

IMAGE FINDINGS

General Features

- Large, "soft" multicystic mass extending from neck into mediastinum
- Variable size (range: 2-20 cm)
- Smooth or lobulated mass with sharp margins
- May be associated with chylothorax
- Usually large, cystic, with variably sized cysts
- Lack of capsule allows tumor to infiltrate surrounding tissues

CT Findings

- Heterogeneous enhancement uncommon
- CECT is best imaging tool to help characterize mass in relation to surrounding structures

MACROSCOPIC FEATURES

General Features

- Lobulated, well-circumscribed mass
- Infiltrative borders commonly seen
- Multicystic cut surface

LYMPHANGIOMA

Key Facts

Clinical Issues

- Neck mass with extension into mediastinum (75% of patients)
- Anterior mediastinal mass (15% of patients)
- Cough
- Dyspnea
- Majority of patients are pediatric, < 2 years of age
- Up to 50% of cases may be present at birth
- Rapid enlargement of mass can be observed following upper respiratory tract infection that blocks lymphatic drainage
- Surgery is usually curative

Image Findings

- Large "soft" multicystic mass extending from neck into mediastinum
- Variable size (range: 2-20 cm)
- Usually large, cystic, with variable sized cysts
- Lack of a capsule allows tumor to infiltrate surrounding tissues

Microscopic Pathology

- Lesions may be of 3 types: Capillary, cavernous, or cystic lymphangioma
- Composed of solid proliferation of small, capillary-sized lymphatic channels
- Lymphoid aggregates present in stroma
- Lumen of lymphatic spaces may be filled with clear proteinaceous fluid containing small lymphocytes
- Walls of dilated lymphatic channels may show smooth muscle hyperplasia
- Coalescence of dilated lymphatic channels leads to formation of large multicystic mass

- Cysts of varying sizes bordered by fibrous walls of varying sizes
- Cystic spaces may be filled with proteinaceous clear fluid
- Lesions composed predominantly of capillary-sized vessels may show solid, spongy cut surface

MICROSCOPIC PATHOLOGY

Histologic Features

- Lesions may be of 3 types: Capillary, cavernous, or cystic lymphangioma
- **Capillary lymphangioma**
  - Composed of solid proliferation of small, capillary-sized lymphatic channels
  - Lymphatic vessels display attenuated layer of endothelium
  - Thin, adventitial layer surrounds lymphatic spaces
  - Lumen of lymphatic spaces may be filled with clear proteinaceous fluid containing small lymphocytes
  - Lymphoid aggregates present in stroma
  - Least common type of mediastinal lymphangioma
- **Cavernous lymphangioma**
  - Characterized by grossly distended lymphatic channels
  - Hemorrhage into lumen may simulate cavernous hemangioma
  - Lymphoid aggregates and lymphoid follicles commonly seen in stroma
  - Can become secondarily inflamed
  - Walls of dilated lymphatic channels may show smooth muscle hyperplasia
- **Cystic lymphangioma (cystic hygroma)**
  - Coalescence of dilated lymphatic channels leads to formation of large multicystic mass
  - Walls of cysts may show fibrosis or sclerosis
  - Walls of cysts may show acute and chronic inflammation
  - Walls of cysts may contain prominent lymphoid follicles
  - Walls of cyst may contain entrapped fat

DIFFERENTIAL DIAGNOSIS

Hemangioma

- Smooth or lobulated mass with sharp margins
- May contain phleboliths in up to 10% of cases
- Responds to steroids and may involute spontaneously

Cystic Teratoma

- Heterogeneous mass with fat and calcifications on imaging studies
- Multiple fluid levels on chest x-ray
- Histologically displays mature elements derived from all 3 germ layers

Bronchogenic Cyst

- Usually unilocular subcarinal mass
- May contain calcifications in the wall
- Cyst lining composed of ciliated columnar epithelium

Multilocular Thymic Cyst

- Usually occurs in older individuals
- Multilocular cystic mass often with firm adhesions to surrounding structures
- Shows prominent inflammation, hemorrhage, fibrosis, and lymphoid follicular hyperplasia in stroma
- Cyst lining is in continuity with dilated Hassall corpuscles

SELECTED REFERENCES

1. Teramoto K et al: Mediastinal cavernous lymphangioma in an adult. Gen Thorac Cardiovasc Surg. 56(2):88-90, 2008
2. Bossert T et al: Giant cystic lymphangioma of the mediastinum. Eur J Cardiothorac Surg. 21(2):340, 2002
3. Oshikiri T et al: Five cases of the lymphangioma of the mediastinum in adult. Ann Thorac Cardiovasc Surg. 7(2):103-5, 2001
4. Charruau L et al: Mediastinal lymphangioma in adults: CT and MR imaging features. Eur Radiol. 10(8):1310-4, 2000
5. Bratu M et al: Cystic hygroma of the mediastinum in children. Am J Dis Child. 119(4):348-51, 1970

LYMPHANGIOMA

Histologic Features

(Left) *Cystic lymphangioma of the mediastinum shows dilated lymphatic spaces filled with homogeneous eosinophilic, proteinaceous material. Notice the walls of the cysts are thickened by fibrosis and contain focal lymphoid infiltrates* ➩. ***(Right)*** *Cystic lymphangioma of the mediastinum shows multiple dilated lymphatic spaces of varying sizes lined by a flattened layer of endothelial cells. The walls of the cyst show fibrosis and scattered lymphoid cells.*

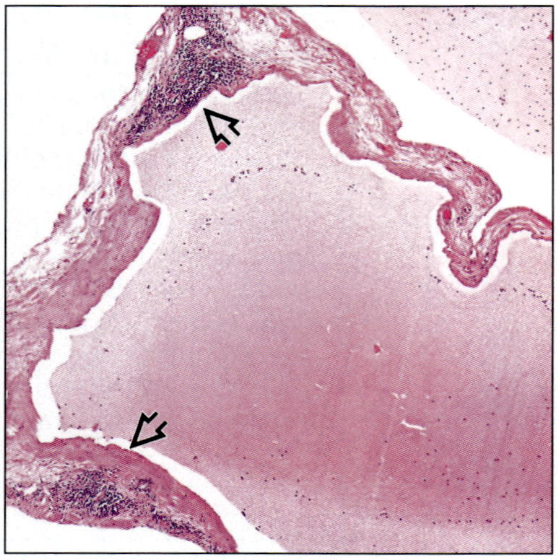

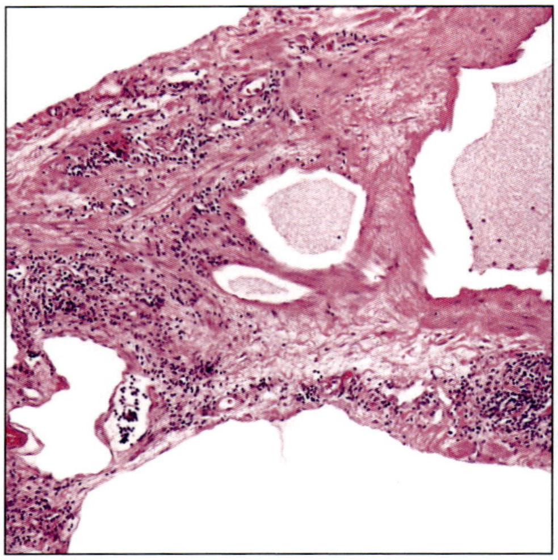

(Left) *Cystic lymphangioma of the mediastinum shows complex, dilated vessel lumens lined by a single layer of flattened endothelial cells. The walls of the vessels are thickened by fibrosis and contain scattered lymphocytes.* ***(Right)*** *High magnification of cystic lymphangioma of the mediastinum shows lymphatic vessels lined by a layer of flattened endothelial cells. One of the vessels contains scattered small lymphocytes in the lumen* ➩.

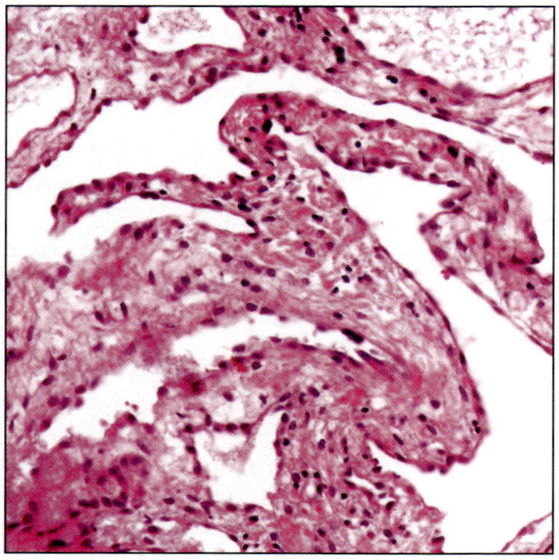

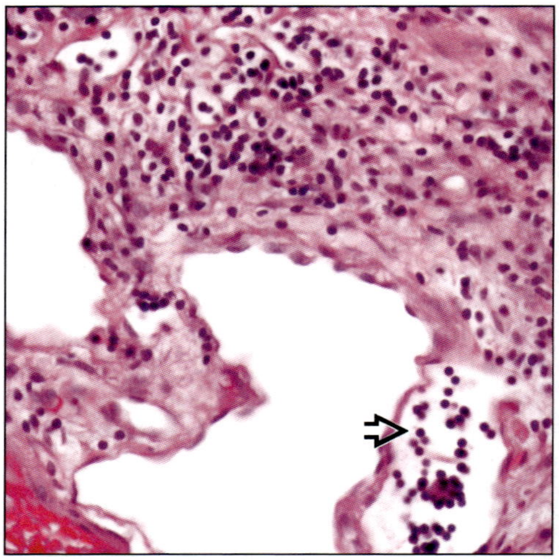

(Left) *Capillary lymphangioma of the mediastinum shows proliferation of small, capillary-sized vessels amid connective tissue stroma. Focal areas like this can be seen occasionally in cystic lymphangiomas of the mediastinum.* ***(Right)*** *Cystic lymphangioma of the mediastinum with fibrosis of the vessel walls shows irregular vascular lumens that contain variably hyalinized stroma with focal areas of stromal edema. A prominent endothelial cell layer is seen lining the vessels.*

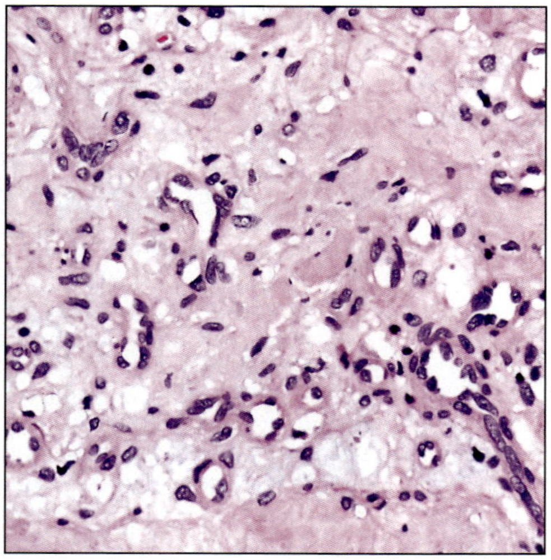

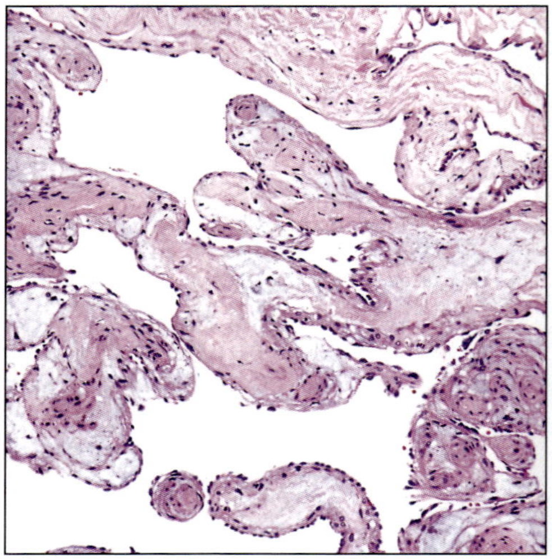

LYMPHANGIOMA

Other Features

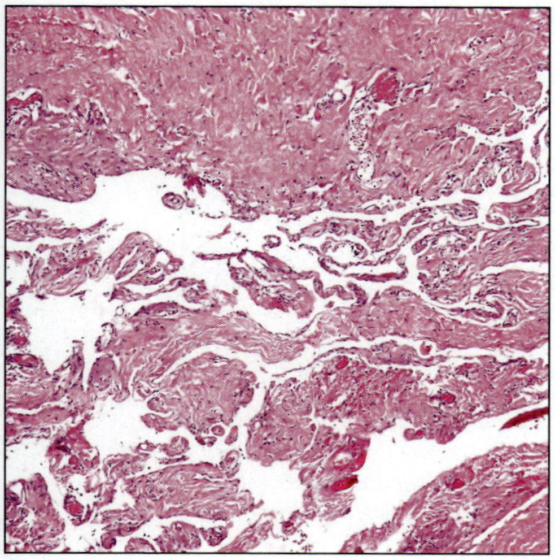
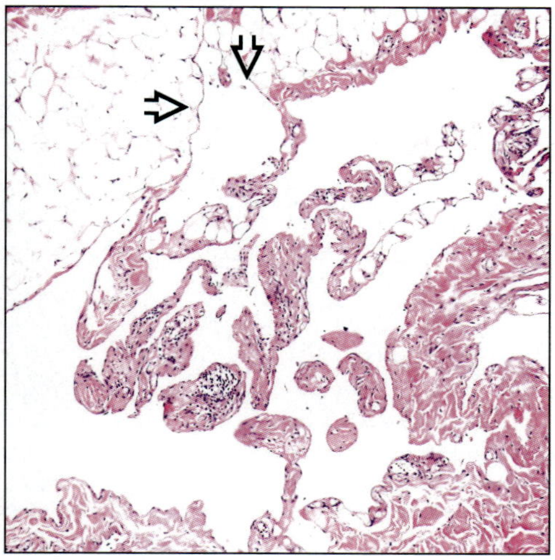

(Left) *Scanning magnification of lymphangioma of the mediastinum with prominent fibrosis shows empty anastomosing vascular channels surrounded by abundant connective tissue. The vascular nature of the lesion can be easily missed on cursory examination.* ***(Right)*** *High magnification of cystic lymphangioma shows complex dilated vascular spaces lined by a single layer of flattened endothelial cells. Notice the vascular spaces dissecting among the fat ➩.*

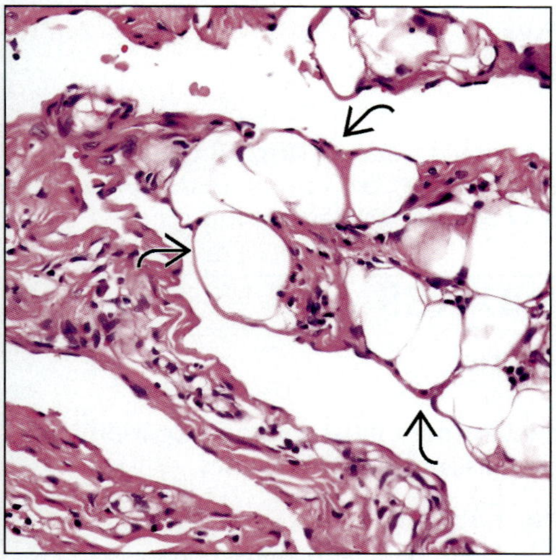
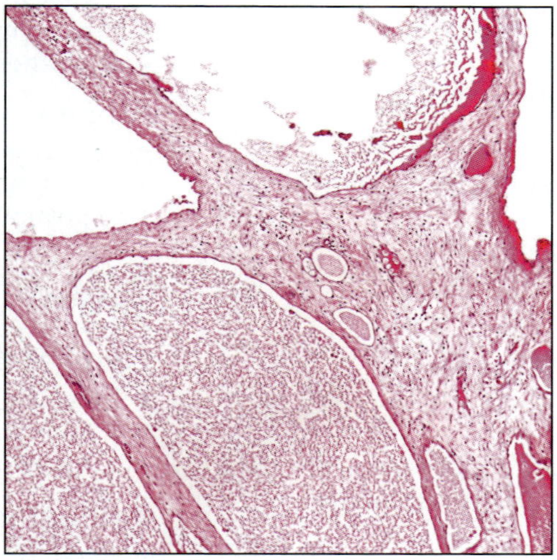

(Left) *Lymphangioma of the mediastinum shows lymphatic spaces containing entrapped mature adipocytes ➩. The adipocytic component may be quite prominent and lead to confusion with an angiolipomatous lesion.* ***(Right)*** *Cystic lymphangioma of the mediastinum shows dilated lymphatic spaces containing eosinophilic proteinaceous material in their lumens. Notice the walls of the dilated vascular spaces are thickened by fibrosis and contain scattered inflammatory cells.*

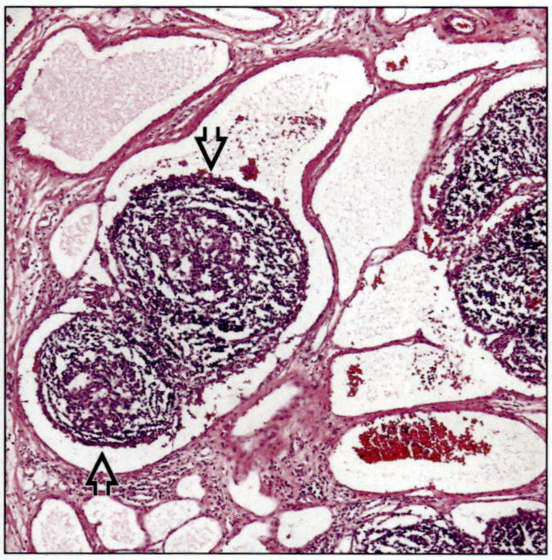
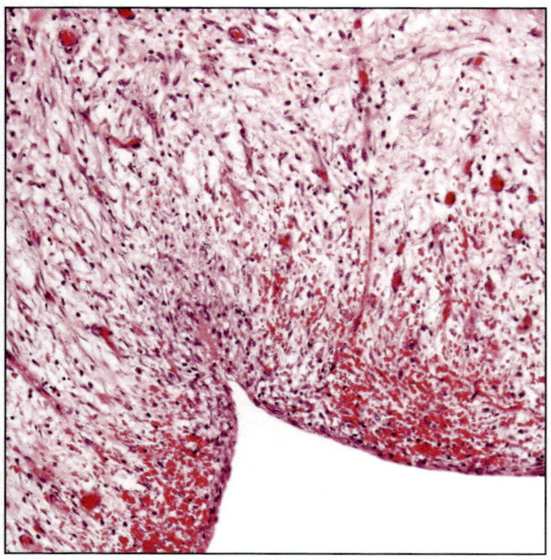

(Left) *Cystic lymphangioma of the mediastinum shows dilated vascular spaces with a few scattered lymphoid follicles with well-formed germinal centers in the stroma ➩.* ***(Right)*** *Cystic lymphangioma of the mediastinum shows thickened wall of a dilated lymphatic vessel with edema, hemorrhage, acute and chronic inflammation, and granulation tissue. Secondary inflammation in mediastinal lymphangiomas may lead to scarring and fibrous adhesions.*

HEMANGIOMA

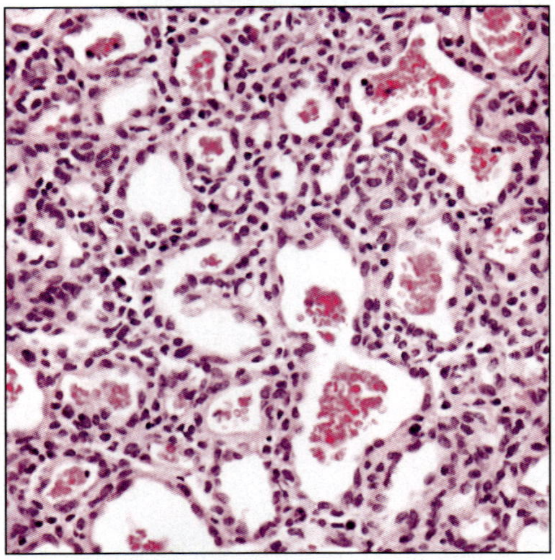

Capillary hemangioma of the mediastinum shows a tightly packed proliferation of small, capillary-sized vessels filled with red blood cells with little intervening stroma.

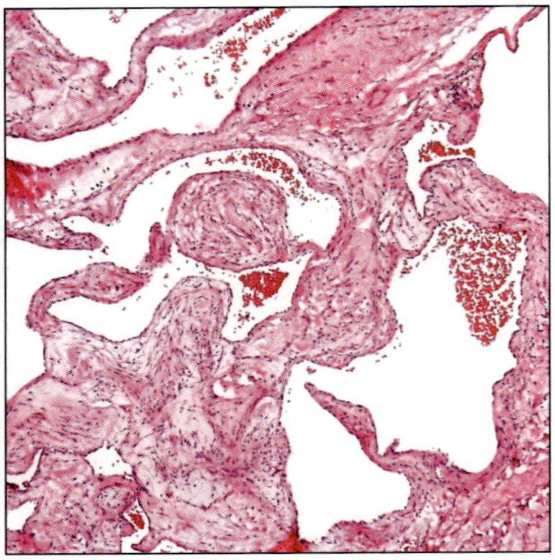

Cavernous hemangioma of the mediastinum shows large, dilated vascular spaces lined by small, flattened endothelial cells containing extravasated red blood cells.

TERMINOLOGY

Synonyms

- Hemangiofibroma, angiomyoma, hemangiomyoma

Definitions

- Benign neoplastic vascular proliferation

CLINICAL ISSUES

Epidemiology

- Incidence
  - Rare tumor
- Age
  - Affects broad age range, from newborns to old age
  - More frequent in children and young adults
- Gender
  - No gender predilection

Site

- Anterior and posterior mediastinum
- Some cases may be diffuse and multifocal (hemangiomatosis)

Presentation

- Dyspnea
- Cough
- Chest pain
- About 15% of patients may be asymptomatic, and lesion is discovered on routine chest x-ray
- Incidental finding at autopsy

Natural History

- Benign lesions that usually produce symptoms through compression
- Rarely invasive, but unencapsulated; may infiltrate mediastinal structures
- Some cases are associated with multiorgan, systemic involvement (hemangiomatosis)
- Some cases may regress spontaneously

Treatment

- Surgical excision
- Sclerotherapy

Prognosis

- Most cases are cured by simple surgical excision
- Expectant approach may be warranted in children due to possibility of spontaneous regression

IMAGE FINDINGS

General Features

- Location
  - Anterior mediastinum most common location
  - Posterior mediastinum in 1/4 of cases

Radiographic Findings

- Smooth or lobulated mass with sharp borders
- Phleboliths can be present in up to 10% of cases

MR Findings

- T1 weighted images may show linear areas of high intensity from stromal fat

CT Findings

- Often heterogeneous lesion with mixed attenuation
- Phleboliths appear as small round or ring-like calcifications with central lucency
- Central enhancement on CECT is very characteristic

MACROSCOPIC FEATURES

General Features

- Well circumscribed and unencapsulated
- Some tumors may show infiltration of adjacent structures
- Cystic and hemorrhagic cut surface

Size

- Variable size: 2-20 cm

HEMANGIOMA

Key Facts

Clinical Issues

- Rare tumor
- Affects broad age range, from newborns to old age
- More frequent in children and young adults
- Anterior and posterior mediastinum
- Some cases may be diffuse and multifocal (hemangiomatosis)
- Dyspnea
- Cough
- Chest pain
- Benign lesions that usually produce symptoms through compression
- Rarely invasive, but unencapsulated; may infiltrate mediastinal structures
- Some cases may regress spontaneously
- Most cases are cured by simple surgical excision

Microscopic Pathology

- **Capillary hemangiomas**
  - Lobular growth pattern separated by thin fibroconnective tissue bands
  - Lobules composed of solid, cellular proliferation of endothelial cells with compressed vascular lumens
  - Rare mitotic figures can occasionally be found
- **Cavernous hemangiomas**
  - Large, ectatic vessels filled with blood seen on scanning magnification
  - Stroma separating the vessels may contain prominent smooth muscle proliferation
  - Areas showing admixture of fibrosis, smooth muscle, and mature fat are commonly seen
  - Cellular proliferation can dissect focally into adjacent fibroadipose tissue

MICROSCOPIC PATHOLOGY

Histologic Features

- **Capillary hemangiomas**
  - Lobular growth pattern separated by thin fibroconnective tissue bands
  - Lobules composed of solid, cellular proliferation of endothelial cells with compressed vascular lumens
  - Cells contain round to oval nuclei with peripheral margination of chromatin and small, eccentric nucleoli
  - Small, compressed, and slit-like capillary vessels identified adjacent to solid areas
  - Rare mitotic figures can occasionally be found
  - Cellular proliferation can dissect focally into adjacent fibroadipose tissue
  - Regressive changes, including hyalinization, cystic changes, and fatty overgrowth, are commonly seen
  - Fibrosis and hyalinization may lead to compartmentalization closely resembling neuroendocrine neoplasm
- **Cavernous hemangiomas**
  - Large, ectatic vessels filled with blood seen on scanning magnification
  - Stroma separating the vessels may contain prominent smooth muscle proliferation
  - Areas showing admixture of fibrosis, smooth muscle, and mature fat are commonly seen
  - Focal inflammatory stromal changes with lymphocytes and plasma cells may be present
  - May contain foci of dystrophic calcification
  - Absence of cellular atypia or mitotic activity

DIFFERENTIAL DIAGNOSIS

Lymphangioma

- Ectatic lymphatics filled with homogeneous proteinaceous eosinophilic material (chyle)
- Inflammatory interstitial lymphoid infiltrate with well-formed follicles and prominent germinal centers in stroma

Thymolipoma

- Mature fat admixed with remnants of thymic tissue with Hassall corpuscles
- Absence of vascular component

Epithelioid Hemangioendothelioma

- Solid proliferation of large, atypical epithelioid cells with enlarged nuclei, prominent nucleoli, and abundant cytoplasm
- Prominent intracytoplasmic vacuoles are seen, sometimes containing red blood cells in their lumens
- Myxoid degeneration of the stroma may simulate cartilaginous matrix
- Atypical cells are strongly positive for FVIII-RAg and CD31

Angiomyolipoma

- Vascular proliferation containing entrapped fat and smooth muscle
- Smooth muscle proliferation is characteristically distributed concentrically around vessel walls

DIAGNOSTIC CHECKLIST

Pathologic Interpretation Pearls

- Mediastinal hemangiomas may often contain heterologous elements, including fat, muscle, and fibrous tissue
- Hemangiomas of capillary type may show solid growth pattern with compressed vascular lumens and scattered mitoses
- Capillary hemangiomas often show infiltrative borders and may invade adjacent structures

SELECTED REFERENCES

1. Yamazaki A et al: Cavernous hemangioma of the anterior mediastinum: case report and 50-year review of Japanese cases. Jpn J Thorac Cardiovasc Surg. 54(5):221-4, 2006
2. Moran CA et al: Mediastinal hemangiomas: a study of 18 cases with emphasis on the spectrum of morphological features. Hum Pathol. 26(4):416-21, 1995

HEMANGIOMA

Capillary Hemangioma

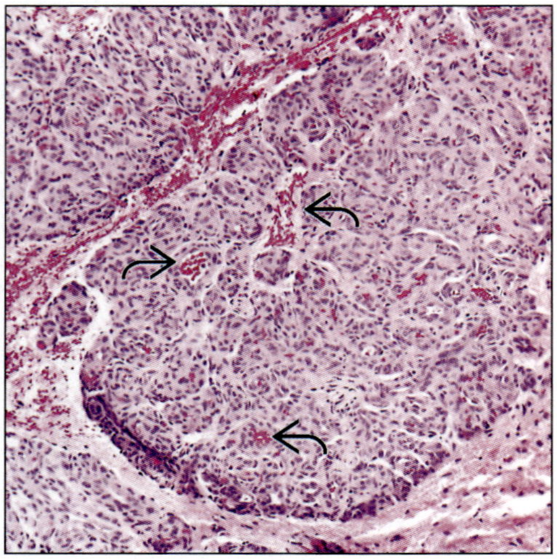

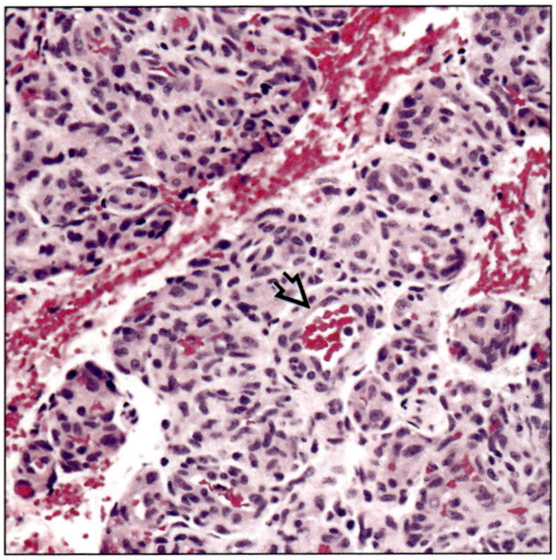

(Left) *Capillary-type hemangioma of the anterior mediastinum shows cellular lobules composed of a proliferation of small round cells with occasional small vessels displaying patent lumens filled with red blood cells* ↪*.* ***(Right)*** *Higher magnification of capillary-type hemangioma of the mediastinum shows solid proliferation of small round, endothelial cells with compressed vascular lumens. Notice the occasional small vessel with patent lumen containing a few red blood cells* ⇨*.*

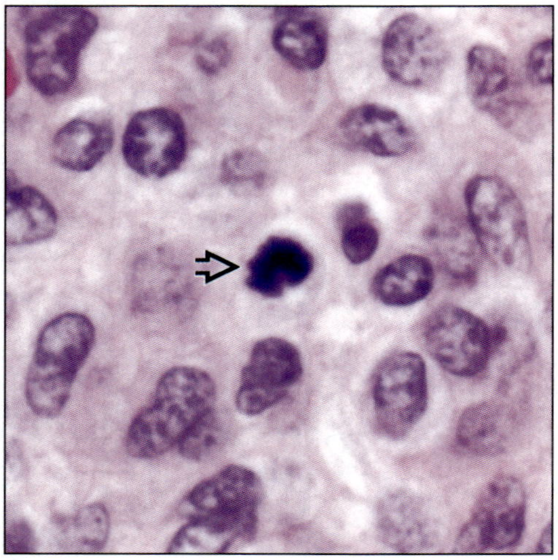

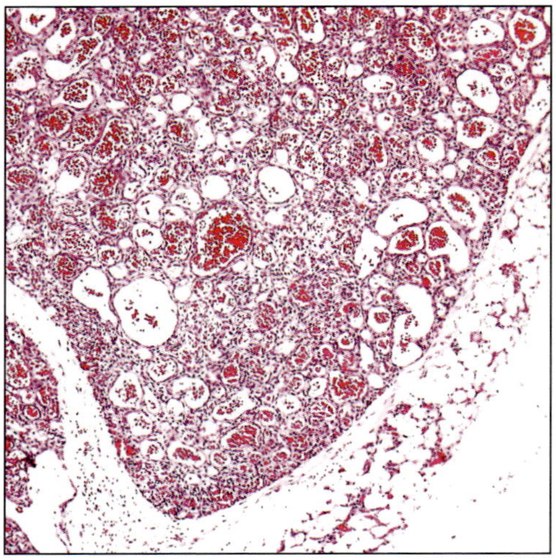

(Left) *High magnification of cellular capillary hemangioma of the mediastinum shows nuclear detail of the endothelial cells with dispersed chromatin and absence of nucleoli or cellular atypia. Notice the single mitotic figure in the center of the field* ⇨*.* ***(Right)*** *Capillary hemangioma of the mediastinum shows numerous scattered small vascular spaces with open lumens containing red blood cells. These lesions can closely resemble lobular capillary hemangiomas of the skin.*

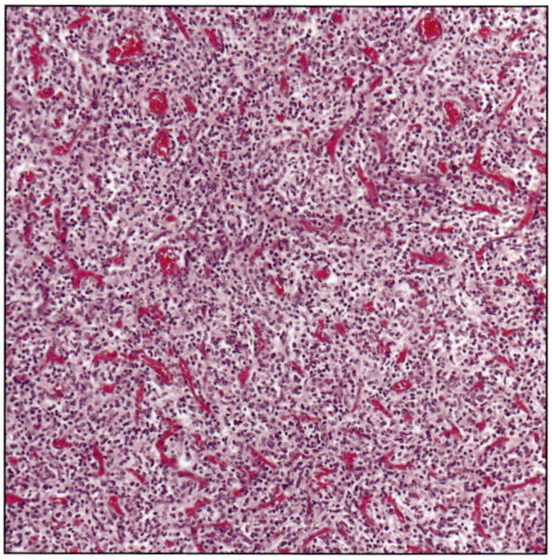

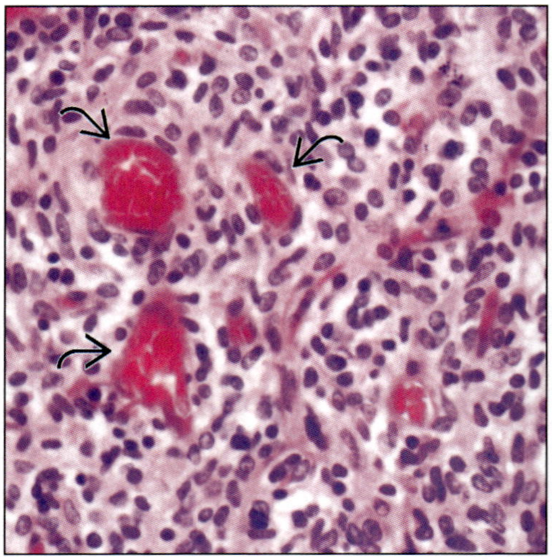

(Left) *Scanning magnification of capillary hemangioma of the mediastinum shows solid sheets of monotonous small, round endothelial cells with numerous compressed, slit-like vascular lumens filled with red blood cells. The lesion may be difficult to recognize as a vascular neoplasm.* ***(Right)*** *High magnification of capillary hemangioma of the mediastinum shows an area with solid growth pattern. Notice a few small vessels with patent lumens are filled with red blood cells* ↪*.*

Cavernous Hemangioma

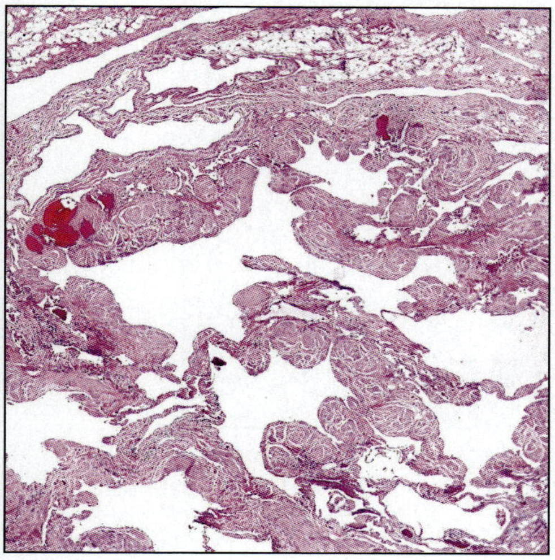

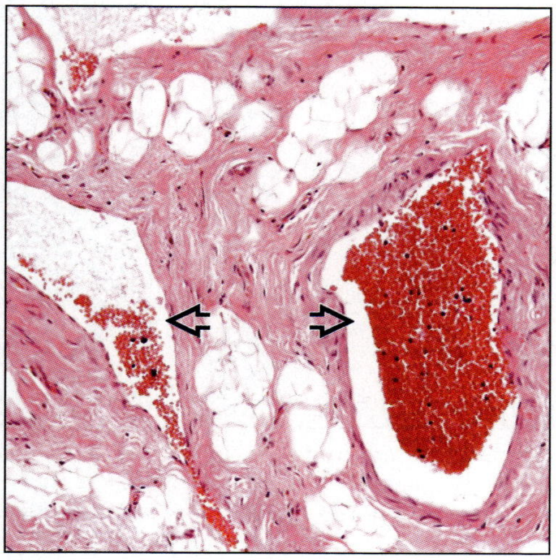

(Left) *Cavernous hemangioma of the anterior mediastinum in a 2-year-old child shows large, dilated, and irregular vascular spaces lined by a flattened layer of endothelial cells and separated by thick, fibrous walls.* ***(Right)*** *Cavernous hemangioma of the anterior mediastinum shows dilated cavernous spaces filled with red blood cells. Notice the extensive fibrosis and entrapment of mature adipose tissue in the walls of the dilated vascular spaces.*

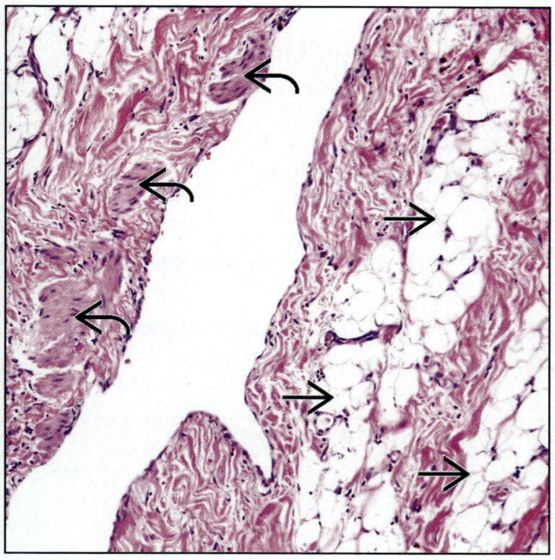

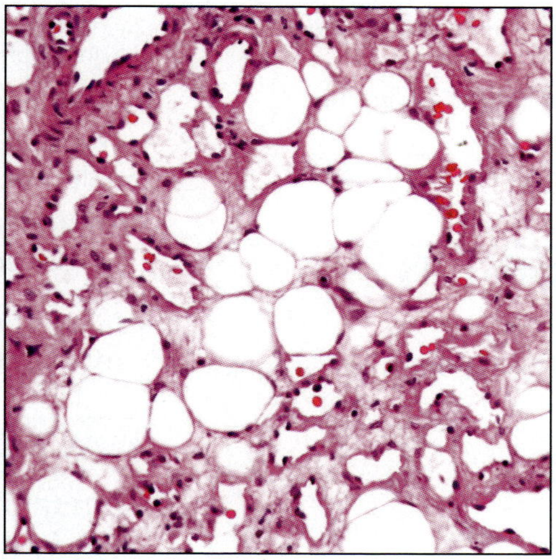

(Left) *Cavernous hemangioma of the anterior mediastinum shows a dilated vascular space lined by a flattened layer of endothelial cells. Notice the walls flanking the vascular space show fibrosis, muscular hyperplasia, and entrapped mature adipose tissue elements.* ***(Right)*** *High magnification of cavernous hemangioma of the mediastinum shows infiltration of the fat at the edges of the lesion by a proliferation of small vascular channels lined by small endothelial cells.*

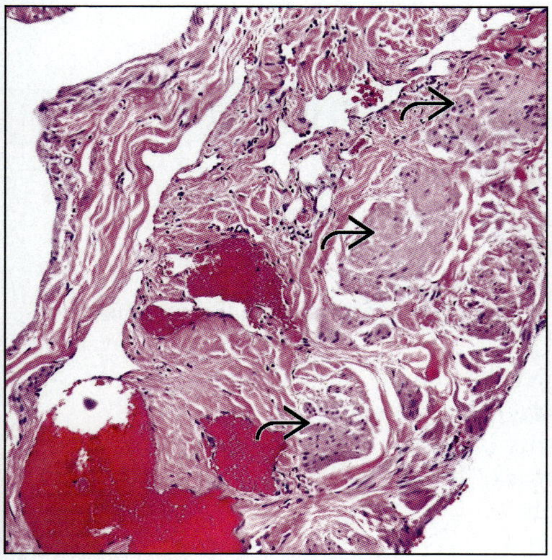

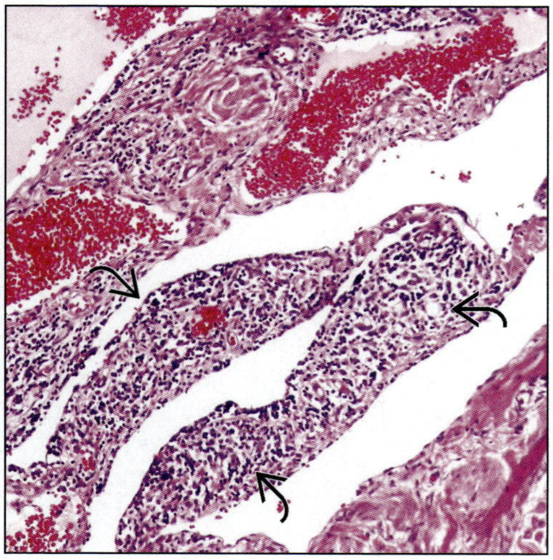

(Left) *Cavernous hemangioma of the mediastinum shows detail of the wall of the vascular spaces showing fibrosis and proliferation of bundles of smooth muscle.* ***(Right)*** *Cavernous hemangioma of the mediastinum shows dilated vascular spaces flanked by connective tissue containing prominent inflammatory cell infiltrate. Notice the inflammatory cells are diffusely scattered throughout and do not form discrete lymphoid follicles with germinal centers.*

PARAGANGLIOMA

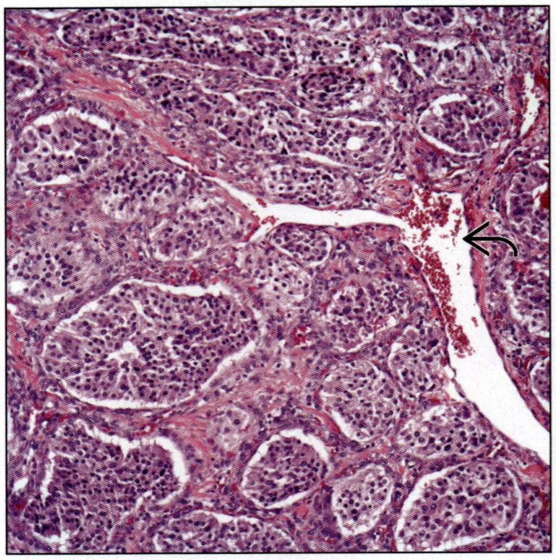

Mediastinal paraganglioma shows the typical nesting pattern of growth. Note the presence of a dilated vascular structure ⮳. These findings are typical for paraganglioma.

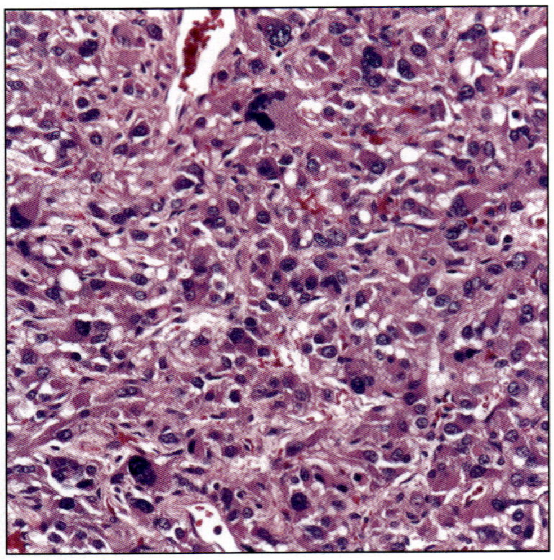

Mediastinal paraganglioma shows the presence of marked nuclear atypia and macronuclei and a lack of mitotic activity.

TERMINOLOGY

Synonyms

- Extraadrenal paraganglioma, carotid body tumor

Definitions

- Neuroendocrine neoplasm

ETIOLOGY/PATHOGENESIS

Etiology

- These tumors may originate from normal paraganglia

CLINICAL ISSUES

Epidemiology

- Incidence
  - Unusual tumors in mediastinal compartment
- Age
  - May occur at any age
  - More common in 3rd decade of life
- Gender
  - No gender predilection
  - Some studies have reported slight predominance in male patients

Site

- Paragangliomas may occur in anterior and posterior mediastinum

Presentation

- Chest pain
- Cough
- Difficulty in swallowing
- Dyspnea
- Headache
- Hypertension
- Diaphoresis
- Part of the multiple endocrine neoplasia (MEN) syndrome
- Some patients may be asymptomatic

Treatment

- Complete surgical resection
- Adjuvant therapy in selected cases

Prognosis

- In majority of cases, complete surgical resection is curative
- In some cases, paragangliomas behave aggressively with metastatic disease leading to death

MACROSCOPIC FEATURES

General Features

- Soft, irregular
- Tan to light brown

Size

- Varies from 2 cm to > 10 cm in diameter

MICROSCOPIC PATHOLOGY

Histologic Features

- So-called zellballen growth pattern
- Nested pattern
- Spindle cell pattern
- Presence of large cells with macronuclei and bizarre shapes
- Granular-like cells may be prominent
- Melanin pigment may also be seen
- Mitotic activity is rare
- Extensive areas of hyalinization may be present
- Ectatic vessels

PARAGANGLIOMA

Key Facts

Terminology
- Synonyms
  - Extraadrenal paraganglioma, carotid body tumor

Clinical Issues
- Incidence
  - May occur at any age
  - More common in 3rd decade of life
  - May occur in anterior and posterior mediastinum
- Symptomatology
  - Dyspnea
  - Headache
  - Hypertension
  - Diaphoresis
  - Part of multiple endocrine neoplasia (MEN) syndrome
- Treatment and prognosis
  - In majority of cases, complete surgical resection is curative

Top Differential Diagnoses
- Neuroendocrine carcinoma
- Ectopic parathyroid tumor
- Thymic carcinoma

Diagnostic Checklist
- Zellballen growth pattern
- Prominent cellular atypia
- Macronuclei
- Rare mitotic activity

Immunohistochemistry

Antibody	Reactivity	Staining Pattern	Comment
Chromogranin-A	Positive	Cytoplasmic	Strongly positive
Synaptophysin	Positive	Not applicable	Strongly positive
CD56	Positive	Cytoplasmic	Strongly positive
S100	Positive	Nuclear	In sustentacular cells
NFP	Positive	Cytoplasmic	In about 50% of cases
Enkephalin	Positive	Cytoplasmic	In about 50% of cases
NSE	Positive	Cytoplasmic	Strongly positive
CK-PAN	Negative		It may be focally positive in some gangliocytic paragangliomas
CK-LMW-NOS	Negative		
CK-HMW-NOS	Negative		

DIFFERENTIAL DIAGNOSIS

Well-differentiated Neuroendocrine Carcinoma (Carcinoid Tumor)
- Neuroendocrine carcinomas generally show positive staining for pan keratin
- Neuroendocrine carcinomas would display mitotic activity
- Paragangliomas and neuroendocrine carcinomas share similar immunophenotype with neuroendocrine markers

Ectopic Parathyroid Tumor
- Generally positive for keratin markers
- Rarely displays cellular atypia of paragangliomas
- Parathyroid tumors generally show positive staining for PTH while paragangliomas are negative

Thymic Carcinoma
- Displays more cellular atypia and mitotic activity
- Generally is negative for neuroendocrine markers
- Growth pattern of thymic carcinoma is not of zellballen type

DIAGNOSTIC CHECKLIST

Clinically Relevant Pathologic Features
- Mitotic rate
- Nuclear features
- Growth pattern

Pathologic Interpretation Pearls
- Zellballen growth pattern
- Prominent cellular atypia
- Macronuclei
- Rare mitotic activity

SELECTED REFERENCES

1. Brown ML et al: Mediastinal paragangliomas: the mayo clinic experience. Ann Thorac Surg. 86(3):946-51, 2008
2. Plaza JA et al: Sclerosing paraganglioma: report of 19 cases of an unusual variant of neuroendocrine tumor that may be mistaken for an aggressive malignant neoplasm. Am J Surg Pathol. 30(1):7-12, 2006
3. Moran CA et al: Mediastinal paragangliomas. A clinicopathologic and immunohistochemical study of 16 cases. Cancer. 72(8):2358-64, 1993

PARAGANGLIOMA

Microscopic Features

(Left) *Mediastinal paraganglioma shows diffuse growth pattern with only a few scattered ectatic blood vessels.* *(Right)* *Mediastinal paraganglioma shows a more vascular differentiation almost mimicking a primary vascular neoplasm. However, note the presence of the neuroendocrine cellular proliferation around the numerous ectatic blood vessels.*

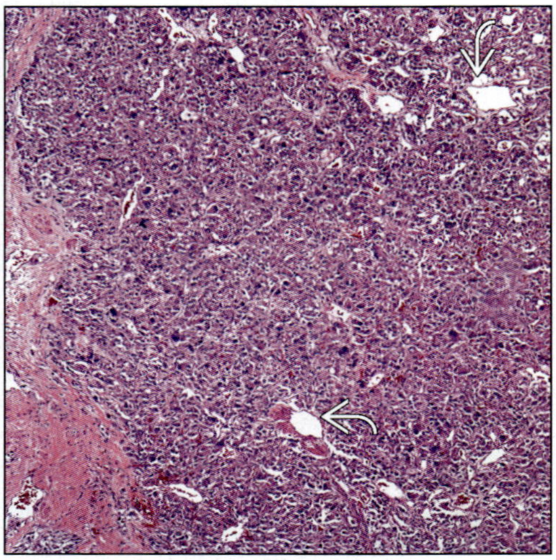

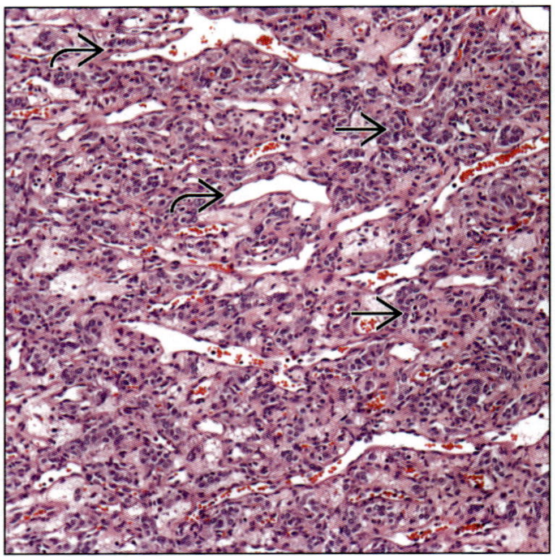

(Left) *Mediastinal paraganglioma shows extensive areas of edematous tissue and only scattered nests of tumor cells. These features may pose a problem in making an unequivocal diagnosis of paraganglioma.* *(Right)* *Mediastinal paraganglioma is shown with extensive areas of fibroconnective tissue. This feature may be seen in several other neuroendocrine tumors, including paragangliomas.*

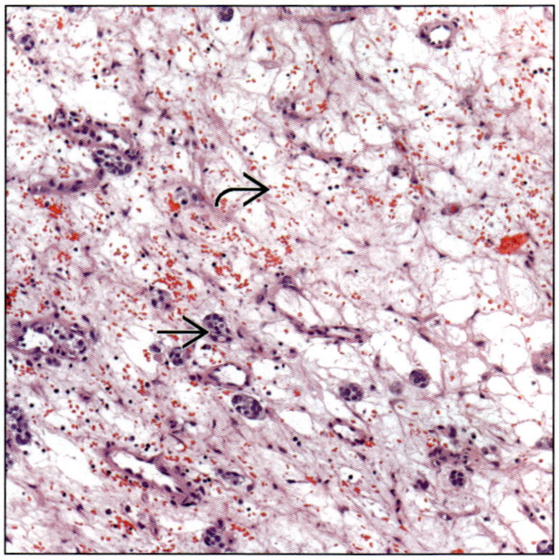

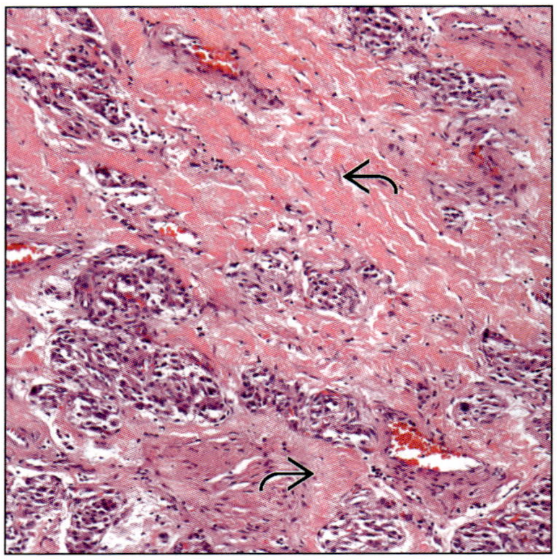

(Left) *Mediastinal paraganglioma shows the presence of extensive areas of collagenization alternating with a prominent vessel proliferation. Similar histological features may be seen in other nonneuroendocrine tumors.* *(Right)* *Mediastinal paraganglioma shows a cellular proliferation composed of rather small cells with a moderate amount of cytoplasm, round nuclei, and inconspicuous nucleoli growing in a nested pattern.*

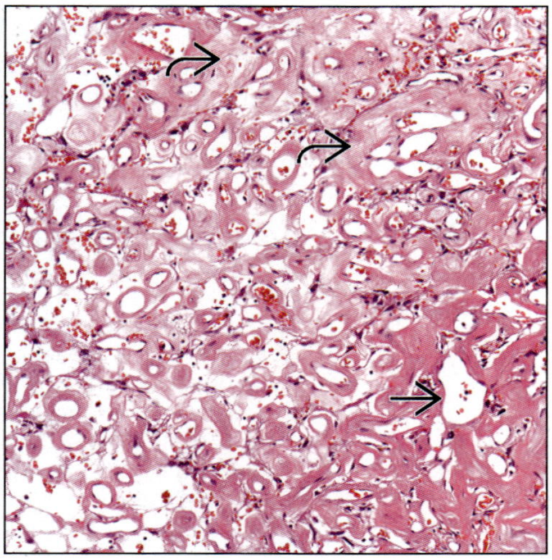

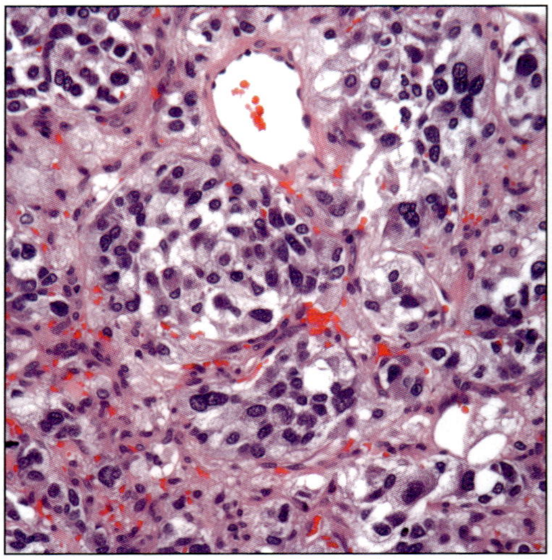

PARAGANGLIOMA

Microscopic Features

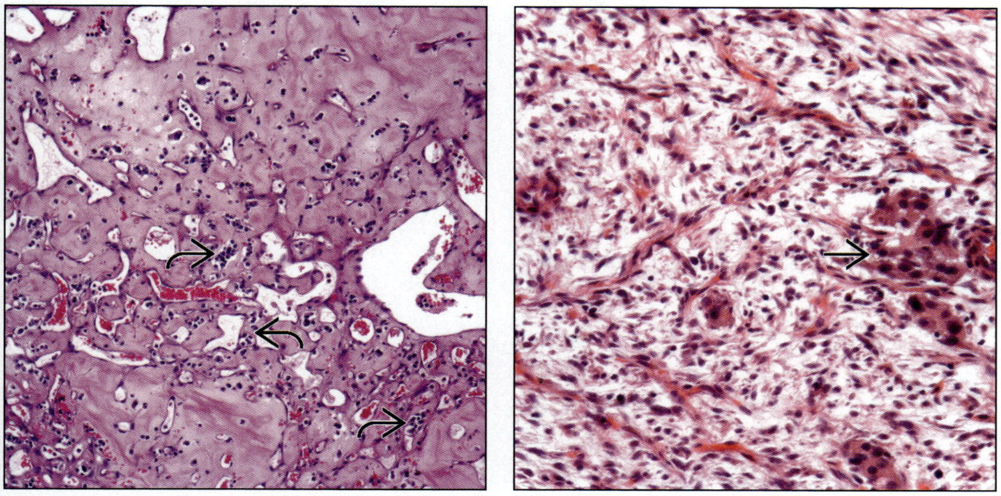

(Left) Dense collagenization with numerous dilated vascular channels mimicking a vascular neoplasm. However, note the presence of clusters of neuroendocrine cells ↪. **(Right)** Spindle cell paraganglioma of the mediastinum in which one is still able to recognize clusters of more conventional neuroendocrine cells →. In the majority of cases of predominant spindle cell component, one is able to identify conventional areas of paraganglioma.

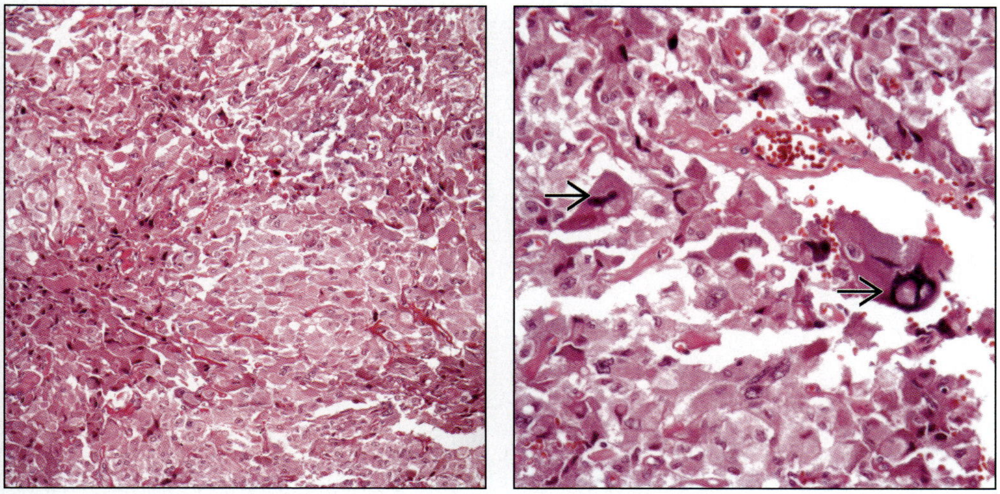

(Left) Mediastinal paraganglioma shows prominent oncocytic and granular cell features. These types of cellular proliferation are unusual and can give rise to a wide differential diagnosis. **(Right)** Mediastinal paraganglioma is shown with oncocytic and granular cell changes. Note the presence of larger cells with ample cytoplasm and bizarre nuclei → but without mitotic activity.

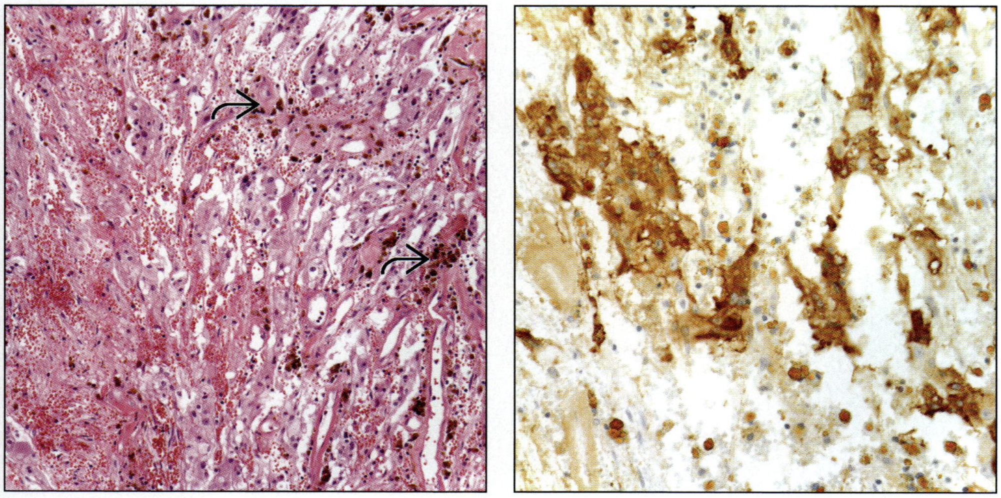

(Left) Mediastinal paraganglioma is shown with extensive areas of hemorrhage and hemosiderin pigment ↪. In such cases, it may be difficult to identify neuroendocrine cells, and the use of immunohistochemistry is required. **(Right)** Chromogranin-A shows positive staining in tumor cells corresponding to a case with extensive hemorrhage. The use of neuroendocrine markers is important in the diagnosis of paragangliomas.

Neoplasms, Malignant, Primary

Epithelial Neoplasms

Germ Cell Tumors

Hematopoietic Malignancies

Mesenchymal Neoplasms

Sympathetic Nervous System Tumors

Other Tumors

Thymoma and Thymic Carcinoma Protocols

OVERVIEW OF MALIGNANT THYMIC NEOPLASMS

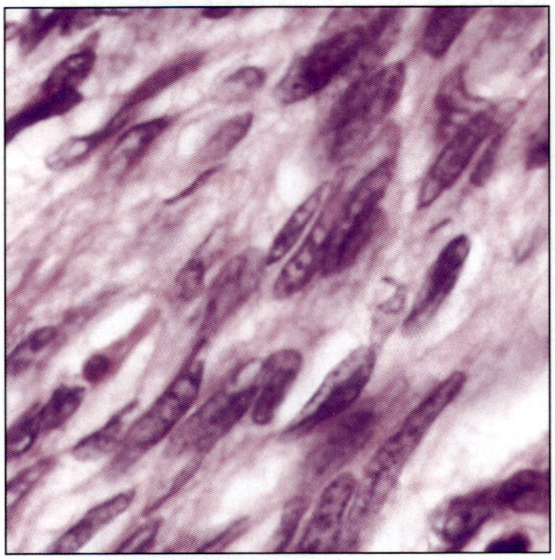

WHO type A thymoma (spindle cell thymoma) shows characteristic cytomorphology of the tumor cells with elongated spindle cells displaying nuclei that contain dispersed chromatin and absence of nucleoli.

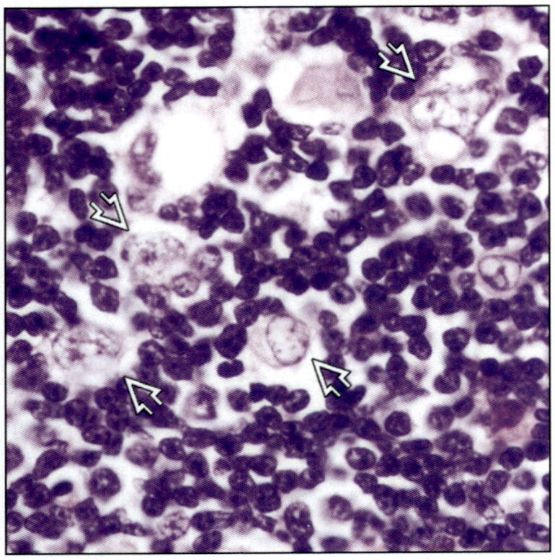

WHO type B thymoma (lymphocyte rich) shows large epithelioid cells ➡ with vesicular nuclei and indistinct rim of amphophilic cytoplasm surrounded by dense population of small lymphocytes.

TERMINOLOGY

Definitions

- Primary malignant thymic neoplasms are derived from thymic epithelium, stroma, germ cells, or lymphoid component and include
  - Primary thymic epithelial neoplasms
    - Well-differentiated primary thymic epithelial neoplasms (thymoma)
    - Moderately differentiated primary thymic epithelial neoplasms (atypical thymoma)
    - Poorly differentiated primary thymic epithelial neoplasms (thymic carcinoma)
  - Thymic lymphoproliferative disorders
    - Hodgkin disease
    - Lymphoblastic lymphoma
    - Mediastinal diffuse large B-cell lymphoma
    - Other types of mediastinal lymphomas
  - Germ cell tumors arising in the mediastinum
    - Teratomatous lesions
    - Seminoma
    - Yolk sac tumor
    - Choriocarcinoma
    - Embryonal carcinoma
  - Neuroendocrine carcinomas of the thymus
    - Well-differentiated neuroendocrine carcinoma (thymic "carcinoid")
    - Moderately differentiated neuroendocrine carcinoma ("atypical carcinoid" of thymus)
    - Poorly differentiated neuroendocrine carcinoma (small cell and large cell neuroendocrine carcinomas)
  - Sarcomas
    - Liposarcoma
    - Leiomyosarcoma
    - Epithelioid hemangioendothelioma
    - Chondrosarcoma
    - Osteosarcoma
    - Chordoma
    - Fibrosarcoma and malignant fibrous histiocytoma
    - Synovial sarcoma
    - Malignant peripheral nerve sheath tumors
    - Rhabdomyosarcoma
    - Alveolar soft parts sarcoma
    - Mesenchymal chondrosarcoma

EPIDEMIOLOGY

Age Range

- Malignant thymic neoplasms affect all age groups but are more common in middle-aged adults (40-50 years)

Incidence

- Rare tumors
  - Metastases to the mediastinum outnumber primary malignancies 9:1

Natural History

- Thymomas are slow-growing tumors; their prognosis is largely dependent on the status of capsular integrity at the time of resection
  - Most thymomas are found in stage I (noninvasive, completely encapsulated)
  - All histologic types have the capability to invade, recur, and metastasize
  - Overall recurrence rate for thymoma is 10% with the mean time to recurrence being 6 years (range: 1-16 years)
  - Survival after recurrence is usually good if adequately treated, with up to 65% 10-year survival after treatment of the recurrence
  - Atypical thymomas (WHO type B3) are associated with a higher incidence and earlier recurrences
  - Increased survival is also closely associated with completeness of excision
    - Incompletely excised tumors are associated with shorter survival

OVERVIEW OF MALIGNANT THYMIC NEOPLASMS

Modified Masaoka Staging for Thymoma

Stage	Description
Stage I	Grossly and microscopically completely encapsulated (including microscopic invasion *into* the capsule)
Stage IIa	Microscopic transcapsular invasion
Stage IIb	Microscopic invasion into thymic or surrounding fat, or grossly adherent but not breaking through mediastinal pleura or pericardium
Stage III	Microscopic invasion of neighboring organs (pericardium, great vessels, lung)
Stage IVa	Pleural or pericardial dissemination
Stage IVb	Hematogenous or lymphatic dissemination

Koga K et al. A review of 79 thymomas: modification of staging system and reappraisal of conventional division into invasive and non-invasive thymoma. Pathol Int. 44:359-367, 1994.

        - Completely excised tumors are associated with a more favorable survival, independent of stage or histology
    - Metastases are rare in thymoma and more often occur in intrathoracic lymph nodes, lung, and pleura
        - Intrathoracic metastases are seen in about 10% of patients with thymoma
        - Distant metastases are extremely rare in thymoma (about 1-2% of patients)
        - Distant metastases are associated with a poor prognosis (average survival after metastases is 1.5-3 years)
        - All histologic types are associated with the potential for metastases
    - Mortality in thymoma is in the order of 10% of patients
        - Thymoma deaths usually occur late in the disease, between 10-15 years after initial diagnosis
- Thymic carcinomas are, in general, highly aggressive tumors with short patient survival and poor response to treatment
    - Low-grade variants of thymic carcinoma (i.e., mucoepidermoid, well-differentiated squamous cell carcinoma) may have a good prognosis
    - High-grade histologic variants (small cell carcinoma, lymphoepithelioma-like carcinoma, clear cell carcinoma) are rapidly fatal and refractory to treatment

CLINICAL IMPLICATIONS

Clinical Presentation

- Majority of mediastinal tumors present with symptoms referable to compression of mediastinal structures by an expanding mass
    - Cough
    - Chest pain
    - Dyspnea
    - Superior vena cava syndrome
- A significant number of thymomas can be asymptomatic and discovered incidentally on routine chest x-rays
- Thymomas are commonly associated with paraneoplastic syndromes, myasthenia gravis in particular

MACROSCOPIC FINDINGS

General Features

- Size
    - Most mediastinal tumors reach a large size before they become symptomatic (> 10 cm in greatest diameter)
        - Thymomas are often discovered as an incidental finding and when they are still small in patients undergoing coronary artery bypass graft surgery
- Sections to be submitted
    - It is recommended to submit at least 1 section per cm of greatest diameter of the lesion
    - Cystic lesions are best sampled extensively to make sure a microscopic focus of burned-out neoplasm in the walls of the cysts is not missed
    - Thymomas require inking and extensive sampling of the capsule for staging and identification of invasion
- Mediastinal compartments
    - Certain types of tumors have a special predilection for the various mediastinal compartments
        - Anterior-superior mediastinum: Thymoma, thymic carcinoma, lymphoma, germ cell tumors, multilocular thymic cysts
        - Middle mediastinum: Lymphomas, Castleman disease, mediastinal cysts, sarcomas, metastases to the mediastinum
        - Posterior mediastinum: Neurogenic tumors, sarcomas, lymphomas

SELECTED REFERENCES

1. Suster S et al: The mediastinum. In Weidner N et al: Modern Surgical Pathology. 2nd ed. Philadelphia: Saunders Elsevier. 454-516, 2009
2. Marchevsky AM et al: Evidence-based pathology and the pathologic evaluation of thymomas: the World Health Organization classification can be simplified into only 3 categories other than thymic carcinoma. Cancer. 112(12):2780-8, 2008
3. Suster S et al: Histologic classification of thymoma: the World Health Organization and beyond. Hematol Oncol Clin North Am. 22(3):381-92, 2008
4. Suster S et al: Thymoma classification: current status and future trends. Am J Clin Pathol. 125(4):542-54, 2006
5. Suster S: Thymic carcinoma: update of current diagnostic criteria and histologic types. Semin Diagn Pathol. 22(3):198-212, 2005

THYMOMA

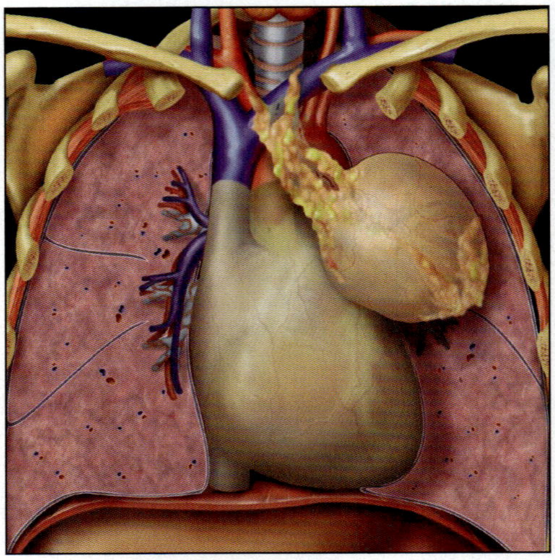

Schematic representation of the chest cavity shows a round to ovoid, well-circumscribed thymoma in the anterior mediastinal compartment on top of the pericardium and protruding onto the left hemithorax.

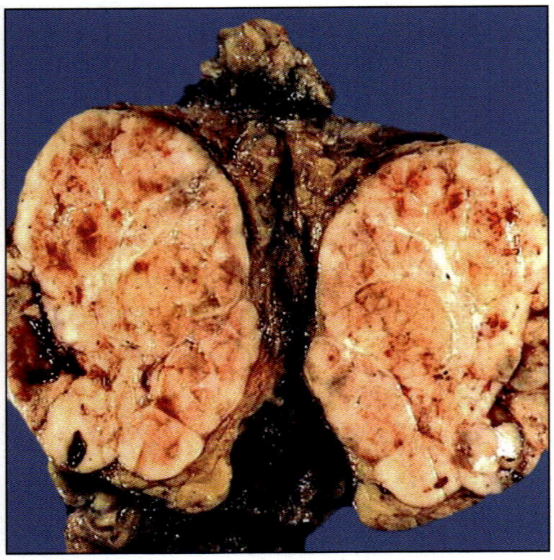

Gross appearance of bisected thymoma shows a well-circumscribed, fleshy, lobulated mass composed of tan-white, homogeneous rubbery tissue with focal areas of congestion and hemorrhage.

TERMINOLOGY

Synonyms

- Primary thymic epithelial neoplasm

Definitions

- Primary thymic epithelial neoplasm composed of thymic epithelial cells admixed in varying proportions with immature T-lymphocytes

ETIOLOGY/PATHOGENESIS

Pathogenesis

- Unknown
- Close association with myasthenia gravis and other autoimmune disorders

CLINICAL ISSUES

Presentation

- Chest pain
- Shortness of breath
- Paraneoplastic syndrome (myasthenia gravis, hypogammaglobulinemia, pure red cell aplasia, etc.)
- Superior vena cava syndrome
- Asymptomatic in up to 30% of cases
- Incidental finding on routine chest x-ray or during coronary artery bypass surgery

Natural History

- Majority of thymomas are very low-grade malignant neoplasms with generally indolent behavior
- Size and status of capsular integrity are 2 important determinant factors for prognosis
- Invasive tumors are associated with more aggressive behavior
- Incompletely excised tumors have tendency to recur locally and spread along chest cavity
- Recurrences can take place many years after initial resection (i.e., > 10-15 years)
- Most common sites for metastases are lung, pleura, and thoracic lymph nodes
- Extrathoracic metastases are extremely rare (< 2% of cases)

Treatment

- Complete surgical excision for noninvasive tumors
- Radiation therapy for incompletely resected tumors
- Surgical excision + postoperative radiation therapy for invasive tumors
- Repeat surgical excision + radiation for recurrent tumors
- Combination chemotherapy for advanced stage and metastatic tumors
- Best chance for cure is complete surgical excision with negative margins

Prognosis

- Most important prognostic factor is clinical staging (Koga modified Masaoka scheme)
- 80-90% survival at 15 years with stages I and II
- 70% survival at 15 years with stage III
- 60% survival at 5 years with stage IV
- Stages I and II include infiltration of capsule and minimal invasion of perithymic fat (collectively regarded as "noninvasive" tumors; confined to anterior mediastinum)
- Stages III and IV include infiltration of adjacent or neighboring structures, implants, and distant metastases (collectively regarded as "invasive")

IMAGE FINDINGS

General Features

- Best diagnostic clue
  - Smooth or lobulated anterior mediastinal mass
- Location
  - Generally anterior mediastinum

THYMOMA

Key Facts

Clinical Issues

- Majority of thymomas are very low-grade malignant neoplasms with generally indolent behavior
- Status of capsular integrity is most important determinant factor for prognosis

Microscopic Pathology

- WHO classification system is based predominantly on cell type, cytologic atypia, and proportion of lymphocytes to epithelial cells: Thymoma type A, AB, B1, B2, B3, and thymic carcinoma
- 2 basic cell types are recognized: Spindle/oval and round/epithelioid
  - Type A thymoma: Composed of oval or spindle cells with scattered nuclear chromatin and inconspicuous or absent nucleoli without mitotic activity
  - Type AB thymoma: Composed of oval or spindle cells identical to those seen in type "A" but admixed with abundant small lymphocytes
  - Type B1 thymoma: Composed of round/epithelioid cells with single small eosinophilic nucleoli and abundant cytoplasm, admixed with numerous small T-lymphocytes
  - Type B2 thymoma: Composed of approximately equal admixture of round epithelial cells and small lymphocytes
  - Type B3 thymoma: Composed of sheets of large epithelioid cells admixed with scant lymphocytes
- Thymic carcinoma (type C thymoma): Characterized by overt cytologic features of malignancy and absence of organotypical thymic features; resembles carcinomas at other sites

  - May also occur in posterior mediastinum
  - May arise ectopically in pulmonary hilum, pleura, or head and neck
- Size
  - Usually between 4-15 cm

Radiographic Findings

- Round or oval anterior mediastinal mass
- Usually centered over heart; best seen on lateral view
- Linear and peripheral calcifications in capsule (10% of patients)

MR Findings

- T1WI: Isointense relative to muscle
- T2WI: Hyperintense, approaching that of fat

CT Findings

- CECT best imaging tool for thymoma
- Oval or lobulated mass within anterior mediastinum
- Homogeneous enhancement is common in small tumors
- Heterogeneous enhancement more common in large tumors
- Thin and linear calcifications seen within capsule in 1/3 of patients
- Cystic changes and necrosis common in larger tumors
- Obliteration of mediastinal fat planes or mediastinal structures seen in invasive tumors

MACROSCOPIC FEATURES

General Features

- Generally well-circumscribed, encapsulated, solid tumor
- Homogeneous tan-white, rubbery tissue on cut surface
- Lobulated cut surface
- May be cystic and multilocular
- May contain calcifications in capsule or within tumor
- Rarely can be multifocal
- Can be ectopically located in posterior mediastinum, lung, neck, or pleura
- Can show areas of necrosis and hemorrhage
- Invasive tumors usually compromise adjacent structures, including large vessels, pericardium, pleura
- Distant metastases are rare

Sections to Be Submitted

- At least 1 section per cm of greatest tumor diameter
- Take additional sections if tumor shows variegated appearance
- Sample solid areas in cyst walls in multicystic tumors
- Always include sections of inked outer surface of specimen
- Coordination with surgeon should be sought to establish "true" margins to be sampled
- Any structures attached to specimen (i.e., pleura, lung, large vessels) should be inked and sampled separately as they represent "true" margins

MICROSCOPIC PATHOLOGY

Histologic Features

- Histologic classification is controversial
- Currently 2 systems are in use: Suster & Moran classification and WHO classification
- Suster & Moran classification: Based on degree of organotypical differentiation, divided into 3-tiered system
  - Well-differentiated (thymoma)
  - Moderately differentiated (atypical thymoma)
  - Poorly differentiated (thymic carcinoma)
- WHO classification is based primarily on cell type, cytologic atypia, and proportion of lymphocytes to epithelial cells
  - WHO type A: Composed of spindle cells without cytologic atypia
  - WHO type AB: Composed of spindle cells admixed with abundant lymphocytes
  - WHO type B1: Composed of round, epithelioid cells admixed with abundant lymphocytes
  - WHO type B2: Composed of round, epithelioid cells admixed with equal amounts of lymphocytes
  - WHO type B3: Composed predominantly of epithelial cells with cytologic atypia

THYMOMA

- WHO classification has a series of other distinctive histologic types that do not fit into the standard categories
  - "Metaplastic" thymoma
  - Multifocal thymoma
  - Microscopic thymoma
  - Micronodular thymoma
  - Anaplastic thymoma
- Older ("traditional") classification by Bernatz et al from Mayo Clinic is still used today by many and divides these tumors based on their cell composition
  - Lymphocyte-rich thymoma
  - Mixed, lymphoepithelial thymoma
  - Epithelial-rich thymoma
  - Spindle cell thymoma

Cytologic Features

- 2 basic cell types are recognized
  - Oval/spindle cells (types A, AB)
  - Round/epithelioid cells (types B1-3)
- Type A thymoma is composed of oval or spindle cells with scattered nuclear chromatin and inconspicuous or absent nucleoli and no mitotic activity
  - Spindle cell thymoma usually contains few lymphocytes
  - Majority of spindle cell thymomas are low grade and encapsulated
  - Invasive or atypical spindle cell thymoma can follow aggressive behavior
  - Distant metastases and death can occur in some cases of spindle cell thymoma
- Type AB thymoma is composed of oval or spindle cells identical to those in type "A" but admixed with abundant small lymphocytes.
  - Spindle cells do not display mitotic activity
  - Lymphocytes admixed with epithelial cells are of T-cell type
  - Tumors usually contain admixture of lymphocyte-rich and lymphocyte-poor areas
  - Tumors may be composed exclusively of lymphocyte-rich areas and be confused for B1 thymoma
- Type B1 thymoma is composed of round/epithelioid cells with single small eosinophilic nucleoli and abundant cytoplasm, admixed with numerous small T-lymphocytes
  - Small lymphocytes predominate and overshadow epithelial cells
  - Contains frequent perivascular spaces and areas of "medullary" differentiation
  - Equivalent to "lymphocyte-rich" or "lymphocyte-predominant" in traditional classification (Mayo Clinic)
- Type B2 thymoma is composed of approximately equal admixture of round epithelial cells and small lymphocytes
  - Epithelial cells may show mild degree of atypia and enlargement of nuclei
  - Admixtures with B1 areas may be seen in about 30% of cases
  - Equivalent to "mixed lymphoepithelial" thymoma of traditional classification (Mayo Clinic)
- Type B3 thymoma is composed of sheets of large epithelioid cells admixed with scant lymphocytes
  - Epithelial cells are characterized by nuclear enlargement with dense chromatin pattern and prominent nucleoli
  - Mitotic figures can be encountered in epithelial cells
  - Cell nuclei show tendency to adopt raisin-like configuration
  - Cytoplasm of tumor cells is usually abundant, eosinophilic, and with sharp cell borders
  - Tendency for epithelial cells to palisade around perivascular spaces
  - Tumor cells can also be oval or spindle with similar nuclear features
- Type A thymomas may exhibit unusual growth patterns
  - Hemangiopericytic growth pattern
  - Micronodular growth pattern with lymphoid B-cell hyperplasia
  - Biphasic pattern with pseudosarcomatous stroma ("metaplastic" thymoma)
  - Skin adnexal-like ("adenoid") growth pattern
  - Sclerosing growth pattern
  - Rosette-forming growth pattern
- Type B thymomas may exhibit unusual features
  - Extensive multilocular thymic cyst-like changes
  - Areas of infarction, hemorrhage, and necrosis
  - Massive infiltration by plasma cells in stroma
  - Clear cell changes
  - "Starry sky" appearance simulating lymphoma
- Type C thymoma (thymic carcinoma) is characterized by overt cytologic evidence of malignancy and absence of organotypical features of thymic differentiation
  - Diagnosis of exclusion
  - Requires demonstration of absence of tumor elsewhere clinically and radiographically

Lymphatic/Vascular Invasion

- Very rare; unknown significance but generally associated with worse prognosis

Margins

- Very difficult to determine without assistance of surgeon
- True resection margins need to be inked or tagged by surgeon before submitting to pathology
- Inked anterior surface does not represent "margin" unless it was invading at time of surgery
- True margins need to be inked for proper assessment

Lymph Nodes

- Thymoma rarely metastasizes to lymph nodes
- Majority of lymph node metastases in thymoma are to mediastinal nodes
- Other intrathoracic lymph nodes may also be involved more rarely by metastatic thymoma

DIFFERENTIAL DIAGNOSIS

Lymphoblastic Lymphoma

- Does not show scattered keratin-positive cells admixed with the immature T-lymphocytes

- Shows rapid growth with sudden onset of symptoms
  - Thymoma is slow-growing tumor with slowly progressive symptoms
- Most common age for lymphoblastic lymphoma is childhood and adolescence
  - Most common age for thymoma is in middle-aged adults; rare in children and adolescents

Acquired Multilocular Thymic Cyst

- Multilocular cysts do not contain discrete areas attached to walls of cysts showing typical type B thymoma
  - Type A thymoma can undergo massive cystic changes, but the cells lining the cysts are spindle cells
- Shows small cuboidal or squamous epithelial cells lining the cysts in continuity with dilated Hassall corpuscles
- Shows prominent lymphoid follicular hyperplasia and severe acute and chronic inflammation with cholesterol cleft granulomas

Hemangiopericytoma/Solitary Fibrous Tumor

- Spindle cells in solitary fibrous tumors are not keratin-positive
- Spindle cells in solitary fibrous tumor are CD34, Bcl-2, and CD99 positive
- Shows characteristic linear pattern of stromal collagenization resulting in deposition of rope-like collagen separating spindle cells
- Devoid of immature T cells
  - Spindle cell thymoma may contain variable number of immature T cells admixed with epithelial cells

Neuroendocrine Carcinomas

- Positive for neuroendocrine markers
  - Rosette-like structures in thymoma are only positive for cytokeratin
- Thymic carcinoids usually show increased mitotic activity and tumor cells necrosis
- Tumor cells in carcinoids show characteristic stippled ("salt and pepper") chromatin pattern
- Other features of thymic carcinoids include a nested growth pattern ("zellballen") and formation of trabeculae, ribbons, and festoons

DIAGNOSTIC CHECKLIST

Clinically Relevant Pathologic Features

- Encapsulation/circumscription
- Presence or absence of cytologic atypia in epithelial cells
- Size of tumor
- Clinical stage
- Presence or absence of myasthenia gravis

Pathologic Interpretation Pearls

- Great variation in histologic appearance due to tumor heterogeneity
- Identification of scattered keratin-positive neoplastic cells in lymphocyte-rich tumors
- Hemorrhage and necrosis may be seen in encapsulated low-grade, well-differentiated tumors; not to be mistaken for ominous sign
- Capsular invasion is most significant prognostic factor
- Rarely, thymoma may be devoid of a capsule; should not be overinterpreted for invasion
- Types A, AB, B1, and B2 in WHO classification observe similar behavior; prognosis is determined by status of capsular integrity
- Type B3 thymoma in WHO classification has slightly more aggressive biologic behavior with frequent invasion at time of diagnosis and earlier recurrences

SELECTED REFERENCES

1. Casey EM et al: Clinical management of thymoma patients. Hematol Oncol Clin North Am. 22(3):457-73, 2008
2. Gupta R et al: Evidence-based pathology and the pathologic evaluation of thymomas: transcapsular invasion is not a significant prognostic feature. Arch Pathol Lab Med. 132(6):926-30, 2008
3. Marchevsky AM et al: Evidence-based pathology and the pathologic evaluation of thymomas: the World Health Organization classification can be simplified into only 3 categories other than thymic carcinoma. Cancer. 112(12):2780-8, 2008
4. Moran CA et al: The World Health Organization (WHO) histologic classification of thymomas: a reanalysis. Curr Treat Options Oncol. 9(4-6):288-99, 2008
5. Rossi G et al: Thymoma classification: does it matter? Histopathology. 53(4):483-4, 2008
6. Suster S et al: Histologic classification of thymoma: the World Health Organization and beyond. Hematol Oncol Clin North Am. 22(3):381-92, 2008
7. Verghese ET et al: Interobserver variation in the classification of thymic tumours--a multicentre study using the WHO classification system. Histopathology. 53(2):218-23, 2008
8. Wick MR: Prognostic factors for thymic epithelial neoplasms, with emphasis on tumor staging. Hematol Oncol Clin North Am. 22(3):527-42, 2008
9. Suster S et al: Thymoma classification: current status and future trends. Am J Clin Pathol. 125(4):542-54, 2006
10. Suster S: Diagnosis of thymoma. J Clin Pathol. 59(12):1238-44, 2006
11. Suster S et al: Problem areas and inconsistencies in the WHO classification of thymoma. Semin Diagn Pathol. 22(3):188-97, 2005
12. Travis WD et al. Pathology and genetics of tumors of the lung, pleura, thymus and heart. In: World Health Organization Classification of Tumors. Lyon: IARC Press. 145-171; 2004
13. Marchevsky AM et al: Protocol for the examination of specimens from patients with thymic epithelial tumors located in any area of the mediastinum. Arch Pathol Lab Med. 127(10):1298-303, 2003
14. Rieker RJ et al: Histologic classification of thymic epithelial tumors: comparison of established classification schemes. Int J Cancer. 98(6):900-6, 2002
15. Moran CA et al: On the histologic heterogeneity of thymic epithelial neoplasms. Impact of sampling in subtyping and classification of thymomas. Am J Clin Pathol. 114(5):760-6, 2000

THYMOMA

Immunohistochemistry

Antibody	Reactivity	Staining Pattern	Comment
AE1/AE3	Positive	Cytoplasmic	Stains only neoplastic thymic epithelial cells
p63	Positive	Nuclear	Stains neoplastic thymic epithelial cells in all histologic types
CK19	Positive	Cytoplasmic	Stains neoplastic cells in all histologic types of thymoma
CD1a	Positive	Cytoplasmic	Stains immature T-lymphocytes
TdT	Positive	Nuclear	Stains immature T-lymphocytes
CD3	Positive	Cytoplasmic	Stains T-lymphocytes
CD99	Positive	Cytoplasmic	Stains immature T-lymphocytes
CD20	Positive	Cytoplasmic	May be positive in spindle cells in thymoma (WHO types A and AB) and also highlights small subpopulation of B-lymphocytes
Bcl-2	Positive	Cytoplasmic	May be positive in spindle cell thymoma (WHO types A and AB)
CD5	Negative	Cytoplasmic	Is negative in epithelial cells of most thymomas, except WHO B3
CD117	Negative	Cytoplasmic	Is negative in epithelial cells of most thymomas; stains germ cells and mast cells within tumor

Histologic Classification Systems for Thymoma

Suster & Moran Classification	WHO 2004 Classification
Well-differentiated thymic epithelial neoplasm (thymoma)	WHO type A (spindle cell)
Well-differentiated thymic epithelial neoplasm (thymoma)	WHO Type AB (spindle cell with abundant lymphocytes)
Well-differentiated thymic epithelial neoplasm (thymoma)	WHO type B1 (lymphocyte-predominant)
Well-differentiated thymic epithelial neoplasm (thymoma)	WHO type B2 (lymphoepithelial)
Moderately differentiated thymic epithelial neoplasm (atypical thymoma)	WHO type B3 (epithelial-rich)
Poorly differentiated thymic epithelial neoplasm (thymic carcinoma)	Thymic carcinoma

Classification of Thymoma According to Grades of Differentiation (Suster & Moran)

Diagnosis	Differentiation Grade	Features
Organotypical thymoma	Well-differentiated thymic neoplasm	Preservation of organotypical features of thymic differentiation; no cytologic evidence of atypia
Atypical thymoma	Moderately differentiated thymic neoplasm	Partial preservation of organotypical features of differentiation of the thymus; mild to moderate cytologic atypia
Thymic carcinoma	Poorly differentiated thymic neoplasm	Loss of organotypical features of differentiation of the thymus; overt cytologic evidence of malignancy

16. Suster S et al: Micronodular thymoma with lymphoid B-cell hyperplasia: clinicopathologic and immunohistochemical study of eighteen cases of a distinctive morphologic variant of thymic epithelial neoplasm. Am J Surg Pathol. 23(8):955-62, 1999
17. Suster S et al: Primary thymic epithelial neoplasms: spectrum of differentiation and histological features. Semin Diagn Pathol. 16(1):2-17, 1999
18. Suster S et al: Thymoma, atypical thymoma, and thymic carcinoma. A novel conceptual approach to the classification of thymic epithelial neoplasms. Am J Clin Pathol. 111(6):826-33, 1999
19. Suster S et al: Thymoma with pseudosarcomatous stroma: report of an unusual histologic variant of thymic epithelial neoplasm that may simulate carcinosarcoma. Am J Surg Pathol. 21(11):1316-23, 1997
20. Suster S et al: Primary thymic epithelial neoplasms showing combined features of thymoma and thymic carcinoma. A clinicopathologic study of 22 cases. Am J Surg Pathol. 20(12):1469-80, 1996
21. Suster S et al: Malignant thymic neoplasms that may mimic benign conditions. Semin Diagn Pathol. 12(1):98-104, 1995
22. Dawson A et al: Observer variation in the histopathological classification of thymoma: correlation with prognosis. J Clin Pathol. 47(6):519-23, 1994
23. Koga K et al: A review of 79 thymomas: modification of staging system and reappraisal of conventional division into invasive and non-invasive thymoma. Pathol Int. 44(5):359-67, 1994
24. Suster S et al: Cystic thymomas. A clinicopathologic study of ten cases. Cancer. 69(1):92-7, 1992
25. Suster S et al: Thymic carcinoma. A clinicopathologic study of 60 cases. Cancer. 67(4):1025-32, 1991
26. Wick MR: Assessing the prognosis of thymomas. Ann Thorac Surg. 50(4):521-2, 1990

Cell Types

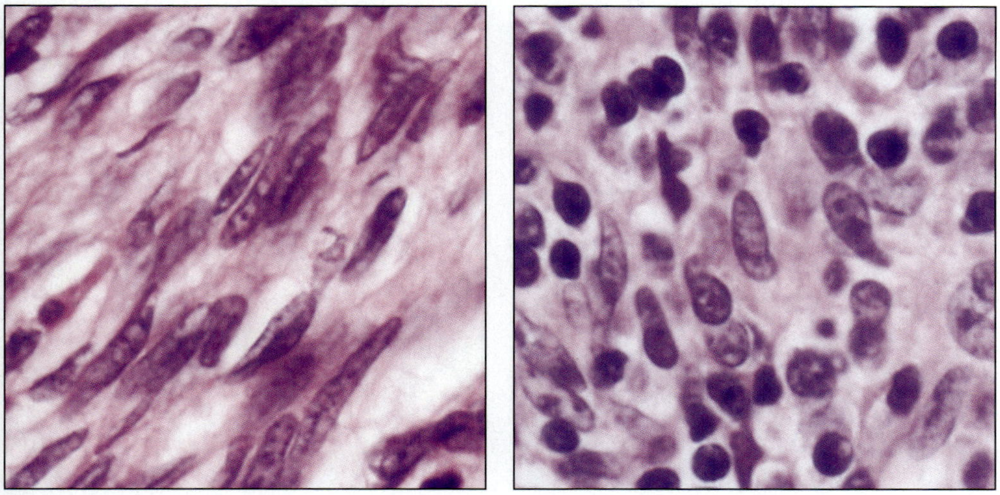

(Left) *Type A thymoma is composed of spindle cells with elongated nuclei showing dispersed chromatin pattern and absent or very inconspicuous nucleoli and an indistinct rim of lightly eosinophilic to amphophilic cytoplasm.* ***(Right)*** *Type AB thymoma is composed of a similar proliferation of spindle cells with elongated nuclei showing dispersed chromatin pattern. The cells are essentially identical to those seen in type A except they are surrounded by abundant lymphocytes.*

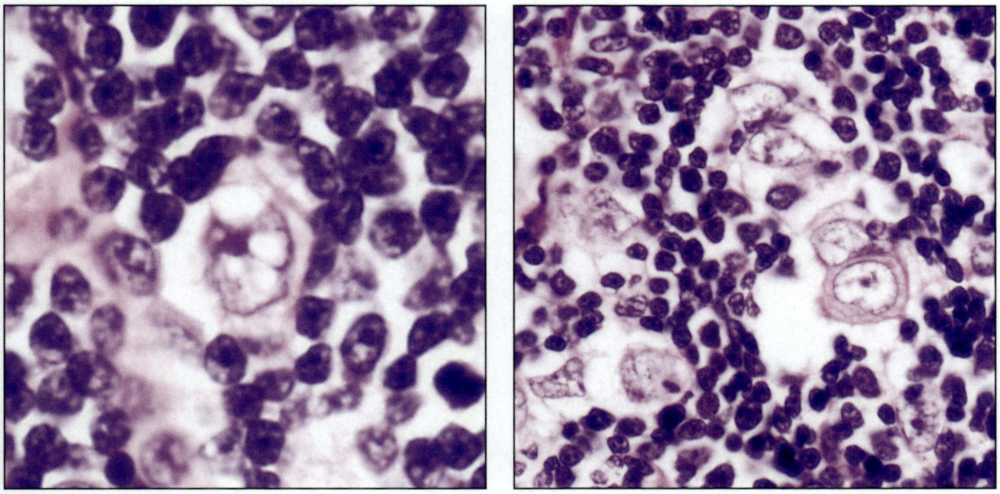

(Left) *Type B1 thymoma is composed of large, round epithelioid cells with large, vesicular nuclei containing single prominent eosinophilic nucleoli and surrounded by an indistinct rim of amphophilic cytoplasm.* ***(Right)*** *Type B2 thymoma shows round epithelioid cells that may be slightly larger than those seen in B1 thymomas but which essentially show similar nuclear features. Notice there are more epithelial cells per lymphocyte than in type B1.*

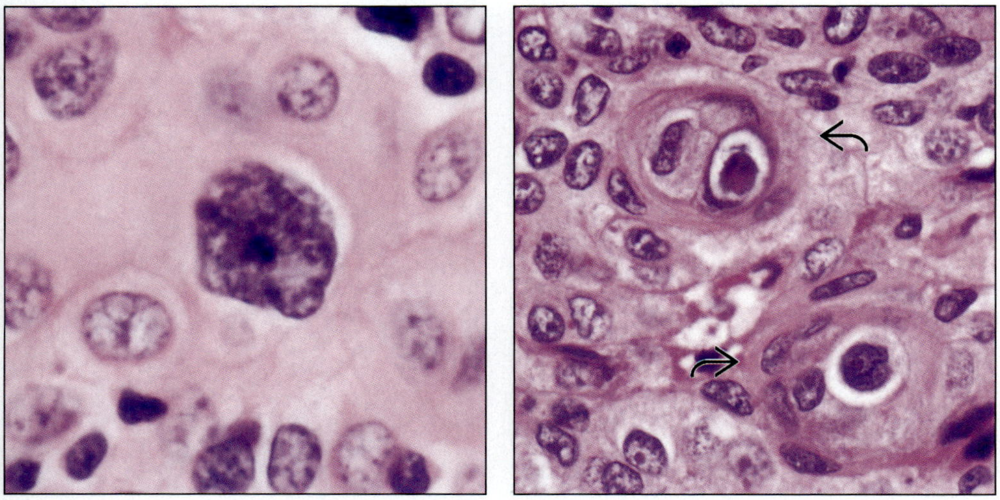

(Left) *Type B3 thymoma shows sheets of large epithelioid to polygonal cells with enlarged nuclei, marked increase in nuclear chromatin, prominent nucleoli, and abundant eosinophilic cytoplasm with sharp cell borders.* ***(Right)*** *Type B3 thymoma may show foci of abortive squamous differentiation, showing large, round to polygonal cells with large nuclei and prominent nucleoli. Notice the tight apposition and moulding of the cells forming abortive squamous eddies* ↷.

THYMOMA

Spindle Cell Thymoma (WHO Type A)

(Left) *Spindle cell thymoma (WHO type A) shows fascicles of bland-appearing spindle cells admixed with a few scattered small lymphocytes.* ***(Right)*** *High-power view of a spindle cell thymoma (WHO type A) shows spindle cells with elongated nuclei that contain scattered chromatin and absence of nucleoli. The cells are characterized by a scant rim of indistinct, amphophilic cytoplasm. This spindle cell proliferation can closely resemble a spindle cell mesenchymal neoplasm.*

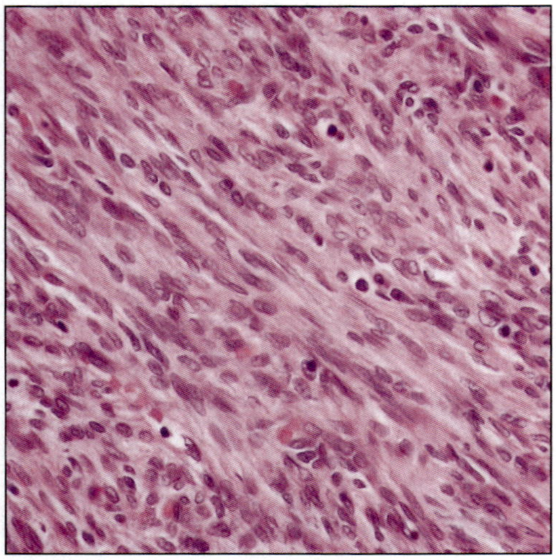

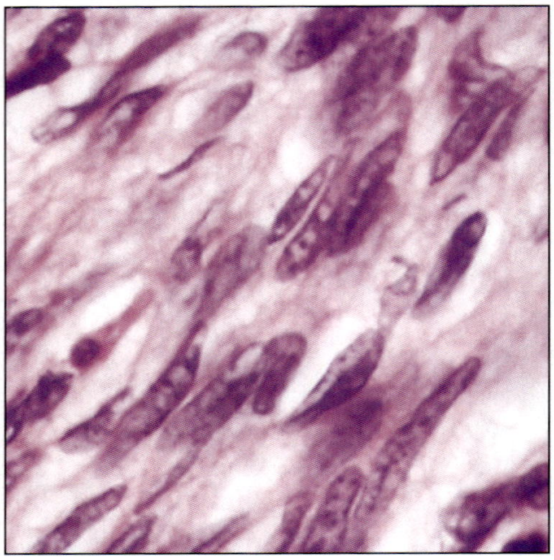

(Left) *A short storiform pattern is appreciated in this example of spindle cell thymoma (WHO type A). Notice the sprinkling of small lymphocytes in the background. This growth pattern can be confused for a fibrohistiocytic neoplasm or a solitary fibrous tumor of the mediastinum.* ***(Right)*** *Spindle cell thymoma (WHO type A) shows a striking microcystic pattern of growth with small, abortive gland-like structures. The microcysts are primarily composed of dilated perivascular spaces.*

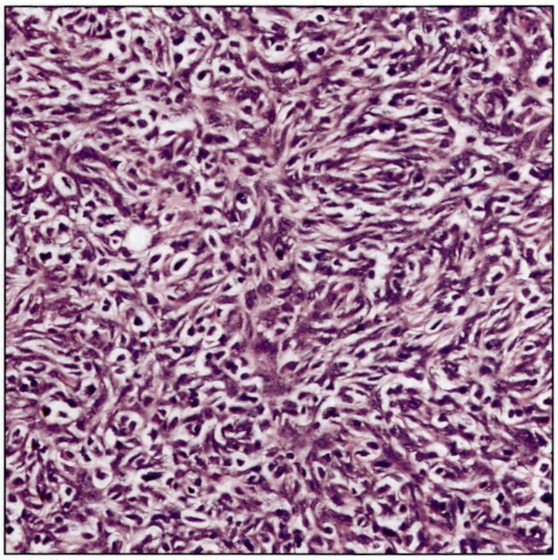

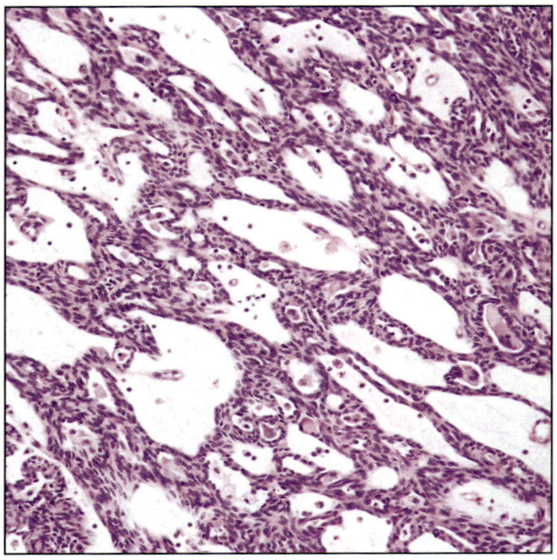

(Left) *Spindle cell thymoma (WHO type A) shows a macrocystic pattern of growth with large, irregular cystic spaces lined by the thymic epithelial cells. The macrocysts are caused by the confluence and coalescence of smaller, dilated perivascular spaces.* ***(Right)*** *Spindle cell thymoma (WHO type A) shows capsular invasion by tumor ⇨. Notice the solid nodule traversing the fibrous capsule of the thymus that is still attached to the underlying main tumor mass by a short pedicle ⇗.*

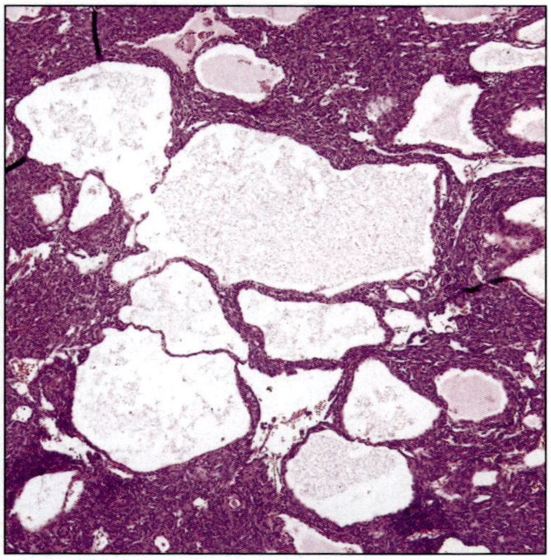

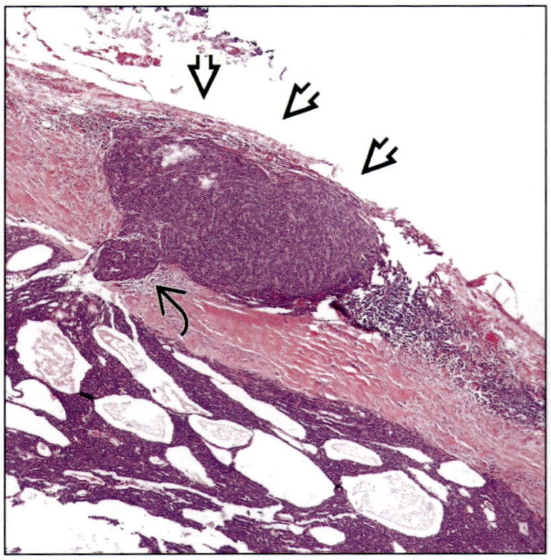

Unusual Variants of Spindle Cell Thymoma

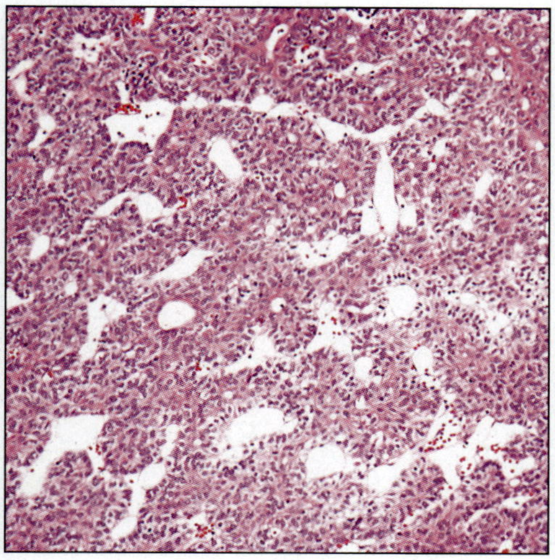
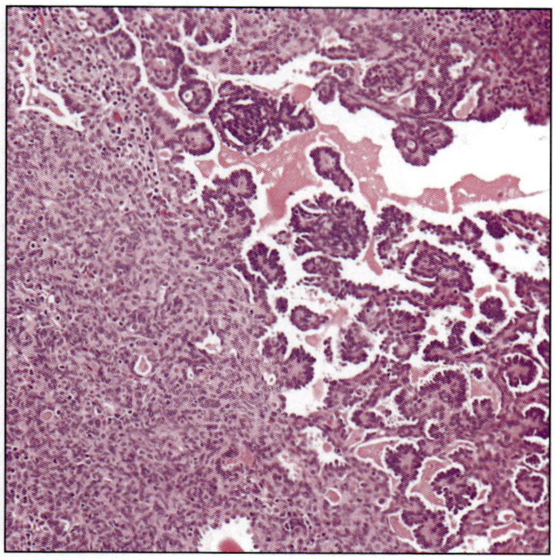

(Left) *Spindle cell thymoma (WHO type A) shows a striking hemangiopericytoma-like vascular pattern. Notice numerous small to medium-sized vascular spaces displaying open lumens and occasional branching of vessels.* ***(Right)*** *Spindle cell thymoma (WHO type A) shows prominent papillary structures (right 1/2 of field) that gradually merge with solid, spindle cell component on the left side. These tumors can be confused for metastatic papillary carcinoma.*

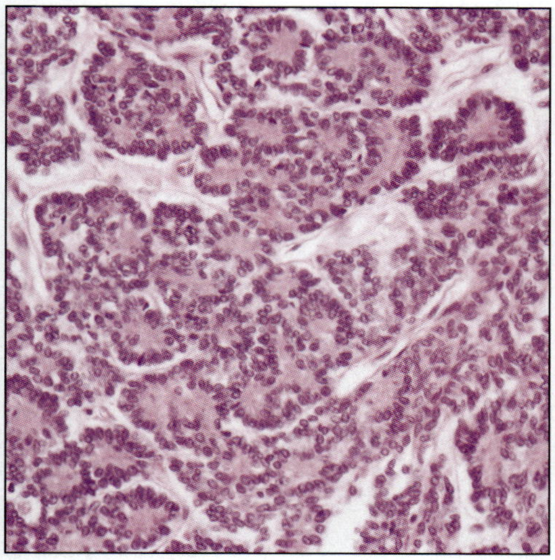
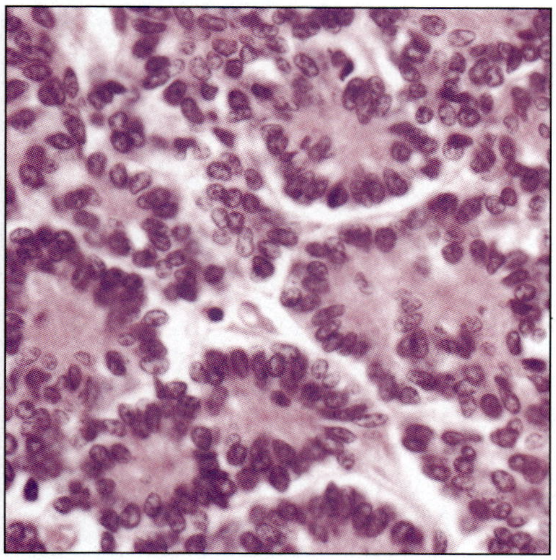

(Left) *Spindle cell thymoma (WHO type A) shows numerous small, rosette-like structures with striking palisading of nuclei in the periphery and central cores containing amorphous material.* ***(Right)*** *High-power view of spindle cell thymoma with epithelial rosettes shows rosette-like structures displaying peripheral palisading of nuclei and central cores containing pink, amorphous material. These tumors may be confused for primary or metastatic neuroendocrine neoplasms.*

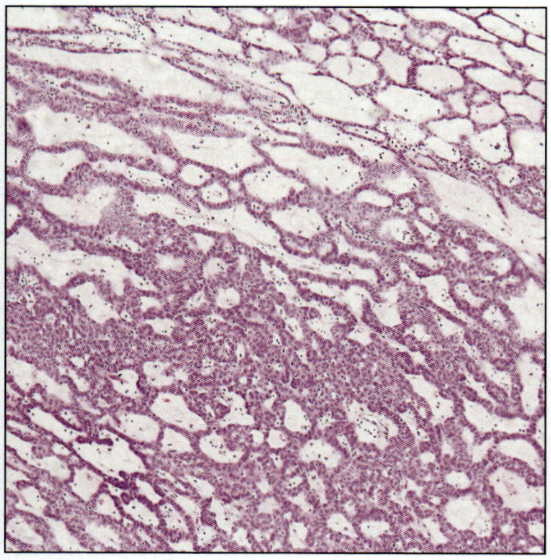
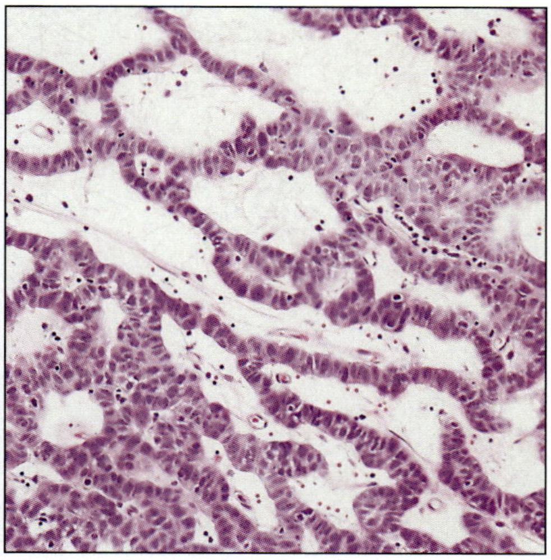

(Left) *Spindle cell thymoma (WHO type A) shows a delicate, lace-like pattern composed of cords and rows of single cells adopting a net-like configuration reminiscent of a benign skin adnexal tumor.* ***(Right)*** *High-power view of spindle cell thymoma shows an adenoid, lace-like arrangement of tumor cells. The cells are oval to spindle and adopt a palisaded appearance. A few scattered small lymphocytes are also present. The image is reminiscent of a benign skin adnexal tumor.*

THYMOMA

Unusual Variants of Spindle Cell Thymoma

*(**Left**) Micronodular thymoma with lymphoid B-cell hyperplasia shows discrete, small nodules against a background of small lymphocytes in the stroma. (**Right**) High power of micronodule in micronodular thymoma shows cells with oval nuclei surrounded by an indistinct rim of amphophilic cytoplasm. The cells surrounding the nodule are polyclonal B-lymphocytes. This image can be confused for a metastatic carcinoma to mediastinal lymph node.*

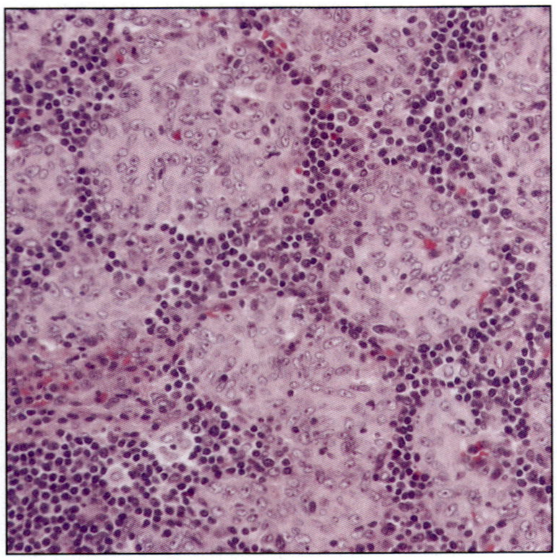

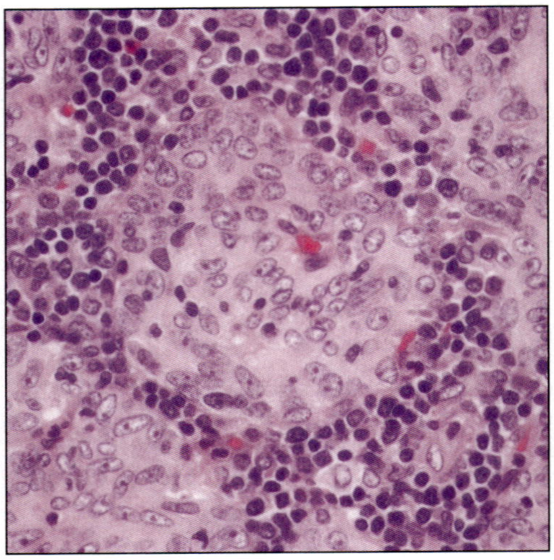

*(**Left**) Micronodular thymoma with lymphoid B-cell hyperplasia shows a hyperplastic lymphoid follicle with reactive germinal center ↪. The solid nodule beneath is composed mainly of spindle to oval cells with scant cytoplasm. (**Right**) Spindle cell thymoma (WHO type A) shows massive dilatation of perivascular spaces with abundant hyalinization and sclerosis. Notice fibroepitheliomatous appearance caused by strands of epithelial cells circumscribing hyalinized stroma.*

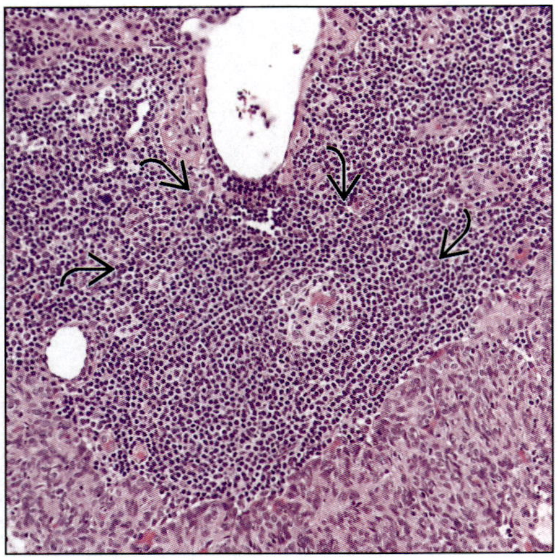

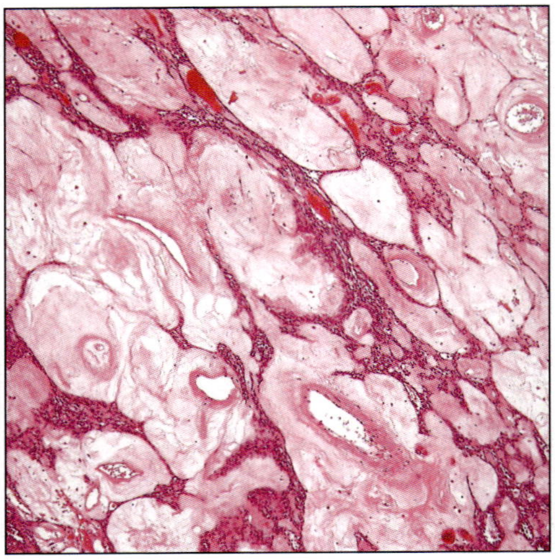

*(**Left**) Rhabdomyomatous variant of thymoma shows a biphasic appearance on scanning magnification. There are strands and cords of oval to spindle epithelial tumor cells circumscribing clusters of large eosinophilic cells. (**Right**) High power of rhabdomyomatous thymoma shows large "rhabdoid" cells in the center characterized by small, oval nuclei surrounded by an ample rim of densely eosinophilic cytoplasm. These cells express desmin and correspond to "myoid" cells of the thymus.*

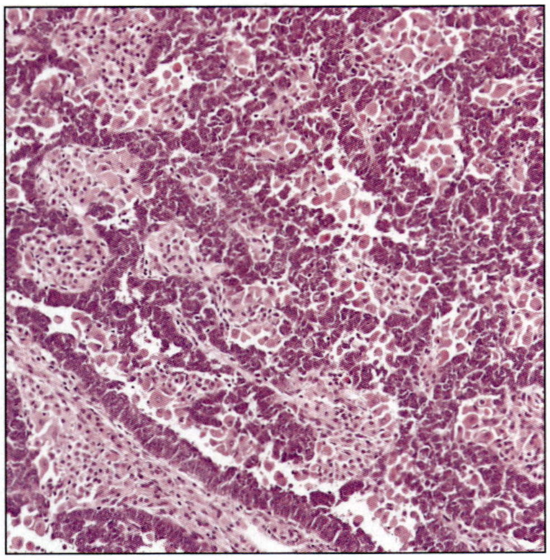

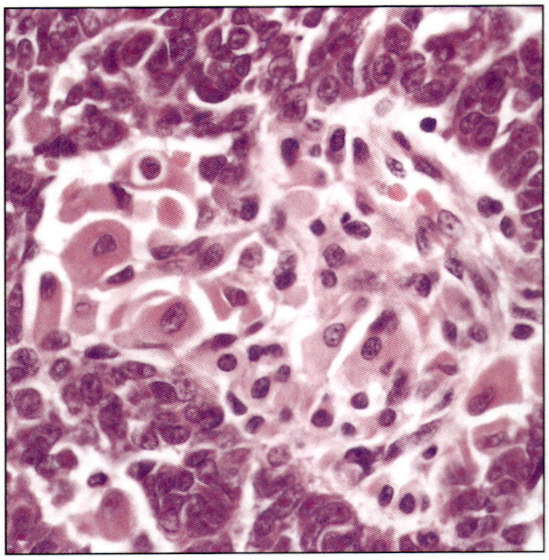

"Metaplastic" Thymoma with Pseudosarcomatous Stroma

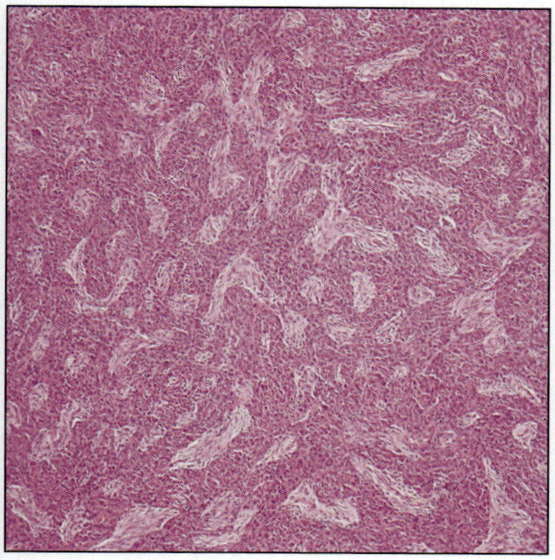

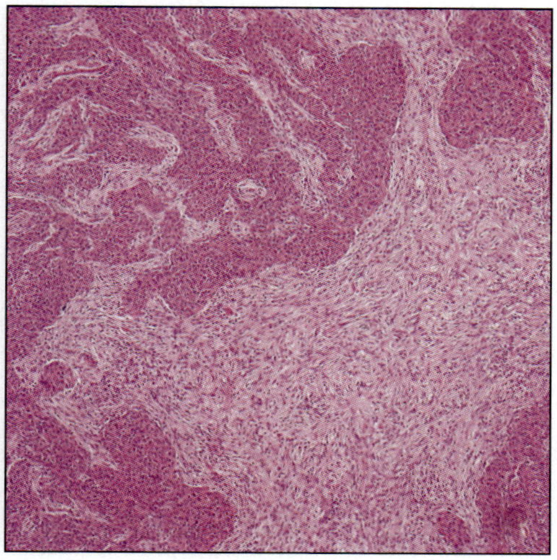

(Left) *Spindle cell thymoma with pseudosarcomatous stroma (so-called "metaplastic" thymoma) shows a sieve-like architecture with anastomosing cords and trabeculae of epithelial tumor cells circumscribing stromal areas containing a spindle cell population.* ***(Right)*** *Thymoma with pseudosarcomatous stroma shows a sharp demarcation between the epithelial component (periphery) and the spindle cell stromal component (center).*

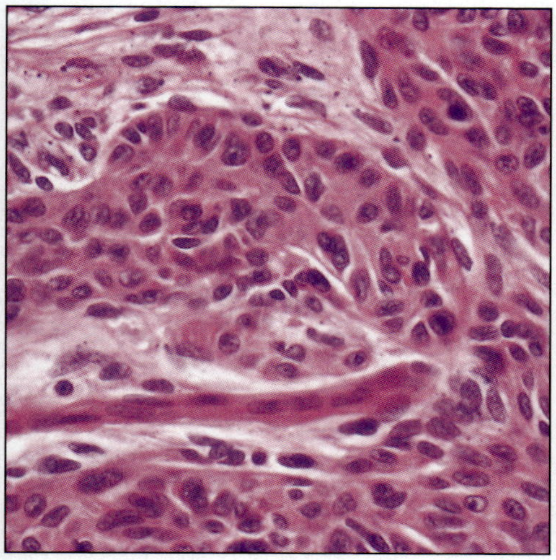

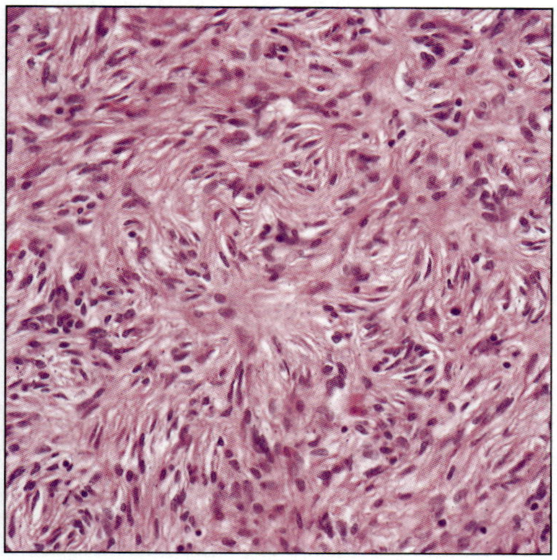

(Left) *High magnification of epithelial component is shown in thymoma with pseudosarcomatous stroma ("metaplastic" thymoma). Notice the large, oval to round nuclei with prominent nucleoli.* ***(Right)*** *High magnification of stromal component of spindle cell thymoma with pseudosarcomatous stroma shows a storiform pattern of growth. Notice the bland appearance of the spindle cells, the absence of nuclear pleomorphism and mitoses, and the lack of necrosis.*

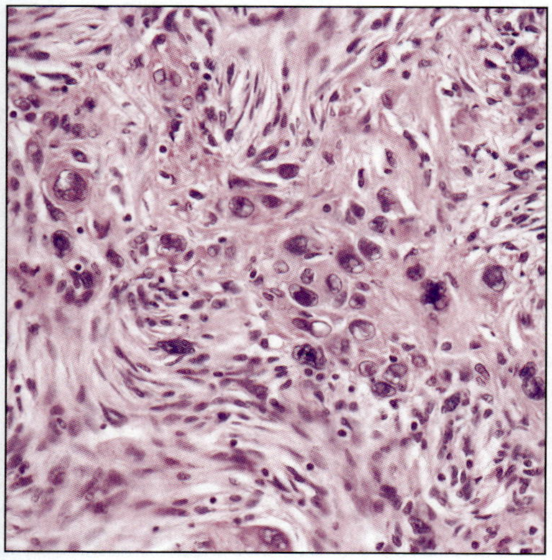

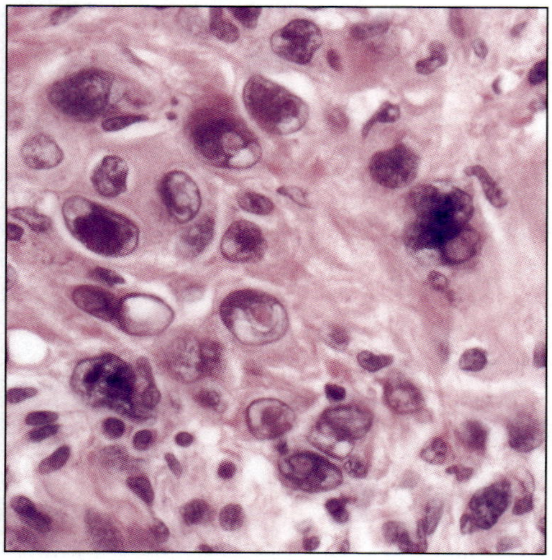

(Left) *Epithelial component in thymoma with pseudosarcomatous stroma ("metaplastic" thymoma) shows marked cytologic atypia in many of the tumor cells. Notice the spindle cell stroma surrounding the tumor cell island lacks mitotic activity or nuclear pleomorphism.* ***(Right)*** *High magnification of atypical epithelial component in thymoma with pseudosarcomatous stroma ("metaplastic" thymoma) shows enlarged tumor cells with large nuclei and prominent nucleoli.*

Lymphocyte-rich Spindle Cell Thymoma (WHO Type AB)

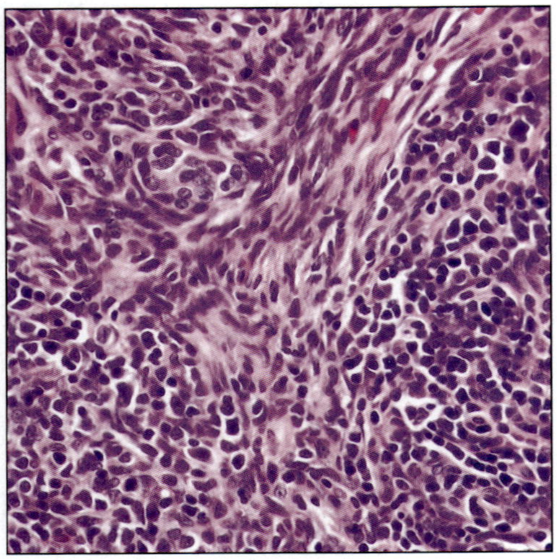
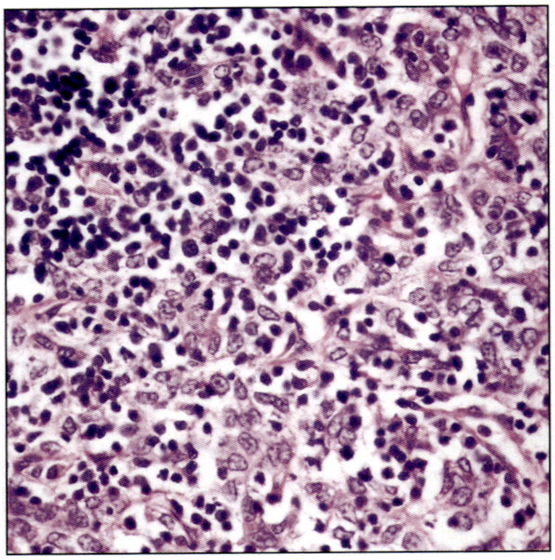

(Left) *Lymphocyte-rich spindle cell thymoma (WHO type AB) shows storiform fascicle of spindle cells (center) with few lymphocytes surrounded by areas containing scattered spindle cells admixed with numerous lymphocytes.* ***(Right)*** *High power of lymphocyte-rich spindle cell thymoma (WHO type AB) shows scattered small spindle epithelial cells admixed with numerous scattered small lymphocytes. The small spindle cells show identical nuclear features to those in the fascicular areas.*

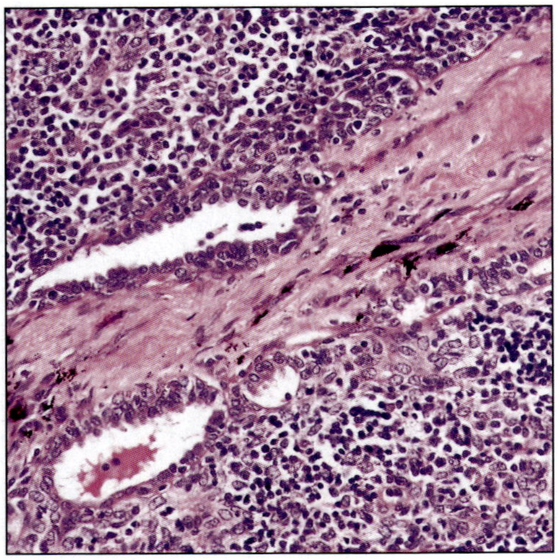
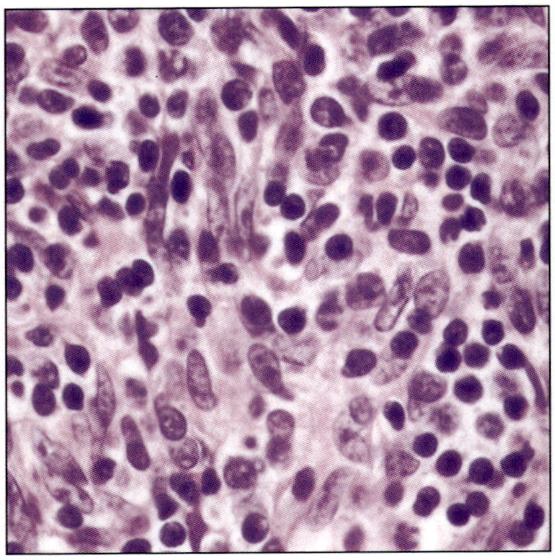

(Left) *Lymphocyte-rich spindle cell thymoma shows focal glandular structures admixed with the spindle cell population. Similar gland-like structures are commonly seen in conventional spindle cell thymoma and should not be confused for metastatic adenocarcinoma.* ***(Right)*** *High power of lymphocyte-rich spindle cell thymoma shows oval to spindle-shaped nuclei with dispersed chromatin and absent or inconspicuous nucleoli identical to those of conventional spindle cell thymoma. Notice abundant lymphocytes.*

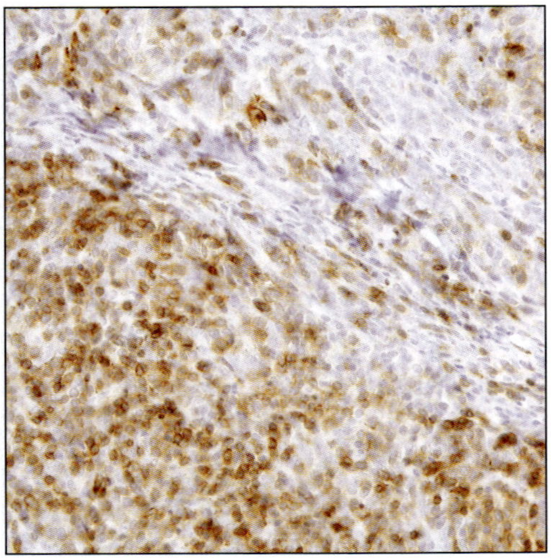
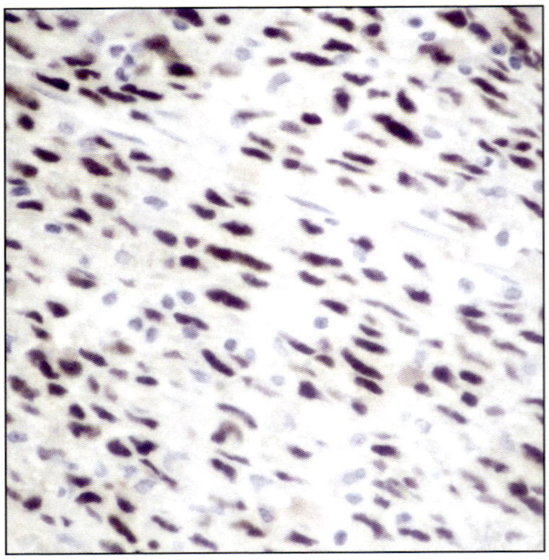

(Left) *Immunohistochemical staining of lymphocyte-rich spindle cell thymoma (WHO type AB) for the lymphoid marker CD1a highlights numerous immature T-lymphocytes admixed with the spindle cells.* ***(Right)*** *Immunohistochemical staining of lymphocyte-rich spindle cell thymoma (WHO type AB) with p63 antibody shows strong nuclear positivity in the spindle thymic epithelial cells. Notice how the stain highlights the elongated, oval to spindle shape of the nuclei in the tumor cells.*

Lymphocyte-rich Thymoma (WHO Type B1)

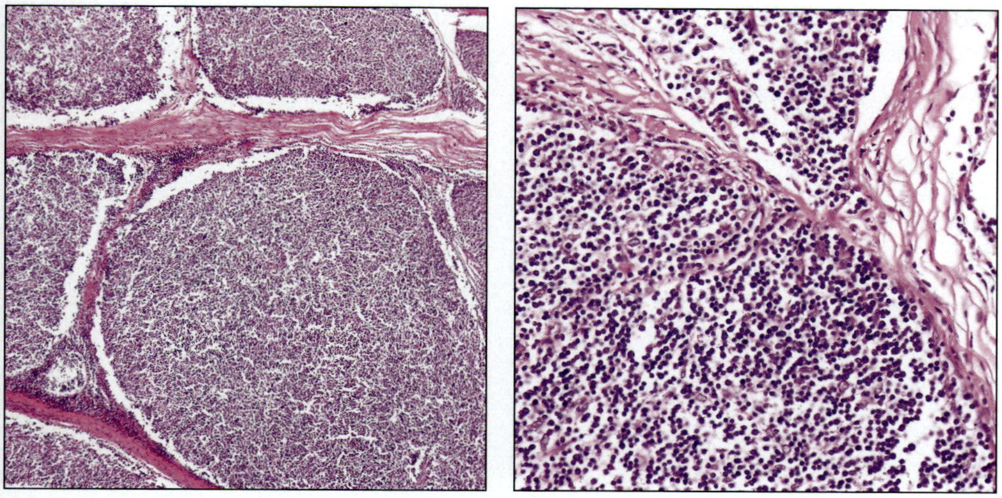

(Left) *Lymphocyte-rich thymoma (WHO type B1) shows round lobules of tumor tissue containing abundant lymphocytes. The lobules are circumscribed by broad bands of fibroconnective tissue.* ***(Right)*** *Higher magnification of round cellular lobule in lymphocyte-rich thymoma (WHO type B1) shows a predominantly lymphoid cell population. The lobules are separated by thin bands of fibrocollagenous tissue. These tumors can be easily mistaken for lymphocytic lymphomas.*

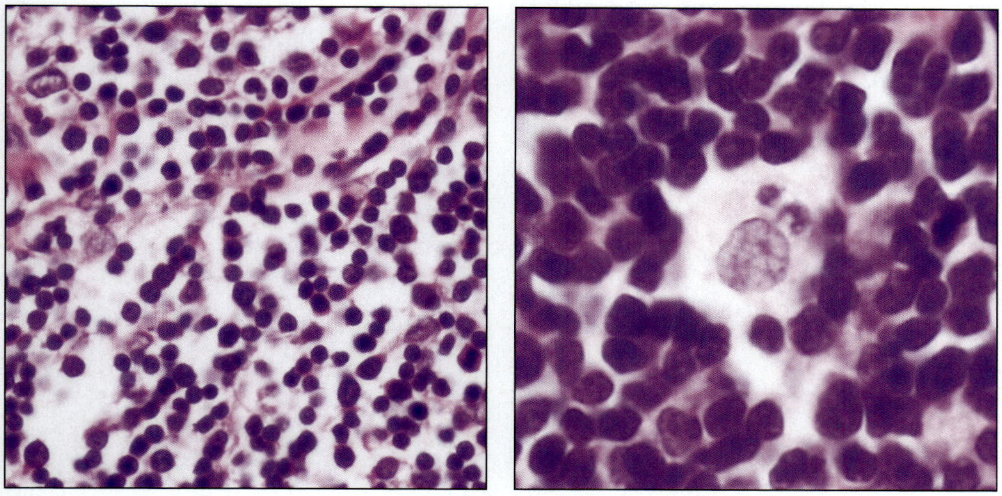

(Left) *High magnification of lymphocyte-rich thymoma (WHO type B1) shows a monotonous population of small lymphocytes with only rare, scattered cells with larger nuclei and an indistinct rim of cytoplasm.* ***(Right)*** *High magnification of lymphocyte-rich thymoma (WHO type B1) shows a large neoplastic epithelial cell in the center surrounded by a dense population of small lymphocytes.*

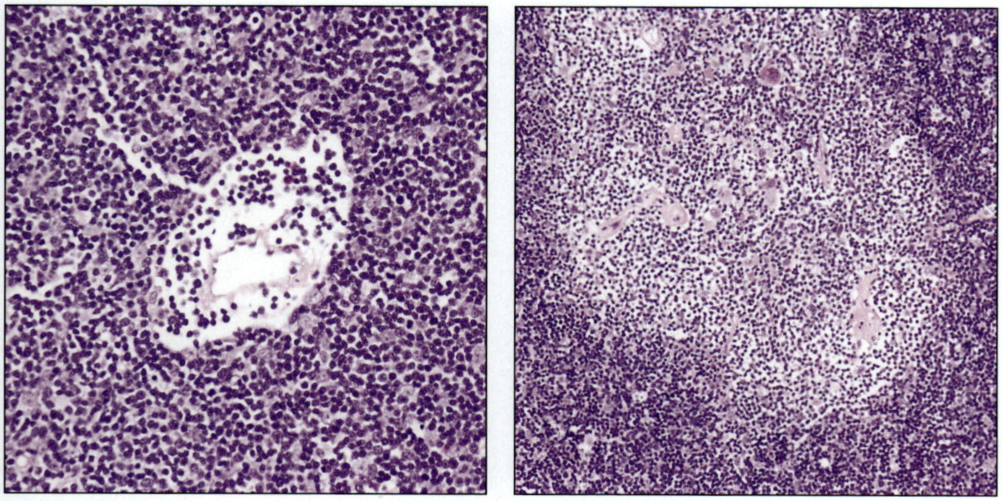

(Left) *Lymphocyte-rich thymoma (WHO type B1) shows a dilated perivascular space (center of the field) filled with scattered small lymphocytes. Notice the small vessel lumen "floating" inside the empty perivascular space.* ***(Right)*** *Lymphocyte-rich thymoma (WHO type B1) shows an area of "medullary" differentiation (center). This area is sparsely cellular and contains fewer lymphocytes than the surrounding parenchyma, as well as areas of hyalinization with abortive Hassall corpuscles.*

THYMOMA

Unusual Features in Lymphocyte-rich Thymoma

(Left) *Lymphocyte-rich thymoma (WHO type B1) shows prominent "starry sky" appearance. These tumors can be easily confused for lymphoblastic lymphoma, which are also often characterized by this histologic appearance.* ***(Right)*** *Lymphocyte-rich thymoma (WHO type B1) shows "starry sky" appearance represented by the large cells surrounded by clear spaces. The "starry sky" appearance is caused by an abundance of tingible-body macrophages.*

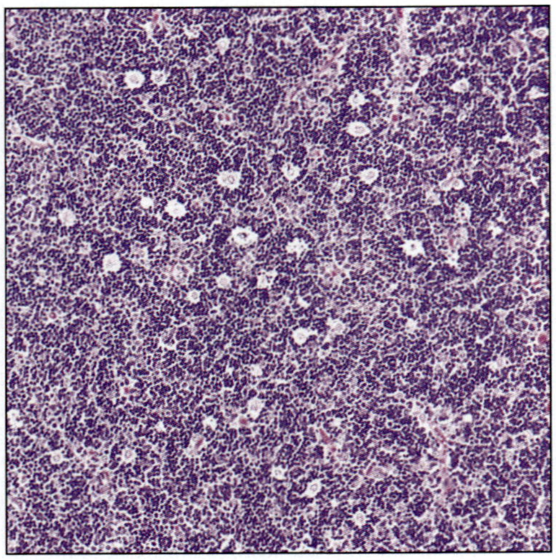

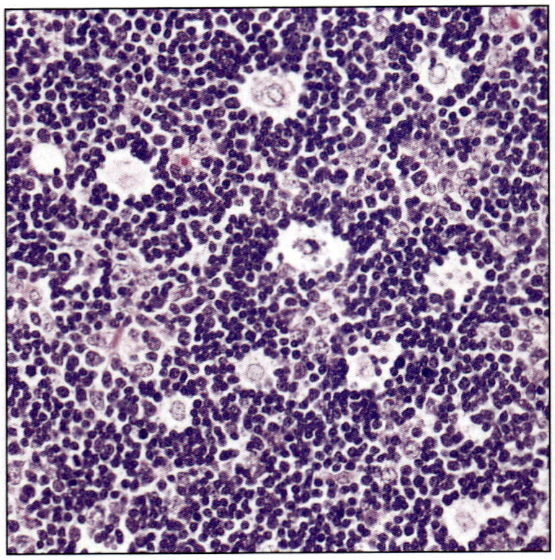

(Left) *Lymphocyte-rich thymoma (WHO type B1) shows well-developed and sharply defined areas resembling the normal cortex* ↪ *circumscribing lighter areas resembling the thymic medulla* ⇨*. Tumors with these features were termed "organoid" and "predominantly cortical" thymoma in prior terminology.* ***(Right)*** *High-power view shows Hassall corpuscle within area of "medullary" differentiation in lymphocyte-rich thymoma (WHO type B1; "organoid" thymoma).*

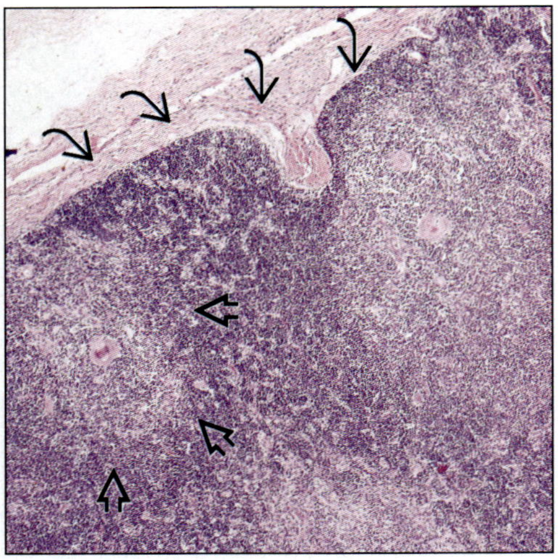

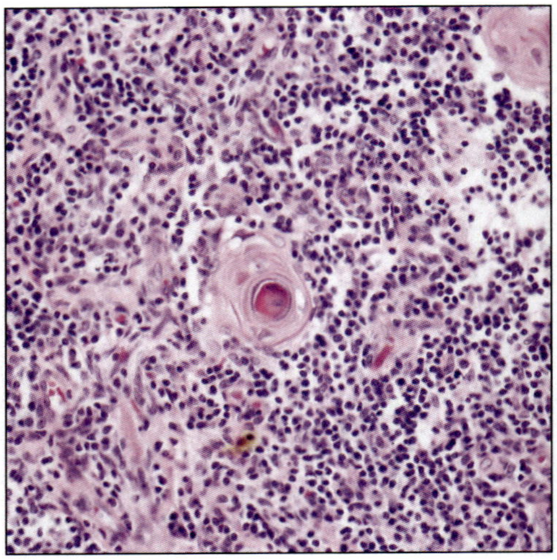

(Left) *Area of necrosis and infarction is seen in lymphocyte-rich (WHO type B1) thymoma. This is caused by vaso-occlusive phenomena in the vicinity of the infarcted areas of tumors with cystic changes. This should not be confused for a sign of malignancy or more aggressive behavior.* ***(Right)*** *Focus of vascular invasion in lymphocyte-rich thymoma (WHO type B2). The significance of this finding is unknown, but it is believed to be associated with more aggressive behavior.*

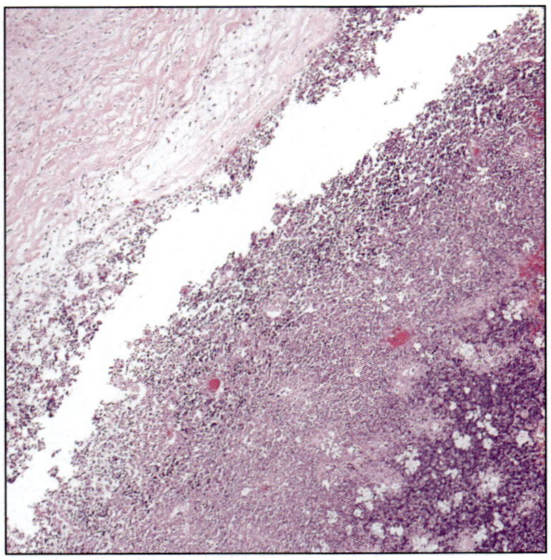

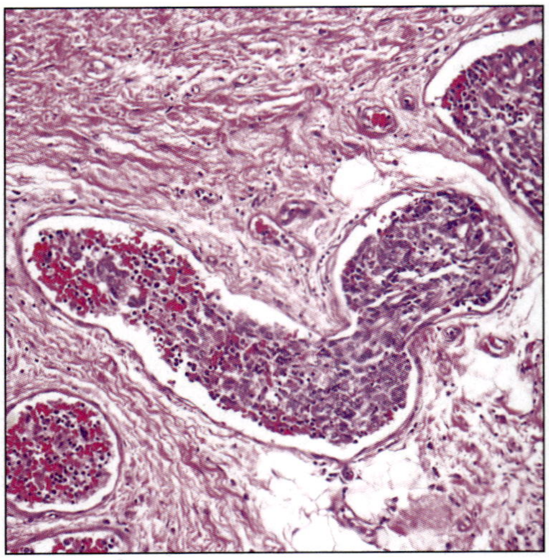

Lymphocyte-rich Thymoma (WHO Type B2)

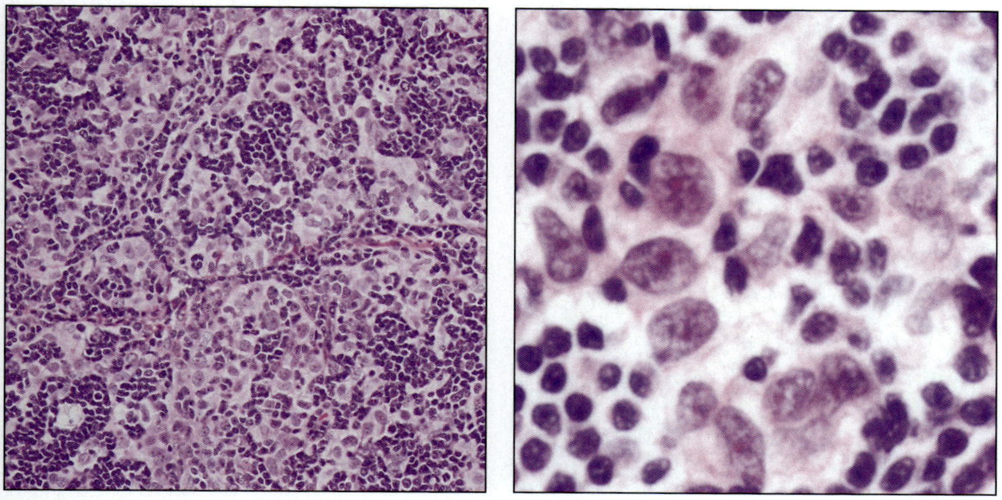

(Left) *Mixed lymphoepithelial (WHO type B2) thymoma shows approximately equal admixture of lymphocytes with neoplastic epithelial cells.* ***(Right)*** *Higher magnification of mixed lymphoepithelial thymoma (WHO type B2) shows abundant large, round to oval epithelial cells displaying vesicular nuclei with prominent eosinophilic nucleoli and indistinct rim of amphophilic cytoplasm. Note the variation in size and shape of the epithelial cells.*

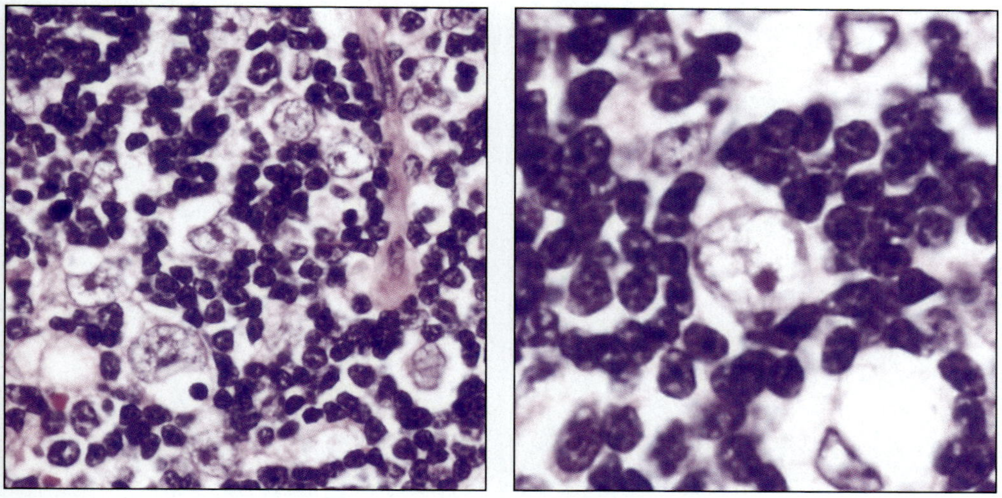

(Left) *Another example of mixed lymphoepithelial thymoma (WHO type B2) shows a large number of thymic epithelial cells admixed with small lymphocytes.* ***(Right)*** *High power of mixed lymphoepithelial thymoma (WHO type B2) shows a large epithelial cell in the center surrounded by small lymphocytes. The large cell in the center of the field shows vesicular nucleus with prominent eosinophilic nucleolus.*

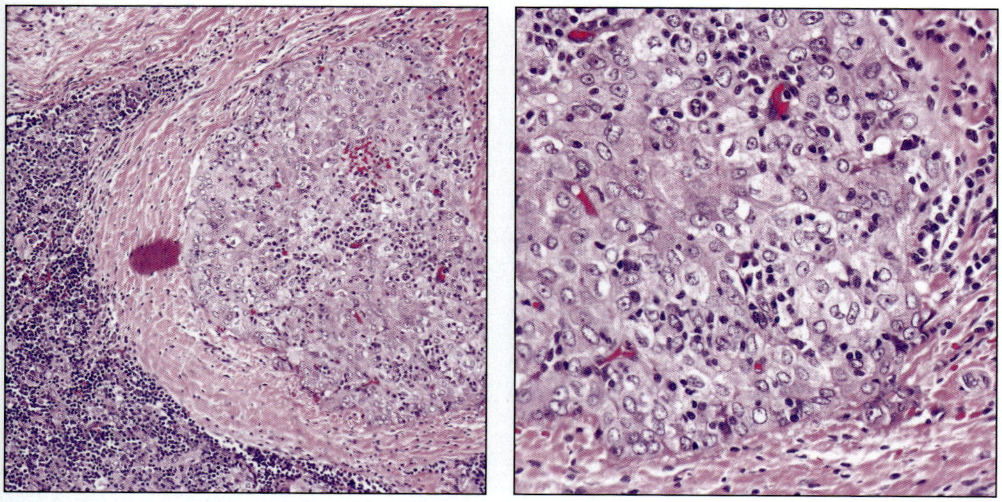

(Left) *Combinations of thymoma WHO type B2 and B3 are seen in approximately 30% of cases. The nodule on the right corresponds to a focus of atypical thymoma (WHO B3). The areas on the left show lymphoepithelial thymoma (WHO type B2) and contain a higher density of small lymphocytes.* ***(Right)*** *Higher magnification from a nodule with atypical thymoma (WHO type B3) in a combined thymoma, type B2 + B3. Notice the large size of the epithelial cells.*

Immunohistochemical Features

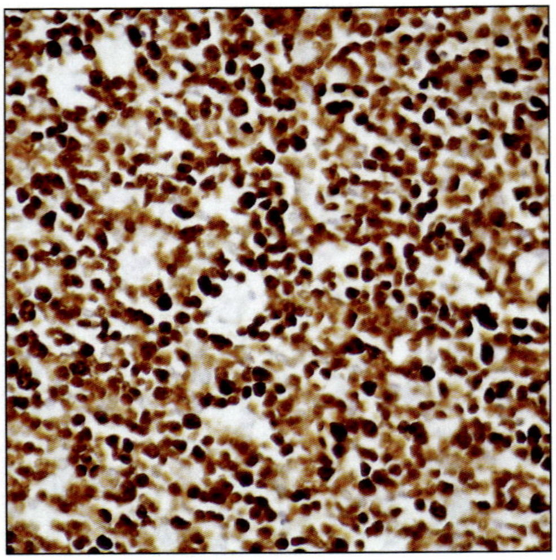
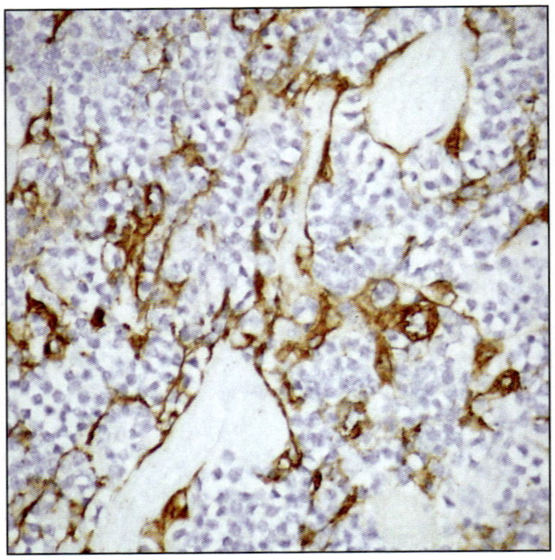

(Left) *Lymphocyte-rich thymoma with "starry sky" appearance simulating lymphoblastic lymphoma shows striking nuclear positivity in small lymphocytes for TdT, not to be confused with lymphoblastic lymphoma.* ***(Right)*** *Immunoperoxidase stain for cytokeratin AE1/AE3 in lymphocyte-rich thymoma simulating lymphoblastic lymphoma shows scattered isolated keratin(+) tumor cells. Identification of keratin(+) cell population is critical for making the correct diagnosis.*

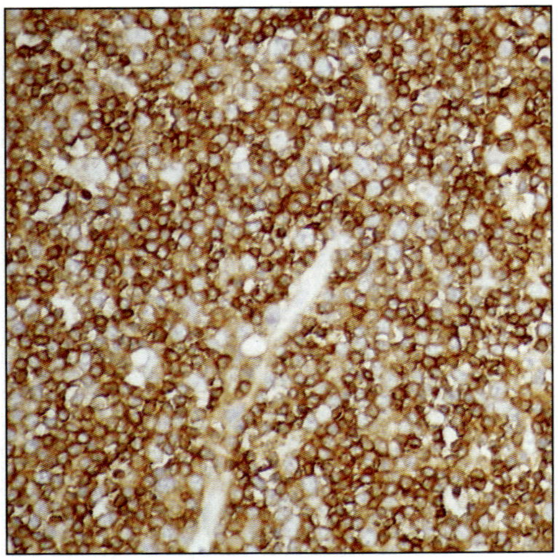
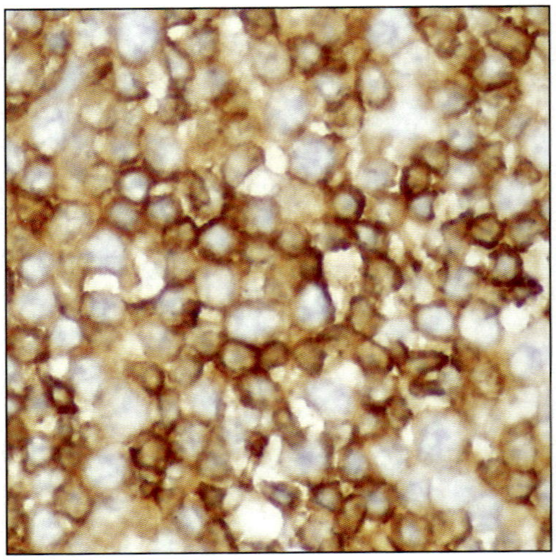

(Left) *Strong membrane positivity for CD3 is observed in this lymphocyte-rich thymoma (WHO type B1). A similar pattern of staining should also be expected for CD1a, a marker of immature T cells.* ***(Right)*** *Positive staining of the tumor cells for CD99 is seen in this lymphocyte-rich thymoma (WHO type B1). CD99 is a marker of T lymphoblasts and can be used in lieu of CD1a or TdT for the demonstration of immature T-lymphoblastic cells in lymphocyte-rich thymomas.*

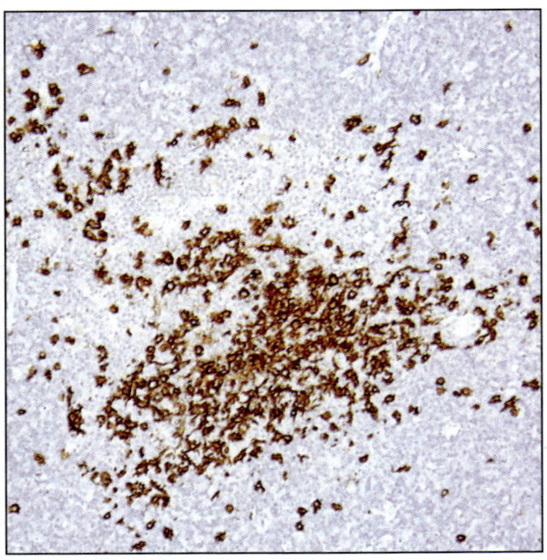
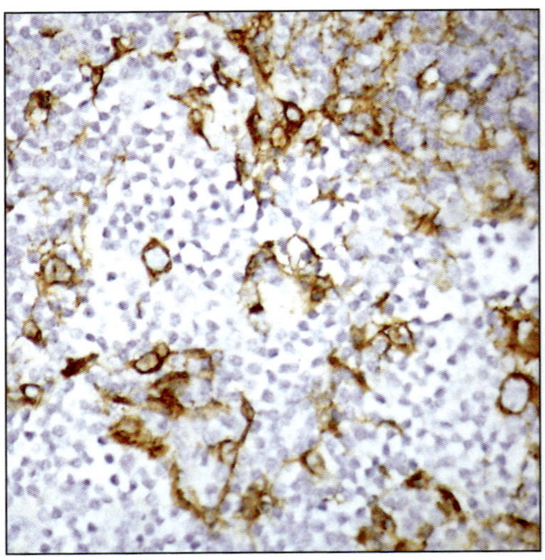

(Left) *Cluster of small lymphocytes is seen to stain with CD20, a B-cell marker. This represents residual islands of the native thymic B-cell lymphoid cell population that can give rise to MALT lymphomas in the thymus.* ***(Right)*** *Lymphocyte-rich thymoma (WHO type B1) shows a network of scattered keratin-positive thymic epithelial cells against a background of small lymphocytes. The distribution of the scattered keratin-positive cells identifies them as the neoplastic epithelial component.*

Microscopic Features

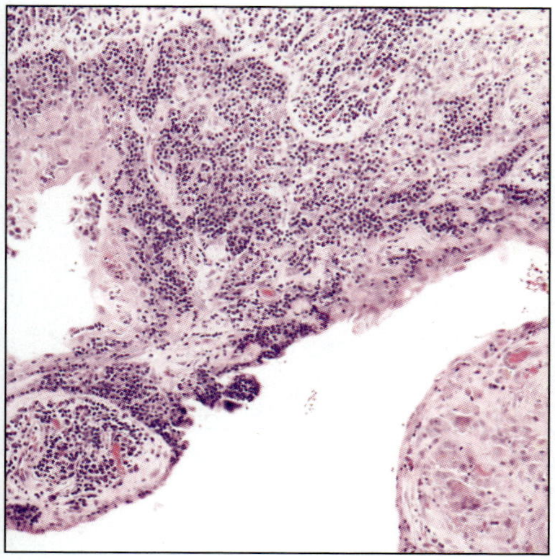

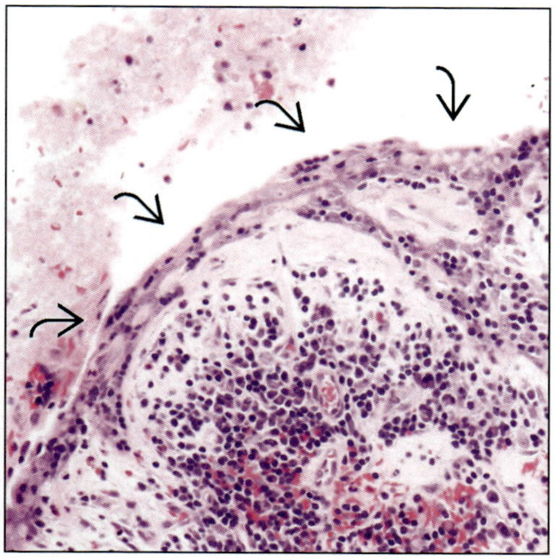

(Left) *Lymphocyte-rich (WHO type B1) thymoma shows secondary multilocular cystic changes in the surrounding, uninvolved residual thymus. The epithelial lining of the cysts is in continuity with dilated Hassall corpuscles and devoid of cytologic atypia.* ***(Right)*** *High power in lymphocyte-rich thymoma shows secondary multilocular thymic cyst-like changes. Notice hemorrhage and inflammation in the wall of the cyst and the flattened squamous epithelial lining.*

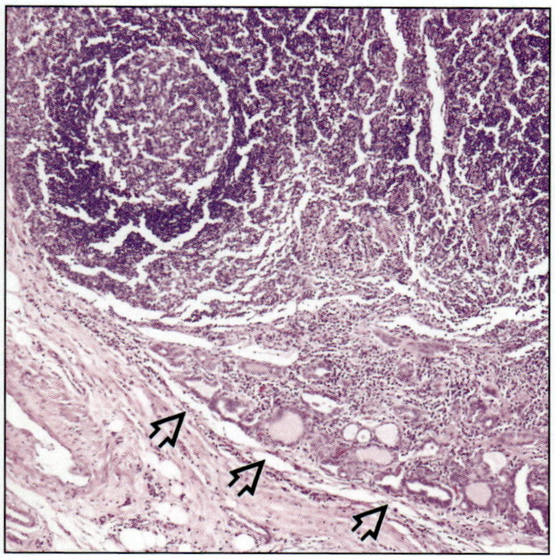

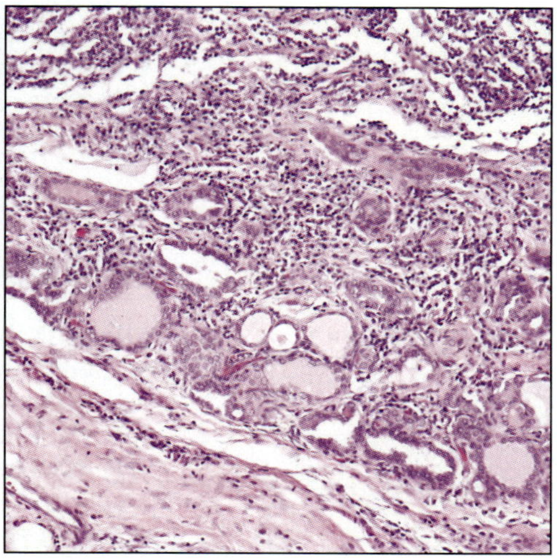

(Left) *Metastasis of spindle cell thymoma to a mediastinal lymph node is seen. Notice the gland-like structures in the lymph node sinus percolating into the node adjacent to a follicle with a germinal center.* ***(Right)*** *High-power view shows lymph node metastasis from spindle cell thymoma (WHO type A) to mediastinal lymph node. Notice solid nests of spindle cells admixed with cyst-like structures within the lymph node sinus.*

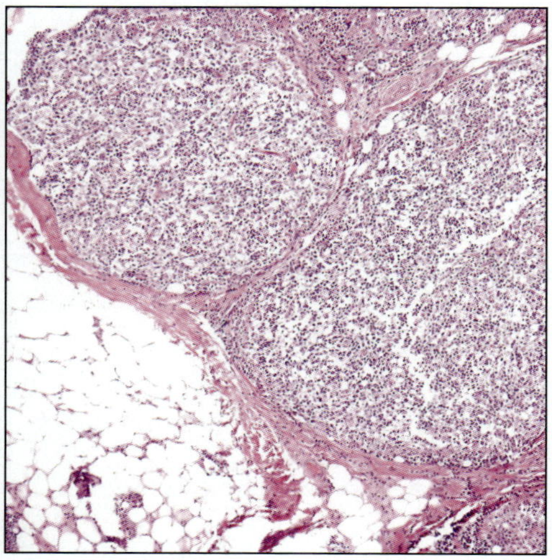

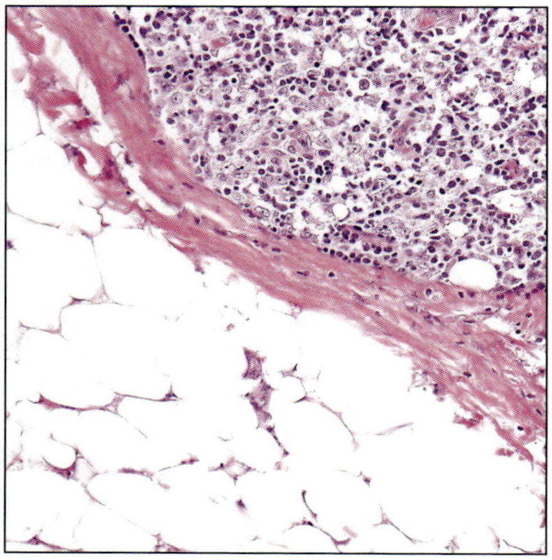

(Left) *Invasion of the capsule into mediastinal fat is noted in this example of mixed lymphoepithelial thymoma (WHO type B2). Notice preservation of the lobular architecture. This focus would be considered as microinvasion (stage IIA) in the modified Masaoka staging by Koga et al. The tumor would be thus classified as "noninvasive" because it does not yet invade neighboring organs.* ***(Right)*** *High-power view shows microinvasive lymphoepithelial thymoma infiltrating perithymic fat.*

ATYPICAL THYMOMA

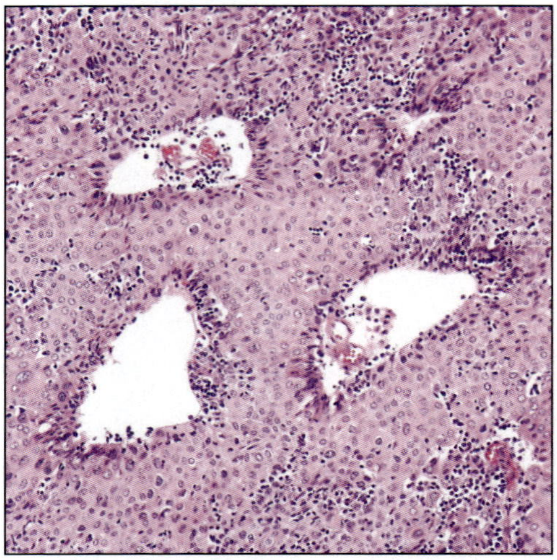

Atypical thymoma (WHO type B3) shows sheets of large, thymic epithelial cells with dilated perivascular spaces and a sprinkling of lymphocytes in the background.

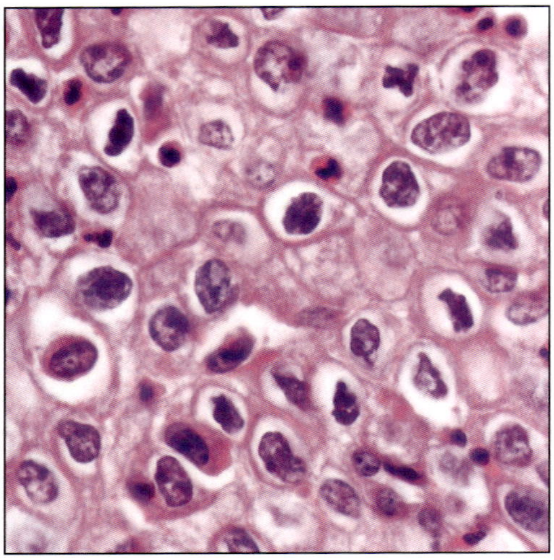

Atypical thymoma (WHO type B3) shows sheets of large, cohesive epithelial cells with enlarged, hyperchromatic nuclei and abundant eosinophilic cytoplasm. Notice sharp cell borders.

TERMINOLOGY

Abbreviations

- Atypical thymoma (AT)

Synonyms

- WHO type B3, polygonal cell thymoma, well-differentiated thymic carcinoma

Definitions

- Moderately differentiated thymic epithelial neoplasm, intermediate between thymoma and thymic carcinoma

CLINICAL ISSUES

Site

- Anterior-superior mediastinum

Presentation

- Cough
- Chest pain
- Dyspnea
- Superior vena cava syndrome
- Frequent association with myasthenia gravis

Treatment

- Surgical excision

Prognosis

- Intermediate between encapsulated thymoma and thymic carcinoma
- Earlier recurrences
- More often invasive at time of presentation

MACROSCOPIC FEATURES

General Features

- Large mass
- Hemorrhage and necrosis are rarely present

Sections to Be Submitted

- 1 section per centimeter of greatest tumor dimension
- Inked margins of resection
- Sections should be taken from periphery of tumor

Size

- Variable; from 3-20 cm

MICROSCOPIC PATHOLOGY

Histologic Features

- Confluent sheets of epithelioid cells with scant lymphocytes
- Prominent perivascular spaces
- Palisading of epithelial tumor cells around perivascular spaces
- Foci of squamous differentiation
- Large epithelioid tumor cells with abundant cytoplasm and sharp cell borders
- Large nuclei with dense chromatin pattern
- "Raisinoid" nuclei with wrinkled nuclear membrane
- Prominent nucleoli
- Scattered mitoses
- Cells may also be spindle or oval, with mild to moderate cytologic atypia
- Cells can show prominent cytoplasmic clearing

DIFFERENTIAL DIAGNOSIS

Well-differentiated Squamous Cell Carcinoma

- Atypical thymoma grows as sheets of uniform tumor cells rather than tumor cell islands
- Squamous cell carcinoma shows more extensive keratinization
- Squamous cell carcinoma does not have dilated perivascular spaces

ATYPICAL THYMOMA

Key Facts

Terminology
- WHO type B3, polygonal cell thymoma, well-differentiated thymic carcinoma
- Moderately differentiated thymic epithelial neoplasm intermediate between thymoma and thymic carcinoma

Microscopic Pathology
- Confluent sheets of epithelioid cells with scant lymphocytes
- Prominent perivascular spaces
- Palisading of epithelial tumor cells around perivascular spaces
- Foci of squamous differentiation
- Large epithelioid tumor cells with abundant cytoplasm and sharp cell borders
- Large nuclei with dense chromatin pattern
- "Raisinoid" nuclei with wrinkled nuclear membrane
- Prominent nucleoli
- Scattered mitoses
- Cells may also be spindle or oval, with mild to moderate cytologic atypia
- Lymphocytes are mainly mature T cells

Top Differential Diagnoses
- Well-differentiated squamous cell carcinoma
- Thymoma, mixed lymphoepithelial (WHO type B2)
- Squamous cell carcinoma of lung origin

Diagnostic Checklist
- Confluent sheets of epithelioid cells with scant lymphocytes
- Perivascular spaces
- Large epithelioid cells with sharp cell borders

Immunohistochemistry

Antibody	Reactivity	Staining Pattern	Comment
CK-PAN	Positive	Cytoplasmic	
p63	Positive	Nuclear	Strongly positive in majority of tumor cells
CD5	Positive	Cytoplasmic	May be positive in a few of the tumor cells
EMA	Positive	Cell membrane & cytoplasm	Focal staining; usually highlights foci of squamous differentiation
CD3	Positive	Cytoplasmic	Stains small lymphocytes
CK5/6	Positive	Cytoplasmic	Positive in tumor cells
CK19	Positive	Cytoplasmic	Positive in tumor cells
Calretinin	Positive	Cytoplasmic	May be positive in a few of the tumor cells
CD1a	Negative	Not applicable	Usually negative in small lymphocytes
CD99	Negative	Not applicable	Usually negative in small lymphocytes

- Lymphocytes in squamous cell carcinoma are B-cell type

Thymoma, Mixed Lymphoepithelial (WHO Type B2)
- B2 thymoma shows more abundant lymphocytes
- Nuclei in B2 thymoma are not as hyperchromatic as in atypical thymoma
- Absence of squamous differentiation in WHO B2 thymoma

Squamous Cell Carcinoma of Lung Origin
- Radiological evidence of lung tumor mass
- Absence of T lymphocytes

DIAGNOSTIC CHECKLIST

Clinically Relevant Pathologic Features
- Extent of invasiveness

Pathologic Interpretation Pearls
- Confluent sheets of epithelioid cells with scant lymphocytes
- Perivascular spaces
- Large epithelioid cells with sharp cell borders

SELECTED REFERENCES

1. Wu M et al: Immunohistochemical detection of p63 and XIAP in thymic hyperplasia and thymomas. Am J Clin Pathol. 131(5):689-93, 2009
2. Suster S et al: Histologic classification of thymoma: the World Health Organization and beyond. Hematol Oncol Clin North Am. 22(3):381-92, 2008
3. Shiraishi J et al: Atypical thymoma (WHO B3) with neuroendocrine differentiation: report of a case. Virchows Arch. 449(2):234-7, 2006
4. Baran JL et al: Atypical thymoma: a report of seven patients. Ann Thorac Surg. 78(2):411-6, 2004
5. Pomplun S et al: Immunohistochemical markers in the differentiation of thymic and pulmonary neoplasms. Histopathology. 40(2):152-8, 2002
6. Kondo K et al: Two cases of repeatedly recurrent atypical thymoma. Chest. 115(1):282-5, 1999
7. Suster S et al: Primary thymic epithelial neoplasms: spectrum of differentiation and histological features. Semin Diagn Pathol. 16(1):2-17, 1999
8. Suster S et al: Thymoma, atypical thymoma, and thymic carcinoma. A novel conceptual approach to the classification of thymic epithelial neoplasms. Am J Clin Pathol. 111(6):826-33, 1999
9. Suster S et al: Thymoma with pseudosarcomatous stroma: report of an unusual histologic variant of thymic epithelial neoplasm that may simulate carcinosarcoma. Am J Surg Pathol. 21(11):1316-23, 1997

ATYPICAL THYMOMA

General Features of Atypical Thymoma

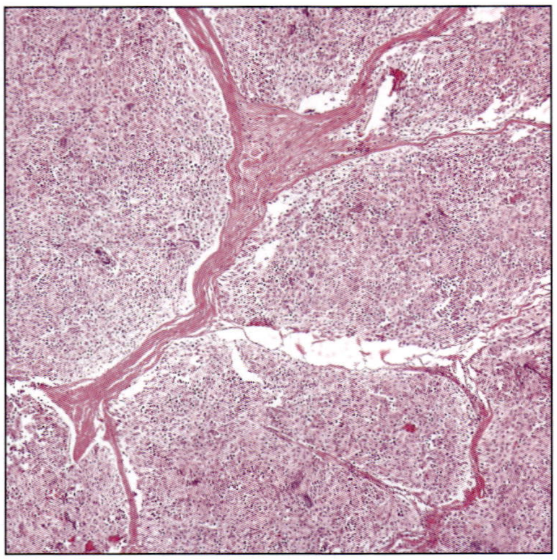

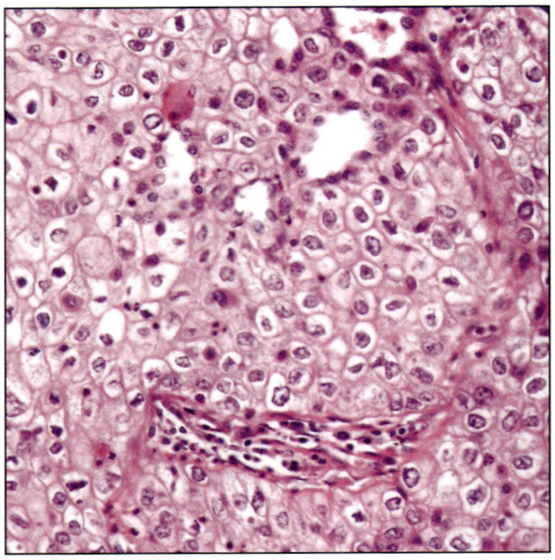

(Left) *Scanning magnification of atypical thymoma (WHO type B3) shows monotonous population of epithelial cells with preservation of lobular architecture and thick fibrous bands separating the tumor cell lobules.* ***(Right)*** *Atypical thymoma (WHO type B3) shows sheets of large, monotonous, round to polygonal epithelial cells with abundant eosinophilic cytoplasm and sharp cell borders. The nuclei of the cells are large, hyperchromatic, and have numerous nuclear irregularities.*

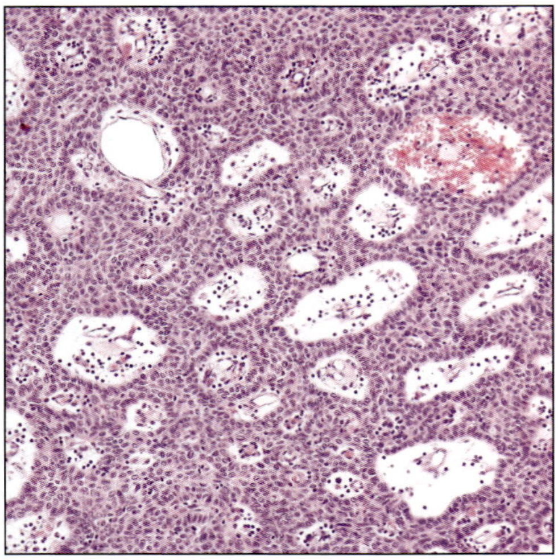

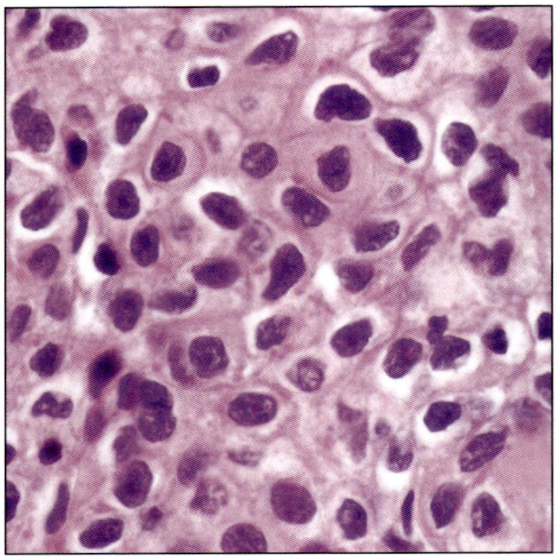

(Left) *Scanning magnification of atypical thymoma (WHO type B3) shows numerous small, dilated perivascular spaces surrounded by a monotonous population of epithelial cells. Notice palisading of epithelial cells around perivascular spaces.* ***(Right)*** *High magnification of atypical thymoma (WHO type B3) shows cells with large, irregular nuclei and dense chromatin pattern. The nuclei are surrounded by an ample rim of eosinophilic cytoplasm and show sharply defined cell borders.*

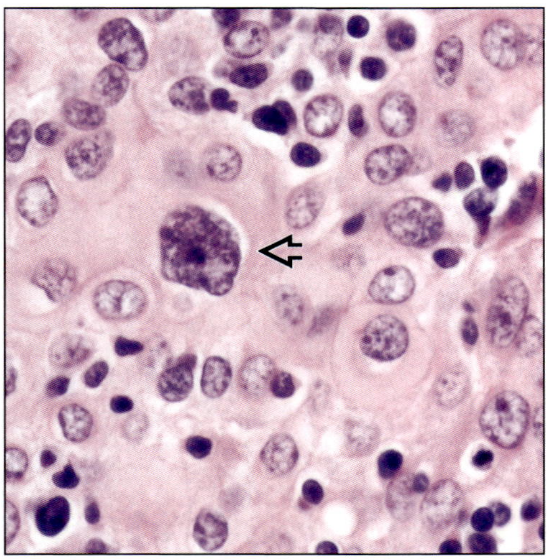

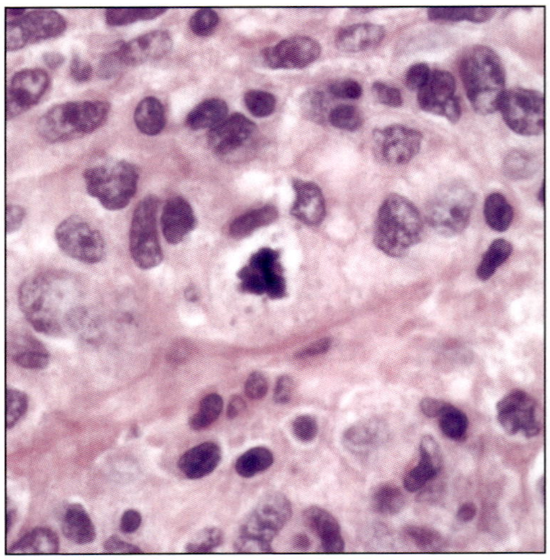

(Left) *High magnification of atypical thymoma (WHO type B3) shows large cells with enlarged nuclei. The cells contain abundant eosinophilic cytoplasm. Notice the large, atypical cell ⇨ with prominent nucleolus and cerebriform nuclear convolutions.* ***(Right)*** *Atypical thymoma (WHO type B3) shows sheets of large epithelioid cells with abundant cytoplasm. The cells show a dense chromatin pattern and eosinophilic nucleoli. Notice the abnormal mitotic figure in the center of the field.*

Nuclear Variation in Atypical Thymoma

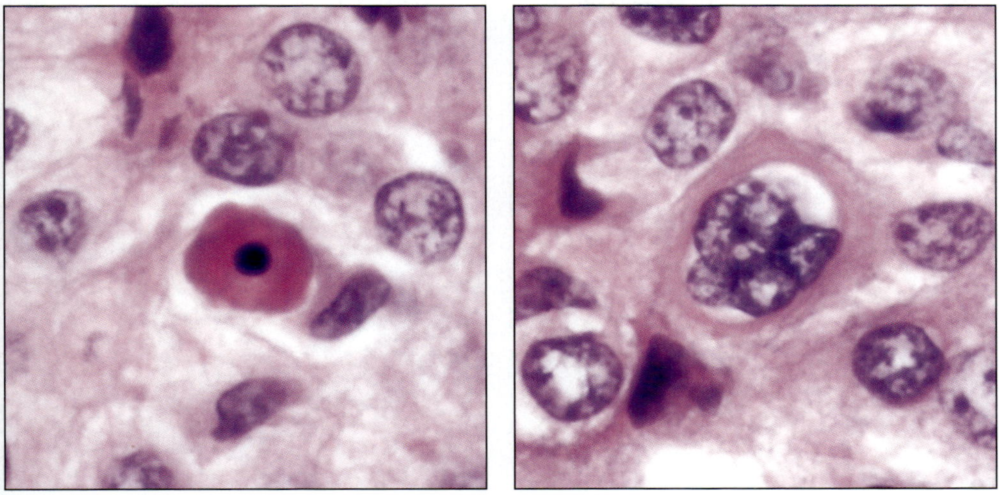

(Left) *Higher magnification of atypical thymoma (WHO type B3) shows round epithelial cells with hyperchromatic nuclei. Notice single-cell keratinization in the center of the field.* ***(Right)*** *High magnification of atypical thymoma (WHO type B3) shows multinucleated cell in the center. The nuclei are large, irregular, hyperchromatic, and overlapping and resemble those of the surrounding mononuclear cells.*

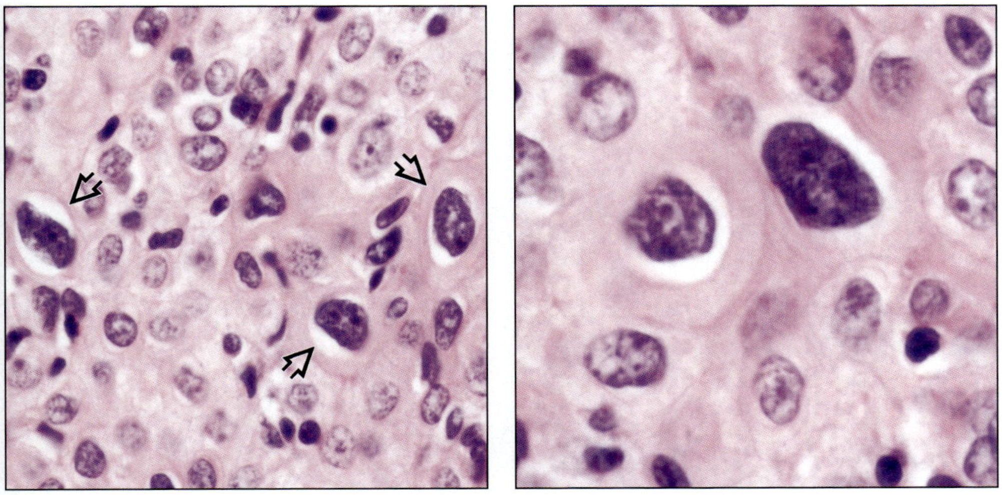

(Left) *Atypical thymoma (WHO type B3) shows numerous large, atypical cells admixed with smaller epithelioid cells. The large cells ➪ show irregular nuclei with dense chromatin pattern, multiple small nucleoli, and irregularities of the nuclear envelope.* ***(Right)*** *Higher magnification of atypical thymoma (WHO type B3) shows large, atypical cells with enlarged, irregular nuclei containing a dense chromatin pattern and multiple, small nucleoli. Notice the clear perinuclear halos.*

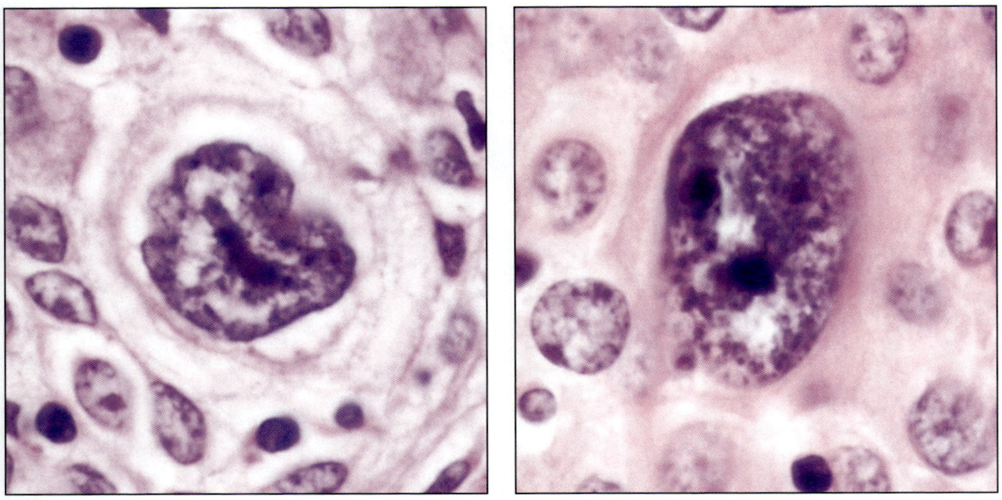

(Left) *High magnification of atypical thymoma (WHO type B3) shows single enlarged nucleus with irregular nuclear contours and single prominent nucleolus.* ***(Right)*** *High magnification of atypical thymoma (WHO type B3) shows a monster cell approximately 4 times the size of the adjoining cells. The large cell shows dense nuclear chromatin and 2 large nucleoli and is surrounded by an ample rim of eosinophilic cytoplasm.*

Atypical Thymoma, Spindle Cell Type

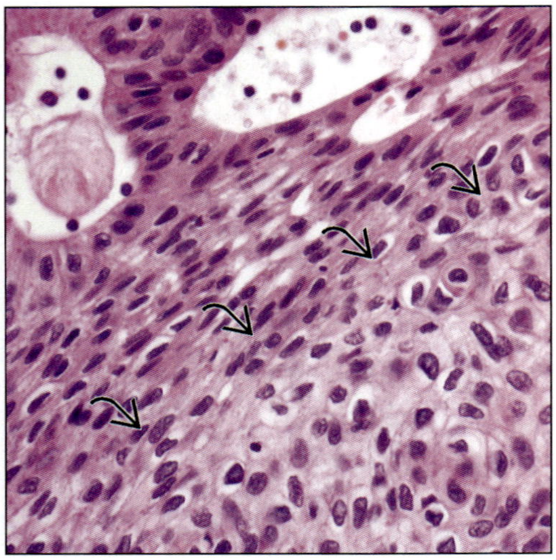

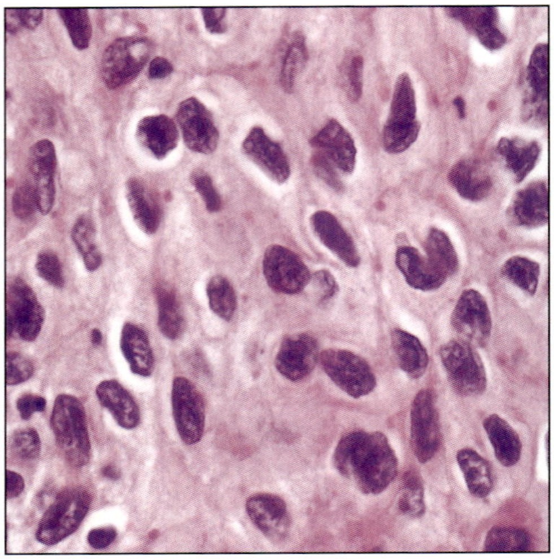

(Left) *Atypical thymoma (WHO type B3) shows transitions between conventional epithelioid areas ➔ and areas showing prominent spindling of the tumor cells (top) beneath 2 small perivascular spaces.* ***(Right)*** *High magnification of atypical thymoma (WHO type B3) shows spindling of the tumor cells. Notice the elongated shape of the cell nuclei and the dense chromatin pattern. Some of the cells contain perinuclear halos and show sharp cell borders.*

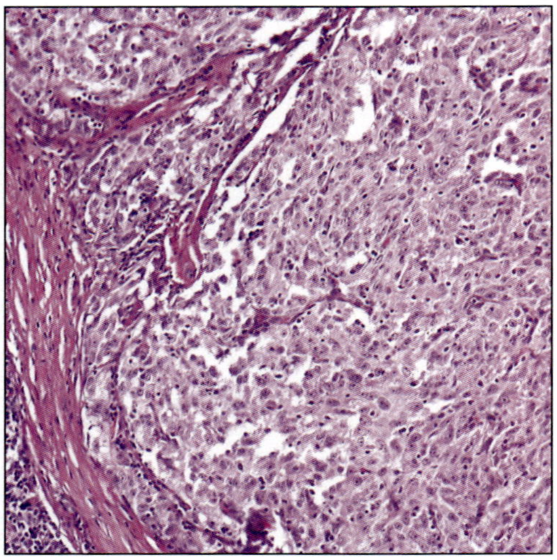

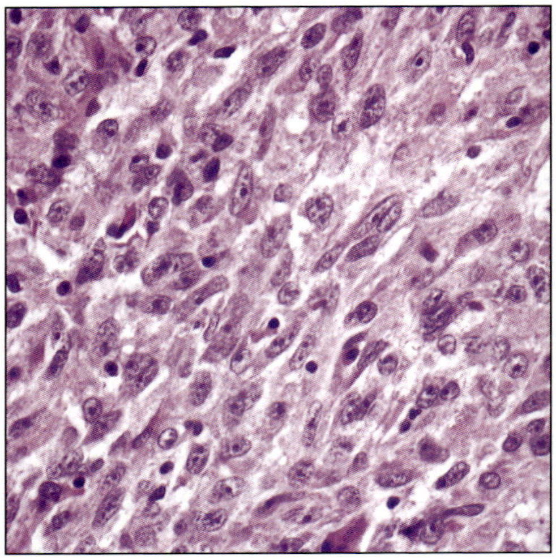

(Left) *Scanning magnification of atypical thymoma (WHO type B3), spindle cell type, shows preserved lobular architecture and sprinkling of small lymphocytes, 2 of the organotypical features of the thymus.* ***(Right)*** *High magnification of atypical thymoma (WHO type B3), spindle cell type, shows relatively uniform population of spindle cells admixed with a few scattered small lymphocytes. The spindle cells display prominent eosinophilic nucleoli.*

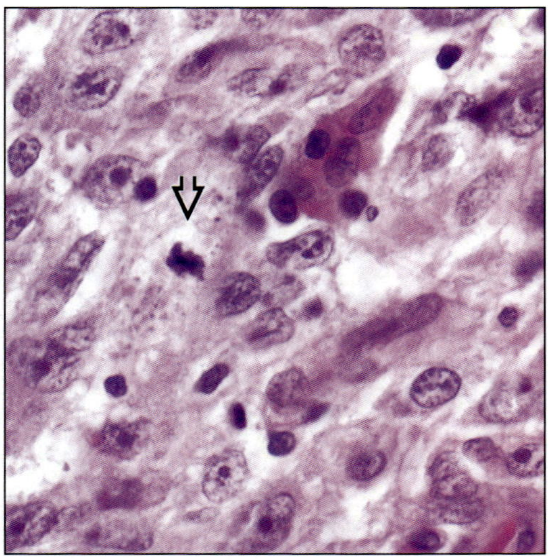

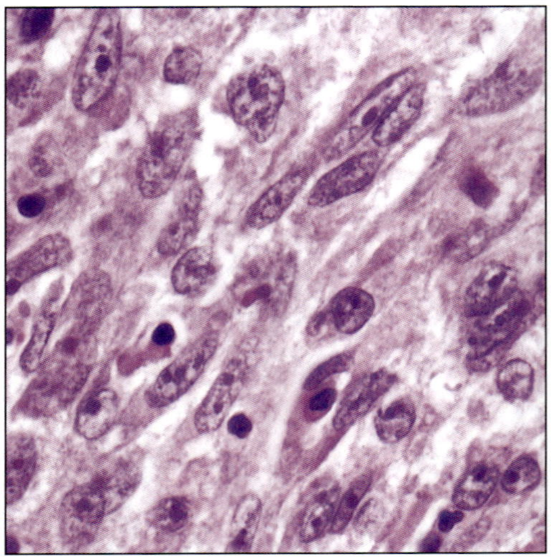

(Left) *High magnification of atypical thymoma (WHO type B3), spindle cell type, shows oval to spindle cells with scattered nuclear chromatin and prominent nucleoli. Notice atypical mitosis toward the center of the field ⇒.* ***(Right)*** *High magnification of atypical thymoma (WHO type B3), spindle cell type, shows population of atypical spindle cells with a few scattered small lymphocytes. The atypical spindle cells show dispersed nuclear chromatin with prominent eosinophilic nucleoli.*

Transitions Between Atypical Thymoma and Other Types

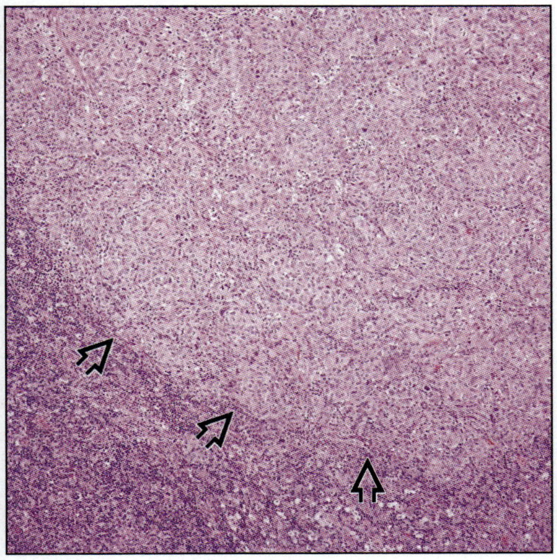

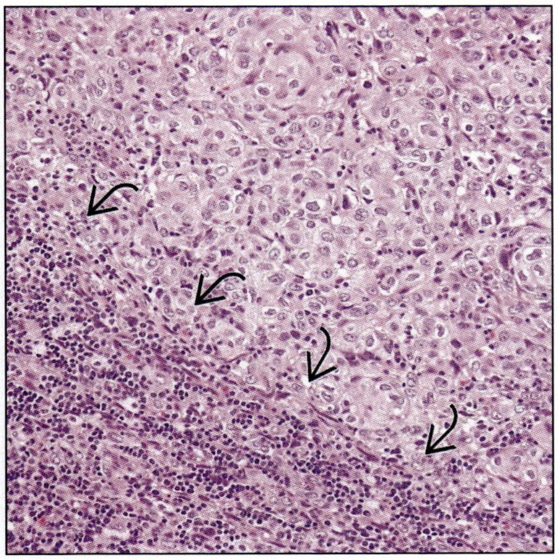

(Left) *Atypical thymoma (WHO type B3) shows transition from adjacent focus of lymphoepithelial thymoma (WHO type B2). Notice the larger cells with fewer lymphocytes in the atypical thymoma component.* ***(Right)*** *High magnification showing interface between atypical thymoma (WHO type B3) (top right) and lymphoepithelial thymoma (WHO type B2) (bottom). Notice the smaller cells with increased number of lymphocytes in the type B2 thymoma component.*

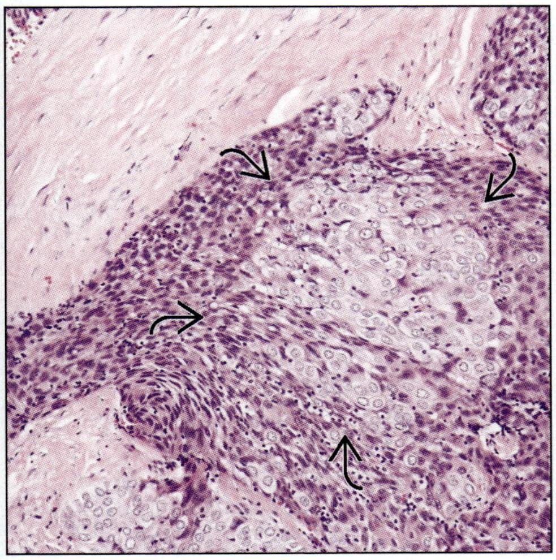

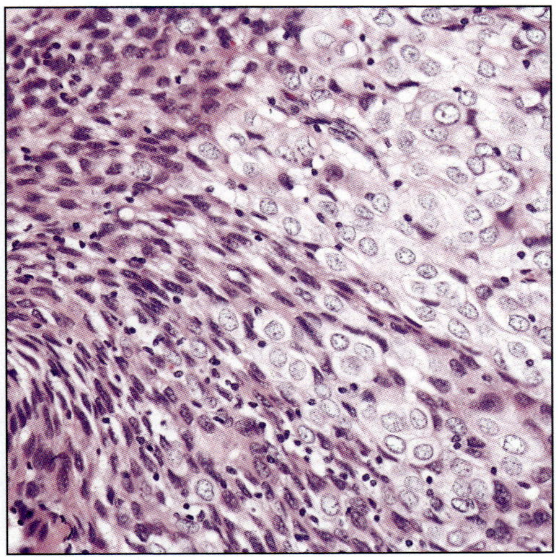

(Left) *Scanning magnification shows transitions between spindle cell thymoma (WHO type A) and atypical thymoma (WHO type B3).* ***(Right)*** *High magnification shows transitions between spindle cell thymoma (WHO type A) (left) and atypical thymoma (WHO type B3) (right). Notice the character of the cells on the right, which are composed of a population of round cells with enlarged nuclei and an abundant rim of pale, lightly eosinophilic cytoplasm.*

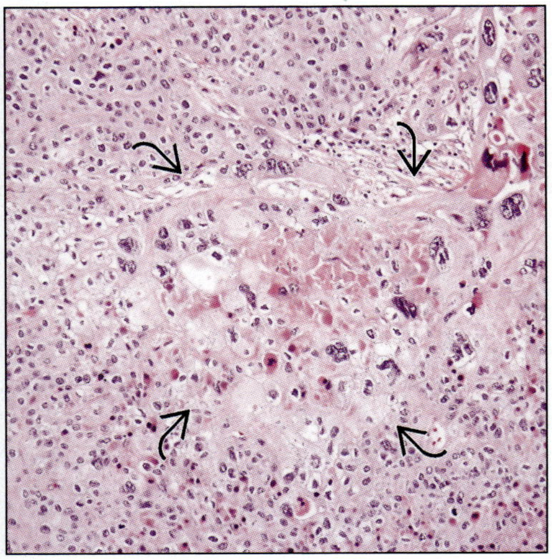

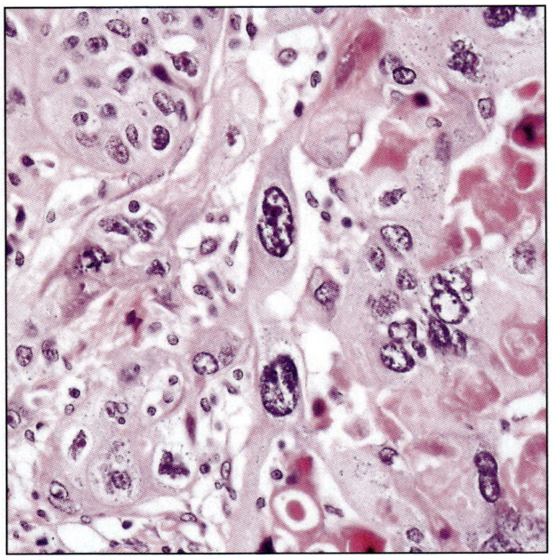

(Left) *Scanning magnification of mediastinal mass shows transitions between atypical thymoma (WHO type B3) and well-differentiated squamous cell carcinoma of the thymus.* ***(Right)*** *High magnification of mediastinal tumor shows transitions between atypical thymoma (left) and well-differentiated squamous cell carcinoma (right). Notice striking nuclear pleomorphism, abnormal mitosis, and abundant single cell keratinization in the squamous cell carcinoma component.*

ATYPICAL THYMOMA

Squamous Foci in Atypical Thymoma

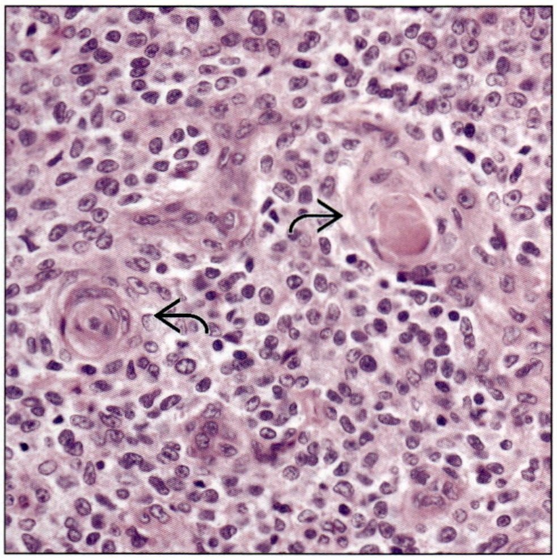
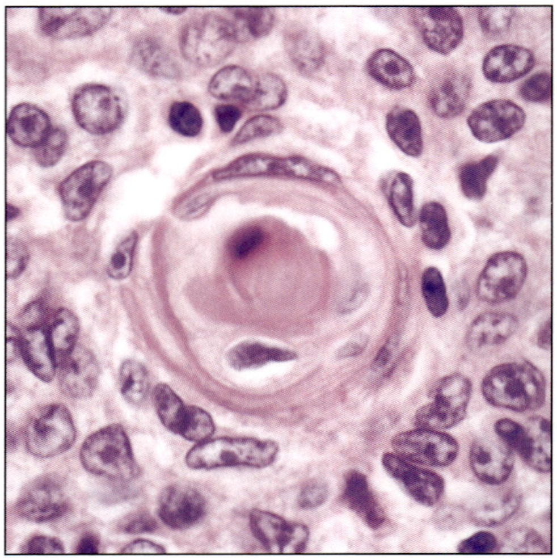

(Left) *Atypical thymoma (WHO type B3) shows foci of squamous differentiation* →. *The small foci of keratinization show concentric arrangement of squamoid cells.* ***(Right)*** *High magnification of focus of keratinization in atypical thymoma (WHO type B3) shows concentric layering of squamoid cells with a small focus of central keratinization. The cells surrounding this focus show enlarged nuclei with prominent nucleoli.*

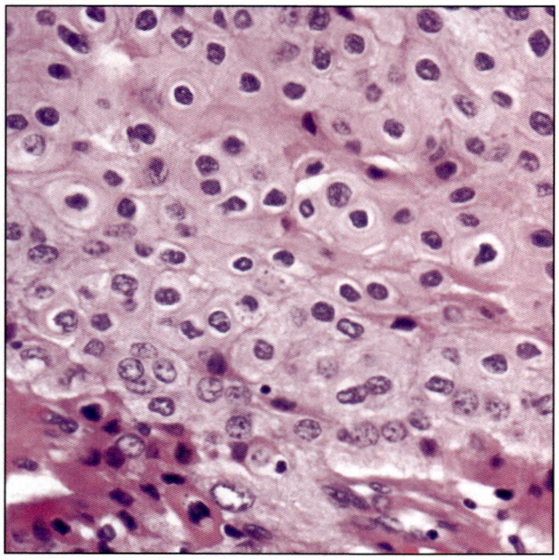
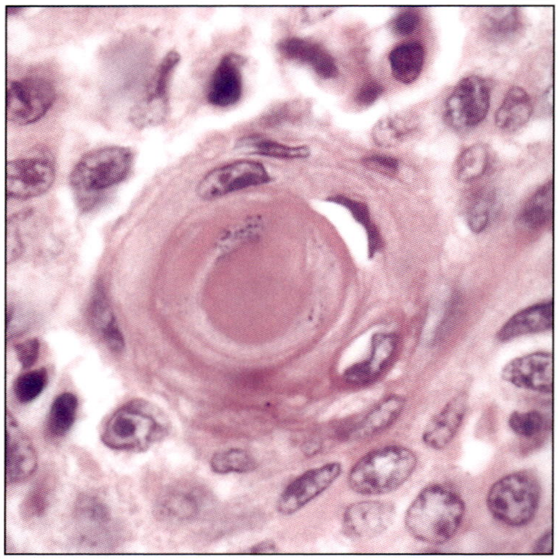

(Left) *Atypical thymoma (WHO type B3) shows striking epidermoid appearance of the tumor cells, with large, epithelioid cells and abundant cytoplasm displaying a pavement-like architecture with sharp cell membranes.* ***(Right)*** *Focus of keratinization in atypical thymoma (WHO type B3) shows concentric layering of epidermoid cells with central focus of keratinization and keratin pearl formation.*

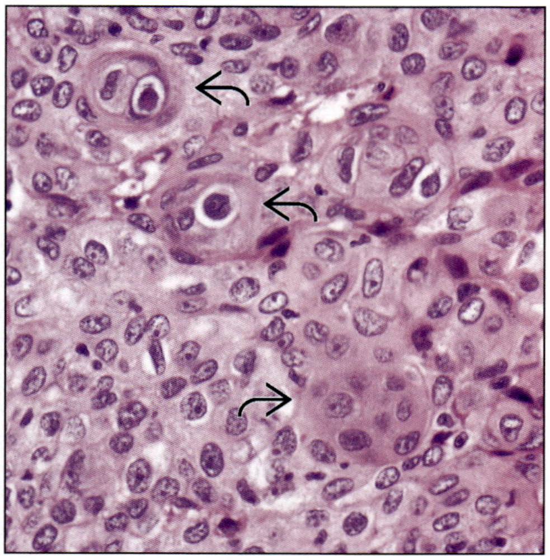
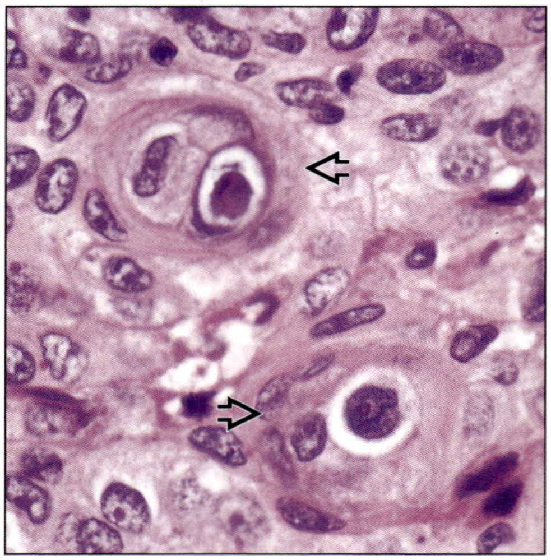

(Left) *Multiple foci of keratinization in atypical thymoma (WHO type B3) show small clusters of tumor cells displaying concentric arrangement of epithelial cells* → *admixed with sheets of epithelioid cells.* ***(Right)*** *High magnification of atypical thymoma (WHO type B3) shows concentric arrangement of squamoid cells displaying enlarged nuclei with prominent nucleoli and surrounded by an ample rim of eosinophilic cytoplasm* ⇨.

Clear Cell Features in Atypical Thymoma

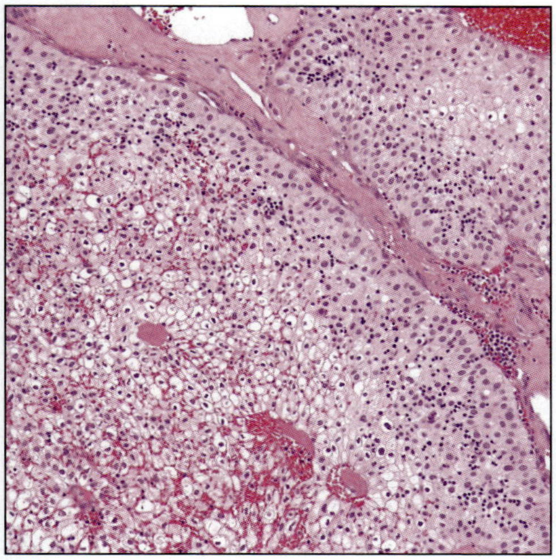
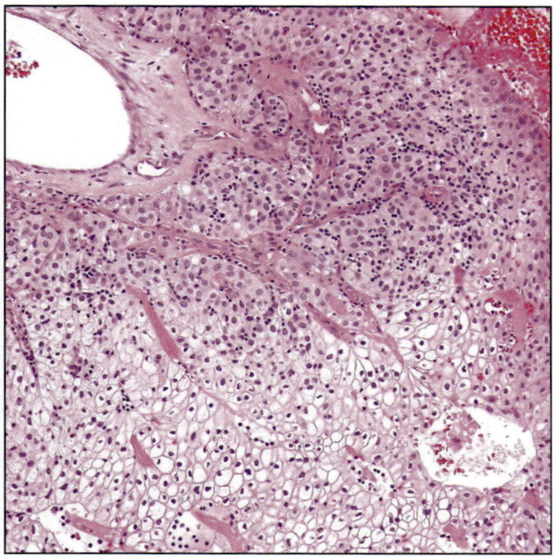

(Left) *Scanning magnification of atypical thymoma (WHO type B3) shows tumor lobules separated by broad bands of connective tissue and displaying prominent clearing of the cytoplasm of the tumor cells.* ***(Right)*** *High magnification of atypical thymoma (WHO type B3) shows conventional areas (top) of monotonous epithelioid cells with abundant eosinophilic cytoplasm merging with areas in which the tumor cells display prominent cytoplasmic clearing (bottom).*

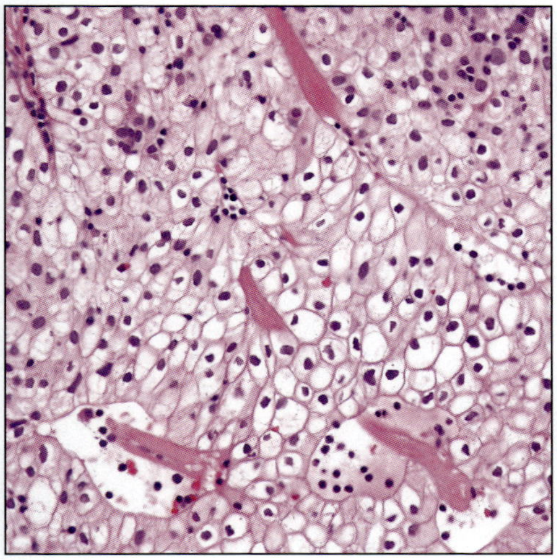
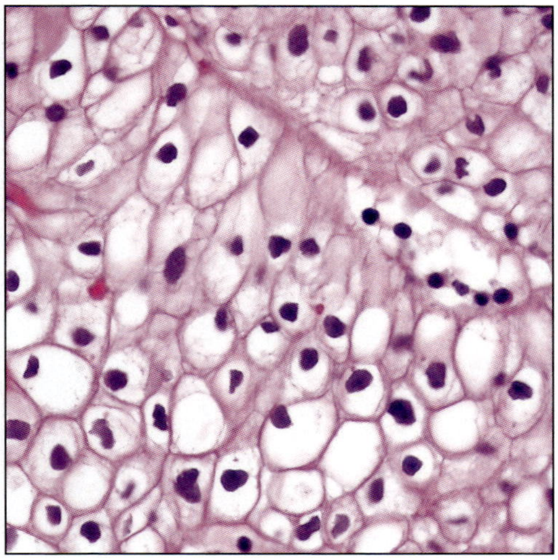

(Left) *Atypical thymoma (WHO type B3) shows sheets of monotonous tumor cells with prominent clearing of the cytoplasm imparting the tissue with a "plant-like" appearance.* ***(Right)*** *High magnification of atypical thymoma (WHO type B3) shows cells with hyperchromatic nuclei with irregular ("raisinoid") nuclear contours and abundant, optically clear cytoplasm bounded by a thick eosinophilic cell membrane.*

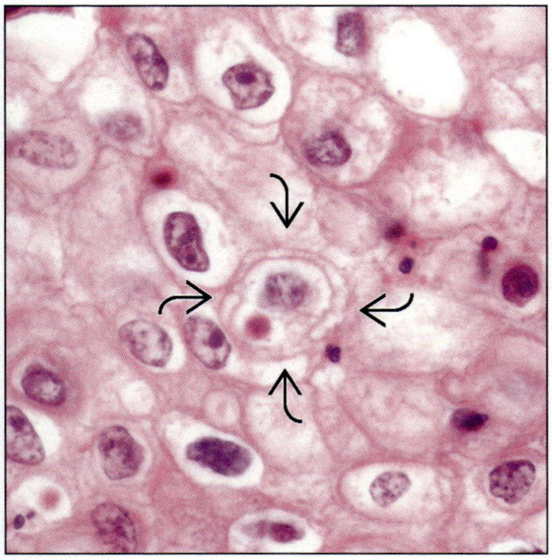
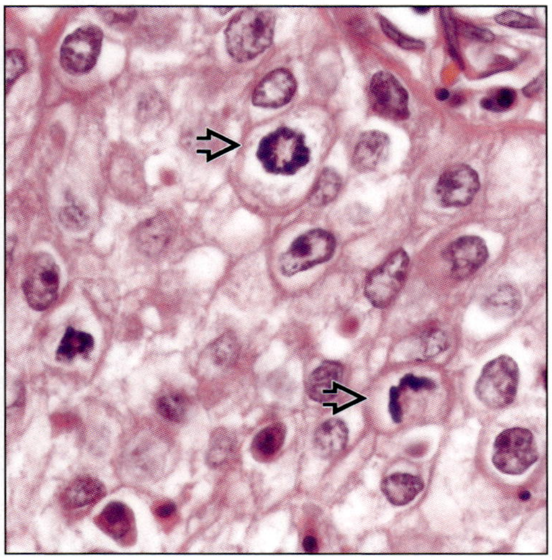

(Left) *Atypical thymoma (WHO type B3) shows prominent clearing of the cytoplasm of the tumor cells. The cell in the center* ➔ *shows a hint of intercellular bridges. Notice the raisin-like appearance of the nuclei in the surrounding cells due to irregularities of the nuclear envelope.* ***(Right)*** *High magnification shows atypical thymoma (WHO type B3) with clearing of the cytoplasm. Notice 2 cells in mitosis* ➔ *and the presence of sharp cytoplasmic cell borders.*

ATYPICAL THYMOMA

Invasive Properties

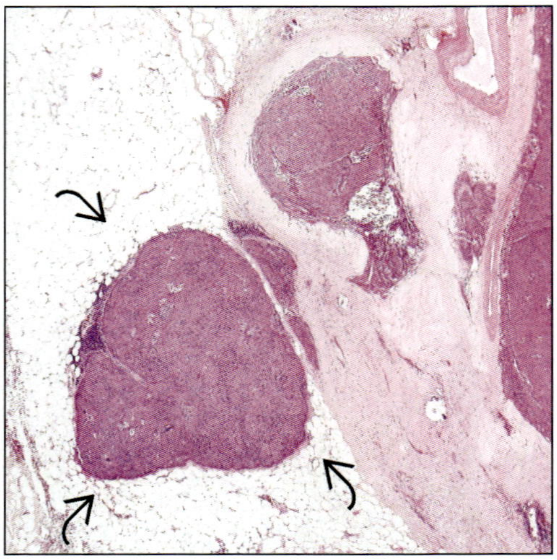

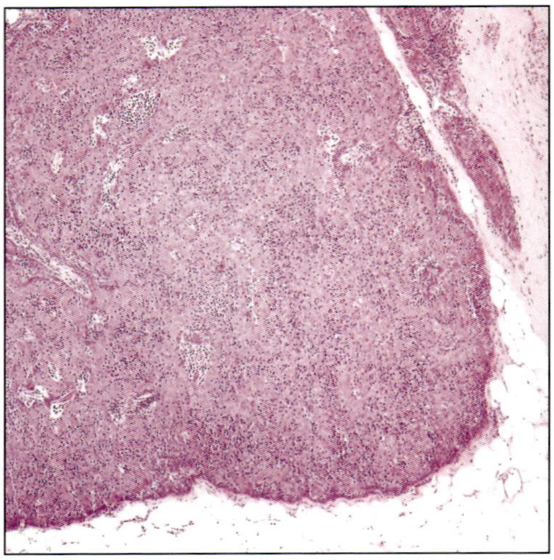

(Left) *Scanning magnification of atypical thymoma (WHO type B3) shows infiltration of the capsule and of mediastinal fat by tumor ➔.* ***(Right)*** *High magnification of invasive atypical thymoma (WHO type B3) shows lobule of tumor cells penetrating into the mediastinal fat. The invasive focus retains the features of the original tumor and shows sheets of monotonous epithelial cells with a sprinkling of small immature lymphocytes.*

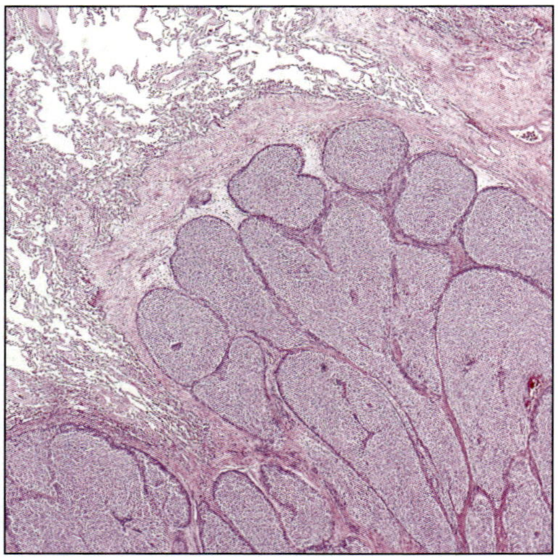

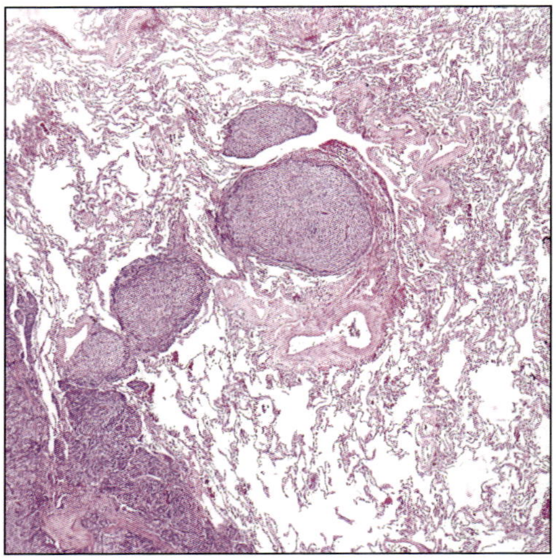

(Left) *Invasive atypical thymoma (WHO type B3) shows small lobules of tumor cells infiltrating the pleural surface and pushing into lung parenchyma.* ***(Right)*** *Infiltration of lung parenchyma by atypical thymoma (WHO type B3) shows small tumor cell islands lying within lung parenchyma. Notice the preservation of the lobular architecture in the tumor cell islands with infiltration and displacement of surrounding air spaces.*

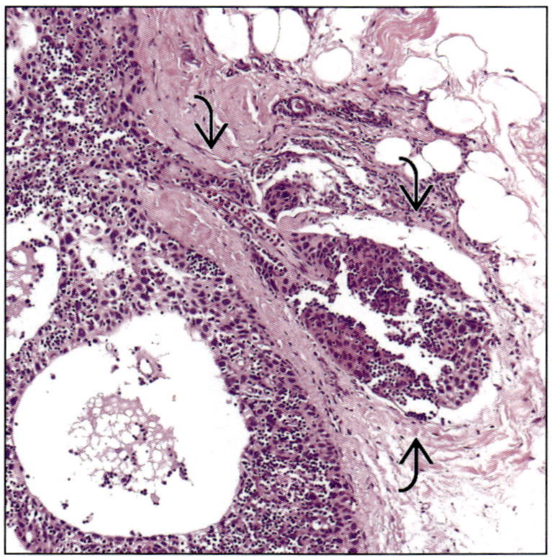

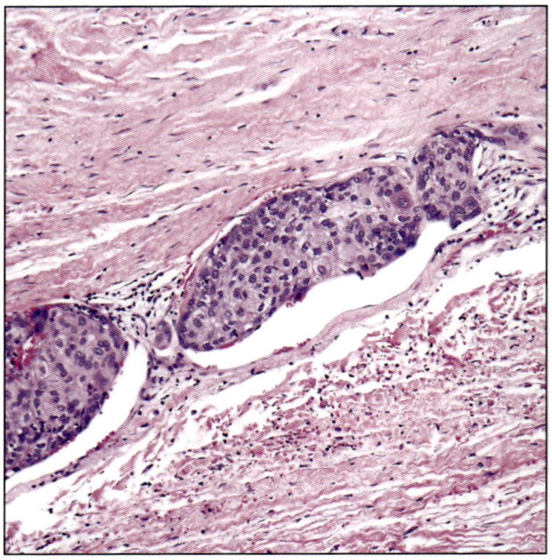

(Left) *Atypical thymoma (WHO type B3) shows through-and-through infiltration of the fibrous capsule by tumor into the adjacent mediastinal fat ➔.* ***(Right)*** *Vascular invasion in atypical thymoma (WHO type B3) is characterized by multiple tumor emboli within the lumen of small vessels. The tumor emboli are composed of large epithelioid cells with abundant cytoplasm that are partially attached to the vessel walls.*

Immunohistochemical Features

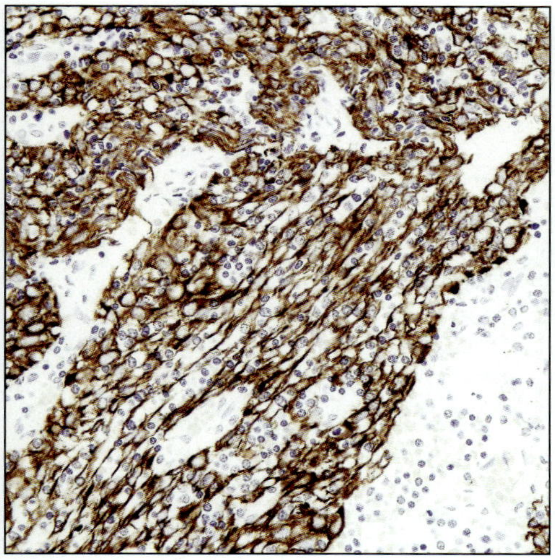
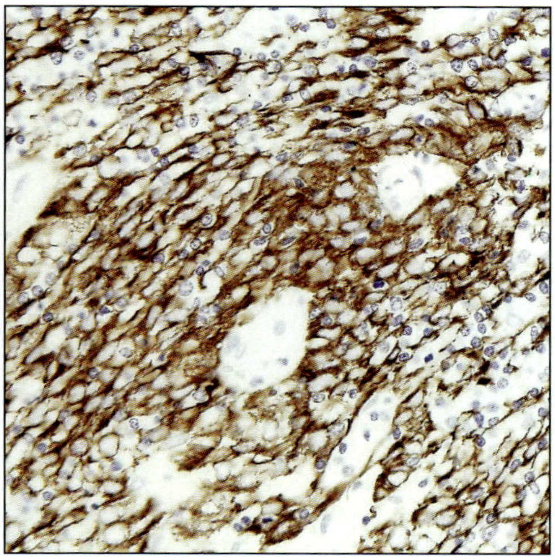

(Left) *Atypical thymoma (WHO type B3) shows strong cytoplasmic positivity in the majority of the tumor cells with cytokeratin AE1/AE3 antibody.* ***(Right)*** *Atypical thymoma (WHO type B3) shows strong positivity of the tumor cells with antibodies against CK19. CK19 intensely stains the majority of primary thymic epithelial neoplasms, including atypical thymoma.*

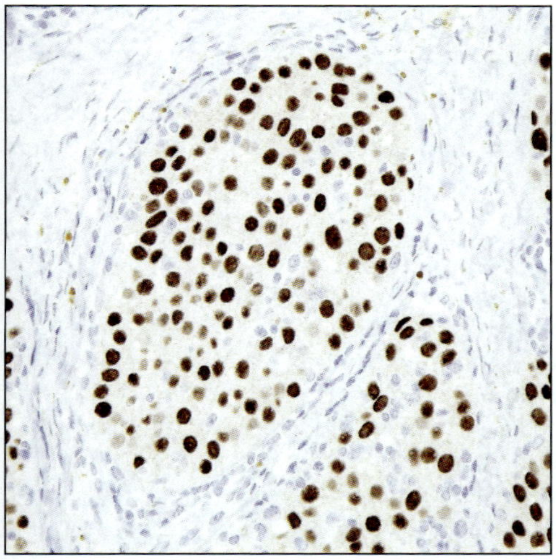
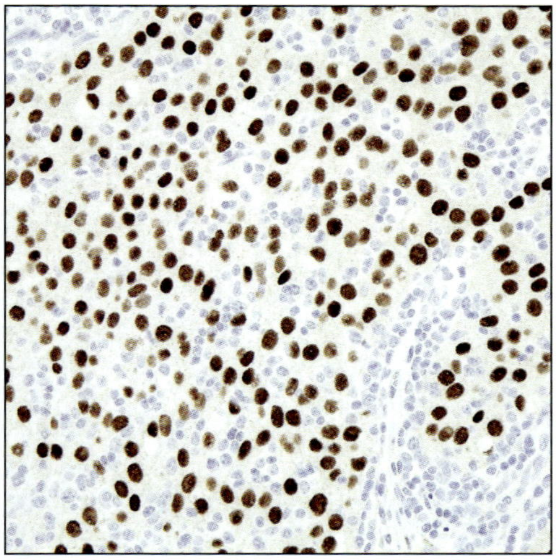

(Left) *Immunohistochemical staining of atypical thymoma (WHO type B3) with p63 shows strong positive nuclear staining of the tumor cells.* ***(Right)*** *Immunohistochemical staining of atypical thymoma (WHO type B3) with the proliferation marker Ki-67 shows strong nuclear staining in a large number of the tumor cells. Proliferative activity is often increased in atypical thymoma.*

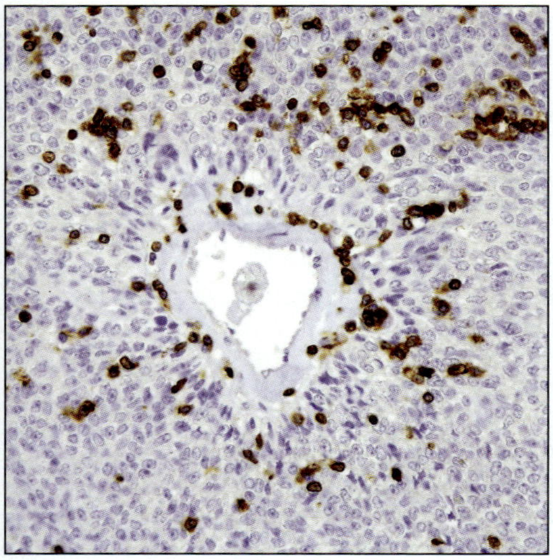
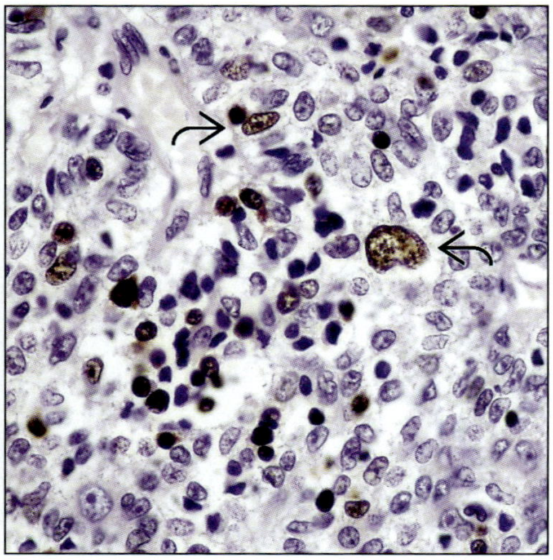

(Left) *Immunohistochemical staining of atypical thymoma (WHO type B3) with CD1a shows a few scattered positive small lymphocytes.* ***(Right)*** *Immunohistochemical staining of atypical thymoma (WHO type B3) with CD5 shows a few positive small lymphocytes, as well as a few positive epithelial cells ⮫. The cells in atypical thymoma can also react with CD5. This marker is therefore not helpful in separating this tumor from thymic carcinoma.*

THYMIC CARCINOMA

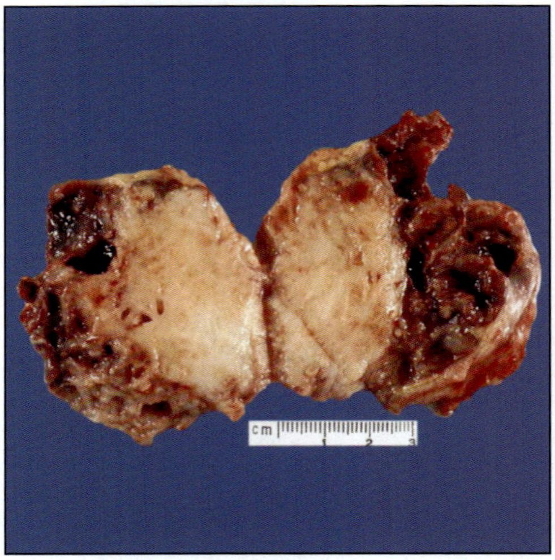

Gross appearance of squamous cell carcinoma of the thymus shows solid tumor surrounded by areas of hemorrhage, necrosis, and cystic degeneration.

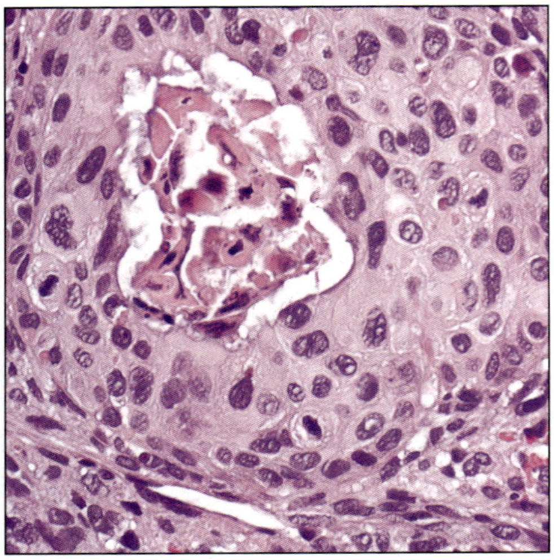

High magnification of thymic squamous cell carcinoma shows well-differentiated focus of keratinization surrounded by large atypical cells with sharp cell borders and occasional intercellular bridges.

TERMINOLOGY

Abbreviations

- Thymic carcinoma (TC)

Synonyms

- Malignant thymoma type II
- WHO type C thymoma
- Poorly differentiated (high-grade) thymic epithelial neoplasm

Definitions

- Primary thymic epithelial neoplasm showing overt cytologic features of malignancy with loss of organotypical features of thymic differentiation

ETIOLOGY/PATHOGENESIS

Pathogenesis

- Unknown
- Some cases may arise from malignant degeneration of preexisting thymoma

CLINICAL ISSUES

Epidemiology

- Incidence
  - Extremely rare neoplasm; accounts for less than 1% of thymic tumors
- Age
  - Affects all age groups but is most frequent between 30-60 years of age
- Gender
  - Slight male predilection (M:F = 1.5:1)

Presentation

- Incidental finding in small subset of cases
- Anorexia
- Weight loss
- Chest pain
- Shortness of breath
- Paraneoplastic syndromes are not seen

Natural History

- Highly aggressive neoplasm; generally refractory to treatment

Treatment

- Options, risks, complications
  - Treatment related to grade and stage
- Surgical approaches
  - Surgical resection may be curative for low-grade, encapsulated lesions
  - Surgical excision may be indicated in larger tumors for debulking or palliation of symptoms
- Adjuvant therapy
  - Radiation and chemotherapy are used in high-grade or high-stage tumors

Prognosis

- Generally poor prognosis.
- High-grade tumors have median survival of 18 months
- Usual sites of metastases include lymph nodes, bone, lung, pleura, liver, and brain

IMAGE FINDINGS

General Features

- Lobulated, marginated, anterior mediastinal mass

Radiographic Findings

- Calcification in 10-40% of cases
- Obscuring of mediastinal fat plane
- Extension to pericardium and pleura
- Extrathymic metastases often present
- Invasion into great vessels and mediastinal structures seen in about 40% of cases

CT Findings

- Best imaging tool for thymic carcinoma

THYMIC CARCINOMA

Key Facts

Clinical Issues
- Generally poor prognosis
- High-grade tumors have median survival of 18 months
- Usual sites of metastases include lymph nodes, bone, lung, pleura, liver, and brain

Macroscopic Features
- Commonly contain areas of hemorrhage and necrosis
- Usually invasive, unencapsulated, and poorly circumscribed
- Cystic degeneration can be seen in some subtypes (basaloid, mucoepidermoid)

Microscopic Pathology
- Closely resembles other types of carcinoma
  - Well-differentiated squamous cell carcinoma of thymus
  - Basaloid carcinoma
  - Mucoepidermoid carcinoma
  - Poorly differentiated, nonkeratinizing (lymphoepithelioma-like) carcinoma
  - Adenocarcinoma of thymus
  - Papillary carcinoma
  - Clear cell carcinoma
  - Spindle cell (sarcomatoid) carcinoma
  - Carcinosarcoma
  - Anaplastic carcinoma

Top Differential Diagnoses
- Atypical thymoma (WHO type B3)
- Metastatic carcinoma of lung
- Metastatic carcinoma from other organs

- Usually heterogeneous enhancement with areas of necrosis
- Unenhanced images for screening purposes followed by contrast-enhanced scans

MACROSCOPIC FEATURES

General Features
- Commonly contain areas of hemorrhage and necrosis
- Usually invasive, unencapsulated, and poorly circumscribed
- Cystic degeneration can be seen in some subtypes (basaloid, mucoepidermoid)

Sections to Be Submitted
- Sections should include tumor with capsule (1 per cm of greatest diameter) as well as infiltrating margins and any included lymph nodes or surrounding structures

MICROSCOPIC PATHOLOGY

Histologic Features
- **Well-differentiated squamous cell carcinoma of thymus**
  - Identical histologic features to squamous cell carcinoma arising at other locations
  - Must 1st rule out metastasis from other organ or occult primary site
  - Stage-by-stage has better prognosis than squamous cell carcinoma of lung with massive mediastinal compromise
- **Basaloid carcinoma**
  - Small hyperchromatic round to oval tumor cells with prominent peripheral palisading of nuclei
  - Often associated with cystic changes; tumor cells can be tracked to lining of cysts
  - Usually associated with low-grade behavior but can also metastasize distantly
- **Mucoepidermoid carcinoma**
  - Admixture of squamous, intermediate, and mucinous cells with cribriform cystic spaces filled with mucin
  - Mucinous cysts and individual mucocytes are highlighted by mucicarmine stains
  - Frequently associated with cystic changes of thymus
  - Most cases are well differentiated; however, moderate and poorly differentiated variants also exist and are associated with more aggressive behavior
- **Poorly differentiated, nonkeratinizing (lymphoepithelioma-like) carcinoma**
  - Most frequent type of thymic carcinoma in Western patients
  - Poorly differentiated tumor cells with large hyperchromatic nuclei with prominent eosinophilic nucleoli and frequent mitotic figures; resembles poorly differentiated carcinoma (lymphoepithelioma) of nasopharynx
  - Large tumor cell islands characterized by central comedo-like areas of necrosis
  - Some cases are characterized by dense lymphoplasmacellular stromal infiltrates; others are devoid of lymphoid stroma
  - Can often show admixtures with areas of spindle cell thymoma (WHO type A)
  - Some cases in children and adolescents may be associated with Epstein-Barr virus
- **Adenosquamous carcinoma**
  - Biphasic glandular and squamous components
  - High-grade tumor usually associated with poor prognosis
  - May harbor "myoid" cell component ("rhabdomyomatous carcinoma of thymus")
- **Adenocarcinoma of thymus**
  - Very rare variant (few cases reported)
  - May be of mucinous and nonmucinous type; mucinous variant resembles "colloid carcinoma" in other organs
  - Metastasis from distant or occult primary must be stringently ruled out before making this diagnosis
- **Papillary carcinoma**

THYMIC CARCINOMA

- Very rare type; very few cases reported in literature
- Often associated with areas of spindle cell thymoma (WHO type A)
- Papillary areas may display very low-grade cytologic features
- **Clear cell carcinoma**
  - Characterized by large cells with abundant clear cytoplasm
  - Can display very aggressive behavior
  - Most cases represent secondary clear cell changes in squamous cell carcinoma
  - Care must be taken to exclude metastasis from clear cell carcinoma of lung, kidney, adrenal, or other organs
- **Spindle cell (sarcomatoid) carcinoma**
  - Composed of highly atypical spindle epithelial cells with high nuclear grade and brisk mitotic activity
  - Majority are seen in association with preexisting areas of spindle cell thymoma (WHO type A)
  - Aggressive behavior with frequent distant metastases
- **Carcinosarcoma**
  - True mixed tumor with both malignant epithelial (carcinomatous) component and malignant sarcomatous component
  - Most frequent sarcomatous component is rhabdomyosarcoma; most frequent carcinomatous component is poorly differentiated adenocarcinoma
  - Highly aggressive tumor with high mortality
- **Anaplastic carcinoma**
  - Bizarre tumor cells with marked nuclear atypia and abnormal mitotic figures
  - Diagnosis of exclusion: Needs demonstration of epithelial lineage of tumor cells by either immunohistochemistry or electron microscopy
  - Rare foci of differentiated squamous carcinoma or adenocarcinoma can be occasionally identified
  - Highly aggressive behavior
- **Neuroendocrine carcinoma**
  - Well, moderately, or poorly differentiated types
- **Other rare types of thymic carcinoma**
  - Rhabdoid carcinoma of thymus: Characterized by eccentric globular eosinophilic cytoplasmic inclusions
  - Hepatoid carcinoma of thymus: Tumor cells resemble hepatocytes
  - Desmoplastic carcinoma of thymus: Characterized by prominent desmoplastic stroma entrapping squamoid elements

Predominant Cell/Compartment Type

- Epithelial

Grade

- Low-grade and high-grade types, depending on degree of cytologic atypia, mitotic activity, and amount of necrosis

ANCILLARY TESTS

Cytology

- As screening tool to confirm presence of malignant cells

Frozen Sections

- To confirm presence of cytologic atypia, mitotic activity, and necrosis; not for definitive diagnosis

Cytogenetics

- Several nonrecurrent chromosomal losses and gains have been reported but are not useful for diagnosis or prognosis

DIFFERENTIAL DIAGNOSIS

Atypical Thymoma (WHO Type B3)

- May be difficult to distinguish from low-grade, well-differentiated squamous cell carcinoma of thymus
  - Should not show marked cytologic atypia or overt features of malignancy
  - Contains perivascular spaces and immature T lymphocytes
  - Usually lacks vascular invasion and necrosis

Metastatic Carcinoma of Lung

- Well-differentiated squamous cell carcinoma of lung can metastasize massively to mediastinal lymph nodes
- Bronchoscopy with bilateral bronchial brushings and washings are necessary to rule out primary bronchial squamous cell carcinoma
- Immunohistochemical stains for TTF-1 may be helpful for identifying pulmonary metastases of adenocarcinoma

Metastatic Carcinoma from Other Organs

- Carcinomas in mediastinum are statistically more likely to represent metastases from other organs rather than primary tumors of thymus
  - Thorough clinical and radiographic examination is required to rule out possibility of occult or late metastasis from distant primary before rendering diagnosis of thymic carcinoma

DIAGNOSTIC CHECKLIST

Clinically Relevant Pathologic Features

- Thymic carcinoma is diagnosis of **exclusion**
- There are no pathognomonic features that can permit a pathologist to make this diagnosis based on histology because tumors resemble carcinomas from other organs
- Demonstration of absence of tumor elsewhere is required for definitive diagnosis

Pathologic Interpretation Pearls

- Islands of poorly differentiated cells with central comedo-like areas of necrosis characterize poorly differentiated nonkeratinizing (lymphoepithelioma-like) squamous cell carcinoma
- Cases showing areas of transition with well-differentiated or atypical thymoma can be seen in a significant number of cases

Immunohistochemistry

Antibody	Reactivity	Staining Pattern	Comment
CK-PAN	Positive	Cytoplasmic	Used to confirm epithelial nature of tumor cells
CD5	Positive	Cytoplasmic	Stains the neoplastic epithelial cells in thymic carcinoma*
C117	Positive	Cell membrane & cytoplasm	Positivity demonstrated in neoplastic epithelial cells in 80% of cases of squamous cell thymic carcinoma in 1 study; up to 20% of pulmonary squamous cell carcinomas may also be positive; not studied in other variants of thymic carcinoma
Chromogranin-A	Positive	Cytoplasmic	Can be focally positive in some cases of nonneuroendocrine-type thymic carcinoma as a result of aberrant differentiation
Ki-67	Positive	Nuclear	Expressed in > 50% of tumor cell nuclei in high-grade tumors; < 10% nuclear positivity in low-grade tumors
Calretinin	Positive	Cytoplasmic	About 30% of thymic carcinomas are positive for calretinin, mesothelin, and CK5/6
CD3	Negative	Not applicable	T-cell markers are generally negative in lymphoid cells of thymic carcinoma; lymphocytes in thymic carcinoma are of B-cell type

**Reactivity depends on type of antibody used. Monoclonal antibody has more specificity but poor sensitivity; polyclonal antibody shows more sensitivity but poor specificity. Other tumors metastatic to mediastinum from other organs can also stain with this antibody, including lung, colon, bladder, and other types. Many variants of thymic carcinoma (such as small cell neuroendocrine carcinoma and poorly differentiated nonkeratinizing squamous cell carcinoma) do not react with this antibody.*

Classification of Thymic Carcinoma According to Histologic Grade

Low-Grade Tumors	High-Grade Tumors
Well-differentiated squamous cell carcinoma	Poorly differentiated, nonkeratinizing (lymphoepithelioma-like) carcinoma
Basaloid carcinoma	Clear cell carcinoma
Well-differentiated mucoepidermoid carcinoma	Poorly differentiated mucoepidermoid carcinoma
Papillary carcinoma	Sarcomatoid (spindle cell) carcinoma
	Carcinosarcoma
	Anaplastic carcinoma
	Adenocarcinoma

SELECTED REFERENCES

1. Marchevsky AM et al: Thymic epithelial neoplasms: a review of current concepts using an evidence-based pathology approach. Hematol Oncol Clin North Am. 22(3):543-62, 2008
2. Moran CA et al: Thymic carcinoma: current concepts and histologic features. Hematol Oncol Clin North Am. 22(3):393-407, 2008
3. Rajan A et al: Treatment of advanced thymoma and thymic carcinoma. Curr Treat Options Oncol. 9(4-6):277-87, 2008
4. Rieker RJ et al: An institutional study on thymomas and thymic carcinomas: experience in 77 patients. Thorac Cardiovasc Surg. 56(3):143-7, 2008
5. Suster S et al: Histologic classification of thymoma: the World Health Organization and beyond. Hematol Oncol Clin North Am. 22(3):381-92, 2008
6. Ra SH et al: Mucinous adenocarcinomas of the thymus: report of 2 cases and review of the literature. Am J Surg Pathol. 31(9):1330-6, 2007
7. Nakagawa K et al: Immunohistochemical KIT (CD117) expression in thymic epithelial tumors. Chest. 128(1):140-4, 2005
8. Suster S: Thymic carcinoma: update of current diagnostic criteria and histologic types. Semin Diagn Pathol. 22(3):198-212, 2005
9. Chalabreysse L et al: Thymic carcinoma: a clinicopathological and immunohistological study of 19 cases. Histopathology. 44(4):367-74, 2004
10. Pan CC et al: KIT (CD117) is frequently overexpressed in thymic carcinomas but is absent in thymomas. J Pathol. 202(3):375-81, 2004
11. Choi WW et al: Adenocarcinoma of the thymus: report of two cases, including a previously undescribed mucinous subtype. Am J Surg Pathol. 27(1):124-30, 2003
12. Pan CC et al: Expression of calretinin and other mesothelioma-related markers in thymic carcinoma and thymoma. Hum Pathol. 34(11):1155-62, 2003
13. Suster S et al: Spindle cell thymic carcinoma: clinicopathologic and immunohistochemical study of a distinctive variant of primary thymic epithelial neoplasm. Am J Surg Pathol. 23(6):691-700, 1999
14. Suster S et al: Primary thymic epithelial neoplasms showing combined features of thymoma and thymic carcinoma. A clinicopathologic study of 22 cases. Am J Surg Pathol. 20(12):1469-80, 1996
15. Suster S et al: Thymic carcinoma. A clinicopathologic study of 60 cases. Cancer. 67(4):1025-32, 1991

Squamous Cell Carcinoma of Thymus

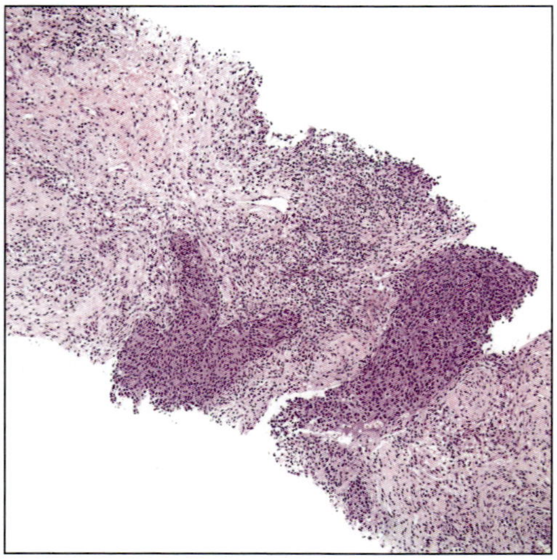

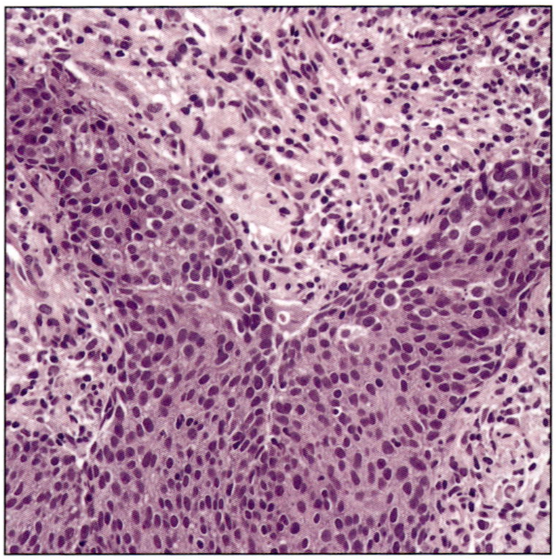

(Left) *Core biopsy of well to moderately differentiated squamous cell carcinoma of the thymus shows connective tissue containing islands of atypical cells. The surrounding stroma shows chronic inflammation and desmoplasia.* ***(Right)*** *High magnification of primary squamous cell carcinoma of the thymus shows islands of large tumor cells with hyperchromatic nuclei and abundant cytoplasm and containing scattered mitotic figures.*

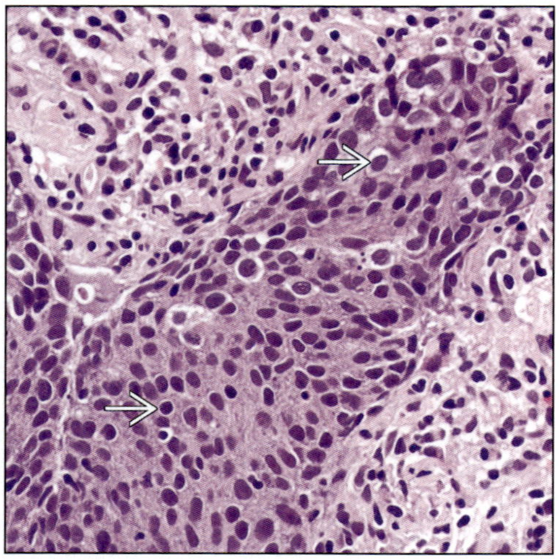

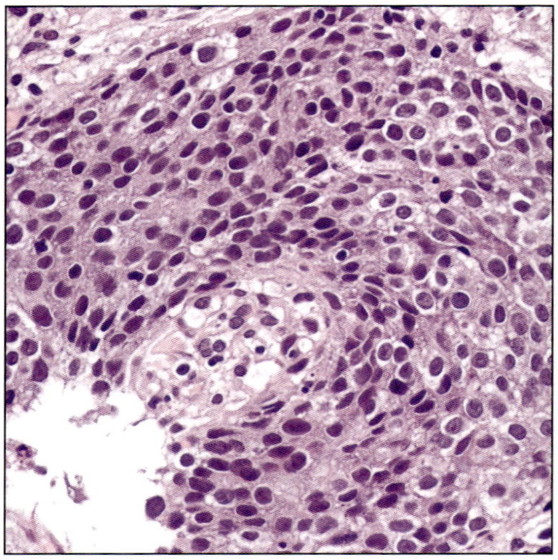

(Left) *Squamous cell carcinoma of the thymus shows a pavement-like arrangement of the tumor cells admixed with numerous apoptotic cells ➡. The tumor cells expressed CK5/6 and p63 by immunohistochemistry, supporting a squamous epithelial origin.* ***(Right)*** *High magnification of well-differentiated squamous cell carcinoma of the thymus shows large cells with sharp cell membranes and focal clearing of the cytoplasm. The tumor cells show a pavement-like architecture.*

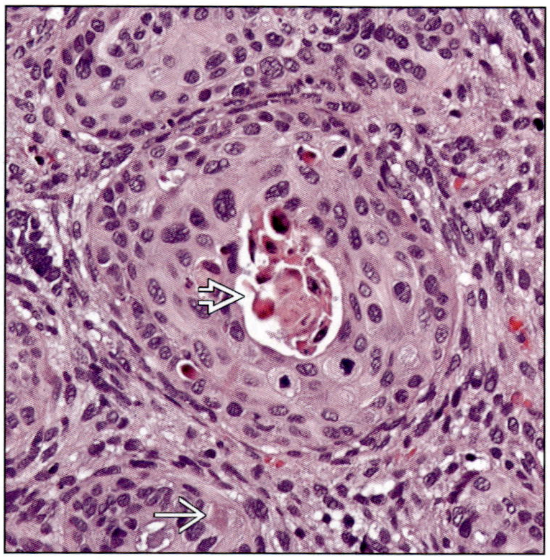

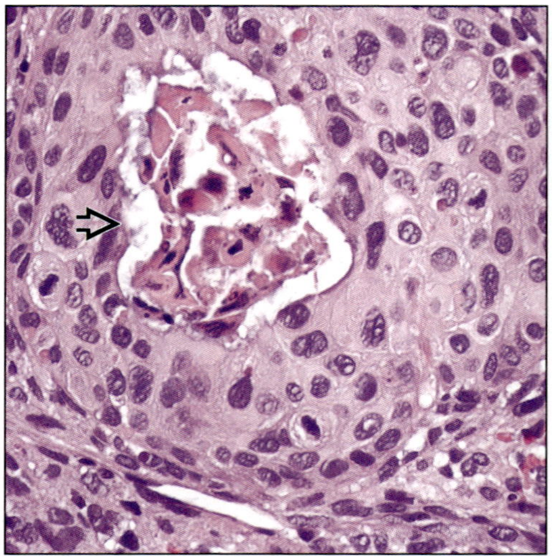

(Left) *Small island of tumor cells in well-differentiated squamous cell carcinoma of the thymus shows foci displaying single cell keratinization ➡ and a central area of horn pearl formation ⇨.* ***(Right)*** *High magnification of focus of keratinization in squamous cell carcinoma of the thymus shows large atypical cells with sharp cell borders and occasional intercellular bridges. Notice central focus of abrupt keratinization ⇨.*

Well-differentiated Mucoepidermoid Carcinoma

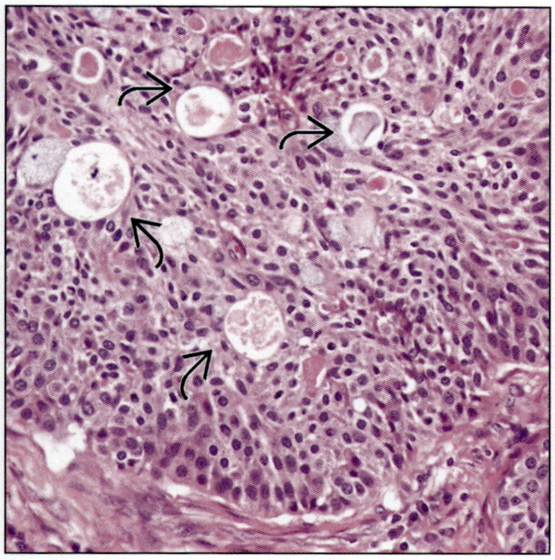

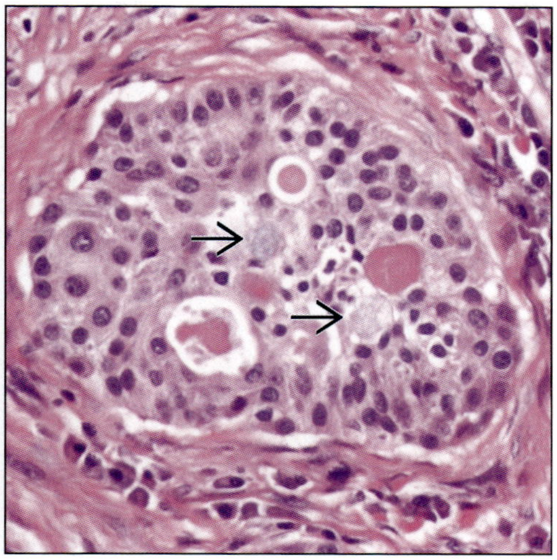

(Left) *Primary mucoepidermoid carcinoma of the thymus shows sheets of squamoid intermediate cells dotted by small mucinous cysts ↪ admixed with scattered individual mucocytes.* ***(Right)*** *High magnification from a small tumor cell island in a well-differentiated mucoepidermoid carcinoma of the thymus shows cohesive squamoid cells with small mucinous cysts and occasional singly scattered mucocytes →.*

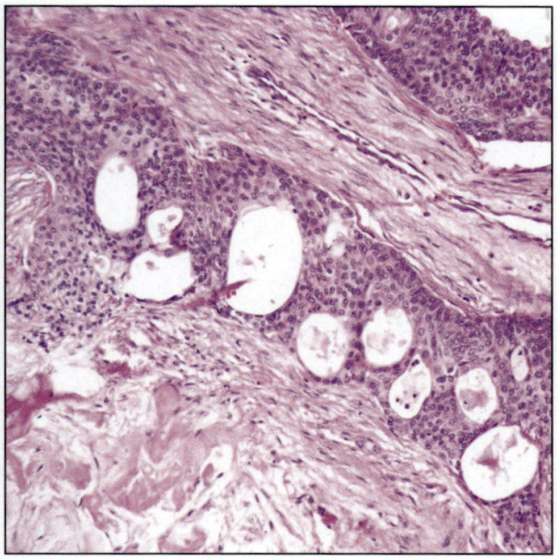

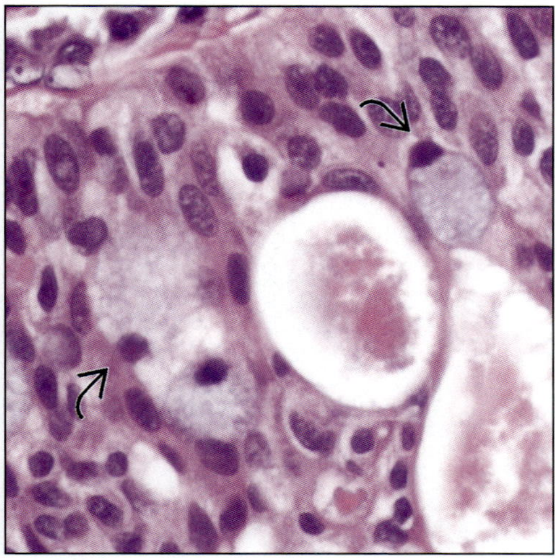

(Left) *Cords of tumor cells with cribriform-like cystic spaces filled with mucin are seen in this example of well-differentiated mucoepidermoid carcinoma of the thymus.* ***(Right)*** *High magnification of well-differentiated mucoepidermoid carcinoma of the thymus shows a cohesive population of squamoid epithelial cells containing mucinous microcysts surrounded by mucocytes that are filled with abundant light bluish mucin content ↪.*

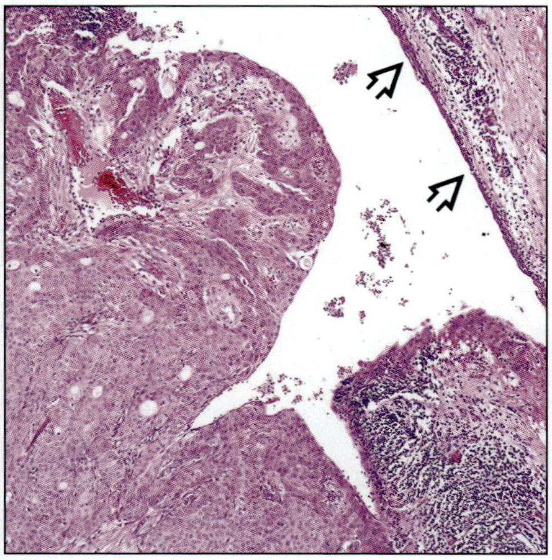

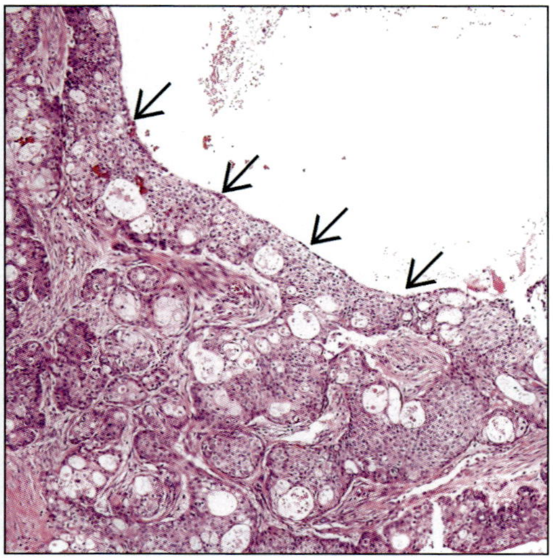

(Left) *Cystic area in moderately differentiated mucoepidermoid carcinoma of the thymus shows a flat cuboidal epithelial lining ⇨ slowly merging with solid sheets of epithelioid tumor cells on the left of the image.* ***(Right)*** *Example of cystic mucoepidermoid carcinoma of the thymus shows dilated cystic lumen (top right) flanked by sheets and lobules of tumor cells displaying mucoepidermoid features →. In some cases, the tumor may originate from the lining of the cyst.*

THYMIC CARCINOMA

Poorly Differentiated Mucoepidermoid Carcinoma

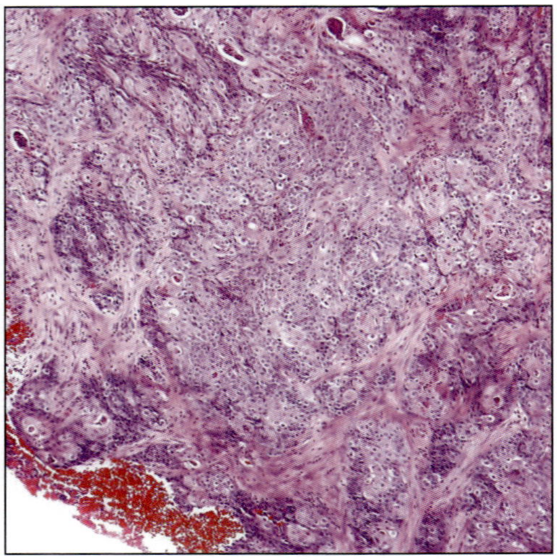

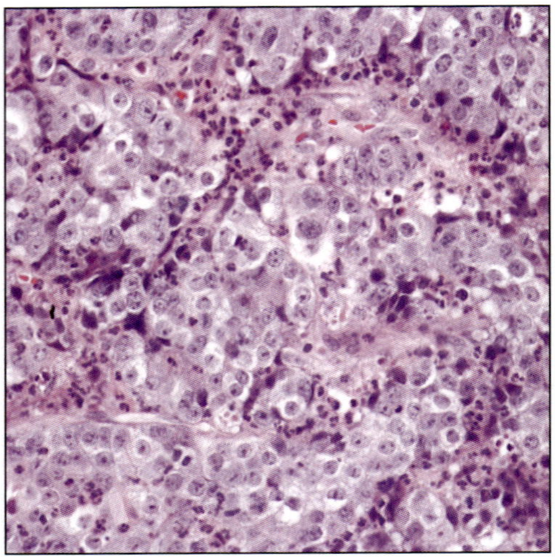

(Left) *Scanning magnification of poorly differentiated mucoepidermoid carcinoma of the thymus shows sheets and small islands of tumor cells embedded in fibrous stroma.* ***(Right)*** *High magnification of poorly differentiated mucoepidermoid carcinoma of the thymus shows sheets of monotonous tumor cells without evidence of luminal differentiation or other distinctive lineage. There is an inflammatory cell infiltrate in the interstitium.*

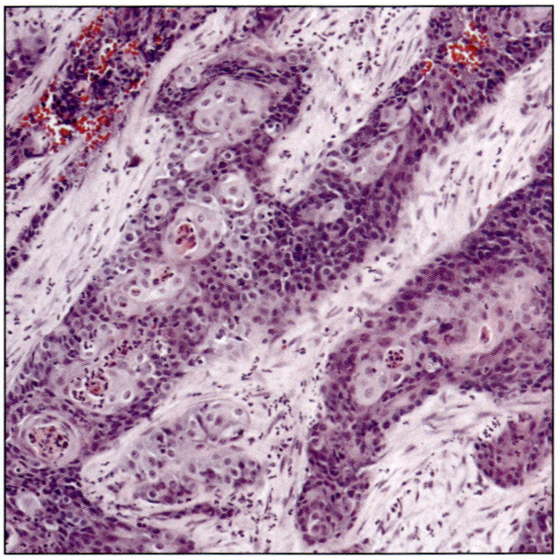

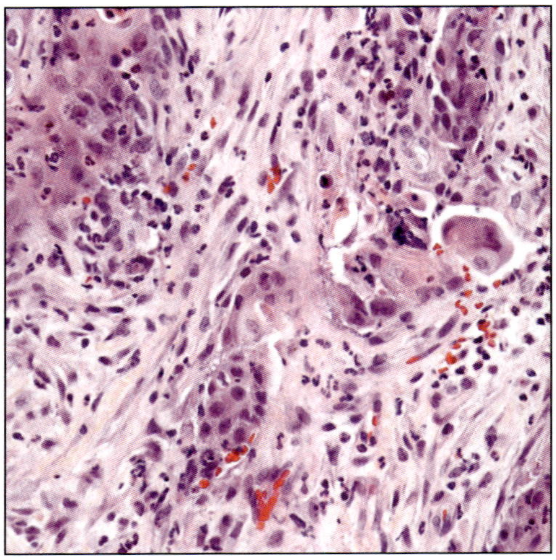

(Left) *Moderate to poorly differentiated mucoepidermoid carcinoma of the thymus shows immature intermediate cells merging with better differentiated epidermoid cells set against a desmoplastic stroma.* ***(Right)*** *High magnification of poorly differentiated mucoepidermoid carcinoma of the thymus shows infiltration of vascular lumens by carcinoma cells. Vascular and lymphatic involvement is a common event in these tumors.*

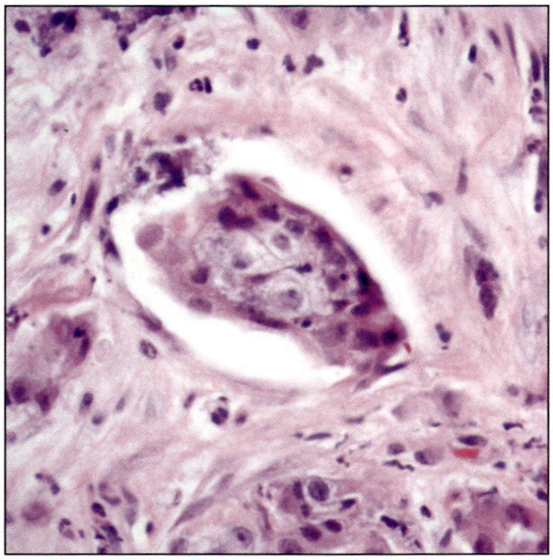

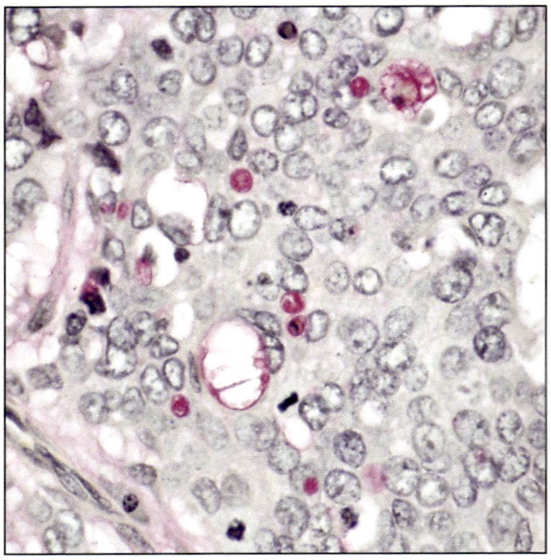

(Left) *High magnification of focus of lymphatic invasion in poorly differentiated mucoepidermoid carcinoma of the thymus is shown. Notice the clearly squamoid appearance of the tumor embolus within the vessel lumen.* ***(Right)*** *Mucicarmine stain in poorly differentiated mucoepidermoid carcinoma of the thymus shows focal cytoplasmic positivity (red) of scattered tumor cells, corresponding to intracellular mucin.*

Basaloid Carcinoma

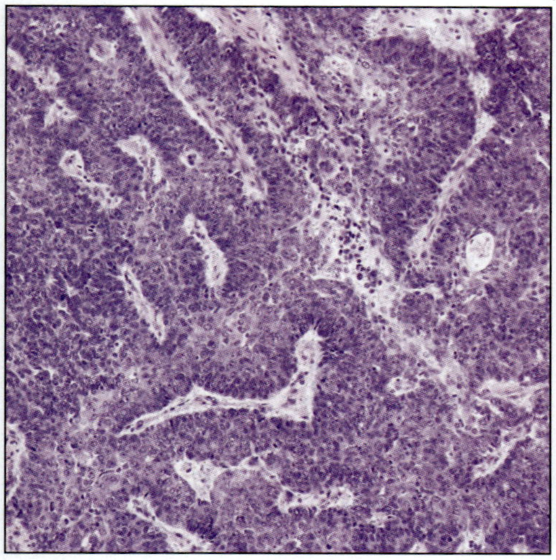
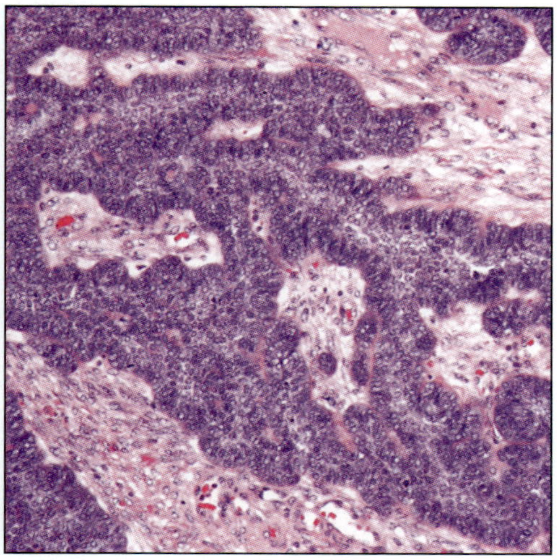

(Left) *Scanning magnification in basaloid carcinoma of the thymus shows anastomosing cords of hyperchromatic tumor cells displaying prominent peripheral palisading of nuclei.* ***(Right)*** *Higher magnification of basaloid carcinoma of the thymus shows a monotonous population of round to oval tumor cells with clear nuclear chromatin and peripheral palisading of nuclei. The striking peripheral palisading of nuclei is reminiscent of basal cell carcinoma of the skin.*

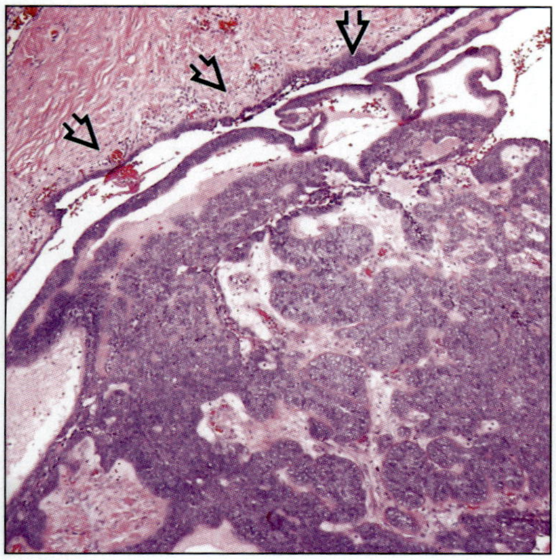
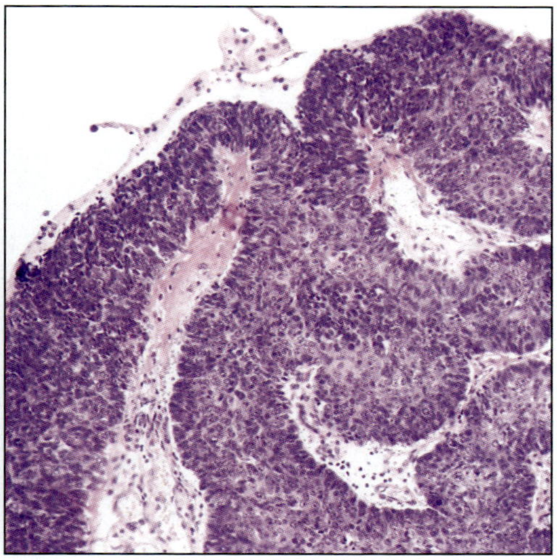

(Left) *Scanning magnification of basaloid carcinoma of the thymus shows early cystic changes that can be seen at the periphery of the lesion* ➩*. The lining of the cysts may or may not contain the same type of epithelium as the solid part of the tumor.* ***(Right)*** *Cords of monotonous tumor cells with peripheral palisading of nuclei are seen in this basaloid carcinoma of the thymus. The tumor cells are quite monotonous, and no nuclear pleomorphism is appreciated.*

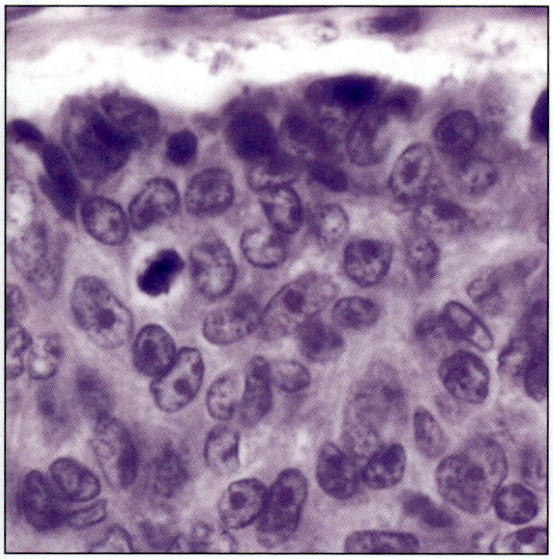
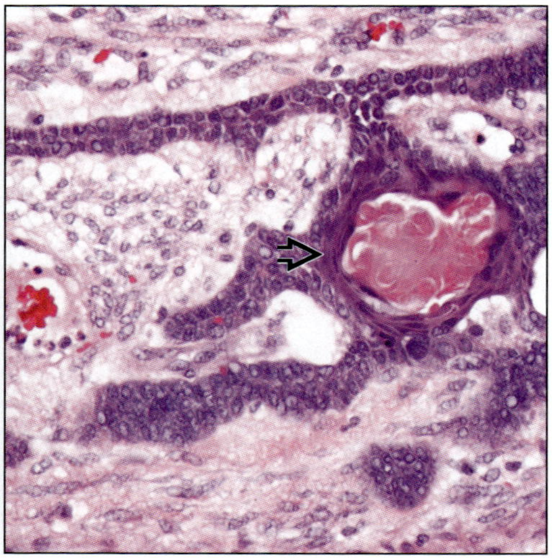

(Left) *Higher magnification of basaloid carcinoma of the thymus shows primitive-appearing round to oval tumor cells, with large oval nuclei and prominent central eosinophilic nucleoli. The tumor shows frequent mitotic figures.* ***(Right)*** *Basaloid carcinoma of the thymus shows a focus of abrupt keratinization* ➩ *with keratin pearl formation in the center of the lumen. The rest of the tumor cells appear as primitive, undifferentiated small cells.*

THYMIC CARCINOMA

Clear Cell Carcinoma of Thymus

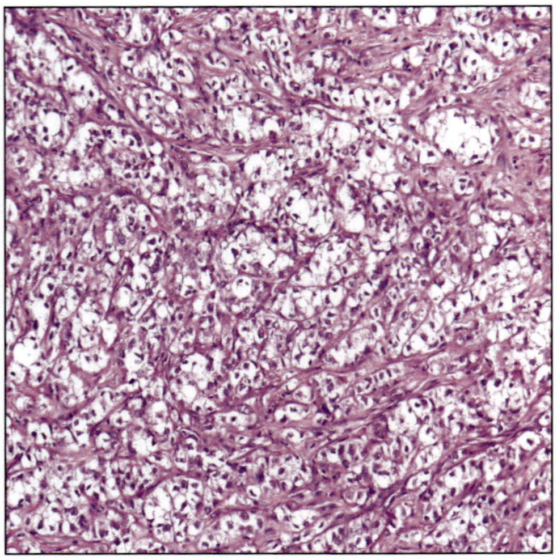
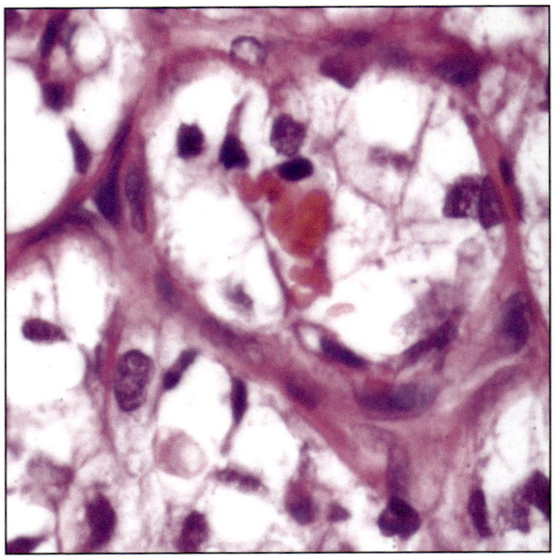

(Left) *Scanning magnification in clear cell carcinoma of the thymus shows sheets of large tumor cells with abundant clear cytoplasm. Tumors with this histologic appearance may closely resemble metastatic clear cell renal cell carcinoma.* ***(Right)*** *High magnification of clear cell carcinoma of the thymus shows large cells with abundant water-clear cytoplasm and centrally placed small nuclei with vesicular chromatin and inconspicuous nucleoli.*

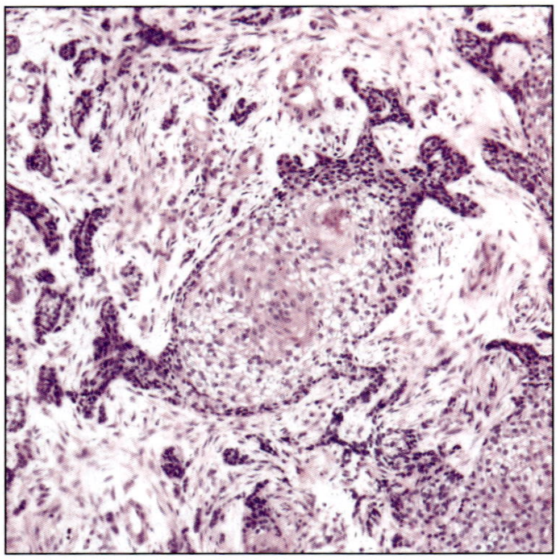
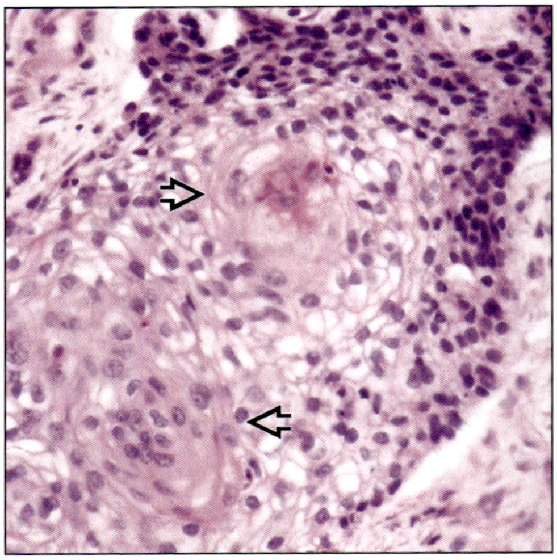

(Left) *Scanning magnification of tumor cell island in clear cell carcinoma of the thymus shows central clearing of the cytoplasm with condensation of dark small nuclei toward the periphery. Notice small infiltrating islands of tumor cells surrounded by desmoplastic stroma.* ***(Right)*** *Higher magnification of clear cell carcinoma of the thymus shows transitions between the clear cells and areas showing more epidermoid features ⇨.*

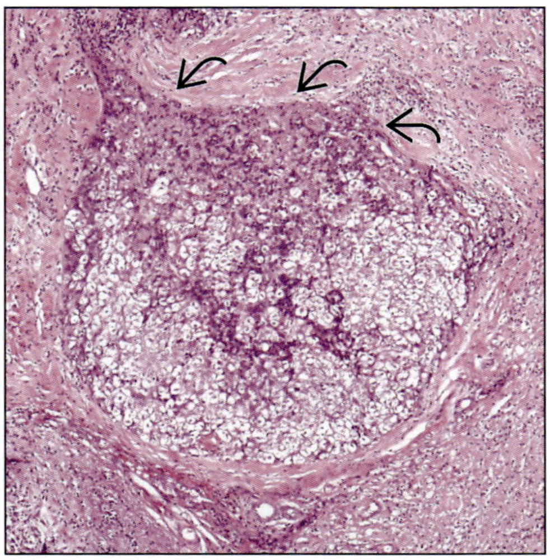
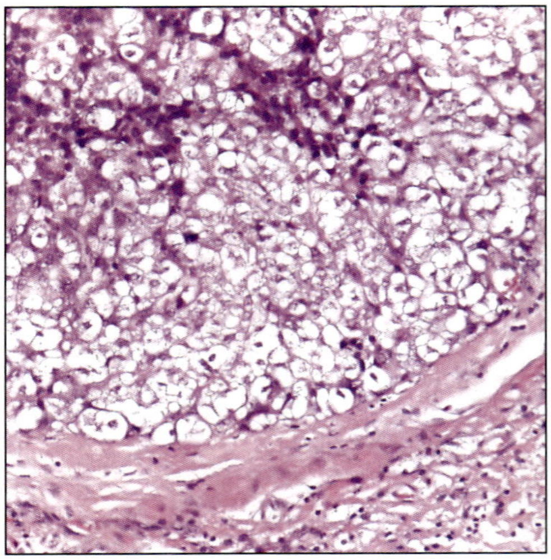

(Left) *Clear cell carcinoma of the thymus shows a well-circumscribed tumor lobule composed of clear tumor cells admixed with cells displaying more conventional eosinophilic cytoplasm ↶. Notice the angulated character of the tumor cell nodule reminiscent of the growth pattern seen in thymoma.* ***(Right)*** *High magnification of clear cell carcinoma of the thymus shows large round tumor cells with abundant water-clear cytoplasm and small centrally placed nuclei.*

Spindle Cell and Sarcomatoid Carcinoma

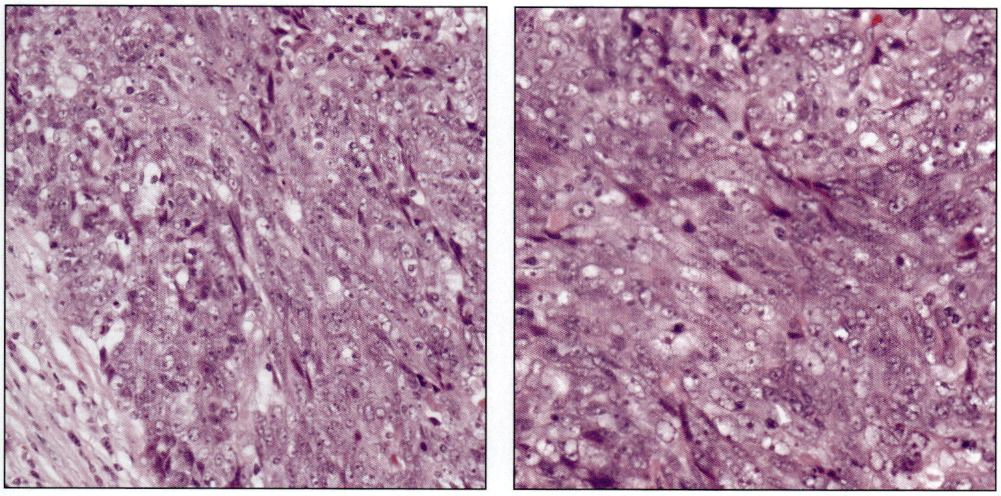

(Left) *Spindle cell (sarcomatoid) carcinoma of the thymus shows dense spindle cell population disposed in longitudinal fascicles with oval nuclei displaying prominent eosinophilic nucleoli.* ***(Right)*** *High magnification of spindle cell carcinoma of the thymus shows round to oval nuclei with vesicular chromatin pattern and prominent, central eosinophilic nucleoli. The cells contain a rim of eosinophilic cytoplasm and display scattered mitotic figures.*

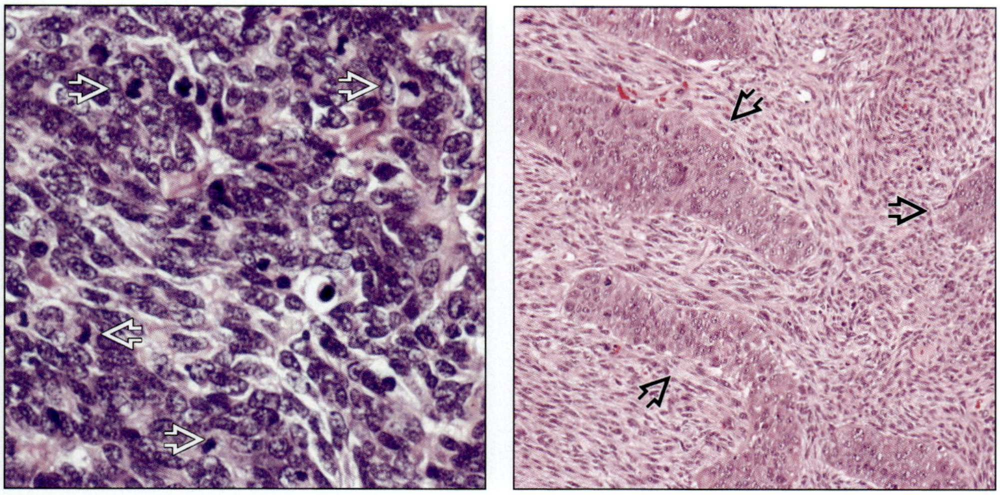

(Left) *High magnification of spindle cell (sarcomatoid) carcinoma of the thymus shows neoplastic spindle cells characterized by oval to spindled hyperchromatic nuclei with occasional small nucleoli and a scant rim of cytoplasm. Notice frequent mitotic figures ⇨.* ***(Right)*** *Carcinosarcoma of the thymus shows a biphasic malignant neoplasm composed of well-defined islands of cohesive epithelial cells ⇨ surrounded by a densely cellular spindle cell stroma.*

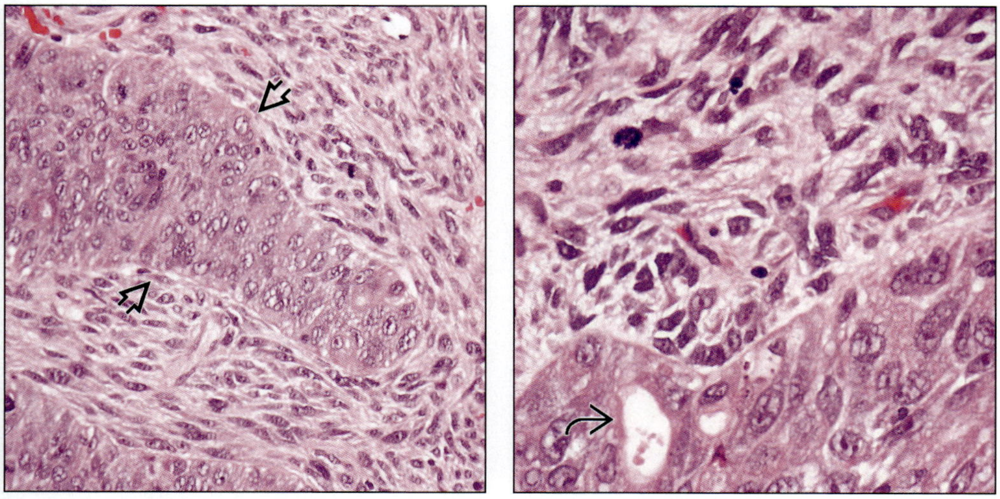

(Left) *High magnification of carcinosarcoma of the thymus shows an island of epithelioid cells ⇨, corresponding to a poorly differentiated carcinomatous component, surrounded by atypical spindle cell, sarcomatous elements.* ***(Right)*** *High magnification of carcinosarcoma of the thymus shows an island of epithelial tumor cells with focal abortive lumen formation ↪. The sarcomatous element in the surrounding stroma is composed of keratin-negative spindle cells.*

Lymphoepithelioma-like Carcinoma of Thymus

(Left) *Lymphoepithelioma-like carcinoma of the thymus shows a cluster of round tumor cell islands with central comedo-like areas of necrosis. Notice the dense lymphoplasmacellular infiltrate surrounding the tumor cell islands, characteristic of this lesion.* ***(Right)*** *Island of tumor cells in lymphoepithelioma-like carcinoma of the thymus shows characteristic comedo-like area of necrosis ⇒. The tumor cells in this lobule are monotonous with numerous mitoses.*

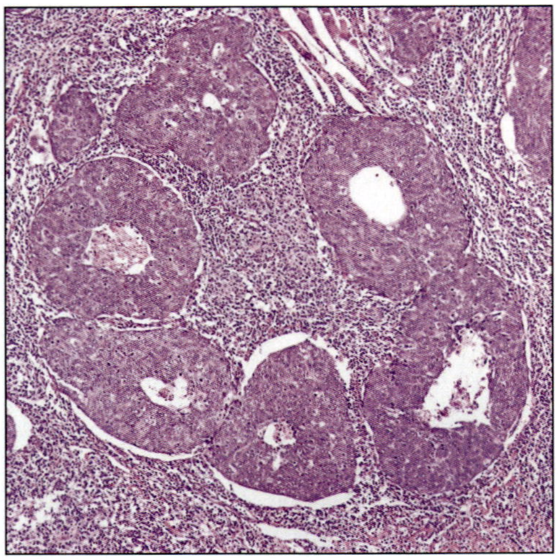

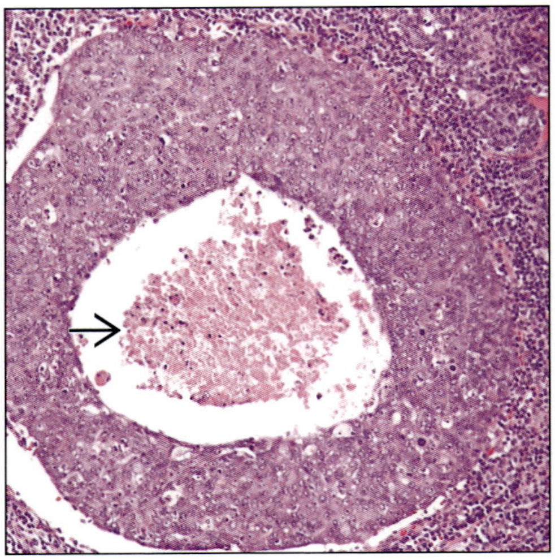

(Left) *High magnification of lymphoepithelioma-like carcinoma of the thymus shows a small island of monotonous tumor cells. Notice focal overlapping of nuclei ⇒ and prominent, mostly centrally placed eosinophilic nucleoli ⇒.* ***(Right)*** *Small islands of lymphoepithelioma-like carcinoma of the thymus shows scattered atypical mitoses ⇒. Notice the dense lymphoplasmacellular infiltration in the surrounding stroma.*

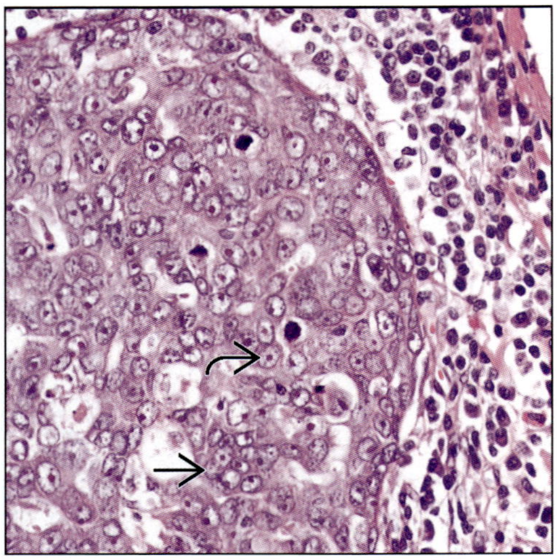

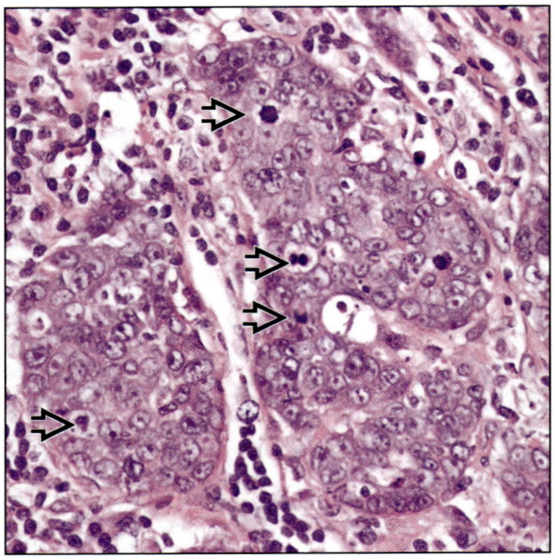

(Left) *Lymphoepithelioma-like carcinoma of the thymus shows nuclear detail of the cells. Notice small round centrally placed nucleoli ⇒ and dense lymphoid infiltrate in the surrounding stroma. The cells in this infiltrate are polyclonal small lymphocytes.* ***(Right)*** *High magnification of lymphoepithelioma-like carcinoma of the thymus shows cells with round to oval nuclei with vesicular chromatin and prominent eosinophilic nucleoli and an indistinct rim of cytoplasm.*

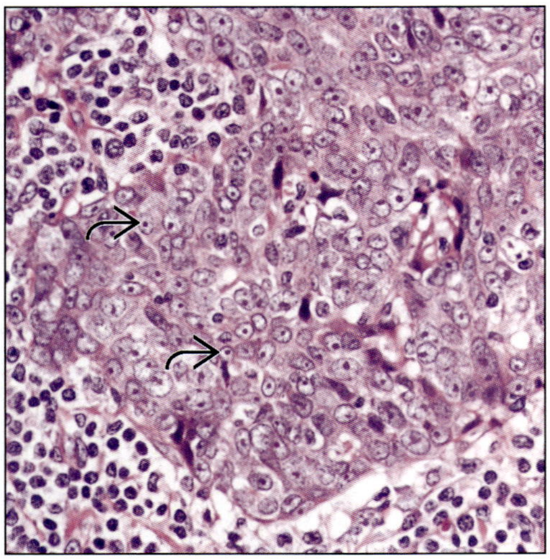

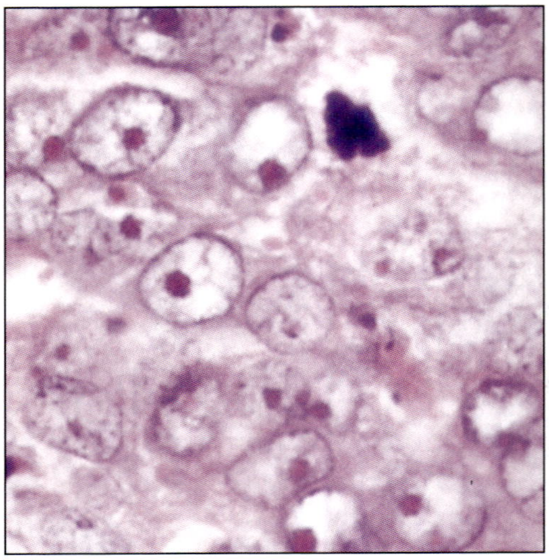

Lymphoepithelioma-like Carcinoma of Thymus

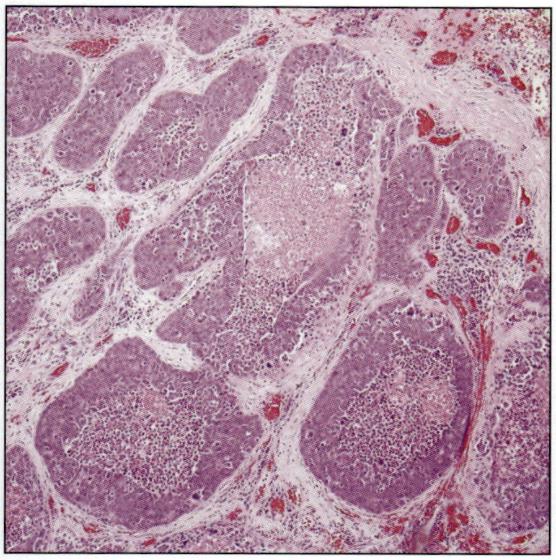
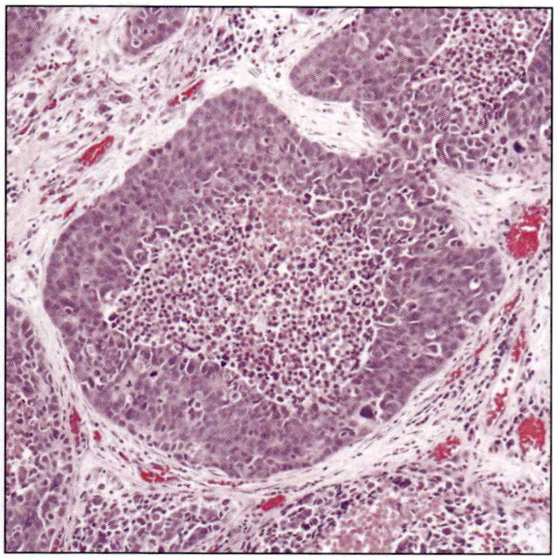

(Left) *Scanning magnification of lymphoepithelioma-like carcinoma of the thymus (poorly differentiated, nonkeratinizing squamous cell carcinoma) shows tumor cell islands with extensive, comedo-like areas of necrosis.* ***(Right)*** *High magnification of lymphoepithelioma-like carcinoma of the thymus shows island of monotonous tumor cells with prominent comedo-like area of necrosis. The central comedo-like areas of necrosis are characteristic for this tumor.*

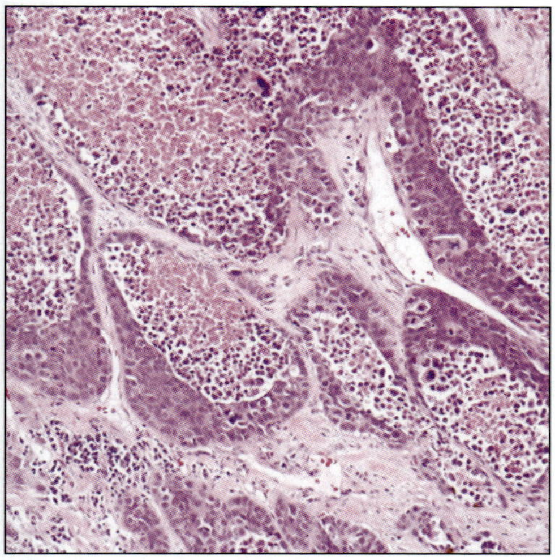
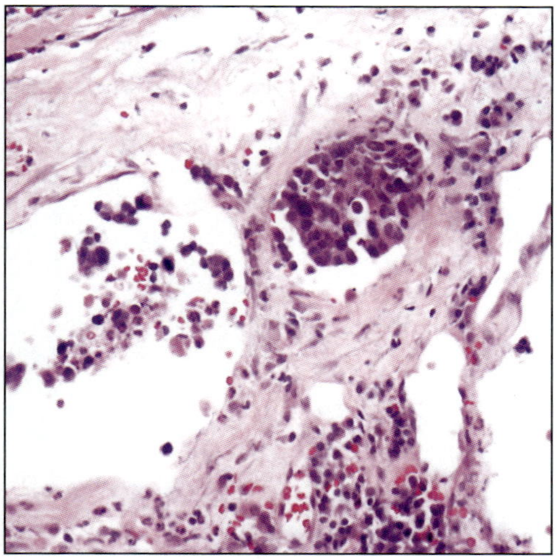

(Left) *Lymphoepithelioma-like carcinoma of the thymus (poorly differentiated, nonkeratinizing squamous cell carcinoma) shows extensive central areas of necrosis within the tumor cell islands.* ***(Right)*** *Focus of vascular invasion is seen in lymphoepithelioma-like carcinoma of the thymus. Vascular invasion is a common finding in these tumors and accounts in part for the highly aggressive clinical behavior of these neoplasms when arising in the thymus.*

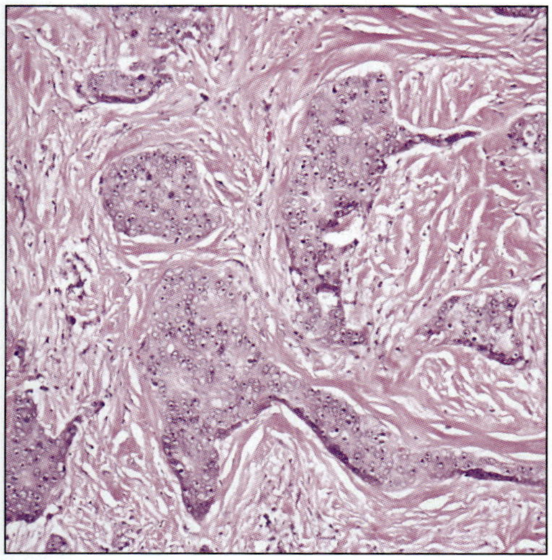
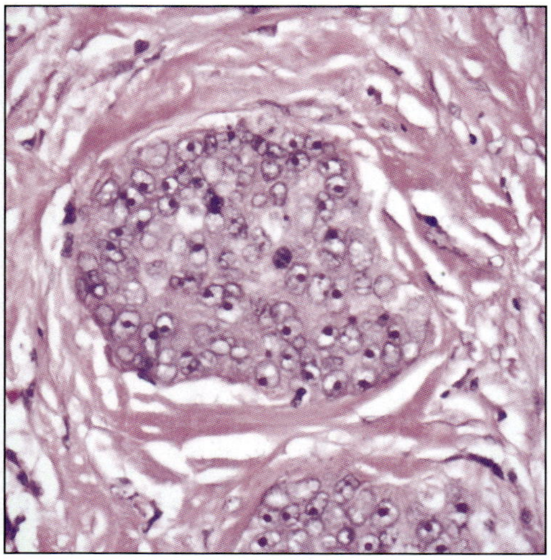

(Left) *Lymphoepithelioma-like carcinoma of the thymus shows islands of tumor cells surrounded by a paucicellular desmoplastic stroma. Not all lymphoepithelioma-like carcinomas of the thymus contain an abundant lymphoid infiltrate; the diagnosis is established based on the cytology of the tumor cells.* ***(Right)*** *High magnification shows a tumor cell island in lymphoepithelioma-like carcinoma of the thymus. Notice the absence of dense lymphoid stromal infiltrate.*

THYMIC CARCINOMA

Anaplastic Carcinoma of Thymus

(Left) *Anaplastic carcinoma of the thymus shows sheets of large atypical tumor cells associated with extensive areas of tumor necrosis. No recognizable architecture is appreciated on scanning magnification.* ***(Right)*** *High magnification of anaplastic carcinoma of the thymus shows bizarre giant tumor cells located toward the center of the field surrounded by smaller, atypical tumor cells. Notice the tripolar mitosis ⇨.*

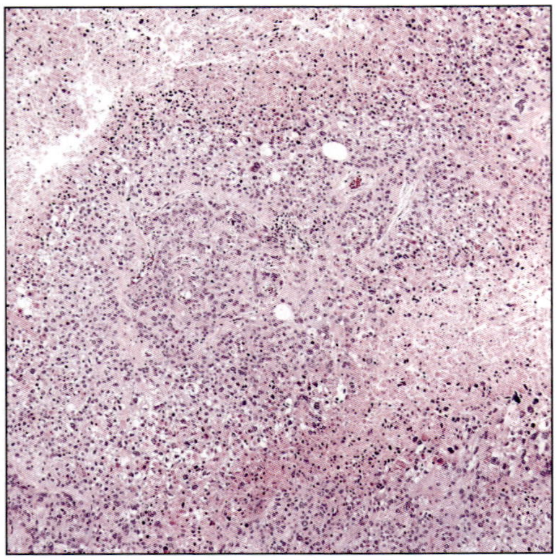

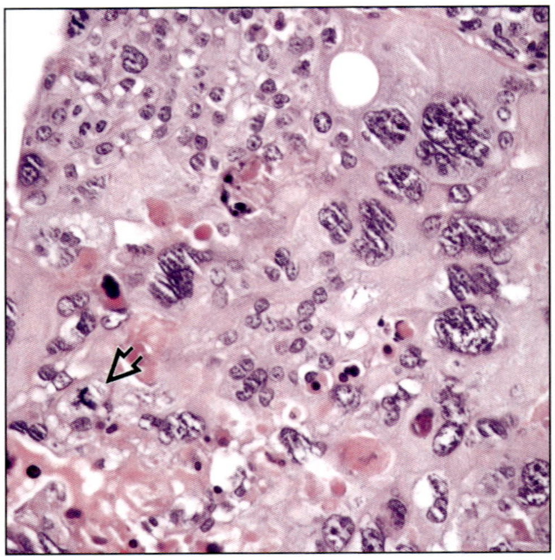

(Left) *High magnification of anaplastic carcinoma of the thymus shows bizarre pleomorphic and multinucleated tumor cells admixed with abundant necrotic and apoptotic cells.* ***(Right)*** *Anaplastic carcinoma of the thymus shows sheets of atypical tumor cells with scattered large, multinucleated and multilobated anaplastic tumor cells ⇨. Notice the total absence of organization or other features of differentiation. Tumors like this can resemble pleomorphic sarcomas.*

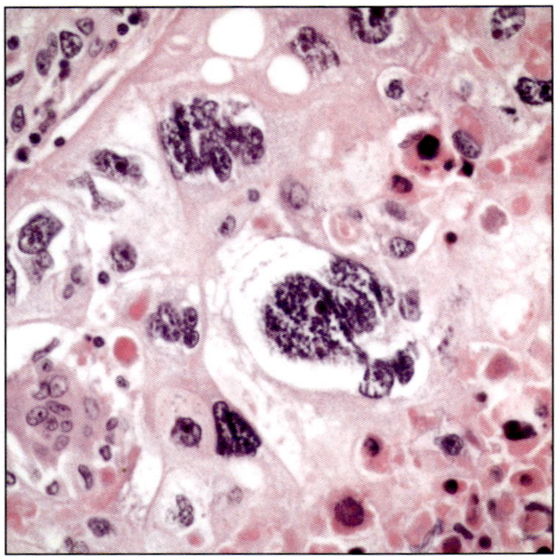

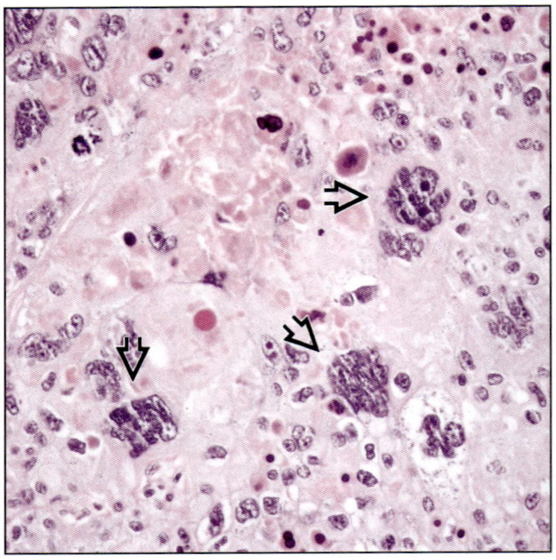

(Left) *High magnification of anaplastic carcinoma of the thymus shows characteristic bizarre, multilobated and multinucleated tumor cells. Notice abnormal mitosis at the bottom of the field ⇨.* ***(Right)*** *High magnification of a bizarre pleomorphic tumor cell ⇨ in anaplastic carcinoma of the thymus shows multiple nuclei with prominent nucleoli and ill-defined cell borders. Notice the extensive areas of necrosis surrounding the multinucleated tumor cell.*

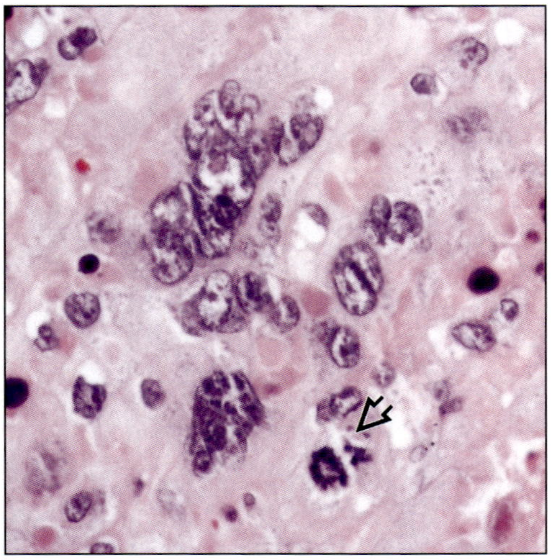

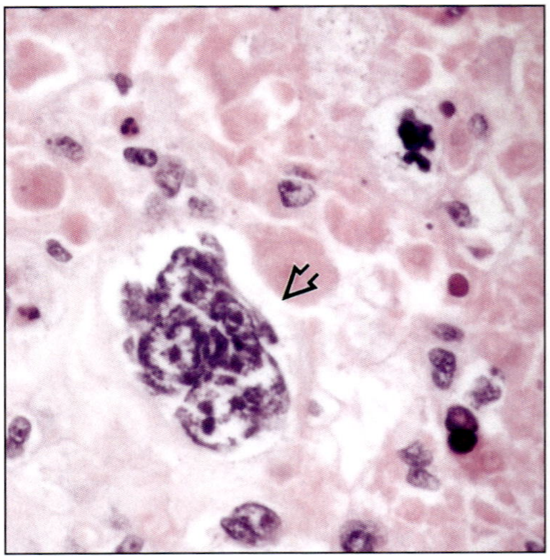

Immunohistochemical Features

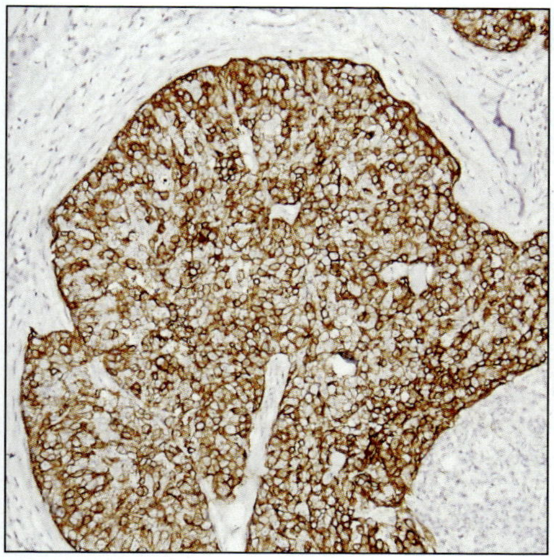
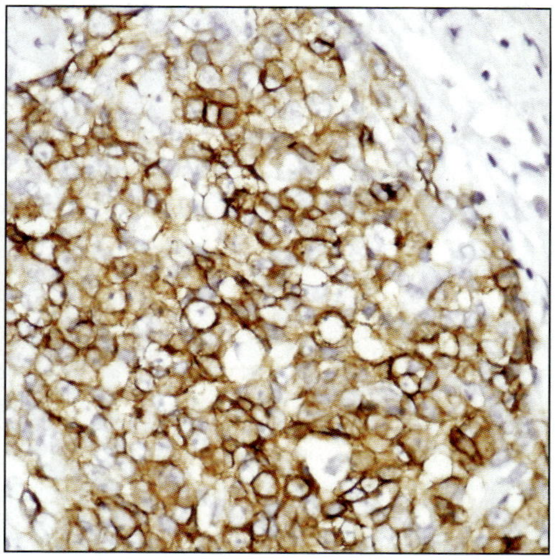

(Left) *Immunohistochemical stain for broad-spectrum cytokeratin AE1/AE3 in lymphoepithelioma-like carcinoma of the thymus shows strong staining in an island of tumor cells.* ***(Right)*** *Immunohistochemical staining for C-Kit (CD117) in primary thymic carcinoma, lymphoepithelioma-like type, shows strong membrane staining of the tumor cells for this antigen. This finding is encountered mostly in thymic tumors of squamous cell lineage.*

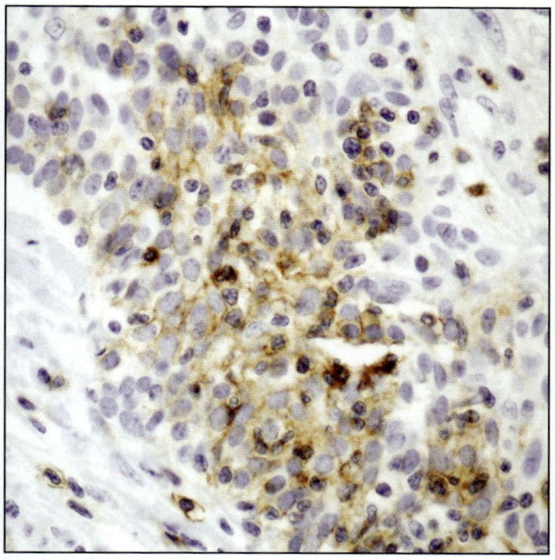
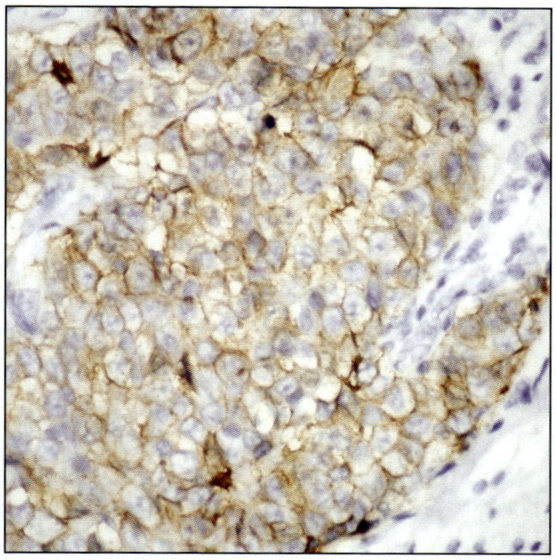

(Left) *Immunohistochemical staining of thymic carcinoma with CD5 shows focal membrane and cytoplasmic staining in some of the tumor cells for this marker. Not all types of thymic carcinoma stain for this marker, and many other types of nonthymic cancers can be positive as well.* ***(Right)*** *Immunohistochemical staining for MOC-31, an epithelium-associated marker, in poorly differentiated thymic carcinoma shows faint staining in a cluster of tumor cells.*

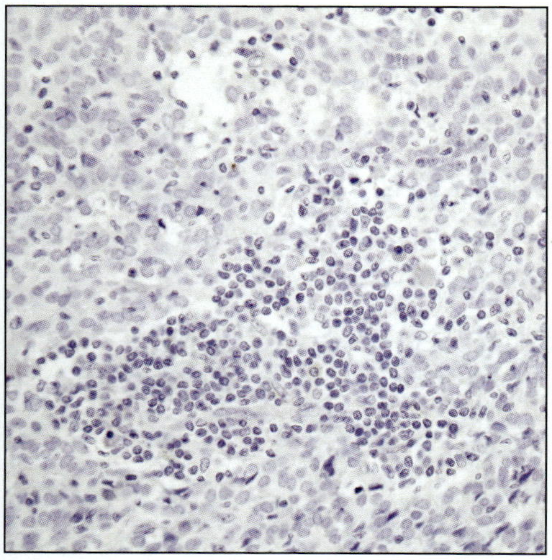
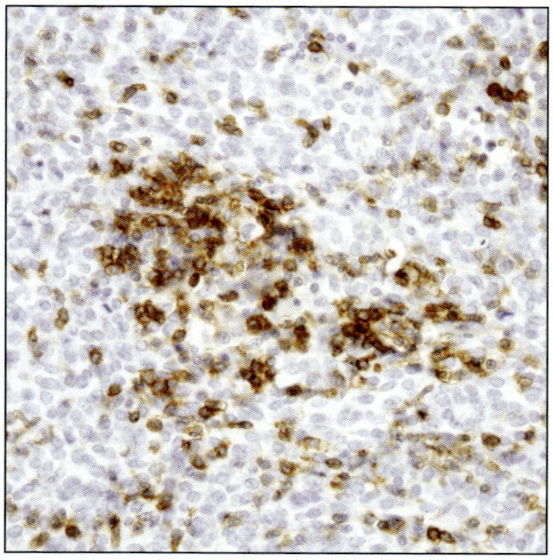

(Left) *Immunohistochemical staining for CD99 in poorly differentiated thymic carcinoma shows complete absence of reactivity in the small lymphocytes admixed with the tumor cells for this marker. CD99 is a marker of immature T lymphoblasts commonly seen in thymomas.* ***(Right)*** *Immunohistochemical staining for CD20 in poorly differentiated thymic carcinoma shows numerous positive small lymphocytes in clusters and scattered singly within the malignant thymic epithelial cell population.*

NEUROENDOCRINE CARCINOMAS OF THE THYMUS

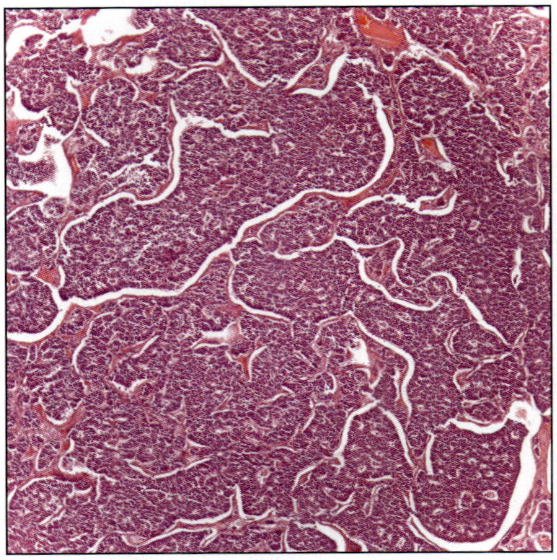

Well-differentiated neuroendocrine carcinoma (carcinoid tumor) shows a cellular proliferation arranged in cords and nests.

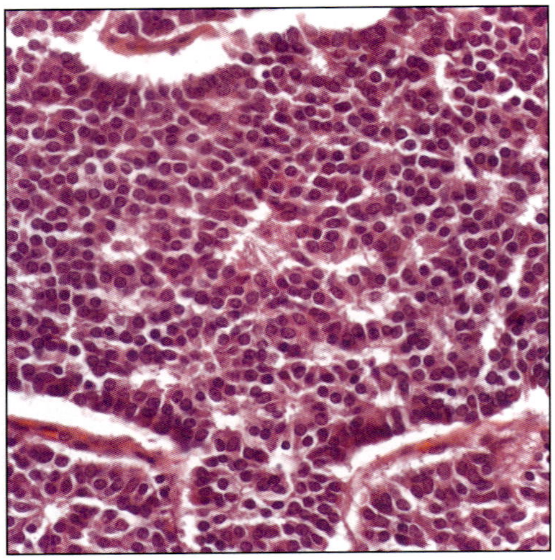

High-power magnification of a well-differentiated neuroendocrine carcinoma (carcinoid tumor) shows a homogeneous cellular proliferation without nuclear atypia or mitotic activity.

TERMINOLOGY

Abbreviations

- Well-differentiated neuroendocrine carcinoma (WDNECa)
- Moderately differentiated neuroendocrine carcinoma (MDNECa)
- Poorly differentiated neuroendocrine carcinoma (PDNECa)

Synonyms

- Carcinoid tumor, atypical carcinoid, small cell carcinoma

Definitions

- Malignant neuroendocrine neoplasms that range from low- to high-grade malignancies

ETIOLOGY/PATHOGENESIS

Etiology

- Probably originating from Kulchitsky cells

CLINICAL ISSUES

Epidemiology

- Incidence
  - Thymic neuroendocrine carcinomas represent approximately 5% of all mediastinal tumors
- Age
  - Neuroendocrine carcinomas can occur in any age group
- Gender
  - No specific gender predilection for thymic neuroendocrine carcinomas

Site

- Anterior mediastinum

Presentation

- Chest pain
- Cough
- Dyspnea
- Cushing syndrome
- Multiple endocrine neoplasia, type II (MEN-II)
- Proximal myopathy
- Polyarthropathy
- Peripheral neuropathy
- Incomplete Sipple syndrome
- ADH secretion
- Eaton-Lambert syndrome
- Hypertrophic osteoarthropathy
- ACTH secretion
- Paraneoplastic syndromes

Treatment

- Complete surgical resection
- Depending on grade of tumor
  - Surgical resection followed by chemotherapy
  - In poorly differentiated tumors (small cell carcinoma): Chemotherapy

Prognosis

- Depends on grade and surgical stage of neoplasm at time of diagnosis
  - WDNECa: 5-year survival approximately 50%
  - MDNECa: 5-year survival approximately 25%
  - PDNECa: 5-year survival 0%

MACROSCOPIC FEATURES

General Features

- Tan to brown color
- Soft consistency
- Well-defined but not encapsulated tumor
- Areas of hemorrhage &/or necrosis may be present
- Minority of cases will present with cystic changes

NEUROENDOCRINE CARCINOMAS OF THE THYMUS

Key Facts

Terminology
- Synonyms: Carcinoid tumor, atypical carcinoid, small cell carcinoma
- Malignant neoplasms that range from low- to high-grade malignancies

Clinical Issues
- Incidence
  - Thymic neuroendocrine carcinomas represent approximately 5% of all mediastinal tumors
  - Can occur at any age
- Symptoms
  - Paraneoplastic syndromes
  - Multiple endocrine neoplasia, type II (MEN-II)
  - Cushing syndrome
- Prognosis depends on grade and surgical stage of neoplasm at time of diagnosis
  - WDNECa: 5-year survival approximately 50%
  - MDNECa: 5-year survival approximately 25%
  - PDNECa: 5-year survival 0%
- Treatment
  - Complete surgical resection
  - Surgical resection followed by chemotherapy in higher grade tumors

Top Differential Diagnoses
- Paraganglioma
- Ectopic parathyroid tumor
- Thymic carcinoma

Diagnostic Checklist
- Nesting growth pattern
- Mitotic activity
- Presence of necrosis

Sections to Be Submitted
- Important to document transitional areas of tumor and normal thymus
- Important to document presence of necrosis &/or hemorrhage

Size
- Variable size from a few cm to > 10 cm in diameter

MICROSCOPIC PATHOLOGY

Histologic Features
- Nesting growth pattern
- Spindle cell growth pattern
- Oncocytic growth pattern
- Pigmented
- Cystic
- Angiomatoid growth pattern

DIFFERENTIAL DIAGNOSIS

Paraganglioma
- Paraganglioma and neuroendocrine carcinomas may share similar immunophenotype in terms of neuroendocrine markers
- Usually negative for keratin markers
- May show presence of prominent nuclear atypia, but mitotic activity is rare

Ectopic Parathyroid Tumor
- May also share similar immunophenotype
- May show the presence of chief and oncocytic cells
- Generally shows positive staining for PTH
- Shows positive staining for PAS

Thymoma
- May show areas that mimic histologically a neuroendocrine tumor
- Generally negative for neuroendocrine markers

Thymic Carcinoma
- Usually negative for neuroendocrine markers
- Histology of thymic carcinoma is different from "neuroendocrine pattern" seen in neuroendocrine tumors

Metastatic Neuroendocrine Carcinoma
- Clinical history is important tool in arriving at specific site of origin
- Use of immunohistochemical studies in some cases may provide a clue for site of origin

DIAGNOSTIC CHECKLIST

Clinically Relevant Pathologic Features
- Nuclear features
- Mitotic rate
- Invasive pattern

Pathologic Interpretation Pearls
- Nesting growth pattern
- Mitotic activity
- Presence of necrosis

SELECTED REFERENCES

1. Moran CA et al: Cystic well-differentiated neuroendocrine carcinoma (carcinoid tumor): a clinicopathologic and immunohistochemical study of two cases. Am J Clin Pathol. 126(3):377-80, 2006
2. Moran CA: Primary neuroendocrine carcinomas of the mediastinum: review of current criteria for histopathologic diagnosis and classification. Semin Diagn Pathol. 22(3):223-9, 2005
3. Moran CA et al: Neuroendocrine carcinomas (carcinoid tumor) of the thymus. A clinicopathologic analysis of 80 cases. Am J Clin Pathol. 114(1):100-10, 2000
4. Moran CA et al: Primary neuroendocrine carcinoma (thymic carcinoid) of the thymus with prominent oncocytic features: a clinicopathologic study of 22 cases. Mod Pathol. 13(5):489-94, 2000

NEUROENDOCRINE CARCINOMAS OF THE THYMUS

Immunohistochemistry

Antibody	Reactivity	Staining Pattern	Comment
CK-HMW-NOS	Positive	Cytoplasmic	Not specific for neuroendocrine tumors
CK-LMW-NOS	Positive	Cytoplasmic	Not specific for neuroendocrine tumors
Chromogranin-A	Positive	Cytoplasmic	
Synaptophysin	Positive	Cytoplasmic	
CD56	Positive	Cytoplasmic	
p53	Positive	Nuclear & cytoplasmic	In < 5% of cases
S100	Positive	Nuclear & cytoplasmic	In some cases
PTH	Positive	Cytoplasmic	Focal in some cases
Calcitonin	Positive	Cytoplasmic	Focal in some cases

Classification of Thymic Neuroendocrine Carcinomas

Traditional Classification	WHO Classification	Moran & Suster Classification
Carcinoid	Well-differentiated neuroendocrine carcinoma	Well-differentiated neuroendocrine carcinoma (low grade)
Atypical carcinoid	Well-differentiated neuroendocrine carcinoma	Moderately differentiated neuroendocrine carcinoma (intermediate grade)
Small cell carcinoma	Poorly differentiated neuroendocrine carcinoma	Poorly differentiated neuroendocrine carcinoma (high grade)

Histological Classification of Thymic Neuroendocrine Carcinomas*

Tumor Type	Histological Feature
Well-differentiated neuroendocrine carcinoma	Well-developed "neuroendocrine pattern"
	Mild cellular atypia
	0-3 mitotic figures x 10 HPF
	Only focal necrosis
Moderately differentiated neuroendocrine carcinoma	Focal preservation of "neuroendocrine pattern"
	Mixture of nesting and diffuse growth patterns
	Moderate cellular atypia
	4-9 mitotic figures x 10 HPF
	Necrosis in form of comedo-like necrosis
Poorly differentiated neuroendocrine carcinoma	Complete loss of "neuroendocrine" growth pattern
	Marked cellular atypia
	> 10 mitotic figures x 10 HPF
	Necrosis

On resected specimens.

5. Moran CA et al: Thymic neuroendocrine carcinomas with combined features ranging from well-differentiated (carcinoid) to small cell carcinoma. A clinicopathologic and immunohistochemical study of 11 cases. Am J Clin Pathol. 113(3):345-50, 2000
6. Klemm KM et al: Primary neuroendocrine carcinomas of the thymus. Semin Diagn Pathol. 16(1):32-41, 1999
7. Moran CA et al: Angiomatoid neuroendocrine carcinoma of the thymus: report of a distinctive morphological variant of neuroendocrine tumor of the thymus resembling a vascular neoplasm. Hum Pathol. 30(6):635-9, 1999
8. Moran CA et al: Spindle-cell neuroendocrine carcinomas of the thymus (spindle-cell thymic carcinoid): a clinicopathologic and immunohistochemical study of seven cases. Mod Pathol. 12(6):587-91, 1999
9. Suster S et al: Thymic carcinoma: spectrum of differentiation and histologic types. Pathology. 30(2):111-22, 1998
10. de Montpréville VT et al: Thymic neuroendocrine carcinoma (carcinoid): a clinicopathologic study of fourteen cases. J Thorac Cardiovasc Surg. 111(1):134-41, 1996
11. Suster S et al: Thymic carcinoid with prominent mucinous stroma. Report of a distinctive morphologic variant of thymic neuroendocrine neoplasm. Am J Surg Pathol. 19(11):1277-85, 1995
12. Suster S et al: Thymic carcinoma. A clinicopathologic study of 60 cases. Cancer. 67(4):1025-32, 1991
13. Wick MR et al: Neuroendocrine neoplasms of the mediastinum. Semin Diagn Pathol. 8(1):35-51, 1991
14. Wick MR et al: Neuroendocrine neoplasms of the thymus. Pathol Res Pract. 183(2):188-99, 1988
15. Wick MR et al: Oat-cell carcinoma of the thymus. Cancer. 49(8):1652-7, 1982

Microscopic Features

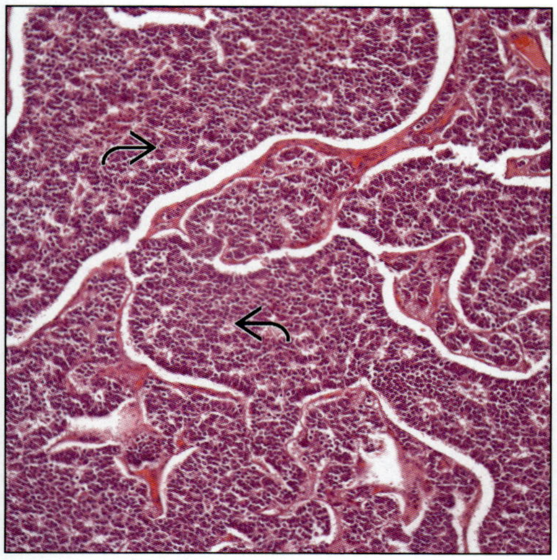

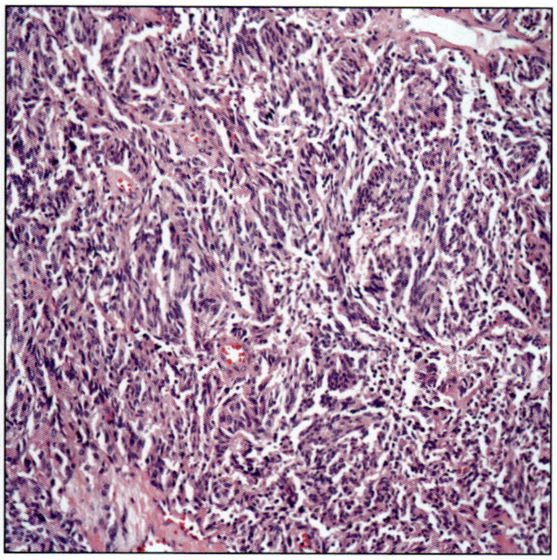

(Left) *Well-differentiated neuroendocrine carcinoma shows a well-organized pattern of growth without the presence of necrosis. Scattered rosettes are present in this tumor.* ***(Right)*** *Well-differentiated neuroendocrine carcinoma with spindle cell features. This histology is also commonly encountered in these tumors. The presence of mitosis and necrosis are important to determine the grade of the tumor.*

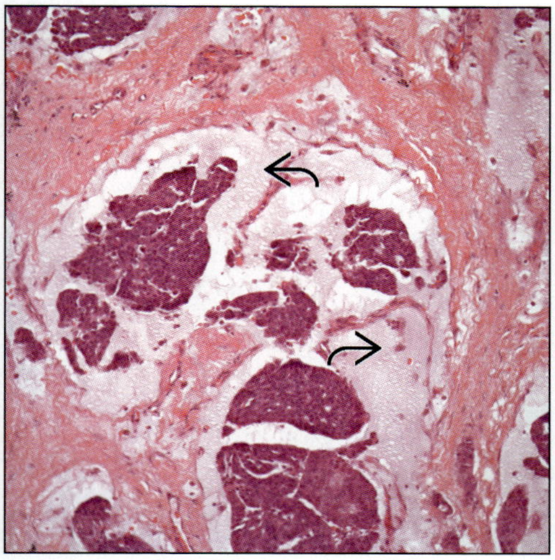

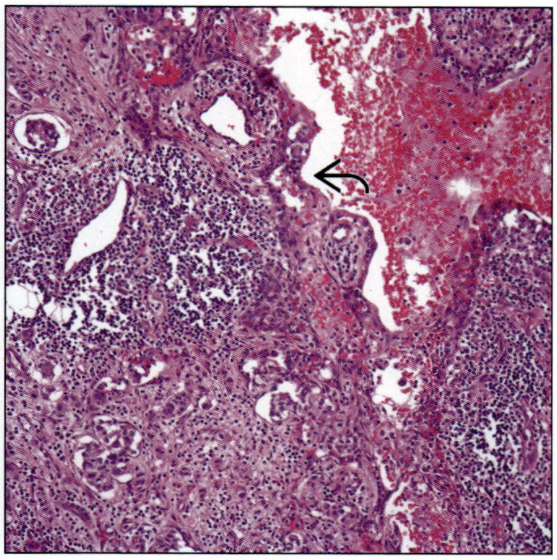

(Left) *Well-differentiated neuroendocrine carcinoma is shown, with prominent mucinous changes in the stroma. This feature is unusual in these tumors in mediastinal location.* ***(Right)*** *Well-differentiated neuroendocrine carcinoma with prominent cystic changes similar to those described in multilocular thymic cysts. The presence of cystic neuroendocrine carcinomas in the mediastinum is rare.*

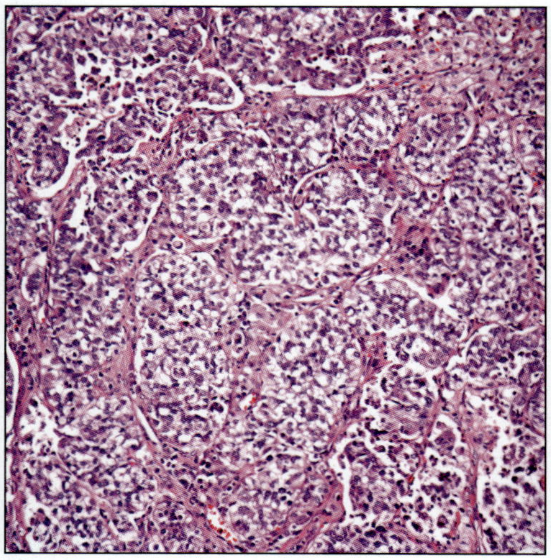

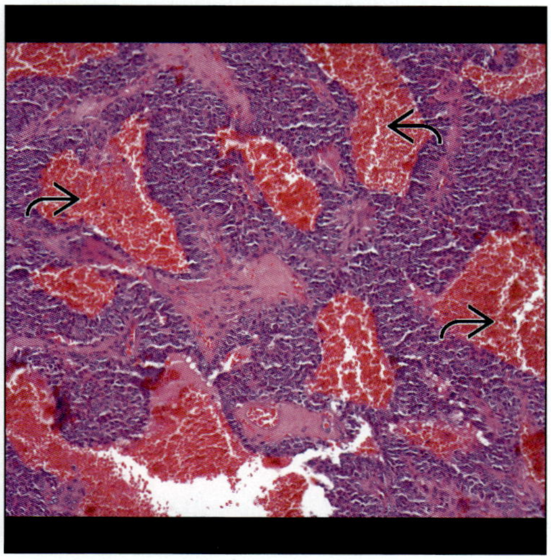

(Left) *Well-differentiated neuroendocrine carcinoma shows striking clear cell features. Still, the tumor shows a subtle nesting pattern of growth.* ***(Right)*** *Well-differentiated neuroendocrine carcinoma is shown with the presence of ectatic spaces containing blood and mimicking a vascular neoplasm. This is the so-called angiomatoid variant of neuroendocrine carcinoma.*

NEUROENDOCRINE CARCINOMAS OF THE THYMUS

Gross and Microscopic Features

(Left) *Thoracic radiograph shows an anterior mediastinal tumor. Superimposed is the actual specimen resected from this patient recapitulating the actual radiological imaging.* ***(Right)*** *Gross photograph shows the bisected anterior mediastinal tumor in the previously displayed radiograph. Note the presence of hemorrhagic areas as well as focal necrotic areas. These are common findings in these tumors.*

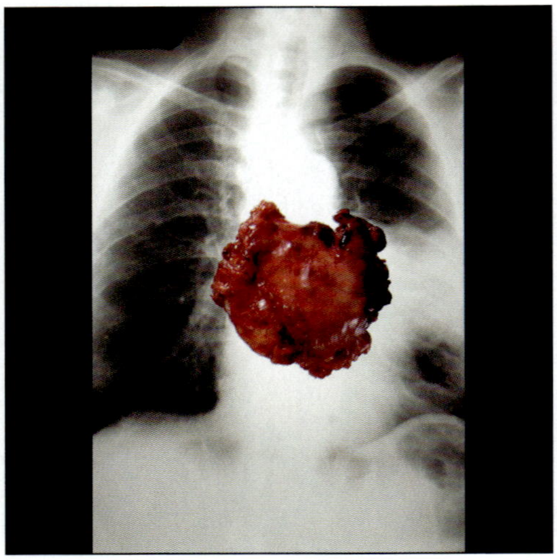

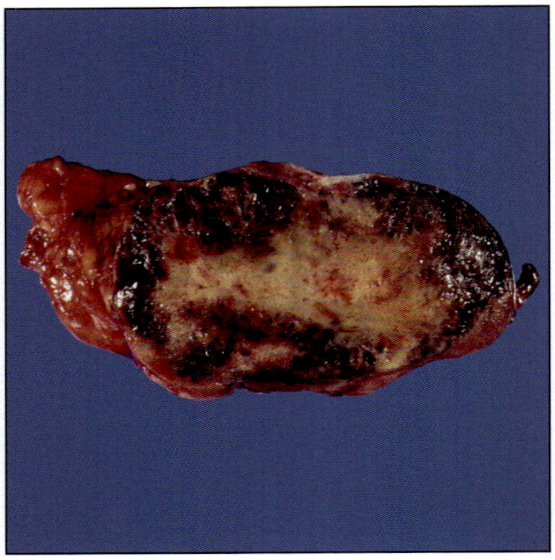

(Left) *Low-power view of moderately differentiated neuroendocrine carcinoma (atypical carcinoid) shows evidence of comedo-like necrosis ↪. This feature by itself is diagnostic of a moderately differentiated tumor.* ***(Right)*** *Moderately differentiated neuroendocrine carcinoma (atypical carcinoid) shows comedo-like necrosis ↪ as well as central calcification →. In addition, note the presence of a more diffuse growth pattern ⇨.*

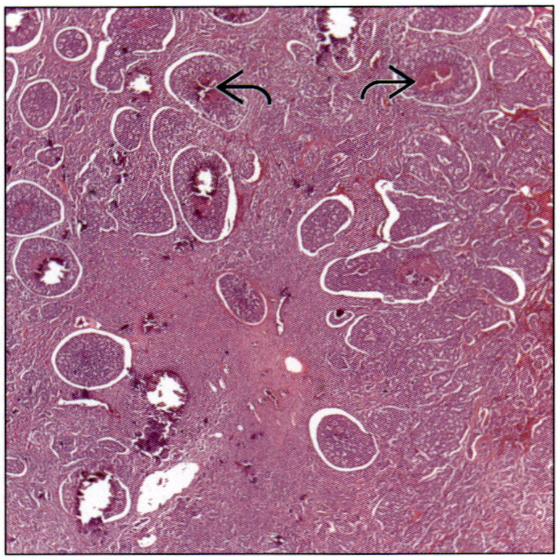

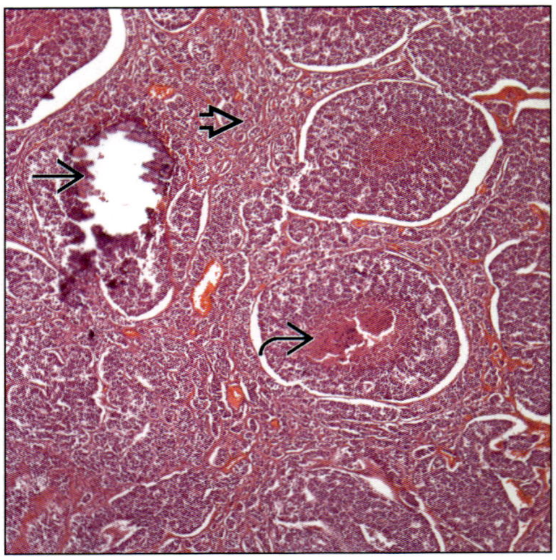

(Left) *Moderately differentiated neuroendocrine carcinoma (atypical carcinoid) shows oncocytic changes and mitotic activity →. The presence of mitotic activity is an important feature for the grading of these tumors.* ***(Right)*** *Spindle cell moderately differentiated neuroendocrine carcinoma shows numerous mitotic figures ↪. A moderately differentiated tumor may be seen in any histological subtype.*

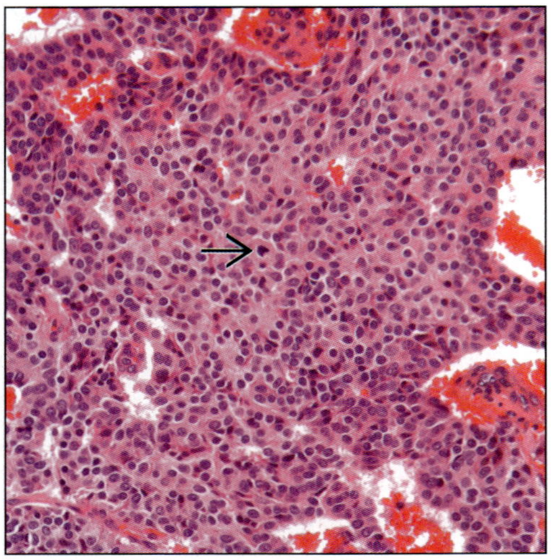

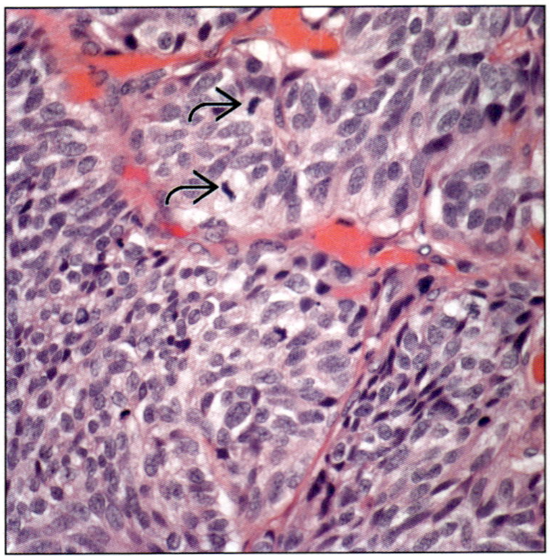

Microscopic Features

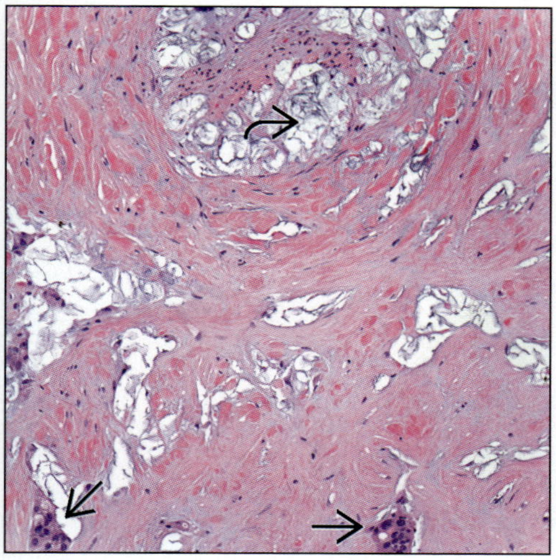

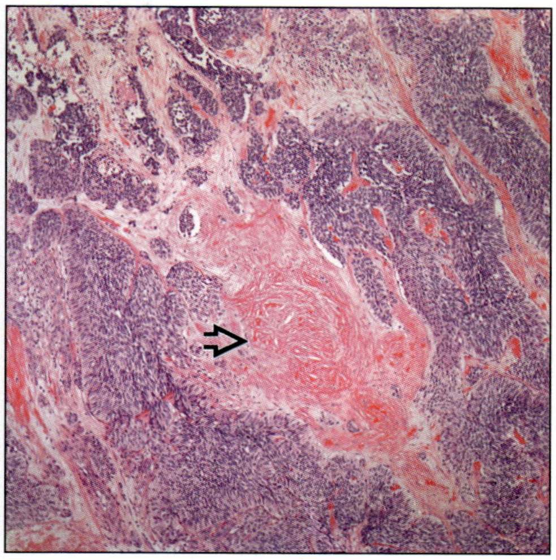

(Left) *Mucinous neuroendocrine carcinoma is shown in which the cellular component is rather scant. The tumor is composed essentially of mucinous material ⇗ and fibroconnective tissue. Note the presence of clusters of neuroendocrine cells ⇒.* ***(Right)*** *Neuroendocrine carcinoma is shown with prominent sclerotic changes ⇨. These changes may be seen in other neuroendocrine mediastinal tumors as well.*

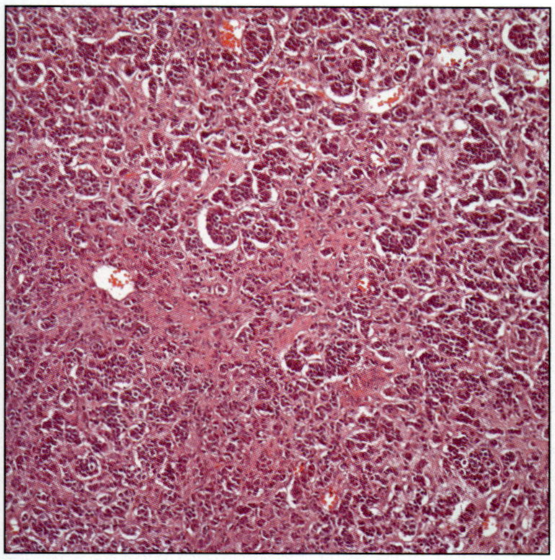

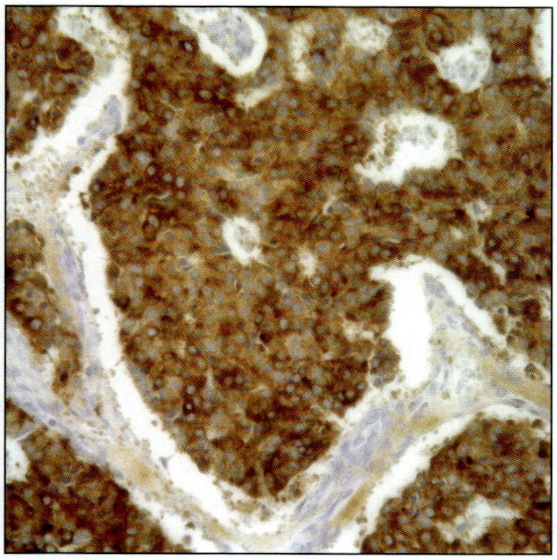

(Left) *Moderately differentiated neuroendocrine carcinoma (atypical carcinoid) shows a loss of the organoid pattern, and the tumor shows a disorganized pattern of growth.* ***(Right)*** *Chromogranin-A shows strong positive staining in neuroendocrine carcinomas; thus, it is a useful marker for these tumors. However, it is important to keep in mind that chromogranin staining may also be positive in other neuroendocrine tumors.*

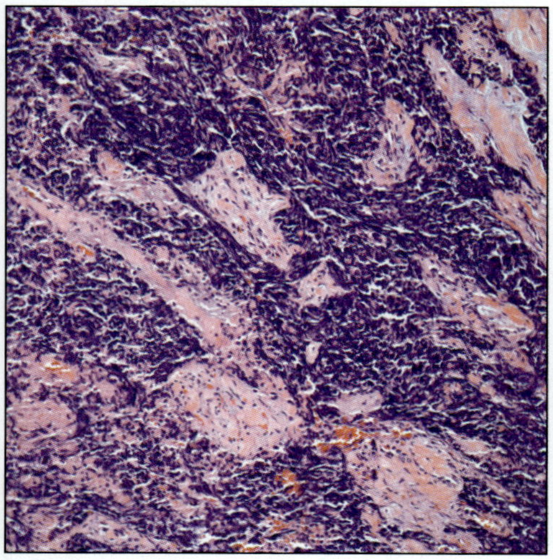

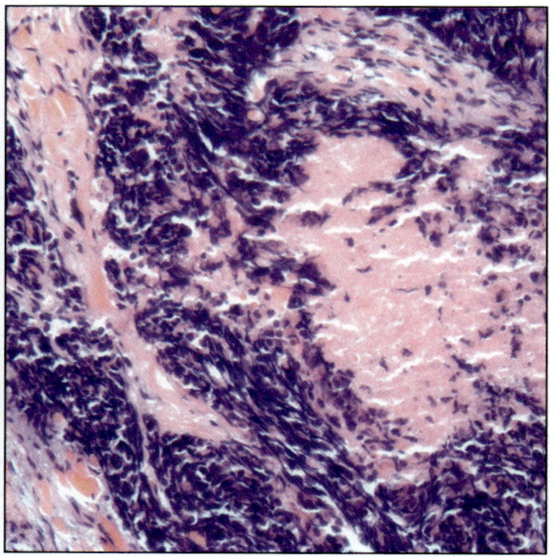

(Left) *High-grade neuroendocrine carcinoma (small cell type) is shown. The features are similar to those seen in small cell carcinomas of the lung. This type of tumor is unusual in the thymus.* ***(Right)*** *Small cell carcinoma of the anterior mediastinum (high-grade neuroendocrine carcinoma) shows the presence of necrosis and crush artifact. The criteria for the diagnosis of this tumor are the same as those for pulmonary small cell carcinoma.*

MEDIASTINAL TERATOMA

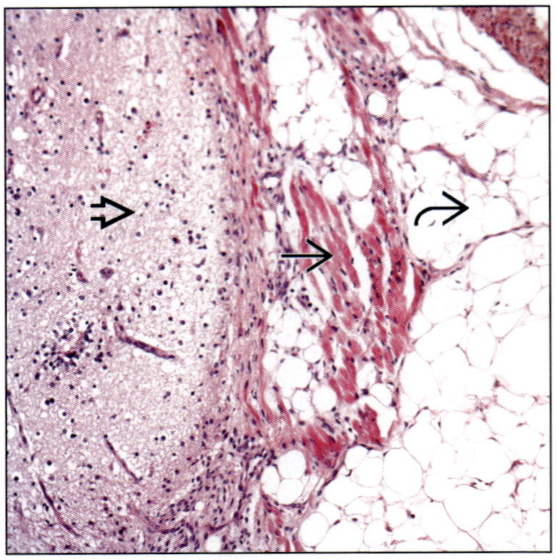

Mediastinal teratoma shows mature glial tissue ⇨ adjacent to fibers of skeletal muscle → and mature adipose tissue ↷. Note that all tissues are mature.

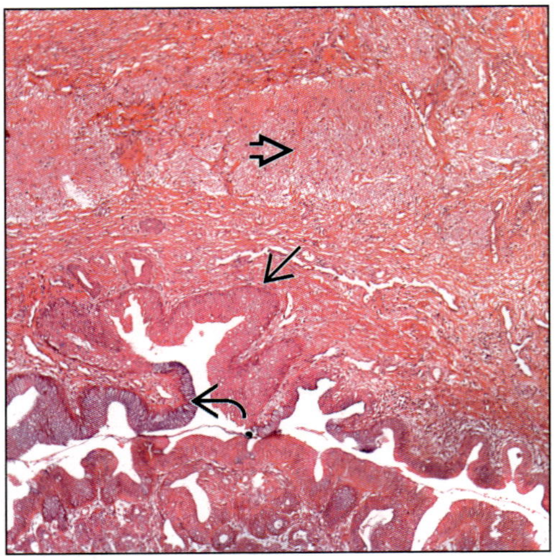

Mediastinal mature teratoma is shown with presence of cystic structures lined by squamous → and glandular epithelium ↶. Mature glial tissue is also present ⇨.

TERMINOLOGY

Definitions

- Neoplasm showing tissues derived from 3 germinal layers
  - At least 2 must be present

ETIOLOGY/PATHOGENESIS

Etiology

- Although an unequivocal explanation for the occurrence of mediastinal germ cell tumors is not available, some authors have proposed the possibility of ectopically misplaced germ cells

CLINICAL ISSUES

Epidemiology

- Incidence
  - Most common germ cell tumors in anterior mediastinum
  - Approximately 45% of all mediastinal germ cell tumors
- Age
  - More common in young individuals
  - Teratomas are most common germ cell tumor in children
- Gender
  - Mature teratomas may be more common in males (approximately 2:1)
  - Teratomas with malignant component may be more common in males

Site

- Teratomas more common in anterior mediastinum
- Posterior mediastinum may be site in unusual cases

Presentation

- Cough
- Chest pain
- Dyspnea
- Hemoptysis
- Klinefelter syndrome
- Hematologic conditions
- Precocious puberty
- Asymptomatic

Treatment

- Surgical approaches
  - Mature teratomas: Complete surgical resection
  - Immature teratomas: Chemotherapy may be used
  - Teratomas with another malignant component: Chemotherapy

Prognosis

- Mature teratomas: Prognosis is good in majority of cases
- Immature teratomas: Depends on clinical stage
- Teratomas with another malignant component: Clinical stage and type and percentage of malignant component are important parameters to determine prognosis

IMAGE FINDINGS

General Features

- Calcification in 20-40% of cases
- Fat-fluid levels are considered classic for teratomas

MACROSCOPIC FEATURES

General Features

- Cyst and solid tumors
- Presence of hair or teeth
- Presence of sebaceous material

Sections to Be Submitted

- Sections from solid and cystic areas must be evaluated

Key Facts

Etiology/Pathogenesis
- Some authors have proposed the possibility of ectopically misplaced germ cells

Clinical Issues
- Incidence
  - Most common germ cell tumors in anterior mediastinum
  - Approximately 45% of all mediastinal germ cell tumors
  - More common in young individuals
  - Most common germ cell tumor in children
  - May be more common in males (approximately 2:1)
  - Teratomas with malignant component may be more common in males
- Symptoms
  - Precocious puberty
  - Hematologic conditions
  - Chest pain
  - Dyspnea
  - Asymptomatic

Macroscopic Features
- Cyst and solid tumors
- Presence of hair or teeth
- Presence of sebaceous material

Microscopic Pathology
- Mature elements derived from 3 germ cell layers
  - Mature teratoma
  - Immature teratoma
  - Teratomas with malignant component

- Reasonable number of sections needs to be submitted for histological evaluation

Size
- Vary in size from a few cm to > 15 cm in diameter

MICROSCOPIC PATHOLOGY

Histologic Features
- Mature teratoma
  - Mature elements derived from 3 germ cell layers
  - Pancreatic tissue is commonly seen
  - Presence of skin adnexa is commonly seen
- Immature teratoma
  - Presence of neural tubules
  - Presence of rosettes
- Teratomas with malignant component
  - Seminoma
  - Yolk sac tumor
  - Embryonal carcinoma
  - Choriocarcinoma
  - Another malignant epithelial component: Adenocarcinoma, etc.
- Presence of malignant mesenchymal component
  - Angiosarcoma
  - Rhabdomyosarcoma
  - Osteosarcoma
  - Chondrosarcoma

Predominant Pattern/Injury Type
- Biphasic

Predominant Cell/Compartment Type
- Germ, nonseminomatous

DIFFERENTIAL DIAGNOSIS

Sarcoma
- Pure malignant mesenchymal neoplasms (sarcomas) do not show other type of epithelial differentiation

Carcinoma
- Strictly malignant epithelial tumors; do not show other germinal layer components

Other Germ Cell Tumor
- Presence of at least 2 different germ cell layers is diagnostic of teratoma

DIAGNOSTIC CHECKLIST

Clinically Relevant Pathologic Features
- Gross appearance

Pathologic Interpretation Pearls
- Presence of following features should help in diagnosis
  - Tissues from different germ cell layers
  - Neural tubules &/or rosettes
  - Malignant mesenchymal components
- Determine percentage of different components: Mature, immature, and malignant

SELECTED REFERENCES

1. Barksdale EM Jr et al: Teratomas in infants and children. Curr Opin Pediatr. 21(3):344-9, 2009
2. El Mesbahi O et al: Chemotherapy in patients with teratoma with malignant transformation. Eur Urol. 51(5):1306-11; discussion 1311-2, 2007
3. Malagón HD et al: Germ cell tumors with sarcomatous components: a clinicopathologic and immunohistochemical study of 46 cases. Am J Surg Pathol. 31(9):1356-62, 2007
4. Romagnani E et al: Mediastinal mature teratoma with an immature component--what about the treatment?. Ann Oncol. 17(10):1602-4, 2006
5. Moeller KH et al: Mediastinal mature teratoma: imaging features. AJR Am J Roentgenol. 169(4):985-90, 1997
6. Moran CA et al: Primary germ cell tumors of the mediastinum: I. Analysis of 322 cases with special emphasis on teratomatous lesions and a proposal for histopathologic classification and clinical staging. Cancer. 80(4):681-90, 1997

MEDIASTINAL TERATOMA

Immunohistochemistry

Antibody	Reactivity	Staining Pattern	Comment
S100	Positive	Nuclear & cytoplasmic	In neural component of mature and immature teratomas
NSE	Positive	Cytoplasmic	In neural or epithelial components
GFAP	Positive	Cytoplasmic	In neural components
CK-PAN	Positive	Cytoplasmic	In epithelial components
Desmin	Positive	Cytoplasmic	In muscle components
MYOD1	Positive	Cytoplasmic	Rhabdomyoblastic differentiation
Myoglobin	Positive	Cytoplasmic	Rhabdomyoblastic differentiation
FVIIIRAg	Positive	Cytoplasmic	Vascular differentiation
CD31	Positive	Cytoplasmic	Vascular differentiation
α-fetoprotein	Positive	Cytoplasmic	If yolk sac or embryonal carcinoma is present
PLAP	Positive	Cytoplasmic	If seminoma is present
HCG	Positive	Cytoplasmic	If choriocarcinoma is present
Chromogranin-A	Positive	Cytoplasmic	If neuroendocrine elements are present
Synaptophysin	Positive	Cytoplasmic	If neuroendocrine or neural elements are present
CD34	Positive	Cytoplasmic	If vascular elements are present
CK5/6	Positive	Cytoplasmic	In squamous elements
p63	Positive	Nuclear	In squamous elements
CEA-M	Positive	Cytoplasmic	In carcinomatous as well as normal glandular elements
PLACEN_LACT	Positive	Cytoplasmic	Germ cell components
CD30	Positive	Golgi zone	If embryonal carcinoma is present
CD117	Positive	Nuclear & cytoplasmic	In seminomatous components

Histological Classification of Mediastinal Teratomas

Tumor	Definition
Mature teratoma	Only mature elements representing different germ layers
Immature teratoma	Mature elements admixed with neural tubules &/or rosettes
Teratoma with malignant component	
Type I	Teratomas with another germ cell component (seminoma, yolk sac tumor, embryonal carcinoma, choriocarcinoma)
Type II	Teratomas with malignant epithelial non-germ cell component (squamous cell carcinoma, adenocarcinoma, small cell carcinoma, etc.)
Type III	Teratoma with malignant mesenchymal component (rhabdomyosarcoma, osteosarcoma, angiosarcoma, etc.)
Type IV	Teratoma with any combination of the above
Mature teratomas	Represent ~ 65% of all cases
Immature teratomas	Represent ~ 5% of all cases
Teratomas with malignant component	Represent ~ 30% of all cases

Clinical Staging of Mediastinal Germ Cell Tumors

Stage	Description
I	Well-circumscribed tumor ± focal adhesions to pleura or pericardium but without microscopic evidence of invasion into adjacent organs
II	Tumor confined to mediastinum with macroscopic &/or microscopic evidence of infiltration into adjacent structures (pleura, pericardium, great vessels)
III	Tumor with metastases
IIIA	Metastases to intrathoracic organs (lymph nodes, lung, etc.)
IIIB	Extrathoracic metastases

MEDIASTINAL TERATOMA

Mature Teratoma

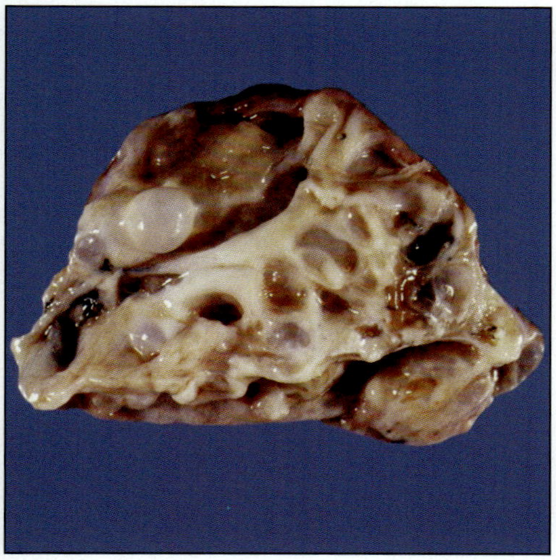

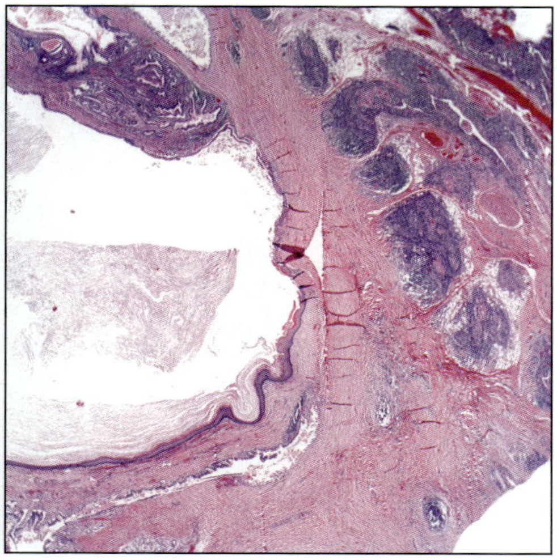

(Left) *Gross photograph shows a mediastinal teratoma. Note the presence of cystic structures admixed with solid areas. Since there are no macroscopic features to separate immature from other possible malignant components, it is very important to properly sample these tumors.* ***(Right)*** *Low-power view shows a mediastinal teratoma displaying cystic structures and solid areas, all of them with mature elements.*

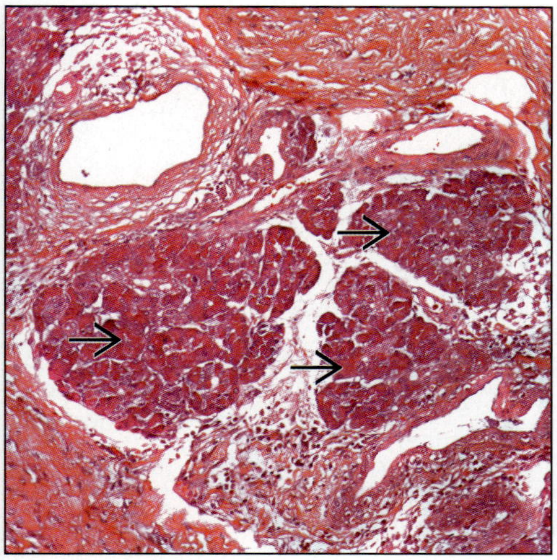

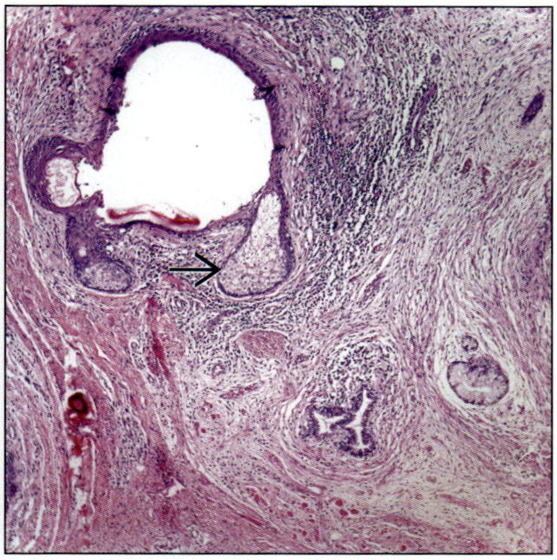

(Left) *Mature teratoma shows acinar structures compatible with pancreas →. Pancreas is a common component in mediastinal teratomas, and in some cases, it may be a functioning pancreas.* ***(Right)*** *Mediastinal mature teratoma shows skin appendages → admixed with other mature cystic elements embedded in a fibroconnective tissue stroma. These structures are invariably present in the great majority of mature teratomas.*

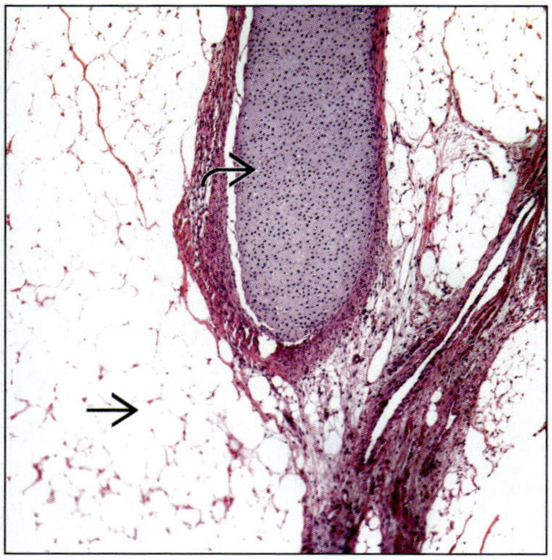

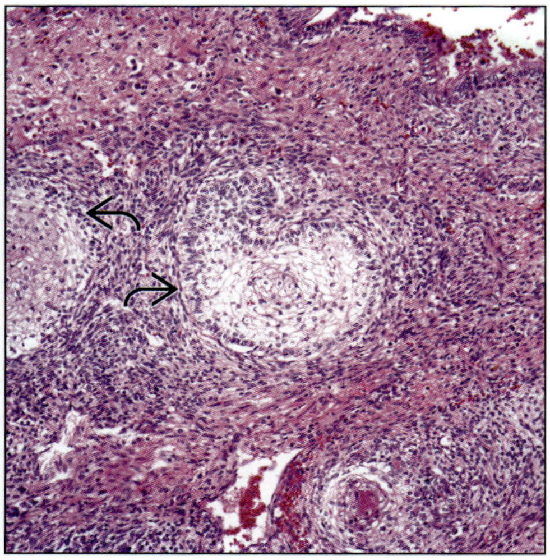

(Left) *Mature teratoma shows 2 classical mature component in these tumors: Mature cartilage ↗ and mature adipose tissue →.* ***(Right)*** *Mature teratoma shows dense fibroconnective tissue with only focal dermal appendages ↗. This feature is commonly seen in mature teratomas.*

MEDIASTINAL TERATOMA

Immature Teratoma

(Left) *Gross photograph shows an immature mediastinal teratoma. Although this particular tumor shows more solid than cystic areas, there is really not a way to separate mature from immature tumors. However, the presence of solid areas should be suspicious for immature or other malignant components. Note the presence of residual thymic gland.* ***(Right)*** *Immature teratoma shows areas of rosette formation and neurotubules embedded in an immature stromal tissue.*

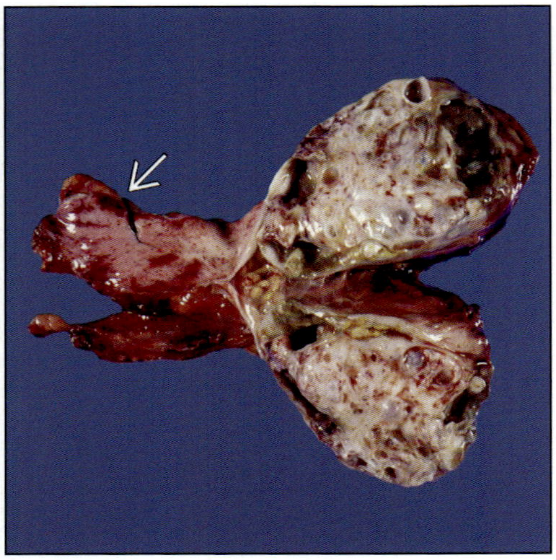

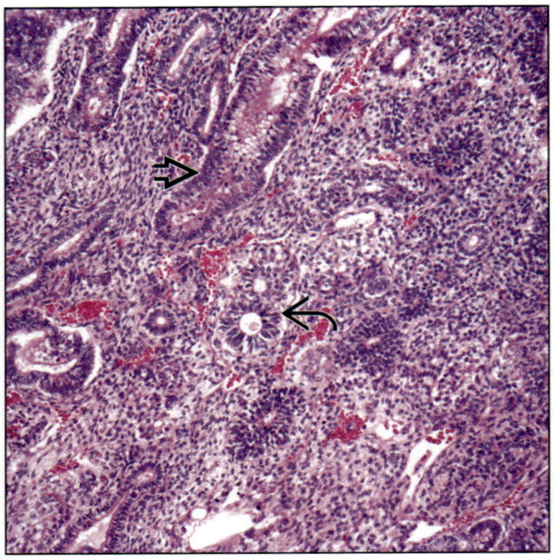

(Left) *Mediastinal immature teratoma shows prominent solid areas with only scattered tubular neural structures.* ***(Right)*** *Closer view shows a mediastinal immature teratoma displaying solid and classical areas of immature neural differentiation. This feature is reminiscent to that seen in cases of neuroblastoma, and often there is more cellular atypia and mitotic activity.*

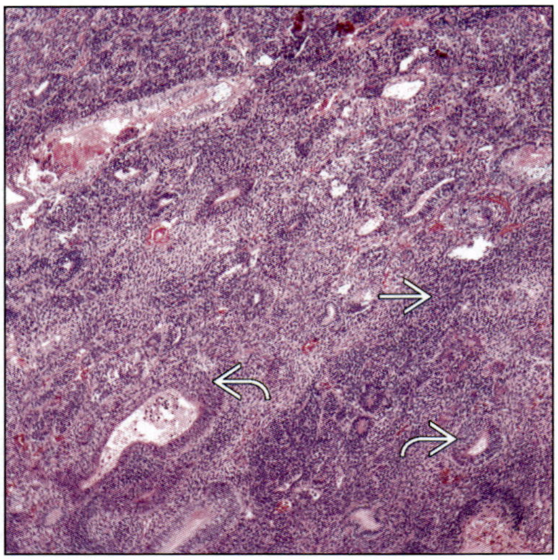

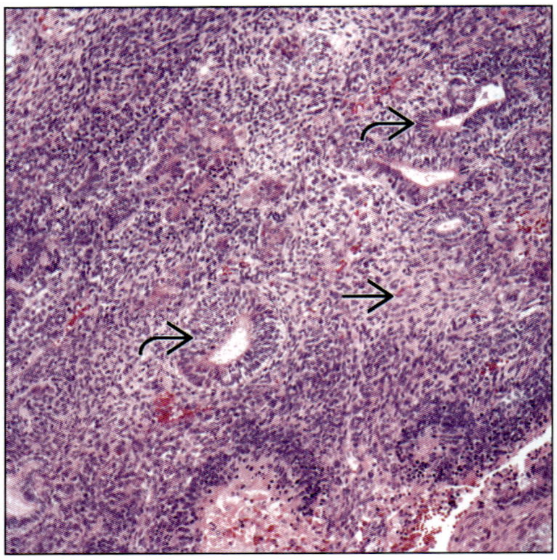

(Left) *Mediastinal immature teratoma is shown with neural rosettes admixed with cartilage. It is common to see mature and immature elements admixed with each other. Pure immature teratomas are extremely rare, if any exist at all.* ***(Right)*** *Solid highly atypical areas of neural tissue admixed with neural rosettes. These histological features are classic for the diagnosis of immature teratoma.*

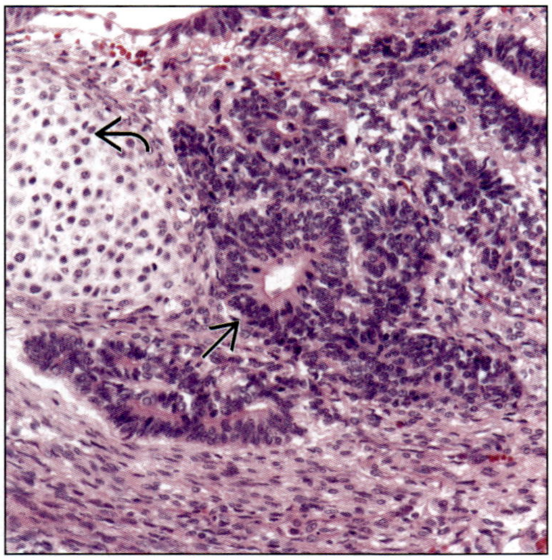

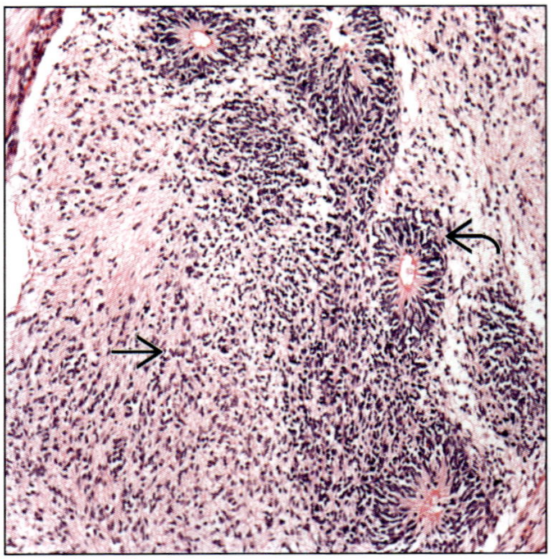

Teratoma with Malignant Component

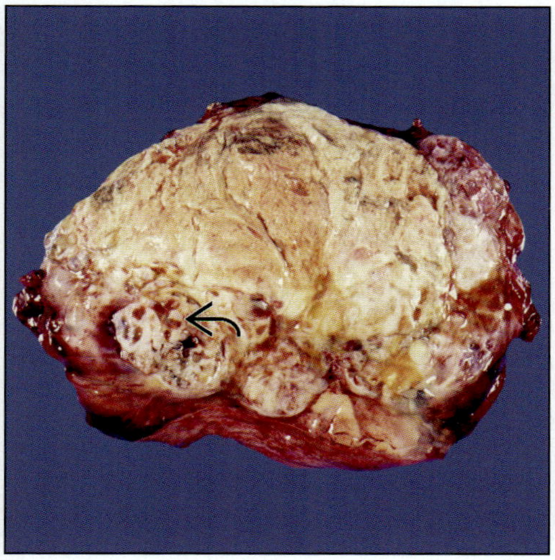
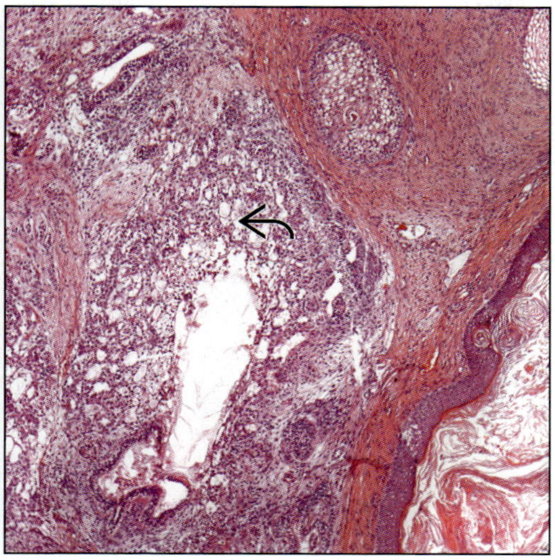

(Left) Gross photograph shows a mediastinal teratoma with a malignant component. Once again, the presence of solid areas should raise the suspicion of a possible malignant component. Ample sampling is crucial for this diagnosis. Note that this tumor also shows cystic areas ⮫. **(Right)** Light microscopy shows a mediastinal teratoma with a malignant component. In this particular case, the malignant component is that of a yolk sac tumor ⮫. This corresponds to type I.

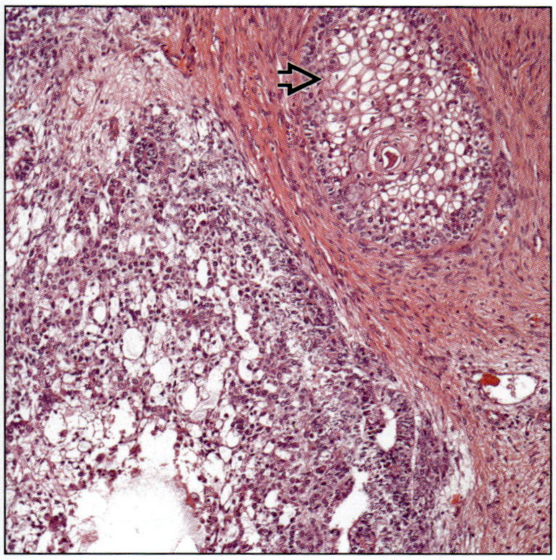
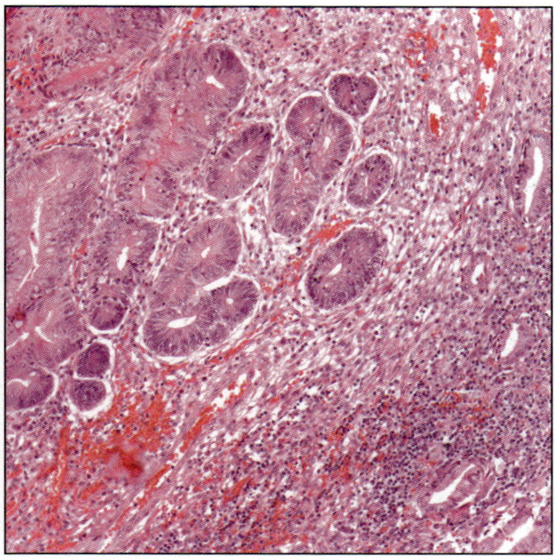

(Left) Closer view shows the yolk sac component of this teratomatous lesion. The tumor also displays mature elements in the form of appendages ⇨. This type of teratoma corresponds to type I, which is a teratoma associated with another germ cell tumor. **(Right)** Mediastinal teratoma is shown with a malignant component. In this case, the malignant component is adenocarcinoma, a malignant epithelial component. This corresponds to type II.

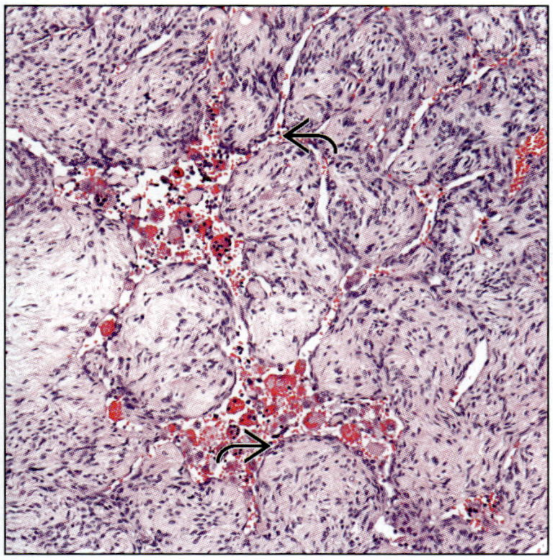
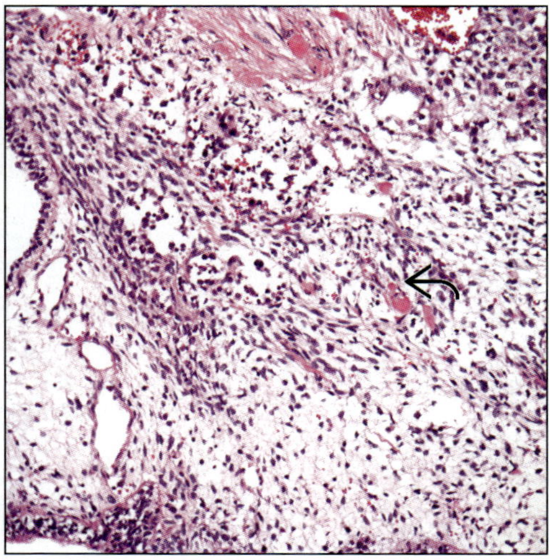

(Left) Type III teratoma with a malignant mesenchymal component. Note the anastomosing vascular channels ⮫ in keeping with angiosarcoma. **(Right)** Mediastinal teratoma is shown with a malignant component of type III. Note the presence of rhabdomyoblastic differentiation ⮫. In some cases, the malignant mesenchymal component may be of the undifferentiated type.

MEDIASTINAL SEMINOMA

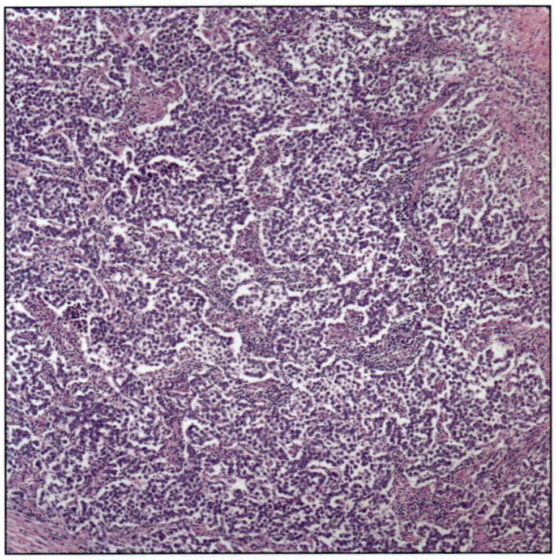

Low-power view of a thymic seminoma is shown with sheets of neoplastic cells with little intervening stroma and scattered inflammatory cells.

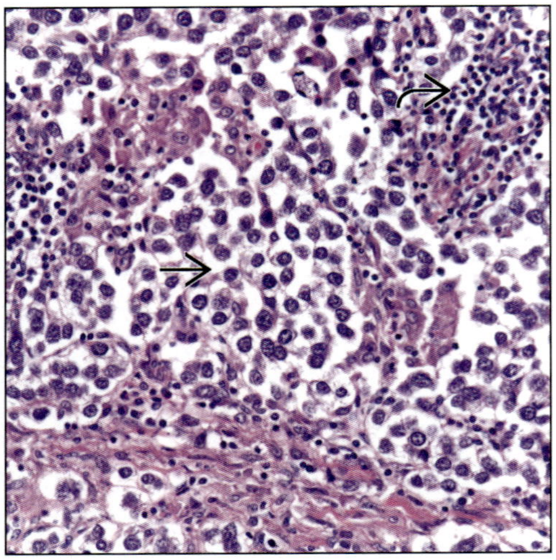

High-power view of a thymic seminoma displays sheets of neoplastic cells ➔ with a discrete inflammatory reaction composed of lymphocytes ➚.

TERMINOLOGY

Synonyms

- Thymic seminoma, germinoma

Definitions

- Malignant germ cell tumor

ETIOLOGY/PATHOGENESIS

Etiology

- Although etiology of these tumors is unknown, some theories have stated that misplaced germ cells in anterior mediastinum may be origin of these tumors

CLINICAL ISSUES

Epidemiology

- Incidence
  - Difficult to determine exact incidence
  - 2nd most common germ cell tumor after teratomas
  - May account for approximately 37% of all germ cell tumors
- Age
  - Majority of tumors occur in young adults between ages of 20 and 30 years
  - Highly unusual in patients < 12 years old
  - Minority of cases in adult patients > 60 years old
- Gender
  - Almost exclusive occurrence in males
  - Only a few cases reported in females

Site

- Anterior mediastinal tumor
- Rarely in posterior mediastinum

Presentation

- Shortness of breath
- Cough
- Chest pain
- Hemoptysis
- Superior vena cava syndrome
- Gynecomastia
- Pulmonic stenosis
- Ventricular septal defect
- Congenital absence of thoracic hemivertebrae
- In some cases, patients may be asymptomatic

Treatment

- Chemotherapy
- Radiation therapy

Prognosis

- Depends on clinical staging
- May be better in younger than in older patients

IMAGE FINDINGS

General Features

- Large, bulky tumors
- Well marginated
- May extend to both sides of the midline

CT Findings

- Homogeneous attenuation equal to soft tissue

MACROSCOPIC FEATURES

General Features

- Large tumors
- Slightly lobulated, firm and tan
- Cystic tumor can occur in < 10% of cases

Size

- Vary in size from a few cm to > 15 cm in greatest dimension

MEDIASTINAL SEMINOMA

Key Facts

Terminology
- Thymic seminoma

Etiology/Pathogenesis
- Probably misplaced germ cells in anterior mediastinum

Clinical Issues
- Incidence
  - May account for approximately 37% of all germ cell tumors
  - Majority of tumors occur in young adults between ages of 20 and 30 years
  - Almost exclusive occurrence in men
- Symptoms
  - Gynecomastia
  - Superior vena cava syndrome
  - Chest pain

Macroscopic Features
- Large tumors
- Cystic tumor can occur in < 10% of cases

Top Differential Diagnoses
- Carcinoma
- Lymphoma
- Melanoma
- Thymoma
- Metastatic seminoma from testicular origin

Diagnostic Checklist
- Sheets of neoplastic cells
- Inflammatory component (lymphocytes)
- Cells with clear or eosinophilic cytoplasm
- PLAP positive immunohistochemical study

MICROSCOPIC PATHOLOGY

Histologic Features
- Sheets or discrete nesting pattern
- Medium-sized cells
- Clear or lightly eosinophilic cytoplasm
- Inflammatory infiltrate (lymphocytes)

Predominant Pattern/Injury Type
- Sheets

Predominant Cell/Compartment Type
- Germ, seminomatous

DIFFERENTIAL DIAGNOSIS

Carcinoma
- Displays lobulation and more cellular pleomorphism
- Positive reaction for PLAP unusual

Lymphoma
- May show extensive areas of fibrosis
- Shows negative staining for CK-LMW-NOS and PLAP

Melanoma
- Shows positive staining for S100 protein and mart-1; negative for keratin and PLAP

Thymoma
- Shows classical features of lobulation and mixed biphasic cellular components

Metastatic Seminoma from Testicular Origin
- Rarely metastasizes as bulky anterior mediastinal tumor
- May metastasize to mediastinal lymph nodes
- Identical histopathological and immunohistochemical features for both tumors (mediastinal and testicular)

DIAGNOSTIC CHECKLIST

Clinically Relevant Pathologic Features
- Age distribution

Pathologic Interpretation Pearls
- Sheets of neoplastic cells
- Inflammatory component (lymphocytes)
- Cells with clear or eosinophilic cytoplasm
- PLAP positive immunohistochemical study

SELECTED REFERENCES

1. Giannis M et al: Cisplatin-based chemotherapy for advanced seminoma: report of 52 cases treated in two institutions. J Cancer Res Clin Oncol. 135(11):1495-500, 2009
2. Sung MT et al: Primary mediastinal seminoma: a comprehensive assessment integrated with histology, immunohistochemistry, and fluorescence in situ hybridization for chromosome 12p abnormalities in 23 cases. Am J Surg Pathol. 32(1):146-55, 2008
3. Malagón HD et al: Germ cell tumors with sarcomatous components: a clinicopathologic and immunohistochemical study of 46 cases. Am J Surg Pathol. 31(9):1356-62, 2007
4. Bedano PM et al: Metachronous intracranial germinoma in a patient with a previous primary mediastinal seminoma. J Clin Oncol. 24(15):2386-7, 2006
5. Miyawaki M et al: [High-dose chemotherapy with peripheral blood stem cell auto transplantation for an intractable case of mediastinal seminoma.] Gan To Kagaku Ryoho. 33(6):845-8, 2006
6. Ravenel JG et al: Primary posterior mediastinal seminoma. AJR Am J Roentgenol. 183(6):1835-7, 2004
7. Takeda S et al: Primary germ cell tumors in the mediastinum: a 50-year experience at a single Japanese institution. Cancer. 97(2):367-76, 2003
8. Chhieng DC et al: Fine-needle aspiration biopsy of nonteratomatous germ cell tumors of the mediastinum. Am J Clin Pathol. 118(3):418-24, 2002
9. Strollo DC et al: Primary mediastinal malignant germ cell neoplasms: imaging features. Chest Surg Clin N Am. 12(4):645-58, 2002

MEDIASTINAL SEMINOMA

Immunohistochemistry

Antibody	Reactivity	Staining Pattern	Comment
PLAP	Positive	Cytoplasmic	
CK8/18/CAM5.2	Positive	Cytoplasmic	
CD117	Positive	Nuclear & cytoplasmic	
HPL	Positive	Cytoplasmic	
CK-PAN	Positive	Cytoplasmic	Weak
Vimentin	Positive	Cytoplasmic	
HCG	Positive	Cytoplasmic	Scattered cells
EMA	Negative		
CEA-M	Negative		
α-fetoprotein	Negative		
CD30	Negative		

Histological, Histochemical, and Molecular Features Associated with Mediastinal Seminomas

Histological Feature	Percentage
Thymic remnants	~ 27% of cases
Noncaseous granulomatous inflammation	~ 46% of cases
Lymphoid hyperplasia	~ 10% of cases
Cystic changes	< 10% of cases
Syncytiotrophoblastic component	< 5% of cases
Necrosis	~ 25% of cases
K-ras-2 genotype	Normal in ~ 90% of cases
Mutation in codon 13	In a few cases
PAS	Positive for intracytoplasmic glycogen
D-PAS	Negative for intracellular mucin
Mucicarmine	Negative for intracellular mucin

Clinical Staging of Mediastinal Germ Cell tumors

Stage	Description
I	Well-circumscribed tumor ± focal adhesions to pleura or pericardium but without microscopic evidence of invasion into adjacent structures
II	Tumor confined to mediastinum with macroscopic &/or microscopic evidence of infiltration into adjacent structures (pleura, pericardium, great vessels)
III	Tumor with metastases
IIIA	With metastases to intrathoracic organs (lymph nodes, lung, etc.)
IIIB	With extrathoracic metastases

10. Bokemeyer C et al: Extragonadal seminoma: an international multicenter analysis of prognostic factors and long term treatment outcome. Cancer. 91(7):1394-401, 2001
11. Moran CA: Germ cell tumors of the mediastinum. Pathol Res Pract. 195(8):583-7, 1999
12. Weidner N: Germ-cell tumors of the mediastinum. Semin Diagn Pathol. 16(1):42-50, 1999
13. Suster S et al: Germ cell tumors of the mediastinum and testis: a comparative immunohistochemical study of 120 cases. Hum Pathol. 29(7):737-42, 1998
14. Moran CA et al: Primary germ cell tumors of the mediastinum: II. Mediastinal seminomas--a clinicopathologic and immunohistochemical study of 120 cases. Cancer. 80(4):691-8, 1997
15. Przygodzki RM et al: Primary mediastinal and testicular seminomas: a comparison of K-ras-2 gene sequence and p53 immunoperoxidase analysis of 26 cases. Hum Pathol. 27(9):975-9, 1996
16. Moran CA et al: Mediastinal seminomas with prominent cystic changes. A clinicopathologic study of 10 cases. Am J Surg Pathol. 19(9):1047-53, 1995
17. Rosado-de-Christenson ML et al: From the archives of the AFIP. Mediastinal germ cell tumors: radiologic and pathologic correlation. Radiographics. 12(5):1013-30, 1992

Gross and Microscopic Features

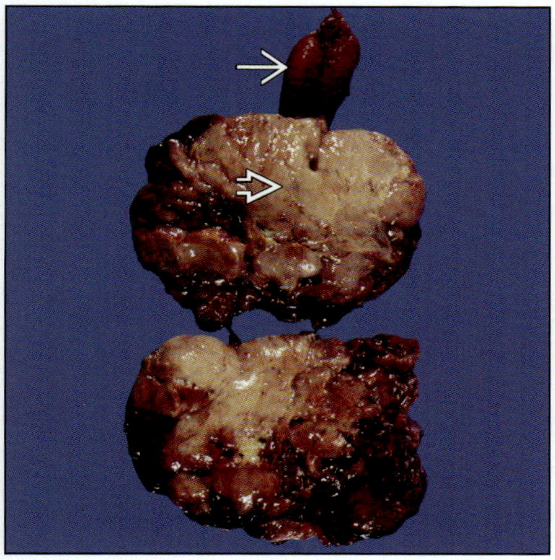
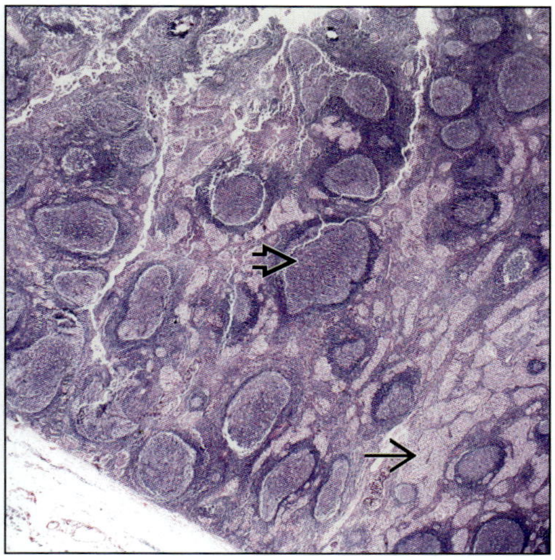

(Left) Gross photograph of a thymic seminoma shows a soft, light brown to tan tumor with a homogeneous fleshy surface ➔. On the upper portion, one can still see grossly identifiable remnants of the thymic gland ➔. *(Right)* Low-power view of a thymic seminoma shows the presence of marked follicular hyperplasia ➔, and within hyperplastic follicles, neoplastic seminoma cells ➔. This pattern can be confused with a mediastinal lymphoma.

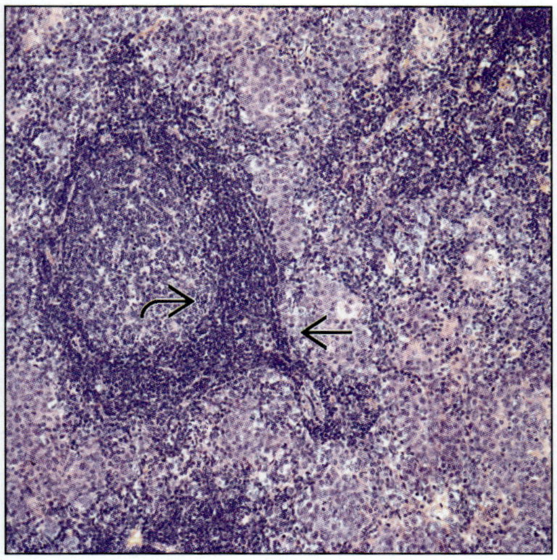
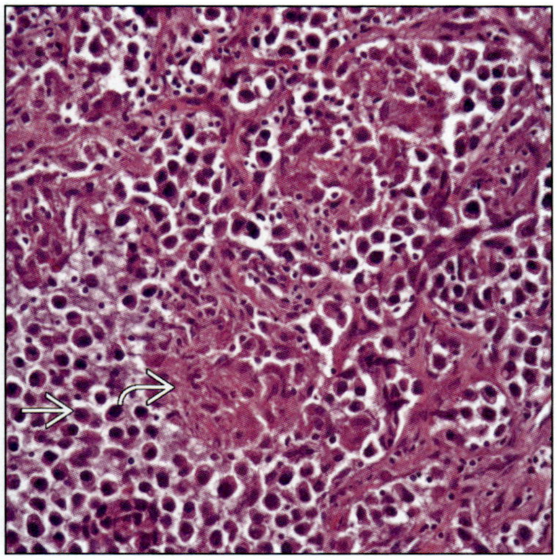

(Left) High-power view of a mediastinal seminoma demonstrates the difference between the 2 populations of cells, clearly distinguishing the neoplastic seminomatous component ➔ from the hyperplastic lymphoid follicle ➔. *(Right)* Higher magnification of a mediastinal seminoma shows close association between the ill-defined granulomas ➔ and the neoplastic cells ➔.

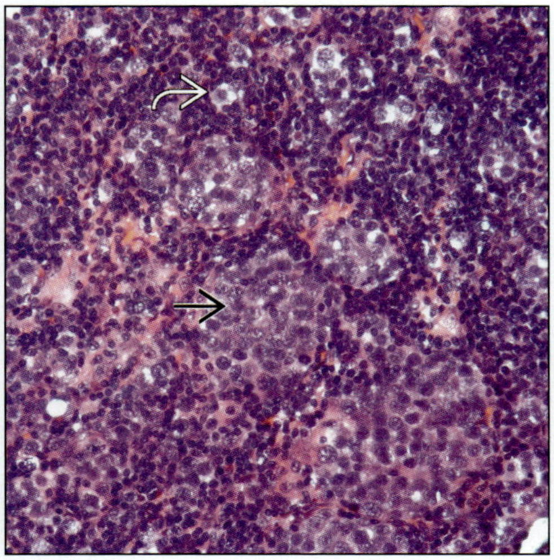
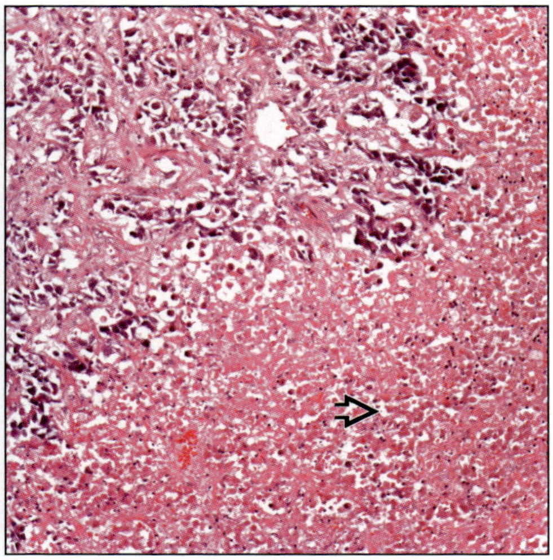

(Left) Thymic seminoma displays numerous clusters of neoplastic cells ➔ embedded in a lymphoid stroma. In some areas of heavy lymphoid component, there are neoplastic cells intimately admixed with lymphocytes ➔. *(Right)* Seminoma with extensive areas of necrosis ➔. In this setting, many times it is difficult to identify classical seminoma cells, thus the need for immunohistochemical studies.

MEDIASTINAL SEMINOMA

Microscopic Features

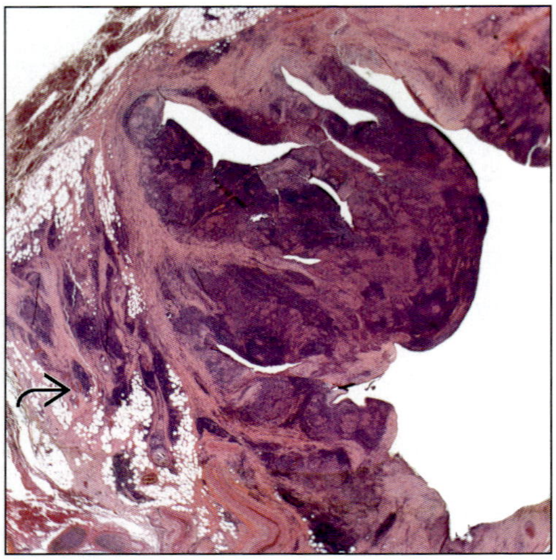

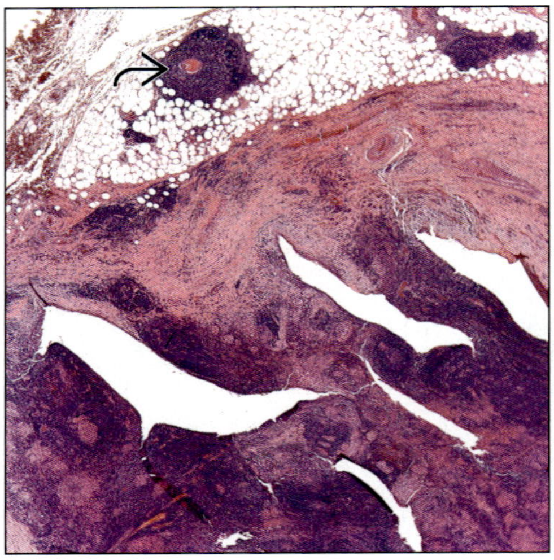

(Left) *Low-power view of a thymic cystic seminoma mimics a benign thymic cystic lesion. Note that the cystic walls show a dense inflammatory reaction admixed with a noncaseous granulomatous reaction and adjacent remnants of thymic tissue* ↪*.* ***(Right)*** *Hematoxylin & eosin shows a cystic seminoma in which the walls are heavily infiltrated by a dense inflammatory reaction, making it difficult to observe the neoplastic cells. Residual thymus is present* ↪*.*

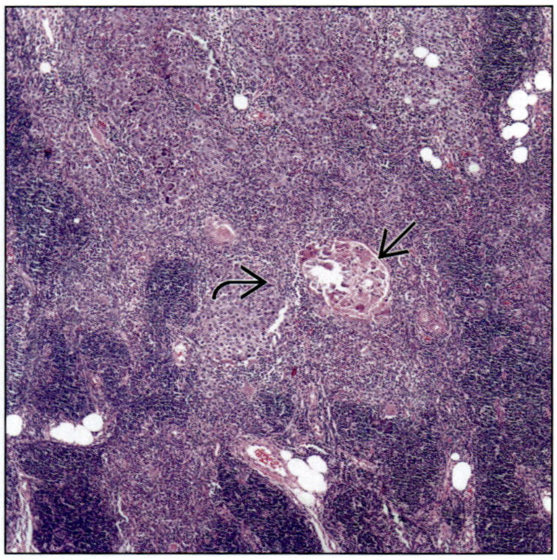

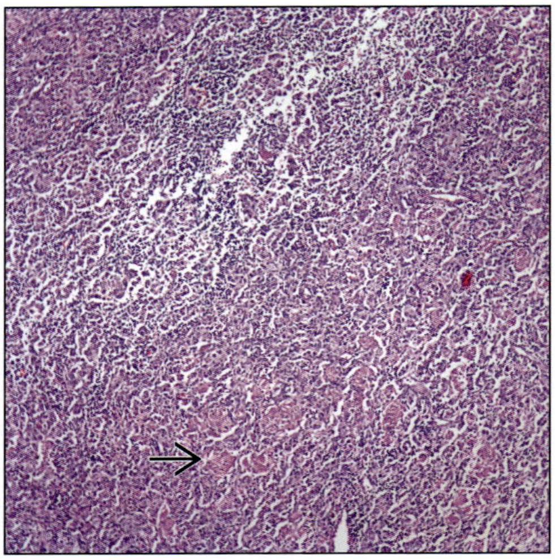

(Left) *Seminoma cells are shown intimately admixed with thymic tissue. Note the presence of a Hassall corpuscle* → *admixed with the neoplastic cells* ↪*.* ***(Right)*** *Low-power view of a thymic seminoma displays sheets of neoplastic cells without any particular growth pattern. Discrete, noncaseous, ill-defined granulomas are present* →*. This pattern can be easily confused with a lymphoma.*

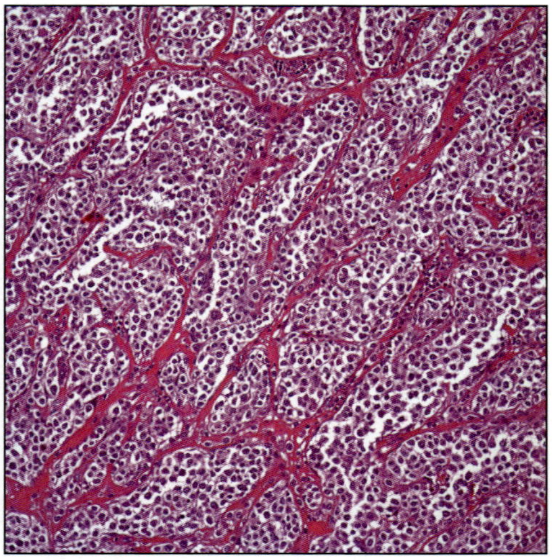

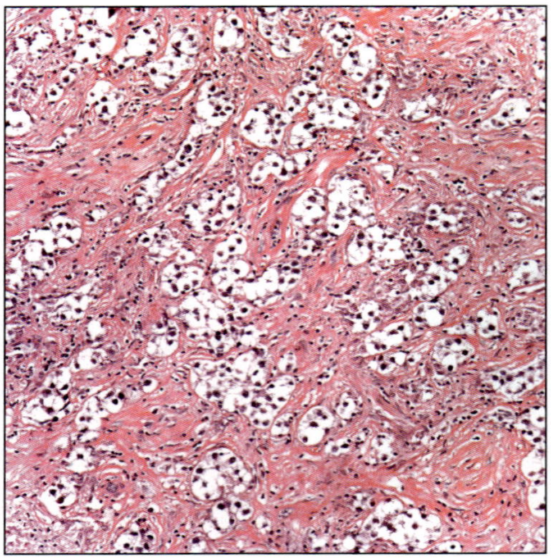

(Left) *Seminoma with a nested growth pattern. Similar primary tumors of the mediastinum may have a similar growth pattern, namely, neuroendocrine carcinomas.* ***(Right)*** *Closer view of a thymic seminoma in which the neoplastic cells display marked clearing of the cytoplasm. The intervening stroma does not show a marked inflammatory reaction.*

Microscopic Features

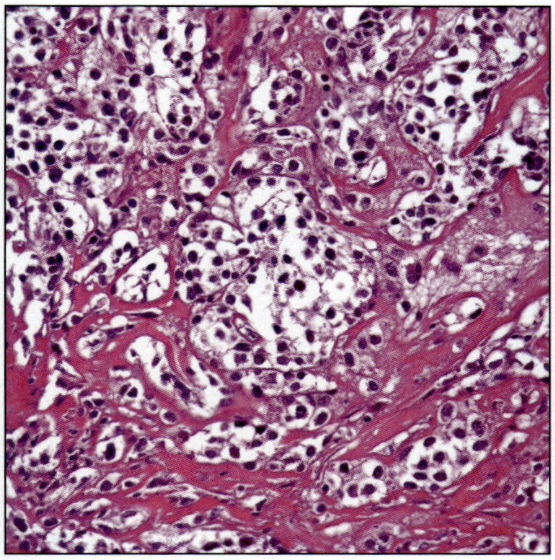

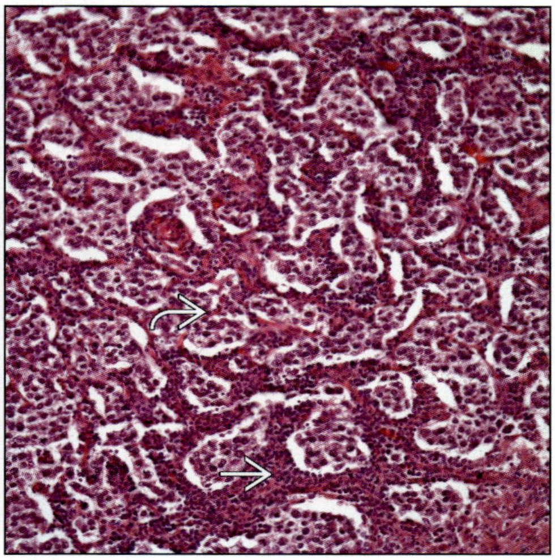

(Left) *Higher magnification of seminoma cells with prominent clear cytoplasm. In these cases, glycogen is more likely to be identified on PAS stains.* ***(Right)*** *Classical growth pattern of seminoma shows islands of tumor cells ↪ separated by thin fibroconnective tissue with inflammatory cells, mainly lymphocytes ➡.*

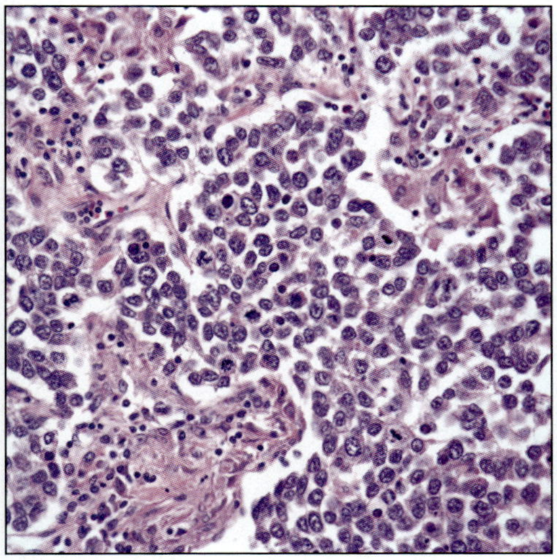

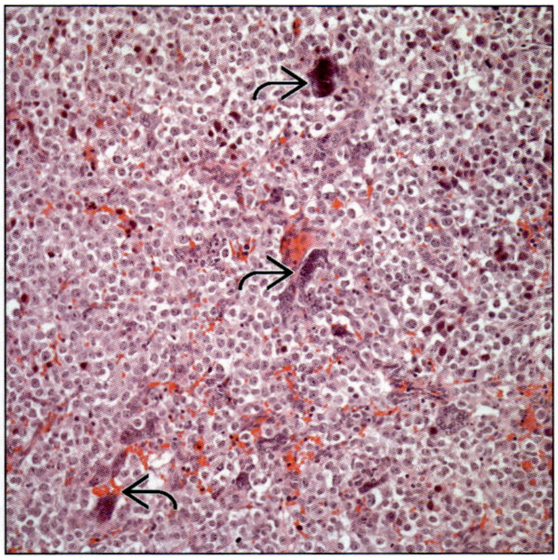

(Left) *The classic appearance of a thymic seminoma is shown in which the cells are oval with light eosinophilic cytoplasm, some with nucleoli and others with numerous chromocenters. Mitotic figures are present. Note the delicate fibroconnective tissue with mild inflammatory infiltrate.* ***(Right)*** *Thymic seminoma shows focal presence of multinucleated syncytiotrophoblastic cells ↪. This is another uncommon feature of these tumors, seen in < 10% of cases.*

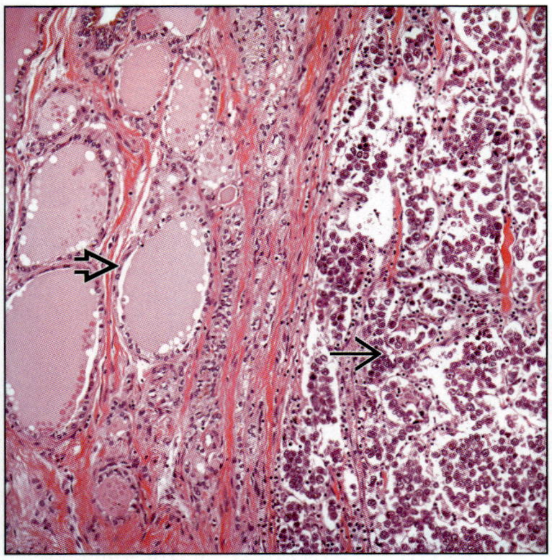

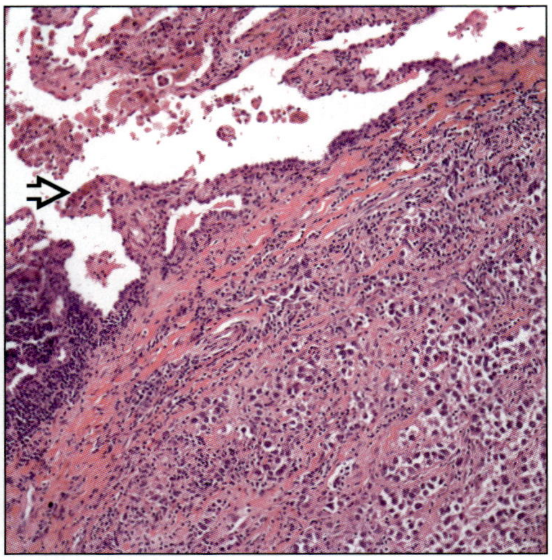

(Left) *Hematoxylin & eosin shows a thymic seminoma invading the thyroid gland. Note the presence of thyroid follicles ⇨ adjacent to areas of seminomatous infiltration →. This is an unusual site of metastatic disease.* ***(Right)*** *Thymic seminoma infiltrates into lung parenchyma ⇨. This is a more common site of spreading of thymic seminomas, which usually infiltrate intrathoracic structures 1st.*

YOLK SAC TUMOR

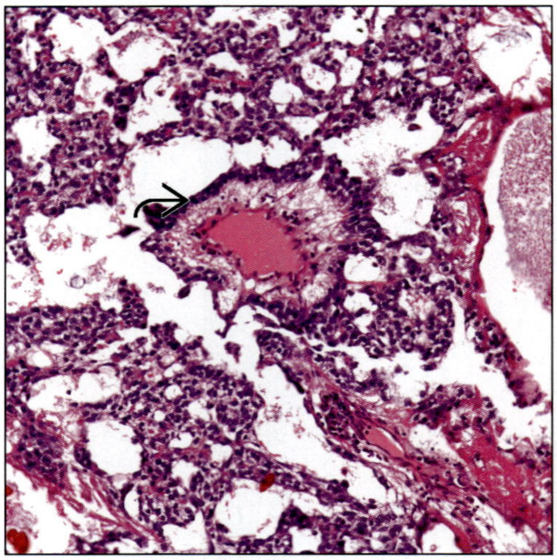

A yolk sac tumor is seen with the typical appearance of a neoplastic cellular proliferation and a Schiller-Duval body ⮫.

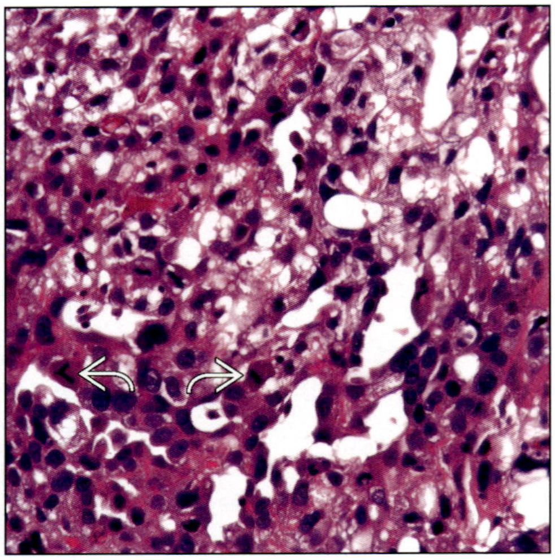

High-power view of a yolk sac tumor shows a reticular growth pattern composed of small cells without much nuclear pleomorphism. Note the presence of mitotic activity ⮫.

TERMINOLOGY

Abbreviations

- Yolk sac tumor (YST)

Synonyms

- Endodermal sinus tumor, infantile-type embryonal carcinoma

Definitions

- Malignant germ cell tumor

ETIOLOGY/PATHOGENESIS

Unknown Etiology

- Some authors have stated the possibility of misplaced germ cells in mediastinum

CLINICAL ISSUES

Epidemiology

- Incidence
  - Most common nonseminomatous germ cell tumor in the mediastinum
  - May account for approximately 20% of all nonteratomatous germ cell tumors in the mediastinum
- Age
  - Tumor is more common in young adults in 3rd decade of life
- Gender
  - Appears to occur predominantly in males

Site

- Anterior mediastinum

Presentation

- Cough
- Difficulty breathing
- Superior vena cava syndrome
- Chest pain
- Klinefelter syndrome
- Sexual precocity
- Idiopathic thrombocytopenia
- Acute megakaryoblastic leukemia
- Malignant histiocytosis
- Patients may also be asymptomatic

Laboratory Tests

- Increased α-fetoprotein in serum

Treatment

- Options, risks, complications
  - Surgery, if possible
  - Chemotherapy, platinum-based

Prognosis

- Poor
  - Survival: ~ 6-24 months

IMAGE FINDINGS

General Features

- Heterogeneous attenuation

MACROSCOPIC FEATURES

General Features

- Significant necrosis and hemorrhage

Sections to Be Submitted

- Approximately 1 section per cm of tumor
- Include transitional areas of thymus (if present) and tumor

Size

- Variable, from a few cm to > 20 cm in diameter
- Rarely, YST may present as cystic anterior mediastinal tumor

Key Facts

Terminology
- Yolk sac tumor (YST)
- Endodermal sinus tumor, infantile type embryonal carcinoma

Clinical Issues
- Most common nonseminomatous germ cell tumor in mediastinum
- May account for ~ 20% of all nonteratomatous germ cell tumors in mediastinum
- Tumor is more common in young adults in 3rd decade of life
- Yolk sac tumors appear predominantly in males

Macroscopic Features
- Variable size from a few cm to over 20 cm in diameter
- Rarely YST may present as cystic anterior mediastinal tumor

Microscopic Pathology
- Reticulated
- Cells growing in multiple communicating channels resembling immature glomeruli (Schiller-Duval bodies)
- Numerous intracellular and extracellular hyaline globules
- Loose reticular network

Top Differential Diagnoses
- Embryonal carcinoma
- Sarcoma
- Metastatic carcinoma
- Multilocular thymic cyst

MICROSCOPIC PATHOLOGY

Histologic Features
- Cells growing in multiple communicating channels resembling immature glomeruli (Schiller-Duval bodies)
- Numerous intracellular and extracellular hyaline globules
- Loose reticular network

Predominant Pattern/Injury Type
- Reticulated

Predominant Cell/Compartment Type
- Germ, nonseminomatous

ANCILLARY TESTS

Histochemistry
- Periodic acid-Schiff
  - Reactivity: Positive
  - Staining pattern
    - Cytoplasmic inclusion
    - Stromal matrix
- Mucicarmine
  - Reactivity: Negative
  - Staining pattern
    - Not applicable
- PAS-diastase
  - Reactivity: Negative
  - Staining pattern
    - Not applicable

Electron Microscopy
- Transmission
  - Large amounts of basal lamina outlining cells
  - Zonula occludens junctions joining cells

DIFFERENTIAL DIAGNOSIS

Embryonal Carcinoma
- Most often shows the presence of nucleoli in tumor cells
- Shows more nuclear pleomorphism
- More often shows abortive gland-like structures
- Most likely shows positive staining for CD30
- Both tumors may show similar immunophenotype

Metastatic Carcinoma
- In metastatic carcinoma of liver origin, it is likely that tumor may show bile while YST does not
- Generally, carcinomas will not show conventional areas of YST
- History of carcinoma is ultimately most reliable information

Sarcoma
- YST with spindle cell morphology also shows conventional areas of YST but will be absent in true sarcomas
- True sarcomas rarely will show positive staining for keratin and generally are negative for AFP
- Positive staining for mesenchymal markers, such as desmin, SMA, and others will be against YST

Multilocular Thymic Cyst
- Similar cystic features
- Does not display any atypical cellular proliferation
- Ample sectioning is important in these cases

Mixed Germ Cell Tumor
- YST is often accompanied by another germ cell tumor
- Most common association is with embryonal carcinoma
- Ample sampling is important in these cases

DIAGNOSTIC CHECKLIST

Clinically Relevant Pathologic Features
- Age distribution

YOLK SAC TUMOR

Immunohistochemistry

Antibody	Reactivity	Staining Pattern	Comment
α-fetoprotein	Positive	Cytoplasmic	
AE1/AE3	Positive	Cytoplasmic	
CEA-M	Positive	Cytoplasmic	
α-1-antitrypsin	Positive	Cytoplasmic	
PLAP	Positive	Cytoplasmic	Variable
EMA	Positive	Cell membrane	Variable
NSE	Positive	Cytoplasmic	Variable
LEU-7	Positive	Cytoplasmic	Variable
CK8/18/CAM5.2	Positive	Cytoplasmic	
CD30	Negative	Not applicable	
HCG	Negative	Not applicable	

Histological Growth Patterns of Yolk Sac Tumor

Histological Pattern	Frequency
Reticular pattern of growth with Schiller-Duval Bodies	Most common
Hepatoid variant	Unusual
Intestinal variant	Unusual
Spindle cell variant	Unusual
Cystic	Unusual

Clinical Staging of Mediastinal Germ Cell Tumors

Stage	Description
I	Well-circumscribed tumor ± focal adhesions to pleura or pericardium and without microscopic evidence of invasion into adjacent structures
II	Tumor confined to mediastinum with macroscopic &/or microscopic evidence of infiltration into adjacent structures, such as pleura, pericardium, and great vessels
III	Tumor metastases
IIIA	With metastases to intrathoracic organs (lymph nodes, lung, etc.)
IIIB	With extrathoracic metastases

- Most common in young men

Pathologic Interpretation Pearls

- Schiller-Duval bodies
- Extracellular and intracellular hyaline bodies

SELECTED REFERENCES

1. Malagón HD et al: Germ cell tumors with sarcomatous components: a clinicopathologic and immunohistochemical study of 46 cases. Am J Surg Pathol. 31(9):1356-62, 2007
2. Moran CA: Germ cell tumors of the mediastinum. Pathol Res Pract. 195(8):583-7, 1999
3. Suster S et al: Germ cell tumors of the mediastinum and testis: a comparative immunohistochemical study of 120 cases. Hum Pathol. 29(7):737-42, 1998
4. Moran CA et al: Hepatoid yolk sac tumors of the mediastinum: a clinicopathologic and immunohistochemical study of four cases. Am J Surg Pathol. 21(10):1210-4, 1997
5. Moran CA et al: Mediastinal yolk sac tumors associated with prominent multilocular cystic changes of thymic epithelium: a clinicopathologic and immunohistochemical study of five cases. Mod Pathol. 10(8):800-3, 1997
6. Moran CA et al: Primary germ cell tumors of the mediastinum: I. Analysis of 322 cases with special emphasis on teratomatous lesions and a proposal for histopathologic classification and clinical staging. Cancer. 80(4):681-90, 1997
7. Moran CA et al: Primary germ cell tumors of the mediastinum: III. Yolk sac tumor, embryonal carcinoma, choriocarcinoma, and combined nonteratomatous germ cell tumors of the mediastinum--a clinicopathologic and immunohistochemical study of 64 cases. Cancer. 80(4):699-707, 1997
8. Moran CA et al: Yolk sac tumors of the mediastinum with prominent spindle cell features: a clinicopathologic study of three cases. Am J Surg Pathol. 21(10):1173-7, 1997

YOLK SAC TUMOR

Gross and Microscopic Features

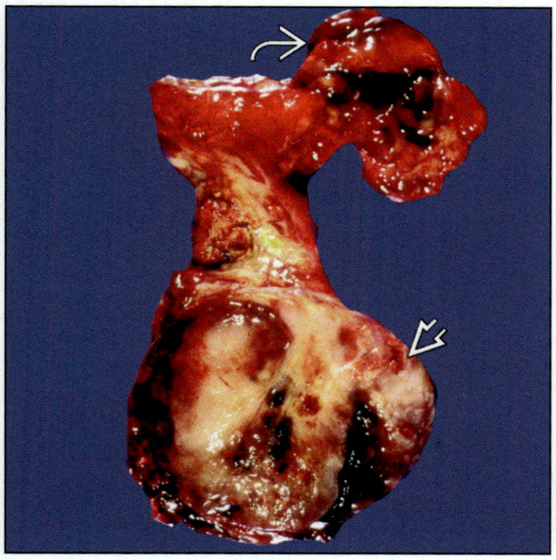

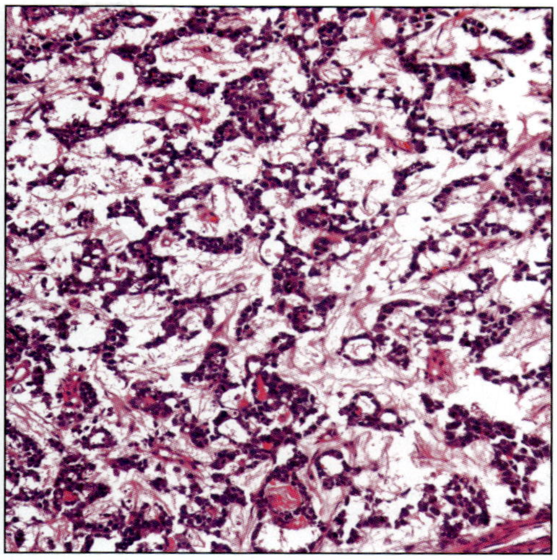

(Left) *Gross photograph shows a mediastinal YST. The tumor is fleshy with focal areas of hemorrhage. Note the presence of a residual portion of thymus.* ***(Right)*** *Yolk sac tumor shows a neoplastic cellular proliferation embedded in a myxoid stroma. The tumor does not show much in terms of cellular atypia or mitotic activity.*

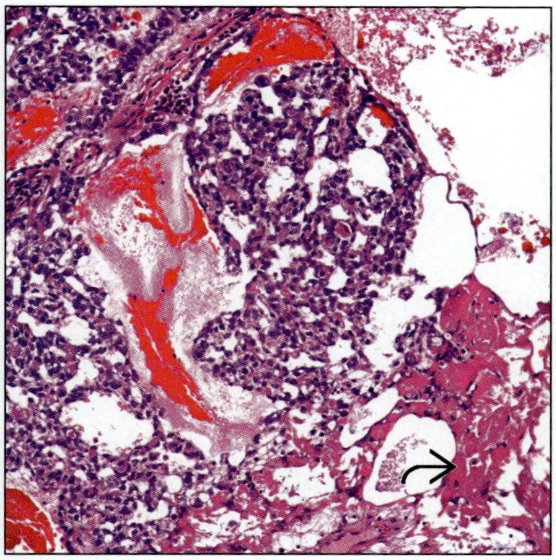

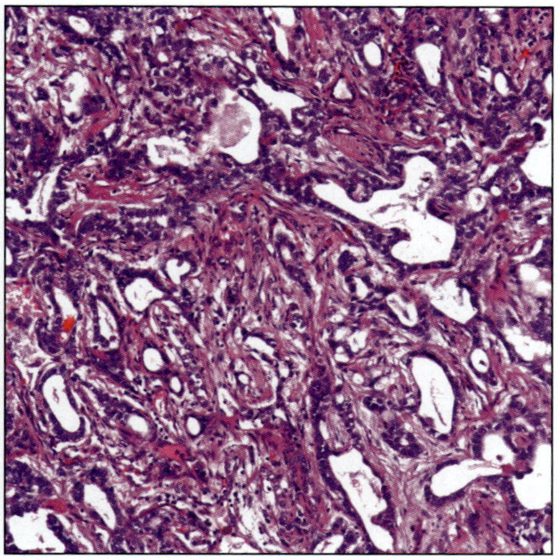

(Left) *Yolk sac tumor shows a neoplastic cellular proliferation composed of rather small cell areas admixed with fibrinoid material.* ***(Right)*** *Yolk sac tumor shows a reticular growth pattern in which there are alternating small pseudoglands lined by low cuboidal neoplastic cells and separated by fibrocollagenous tissue.*

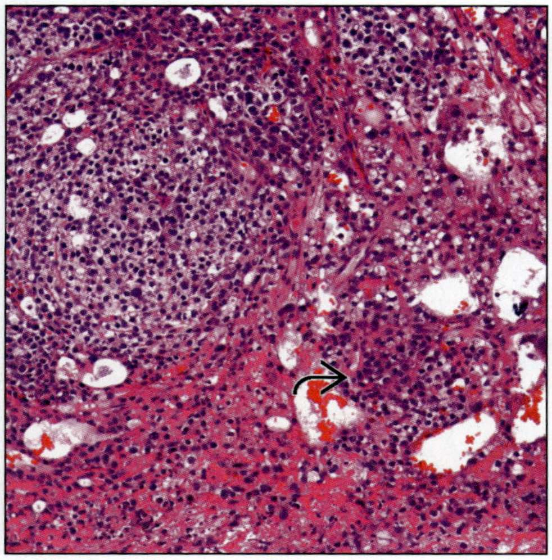

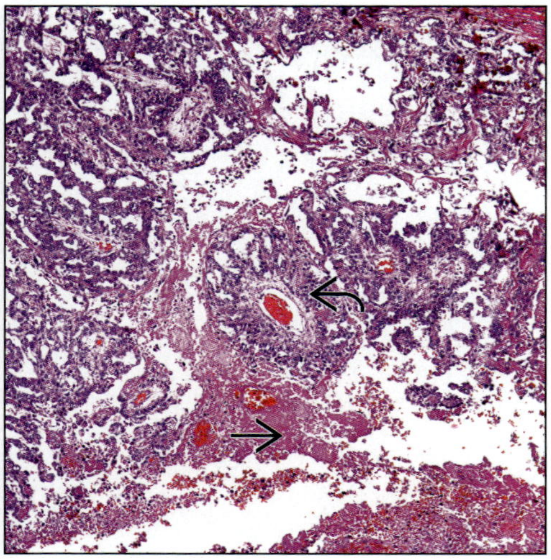

(Left) *Yolk sac tumor with an area in which the neoplastic cell acquires a clear cytoplasm. In some areas, the tumor cells are admixed with fibrinoid inflammatory material.* ***(Right)*** *Yolk sac tumor with more conventional areas and presence of necrosis. Note the presence of a Schiller-Duval body. These features are typical of yolk sac tumor.*

YOLK SAC TUMOR

Microscopic Features

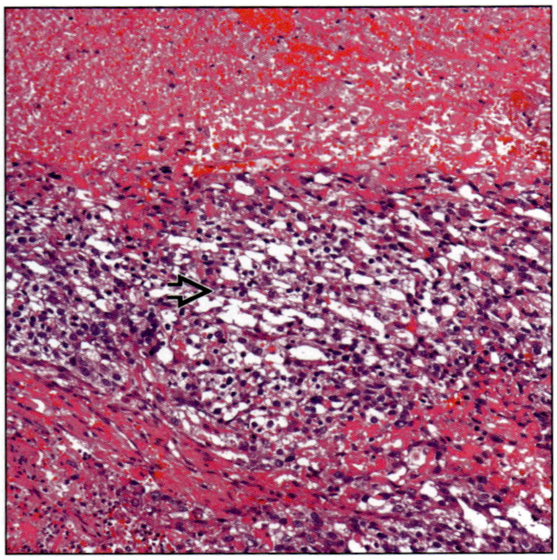
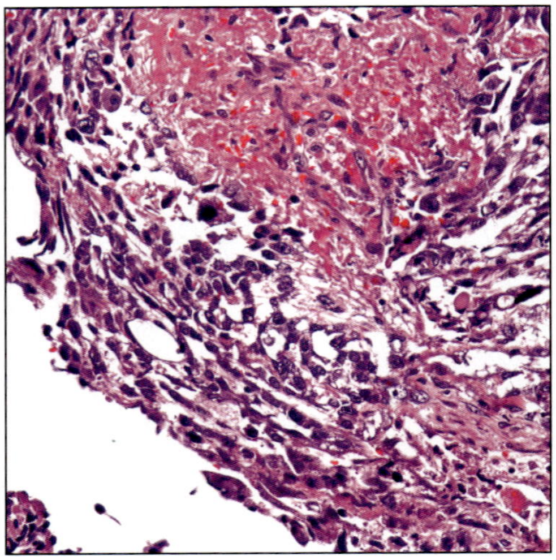

(Left) *Yolk sac tumor with extensive areas of necrosis. However, one is still able to recognize a neoplastic cellular proliferation composed of rather smaller cells.* ***(Right)*** *Yolk sac tumor with marked spindle cell component and necrosis. This type of growth pattern can easily be missed for a mesenchymal neoplasm.*

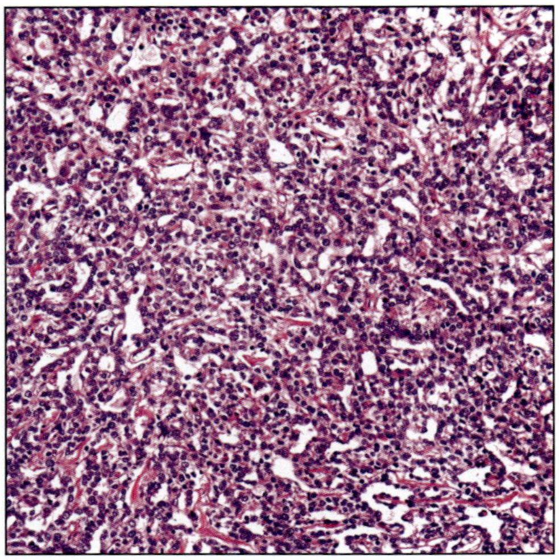
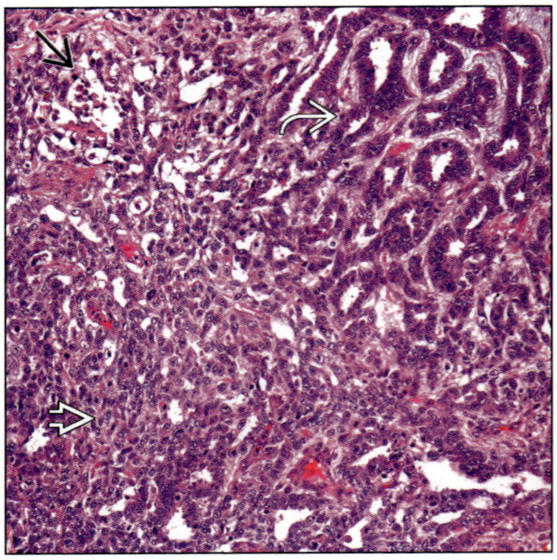

(Left) *Yolk sac tumor with more solid areas. The neoplastic cellular proliferation is composed of small cells without any particular growth pattern.* ***(Right)*** *In some cases of yolk sac tumor, solid areas can alternate with more glandular components. However, note the presence of more conventional areas.*

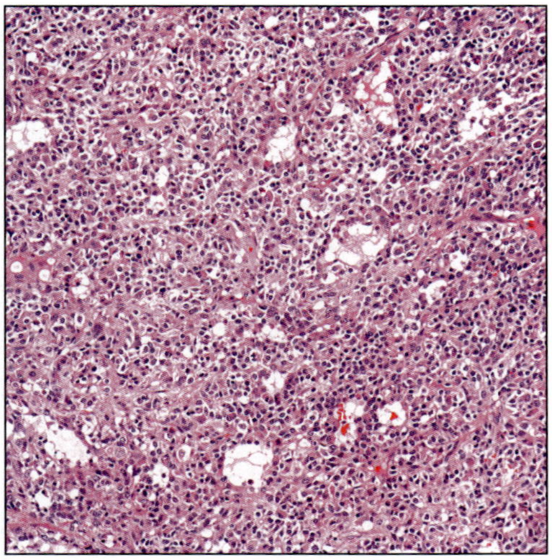
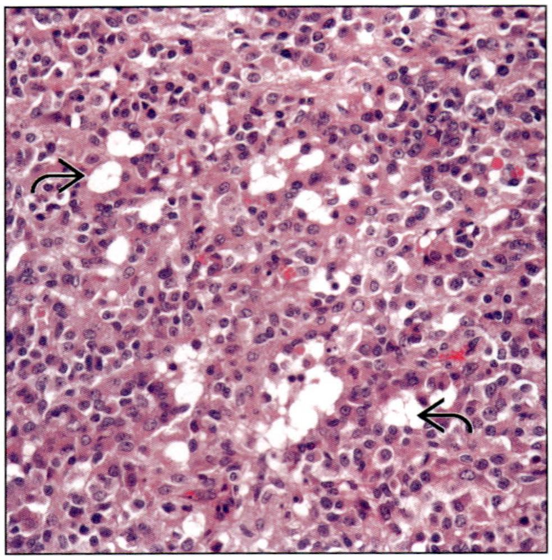

(Left) *Yolk sac tumor shows a homogeneous cellular proliferation of medium-sized cells with eosinophilic cytoplasm. This is the so-called hepatoid variant.* ***(Right)*** *Yolk sac tumor with a more solid pattern composed of medium-sized cells with round nuclei and eosinophilic cytoplasm. This is the so-called hepatoid variant. Some areas resemble fat droplets.*

Microscopic Features

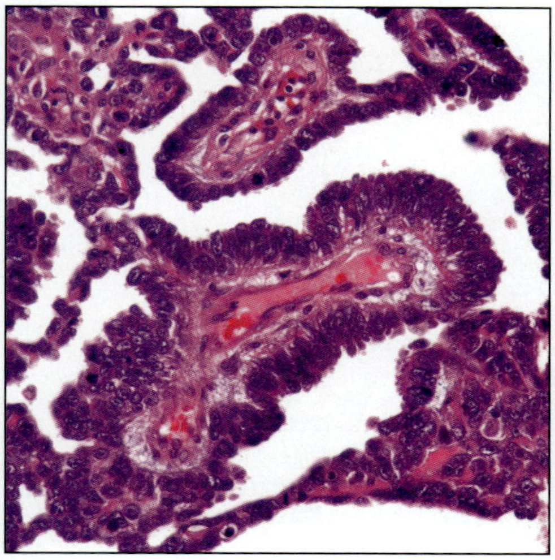

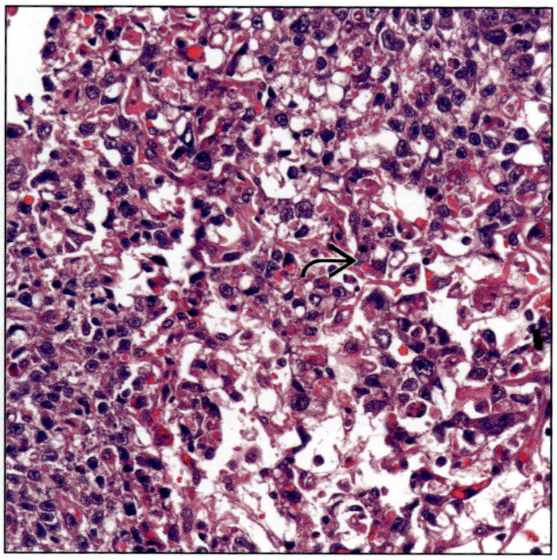

(Left) *Yolk sac tumor with papillary-like structures resembling intestinal villi. This represents the so-called intestinal variant of this tumor.* ***(Right)*** *In other areas, the tumor shows more conventional areas of yolk sac tumor, mainly the presence of intra- and extracellular hyaline globules.*

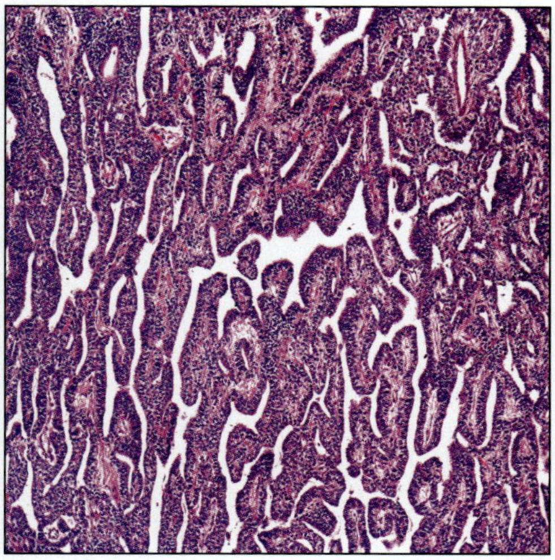

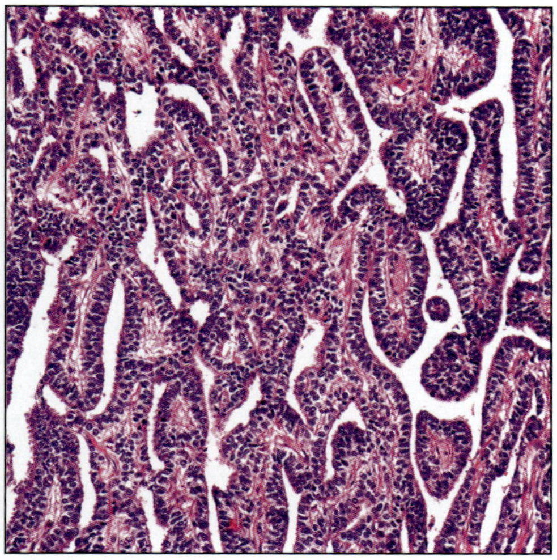

(Left) *Yolk sac tumor with a prominent pseudoglandular formation. There appears to be anastomosing glandular structures.* ***(Right)*** *Higher magnification shows these pseudoglands to be lined by a low cuboidal type of neoplastic cells. There is very little intervening stroma, and no vasculature is identified.*

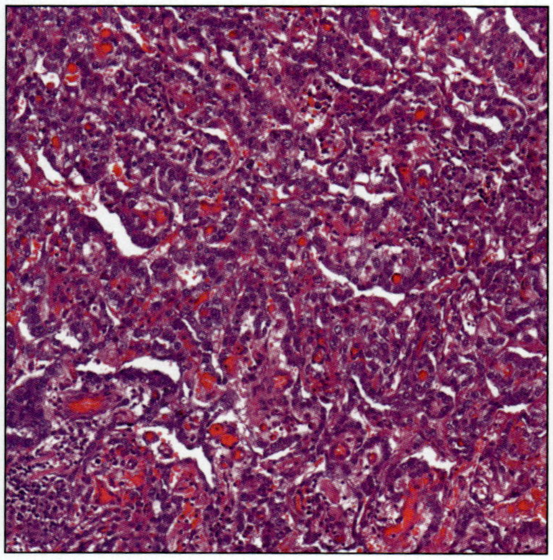

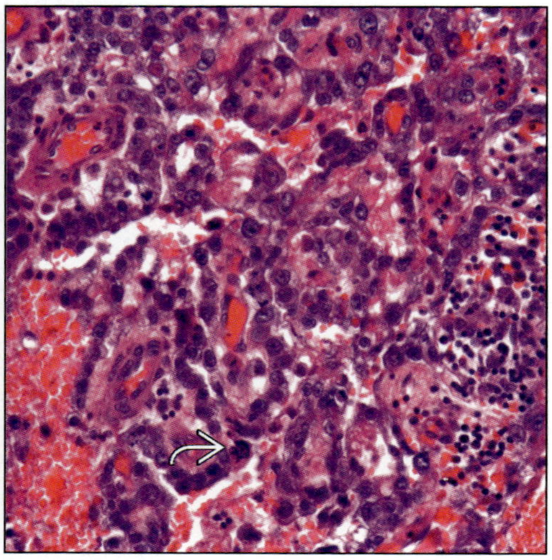

(Left) *Yolk sac tumor with prominent tubular formation, which is separated by thin fibrocollagenous tissue. There is not a well-defined growth pattern.* ***(Right)*** *Higher magnification shows that the neoplastic cells are rather small and homogeneous. However, a few mitotic figures can still be identified.*

CHORIOCARCINOMA

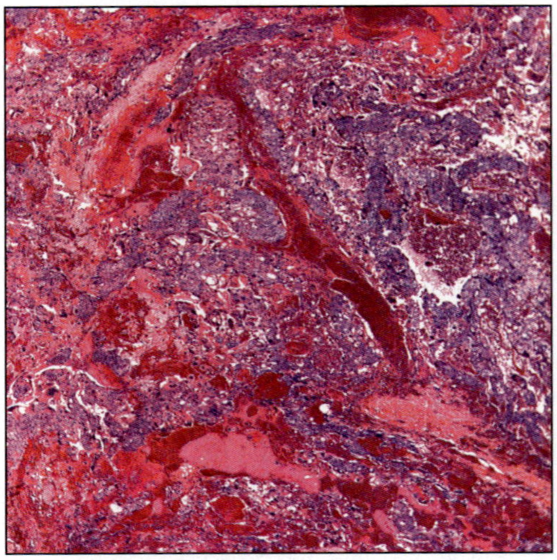

Primary mediastinal choriocarcinoma is seen with areas of hemorrhage admixed with neoplastic cellular proliferation without a specific growth pattern.

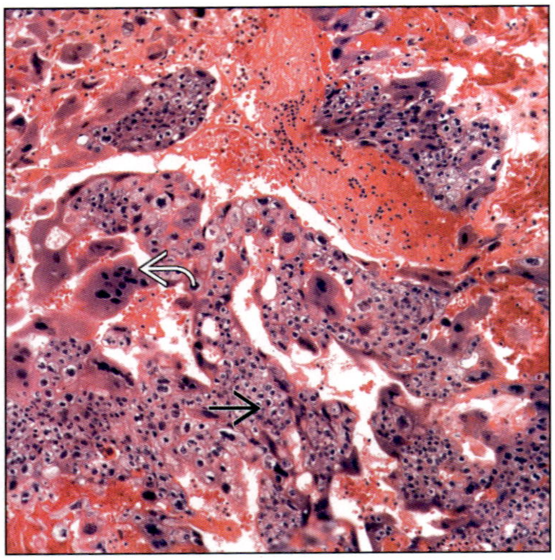

Choriocarcinoma with areas of hemorrhage admixed with a biphasic cellular proliferation is composed of large multinucleated cells (syncytiotrophoblast) and round cells (cytotrophoblast).

TERMINOLOGY

Synonyms
- Chorioepithelioma

Definitions
- Malignant germ cell tumor

ETIOLOGY/PATHOGENESIS

Etiology
- Misplaced germ cells in mediastinum
- Unknown etiology

CLINICAL ISSUES

Epidemiology
- Incidence
  - May represent the least common of all germ cell tumors in mediastinum
  - Accounts for < 5% of all germ cell tumors of mediastinum
- Age
  - More common in 3rd and 4th decades of life
- Gender
  - More common in males

Presentation
- Cough
- Dyspnea
- Gynecomastia
- Chest pain
- Superior vena cava syndrome

Laboratory Tests
- Increased hCG in serum

Treatment
- Chemotherapy
- Surgical debulking if necessary

Prognosis
- Poor
- Usually patients die within 12-18 months
- Most patients at time of diagnosis already have widespread metastatic disease

IMAGE FINDINGS

General Features
- Location
  - Anterior mediastinal mass
  - No pathognomonic features to separate choriocarcinoma from other nonseminomatous germ cell tumors

MACROSCOPIC FEATURES

General Features
- Large bulky tumors
- Extensive areas of hemorrhage and necrosis

Sections to Be Submitted
- Due to presence of extensive necrosis and hemorrhage, extensive sampling is required

Size
- Varies from a few cm to large tumors of > 10 cm in diameter

MICROSCOPIC PATHOLOGY

Histologic Features
- Hemorrhage
- Necrosis
- Cytotrophoblast
- Syncytiotrophoblast
- Marked nuclear atypia

CHORIOCARCINOMA

Key Facts

Terminology
- Chorioepithelioma

Clinical Issues
- Incidence
  - May represent the least common of all germ cell tumors in mediastinum
  - Represents < 5% of all germ cell tumors of mediastinum
  - Choriocarcinomas appear to be more common in 3rd and 4th decade of life
  - Choriocarcinomas are more common in men
- Symptoms
  - Cough
  - Dyspnea
  - Gynecomastia
  - Chest pain
  - Superior vena cava syndrome
- Laboratory findings
  - Increase HCG in serum

Image Findings
- Anterior mediastinal mass

Macroscopic Features
- Large bulky tumors
- Extensive areas of hemorrhage and necrosis

Microscopic Pathology
- Hemorrhage
- Necrosis
- Cytotrophoblast
- Syncytiotrophoblast
- Pleomorphism
- Mitotic activity

Predominant Pattern/Injury Type
- Hemorrhagic

Predominant Cell/Compartment Type
- Germ, nonseminomatous

DIFFERENTIAL DIAGNOSIS

Pleomorphic Carcinoma (PC) of Lung Origin
- Primary lung carcinomas may express hCG just like choriocarcinomas
- Choriocarcinomas are usually tumors of younger patients in contrast to lung carcinoma
- Choriocarcinomas are bulky anterior mediastinal masses, which may spread to lung
- Lung carcinoma presents predominantly with a lung mass
- Pleomorphic carcinoma is more common in older individuals
- Pleomorphic carcinoma may show ectopic production of hCG
- PC shows sarcomatous component with multinucleated giant cells
- Choriocarcinoma shows presence of cyto- and syncytiotrophoblastic cells

Metastatic Choriocarcinoma of Gonadal Origin
- Histology in both primary and metastatic disease is similar
- Immunophenotype of both tumors is the same
- In some cases of primary testicular choriocarcinoma, tumor may have undergone regression "burned-out"
- It would be unusual for metastases to present with bulky anterior mediastinal mass
- Clinical history would be very important

Thymic Carcinoma
- Most thymic carcinomas do not show marked pleomorphism present in choriocarcinomas
- Presence of cyto- and syncytiotrophoblastic components are not present in thymic carcinoma
- Positive staining for hCG would be unusual in thymic carcinoma

Giant Cell Carcinoma
- Usually shows malignant multinucleated giant cells not of syncytiotrophoblastic type of choriocarcinoma
- Commonly shows cannibalism by giant cells
- May show ectopic production of hCG
- Does not show presence cytotrophoblastic component

Mixed Germ Cell Tumor
- Choriocarcinoma may be component of another germ cell tumor
- Extensive sampling is required in order to properly rule out mixed germ cell tumor
- Presence of high hGC in serum should prompt search for choriocarcinomatous component

DIAGNOSTIC CHECKLIST

Clinically Relevant Pathologic Features
- Gross appearance
- Increase HCG in serum

Pathologic Interpretation Pearls
- Hemorrhage and necrosis
- Presence of cyto- and syncytiotrophoblastic cells
- Positive staining for hCG
- Marked pleomorphism
- Anterior mediastinal mass

SELECTED REFERENCES

1. Moran CA: Germ cell tumors of the mediastinum. Pathol Res Pract. 195(8):583-7, 1999
2. Weidner N: Germ-cell tumors of the mediastinum. Semin Diagn Pathol. 16(1):42-50, 1999

CHORIOCARCINOMA

Immunohistochemistry

Antibody	Reactivity	Staining Pattern	Comment
CK8/18/CAM5.2	Positive	Cytoplasmic	
α-fetoprotein	Positive	Cytoplasmic	Only focal in some cases
CEA-M	Positive	Cytoplasmic	Only focal in some cases
EMA	Positive	Cell membrane	Focal
HPL	Positive	Cytoplasmic	Focal in some cases
CK-PAN	Positive	Cytoplasmic	
Vimentin	Positive	Cytoplasmic	
HCG-α	Positive	Cytoplasmic	
HCG-β	Positive	Cytoplasmic	
CD15	Negative		May show focal positive cells in some cases
PLAP	Negative		May be focally positive in some cases
CD30	Negative		
TTF-1	Negative		
S100	Negative		
CDX-2	Negative		
Calretinin	Negative		

Histochemical Features of Choriocarcinomas

Histochemical Stain	Result
Mucicarmine	Negative for intracellular mucin
D-PAS	Negative for intracellular mucin
PAS	Focally positive in cytotrophoblastic component in some cases

Clinical Staging of Mediastinal Germ Cell Tumors

Stage	Tumor Extension
I	Well-circumscribed tumor ± focal adhesions to pleura or pericardium and without microscopic evidence of invasion into adjacent structures
II	Tumor confined to mediastinum with macroscopic &/or microscopic evidence of infiltration into adjacent structures, such as pleura, pericardium, and great vessels
III	Tumor with metastases
IIIA	With metastases to intrathoracic organs (lymph nodes, lung, etc.)
IIIB	With extrathoracic metastases

3. Suster S et al: Germ cell tumors of the mediastinum and testis: a comparative immunohistochemical study of 120 cases. Hum Pathol. 29(7):737-42, 1998
4. Moran CA et al: Primary germ cell tumors of the mediastinum: III. Yolk sac tumor, embryonal carcinoma, choriocarcinoma, and combined nonteratomatous germ cell tumors of the mediastinum--a clinicopathologic and immunohistochemical study of 64 cases. Cancer. 80(4):699-707, 1997
5. Moran CA et al: Primary mediastinal choriocarcinomas: a clinicopathologic and immunohistochemical study of eight cases. Am J Surg Pathol. 21(9):1007-12, 1997
6. Narushima M et al: [A case of primary anterior mediastinal choriocarcinoma.] Nihon Kyobu Shikkan Gakkai Zasshi. 28(2):374-8, 1990
7. Taccagni GL et al: Mixed germ cell tumour of the mediastinum (seminoma, embryonal carcinoma, choriocarcinoma and teratoma). Light and electron microscopic cytology and histological investigation. Pathol Res Pract. 185(4):506-10; discussion 511-3, 1989
8. Kathuria S et al: Primary choriocarcinoma of mediastinum with immunohistochemical study and review of the literature. J Surg Oncol. 34(1):39-42, 1987
9. Knapp RH et al: Malignant germ cell tumors of the mediastinum. J Thorac Cardiovasc Surg. 89(1):82-9, 1985
10. Hsueh YS et al: Primary mediastinal choriocarcinoma in a man with an abnormal chromosome. South Med J. 77(11):1466-9, 1984
11. Connolly CE et al: Brief report: primary choriocarcinoma of the mediastinum. Ir J Med Sci. 148(1):20-2, 1979
12. Luna MA et al: Germ-cell tumors of the mediastinum, postmortem findings. Am J Clin Pathol. 65(4):450-4, 1976

CHORIOCARCINOMA

Gross and Microscopic Features

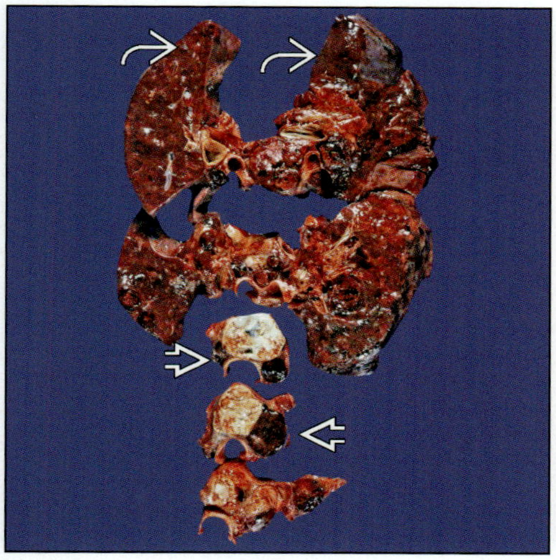
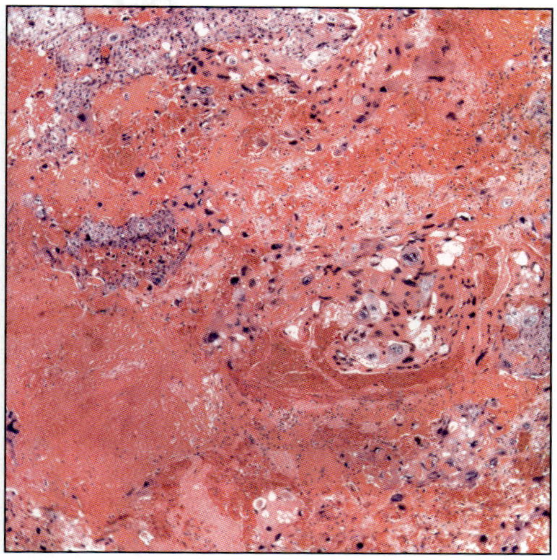

(Left) *Gross photograph of a primary mediastinal choriocarcinoma (autopsy material). Note the presence of a bulky fleshy and hemorrhagic tumor mass ⇨. Adjacent lungs do not show evidence of metastatic disease ↷.* ***(Right)*** *Extensive areas of hemorrhage with clusters of neoplastic cells are shown. Some of the neoplastic cells are multinucleated and of the syncytiotrophoblastic type, while the majority represent cytotrophoblastic cells.*

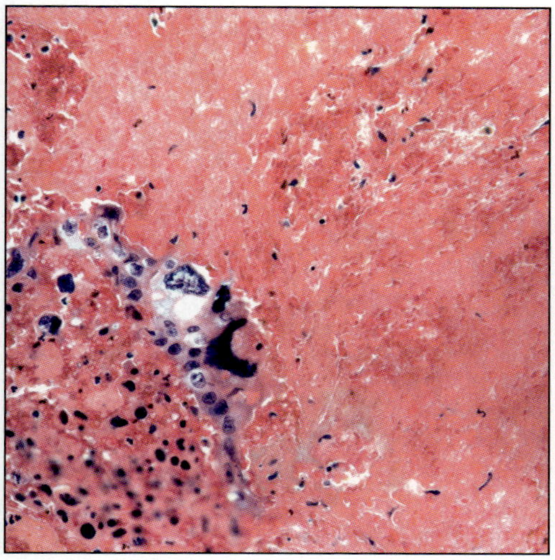
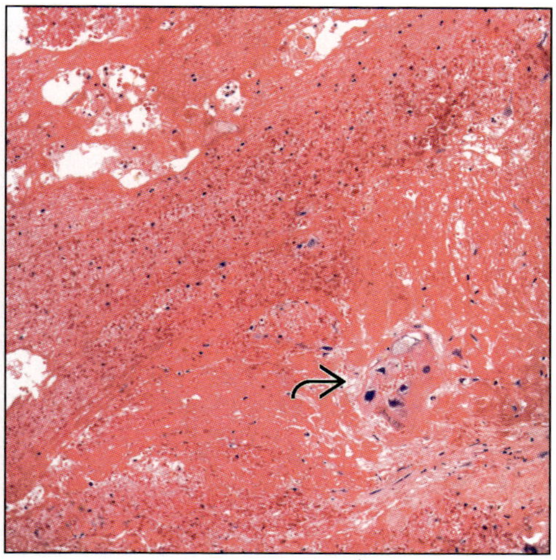

(Left) *Extensive areas of hemorrhage contain a cluster of neoplastic cells of the cytotrophoblastic and syncytiotrophoblastic type.* ***(Right)*** *Choriocarcinoma is shown with extensive areas of hemorrhage, which at times may obscure the neoplastic nature of the process. Here, only a cluster of neoplastic cells ↷ floating in the hemorrhage is observed.*

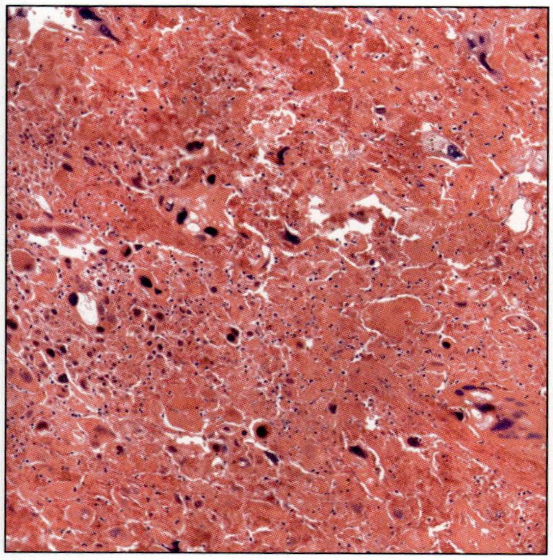
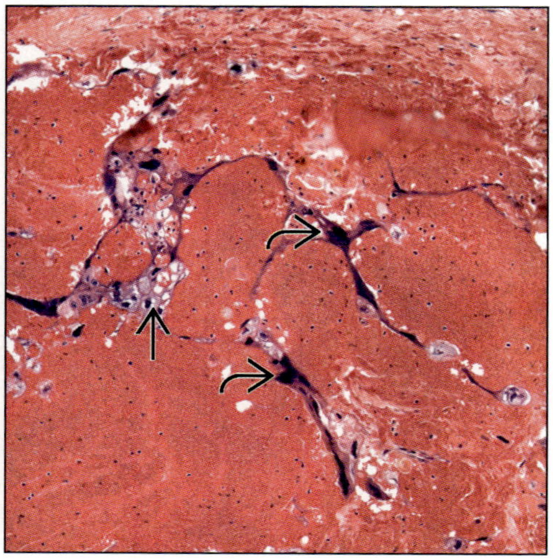

(Left) *Choriocarcinoma with areas of hemorrhage shows single cells distributed haphazardly. Note the marked nuclear pleomorphism. These features are also suggestive of choriocarcinoma.* ***(Right)*** *Choriocarcinoma with areas of hemorrhage is shown, but one is still able to recognize 2 different populations of tumors cells. The giant cells represent syncytiotrophoblasts ↷, and the round cells represent cytotrophoblasts →.*

CHORIOCARCINOMA

Variant Microscopic Features

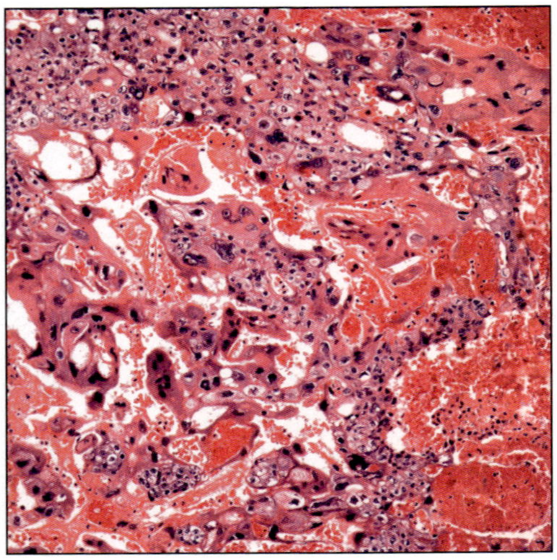

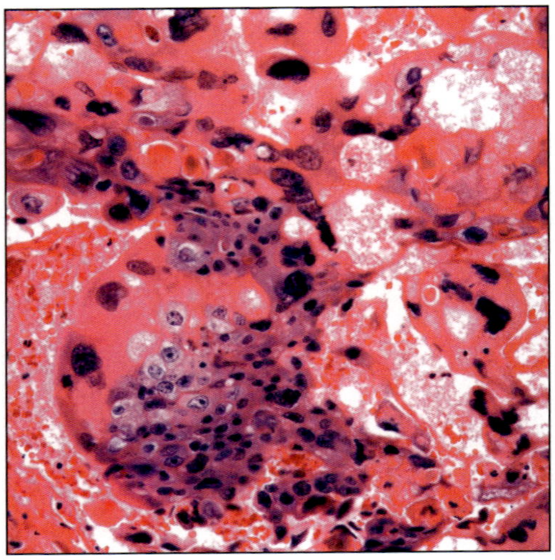

*(**Left**) Choriocarcinoma with presence of 2 distinct cellular proliferations is composed of round cells with clear cytoplasm and multinucleated giant cells. More nuclear pleomorphism is present in the giant cells. (**Right**) Choriocarcinoma with mononucleated and multinucleated cells shows vague squamoid features. The tumor shows a subtle deciduoid-like appearance.*

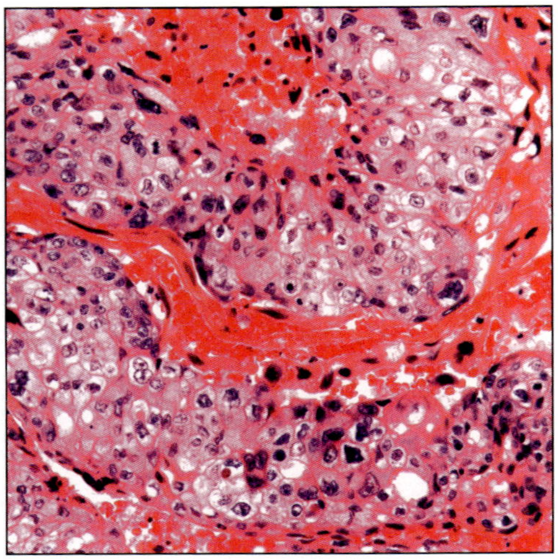

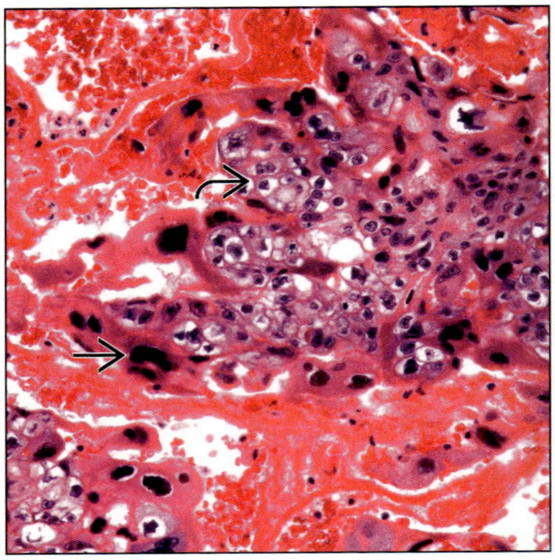

*(**Left**) Cords of neoplastic cells, predominantly of the cytotrophoblastic type, are composed of medium-sized cells with round nuclei and prominent nucleoli. Scattered larger cells are also present. (**Right**) More conventional areas composed of cytotrophoblastic ↪ and syncytiotrophoblastic → cells are seen embedded in a fibrinoid hemorrhagic background, typical of choriocarcinoma.*

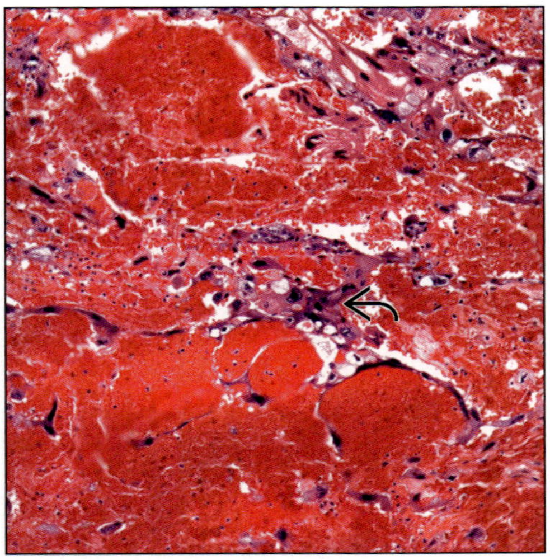

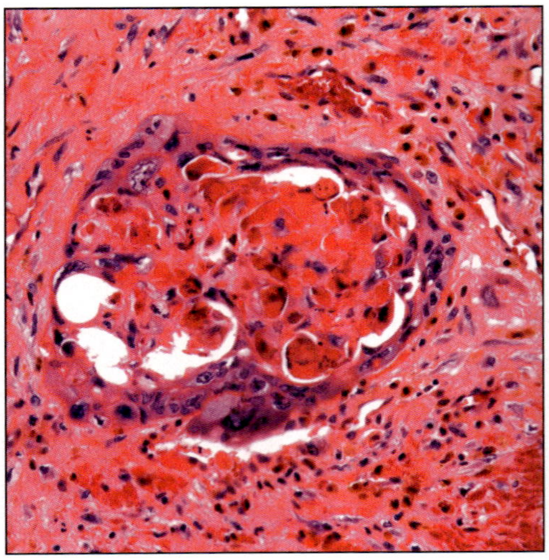

*(**Left**) Choriocarcinoma with extensive areas of hemorrhage. However, conventional neoplastic cellular proliferation is also present ↪. (**Right**) Choriocarcinoma with focal cystic areas. However, the cellular proliferation is composed of mononuclear and multinucleated cells, typical of choriocarcinoma.*

CHORIOCARCINOMA

Variant Microscopic Features

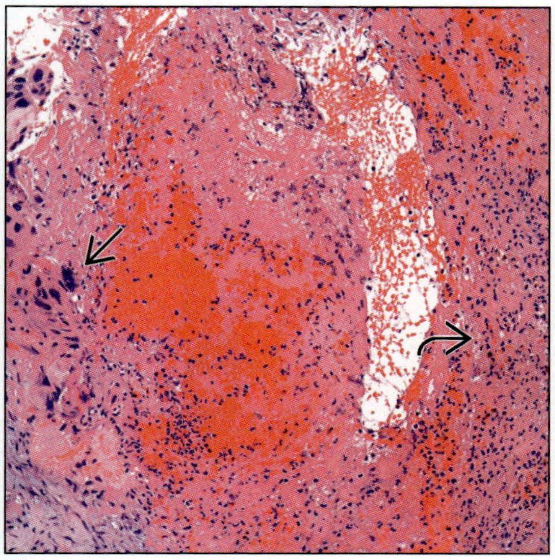

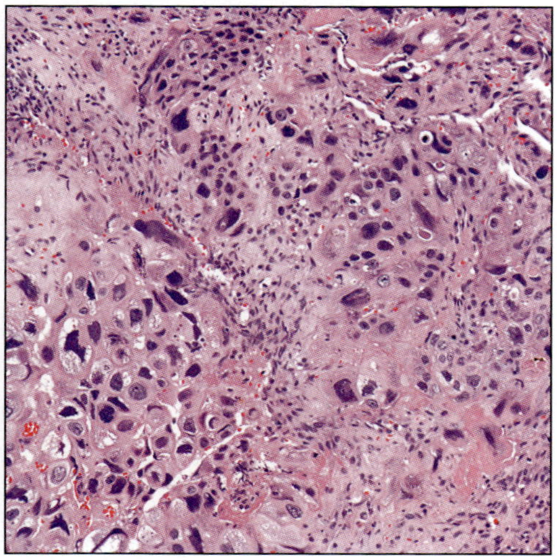

(Left) *Choriocarcinoma is shown with extensive fibrinoid necrosis and prominent inflammatory cells* ↪*. However, the presence of a neoplastic process composed of multinucleated giant cells is apparent* →*.* ***(Right)*** *In some areas, the tumoral cells are more viable without evidence of necrosis or hemorrhage. Nevertheless, the dual neoplastic population of cells is still present.*

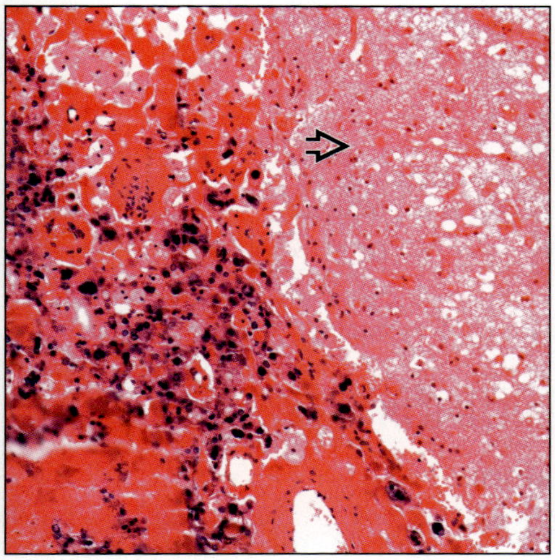

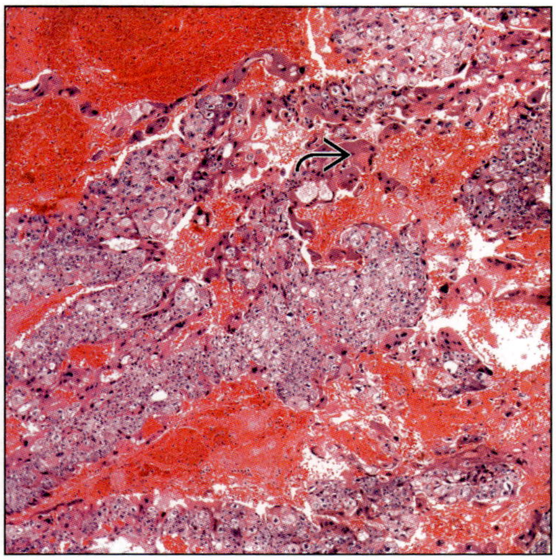

(Left) *Metastatic mediastinal choriocarcinoma to the brain* ⇨*. The histology of the mediastinal tumor is similar to the metastatic tumor.* ***(Right)*** *Choriocarcinoma with extensive hemorrhage and predominantly syncytial cells (mononuclear cells) with clear cytoplasm. Only scattered syncytiotrophoblastic cells are present* ↪*.*

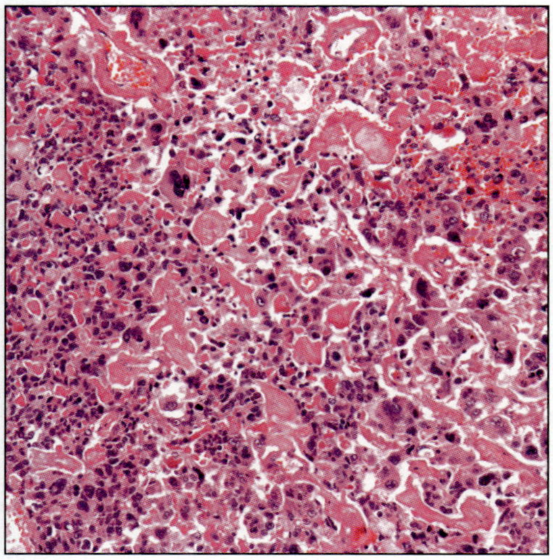

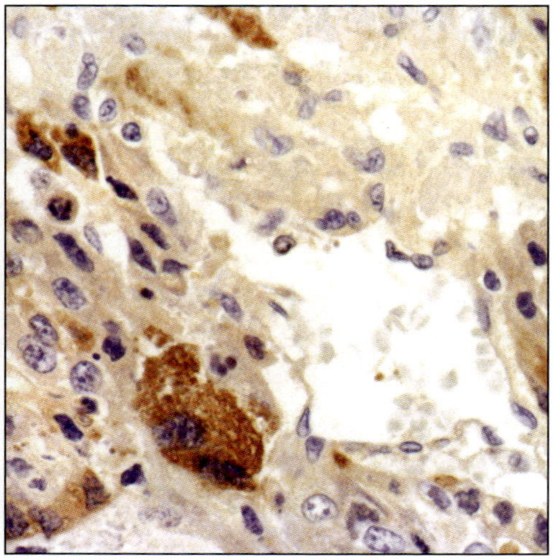

(Left) *Choriocarcinoma shows a dual neoplastic cellular proliferation composed of round mononuclear cells and multinucleated giant cells admixed with areas containing amorphous material.* ***(Right)*** *hCG immunohistochemical stain shows positive reaction in tumor cells, mainly in the syncytiotrophoblastic cells. The cytotrophoblastic cells (round cells) show only weakly focal positive staining.*

EMBRYONAL CARCINOMA

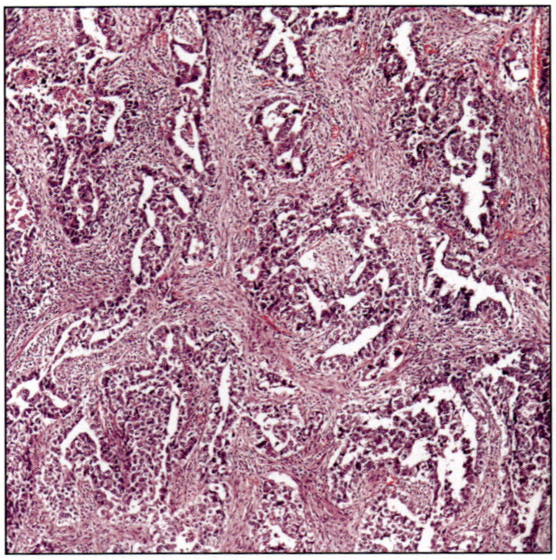

Embryonal carcinoma shows the typical glandular arrangement of neoplastic cells separated by inflamed fibroconnective tissue.

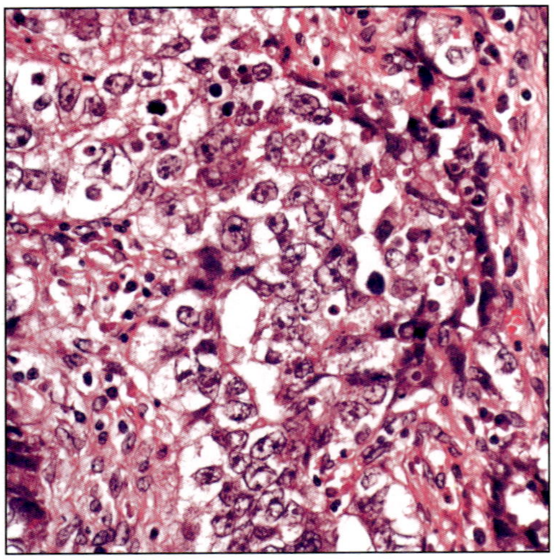

Closer view of the neoplastic cells shows medium-sized cells with round to oval vesiculated nuclei and prominent nucleoli. These features are typical of embryonal carcinoma.

TERMINOLOGY

Abbreviations

- Embryonal carcinoma (EC)

Synonyms

- Embryonal carcinoma adult type

Definitions

- Malignant germ cell tumor

ETIOLOGY/PATHOGENESIS

Etiology

- Although a definitive etiology is unknown, misplaced germ cells in mediastinum may be the origin of these tumors

CLINICAL ISSUES

Epidemiology

- Incidence
  - Unusual tumor in its pure form
  - More often accompanied with another germ cell tumor, mainly yolk sac tumor
  - May account for no more than 10% of all germ cell tumors of mediastinum
- Age
  - Tumor is more common in young adults
  - More common in 3rd decade of life
  - Unusual in older individuals
- Gender
  - More common in males
  - Unusual cases in females have been described

Presentation

- Chest pain
- Cough
- Dyspnea
- Klinefelter syndrome
- Hematologic dyscrasias
- Chromosomal abnormalities

Treatment

- Chemotherapy
- Cis platinum-based therapy
- Surgical debulking if appropriate

Prognosis

- Poor
- May depend on clinical staging

IMAGE FINDINGS

General Features

- Anterior mediastinal tumor
- Bulky tumor indistinguishable from other nonteratomatous germ cell tumors

MACROSCOPIC FEATURES

General Features

- Large, ill-defined tumors
- Extensive necrosis and hemorrhage

Sections to Be Submitted

- Extensive sampling is required
- Possible sites of involvement
  - Lung
  - Pericardium
  - Lymph nodes
  - Diaphragm

Size

- Variable from a few cm to > 10 cm in diameter

EMBRYONAL CARCINOMA

Key Facts

Terminology
- Embryonal carcinoma adult type

Clinical Issues
- Incidence
  - Unusual tumor in its pure form
  - More often accompanied with another germ cell tumor, mainly yolk sac tumor
  - May account for no more than 10% of all mediastinal germ cell tumors
  - More common in young adults; unusual in older individuals
  - More common in 3rd decade of life
  - More common in males
- Symptoms
  - Chest pain
  - Cough
  - Dyspnea
  - Klinefelter syndrome
  - Hematologic dyscrasias
  - Chromosomal abnormalities

Microscopic Pathology
- Gland-like appearance
- Sheets of neoplastic cells
- Primitive cellular proliferation
- Cells with prominent nucleoli
- Extensive necrosis
- Prominent cellular atypia and mitotic activity

Top Differential Diagnoses
- Anaplastic large cell lymphoma
- Metastatic adenocarcinoma of lung origin

MICROSCOPIC PATHOLOGY

Histologic Features
- Gland-like appearance
- Sheets of neoplastic cells
- Primitive cellular proliferation
- Cells with prominent nucleoli
- Extensive necrosis
- Prominent cellular atypia and mitotic activity

Predominant Pattern/Injury Type
- Necrosis

Predominant Cell/Compartment Type
- Germ, nonseminomatous

ANCILLARY TESTS

Electron Microscopy
- Transmission
  - Intercellular junctions and desmosomes
  - Tight junctions and telolysosomes

DIFFERENTIAL DIAGNOSIS

Metastatic Adenocarcinoma of Lung Origin
- Glands in adenocarcinoma are better formed
- Glands in adenocarcinoma may show positive intracellular mucin
- Adenocarcinoma of lung origin may show positive staining for TTF-1
- Lung adenocarcinomas are more common in older patients unlike young age in EC
- Would be highly unusual for lung adenocarcinoma to show positive staining for CD30

Seminoma
- Seminomas show more cohesive growth pattern
- Seminomas rarely show extensive areas of necrosis
- EC may show positive staining for CD30 while negative in seminomas
- EC shows more prominent nuclear atypia and mitotic activity

Yolk Sac Tumor
- YST and EC may show similar histopathological pattern
- YST and EC may show similar immunophenotype
- Presence of prominent nucleoli in EC may help in separating these tumors

Mixed Germ Cell Tumor
- Extensive sampling is of utmost importance
- EC is often accompanied with another germ cell tumor, namely yolk sac tumor

Thymic Carcinoma
- Some high-grade carcinomas of thymus may share some histopathological features
- Thymic carcinoma does not show staining for α-fetoprotein or CD30

Anaplastic Large Cell Lymphoma
- Anaplastic large cell lymphoma and EC may show positive staining for CD30 and EMA/MUC1
- Does not show positive staining for α-fetoprotein

DIAGNOSTIC CHECKLIST

Clinically Relevant Pathologic Features
- Gross appearance
- Extensive areas of hemorrhage and necrosis
- Bulky, slightly lobulated tumor

Pathologic Interpretation Pearls
- Gland-like growth pattern
- Embryonic type of epithelium
- Prominent nucleoli
- Nuclear pleomorphism and mitotic activity
- Extensive necrosis

EMBRYONAL CARCINOMA

Immunohistochemistry

Antibody	Reactivity	Staining Pattern	Comment
α-fetoprotein	Positive	Cytoplasmic	Also positive in yolk sac tumors
PLAP	Positive	Cytoplasmic	In some cases, patchy and focal
NSE	Positive	Cytoplasmic	Not specific
LEU-7	Positive	Cytoplasmic	In some cases
Vimentin	Positive	Cytoplasmic	
CK-PAN	Positive	Cytoplasmic	Also positive in other epithelial tumors
CK8/18/CAM5.2	Positive	Cytoplasmic	Also positive in other epithelial tumors
CD30	Positive	Golgi zone	Not in all cases; also positive in anaplastic large cell lymphoma
EMA	Positive	Cell membrane	Positive in other epithelial tumors
CEA-M	Negative		
TTF-1	Negative		
CD15	Negative		
CD5	Negative		
HPL	Negative		May be focally positive in some cases
CD20	Negative		
ALK1	Negative		

Clinical Staging of Germ Cell Tumors of Mediastinum

Stage	Description
I	Well-circumscribed tumor ± focal adhesions to pleura or pericardium and without microscopic evidence of invasion into adjacent structures
II	Tumor confined to mediastinum with macroscopic &/or microscopic evidence of infiltration into adjacent structures, such as pleura, pericardium, and great vessels
III	Tumor with metastases
IIIA	With metastases to intrathoracic organs (lymph nodes, lung, etc.)
IIIB	With extrathoracic metastases

Histochemical Features of Embryonal Carcinoma

Histochemical Stain	Result
PAS	Positive for intracellular glycogen
Mucicarmine	Negative for intracellular mucin
D-PAS	Negative for intracellular mucin

SELECTED REFERENCES

1. Moran CA: Germ cell tumors of the mediastinum. Pathol Res Pract. 195(8):583-7, 1999
2. Weidner N: Germ-cell tumors of the mediastinum. Semin Diagn Pathol. 16(1):42-50, 1999
3. el-Khatib M et al: Embryonal carcinoma of the anterior mediastinum. AJR Am J Roentgenol. 170(3):722, 1998
4. Suster S et al: Germ cell tumors of the mediastinum and testis: a comparative immunohistochemical study of 120 cases. Hum Pathol. 29(7):737-42, 1998
5. Moran CA et al: Primary germ cell tumors of the mediastinum: I. Analysis of 322 cases with special emphasis on teratomatous lesions and a proposal for histopathologic classification and clinical staging. Cancer. 80(4):681-90, 1997
6. Moran CA et al: Primary germ cell tumors of the mediastinum: III. Yolk sac tumor, embryonal carcinoma, choriocarcinoma, and combined nonteratomatous germ cell tumors of the mediastinum--a clinicopathologic and immunohistochemical study of 64 cases. Cancer. 80(4):699-707, 1997
7. Motoyama T et al: Fine needle aspiration cytology of primary mediastinal germ cell tumors. Acta Cytol. 39(4):725-32, 1995
8. Lakhkar BN et al: Primary mediastinal embryonal cell carcinoma. Indian J Chest Dis Allied Sci. 33(1):35-8, 1991
9. Taccagni GL et al: Mixed germ cell tumour of the mediastinum (seminoma, embryonal carcinoma, choriocarcinoma and teratoma). Light and electron microscopic cytology and histological investigation. Pathol Res Pract. 185(4):506-10; discussion 511-3, 1989
10. Knapp RH et al: Malignant germ cell tumors of the mediastinum. J Thorac Cardiovasc Surg. 89(1):82-9, 1985

Gross and Microscopic Features

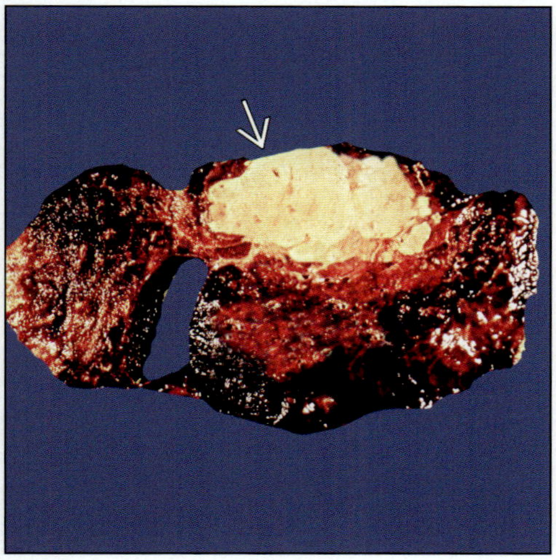

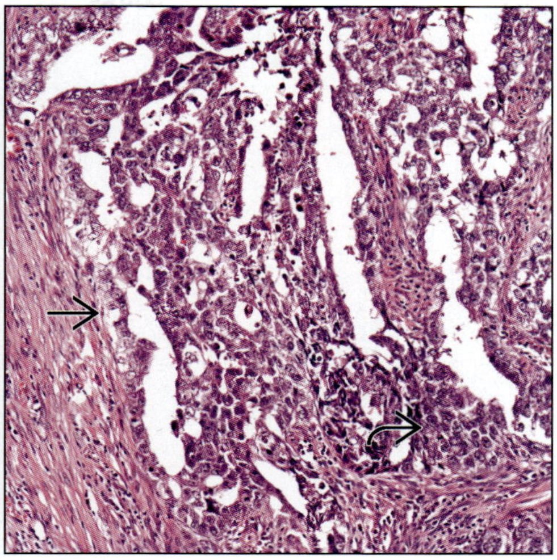

(Left) *Gross photograph shows a fairly well-circumscribed but not encapsulated tumor mass* ➔ *involving the thymic gland. The tumor is yellowish and lacks extensive areas of necrosis or hemorrhage.* ***(Right)*** *This embryonal carcinoma shows typical features of pseudoglandular* → *appearance and solid areas* ↷*. These features are invariably seen in this tumor.*

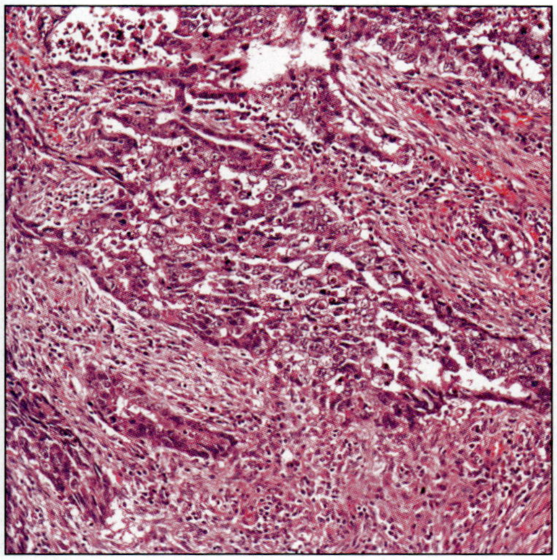

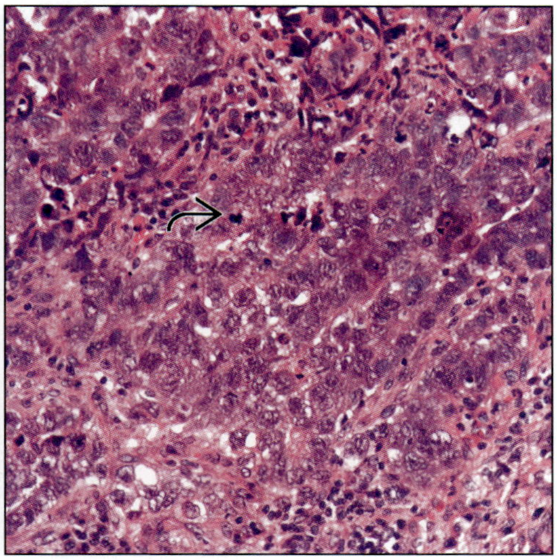

(Left) *Embryonal carcinoma shows neoplastic glandular structures dissecting fibroconnective tissue. This pattern can be seen in adenocarcinomas.* ***(Right)*** *This embryonal carcinoma shows solid areas. The neoplastic cells show medium-sized cells with eosinophilic cytoplasm, round vesiculated nuclei, and prominent nucleoli. Atypical mitotic figures are present* ↷*.*

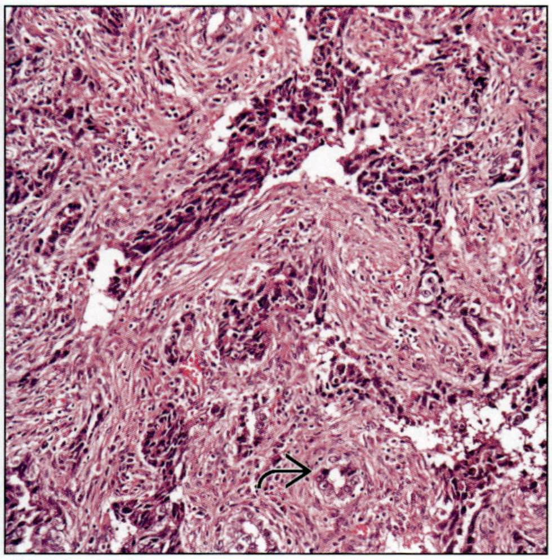

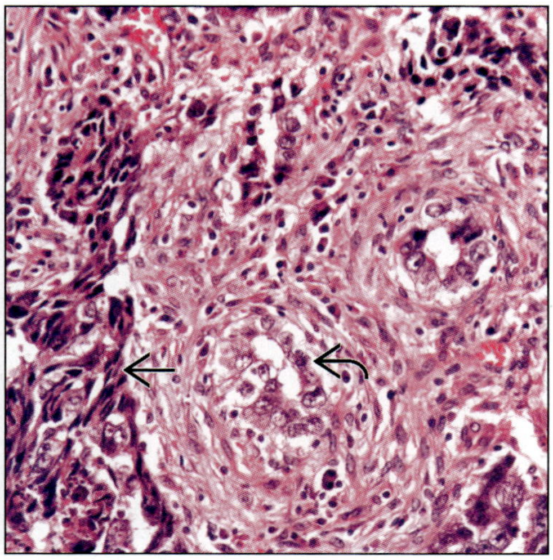

(Left) *Islands of tumor cells are dissecting fibroconnective tissue, giving the appearance of an epithelial neoplasm, namely squamous cell carcinoma. Note that the small glandular structures* ↷ *are more in keeping with embryonal carcinoma.* ***(Right)*** *Higher magnification shows the contrast between the glandular structures* ↷ *and the compressed islands of tumor cells* →*.*

EMBRYONAL CARCINOMA

Microscopic Features

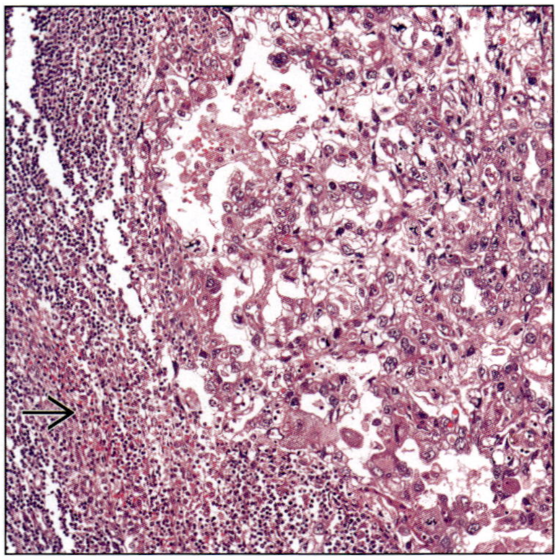

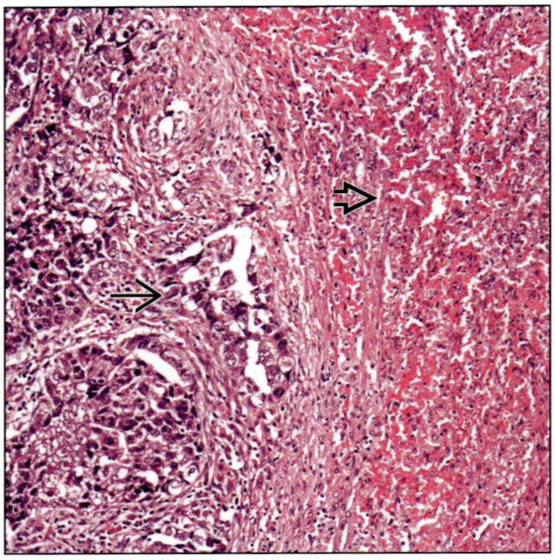

(Left) *In some cases, embryonal carcinoma may not show areas of necrosis but rather an inflammatory reaction composed mainly of lymphocytes and plasma cells →.* ***(Right)*** *A common feature of embryonal carcinoma is the presence of extensive areas of necrosis ⇨. Note the transition areas with tumor cells →.*

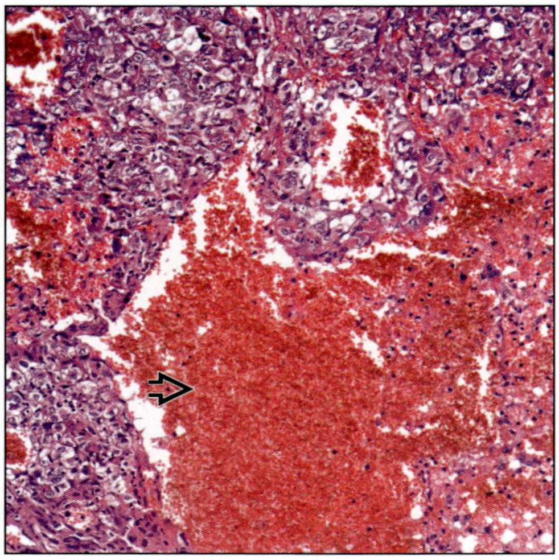

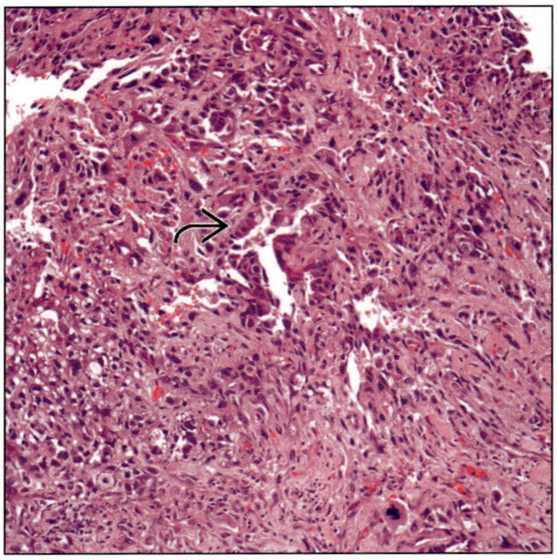

(Left) *Embryonal carcinoma may also show extensive areas of hemorrhage ⇨, which in some cases may obscure the nature of the neoplasm.* ***(Right)*** *Fibroconnective tissue infiltrated by neoplastic cells, which are in sheets and in focal areas, are seen forming pseudoglandular structures ↪. This pattern can be confused for adenocarcinoma.*

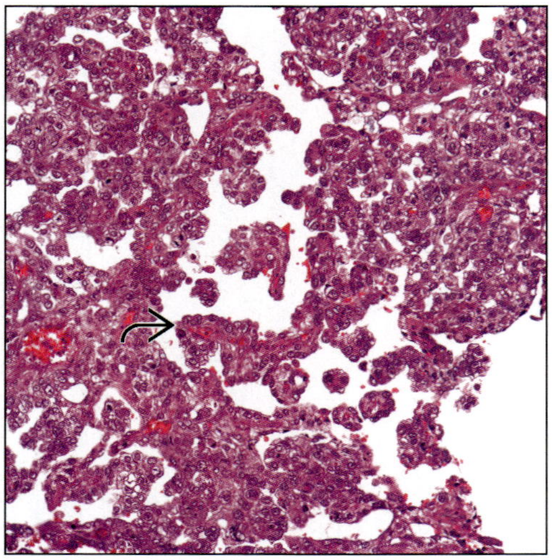

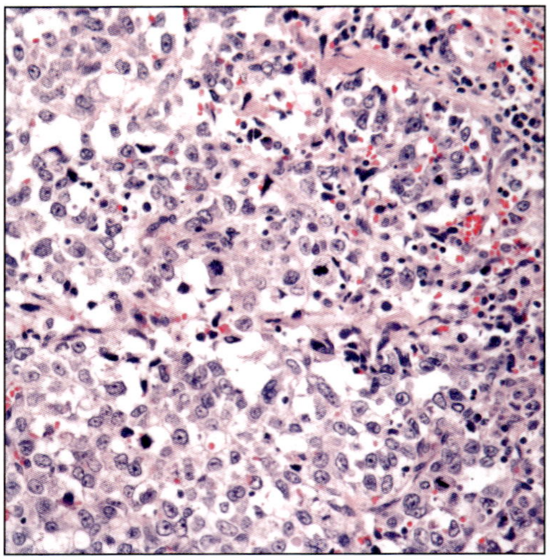

(Left) *Embryonal carcinoma shows cords of neoplastic cells, and in focal areas, these cords acquire a pseudopapillary appearance ↪.* ***(Right)*** *Embryonal carcinoma with a solid growth pattern is composed of medium-sized cells with prominent nucleoli. Numerous mitotic figures are easily identified.*

Microscopic Features

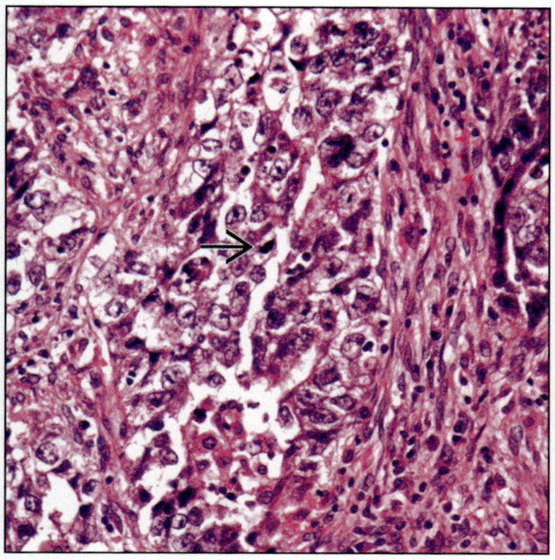

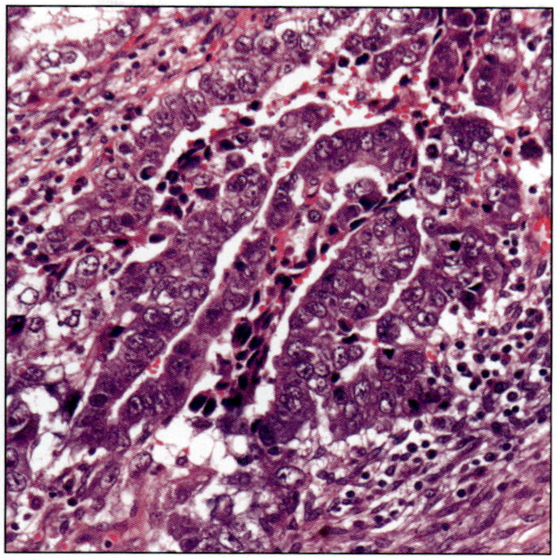

(Left) *This closer view shows neoplastic cells of embryonal carcinoma that are medium sized with round to oval vesiculated nuclei and prominent nucleoli. Mitoses are easily identified* ➔. ***(Right)*** *High magnification shows neoplastic cells arranged in cords with little intervening stroma. No necrosis is present, but atypical mitotic figures are seen.*

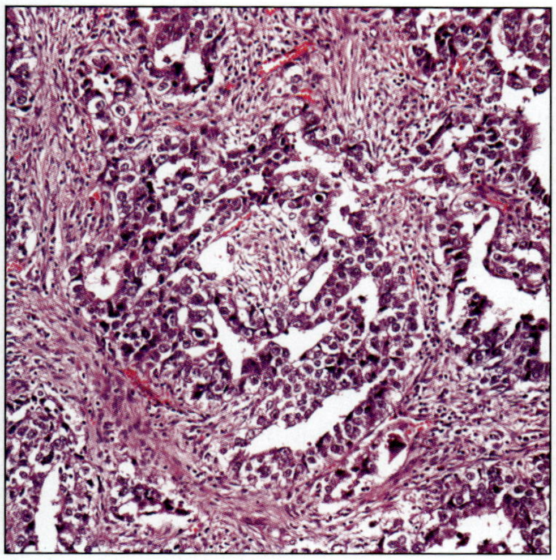

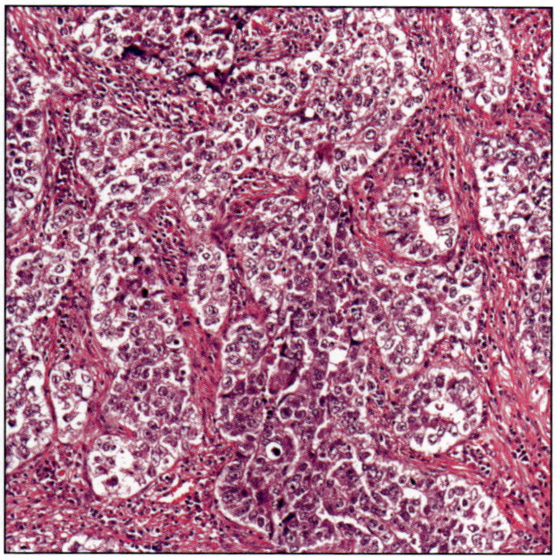

(Left) *Embryonal carcinoma shows a back-to-back glandular-like appearance. Note that the neoplastic cells have prominent nucleoli and a vesicular cytoplasm.* ***(Right)*** *Embryonal carcinoma with a pseudoglandular arrangement. The cells show a clear cytoplasm; even at this magnification, it is easy to observe nuclear atypia and mitotic activity.*

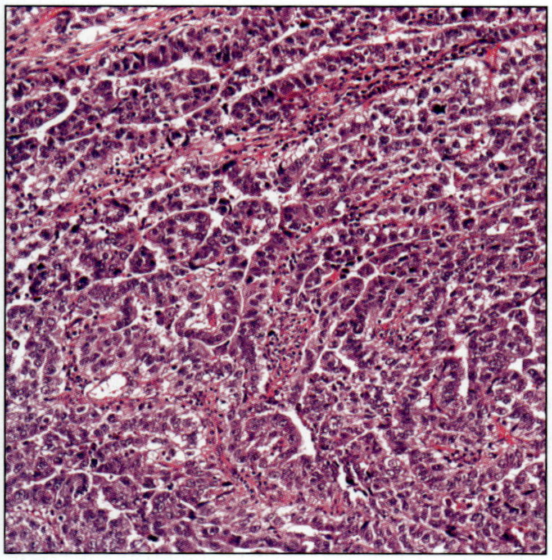

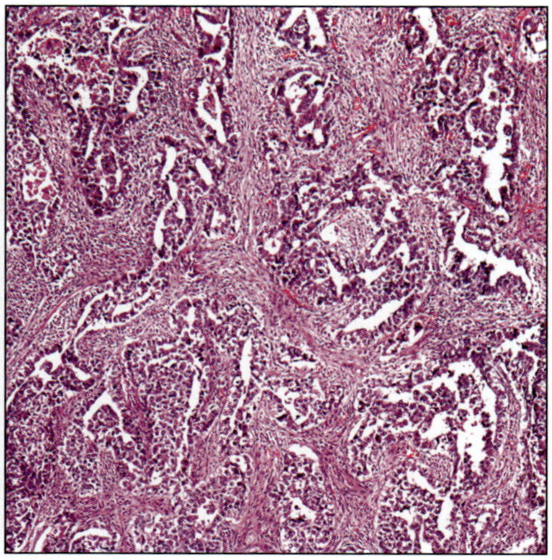

(Left) *Embryonal carcinoma shows cords and a pseudoglandular arrangement of neoplastic cells. This appearance can easily be confused with a metastatic carcinoma.* ***(Right)*** *Embryonal carcinoma shows the classical glandular appearance in which glands are separated by bands of fibroconnective tissue.*

HODGKIN LYMPHOMA OF THE MEDIASTINUM

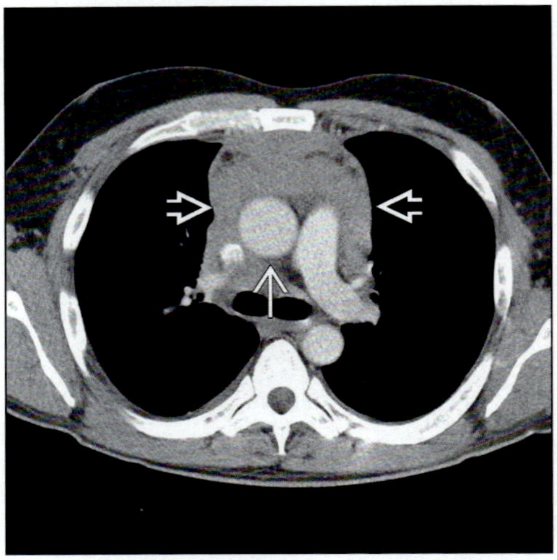

Axial contrast-enhanced CT shows a soft tissue anterior mediastinal mass ➡, which surrounds the aorta ➡ and other vascular structures without obstruction. This is typical of Hodgkin lymphoma.

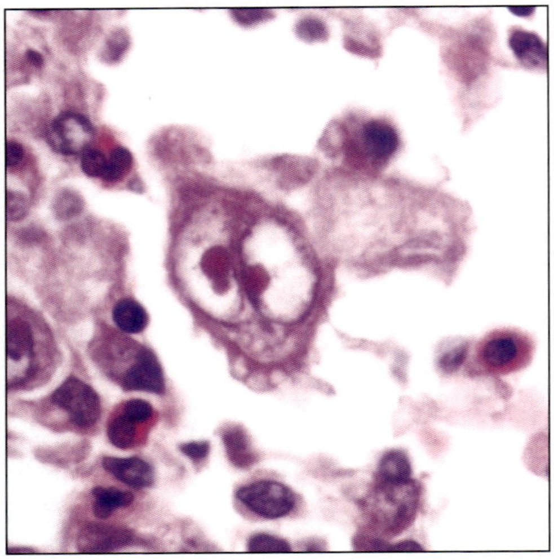

Classical Reed-Sternberg cell is seen in Hodgkin lymphoma (center of the field). Notice the large nuclei with prominent "owl-eyed" nucleoli and scattered eosinophils surrounding them.

TERMINOLOGY

Abbreviations

- Hodgkin lymphoma (HL)

Synonyms

- Hodgkin disease
- Classical Hodgkin lymphoma (CHL)

Definitions

- Malignant proliferation of CD30/CD15(+) lymphoreticular cells of B-cell lineage intimately admixed with other reactive cellular elements arising within mediastinal lymph nodes &/or thymus

CLINICAL ISSUES

Presentation

- Asymptomatic in about 50% of patients (incidental finding on chest x-ray or CT scan)
- More frequent in young patients; female predilection
- Chest pain and dyspnea
- Advanced cases may present with superior vena cava syndrome
- Fever and night sweats (type B symptoms) present in about 30% of patients
- Disease may involve mediastinal lymph nodes, thymus, or both

Treatment

- Radiation therapy is effective for patients in stages I and II
- Advanced stages and bulky mediastinal disease require combination chemotherapy

Prognosis

- Mediastinal HL is a curable disease for patients with stages I or II disease
- Approximately 95% of patients with stage IA or IIA disease and small tumor burden will be alive and free of disease at 10 years
- Patients who fail chemotherapy for advanced disease and suffer relapse have poor prognosis

IMAGE FINDINGS

General Features

- Chest x-rays show solid, lobulated anterior mediastinal mass
- Tumors can show multicystic changes on imaging studies
- Prevascular and paratracheal lymph nodes are most commonly affected

CT Findings

- Multiple rounded soft tissue masses or bulky soft tissue masses
- Displacement, compression, and invasion of mediastinal or chest wall structures

MACROSCOPIC FEATURES

General Features

- HL may involve mediastinal lymph nodes or thymus proper
- When involving thymus, tumor tends to be well circumscribed and encapsulated
- Nodular, gray-white, homogeneous and rubbery tissue on cut section
- When involving thymus, tumor may show prominent cystic changes

Sections to Be Submitted

- 1 block per cm of largest tumor diameter
- In cystic lesions, sample amply solid areas in cyst walls

HODGKIN LYMPHOMA OF THE MEDIASTINUM

Key Facts

Clinical Issues
- Asymptomatic in about 50% of patients (incidental finding on chest x-ray or CT scan)
- More frequent in young patients; female predilection
- Chest pain and dyspnea
- Fever and night sweats (type B symptoms) present in about 30% of patients

Macroscopic Features
- HL may involve mediastinal lymph nodes or thymus proper
- When involving thymus, tumor tends to be well circumscribed and encapsulated
- When involving thymus, cystic changes may be prominent in tumor

Microscopic Pathology
- Nodular sclerosing subtype is most common variant encountered in mediastinum
- Ill-defined, cellular nodules separated by broad bands of fibrous tissue
- Admixture of small lymphocytes, plasma cells, eosinophils, histiocytes, and Reed-Sternberg cells and their variants
- "Syncytial" variant of HL shows sheets of "lacunar" Reed-Sternberg cells surrounding areas of necrosis
- Classical Reed-Sternberg cells are large, binucleated, and display characteristic "owl-eyed" large eosinophilic nucleoli
- Mononuclear variants (Hodgkin cells) have large single nucleus with prominent eosinophilic nucleolus

MICROSCOPIC PATHOLOGY

Histologic Features
- Nodular sclerosing subtype is most common variant encountered in mediastinum
  - Ill-defined, cellular nodules separated by broad bands of fibrous tissue
  - Admixture of small lymphocytes, plasma cells, eosinophils, histiocytes, and Reed-Sternberg cells and their variants
  - Epithelial-lined cysts containing solid areas with characteristic lymphoreticular proliferation in cyst walls
  - Entrapped, hyperplastic thymic epithelium can be encountered within tumor in cases arising in thymus
  - Sclerosis can be massive, resulting in large expanses of acellular collagenous stroma with small islands containing characteristic tumor cells
  - Pattern of sclerosis may be fine and reticular, resulting in "compartmentalization" of tumor cells reminiscent of diffuse large B-cell lymphoma of mediastinum with sclerosis
- Syncytial variant of nodular sclerosis Hodgkin lymphoma
  - Sheets of "lacunar" Reed-Sternberg cells surrounding areas of necrosis

Cytologic Features
- Identification of Reed-Sternberg cells is required for diagnosis
  - Classical Reed-Sternberg cells are large, binucleated, and display characteristic "owl-eyed" large eosinophilic nucleoli
  - Mononuclear variants (Hodgkin cells) have large single nucleus with prominent eosinophilic nucleolus
  - "Lacunar" Reed-Sternberg cells are characterized by clear halo surrounding nucleus
  - Reed-Sternberg cells may show bizarre forms due to extensive degenerative changes
    - Anaplastic tumor cells with abundant cytoplasm reminiscent of pleomorphic high-grade sarcoma
    - Degenerating cells with pyknotic, hyperchromatic nuclei ("mummy" cells)

ANCILLARY TESTS

Immunohistochemistry
- Reed-Sternberg cells and their variants are positive for CD30 and CD15
- Reed-Sternberg cells are negative for CD3, CD20, and CD45

DIFFERENTIAL DIAGNOSIS

Germ Cell Tumor
- Seminoma, embryonal carcinoma, yolk sac tumor
- Elevated oncofetal proteins (AFP, PLAP, HCG, etc.) in serum
- Absence of regional or generalized lymphadenopathy
- Absence of Reed-Sternberg cells

Thymoma
- Epithelial cells in thymoma are devoid of cytologic atypia or multinucleation
- Monotonous lymphoid cell infiltrate (immature T cells) seen in thymoma
- Absence of Reed-Sternberg cells in thymoma
- Large epithelioid cells in thymoma stain for cytokeratin rather than for CD30

Diffuse Large Cell Lymphoma (DLCL) of Mediastinum
- Pattern of sclerosis in DLCL is characterized by small compartments rather than large lobules
- Neoplastic cell population is more uniform than in HL, without eosinophils, histiocytes, and plasma cells
- Atypical tumor cells in DLCL are positive for CD20 and CD45 and negative for CD15 and CD30

HODGKIN LYMPHOMA OF THE MEDIASTINUM

Immunohistochemistry

Antibody	Reactivity	Staining Pattern	Comment
CD30	Positive	Cell membrane & cytoplasm	Membranous and dot-like, paranuclear cytoplasmic positivity is distinctive pattern of staining for RS cells
CD15	Positive	Cell membrane & cytoplasm	Not as sensitive as CD30 for RS cells; can stain many other types of cells (i.e., granulocytes, etc.)
pax-5	Positive	Nuclear	Pax-5 nuclear staining of Hodgkin cells is helpful to demonstrate B-cell lineage and distinguish HL from CD30/CD15(+), CD45/CD20(-) peripheral T-cell lymphoma
CD3	Negative	Not applicable	CD3 helps rule out peripheral T-cell lymphoma, especially when there is atypical medium-sized population of lymphocytes in background
CD20	Negative	Not applicable	CD20 is usually negative in Reed-Sternberg cells; most CD30(+) large cell lymphomas of mediastinum are of B-cell type (CD20[+])
CD45	Negative	Not applicable	Reed-Sternberg cells are CD45 negative, unlike diffuse large B-cell lymphoma in which cells are always positive

Anaplastic Large Cell Lymphoma (ALCL)

- Tumor cells in ALCL can look indistinguishable from Reed-Sternberg cells
- Cell population in ALCL is more uniform and homogeneous
- Nodularity and sclerosis are not prominent features of ALCL
- Tumor cells in ALCL are CD30(+) but CD15(-)
- Tumor cells in ALCL may type as either T or B, and may be ALK1 positive
- ALCL can be confused for "syncytial" variant of HL; confirmation by immunohistochemistry is recommended

DIAGNOSTIC CHECKLIST

Clinically Relevant Pathologic Features

- Age distribution
  - Younger age group (children and adolescents)
- Gross appearance
  - Multinodular, lobulated, and infiltrative mass
  - Frequently displays prominent multicystic changes
  - Homogeneous, fleshy cut surface
- Invasive pattern
  - Often infiltrates adjacent organs (lung, pleura, pericardium)
  - Painless cervical and supraclavicular lymphadenopathy
- Nuclear features
  - Diagnosis based on identification of Reed-Sternberg cells
  - HL has large mono- or multinucleated cells with single or multiple prominent eosinophilic nucleoli
- Immunohistochemistry
  - Reed-Sternberg cells positive for CD30 and CD15

Pathologic Interpretation Pearls

- Reed-Sternberg cells must be present in appropriate milieu for diagnosis
- Diagnosis is best confirmed by immunohistochemistry
- Tumors can undergo extensive stromal sclerosis or massive cystic changes that will mask underlying disease

SELECTED REFERENCES

1. Suster S et al: The Mediastinum. In Weidner et al: Modern Surgical Pathology. 2nd ed. Philadelphia: Saunders Elsevier. 454-516; 2009
2. Ng AK et al: Long-term results of a prospective trial of mantle irradiation alone for early-stage Hodgkin's disease. Ann Oncol. 17(11):1693-7, 2006
3. Krasin MJ et al: Patterns of treatment failure in pediatric and young adult patients with Hodgkin's disease: local disease control with combined-modality therapy. J Clin Oncol. 23(33):8406-13, 2005
4. Brice P et al: Advanced Hodgkin disease with large mediastinal involvement can be treated with eight cycles of chemotherapy alone after a major response to six cycles of chemotherapy: a study of 82 patients from the Groupes d'Etudes des Lymphomes de l'Adulte H89 trial. Cancer. 92(3):453-9, 2001
5. Enrici RM et al: Long-term results of 60 patients with pathologic stage I & IIA Hodgkin's disease treated with exclusive mantle radiation therapy. Eur J Haematol. 63(2):126-33, 1999
6. Glick RD et al: Lymphomas of the anterior mediastinum. Semin Pediatr Surg. 8(2):69-77, 1999
7. Higgins JP et al: CD30 expression is common in mediastinal large B-cell lymphoma. Am J Clin Pathol. 112(2):241-7, 1999
8. Roth SL et al: Contiguous pattern spreading in patients with Hodgkin's disease. Radiother Oncol. 47(1):7-16, 1998
9. Suzuki K et al: Isolated mediastinal Hodgkin's disease mimicking thymoma: report of a case. Surg Today. 28(2):213-6, 1998
10. Hughes-Davies L et al: Stage IA-IIB Hodgkin's disease: management and outcome of extensive thoracic involvement. Int J Radiat Oncol Biol Phys. 39(2):361-9, 1997
11. Luker GD et al: Mediastinal Hodgkin disease in children: response to therapy. Radiology. 189(3):737-40, 1993
12. Orlandi E et al: Residual mediastinal widening following therapy in Hodgkin's disease. Hematol Oncol. 8(3):125-31, 1990
13. Farah R et al: Management of stage I and II Hodgkin's disease. Hematol Oncol Clin North Am. 3(2):253-63, 1989
14. Moormeier JA et al: The staging of Hodgkin's disease. Hematol Oncol Clin North Am. 3(2):237-51, 1989

Nodular Sclerosing Hodgkin Lymphoma

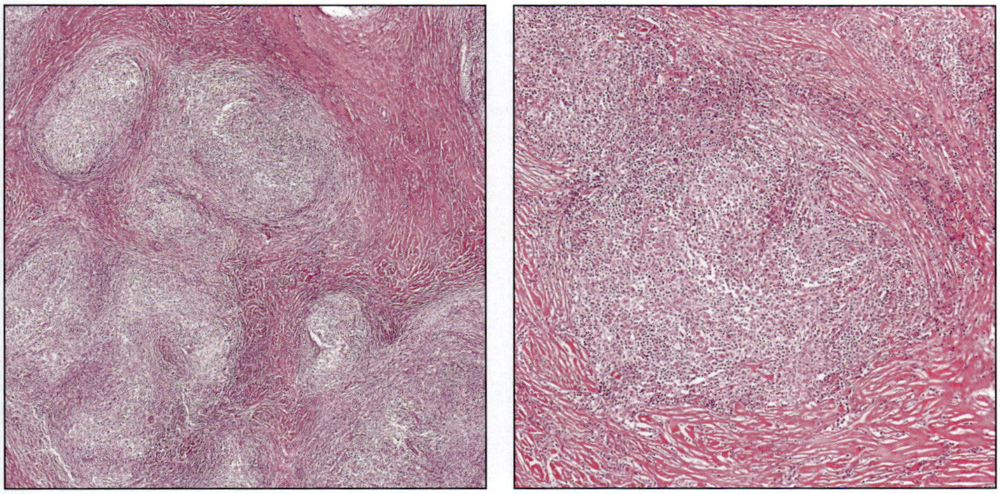

(Left) *Scanning magnification is seen in typical example of nodular sclerosis Hodgkin lymphoma. There are several round cellular nodules separated by broad bands of dense fibroconnective tissue. Nodules are ill defined and of varying sizes.* ***(Right)*** *High magnification of nodular sclerosis Hodgkin lymphoma shows a round cellular nodule containing a mixed population of cells and surrounded by dense fibroconnective tissue. The cell population within the nodule appears to be mixed.*

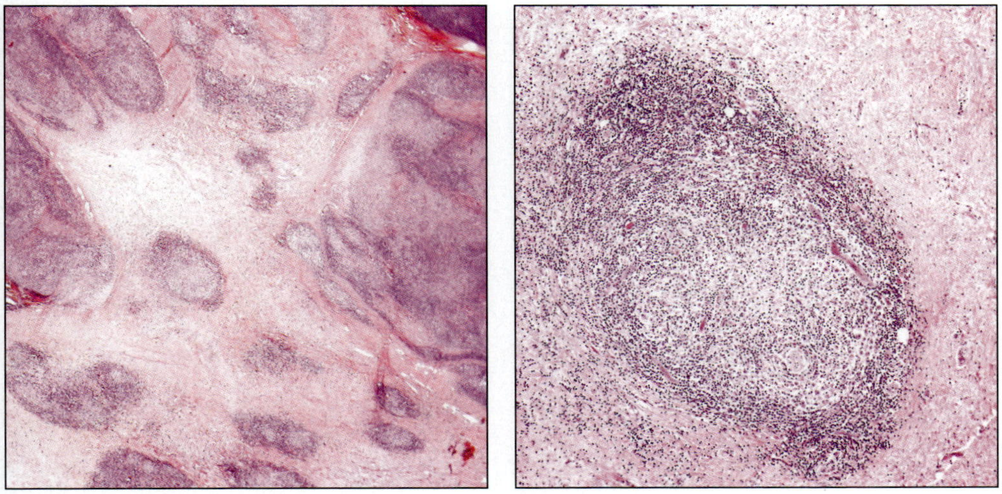

(Left) *Scanning magnification of nodular sclerosis Hodgkin lymphoma shows more advanced fibrosis separating smaller nodules and creating large expanses of acellular connective tissue. A similar picture may be seen in other sclerosing tumors, such as seminoma.* ***(Right)*** *High power of nodular sclerosis Hodgkin lymphoma shows a cellular nodule composed of an atypical cell population admixed with small lymphocytes, plasma cells, and eosinophils and surrounded by dense fibrous tissue.*

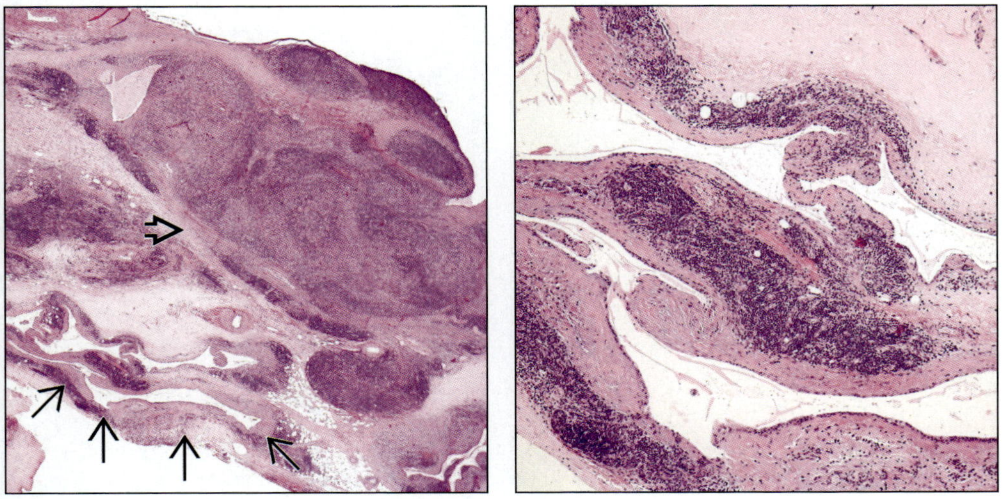

(Left) *Cystic Hodgkin lymphoma shows a solid cellular nodule with neoplastic components* ⇨ *in the wall of a large cyst and several smaller dilated cystic spaces noted toward the bottom of the field* →*.* ***(Right)*** *The cystic spaces in cystic Hodgkin lymphoma are lined by a single layer of simple cuboidal epithelium. The walls of the cysts harbor a dense lymphoid infiltrate containing lymphocytes, plasma cells, histiocytes, eosinophils, and scattered Reed-Sternberg cells.*

Nodular Sclerosing Hodgkin Lymphoma

(Left) *Nodular sclerosis Hodgkin lymphoma of the mediastinum shows sharp delineation of the round cellular nodule from the surrounding connective tissue, with sharp circumscription from the surrounding bands of fibrous tissue.* ***(Right)*** *High magnification of nodular sclerosis Hodgkin lymphoma shows a dense lymphoid cell population punctuated by larger cells with clear halos ("lacunar" cells). Notice the large nuclei and prominent eosinophilic nucleoli within the "lacunar" cells.*

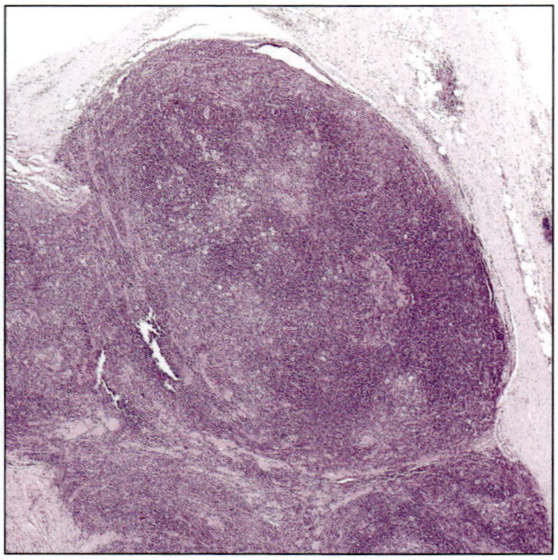

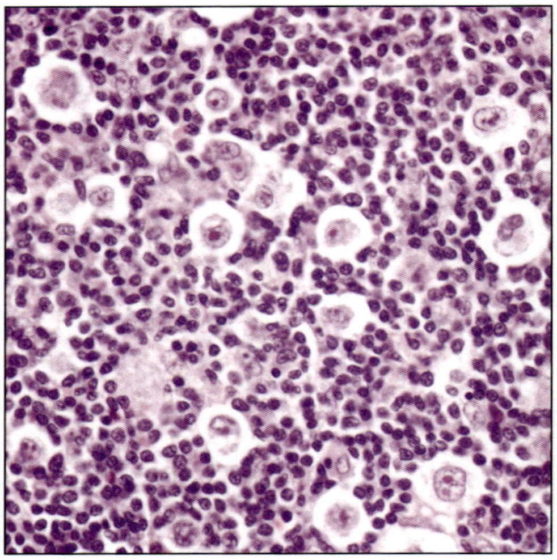

(Left) *High magnification of nodular sclerosis Hodgkin lymphoma shows a characteristic mononuclear Reed-Sternberg cell. Notice large nucleus with clear halo and large, prominent single eosinophilic nucleolus.* ***(Right)*** *Higher magnification of nodular sclerosis Hodgkin lymphoma shows a classical binucleated Reed-Sternberg cell. Notice the 2 large nuclei, each containing a single prominent eosinophilic nucleolus. The surrounding cell population is composed primarily of small lymphocytes.*

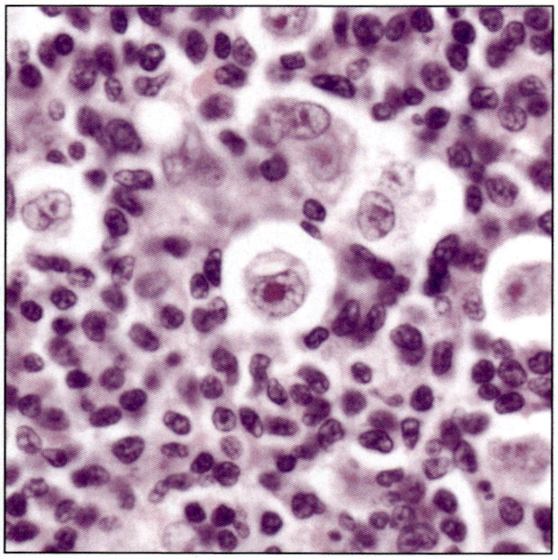

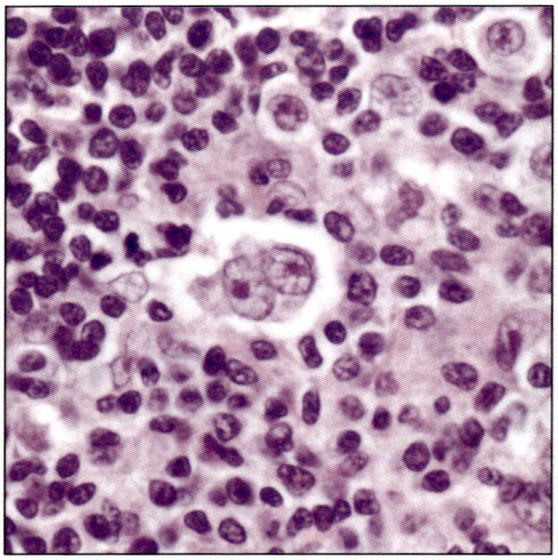

(Left) *Nodular sclerosis Hodgkin lymphoma is seen involving the thymus. Notice entrapped hyperplastic thymic epithelium ⇨ circumscribing the lymphoid cellular proliferation underneath with scattered prominent eosinophils.* ***(Right)*** *High magnification of nodular sclerosis Hodgkin lymphoma involving the thymus shows a mixed cell population with small lymphocytes, abundant eosinophils, and scattered mononuclear and binucleated Reed-Sternberg cells.*

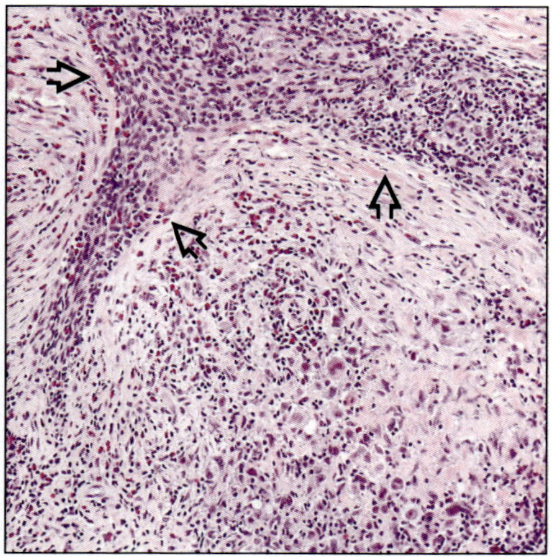

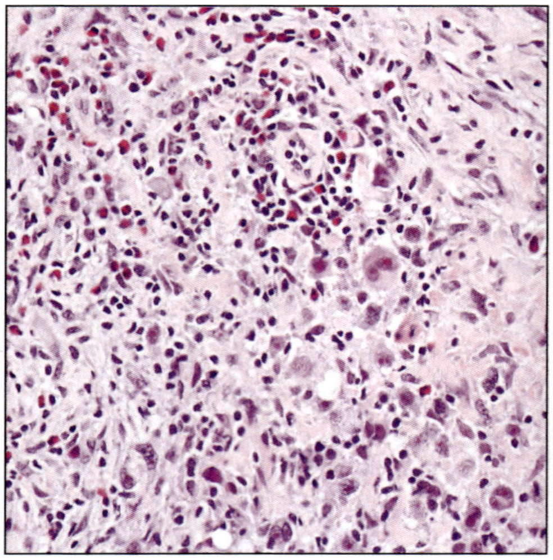

Reed-Sternberg and Hodgkin Cells

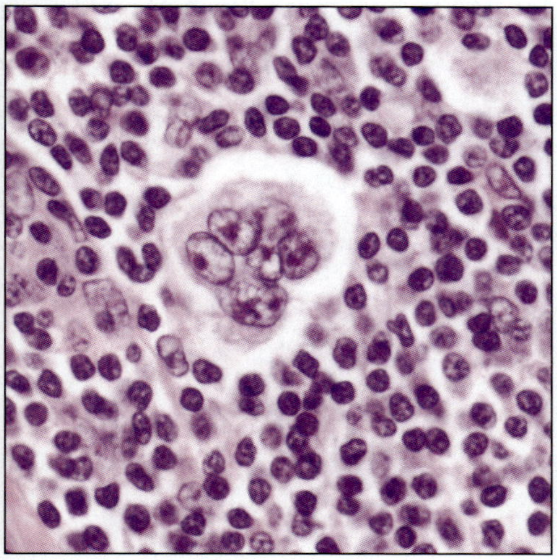

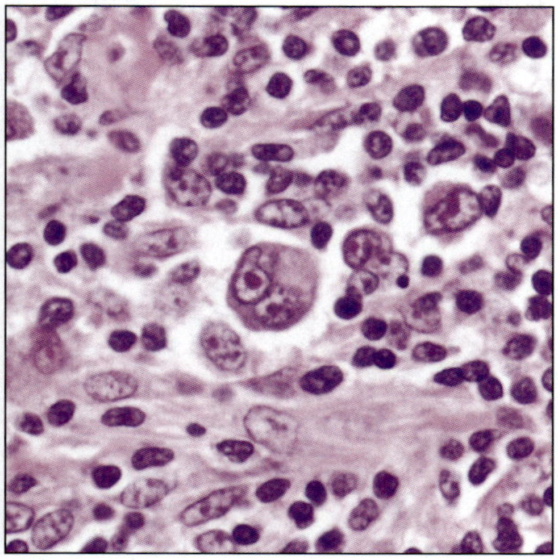

(Left) *Nodular sclerosis Hodgkin lymphoma shows a Reed-Sternberg cell containing 6 nuclei (center of the field), each harboring a large, prominent eosinophilic nucleolus; the nuclei are surrounded by an indistinct rim of amphophilic cytoplasm.* ***(Right)*** *Nodular sclerosis Hodgkin disease shows typical binucleated Reed-Sternberg cell with the characteristic "owl-eyed" nucleoli. Notice a few mononuclear variants of Reed-Sternberg cells (Hodgkin cells) lying in the vicinity.*

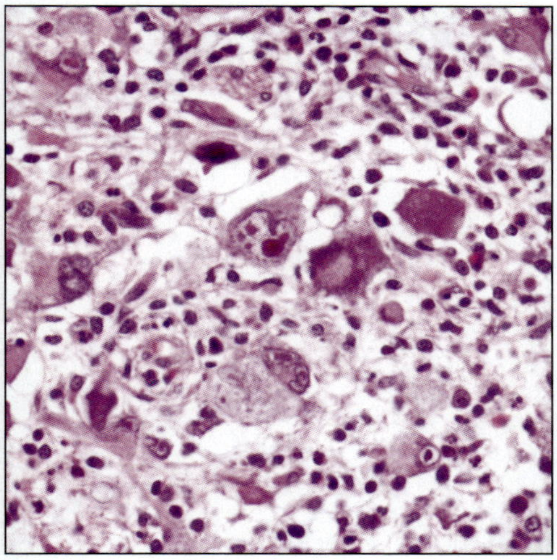

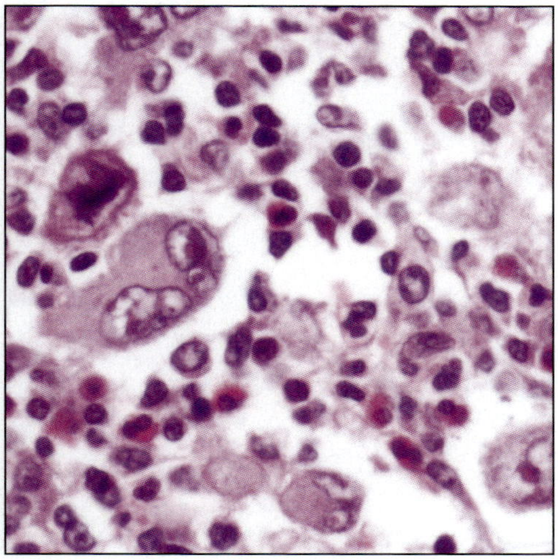

(Left) *Pleomorphic type of Reed-Sternberg cells in nodular sclerosis Hodgkin lymphoma shows bizarre shapes, abundant dense eosinophilic cytoplasm, and prominent eosinophilic nucleoli surrounded by a mixed lymphoid cell population.* ***(Right)*** *Another example of anaplastic morphology in Hodgkin lymphoma shows large, bizarre tumor cells, some of which contain multiple nuclei with prominent eosinophilic nucleoli. Notice the eosinophils surrounding the large atypical cells.*

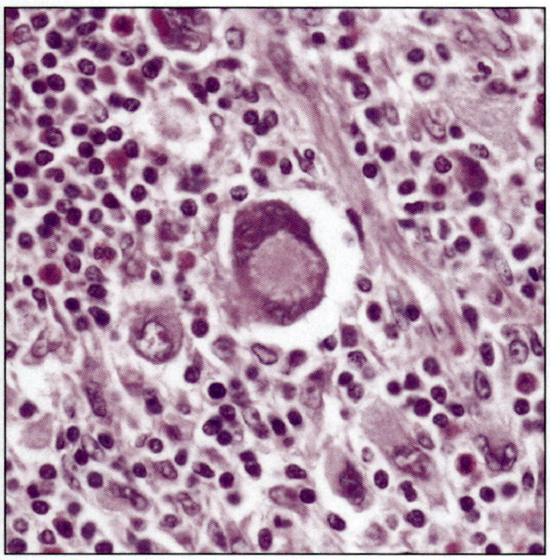

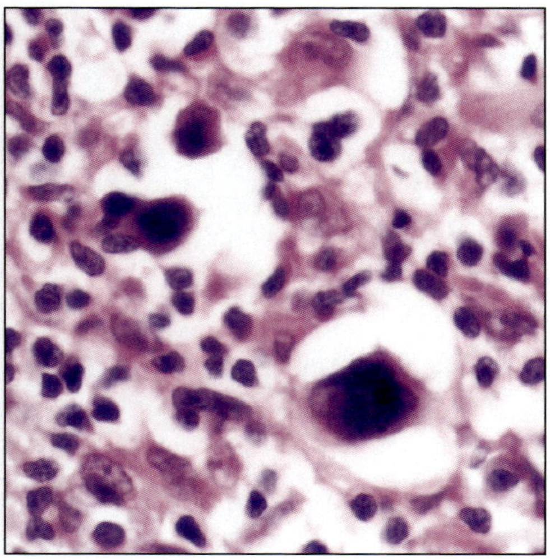

(Left) *Nodular sclerosis Hodgkin lymphoma shows a degenerating multinucleated Reed-Sternberg cell (center of the field) displaying abundant cytoplasm reminiscent of atypical cells seen in high-grade pleomorphic sarcomas ("malignant fibrous histiocytoma").* ***(Right)*** *Nodular sclerosis Hodgkin lymphoma shows hyperchromatic nuclei ("mummy" cells) present in Reed-Sternberg cells. The surrounding cell population is composed of lymphocytes, histiocytes, and plasma cells.*

HODGKIN LYMPHOMA OF THE MEDIASTINUM

Variants of Mediastinal Hodgkin Lymphoma

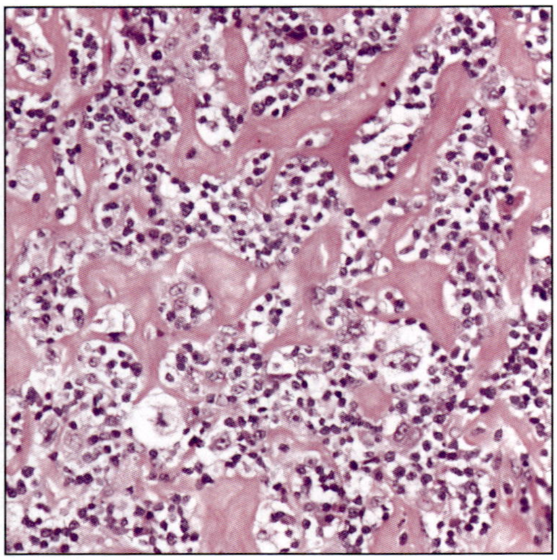
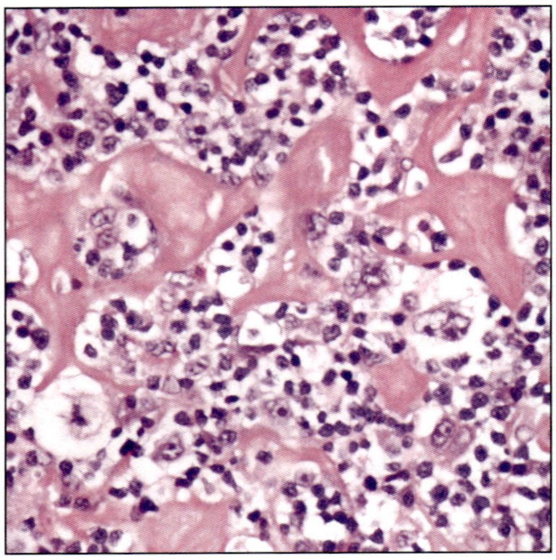

(Left) *Nodular sclerosis Hodgkin lymphoma (HL) with unusual pattern of fine interstitial sclerosis in mediastinal Hodgkin disease resulting in compartmentalization effect reminiscent of diffuse large B-cell lymphoma of mediastinum. Note fine bands of fibrous tissue separating the lymphoid cell population.* ***(Right)*** *High magnification of nodular sclerosis HL shows small islands of lymphoid cells with a few large, atypical mono- and multinucleated Reed-Sternberg cells.*

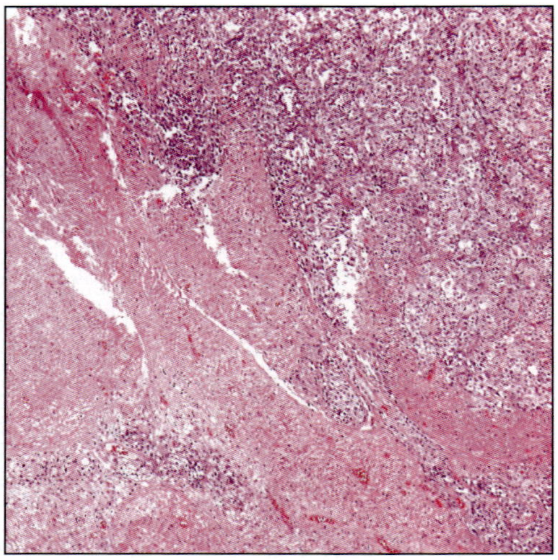
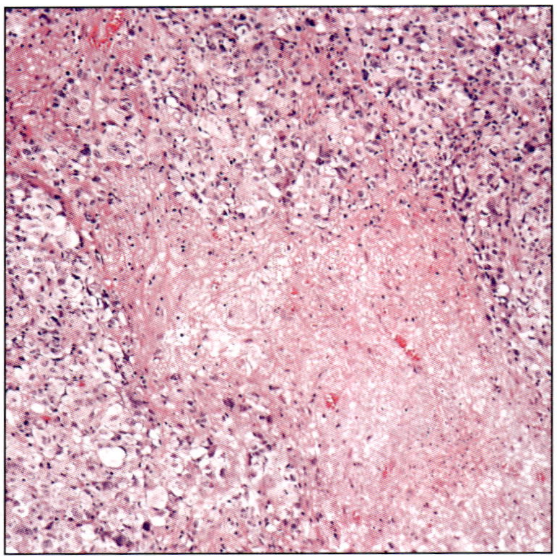

(Left) *Syncytial variant of Hodgkin lymphoma of the mediastinum shows solid cellular areas (top right) separated from extensive areas of tumor cell necrosis (bottom half). The cells in the cellular areas form solid sheets and circumscribe the areas of necrosis.* ***(Right)*** *Syncytial variant of Hodgkin lymphoma of the mediastinum shows sheets of large, atypical mononuclear cells surrounding a central, irregular area of necrosis. Notice the monotonous nature of the mononuclear cells.*

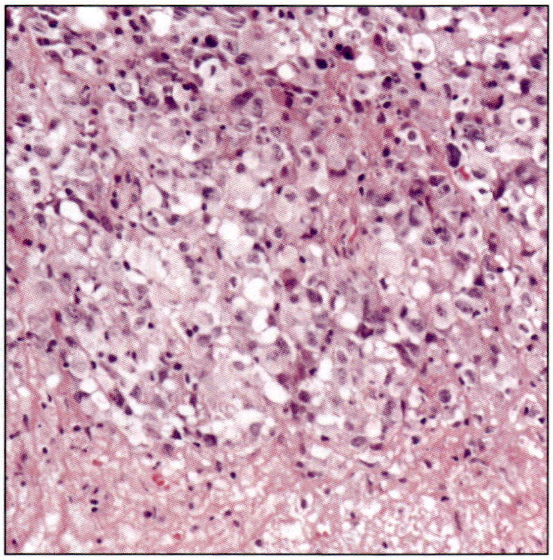
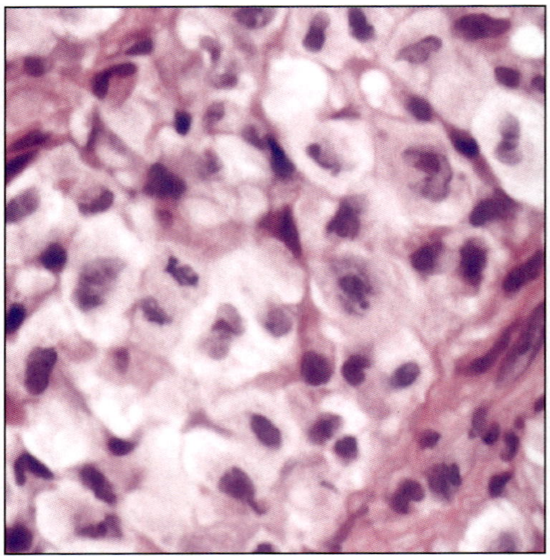

(Left) *High magnification of syncytial variant of Hodgkin lymphoma shows solid cellular areas composed of an atypical cell population. Notice the uniformity and monotony of the tumor cell population. Such areas can closely resemble diffuse large B-cell lymphoma of the mediastinum.* ***(Right)*** *Higher magnification of syncytial variant of Hodgkin lymphoma shows solid sheets of mononuclear lacunar Reed-Sternberg cells with enlarged nuclei and prominent clear cytoplasmic halos.*

Immunohistochemical Features

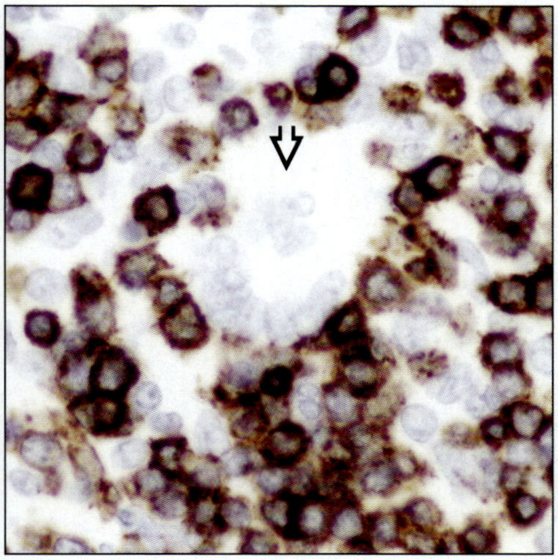

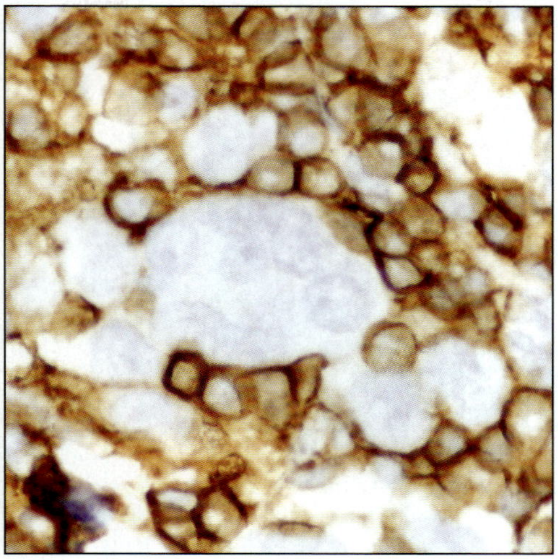

(Left) *Immunoperoxidase stain for CD3 highlights small T-lymphocytes in Hodgkin lymphoma. Notice the rosette-like distribution of CD3(+) T-lymphocytes around a Reed-Sternberg cell.* ***(Right)*** *Immunohistochemical staining of Hodgkin lymphoma of the mediastinum for CD45 shows staining of the small lymphocytes in the periphery but negative staining of the large, multinucleated Reed-Sternberg cell in the center of the field.*

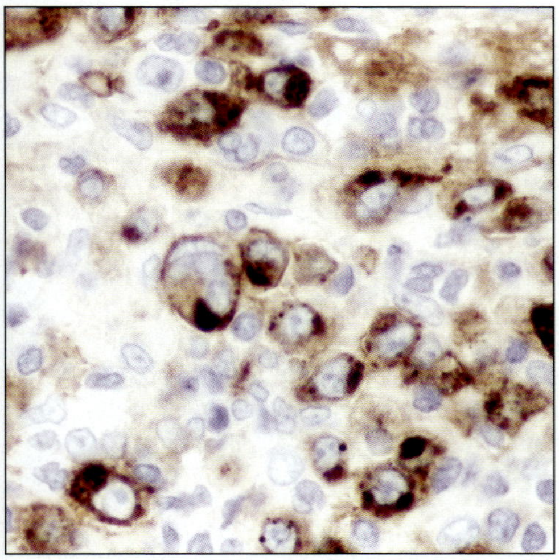

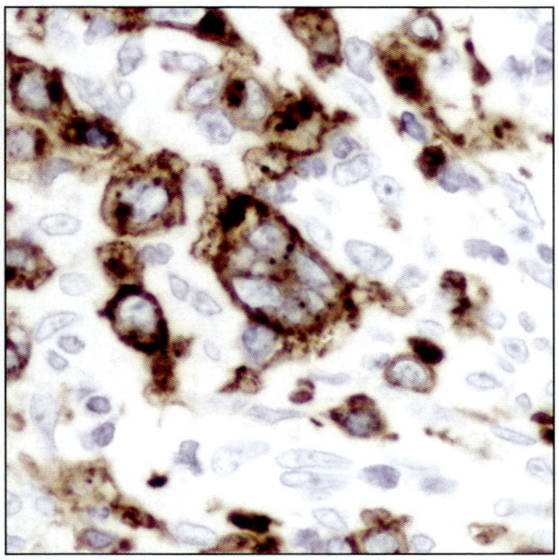

(Left) *Immunohistochemical staining of Hodgkin lymphoma shows positivity for CD15 (Leu-M1) in scattered Reed-Sternberg cells. Notice that the staining pattern is both membranous and paranuclear, with Golgi zone distribution.* ***(Right)*** *Immunohistochemical staining shows positivity of Reed-Sternberg cells in Hodgkin lymphoma for CD30. Notice the membrane and dot-like paranuclear pattern of staining of the large, multinucleated Reed-Sternberg cell in the center of the field.*

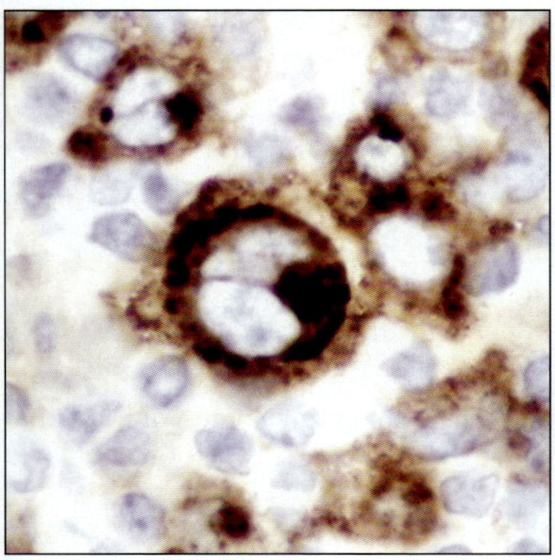

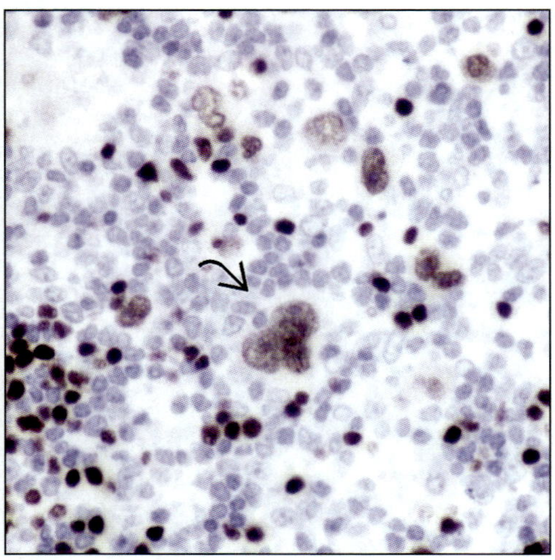

(Left) *Immunoperoxidase stain shows membranous, cytoplasmic, and dot-like paranuclear positivity for CD30 in large, binucleated Reed-Sternberg cell in the center of the field in classical Hodgkin lymphoma.* ***(Right)*** *Immunohistochemical staining for Pax-5 shows positive nuclear staining in Reed-Sternberg cells in classical Hodgkin lymphoma. This serves to identify these cells as of B-cell lineage in equivocal cases and supports a diagnosis of HL over that of T-cell lymphoma.*

DIFFUSE LARGE CELL LYMPHOMA OF THE MEDIASTINUM

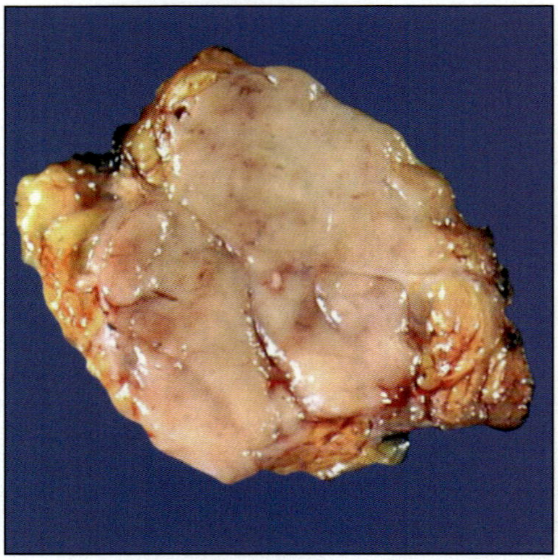

Gross photograph of mediastinal diffuse large cell lymphoma shows an ill-defined mass with tan-white, lobulated, and homogeneous cut surface.

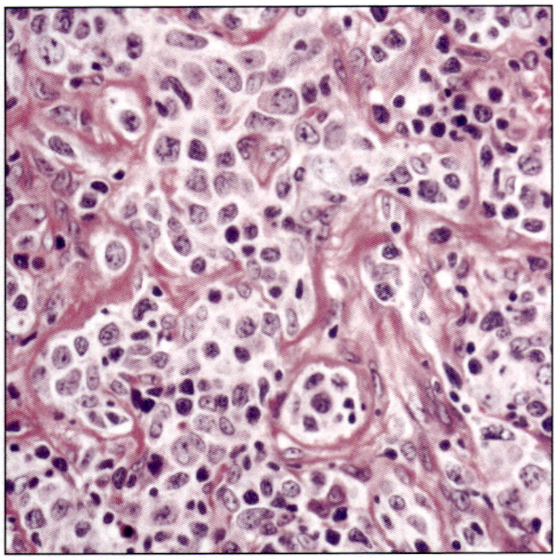

The histologic appearance of mediastinal diffuse large cell lymphoma is characterized by small islands or nests of large tumor cells separated by thin, collagenized, fibrous septa.

TERMINOLOGY

Abbreviations

- Diffuse large cell lymphoma of the mediastinum (DLCLM)

Synonyms

- Mediastinal large B-cell lymphoma (MLBCL); mediastinal diffuse large cell lymphoma (MDLCL); diffuse large cell lymphoma with sclerosis

Definitions

- Primary large cell lymphoma arising from native thymic lymphoid B-cell population

ETIOLOGY/PATHOGENESIS

Pathogenesis

- Derived from extranodal, mucosa-associated, native lymphoid cell population originating in medullary compartment of thymus
- In some cases, may represent progression from extranodal marginal zone B-cell lymphoma (MALToma) of thymus
- Gene expression profiling has demonstrated 30% similarity of gene expression with classical Hodgkin lymphoma

CLINICAL ISSUES

Epidemiology

- Incidence
  - Represents about 6% of all large cell lymphomas in adults
  - Represents about 25% of all childhood non-Hodgkin lymphomas
- Age
  - Most commonly occurs in young adults (range: 15-73; median: 32)
  - Can also occur in children and adolescents
- Gender
  - Predilection for women

Presentation

- Distinctive clinicopathologic syndrome
  - Predominantly affects women in 3rd decade of life
  - Presents with rapidly growing, large (> 10 cm in diameter), infiltrative anterior mediastinal mass
  - Rarely involves peripheral lymph nodes, bone marrow, or other lymphoid organs
  - Commonly presents with superior vena cava syndrome, pleural effusion, and airway obstruction
  - Relapses involve variety of extrathoracic sites, including kidneys, adrenals, liver, and central nervous system

Treatment

- Combination chemotherapy ± radiation therapy

Prognosis

- Despite high-grade histology and aggressive presentation, DLCLMs respond well to combination chemotherapy
- Recent studies have shown remission rates of nearly 80% and disease-free survival of 60% at 3 years

IMAGE FINDINGS

Radiographic Findings

- Mediastinal widening with pleural effusion

CT Findings

- Large mediastinal mass obscuring borders of heart and great vessels
- Infiltration of lung or pericardium
- Pleural effusion

DIFFUSE LARGE CELL LYMPHOMA OF THE MEDIASTINUM

Key Facts

Clinical Issues

- Predominantly affects women in 3rd decade of life
- Presents with rapidly growing, large (> 10 cm in diameter), infiltrative anterior mediastinal mass
- Rarely involves peripheral lymph nodes, bone marrow, or other lymphoid organs
- Commonly presents with superior vena cava syndrome, pleural effusion, and airway obstruction
- Relapses involve a variety of extrathoracic sites, including kidneys, adrenals, liver, and central nervous system

Microscopic Pathology

- Nuclei may show great variability, from centroblastic to immunoblastic morphology
- Nuclear pleomorphism with bizarre forms can often be found
- Crushing artifact is common finding in small endoscopic biopsies or core needle biopsies
- Stromal sclerosis may be fine and delicate or coarse, separating tumor cells into small nests
- Consistent B-cell phenotype: CD19(+), CD20(+), CD22(+), CD79-α(+)
- Other markers: May show CD30(+) when using heat-induced epitope retrieval techniques; generally Bcl-6(+), variably Bcl-2(+)
- Negative markers: Ig, CD5, CD15, CD21, CD30 (in multinucleated tumor cells), EBV
- Other lymphoid markers: CD45(+), HLA-DR(+), IgG or IgA(+), may show κ or λ light chain restriction

MACROSCOPIC FEATURES

General Features

- Bulky mediastinal disease with infiltration of lung, pleura, pericardium, and chest wall
- Homogeneous rubbery cut surface; may show areas of hemorrhage and necrosis

MICROSCOPIC PATHOLOGY

Histologic Features

- Most cases are characterized by sheets of large lymphoid cells with prominent nucleoli and pale cytoplasm
- May show unusual histologic features, including following subtypes
  - Clear cell mediastinal lymphoma
    - Sheets of large CD20(+) lymphoid cells with large nuclei and prominent nucleoli surrounded by ample rim of water-clear cytoplasm
    - Clear cell lymphoma may resemble metastases of renal cell carcinoma and other clear cell malignant neoplasms
  - Spindle cell mediastinal lymphoma
    - Sheets or fascicles of CD20(+) spindle cells with elongated, hyperchromatic nuclei
    - May show a prominent "storiform" pattern resembling malignant fibrohistiocytic neoplasms
    - Spindle cell lymphoma may be confused for a variety of spindle cell sarcomas
  - Pleomorphic mediastinal large cell lymphoma
    - Sheets of bizarre CD20(+) pleomorphic tumor cells with atypical multinucleated and multilobated cells
    - Pleomorphic large cell lymphoma may resemble variety of high-grade pleomorphic sarcomas
  - Large cell mediastinal lymphoma with marked tropism for germinal centers ("germinotropic lymphoma")
    - Clusters of large, CD20(+) atypical lymphoid cells encroaching on germinal centers and replacing follicular center cells
    - Irregular replacement of follicles by large, atypical lymphoid cells in fashion reminiscent of progressive transformation of germinal centers
    - Atypical lymphoid cells are found within lymphoid follicles without involvement of interfollicular areas
    - Germinotropic lymphoma may be confused for mediastinal seminoma, metastatic carcinoma, or melanoma
  - Signet ring cell mediastinal lymphoma
    - Sheets or singly scattered CD20(+) lymphoid cells displaying prominent signet-ring cell features are seen admixed with lymphoid cells
    - Signet-ring cell lymphoma may be confused for liposarcoma or metastases of signet-ring cell carcinoma
  - Mediastinal large B-cell lymphoma with Hodgkin-like or anaplastic large cell lymphoma-like features
    - Sheets of large anaplastic CD20(+) lymphoid cells with indented nuclei and prominent eosinophilic nucleoli
    - Sheets of Reed-Sternberg-like multinucleated or multilobated B-lymphoid cells with prominent eosinophilic nucleoli
    - Tumor cells may be positive for CD30 but are also positive for CD20 and are negative for ALK1 and T-cell markers
  - Diffuse large B-cell lymphoma with sclerosis
    - Nests of large, atypical CD20(+) lymphocytes surrounded by variable degrees of stromal collagenization, creating a "compartmentalized" growth pattern
    - Stromal sclerosis may be fine and delicate or coarse, separating tumor cells into small nests
    - Advanced stages of collagenization may show extensive paucicellular stromal sclerosis with few residual atrophic tumor cells
    - Nests of tumor cells separated by fibrous septa may be confused for carcinoma or melanoma

- Other unusual histologic features
  - Residual thymic epithelial islands may show hyperplastic features and undergo cystic changes
  - Sheets of atypical B lymphocytes may show degenerative changes, resulting in "pseudoalveolar" growth pattern
  - Tumor cells may show angiocentric distribution around vessel walls with plugging of vessel wall lumen
  - Some cases show overlapping morphologic and genetic features with Hodgkin lymphoma (so-called gray-zone lymphoma)

Cytologic Features

- Nuclei may show great variability, from centroblastic to immunoblastic morphology
- Nuclear pleomorphism with bizarre forms can often be found
- Reed-Sternberg-like cells and small multinucleated or multilobated cells can also be seen
- Cells can be spindled, signet-ring, clear, or pleomorphic
- Crushing artifact is common finding in small endoscopic biopsies or core needle biopsies
- Tumors involving thymus may contain entrapped benign thymic epithelial elements
- Tumor cell necrosis is frequent finding in large tumors
- Tumor cells often show extensive infiltration of adjacent structures, with sparing and preservation of mediastinal fat

ANCILLARY TESTS

Immunohistochemistry

- Consistent B-cell phenotype: CD19(+), CD20(+), CD22(+), CD79-α(+)
- Other lymphoid markers: CD45(+), HLA-DR(+), IgG, or IgA(+)
- Other markers: May show weak CD30 positivity when using heat-induced epitope retrieval techniques; generally Bcl-6(+), variably Bcl-2(+)
- Negative markers: Ig, EBV, CD5, CD15, CD21, CD30 (in multinucleated tumor cells)
- Immunoexpression of MAL is seen in 50% of cases
- May show κ or λ light chain restriction

Molecular Genetics

- Frequent chromosomal gains: 2p, 6p, 7q, 9p, 12, and X
- Most important cytogenetic abnormality is gain of chromosome arm 9p observed in up to 75% of cases, leading to overexpression of c-REL
- Aberrations of chromosome X are seen in up to 87% of cases
- Bcl-2 rearrangements observed in up to 30% of cases
- Overexpression of *MAL* gene is believed to be specific for MDLCL although it is shared with classic Hodgkin lymphoma
- Immunoglobulin gene rearrangements are present
- Absence of Epstein-Barr virus (EBV) genome
- Gene expression profiling shows close similarities with classical Hodgkin lymphoma

DIFFERENTIAL DIAGNOSIS

Thymic Carcinoma and Metastatic Carcinoma

- Tumor cells are cohesive and positive for epithelial markers (cytokeratins, etc.) in thymic carcinoma
- Metastatic renal cell carcinoma is positive for cytokeratins, EMA, CD10, and vimentin
- Thymic carcinoma and metastatic carcinoma tend to occur at older age

Anaplastic Large Cell Lymphoma (ALCL)

- Sclerosis and compartmentalization are not features of ALCL
- Immunophenotype of ALCL is CD30(+), ALK1(+)
- Staining for CD30 in neoplastic cells is stronger and more diffuse in ALCL than in MDLCL
- ALCL is characterized by t(2;5) translocation

Hodgkin Lymphoma

- Mixed cell infiltrate with eosinophils, plasma cells, and small lymphocytes
- Reed-Sternberg cells are CD15/CD30(+) and negative for CD19, CD20, and CD22

Metastatic Amelanotic Malignant Melanoma

- Melanoma cells are positive for S100 protein and other melanocytic markers (HMB-45, Melan-A, tyrosinase, etc.)
  - Melanoma cells are negative for CD20 and CD45

Mediastinal Seminoma

- Tumor cells have large vesicular nuclei with prominent irregular nucleoli due to presence of nucleolonemata
- Tumor cells are positive for PLAP, OCT4, and D2-40, and negative for CD20 and CD45

Sarcoma

- Usually occurs in older age group than MDLCL
- Pleomorphic sarcomas are negative for lymphoid markers (CD20, CD45)

DIAGNOSTIC CHECKLIST

Clinically Relevant Pathologic Features

- Age distribution
  - Young adults (3rd-4th decades)
- Gross appearance
  - Large bulky masses with extensive infiltration of local structures (lung, pleura, pericardium, diaphragm, etc.)
- Metastatic distribution
  - Unusual distribution of extrathoracic metastases: Kidneys, adrenals, liver, pancreas, ovaries, CNS

Pathologic Interpretation Pearls

- Core biopsies are often difficult to diagnose due to distortion by sclerosis or necrosis
- Care must be taken not to misinterpret keratin-positive, entrapped, residual thymic epithelium for evidence of carcinoma on small biopsies
- Nested, compartmentalized appearance should not be mistaken for other types of tumors

Immunohistochemistry

Antibody	Reactivity	Staining Pattern	Comment
CD20	Positive	Cell membrane	Strongly positive in all cases of MDLCL
CD45	Positive	Cytoplasmic	Positive in majority of cases of MDLCL
CD19	Positive	Cytoplasmic	Positive in majority of cases of MDLCL
CD22	Positive	Cytoplasmic	Positive in majority of cases of MDLCL
CD79-α	Positive	Cytoplasmic	Positive in all cases of MDLCL
HLA-DR	Positive	Cytoplasmic	Positive in majority of cases of MDLCL
Bcl-2	Positive	Nuclear	Positive in majority of cases of MDLCL
Bcl-6	Positive	Nuclear	Positive in majority of cases of MDLCL
CD5	Negative	Not applicable	Helpful for differentiating MDLCL from follicular lymphoma
CD10	Negative	Not applicable	May be positive in 50% of MDLCL
CD15	Negative	Not applicable	Helpful for differentiating MDLCL from Hodgkin lymphoma
CD21	Negative	Not applicable	Helpful for differentiating MDLCL from conventional nodal-based DLCL
ALK1	Negative	Not applicable	Useful for differentiating MDLCL from ALCL
CD30	Equivocal	Cytoplasmic	Positivity in MDLCL is weak and cytoplasmic, rather than strong and paranuclear as in ALCL

- High level of suspicion should exist in proper clinicopathologic context
  - Young female
  - Rapidly growing and extensively invasive anterior mediastinal mass
  - No peripheral lymphadenopathy
- Immunohistochemical stains are critical for diagnosis
  - CD20/CD45(+)
  - May be weakly and focally positive for CD30 using heat-induced epitope retrieval
  - Negative for CD5, CD10, CD15, CD21
  - Negative for other markers of differentiation (keratins, CEA, EMA, S100 protein, HMB-45, PLAP, etc.)
  - Overexpression of *MAL* gene is seen in 50% of cases and is considered specific for MDLCL, but it can also be observed in 30% of nodular sclerosing Hodgkin lymphoma
- Molecular studies may be of limited value
  - No rearrangements of T-cell receptor β chain gene constant region
  - No distinctive cytogenetic chromosomal translocations
  - May show Ig heavy or light chain gene rearrangements
  - Absence of t(2;5) may help to distinguish MDLCL from ALCL in equivocal cases

SELECTED REFERENCES

1. Faris JE et al: Primary mediastinal large B-cell lymphoma. Clin Adv Hematol Oncol. 7(2):125-33, 2009
2. Fietz T et al: Treatment of primary mediastinal large B cell lymphoma with an alternating chemotherapy regimen based on high-dose methotrexate. Ann Hematol. 88(5):433-9, 2009
3. Dunphy CH et al: Primary mediastinal B-cell lymphoma: detection of BCL2 gene rearrangements by PCR analysis and FISH. J Hematop. 1(2):77-84, 2008
4. Massoud M et al: Primary mediastinal large B-cell lymphomas treated with dose-intensified CHOP alone or CHOP combined with radiotherapy. Leuk Lymphoma. 49(8):1510-5, 2008
5. Rodríguez J et al: Primary mediastinal B-cell lymphoma: treatment and therapeutic targets. Leuk Lymphoma. 49(6):1050-61, 2008
6. Kimm LR et al: Frequent occurrence of deletions in primary mediastinal B-cell lymphoma. Genes Chromosomes Cancer. 46(12):1090-7, 2007
7. Mazzarotto R et al: Primary mediastinal large B-cell lymphoma: results of intensive chemotherapy regimens (MACOP-B/VACOP-B) plus involved field radiotherapy on 53 patients. A single institution experience. Int J Radiat Oncol Biol Phys. 68(3):823-9, 2007
8. Renné C et al: High expression of several tyrosine kinases and activation of the PI3K/AKT pathway in mediastinal large B cell lymphoma reveals further similarities to Hodgkin lymphoma. Leukemia. 21(4):780-7, 2007
9. Kolonić SO et al: Primary mediastinal large B-cell lymphoma: a single-center study of clinicopathologic characteristics. Int J Hematol. 83(4):331-6, 2006
10. Hamlin PA et al: Primary mediastinal large B-cell lymphoma: optimal therapy and prognostic factor analysis in 141 consecutive patients treated at Memorial Sloan Kettering from 1980 to 1999. Br J Haematol. 130(5):691-9, 2005
11. Traverse-Glehen A et al: Mediastinal gray zone lymphoma: the missing link between classic Hodgkin's lymphoma and mediastinal large B-cell lymphoma. Am J Surg Pathol. 29(11):1411-21, 2005
12. Pileri SA et al: Pathobiology of primary mediastinal B-cell lymphoma. Leuk Lymphoma. 44 Suppl 3:S21-6, 2003
13. Savage KJ et al: The molecular signature of mediastinal large B-cell lymphoma differs from that of other diffuse large B-cell lymphomas and shares features with classical Hodgkin lymphoma. Blood. 102(12):3871-9, 2003
14. Suster S: Primary large-cell lymphomas of the mediastinum. Semin Diagn Pathol. 16(1):51-64, 1999
15. Suster S et al: Pleomorphic large cell lymphomas of the mediastinum. Am J Surg Pathol. 20(2):224-32, 1996
16. Suster S: Large cell lymphoma of the mediastinum with marked tropism for germinal centers. Cancer. 69(12):2910-6, 1992

DIFFUSE LARGE CELL LYMPHOMA OF THE MEDIASTINUM

Mediastinal Large Cell Lymphoma with Sclerosis

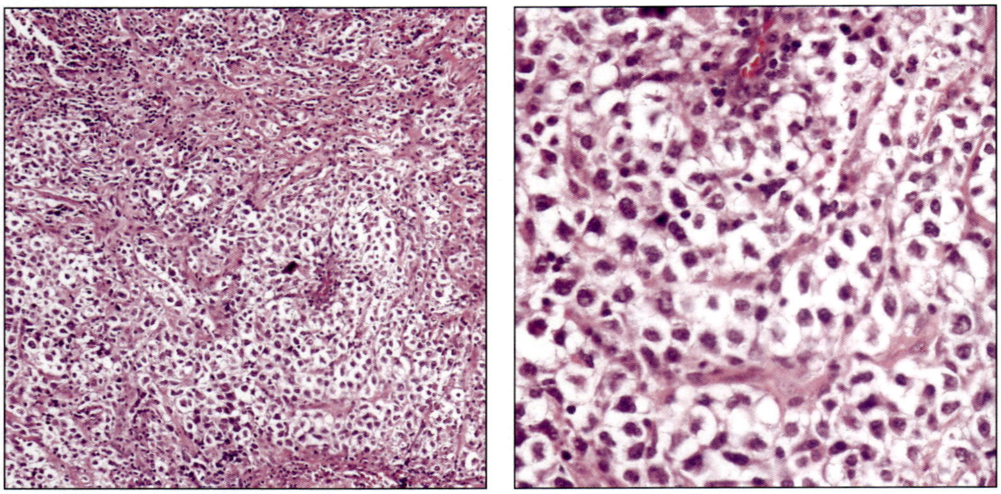

(Left) *Mediastinal diffuse large cell lymphoma with sclerosis shows sheets and ill-defined nests of large, discohesive tumor cells separated by thin strands of fibroconnective tissue.* ***(Right)*** *Higher magnification of mediastinal diffuse large cell lymphoma shows discrete small nests of tumor cells separated by thin fibrovascular septa, resulting in a "compartmentalized" appearance. A similar appearance can be observed in metastatic amelanotic malignant melanoma.*

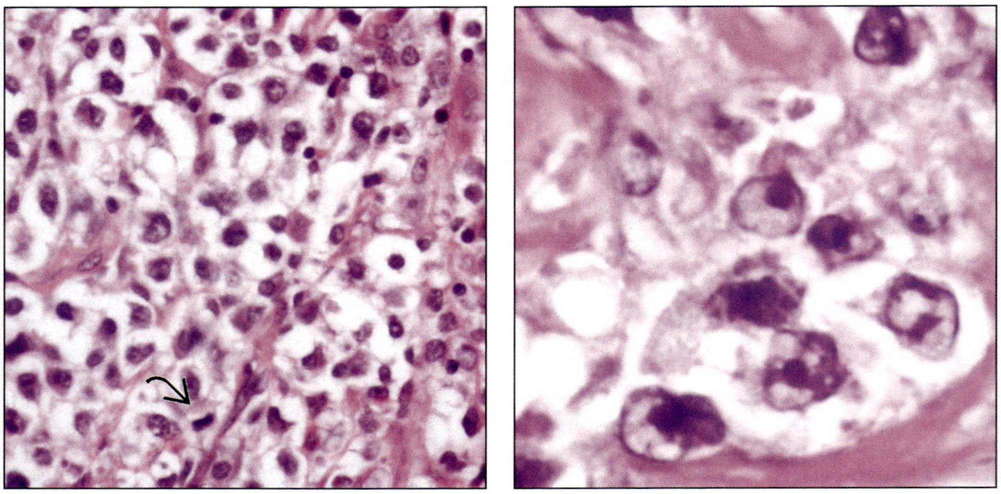

(Left) *High magnification of mediastinal diffuse large cell lymphoma with sclerosis shows large lymphoid cells surrounded by a clear halo with occasional scattered mitotic figures ➔.* ***(Right)*** *Higher magnification of mediastinal diffuse large cell lymphoma with sclerosis shows large, atypical lymphoid cells with vesicular nuclei and prominent single eosinophilic nucleoli. The cells are surrounded by an ample rim of clear or amphophilic cytoplasm.*

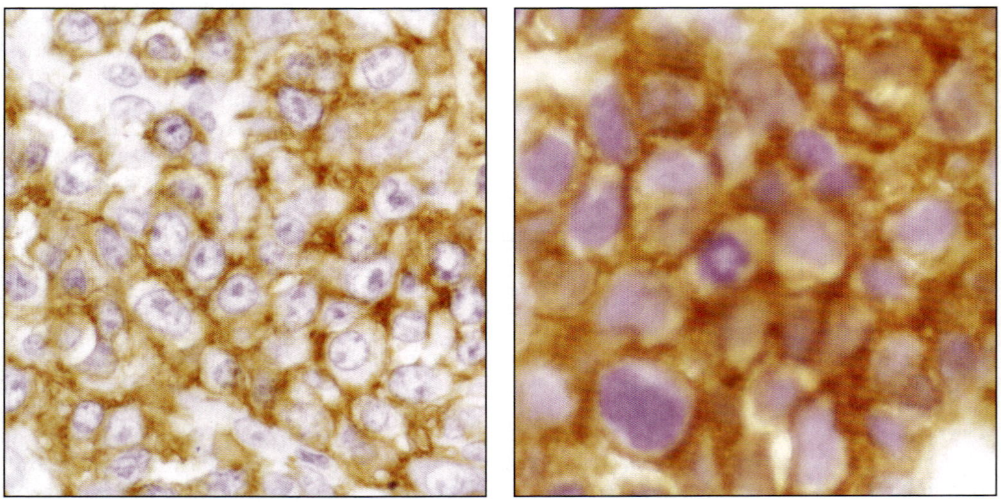

(Left) *Immunohistochemical stain for CD20 shows positive membrane staining in the large, atypical lymphoid cells in mediastinal diffuse large B-cell lymphoma.* ***(Right)*** *Immunohistochemical staining for CD45 (leukocyte common antigen) shows strong positivity of the tumor cells in mediastinal diffuse large B-cell lymphoma. Positivity for this marker, together with CD20 positivity and negative staining for CD15/CD30, is helpful for distinguishing this tumor from mediastinal Hodgkin lymphoma in equivocal cases.*

Mediastinal Large Cell Lymphoma with Sclerosis

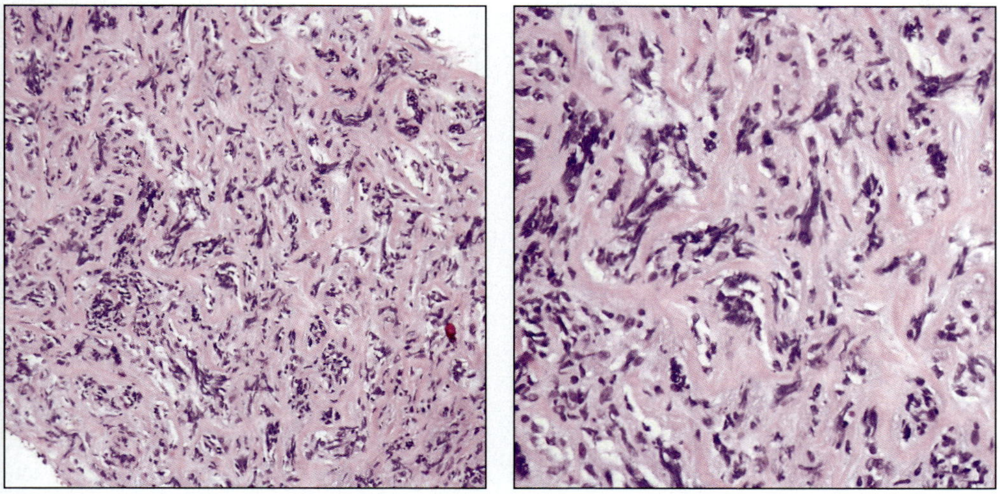

(Left) *Core biopsy of a large anterior mediastinal mass came from a patient with mediastinal diffuse large cell lymphoma with sclerosis. Note the abundant fibrous tissue containing mainly crushed and distorted cells.* ***(Right)*** *Higher magnification of core biopsy of anterior mediastinal mass in a patient with diffuse large cell lymphoma with sclerosis shows numerous crushed cells embedded in fibrous tissue. This picture is highly suggestive of mediastinal lymphoma in the proper clinical setting.*

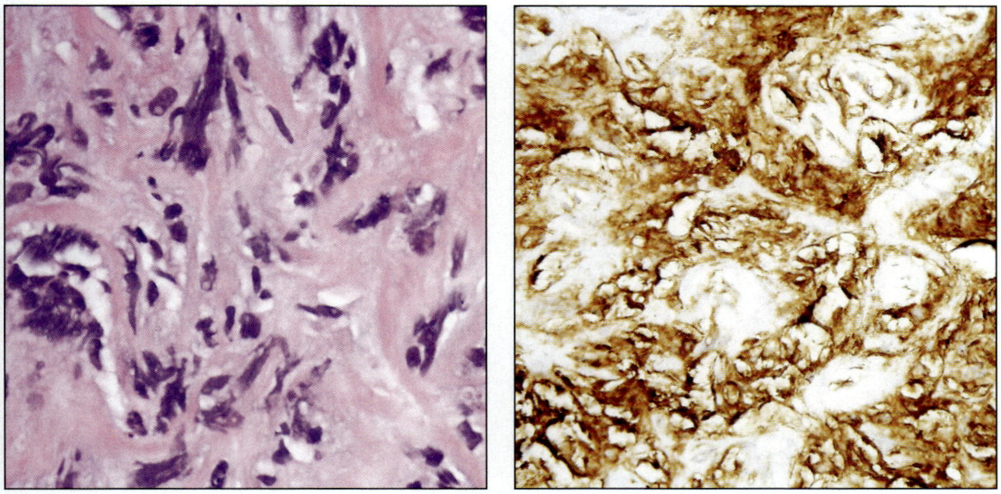

(Left) *Higher magnification of mediastinal diffuse large cell lymphoma core biopsy shows extensively distorted cells, mainly composed of crushed lymphocytes surrounded by dense collagenous tissue. Biopsies like this may be very hard to interpret due to the extensive tissue distortion that precludes evaluation of nuclear detail.* ***(Right)*** *Immunohistochemical staining for CD20 in a core biopsy of mediastinal diffuse large B-cell lymphoma shows strong positivity of the crushed tumor cells.*

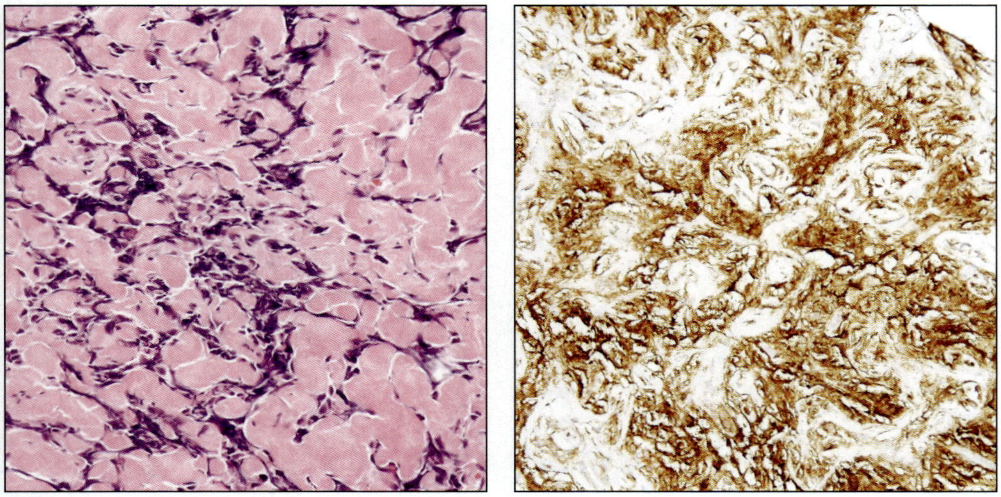

(Left) *Extensive distortion of tumor cells is seen in this mediastinal biopsy from a patient with mediastinal diffuse large B-cell lymphoma with sclerosis. The sclerosis in this case takes the form of small rounded balls of collagen that crush and distort the surrounding tumor cells.* ***(Right)*** *Immunohistochemical staining with CD20 in mediastinal diffuse large B-cell lymphoma highlights the lymphoid cells lying between the collagen bundles.*

DIFFUSE LARGE CELL LYMPHOMA OF THE MEDIASTINUM

Mediastinal Diffuse Large Cell Lymphoma

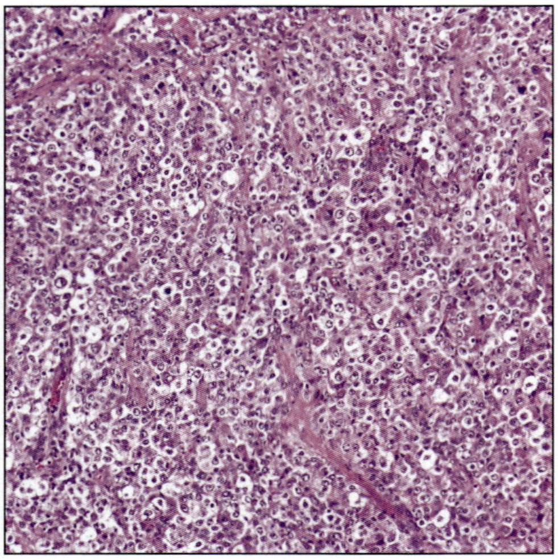
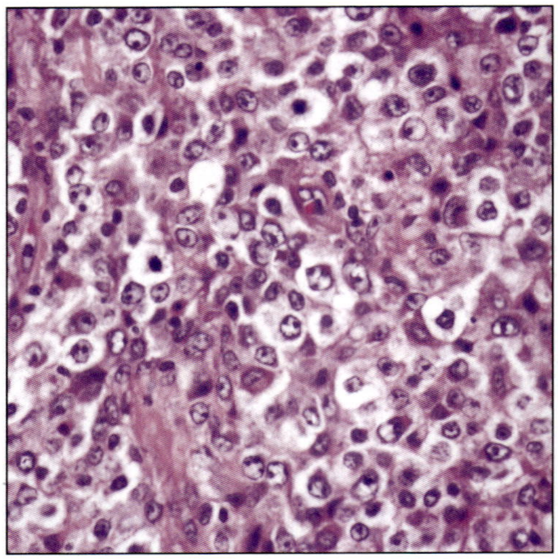

(Left) *Mediastinal diffuse large B-cell lymphoma shows sheets of large, atypical lymphoid cells with very little intervening stroma. Striking sclerosis and compartmentalization are not features seen in this case.* ***(Right)*** *Mediastinal diffuse large B-cell lymphoma shows sheets of large, atypical lymphoid cells. Cases devoid of stromal sclerosis, such as this, are more readily recognizable as a malignant lymphoma on routine histopathologic examination than those with prominent sclerotic fibrous bands.*

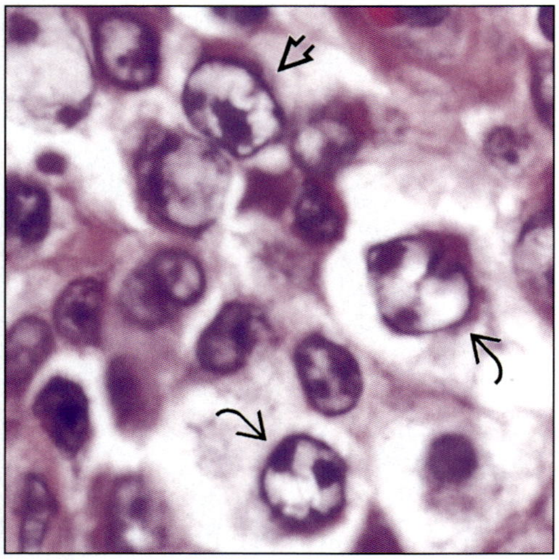
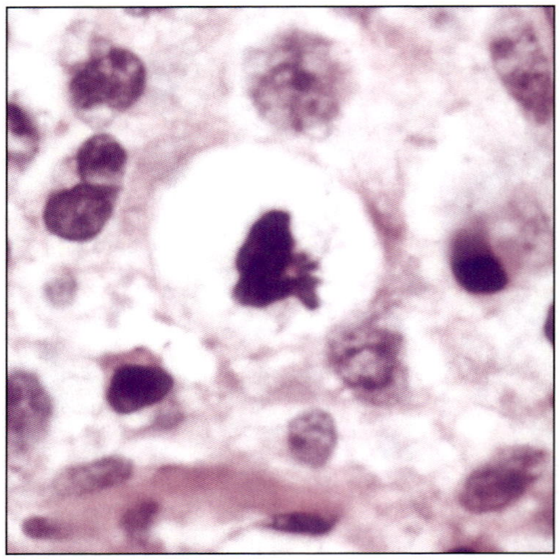

(Left) *High magnification from mediastinal diffuse large B-cell lymphoma shows atypical lymphoid cells. Some of the cells contain a single prominent nucleolus ➢; others show multiple nucleoli ↷.* ***(Right)*** *High magnification from mediastinal diffuse large B-cell lymphoma shows large, atypical lymphoid cells and an abnormal mitotic figure (center). Mitotic activity may vary in these tumors from minimal to > 10 mitoses per 10 high-power fields.*

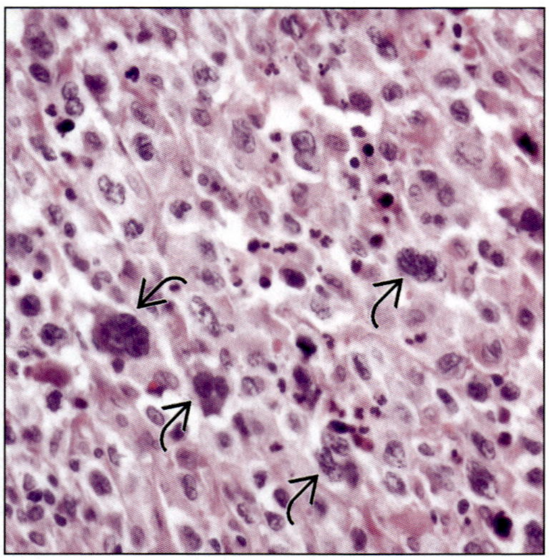
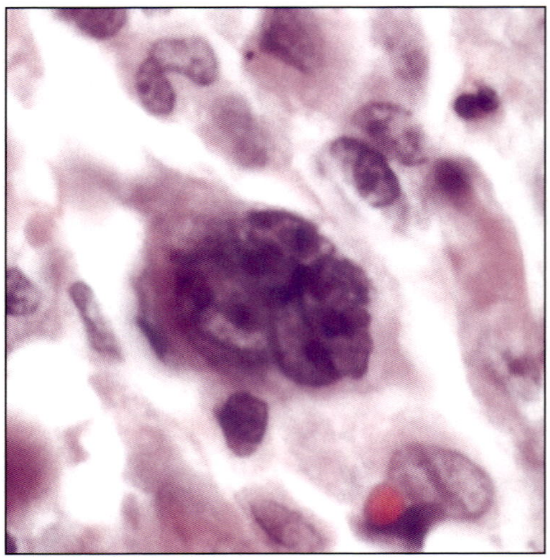

(Left) *Mediastinal diffuse large B-cell lymphoma shows sheets of atypical lymphoid cells containing a few scattered, larger, multinucleated cells ↷.* ***(Right)*** *High magnification from mediastinal diffuse large B-cell lymphoma shows a large multinucleated tumor cell. The cell is characterized by multiple overlapping nuclei with prominent eosinophilic nucleoli and is surrounded by a scant rim of amphophilic cytoplasm. These cells display a close resemblance to Reed-Sternberg cells.*

Pleomorphic Mediastinal Lymphoma

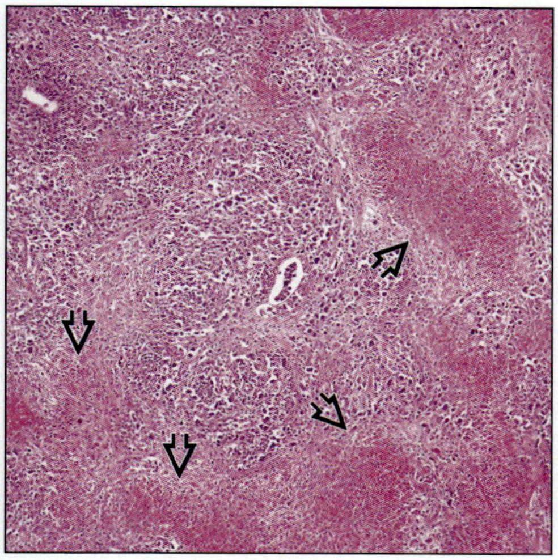

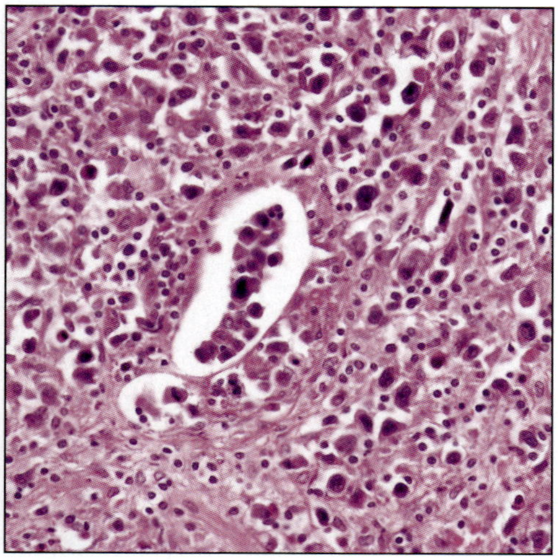

(Left) *Pleomorphic mediastinal diffuse large B-cell lymphoma shows extensive areas of necrosis ⮚. The residual tumor cell population shows marked nuclear pleomorphism.* ***(Right)*** *Pleomorphic mediastinal large B-cell lymphoma shows large tumor cells with bizarre hyperchromatic nuclei. The size of the pleomorphic tumor cells is at least 4x that of a normal immunoblast. For comparison, note the smaller atypical lymphocytes scattered in the vicinity.*

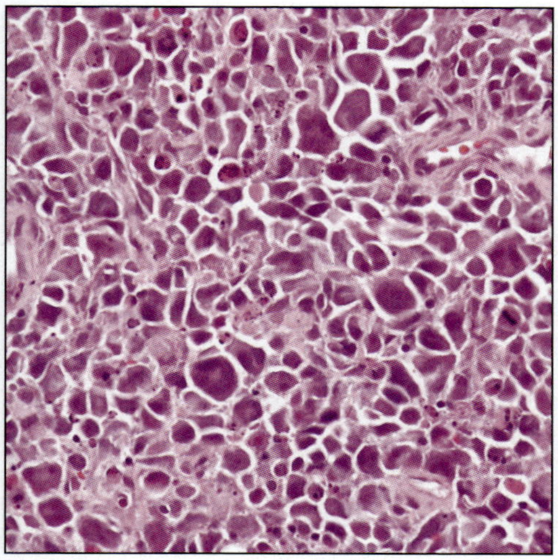

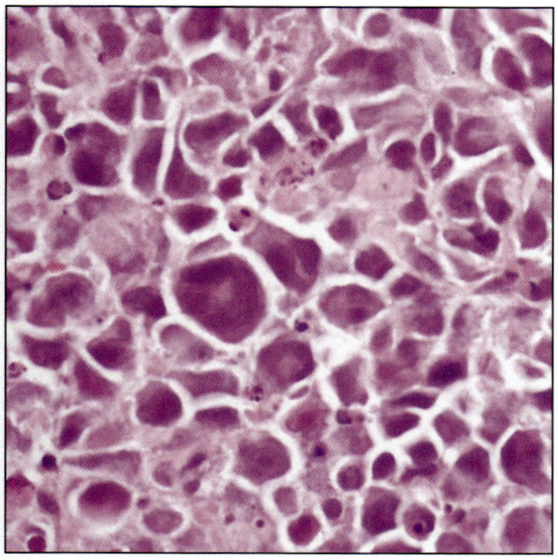

(Left) *Pleomorphic mediastinal B-cell lymphoma shows population of bizarre tumor cells simulating a pleomorphic high-grade sarcoma (a.k.a. "malignant fibrous histiocytoma"). The large size of the tumor cells is uncharacteristic of lymphoma.* ***(Right)*** *High magnification of pleomorphic mediastinal large cell lymphoma shows atypical nuclear features, including bizarre pleomorphic nuclei, occasional "tadpole" cells, and bizarre multinucleated cells.*

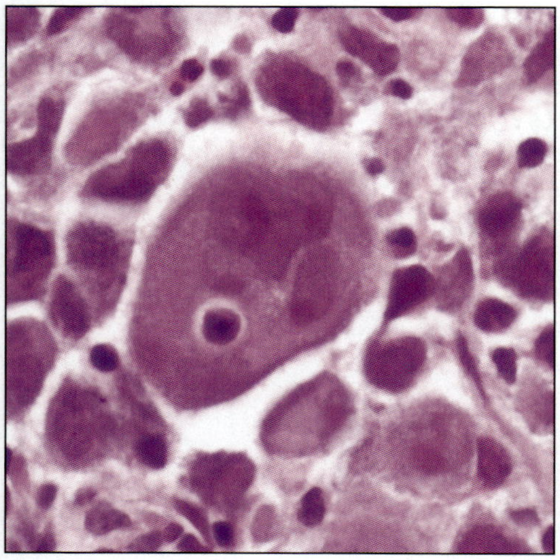

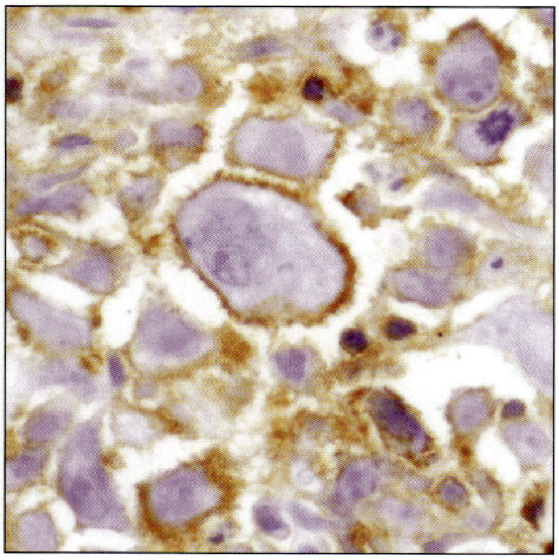

(Left) *High magnification of pleomorphic mediastinal large B-cell lymphoma shows a large tumor cell (center) with multiple nuclei and phagocytosis of a small lymphocyte (emperipolesis). Similar cells are a common finding in "fibrohistiocytic" sarcomas.* ***(Right)*** *Immunohistochemical staining for CD20 in mediastinal pleomorphic large cell lymphoma shows nice membrane staining of the tumor cells, including the bizarre multinucleated cell in the center.*

DIFFUSE LARGE CELL LYMPHOMA OF THE MEDIASTINUM

ALCL-like Mediastinal B-cell Lymphoma

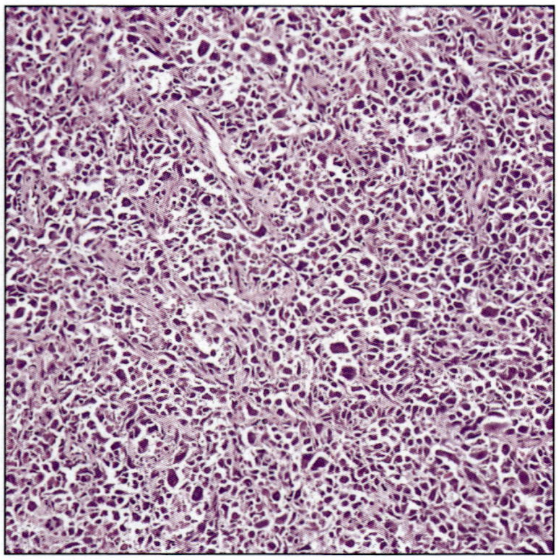

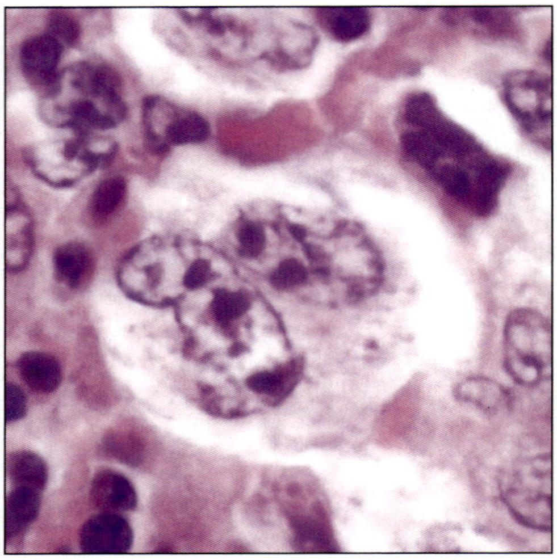

(Left) *Mediastinal diffuse large B-cell lymphoma resembling anaplastic large cell lymphoma (ALCL) shows a population of tumor cells that contains scattered larger cells admixed with smaller atypical lymphocytes.* ***(Right)*** *High magnification of large tumor cells in mediastinal diffuse large B-cell lymphoma shows cells with kidney-shaped nuclei containing a vesicular chromatin pattern and multiple large eosinophilic nucleoli closely resembling Reed-Sternberg cells.*

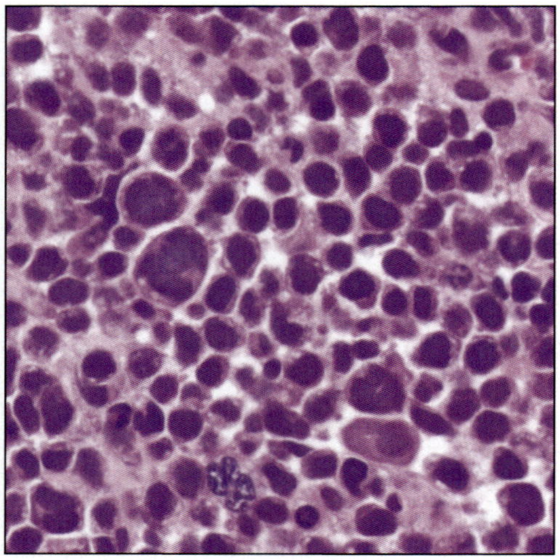

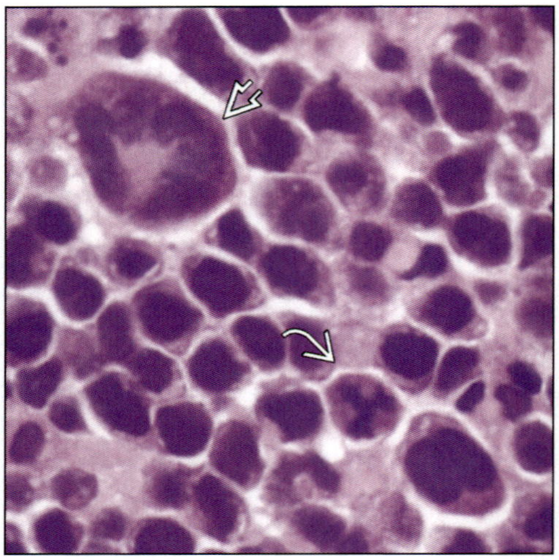

(Left) *Mediastinal large cell lymphoma that resembles anaplastic large cell lymphoma (ALCL) shows hyperchromatic tumor cells admixed with smaller atypical lymphocytes resembling a metastasis from an anaplastic carcinoma.* ***(Right)*** *High magnification of mediastinal diffuse large B-cell lymphoma resembling anaplastic large cell lymphoma (ALCL) shows tumor cells with irregular, horseshoe-shaped nuclei ⇨ similar to those seen in ALCL. Notice the tripolar mitosis ➙.*

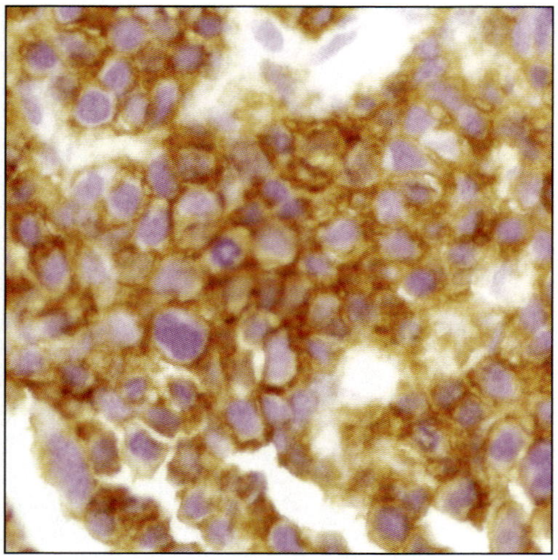

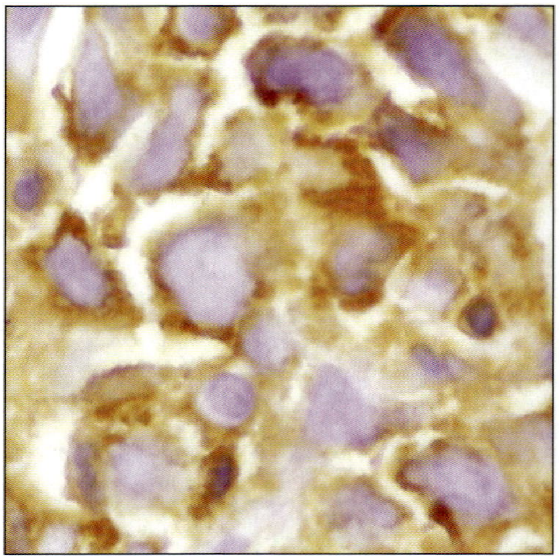

(Left) *Mediastinal large cell lymphoma resembling anaplastic large cell lymphoma (ALCL) shows strong membrane positivity for CD20 antibody by immunohistochemistry. The tumor cells in this case were negative for CD30, ALK1, and a variety of T-cell markers.* ***(Right)*** *Immunohistochemical staining for CD20 in mediastinal large B-cell lymphoma resembling anaplastic large cell lymphoma (ALCL) is shown. This marker labels the large, anaplastic, and Reed-Sternberg-like cells.*

Clear Cell Mediastinal Lymphoma

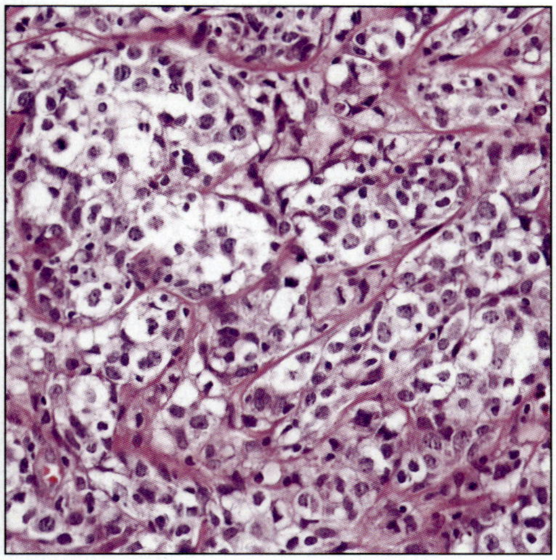
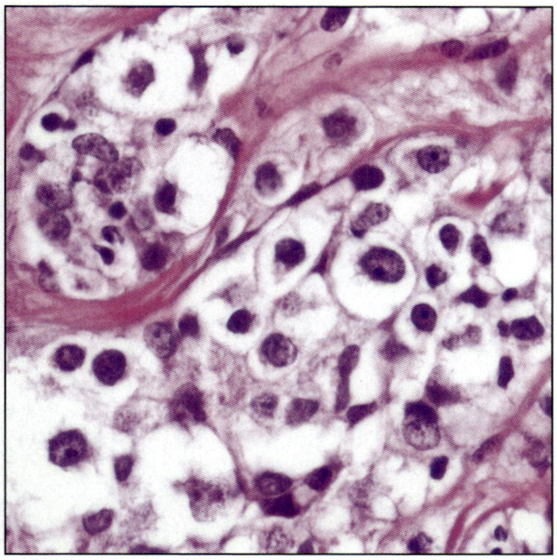

(Left) *Clear cell mediastinal large cell lymphoma shows nests of large tumor cells separated by thin fibrous bands. Notice the abundant water-clear, empty cytoplasm that surrounds the nuclei of the tumor cells.* ***(Right)*** *High magnification of mediastinal diffuse large cell lymphoma, clear cell type, shows nests of tumor cells with abundant clear cytoplasm, simulating a metastasis from clear cell renal cell carcinoma or some other type of clear cell carcinoma.*

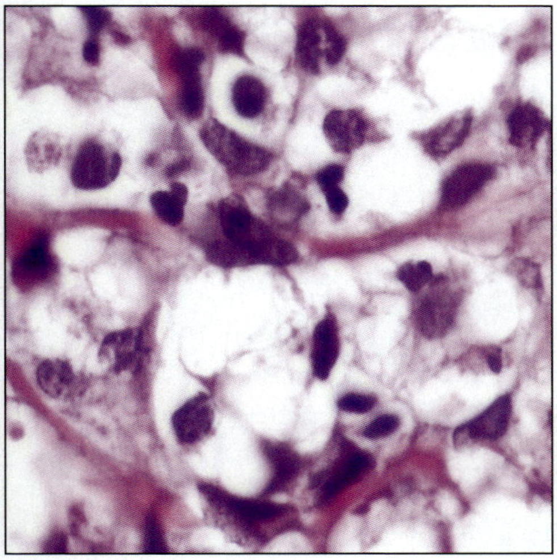
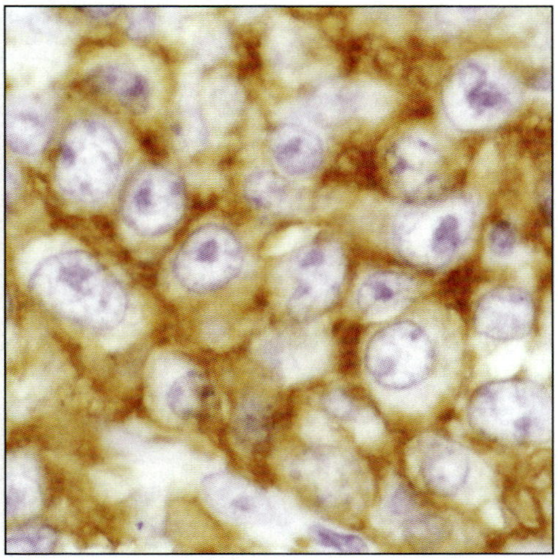

(Left) *High magnification of mediastinal diffuse large B-cell lymphoma, clear cell type, shows nuclear detail of the tumor cells, which are surrounded by abundant clear cytoplasmic rims. It may be very difficult to distinguish this image from a metastasis of clear cell renal cell carcinoma without the use of special stains.* ***(Right)*** *Immunohistochemical staining for CD20 in mediastinal diffuse large B-cell lymphoma, clear cell type, shows membrane positivity in the tumor cells.*

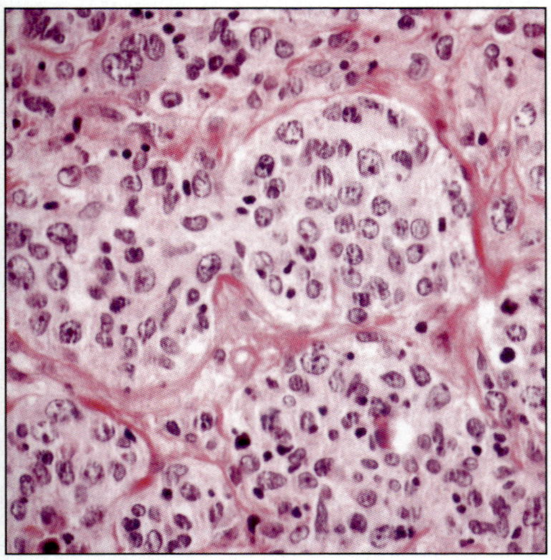
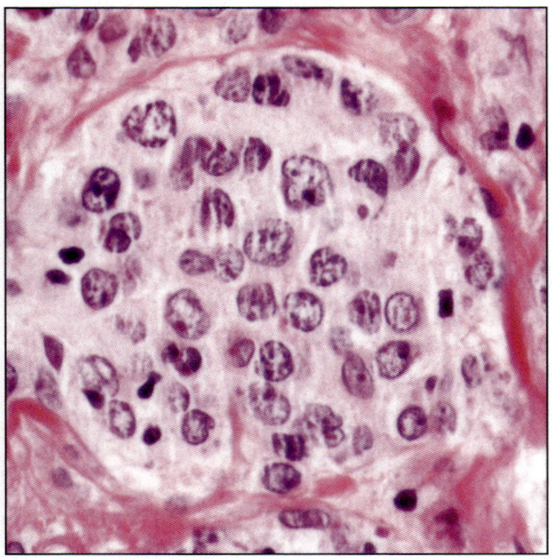

(Left) *Mediastinal diffuse large B-cell lymphoma with sclerosis, clear cell type, shows compartmentalizing effect created by thin bands of fibrous tissue. Notice the abundant clear cytoplasm surrounding the tumor cells.* ***(Right)*** *High magnification of an island of tumor cells in mediastinal diffuse large B-cell lymphoma, clear cell type, shows atypical lymphoid cells surrounded by an indistinct rim of clear or amphophilic cytoplasm. The nested appearance of the cells is reminiscent of melanoma.*

DIFFUSE LARGE CELL LYMPHOMA OF THE MEDIASTINUM

Germinotropic Mediastinal Lymphoma

(Left) *Mediastinal diffuse large B-cell lymphoma with marked tropism for germinal centers ("germinotropic lymphoma") shows irregular replacement of lymphoid follicles and germinal centers ⇨ by clusters and nests of large tumor cells →.* ***(Right)*** *Mediastinal large cell lymphoma with marked tropism for germinal centers ("germinotropic lymphoma") shows progressive and gradual replacement of the germinal center in the lymphoid follicle by discrete clusters and islands of large tumor cells ⇨.*

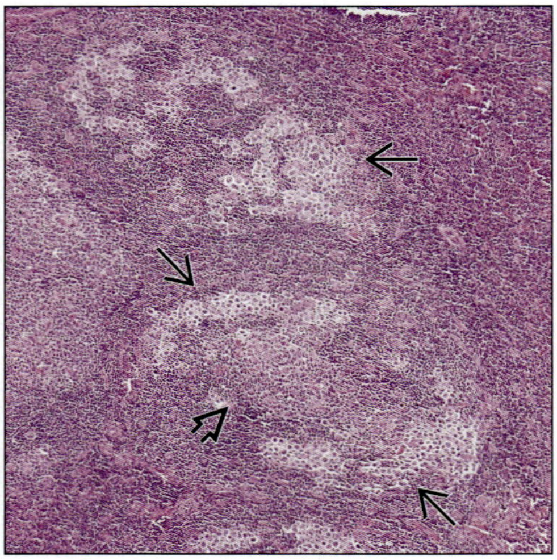

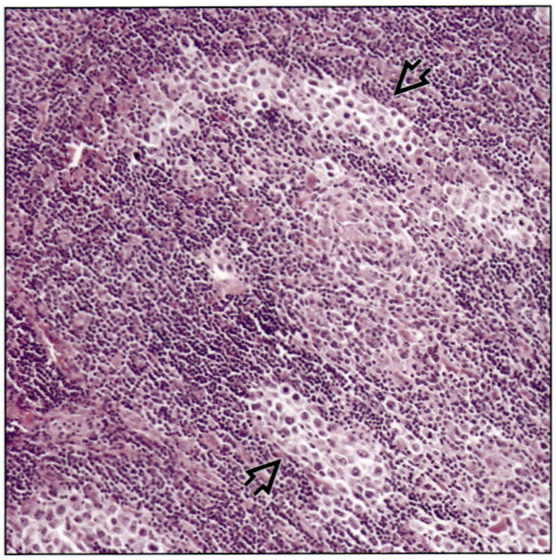

(Left) *High magnification of mediastinal large cell lymphoma with marked tropism for germinal centers ("germinotropic lymphoma") shows a cluster of large, atypical lymphoid cells disrupting the follicle mantle zone.* ***(Right)*** *High magnification in mediastinal large B-cell lymphoma with marked tropism for germinal centers ("germinotropic lymphoma") shows large, atypical lymphoid cells with irregular nuclei and prominent eosinophilic nucleoli surrounded by a scant rim of cytoplasm.*

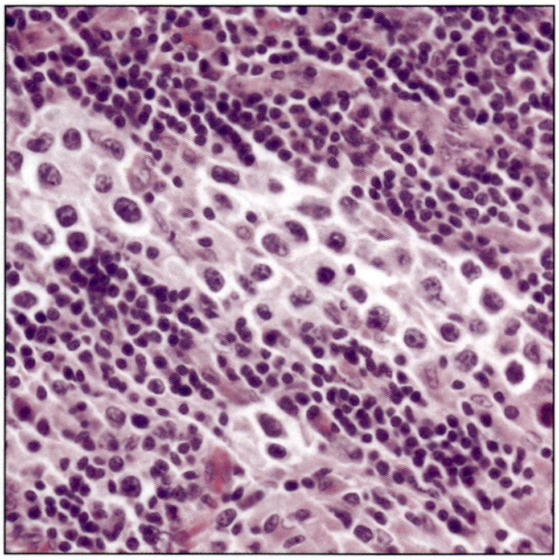

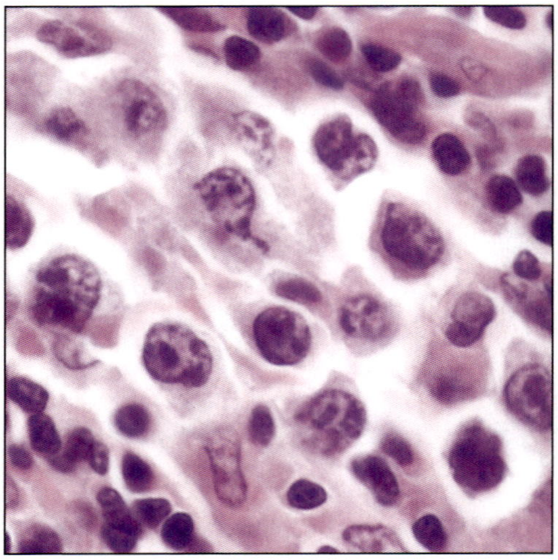

(Left) *Mediastinal large B-cell lymphoma with marked tropism for germinal centers ("germinotropic lymphoma") shows almost complete replacement of the follicle by sheets and clusters of large, atypical lymphoid cells. A similar morphologic appearance can be observed in mediastinal seminoma.* ***(Right)*** *Higher magnification of mediastinal large B-cell lymphoma with marked tropism for germinal centers shows progressive replacement of the germinal center by tumor cells.*

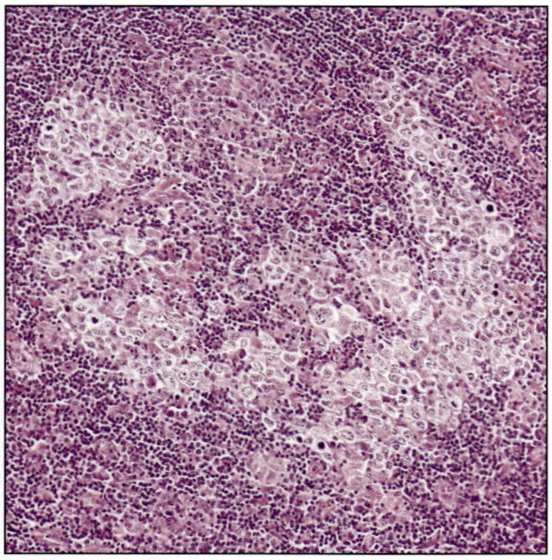

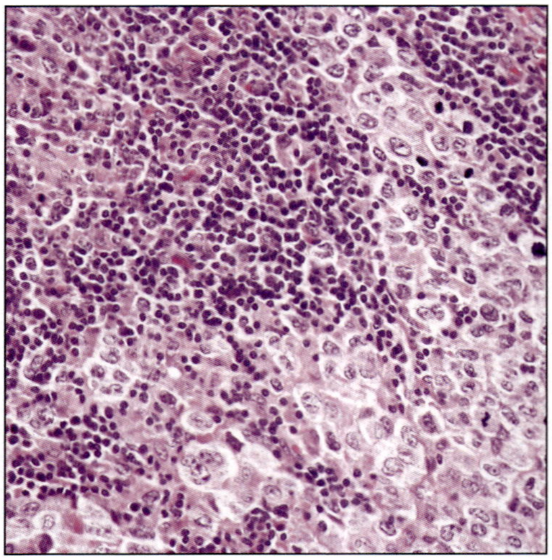

Spindle Cell and Signet Ring Cell Mediastinal Lymphoma

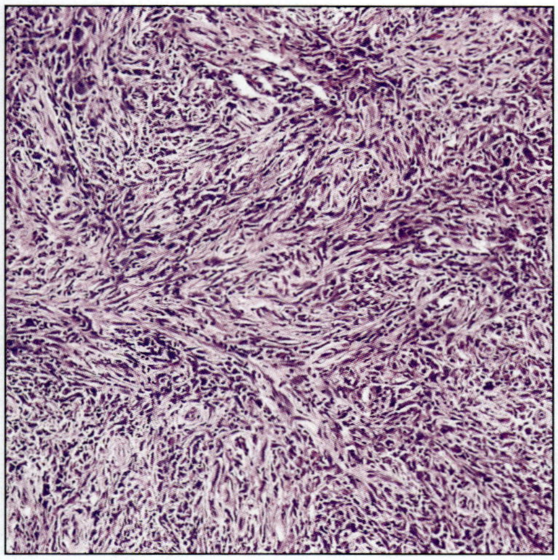
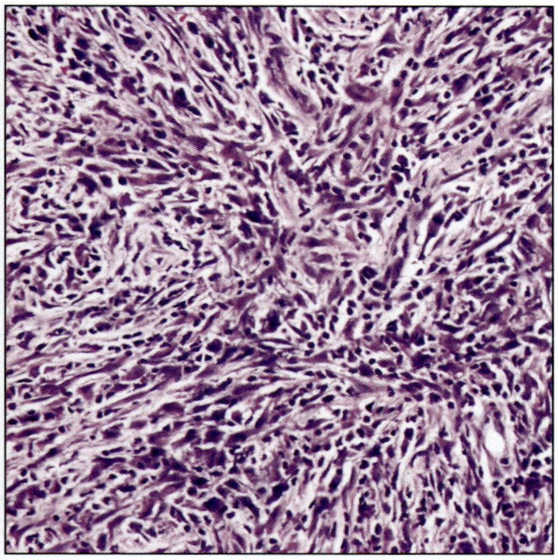

(Left) *Mediastinal diffuse large B-cell lymphoma, spindle cell type, shows atypical spindle cell proliferation that on scanning magnification closely resembles a spindle cell sarcoma.* ***(Right)*** *Mediastinal diffuse large B-cell lymphoma with sarcomatoid appearance shows fascicles of atypical spindle cells with a vague storiform pattern, simulating a malignant fibrohistiocytic tumor. Tumors like this can be easily mistaken for a variety of spindle cell sarcomas.*

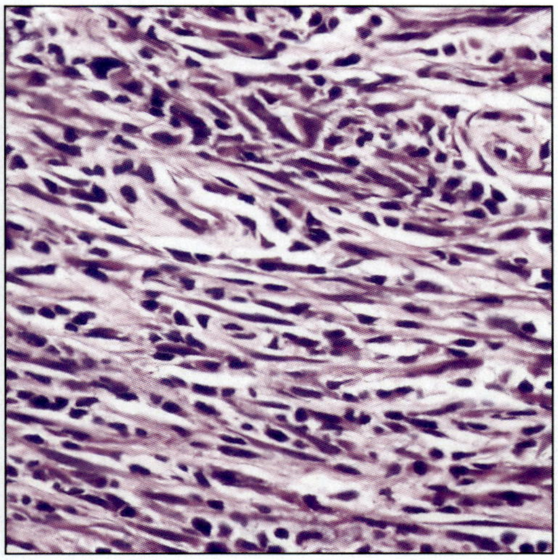
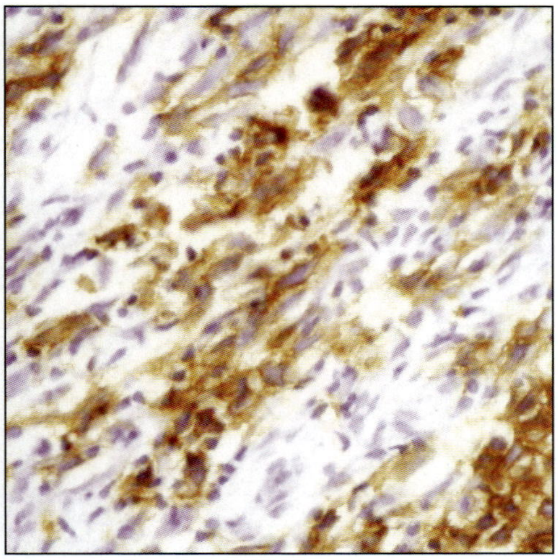

(Left) *High magnification of mediastinal diffuse large B-cell lymphoma with prominent spindling of the tumor cells shows fascicular appearance of elongated spindle cells admixed with small lymphocytes, simulating a spindle cell sarcoma.* ***(Right)*** *Immunohistochemical staining for CD20 in mediastinal diffuse large cell lymphoma with prominent spindling of the tumor cells shows positive staining of elongated, spindle tumor cells for this antibody.*

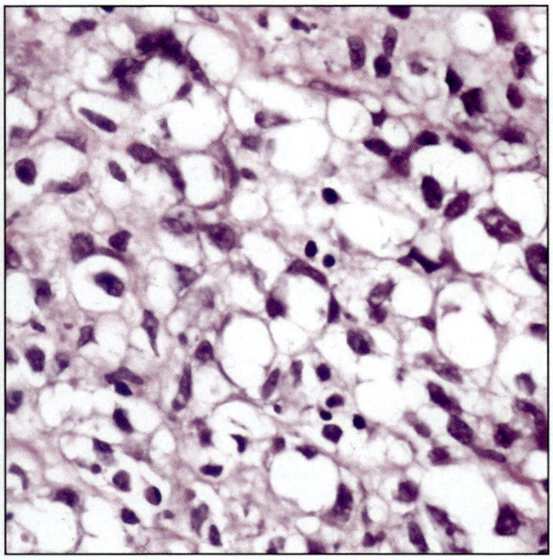
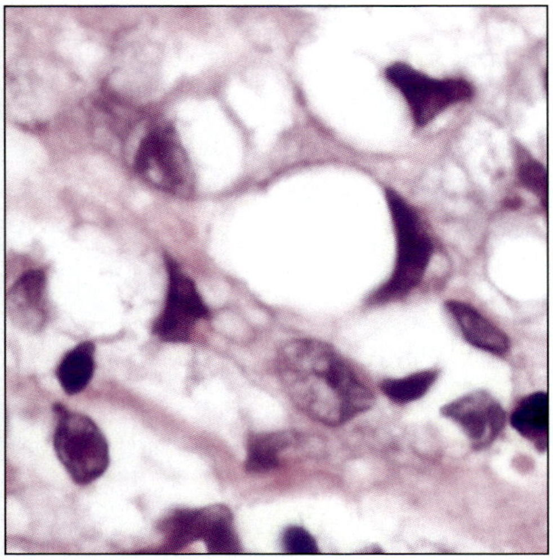

(Left) *Mediastinal diffuse large B-cell lymphoma with signet ring cells shows sheets of large vacuolated cells that resemble adipocytes admixed with a few scattered small lymphocytes. The morphologic appearance depicted here may closely simulate a liposarcoma.* ***(Right)*** *Higher magnification of mediastinal lymphoma shows a few signet ring cell lymphocytes with large hyperchromatic nuclei displaced to the periphery. The cells were CD20(+).*

Unusual Features in Mediastinal Large Cell Lymphoma

*(**Left**) Mediastinal diffuse large B-cell lymphoma shows extensive pattern of stromal sclerosis. (**Right**) High magnification of mediastinal diffuse large B-cell lymphoma with sclerosis shows extensive stromal deposition of collagen surrounding the lymphoid tumor cells. Tumors with these features may be confused for idiopathic sclerosing mediastinitis or for a sclerosing epithelioid fibrosarcoma arising in the mediastinum.*

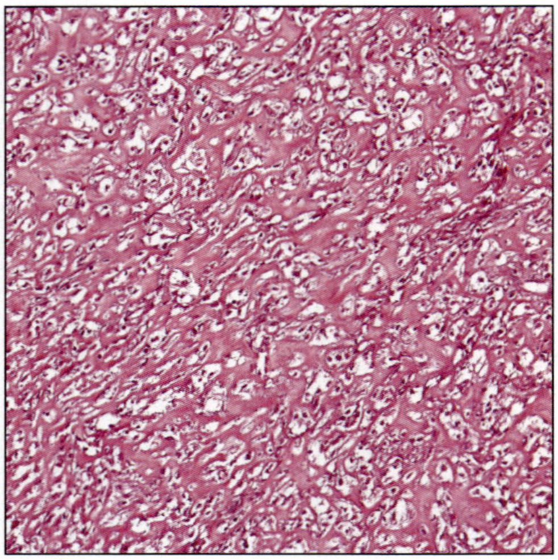

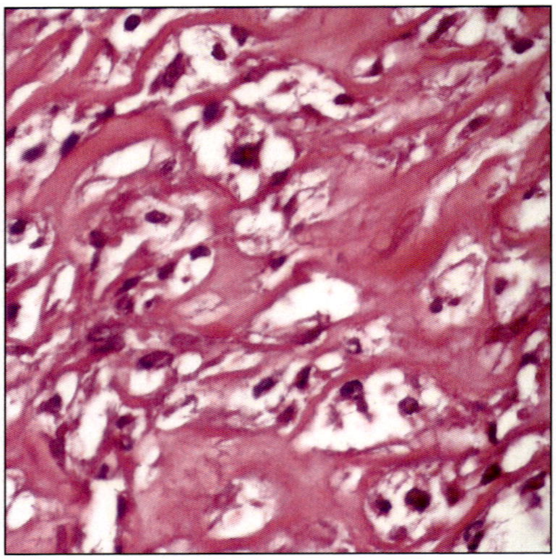

*(**Left**) The concentric pattern of stromal sclerosis in mediastinal diffuse large B-cell lymphoma, as seen in this biopsy, can resemble a solitary fibrous tumor of the mediastinum due to the rope-like pattern of distribution of the collagen fibers. (**Right**) High magnification of mediastinal diffuse large B-cell lymphoma with sclerosis shows concentric pattern of collagen deposition. Notice the perivascular distribution of the sclerosis and a few scattered residual lymphocytes.*

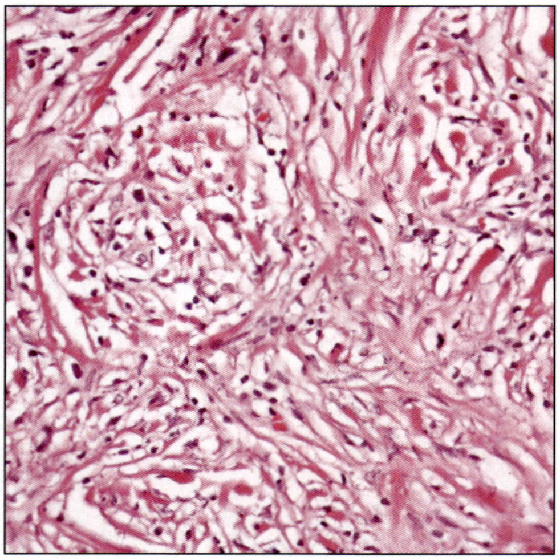

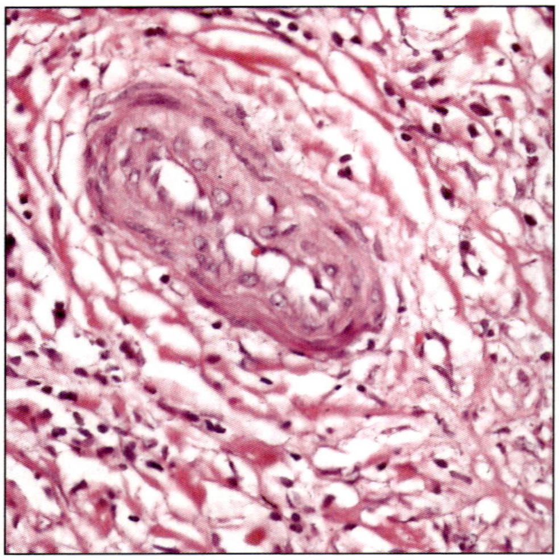

*(**Left**) Mediastinal diffuse large B-cell lymphoma shows entrapped residual thymic epithelium within the tumor ⇨. Notice the elongated character of the thymic epithelial rests. Positive keratin stains may lead to confusion with thymoma or carcinoma in such cases. (**Right**) Mediastinal diffuse large cell lymphoma with cystic changes shows dilatation of entrapped thymic epithelium resulting in large cystic spaces. Fortunately, this is usually only a focal event in these tumors.*

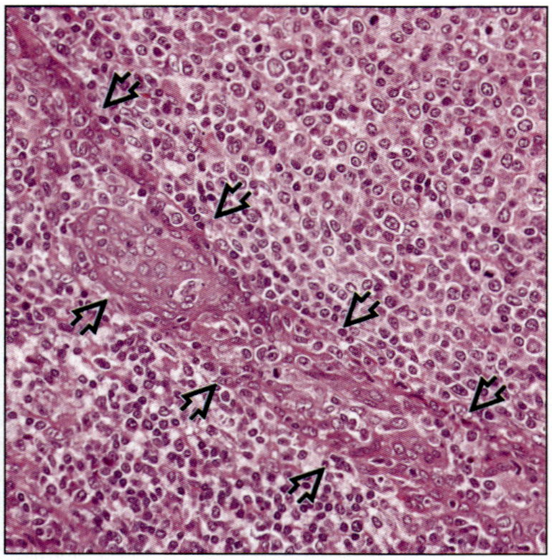

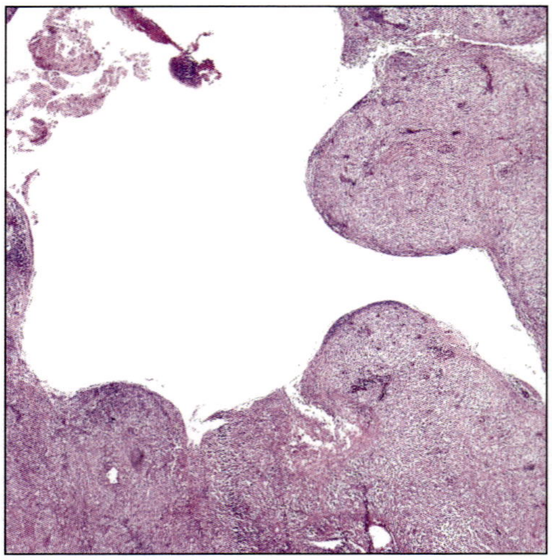

Unusual Features in Mediastinal Large Cell Lymphoma

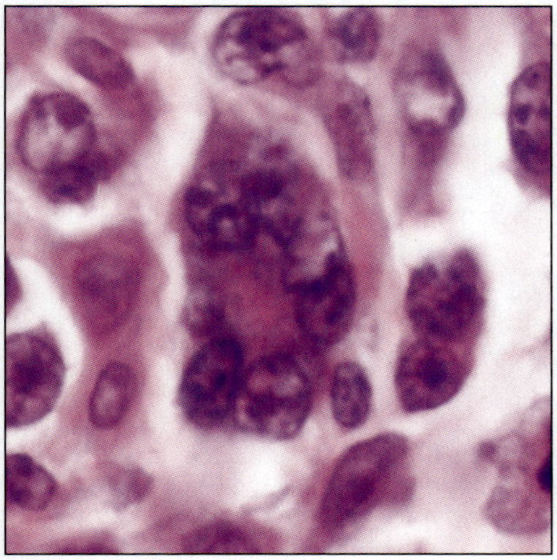
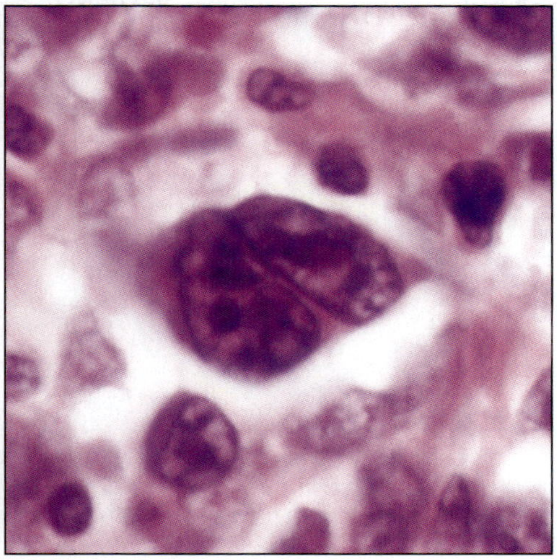

(Left) *Mediastinal large B-cell lymphoma may show a wide spectrum of cells, including multinucleated cells with wreath-like disposition of nuclei (center) that can sometimes resemble Touton giant cells.* ***(Right)*** *Mediastinal diffuse large B-cell lymphoma shows classical binucleate Reed-Sternberg-like cells. This cell was positive for CD20 and negative for CD15 and CD30. The rest of the tumor marked as a conventional diffuse large B-cell lymphoma.*

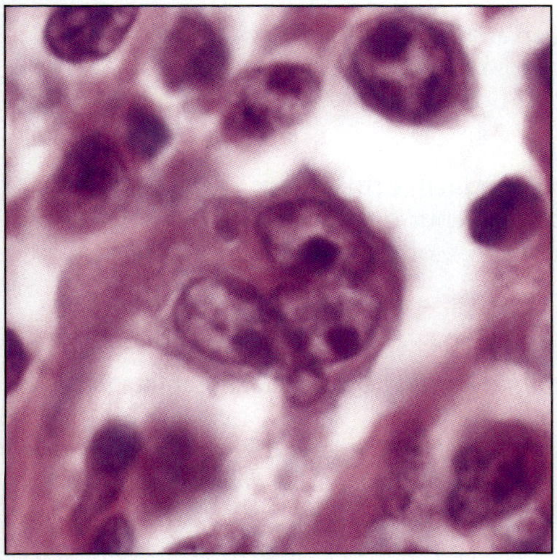
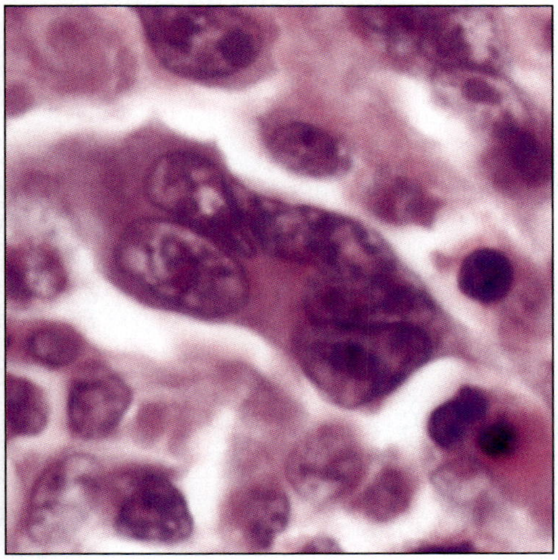

(Left) *Mediastinal diffuse large B-cell lymphoma shows a Reed-Sternberg-like cell with 3 nuclei, each displaying a prominent eosinophilic nucleolus. The milieu of this tumor, however, was incompatible with Hodgkin lymphoma and showed abundant large immunoblastic cells with B-cell phenotype.* ***(Right)*** *Mediastinal diffuse large B-cell lymphoma shows bizarre, multinucleated, CD20(+) cells with atypical nuclei and prominent eosinophilic nucleoli.*

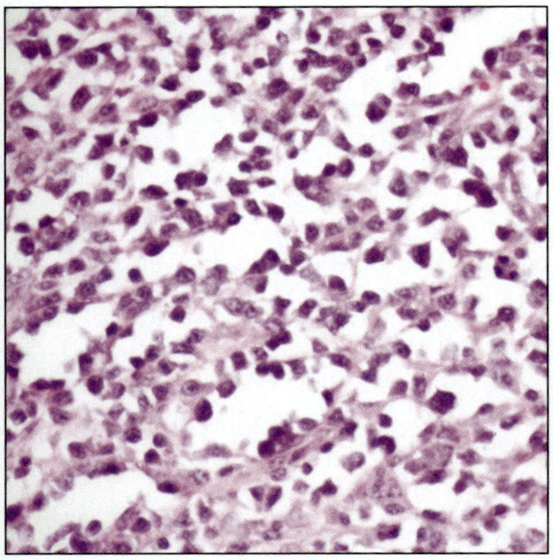
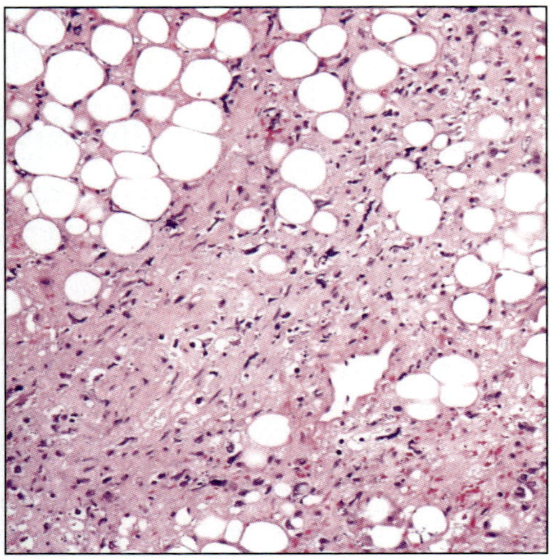

(Left) *Mediastinal large B-cell lymphoma shows an unusual architectural pattern characterized by artifactual separation of the tumor cells, resulting in a pseudoalveolar pattern of growth. Tumors like this can be mistaken for metastases of alveolar rhabdomyosarcoma to the mediastinum.* ***(Right)*** *Mediastinal diffuse large B-cell lymphoma with sclerosis shows a distinctive pattern of infiltration of mediastinal fat with preservation and sparing of the adipocytes.*

LYMPHOBLASTIC LYMPHOMA

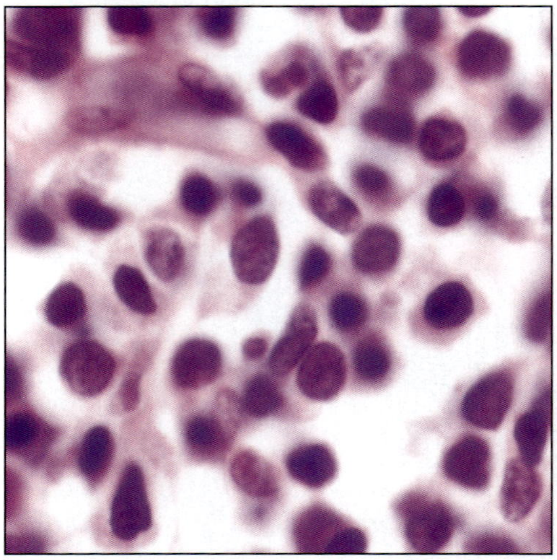

High magnification of nonconvoluted T-lymphoblastic lymphoma of the mediastinum shows primitive nuclei with dense chromatin pattern and with smooth nuclear contours.

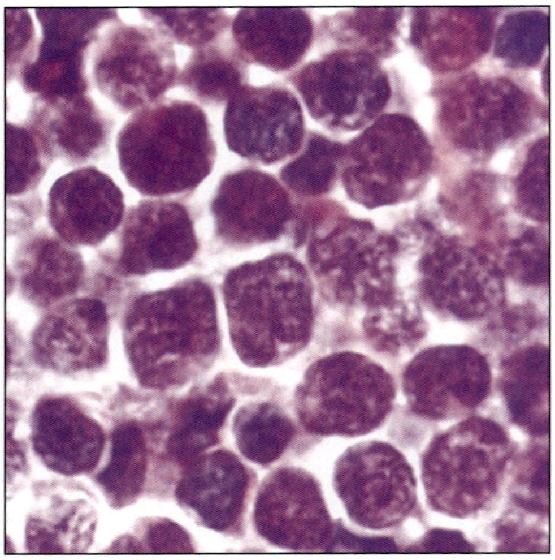

High magnification of T-lymphoblastic lymphoma of the mediastinum, convoluted type, shows primitive nuclei with deep nuclear convolutions and nuclear membrane irregularities.

TERMINOLOGY

Abbreviations

- Lymphoblastic lymphoma (LBL)

Synonyms

- Lymphoblastic lymphoma/leukemia, lymphoma of precursor lymphocytes

Definitions

- Diffuse lymphoma of immature or precursor lymphocytes, predominantly of T-cell type

ETIOLOGY/PATHOGENESIS

Pathogenesis

- Neoplastic proliferation of blastic precursor lymphocytes
- Associations with prior radiation, Down syndrome, and other genetic diseases have been noted
- Phenotype can be either of T-precursor cell type or B-precursor cell type

CLINICAL ISSUES

Epidemiology

- Incidence
  - Occurs more commonly in children than in adults
    - Incidence in children is about 3 cases per 100,000 population
    - 75% of affected children are under 15 years of age
    - Peak incidence in children is between 2-5 years old
    - More frequent in males than females
  - Also affects men in 3rd decade of life
  - Can rarely occur in older individuals over age of 60 years

Site

- Anterior superior and middle mediastinum
- Supradiaphragmatic, supraclavicular, cervical, and axillary lymph nodes

Presentation

- Rapidly enlarging mediastinal mass
- Aggressive clinical course
  - Rapid progression, often with superior vena cava syndrome
  - Frequent relapses
  - Short survival
  - Generally diagnosed in advanced stages (stage III or IV)
  - Dissemination to other organs is common
    - Central nervous system (most common site of relapse)
    - Skin, testes, eyes, kidneys, breast, and lungs
    - Bone marrow involvement occurs early in disease
    - Leukemic phase with circulating blasts in peripheral blood occurs shortly after initial diagnosis

IMAGE FINDINGS

General Features

- Location
  - Superior mediastinal nodes (prevascular and paratracheal)

Radiographic Findings

- Bulky mediastinal bilateral hilar lymphadenopathy
- Pleural effusion may be seen due to lymphatic or venous obstruction

CT Findings

- Contrast-enhanced computed tomography (CECT) is imaging modality of choice
- Slight to moderate uniform enhancement following intravenous contrast

LYMPHOBLASTIC LYMPHOMA

Key Facts

Etiology/Pathogenesis
- Neoplastic proliferation of blastic precursor lymphocytes

Clinical Issues
- Occurs more commonly in children than in adults
- Anterior superior and middle mediastinum
- Rapidly enlarging mediastinal mass
- Aggressive clinical course

Microscopic Pathology
- Diffuse sheets of immature lymphoid cells
- Infiltration of lymph node capsule and mediastinal fat with "single file" arrangement of tumor cells
- "Starry sky" appearance due to numerous tingible body macrophages
- Crush artifact
- Lymphoblasts show large immature nuclei with dense chromatin and small inconspicuous or absent nucleoli
- Lymphoblasts can be convoluted or nonconvoluted
- Almost all precursor lymphocytes (T and B) express nuclear enzyme, terminal deoxynucleotidyl transferase (TdT)
- Precursor lymphocytes also express CD34 and CD99

Top Differential Diagnoses
- Burkitt lymphoma
- B-cell chronic lymphocytic leukemia/small lymphocytic lymphoma
- Lymphocyte-rich thymoma (WHO type B1)
  - Most important test is immunoperoxidase stain for pancytokeratin to identify scattered neoplastic thymic epithelial cells

MICROSCOPIC PATHOLOGY

Histologic Features
- Diffuse sheets of immature lymphoid cells
- "Pseudonodular" pattern due to compartmentalization by thin strands of fibrous tissue
- Infiltration of lymph node capsule and mediastinal fat with "single file" arrangement of tumor cells
- "Starry sky" appearance due to numerous tingible body macrophages
- Crush artifact
- Occasional spared, residual lymphoid follicles with germinal centers may become entrapped by lymphoblastic proliferation

Cytologic Features
- Lymphoblasts show large immature nuclei with dense chromatin and small, inconspicuous or absent nucleoli
  - Lymphoblastic cells show high nuclear-to-cytoplasmic ratio
- Lymphoblasts can be convoluted or nonconvoluted
  - Convoluted lymphoblasts show multiple, complex nuclear indentations
  - Nonconvoluted lymphoblasts show smooth nuclear contours
- Frequent mitotic figures

ANCILLARY TESTS

Immunohistochemistry
- Almost all precursor lymphocytes (T and B) express the nuclear enzyme terminal deoxynucleotidyl transferase (TdT)
- Precursor lymphocytes also express CD34 and CD99
- 90% of cases correspond to T-cell precursor lymphoblasts and express CD3 and CD43
- 10% of cases correspond to B-cell precursor lymphoblasts and express CD10, CD19, CD20, CD22, and CD79a

Cytogenetics
- Various cytogenetic abnormalities
  - Favorable prognosis: t(12;21)(p13;q22)
  - Intermediate prognosis: t(1;19)(q23;p13)
  - Poor prognosis: t(9;22)(q34;q11), BCR/ABL, t(v;11q23)

Electron Microscopy
- Round to oval cells with smooth surfaces and no cytoplasmic processes
- Convoluted nuclei with deep indentations and scant cytoplasm with few organelles

Molecular Diagnosis
- t(12;21) is most frequent translocation in B-precursor ALL in children (25% of cases)
  - Molecular demonstration of fusion of TEL at 12p13 to AML1 at 21q22
- t(9;22) is frequently demonstrated in T-precursor ALL in adults (30% of cases)
  - Molecular demonstration of BCR/ABL

DIFFERENTIAL DIAGNOSIS

Burkitt Lymphoma
- Also occurs in children and shows diffuse sheets of immature lymphoid cells
- Burkitt lymphoma cells have round nonconvoluted nuclei with multiple prominent nucleoli and basophilic cytoplasm
- "Starry sky" pattern may be prominent in both Burkitt and lymphoblastic lymphoma
- Lymphocytes are negative for TdT and CD99
- Lymphocytes are positive for CD10, CD20, and CD45
- Lymphocytes in Burkitt lymphoma show κ/λ light chain restriction

B-cell Chronic Lymphocytic Leukemia/Small Lymphocytic Lymphoma
- B-cell CLL/small lymphocytic lymphoma occurs mostly in elderly patients rather than in children

LYMPHOBLASTIC LYMPHOMA

Immunohistochemistry

Antibody	Reactivity	Staining Pattern	Comment
TdT	Positive	Nuclear	All LBLs show nuclear positivity for TdT regardless of whether they are of T- or B-cell lineage
CD99	Positive	Cell membrane & cytoplasm	All LBLs express CD99: Caution should be exercised not to mistake this finding for evidence of a small round blue cell tumor in the Ewing/PNET family
CD43	Positive	Cell membrane & cytoplasm	Most LBL of either T- or B-cell lineage express cytoplasmic CD43
CD1a	Positive	Cytoplasmic	Positive in T-cell precursor LBL
CD3	Positive	Cytoplasmic	Positive in T-cell precursor LBL
CD10	Positive	Cytoplasmic	May be positive in both T- and B-cell precursor LBL
CD19	Positive	Cytoplasmic	Positive in B-cell precursor LBL
CD20	Positive	Cytoplasmic	Positive in B-cell precursor LBL
CD22	Positive	Cytoplasmic	Positive in B-cell precursor LBL
CD45	Negative	Not applicable	Usually negative in LBL by immunohistochemistry but may be detected by flow cytometry

- Cells are small and uniform, and mitoses are rare
- No "starry sky" appearance or crush artifact
- Cells show CD5(+) mature B-cell phenotype as well as κ/λ light chain restriction
- Cells are negative for TdT and CD99

Lymphocyte-rich Thymoma (WHO Type B1)

- B1 thymoma can show similar histology to lymphoblastic lymphoma due to high content of immature T-lymphocytes
- Lymphocytes in B1 thymoma are also positive for TdT and CD99
- B1 thymoma may also show "starry sky" appearance simulating lymphoblastic lymphoma
- B1 thymoma is usually lobulated and does not infiltrate capsule or perithymic fat in single file arrangement
- Clinically, tumors are slow growing and do not present clinically with rapid growth and widespread infiltration of surrounding structures
- Flow cytometry studies may mistakenly be misinterpreted as lymphoblastic lymphoma due to high content of immature T-lymphoblasts
- Most important test is immunoperoxidase stain for pancytokeratin to identify scattered neoplastic thymic epithelial cells

DIAGNOSTIC CHECKLIST

Clinically Relevant Pathologic Features

- Age distribution
  - More common in children and young adults
  - Rarely can occur in older adults
- Clinical presentation
  - Rapidly growing mediastinal mass
  - Shortness of breath, chest pain, and superior vena cava syndrome
  - Often presents as medical emergency
- Histologic findings
  - Sheets of primitive lymphoid cells with dispersed chromatin pattern and inconspicuous or absent nucleoli
  - "Starry sky" appearance and crush artifact
  - Infiltration of mediastinal fat with preservation of fat cells
  - High mitotic activity
  - Prominent nuclear convolutions in high percentage of cases
- Special studies
  - Nuclear TdT positivity and membranous CD99 positivity in tumor cells
  - Absence of keratin(+) epithelial cells admixed with lymphoid cell infiltrate
  - Molecular demonstration of t(12;21) or t(9;22)

Pathologic Interpretation Pearls

- Large diffusely infiltrative "small blue cell tumor" in mediastinal location in a child
- Cells with primitive nuclei with scant cytoplasm and absent or inconspicuous nucleoli
- TdT/CD99 positivity in absence of keratin(+) cells in background

SELECTED REFERENCES

1. Dabaja BS et al: The role of local radiation therapy for mediastinal disease in adults with T-cell lymphoblastic lymphoma. Cancer. 94(10):2738-44, 2002
2. Thomas DA et al: Lymphoblastic lymphoma. Hematol Oncol Clin North Am. 15(1):51-95, vi, 2001
3. Glick RD et al: Lymphomas of the anterior mediastinum. Semin Pediatr Surg. 8(2):69-77, 1999
4. Suster S: Primary large-cell lymphomas of the mediastinum. Semin Diagn Pathol. 16(1):51-64, 1999
5. Kirn D et al: Large-cell and immunoblastic lymphoma of the mediastinum: prognostic features and treatment outcome in 57 patients. J Clin Oncol. 11(7):1336-43, 1993
6. Garand R et al: Comparison of outcome, clinical, laboratory, and immunological features in 164 children and adults with T-ALL. The Groupe d'Etude Immunologique des Leucémies. Leukemia. 4(11):739-44, 1990

Histologic Features

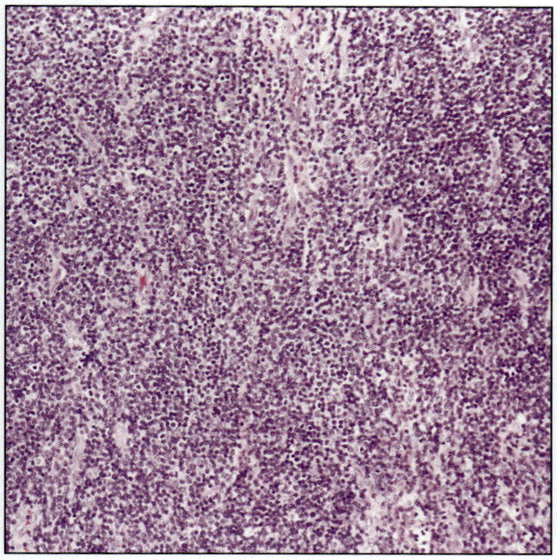

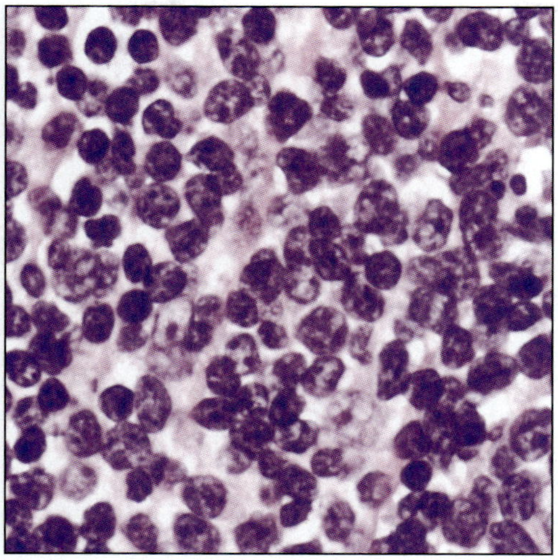

(Left) *Scanning magnification of lymphoblastic lymphoma of the mediastinum shows sheets of small hyperchromatic lymphoid cells.* ***(Right)*** *High magnification of lymphoblastic lymphoma of the mediastinum shows primitive lymphoid cells with round to oval nuclei, a dense chromatin pattern, and absent or inconspicuous nucleoli surrounded by a scant rim of amphophilic cytoplasm. The absence of nucleoli and primitive appearance of the nuclei are characteristic of this tumor.*

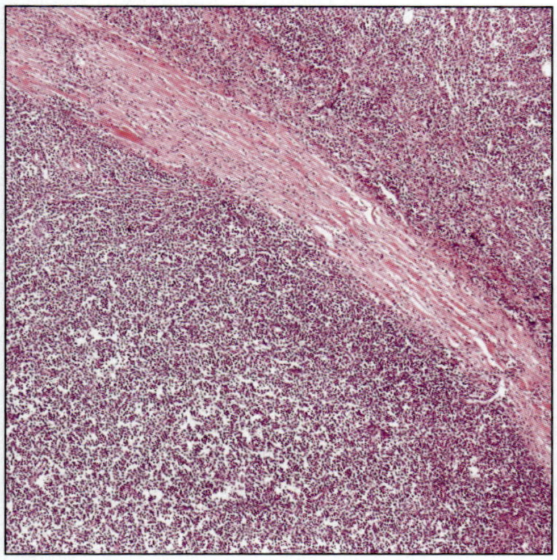

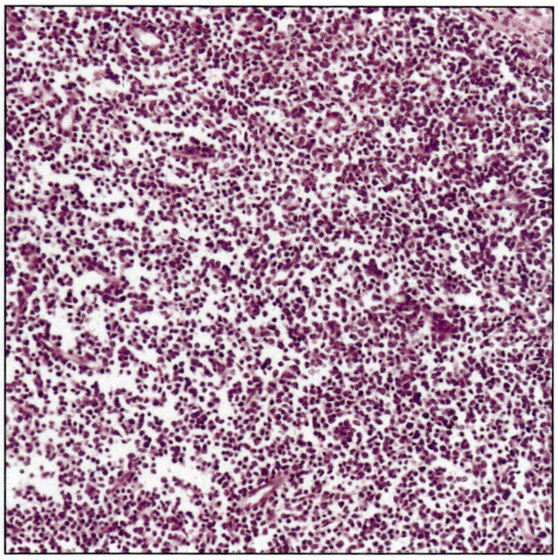

(Left) *Lymphoblastic lymphoma of mediastinum shows a dense fibrous connective tissue band separating the tumor into pseudolobules. The pseudolobular appearance is reminiscent of the architecture typically seen in lymphocyte-rich thymoma. Absence of keratin-positive cells serves to distinguish it from thymoma.* ***(Right)*** *High magnification of lymphoblastic lymphoma of the mediastinum shows sheets of monotonous lymphoid cells without any intervening stroma.*

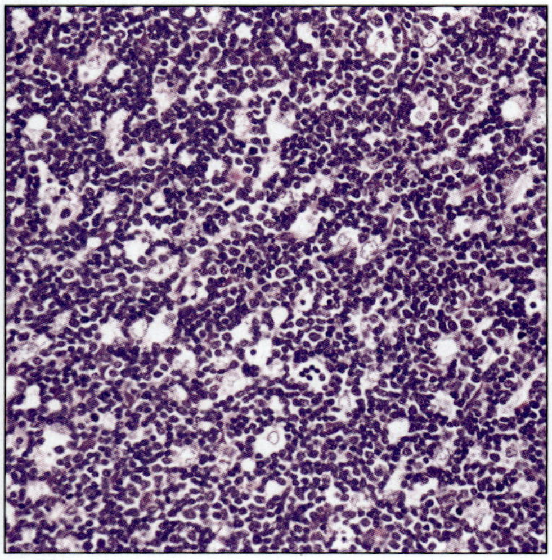

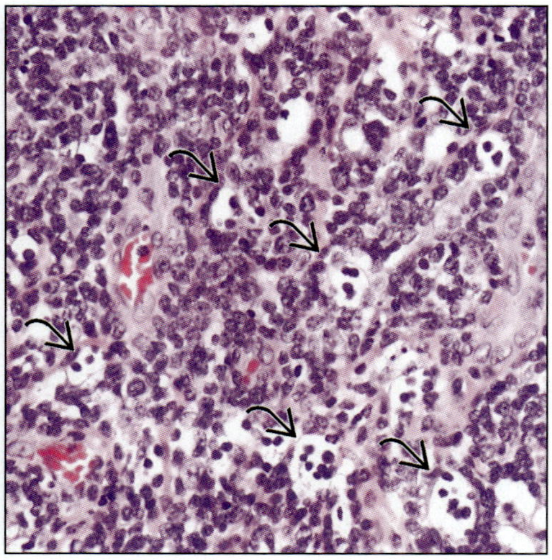

(Left) *Lymphoblastic lymphoma of the mediastinum shows a prominent "starry sky" appearance due to tingible body macrophages. A similar appearance can be observed in cases of lymphocyte-rich thymoma and in thymus glands undergoing stress involution.* ***(Right)*** *High magnification of lymphoblastic lymphoma shows "starry sky" appearance due to multiple tingible body macrophages ↷. The surrounding population is composed of immature T-lymphoblasts.*

LYMPHOBLASTIC LYMPHOMA

Special Histologic Features

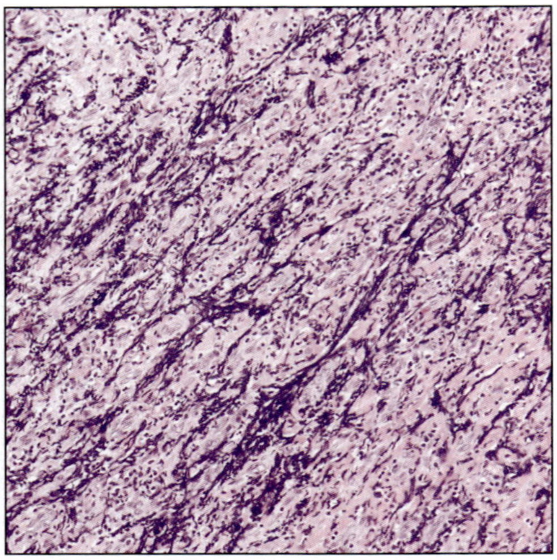
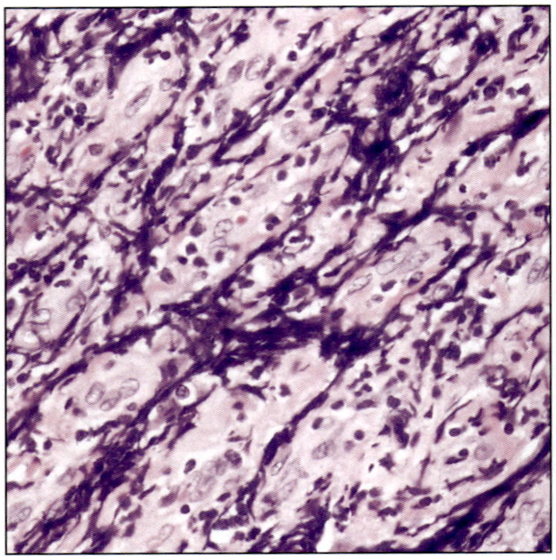

(Left) *Typical appearance of lymphoblastic lymphoma of the mediastinum in a core needle biopsy sample shows distortion of the tumor cells due to "crush" artifact. Biopsies like this may be difficult to distinguish from other types of lymphomas or metastatic carcinoma.* ***(Right)*** *High magnification shows lymphoblastic lymphoma with extensive distortion due to "crush" artifact. Notice the purplish blue streaking of the nuclear chromatin in the stroma separating a few viable cells.*

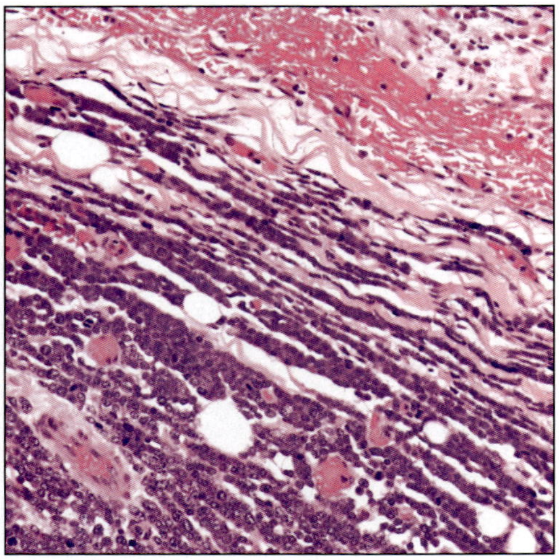
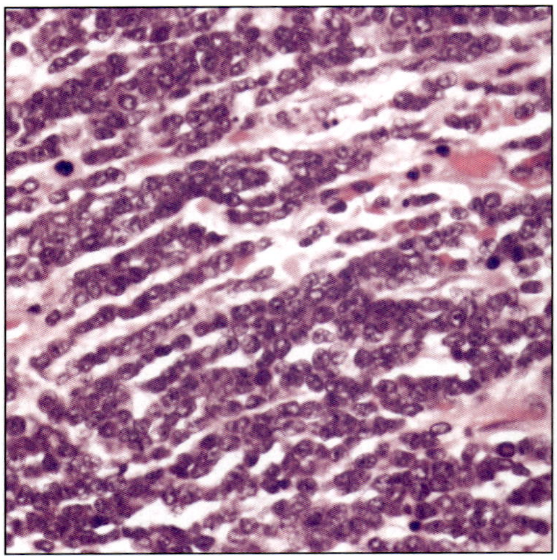

(Left) *Section taken from the periphery of a lymphoblastic lymphoma of the mediastinum shows a linear, single file arrangement of the tumor cells reminiscent of metastatic invasive lobular carcinoma of the breast.* ***(Right)*** *High magnification of lymphoblastic lymphoma of the mediastinum shows a "single file" pattern of infiltration of the tumor cells. Notice the primitive appearance of the nuclei and the absence of "molding" of the tumor cells.*

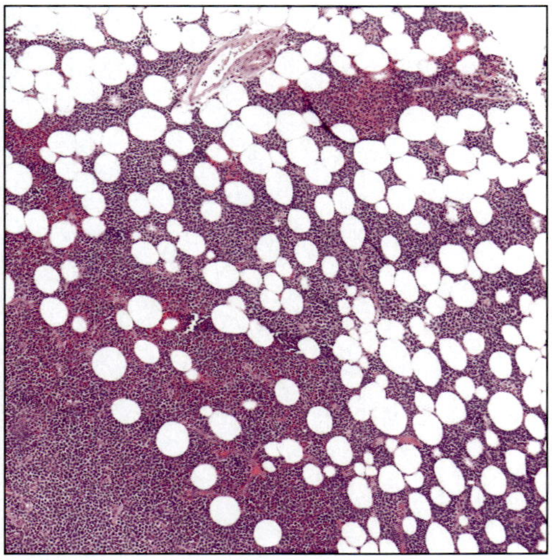
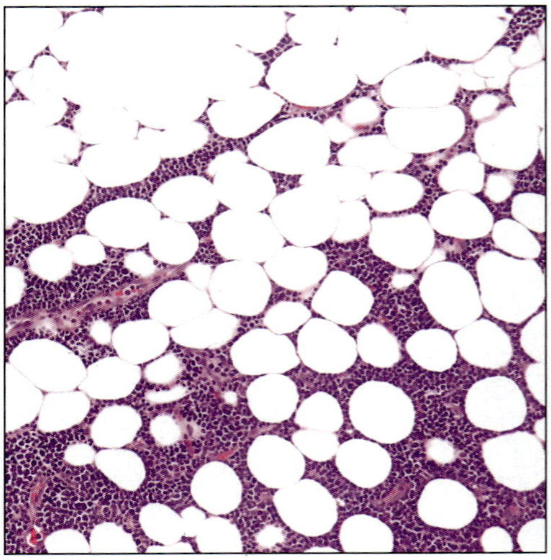

(Left) *Lymphoblastic lymphoma of the mediastinum shows characteristic pattern of infiltration of mediastinal fat at the periphery of the lesion. The tumor cells infiltrate and encircle the adipocytes without destroying them.* ***(Right)*** *High magnification of lymphoblastic lymphoma of the mediastinum shows infiltration with preservation of mediastinal fat. This feature can help separate lymphoblastic lymphoma from lymphocyte-rich thymoma on frozen sections.*

Immunohistochemical Features

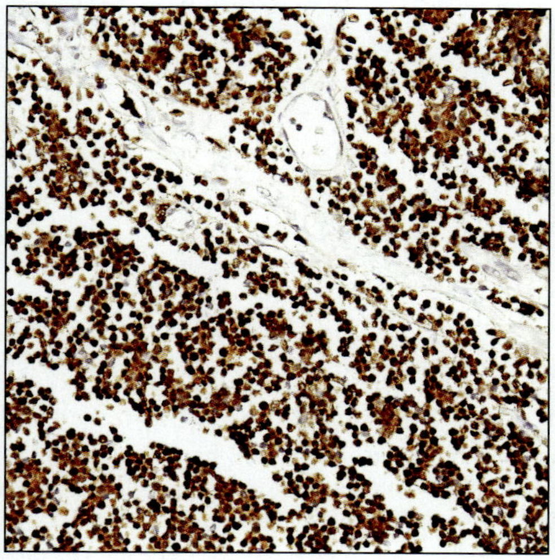

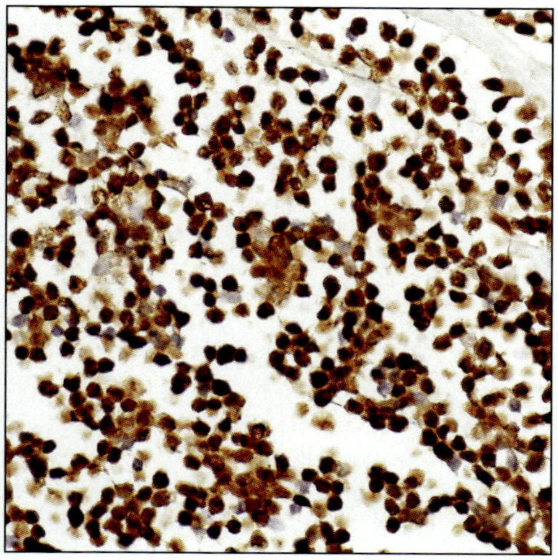

*(**Left**) Immunohistochemical staining of lymphoblastic lymphoma of the mediastinum for TdT shows strong nuclear positivity in the majority of tumor cells. (**Right**) High magnification of lymphoblastic lymphoma of the mediastinum shows positive nuclear staining of the tumor cells with antibodies for TdT. Absence of keratin-positive cells admixed with the lymphoid cells in this sample will allow accurate distinction of this tumor from a lymphocyte-rich thymoma.*

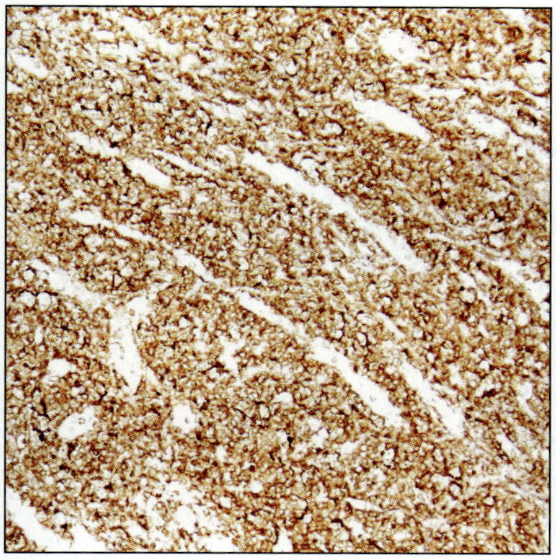

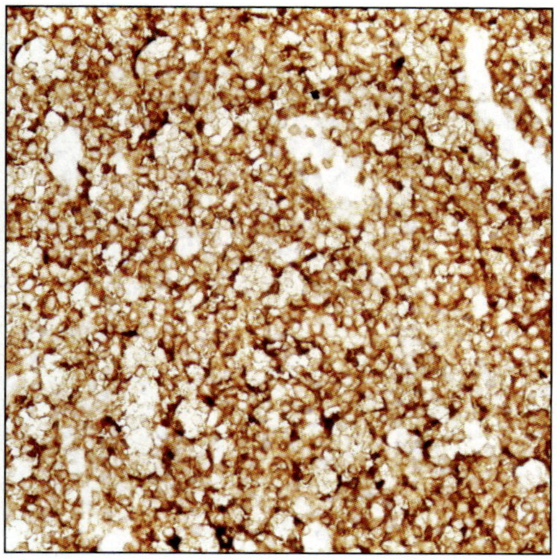

*(**Left**) Immunoperoxidase stain for CD3 in mediastinal lymphoblastic lymphoma shows strong positivity in all the tumor cells. The CD3 positivity together with TdT nuclear positivity identifies this tumor as a T-lymphoblastic lymphoma/leukemia. (**Right**) Immunohistochemical staining for CD99 in mediastinal lymphoblastic lymphoma shows cytoplasmic positivity of the tumor cells. CD99 strongly labels immature T-lymphoblasts and can be used in lieu of TdT.*

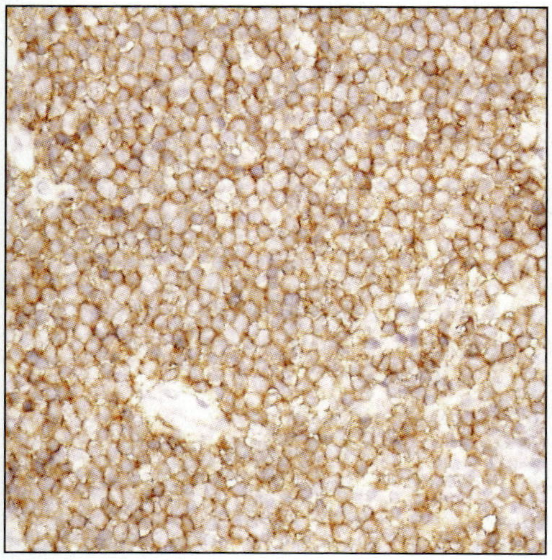

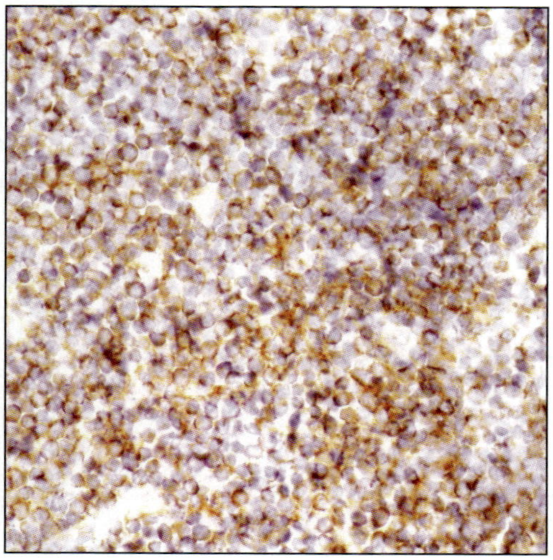

*(**Left**) Immunohistochemical staining for CD43 in T-lymphoblastic lymphoma of the mediastinum shows strong membrane staining in the tumor cells. This marker is associated with a more aggressive biologic behavior. (**Right**) Immunohistochemical staining with CD10 in mediastinal lymphoblastic lymphoma shows positive cytoplasmic staining of the tumor cells. CD10 positivity can be observed in lymphoblastic lymphoma of both B- and T-cell lineage.*

MALT LYMPHOMA OF THE THYMUS

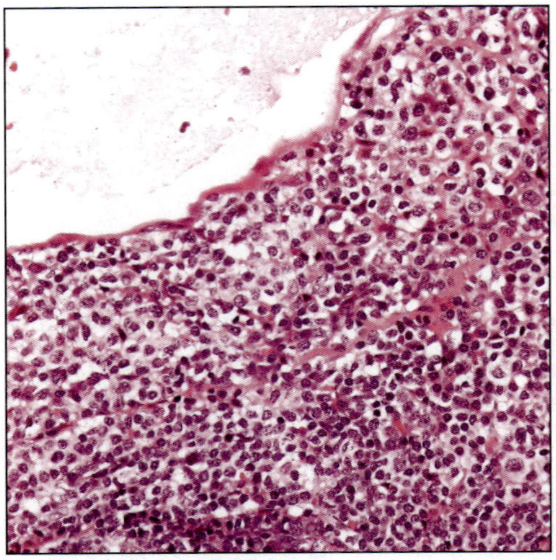

MALT lymphoma of the thymus shows sheets of small lymphoid cells with clear perinuclear halos cuffing a dilated cystic space. The cystic space is lined by a layer of flattened cuboidal epithelium.

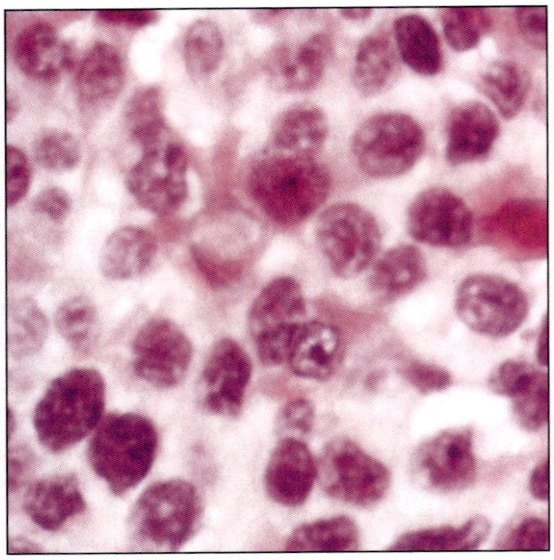

High magnification of MALT lymphoma of the thymus shows monotonous proliferation of lymphocytes with minimal nuclear irregularities. Some of the lymphocytes display clear perinuclear halos.

TERMINOLOGY

Abbreviations

- Mucosa-associated lymphoid tissue lymphoma (MALT lymphoma)

Synonyms

- Marginal zone B-cell lymphoma
- Monocytoid B-cell lymphoma
- Parafollicular B-cell lymphoma

Definitions

- Low-grade lymphoma derived from distinct native population of thymic postgerminal center stage parafollicular B cells

ETIOLOGY/PATHOGENESIS

Pathogenesis

- Believed to represent thymic counterpart of distinctive type of extranodal marginal zone lymphoma of mucosa-associated lymphoid tissue (MALToma)

CLINICAL ISSUES

Site

- Anterior-superior mediastinum

Presentation

- Asymptomatic (> 50% of cases)
- Chest pain and shortness of breath in larger lesions
- Indolent growth with protracted clinical course (> 80% 5-year survival)
- Often associated with Sjögren syndrome and polyclonal hypergammaglobulinemia
- Predilection for middle-aged females

Treatment

- Surgical excision
- Postoperative chemotherapy in some cases

Prognosis

- Generally excellent prognosis with long-term survival
- Some cases may give rise to development of diffuse large cell lymphoma

MACROSCOPIC FEATURES

General Features

- Diffusely enlarged thymus with homogeneous rubbery cut surface
- May display secondary cystic changes

Sections to Be Submitted

- One section per cm of largest diameter
- Submit fresh tissue for flow cytometry and cytogenetics

Size

- 5-10 cm in greatest dimension

MICROSCOPIC PATHOLOGY

Histologic Features

- Monotonous proliferation of small lymphoid cells in interfollicular distribution
- Lymphoid cell population is admixed with reactive, hyperplastic lymphoid follicles
- Lymphoid cells infiltrate residual epithelial structures (i.e., Hassall corpuscles), creating lymphoepithelial lesions
- Residual thymic epithelium may undergo cystic degeneration resulting in multiple thymic cysts
- Small lymphocytes can infiltrate surrounding perithymic fat at edges of lesion
- Colonization of germinal centers by neoplastic small mantle zone lymphocytes

MALT LYMPHOMA OF THE THYMUS

Key Facts

Terminology
- Low-grade lymphoma derived from distinct native population of thymic postgerminal center stage parafollicular B cells

Etiology/Pathogenesis
- Believed to represent thymic counterpart of distinctive type of extranodal marginal zone lymphoma of mucosa-associated lymphoid tissue (MALToma)

Clinical Issues
- Generally excellent prognosis with long-term survival
- Some cases may give rise to development of diffuse large cell lymphoma
- Indolent growth with protracted clinical course

Microscopic Pathology
- Monotonous proliferation of small lymphoid cells in interfollicular distribution
- Lymphoid cell population is admixed with reactive, hyperplastic lymphoid follicles
- Lymphoid cells infiltrate residual epithelial structures (i.e., Hassall corpuscles), creating lymphoepithelial lesions
- Residual thymic epithelium may undergo cystic degeneration resulting in multiple thymic cysts
- Small lymphocytes can infiltrate surrounding perithymic fat at edges of lesion
- Lymphoid cells display slightly irregular nuclei surrounded by clear cytoplasmic halos
- Lymphoid cells may display plasmacytoid features
- Rare mitotic figures may be present

Cytologic Features
- Lymphoid cells display slightly irregular nuclei surrounded by clear cytoplasmic halos
- Lymphoid cells often display plasmacytoid features
- Rare mitotic figures may be present

ANCILLARY TESTS

Immunohistochemistry
- Positive for CD11c, CD19, CD20, CD22, CD24, CD43, CD79-α, Bcl-2, Pax-5, and IgA
- Negative for CD5, CD10, CD21, CD23, CD25, CD35, cyclin-D1, Bcl-6, and *AP12-MALT1* gene fusion

DIFFERENTIAL DIAGNOSIS

Thymic Lymphoid Hyperplasia
- Most often associated with autoimmune disorders such as myasthenia gravis
- Preservation of normal underlying corticomedullary architecture of thymus
- Absence of lymphoepithelial lesions
- Absence of monocytoid B-cell population surrounding follicles
- Absence of infiltration of perithymic fat by small lymphocytes

Small Lymphocytic Lymphoma/Chronic Lymphocytic Leukemia
- Characterized by diffuse effacement of underlying architecture without follicles or germinal centers
- May show lymphoplasmacytic differentiation
- Absence of clear perinuclear halos in lymphoid cells
- Absence of lymphoepithelial lesions
- Neoplastic lymphocytes are positive for CD5 and CD23

Follicular Lymphoma
- Enlarged follicles showing uniform population of transformed germinal center cells
- Absence of significant monocytoid interfollicular B-cell population
- Absence of lymphoepithelial lesions
- Cells within follicles are strongly positive for Bcl-2, CD10, and Bcl-6

DIAGNOSTIC CHECKLIST

Clinically Relevant Pathologic Features
- Usually asymptomatic; discovered incidentally on routine chest x-rays
- Indolent lesion with slow evolution and good prognosis

Pathologic Interpretation Pearls
- Enlargement of thymus with prominent lymphoid follicles but with effacement of underlying native architecture
- Gross and microscopic cystic changes
- Lymphoepithelial lesions
- Monotonous interfollicular population of lymphoid cells with monocytoid features

SELECTED REFERENCES

1. Braham E et al: Thymic marginal zone B-cell lymphoma of mucosa-associated lymphoid tissue-type in a patient with Sjögren's syndrome and cryoglobulinaemia. Pathology. 41(7):701-3, 2009
2. Inagaki H et al: Primary thymic extranodal marginal-zone B-cell lymphoma of mucosa-associated lymphoid tissue type exhibits distinctive clinicopathological and molecular features. Am J Pathol. 160(4):1435-43, 2002
3. Parrens M et al: Mucosa-associated lymphoid tissue of the thymus hyperplasia vs lymphoma. Am J Clin Pathol. 117(1):51-6, 2002
4. McCluggage WG et al: Low-grade B-cell lymphoma of mucosa-associated lymphoid tissue (MALT) of thymus. Hum Pathol. 31(2):255-9, 2000
5. Suster S et al: Malignant thymic neoplasms that may mimic benign conditions. Semin Diagn Pathol. 12(1):98-104, 1995

MALT LYMPHOMA OF THE THYMUS

Microscopic Features

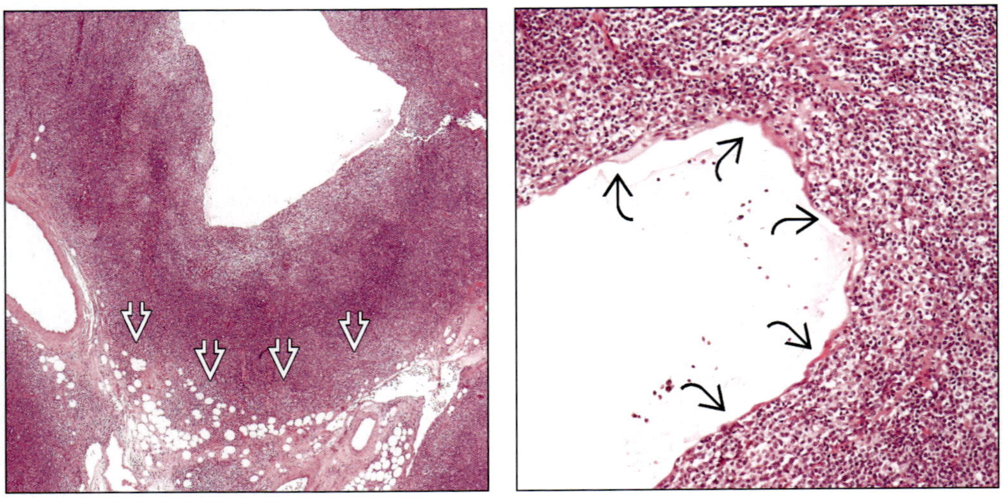

(Left) *Scanning magnification in MALT lymphoma of the thymus shows cystically dilated spaces surrounded by a dense, monotonous lymphoid cell population. The lymphocytes are not confined to the thymus and are seen percolating into the surrounding fat →.* ***(Right)*** *MALT lymphoma of the thymus shows a dilated cystic space lined by a single layer of flattened cuboidal epithelium →. The cyst is surrounded by monotonous sheets of small lymphocytes.*

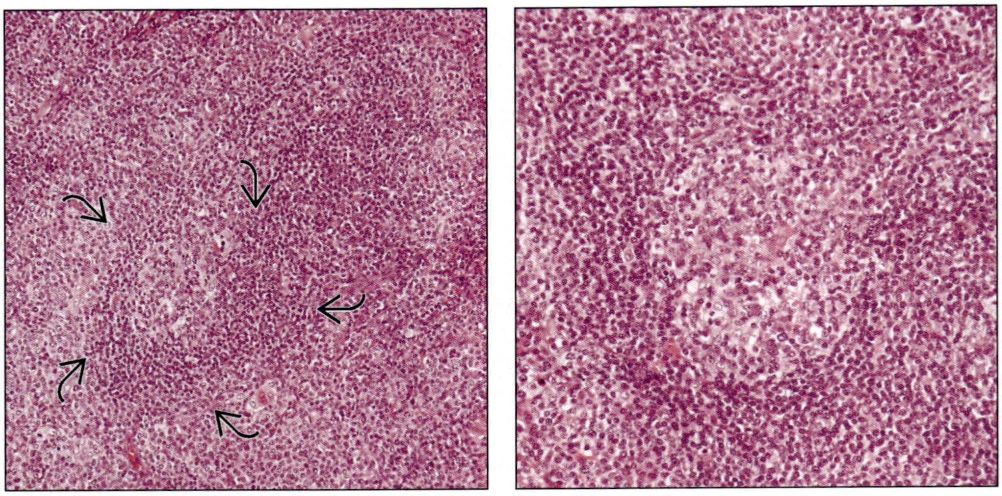

(Left) *MALT lymphoma of the thymus shows sheets of monotonous small lymphocytes circumscribing a lymphoid follicle with a reactive germinal center →. The lymphoid cells surrounding the lymphoid follicle show striking perinuclear clearing.* ***(Right)*** *High-power magnification of MALT lymphoma of the thymus shows a lymphoid follicle with a reactive germinal center surrounded by a monotonous population of small lymphocytes.*

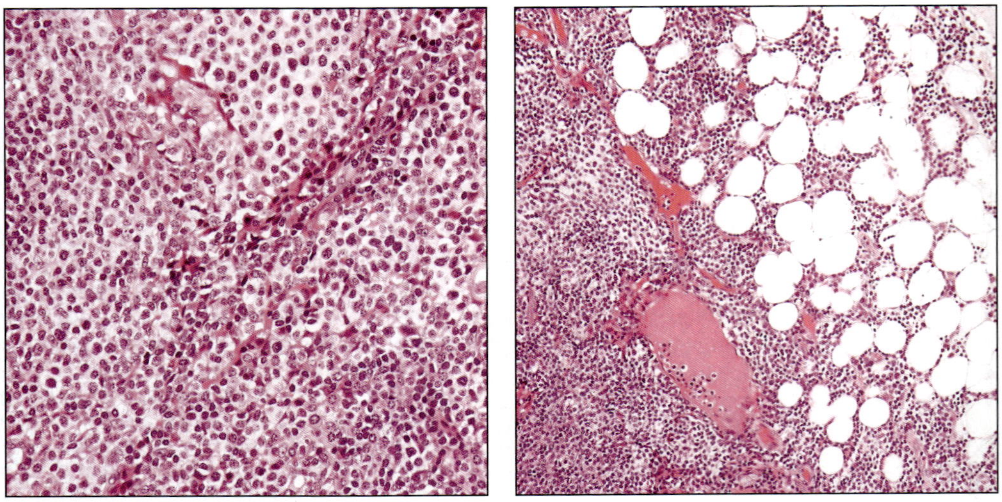

(Left) *High magnification of MALT lymphoma of the thymus shows sheets of monotonous lymphoid cells with minimal nuclear irregularities. Notice the spacing between the cells caused by clear, perinuclear halos.* ***(Right)*** *Scanning magnification in MALT lymphoma of the thymus shows infiltration of perithymic adipose tissue by small lymphocytes. Notice percolation of small lymphocytes among the fat cells with preservation of the normal fat.*

Microscopic Features

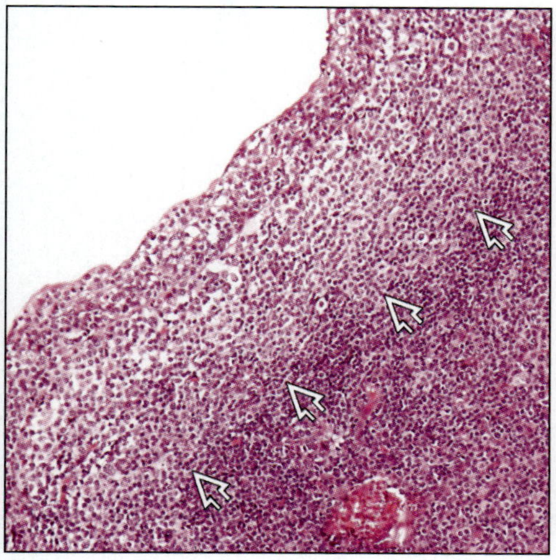

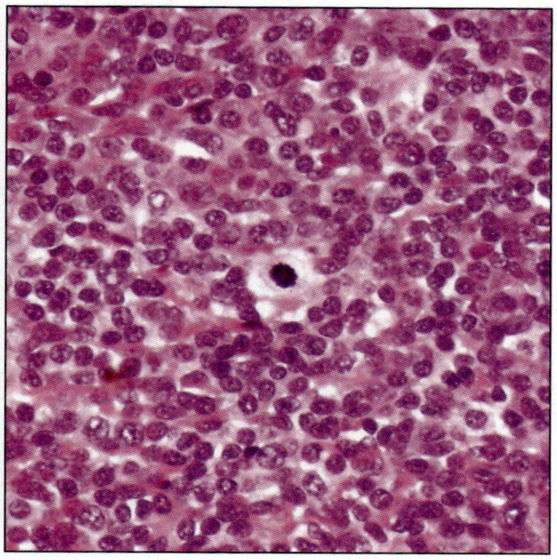

(Left) *Scanning magnification of MALT lymphoma of the thymus shows a band ➔ of monotonous lymphoid cells against the lining of a cystic cavity (top left). Notice the lighter staining quality of neoplastic lymphocytes above the arrows due to an abundance of cytoplasm in the tumor cells.* ***(Right)*** *MALT lymphoma of the thymus shows sheets of monotonous small lymphocytes. Notice the rare mitotic figure in the center of the field.*

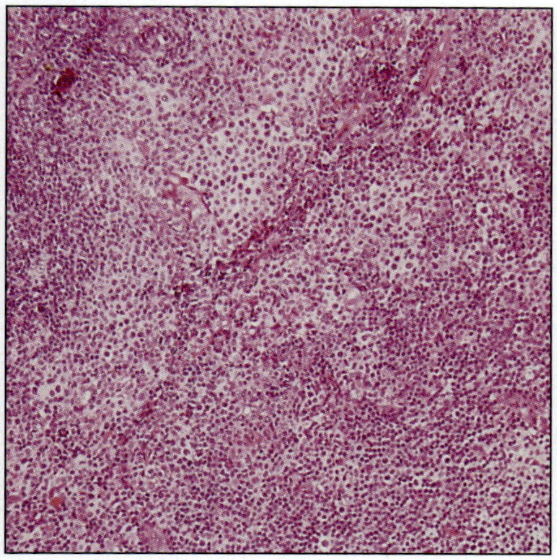

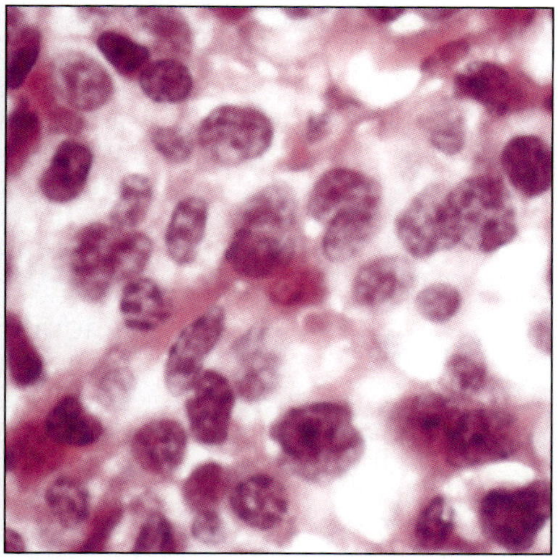

(Left) *MALT lymphoma of the thymus shows sheets of monotonous lymphoid cells with distinctive "fried egg" appearance due to clear perinuclear halos surrounding the individual tumor cells.* ***(Right)*** *High magnification of MALT lymphoma of the thymus shows population of monotonous small lymphocytes with minimal nuclear irregularities and dispersed nuclear chromatin pattern. The cells are separated from each other by an ample rim of amphophilic cytoplasm.*

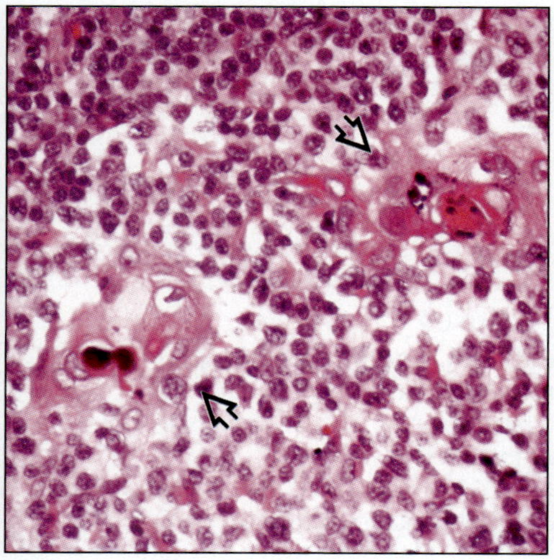

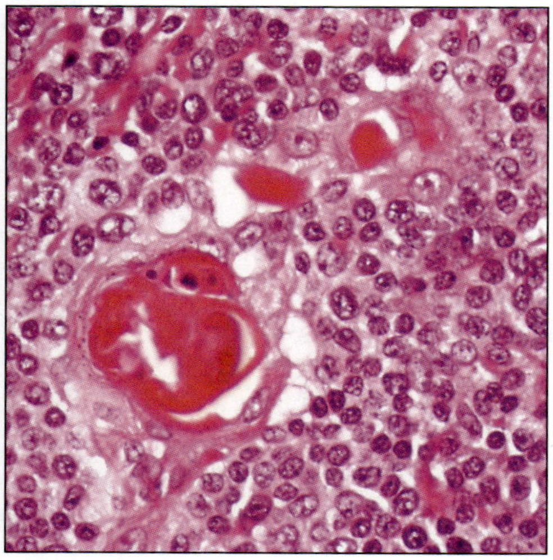

(Left) *MALT lymphoma of the thymus shows entrapment of Hassall corpuscles by dense lymphoid cell infiltrate creating characteristic lymphoepithelial lesions ➔.* ***(Right)*** *High magnification of MALT lymphoma of the thymus shows distinctive lymphoepithelial lesion. Notice entrapment of Hassall corpuscle (center) by the dense lymphoid cell population with infiltration and percolation of individual small lymphocytes into the epithelium.*

LIPOSARCOMA

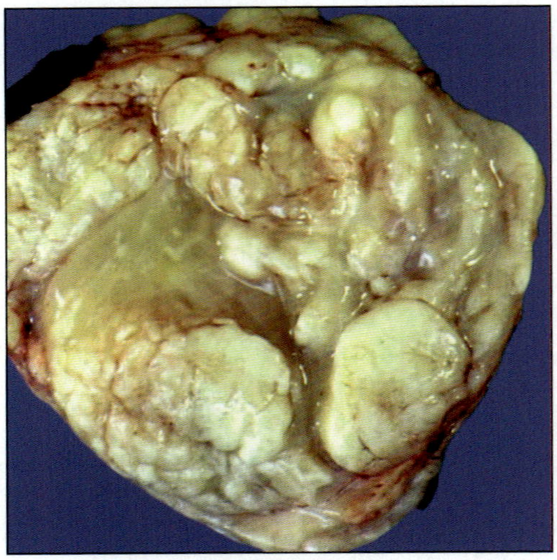

Gross appearance of dedifferentiated liposarcoma of the mediastinum shows a well-circumscribed, lobulated mass with an admixture of fleshy white (dedifferentiated) and myxoid (well-differentiated) areas.

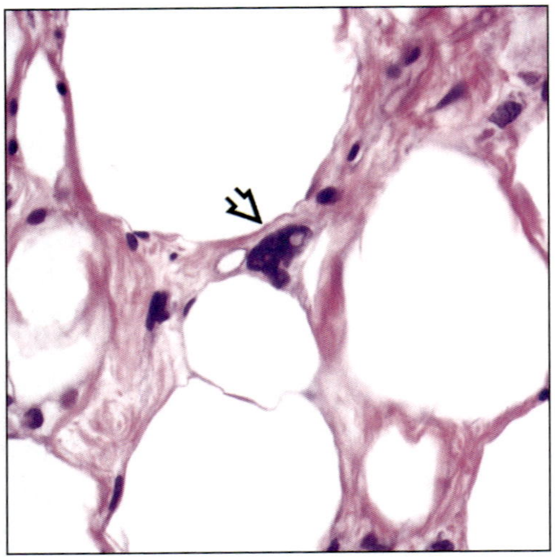

Histologic appearance of well-differentiated liposarcoma of the anterior mediastinum shows atypical lipoblast ⇨ surrounded by normal-appearing adipocytic cells.

TERMINOLOGY

Abbreviations

- Liposarcoma (LS)

Synonyms

- Atypical lipomatous tumor

Definitions

- Malignant neoplastic proliferation of adipocytic cells

CLINICAL ISSUES

Epidemiology

- Incidence
  - Rare tumor
- Age
  - Broad age range; children to adults (mean: 43 years)
- Gender
  - Slight predilection for males

Site

- Anterior and posterior mediastinum
- More common in anterior mediastinum

Presentation

- Cough
- Dyspnea
- Chest pain
- Asymptomatic in up to 1/3 of patients
- May be an incidental finding on routine chest x-ray or at autopsy

Treatment

- Surgical excision

Prognosis

- Depends on stage and histologic type
- Recurrences in 33% of cases
- Large, infiltrative, and unresectable tumors are associated with worse prognosis
- Myxoid/round cell, dedifferentiated and pleomorphic liposarcomas are associated with more aggressive behavior
- Round cell and pleomorphic liposarcomas are associated with distant metastases and high mortality
- Well-differentiated liposarcomas can recur 15-20 years after initial diagnosis

MACROSCOPIC FEATURES

General Features

- Well-differentiated tumors are lobulated, well circumscribed, and thinly encapsulated with a soft, yellowish cut surface
- Poorly differentiated tumors are irregular, infiltrative, with yellow-white firm cut surfaces and areas of hemorrhage and necrosis

Sections to Be Submitted

- 1 section per centimeter of largest tumor diameter
- Additional sections must be submitted in tumors suspected of corresponding to dedifferentiated liposarcomas to identify lipogenic elements

Size

- 5-30 cm

MICROSCOPIC PATHOLOGY

Histologic Features

- **Well-differentiated, lipoma-like liposarcoma/ atypical lipomatous tumor**
  - Sheets of mature-appearing adipocytes ± scattered atypical lipoblastic cells
  - Areas of densely collagenized stroma containing atypical lipoblasts and spindle cells
  - Thymoliposarcoma is characterized by admixture of normal thymus with atypical lipomatous areas
  - Scattered lymphoid aggregates or lymphoid follicles

LIPOSARCOMA

Key Facts

Clinical Issues
- Rare tumor
- Broad age range; from children to adults (mean age: 43 years)
- Anterior and posterior mediastinum
- Dyspnea
- Chest pain
- Recurrences in 33% of cases
- Myxoid/round cell, dedifferentiated, and pleomorphic liposarcomas are associated with more aggressive behavior

Microscopic Pathology
- Well-differentiated, lipoma-like liposarcoma/atypical lipomatous tumor
- Myxoid/round cell liposarcoma
- Dedifferentiated liposarcoma
- Pleomorphic liposarcoma

Ancillary Tests
- Lipoblasts and atypical cells in well-differentiated lipoma-like liposarcoma and dedifferentiated liposarcoma are positive for MDM2 and CDK4
- Well-differentiated liposarcoma and dedifferentiated liposarcoma show amplification of *MDM2* at 12q14-15 region
- Myxoid liposarcoma shows TSL-CHOP translocation in t(12;16)(q13;p11)

Top Differential Diagnoses
- Lipoma and thymolipoma
- Low-grade spindle cell tumors
- High-grade pleomorphic sarcomas
- Small round blue cell tumors

- **Myxoid/round cell liposarcoma**
  - Scattered small, stellate or round cells embedded in abundant myxoid matrix
  - Prominent arborizing ("chicken wire") vascular pattern of small branching vessels in stroma
  - Round cell variant characterized by increased cellularity with emergence of dense sheets of primitive, hyperchromatic small round cells
  - "Pulmonary-edema" pattern with dilated spaces filled with serum may be seen in these tumors
- **Dedifferentiated liposarcoma**
  - Well-differentiated liposarcoma that shows emergence of nonlipogenic atypical spindle cell component
  - Low-grade dedifferentiated component shows bland-appearing spindle cell proliferation with low mitotic rate
  - High-grade dedifferentiated component shows pleomorphic tumor cells with atypical mitoses simulating malignant fibrous histiocytoma
  - Dedifferentiated component may be heterologous (i.e., rhabdo-, leio-, or osteosarcomatous)
  - Dedifferentiated component may show foci of spindle cells showing a distinctive whorling pattern that resembles meningioma
- **Pleomorphic liposarcoma**
  - High-grade pleomorphic sarcoma with focal areas containing lipoblastic elements
  - Bizarre lipoblasts and multinucleated floret-type giant cells
- **Pleomorphic myxoid liposarcoma**
  - Shows areas of myxoid liposarcoma admixed with pleomorphic tumor cells
  - More aggressive behavior than conventional myxoid liposarcoma
  - Rare morphologic variant more often seen in mediastinum

Cytologic Features
- Majority of cells in well-differentiated liposarcoma resemble normal mature adipocytes
- Well-differentiated liposarcoma may contain atypical, multinucleated adipocytes
- Well-differentiated liposarcoma often contains floret-type multinucleated cells
- Sclerosing areas in well-differentiated liposarcoma contain floret-type cells and bland-appearing spindle stromal cells
- Lipoblasts may vary from small, signet-ring lipoblasts to multivacuolated adipocytes with multiple enlarged, atypical nuclei
- Round cell liposarcoma shows primitive small round blue cells with scant cytoplasm
- Pleomorphic liposarcoma contains bizarre, anaplastic and multinucleated atypical lipoblastic cells

ANCILLARY TESTS

Immunohistochemistry
- Mature adipocytes are S100 protein positive
- Lipoblasts and atypical cells in well-differentiated lipoma-like liposarcoma and dedifferentiated liposarcoma are MDM2 and CDK4 positive

Cytogenetics
- Supernumerary ring and giant marker chromosomes are seen in well-differentiated and dedifferentiated liposarcoma
- Random and nonrandom telomeric association can also be seen in well-differentiated liposarcoma
- Characteristic t(12;16)(q13;p11) is present in > 90% of myxoid and round cell liposarcomas
  - t(12;16) in myxoid/round cell liposarcoma leads to fusion of *CHOP* and *FUS* genes with generation of a FUS/DDIT3 hybrid protein
- Variant chromosomal translocation t(12;22)(q13;q12) is also present in myxoid liposarcoma in which *DDIT3* fuses with *EWS*
- No distinctive cytogenetic markers have been observed in pleomorphic liposarcoma

Cytogenetic Abnormalities in Adipocytic Neoplasms

Tumor Type	Cytogenetic Abnormality	Testing Method
Well-differentiated liposarcoma/atypical lipomatous tumor	*MDM2* amplification	Immunohistochemistry, FISH, Southern blotting, comparative genomic hybridization
Myxoid/round cell liposarcoma	CHOP; *FUS/DDIT3* fusion product	FISH, PCR, Southern blotting
Low-grade dedifferentiated liposarcoma	*MDM2* amplification (in both well-differentiated and low-grade dedifferentiated cells)	Immunohistochemistry, FISH
High-grade dedifferentiated liposarcoma	*MDM2* amplification (only in well-differentiated component)	Immunohistochemistry, FISH
Pleomorphic liposarcoma	*MDM2* amplification (in only 1/3 of cases)	Immunohistochemistry, FISH

Molecular Diagnostics

- FISH for *MDM2* shows consistent amplification in 12q14-15 in well-differentiated and dedifferentiated liposarcomas
- Neighboring genes such as *CDK4*, *SAS*, and *HMGIC* can also be amplified in well-differentiated and dedifferentiated liposarcomas
- 12q14-15 amplification is not observed in benign tumors and may serve to distinguish well-differentiated liposarcoma from lipoma
- FISH for detection of *FUS/DDIT3* fusion product is helpful in confirming diagnosis of myxoid/round cell liposarcoma
- Amplification of *MDM2* can be observed in about 1/3 of pleomorphic liposarcomas

DIFFERENTIAL DIAGNOSIS

Lipoma and Thymolipoma

- Mediastinal lipomas are small and well-circumscribed, completely encapsulated lesions
  - Absence of areas of sclerosis, lipoblasts, floret-type multinucleated cells, or signet ring lipoblastic cells
- Thymolipoma shows admixture of mature adipose tissue with entrapped involuted thymic remnants

Low-Grade Spindle Cell Tumors

- May be difficult to distinguish from low-grade dedifferentiated liposarcoma
  - Low-grade dedifferentiated liposarcoma is positive for MDM2 or CDK4
- Low-grade spindle cell sarcomas of mediastinum lack well-differentiated adipocytic component
- Solitary fibrous tumors are positive for CD34 and Bcl-2
- Schwannomas and neurofibromas are S100 protein(+)
- Spindle cell thymomas are positive for cytokeratin
- Leiomyomas and low-grade leiomyosarcomas are positive for desmin and smooth muscle actin

High-Grade Sarcomas

- May be difficult to distinguish from high-grade dedifferentiated liposarcoma or pleomorphic liposarcoma
- Nonlipogenic high-grade sarcomas lack lipoblastic cells or well-differentiated adipocytic components

Small Round Blue Cell Tumors

- May be confused with round cell liposarcoma
- Small round blue cell tumors (Ewing/PNET, small desmoplastic round blue cell tumor, neuroblastoma, rhabdomyosarcoma) usually lack myxoid stroma
- Ewing/PNET are positive for CD99 (c-mic2)
- Small desmoplastic round blue cell tumors are polyphenotypic (positive for vimentin, cytokeratin, desmin, synaptophysin, EMA, and other markers)
- Neuroblastoma is positive for NSE
- Rhabdomyosarcoma is positive for desmin, Myo-D1, and myogenin
- Small round blue cell tumors lack CHOP translocation

DIAGNOSTIC CHECKLIST

Clinically Relevant Pathologic Features

- Histologic tumor type influences biologic behavior
- Myxoid/round cell liposarcoma and pleomorphic liposarcoma have worse prognosis
- Assessment of margins & adequacy of excision may be very difficult to asses in well-differentiated neoplasms

Pathologic Interpretation Pearls

- Well-differentiated adipocytic tumors in mediastinum are best regarded as well-differentiated liposarcoma irrespective of histology
- Extensive sampling may be required to identify low-grade, well-differentiated liposarcomatous component in dedifferentiated liposarcomas

SELECTED REFERENCES

1. Alaggio R et al: Liposarcomas in young patients: a study of 82 cases occurring in patients younger than 22 years of age. Am J Surg Pathol. 33(5):645-58, 2009
2. Coulibaly B et al: Recurrent dedifferentiated liposarcoma of mediastinum involving lung and pleura. Interact Cardiovasc Thorac Surg. 9(4):741-2, 2009
3. Fukai R et al: A dedifferentiated liposarcoma of the anterior mediastinum. Int J Clin Oncol. 14(2):174-7, 2009
4. Hahn HP et al: Primary mediastinal liposarcoma: clinicopathologic analysis of 24 cases. Am J Surg Pathol. 31(12):1868-74, 2007
5. Adachi T et al: Immunoreactivity of p53, mdm2, and p21WAF1 in dedifferentiated liposarcoma: special emphasis on the distinct immunophenotype of the well-differentiated component. Int J Surg Pathol. 9(2):99-109, 2001
6. Klimstra DS et al: Liposarcoma of the anterior mediastinum and thymus. A clinicopathologic study of 28 cases. Am J Surg Pathol. 19(7):782-91, 1995

Well-differentiated Liposarcoma of the Mediastinum

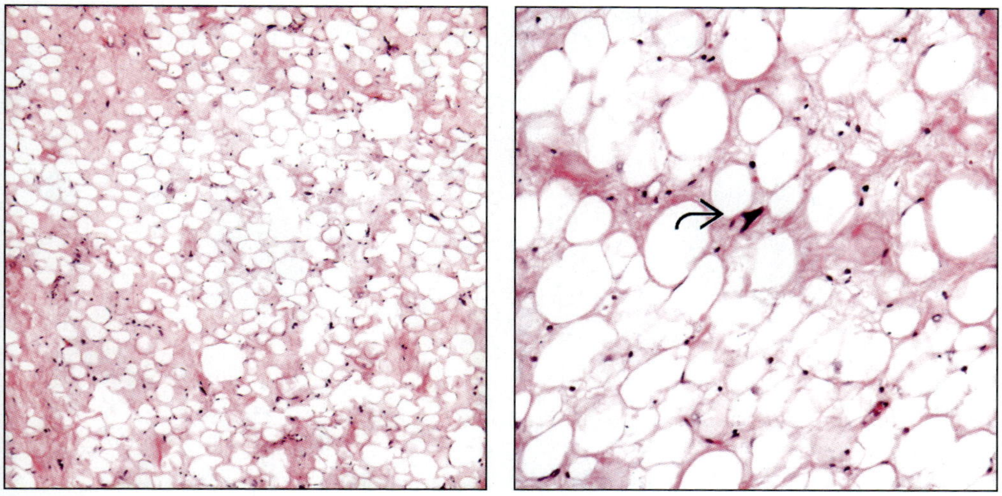

(Left) *Scanning magnification of well-differentiated lipoma-like liposarcoma/atypical lipomatous tumor of the mediastinum shows a monotonous, evenly spaced population of mature, normal-appearing adipocytes. The lesion resembles a lipoma.* ***(Right)*** *Higher magnification of well-differentiated lipoma-like liposarcoma/atypical lipomatous tumor of the mediastinum shows a rare atypical cell → admixed with the surrounding normal-appearing, mature adipocytic cells.*

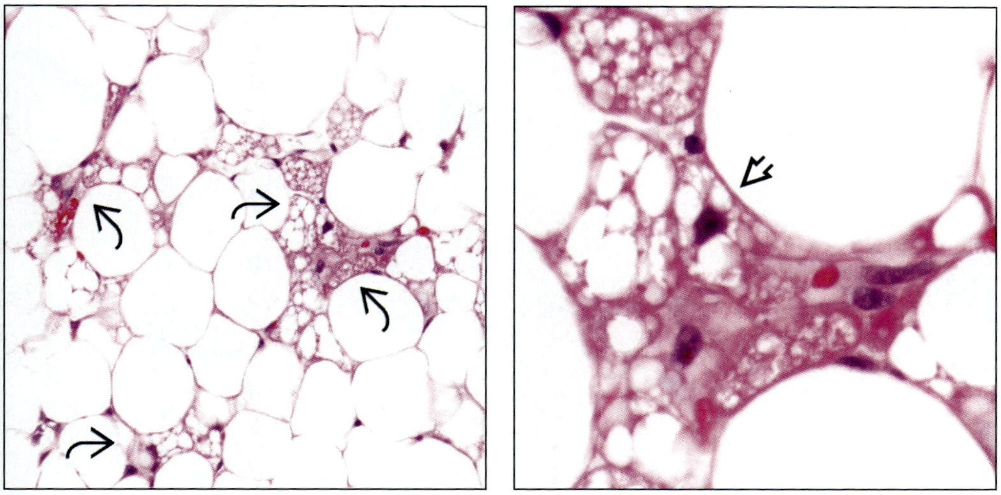

(Left) *Scanning magnification of well-differentiated lipoma-like liposarcoma/atypical lipomatous tumor of the mediastinum shows uniform population of mature adipocytes admixed with a few multivacuolated adipocytes →.* ***(Right)*** *High magnification of well-differentiated lipoma-like liposarcoma/atypical lipomatous tumor of the mediastinum shows multivacuolated lipoblasts. Notice slightly atypical nuclei surrounded by multiple cytoplasmic vacuoles ⇨.*

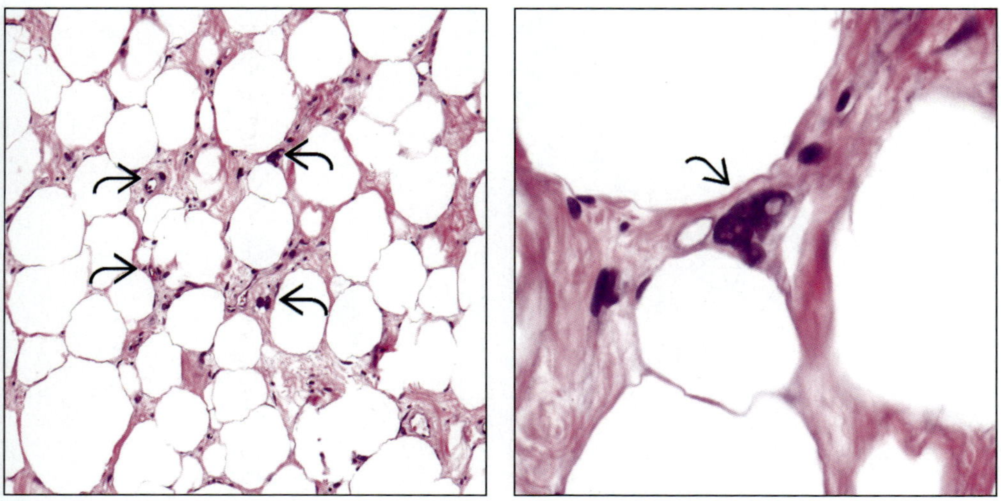

(Left) *Scanning magnification of well-differentiated lipoma-like liposarcoma/atypical lipomatous tumor of the mediastinum shows uniform population of normal-appearing fat with a few scattered larger, atypical cells →.* ***(Right)*** *High magnification of well-differentiated lipoma-like liposarcoma/atypical lipomatous tumor of the mediastinum shows mature adipocytes surrounding a large, atypical lipoblastic cell →. Notice the dense nuclear chromatin and irregularly shaped nucleus.*

LIPOSARCOMA

Cytology of Well-differentiated Liposarcoma

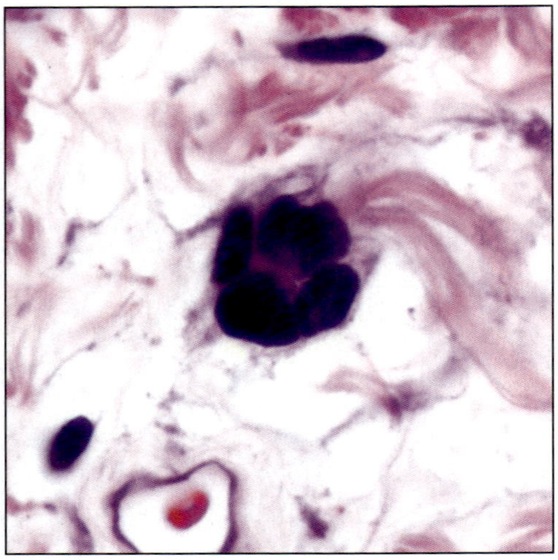
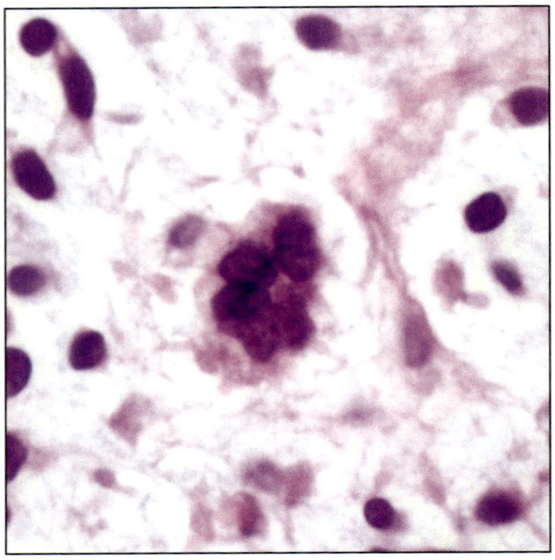

(Left) *Floret-type atypical cell in mediastinal well-differentiated lipoma-like liposarcoma shows multiple large, hyperchromatic nuclei disposed toward the periphery, resembling the petals of a flower.* ***(Right)*** *Another variation on the theme of the floret-type multinucleated lipoblast in mediastinal liposarcoma shows multiple nuclei surrounded by multivacuolated cytoplasm. These cells are common in well-differentiated lipoma-like liposarcoma/atypical lipomatous tumor.*

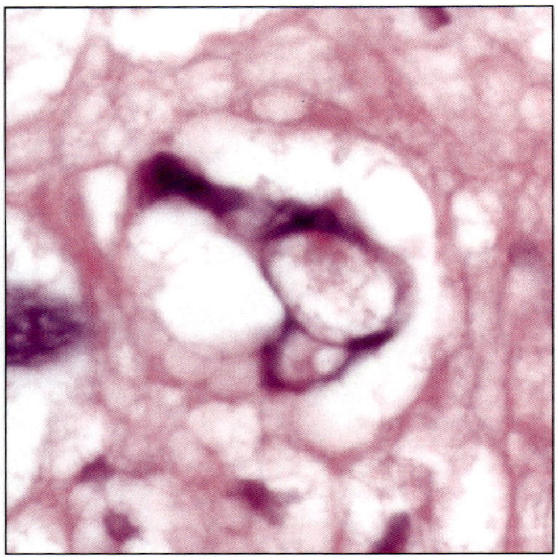
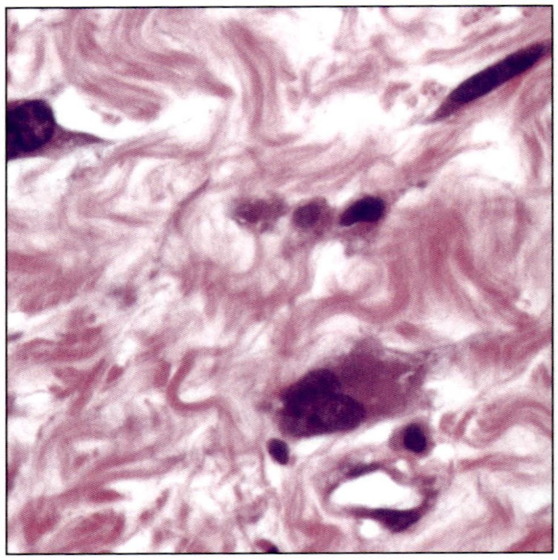

(Left) *Large multivacuolated lipoblast in well-differentiated lipoma-like liposarcoma/ atypical lipomatous tumor of the mediastinum shows multiple large cytoplasmic and intranuclear vacuoles.* ***(Right)*** *Lipoblastic cell in the sclerosing portion of a well-differentiated lipoma-like liposarcoma/ atypical lipomatous tumor of the mediastinum shows multinucleation with a single intranuclear vacuole but devoid of any discernible cytoplasmic vacuolization.*

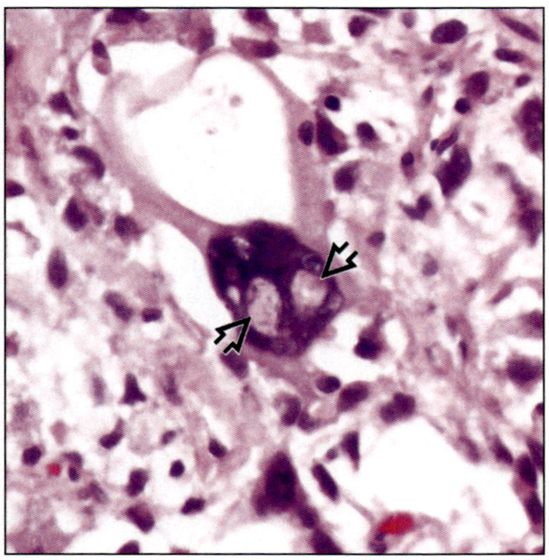
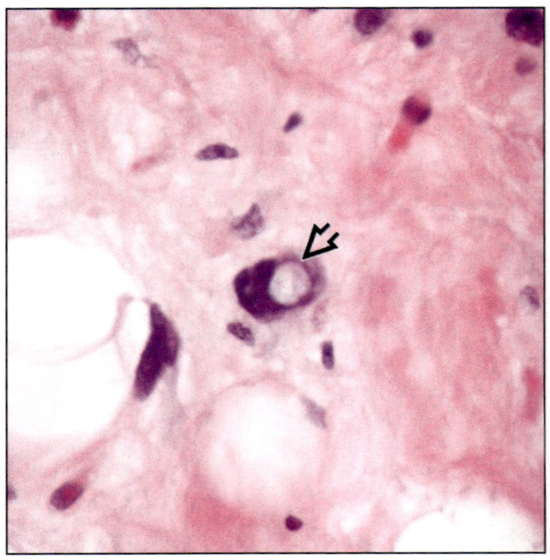

(Left) *Atypical lipoblastic cell in a well-differentiated lipoma-like liposarcoma of the mediastinum is characterized by a single, large, atypical nucleus with dense chromatin pattern and multiple intranuclear vacuoles caused by invaginations of the cytoplasm (pseudoinclusions)* ⇨. ***(Right)*** *Sclerosing portion of well-differentiated lipoma-like liposarcoma of the mediastinum shows a signet ring cell lipoblast containing a single cytoplasmic vacuole that displaces the nucleus to the periphery* ⇨.

Sclerosing Well-differentiated Liposarcoma

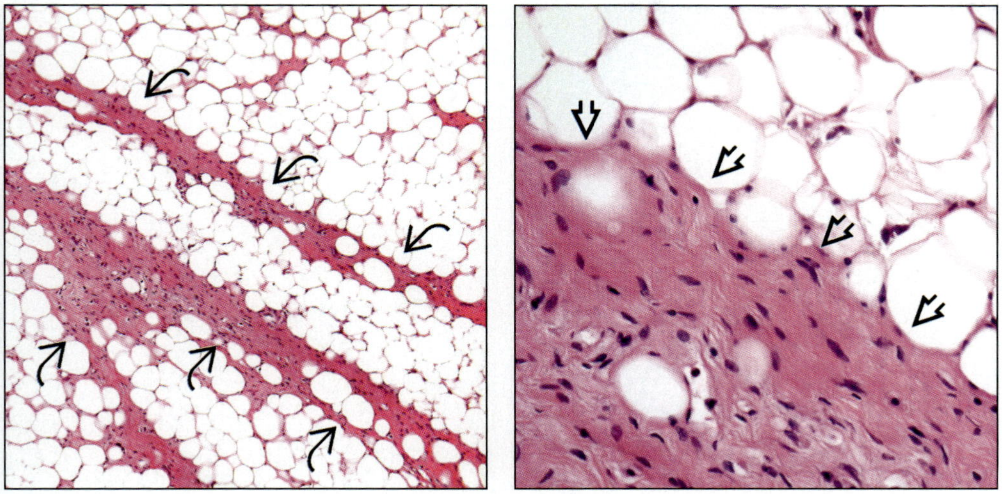

(Left) *Sclerosing well-differentiated lipoma-like liposarcoma of the mediastinum shows thin fibrous bands dissecting the fatty tissue* ➚. ***(Right)*** *High magnification of sclerosing portion of well-differentiated lipoma-like liposarcoma/atypical lipomatous tumor of the mediastinum* ➯ *shows dense collagen deposition with numerous small, hyperchromatic spindle cells admixed with small, round, more primitive cells.*

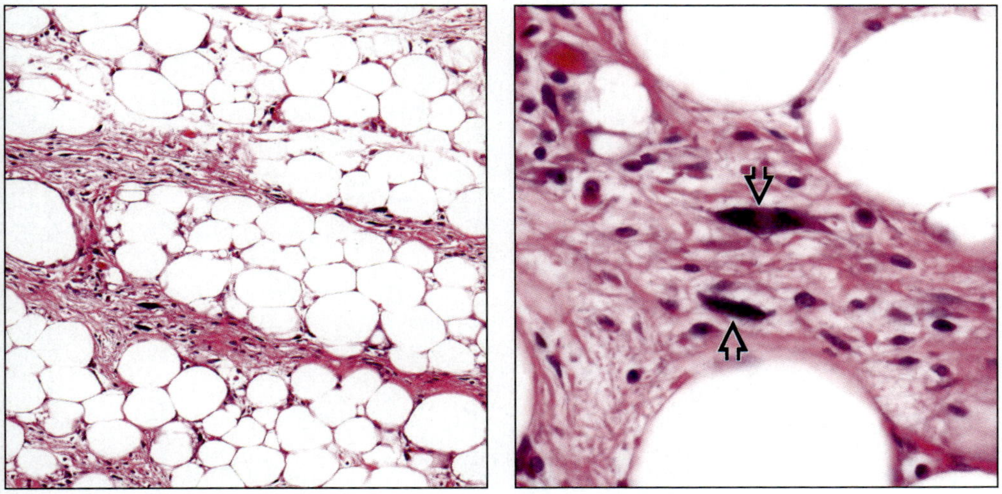

(Left) *Scanning magnification of well-differentiated lipoma-like liposarcoma/atypical lipomatous tumor of the mediastinum with sclerosis shows dense fibrous bands dissecting in-between the adipocytes that contain atypical, hyperchromatic cells.* ***(Right)*** *Higher magnification of well-differentiated lipoma-like liposarcoma of the mediastinum with sclerosis shows atypical spindle cells lying within the area of sclerosis. The atypical cells display large hyperchromatic nuclei* ➯.

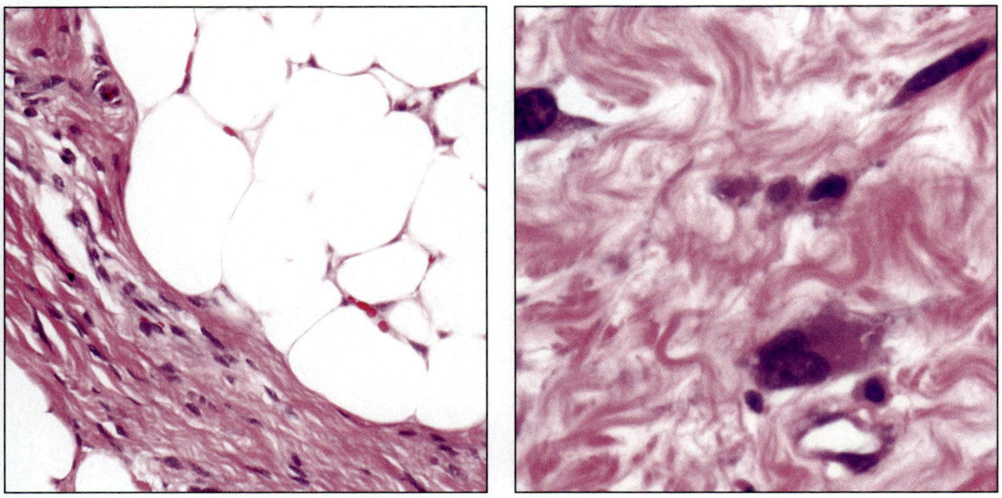

(Left) *Area of sclerosis within well-differentiated lipoma-like liposarcoma/atypical lipomatous tumor of the mediastinum shows a well-defined band of stromal fibrosis that is sharply separated from the surrounding adipose tissue.* ***(Right)*** *High magnification of area of fibrosis in a well-differentiated lipoma-like liposarcoma/atypical lipomatous tumor of the mediastinum shows scattered atypical spindle and lipoblastic cells with enlarged, hyperchromatic nuclei.*

LIPOSARCOMA

Dedifferentiated Liposarcoma

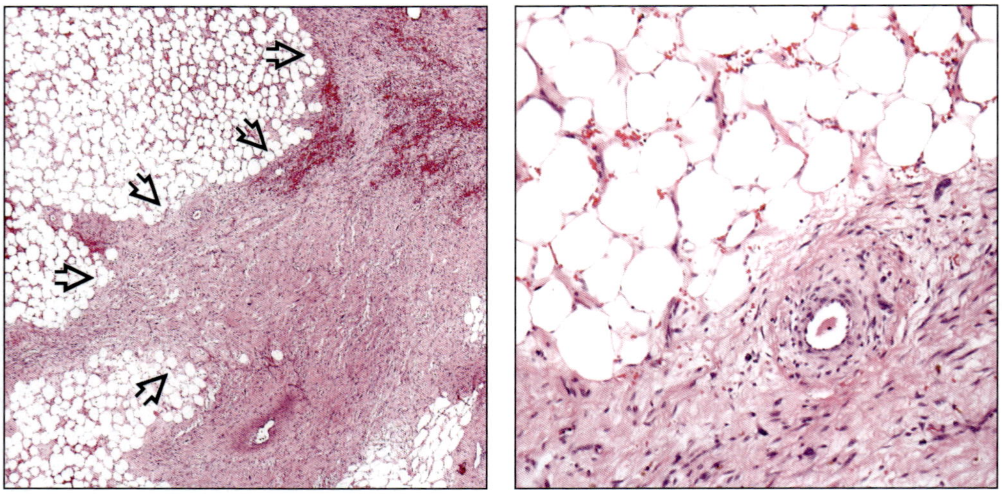

(Left) *Scanning magnification of low-grade dedifferentiated liposarcoma of the mediastinum shows well-differentiated lipoma-like liposarcoma merging with solid areas containing an atypical spindle cell population* ⇨. ***(Right)*** *Higher magnification in low-grade dedifferentiated liposarcoma of the mediastinum shows mature adipose elements (top) merging with a more solid, spindle cell population (bottom). Notice the low-grade appearance of the spindle cells in the dedifferentiated areas.*

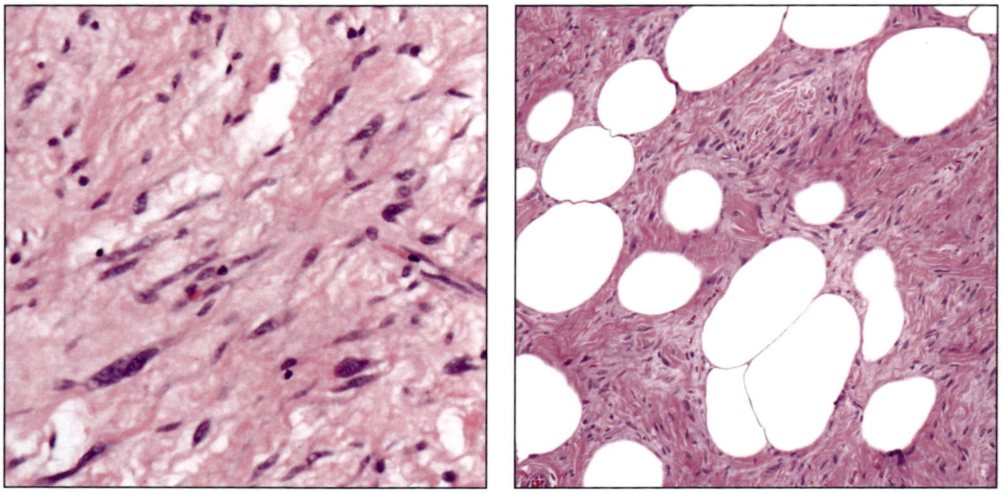

(Left) *Higher magnification of low-grade dedifferentiated liposarcoma of the mediastinum shows mildly atypical spindle cell population embedded in heavily hyalinized stroma.* ***(Right)*** *Area of dedifferentiated liposarcoma of the mediastinum shows spindle cell proliferation with smooth muscle differentiation percolating in-between the normal residual adipose tissue in the tumor. The smooth muscle most likely is an expression of aberrant differentiation in these tumors.*

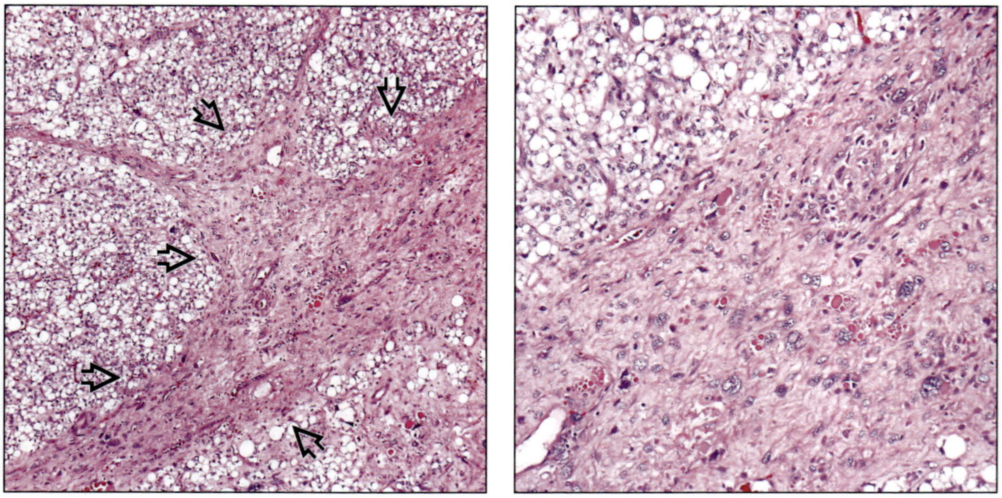

(Left) *Scanning magnification in high-grade dedifferentiated liposarcoma of the mediastinum shows preserved mature-appearing areas of lipoma-like liposarcoma surrounding irregular fibrous strands that contain a population of bizarre, pleomorphic tumor cells* ⇨. ***(Right)*** *High magnification of high-grade dedifferentiated liposarcoma shows a population of bizarre, atypical tumor cells that closely resemble a malignant fibrous histiocytoma.*

Myxoid Liposarcoma

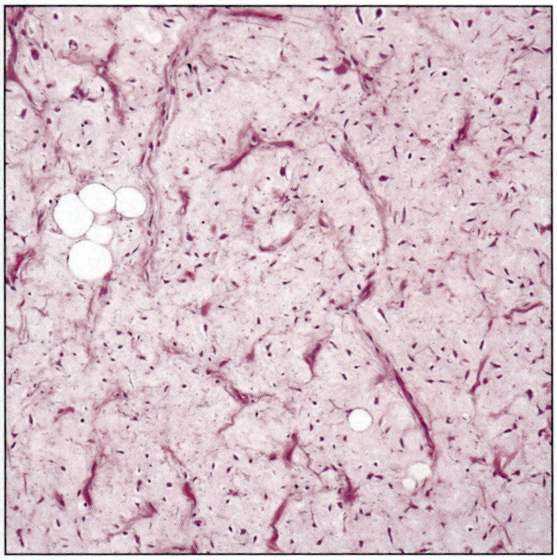

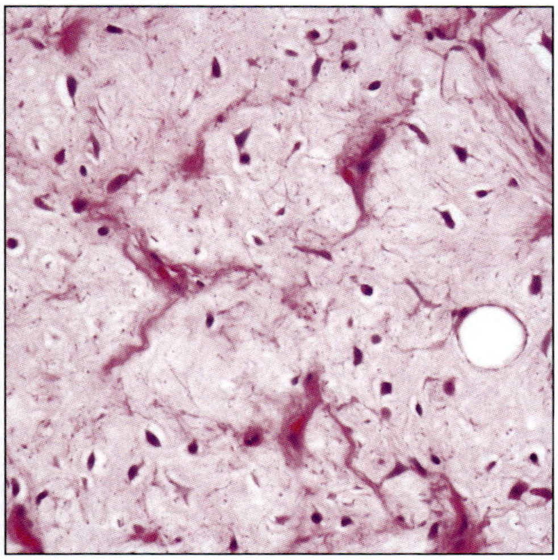

(Left) *Scanning magnification of myxoid liposarcoma of the mediastinum shows a population of small round or stellate cells embedded in abundant myxoid matrix. Notice the arborizing capillary network scattered in the myxoid stroma.* ***(Right)*** *High magnification of myxoid liposarcoma of the mediastinum shows small, primitive, spindle to stellate, hyperchromatic cells suspended in an abundant myxoid matrix. Notice the small branching vessels displaying a "chicken wire" configuration.*

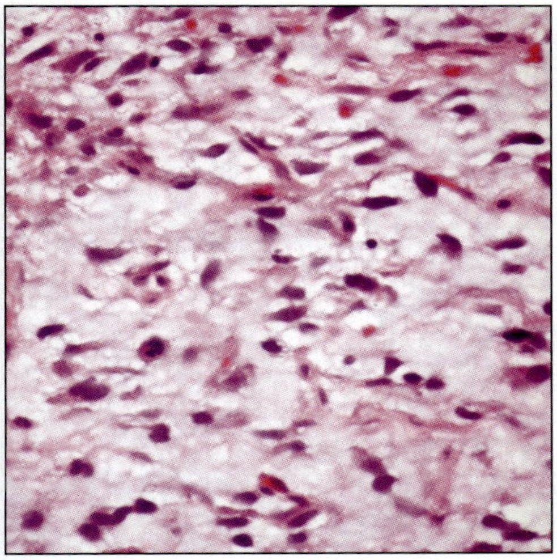

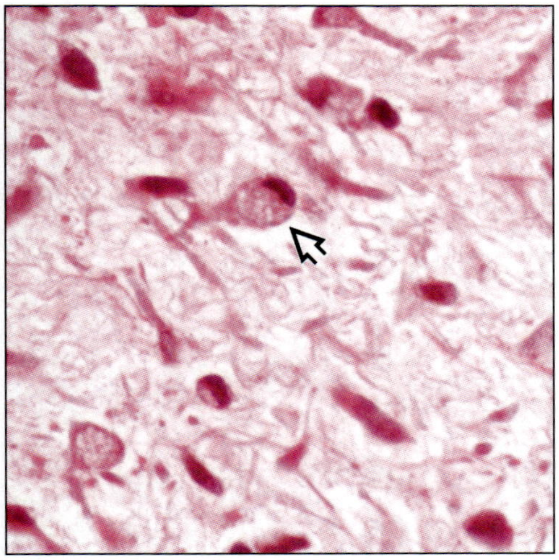

(Left) *Myxoid liposarcoma of the mediastinum shows a population of small round cells and short, hyperchromatic spindle cells lying within a myxoid stroma.* ***(Right)*** *High magnification of myxoid liposarcoma of the mediastinum shows small, round, and spindle cells suspended in abundant myxoid stroma. A few of the cells show a prominent single intracytoplasmic vacuole that pushes the nucleus to the periphery, adopting a signet ring cell appearance* ⮚.

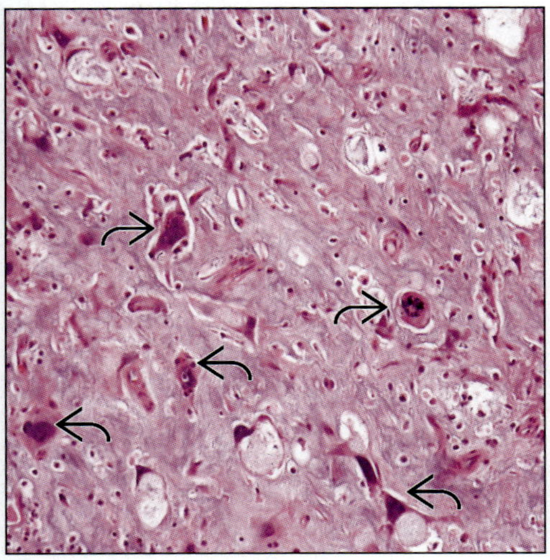

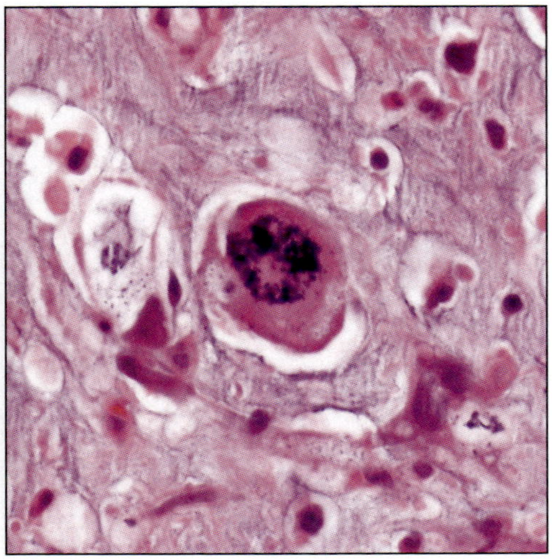

(Left) *Myxoid liposarcoma of the mediastinum with pleomorphic tumor cells shows scattered small cells, abundant myxoid stroma, and a few larger, atypical tumor cells* ⮫. ***(Right)*** *Myxoid pleomorphic liposarcoma of the mediastinum shows a large, atypical tumor cell with an abnormal mitosis (center), surrounded by abundant myxoid matrix. These tumors have been shown to occur with more frequency in the anterior mediastinum and behave more aggressively.*

LIPOSARCOMA

Round Cell Liposarcoma

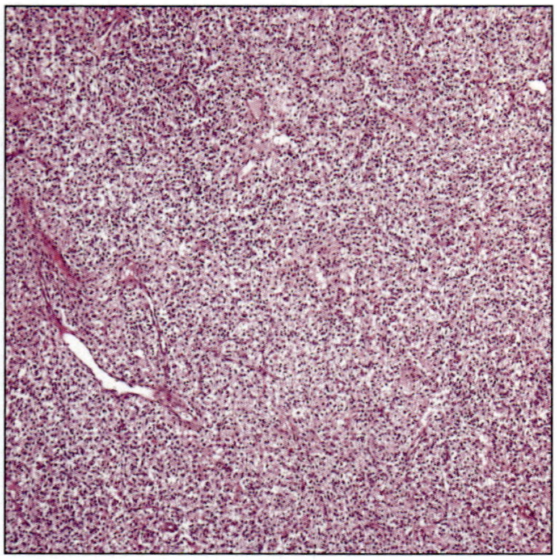

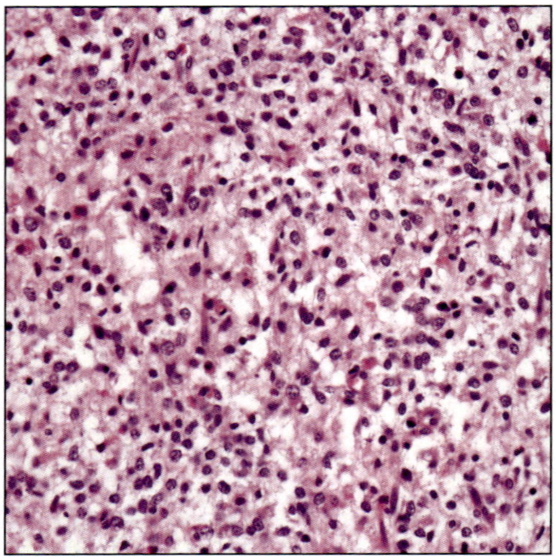

(Left) *Round cell liposarcoma of the mediastinum shows a hypercellular small round cell population without any discernible histologic growth pattern. Tumors with these features can be confused for other small round blue cell tumors, including lymphomas, rhabdomyosarcoma, Ewing/PNET, etc.* ***(Right)*** *High magnification of round cell liposarcoma of the mediastinum shows a monotonous population of primitive small round blue cells. The tumor is very cellular and contains hardly any stroma.*

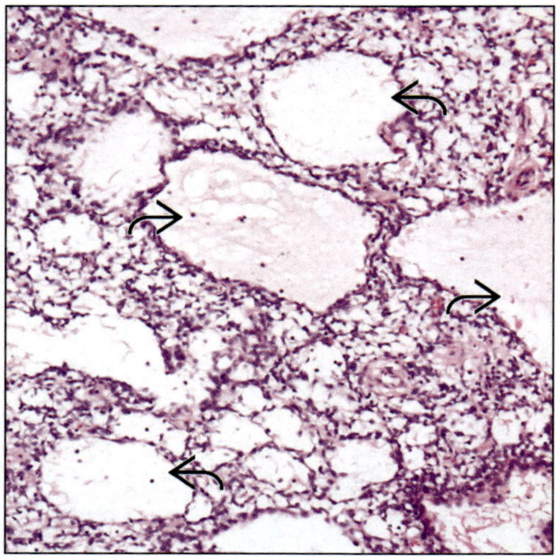

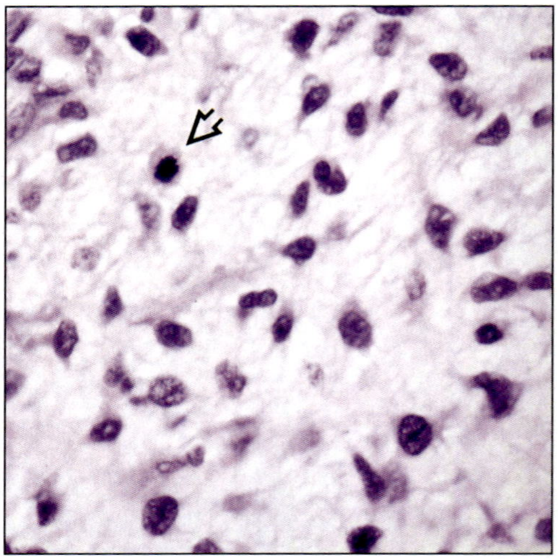

(Left) *Pulmonary edema-like pattern of growth in round cell liposarcoma of the mediastinum is characterized by dilated cystic spaces filled with serum* ↷ *and surrounded by the small round blue cells.* ***(Right)*** *High magnification of round cell liposarcoma of the mediastinum shows a primitive-appearing small round blue cell population embedded in abundant, lightly staining myxoid stroma. The cells have hyperchromatic nuclei; notice the mitotic figure* ⇨*.*

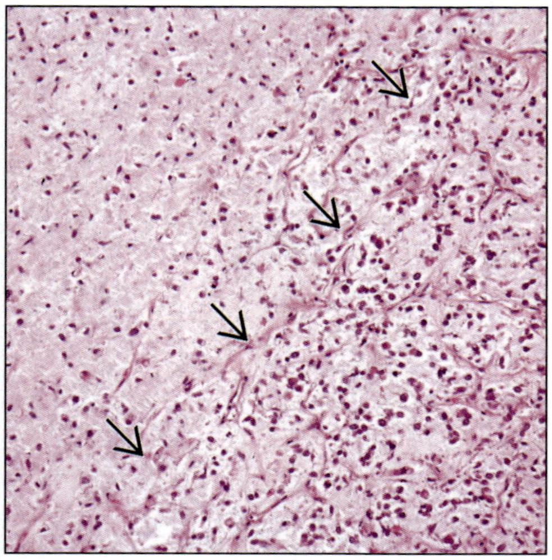

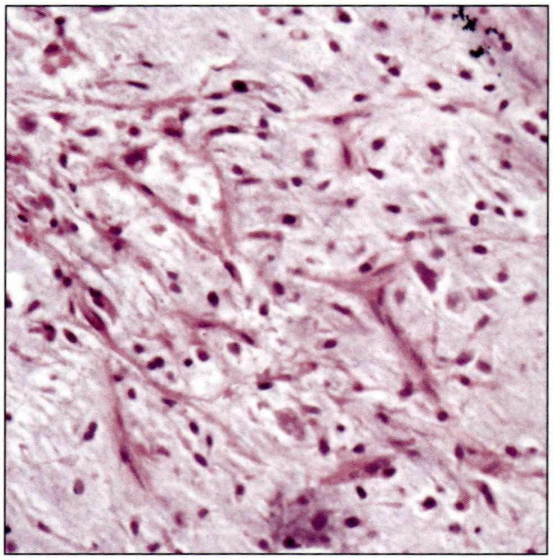

(Left) *Transitions between myxoid liposarcoma and areas with increased cellularity (round cell liposarcoma) are present in this example of round cell liposarcoma of the mediastinum. Notice the gradual increase of cellularity toward the right side of the field* →*.* ***(Right)*** *Residual plexiform pattern of vessels ("chicken wire") is noted focally in a round cell liposarcoma of the anterior mediastinum. Notice, however, the increase in the number of small round and spindle cells in the background.*

Pleomorphic Liposarcoma

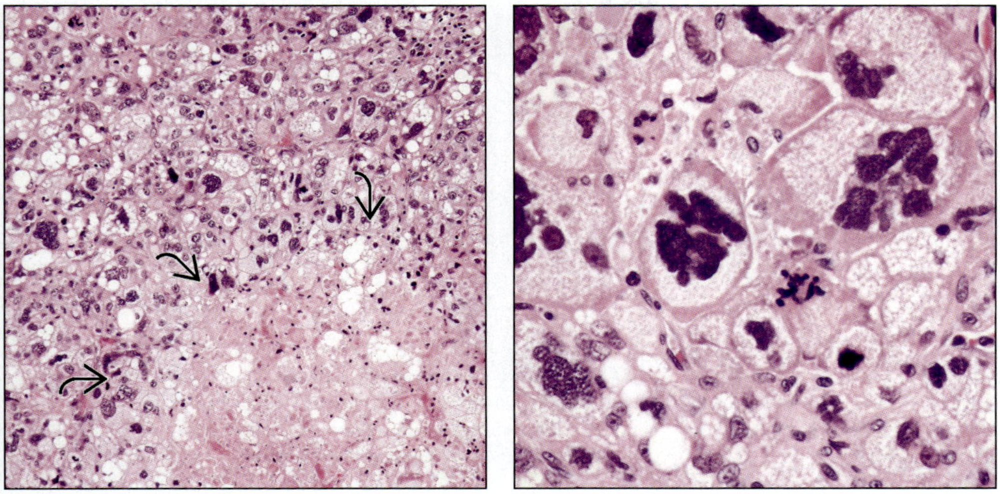

(Left) *Pleomorphic liposarcoma of the mediastinum shows a population of bizarre tumor cells surrounding an area of necrosis ➔. The viable areas of the tumor resemble a pleomorphic high-grade sarcoma.* ***(Right)*** *High magnification from a cellular area of the tumor in pleomorphic liposarcoma shows bizarre, pleomorphic cells with multiple or multilobated nuclei and scattered abnormal mitotic figures. Notice the prominent cytoplasmic vacuoles in the tumor cells.*

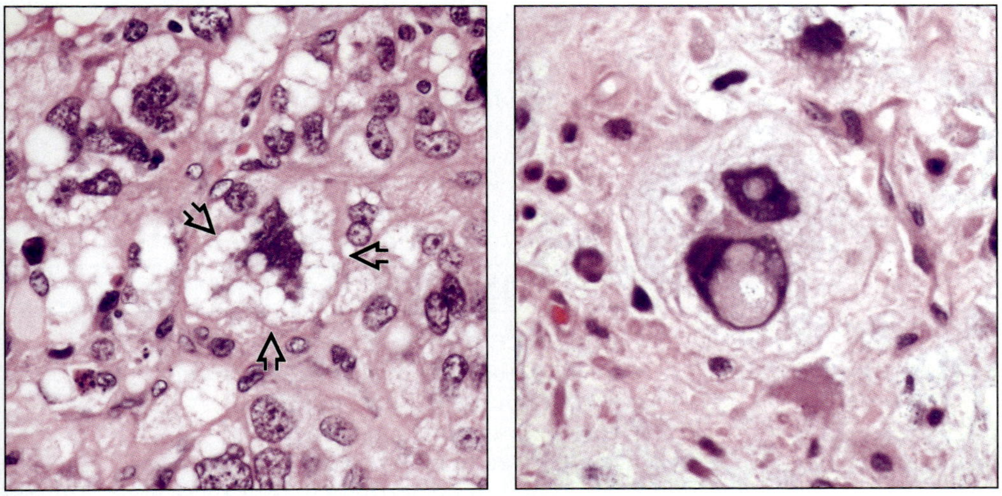

(Left) *High magnification in pleomorphic liposarcoma of the mediastinum shows a pleomorphic tumor cell ➔ with large, hyperchromatic nucleus. Notice nuclear scalloping by multiple fatty vacuoles in the cytoplasm; the latter is evidence of lipoblastic differentiation and serves to separate these tumors from MFH.* ***(Right)*** *High magnification of a tumor cell in pleomorphic liposarcoma shows multiple nuclei surrounded by abundant vacuolated cytoplasm. Notice the intranuclear vacuoles.*

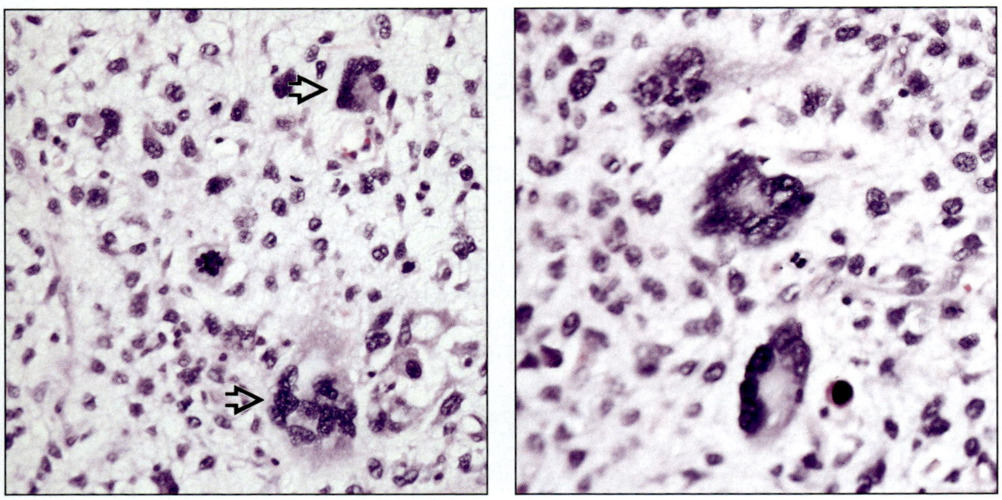

(Left) *Example of myxoid/round cell liposarcoma with pleomorphic tumor cells shows scattered, bizarre multinucleated cells ➔ set against a myxoid background. Notice also small round blue cells corresponding to the round cell liposarcoma component.* ***(Right)*** *High magnification of myxoid/round cell liposarcoma of the mediastinum with pleomorphic component shows bizarre, multinucleated lipoblastic tumor cells with dark-staining nuclei.*

LEIOMYOSARCOMA

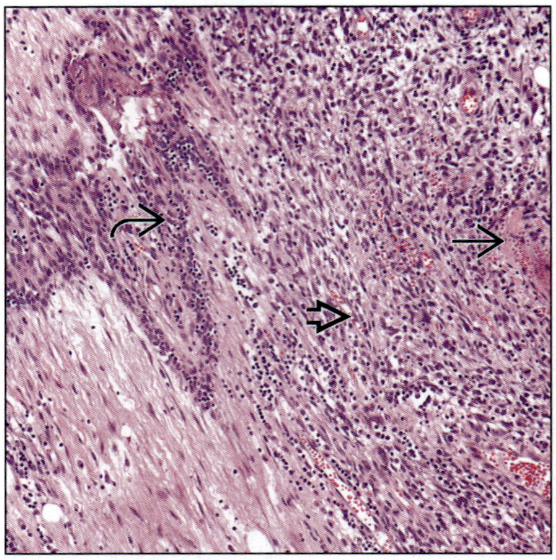

Mediastinal leiomyosarcoma shows a malignant spindle cell proliferation ⇨ with areas of necrosis →. Note the presence of residual thymic epithelium ↪.

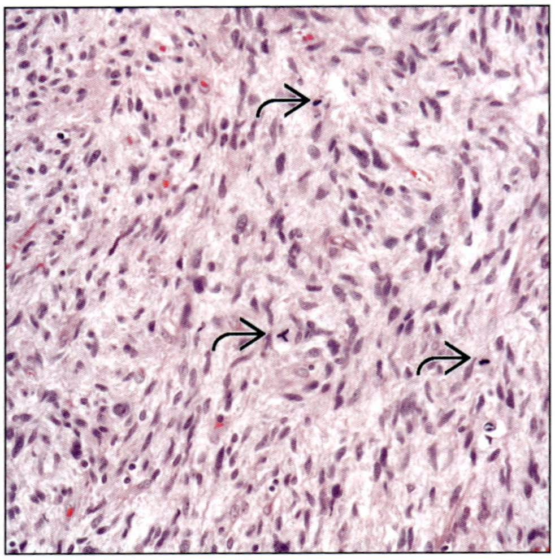

Mediastinal leiomyosarcoma shows prominent nuclear atypia and numerous mitotic figures ↪. These features are similar to those tumors occurring in soft tissues.

TERMINOLOGY

Abbreviations

- Leiomyosarcoma (LMS)

Synonyms

- Malignant smooth muscle tumor

Definitions

- Malignant mesenchymal neoplasm of smooth muscle origin

CLINICAL ISSUES

Epidemiology

- Incidence
  - Unusual tumor in mediastinal compartment
- Age
  - More common in adults
  - Range: 25-70 years old
- Gender
  - There is no gender predilection although LMS may be slightly more common in males

Site

- Tumor may appear in anterior or posterior mediastinum

Presentation

- Chest pain
- Dyspnea
- Cough
- General malaise
- Pleural effusion
- Asymptomatic

Treatment

- Surgical approaches
  - Complete surgical resection of tumor
- Adjuvant therapy
  - Depending on surgical staging, radiation or chemotherapy may be considered

Prognosis

- Depends on staging of tumor
  - Patients with advanced stage may follow a more aggressive behavior
  - Patients with more limited disease (early stage) may follow a more favorable outcome

MACROSCOPIC FEATURES

General Features

- Well-defined but not encapsulated tumors
- Rubbery tumor mass at cut surface
- May show cystic changes
- Light brown to tan in color
- Necrosis &/or hemorrhage may be present

Size

- Varies from 5 cm to > 12 cm in greatest diameter

MICROSCOPIC PATHOLOGY

Histologic Features

- Solid spindle cellular proliferation
- Spindle cells with cigar-like nuclei and eosinophilic cytoplasm
- Variable nuclear atypia depending on degree of differentiation (grade of tumor)
- Variable mitotic activity depending on degree of differentiation (grade of tumor)

DIFFERENTIAL DIAGNOSIS

Solitary Fibrous Tumor

- Tumor shows different growth patterns
- Immunohistochemical studies for CD34 and Bcl-2 are commonly seen positive

LEIOMYOSARCOMA

Key Facts

Clinical Issues

- Incidence
  - More common in adults
  - Range: 25-70 years of age
- Anatomic site
  - Tumor may appear in anterior or posterior mediastinum
- Treatment
  - Complete surgical resection of tumor
  - Depending on surgical staging, radiation or chemotherapy may be considered
- Symptoms
  - Chest pain
  - Dyspnea
  - Cough
  - Pleural effusion
  - Asymptomatic

Microscopic Pathology

- Solid spindle cellular proliferation
- Spindle cells with cigar-like nuclei and eosinophilic cytoplasm
- Variable nuclear atypia depending on degree of differentiation (grade of tumor)

Top Differential Diagnoses

- Solitary fibrous tumor
- Monophasic synovial sarcoma
- Spindle cell thymoma
- Metastatic leiomyosarcoma

Immunohistochemistry

Antibody	Reactivity	Staining Pattern	Comment
Actin-HHF-35	Positive	Cytoplasmic	In the majority of cases
Desmin	Positive	Cytoplasmic	In high-grade tumors, it may be negative
Caldesmon	Positive	Cytoplasmic	In better differentiated tumors
Vimentin	Positive	Cytoplasmic	Not specific
AE1/AE3	Negative		May be positive in some cases
MYOD1	Negative		
Myoglobin	Negative		
CD34	Negative		
EMA	Negative		

- Immunohistochemical stains for muscle differentiation are usually negative

Monophasic Synovial Sarcoma

- Generally shows negative staining for muscle markers
- Shows positive staining for EMA &/or keratin

Spindle Cell Thymoma

- Shows lymphocytes
- Lacks increased mitotic activity
- Shows negative staining for muscle markers

Metastatic Leiomyosarcoma

- Clinical and radiological evaluation are of utmost importance
- Clinical history of previous LMS in soft tissue would lead to correct interpretation

Leiomyoma

- Grossly, leiomyomas do not show areas of necrosis &/ or hemorrhage
- Lacks the presence of increased mitotic activity &/or cellular atypia
- Both tumors may show similar immunophenotype

DIAGNOSTIC CHECKLIST

Clinically Relevant Pathologic Features

- Mitotic rate

Pathologic Interpretation Pearls

- Solid spindle cellular proliferation
- Cigar-like nucleus
- Subtle storiform pattern with cross sections of tumor at right angles

SELECTED REFERENCES

1. Conner WC et al: Surgical management of leiomyosarcoma of the mediastinum. Ann Thorac Surg. 77(1):334-6, 2004
2. Eroğlu A et al: Primary leiomyosarcoma of the anterior mediastinum. Eur J Cardiothorac Surg. 21(5):943-5, 2002
3. Auliac JB et al: [Mediastinal leiomyosarcoma.] Rev Mal Respir. 16(2):210-3, 1999
4. Moran CA et al: Primary leiomyosarcomas of the lung: a clinicopathologic and immunohistochemical study of 18 cases. Mod Pathol. 10(2):121-8, 1997
5. Moran CA et al: Malignant smooth muscle tumors presenting as mediastinal soft tissue masses. A clinicopathologic study of 10 cases. Cancer. 74(8):2251-60, 1994
6. Van Schil PE et al: Primary mediastinal leiomyosarcoma. Thorac Cardiovasc Surg. 41(6):377-8, 1993

LEIOMYOSARCOMA

Microscopic Features

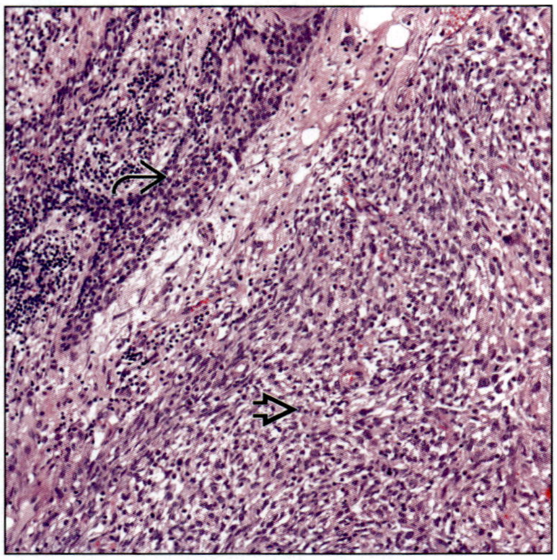
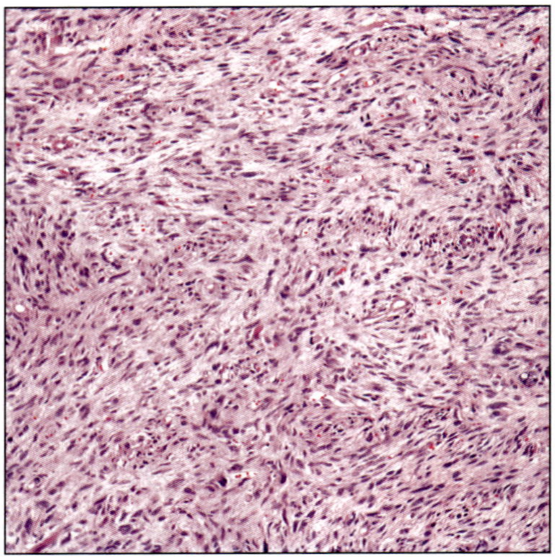

(Left) *Mediastinal leiomyosarcoma shows a malignant spindle cell proliferation. Also note the presence of residual thymic epithelium.* ***(Right)*** *Mediastinal leiomyosarcoma is shown with a solid spindle cellular proliferation and vague storiform pattern. The tumor shows marked nuclear atypia; however, this pattern may also be seen in some other high-grade sarcomas.*

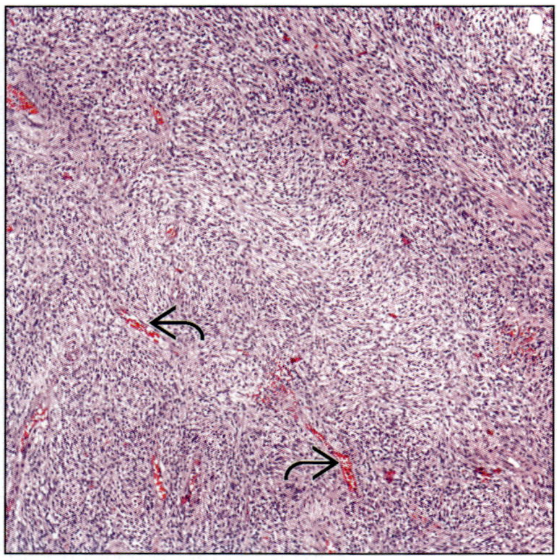
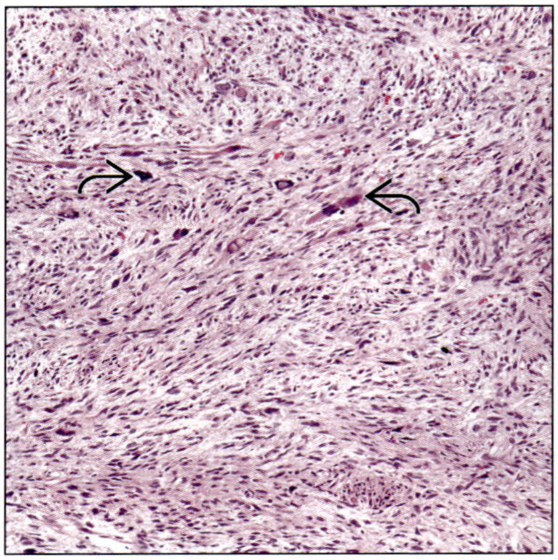

(Left) *Leiomyosarcoma with the typical fascicular growth pattern. Scattered blood vessels are also present.* ***(Right)*** *Mediastinal leiomyosarcoma displays cellular pleomorphism and prominent nuclear atypia; this pattern is highly suggestive of leiomyosarcoma. These features are more commonly seen in high-grade tumors.*

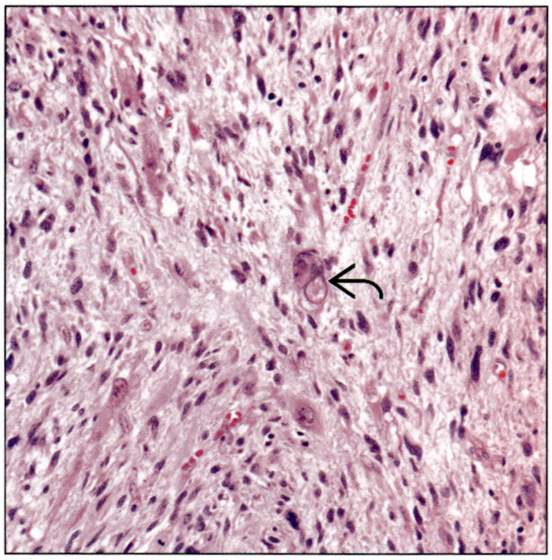
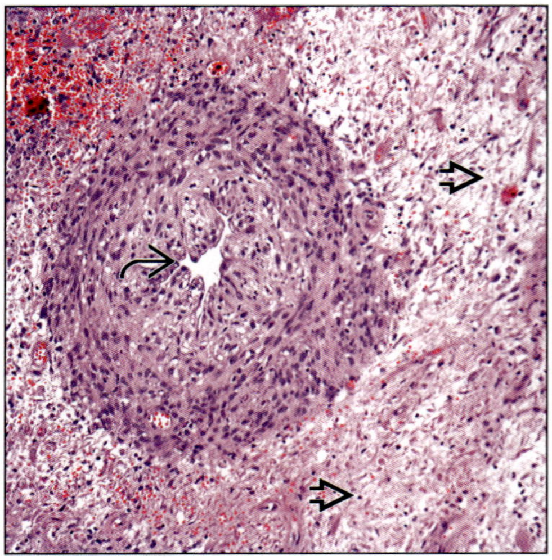

(Left) *High-power view shows prominent nuclear atypia, binucleated cells with intracytoplasmic inclusions in association with a spindle cell proliferation. These features are of high-grade tumors.* ***(Right)*** *High-grade leiomyosarcoma shows areas of degeneration and necrosis. Note the thin-walled vessel surrounded by the tumor.*

Microscopic Features

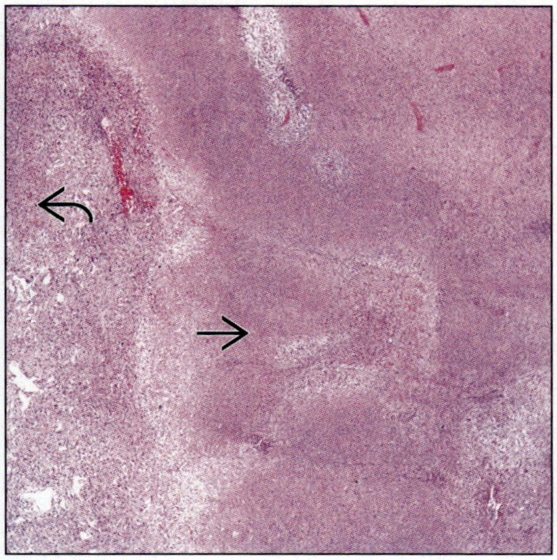
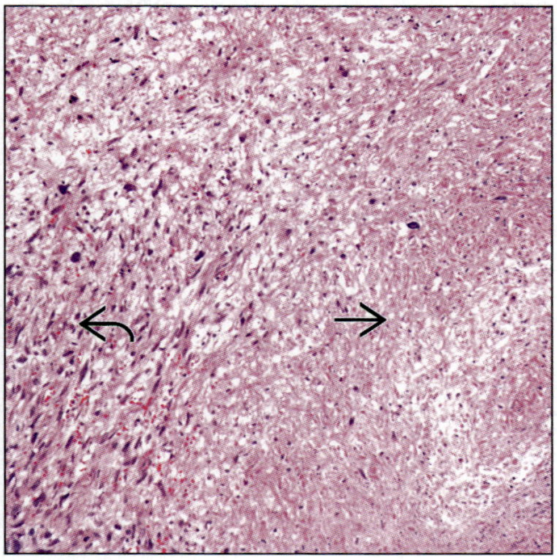

(Left) *Mediastinal leiomyosarcoma shows extensive areas of necrosis →. Areas of viable tumor are also present ↪. In some cases, extensive necrosis may obscure the true nature of the neoplasm. The presence of necrosis is a feature of high-grade tumors.* ***(Right)*** *High-power view shows a malignant spindle cellular proliferation ↪ admixed with extensive necrosis →. These features are diagnostic of a high-grade sarcoma.*

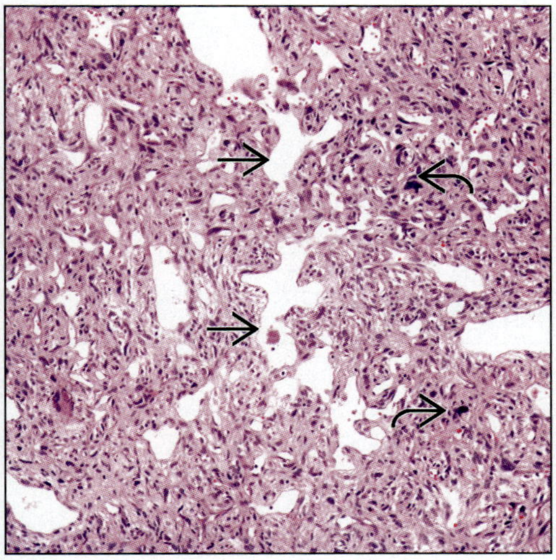
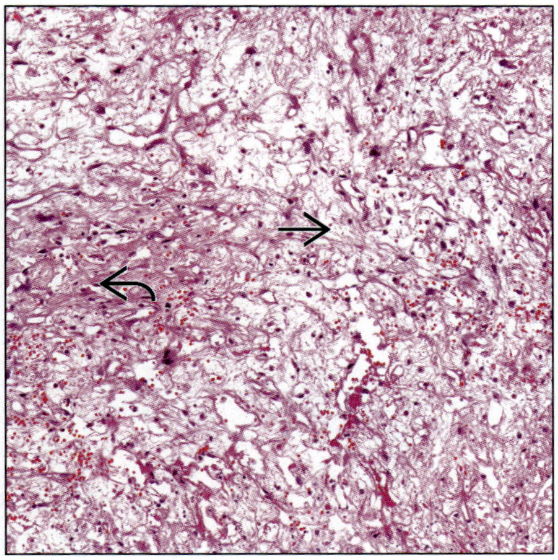

(Left) *Mediastinal leiomyosarcoma shows prominent vascular channels → mimicking a hemangiopericytoma. Note the nuclear atypia ↪. The HPC pattern is commonly seen in leiomyosarcomas.* ***(Right)*** *Some cases of mediastinal leiomyosarcoma may show extensive fibrinous necrosis → with only focal areas of an atypical cellular proliferation ↪, making the diagnosis more difficult.*

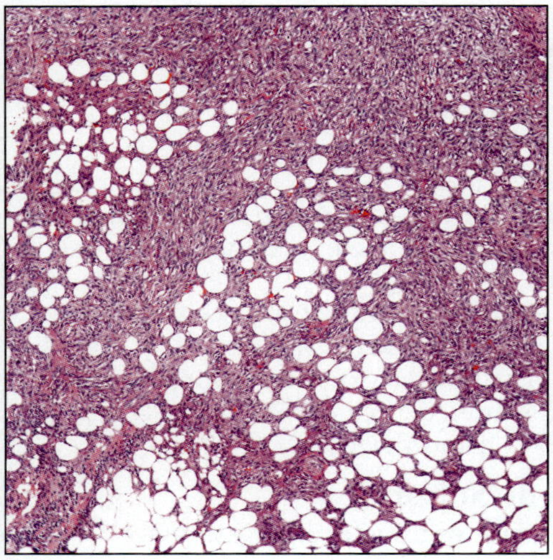
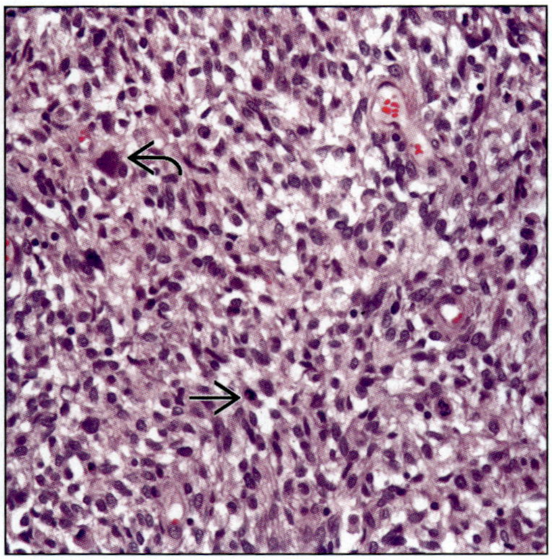

(Left) *Mediastinal leiomyosarcoma is seen infiltrating mediastinal adipose tissue. This feature may be seen in some other tumors, mainly of epithelial origin, such as thymoma.* ***(Right)*** *High-power view of a high-grade leiomyosarcoma shows nuclear atypia, scattered multinucleated giant cells ↪, and mitotic figures →.*

SYNOVIAL SARCOMA

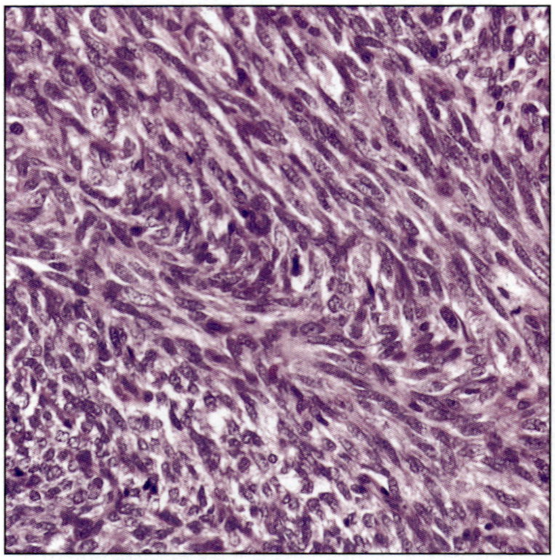

Monophasic spindle cell variant of synovial sarcoma of the mediastinum shows a monotonous population of atypical spindle cells with scant stroma.

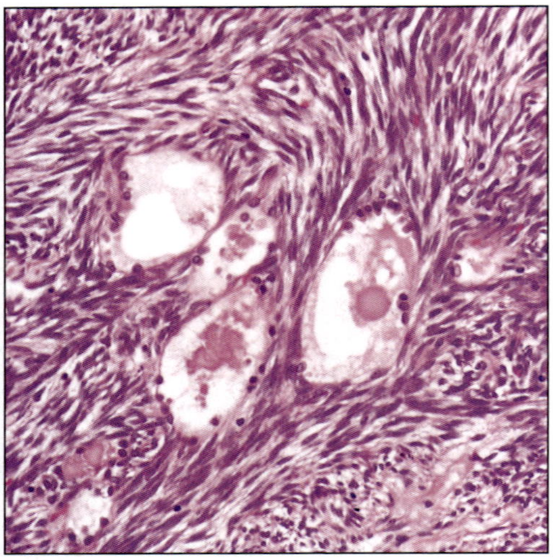

Biphasic variant of synovial sarcoma of the mediastinum shows admixture of well-formed glandular structures with a monotonous population of atypical spindle cells.

TERMINOLOGY

Abbreviations

- Synovial sarcoma (SS)

Synonyms

- Primary carcinoma of soft tissue

Definitions

- Primary malignant epithelial neoplasm arising from soft tissues

ETIOLOGY/PATHOGENESIS

Pathogenesis

- Unknown; unrelated to synovium or synovial cells
- Pluripotential mesenchymal cells capable of aberrant epithelial differentiation

CLINICAL ISSUES

Epidemiology

- Incidence
  - Rare tumor
- Age
  - Broad age range: 3-83 years
  - Predilection for young adults (median: 35 years)
- Gender
  - Female predilection (2:1)

Site

- May involve all mediastinal compartments: Anterior, middle, and posterior

Presentation

- Cough
- Chest pain
- Pleural effusion
- Shortness of breath
- Neck or back pain

Treatment

- Surgical excision

Prognosis

- Aggressive behavior similar to soft tissue counterpart
- Local recurrences and distant metastases to lung, lymph nodes, liver, and epidural space

IMAGE FINDINGS

General Features

- Tumors may present as well circumscribed or infiltrative masses with focal calcifications

CT Findings

- Well-circumscribed mediastinal mass with low attenuation
- Pleural effusion

MACROSCOPIC FEATURES

General Features

- Usually well-circumscribed, fleshy tumors surrounded by thin, fibrous capsule
- May be infiltrative and extend into surrounding structures, such as lung, pleura, pericardium, chest wall, and ribs
- Cut section shows gray-white to tan, homogeneous soft tissue with gelatinous consistency
- Some cases may undergo extensive cystic changes
- May contain scattered calcifications
- Can show focal hemorrhage and necrosis

Sections to Be Submitted

- 1 section per each centimeter of largest tumor diameter

Key Facts

Clinical Issues
- Predilection for young adults (median: 35 years)
- Female predilection (2:1)
- Aggressive behavior similar to soft tissue counterpart

Microscopic Pathology
- Uniform and monotonous proliferation of atypical oval to spindle cells with minimal stroma
- Glandular structures may be very focal or may predominate
- Fascicular growth pattern with "herringbone" appearance is most common histologic pattern of growth
- Many tumors show, at least focally, a prominent hemangiopericytomatous growth pattern
- Other growth patterns include storiform, palisading, and sclerosing
- Stromal changes may include fibrosis, calcifications, and myxoid changes

Ancillary Tests
- Pattern of cytokeratin positivity in monophasic spindle cell tumors is usually weak and focal (patchy)
- Spindle cells
  - Strongly and diffusely stain for Bcl-2
  - Usually stain for CD99
  - May be positive for S100 protein in 30% of cases
  - Are negative for actin, desmin, CD34, HMB-45, CEA, MOC-31, and p63
- (X;18)(p11;q11) translocation is characteristically present in > 80% of cases

Size
- 5-20 cm

MICROSCOPIC PATHOLOGY

Histologic Features
- **Monophasic (spindle cell) synovial sarcoma**
  - Uniform and monotonous proliferation of atypical oval to spindle cells with minimal stroma
  - Spindle cells show vesicular or hyperchromatic nuclei with coarse chromatin pattern and inconspicuous nucleoli
  - Mitotic activity may vary from low (1 mitosis per 10 HPF) to high (> 10 mitoses per 10 HPF)
  - Fascicular growth pattern with "herringbone" appearance is most common histologic pattern of growth
  - Many tumors show, at least focally, a prominent hemangiopericytomatous growth pattern
  - Other growth patterns include storiform, palisading, sclerosing, nesting, and rhabdoid
  - Stromal changes may include fibrosis, calcifications, and myxoid changes
  - "Poorly differentiated" variant characterized by round cell, epithelioid morphology rather than spindle cells
  - Some tumors can show prominent hemorrhage and necrosis
  - Secondary cystic changes are often seen in monophasic tumors
- **Biphasic synovial sarcoma**
  - Shows admixture of well-formed glandular structures and spindle cells
  - Spindle cell component surrounding glands has identical features to those seen in monophasic variant
  - Glandular structures may be very focal or may predominate
  - Glandular structures are lined by large, round to polygonal or columnar epithelial cells
  - Glandular cells are round to oval nuclei with abundant eosinophilic cytoplasm
  - Glands may contain dense, homogeneous eosinophilic secretions in lumen
  - Glandular structures may adopt tubulo-papillary pattern with intraluminal papillary infoldings
  - Glandular structures can display prominent cytoplasmic clearing of tumor cells

ANCILLARY TESTS

Immunohistochemistry
- All biphasic tumors show strong keratin positivity in the glandular component
- Monophasic tumors are frequently, but not always, positive for cytokeratin stains
- Pattern of cytokeratin positivity in monophasic spindle cell tumors is usually weak and focal (patchy)
- Epithelial membrane antigen (EMA) shows similar pattern and distribution as cytokeratin
- Low molecular weight cytokeratins are more sensitive than broad-spectrum cytokeratins for monophasic tumors
- Spindle cells
  - Strongly express vimentin
  - Strongly and diffusely stain for Bcl-2
  - Usually stain for CD99
  - May be positive for calretinin and calponin
  - May be positive for S100 protein in 30% of cases
  - Negative for actin, desmin, CD34, HMB-45, CEA, MOC-31, and p63

Cytogenetics
- (X;18)(p11;q11) translocation characteristically present in > 80% of cases
- Other complex translocations may be found infrequently
- FISH and Rt-PCR are useful for detecting translocations in paraffin-embedded tissues
- 2/3 contain an *SYT/SSX1* fusion
- 1/3 contain an *SYT/SSX2* fusion
- Rare cases may show an *SYT/SSX4* fusion

- Cases with *SYT/SSX2* fusion are associated with better prognosis

Electron Microscopy

- Glandular epithelial component shows similar features to adenocarcinoma
- Monophasic spindle cell component shows closely apposed cell membranes, frequent desmosomal junctions, and occasional surface microvilli
- Monophasic spindle cell component does not contain abundant rough endoplasmic reticulum or other features of fibroblastic cells

DIFFERENTIAL DIAGNOSIS

Metastatic Adenocarcinoma

- Clinical history is helpful for diagnosis
- Metastatic adenocarcinoma will usually not contain stromal, atypical spindle cell component

Pulmonary Blastoma

- Only rarely will secondarily involve mediastinum, but bulk of tumor will be centered in lung
- Cells lining glands in pulmonary blastoma show subnuclear clearing simulating fetal lung
- Most biphasic pulmonary blastomas are characterized by squamoid morules located at base of glands
- Spindle cell component in pulmonary blastoma is negative for epithelial markers (keratin, EMA)

Thymic Carcinosarcoma

- Spindle cell component in thymic carcinosarcoma is negative for epithelial markers (keratin, EMA)
- Glandular component in thymic carcinosarcoma displays pronounced nuclear atypia
- Negative for t(X;18) translocation

Biphasic Pleural Mesothelioma

- Usually grows as diffuse, plaque-like process covering pleural surface, rather than discrete, well-circumscribed tumor mass
- Spindle cell component in pleural mesothelioma shows marked cytologic atypia and nuclear pleomorphism
- Spindle cells in pleural mesothelioma are negative for Bcl-2 and CD99

Spindle Cell Thymoma

- Slow-growing tumor that is usually encapsulated and noninvasive
- Absence of cytologic atypia or mitotic activity in spindle cells
- Lobular architecture with fibrous bands separating lobules
- Presence of immature T lymphocytes
- Spindle cells are negative for vimentin, CD99, and Bcl-2

Spindle Cell Thymic Carcinoma

- Marked cytologic atypia, nuclear pleomorphism, and mitotic activity
- Spindle cells are negative for Bcl-2 and CD99
- Absence of t(X;18) translocation

Malignant Peripheral Nerve Sheath Tumor

- Commonly arises in background of neurofibromatosis
- Grossly associated with nerve trunks
- Spindle cells are negative for cytokeratins and CD99
- Electron microscopy shows complex interdigitating cytoplasmic processes invested by basal lamina material
- Absence of t(X;18) translocation

Solitary Fibrous Tumor

- Usually shows variegation in growth patterns within same tumor and lack of uniformity of cell population
- Commonly shows variable degrees of stromal fibrosis, including characteristic, rope-like deposition of keloidal collagen
- Spindle cells are positive for CD34
- Spindle cells are negative for cytokeratins and EMA
- Absence of t(X;18) translocation

Metastasis of Synovial Sarcoma of Soft Tissue to Mediastinum

- Clinical history is only means for making this distinction

DIAGNOSTIC CHECKLIST

Pathologic Interpretation Pearls

- Uniform and monotonous population of cells with minimal nuclear pleomorphism
- Prominent "herringbone" and hemangiopericytic growth pattern
- Cytokeratin and EMA staining usually focal and patchy; may be difficult to demonstrate
- Strong and diffuse positivity for Bcl-2 is seen in almost all cases

SELECTED REFERENCES

1. Katakura H et al: Mediastinal synovial sarcoma. Thorac Cardiovasc Surg. 57(3):183-5, 2009
2. Jeganathan R et al: Primary mediastinal synovial sarcoma. Ulster Med J. 76(2):109-11, 2007
3. Suster S et al: Primary synovial sarcomas of the mediastinum: a clinicopathologic, immunohistochemical, and ultrastructural study of 15 cases. Am J Surg Pathol. 29(5):569-78, 2005
4. Gotoh M et al: Synovial sarcoma of the mediastinum: report of a case. Surg Today. 34(6):521-4, 2004
5. Yano M et al: SYT-SSX fusion genes in synovial sarcoma of the thorax. Lung Cancer. 44(3):391-7, 2004
6. Trupiano JK et al: Mediastinal synovial sarcoma: report of two cases with molecular genetic analysis. Ann Thorac Surg. 73(2):628-30, 2002
7. Suster S et al: Expression of bcl-2 oncoprotein in benign and malignant spindle cell tumors of soft tissue, skin, serosal surfaces, and gastrointestinal tract. Am J Surg Pathol. 22(7):863-72, 1998
8. Witkin GB et al: A biphasic tumor of the mediastinum with features of synovial sarcoma. A report of four cases. Am J Surg Pathol. 13(6):490-9, 1989

Monophasic Spindle Cell Type

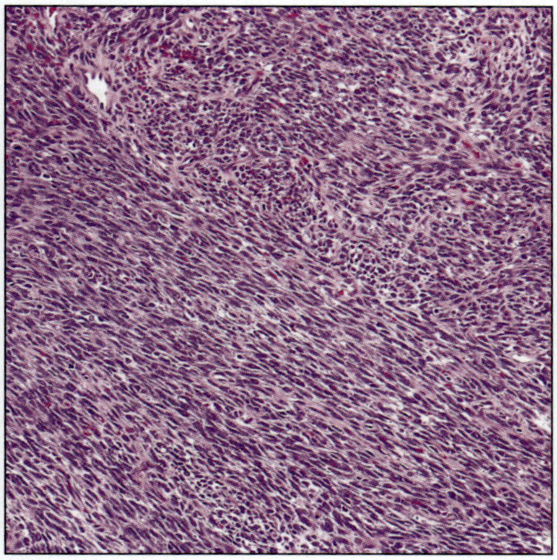
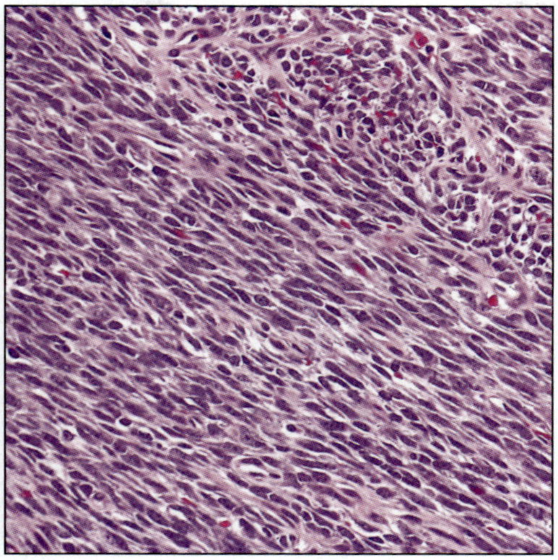

(Left) *Scanning magnification of monophasic spindle cell synovial sarcoma of the mediastinum shows a monotonous population of atypical spindle cells with a fascicular growth pattern.* ***(Right)*** *Monophasic spindle cell synovial sarcoma of the mediastinum shows a monotonous population of atypical spindle cells. This histologic picture can be seen in a wide variety of other spindle cell sarcomas, including fibrosarcoma and malignant peripheral nerve sheath tumor.*

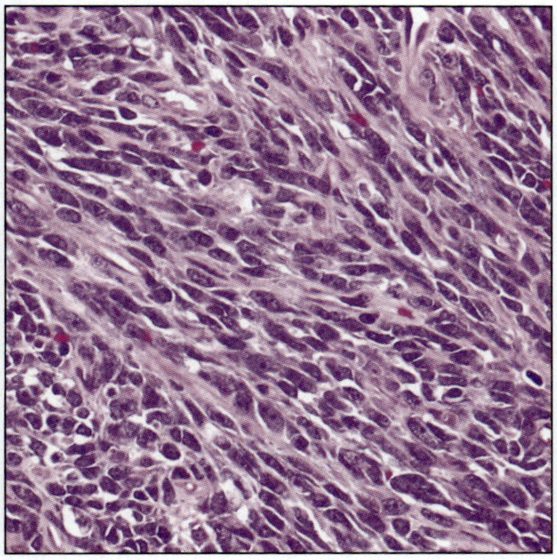
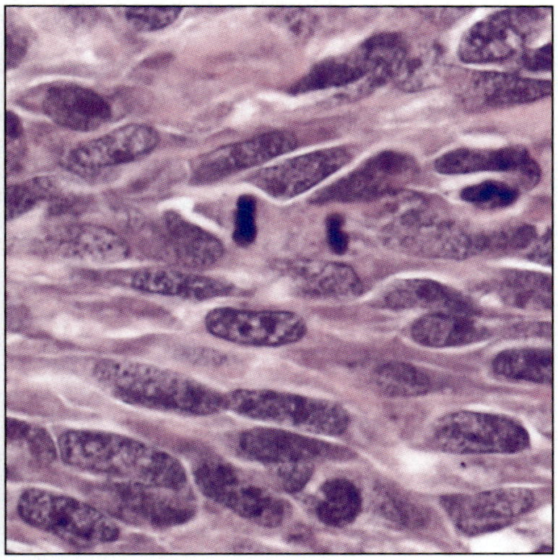

(Left) *Higher magnification of spindle cell monophasic synovial sarcoma of the mediastinum shows a monotonous population of atypical spindle cells. Notice the absence of stroma and the uniform appearance of the spindle cells.* ***(Right)*** *High magnification of monophasic synovial sarcoma of the mediastinum shows atypical spindle cells with tapered ends, small nucleoli, and a scattered chromatin pattern that is surrounded by a scant rim of cytoplasm and contains scattered mitotic figures.*

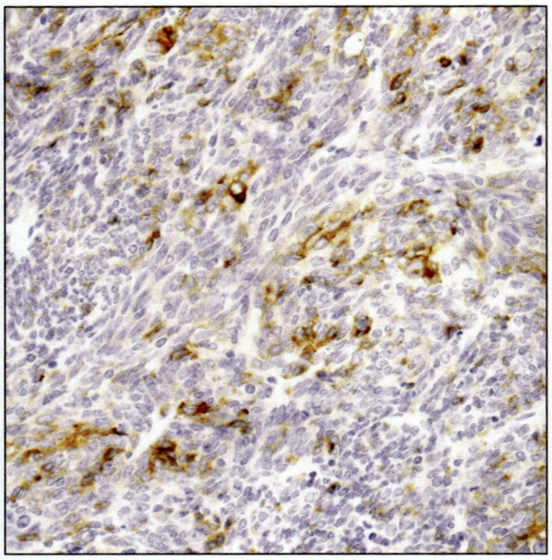
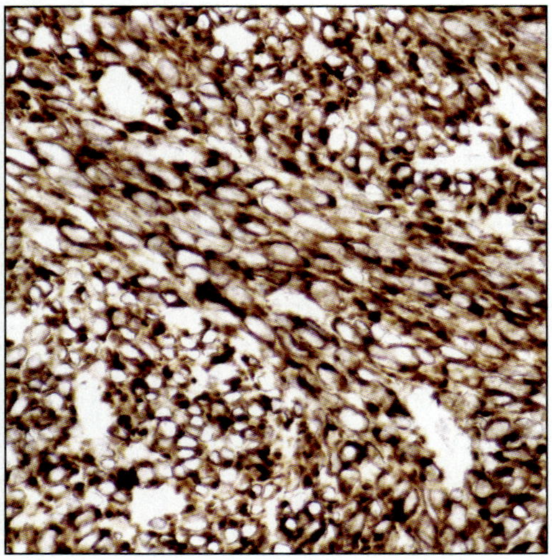

(Left) *Immunohistochemical staining for AE1/AE3 cytokeratin in monophasic spindle cell synovial sarcoma of the mediastinum shows spotty positivity in scattered tumor cells, a distinctive staining pattern for this tumor.* ***(Right)*** *Immunohistochemical staining of spindle cell synovial sarcoma of the mediastinum for BCL2 oncogene shows strong cytoplasmic staining of virtually every cell with this antibody. This diffuse pattern of staining is distinctive for this tumor.*

SYNOVIAL SARCOMA

"Herringbone" Growth Pattern

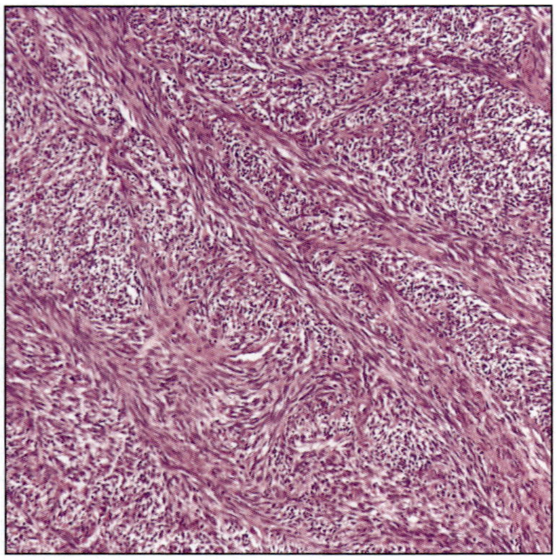

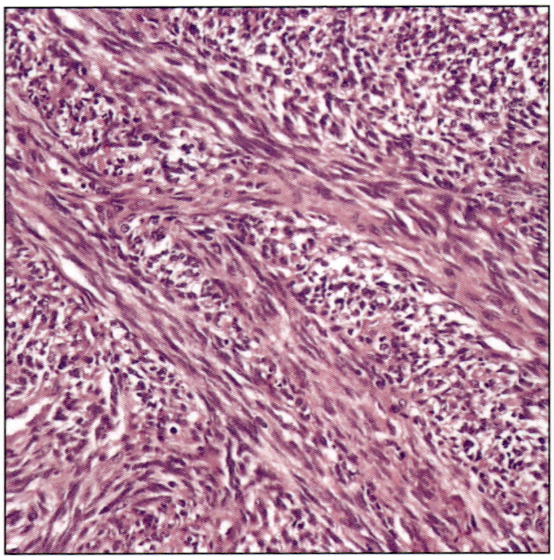

(Left) *Scanning magnification of monophasic synovial sarcoma of the mediastinum shows prominent "herringbone" pattern of growth, with short fascicles of spindle cells intersecting longer, longitudinal fascicles at acute angles.* ***(Right)*** *High magnification of monophasic synovial sarcoma of the mediastinum with prominent "herringbone" pattern shows a monotonous population of atypical spindle cells forming intersecting fascicles that appear to be cut at right angles.*

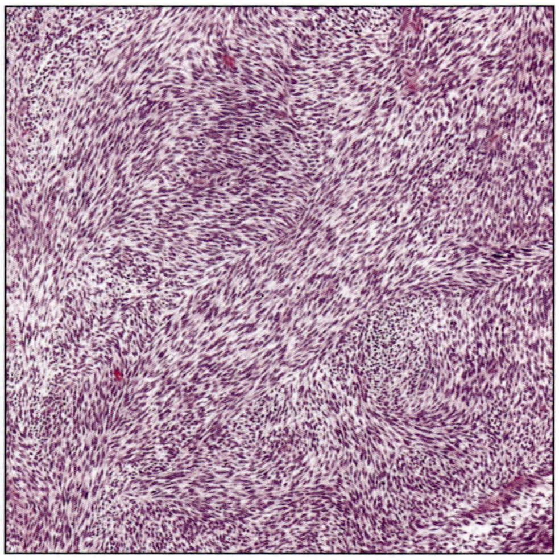

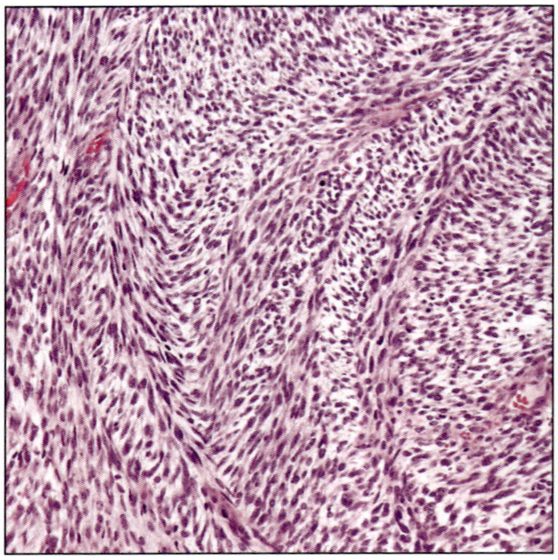

(Left) *Monophasic synovial sarcoma of the mediastinum with a prominent "herringbone" pattern of growth shows short fascicles of monotonous atypical spindle cells intersecting one another. This image is virtually indistinguishable from that of a malignant peripheral nerve sheath tumor.* ***(Right)*** *High magnification in monophasic synovial sarcoma of the mediastinum with prominent "herringbone" pattern shows a monotonous population of atypical spindle cells intersecting one another at acute angles.*

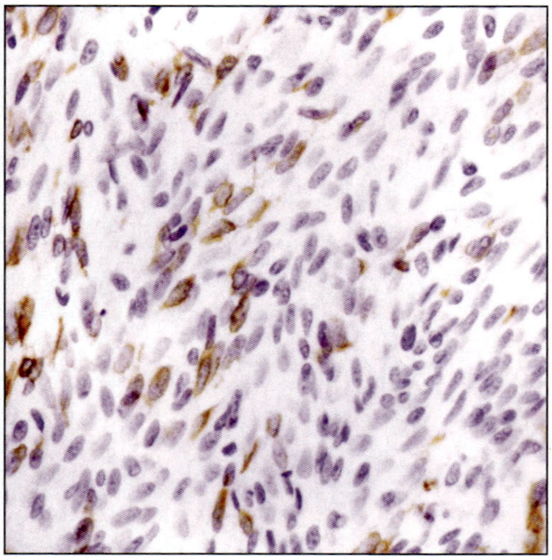

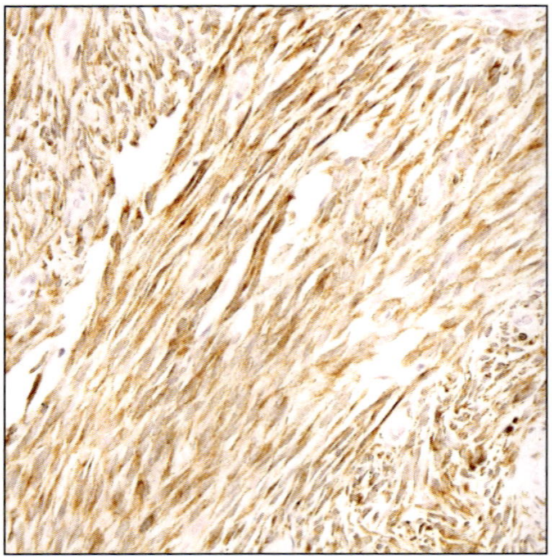

(Left) *Immunohistochemical staining for cytokeratin AE1/AE3 in monophasic synovial sarcoma of the mediastinum with prominent "herringbone" pattern shows scattered keratin-positive spindle cells.* ***(Right)*** *Immunohistochemical staining for BLC2 oncogene of monophasic synovial sarcoma of the mediastinum with prominent "herringbone" pattern shows strong and diffuse positivity in the majority of the tumor cells.*

Hemangiopericytic Growth Pattern

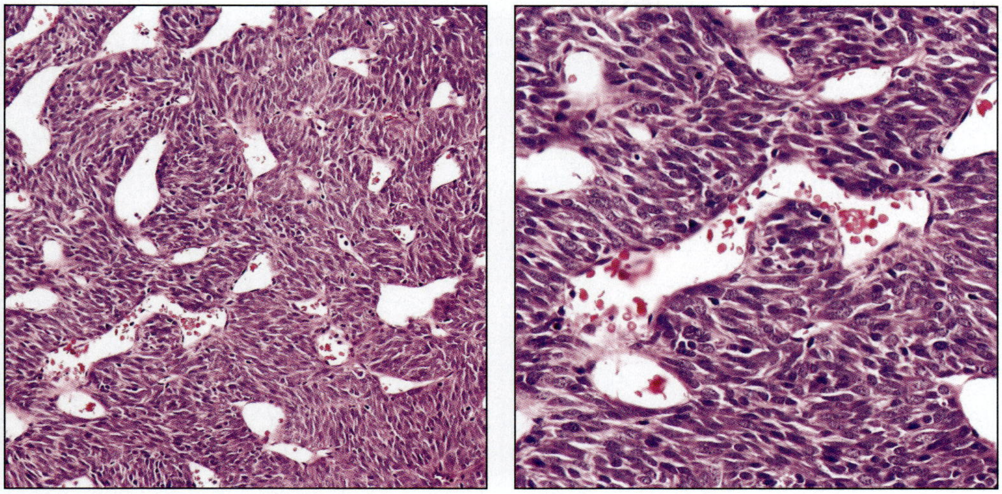

(Left) *Scanning magnification of monophasic synovial sarcoma of the mediastinum with a prominent hemangiopericytic growth pattern shows a dense spindle cell population flanking small, dilated vascular spaces with open lumens.* ***(Right)*** *Monophasic synovial sarcoma of the mediastinum with a prominent hemangiopericytic growth pattern shows branching small to medium vessels with open lumens, a histologic picture indistinguishable from hemangiopericytoma.*

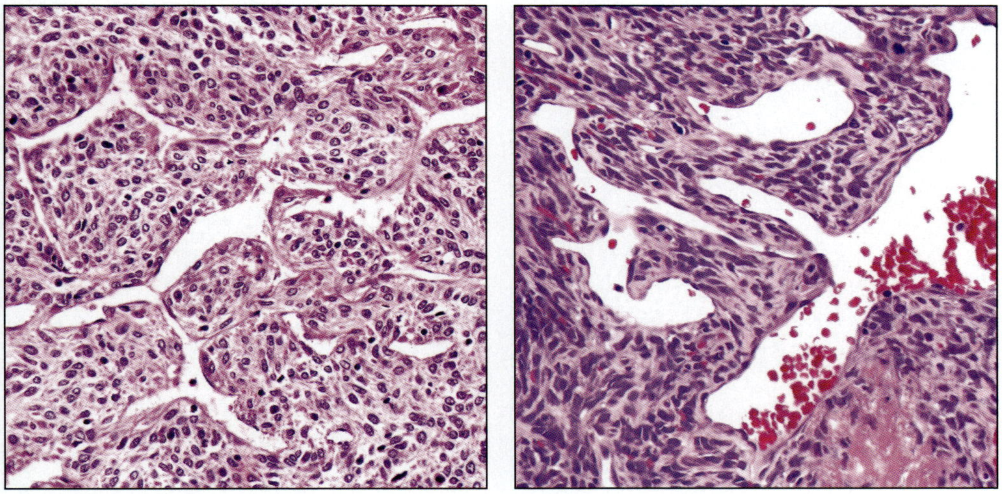

(Left) *Monophasic synovial sarcoma of the mediastinum with a prominent hemangiopericytomatous growth pattern shows vascular spaces that appear to branch at right angles. Tumors like this can be easily mistaken for solitary fibrous tumors.* ***(Right)*** *Monophasic synovial sarcoma of the mediastinum with a prominent hemangiopericytic growth pattern shows branching vessels with open lumens and a complex, antler-like or "staghorn" pattern of growth.*

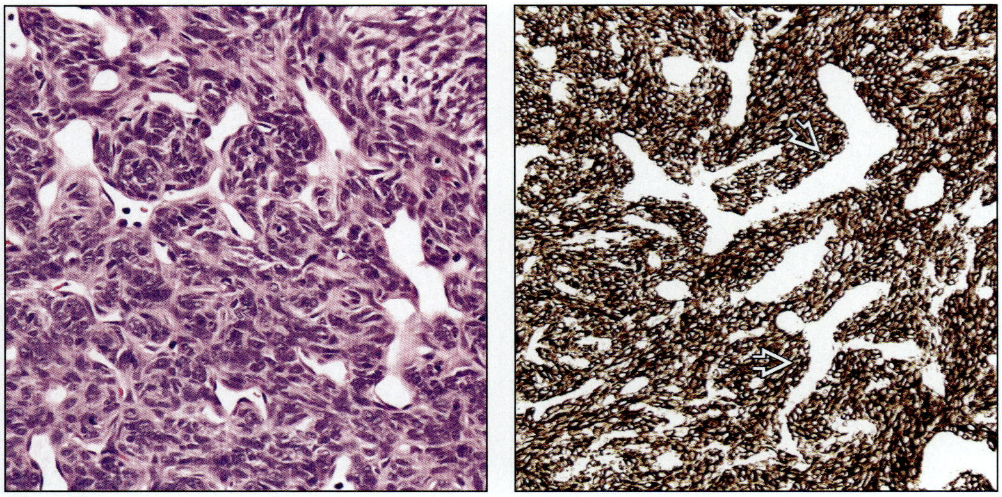

(Left) *Monophasic synovial sarcoma of the mediastinum with a prominent hemangiopericytic growth pattern shows multiple small vessels with open lumens and a complex branching luminal pattern.* ***(Right)*** *Immunohistochemical staining for vimentin in monophasic synovial sarcoma of the mediastinum shows strong positivity of the tumor cells and highlights the prominent branching hemangiopericytoma-like vessels in the background* ➪.

SYNOVIAL SARCOMA

Storiform Growth Pattern

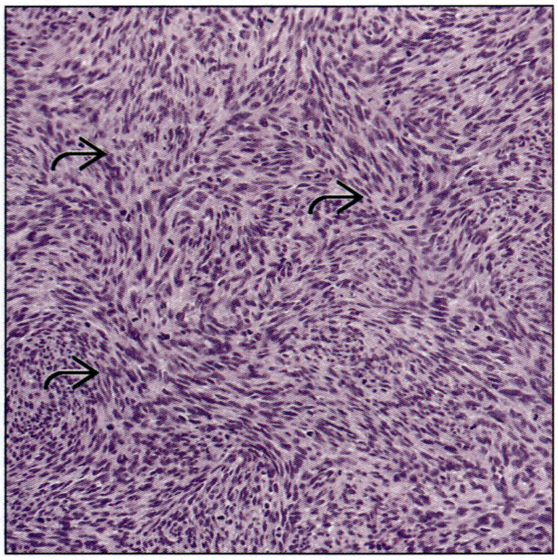

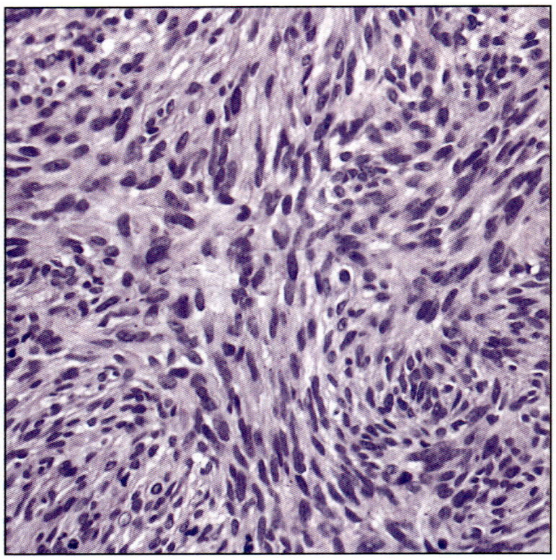

(Left) *Scanning magnification of monophasic synovial sarcoma of the mediastinum with prominent storiform growth pattern shows interlacing fascicles of spindle cells with a pinwheel distribution ↷. Tumors with these features are easily mistaken for "malignant fibrous histiocytoma."* ***(Right)*** *High magnification of monophasic synovial sarcoma of the mediastinum with prominent storiform pattern shows detail of storiform (mat-like) fascicle of spindle cells.*

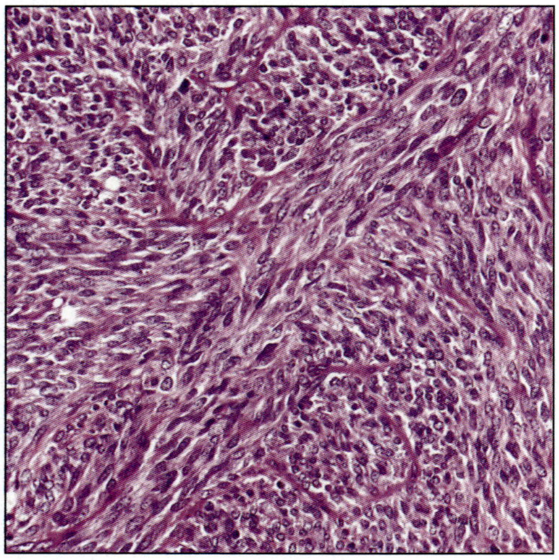

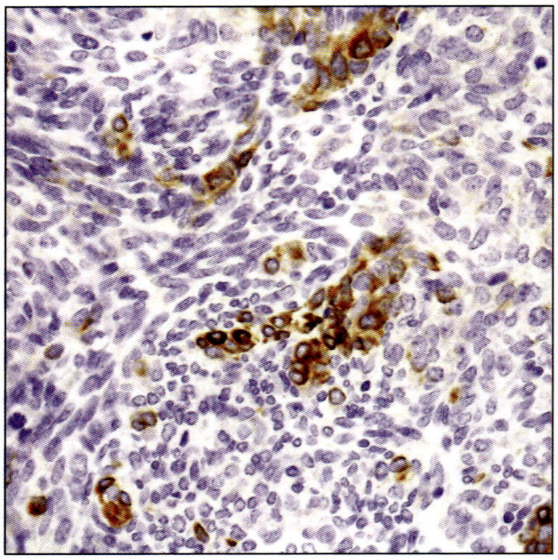

(Left) *Scanning magnification of monophasic synovial sarcoma of the mediastinum with prominent storiform pattern shows atypical spindle cells that seem to be radiating from a central spoke in a pinwheel fashion reminiscent of "fibrohistiocytic" tumors.* ***(Right)*** *Immunohistochemical staining for broad-spectrum cytokeratin (keratin AE1/AE3) in monophasic synovial sarcoma of the mediastinum with prominent storiform pattern shows focal staining of the tumor cells.*

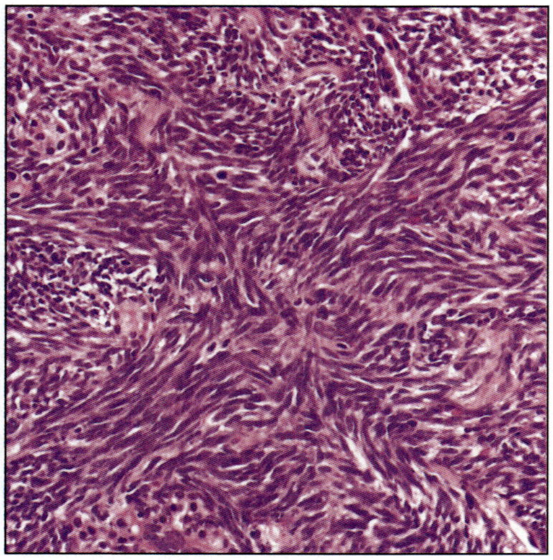

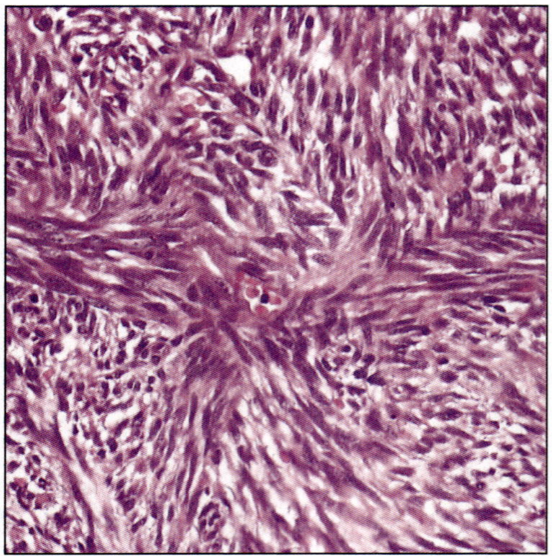

(Left) *Scanning magnification of monophasic synovial sarcoma of the mediastinum with prominent storiform pattern shows striking storiform architecture. The uniformity of the tumor cells, absence of pleomorphism, and significant mitotic activity bear a superficial resemblance to dermatofibrosarcoma protuberans in this tumor.* ***(Right)*** *High magnification of monophasic synovial sarcoma of the mediastinum with prominent storiform pattern shows a bland appearance and monotony of the tumor cells.*

Unusual Growth Patterns

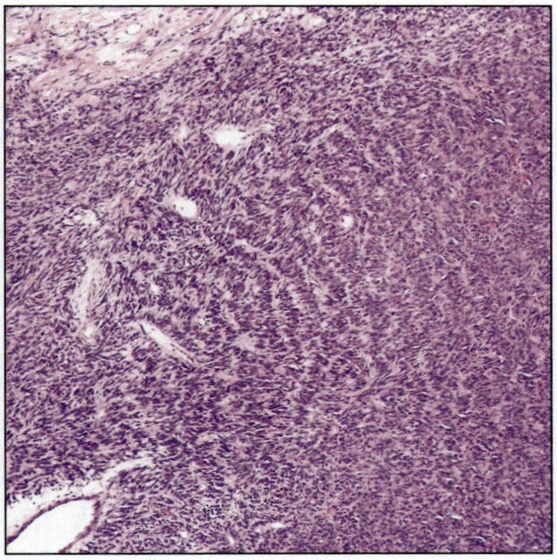
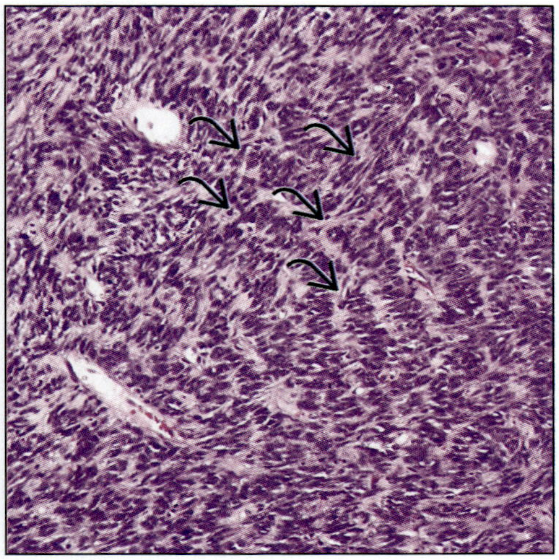

(Left) *Scanning magnification shows monophasic, spindle cell synovial sarcoma of the mediastinum characterized by striking nuclear palisading of the cells. Tumors with these features can closely resemble malignant peripheral nerve sheath tumors.* ***(Right)*** *Higher magnification of monophasic synovial sarcoma of the mediastinum shows striking palisading of nuclei ➔. The tumor cells are quite monotonous and merge imperceptibly with more traditional fascicular areas in the vicinity.*

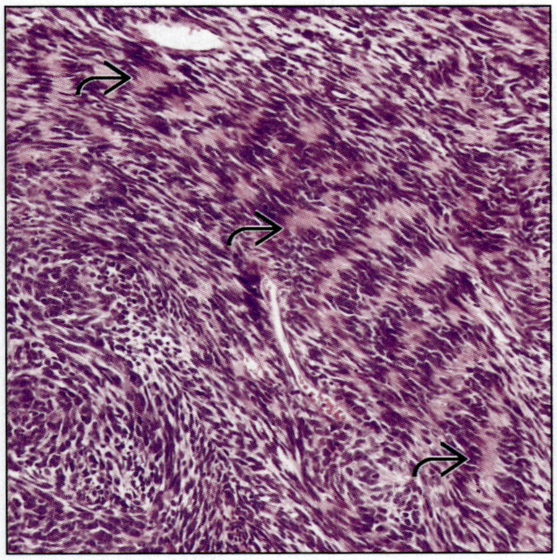
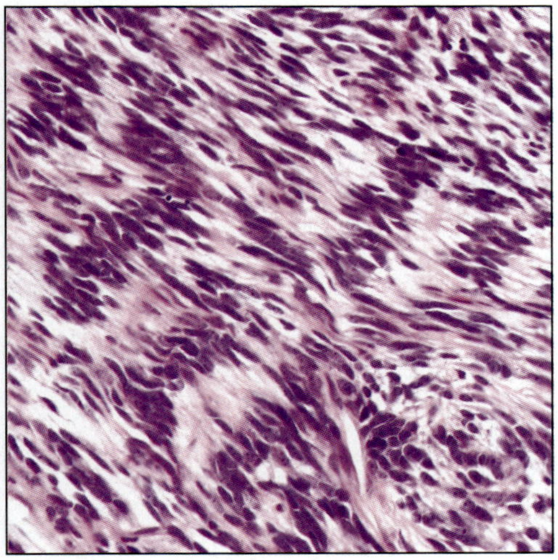

(Left) *Scanning magnification of monophasic synovial sarcoma of the mediastinum with striking palisading of tumor cells shows structures that are reminiscent of Verocay bodies ➔.* ***(Right)*** *High magnification of monophasic synovial sarcoma of the mediastinum with striking palisading shows detail of nuclear palisades resembling Verocay bodies. Tumors with these features can be easily mistaken for malignant peripheral nerve sheath tumors.*

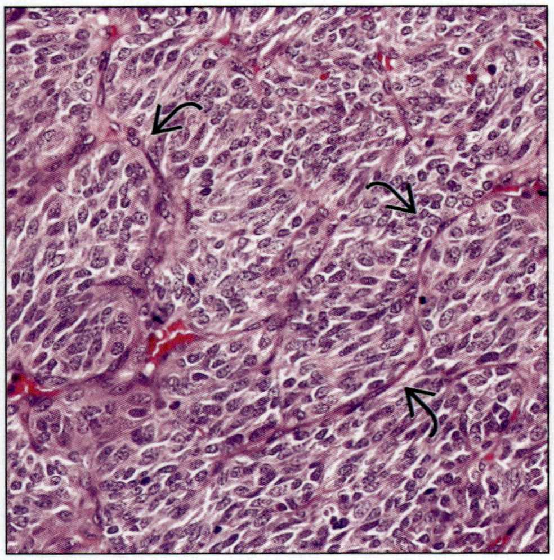
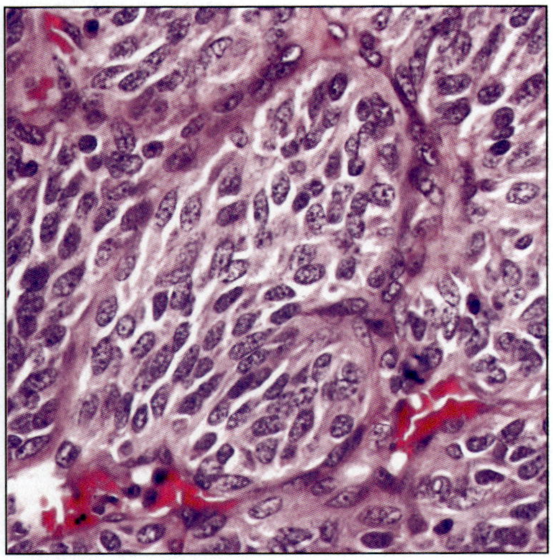

(Left) *Monophasic synovial sarcoma of the mediastinum with prominent "nesting" pattern shows discrete nests of tumor cells separated by thin fibrovascular septae ➔. Tumors with these features can closely resemble metastatic malignant melanoma to the mediastinum.* ***(Right)*** *High magnification of monophasic synovial sarcoma of the mediastinum with a prominent "nesting" pattern shows a monotonous population of spindle tumor cells surrounded by a thin fibrovascular septa.*

SYNOVIAL SARCOMA

Poorly Differentiated Synovial Sarcoma

(Left) *Scanning magnification of poorly differentiated synovial sarcoma of the mediastinum is characterized by sheets of monotonous round, epithelioid tumor cells. These tumors can be mistaken for a variety of small round blue cell tumors.* ***(Right)*** *High magnification of poorly differentiated synovial sarcoma of the mediastinum shows round tumor cells with small, uniform nuclei with minimal nuclear atypia, surrounded by a clear cytoplasmic halo.*

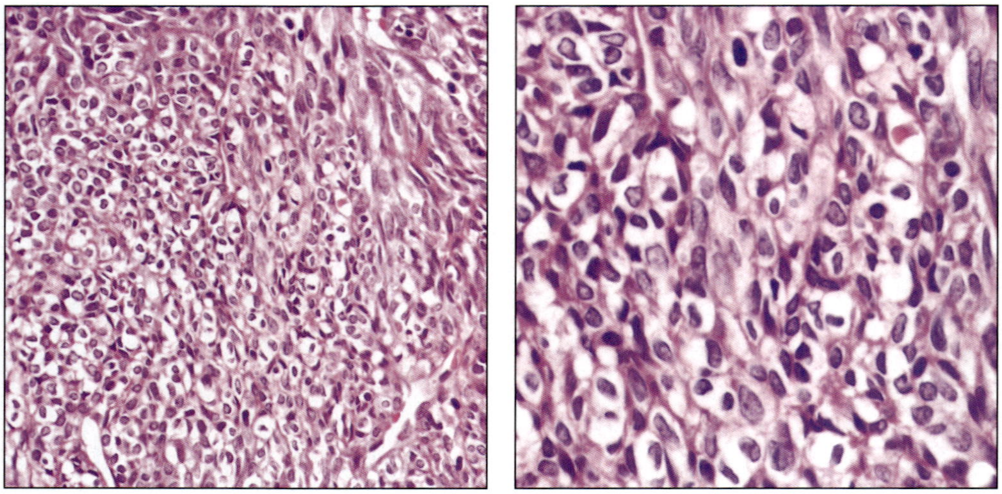

(Left) *Scanning magnification of poorly differentiated synovial sarcoma of the mediastinum shows ill-defined lobules* → *composed of round, epithelioid tumor cells admixed with a few spindle cells in the background. The tumor bears a superficial resemblance to epithelioid malignant peripheral nerve sheath tumors.* ***(Right)*** *Higher magnification of poorly differentiated synovial sarcoma of the mediastinum shows a monotonous population of bland-appearing, small round blue cells.*

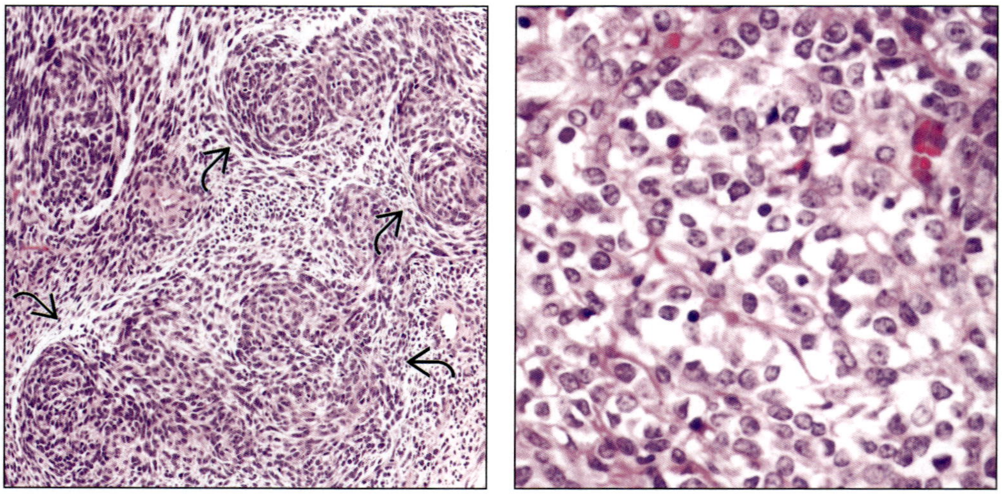

(Left) *Poorly differentiated synovial sarcoma of the mediastinum, rhabdoid cell variant, shows sheets of small round blue cells displaying prominent eosinophilic cytoplasmic inclusions indistinguishable from those seen in rhabdoid tumors.* ***(Right)*** *Higher magnification of poorly differentiated synovial sarcoma of the mediastinum, rhabdoid type, shows rhabdoid cells characterized by nuclei displaced to the periphery by globular cytoplasmic accumulations of intermediate filaments* →.

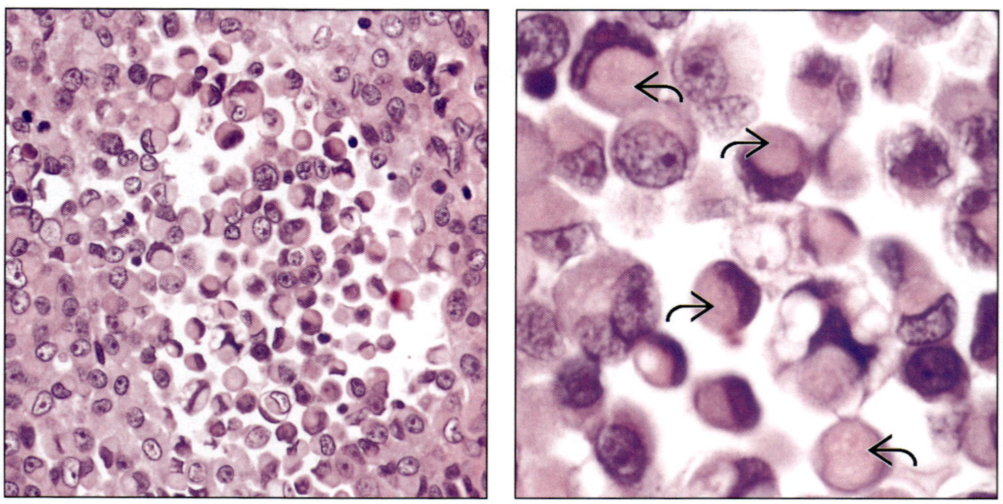

Unusual Stromal Features

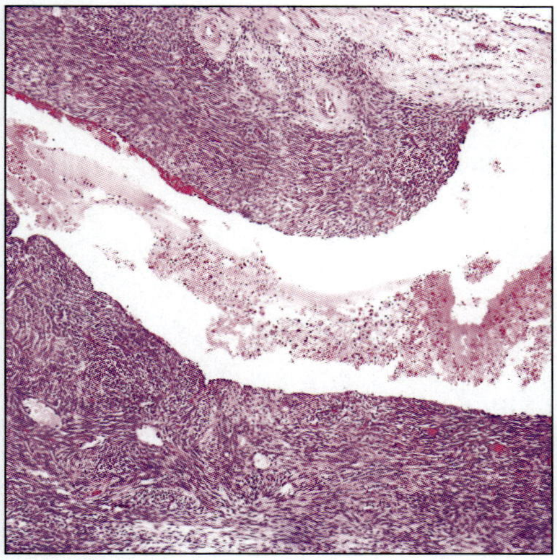

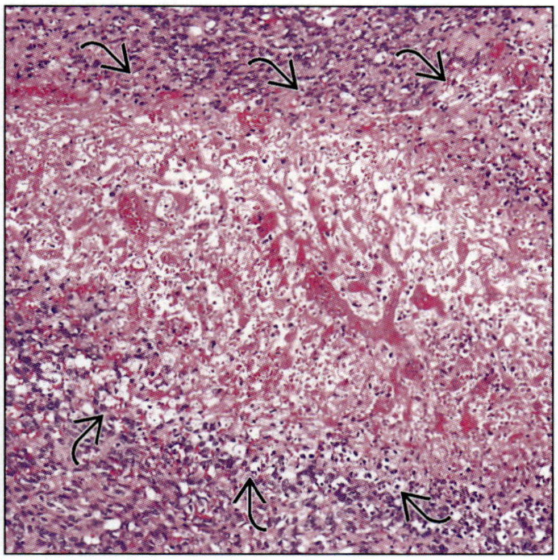

(Left) *Monophasic synovial sarcoma of the mediastinum with secondary cystic changes shows a large cystic space flanked by a dense spindle cell population. The tumors can show massive, gross cystic changes and be mistaken clinically for cystic teratomas.* ***(Right)*** *Focal areas of necrosis* ↪ *are seen in poorly differentiated synovial sarcoma of the mediastinum. Necrosis is not a common feature of mediastinal synovial sarcoma and is often associated with a more aggressive behavior.*

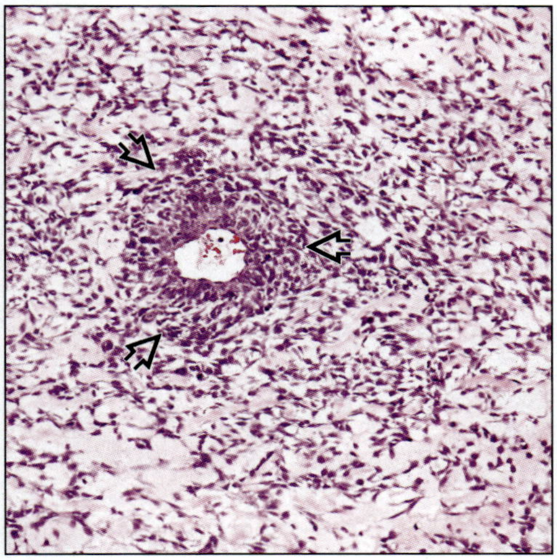

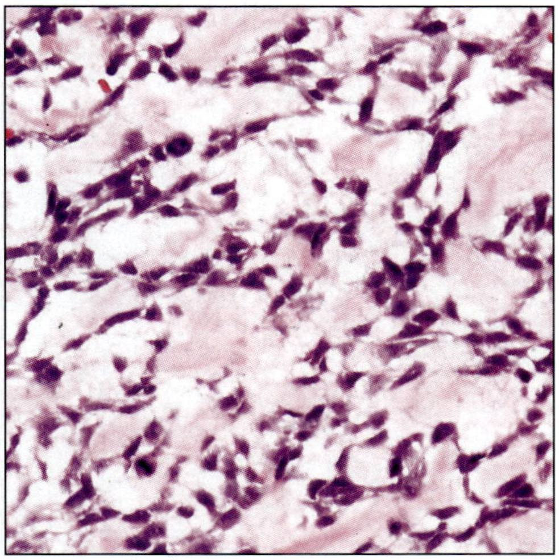

(Left) *Prominent myxoid stromal changes are seen in this monophasic synovial sarcoma of the mediastinum. Tumors with these features may be confused with fibromyxoid sarcomas and myxoid malignant fibrous histiocytoma. Notice perivascular cuffing by the tumor cells* ⇨. ***(Right)*** *High magnification of monophasic synovial sarcoma of the mediastinum with prominent myxoid stromal changes shows a lightly staining myxoid matrix separating the spindle tumor cells.*

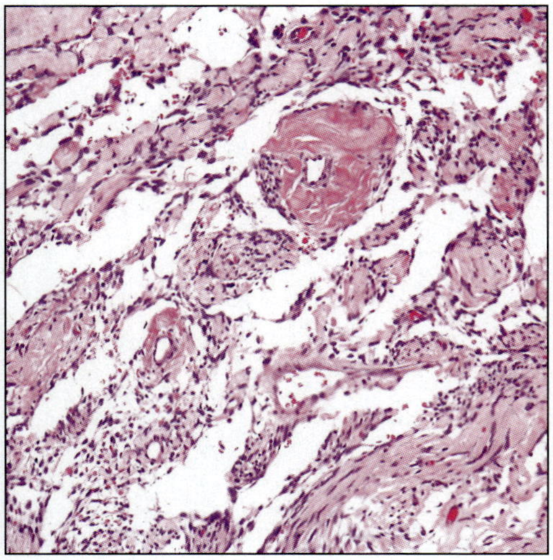

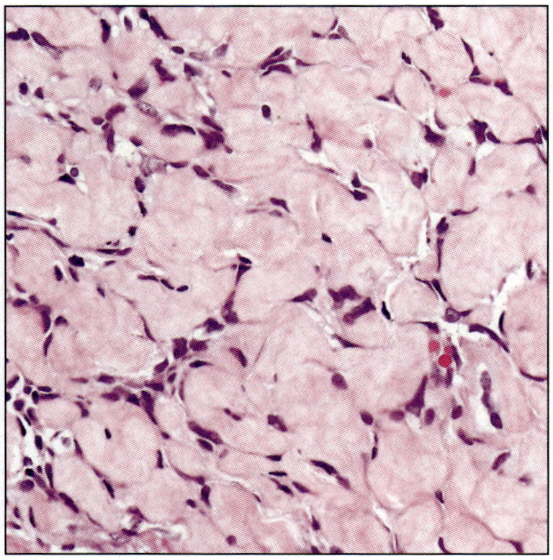

(Left) *Monophasic synovial sarcoma of the mediastinum shows artifactual clefting and separation of the stroma resulting in a pseudovascular appearance that may be mistaken for a malignant vascular neoplasm (i.e., angiosarcoma).* ***(Right)*** *Monophasic synovial sarcoma of the mediastinum shows extensive stromal collagenization resulting in scattered spindle cells separated by hyalinized matrix. Tumors with these features may be mistaken for fibrosarcoma or solitary fibrous tumors.*

SYNOVIAL SARCOMA

Biphasic Type

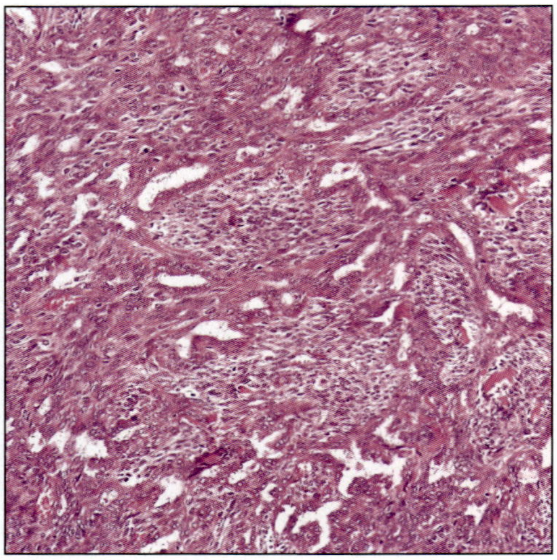
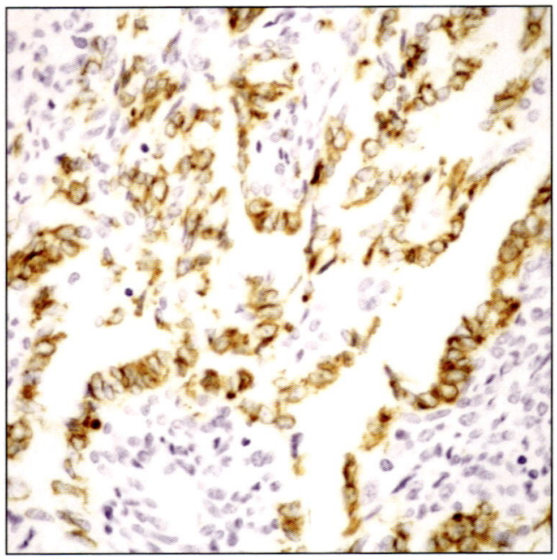

(Left) *Biphasic synovial sarcoma of the mediastinum shows evenly dispersed small glands with open lumens separated by dense, atypical spindle cell stroma.* ***(Right)*** *Immunohistochemical staining for cytokeratin AE1/AE3 antibody in biphasic synovial sarcoma of the mediastinum highlights the cells lining the glandular spaces. The glandular cells in biphasic synovial sarcoma stain very strongly for cytokeratin, unlike the spindle cells that generally display only focal positivity.*

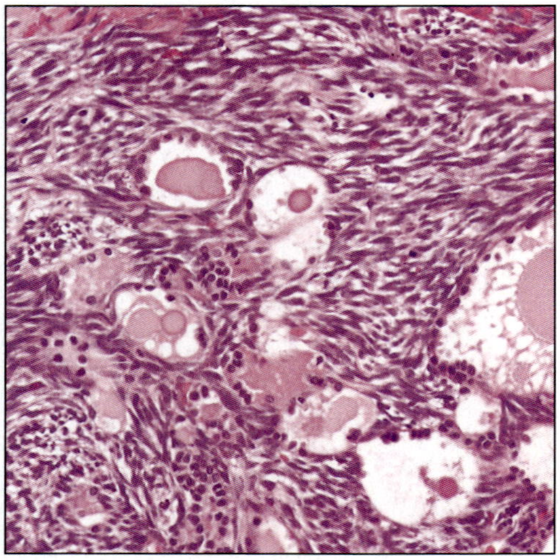
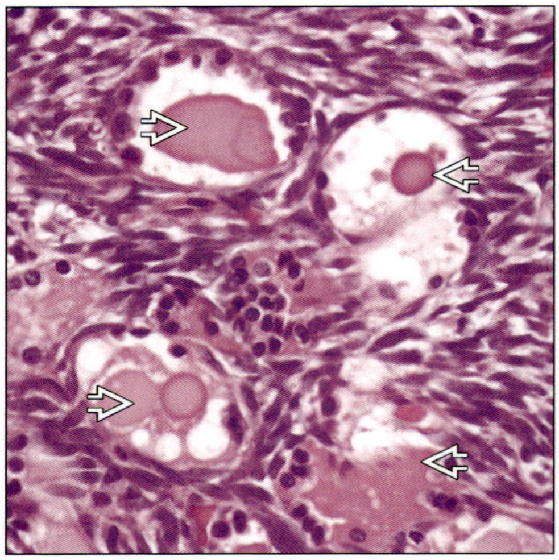

(Left) *Biphasic synovial sarcoma of the mediastinum is composed of small glands lined by small cuboidal or hobnailed tumor cells and are seen with proteinaceous secretions in their lumens. Notice the monotonous spindle cell proliferation surrounding the glands.* ***(Right)*** *High magnification of biphasic synovial sarcoma of the mediastinum shows small glands lined by hobnailed cells and displaying eosinophilic proteinaceous secretions in their lumens* ⇨*.*

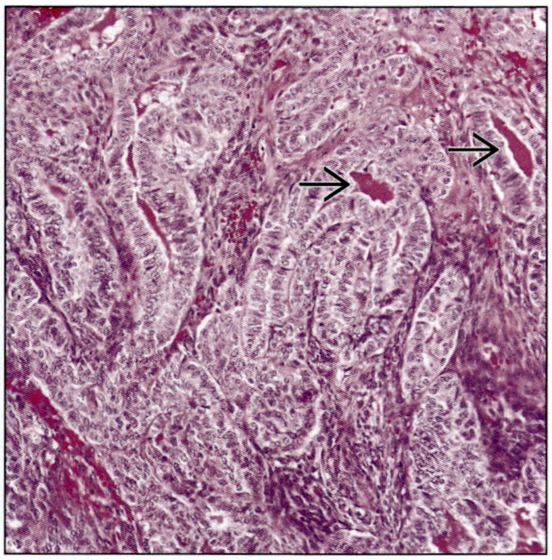
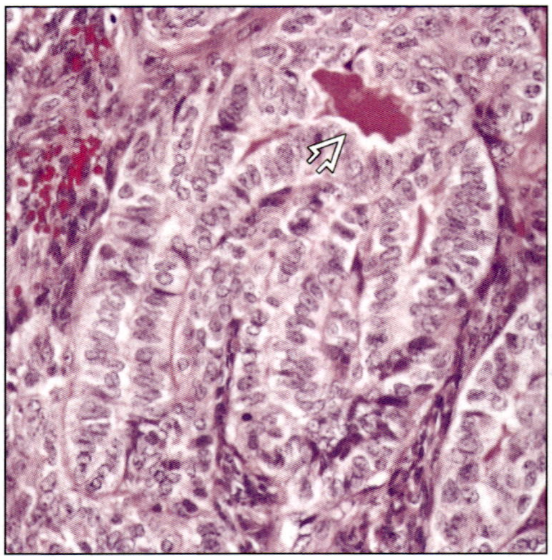

(Left) *Biphasic synovial sarcoma of the mediastinum shows large glandular structures with collapsed lumens lined by tall columnar cells. Notice the residual abortive glandular lumens filled with eosinophilic secretion* →*.* ***(Right)*** *High magnification of biphasic synovial sarcoma of the mediastinum shows collapsed glandular structures lined by tall columnar cells with clear cytoplasm. Notice the residual small lumen filled with proteinaceous material in one of the glands* ⇨*.*

Biphasic Type

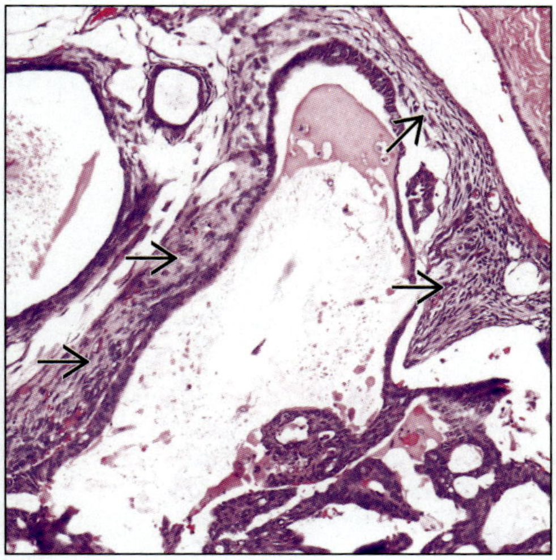
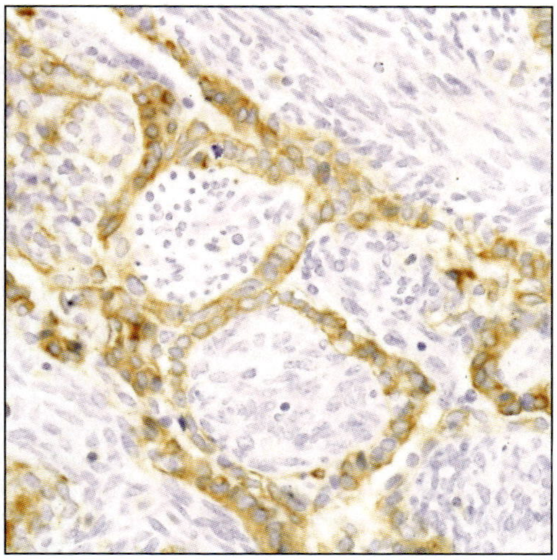

(Left) *Biphasic synovial sarcoma of the mediastinum shows intestinal-type glands with dilated lumens and mucinous luminal contents. Cases like this can be easily mistaken for metastases from adenocarcinomas of enteric origin, except for the fact that the glands are surrounded by a thin layer of atypical spindle cells.* ***(Right)*** *Immunohistochemical staining for cytokeratin AE1/AE3 in biphasic synovial sarcoma of the mediastinum shows negative staining of the spindle cells.*

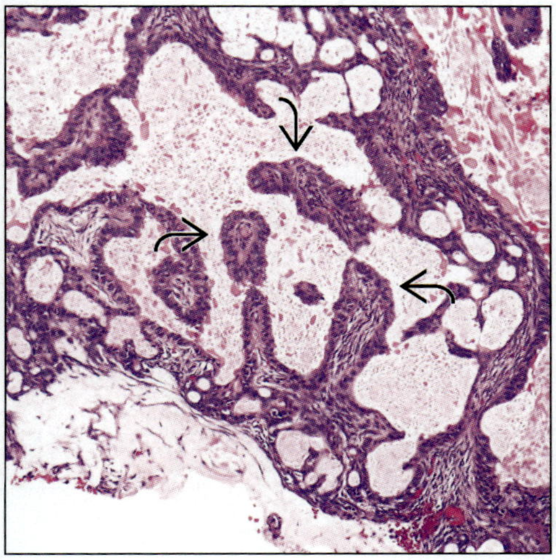
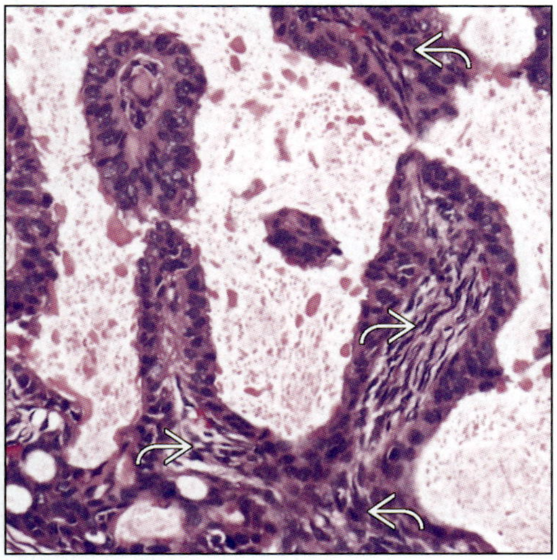

(Left) *Scanning magnification of biphasic synovial sarcoma of the mediastinum with intestinal-type glands shows focal papillary formations protruding into the lumen of the dilated glands.* ***(Right)*** *High magnification of biphasic synovial sarcoma of the mediastinum with intestinal-type glands shows papillary formation protruding into the lumen of the glandular spaces. Notice the spindle cell stroma in the cores of the papillae and the mucinous content in the lumen.*

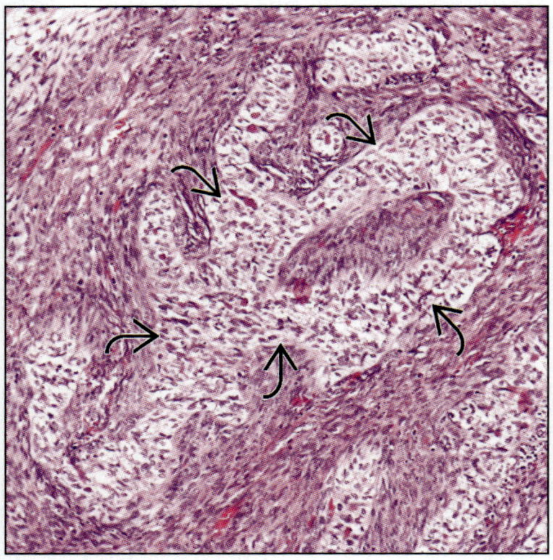
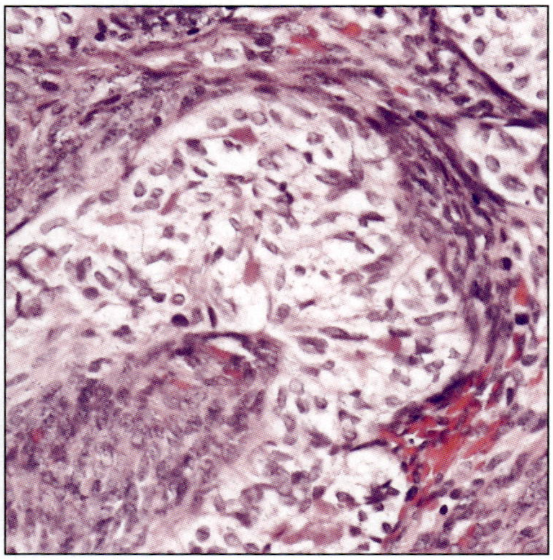

(Left) *Scanning magnification of unusual variant of biphasic synovial sarcoma of the mediastinum shows areas characterized by clear cells surrounded by a dense, monotonous, atypical spindle cell proliferation.* ***(Right)*** *Higher magnification of unusual variant of biphasic synovial sarcoma of the mediastinum shows islands of large, clear cells with abundant water-clear cytoplasm surrounded by a dense, monotonous, atypical spindle cell population.*

NEUROFIBROMA

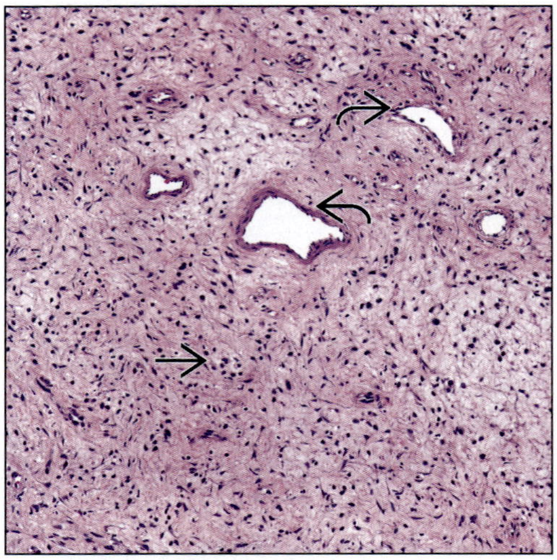

Mediastinal neurofibroma shows a classic spindle cell proliferation ➡ embedded in a rather loose fibroconnective tissue admixed with dilated vascular structures ↪.

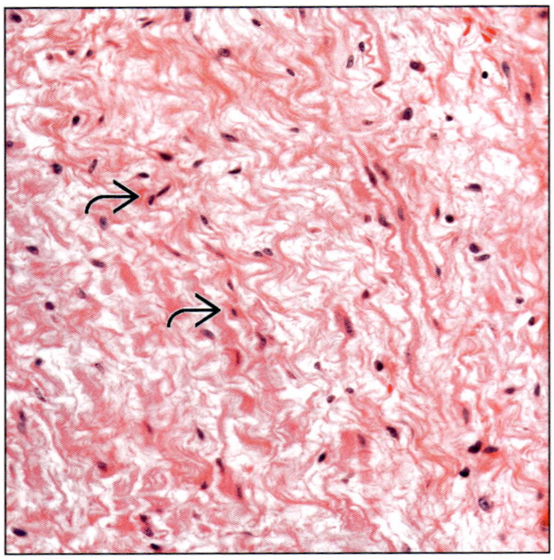

High-power view of a mediastinal neurofibroma shows a spindle cell proliferation ↪ admixed with fibrocollagenous tissue. Note the absence of cellular pleomorphism.

TERMINOLOGY

Abbreviations

- Neurofibroma (NF)

Definitions

- Benign neural neoplasm

ETIOLOGY/PATHOGENESIS

Pathogenesis

- Proliferation of perineural fibroblasts, Schwann cells, and neurites

CLINICAL ISSUES

Epidemiology

- Incidence
  - One of most common neural tumors
- Age
  - Usually adults in 3rd or 4th decade of life
- Gender
  - No apparent gender predilection

Site

- Posterior mediastinum

Presentation

- Chest pain
- Dyspnea
- Cough
- Neurofibromatosis (von Recklinghausen disease)
- Some patients may be asymptomatic

Treatment

- Surgical approaches
  - Complete surgical resection

Prognosis

- Good

MACROSCOPIC FEATURES

General Features

- Well circumscribed but not encapsulated
- Light tan in color

Sections to Be Submitted

- In cases of patients with history of neurofibromatosis, careful sampling to rule out sarcoma

Size

- Variable size
- May be up to or > 10 cm in diameter

MICROSCOPIC PATHOLOGY

Histologic Features

- Spindle cell proliferation
- Wavy nuclei and pointed ends
- Loose fibroconnective tissue
- Absent mitotic activity
- In some cases, stroma may be myxoid
- Occasional Wagner-Meissner bodies may be seen
- Pacini corpuscles may be seen
- Mucin-producing glands may be seen focally
- Melanin pigment may be present

DIFFERENTIAL DIAGNOSIS

Schwannoma

- Shows presence of Verocay bodies in contrast to NF
- S100 protein is generally strongly positive in schwannomas in contrast to NF

Neurofibrosarcoma

- Usually shows presence of increased mitotic activity
- May also show presence of areas of necrosis, which would be unusual in NF

NEUROFIBROMA

Key Facts

Terminology
- Neurofibroma (NF)

Etiology/Pathogenesis
- Proliferation of perineural fibroblasts, Schwann cells, and neurites

Clinical Issues
- One of most common neural tumors
- Usually adults in 3rd or 4th decade of life
- Location
  - Posterior mediastinum
- Symptoms
  - Chest pain
  - Dyspnea
  - Cough
  - Neurofibromatosis
  - Some patients may be asymptomatic
- Treatment
  - Complete surgical resection
- Prognosis
  - Good

Top Differential Diagnoses
- Schwannoma
- Neurofibrosarcoma
- Ganglioneuroma
- Solitary fibrous tumor
- Leiomyoma

Diagnostic Checklist
- Spindle cell proliferation without mitotic activity
- Loose fibrocollagenous or myxoid stroma

Immunohistochemistry

Antibody	Reactivity	Staining Pattern	Comment
S100	Positive	Nuclear & cytoplasmic	May be focal and weak
NFP	Positive	Nuclear & cytoplasmic	May be focal and weak
NSE	Positive	Cytoplasmic	Not specific
CD34	Negative		May be positive in vascular spaces
AE1/AE3	Negative		
Actin-HHF-35	Negative		May show focal positive staining around vessels

Ganglioneuroma
- Generally has presence of ganglion cells in contrast to NF, which lacks their presence

Solitary Fibrous Tumor
- Usually shows different growth pattern in same tumor
- Usually positive for CD34 and Bcl-2, which are negative in NF

Leiomyoma
- Both tumors may show similar histological features with lack of mitotic activity
- Shows positive staining for actin, whereas NF is negative
- Leiomyoma in posterior mediastinum is rare

DIAGNOSTIC CHECKLIST

Clinically Relevant Pathologic Features
- Mitotic rate
- Nuclear features

Pathologic Interpretation Pearls
- Spindle cell proliferation without mitotic activity
- Loose fibrocollagenous or myxoid stroma

SELECTED REFERENCES

1. Cardillo G et al: Surgical treatment of benign neurogenic tumours of the mediastinum: a single institution report. Eur J Cardiothorac Surg. 34(6):1210-4, 2008
2. Patel VS et al: Intrathoracic peripheral nerve sheath tumors in patients with neurofibromatosis type 1 (von Recklinghausen disease). J Thorac Cardiovasc Surg. 131(3):736-7, 2006
3. Saito H et al: Mediastinal neurofibroma originating from the left intrathoracic phrenic nerve: report of a case. Surg Today. 34(11):950-3, 2004
4. Takeda S et al: Intrathoracic neurogenic tumors--50 years' experience in a Japanese institution. Eur J Cardiothorac Surg. 26(4):807-12, 2004
5. Takeda S et al: Posterior mediastinal mass in patients with von Recklinghausen's disease. Respiration. 67(2):234-7, 2000
6. Marchevsky AM: Mediastinal tumors of peripheral nervous system origin. Semin Diagn Pathol. 16(1):65-78, 1999
7. Voets AJ et al: Mediastinal neurofibroma as a cause of unilateral diaphragm paralysis in von Recklinghausen's disease. Intensive Care Med. 25(11):1336-7, 1999
8. Strollo DC et al: Primary mediastinal tumors: part II. Tumors of the middle and posterior mediastinum. Chest. 112(5):1344-57, 1997
9. Sugio K et al: Neurogenic tumors of the mediastinum originated from the vagus nerve. Eur J Surg Oncol. 21(2):214-6, 1995

NEUROFIBROMA

Gross and Microscopic Features

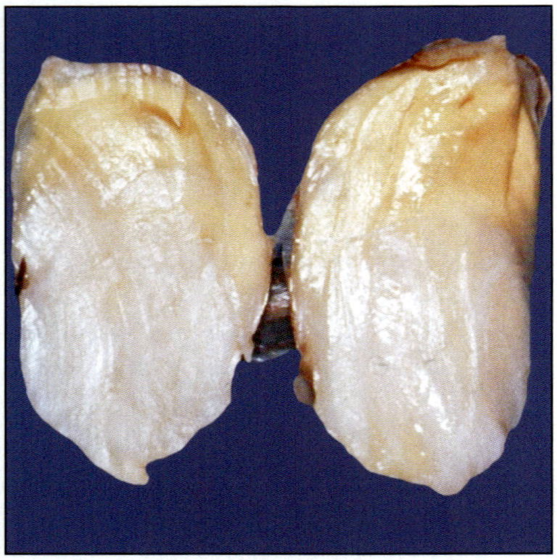

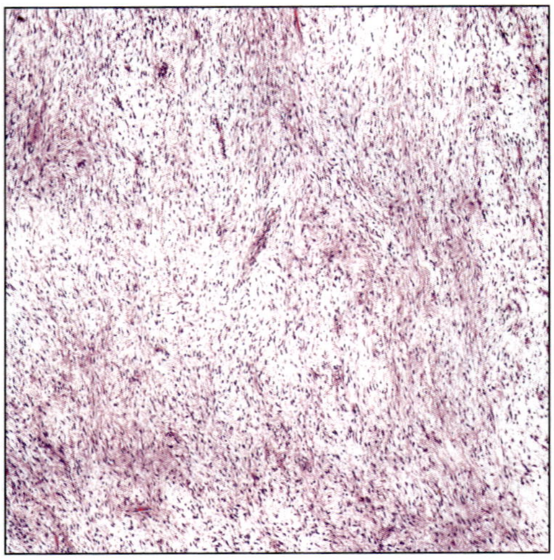

__(Left)__ Mediastinal neurofibromas are usually well-circumscribed tumors of whitish color and homogeneous surface. Note the absence of necrosis &/or hemorrhage; such features should alert one to the possibility of malignancy. __(Right)__ Neurofibroma shows a monotonous bland spindle cell proliferation with scattered compressed blood vessels. No necrosis or hemorrhage is normally seen in these tumors.

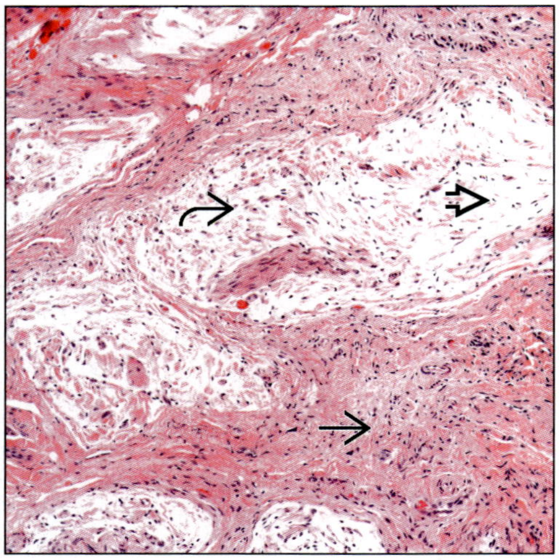

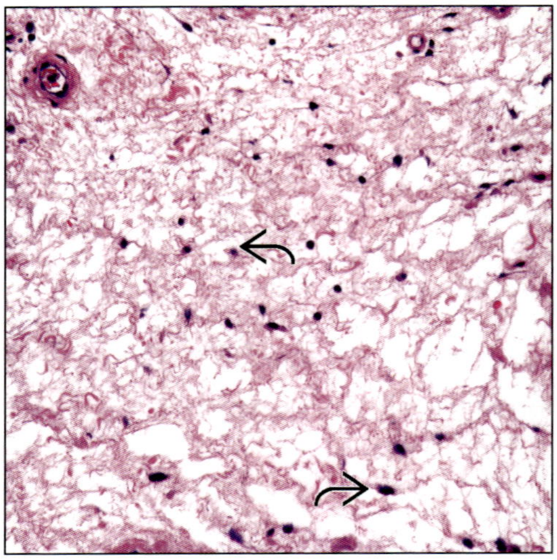

__(Left)__ In some cases, neurofibromas may adopt a rather lobular growth pattern ↷ in which lobules are separated by fibrocollagenous tissue →. A subtle myxoid change may be seen in some areas ⇨. __(Right)__ Mediastinal neurofibroma is shown with prominent myxoid changes and very little cellular component. However, the spindle cells are still recognizable ↷, and the tumor does not show necrosis &/or hemorrhage.

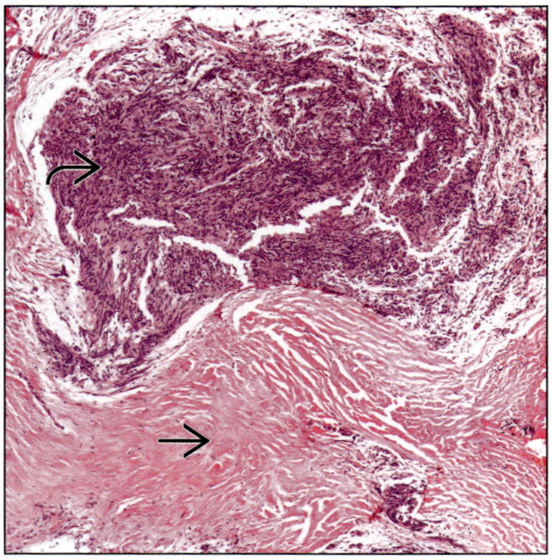

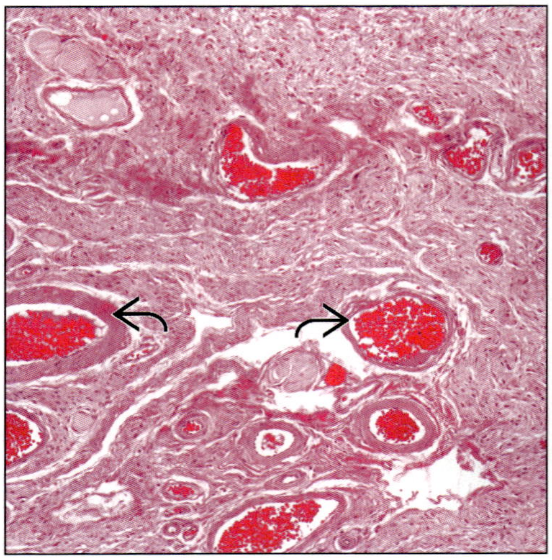

__(Left)__ Mediastinal neurofibroma shows extensive dense fibrocollagen →, and the neurofibroma is composed of a rather solid spindle cellular proliferation ↷. Some of these cellular areas can be confused for malignancy. __(Right)__ Mediastinal neurofibroma is shown with extensive areas of vascular dilatation ↷ almost mimicking a vascular neoplasm such as cavernous hemangioma.

NEUROFIBROMA

Microscopic Features

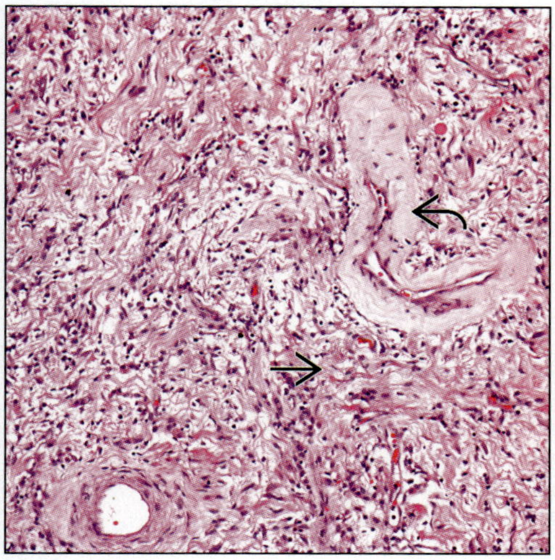
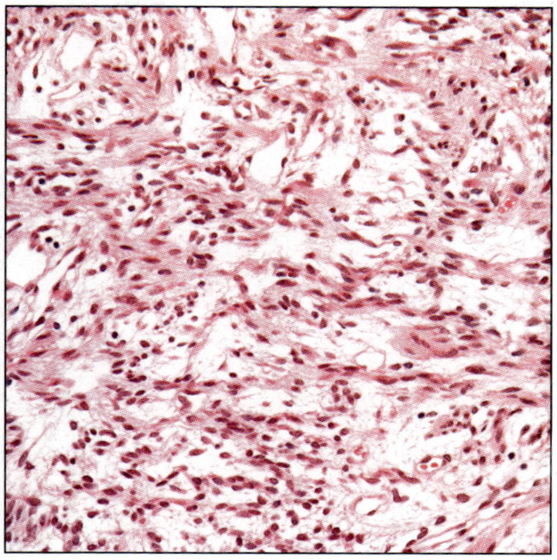

(Left) *Neurofibroma shows compressed blood vessels ↪. Note the perivascular collagenization of the vessels as well as the spindle cellular proliferation → admixed with some inflammatory cells.* ***(Right)*** *Mediastinal neurofibroma shows predominantly spindle cellular proliferation with loose fibroconnective tissue and focal myxoid changes. Note the absence of cellular pleomorphism.*

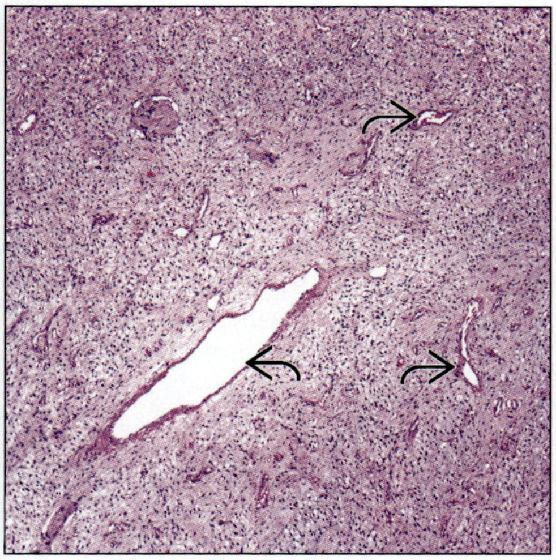
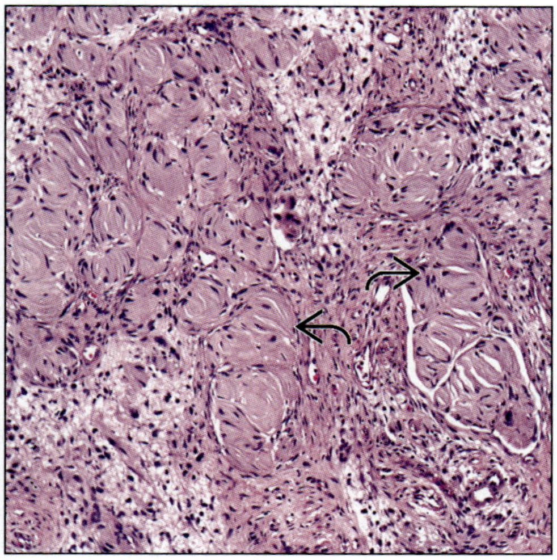

(Left) *Mediastinal neurofibroma shows a spindle cellular proliferation in a more solid growth pattern. Note the presence of several blood vessels of different sizes ↪.* ***(Right)*** *Mediastinal neurofibroma is shown with the presence of Wagner-Meissner bodies ↪. In general, the presence of Wagner-Meissner bodies is not a common finding and may help in the diagnosis.*

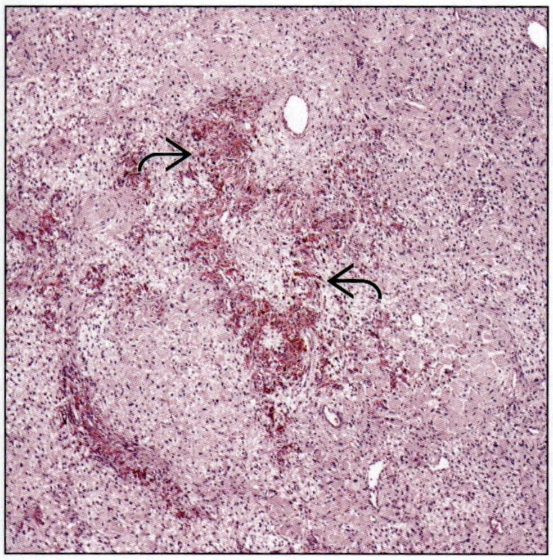
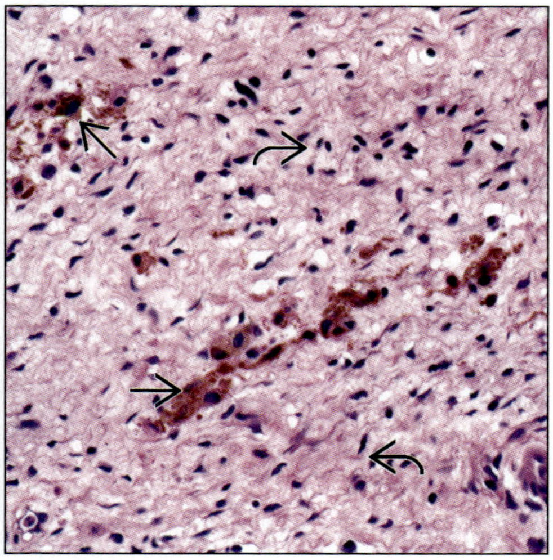

(Left) *Mediastinal neurofibroma is shown with focal areas of melanin pigment ↪. This feature may be mistaken for melanoma; however, neurofibromas lack cellular atypia &/or mitotic figures.* ***(Right)*** *High power shows a mediastinal neurofibroma in which the melanin pigment → is more focal. Note the classical histological features of neurofibroma ↪.*

PERIPHERAL NERVE SHEATH TUMOR

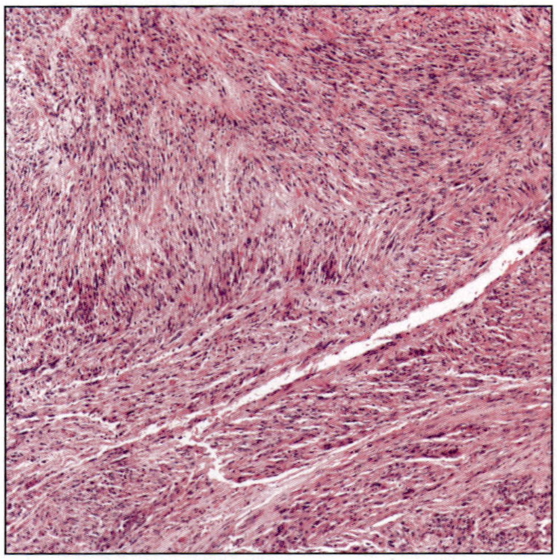

Mediastinal peripheral nerve sheath tumor shows a solid spindle cell proliferation with a vague herringbone-like pattern of growth.

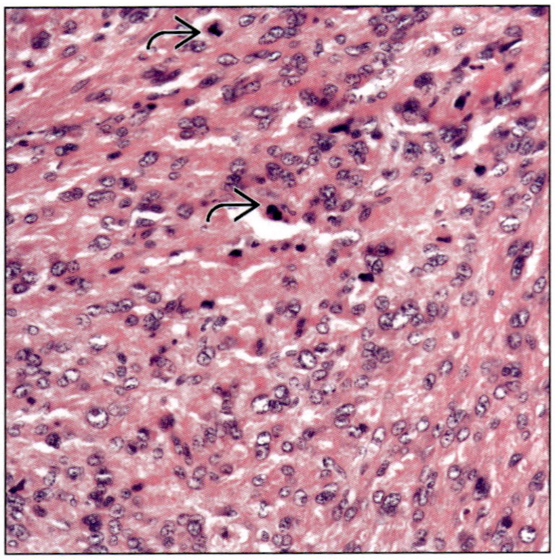

High-power view of a mediastinal peripheral nerve sheath tumor shows more epithelioid areas with cellular pleomorphism, nuclear atypia, and mitotic activity ➔.

TERMINOLOGY

Abbreviations

- Peripheral nerve sheath tumor (PNST)

Synonyms

- Malignant schwannoma, neurofibrosarcoma, neurogenic sarcoma

Definitions

- Malignant tumor of neural sheath origin

ETIOLOGY/PATHOGENESIS

Etiology

- These tumors may occur as manifestation of neurofibromatosis (von Recklinghausen disease)
- PNST may also occur post radiation

CLINICAL ISSUES

Epidemiology

- Incidence
  - Unusual in mediastinal location
  - May account for approximately 5% of all mediastinal tumors
- Age
  - More common in adults in 3rd, 4th, and 5th decades of life
- Gender
  - No apparent gender predilection
  - Patients with neurofibromatosis are commonly male and young adults

Site

- More common in posterior mediastinum but can also occur in anterior mediastinum

Presentation

- Chest pain
- Cough
- Dyspnea
- Neurofibromatosis

Treatment

- Surgical approaches
  - Complete surgical resection
- Adjuvant therapy
  - Radiation &/or chemotherapy will be determined on individual basis and depending on extent of tumor at time of diagnosis

Prognosis

- Tumors follow aggressive behavior, and prognosis is poor
- Worse prognosis in patients with neurofibromatosis

MACROSCOPIC FEATURES

General Features

- Lobulated large but not encapsulated tumors
- Light tan in color
- Areas of necrosis and hemorrhage may be seen

Size

- Usually > 5 cm in diameter

MICROSCOPIC PATHOLOGY

Histologic Features

- Solid spindle cellular proliferation
- Wavy or comma-shaped nuclei
- Nuclear palisading
- Tactoid differentiation
- Cellular pleomorphism with mitotic activity
- Areas of hemorrhage &/or necrosis may be seen
- Perivascular hyalinization

Key Facts

Terminology
- Peripheral nerve sheath tumor (PNST)
- Synonyms: Malignant schwannoma, neurofibrosarcoma, neurogenic sarcoma

Clinical Issues
- These tumors are more common in posterior mediastinum but can also occur in anterior mediastinum
- Symptoms
  - Chest pain
  - Cough
  - Dyspnea
  - Neurofibromatosis
- Prognosis
  - These tumors follow aggressive behavior, and prognosis is poor
  - Worse prognosis in patients with neurofibromatosis
- Incidence
  - Unusual in mediastinal location
  - May account for approximately 5% of all mediastinal tumors

Top Differential Diagnoses
- Neurofibroma
- Leiomyosarcoma
- Solitary fibrous tumor

Diagnostic Checklist
- Solid spindle cellular proliferation
- Perivascular hyalinization
- Hemorrhage &/or necrosis
- Nuclear atypia and mitotic activity

Immunohistochemistry

Antibody	Reactivity	Staining Pattern	Comment
S100	Positive	Nuclear	In < 50% of cases and focal
NFP	Positive	Cytoplasmic	In some cases and not specific
NSE	Positive		In some cases and not specific
Vimentin	Positive	Cytoplasmic	Not specific
CD34	Positive		
Actin-HHF-35	Negative		
Desmin	Negative		
Bcl-2	Negative		

- Heterologous elements may be seen
  - Muscle, cartilage, bone

DIFFERENTIAL DIAGNOSIS

Neurofibroma
- Does not show increase in mitotic activity or cellular pleomorphism
- Rarely shows areas of necrosis, and when present, they are focal

Leiomyosarcoma
- Does not show nuclear palisading or tactoid differentiation
- Commonly shows positive staining for muscle markers in contrast to PNST

Solitary Fibrous Tumor
- Shows more than 1 growth pattern in same tumor
- Commonly shows positive staining for CD34 and Bcl-2 in contrast to PNST

DIAGNOSTIC CHECKLIST

Clinically Relevant Pathologic Features
- Mitotic rate
- Invasive pattern
- Nuclear features

Pathologic Interpretation Pearls
- Solid spindle cellular proliferation
- Palisading of nuclei
- Tactoid differentiation
- Perivascular hyalinization
- Hemorrhage &/or necrosis
- Nuclear atypia and mitotic activity

SELECTED REFERENCES

1. Shimizu J et al: A case of intrathoracic giant malignant peripheral nerve sheath tumor in neurofibromatosis type I (von Recklinghausen's disease). Ann Thorac Cardiovasc Surg. 14(1):42-7, 2008
2. Patel VS et al: Intrathoracic peripheral nerve sheath tumors in patients with neurofibromatosis type 1 (von Recklinghausen disease). J Thorac Cardiovasc Surg. 131(3):736-7, 2006
3. Takeda S et al: Intrathoracic neurogenic tumors--50 years' experience in a Japanese institution. Eur J Cardiothorac Surg. 26(4):807-12, 2004

Gross and Microscopic Features

*(**Left**) Mediastinal PNST shows areas of hemorrhage ➔ and possibly necrosis. In addition, more viable areas of tumor show a fish-flesh-like appearance ➔. These features are of great importance and should be sampled properly. (**Right**) Low-power view shows a mediastinal PNST displaying a spindle cell proliferation arranged in fascicle with a vague storiform pattern. In some areas there is an appearance of clear cells ➔, possibly an artifact of fixation.*

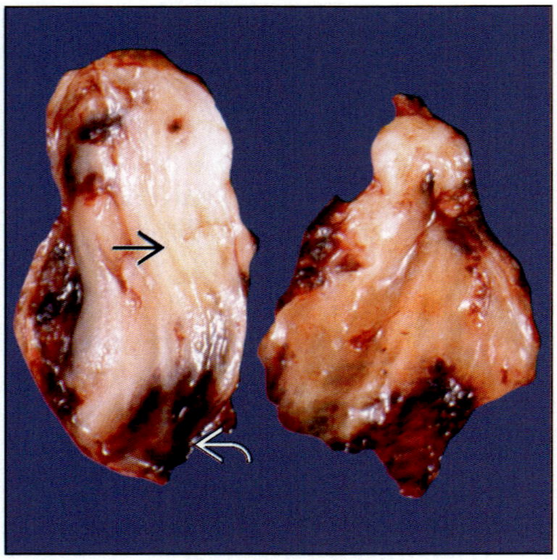

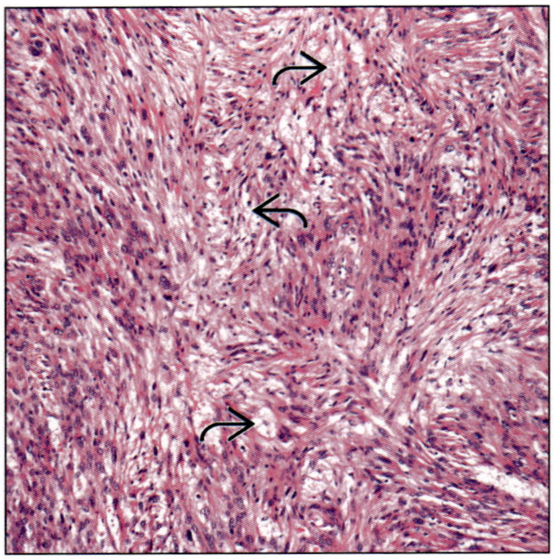

*(**Left**) Mediastinal PNST shows hypo- ➔ and hypercellular ➔ areas. The hypocellular areas show dense fibrocollagenous tissue, while the hypercellular areas show a more epithelioid cellular proliferation. (**Right**) Mediastinal PNST is shown with prominent arrangement of tumor cells around vascular structures ➔. This feature in particular is very common in these tumors and should alert one to the possibility of PNST. Adjacent areas are hypocellular.*

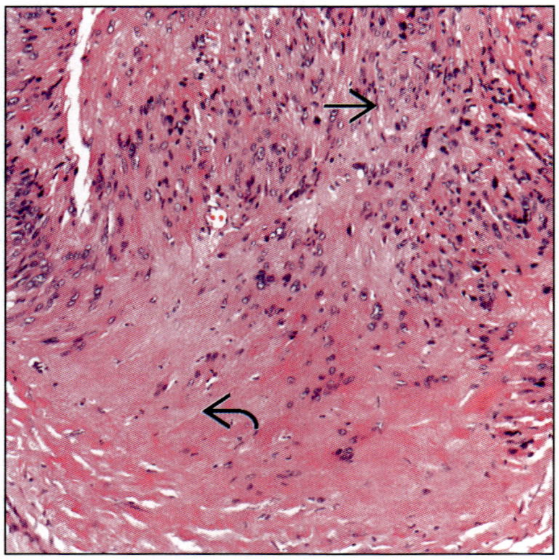

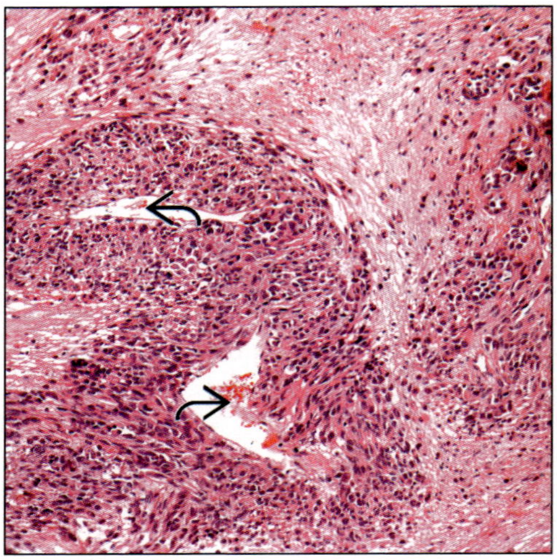

*(**Left**) The presence of perivascular hyalinization and tumor arrangement around vascular structures is a common feature of PNST. Note the concentric arrangement of tumor cells around blood vessels ➔ and the adjacent tumor necrosis ➔. (**Right**) PNST displays extensive areas of necrosis ➔ merging with a viable tumor ➔. The tumor has a vague myxoid appearance with an ectatic vascular structure ➔.*

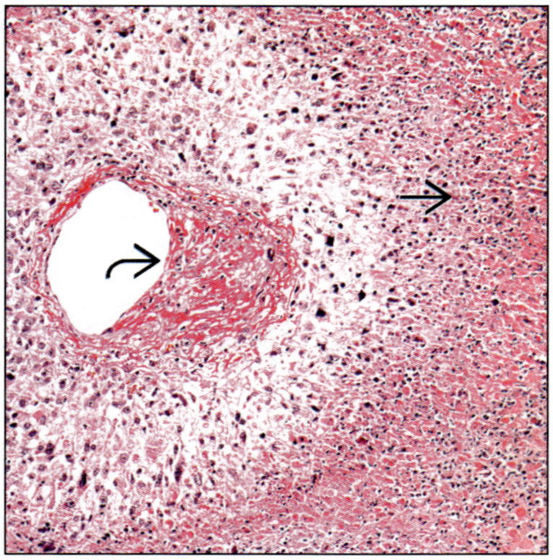

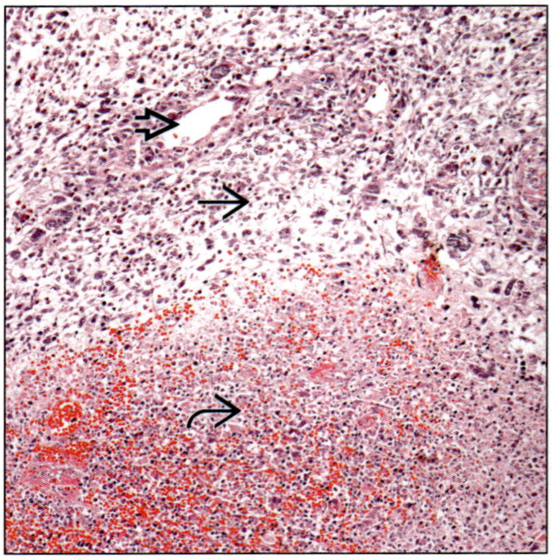

Microscopic Features

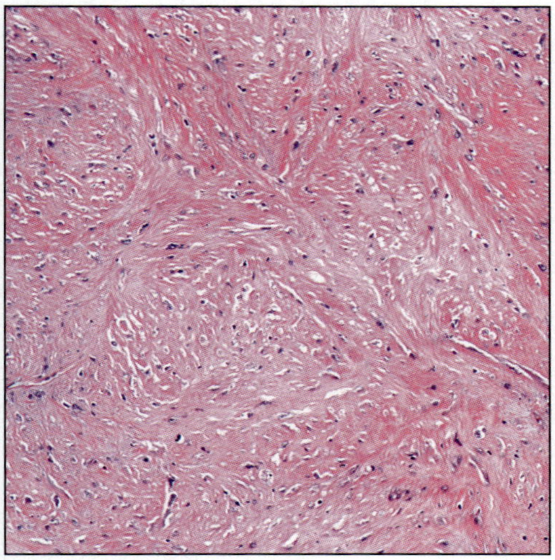

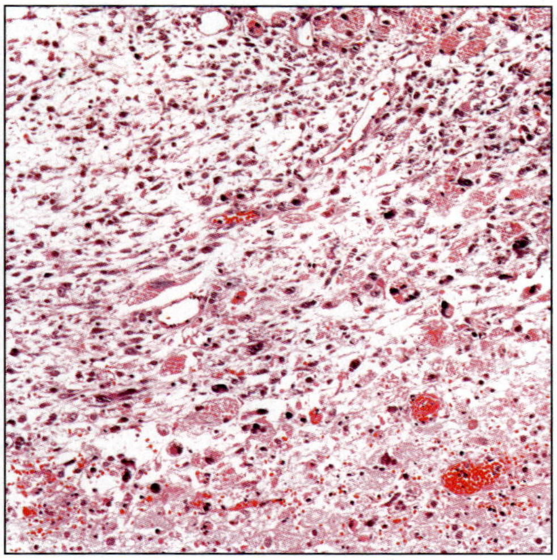

(Left) *Extensive areas of dense collagenization may be present in mediastinal peripheral nerve sheath tumor, which may obscure the true nature of the neoplasm. However, in most of the cases, these areas are only focal.* ***(Right)*** *Mediastinal PNST is shown with marked cellular and nuclear pleomorphism. Pyknotic nuclei, as well as mitotic figures, are present.*

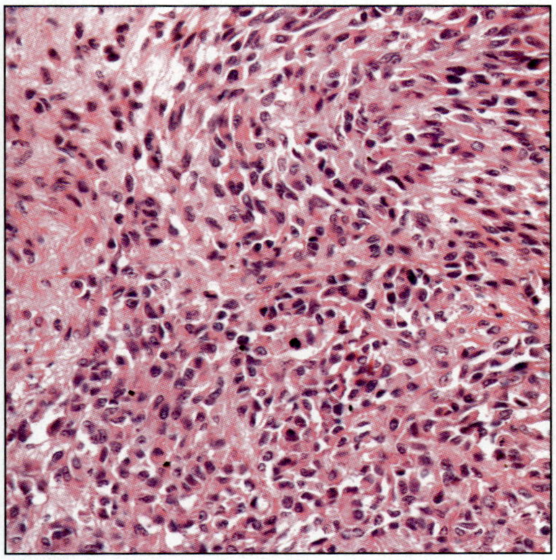

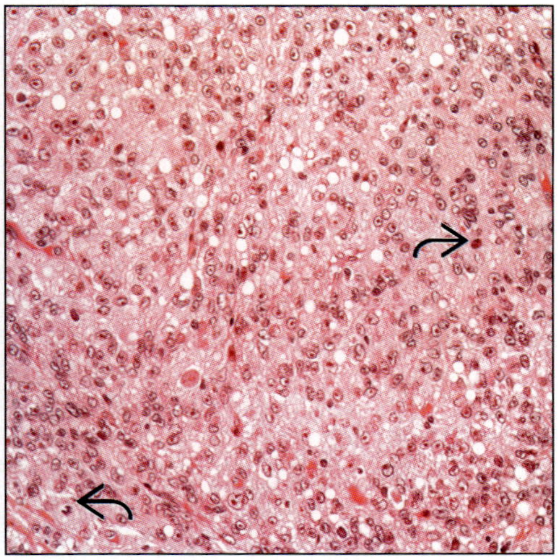

(Left) *High-power view shows an epithelioid PNST composed of oval cells arranged in a subtle nested pattern. This growth pattern can be easily confused with a tumor of epithelial origin.* ***(Right)*** *Epithelioid PNST is composed of oval cells with moderate light eosinophilic cytoplasm and prominent nucleoli. Mitotic figures ↷ are easily encountered. Note that the neoplastic cellular proliferation has vague epithelioid features.*

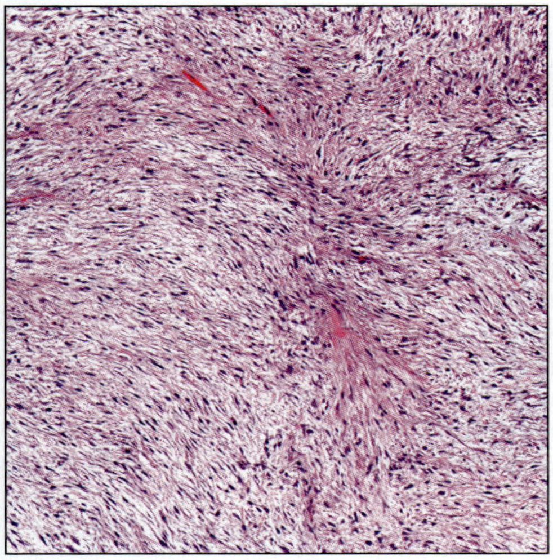

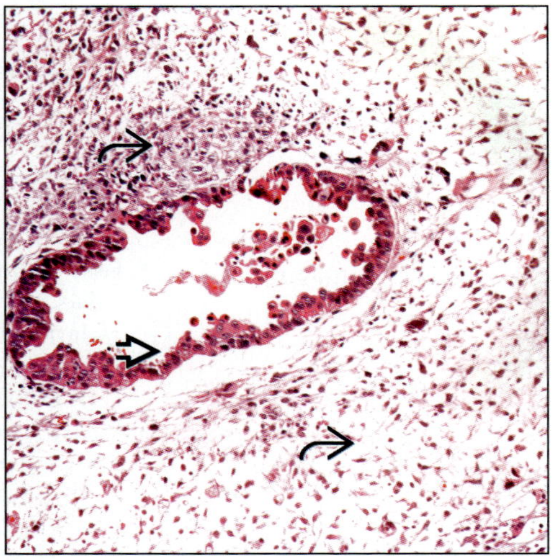

(Left) *In some cases of PNST, the cellularity closely mimics that of benign neurofibroma. In this case there is no evidence of necrosis and hemorrhage.* ***(Right)*** *PNST shows glandular differentiation. The neoplastic cellular proliferation ↷ around the glandular structure ⇨ shows myxoid changes, as well as nuclear atypia and mitotic figures.*

SOLITARY FIBROUS TUMOR/FIBROSARCOMA

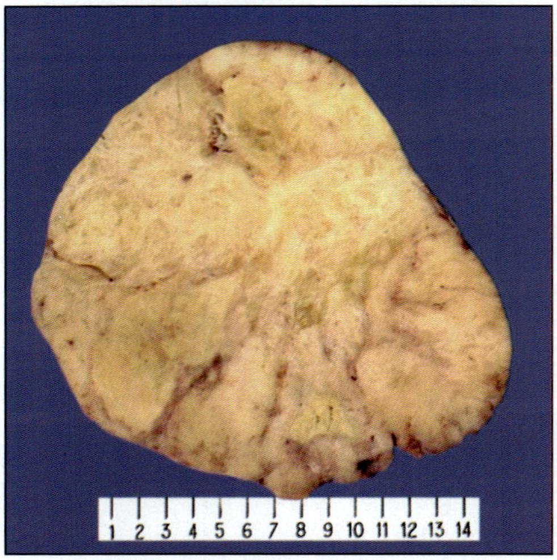

Gross appearance of solitary fibrous tumor of the mediastinum shows a well-circumscribed mass with a lobulated, tan-white homogeneous cut surface and focal areas of necrosis.

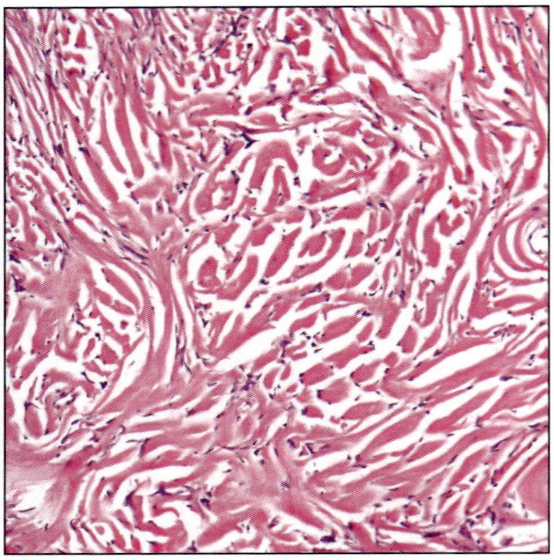

Characteristic histologic appearance of solitary fibrous tumor shows parallel linear arrays of rope-like collagen strands flanked by small, bland-appearing spindle cells.

TERMINOLOGY

Abbreviations

- Solitary fibrous tumor (SFT)

Synonyms

- Localized fibrous tumor, malignant solitary fibrous tumor, mediastinal fibroma, mediastinal fibrosarcoma, hemangiopericytoma, fibrous mesothelioma

Definitions

- Neoplastic, tumor-forming proliferation of dendritic fibroblasts

CLINICAL ISSUES

Site

- Most common mesenchymal spindle cell tumor of anterior mediastinum
- May also occur in posterior and middle mediastinal compartments

Presentation

- Cough
- Chest pain
- Dyspnea
- Hypoglycemia
- Asymptomatic
- May be discovered incidentally on routine imaging studies

Treatment

- Surgical excision

Prognosis

- Majority of cases reported in mediastinum behaved more aggressively than those at other locations
- Large and poorly circumscribed tumors may recur, metastasize, and kill patient
- Histology may not show strict correlation with prognosis
- In general, cytologic atypia, mitotic activity, necrosis, and invasion are associated with aggressive behavior

MACROSCOPIC FEATURES

General Features

- Most tumors are well circumscribed, firm, and lobulated
- Larger tumors are usually infiltrative and adherent to lung and pleura
- May be attached to thymus by a short fibrous pedicle
- Tan-gray, whorled appearance on cut surface
- Larger tumors may show areas of hemorrhage and necrosis
- Gross cystic changes can also be seen on cut surface

Size

- 4-25 cm

MICROSCOPIC PATHOLOGY

Histologic Features

- Tumors are characterized by large variegation of histologic growth patterns that may resemble other types of spindle cell tumors
- **Fascicular pattern**
  - Fascicles of bland-appearing spindle cells with small, dark nuclei generally devoid of mitotic activity
  - Fascicles may resemble those seen in smooth muscle or neural tumors
- **Storiform pattern**
  - Usually shows short storiform pattern resembling "fibrohistiocytic" tumors
  - Storiform pattern is usually only focal and admixed with other areas
- **Hemangiopericytic pattern**

Key Facts

Clinical Issues

- Most common mesenchymal spindle cell tumor of anterior mediastinum
- Cough
- Chest pain
- Dyspnea
- Hypoglycemia
- May be discovered incidentally on routine imaging studies
- Majority of cases reported in mediastinum behaved more aggressively than those at other locations

Microscopic Pathology

- Fascicles of bland-appearing spindle cells with small dark nuclei generally devoid of mitotic activity
- Usually shows short storiform pattern resembling "fibrohistiocytic" tumors
- Small to medium-sized branching vessels with open lumens and "staghorn" appearance
- Hypercellular areas with increased number of nuclei are seen alongside hypocellular areas
- Haphazard distribution of spindle cells separated by keloidal-like strands of collagen
- Large dilated vessels are seen surrounded by dense collagenous tissue
- Advanced cases may show extensive areas of sclerosis and collagenization
- Tumors cells are strongly positive for CD34, Bcl-2, vimentin, and CD99
- Tumor cells are generally negative for cytokeratins, SMA, desmin, S100 protein, and other differentiation markers

  - Small to medium-sized branching vessels with open lumens and "staghorn" appearance
  - Tumors with these features were commonly labeled hemangiopericytoma in previous years
- **Alternating hypo- and hypercellular areas**
  - Hypercellular areas with increased number of nuclei are seen alongside hypocellular areas
  - This growth pattern may resemble malignant peripheral nerve sheath tumors or synovial sarcoma
- **Neural-like growth pattern**
  - Fascicles composed of wavy nuclei, areas with focal palisading of nuclei, and areas resembling Verocay bodies
  - This growth pattern can be easily confused for schwannian neoplasms
- **"Herringbone" pattern**
  - Short fascicles of spindle cells are seen emanating from central area reminiscent of a herring bone
  - This growth pattern can simulate fibrosarcoma, malignant peripheral nerve sheath tumor, and synovial sarcoma
- **"Patternless" pattern**
  - Haphazard distribution of spindle cells separated by keloidal-like strands of collagen
  - Thin, rope-like strands of keloidal collagen, usually showing parallel distribution, are characteristic of these tumors
- **Dense hypercellular pattern**
  - Densely packed sheets of spindle cells with little intervening stroma
  - This growth pattern closely resembles monophasic synovial sarcoma
- **Epithelioid growth pattern**
  - Sheets or nests of round, epithelioid cells with round nuclei
  - This pattern may be confused for melanoma and metastatic carcinoma
- **Angiofibromatous pattern**
  - Large dilated vessels are seen surrounded by dense collagenous tissue
  - Advanced cases may show extensive areas of sclerosis and collagenization
- **Unusual stromal changes**
  - Stromal calcification, metaplastic bone formation, cartilaginous differentiation
  - Extensive degeneration of collagen simulating tumor necrosis
  - Cystic degeneration of the stroma
  - Hemorrhage and necrosis
  - Stromal myxoid changes may be prominent and extensive
  - Irregular stellate deposits of dense collagen (so-called amianthoid fibers)

Cytologic Features

- Spindle cells are usually small and bland appearing with evenly dispersed chromatin and absent or inconspicuous nucleoli
- Mitotic activity is generally very low (< 3 per 10 HPF)
- Giant cells of osteoclast-type or multinucleated tumor cells may be seen
- Malignant cases may show marked nuclear pleomorphism and high mitotic activity
- Cells may rarely adopt round, epithelioid appearance with abundant rim of eosinophilic cytoplasm

Ancillary Techniques

- Immunohistochemistry
  - Tumors cells are strongly positive for CD34, Bcl-2, and vimentin
  - Tumor cells are positive for CD99
  - Tumor cells are generally negative for cytokeratins, SMA, desmin, S100 protein, and other differentiation markers
- Electron microscopy
  - Limited role in diagnosis
  - Ultrastructural features of fibroblastic cells with dendritic cytoplasmic prolongations
- Cytogenetics
  - No known recurrent cytogenetic abnormalities
- Molecular pathology
  - So far plays no role for diagnosis
  - No distinctive alterations have been demonstrated to date

SOLITARY FIBROUS TUMOR/FIBROSARCOMA

Immunohistochemistry

Antibody	Reactivity	Staining Pattern	Comment
CD34	Positive	Cytoplasmic	Stains 60-90% of cases
Bcl-2	Positive	Cytoplasmic	Stains 90-100% of cases
CD99	Positive	Cytoplasmic	Stains 60-70% of cases
Vimentin	Positive	Cytoplasmic	Stains 100% of cases
AE1/AE3	Negative	Not applicable	Should not be positive in these tumors
Desmin	Negative	Not applicable	Negative in tumor cells
S100	Negative	Not applicable	Should not be positive in tumor cells
SMAD4	Equivocal	Cytoplasmic	May stain a few cells, particularly in tangentially cut vessel walls

DIFFERENTIAL DIAGNOSIS

Hemangiopericytoma

- Older term used to designate tumors with distinctive branching pattern of vessels
- Term "hemangiopericytoma" has been replaced by "solitary fibrous tumor" as most such cases represent examples of SFT cases
- Hemangiopericytoma and SFT are currently regarded as synonymous terms in soft tissue locations

Synovial Sarcoma

- High cellularity with marked cytologic atypia and variable mitotic activity
- Monotonous spindle cell population with very scant connective tissue stroma
- Tumor cells show focal cytokeratin and EMA positivity
- Show distinctive t(X;18) translocation
- May be very difficult to distinguish from SFT in some cases, requiring molecular studies for confirmation

Peripheral Nerve Sheath Tumors

- Fascicular proliferation composed of spindle cells with wavy nuclei
- Association with neurofibromatosis and with nerve trunks
- S100 protein positivity in spindle cells
- Complex, interdigitating slender dendritic prolongations seen on ultrastructural examination

Spindle Cell Thymoma

- Fascicular spindle cell proliferation separated by broad fibrous bands into lobules
- Usually shows minor component of scattered, small T lymphocytes
- May display rosette-like structures or microcystic growth pattern
- Spindle cells are positive for cytokeratins and negative for CD34

Sarcomatoid Malignant Mesothelioma

- Atypical spindle cell proliferation with marked nuclear pleomorphism and high mitotic activity
- Focal positivity of spindle cells for keratin and calretinin
- Diffuse growth pattern with spread along pleural surface
- Occupational history of previous asbestos exposure

Pleomorphic High-Grade Sarcoma

- Histologic appearance can be indistinguishable from that of malignant solitary fibrous tumors
- Lacks well-preserved areas showing features of solitary fibrous tumors
- Lacks cells positive for CD34 and Bcl-2

DIAGNOSTIC CHECKLIST

Clinically Relevant Pathologic Features

- Well-circumscribed mass in anterior mediastinum
- History of hypoglycemia or clubbing of fingers

Pathologic Interpretation Pearls

- Bland-appearing spindle cell population with variegation of histologic growth patterns within same tumor
- Prominent hemangiopericytomatous growth pattern admixed with other growth patterns
- Prominent vascularity of stroma with perivascular hyalinization and sclerosis
- Striking, "rope-like" linear deposition of keloidal collagen flanking the spindle cells

SELECTED REFERENCES

1. Eguchi T et al: A solitary fibrous tumor arising from the thymus. Interact Cardiovasc Thorac Surg. 11(3):362-3, 2010
2. Suehisa H et al: Solitary fibrous tumor of the mediastinum. Gen Thorac Cardiovasc Surg. 58(4):205-8, 2010
3. De Raet J et al: Malignant giant solitary fibrous tumor of the mediastinum. J Thorac Oncol. 3(9):1068-70, 2008
4. Gannon BR et al: Solitary fibrous tumor of the anterior mediastinum: a rare extrapleural neoplasm. Tumori. 93(5):508-10, 2007
5. Iwata T et al: Solitary fibrous tumor of the thymus with local invasiveness and pleural dissemination: report of a case. Ann Thorac Cardiovasc Surg. 13(3):198-202, 2007
6. Shiraishi T et al: Mediastinal solitary fibrous tumor: report of a case with direct invasion to the trachea. Thorac Cardiovasc Surg. 52(2):110-2, 2004
7. Marchevsky AM et al: Mediastinal epithelioid solitary fibrous tumor. Arch Pathol Lab Med. 127(4):e212-5, 2003
8. Moran CA et al: The spectrum of histologic growth patterns in benign and malignant fibrous tumors of the pleura. Semin Diagn Pathol. 9(2):169-80, 1992
9. Witkin GB et al: Solitary fibrous tumor of the mediastinum. A report of 14 cases. Am J Surg Pathol. 13(7):547-57, 1989

Fascicular Growth Patterns

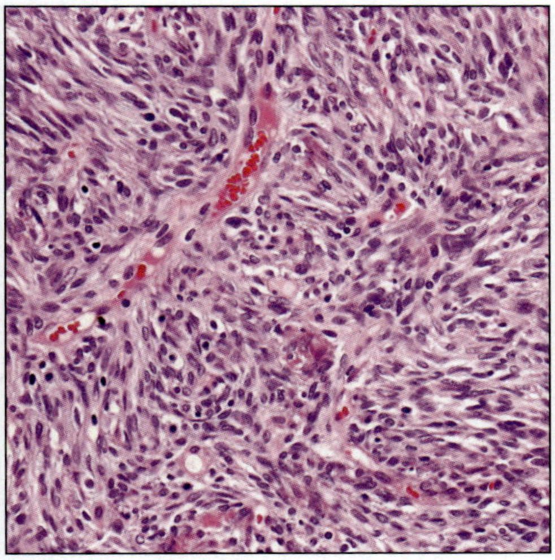

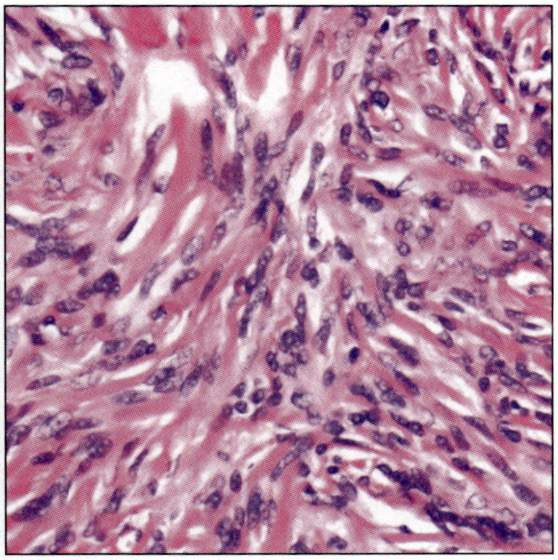

(Left) *Solitary fibrous tumor of the mediastinum shows a vague storiform pattern with overlapping fascicles of spindle cells that appear to emanate from a central spoke. The morphologic appearance of this tumor is reminiscent of a "fibrohistiocytic" neoplasm.* ***(Right)*** *High magnification of a solitary fibrous tumor of the mediastinum with a storiform growth pattern shows a bland-appearing spindle cell population separated by thin linear strands of keloidal collagen.*

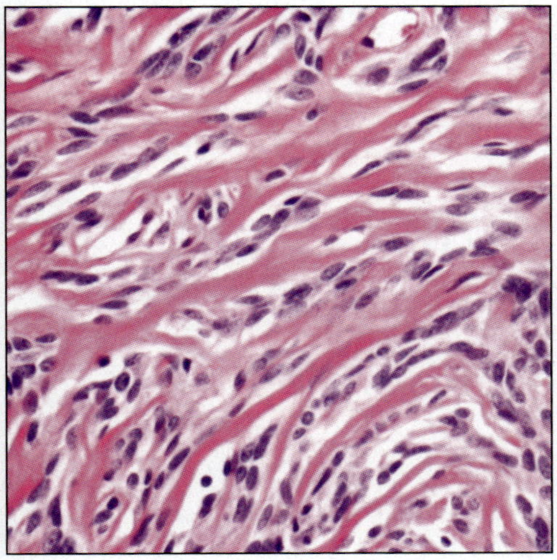

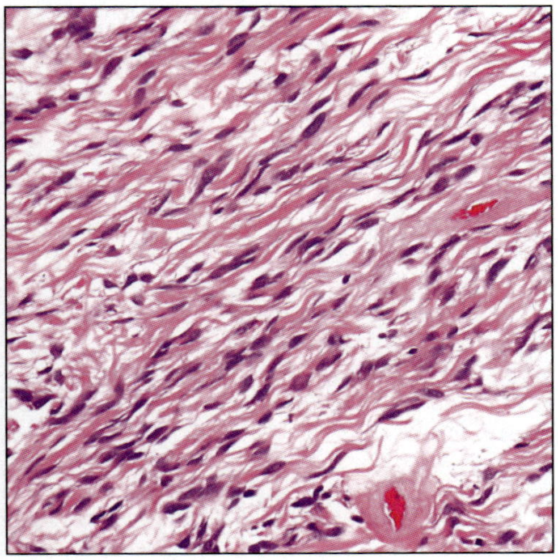

(Left) *High magnification of solitary fibrous tumor of the mediastinum shows characteristic histologic appearance composed of bland spindle cells flanked by thin, rope-like strands of collagen disposed in parallel linear arrays.* ***(Right)*** *Solitary fibrous tumor of the anterior mediastinum shows fascicles of spindle cells lying within loose connective tissue stroma. Notice the prominent wavy appearance of the spindle cells, reminiscent of that commonly observed in schwannian tumors.*

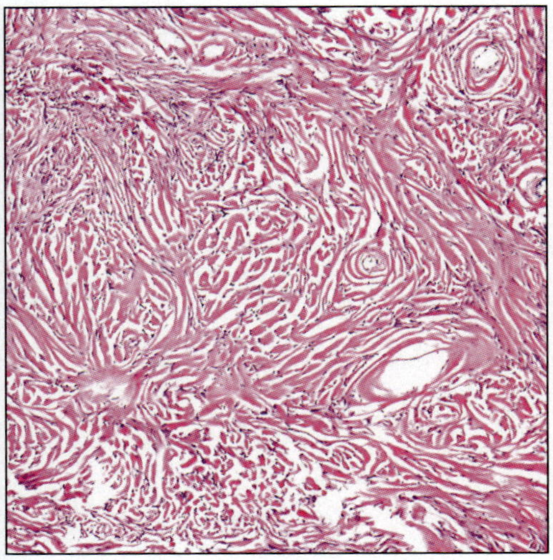

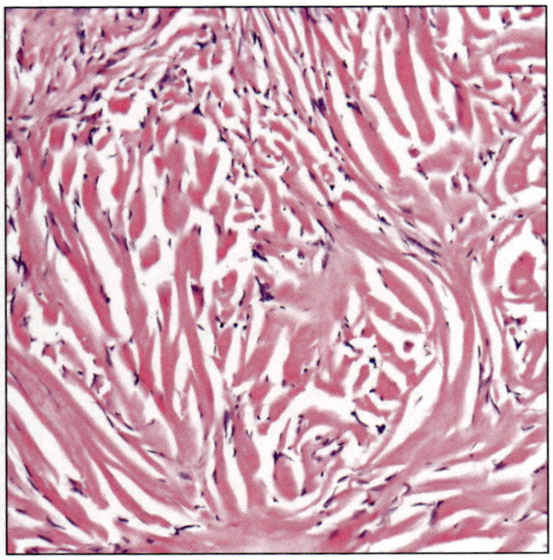

(Left) *Characteristic low-power appearance of a solitary fibrous tumor shows parallel arrays of thin, rope-like strands of keloidal collagen flanked by small spindle cells. This has often been referred to as the "patternless" pattern of growth in these tumors.* ***(Right)*** *High magnification of a solitary fibrous tumor shows a "patternless" pattern characterized by parallel, linear arrays of thin keloidal collagen separating the tumor cells. This pattern of growth is fairly typical for this tumor.*

Other Growth Patterns

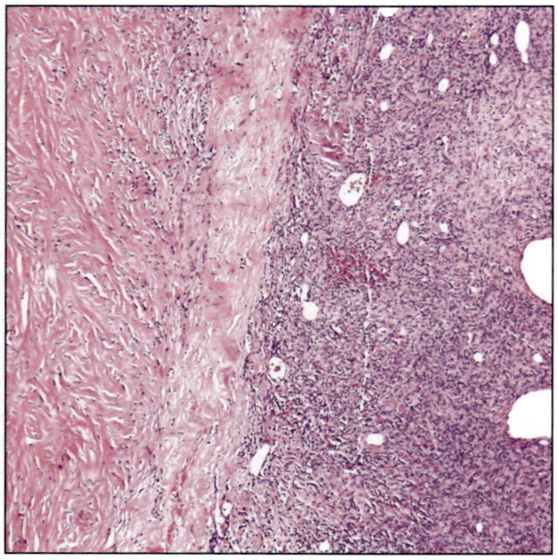

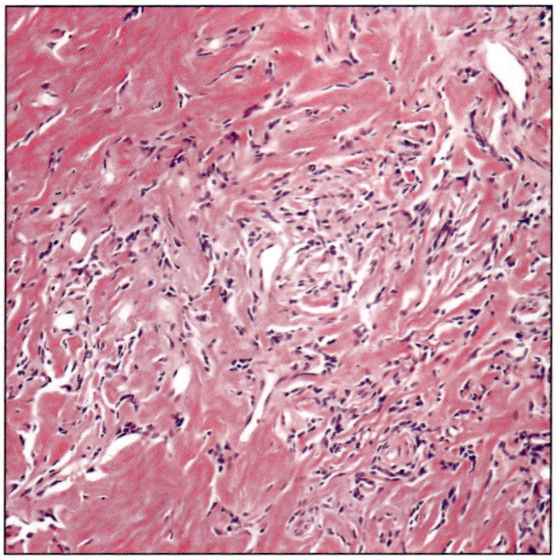

(Left) *Scanning magnification in solitary fibrous tumor of the mediastinum shows an abrupt transition between the hypercellular area (right) and hypocellular, sclerotic area (left). Alternating cellular and hypocellular areas is a common theme in these tumors.* ***(Right)*** *Solitary fibrous tumor of the mediastinum shows a scant spindle cell population admixed with areas of stromal sclerosis. Notice the irregular distribution of the areas of sclerosis with haphazard arrangement of the spindle cells.*

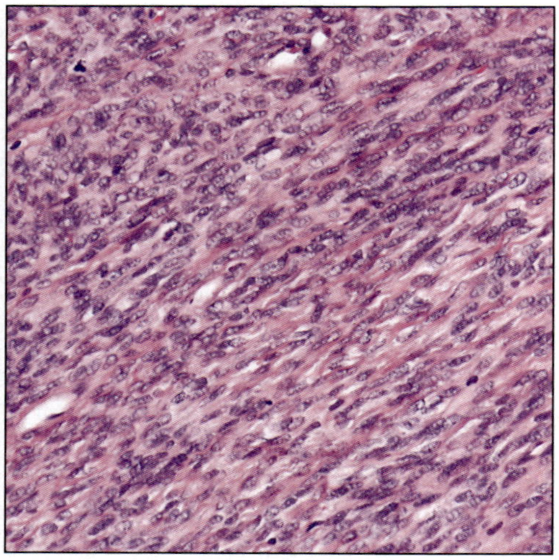

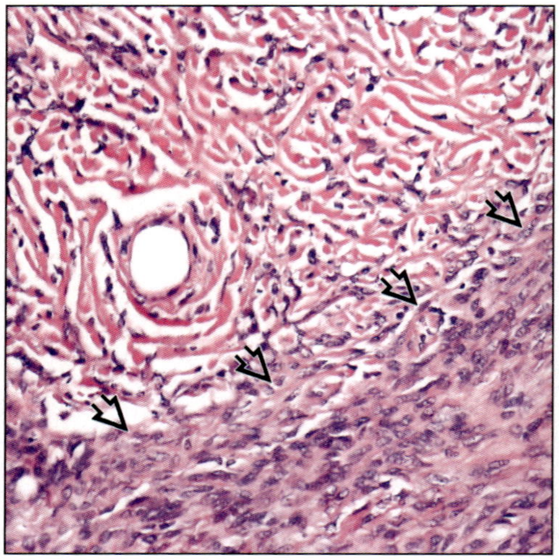

(Left) *Solitary fibrous tumor of the mediastinum shows a solid, hypercellular pattern of growth with sheets of monotonous spindle cells with little intervening stroma. Tumors with this appearance can be easily mistaken for synovial sarcoma.* ***(Right)*** *High magnification of a solitary fibrous tumor with a solid hypercellular growth pattern shows a transition with a more classic sclerosing pattern (top) displaying the characteristic rope-like strands of collagen.*

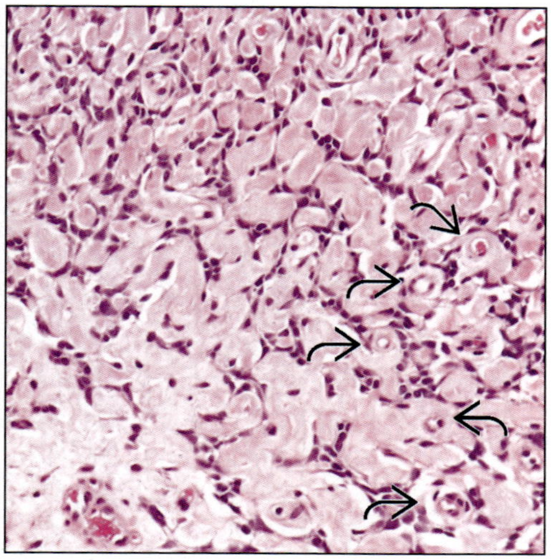

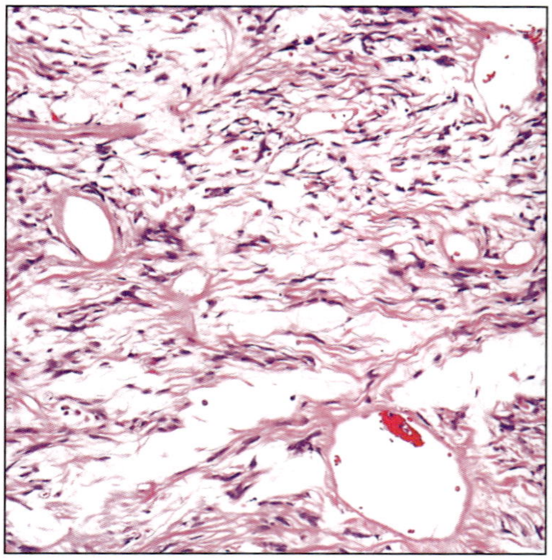

(Left) *Solitary fibrous tumor of the mediastinum shows a micronodular pattern of sclerosis with dense collagen deposition around small vessels . The spindle tumor cells appear compressed and evenly dispersed around these micronodular structures.* ***(Right)*** *Solitary fibrous tumor of the mediastinum shows prominent myxoid stromal deposition. Tumors with this morphologic appearance may be mistaken for myxofibrosarcoma, myxoid neurofibroma, or myxoid MFH.*

Other Growth Patterns

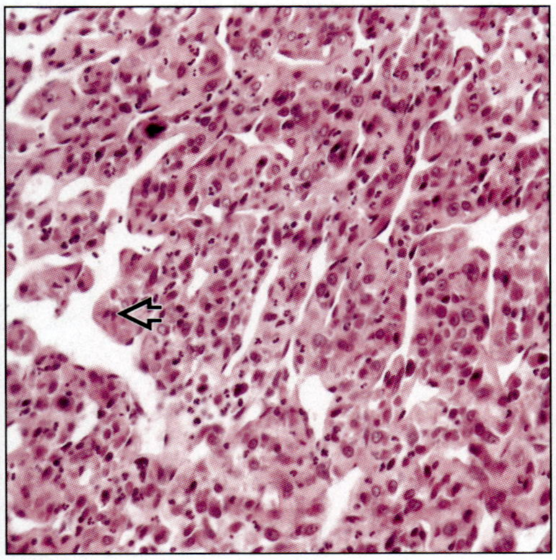

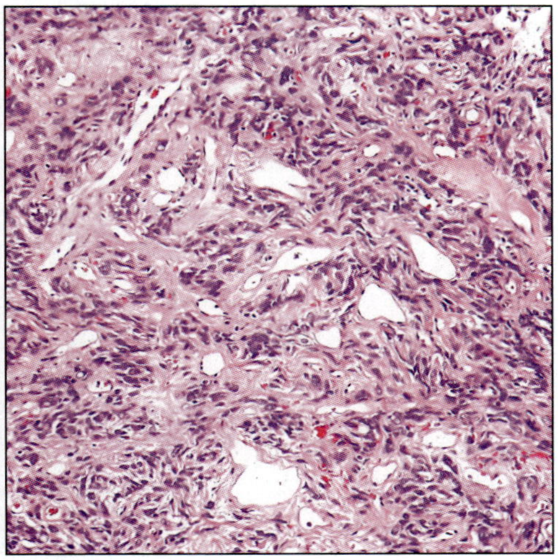

(Left) *Solitary fibrous tumor of the mediastinum shows a striking hemangiopericytic pattern of growth, with numerous slit-like vessels that appear to show complex branching of their lumens. Some of the vessels may adopt an antler-like (or "staghorn") configuration* ⇨. ***(Right)*** *Solitary fibrous tumor of the mediastinum shows prominent hemangiopericytic pattern of growth characterized by numerous small vessels with open lumens surrounded by a dense spindle cell population.*

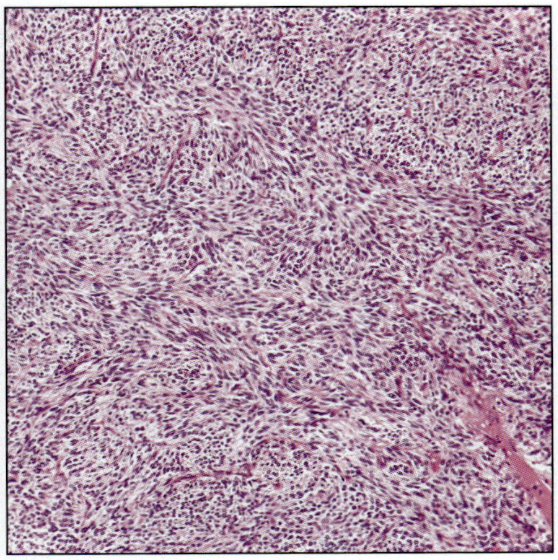

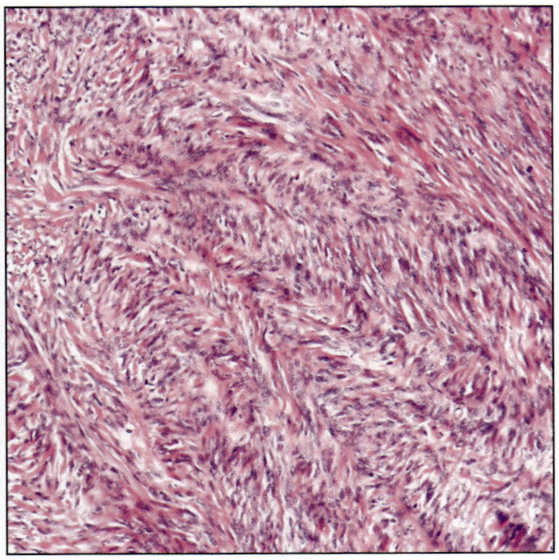

(Left) *Solitary fibrous tumor of the mediastinum with prominent "herringbone" pattern of growth shows a dense population of spindle cells with short fascicles that appear to be branching off from central spokes.* ***(Right)*** *High magnification of solitary fibrous tumor of the mediastinum shows a prominent "herringbone" pattern of growth. Tumors with these features can resemble other soft tissue sarcomas such as malignant peripheral nerve sheath tumors and synovial sarcoma.*

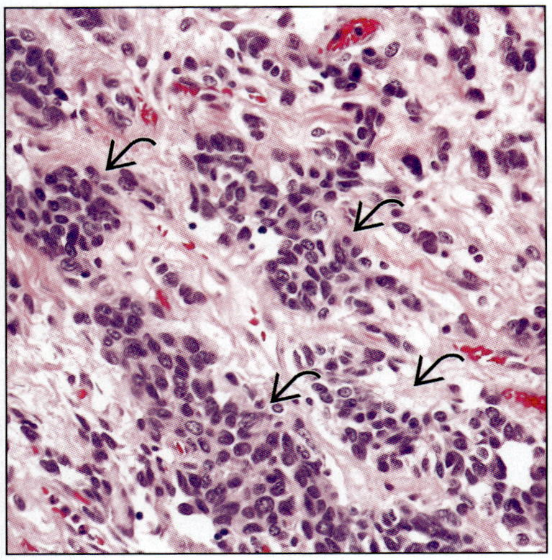

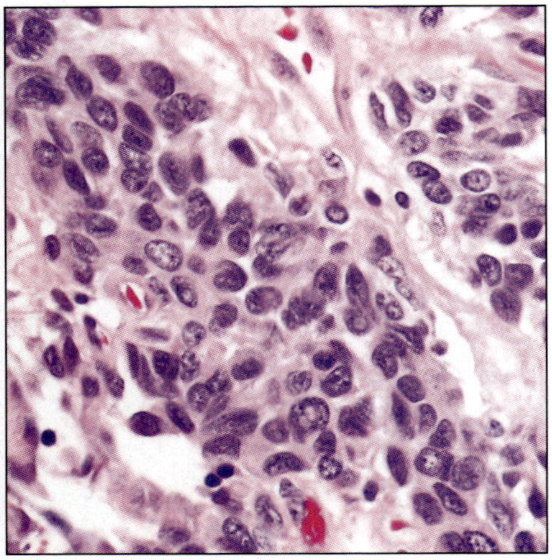

(Left) *Solitary fibrous tumor, epithelioid variant, shows nests of round tumor cells with large, round nuclei surrounded by a rim of lightly eosinophilic cytoplasm* ↗. *This histologic appearance is quite rare in solitary fibrous tumor and may cause confusion with a malignant epithelial neoplasm.* ***(Right)*** *High magnification of solitary fibrous tumor of the mediastinum with epithelioid features shows nests of large epithelioid cells with large, round nuclei surrounded by eosinophilic cytoplasm.*

Immunohistochemical Features

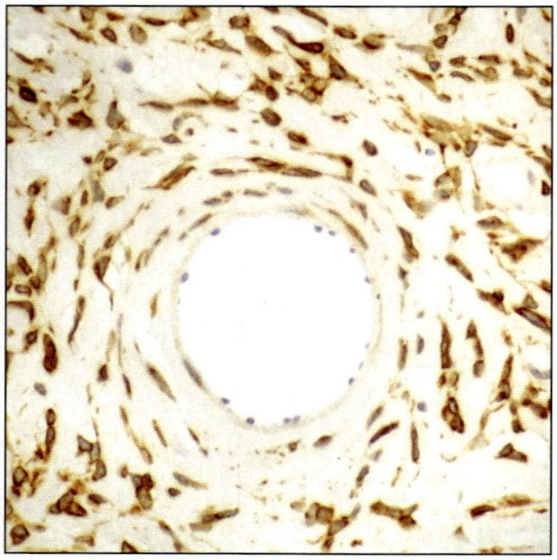
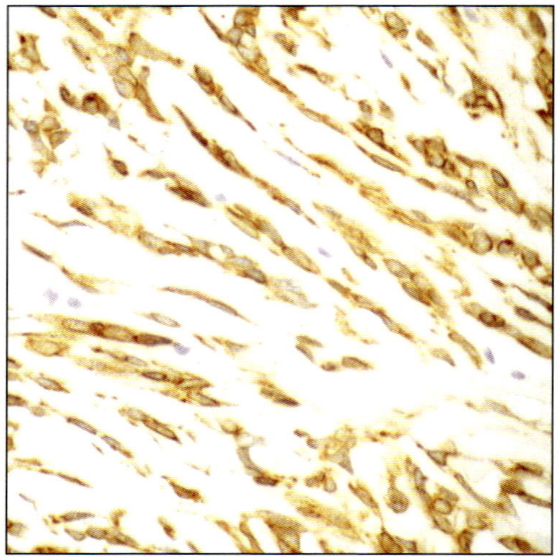

(Left) *Immunohistochemical staining for CD34 in solitary fibrous tumor of the mediastinum shows positivity of the spindle cells in a targetoid distribution around a dilated, small blood vessel.* ***(Right)*** *Immunohistochemical staining for CD34 in solitary fibrous tumor of the mediastinum shows positivity in parallel arrays of spindle cells corresponding to the cells that are seen flanking the rope-like strands of collagen characteristic of this tumor.*

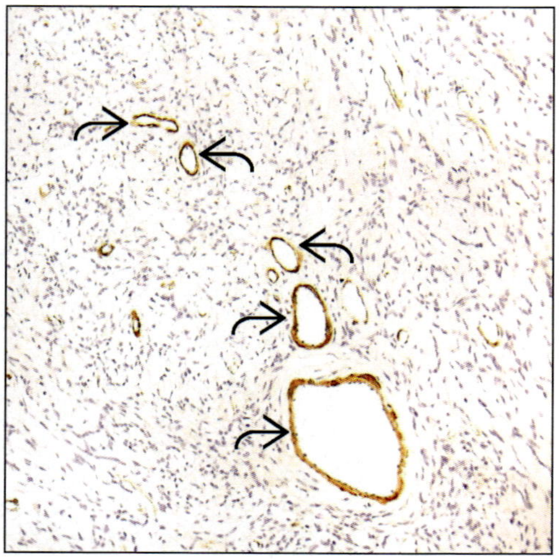
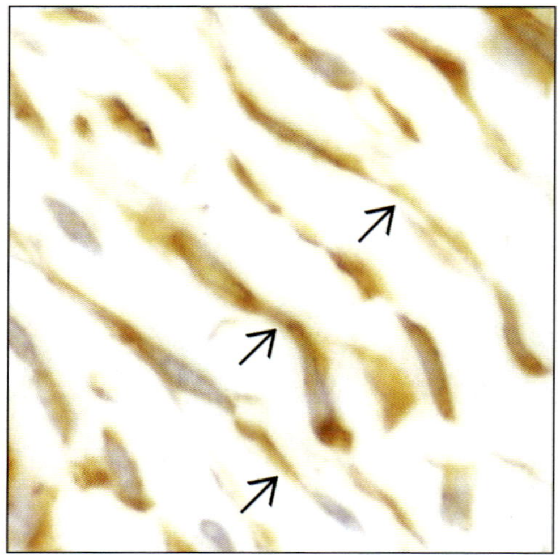

(Left) *Immunohistochemical staining for smooth muscle actin (SMA) in solitary fibrous tumor of the mediastinum shows strong positivity in vessel walls but negative staining in the spindle tumor cells.* ***(Right)*** *High magnification shows immunohistochemical staining of the spindle cells in solitary fibrous tumor of the mediastinum for CD34. Notice the slender dendritic cytoplasmic prolongations that taper off gradually and interconnect with the cell processes from adjoining cells.*

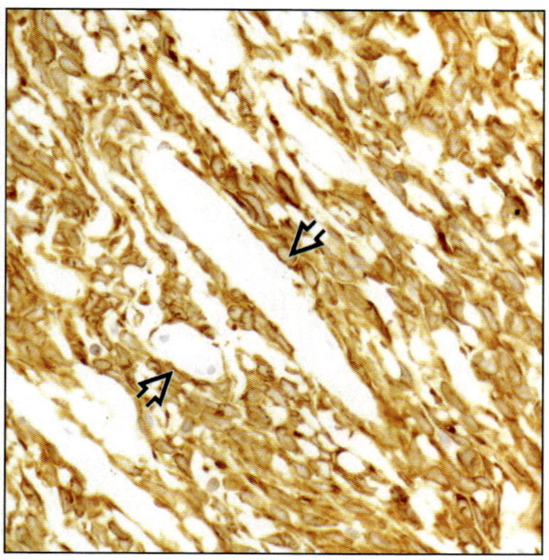
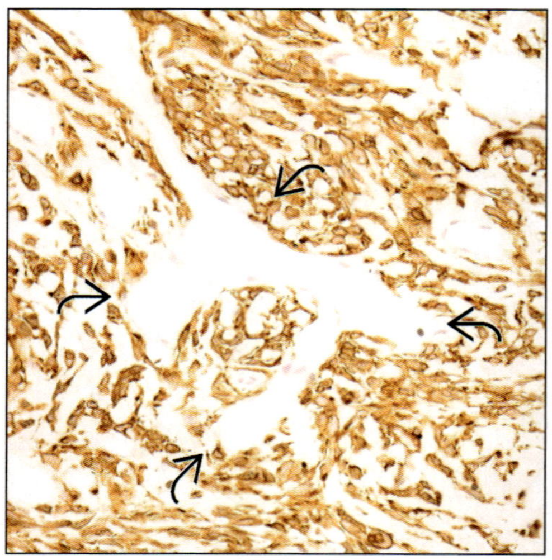

(Left) *Immunohistochemical staining for BCL2 oncogene in solitary fibrous tumor of the mediastinum shows strong cytoplasmic positivity in the majority of the tumor cells for this marker. Notice the empty vessel lumens and absence of staining of vascular endothelium.* ***(Right)*** *Immunohistochemical staining for BCL2 oncogene in solitary fibrous tumor of the mediastinum shows the branching, antler-like blood vessel outlined by the positive tumor cells.*

Other Features

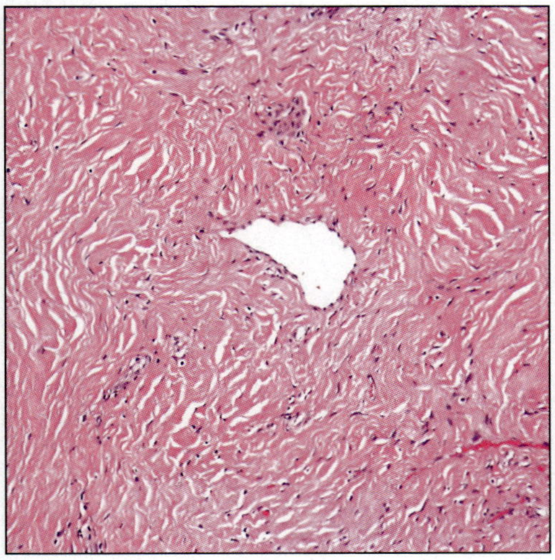

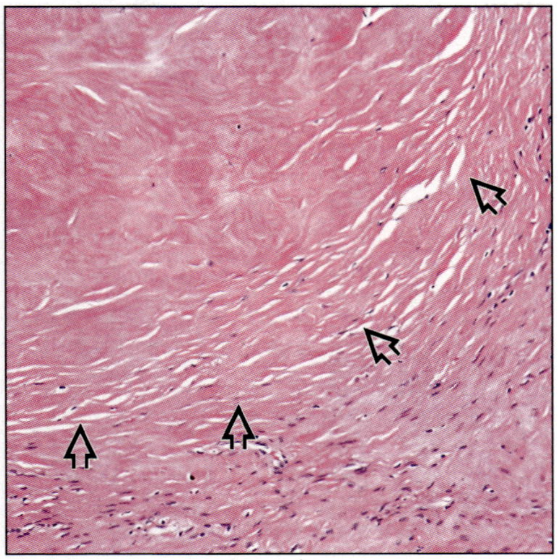

(Left) *Advanced stage of sclerosis in solitary fibrous tumor of the mediastinum shows abundant collagen deposition. Notice the cells are compressed by the collagen and appear as small, round dots in the background rather than spindle cells.* ***(Right)*** *Solitary fibrous tumor of the mediastinum shows a more advanced degree of stromal sclerosis, with dense, homogeneous acellular areas resembling amyloid deposits ➢. Notice the residual scattered spindle cells (bottom).*

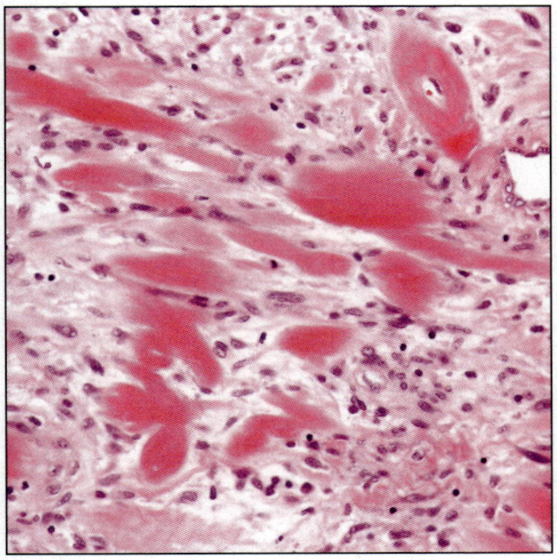

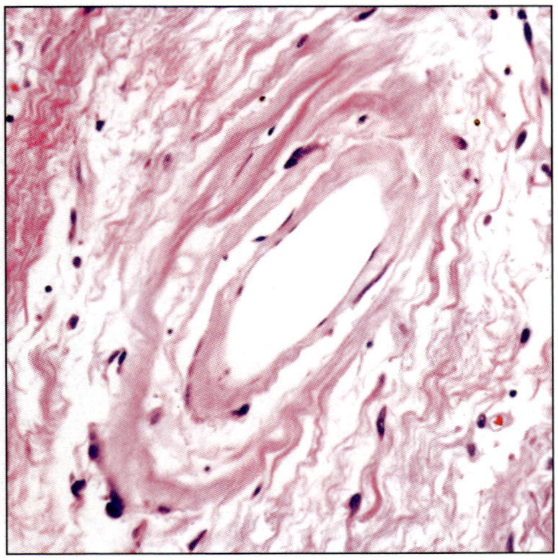

(Left) *Solitary fibrous tumor of the mediastinum shows focal deposits of thick, keloidal collagen bundles. Extensive deposition of collagen fibers in the stroma may result in a histologic picture reminiscent of sclerosing mediastinitis.* ***(Right)*** *Solitary fibrous tumor of the mediastinum shows dilated vessels with prominent perivascular hyalinization imparting the lesion with an angiofibromatous appearance. Foci like this are commonly observed in areas of stromal sclerosis.*

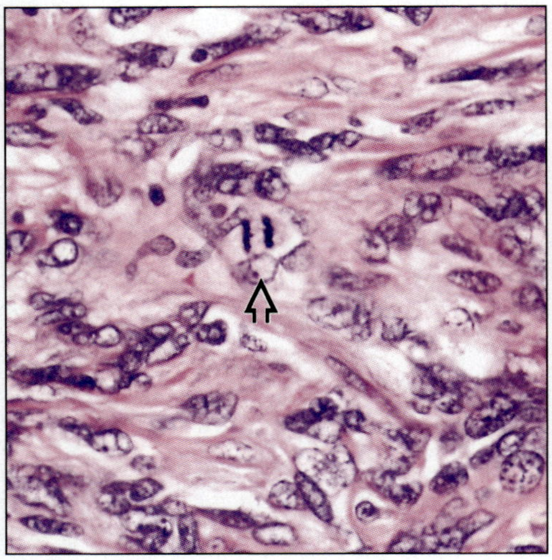

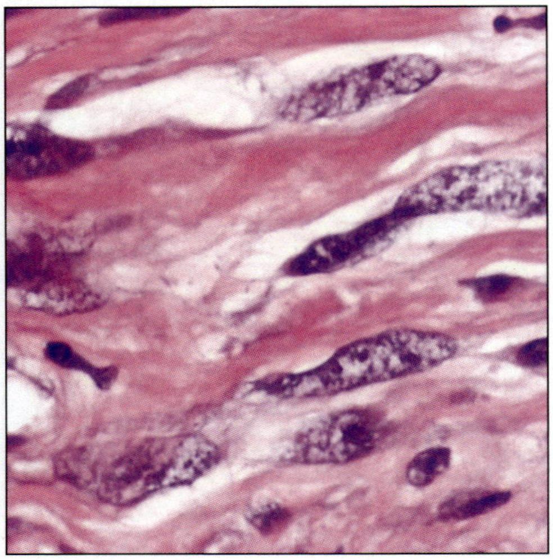

(Left) *High magnification in a solitary fibrous tumor of the mediastinum shows spindle cell population with minimal nuclear pleomorphism. Scattered mitoses can be commonly observed ➢ but are usually < 3 per 10 HPF.* ***(Right)*** *Higher magnification in a solitary fibrous tumor of the mediastinum shows bland-appearing spindle cells embedded in a collagenous stroma. The cells show features indistinguishable from those of conventional fibroblasts.*

SOLITARY FIBROUS TUMOR/FIBROSARCOMA

Malignant Solitary Fibrous Tumor

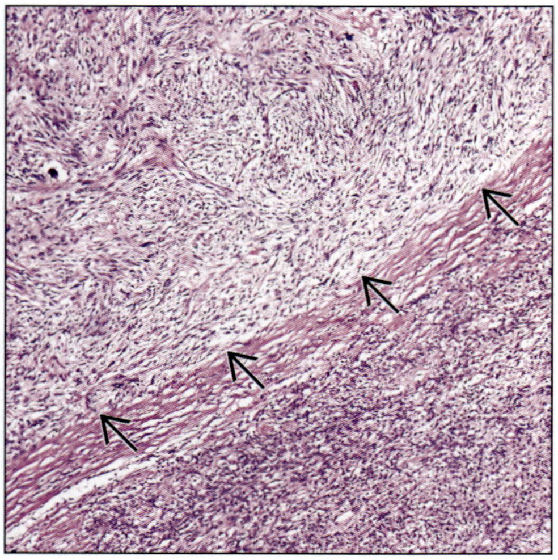
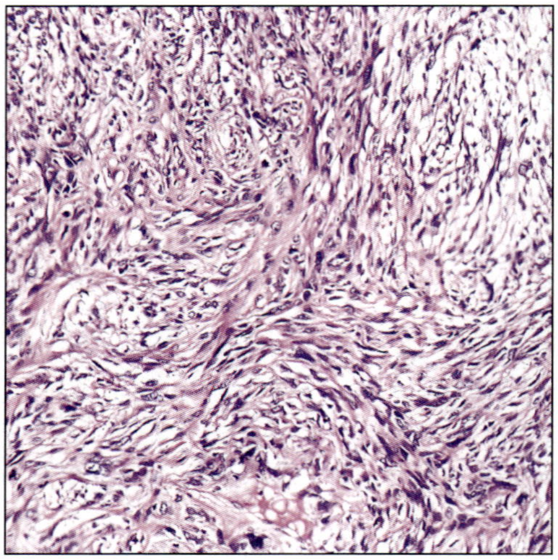

(Left) *Scanning magnification of malignant solitary fibrous tumor of the mediastinum shows transitions between the well-differentiated area in the bottom and a high-grade poorly differentiated area → at the top containing more pronounced nuclear pleomorphism and increased mitotic activity.* ***(Right)*** *Malignant solitary fibrous tumor of the mediastinum shows an area with a striking storiform pattern simulating the appearance of a malignant fibrous histiocytoma (MFH).*

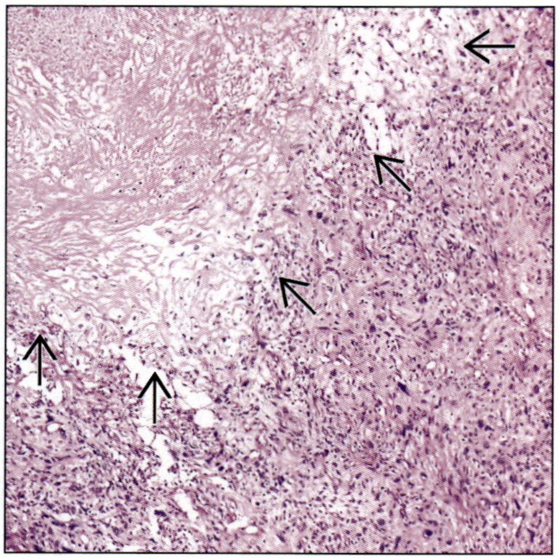
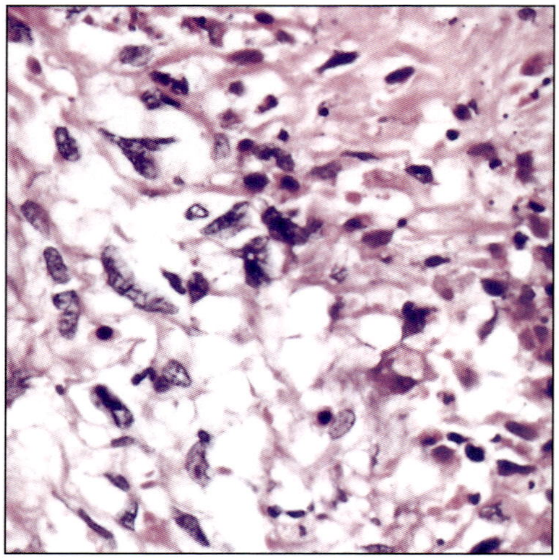

(Left) *Malignant solitary fibrous tumor of the mediastinum shows an area of tumor necrosis → with irregular, jagged borders, surrounded by a highly atypical spindle and pleomorphic tumor cell population.* ***(Right)*** *Higher magnification shows the interphase between the tumor and a focus of necrosis in a malignant solitary fibrous tumor of the mediastinum. Notice the marked cytologic atypia of the spindle tumor cells displaying irregular, hyperchromatic nuclei.*

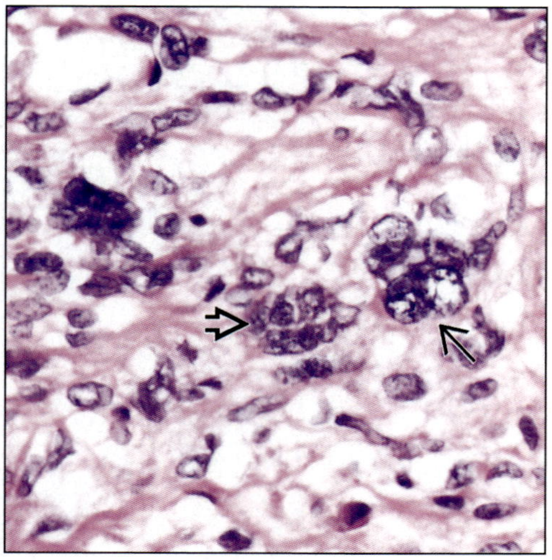
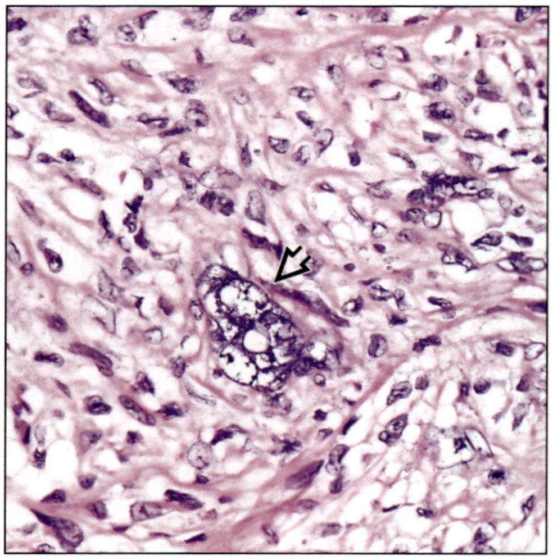

(Left) *Marked nuclear pleomorphism is displayed by the tumor cells in this example of malignant solitary fibrous tumor of the mediastinum. Notice that some of the cells show multilobated nuclei →, while others are multinucleated ⇨.* ***(Right)*** *Malignant solitary fibrous tumor of the mediastinum shows an atypical spindle cell population embedded in collagenous stroma, containing scattered large, pleomorphic tumor cells with bizarre nuclei that display a vesicular chromatin pattern ⇨.*

Malignant Solitary Fibrous Tumor

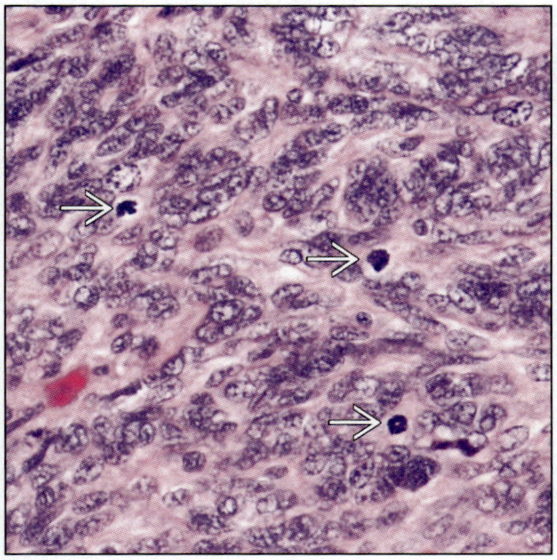
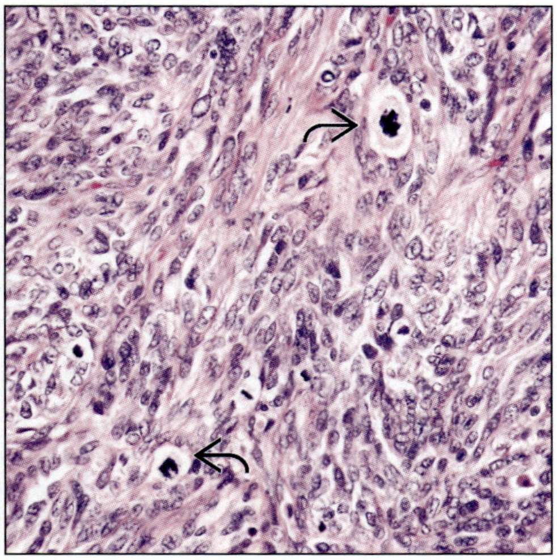

(Left) *Malignant solitary fibrous tumor of the mediastinum shows a monotonous, highly cellular spindle tumor cell population that closely resembles a monophasic synovial sarcoma. Notice the frequent mitoses scattered throughout the field ➔.* ***(Right)*** *Malignant solitary fibrous tumor of the mediastinum shows a highly cellular atypical spindle cell population adopting a fascicular pattern of growth and containing scattered abnormal mitotic figures ⮫.*

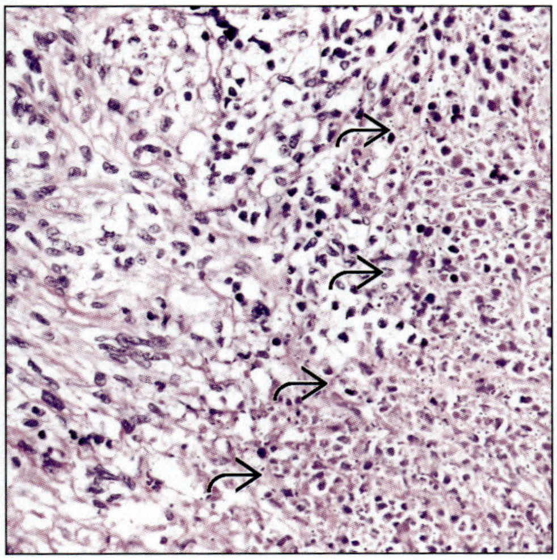
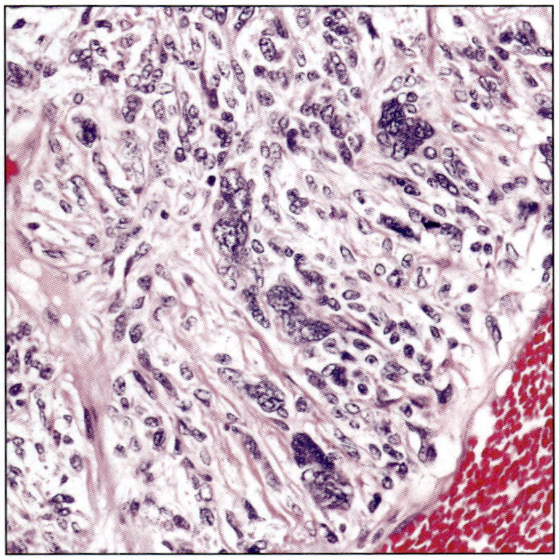

(Left) *Malignant solitary fibrous tumor of the mediastinum shows atypical tumor cell population (left) containing areas of coagulation necrosis ⮫.* ***(Right)*** *Malignant solitary fibrous tumor of the mediastinum shows an atypical spindle tumor cell population admixed with numerous larger, bizarre, multilobated and multinucleated tumor cells. The appearance of this tumor is reminiscent of that of a pleomorphic high-grade sarcoma (a.k.a. malignant fibrous histiocytoma).*

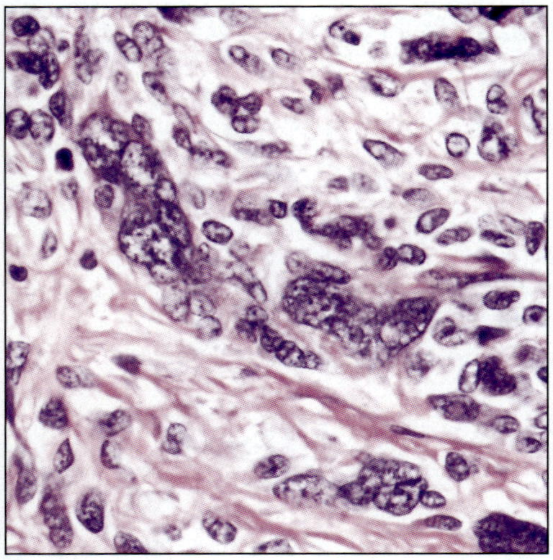
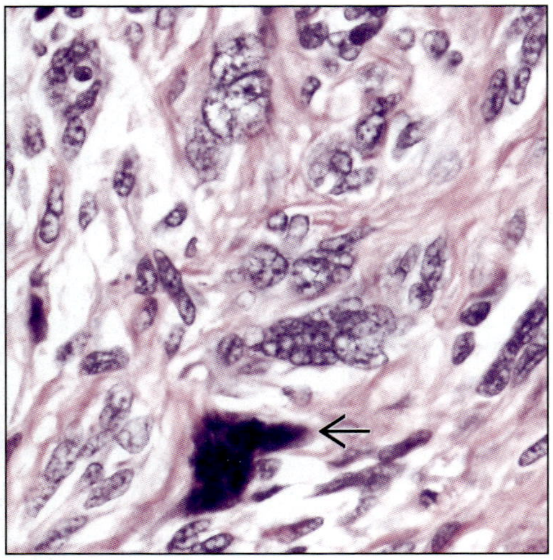

(Left) *Malignant solitary fibrous tumor of the mediastinum shows multiple large tumor cells with multiple hyperchromatic nuclei. Contrast this with the smaller, bland-appearing cells observed in the background.* ***(Right)*** *Malignant solitary fibrous tumor of the mediastinum shows atypical multinucleated tumor cells scattered between the atypical spindle cells. Notice the multinucleated tumor cell at the bottom with darkly stained basophilic nuclei ➔.*

EPITHELIOID HEMANGIOENDOTHELIOMA

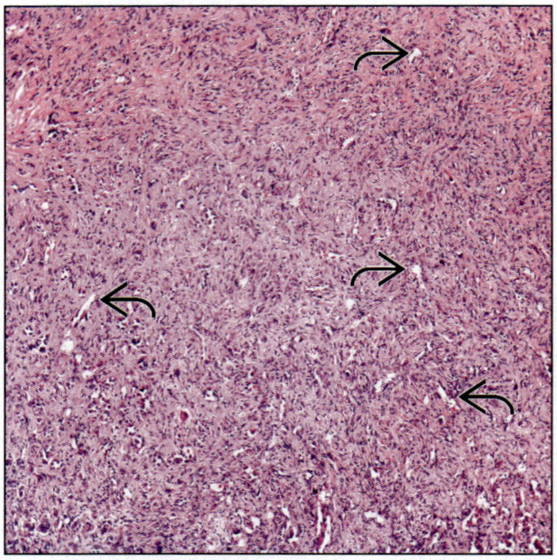

Mediastinal EH displays a solid neoplastic cellular proliferation. However, note the presence, even at this magnification, of several slits ⇾ that may represent vascular spaces.

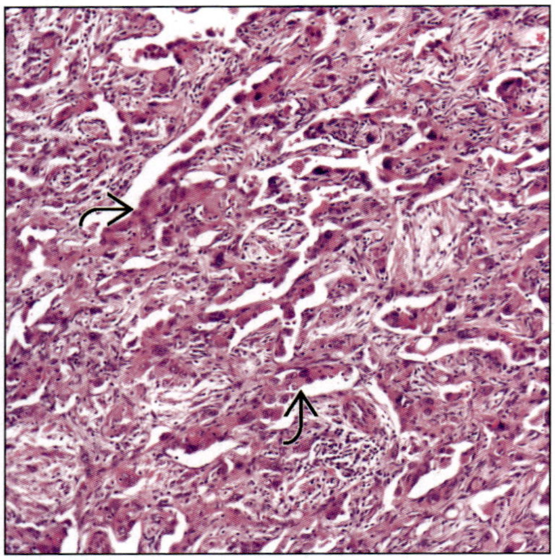

High-power view shows a mediastinal EH in which the tumor shows prominent vascular channels lined by atypical endothelial cells ⇾. This feature is typical for the diagnosis of EH.

TERMINOLOGY

Abbreviations

- Epithelioid hemangioendothelioma (EH)

Definitions

- Vascular neoplasm of intermediate malignant potential

ETIOLOGY/PATHOGENESIS

Etiology

- Although well known to be tumor of vascular origin, its etiology is still unknown

CLINICAL ISSUES

Epidemiology

- Incidence
  - Unusual tumor in mediastinal compartment
  - May account for < 1% of all mediastinal tumors
- Age
  - Wide range from younger patients < 20 years old to older patients > 60 years old
- Gender
  - No apparent gender predilection
    - However, in some series of cases there has been slight male predominance
- Ethnicity
  - No apparent ethnic predilection

Presentation

- Chest pain
- Cough
- Dyspnea
- Asymptomatic

Treatment

- Surgical approaches
  - Complete resection of tumor
- Adjuvant therapy
  - Radiation &/or chemotherapy may be considered depending on extent of tumor at time of diagnosis

Prognosis

- Tumor may follow protracted course with recurrences
- In some cases, may follow rapid course with metastatic disease within thoracic cavity or outside of thorax

MACROSCOPIC FEATURES

General Features

- Well circumscribed, encapsulated
- Some tumors may be locally infiltrative

Size

- Tumors may vary in size from 3 cm to > 10 cm in diameter

MICROSCOPIC PATHOLOGY

Histologic Features

- Nests and cords of medium-sized round to oval epithelioid cells
- Inconspicuous nucleoli
- Cytoplasmic vacuolization
- Rare mitotic activity with no more than 1 x 10 HPF
- Basophilic myxoid matrix resembling hyaline cartilage
- Collagenized stroma
- Necrosis is rare, and when present, it is focal

DIFFERENTIAL DIAGNOSIS

Chordoma

- May show chondromyxoid matrix
- Negative for vascular markers (CD34, CD31, Factor VIII)

EPITHELIOID HEMANGIOENDOTHELIOMA

Key Facts

Terminology

- Epithelioid hemangioendothelioma (EH)

Clinical Issues

- Incidence
  - Unusual tumor in mediastinal compartment
  - May account for < 1% of all mediastinal tumors
  - May affect individuals ranging from 20 to > 60 years of age
  - Some series have reported slight male predominance for occurrence of this tumor
- Symptoms
  - Chest pain
  - Cough
  - Dyspnea
  - Asymptomatic
- Prognosis
  - Tumor may follow protracted course with recurrences
  - In some cases, it may follow rapid course with metastatic disease in or outside of thorax

Top Differential Diagnoses

- Chordoma
- Myxoid chondrosarcoma
- Seminoma
- Thymic carcinoma

Diagnostic Checklist

- Cords of epithelioid cells
- Low mitotic rate of no more than 1-2 x 10 HPF
- Chondromyxoid stroma
- Absent necrosis, and if present, it would be focal

Immunohistochemistry

Antibody	Reactivity	Staining Pattern	Comment
CD31	Positive	Cytoplasmic	Strong reaction in epithelioid cells
FVIIIRAg	Positive	Cytoplasmic	Strong reaction in epithelioid cells
Vimentin	Positive	Cytoplasmic	
CD34	Positive	Cytoplasmic	Only in a few cases, and it is focal
CK8/18/CAM5.2	Negative		It may be focally positive in some cases
Actin-HHF-35	Negative		
Desmin	Negative		
S100	Negative		

Myxoid Chondrosarcoma

- May have presence of well-formed cartilage while EH does not
- Positive for S100 protein while EH is not
- Negative for vascular markers

Seminoma

- Unusual for seminomas to show chondromyxoid matrix
- Positive for keratin and PLAP while that would be unusual for EH
- Seminomas are negative for vascular markers

Thymic Carcinoma

- Shows more cellular atypia and mitotic activity than EH
- Generally negative for vascular markers and positive for epithelial markers, in contrast to EH

DIAGNOSTIC CHECKLIST

Clinically Relevant Pathologic Features

- Mitotic rate
  - In EH, mitotic rate is low or absent (1 x 10 HPF)
- Cytoplasmic features
  - In some cases, it is possible to identify presence of red cells being engulfed by epithelioid cells

Pathologic Interpretation Pearls

- Cords of epithelioid cells
- Low mitotic rate of no more than 1-2 x 10 HPF
- Chondromyxoid stroma
- Absent necrosis, and if present, it would be focal

SELECTED REFERENCES

1. Suster S et al: Epithelioid hemangioendothelioma of the anterior mediastinum. Clinicopathologic, immunohistochemical, and ultrastructural analysis of 12 cases. Am J Surg Pathol. 18(9):871-81, 1994
2. Weidner N: Atypical tumor of the mediastinum: epithelioid hemangioendothelioma containing metaplastic bone and osteoclastlike giant cells. Ultrastruct Pathol. 15(4-5):481-8, 1991
3. Lamovec J et al: Epithelioid hemangioendothelioma of the anterior mediastinum with osteoclast-like giant cells. Light microscopic, immunohistochemical, and electron microscopic study. Am J Clin Pathol. 93(6):813-7, 1990

EPITHELIOID HEMANGIOENDOTHELIOMA

Microscopic Features

(Left) *Mediastinal EH shows a solid neoplastic cellular proliferation in which there are several vascular channels* → *that are readily visible, which should raise the suspicion of a vascular neoplasm.* ***(Right)*** *Mediastinal EH shows a prominent spindle cell component with some vascular spaces* →*. These particular features may be seen in other neoplasms not necessarily of vascular origin.*

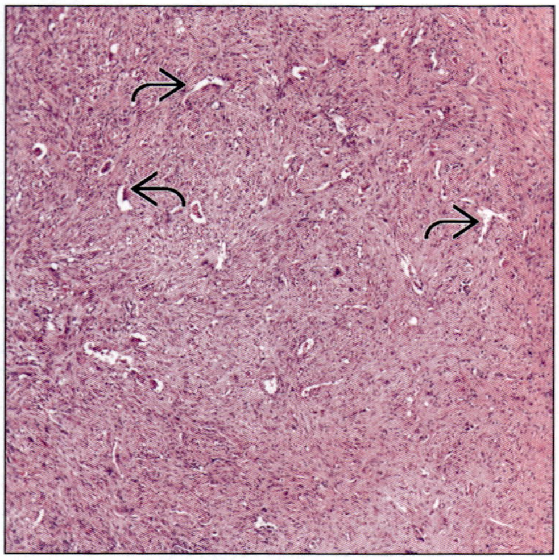

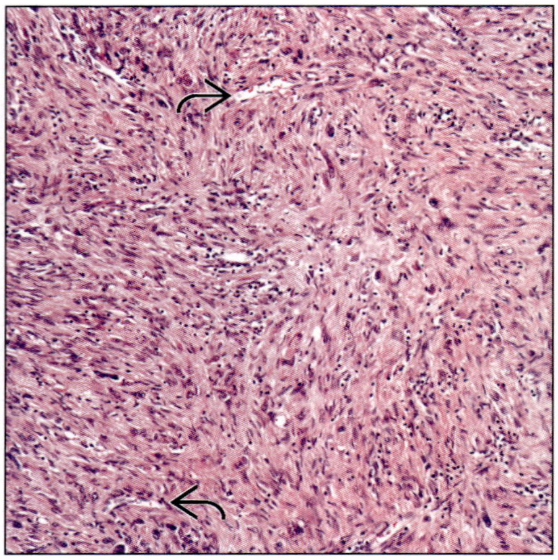

(Left) *Mediastinal EH is shown in which the neoplastic cellular proliferation is embedded in a myxoid or chondromyxoid background* →*. These features, although common in other organs, are not so common in the mediastinum.* ***(Right)*** *Mediastinal EH shows the presence of numerous large multinucleated giant cells* →*. This feature is rather common in mediastinal EH.*

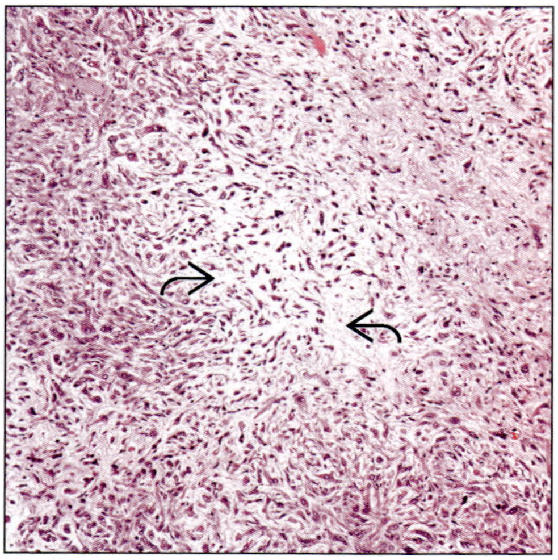

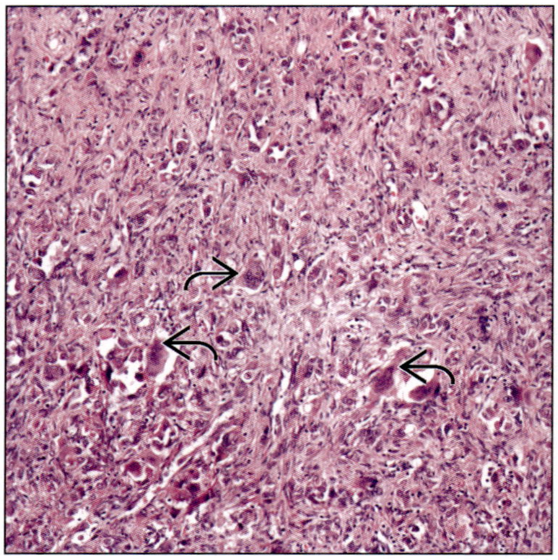

(Left) *Mediastinal EH shows more conventional features of a vascular tumor, namely the presence of anastomosing vascular channels. However, similar features may be seen in angiosarcomas.* ***(Right)*** *Mediastinal EH is shown in which the interanastomosing vascular channels are dissecting fibroconnective tissue. This histological pattern may be seen in other mediastinal tumors.*

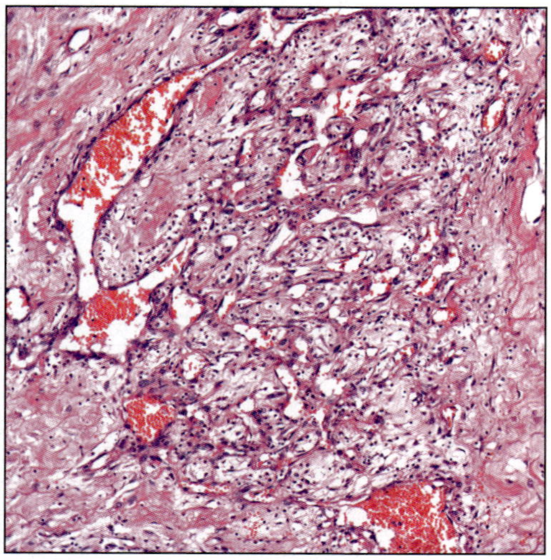

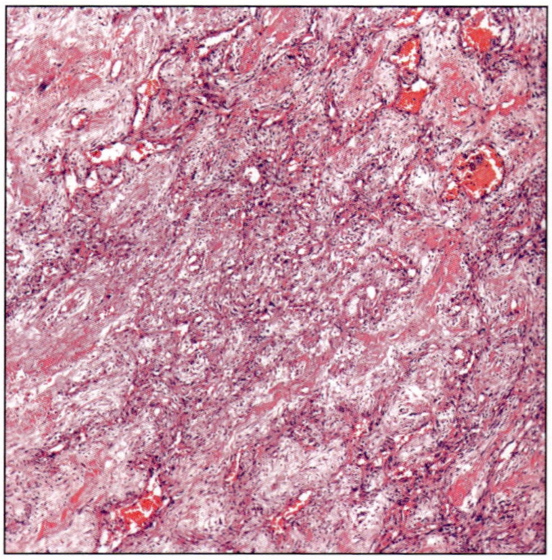

Microscopic Features

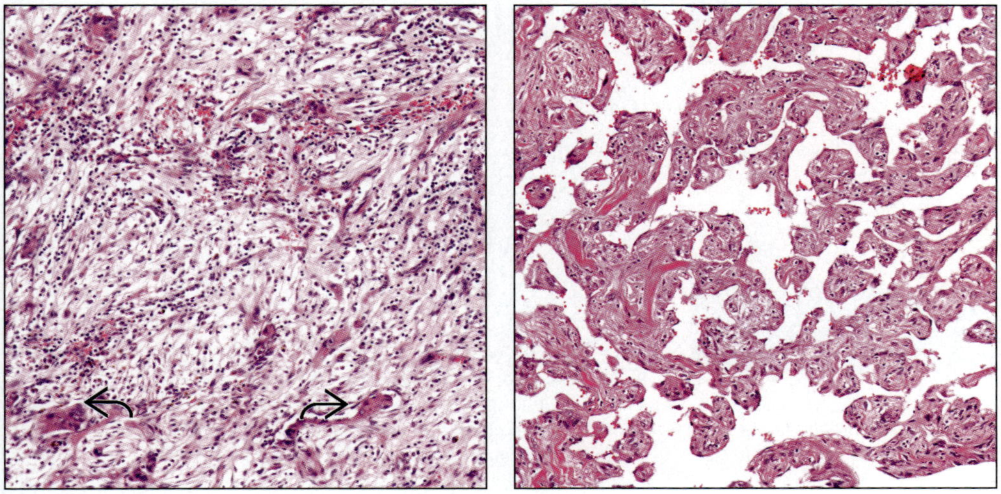

(Left) *Mediastinal EH is shown with prominent loose fibroconnective tissue and inflammatory reaction. Note the presence of vascular channels lined by atypical endothelium ↪.* ***(Right)*** *Mediastinal EH displays a pseudopapillary growth pattern. These structures in fact represent vascular channels. This feature may be seen in low-grade angiosarcomas.*

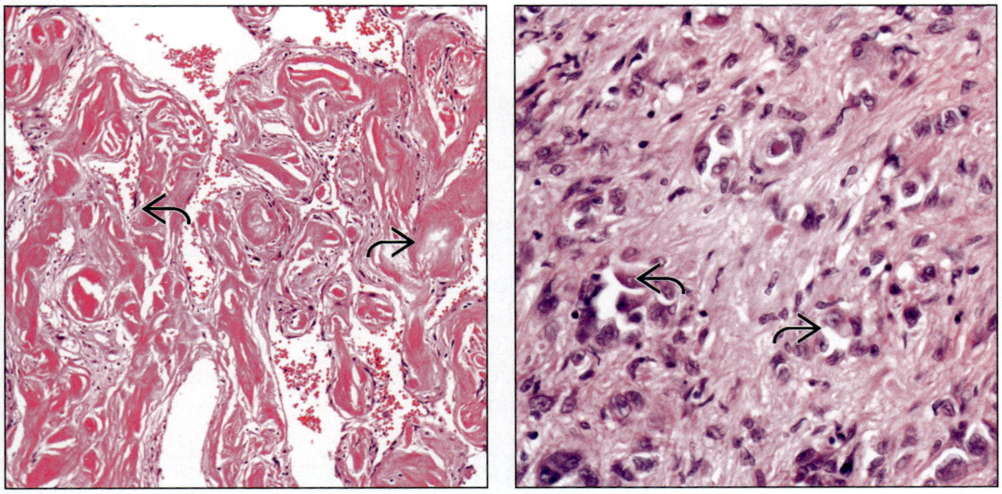

(Left) *Mediastinal EH is shown with extensive hyalinization ↪. This feature, although unusual, may be seen in mediastinal EH and may make the diagnosis difficult.* ***(Right)*** *High-power magnification shows a mediastinal EH in which there are numerous vascular structures lined by neoplastic endothelial cells ↪. However, mitotic activity is absent.*

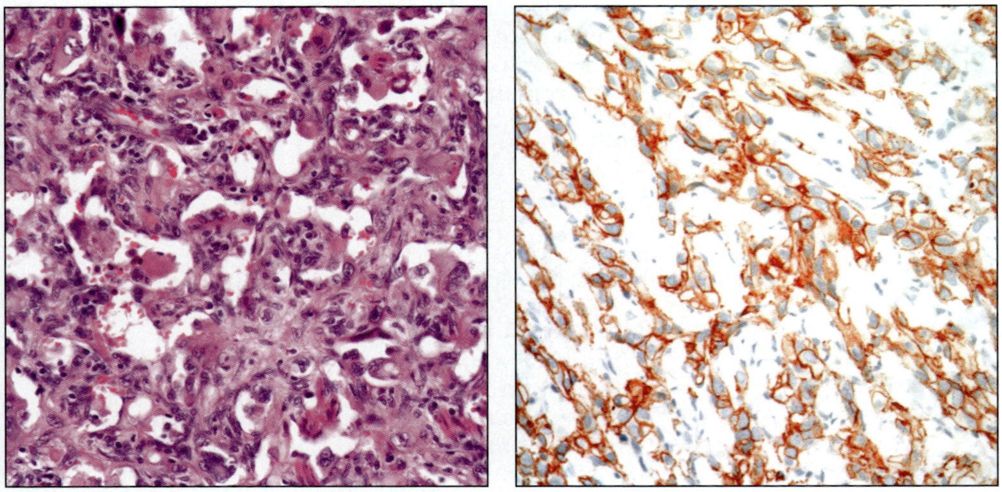

(Left) *Mediastinal EH shows a complex arrangement of vascular structures with an atypical endothelial cellular proliferation. Note the absence of necrosis and hemorrhage or marked nuclear pleomorphism.* ***(Right)*** *Mediastinal EH shows a strong positive reaction in neoplastic cells for a vascular marker (CD31). These immunohistochemical markers are of help in corroborating the vascular nature of the neoplasm.*

MESENCHYMAL CHONDROSARCOMA

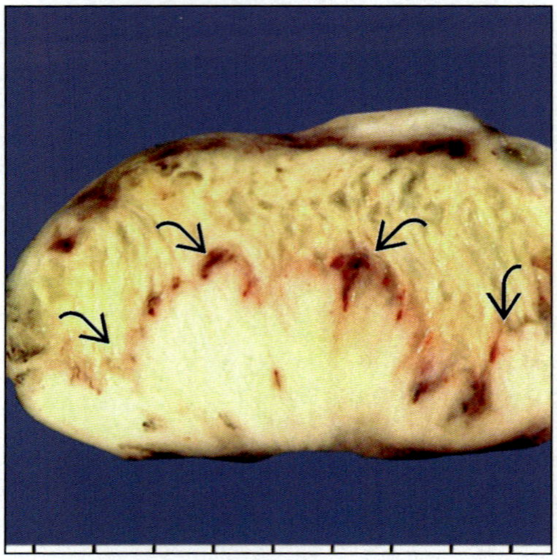

Gross appearance of mesenchymal chondrosarcoma of the mediastinum shows a well-circumscribed mass with a fleshy cut surface and areas of immature cartilage formation ➔.

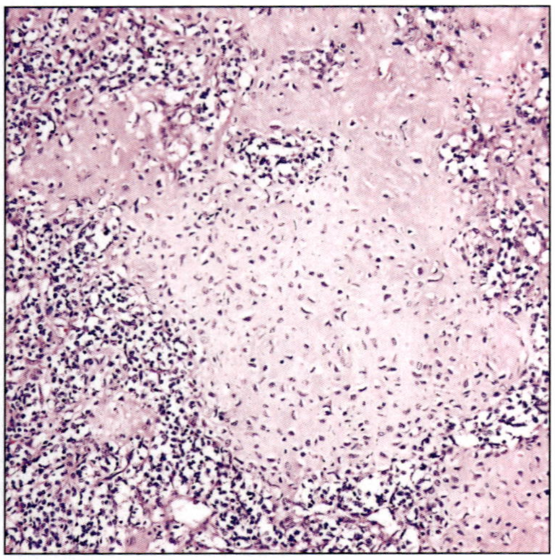

Classical histologic appearance of mesenchymal chondrosarcoma shows an island of immature cartilage (center) and abrupt transitions with surrounding small round blue cells.

TERMINOLOGY

Abbreviations

- Mesenchymal chondrosarcoma (MC)

Definitions

- Biphasic malignant neoplasm composed of primitive neoplastic small round blue cell population admixed with islands of mature cartilage

ETIOLOGY/PATHOGENESIS

Pathogenesis

- Originally believed to represent a variant of chondrosarcoma due to presence of mature cartilage
- Currently regarded as closely related to primitive neuroectodermal tumors (PNET) or Ewing sarcoma

CLINICAL ISSUES

Epidemiology

- Incidence
  - Extremely rare tumor
- Age
  - Predilection for young adults (15-35 years)
  - May also occur in young children
- Gender
  - Slight female predilection

Presentation

- Back pain
- Dyspnea
- More often asymptomatic
- Incidental finding on routine chest x-rays

Treatment

- Surgical approaches
  - Complete surgical excision
- Adjuvant therapy
  - Radiation and chemotherapy

Prognosis

- Aggressive malignancy
- Approximately 50% 5-year survival rate
- Metastasizes in a high percentage of cases
- Metastases are most common to lung

IMAGE FINDINGS

General Features

- Well-defined soft tissue mass in paraspinal location
- May protrude into or involve posterior mediastinum
- Irregular radiopaque stippling due to focal calcifications

MACROSCOPIC FEATURES

General Features

- Well-circumscribed, multilobated soft tissue mass
- Cut surface shows fleshy, gray-white homogeneous tissue with calcified and cartilaginous foci
- May contain small foci of hemorrhage and necrosis

Size

- Variable
- Average: 5-8 cm

MICROSCOPIC PATHOLOGY

Histologic Features

- Sheets of primitive round, oval, or spindle cells
- Foci of cartilaginous differentiation showing abrupt transitions with surrounding round/spindle cells
  - Cartilaginous foci are composed of mature hyaline cartilage
  - Cartilaginous foci may show areas of calcification or ossification

Key Facts

Clinical Issues
- Extremely rare tumor
- Predilection for young adults (15-35 years)
- Slight female predilection
- Incidental finding on routine chest x-rays
- Aggressive malignancy
- Approximately 50% 5-year survival rate

Macroscopic Features
- Well-circumscribed, multilobated soft tissue mass
- Cut surface shows fleshy, gray-white homogeneous tissue with calcified and cartilaginous foci
- May contain small foci of hemorrhage and necrosis
- Average size: 5-8 cm

Microscopic Pathology
- Sheets of primitive round, oval, or spindle cells
- Foci of cartilaginous differentiation showing abrupt transitions with surrounding round/spindle cells
- Cartilaginous foci may often show areas of calcification and ossification
- Primitive spindle cell component may adopt a prominent hemangiopericytic growth pattern
- Undifferentiated tumor cell component
  - Usually negative for S100 protein
  - Shows CD99 membranous positivity
- Primitive small round/spindle cell component shows positivity for SOX9
- Some cases show t(11;22)(q24;q12) translocation typical of the Ewing sarcoma/primitive neuroectodermal tumor family

- Primitive spindle cell component may adopt a prominent hemangiopericytic growth pattern
- Tumor may contain areas of hemorrhage and necrosis

Cytologic Features
- Primitive cells may have round or ovoid, elongated and hyperchromatic nuclei with scant cytoplasm
- Primitive tumor cells usually display low mitotic activity

ANCILLARY TESTS

Immunohistochemistry
- Cartilaginous areas show strong positive staining for S100 protein
- Undifferentiated tumor cell component
  - Usually negative for S100 protein
  - Shows CD99 membranous positivity
- May show focal positivity for CD57 or NSE
- Primitive small round/spindle cell component shows positivity for SOX9

Cytogenetics
- Some cases show t(11;22)(q24;q12) translocation typical of Ewing sarcoma/primitive neuroectodermal tumor family

Electron Microscopy
- Undifferentiated cells have scant cytoplasmic organelles
- Tumor cells show closely apposed cell membranes and desmosome-type junctions

DIFFERENTIAL DIAGNOSIS

Ewing Sarcoma/Primitive Neuroectodermal Tumor
- Lack foci of cartilaginous differentiation or ossification
- Generally more aggressive lesions, with invasion and destruction of adjacent structures

Hemangiopericytoma/Solitary Fibrous Tumor
- Usually lacks foci of cartilaginous differentiation
- Strong CD34 and Bcl-2 positivity

Synovial Sarcoma
- Positive for epithelial markers (cytokeratin, EMA)
- (X;18) translocation

DIAGNOSTIC CHECKLIST

Clinically Relevant Pathologic Features
- Paraspinal or posterior mediastinal mass in young patients
- Well-circumscribed lesion with stippled calcifications
- Slow, indolent growth

Pathologic Interpretation Pearls
- Biphasic appearance with primitive small round blue cell component admixed with cartilaginous foci
- Sheets of dense small round blue cells or hyperchromatic spindle cells with abrupt transitions with cartilaginous foci
- Prominent hemangiopericytomatous growth pattern

SELECTED REFERENCES

1. Fanburg-Smith JC et al: Reappraisal of mesenchymal chondrosarcoma: novel morphologic observations of the hyaline cartilage and endochondral ossification and beta-catenin, Sox9, and osteocalcin immunostaining of 22 cases. Hum Pathol. 41(5):653-62, 2010
2. Wehrli BM et al: Sox9, a master regulator of chondrogenesis, distinguishes mesenchymal chondrosarcoma from other small blue round cell tumors. Hum Pathol. 34(3):263-9, 2003
3. Chetty R: Extraskeletal mesenchymal chondrosarcoma of the mediastinum. Histopathology. 17(3):261-3, 1990
4. Sato N et al: An ultrastructural study of extraskeletal mesenchymal chondrosarcoma. Acta Pathol Jpn. 34(6):1355-63, 1984

MESENCHYMAL CHONDROSARCOMA

Principal Histologic Features

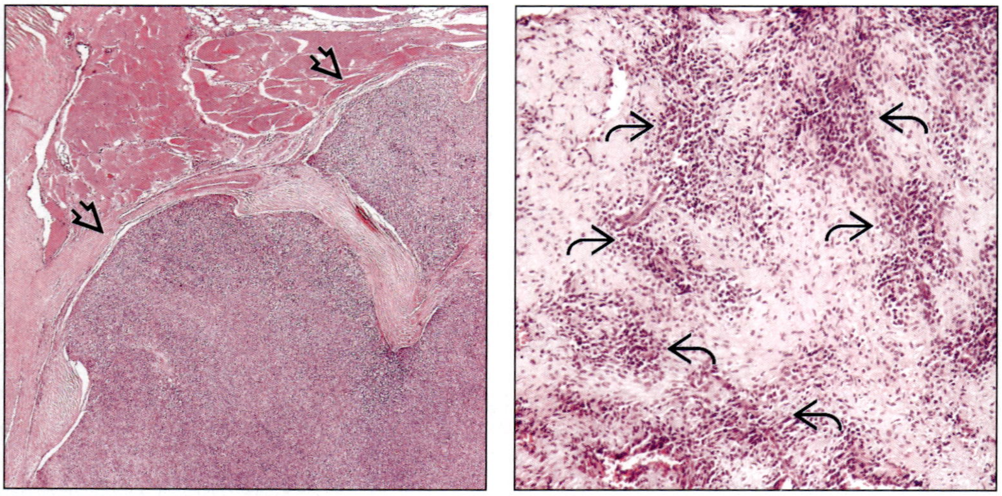

(Left) *Scanning magnification of a mesenchymal chondrosarcoma of the mediastinum shows sharp circumscription from surrounding skeletal muscle and displays a marked lobular configuration →. The tumor resembles a "small round blue cell tumor."* ***(Right)*** *Central portion of mesenchymal chondrosarcoma of the mediastinum shows irregular, pale-staining areas with an immature chondroid matrix circumscribing more cellular areas → that are composed of primitive, small round blue cells.*

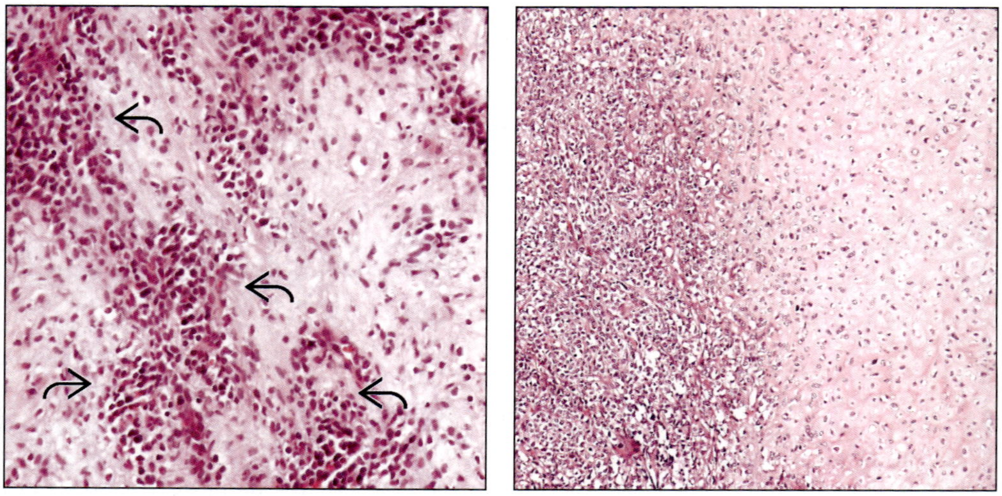

(Left) *High magnification from the central portion of mesenchymal chondrosarcoma of the mediastinum shows a monotonous and primitive small round blue cell population → circumscribing pale, paucicellular areas composed of immature chondroid matrix.* ***(Right)*** *High magnification of mesenchymal chondrosarcoma of the mediastinum shows an abrupt transition between a primitive small round blue cell population (left) and well-formed cartilaginous elements (right).*

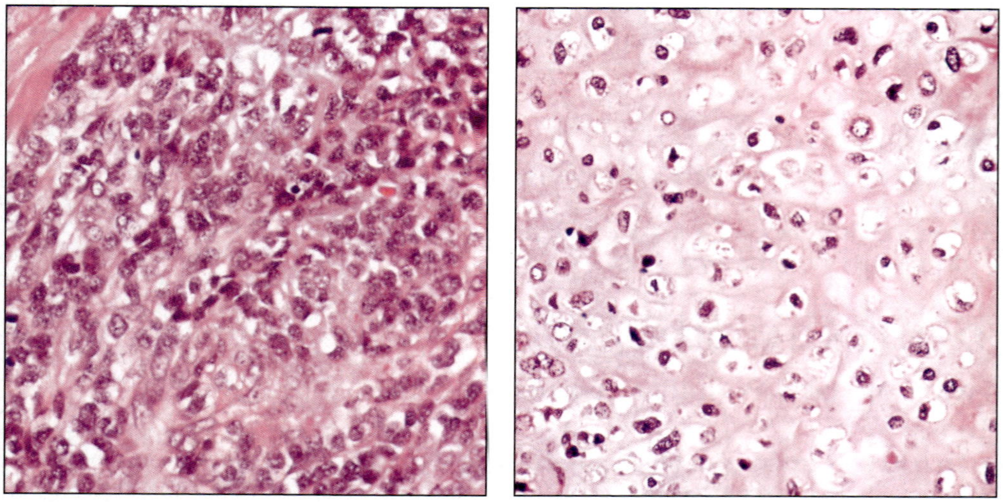

(Left) *High magnification of mesenchymal chondrosarcoma of mediastinum shows monotonous, primitive small round blue cell population. The cells are indistinguishable from other round blue cell tumors such as Ewing sarcoma/PNET, embryonal rhabdomyosarcoma, neuroblastoma, and lymphoblastic lymphoma.* ***(Right)*** *High magnification of mesenchymal chondrosarcoma of mediastinum shows details of cartilaginous elements within the tumor, with mature chondrocytes suspended within empty lacunae.*

MESENCHYMAL CHONDROSARCOMA

Other Histologic Features

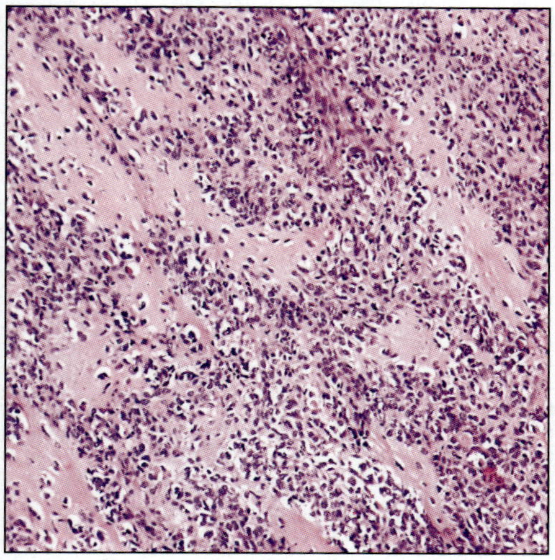

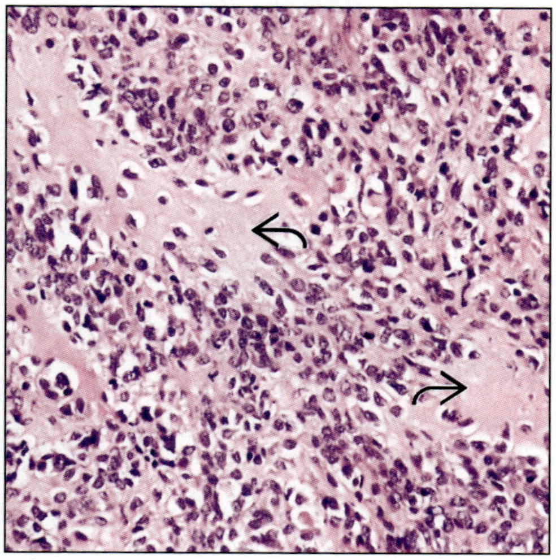

(Left) *Scanning magnification of mesenchymal chondrosarcoma of the mediastinum shows characteristic biphasic appearance with paucicellular areas displaying immature matrix deposition flanked by more cellular areas composed of small round blue cell population.* ***(Right)*** *High magnification of a mesenchymal chondrosarcoma of the mediastinum shows primitive population of small round blue cells circumscribing paucicellular areas with immature hyaline matrix.*

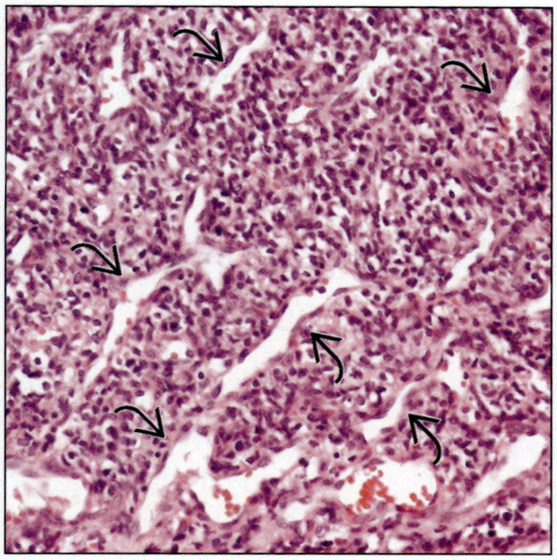

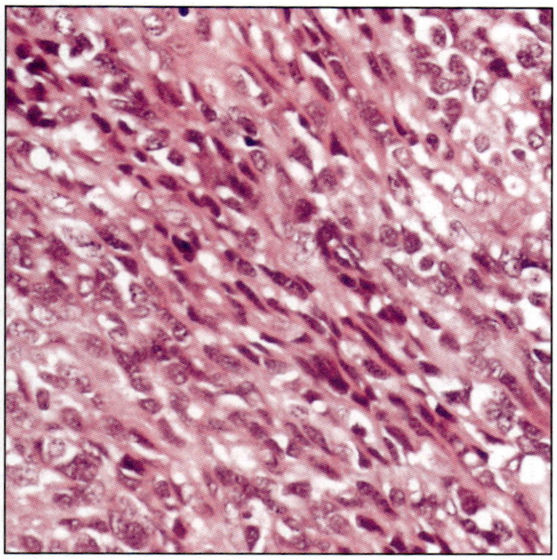

(Left) *Mesenchymal chondrosarcoma of the mediastinum shows branching small vessels surrounded by small round blue cell population. This appearance can resemble other soft tissue tumors with a prominent hemangiopericytic growth pattern.* ***(Right)*** *High magnification of mesenchymal chondrosarcoma of mediastinum shows atypical spindle cell population (center) admixed with primitive small round blue cells.*

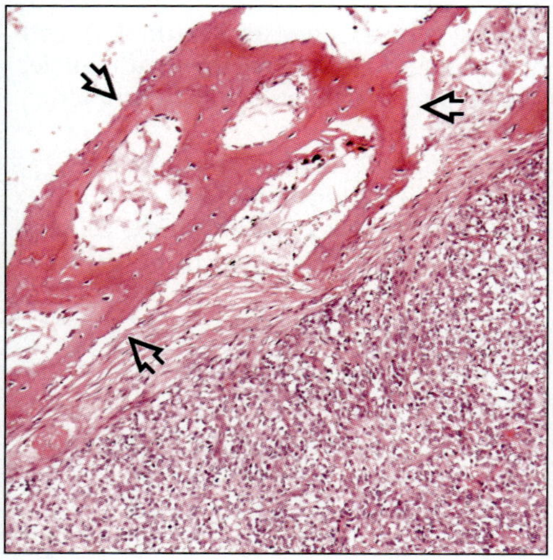

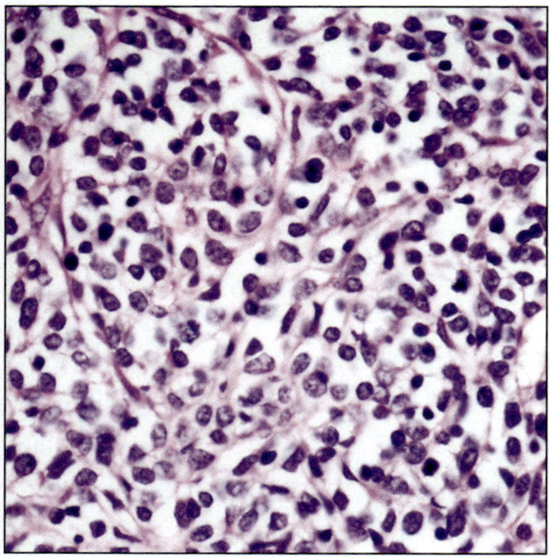

(Left) *Mesenchymal chondrosarcoma of the mediastinum shows prominent metaplastic bone formation.* ***(Right)*** *Mesenchymal chondrosarcoma of the mediastinum shows a monotonous population of primitive small round blue cells. The tumor can be mistaken for a number of other small round blue cell tumors in this location, including extraskeletal Ewing sarcoma/PNET, desmoplastic small round blue cell tumor, neuroblastoma, and others.*

CHORDOMA

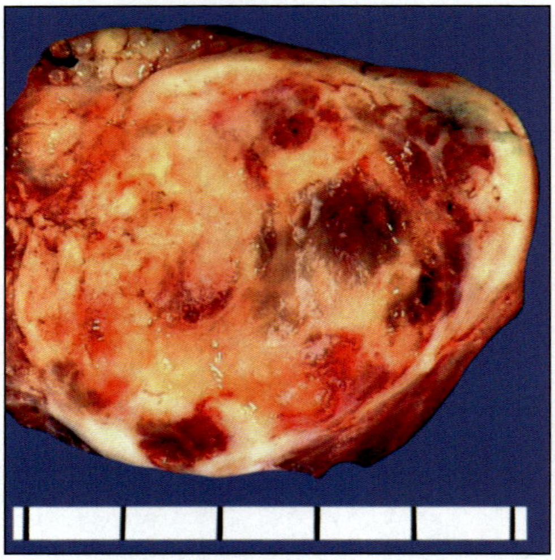

Gross appearance of posterior mediastinal chordoma shows a well-circumscribed and encapsulated tumor mass with soft, gelatinous areas alternating with more solid whitish areas.

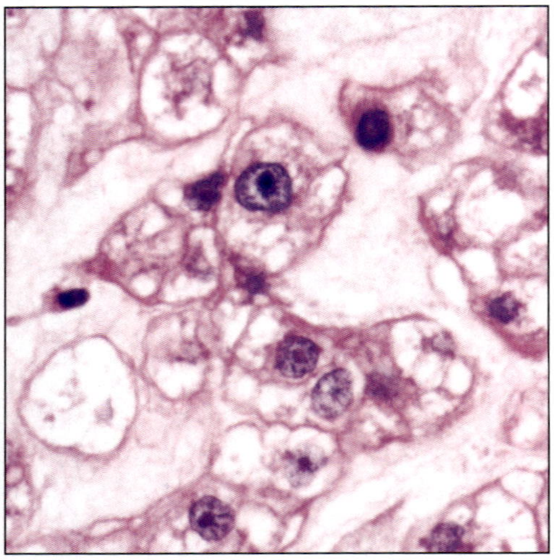

Characteristic histologic appearance of mediastinal chordoma shows clusters of large, epithelioid cells with abundant, bubbly vacuolated cytoplasm.

TERMINOLOGY

Definitions

- Malignant neoplasm presumed to be derived from remnants of embryonic notochord

CLINICAL ISSUES

Site

- Posterior mediastinum
- Paravertebral location involving soft tissue without involvement or destruction of bone

Presentation

- Chest pain, shortness of breath, pleural effusion, backache; may be an incidental finding
- Usually slow-growing neoplasms, often asymptomatic

Treatment

- Surgical excision

Prognosis

- May behave aggressively with frequent recurrences and metastasis; occasional patient deaths due to tumor
- Small, well-circumscribed cases amenable to complete excision; may show long-term, disease-free survival

IMAGE FINDINGS

General Features

- CT scans show well-circumscribed posterior mediastinal mass without evidence of vertebral involvement or destruction

MACROSCOPIC FEATURES

General Features

- Well-circumscribed, encapsulated mass
- Soft, gelatinous, often hemorrhagic cut surface

Sections to Be Submitted

- 1 section per centimeter of largest tumor diameter

Size

- 6-12 cm

MICROSCOPIC PATHOLOGY

Histologic Features

- Striking lobular growth pattern
- Cords and strands of large tumor cells with abundant cytoplasm
- Abundant myxoid stroma
- "Chondroid" chordoma is characterized by areas containing immature chondroid matrix
- "Dedifferentiated" chordoma is characterized by areas containing an atypical spindle cell population

Cytologic Features

- Classical chordoma cells are large and epithelioid with abundant cytoplasm and large hyperchromatic nuclei
- Cells may be small and stellate with hyperchromatic nuclei and scant cytoplasm
- Cells can display abundant "bubbly" (vacuolated) cytoplasm (so-called physaliphorous cells)
- "Dedifferentiated" areas show atypical spindle cells with hyperchromatic nuclei and frequent mitoses

ANCILLARY TESTS

Histochemistry

- PAS stain with diastase will demonstrate intracellular glycogen in tumor cells
- Alcian blue at pH 2.5 demonstrates abundant hyaluronic acid in stroma

CHORDOMA

Key Facts

Clinical Issues
- Chest pain
- Shortness of breath
- Backache
- Usually are slow-growing neoplasms that may often be asymptomatic
- May behave aggressively with frequent recurrences & metastasis and occasional patient deaths from tumor
- Posterior mediastinal location

Image Findings
- CT scans show a well-circumscribed posterior mediastinal mass without evidence of vertebral involvement or destruction

Microscopic Pathology
- Cords and strands of large tumor cells with abundant cytoplasm
- Abundant myxoid stroma
- Classical chordoma cells are large & epithelioid with abundant cytoplasm & large hyperchromatic nuclei
- Cells may be small and stellate with hyperchromatic nuclei and scant cytoplasm
- Cells can display abundant "bubbly" (vacuolated) cytoplasm (so-called physaliphorous cells)
- "Dedifferentiated" areas show atypical spindle cells with hyperchromatic nuclei and frequent mitoses
- Cells are strongly positive for low molecular weight cytokeratin
- Cells are strongly positive for EMA
- Cells are strongly positive for S100 protein

Immunohistochemistry
- Cells are strongly positive for low molecular weight cytokeratin, epithelial membrane antigen (EMA), S100 protein
- Cells are negative for CEA, SMA, desmin, and other differentiation markers

Electron Microscopy
- Closely apposed cell membranes joined by frequent desmosomes with small tonofilaments
- May form microglandular lumens lined by short, immature microvilli
- Scant organelles, including ribosomes, Golgi apparati, glycogen granules, and abundant intermediate filaments

DIFFERENTIAL DIAGNOSIS

Metastatic Mucinous Carcinoma
- Usually forms glandular structures rather than displaying cord-like growth pattern
- Cytoplasm is uniformly distended by mucin rather than showing multivacuolation
- Intracytoplasmic mucin can be demonstrated with PAS and mucicarmine stains
- Tumor cells are positive for cytokeratin and EMA, but negative for S100 protein

Extraskeletal Myxoid Chondrosarcoma
- Characteristic cord-like, single file pattern of growth of small tumor cells embedded in abundant myxoid stroma
- Absence of large, multivacuolated "physaliphorous" cells
- Tumor cells are negative for cytokeratin and EMA

Well-differentiated Chondrosarcoma
- May be mistaken with "chondroid" chordoma
- Absence of large, vacuolated chordoma cells embedded in myxoid stroma
- Tumor cells are negative for keratins and EMA

Epithelioid Hemangioendothelioma
- Sheets, cords, and small islands of large epithelioid cells with prominent cytoplasmic vacuoles
- Vacuoles often contain single red blood cells indicating abortive vascular lumen formation
- Tumor cells are positive for FVIIIRAg and CD31 vascular markers

High-Grade Spindle Cell Sarcoma
- May have similar morphologic appearance as "dedifferentiated" chordoma
- Will not show transitions with areas of more conventional chordomatous elements
- Extensive sampling is indicated to rule out chordomatous elements

DIAGNOSTIC CHECKLIST

Clinically Relevant Pathologic Features
- Small, well-circumscribed and encapsulated lesions may be completely excised with favorable outcome
- Infiltrative, poorly circumscribed, and incompletely excised lesions may show multiple recurrences and metastases
- Tumors with high-grade areas of "dedifferentiation" will follow highly aggressive behavior

SELECTED REFERENCES

1. Soudack M et al: Imaging features of posterior mediastinal chordoma in a child. Pediatr Radiol. 37(5):492-7, 2007
2. Horn KD et al: Cytokeratin immunophenotyping of an unusual cervical vertebral chordoma with extensive chondroid foci and perilaryngeal recurrence: a case report with review of the literature. Am J Otolaryngol. 22(6):428-34, 2001
3. Roeyen G et al: Chordoma of the mediastinum. Eur J Surg Oncol. 25(2):224-5, 1999
4. Suster S et al: Chordomas of the mediastinum: clinicopathologic, immunohistochemical, and ultrastructural study of six cases presenting as posterior mediastinal masses. Hum Pathol. 26(12):1354-62, 1995

CHORDOMA

Classical Growth Pattern

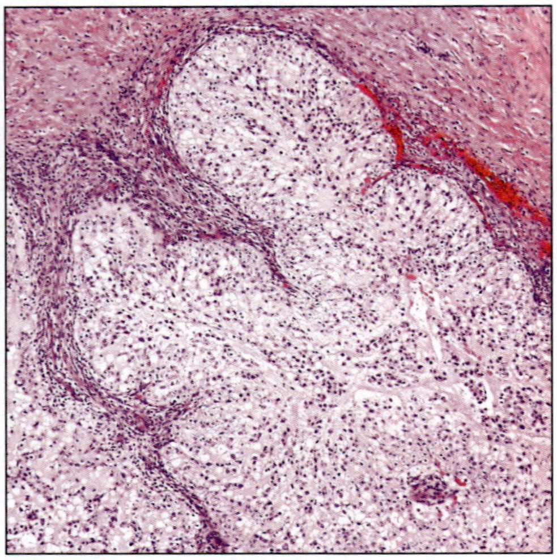

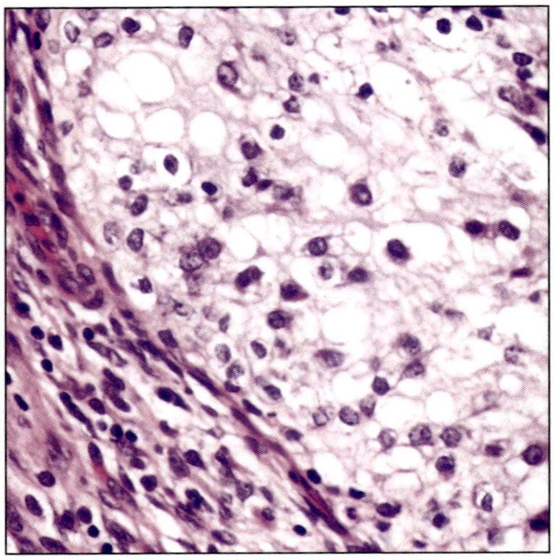

(Left) *Typical scanning magnification of mediastinal chordoma with striking lobular appearance shows irregular lobules of tumor cells with solid architecture surrounded by thick bands of fibrous stroma.* ***(Right)*** *Higher magnification of mediastinal chordoma shows sheets of large clear cells with small, hyperchromatic nuclei surrounded by abundant clear cytoplasm. The tumors with this pattern can resemble a metastasis from a clear cell carcinoma such as metastatic renal cell carcinoma.*

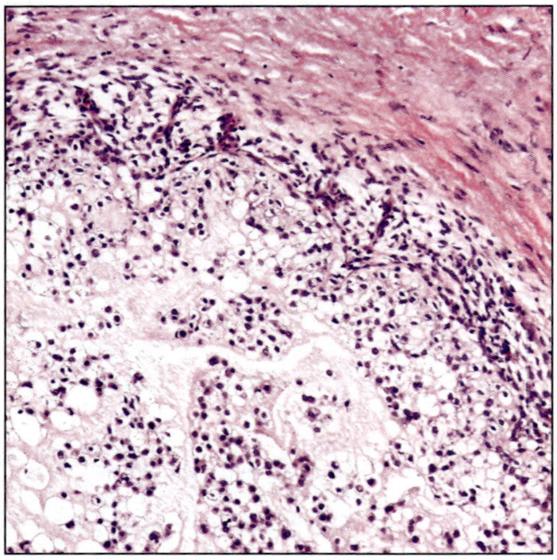

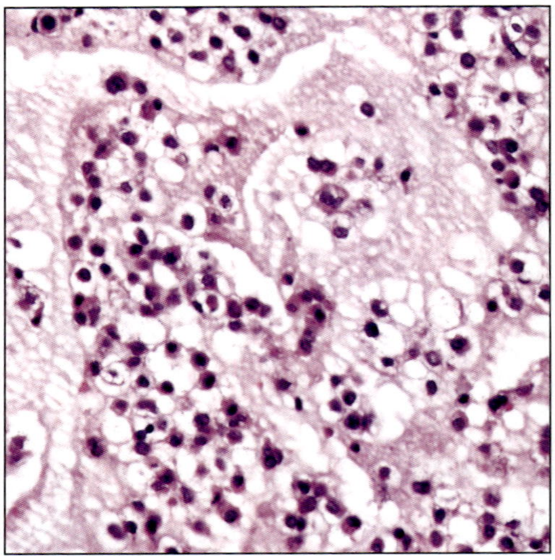

(Left) *Scanning magnification of mediastinal chordoma shows a lobular configuration separated by thick connective tissue bands and a monotonous tumor cell population with abundant background myxoid stroma.* ***(Right)*** *Higher magnification of mediastinal chordoma shows monotonous tumor cell population composed of round cells with hyperchromatic nuclei surrounded by clear cytoplasmic halos. The tumor cells are embedded in abundant lightly staining myxoid stroma.*

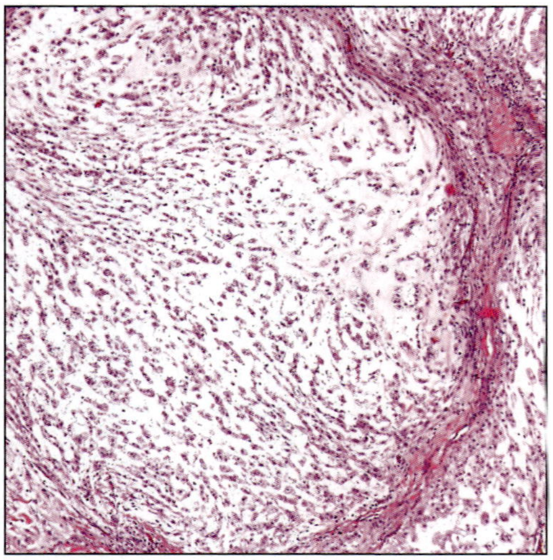

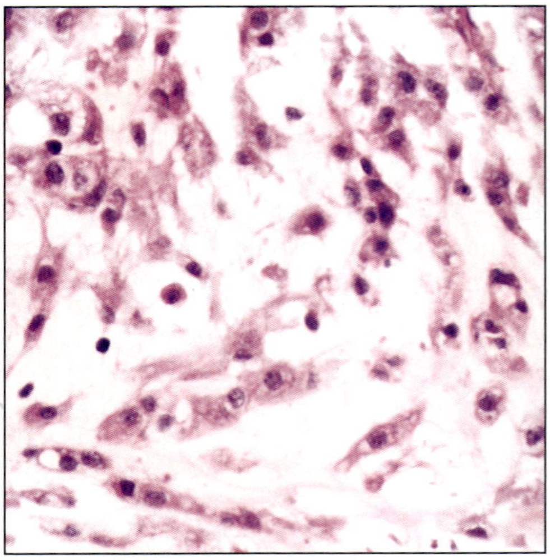

(Left) *Scanning magnification of mediastinal chordoma shows a lobular configuration separated by thin fibrous bands and containing a uniform small cell population set against a lightly staining myxoid stroma.* ***(Right)*** *High magnification of mediastinal chordoma shows a monotonous population of small tumor cells with small round nuclei and a scant rim of eosinophilic cytoplasm suspended in a myxoid stroma. Notice the cording and single-file configuration of the tumor cells.*

Cell Types

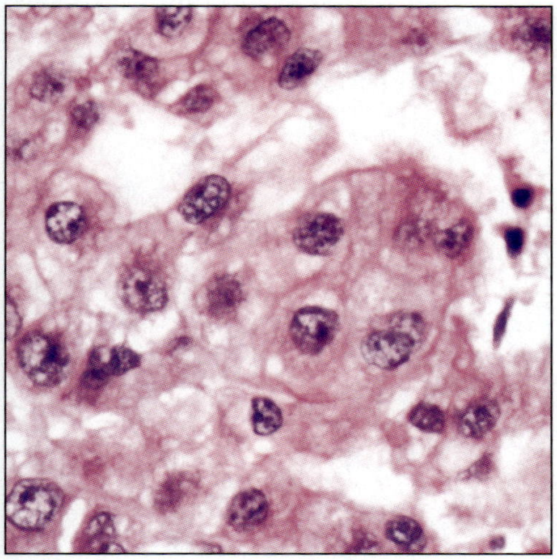

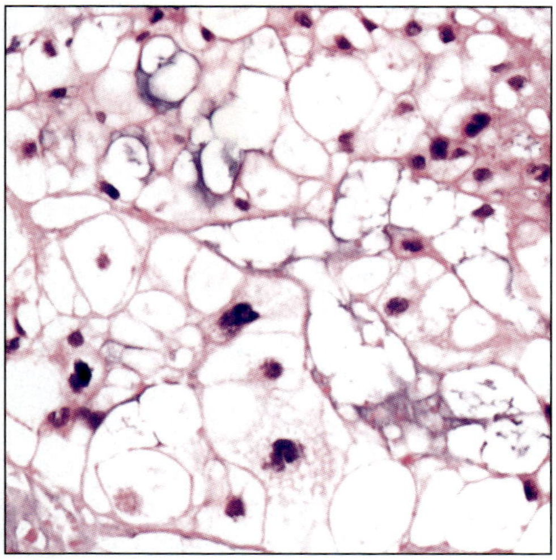

(Left) *Clusters of large, epithelioid cells are seen in the mediastinal chordoma. The cells have large, vesicular nuclei with small nucleoli and are surrounded by abundant, finely granular eosinophilic cytoplasm.* ***(Right)*** *High magnification of mediastinal chordoma shows cells with small, darkly staining nuclei without significant nuclear atypia, surrounded by abundant clear, amphophilic cytoplasm that is bordered by sharply delineated cell membranes.*

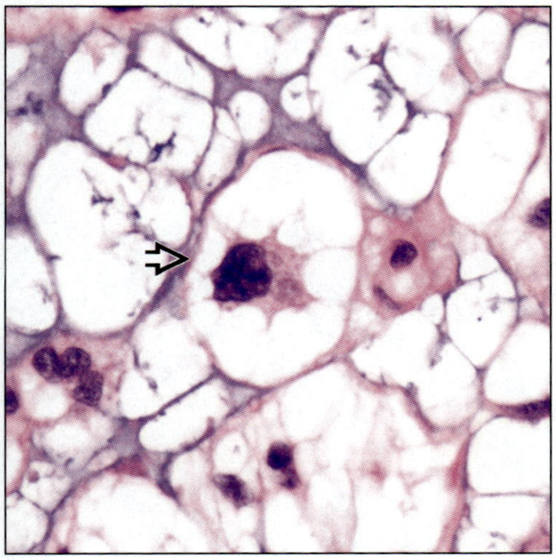

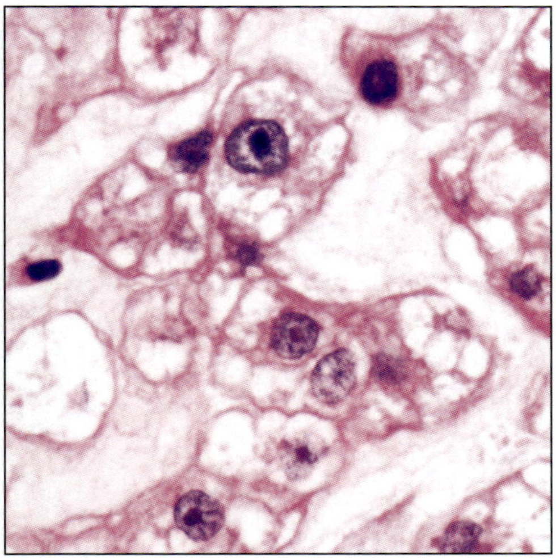

(Left) *Physaliphorous cell in mediastinal chordoma ⇨ shows a centrally placed nucleus with scalloping of the nuclear envelope and multiple clear intracytoplasmic vacuoles.* ***(Right)*** *Physaliphorous cells in mediastinal chordoma show "bubbly" appearance of the cytoplasm due to multiple cytoplasmic vacuoles. Identification of these cells can be extremely helpful for diagnosis as this represents one of the distinctive morphologic features commonly observed in these tumors.*

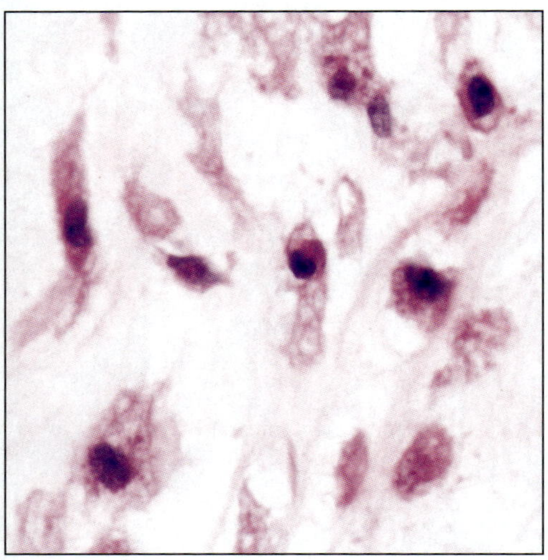

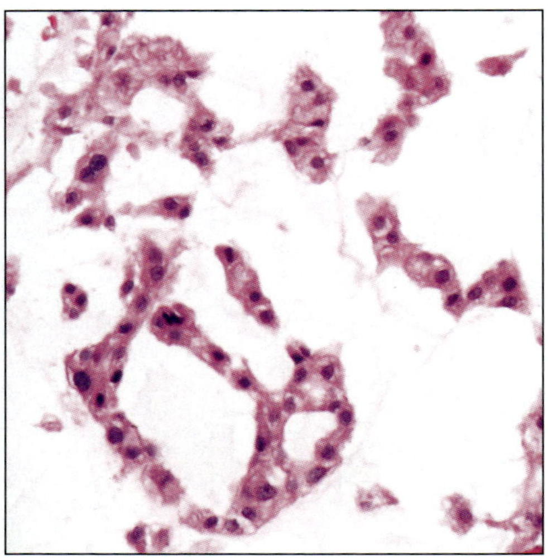

(Left) *Small stellate cells are seen in this example of mediastinal chordoma. The cells are characterized by small round nuclei with a dense chromatin pattern and scant nuclear detail, surrounded by a scant rim of eosinophilic cytoplasm.* ***(Right)*** *Small dark cells are seen in this example of mediastinal chordoma. Notice the striking "cording" pattern of the tumor cells, which form short cords or trabeculae of tumor cells disposed in single file and embedded in a myxoid stroma.*

CHORDOMA

Other Features

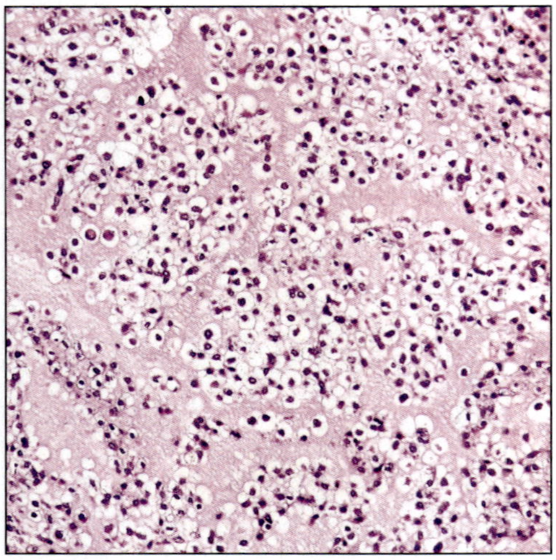

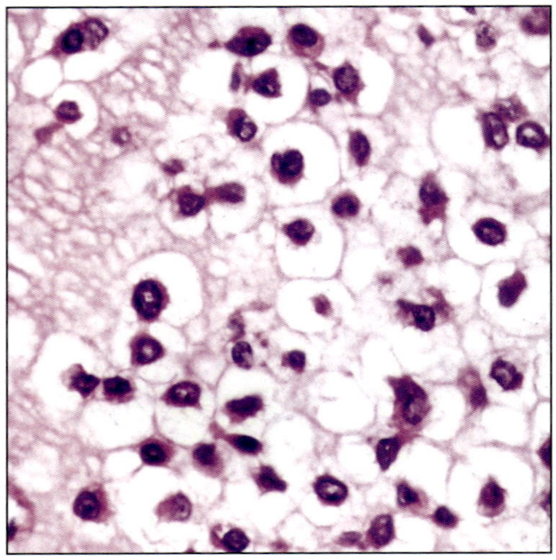

(Left) *Scanning magnification of mediastinal chordoma with a striking cartilaginous appearance shows sheets of tumor cells that appear to be suspended in cartilaginous lacunae closely simulating mature cartilage.* ***(Right)*** *High magnification of mediastinal chordoma with cartilaginous appearance shows sheets of large tumor cells with round, regular nuclei surrounded by clear cytoplasmic halos. The tumor cell nuclei appear to be suspended in cartilaginous lacunae.*

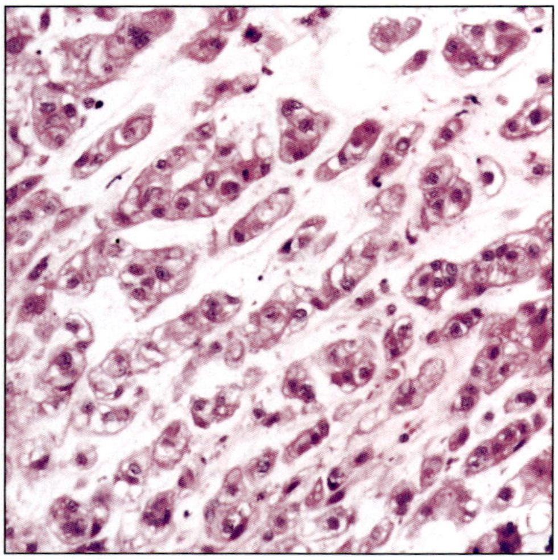

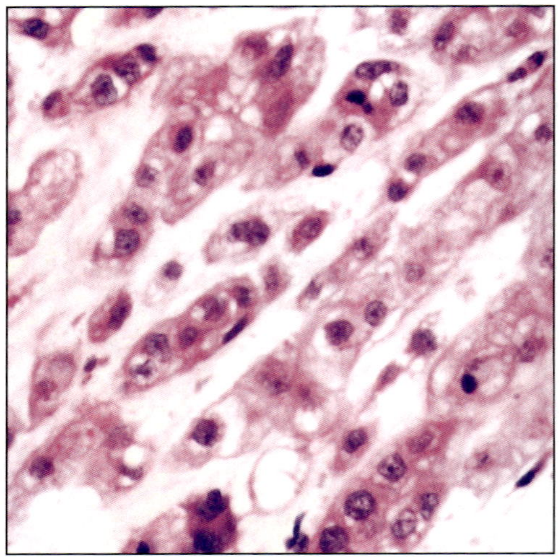

(Left) *Striking cord-like architecture is seen in this example of mediastinal chordoma. This cord-like arrangement of tumor cells is quite distinctive and highly characteristic of these tumors.* ***(Right)*** *High magnification of mediastinal chordoma with cord-like architecture shows cohesive epithelioid cells with single-file arrangement. The epithelioid cells contain small, round nuclei with small, inconspicuous nucleoli and are surrounded by an ample rim of lightly eosinophilic cytoplasm.*

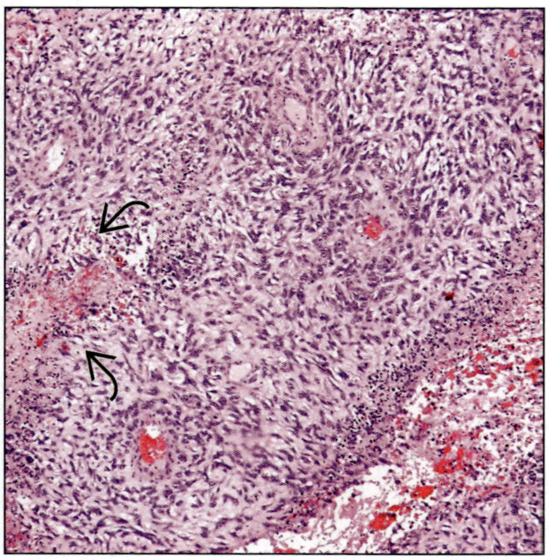

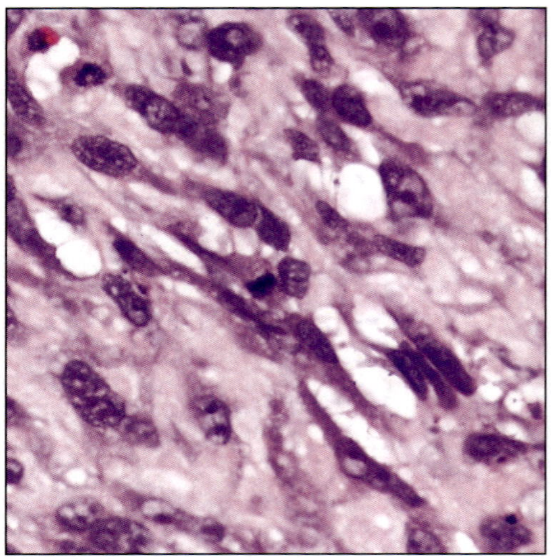

(Left) *"Dedifferentiated" chordoma of the mediastinum shows sheets of atypical tumor cells with perivascular distribution and small foci of necrosis ➔. The morphologic appearance in this area is that of a high-grade spindle cell sarcoma.* ***(Right)*** *High magnification of "dedifferentiated" chordoma of the mediastinum shows highly atypical and hyperchromatic spindle cells with dark-staining nuclei with prominent nucleoli and scattered mitoses embedded in a myxoid stroma.*

Immunohistochemical Features

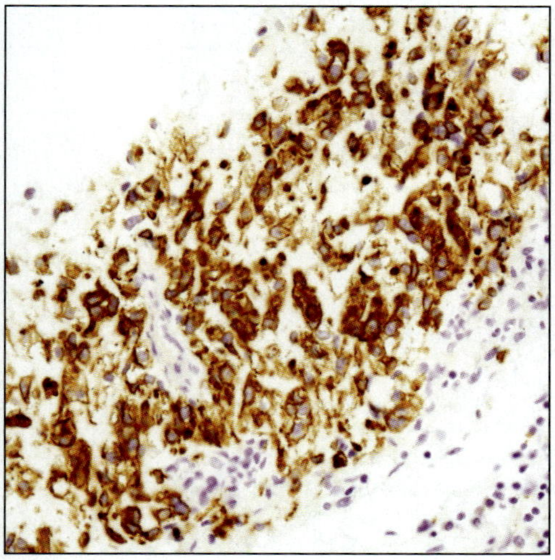
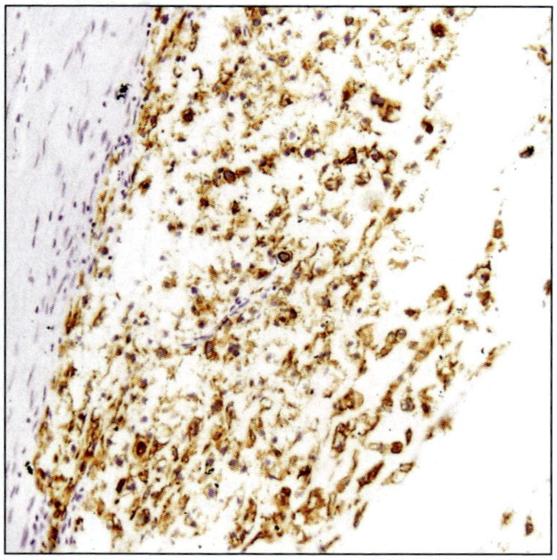

(Left) *Immunohistochemical staining for low molecular weight cytokeratin (CAM5.2) in mediastinal chordoma shows strong cytoplasmic positivity of the tumor cells for this antibody.* ***(Right)*** *Immunohistochemical staining for epithelial membrane antigen (EMA) in mediastinal chordoma shows strong membrane and cytoplasmic staining in the majority of the tumor cells for this antibody. Staining for EMA, however, can be patchy and focal in some of these tumors.*

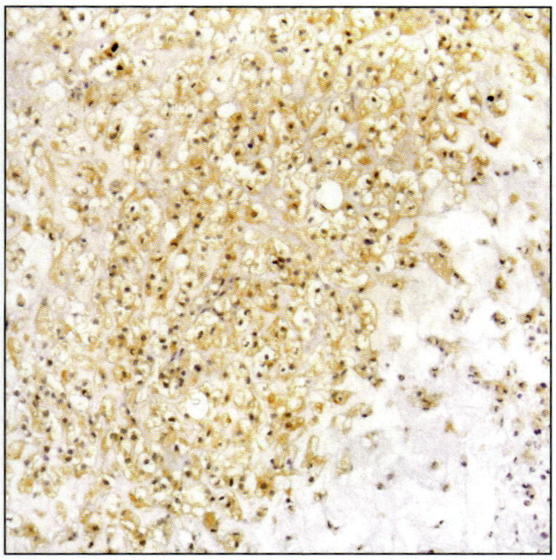
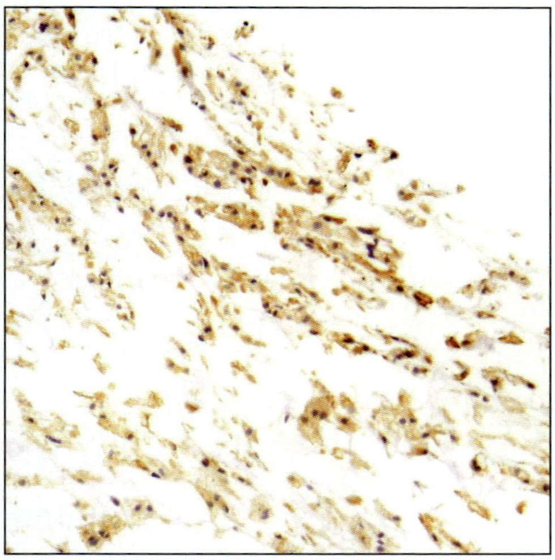

(Left) *Immunohistochemical staining for S100 protein in mediastinal chordoma shows nuclear and cytoplasmic positivity in the majority of the tumor cells in this example with a diffuse growth pattern.* ***(Right)*** *Immunohistochemical staining for S100 protein in mediastinal chordoma with striking cord-like pattern of growth shows nuclear and cytoplasmic positivity in the small tumor cells comprising the cords. The S100 positivity helps to separate these tumors from metastases of carcinoma.*

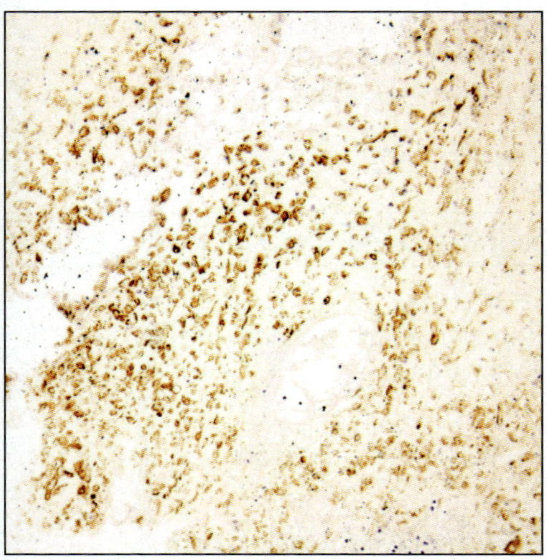
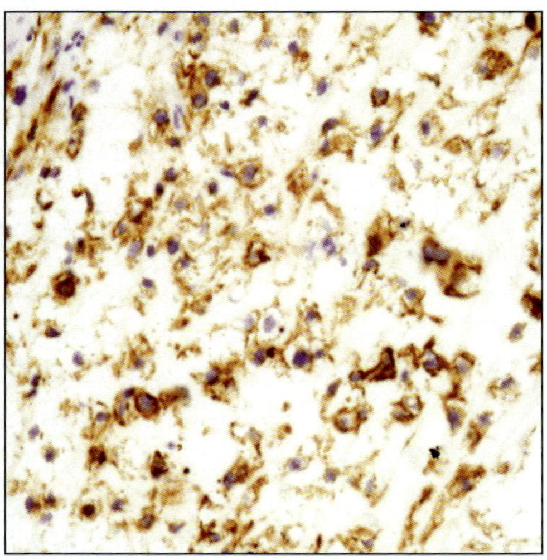

(Left) *Immunohistochemical staining of "dedifferentiated" component in mediastinal chordoma shows strong positivity of the tumor cells for this antibody.* ***(Right)*** *Immunohistochemical staining of tumor cells for pancytokeratin in "dedifferentiated" component of mediastinal chordoma shows cytoplasmic staining of the tumor cells. The "dedifferentiated" areas are usually negative for S100, and the diagnosis depends on identifying areas of more conventional chordoma.*

ALVEOLAR SOFT PART SARCOMA

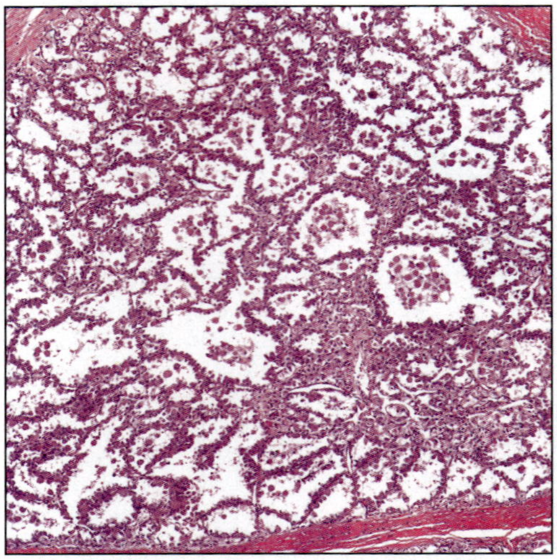

Low-power view shows an alveolar soft part sarcoma with a neoplastic cellular proliferation arranged in an alveolar growth pattern almost mimicking alveolated lung tissue.

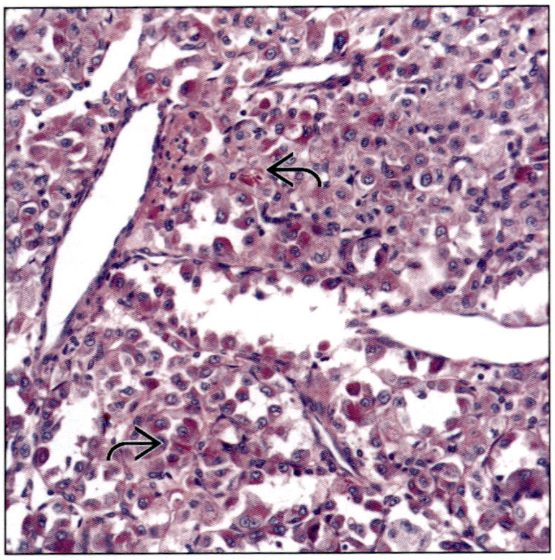

Periodic acid-Schiff shows the characteristic intracellular crystals ➔ typical of alveolar soft part sarcoma. This feature is almost invariably present in all cases.

TERMINOLOGY

Definitions

- Malignant neoplasm of soft tissues

ETIOLOGY/PATHOGENESIS

Etiology

- Although it has been speculated in the past as possible neurogenic or myogenic origin, its etiology remains unknown

CLINICAL ISSUES

Epidemiology

- Incidence
  - Extremely rare tumor in mediastinal compartment
- Age
  - Appears to be more common in young adults in 3rd decade of life
- Gender
  - No gender predilection

Site

- More common in soft tissues of extremities &/or head and neck
- Anterior or posterior mediastinum

Presentation

- Chest pain
- Dyspnea
- Cough
- Asymptomatic

Treatment

- Chemotherapy
- Radiation therapy
- Surgical resection

Prognosis

- Variable
- Tumor can metastasize
- Short- and long-term survivals have been reported

MACROSCOPIC FEATURES

General Features

- Fleshy, soft, and hemorrhagic tumor mass

Size

- Varies in size and can be > 10 cm in diameter

MICROSCOPIC PATHOLOGY

Histologic Features

- Alveolated growth pattern
- Large polygonal cells
- Well-defined cell borders
- Ample cytoplasm
- Eccentrically placed nuclei
- Mild to moderate nuclear atypia
- Mitoses are rare
- Intracytoplasmic crystals

DIFFERENTIAL DIAGNOSIS

Rhabdomyosarcoma

- Positive for muscle markers, including MYOD1, myoglobin, and desmin

Melanoma

- Positive for S100, HMB-45, and mart-1

Paraganglioma

- Positive for neuroendocrine markers, such as chromogranin-A and synaptophysin

ALVEOLAR SOFT PART SARCOMA

Key Facts

Clinical Issues

- Incidence
  - Extremely rare tumor in mediastinal compartment
  - Appears to be more common in young adults in 3rd decade of life
  - More common in soft tissues of extremities &/or head and neck
- Symptoms
  - Chest pain
  - Dyspnea
  - Cough
  - Asymptomatic

Top Differential Diagnoses

- Rhabdomyosarcoma
  - Positive for muscle markers, including MYOD1, myoglobin, and desmin
- Melanoma
  - Positive for S100, HMB-45, and mart-1
- Paraganglioma
  - Positive for neuroendocrine markers, such as chromogranin-A and synaptophysin
- Thymic carcinoma
  - Carcinomas usually will show positive staining for epithelial markers, such as keratins and EMA/MUC1

Diagnostic Checklist

- Alveolar growth pattern
- Large cells with ample cytoplasm
- Presence of intracytoplasmic crystals, especially using PAS histochemical stains
- Mitotic figures are rare

Immunohistochemistry

Antibody	Reactivity	Staining Pattern	Comment
Myoglobin	Positive	Cytoplasmic	Focal in some cases
CK-PAN	Negative		Positive in tumors of epithelial origin
Desmin	Negative		Mainly positive in tumors of muscle origin
S100	Negative		Mainly positive in tumors of neural origin
Actin-HHF-35	Negative		
CK5/6	Negative		
CK8/18/CAM5.2	Negative		
NFP	Negative		
Synaptophysin	Negative		Positive in tumors of neuroendocrine differentiation
Chromogranin-A	Negative		Positive in tumors of neuroendocrine differentiation

Histochemical Features of Alveolar Soft Part Sarcomas

Histochemical Stain	Result
Mucicarmine	Negative
D-PAS	Negative
PAS	Highlight the presence of cytoplasmic crystals

Thymic Carcinoma

- Carcinomas usually will show positive staining for epithelial markers, such as keratins and EMA/MUC1

DIAGNOSTIC CHECKLIST

Clinically Relevant Pathologic Features

- Cytoplasmic features

Pathologic Interpretation Pearls

- Alveolar growth pattern
- Large cells with ample cytoplasm
- Presence of intracytoplasmic crystals
- Mitotic figures are rare

SELECTED REFERENCES

1. Daigeler A et al: Alveolar soft part sarcoma: clinicopathological findings in a series of 11 cases. World J Surg Oncol. 6:71, 2008
2. Folpe AL et al: Alveolar soft-part sarcoma: a review and update. J Clin Pathol. 59(11):1127-32, 2006
3. Anderson ME et al: Alveolar soft part sarcoma: a rare and enigmatic entity. Clin Orthop Relat Res. 438:144-8, 2005
4. Gupta S et al: Alveolar soft part sarcoma: a rare entity with unique cytomorphological features. Cytopathology. 14(1):40-1, 2003
5. van Ruth S et al: Alveolar soft part sarcoma. a report of 15 cases. Eur J Cancer. 38(10):1324-8, 2002
6. Flieder DB et al: Primary alveolar soft-part sarcoma of the mediastinum: a clinicopathological and immunohistochemical study of two cases. Histopathology. 31(5):469-73, 1997

Microscopic Features

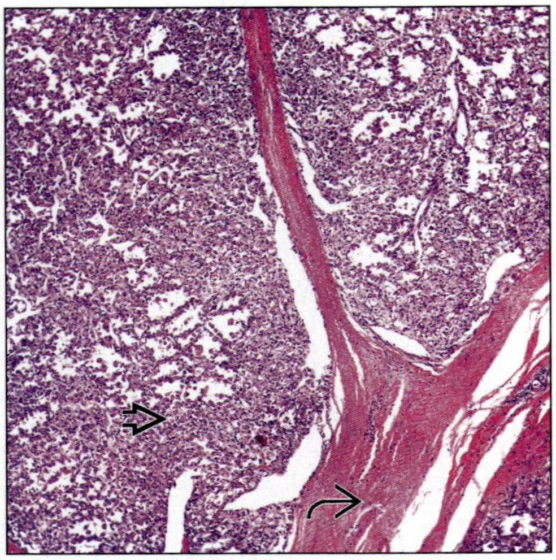

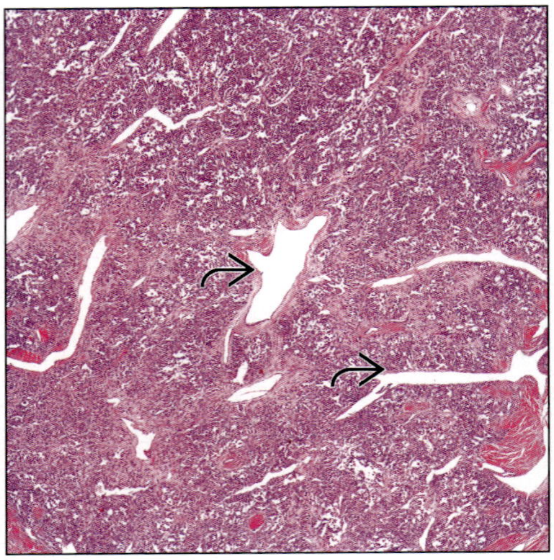

(Left) *Low-power view of alveolar soft part sarcoma shows slight lobulation. The tumor cells → are separated by thick bands of fibrocollagenous tissue →.* ***(Right)*** *Alveolar soft part sarcoma displays prominent ectatic vessels →. The presence of these ectatic vessels may mimic hemangiopericytoma; however, the cellular proliferation would be unusual for hemangiopericytoma.*

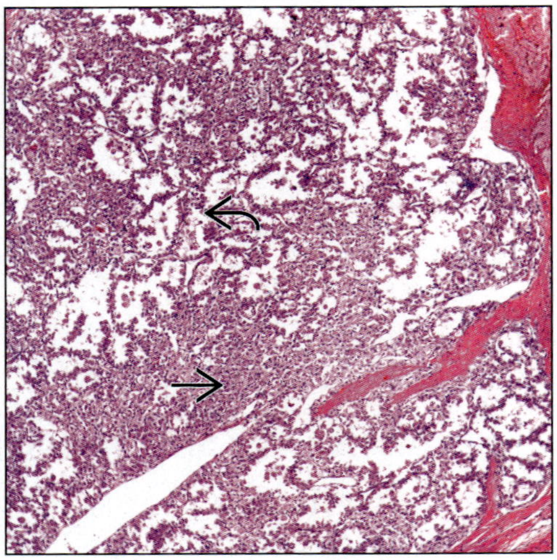

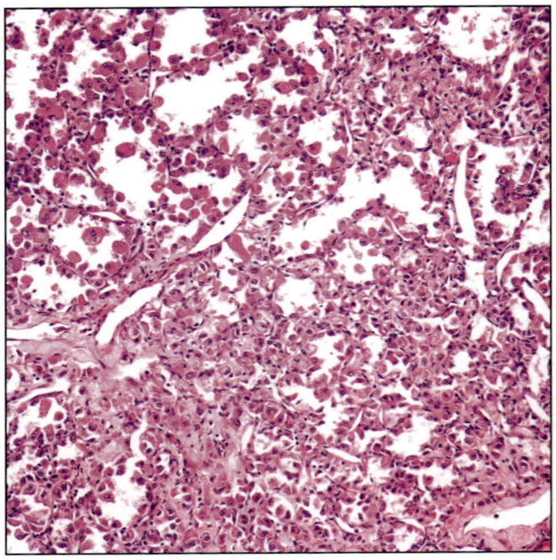

(Left) *Alveolar soft part sarcoma is shown with the characteristic alveolar growth pattern → and only focal solid areas →.* ***(Right)*** *Closer view shows the cellular proliferation in alveolar soft part sarcoma. In addition to the alveolar growth pattern, the cells are round to oval with moderate amounts of eosinophilic cytoplasm, round nuclei, and inconspicuous nucleoli. Increased mitotic activity in this tumor is unusual.*

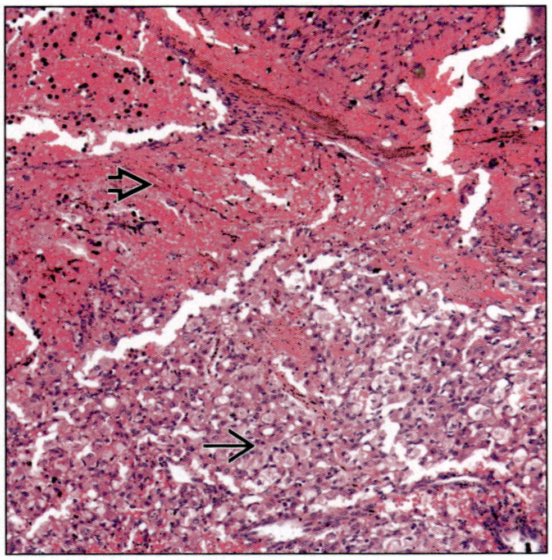

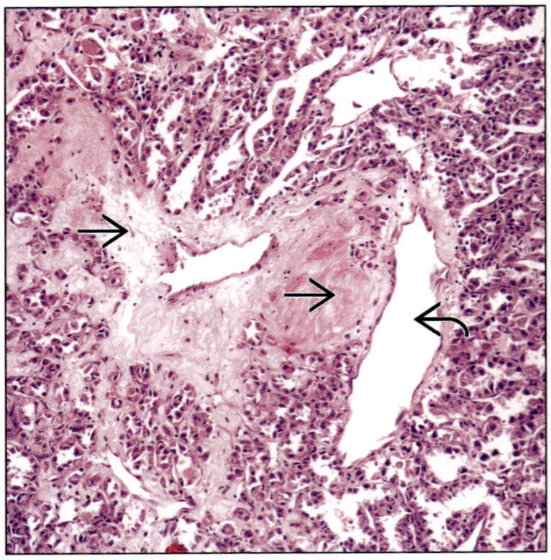

(Left) *Alveolar soft part sarcoma is shown with transition between areas of extensive hemorrhage → and more viable areas of tumor. Note that the tumor does not show the typical alveolated growth pattern →.* ***(Right)*** *Another characteristic of alveolar soft part sarcoma is the presence of ectatic vessels → with perivascular hyalinization →. This pattern may be confused with paragangliomas.*

Microscopic Features

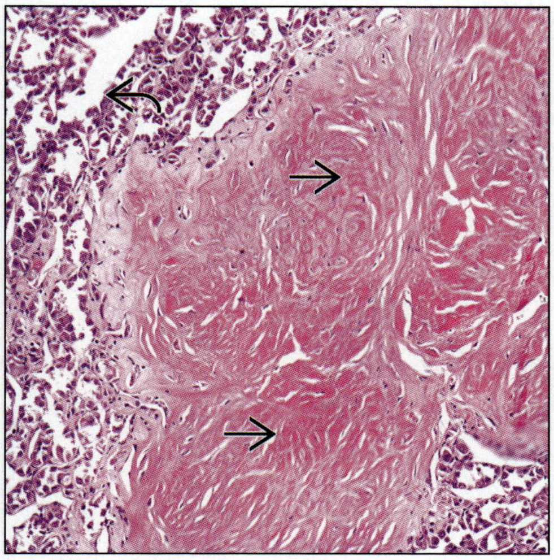
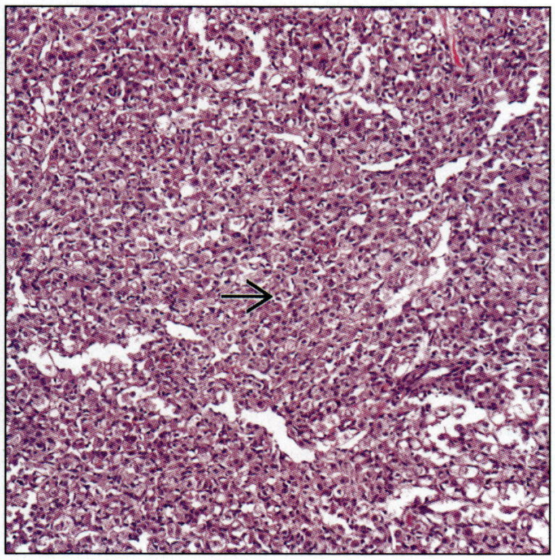

(Left) *Alveolar soft part sarcoma shows extensive stromal hyalinization* → *with only focal areas of viable tumor* ↪. *Although this feature may also be seen in neuroendocrine tumors, it may be seen focally in alveolar soft part sarcoma.* **(Right)** *Alveolar soft part sarcoma is shown with prominent solid growth pattern* →. *In most of the cases, solid areas of tumor may be seen in association with the more typical alveolar growth pattern.*

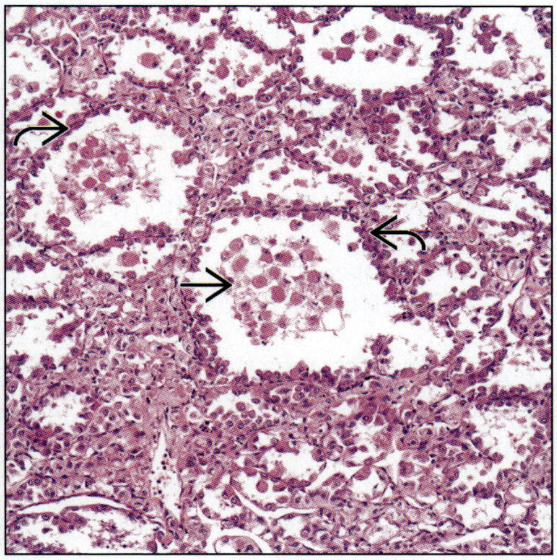
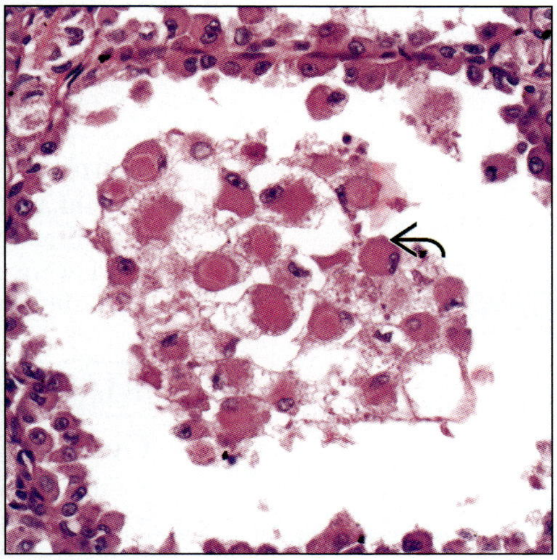

(Left) *Hematoxylin & eosin shows alveolar soft part sarcoma with prominent alveolar-like structures* ↪ *containing malignant cells* →. **(Right)** *High-power magnification of neoplastic cells in alveolar soft part sarcoma is shown with rhabdomyoblastic-like appearance* ↪. *These cytological features can be easily confused with true rhabdomyoblasts and the tumor interpreted as rhabdomyosarcoma. This cellular proliferation is unusual in alveolar soft part sarcoma.*

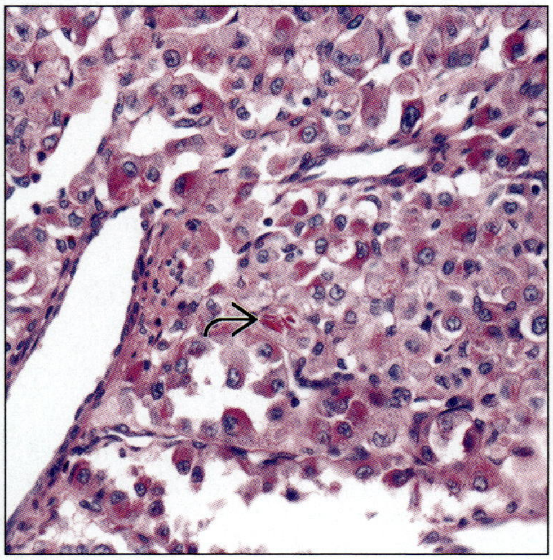
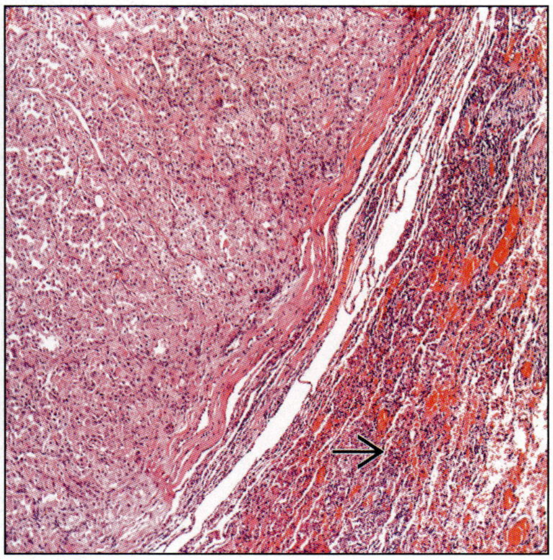

(Left) *Periodic acid-Schiff shows a high-power view of the cytoplasmic crystals* ↪ *that are commonly identified in cases of alveolar soft part sarcoma. The use of PAS histochemical stain facilitates its identification.* **(Right)** *Hematoxylin & eosin shows metastasis from an alveolar soft part sarcoma to the lung. Note the rim of alveolated lung parenchyma* →. *The tumor shows similar features to the original tumor, and lung is a common site of metastasis.*

RHABDOMYOSARCOMA

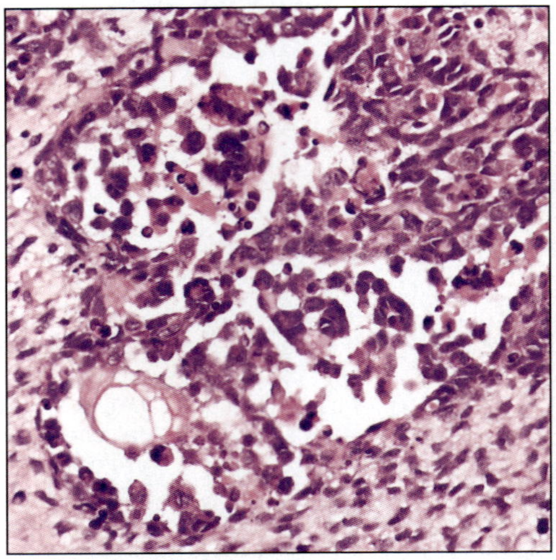

Alveolar rhabdomyosarcoma of the anterior mediastinum shows sheets of primitive small round blue cells with prominent retraction artifact resulting in an "alveolar" appearance.

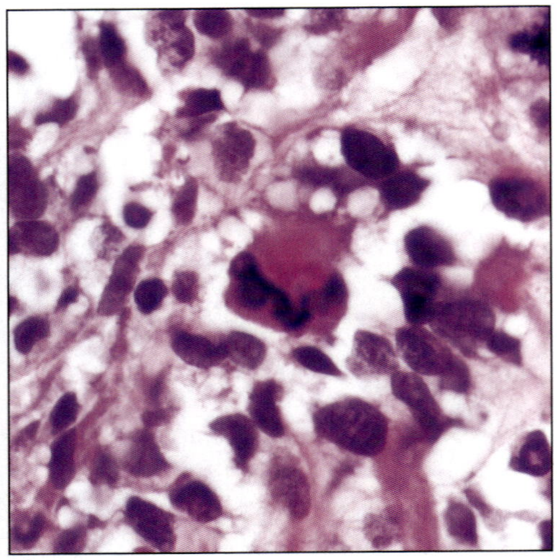

High magnification of alveolar rhabdomyosarcoma of the mediastinum shows a large multinucleated cell in the center displaying hyperchromatic nuclei and abundant pink cytoplasm.

TERMINOLOGY

Abbreviations

- Rhabdomyosarcoma (RMS)

Definitions

- Primary malignant neoplasm of mediastinum showing features of striated muscle differentiation

ETIOLOGY/PATHOGENESIS

Pathogenesis

- Pure cases may arise from totipotential stem cells within mediastinal soft tissue
- Cases associated with teratomatous elements may arise from somatic transformation of germ cells
- Cases associated with thymic carcinosarcomatous elements may arise from native thymic myoid cells

CLINICAL ISSUES

Site

- Anterior mediastinum

Presentation

- Cough
- Chest pain
- Dyspnea
- Pleural effusion
- Mostly affects young adults (mean: 23 years)

Treatment

- Surgical excision
- Adjuvant chemotherapy and radiation therapy

Prognosis

- Highly aggressive tumors with short survival time
- Rapid recurrence and metastases generally within 1st 6 months after diagnosis
- Metastases most often involve lymph nodes but may also involve lung, pleura, bone, and abdominal viscera

IMAGE FINDINGS

General Features

- Solid, unencapsulated expansile lesion with poorly defined, infiltrative borders
- CT scans show large homogeneous mass displacing midline structures with pleural effusion

MACROSCOPIC FEATURES

General Features

- Firm, poorly circumscribed, and infiltrative mass
- Homogeneous, tan-gray cut surface
- Areas of hemorrhage and necrosis

Size

- 4-12 cm

MICROSCOPIC PATHOLOGY

Histologic Features

- Tumors may appear de novo in pure form, or may be associated with germ cell, teratomatous, or carcinomatous elements
- Pure, de novo tumors may show varied histology
- **Embryonal rhabdomyosarcoma**
  - Sheets of "small round blue cells" with hyperchromatic nuclei and scant eosinophilic cytoplasm
  - Scattered immature rhabdomyoblasts characterized by comma-shaped cells with small, dark nuclei and bright pink rim of cytoplasm
  - Spindle cell variant of embryonal rhabdomyosarcoma is composed of atypical spindle cells set against myxoid stroma

Key Facts

Clinical Issues

- Anterior mediastinum
- Cough
- Chest pain
- Dyspnea
- Pleural effusion
- Highly aggressive tumors with short survival

Microscopic Pathology

- Sheets of "small round blue cells" with hyperchromatic nuclei and scant eosinophilic cytoplasm
- Spindle cell variant of embryonal rhabdomyosarcoma is composed of fascicular proliferation of atypical spindle cells against myxoid stroma
- Artifactual clefting of nests of small blue cells from periphery results in striking "alveolar" pattern
- Scattered multinucleated tumor cells with large hyperchromatic nuclei are seen admixed with small blue tumor cells
- Bizarre atypical cells with large, pleomorphic, and irregular nuclei are seen in pleomorphic variant of rhabdomyosarcoma

Ancillary Tests

- Tumor cells are positive for desmin, Myo-D1, and myogenin
- Tumor cells may aberrantly express cytokeratin, NSE, and S100 protein
- Electron microscopy will show thick and thin filaments with Z-bands
- PAX3/FKHR and PAX7/FKHR fusion product can be detected by FISH in alveolar rhabdomyosarcoma

- **Alveolar rhabdomyosarcoma**
  - Solid sheets of "small round blue cells" supported by delicate fibrovascular stroma
  - Artifactual clefting of nests of small blue cells from periphery results in striking "alveolar" pattern
  - Scattered multinucleated tumor cells with large hyperchromatic nuclei are seen admixed with small blue tumor cells
- **Pleomorphic rhabdomyosarcoma**
  - Bizarre atypical cells with large, pleomorphic, and irregular nuclei surrounded by abundant eosinophilic cytoplasm
  - Cells may show slender, tapering cytoplasmic processes resembling racquet cells
  - Only rarely will cells display cytoplasmic cross-striations

Cytologic Features

- Small round blue cells show primitive cytologic appearance with hyperchromatic nuclei devoid of nuclear detail
- High mitotic activity is the norm
- Multinucleated tumor cells in alveolar rhabdomyosarcoma usually assume wreath-like configuration with nuclei in periphery
- Tumor cells in pleomorphic rhabdomyosarcoma rarely if ever display cross striations in cytoplasm

ANCILLARY TESTS

Immunohistochemistry

- Tumor cells may be focally positive for S100 protein, cytokeratin, NSE, and SMA
- Tumor cells strongly show nuclear expression of skeletal muscle transcription factors, Myo-D1, and myogenin
- Tumor cells are positive for desmin and vimentin

Cytogenetics

- Allelic losses in chromosome 11p15 are seen in embryonal rhabdomyosarcomas
- Complex structural and numerical chromosomal changes are seen in embryonal rhabdomyosarcoma, including extra copies of chromosomes 2, 8, and 13
- Specific translocation t(2;13)(q35;q14) is associated with alveolar rhabdomyosarcoma and gives rise to PAX3/FKHR and PAX7/FKHR fusion proteins

Electron Microscopy

- Parallel arrays of microfilaments and ribosomes (myosin-ribosome complexes) are seen in earliest stages of differentiation
- Bundles of thick and thin filaments with focal condensations (Z-bands) characterize mature tumors

DIFFERENTIAL DIAGNOSIS

Small Round Blue Cell Tumors

- Lymphoblastic lymphoma shows positivity for CD3, CD1a, TdT, and CD99 and is negative for skeletal muscle transcription factors
- Lymphocyte-rich thymoma shows positivity for cytokeratin and p63 and is negative for skeletal muscle transcription factors
- Small cell neuroendocrine carcinoma shows positivity for cytokeratin, chromogranin, and synaptophysin and is negative for skeletal muscle transcription factors
- PNET/Ewing sarcoma shows strong positivity for CD99 and is negative for skeletal muscle transcription factors

SELECTED REFERENCES

1. Malagón HD et al: Germ cell tumors with sarcomatous components: a clinicopathologic and immunohistochemical study of 46 cases. Am J Surg Pathol. 31(9):1356-62, 2007
2. Suster S et al: Rhabdomyosarcomas of the anterior mediastinum: report of four cases unassociated with germ cell, teratomatous, or thymic carcinomatous components. Hum Pathol. 25(4):349-56, 1994

RHABDOMYOSARCOMA

Embryonal Rhabdomyosarcoma

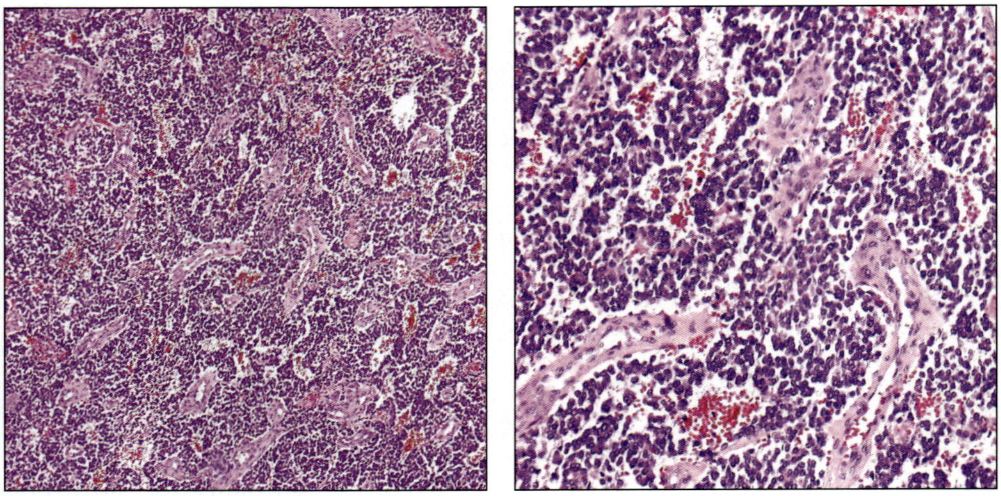

(Left) *Scanning magnification of embryonal rhabdomyosarcoma of the anterior mediastinum in a 19-year-old man shows sheets of "small round blue cells"separated by a well-vascularized stroma without any distinctive architectural growth pattern.* ***(Right)*** *High magnification of embryonal rhabdomyosarcoma of the anterior mediastinum in a 19-year-old man shows a monotonous population of discohesive small round blue cells separated by thin strands of fibrovascular stroma.*

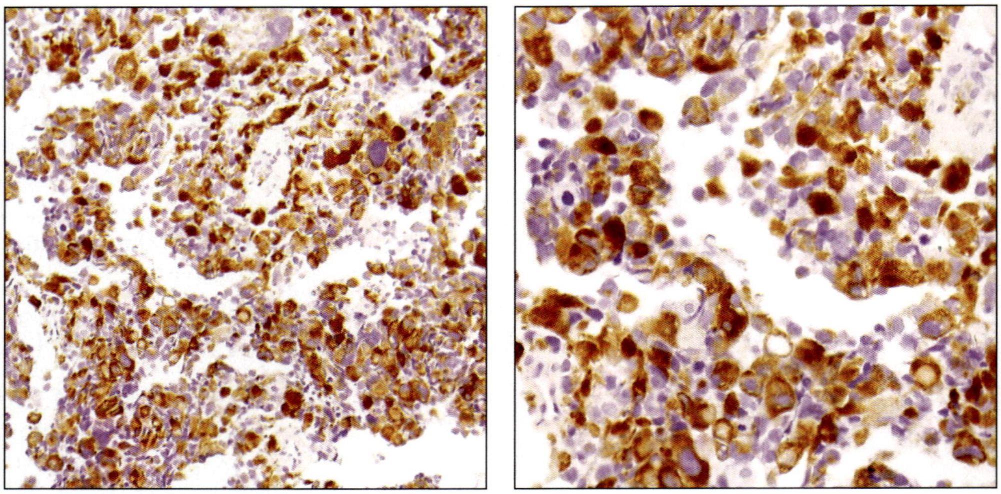

(Left) *Immunohistochemical staining of embryonal rhabdomyosarcoma of the anterior mediastinum with the striated muscle-specific transcription factor, Myo-D1, shows nuclear staining of the tumor cells for this antigen.* ***(Right)*** *Immunohistochemical staining of embryonal rhabdomyosarcoma of the anterior mediastinum for desmin shows strong cytoplasmic staining of the tumor cells for this marker, indicative of myogenic differentiation of the tumor cells.*

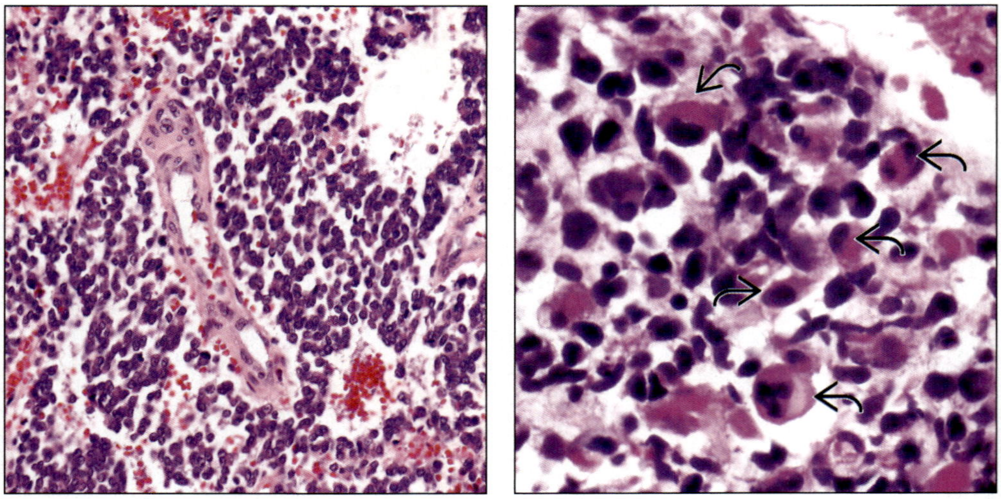

(Left) *Scanning magnification of embryonal rhabdomyosarcoma of the mediastinum shows monotonous proliferation of small round blue cells with scant pink cytoplasm. This tumor can resemble lymphoblastic lymphoma, small cell carcinoma, and Ewing sarcoma/PNET by morphology.* ***(Right)*** *High magnification of embryonal rhabdomyosarcoma shows small round blue cells admixed with slightly larger cells containing abundant, eccentric pink cytoplasm, typical of rhabdomyoblasts ↷.*

Spindle Cell Embryonal Rhabdomyosarcoma

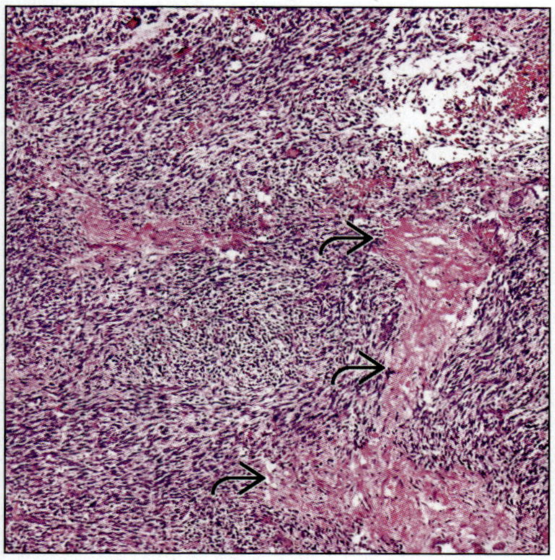
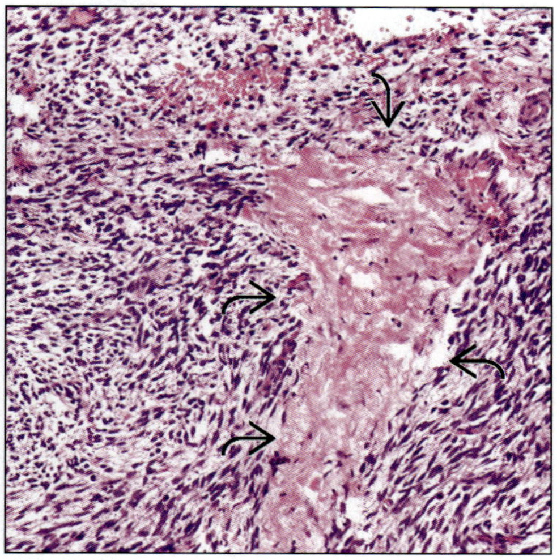

(Left) *Embryonal rhabdomyosarcoma of the anterior mediastinum in a 21-year-old man is characterized by dense spindle cell proliferation with focal areas of necrosis →. The spindle cells show focal whorling and a fascicular pattern of growth.* ***(Right)*** *Embryonal rhabdomyosarcoma of the mediastinum (spindle cell type) shows fascicles of atypical spindle cells circumscribing an area of necrosis →. This tumor can be confused for a variety of other spindle cell sarcomas.*

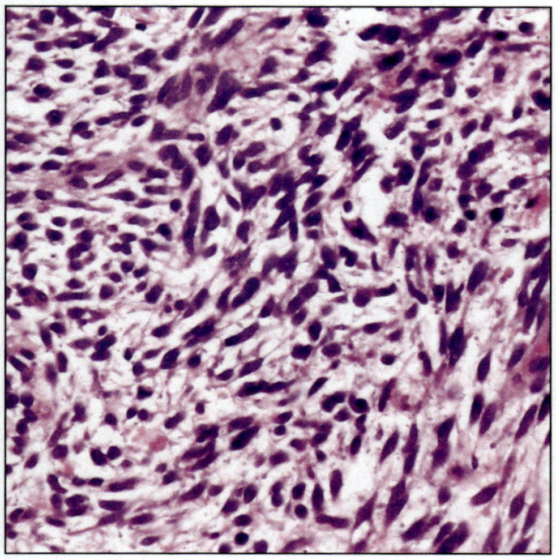
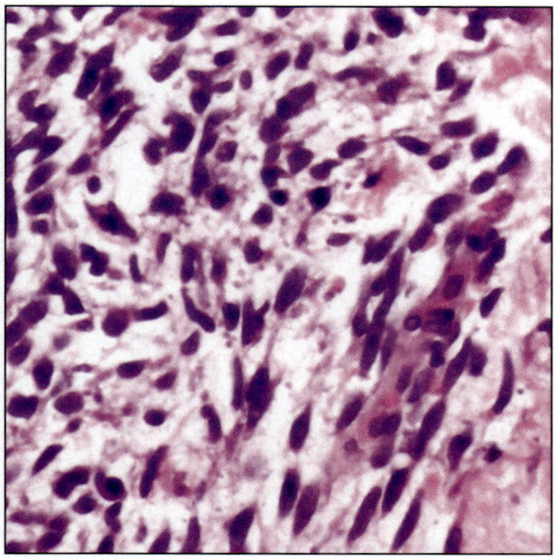

(Left) *High magnification of embryonal rhabdomyosarcoma of the mediastinum (spindle cell variant) shows haphazardly arranged fascicles of hyperchromatic spindle cells containing a few scattered mitoses and with little intervening stroma.* ***(Right)*** *High magnification of embryonal rhabdomyosarcoma of the mediastinum (spindle cell type) shows small spindle cells with dark, hyperchromatic nuclei surrounded by a scant rim of amphophilic cytoplasm.*

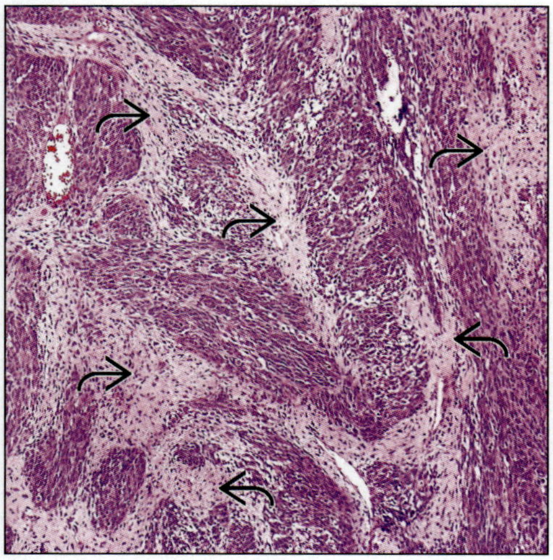
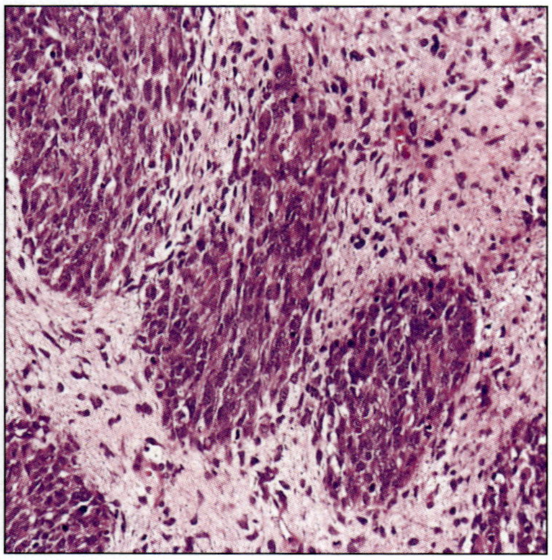

(Left) *Embryonal rhabdomyosarcoma of the anterior mediastinum (spindle cell type) shows dense fascicles of tightly packed spindle cells separated by strands of myxoid stroma →.* ***(Right)*** *Embryonal rhabdomyosarcoma of the anterior mediastinum, spindle cell type, shows fascicles of spindle cells separated by abundant myxoid stroma. Notice the spindle cells contain dark nuclei and are surrounded by a scant rim of amphophilic cytoplasm.*

RHABDOMYOSARCOMA

Alveolar Rhabdomyosarcoma

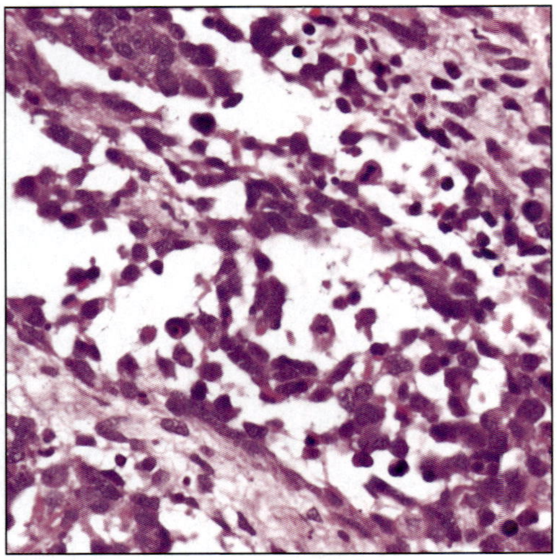
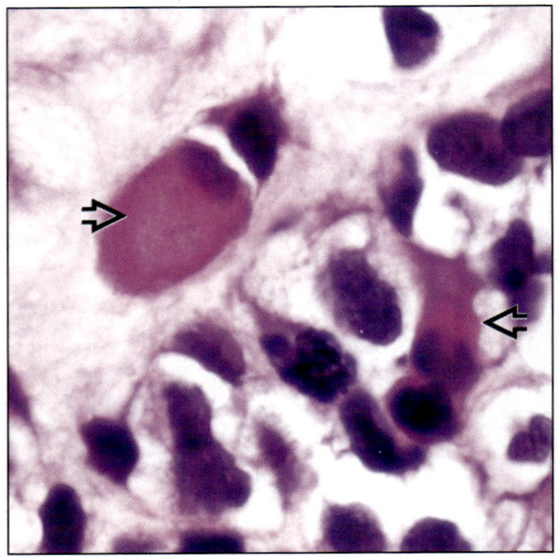

(Left) *Alveolar rhabdomyosarcoma of the anterior mediastinum shows a population of small round blue cells with characteristic artifactual separation of the tumor cells from the surrounding stroma resembling alveolar lumens.* ***(Right)*** *High magnification of alveolar rhabdomyosarcoma of the anterior mediastinum shows primitive cells with abundant globular, eccentric, and deeply staining pink cytoplasm reminiscent of developing embryonal rhabdomyoblasts ⇨.*

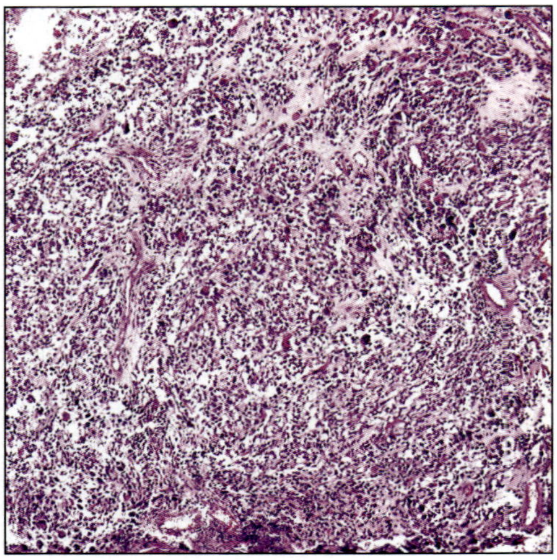
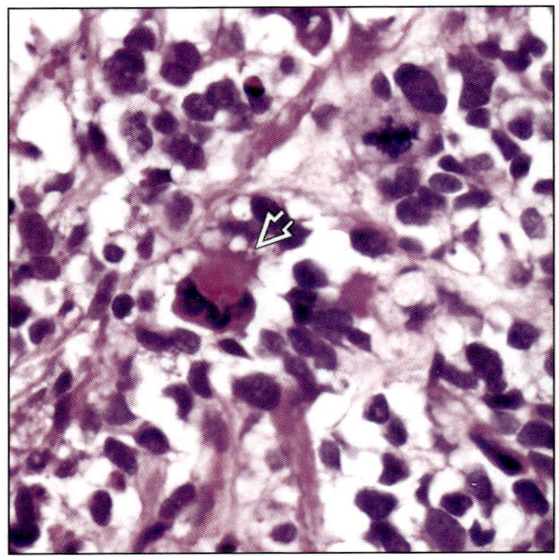

(Left) *Solid variant of alveolar rhabdomyosarcoma of the mediastinum shows compact sheets of small round blue cells without the characteristic alveolar retraction artifact.* ***(Right)*** *High magnification of solid variant of alveolar rhabdomyosarcoma of the mediastinum shows larger cells with marked nuclear pleomorphism and scattered pleomorphic, multinucleated giant cells with abundant pink cytoplasm ➡. The greater variability of the size and shape of the cells characterizes this tumor.*

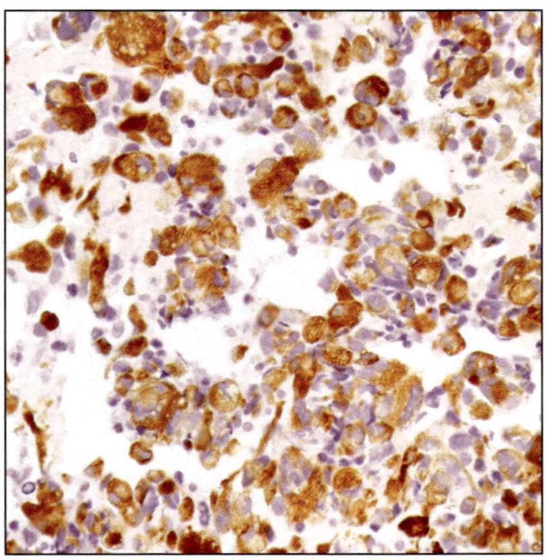
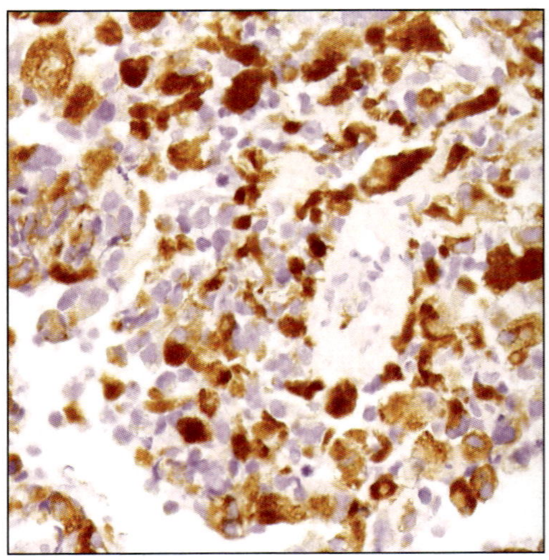

(Left) *Immunohistochemical staining for desmin in alveolar rhabdomyosarcoma of the mediastinum (solid variant) shows strong cytoplasmic staining of the tumor cells for this antibody.* ***(Right)*** *Immunohistochemical staining of alveolar rhabdomyosarcoma of the mediastinum for the skeletal muscle-specific transcription factor, myogenin, shows strong nuclear positivity in the tumor cells. The skeletal muscle transcription factors, myogenin and Myo-D1, are highly specific for these tumors.*

Pleomorphic Rhabdomyosarcoma

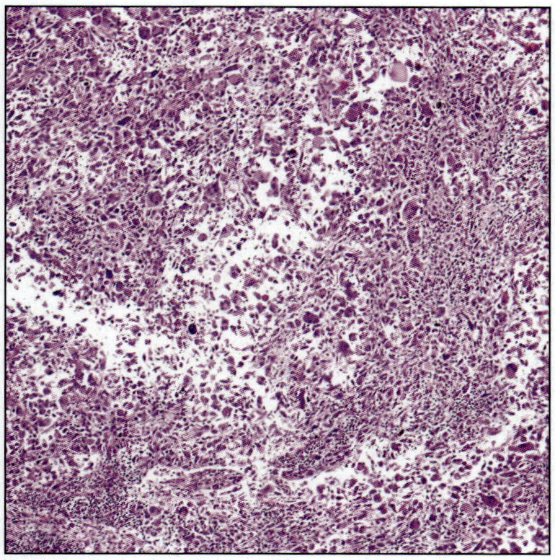
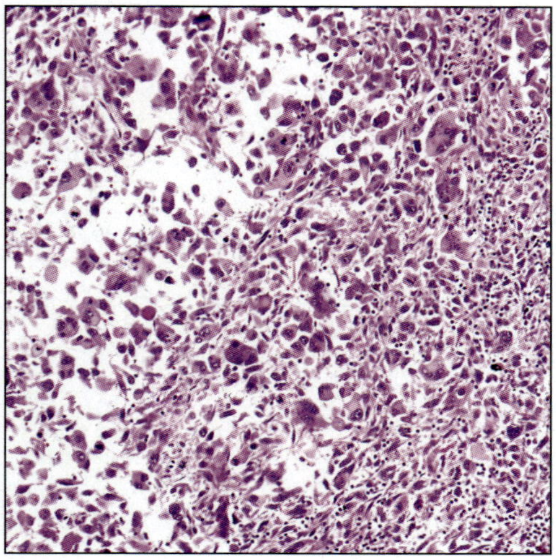

(Left) *Scanning magnification of pleomorphic rhabdomyosarcoma of the mediastinum shows sheets of large, pleomorphic tumor cells admixed with smaller cells with scant intervening stroma.* **(Right)** *Scanning magnification of pleomorphic rhabdomyosarcoma of the mediastinum shows sheets of small cells admixed with larger, pleomorphic tumor cells. Tumors with these features may resemble a variety of other neoplasms, including liposarcoma, MFH, and anaplastic carcinoma.*

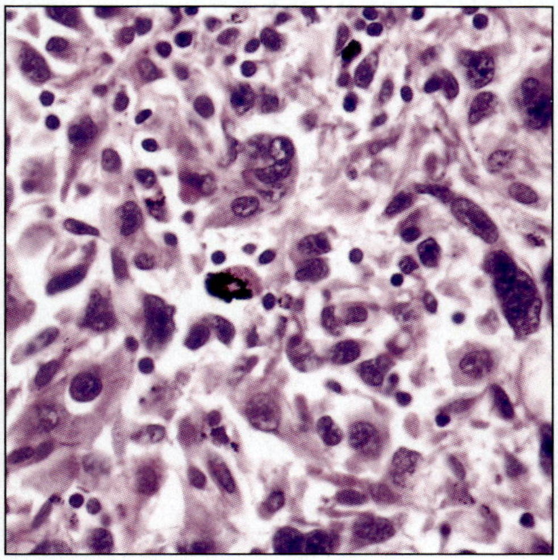
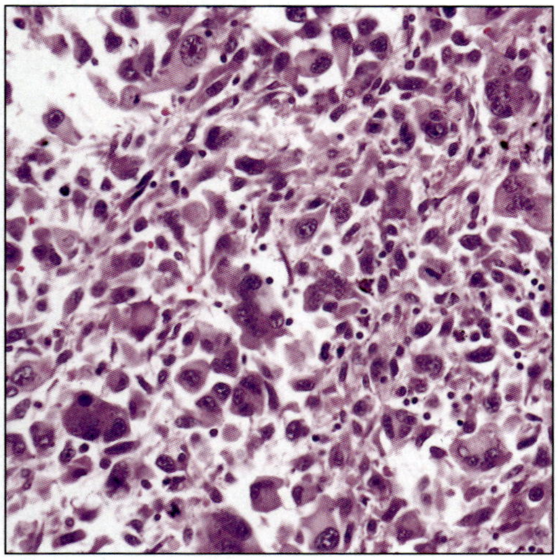

(Left) *High magnification of pleomorphic rhabdomyosarcoma of the mediastinum shows bizarre, pleomorphic tumor cells admixed with smaller, more primitive tumor cells, and a sprinkling of inflammatory cells in the background. Tumors like this can resemble anaplastic carcinomas.* **(Right)** *High magnification of pleomorphic liposarcoma of the mediastinum shows sheets of small atypical cells admixed with scattered larger, pleomorphic cells with bizarre nuclei.*

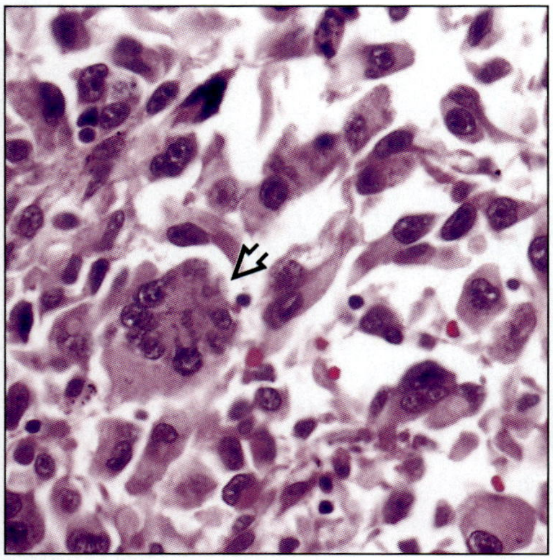
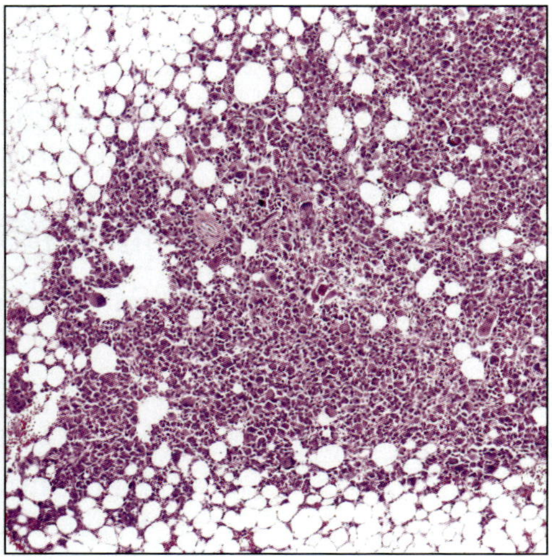

(Left) *High magnification of pleomorphic rhabdomyosarcoma of the mediastinum shows a discohesive population of tumor cells, including spindle cells, "strap" cells, and large multinucleated tumor cells ⇨ with a Touton-like appearance. Tumors like this can resemble malignant fibrous histiocytoma and pleomorphic liposarcoma.* **(Right)** *Pleomorphic rhabdomyosarcoma of the mediastinum shows infiltration of mediastinal fat by the tumor cells.*

GANGLIONEUROMA

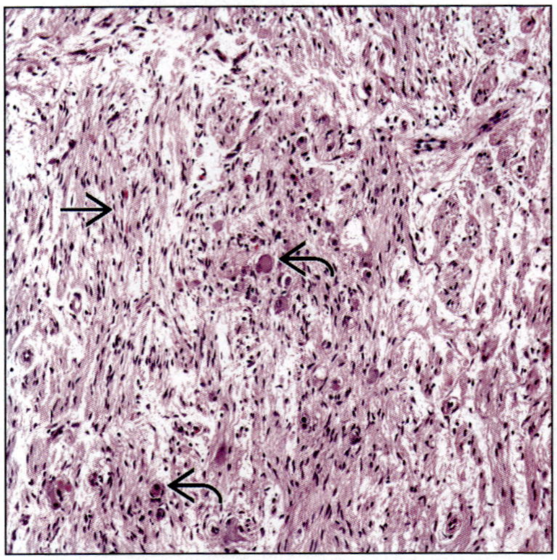

Ganglioneuroma shows a bland spindle cellular proliferation ➙ with scattered larger cells ➙ representing ganglion cells. Both components are essential for the diagnosis.

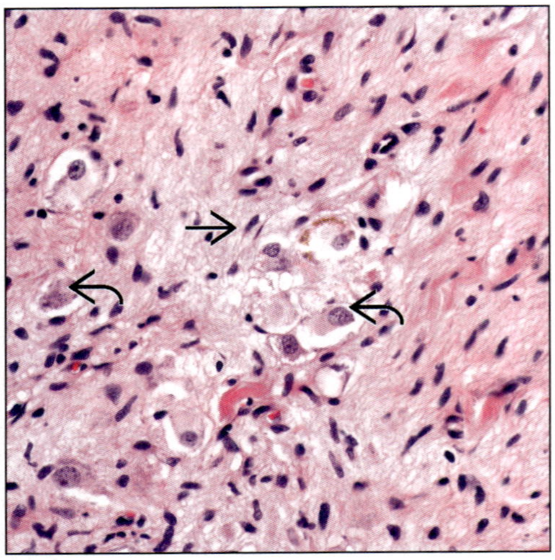

Higher power view of a mediastinal ganglioneuroma displays a spindle cell proliferation ➙ admixed with numerous larger cells with prominent nucleoli (ganglion cells) ➙.

TERMINOLOGY

Abbreviations

- Ganglioneuroma (GN)

Definitions

- Benign tumor of neural origin

ETIOLOGY/PATHOGENESIS

Etiology

- There is no definitive etiology for this neoplasm

CLINICAL ISSUES

Epidemiology

- Incidence
    - Unusual tumors representing a small percentage of mediastinal tumors
- Age
    - More common in younger patients

Site

- GN is more common in posterior mediastinum

Presentation

- Shortness of breath
- Chest pain
- Horner syndrome
- Neurofibromatosis

Treatment

- Surgical approaches
    - Complete surgical resection

Prognosis

- Good

MACROSCOPIC FEATURES

General Features

- Well circumscribed and encapsulated
- Firm, gray to yellowish
- Cut surface shows whitish smooth or whorled appearance
- Areas of necrosis and hemorrhage are generally absent

Size

- Tumors vary in size from 1 cm to > 10 cm in greatest dimension

MICROSCOPIC PATHOLOGY

Histologic Features

- Mature ganglion cells embedded in loose fibrocollagenous or subtle spindle cell stroma
- Proliferation of Schwann cells, nerve fibers, and ganglion cells
- Nissl granules may be seen in some cases in ganglion cells

Cytologic Features

- Mature ganglion cells

DIFFERENTIAL DIAGNOSIS

Schwannoma

- Classically shows Antoni A and B areas while these would be unusual in GN
- It would be unusual for Schwannoma to show numerous ganglion cells

Neurofibroma

- Spindle cell component of neurofibroma is similar to that of GN
- Neurofibromas lack the presence of ganglion cells

GANGLIONEUROMA

Key Facts

Terminology
- Ganglioneuroma (GN)
- Benign tumor of neural origin

Clinical Issues
- Incidence
  - Tumor is more common in young patients
- Location
  - More common in posterior mediastinum
- Symptomatology
  - Chest pain
  - Horner syndrome
  - Shortness of breath
  - Neurofibromatosis
- Treatment
  - Surgical resection
- Prognosis
  - Good
- Clinical features
  - Tumor is more common in younger patients
  - More common in posterior mediastinum
- Shortness of breath
- Symptoms
  - Shortness of breath
  - Chest pain
  - Horner syndrome
  - Neurofibromatosis

Top Differential Diagnoses
- Schwannoma
- Neurofibroma
- Ganglioneuroblastoma
- Solitary fibrous tumor

Immunohistochemistry

Antibody	Reactivity	Staining Pattern	Comment
S100	Positive	Nuclear & cytoplasmic	May be only focal staining
NFP	Positive	Cytoplasmic	Variable staining intensity
NSE	Positive	Cytoplasmic	Positive in ganglion cells
CD56	Positive	Cytoplasmic	May be focal
CK-LMW-NOS	Negative		May be positive in entrapped epithelial structures
EMA	Negative		May be positive in entrapped epithelial structures
Chromogranin-A	Negative		
Synaptophysin	Negative		
CK-PAN	Negative		May be positive in entrapped epithelial structures
CD34	Negative		
Bcl-2	Negative		

Ganglioneuroblastoma
- Shows neuroblastomatous component, which is absent in GN

Solitary Fibrous Tumor
- May show different growth pattern, including HPC, which will be unusual in GN
- Presence of hypo- and hypercellular areas is commonly seen in soft tissue tumor
- Shows positive staining for CD34 &/or Bcl-2 while GN is negative

DIAGNOSTIC CHECKLIST

Clinically Relevant Pathologic Features
- Nuclear features

Pathologic Interpretation Pearls
- Presence of mature ganglion cells embedded in loose fibrocollagenous stroma
- Absence of mitotic activity
- Spindle cell component may be subtle

SELECTED REFERENCES

1. Di Cataldo A et al: Mediastinal ganglioneuroma: a rare and often asymptomatic tumour. A case report. Chir Ital. 57(3):403-5, 2005
2. Modha A et al: Presacral ganglioneuromas. Report of five cases and review of the literature. J Neurosurg Spine. 2(3):366-71, 2005
3. Tanaka O et al: Neurogenic tumors of the mediastinum and chest wall: MR imaging appearance. J Thorac Imaging. 20(4):316-20, 2005
4. Lonergan GJ et al: Neuroblastoma, ganglioneuroblastoma, and ganglioneuroma: radiologic-pathologic correlation. Radiographics. 22(4):911-34, 2002
5. Albonico G et al: Ganglioneuroma of parapharyngeal region. Arch Pathol Lab Med. 125(9):1217-8, 2001
6. Marchevsky AM: Mediastinal tumors of peripheral nervous system origin. Semin Diagn Pathol. 16(1):65-78, 1999
7. Mondal A: Cytopathology of neuroblastoma, ganglioneuroblastoma and ganglioneuroma. J Indian Med Assoc. 93(9):340-3, 1995
8. Gale AW et al: Neurogenic tumors of the mediastinum. Ann Thorac Surg. 17(5):434-43, 1974
9. Battisti C et al: [Multiple ganglioneuromas of the mediastinum associated with Recklinghausen's disease in an 8-year-old body.] Arch Chir Torac Cardiovasc. 25(4):301-23, 1968

GANGLIONEUROMA

Gross and Microscopic Features

(Left) *A tumor mass with a yellowish color and firm consistency is depicted. The tumor is well circumscribed and slightly lobulated. These features are in keeping with a ganglioneuroma.* ***(Right)*** *Low power of a mediastinal ganglioneuroma shows a spindle cellular proliferation → admixed with ectatic vessels ⇨ and areas with numerous ganglion cells ↷.*

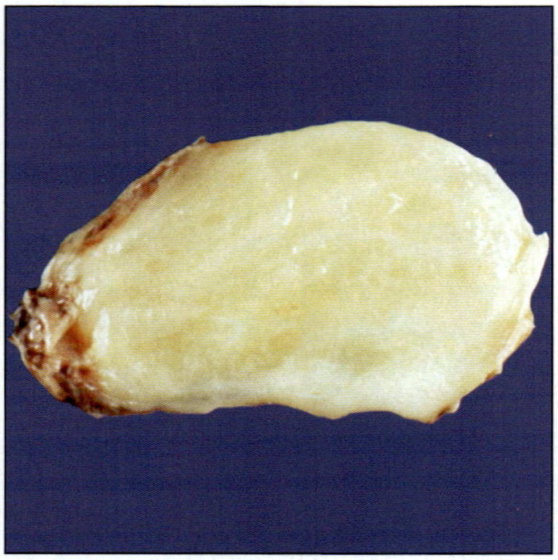

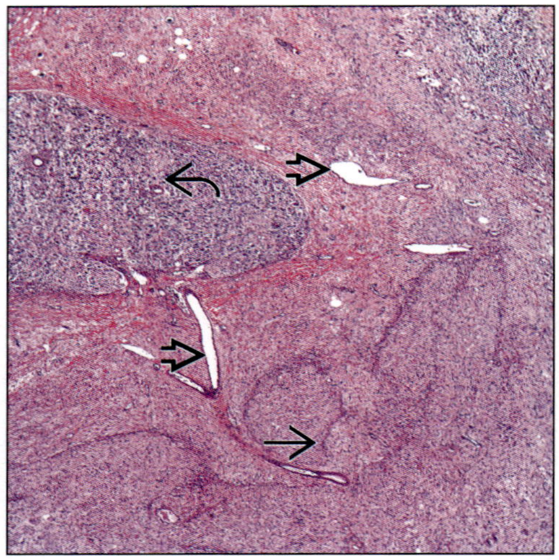

(Left) *Mediastinal ganglioneuroma is shown with prominent ganglion cell component ↷. A 2nd smaller tumor is present with similar histological features →.* ***(Right)*** *Ganglioneuroma shows focal areas of calcification ⇨ in addition to the common histological features of spindle cells and the presence of ganglion cells ↷.*

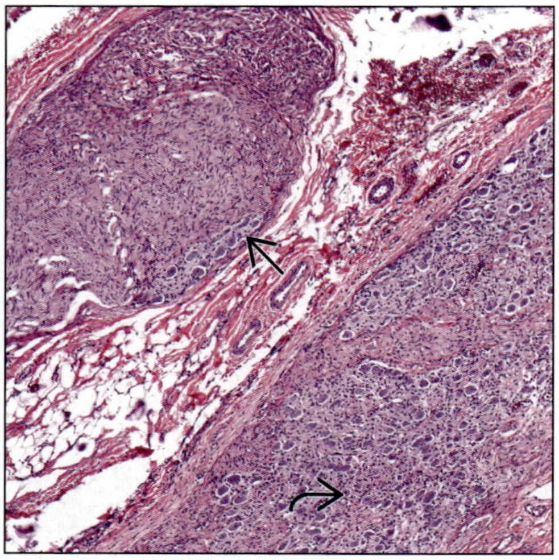

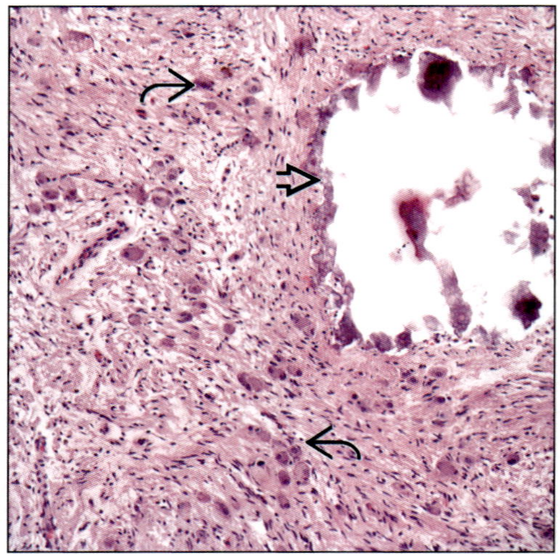

(Left) *In some cases of ganglioneuroma, the diagnosis may not be readily recognized. The tumor may show extensive areas of collagen → and adipose ⇨ tissue with an entrapped nerve ↷.* ***(Right)*** *High-power view shows ganglioneuroma in which the tumor shows extensive areas of collagen deposition and adipose tissue. These features may be easily encountered in hamartomatous lesions.*

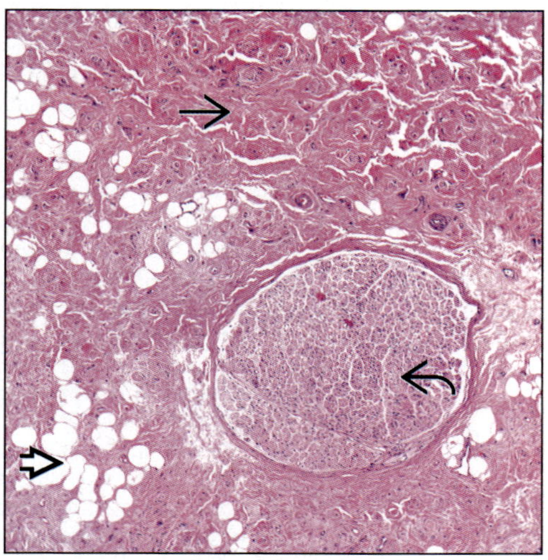

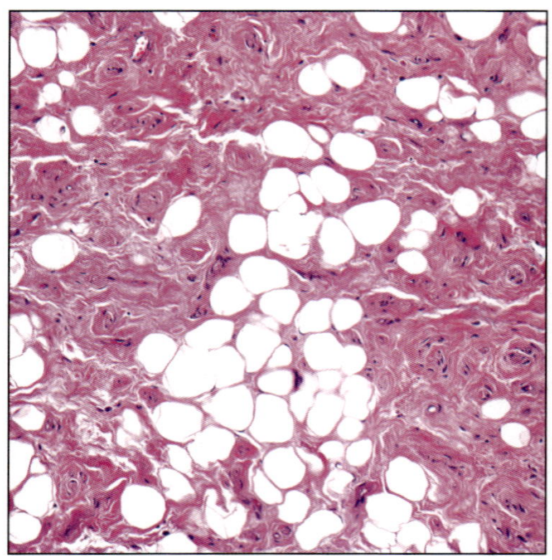

GANGLIONEUROMA

Microscopic Features

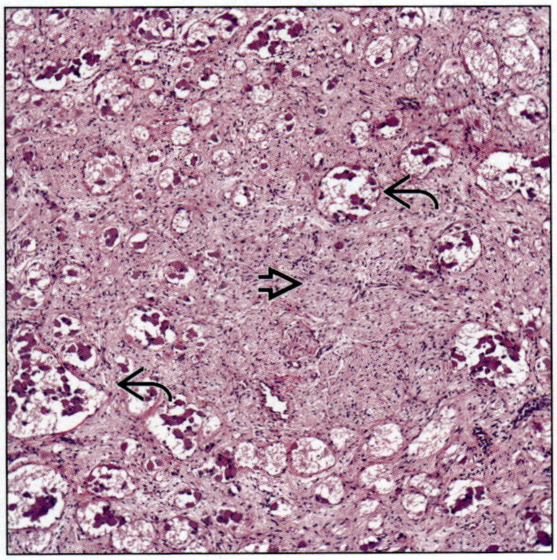

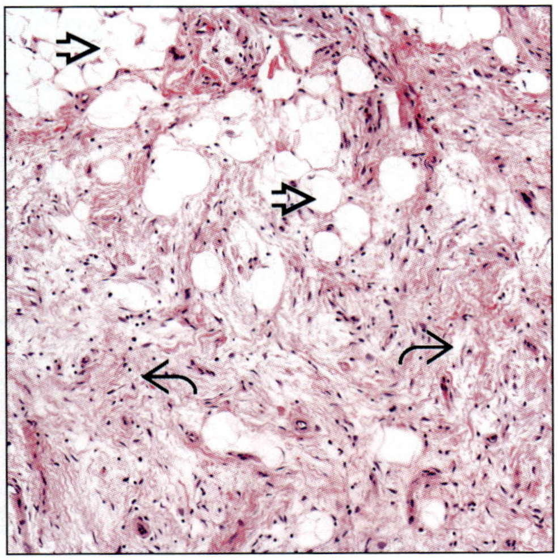

(Left) *Mediastinal ganglioneuroma is shown with a vague alveolar pattern* ↷ *admixed with solid areas* ⇨. *The alveolar-like areas are composed of ganglion cells, while the solid areas are composed of spindle cells.* ***(Right)*** *In some cases of ganglioneuroma, the predominant component may be the neuromatous elements* ↷ *with only scattered ganglion cells and focal myxoid changes admixed with adipose tissue* ⇨, *as is depicted here.*

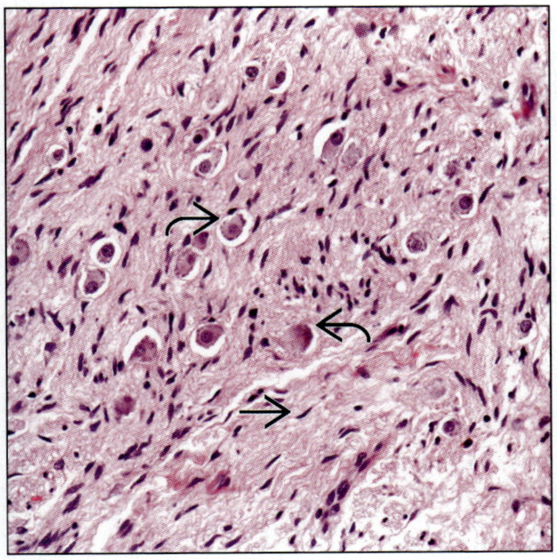

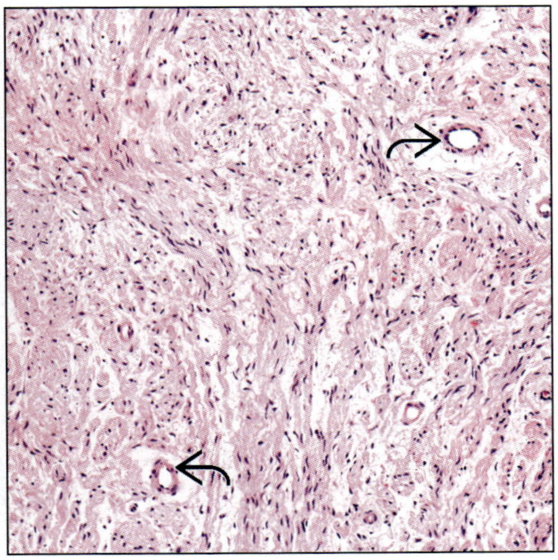

(Left) *Classical histological features of ganglioneuroma are shown in which the tumor shows dual populations of cells. The larger cells represent ganglion cells* ↷, *while the spindle cells represent the neuromatous component* →. ***(Right)*** *Ganglioneuroma shows areas resembling loose fibroconnective tissue or possibly smooth muscle. The predominant cell component is neuromatous with scattered blood vessels* ↷.

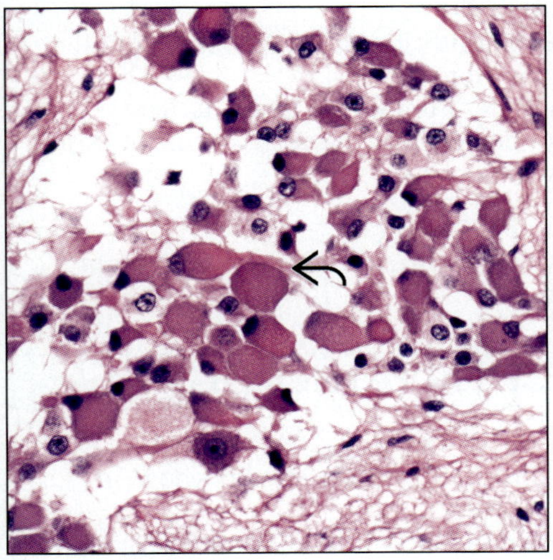

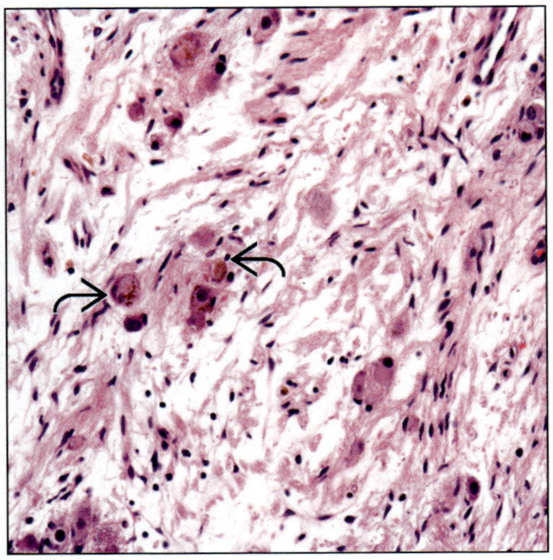

(Left) *High-power view shows the ganglion cells* ↷ *in a ganglioneuroma. This group of ganglion cells can easily be confused with muscle cells like the ones present in tumors with rhabdomyoblastic differentiation.* ***(Right)*** *High-power view shows a ganglioneuroma in which ganglion cells are embedded in a rather myxoid or loose fibroconnective tissue. Note the presence of pigment in the ganglion cells* ↷ *representing Nissl substance.*

NEUROBLASTOMA/GANGLIONEUROBLASTOMA

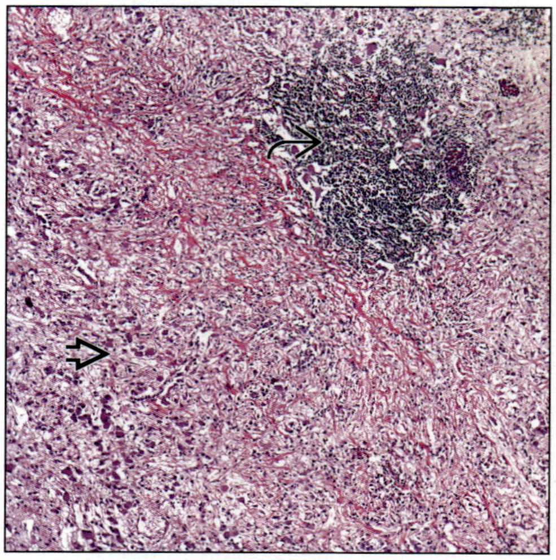

Low-power view shows a ganglioneuroblastoma with predominant ganglioneuromatous component ⇨. Note the presence of the small cluster of cells representing the neuroblastomatous component ⤻.

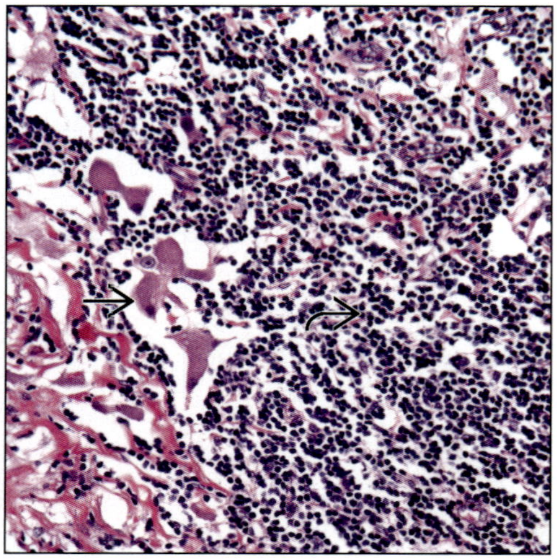

High-power view shows the neuroblastomatous ⤻ component in a GNB. Note that in the periphery there are still identifiable ganglion cells →.

TERMINOLOGY

Abbreviations

- Neuroblastoma (NB), ganglioneuroblastoma (GNB)

Synonyms

- Differentiating neuroblastoma and immature ganglioneuroma both synonyms for GNB

Definitions

- Malignant neoplasm composed of immature neural elements (NB) that may be admixed with ganglioneuromatous component (GNB)

ETIOLOGY/PATHOGENESIS

Etiology

- GNB is believed to represent a transitional tumor of sympathetic cell orgin
- NB is a tumor believed to be of neural crest orgin

CLINICAL ISSUES

Epidemiology

- Incidence
  - Unusual tumors in mediastinal compartment
- Age
  - Tumor more common in younger individuals
  - Usually in patients < 15 years old
- Gender
  - No gender predilection
  - NB may be more commonly seen in male patients

Site

- NB and GNB are usually in posterior mediastinum
- Unusual cases may be in anterior mediastinum

Presentation

- Chest pain
- Paraplegia
- Horner syndrome
- Chronic diarrhea
- Various congenital anomalies
- Asymptomatic

Treatment

- Surgical approaches
  - Complete surgical removal of tumor
- Adjuvant therapy
  - Radiation &/or chemotherapy in advanced cases

Prognosis

- Depends largely on clinical stage of patient at time of diagnosis
- Also depends on degree of differentiation of tumor
- Children appear to have more favorable outcome

MACROSCOPIC FEATURES

General Features

- Lobulated neoplasm with "dumbbell" configuration
- Gray to tan in color
- Consistency varies from soft to hard and fleshy
- Focal areas of hemorrhage, necrosis, or calcification may be present

Size

- Tumors may vary in size from 2 cm to > 10 cm in greatest diameter

MICROSCOPIC PATHOLOGY

Histologic Features

- Small round blue cell proliferation embedded in neuropil
- Variable presence of ganglion cells or precursors in GNB

NEUROBLASTOMA/GANGLIONEUROBLASTOMA

Key Facts

Terminology
- Neuroblastoma (NB), ganglioneuroblastoma (GNB)
- Differentiating neuroblastoma and immature ganglioneuroma both synonyms for GNB
- Malignant neoplasm composed of immature neural elements (NB) that may be admixed with ganglioneuromatous component (GNB)

Etiology/Pathogenesis
- GNB is believed to represent a transitional tumor of sympathetic cell orgin
- NB is a tumor believed to be of neural crest orgin

Clinical Issues
- Tumor is more common in younger individuals
- Usually in patients < 15 years of age
- NB and GNB are usually in posterior mediastinum
- Prognosis
  - Depends on clinical stage at time of diagnosis
  - Depends on degree of differentiation of tumor
  - Children appear to have more favorable outcome

Top Differential Diagnoses
- Neuroblastoma
- Ganglioneuroma (GN)
- Rhabdomyosarcoma
- Ewing sarcoma/PNET

Diagnostic Checklist
- Small round blue cell tumor
- Areas of neuropil
- Presence of ganglion cells or precursors

Immunohistochemistry

Antibody	Reactivity	Staining Pattern	Comment
NSE	Positive	Cytoplasmic	Strong staining
Synaptophysin	Positive	Cytoplasmic	May be only focal weak staining
Chromogranin-A	Positive	Cytoplasmic	
NB84	Positive	Cytoplasmic	Sensitive marker but not specific
CD99	Negative		Useful for differential diagnosis with other small blue cell tumors
CK-PAN	Negative		
Desmin	Negative		

Molecular Studies

Study	Result	Comment
N-myc gene	Amplification	Correlates with better prognosis
DNA analysis	Hyperploidy	Correlates with better prognosis
TRK gene	High expression	Correlates with better prognosis

- Nuclear pleomorphism and increased mitotic activity are not common but vary according to degree of differentiator
- Areas of hemorrhage, necrosis, and calcification may be present
- Neural rosettes of Homer-Wright may be present

DIFFERENTIAL DIAGNOSIS

Neuroblastoma
- Shows similar histological features as those of GNB but lacks the presence of ganglion cells

Ganglioneuroma (GN)
- Presence of small round blue cell component is characteristic of GNB and is absent in GN

Rhabdomyosarcoma
- GNB shows presence of areas of tumor cells embedded in neuropil, which is not a feature of rhabdomyosarcoma
- Positive for muscle markers, while GNB is negative

Ewing Sarcoma/PNET
- Neoplastic cells embedded in neuropil is a feature of GNB and is absent in PNET
- Contrary to GNB, PNET has specific translocation by molecular analysis

DIAGNOSTIC CHECKLIST

Pathologic Interpretation Pearls
- Small round blue cell tumor
- Areas of neuropil
- Presence of ganglion cells or precursors

SELECTED REFERENCES

1. Adam A et al: Ganglioneuroblastoma of the posterior mediastinum: a clinicopathologic review of 80 cases. Cancer. 47(2):373-81, 1981

NEUROBLASTOMA/GANGLIONEUROBLASTOMA

Gross and Microscopic Features

__(Left)__ In this surgically resected GNB, the tumor shows a slightly lobular appearance surrounded by membranous tissue. The cut surface appears white and smooth. The gross features of GNB and NB may be similar, and histological examination is required to separate these 2 tumors. __(Right)__ Low-power view of a GNB shows a slightly lobular appearance separated by thin fibroconnective tissue. The tumor appears to be rich in neuropil ➔; such a feature is helpful in the diagnosis.

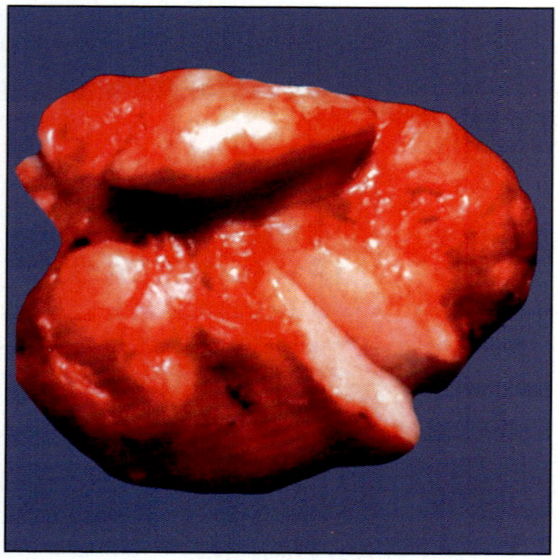

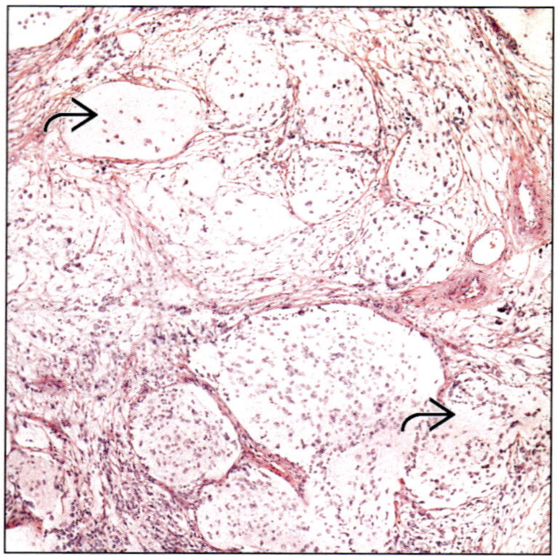

__(Left)__ Mediastinal GNB is shown with sheets of small round blue cells without any particular growth pattern. There are several ectatic blood vessels containing fresh blood. Note that the presence of neuropil is not marked. __(Right)__ Mediastinal GNB shows a cellular proliferation composed of small cells and larger cells with eccentrically placed nuclei, which represent ganglion cell precursors ➔. The identification of ganglion cells is essential in the diagnosis of GNB.

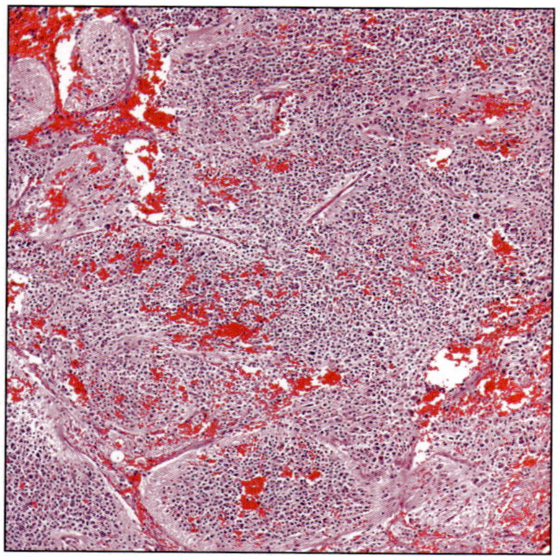

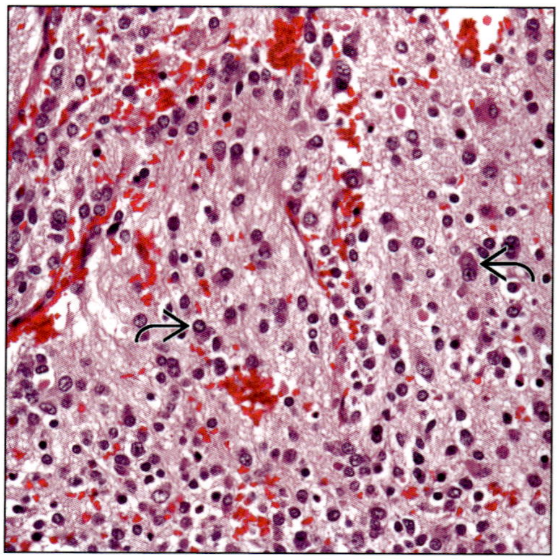

__(Left)__ Higher magnification shows ganglion cell precursors ➔ and more conventional small cells. This image could be mistaken for a mesenchymal neoplasm. __(Right)__ Mediastinal GNB shows a predominantly neuroblastomatous component. In some cases of GNB, the presence of a ganglion cell or its precursor may be more focal. This particular pattern may be seen in the so-called small round blue cell tumors.

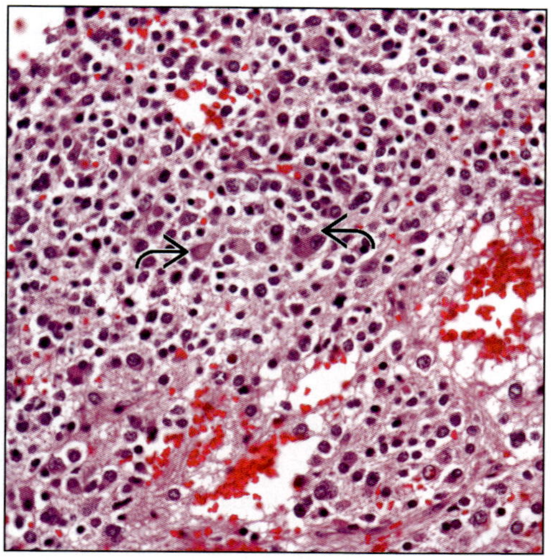

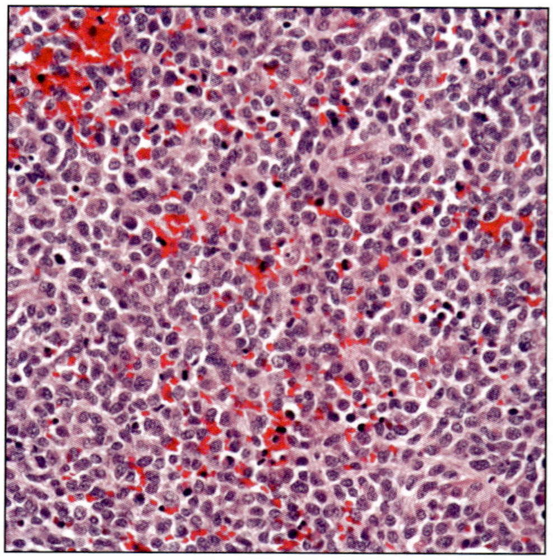

Microscopic Features

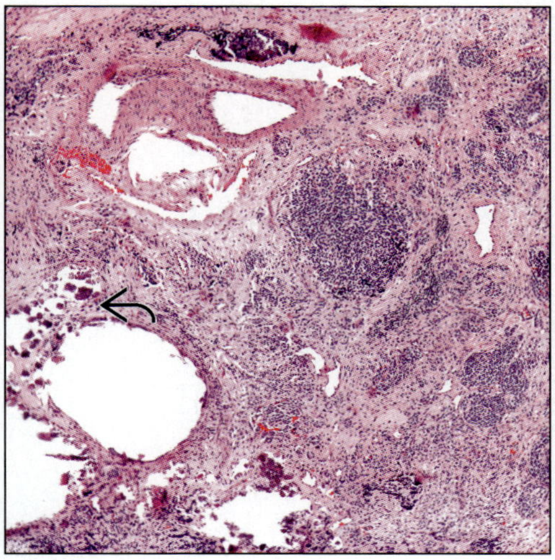

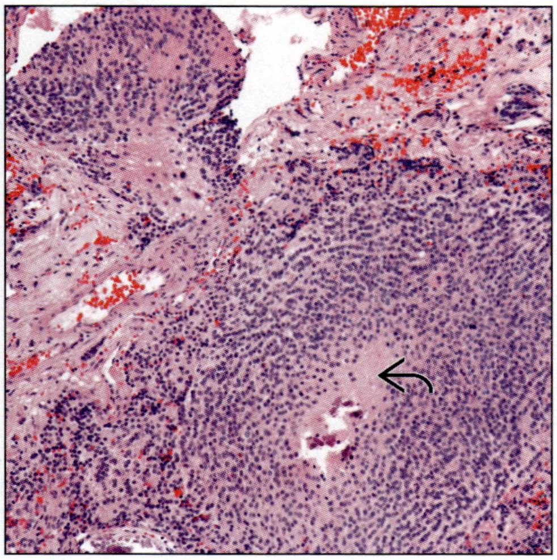

(Left) *Mediastinal neuroblastoma shows a neoplastic cellular proliferation composed of small round blue cells. The tumor shows 2 uncommon features: Cystic changes and calcifications →.* ***(Right)*** *Higher magnification shows a mediastinal NB with a concentric disposition of the tumor cells around a blood vessel. In the center, one can still see the presence of neuropil →.*

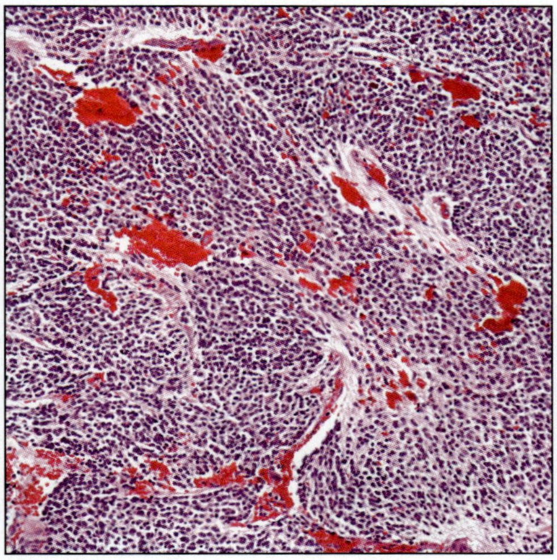

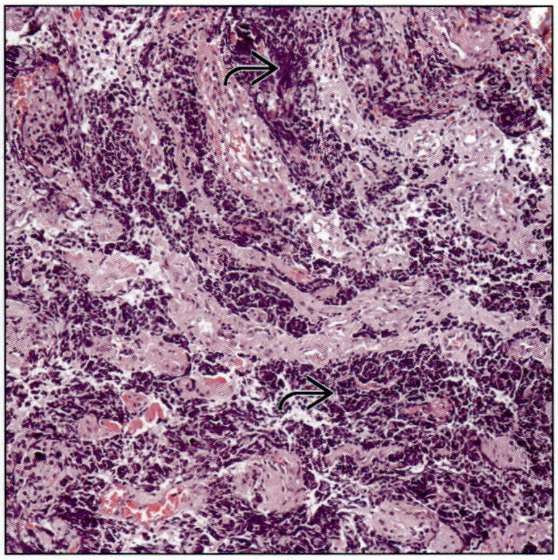

(Left) *Mediastinal NB shows sheets of cells with focal subtle nested areas. In addition, note that the presence of neuropil is not as obvious as it may be in some other cases.* ***(Right)*** *Mediastinal NB shows marked crush artifact →. The presence of crush artifact is commonly seen in small cell carcinomas. Therefore, in this setting, the use of immunohistochemical studies is helpful in leading to the correct interpretation.*

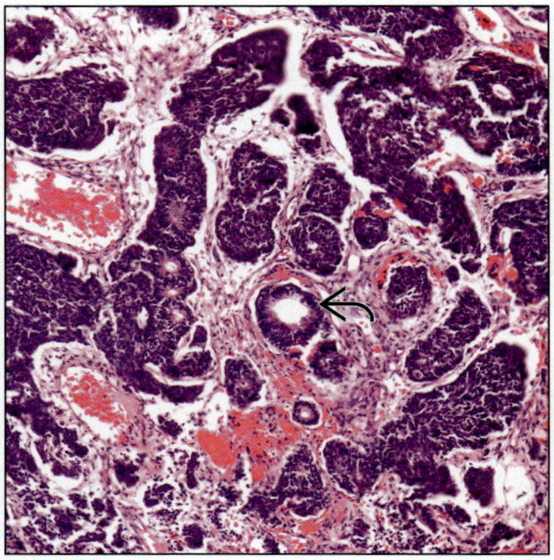

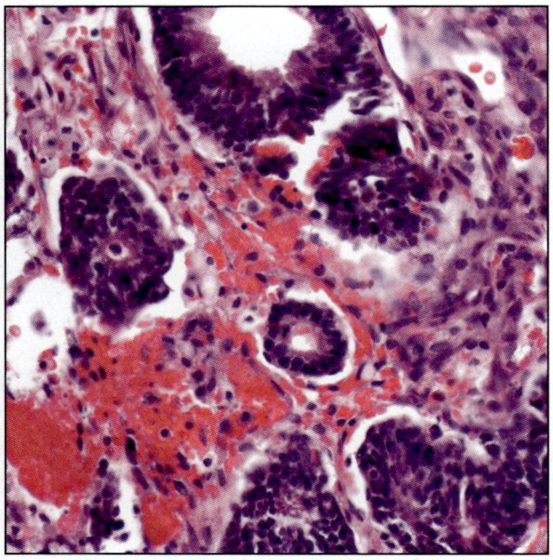

(Left) *Mediastinal NB dissecting fibroconnective tissue in a nested pattern is shown. The presence of rosettes → can be identified and is an important feature in the diagnosis of NB. However, this pattern may also be seen in neuroendocrine carcinomas; thus, immunohistochemical studies would be helpful.* ***(Right)*** *Higher magnification of NB shows rosette-like structures embedded in fibroconnective tissue. This feature may be helpful in the diagnosis of neuroblastoma.*

EPENDYMOMA

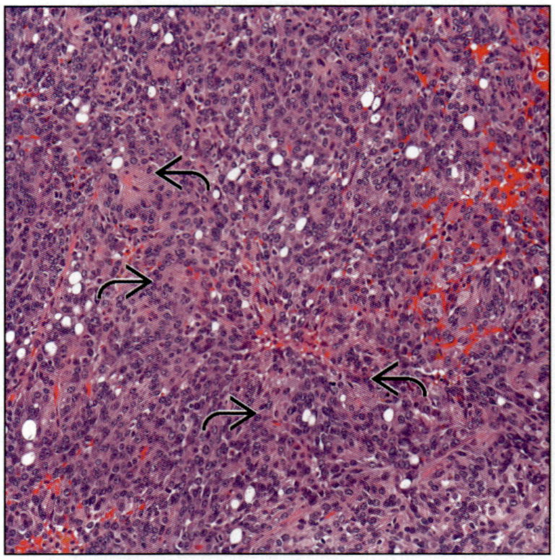

Low-power view shows a mediastinal ependymoma with a solid cellular proliferation and the formation of rosettes ⇗. Note the presence of a rather homogeneous cellular proliferation.

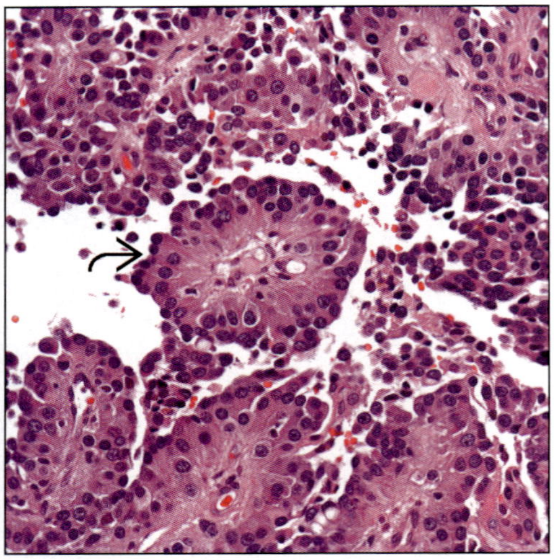

Higher magnification of a mediastinal ependymoma shows ependymal rosettes ⇗. This feature is important in the diagnosis of ependymoma.

TERMINOLOGY

Synonyms

- Myxopapillary ependymoma

Definitions

- Neural neoplasm of possible intermediate malignant potential when in mediastinum

ETIOLOGY/PATHOGENESIS

Pathogenesis

- Probably derived from paravertebral ependymal rests

CLINICAL ISSUES

Epidemiology

- Incidence
  - Ependymomas in mediastinum are very rare
- Age
  - More common in adults with wide range of ages
- Gender
  - No gender predilection

Site

- More common in posterior mediastinum

Presentation

- Cough
- Chest pain
- Dyspnea
- Asymptomatic

Treatment

- Surgical approaches
  - Complete surgical resection

Prognosis

- Mediastinal ependymomas may follow a prolonged and indolent clinical course
- Metastasis to lymph nodes may occur

MACROSCOPIC FEATURES

General Features

- Tumors are well circumscribed with glistening surface
- On cut surface, they are solid, but cystic changes may be seen
- Necrosis and hemorrhage may be seen
- Tan to gray in color

Size

- Variable size; may be > 7 cm in diameter

MICROSCOPIC PATHOLOGY

Histologic Features

- Solid, fairly uniform cellular proliferation that displays moderate atypia
- Cells with finely stippled to vesicular chromatin
- Perivascular pseudorosettes
- Interanastomosing ependymal tubules
- True ependymal rosettes and canals with ciliated cells
- Pseudopapillary areas
- Occasional psammoma bodies may be seen
- Mitotic activity is variable and can range from 1 to > 5 x 10 HPF
- Necrosis and hemorrhage may be present also in variable proportions, focal or extensive

DIFFERENTIAL DIAGNOSIS

Schwannoma

- Does not show increased mitotic activity
- Does not show presence of true ependymal rosettes
- Negative for GFAP

Neuroendocrine Carcinoma

- Negative for GFAP and strongly positive for keratin

EPENDYMOMA

Key Facts

Terminology
- Neural neoplasm of possible intermediate malignant potential when in mediastinum

Etiology/Pathogenesis
- Probably derived from paravertebral ependymal rests

Clinical Issues
- Incidence
  - Ependymomas arising in mediastinum are rare
  - More common in adults with a wide range of ages
  - More common in posterior mediastinum
- Symptoms
  - Cough
  - Chest pain
  - Dyspnea
  - Asymptomatic
- Prognosis
  - Mediastinal ependymomas may follow a prolonged clinical course
  - Metastasis to lymph nodes may occur

Top Differential Diagnoses
- Schwannoma
- Neuroendocrine carcinoma
- Metastatic melanoma

Diagnostic Checklist
- Solid cellular proliferation
- True ependymal rosettes
- Pseudopapillary areas
- Variable mitotic rate

Immunohistochemistry

Antibody	Reactivity	Staining Pattern	Comment
GFAP	Positive	Cytoplasmic	Strong positive staining
S100	Negative		May show focal and weak positivity
CK-PAN	Negative		May be occasionally focally positive
Chromogranin-A	Negative		
Synaptophysin	Negative		
HMB-45	Negative		

- Shows positive staining for neuroendocrine markers (chromogranin &/or synaptophysin)
- True ependymal rosettes are not seen in neuroendocrine carcinomas

Metastatic Melanoma
- True ependymal rosettes are not seen in melanomas
- Strong positive staining for S100 protein &/or HMB-45
- Shows negative staining for GFAP

DIAGNOSTIC CHECKLIST

Pathologic Interpretation Pearls
- Solid cellular proliferation
- True ependymal rosettes
- Pseudopapillary areas
- Variable mitotic rate

GRADING

Anaplastic Ependymoma
- This designation has been given to tumors with increased mitotic activity, necrosis, and cellular atypia

SELECTED REFERENCES

1. Mori T et al: A case of primary mediastinal ependymoma. Ann Thorac Cardiovasc Surg. 15(5):332-5, 2009
2. Estrozi B et al: Myxopapillary ependymoma of the posterior mediastinum. Ann Diagn Pathol. 10(5):283-7, 2006
3. Satti M et al: Mediastinal myxopapillary ependymoma primary or late metastases of paracoccygeal ependymoma: a case report. Ann Diagn Pathol. 9(4):215-8, 2005
4. Neumann DP et al: Magnetic resonance imaging of a mediastinal ependymoma. Conn Med. 62(9):527-30, 1998
5. Wilson RW et al: Primary ependymoma of the mediastinum: a clinicopathologic study of three cases. Ann Diagn Pathol. 2(5):293-300, 1998
6. Nobles E et al: Mediastinal ependymoma. Hum Pathol. 22(1):94-6, 1991
7. Doglioni C et al: Ependymoma of the mediastinum. Arch Pathol Lab Med. 112(2):194-6, 1988

Microscopic Features

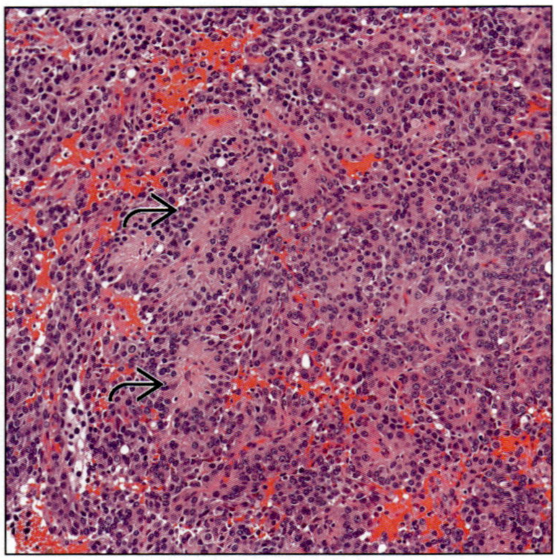

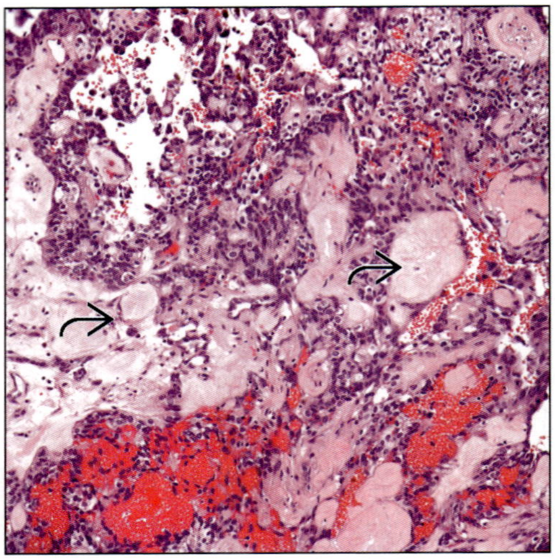

(Left) *Mediastinal ependymoma displays prominent rosettes. This type of differentiation is highly suggestive of a neural neoplasm.* ***(Right)*** *Mediastinal ependymoma displays extensive areas of hyalinization admixed with a cellular proliferation arranged in a papillary-like growth pattern.*

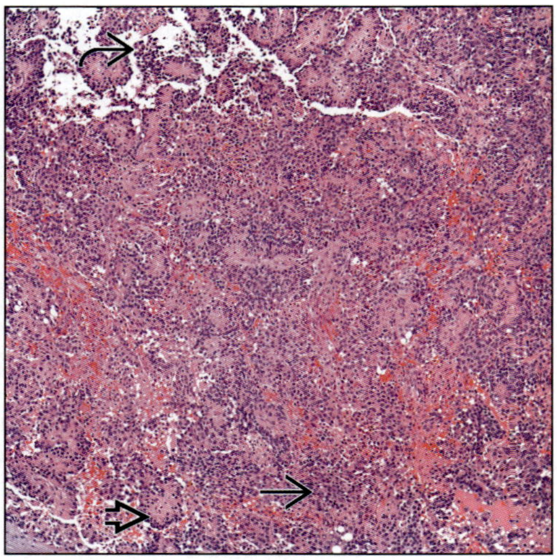

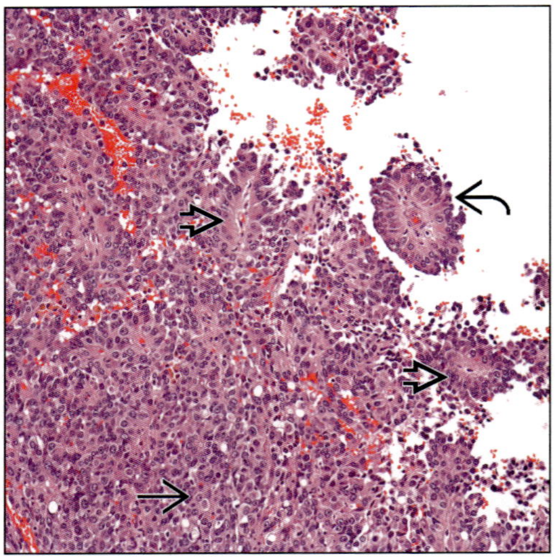

(Left) *Mediastinal ependymoma displays solid areas, rosettes, and papillary-like areas. This constellation of features makes the diagnosis easier.* ***(Right)*** *Higher magnification of mediastinal ependymoma is shown with solid areas of a homogeneous cellular proliferation, areas of papillary-like structures, and ependymal rosettes.*

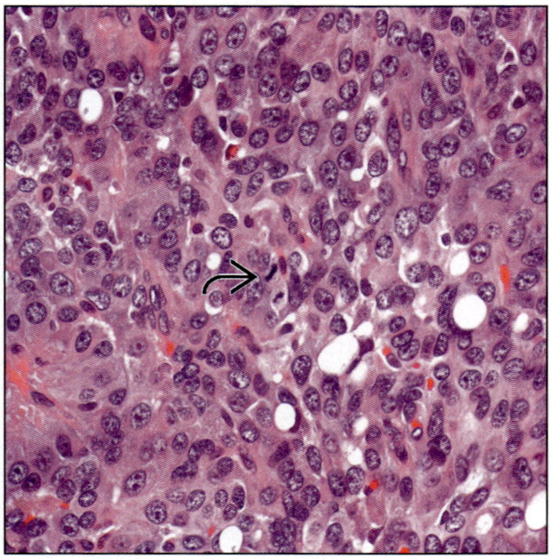

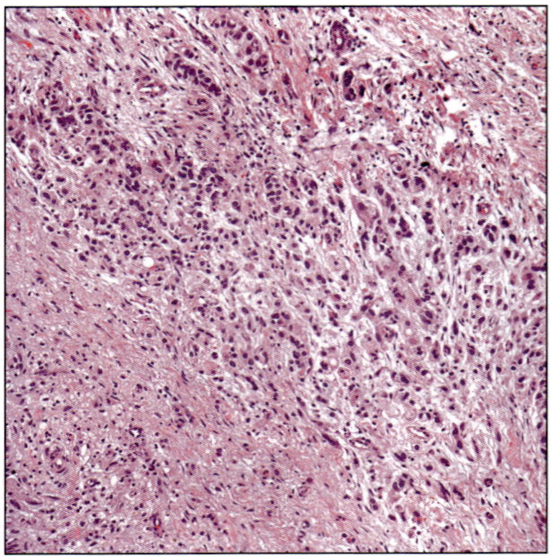

(Left) *High-power view shows a solid area in a mediastinal ependymoma with a rather homogeneous cellular proliferation. There is moderate nuclear pleomorphism and mitotic activity.* ***(Right)*** *Mediastinal ependymoma is shown with myxoid changes and a cellular proliferation without a particular growth pattern. This feature may also be seen in other more common tumors like carcinomas.*

Microscopic Features

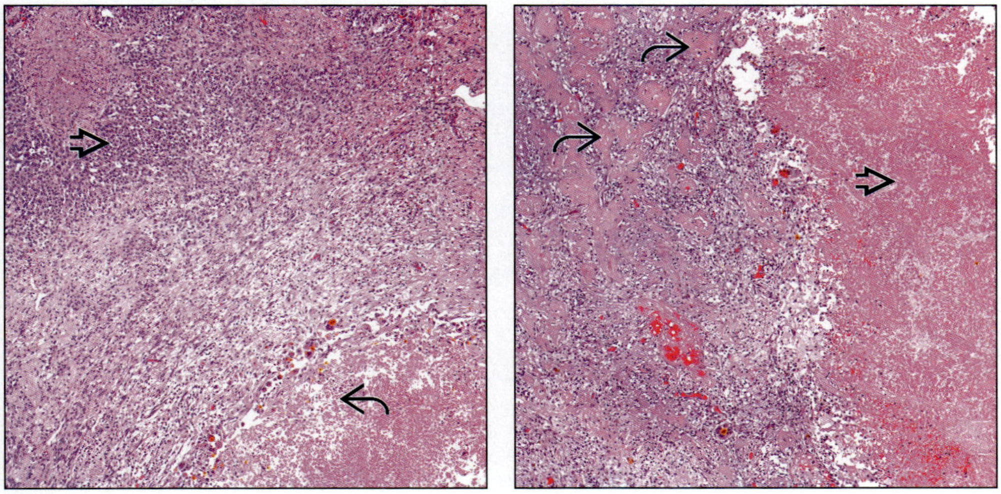

(Left) *Mediastinal ependymoma shows areas of viable tumor* ⇨ *embedded in fibroconnective tissue with chronic inflammation. Note the presence of a necrotic* ↪ *area that in some cases may obscure the neoplastic proliferation.* **(Right)** *Mediastinal ependymoma is seen with areas of hemorrhage* ⇨ *and adjacent areas of a neoplastic cellular proliferation admixed with fibrinoid material* ↪.

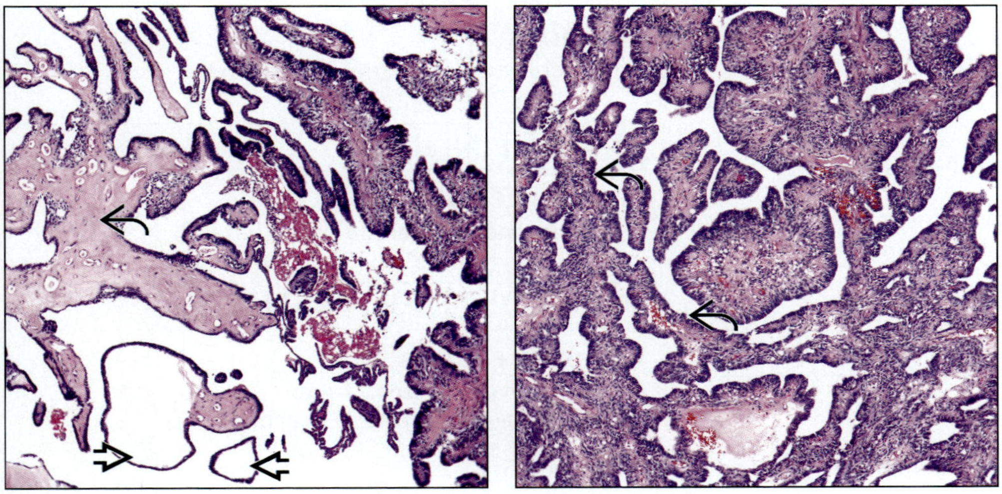

(Left) *Mediastinal ependymoma with prominent papillary-like structures and areas of hyalinization* ↪ *is shown. Some of these papillary-like structures may be devoid of fibrovascular cores* ⇨. **(Right)** *Mediastinal ependymoma is shown with papillary features in which there are anastomosing papillary structures* ↪ *with a more complex pattern. Inside these papillary structures there is a homogeneous cellular proliferation.*

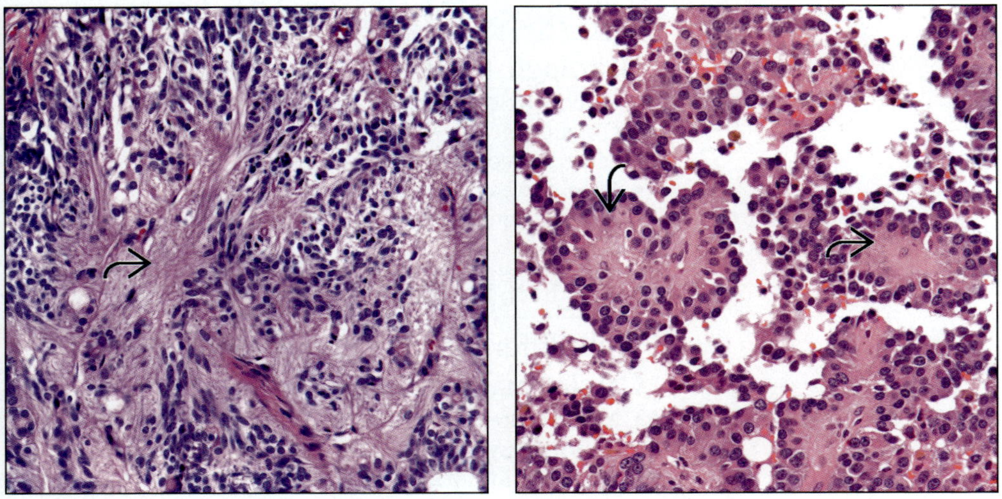

(Left) *Mediastinal ependymoma with prominent neuropil* ↪ *contents is admixed with a small cellular proliferation. These features may also be seen in neuroblastomas.* **(Right)** *Mediastinal ependymoma is shown with prominent ependymal rosettes* ↪. *This feature is helpful in the diagnosis of ependymoma.*

ECTOPIC PARATHYROID TUMOR

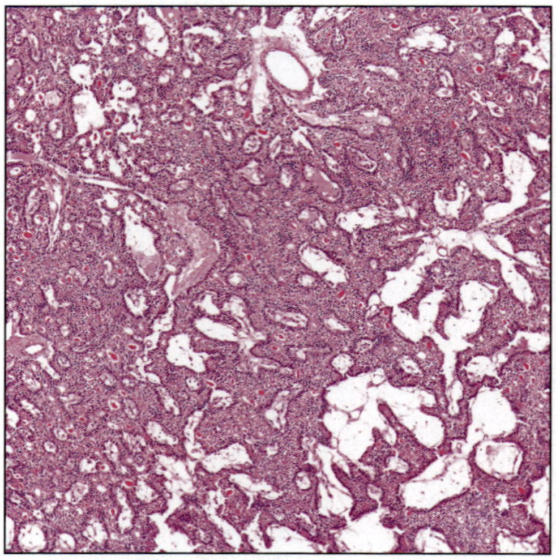

Low-power view shows an ectopic parathyroid adenoma of the mediastinum. The histology recapitulates the features of a normal parathyroid tissue.

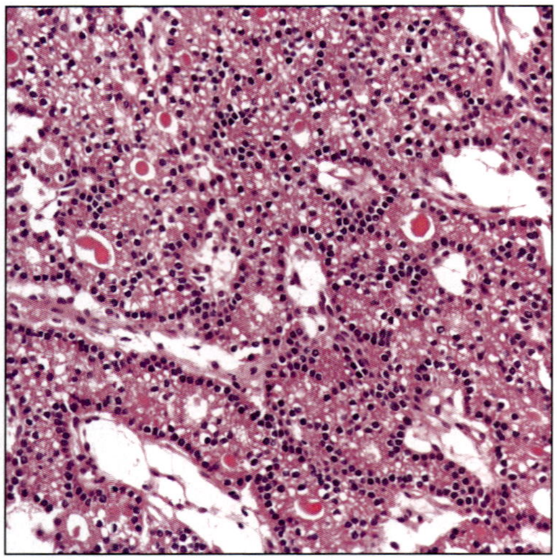

High-power view of a parathyroid adenoma of the mediastinum is shown. The tumor shows a striking neuroendocrine morphology with a homogeneous cellular proliferation.

TERMINOLOGY

Definitions

- Neuroendocrine tumors of mediastinum

ETIOLOGY/PATHOGENESIS

Developmental Anomaly

- Misplacement of normal glands in anterior mediastinum

CLINICAL ISSUES

Epidemiology

- Incidence
  - Among rarest neuroendocrine tumors in mediastinum
- Age
  - Usually in adults
- Gender
  - No gender predilection

Site

- Anterior mediastinum

Presentation

- Chest pain
- Cough
- Dyspnea
- Hyperparathyroidism
- Kidney stones

Laboratory Tests

- Calcium, phosphorus

Treatment

- Surgical approaches
  - Complete surgical resection
- Adjuvant therapy
  - In cases of ectopic parathyroid carcinoma

Prognosis

- Good in cases of parathyroid adenoma

IMAGE FINDINGS

General Features

- Anterior mediastinal tumor

MACROSCOPIC FEATURES

General Features

- Light brown, soft tissue tumor
- Hemorrhage and necrosis may be present

Size

- Variable and can reach over 10 cm in diameter

MICROSCOPIC PATHOLOGY

Histologic Features

- Oncocytic cellular proliferation
- Chief cells
- Mixed oncocytic and chief cells
- Mild nuclear atypia
- Mitotic figures in cases of carcinoma

DIFFERENTIAL DIAGNOSIS

Well-differentiated Neuroendocrine Carcinoma (Carcinoid Tumor)

- Neuroendocrine carcinoma and ectopic parathyroid tumors may share similar immunophenotype
- Parathyroid hormone immunohistochemistry is more commonly seen in ectopic parathyroid tumors

ECTOPIC PARATHYROID TUMOR

Key Facts

Clinical Issues
- Incidence
  - Among the rarest neuroendocrine tumors in mediastinum
  - Usually in adults
- Symptoms
  - Chest pain
  - Cough
  - Dyspnea
  - Hyperparathyroidism
  - Kidney stones

Top Differential Diagnoses
- Well-differentiated neuroendocrine carcinoma (carcinoid tumor)
  - Neuroendocrine carcinoma and ectopic parathyroid tumors may share similar immunophenotype
  - Parathyroid hormone immunohistochemistry is more commonly seen in ectopic parathyroid tumors
- Paraganglioma
  - Generally negative for keratin stains
- Thymic carcinoma
  - Negative for neuroendocrine markers, including parathyroid hormone

Diagnostic Checklist
- Symptom complex
- Oncocytic cellular proliferation
- Chief cells
- Mixed oncocytic and chief cells
- In adenomas, lack of mitotic activity
- In carcinomas, presence of mitosis, hemorrhage, &/or necrosis

Immunohistochemistry

Antibody	Reactivity	Staining Pattern	Comment
CK-PAN	Positive	Cytoplasmic	Not specific
CK8/18/CAM5.2	Positive	Cytoplasmic	Not specific
Chromogranin-A	Positive	Cytoplasmic	Also positive in other neuroendocrine tumors
Synaptophysin	Positive	Cytoplasmic	Also positive in other neuroendocrine tumors
PTH	Positive	Cytoplasmic	Has been focally positive in other neuroendocrine tumors

Histochemical Features of Ectopic Mediastinal Parathyroid Tumors

Histochemical Stain	Result
PAS	Positive
Mucicarmine	Negative
D-PAS	Negative

- Clinical presence of disturbances in calcium metabolism are more in keeping with parathyroid tumors
- PAS is more likely to show positive staining in parathyroid tumors

Paraganglioma
- Generally negative for keratin stains
- Show more nuclear pleomorphism

Thymic Carcinoma
- Negative for neuroendocrine markers, including parathyroid hormone

DIAGNOSTIC CHECKLIST

Clinically Relevant Pathologic Features
- Symptom complex

Pathologic Interpretation Pearls
- Oncocytic cellular proliferation
- Chief cells
- Mixed oncocytic and chief cells
- In adenomas, lack of mitotic activity
- In carcinomas, presence of mitosis, hemorrhage, &/or necrosis

SELECTED REFERENCES

1. Burger AE et al: Thoracoscopic excision of mediastinal parathyroid adenomas: a report of two cases. Ann R Coll Surg Engl. 90(2):W1-5, 2008
2. Ravipati NB et al: Anterior mediastinotomy for parathyroidectomy. Am J Surg. 195(6):799-802, 2008
3. Righi A et al: Mediastinal parathyroid carcinoma with tumor implants in a child: a unique occurrence. Int J Surg Pathol. 16(4):458-60, 2008
4. Yun JS et al: Giant posterior mediastinal parathyroid adenoma. Thyroid. 18(4):475-6, 2008
5. Birdas TJ et al: Mediastinal parathyroid adenoma. Ann Thorac Surg. 79(3):1097, 2005
6. Moran CA et al: Primary parathyroid tumors of the mediastinum: a clinicopathologic and immunohistochemical study of 17 cases. Am J Clin Pathol. 124(5):749-54, 2005
7. Moran CA: Primary neuroendocrine carcinomas of the mediastinum: review of current criteria for histopathologic diagnosis and classification. Semin Diagn Pathol. 22(3):223-9, 2005

ECTOPIC PARATHYROID TUMOR

Microscopic Features

*(**Left**) Ectopic parathyroid adenoma in the mediastinum is shown with remnants of thymic tissue → in the periphery of the tumor. The tumor itself appears well circumscribed and homogeneous. (**Right**) Ectopic parathyroid adenoma shows 2 cell populations composed of chief cells → and oncocytic cells ↷. These histological features recapitulate the normal cells of the parathyroid glands.*

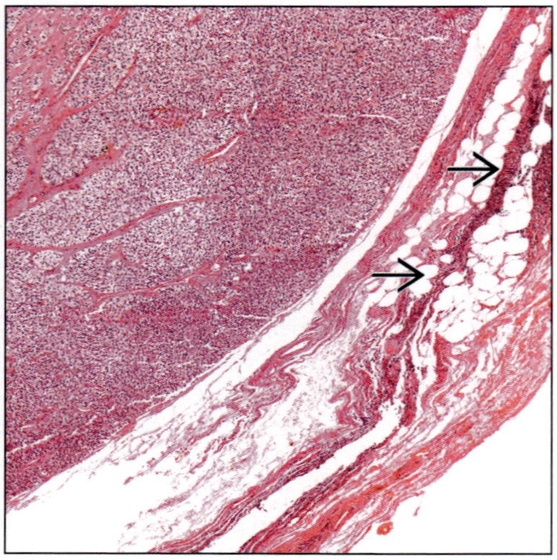

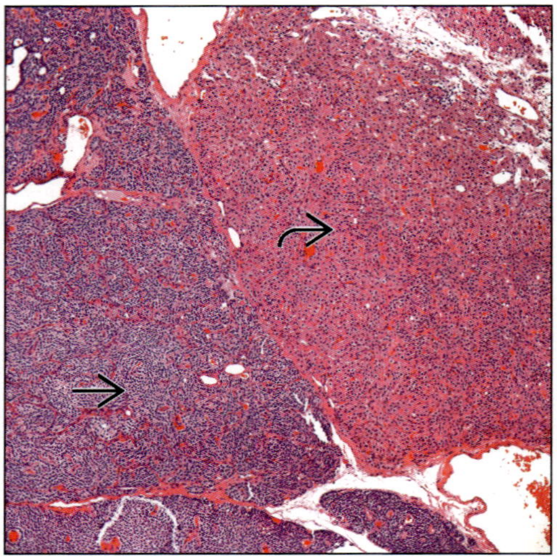

*(**Left**) Ectopic parathyroid adenoma in the mediastinum shows prominent chief cells composed of round cells with clear cytoplasm, round nuclei, and inconspicuous nucleoli. The cellular proliferation is homogeneous without necrosis or mitotic activity. (**Right**) Ectopic parathyroid adenoma of the mediastinum is seen with an edematous component ↷ in the background. Note the presence of islands of tumor cells ⇨ floating in the edematous component.*

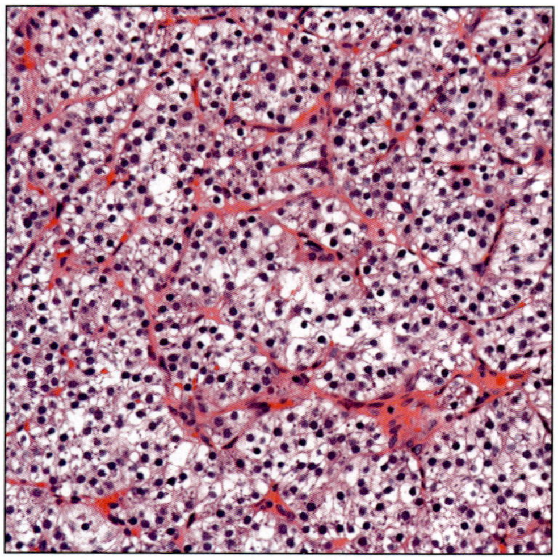

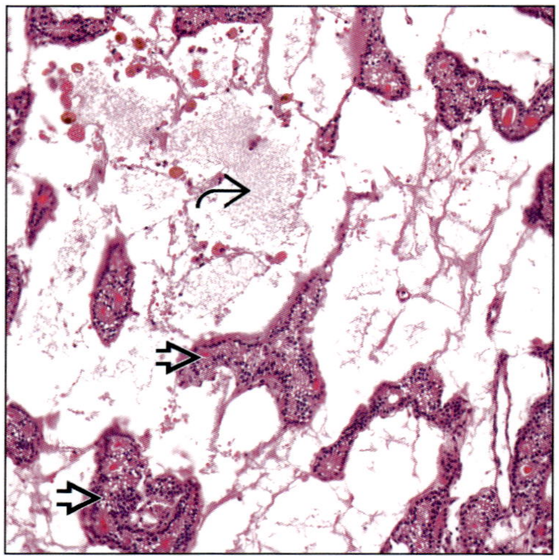

*(**Left**) Ectopic parathyroid adenoma in the mediastinum with angiectatic-like features is composed of large spaces filled with blood ↷ or acellular colloid material →. Similar features have been described in neuroendocrine carcinomas of the thymus. (**Right**) Ectopic parathyroid adenoma in the mediastinum is shown with extensive hyalinization ↷ of the stroma and only small islands of tumor cells. Similar features have been described in paragangliomas.*

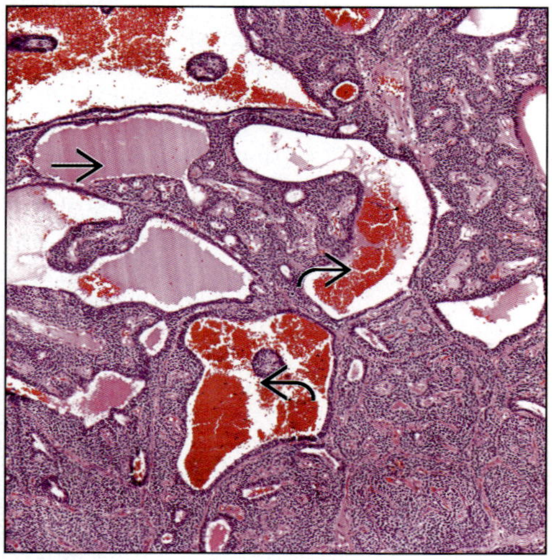

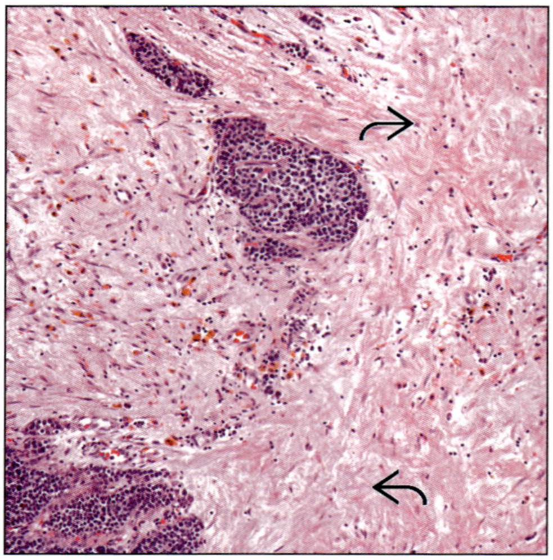

Microscopic Features

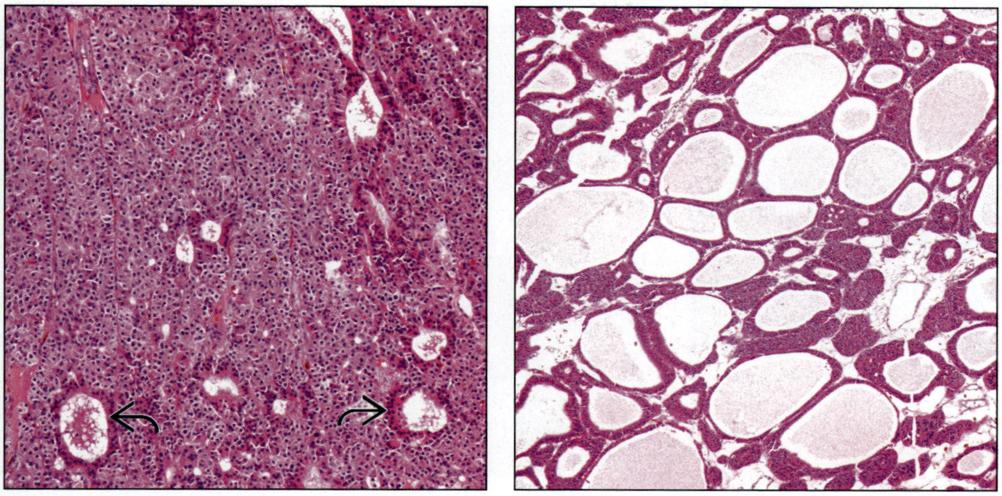

(Left) *Ectopic parathyroid adenoma shows a prominent solid growth pattern with only focal areas of pseudoglandular component* ↪*. In addition, the cellular proliferation has prominent oncocytic features.* ***(Right)*** *Ectopic parathyroid adenoma shows a pseudoglandular or alveolar growth pattern. Also note the prominent oncocytic features of the cellular proliferation.*

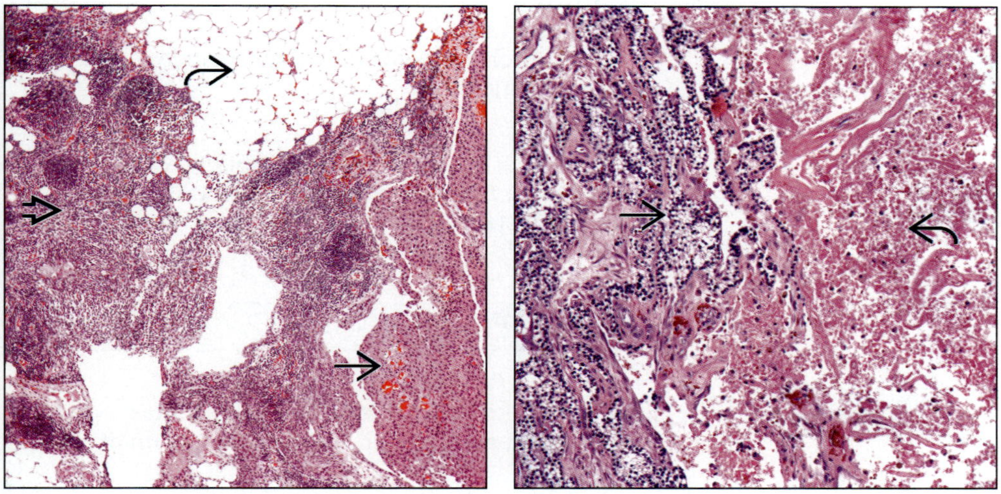

(Left) *Ectopic parathyroid carcinoma of the mediastinum shows areas of residual thymic tissue* ⇨*, including mature adipose tissue* ↪ *and an area of an atypical epithelial cellular proliferation* →*.* ***(Right)*** *Ectopic parathyroid carcinoma shows areas of necrosis* ↪ *alternating with viable areas of parathyroid* →*. The presence of necrosis is an important feature in cases of parathyroid carcinoma.*

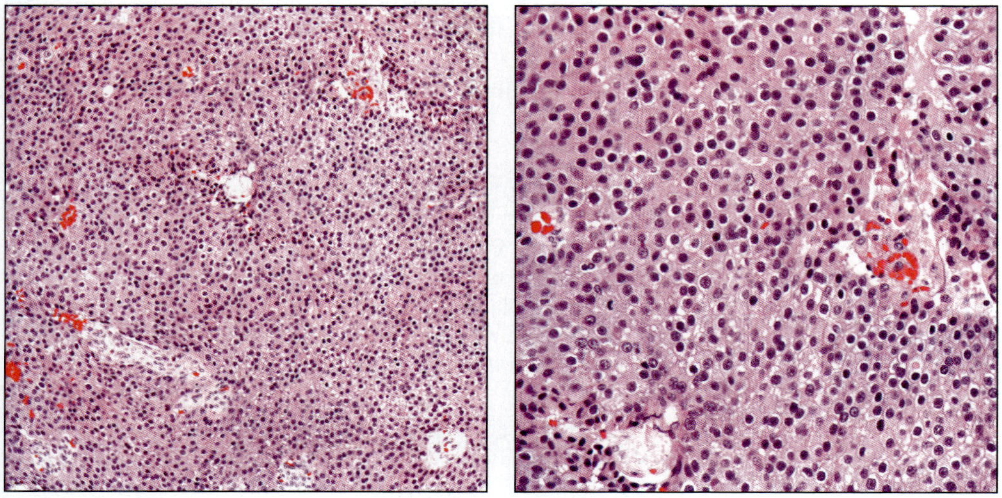

(Left) *High-power view of an ectopic parathyroid carcinoma of the mediastinum shows sheets of epithelial cells with a homogeneous growth pattern. Such cellular proliferation may be seen in other thymic epithelial tumors.* ***(Right)*** *High-power view of an ectopic parathyroid carcinoma is shown with a cellular proliferation displaying cells with irregular nuclear contours and mitotic activity. Mitoses and necrosis are features of carcinomas.*

ECTOPIC THYROID TUMOR

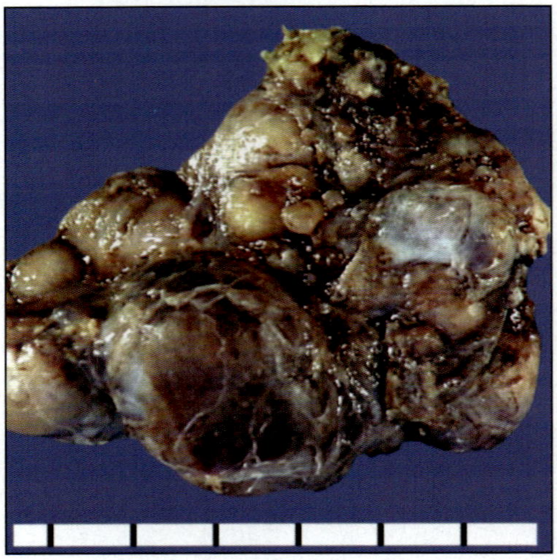

Gross appearance of ectopic mediastinal goiter shows a tan-brown, multinodular mass covered by a thin, shiny capsule, with confluence of multiple, soft nodules of varying sizes.

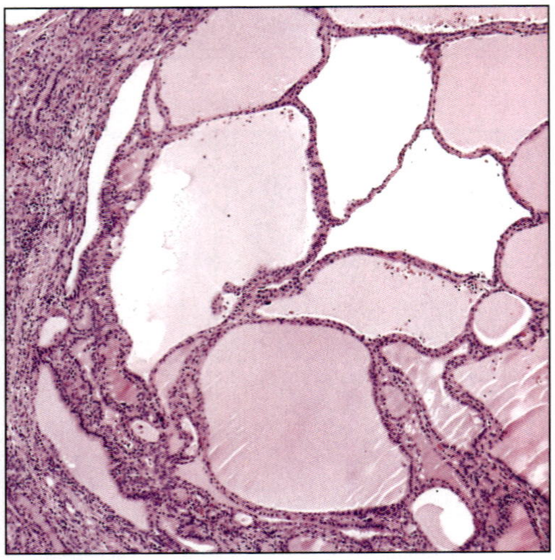

Histologic appearance of mediastinal hyperplastic goiter shows distended follicles filled with colloid, forming an ill-defined nodule.

TERMINOLOGY

Definitions

- Proliferation of thyroid tissue originating from displaced or ectopically located elements in mediastinum

ETIOLOGY/PATHOGENESIS

Developmental Anomaly

- May result from abnormal migration during embryogenesis

CLINICAL ISSUES

Epidemiology

- Incidence
  - Develops in 5% of persons worldwide
- Age
  - Adults
  - Increases in frequency with advancing age
- Gender
  - More common in females (M:F = 1:3)

Site

- Anterior superior mediastinum; rarely in posterior mediastinum

Presentation

- Shortness of breath
- Cough & dysphagia due to compression of esophagus
- Dyspnea, wheezing, and stridor due to compression of trachea
- Dysphonia may occur due to compression of recurrent laryngeal nerve
- Often asymptomatic and discovered incidentally on routine chest x-rays
- Most patients are mildly hypothyroid or euthyroid

Treatment

- Surgical excision
- Observation is recommended for small lesions or in elderly patients

Prognosis

- Majority of lesions are cured by simple excision
- Malignant tumors may recur and metastasize
- In rare instances, histologically benign lesion can recur and invade local structures

IMAGE FINDINGS

General Features

- Tracheal deviation at level of thoracic outlet
- Involvement of superior mediastinum, with extension into neck
- High attenuation due to natural iodine
- Regions of low attenuation due to colloid cysts
- Coarse calcifications in cyst walls in up to 75% of cases
- Enhances strongly with IV contrast
- I-123 and I-131 are diagnostic but often unnecessary
- Best imaging tool is chest x-ray with confirmation by CT scan

MACROSCOPIC FEATURES

General Features

- Generally well circumscribed, encapsulated, and multilobulated
- Malignant neoplasms may be poorly circumscribed and infiltrate adjacent structures

MICROSCOPIC PATHOLOGY

Histologic Features

- **Thyroid tumors**
  - Thyroid nodular hyperplasia

Key Facts

Clinical Issues
- Anterior superior mediastinum; rarely in posterior mediastinum
- Shortness of breath
- Symptoms of hyperparathyroidism
- May be asymptomatic and discovered incidentally on routine chest x-rays
- Majority of lesions are cured by simple excision
- Malignant tumors may recur and metastasize

Macroscopic Features
- Generally well circumscribed, encapsulated, and multilobulated
- Malignant neoplasms may be poorly circumscribed and infiltrate adjacent structures

Microscopic Pathology
- Hyperplastic thyroid nodules are ill-defined, unencapsulated, and composed of normal follicular structures
- May contain focal papillary structures, calcifications, and intraluminal follicular proliferations (Sanderson polsters)
- Rarely, follicular or papillary carcinoma may arise from ectopic thyroid elements
- Follicular carcinoma shows follicles with invasion of capsule and blood vessels
- Papillary carcinoma is characterized by usual nuclear features of this tumor in thyroid
- Medullary carcinoma, anaplastic carcinoma, and poorly differentiated ("insular") carcinoma can also arise in mediastinum

    - Ill-defined, unencapsulated nodules composed of normal follicular structures
    - May show abundant regressive changes, including fibrous pseudocapsule, hemorrhage, and cystic degeneration
    - May contain focal papillary structures, calcifications, and intraluminal follicular proliferations (Sanderson polsters)
    - Rare cases may show local recurrence and infiltration of surrounding soft tissues
  - Thyroid carcinoma
    - Rarely, follicular or papillary carcinoma may arise from displaced thyroid elements
    - Follicular carcinoma shows follicles with invasion of capsule and blood vessels
    - Papillary carcinoma is characterized by usual nuclear features of this tumor in thyroid
    - Medullary carcinoma, anaplastic carcinoma, and poorly differentiated ("insular") carcinoma can also arise in mediastinum
    - Well-differentiated thyroid follicular and papillary neoplasms are positive for thyroglobulin and TTF-1

DIFFERENTIAL DIAGNOSIS

Mediastinal Paraganglioma
- Prominent nesting pattern (Zellballen) with fibrovascular septa
- May show nucleomegaly with atypia but no mitotic activity
- Stains positively for neuroendocrine markers (chromogranin, synaptophysin) but is negative for cytokeratins, thyroglobulin, and TTF-1

Neuroendocrine Carcinomas
- Well-differentiated neuroendocrine carcinoma (carcinoid tumor) can show nesting, solid, acinar, or trabecular pattern
- Cells can be very uniform and closely resemble thyroid or parathyroid neoplasms
- Tumor cells are positive for neuroendocrine markers but negative for thyroglobulin or TTF-1

Metastases of Clear Cell Tumors
- Metastatic clear cell carcinomas can in some instances resemble thyroid tumors
- Clinical history is indispensable for adequate interpretation
- Special stains for thyroglobulin or TTF-1 may be of help in identifying correct cell type

Teratomatous Lesions
- Usually contain elements derived from all 3 germ cell layers, including neural, epithelial, and mesenchymal components
- Teratomas only rarely display mature thyroid epithelium

DIAGNOSTIC CHECKLIST

Pathologic Interpretation Pearls
- Residual, normal, involuting thymus is often present in vicinity of tumor
- Ectopic thyroid lesions in mediastinum are more likely to be benign and hyperplastic

SELECTED REFERENCES

1. Hedayati N et al: The clinical presentation and operative management of nodular and diffuse substernal thyroid disease. Am Surg. 68(3):245-51; discussion 251-2, 2002
2. Dominguez-Malagon H et al: Ectopic poorly differentiated (insular) carcinoma of the thyroid. Report of a case presenting as an anterior mediastinal mass. Am J Clin Pathol. 104(4):408-12, 1995
3. Spinner RJ et al: Thoracic intrathymic thyroid. Ann Surg. 220(1):91-6, 1994
4. Kozol RA et al: Management of ectopic thyroid nodules. Surgery. 114(6):1103-6; discussion 1106-7, 1993
5. Wick MR: Mediastinal cysts and intrathoracic thyroid tumors. Semin Diagn Pathol. 7(4):285-94, 1990

ECTOPIC THYROID TUMOR

Benign Ectopic Mediastinal Thyroid

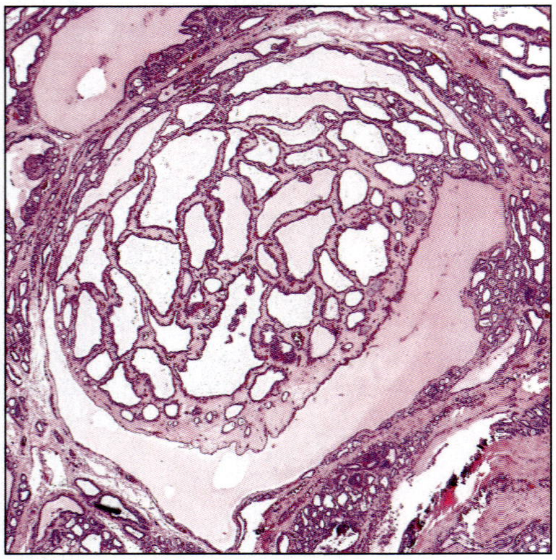

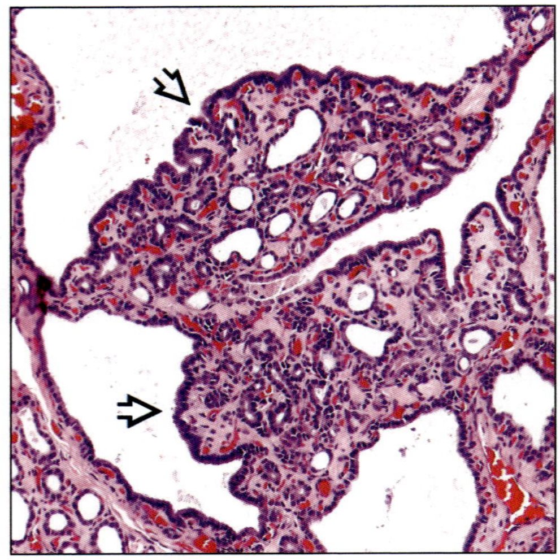

(Left) *Ectopic thyroid tissue in the mediastinum shows features of nodular hyperplasia, with well-circumscribed but unencapsulated nodules composed of dilated thyroid follicles of varying sizes.* ***(Right)*** *High magnification of a dilated follicle in the ectopic mediastinal thyroid shows proliferation of small follicles. These structures (Sanderson polsters) are quite distinctive for nodular hyperplasia of the thyroid.*

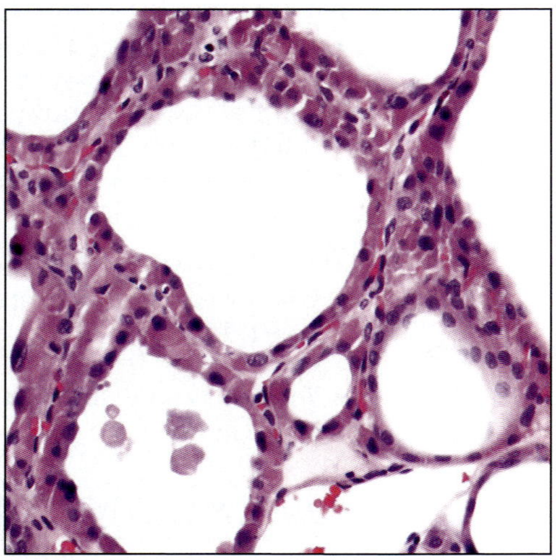

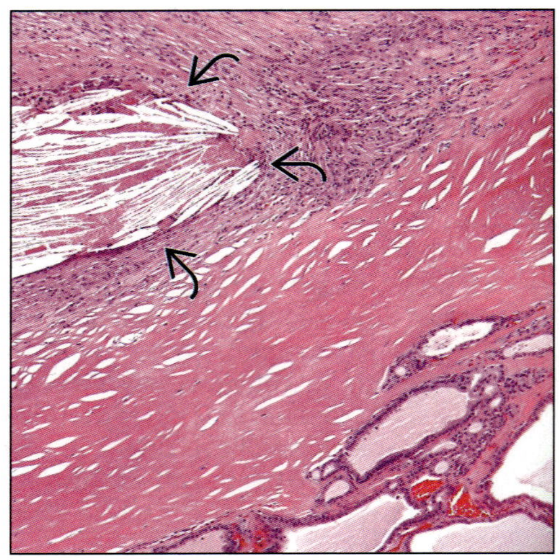

(Left) *Hyperplastic nodule in ectopic thyroid arising in the mediastinum shows prominent oxyphilic (Hurthle cell) changes of the follicular cells. The ectopic thyroid may give rise to hyperplastic nodules with Hurthle cell changes, Hurthle cell adenoma, or Hurthle cell carcinoma.* ***(Right)*** *Mediastinal goiter shows extensive degenerative changes, including marked sclerosis and hyalinization, chronic inflammation, and cholesterol cleft granuloma.*

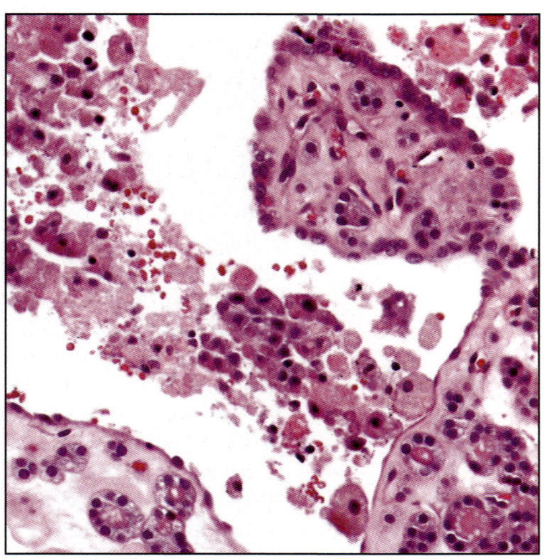

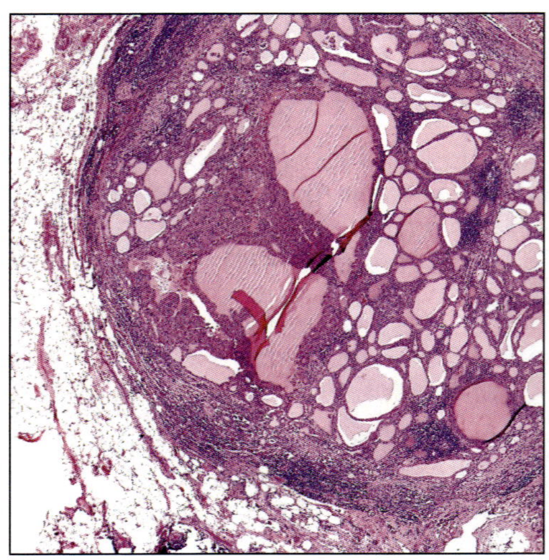

(Left) *Longstanding hyperplastic nodule in mediastinal goiter shows prominent cystic degeneration within one of the nodules, resulting in a dilated cystic cavity containing scattered follicular structures, chronic inflammation, and hemosiderin-laden macrophages.* ***(Right)*** *Recurrent hyperplastic thyroid nodule is seen infiltrating the mediastinal fat in a patient who was previously operated on for nodular hyperplasia of the thyroid originating in the mediastinum.*

Malignant Tumors

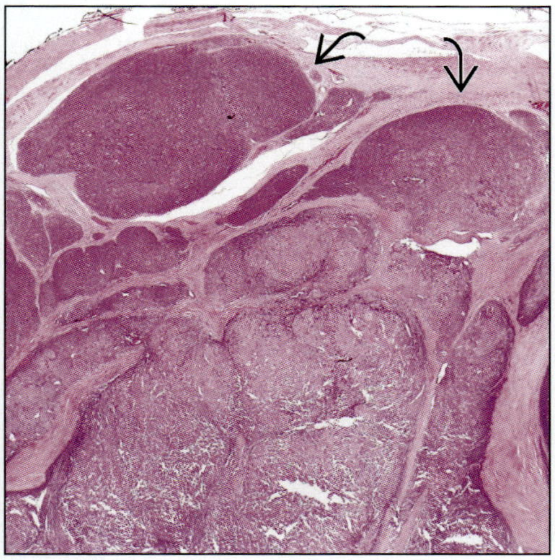

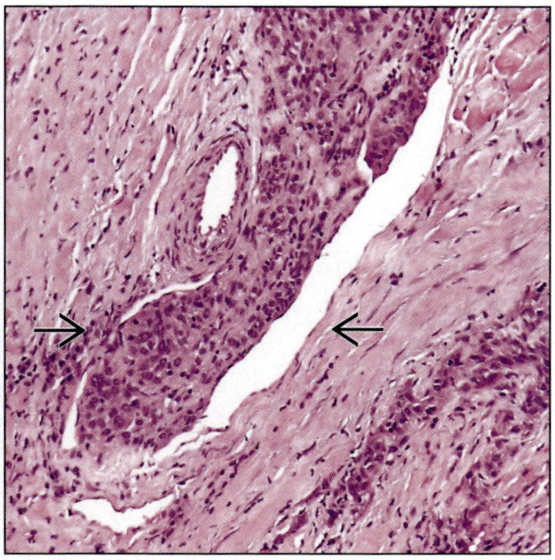

(Left) *Follicular carcinoma of the thyroid arising in ectopic thyroid in the mediastinum shows infiltration of the capsule and surrounding mediastinum by irregular lobules of thyroid follicular tumor cells ⮫.* ***(Right)*** *High magnification of invasive follicular carcinoma of the thyroid arising in ectopic mediastinal thyroid shows focus of vascular invasion →. These tumors in ectopic location show identical features as their counterparts in the normal location.*

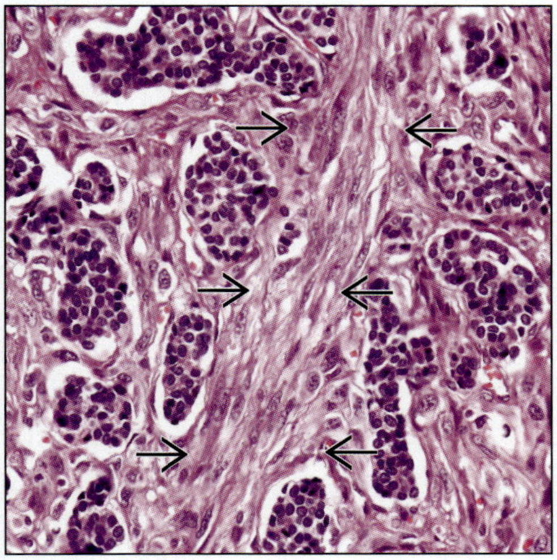

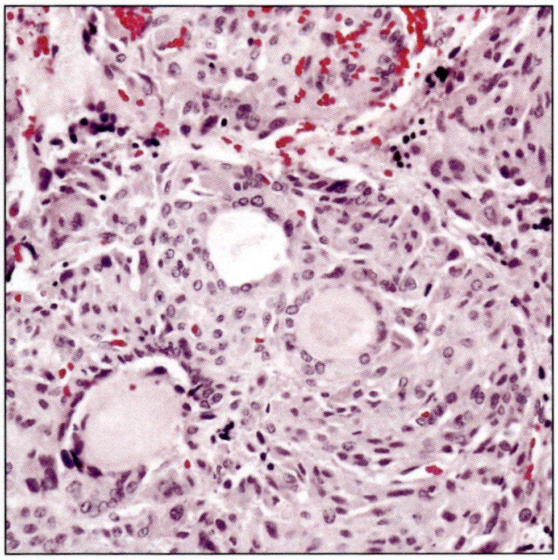

(Left) *Poorly differentiated follicular carcinoma of the thyroid arising in longstanding mediastinal goiter shows focal anaplastic transformation displaying atypical spindle cell proliferation infiltrating between the follicles →.* ***(Right)*** *Ectopic mediastinal thyroid shows focus of medullary thyroid carcinoma arising from the ectopic thyroid parenchyma. The cells in this tumor reacted positively with antibodies for calcitonin, chromogranin, and CEA.*

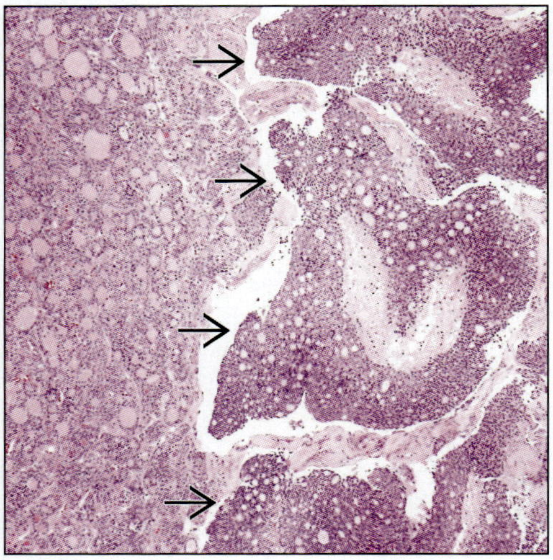

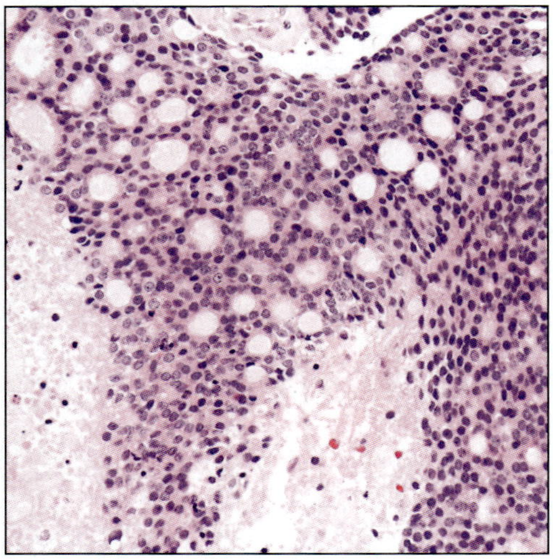

(Left) *Focus of poorly differentiated (so-called insular) carcinoma is seen adjacent to hyperplastic ectopic mediastinal thyroid →.* ***(Right)*** *High magnification of focus of poorly differentiated (so-called insular) carcinoma arising in ectopic mediastinal thyroid shows a population of primitive follicular cells with a prominent microcystic or cribriform pattern surrounding areas of necrosis.*

PROTOCOL FOR THYMOMA AND THYMIC CARCINOMA SPECIMEN EXAMINATION

Thymus: Resection

Surgical Pathology Cancer Case Summary (Checklist)

Specimen

___ Thymus
___ Thymus and other (specify): ____________________________
___ Not specified

Procedure

___ Thymectomy
___ Partial thymectomy
___ Other (specify): ____________________________
___ Not specified

Specimen Integrity

___ Intact
___ Disrupted
___ Indeterminate

Specimen Weight

Specify: _________ grams

Tumor Size

Greatest dimension: _________ cm
*Additional dimensions: _________ x _________ cm
___ Cannot be determined

Histologic Type

Thymoma (specify)

___ Type A thymoma
___ Type AB thymoma
___ Type B1 thymoma
___ Type B2 thymoma
___ Other (specify): ____________________________

Thymic carcinoma (specify)

___ Squamous cell carcinoma
___ Basaloid carcinoma
___ Mucoepidermoid carcinoma
___ Lymphoepithelioma-like carcinoma
___ Sarcomatoid carcinoma
___ Clear cell carcinoma
___ Adenocarcinoma
___ Well-differentiated neuroendocrine carcinoma, typical carcinoid
___ Well-differentiated neuroendocrine carcinoma, atypical carcinoid
___ Poorly differentiated neuroendocrine carcinoma, large cell neuroendocrine carcinoma
___ Poorly differentiated neuroendocrine carcinoma, small cell carcinoma, neuroendocrine type
___ Other (specify): ____________________________

___ **Other (specify):** ____________________________

Tumor Extension

___ Not applicable
___ Not identified
___ Cannot be assessed
___ Pulmonary parenchyma
*Specify lobe(s) of lung: ____________________________
___ Pleura
*Specify location: ____________________________
___ Pericardium

____ Diaphragm

____ Other (specify): ____________________

Margins

____ Cannot be assessed

____ Margins uninvolved by tumor

Distance of tumor from closest margin: _______ mm

____ Margin(s) involved by tumor

Specify margin(s): ____________________

Treatment Effect

____ Not applicable

____ Cannot be determined

____ Not identified

____ Present (specify: _______ % residual viable tumor)

Lymph-Vascular Invasion

____ Not identified

____ Present

____ Indeterminate

Regional Lymph Nodes

____ Cannot be assessed

____ No regional lymph node metastasis

____ Regional lymph node metastasis

____ No nodes submitted or found

Number of lymph nodes examined

Specify: _______

____ Number cannot be determined (explain): ____________________

Number of lymph nodes involved

Specify: _______

____ Number cannot be determined (explain): ____________________

Pathologic Staging for Thymomas (Modified Masaoka Stage) *(applies only to thymomas)*

____ Stage I: Grossly and microscopically encapsulated (includes microscopic invasion into, but not through, the capsule)

____ Stage IIa: Microscopic transcapsular invasion

____ Stage IIb: Macroscopic capsular invasion

____ Stage III: Macroscopic invasion of neighboring organs

____ Stage IVa: Pleural or pericardial dissemination

____ Stage IVb: Hematogenous or lymphatic dissemination

____ Cannot be determined

Implants/Distant Metastasis *(select all that apply)*

____ Cannot be assessed

____ Not identified

Specify site(s)

____ Pleura

____ Pericardium

____ Other (specify): ____________________

Pathologic Staging for Thymic Carcinomas (pTNM) *(does not apply to thymomas)*

TNM descriptors (required only if applicable) (select all that apply)

____ m (multiple primary tumors)

____ r (recurrent)

____ y (post-treatment)

Primary tumor (pT)

____ pTX: Primary tumor cannot be assessed

____ pT0: No evidence of primary tumor

____ pT1: Tumor completely encapsulated

___ pT2: Tumor invades pericapsular connective tissue

___ pT3: Tumor invades neighboring structures, such as pericardium, mediastinal pleura, thoracic wall, great vessels, and lung

___ pT4: Tumor with pleural or pericardial dissemination

Regional lymph nodes (pN)

___ pNX: Regional lymph nodes cannot be assessed

___ pN0: No regional lymph node metastases

___ pN1: Metastasis in anterior mediastinal lymph nodes

___ pN2: Metastasis in other intrathoracic lymph nodes, excluding anterior mediastinal lymph nodes

___ pN3: Metastasis in scalene &/or supraclavicular lymph nodes

Distant metastasis (pM)

___ Not applicable

___ pM1: Distant metastasis

*Specify site(s), if known: ___________________________

*Additional Pathologic Findings *(select all that apply)*

*___ Age-appropriate involution changes

*___ Fibrosis

*___ Cortical hyperplasia

*___ Cystic changes in tumor

*___ Cystic changes in adjacent thymus

*___ Other (specify): ___________________________

*Ancillary Studies

*___ Immunohistochemical staining

*Specify results: ___________________________

*Protocol applies to thymic epithelial tumors located in any area of mediastinum. *Data elements with asterisks are not required. However, these elements may be clinically important but are not yet validated or regularly used in patient management. Adapted with permission from College of American Pathologists, "Protocol for the Examination of Specimens from Patients with Thymoma and Thymic Carcinoma." Web posting date: February 2011, www.cap.org.*

Other Benign/Reactive Conditions

THYMOLIPOMA

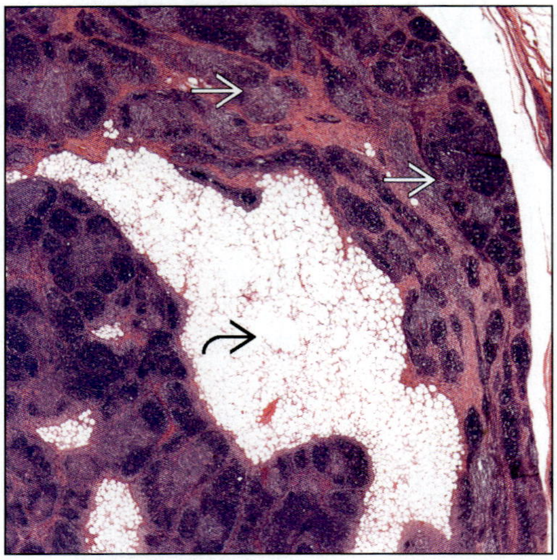

Thymolipoma shows areas of thymic tissue ➔ and areas of adipose tissue ⇗. The presence of these 2 components are essential for the diagnosis.

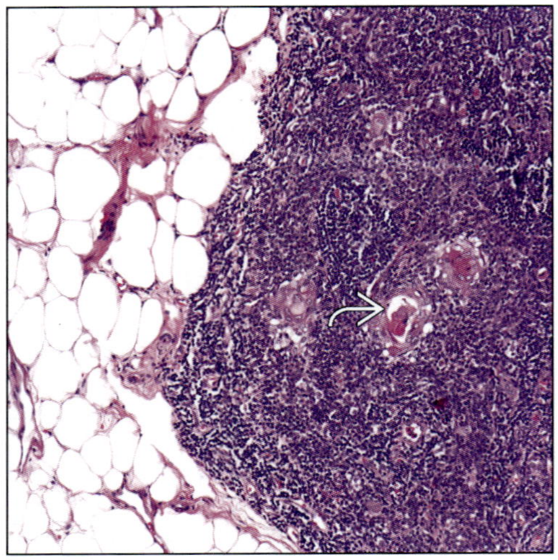

Thymolipoma shows the classic mixture of mature adipose tissue admixed with thymic tissue. Note the presence of Hassall corpuscles ⇗.

TERMINOLOGY

Synonyms

- Thymic lipoma

Definitions

- Benign thymic tumor composed of mature adipose tissue

ETIOLOGY/PATHOGENESIS

Etiology

- May represent overgrowth of adipose tissue in hyperplastic gland, closely related to hamartomatous lesion
  - However, definite etiology is not defined

CLINICAL ISSUES

Epidemiology

- Incidence
  - Unusual thymic tumor that accounts for < 5% of all thymic neoplasms
- Age
  - Can occur in any age group
  - More common in young adults
- Gender
  - No gender predisposition

Site

- Anterior mediastinum

Presentation

- Cough
- Chest pain
- Dyspnea
- Tachypnea
- Myasthenia gravis in some cases
- Asymptomatic

Treatment

- Complete surgical resection

Prognosis

- Complete surgical resection is curative

IMAGE FINDINGS

CT Findings

- Fat attenuation is present in most cases

MACROSCOPIC FEATURES

General Features

- Large tumor mass
- Yellowish or light brown in color
- Slightly lobulated

Size

- Variable size from a few cm to > 10 cm in diameter

MICROSCOPIC PATHOLOGY

Histologic Features

- Mature adipose tissue
- Remnants of thymic tissue
- Dilatation of Hassall corpuscles
- Striated muscle cells may be seen in unusual cases

DIFFERENTIAL DIAGNOSIS

Liposarcoma

- Adipose tissue in liposarcomas shows more atypia
  - Thymolipoma show admixture of thymic tissue and adipose tissue
- Liposarcomas lack presence of dilated Hassall corpuscles

THYMOLIPOMA

Key Facts

Terminology
- Thymic lipoma
- Benign thymic tumor composed of mature adipose tissue

Clinical Issues
- Incidence
  - Unusual thymic tumor that accounts for < 5% of all thymic tumors
  - Thymolipoma can occur at any age
- Symptoms
  - Cough
  - Dyspnea
  - Tachypnea
  - Myasthenia gravis in some cases
  - Asymptomatic
- Treatment
  - Complete surgical resection

Macroscopic Features
- Large tumor mass
- Yellowish or light brown in color
- Slightly lobulated
- Variable size from a few cm to > 10 cm in diameter

Microscopic Pathology
- Dilatation of Hassall corpuscles
- Remnants of thymic tissue
- Mature adipose tissue

Top Differential Diagnoses
- Liposarcoma
- Thymic hyperplasia
- Thymoma
- Involuted thymic tissue

Immunohistochemistry

Antibody	Reactivity	Staining Pattern	Comment
CK-PAN	Positive	Cytoplasmic	Thymic tissue component
CK5/6	Positive	Cytoplasmic	Thymic tissue component
AE1/AE3	Positive	Cytoplasmic	
S100	Positive	Nuclear	Adipose tissue component
Vimentin	Positive	Cytoplasmic	
CD45	Positive	Cytoplasmic	Thymic tissue component
CD20	Positive	Cytoplasmic	Thymic tissue component
CD45RO	Positive	Cytoplasmic	Thymic tissue component

Thymic Hyperplasia
- Thymolipoma always has areas of mature adipose tissue
- Thymic hyperplasia shows abundant thymic tissue with lymphoid hyperplasia and germinal centers

Thymoma
- Would not show presence of extensive areas of mature adipose tissue
- Presence of Hassall corpuscles is unusual in majority of thymomas

Involuted Thymic Tissue
- Thymolipoma presents as a mass
- In involutional changes of thymic gland, presence of adipose tissue is not extensive

DIAGNOSTIC CHECKLIST

Clinically Relevant Pathologic Features
- Gross appearance

Pathologic Interpretation Pearls
- Mixture of thymic and mature adipose tissue
- Absence of atypia in adipose tissue
- Presence of Hassall corpuscles

SELECTED REFERENCES

1. Kondo T et al: Thymolipoma, report of a case suggesting an origin from thymic true hyperplasia. Int J Surg Pathol. 18(6):526-9, 2010
2. Hudacko R et al: Thymolipoma: clues to pathogenesis revealed by cytogenetics. Ann Diagn Pathol. 13(3):185-8, 2009
3. Damadoglu E et al: Mediastinal thymolipoma: an analysis of 10 cases. Respirology. 12(6):924-7, 2007
4. Gannon BR et al: Mediastinal thymolipoma: a rare occurrence with striated myoid cells. Tumori. 93(2):198-200, 2007
5. Tsukioka T et al: Thymolipoma associated with myasthenia gravis. Gen Thorac Cardiovasc Surg. 55(1):26-8, 2007
6. Moran CA et al: Thymolipoma: clinicopathologic review of 33 cases. Mod Pathol. 8(7):741-4, 1995
7. Toyama T et al: Pathogenesis of thymolipoma: report of three cases. Surg Today. 25(1):86-8, 1995
8. Rosado-de-Christenson ML et al: Thymolipoma: analysis of 27 cases. Radiology. 193(1):121-6, 1994
9. Iseki M et al: Thymolipoma with striated myoid cells. Histological, immunohistochemical, and ultrastructural study. Am J Surg Pathol. 14(4):395-8, 1990
10. Nishimura O et al: Thymolipoma: a report of three cases. Jpn J Surg. 20(2):234-7, 1990

THYMOLIPOMA

Gross and Microscopic Features

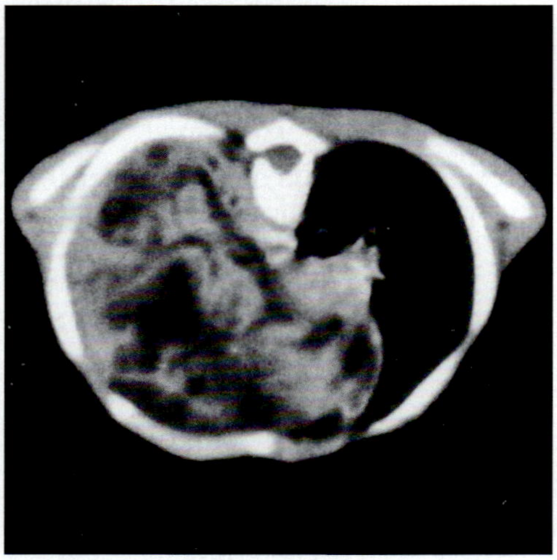

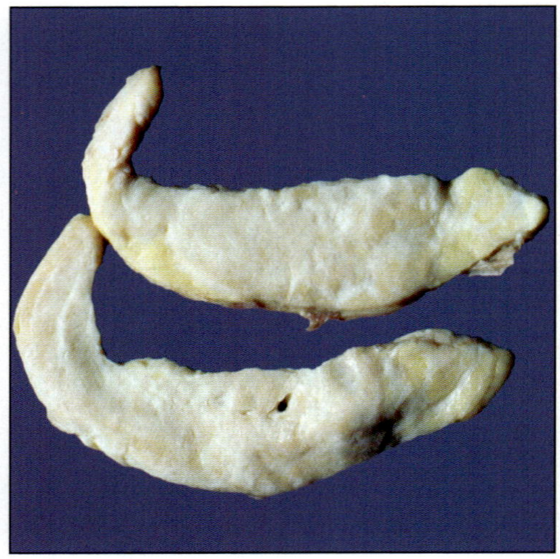

(Left) *CT scan of the thorax shows a large anterior mediastinal mass. The size of thymolipoma varies, and in some cases, the tumor may reach large proportions.* ***(Right)*** *Gross photograph of a thymolipoma shows a rather firm consistency. Note the yellowish areas and the presence of whitish areas, most probably representing areas of adipose and possibly fibrous tissue. Intermixed with these areas, residual thymic tissue may be present.*

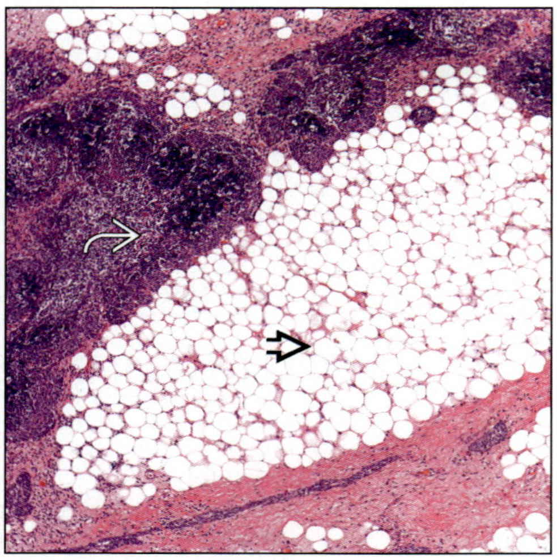

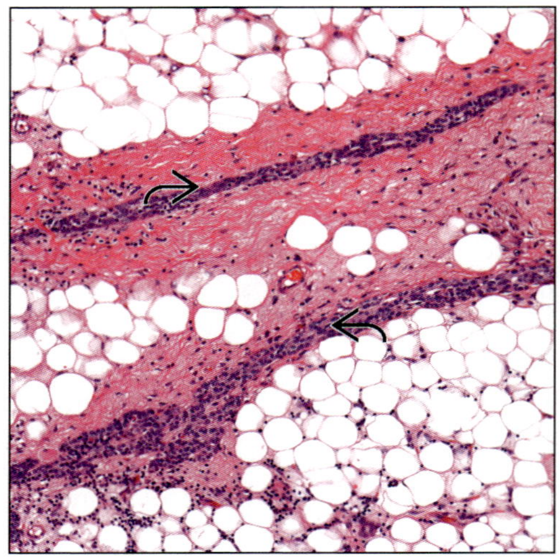

(Left) *Thymolipoma shows extensive areas of mature adipose tissue adjacent to areas of thymic tissue. In some cases, both of these components may be present in almost equal amounts.* ***(Right)*** *In some cases of thymolipoma, the presence of thymic tissue may be very minimal with only residual strands of thymic epithelium.*

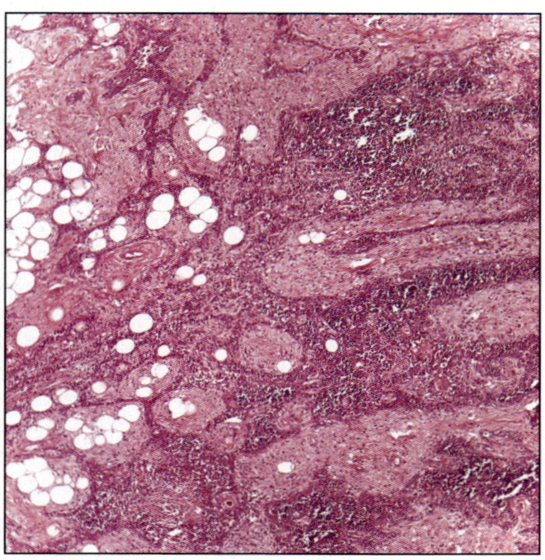

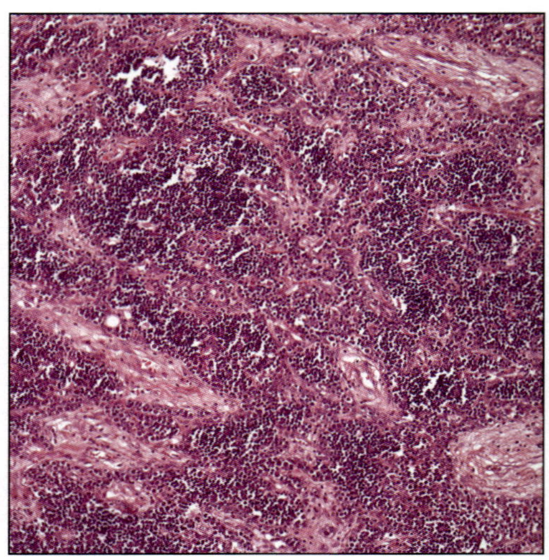

(Left) *Thymolipoma shows extensive areas of fibroconnective tissue admixed with thymic tissue and only a minor component of adipose tissue. Some of these cases have been designated as thymofibrolipoma to describe the components of the tumor.* ***(Right)*** *Hematoxylin & eosin shows thymic tissue and areas of fibroconnective tissue in which no adipose tissue component is present. These histological changes may be seen in cases of thymic hyperplasia.*

Microscopic Features

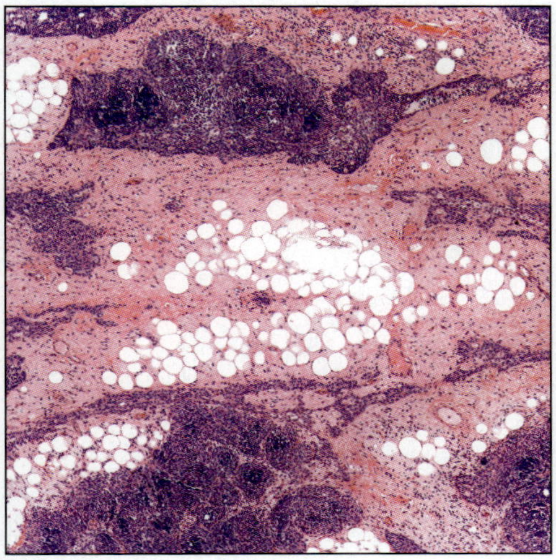

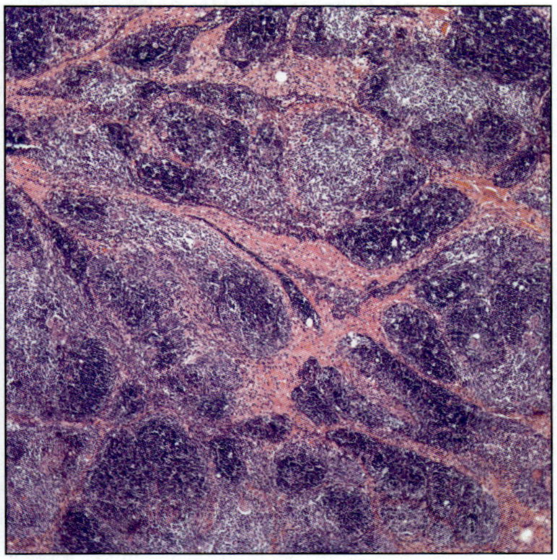

(Left) *Thymolipoma is shown with distinct thymic, adipose, and fibroconnective tissue components. This so-called thymofibrolipoma is due to the marked presence of fibrous component. The designation of thymofibrolipoma does not have any prognostic significance.* ***(Right)*** *Thymic component in a thymolipoma shows a subtle lobulation. This feature can be easily confused for a thymoma due to the lobulation. Thus, a complete examination of the lesion must be performed.*

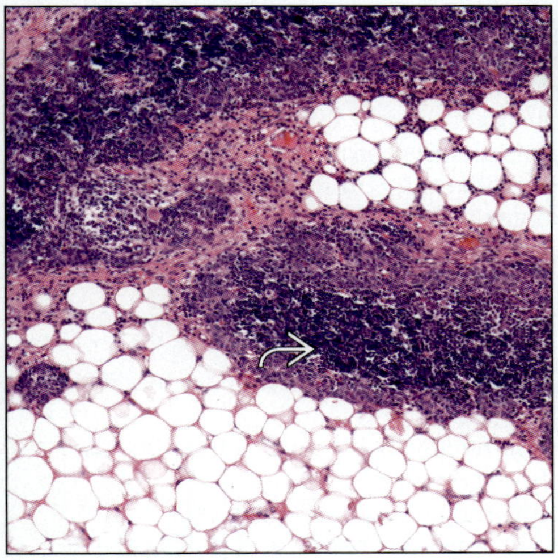

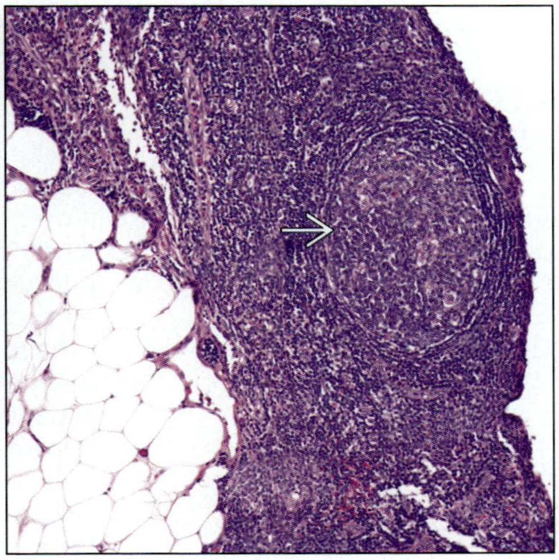

(Left) *Thymolipoma shows areas of residual thymic tissue that, in some areas, almost displays well-demarcated corticomedullary areas →. However, there are extensive areas of mature adipose tissue present.* ***(Right)*** *Thymic component of a thymolipoma shows lymphoid hyperplasia with the presence of germinal centers →. Such a feature is commonly associated with cases of myasthenia gravis; however, the presence of germinal centers can be seen without such an association.*

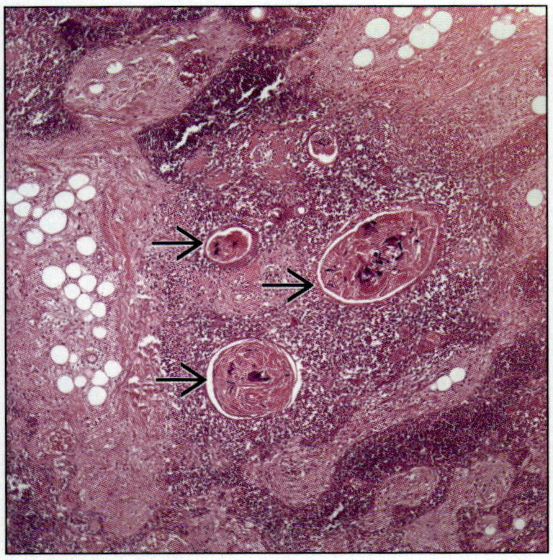

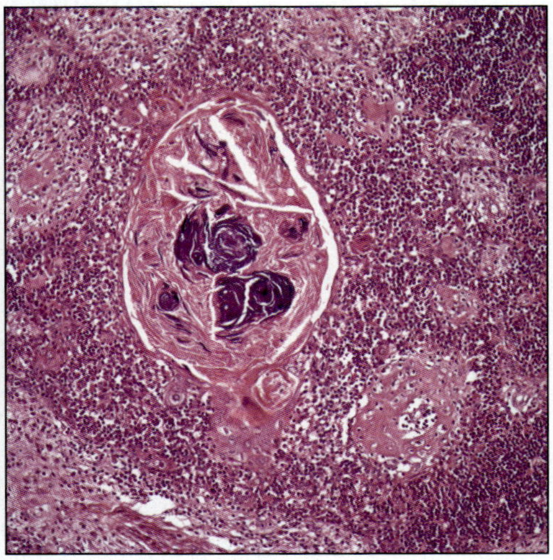

(Left) *Thymolipoma with the characteristic histology shows dilated spaces →. At this magnification, they may be suspicious for another type of pathology.* ***(Right)*** *Higher magnification of the dilated spaces shows keratinization and central calcification. These structures represent dilated and calcified Hassall corpuscles. This is a common occurrence in cases of thymolipoma and has no prognostic significance.*

CASTLEMAN DISEASE

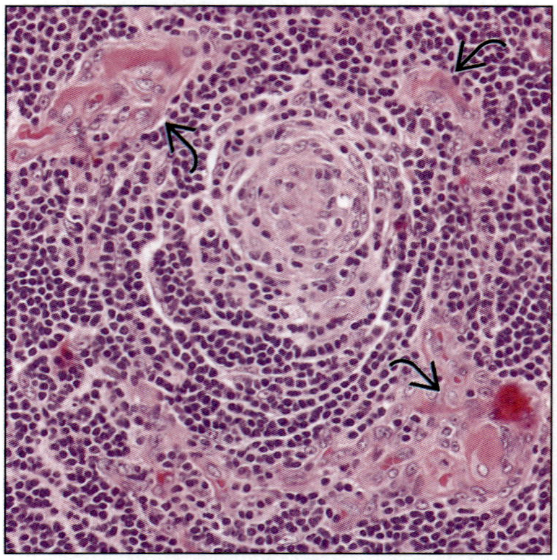

Histologic appearance of Castleman disease, hyaline-vascular type, shows lymphoid follicle with sclerosis and scattered small vessels with hyalinized walls ➔.

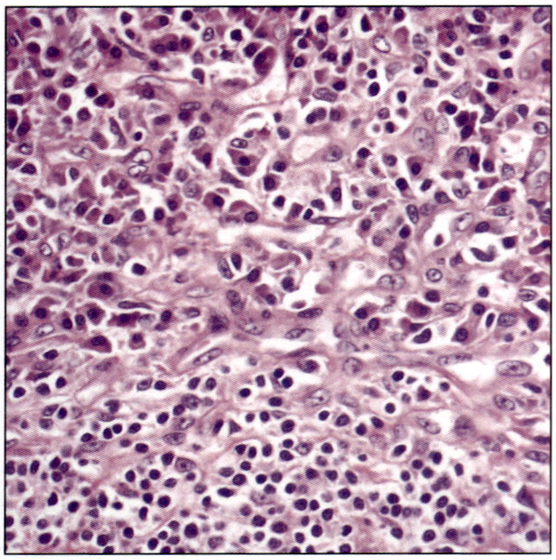

Histologic appearance of Castleman disease, plasma cell type, shows a dense population of mature plasma cells in the interfollicular areas surrounding a lymphoid follicle.

TERMINOLOGY

Synonyms

- Giant lymph node hyperplasia, angiofollicular lymph node hyperplasia, angiomatous lymphoid hamartoma

Definitions

- Heterogeneous group of disorders characterized by lymph nodal enlargement and lymphoid hyperplasia with stromal changes

ETIOLOGY/PATHOGENESIS

Pathogenesis

- Unknown etiology and pathogenesis
- Some cases of plasma cell variant may be related to infection with HHV8 (Kaposi sarcoma-associated herpes virus)
- Some cases are associated with autoimmune diseases such as Wiskott-Aldrich syndrome and AIDS

CLINICAL ISSUES

Epidemiology

- Incidence
  - Affects males and females equally
  - Most common in 3rd decade of life
  - May also affect children and elderly patients

Site

- Most common location is anterior mediastinum
- May also involve middle and posterior mediastinum

Presentation

- Localized type
  - Broad age range
  - Most common histologic features are those of hyaline-vascular type
  - Presents as large mass involving lymph node or lymph node group
  - Compression of airways leads to shortness of breath
  - Compression of vascular structures can lead to esophageal varices
  - Most patients are asymptomatic, and mass is discovered incidentally on routine x-rays
- Multicentric type
  - Most often found in setting of HIV and HHV8 infection
  - Most cases histologically correspond to plasma cell variant
  - B symptoms (fever, night sweats) occur in 95% of patients
  - Hepatosplenomegaly, body cavity effusions, skin rash can also be seen
  - Elevated erythrocyte sedimentation rate, LDH, IL-6, thrombocytopenia, and polyclonal hypergammaglobulinemia are common

Treatment

- Localized cases are cured with simple surgical excision
- Multicentric cases require combination chemotherapy and steroid treatment

MICROSCOPIC PATHOLOGY

Histologic Features

- **Hyaline-vascular type**
  - Most common type encountered in mediastinum
  - Characterized by follicular abnormalities and interfollicular hypervascularity
  - Enlarged follicles with thickened mantle zones and almost complete obliteration of germinal centers
  - Enlarged follicles containing 2 or more germinal centers
  - Small, burned-out follicles with atrophy of germinal centers

Key Facts

Clinical Issues

- Most common in 3rd decade of life
- Localized type
  - Presents as large mass involving lymph node or lymph node group
  - Many patients are asymptomatic, and mass is discovered incidentally on chest x-rays
- Multicentric type
  - Most often encountered in setting of HIV and HHV8 infection
  - Multicentric cases are symptomatic and require combination chemotherapy and steroids

Microscopic Pathology

- Hyaline-vascular type is most common type encountered in mediastinum
  - Characterized by follicular abnormalities and interfollicular hypervascularity
  - Enlarged follicles with thickened mantle zones and almost complete obliteration of germinal centers
  - Enlarged follicles containing 2 or more germinal centers
  - Concentric layering of mantle zone lymphocytes around follicles ("onion skin" appearance)
  - Increased number of vessels in interfollicular spaces admixed with lymphocytes, plasma cells, plasmacytoid monocytes, and immunoblasts
- Plasma cell type is most common type seen in multicentric disease but may also be localized
  - Most characteristic feature is distention of interfollicular spaces by sheets of polyclonal plasma cells

  - Focal hyalinization of atrophic follicles simulating Hassall corpuscles
  - Concentric layering of mantle zone lymphocytes around follicles ("onion skin" appearance)
  - Replacement of follicles by pale, epithelioid cells admixed with small vessels with hyalinized walls
  - Tangentially cut vessels seen penetrating germinal center ("lollipop sign")
  - Increased number of vessels in interfollicular spaces admixed with lymphocytes, plasma cells, plasmacytoid monocytes, and immunoblasts
  - Hyalinization of interfollicular areas with dense bands of sclerosis
  - Prominence of follicular dendritic cells in follicles
  - Cases with dysplastic dendritic follicular cells may develop into follicular dendritic cell sarcomas
  - "Stroma-rich" variant is characterized by massive replacement of interfollicular areas by sclerotic vessels and spindle cells
- **Plasma cell type**
  - Most common type seen in multicentric disease but may also be localized
  - Closely associated with HIV and HHV8 infections
  - Most characteristic feature is distention of interfollicular spaces by sheets of polyclonal plasma cells
  - Follicles may be normal or show some features seen in hyaline-vascular variant
  - Large, atypical plasmablastic cells are present in mantle zones in HHV8(+) cases
  - Kaposi sarcoma and malignant lymphomas can develop from or coexist in lymph nodes with plasma cell type

ANCILLARY TESTS

Immunohistochemistry

- Plasma cells and B cells in both types are polyclonal
- Follicular dendritic cells within germinal centers of hyaline-vascular type are positive for CD21, CD23, and CD35
- Positive HHV8 staining is seen in mantle zone and interfollicular lymphocytes in most cases of plasma cell type
- Some cases of HHV8(+) multicentric Castleman disease may contain a monoclonal plasma cell population

DIFFERENTIAL DIAGNOSIS

Reactive Follicular Hyperplasia

- Reactive follicles are large, with polarization of mantle zones and tingible body macrophages in germinal centers
- No hyalinized small vessels or interfollicular plasmacytosis is seen

Follicular Lymphoma

- Neoplastic follicles are composed of monotonous population of abnormal lymphocytes
- Interfollicular areas are diminished, and there is no evidence of prominent mantle zones
- Neoplastic follicles are monoclonal and stain strongly positive for Bcl-2

SELECTED REFERENCES

1. Nistor C et al: A rare case of unicentric plasma cell type Castleman's disease in the mediastinum. Pneumologia. 59(1):32-5, 2010
2. Erdogan A et al: Posterior mediastinal localization of Castleman's disease: report of a case. Surg Today. 34(9):772-3, 2004
3. Cioffi U et al: Hyaline vascular Castleman's disease of the mediastinum. Int Surg. 84(2):115-7, 1999
4. Moon WK et al: Castleman's disease of the mediastinum: MR imaging features. Clin Radiol. 49(7):466-8, 1994
5. Geary CG et al: Giant lymph node hyperplasia of the mediastinum and refractory anaemia. J Clin Pathol. 31(8):757-60, 1978
6. Keller AR et al: Hyaline-vascular and plasma-cell types of giant lymph node hyperplasia of the mediastinum and other locations. Cancer. 29(3):670-83, 1972

CASTLEMAN DISEASE

Hyaline-Vascular Type

__(Left)__ Scanning magnification of hyaline-vascular Castleman disease of the mediastinum shows preserved but distorted lymph node architecture with numerous scattered lymphoid follicles, some of which have burned-out germinal centers. ***(Right)*** *High magnification of Castleman disease, hyaline-vascular type, shows characteristic abnormal follicle with hyalinized germinal center replaced by large, epithelioid cells and surrounded by a thick mantle zone of lymphocytes.*

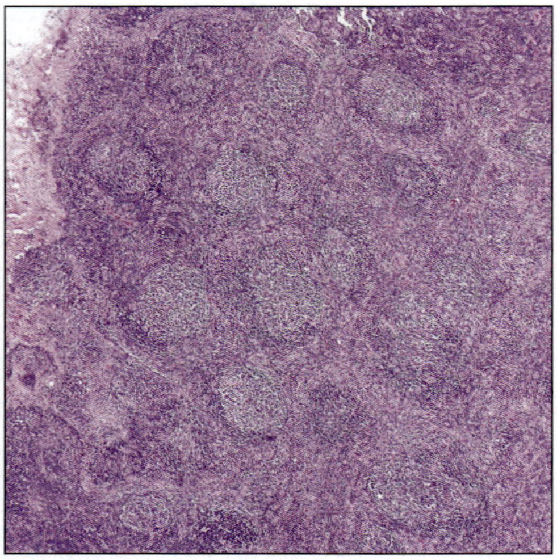

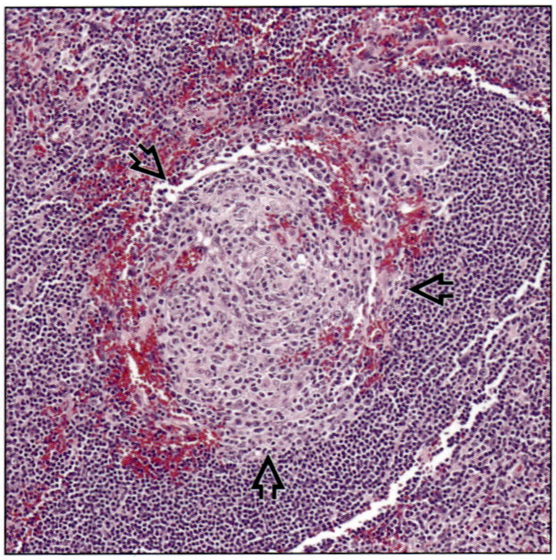

__(Left)__ Scanning magnification of Castleman disease of the mediastinum, hyaline-vascular type, shows multiple lymphoid follicles of various sizes, some of which contain multiple germinal centers. ***(Right)*** *High magnification of abnormal lymphoid follicle in Castleman disease of the mediastinum, hyaline-vascular type, shows burned-out germinal center with small venules traversing the mantle zone and penetrating into the germinal center.*

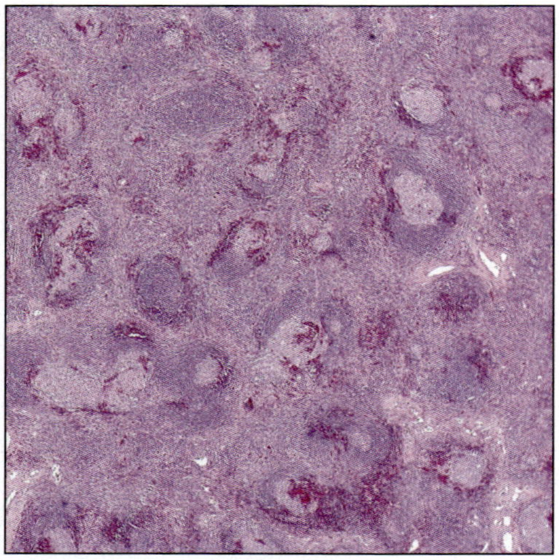

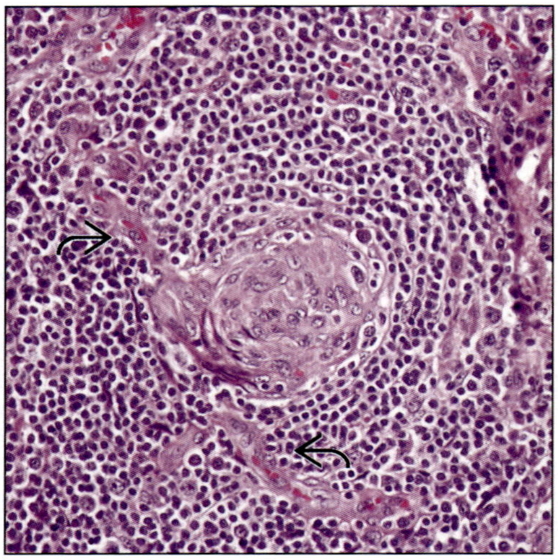

__(Left)__ Scanning magnification of Castleman disease of the mediastinum, hyaline-vascular type, shows multiple nodules with partially hyalinized germinal centers and prominent vascular proliferation in the interfollicular areas. ***(Right)*** *High magnification of an abnormal follicle in Castleman disease of the mediastinum, hyaline-vascular type, shows hyalinization of germinal center and parallel, concentric arrangement of small lymphocytes in the mantle zone ("onion skinning").*

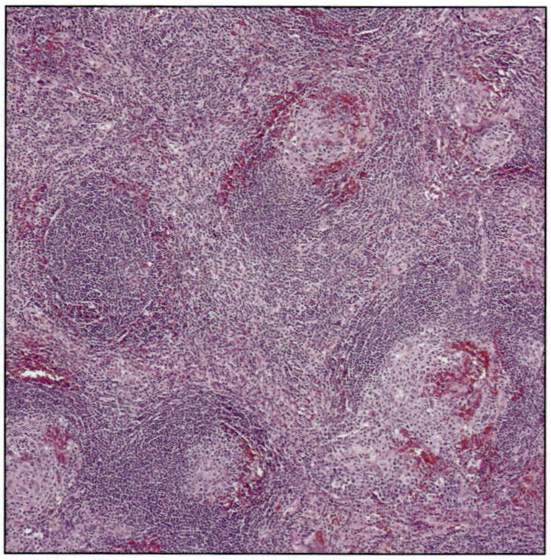

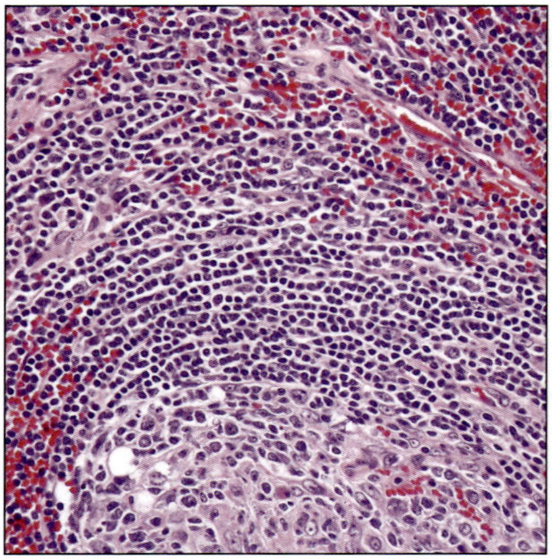

Hyaline-Vascular Type

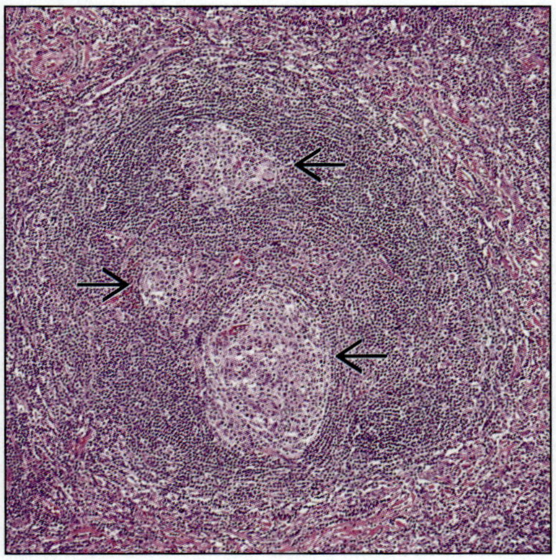
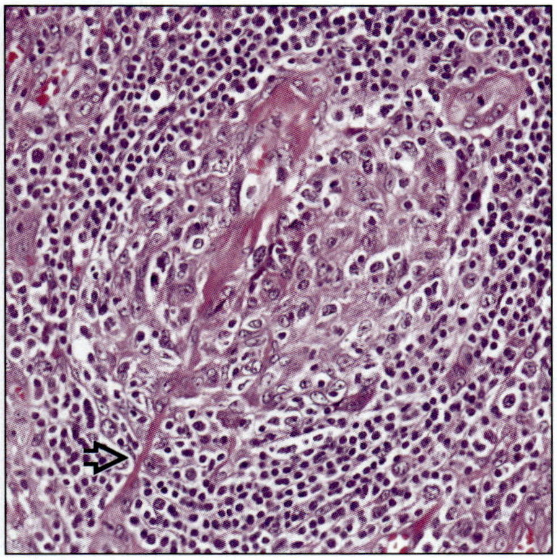

(Left) *Abnormal follicle in Castleman disease of the mediastinum, hyaline-vascular type, shows 3 germinal centers ➔, all located within the same follicle.* ***(Right)*** *High magnification of abnormal follicle in Castleman disease of the mediastinum, hyaline-vascular type, shows a burned-out germinal center traversed by a thin capillary with sclerosis of the vessel wall. Notice that part of the vessel ➢ completely crosses the mantle zone into the interfollicular area.*

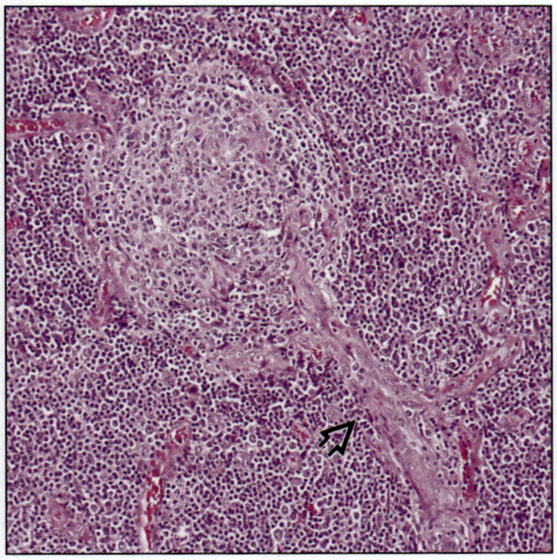
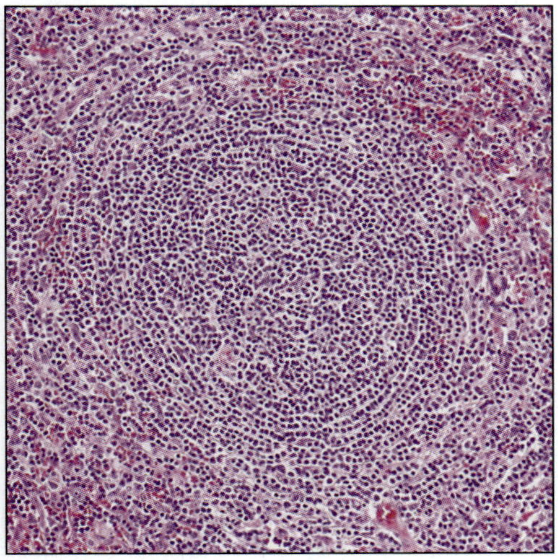

(Left) *High magnification of abnormal lymphoid follicle in Castleman disease of the mediastinum, hyaline-vascular type, shows "lollipop" sign, characterized by a longitudinally cut vessel with hyalinized walls penetrating into the germinal center, simulating the handle of a lollipop ➢.* ***(Right)*** *High magnification of a small, burned-out lymphoid follicle in Castleman disease, hyaline-vascular type, shows a concentric arrangement of lymphocytes with complete absence of the germinal center.*

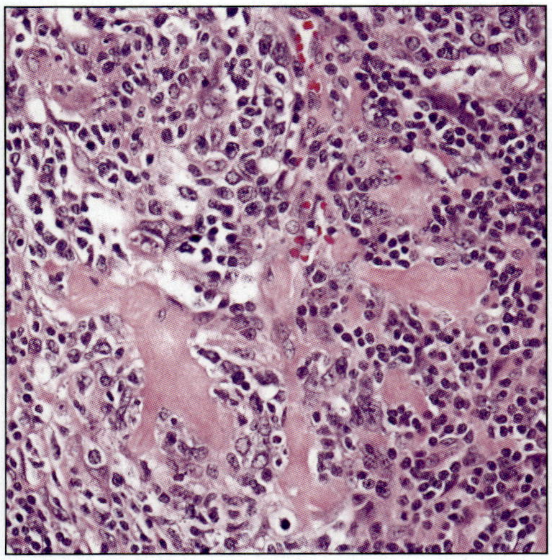
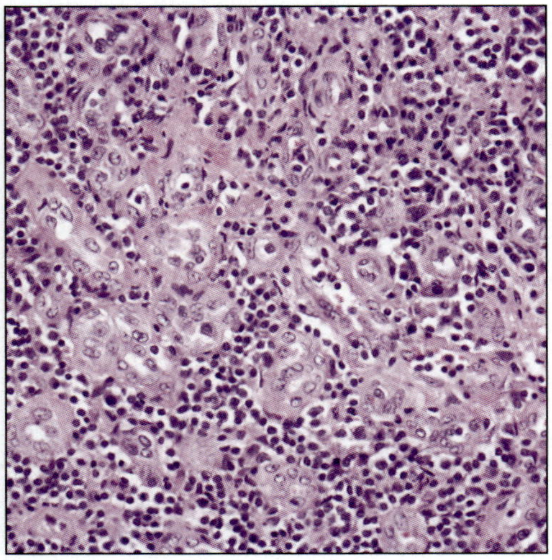

(Left) *High magnification of interfollicular areas in Castleman disease of the mediastinum, hyaline-vascular type, shows stromal sclerosis and hyalinization surrounded by small lymphocytes and occasional immunoblasts.* ***(Right)*** *High magnification of interfollicular areas in Castleman disease of the mediastinum, hyaline-vascular type, shows characteristic interfollicular hypervascularity with numerous small, post-capillary venules with reactive endothelial cells.*

CASTLEMAN DISEASE

Unusual Features in Hyaline-Vascular Type

(Left) *This abnormally large follicle is seen in Castleman disease of the mediastinum, hyaline-vascular type. The enlarged follicle shows an indistinct mantle zone and germinal center.* ***(Right)*** *Burned-out small follicle in Castleman disease of the mediastinum, hyaline-vascular type, shows focal hyalinization in residual follicle →. Areas like this have been mistaken in some cases for Hassall corpuscles, leading to an incorrect diagnosis of lymphocyte-rich thymoma.*

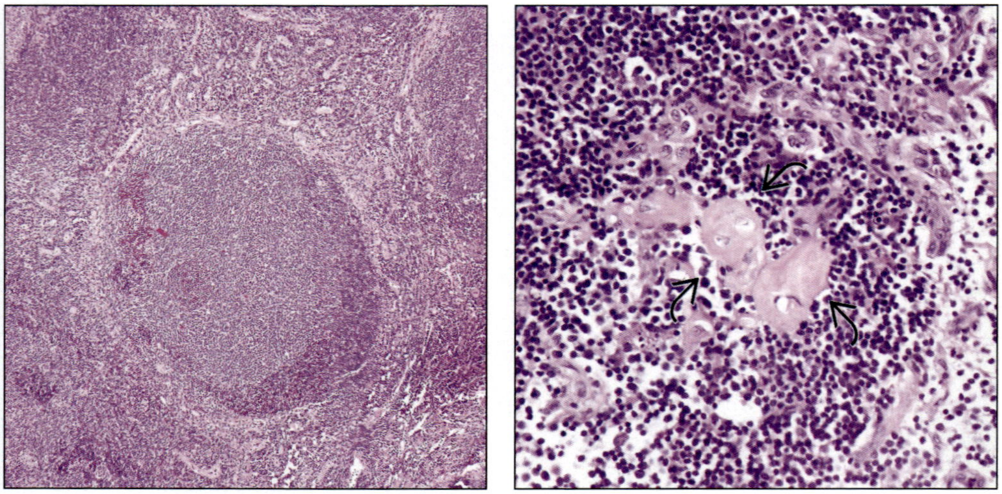

(Left) *Abnormal, dysplastic follicular reticulum cells are seen in a burned-out follicle in Castleman disease of the mediastinum, hyaline-vascular type. Dysplastic or atypical reticulum cells can be found in the follicles or in the interfollicular areas of the nodes and may give rise to reticulum cell sarcomas.* ***(Right)*** *High magnification of abnormal follicle in Castleman disease of the mediastinum, hyaline-vascular type, shows large, hyperchromatic reticulum cells →.*

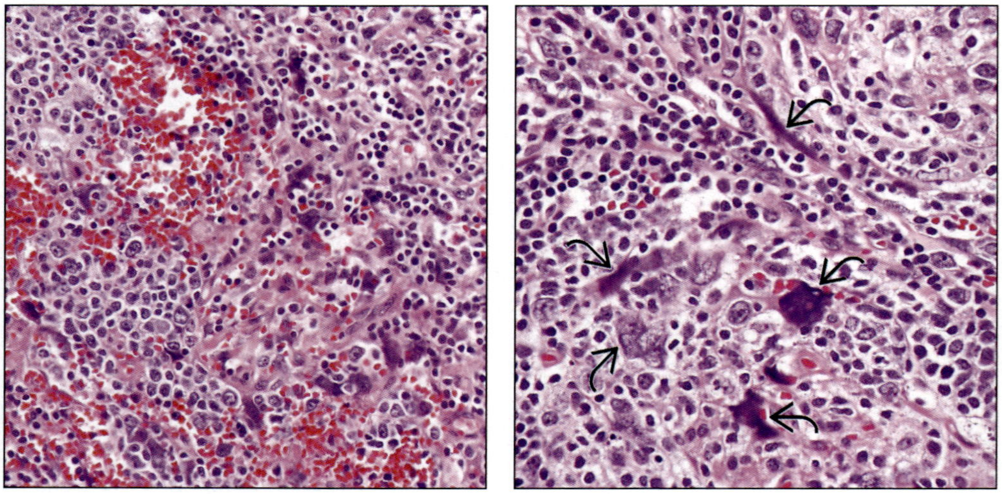

(Left) *Castleman disease of the mediastinum shows a focus of Kaposi sarcoma → in the interfollicular areas arising in association with Castleman disease. Notice the abnormal follicle at the bottom with a hyalinized vessel → traversing the mantle zone into the germinal center.* ***(Right)*** *Higher magnification of the focus of Kaposi sarcoma arising in Castleman disease shows spindle cell proliferation with slit-like vascular spaces containing extravasated red blood cells.*

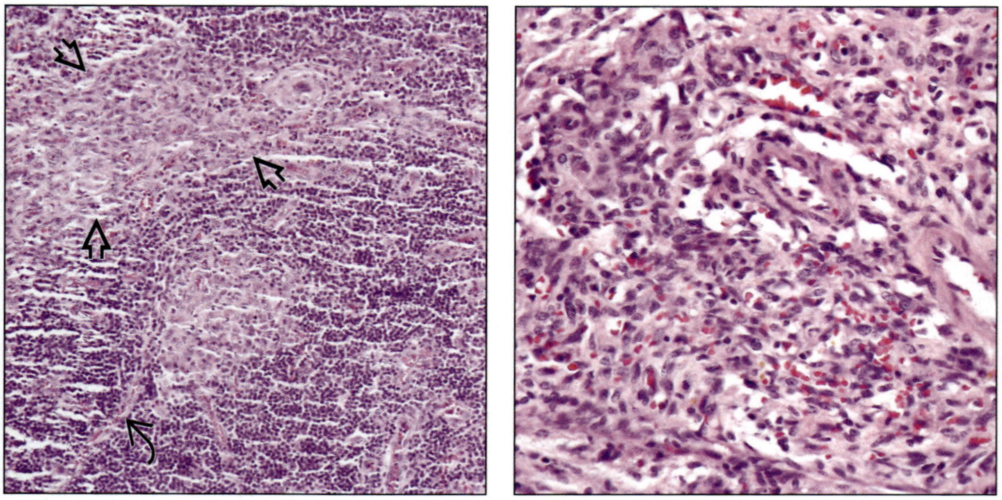

Plasma Cell Type

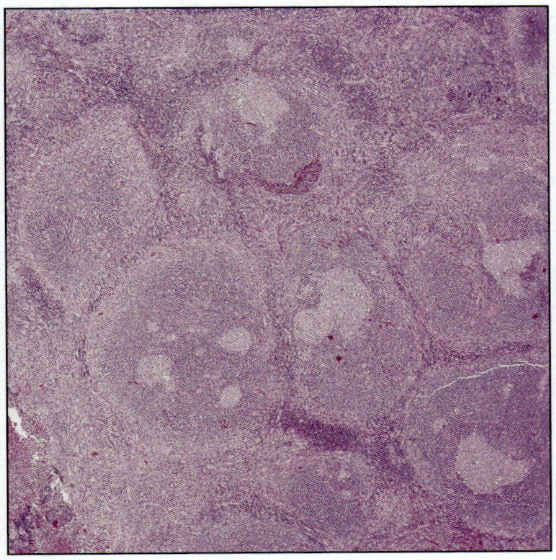

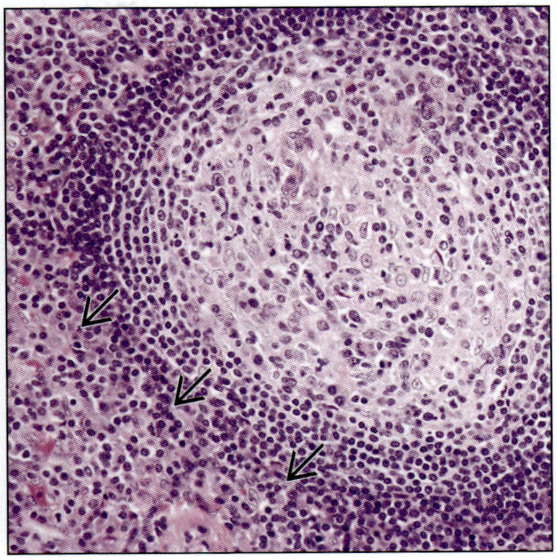

(Left) *Scanning magnification of Castleman disease, plasma cell type, shows numerous, enlarged lymphoid follicles surrounded by a monotonous population of plasma cells in the interfollicular areas.* ***(Right)*** *Higher magnification of Castleman disease, plasma cell type, shows abnormal follicle with hyalinized germinal center and concentric "onion skinning" of mantle zone lymphocytes. Notice the interfollicular area is composed of sheets of mature plasma cells →.*

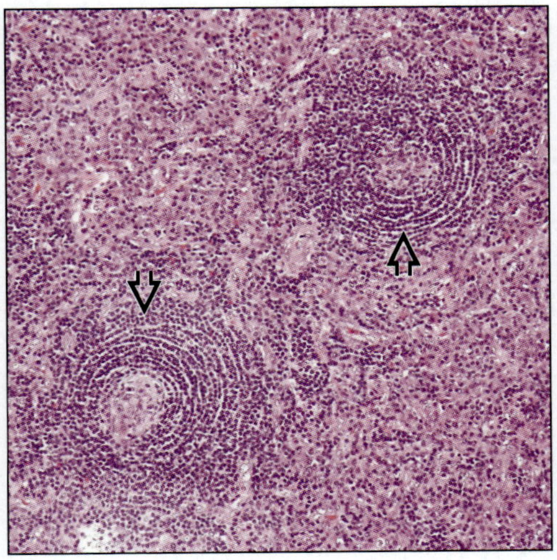

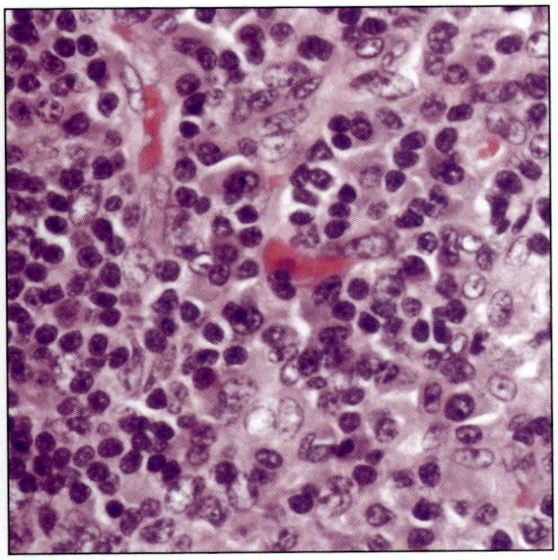

(Left) *Scanning magnification in Castleman disease, plasma cell type, shows 2 small, burned-out follicles with hyalinized germinal centers and "onion skin" mantle zones ⇒ surrounded by a dense plasma cell population in the interfollicular areas.* ***(Right)*** *High magnification of interfollicular area in Castleman disease, plasma cell type, shows sheets of mature plasma cells. Immunohistochemical studies showed that the plasma cells exhibited polyclonality.*

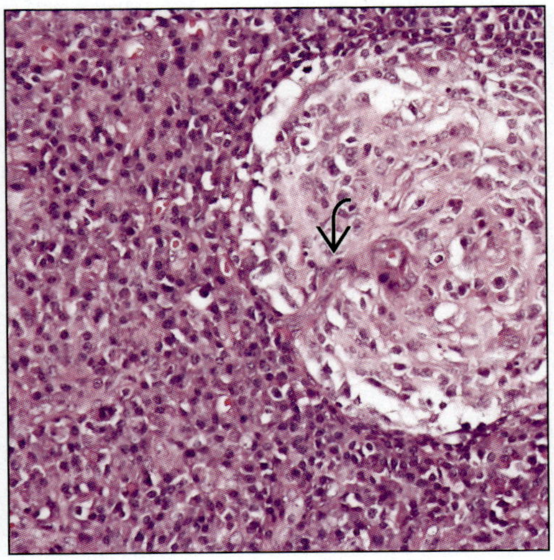

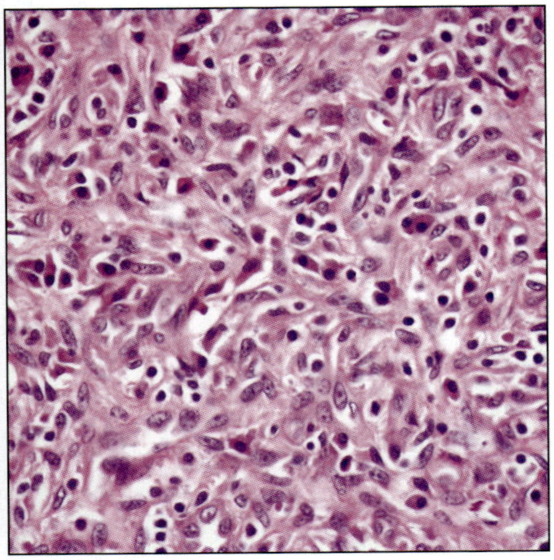

(Left) *Castleman disease, plasma cell type, shows an atrophic, burned-out follicle with a hyalinized germinal center containing a sclerosed vessel →. Notice sheets of monotonous mature plasma cells in the interfollicular areas and absence of mantle zone lymphocytes.* ***(Right)*** *Stroma-rich variant of Castleman disease shows expanded interfollicular areas composed of mature plasma cells admixed with spindle cells. The spindle cells may be of myoid or dendritic reticulum cell lineage.*

BENIGN MEDIASTINAL FOREGUT CYST

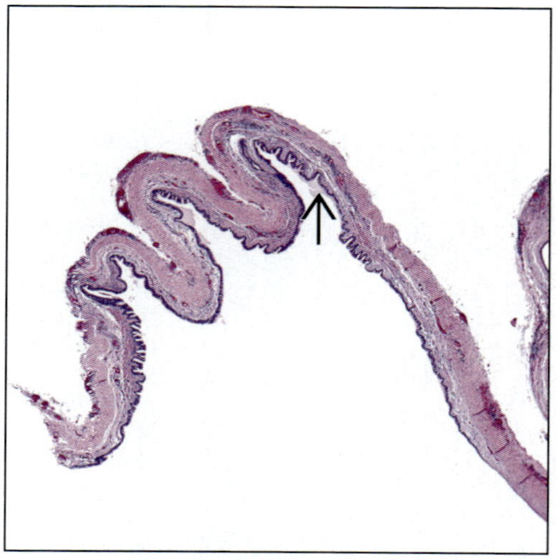

Low-power view shows a mediastinal cyst composed of a strip of fibroconnective tissue with an epithelial lining ⇒.

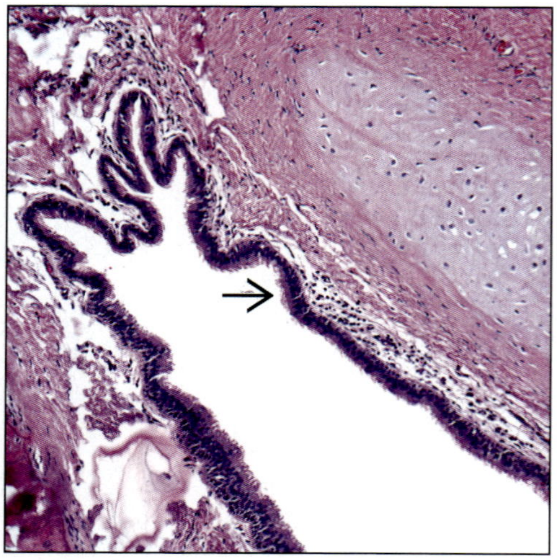

Bronchogenic cyst shows classical features of a lining of respiratory epithelium ⇒ and the presence of cartilage. These 2 components are important in the diagnosis.

TERMINOLOGY

Definitions

- Benign cystic tumors that are classified depending on epithelial lining

ETIOLOGY/PATHOGENESIS

Developmental Anomaly

- So-called foregut cysts may arise due to abnormality during early gestational process in which laryngotracheal groove appears in ventral median aspect of primitive pharynx
  - Eventually develops into trachea and bronchial tree

CLINICAL ISSUES

Epidemiology

- Incidence
  - Unusual benign tumors that may account for 10-20% of all mediastinal tumors
- Age
  - Mediastinal cysts are more common in children
    - However, may also occur in adults
- Gender
  - No predilection

Site

- More commonly seen in anterior and middle mediastinal compartment

Presentation

- Chest pain
- Cough
- Dyspnea
- Asymptomatic

Treatment

- Surgical approaches
  - Complete surgical resection

Prognosis

- Good

MACROSCOPIC FEATURES

General Features

- Unilocular cystic tumors covered by glistening surface

Sections to Be Submitted

- Numerous sections need to be submitted in order to identify specific epithelium to properly classify cyst

Size

- Variable size from a few cm to > 10 cm in diameter

MICROSCOPIC PATHOLOGY

Histologic Features

- Unilocular cyst, which may be lined by different types of epithelium
  - Respiratory epithelium
  - Columnar epithelium
  - Squamous epithelium
  - Mesothelial lining

DIFFERENTIAL DIAGNOSIS

Multilocular Thymic Cyst

- By definition, multilocular thymic cyst is multiloculated cyst in contrast to unilocular aspect of other thymic cyst
- Presence of specific epithelium will lead to correct interpretation

Key Facts

Terminology
- Benign cystic tumors that are classified depending on epithelial lining

Etiology/Pathogenesis
- So-called foregut cysts believed to arise due to abnormality during early gestational process in which laryngotracheal groove appears in ventral median aspect of primitive pharynx
  - Eventually develop into trachea and bronchial tree

Clinical Issues
- Incidence
  - Accounts for approximately 10-20% of all mediastinal tumors
  - More common in children
  - More common in anterior mediastinum
- Symptoms
  - Chest pain
  - Cough
  - Dyspnea
  - Asymptomatic

Top Differential Diagnoses
- Multilocular thymic cyst
- Cystic thymoma

Diagnostic Checklist
- Identification of specific type of epithelium
  - Mesothelial
  - Respiratory
  - Columnar

Clinicopathological Features of Mediastinal Cysts

Cyst	Type of Epithelium	Incidence	Origin	Comment
Bronchogenic cyst	Respiratory epithelium	Most common; about 40-50% of all cysts	Congenital, unilocular	Occurs at any age
Esophageal cyst	Squamous epithelium	Less common than bronchogenic cyst	Congenital, unilocular	More common in children and young adults; may be more common in males
Enteric cyst	Columnar epithelium	Less common than bronchogenic cyst	Congenital, unilocular	More common in children but can occur in adults; commonly seen in posterior mediastinum; patients with vertebral abnormalities
Thymic cyst	Variable lining that may show low cuboidal and squamous epithelium	Rare	Congenital, unilocular	Occurs mainly in children
Pericardial cyst	Mesothelial lining	Common	Congenital, unilocular, pericardium	More common in adults
Mesothelial cyst	Mesothelial lining	Common	Congenital, unilocular	More common in adults

Cystic Thymoma
- Presence of solid areas composed of epithelial cells and lymphocytes will be unusual for unilocular thymic cyst

Other Malignant Neoplasms
- Some germ cell tumors and mucoepidermoid carcinomas have been reported in association with cystic changes
- Careful gross evaluation is important
- Histological evaluation of numerous sections with special emphasis toward solid areas associated with cyst

DIAGNOSTIC CHECKLIST

Clinically Relevant Pathologic Features
- Gross appearance
- Tissue distribution
- Age distribution

Pathologic Interpretation Pearls
- Identification of specific type of epithelium
  - Mesothelial
  - Respiratory
  - Columnar

SELECTED REFERENCES

1. McAdams HP et al: Bronchogenic cyst: imaging features with clinical and histopathologic correlation. Radiology. 217(2):441-6, 2000
2. Davis RD Jr et al: Primary cysts and neoplasms of the mediastinum: recent changes in clinical presentation, methods of diagnosis, management, and results. Ann Thorac Surg. 44(3):229-37, 1987
3. Ovrum E et al: Mediastinal tumours and cysts. A review of 91 cases. Scand J Thorac Cardiovasc Surg. 13(2):161-8, 1979
4. Reed JC et al: Morphologic analysis of foregut cysts in the thorax. Am J Roentgenol Radium Ther Nucl Med. 120(4):851-60, 1974

BENIGN MEDIASTINAL FOREGUT CYST

Gross and Microscopic Features

(Left) *Mediastinal foregut cyst is shown surrounded by membranous tissue and hemorrhage. Histopathologic evaluation of the cyst lining is required to establish the correct diagnosis.* ***(Right)*** *Bronchogenic cyst shows respiratory epithelium and a lymphoid aggregate with germinal center. These features are commonly seen in these cysts.*

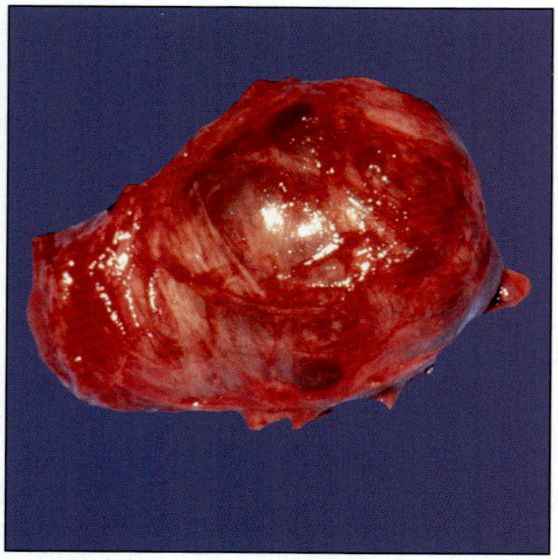

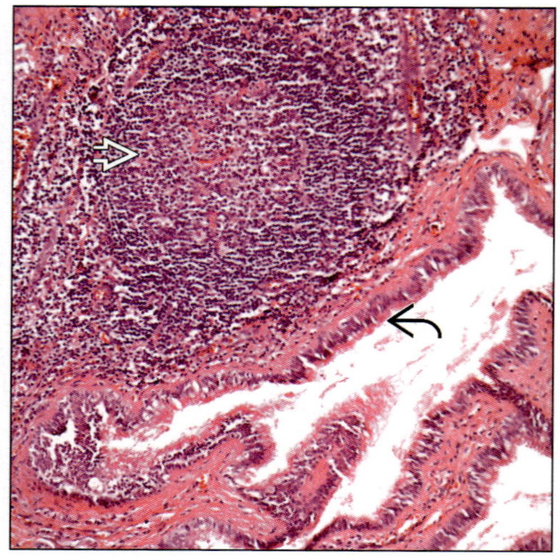

(Left) *Higher magnification of a bronchogenic cyst shows cartilage and a cystic structure lined by respiratory type of epithelium. Note the presence of cilia in the respiratory epithelium.* ***(Right)*** *High-power view shows respiratory epithelium in a bronchogenic cyst. The respiratory epithelium does not show any atypical changes but shows a transition toward a flattened attenuated epithelium.*

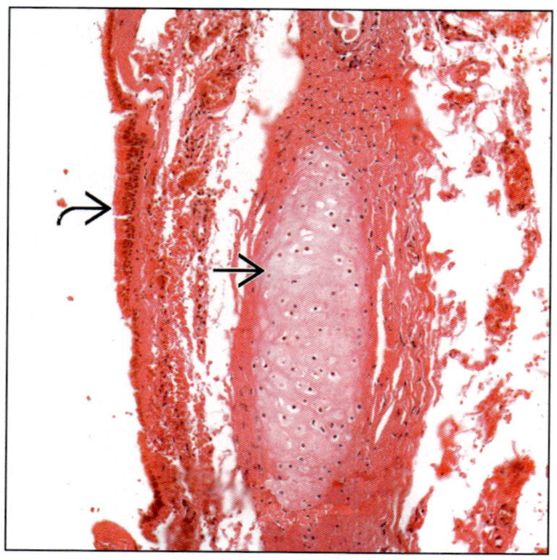

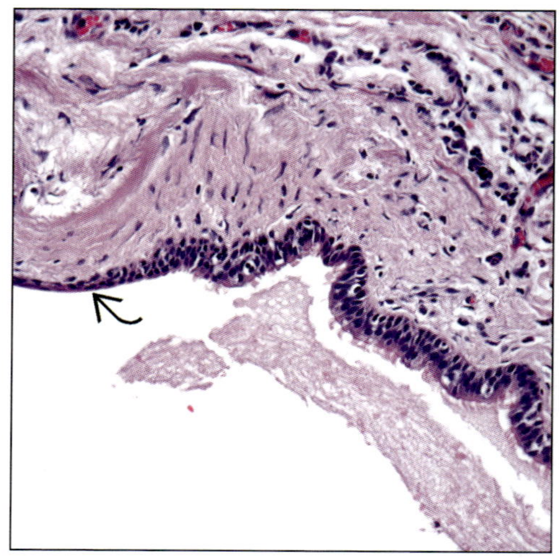

(Left) *Mediastinal cyst composed of dense fibroconnective tissue shows cystic structure lined by an epithelium with tall columnar cells. The cyst wall shows mild inflammatory changes.* ***(Right)*** *High-power view shows the epithelium lining a mediastinal cyst, which is composed of a mucinous type of epithelium. This finding is diagnostic of an enteric cyst.*

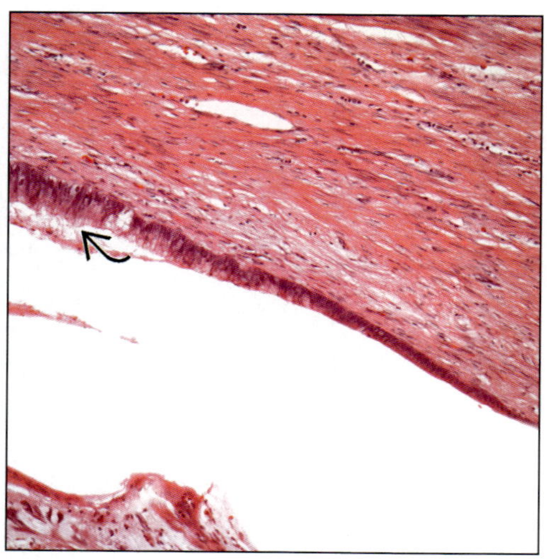

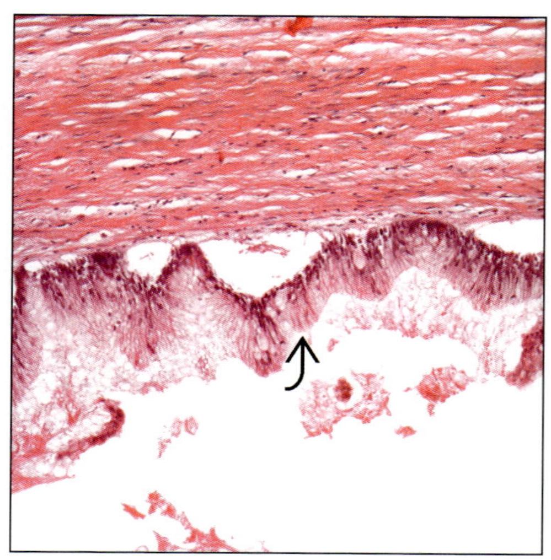

Microscopic Features

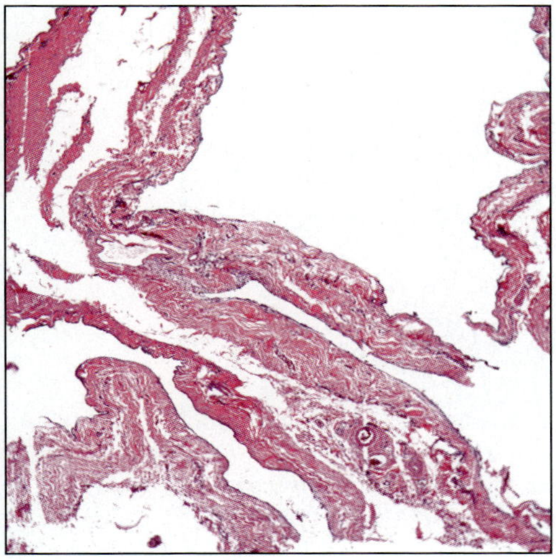

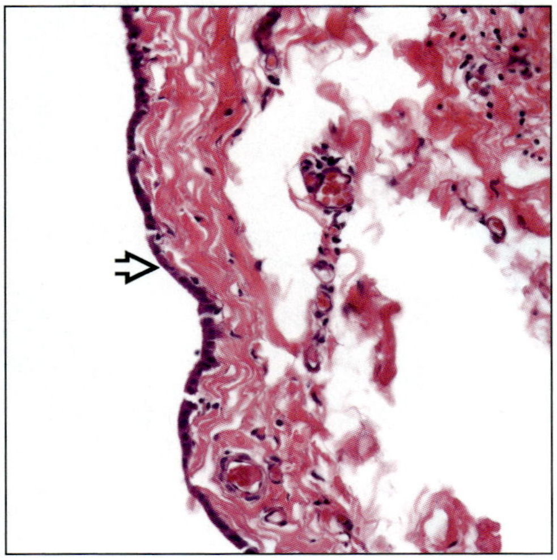

(Left) *Mediastinal cyst is shown composed of several strips of fibroconnective tissue lined by an attenuated epithelium. The cyst wall shows only mild inflammatory changes.* ***(Right)*** *Higher magnification shows the epithelium of a mediastinal cyst. The lining is a low type of cuboidal epithelium, and these findings are consistent with a mesothelial cyst.*

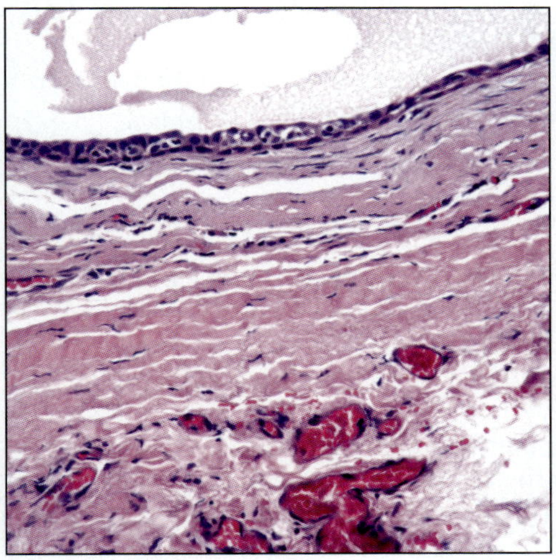

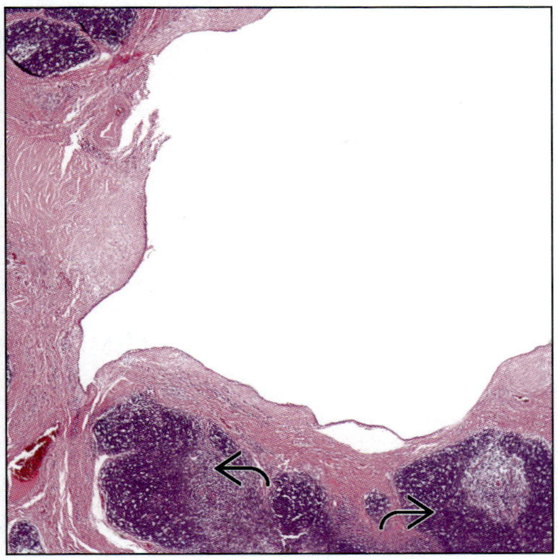

(Left) *This mesothelial cyst is composed of flattened epithelium without atypia and underlying fibroconnective tissue with minimal inflammatory changes.* ***(Right)*** *Mediastinal cyst in which there is an obvious presence of thymic tissue. In addition, the cyst appears uniloculated and lined by a flattened type of epithelium.*

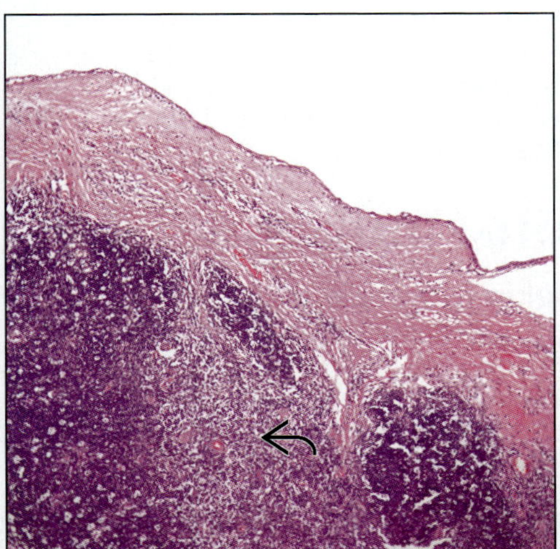

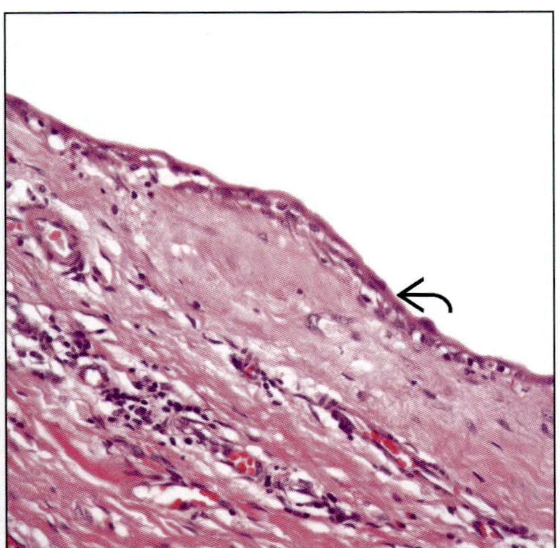

(Left) *High magnification shows a mediastinal cyst with obvious presence of thymic tissue and a cystic structure lined by a flattened type of epithelium. These features are consistent with a thymic cyst.* ***(Right)*** *High magnification shows the epithelium lining a mediastinal cyst, which is composed of a low cuboidal type without atypia. Note the presence of mild inflammatory changes in the wall of the cyst.*

ACQUIRED MULTILOCULAR THYMIC CYST

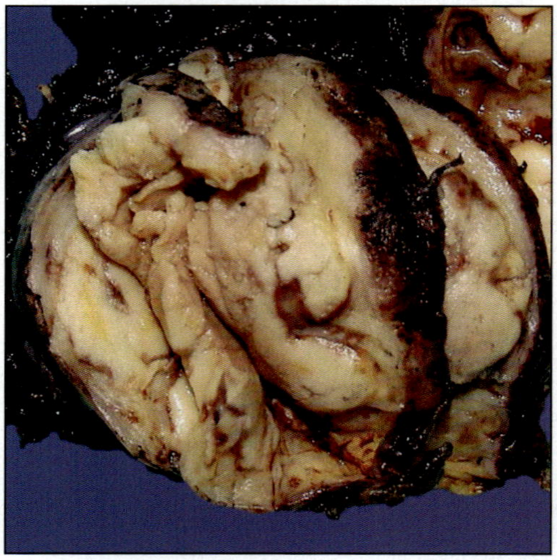

Gross appearance of multilocular thymic cyst shows a well-circumscribed cystic mass with hemorrhage in the walls of the cyst.

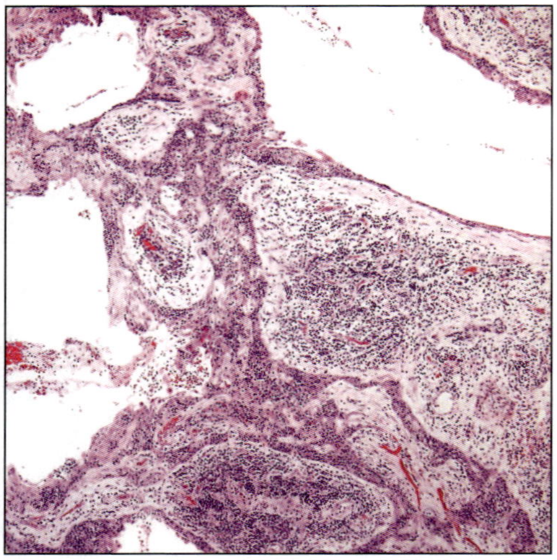

Histologic appearance of multilocular thymic cyst shows cystic cavities lined by a thin layer of epithelium in continuity with strands of hyperplastic thymic epithelium.

TERMINOLOGY

Abbreviations
- Acquired multilocular thymic cyst (AMTC)

Synonyms
- Lymphoepithelial thymic cyst

Definitions
- Acquired reactive process that results in cystic dilatation of thymic epithelium

ETIOLOGY/PATHOGENESIS

Pathogenesis
- Acquired reactive process resulting from underlying infectious or inflammatory stimulus

CLINICAL ISSUES

Presentation
- Chest pain
- Dyspnea
- Chest fullness
- Associated with AIDS in children

Treatment
- Surgical excision

Prognosis
- Excellent prognosis
- Generally cured by complete surgical excision
- Rare cases can recur when incompletely excised

MACROSCOPIC FEATURES

General Features
- Large, multilocular cystic structure
- Cysts may contain clear or hemorrhagic fluid
- May show fibrous adhesions to pleura and pericardium

Sections to Be Submitted
- At least 1 section per centimeter of greatest diameter
- Submit all solid areas in the walls of cysts

Size
- 3-25 cm in diameter

MICROSCOPIC PATHOLOGY

Histologic Features
- Cystic spaces lined by flat, cuboidal to squamous epithelium
  - Squamous epithelium may show pseudoepitheliomatous hyperplasia
  - Lining of cysts can be traced to dilated Hassall corpuscles
- Prominent stromal hemorrhage, fibrosis, and chronic inflammation in wall of cysts
- Prominent granulation tissue and cholesterol-cleft granulomas in stroma
- Prominent lymphoid follicular hyperplasia
- Residual thymus showing branching, elongated strands of thymic epithelium

DIFFERENTIAL DIAGNOSIS

Cystic Hodgkin Lymphoma
- Microscopic islands containing Reed-Sternberg cells should be present
- Positive identification of Reed-Sternberg cells with antibodies to CD30/CD15 required for diagnosis of Hodgkin disease

Cystic Seminoma
- Microscopic islands containing seminoma cells should be present

ACQUIRED MULTILOCULAR THYMIC CYST

Key Facts

Etiology/Pathogenesis

- Acquired reactive process resulting from underlying infectious or inflammatory stimulus

Clinical Issues

- Generally cured by complete surgical excision
  - Rare cases can recur when incompletely excised
- Chest pain
- Dyspnea
- Often seen in children with AIDS

Macroscopic Features

- Large, multilocular cystic structure
- May show fibrous adhesions to pleura and pericardium
- 3-25 cm in diameter

Microscopic Pathology

- Cystic spaces lined by flat, cuboidal to squamous epithelium
  - Squamous epithelium may show pseudoepitheliomatous hyperplasia
  - Lining of cysts can be traced to dilated Hassall corpuscles
- Prominent stromal hemorrhage, fibrosis, and chronic inflammation in wall of cysts
- Prominent granulation tissue and cholesterol cleft granulomas in stroma
- Prominent lymphoid follicular hyperplasia
- Residual thymus showing branching, elongated strands of thymic epithelium

- Positive identification of seminoma cells using PLAP, D2-40, or C-Kit
- Cystic seminomas may also contain abundant epithelioid granulomas that can overshadow the neoplastic elements

Cystic Thymoma

- Solid, confluent areas showing features of thymoma should be present in walls of cyst
- Identification of keratin(+) cells amidst immature CD1a/CD3(+) thymocytes required for diagnosis of thymoma
- Cysts may also result from massive dilatation and confluence of perivascular spaces

Cystic Teratoma

- Heterologous elements should be identified in walls of cyst (i.e., cartilage, glial tissue, squamous or glandular epithelium, etc.)
- May contain immature neural elements (immature teratoma)

MALT Lymphoma of Thymus

- Cystic spaces in MALT lymphoma show infiltration of small lymphocytes into epithelial lining of cyst
- Monotonous population of monocytoid B cells is present surrounding lymphoid follicles in MALT lymphoma
- Infiltration of Hassall corpuscles by lymphocytes create lymphoepithelial lesions in MALT lymphoma

Thymic Carcinoma

- Cystic mucoepidermoid carcinoma will show solid areas exhibiting epidermoid features and mucocytes in the walls of cysts
- Basaloid carcinoma of thymus will show cystic dilatation of tumor cell islands that are lined by atypical, basaloid cells
- Secondary MTC-like changes can be observed in surrounding, uninvolved thymic parenchyma in any type of thymic carcinoma

DIAGNOSTIC CHECKLIST

Clinically Relevant Pathologic Features

- Multiple cysts lined by epithelium that is in continuity with cystically dilated Hassall corpuscles
- Cyst walls show prominent fibrosis and chronic inflammation
- Many cases also show prominent lymphoid follicular hyperplasia
- Cases with pseudoepitheliomatous hyperplasia of lining epithelium may be confused for invasive squamous cell carcinoma arising in a cyst

Pathologic Interpretation Pearls

- Most important feature is to make sure that malignant thymic neoplasm with secondary cystic changes (such as thymoma, lymphoma, or seminoma) has been ruled out by thorough sampling

SELECTED REFERENCES

1. Izumi H et al: Multilocular thymic cyst associated with follicular hyperplasia: clinicopathologic study of 4 resected cases. Hum Pathol. 36(7):841-4, 2005
2. Choi YW et al: Idiopathic multilocular thymic cyst: CT features with clinical and histopathologic correlation. AJR Am J Roentgenol. 177(4):881-5, 2001
3. Chhieng DC et al: Multilocular thymic cyst with follicular lymphoid hyperplasia in a male infected with HIV. A case report with fine needle aspiration cytology. Acta Cytol. 43(6):1119-23, 1999
4. Kontny HU et al: Multilocular thymic cysts in children with human immunodeficiency virus infection: clinical and pathologic aspects. J Pediatr. 131(2):264-70, 1997
5. Mishalani SH et al: Multilocular thymic cyst. A novel thymic lesion associated with human immunodeficiency virus infection. Arch Pathol Lab Med. 119(5):467-70, 1995
6. Suster S et al: Multilocular thymic cyst: an acquired reactive process. Study of 18 cases. Am J Surg Pathol. 15(4):388-98, 1991
7. Suster S et al: Multilocular thymic cysts with pseudoepitheliomatous hyperplasia. Hum Pathol. 22(5):455-60, 1991

ACQUIRED MULTILOCULAR THYMIC CYST

General Features

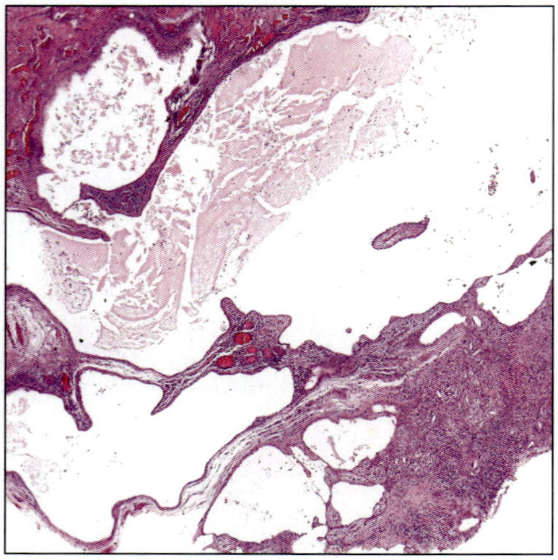

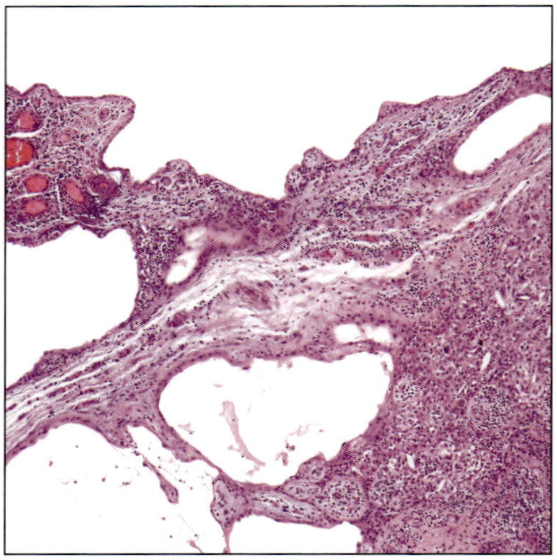

(Left) *Scanning magnification of multilocular thymic cyst shows large cystic spaces delineating multilocular cavities lined by a single layer of epithelium. The walls of the cysts contain a heavy inflammatory infiltrate.* ***(Right)*** *Higher magnification of a multilocular thymic cyst shows dense lymphoid infiltrates in the walls of the cysts. The cysts vary in size and shape, and some of the larger cysts appear to result from the confluence of smaller cysts.*

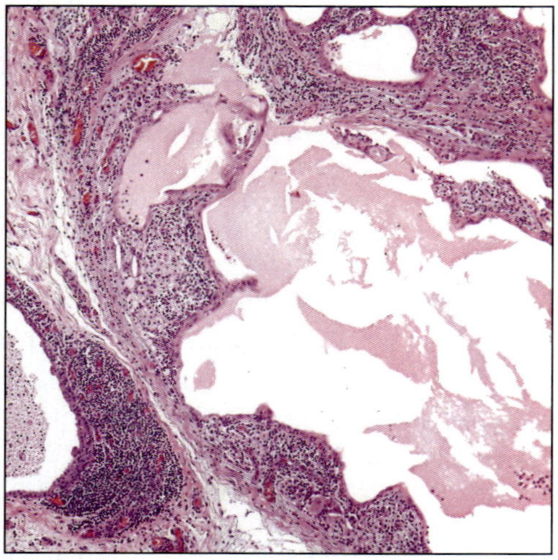

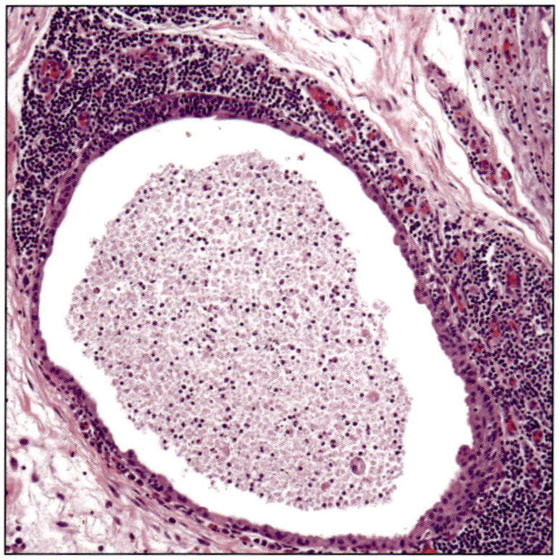

(Left) *A multilocular thymic cyst shows multiple irregular cystic spaces lined by epithelium and containing proteinaceous debris in their lumens.* ***(Right)*** *High magnification from a multilocular thymic cyst shows a lumen filled with proteinaceous debris admixed with inflammatory cells. The cyst wall is lined by a thin layer of cuboidal epithelium and is surrounded by dense inflammatory infiltrate composed primarily of small lymphocytes and admixed with occasional plasma cells and histiocytes.*

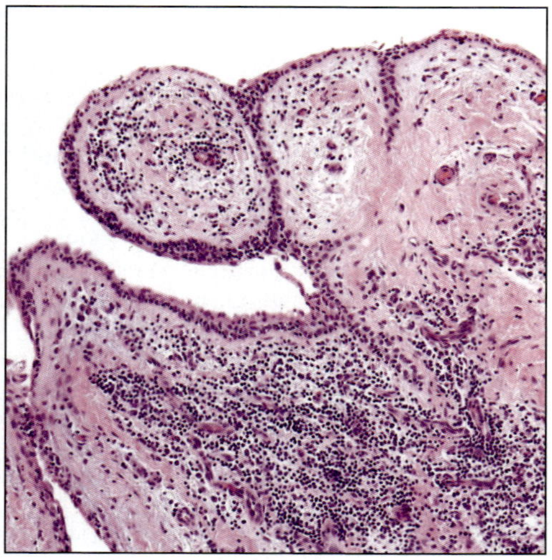

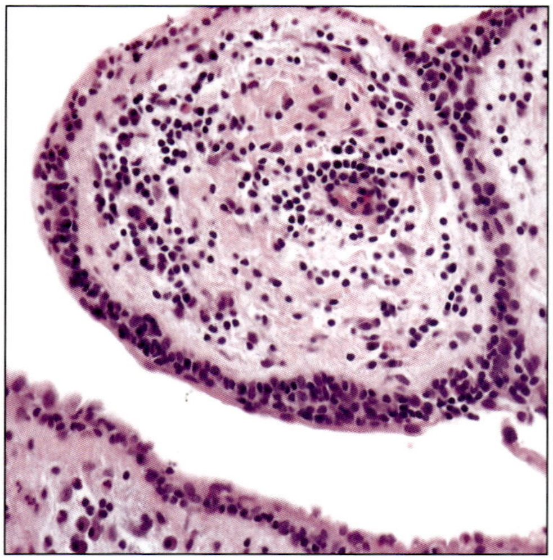

(Left) *Wall of a cyst in a patient with a multilocular thymic cyst shows polypoid protrusion into the lumen by epithelium-lined stroma with features of granulation tissue.* ***(Right)*** *High magnification of polypoid intraluminal invagination of the cyst wall in a multilocular thymic cyst shows a thin layer of stratified, cuboidal epithelium circumscribing an area of granulation tissue with fibroblastic proliferation, scattered inflammatory cells, and small vessels.*

Residual Thymic Epithelium

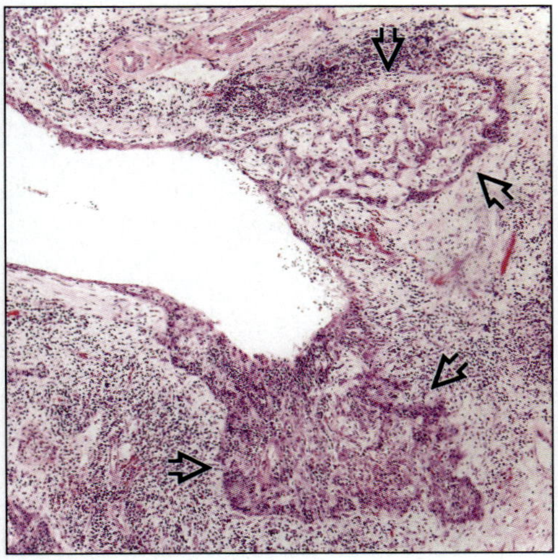

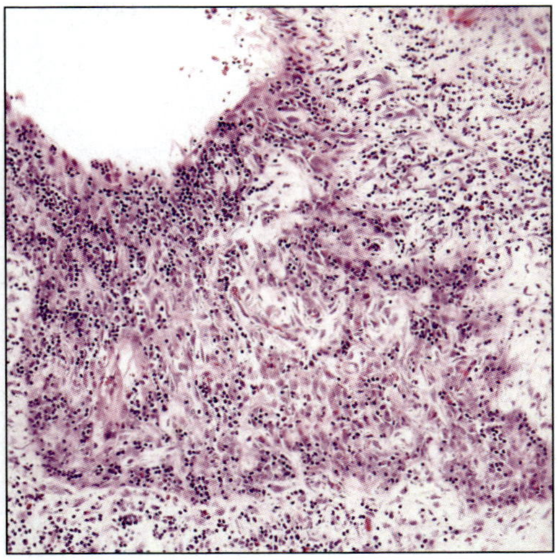

(Left) *Multilocular thymic cyst shows cystic dilatation lined by a thin layer of simple epithelium that can be traced back to residual thymic epithelial elements in the wall of the cyst.* ***(Right)*** *High magnification of cyst wall in a multilocular thymic cyst shows the epithelial lining of the cyst in continuity with residual focus of involuting thymic epithelium within the wall of the cyst. Note that the strands of thymic epithelial cells are intimately admixed with small lymphocytes.*

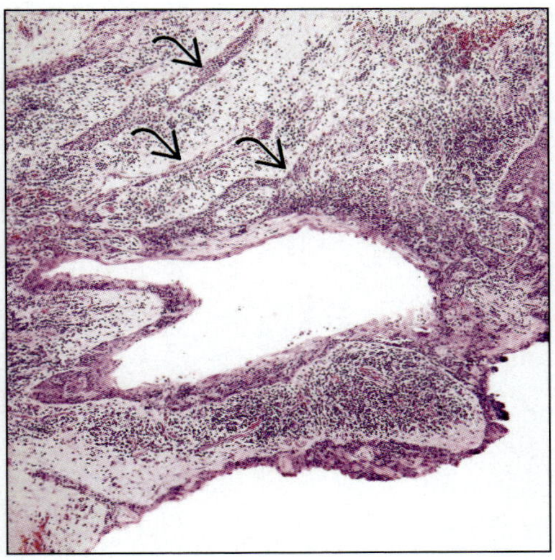

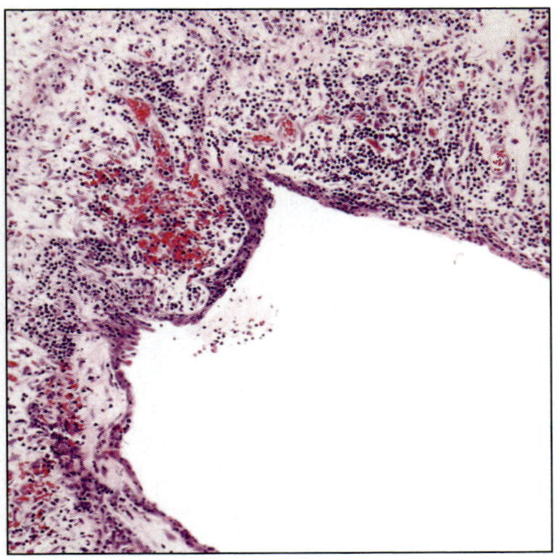

(Left) *Scanning magnification of the cyst wall in a multilocular thymic cyst shows transition between the lining epithelium and strands of residual thymic epithelium. Note that the residual thymic epithelium entrapped in the wall shows a tendency to elongate and branch out into thin strands within the cyst wall.* ***(Right)*** *High magnification of cyst wall in a multilocular thymic cyst shows a thin layer of lining epithelium surrounded by abundant inflammatory infiltrate in the wall of the cyst.*

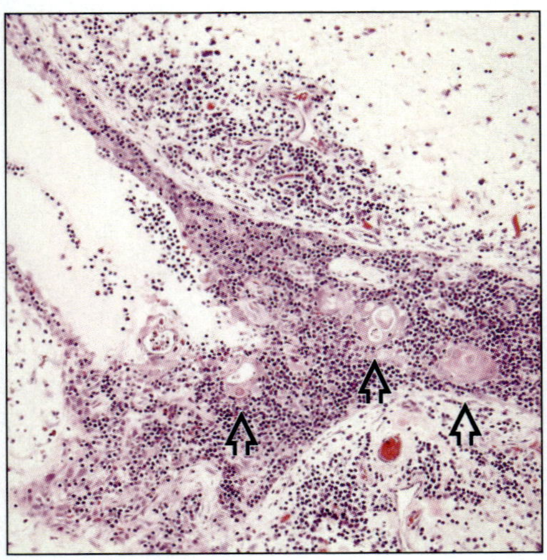

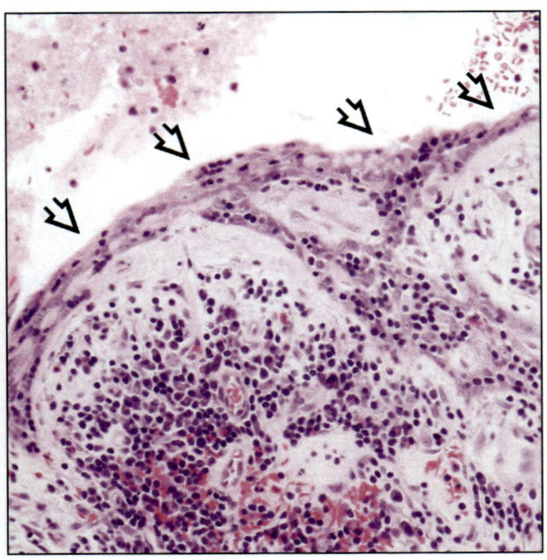

(Left) *High magnification of the cyst wall in a multilocular thymic cyst shows the origin of the cyst lining the epithelium from dilated Hassall corpuscles.* ***(Right)*** *High magnification of cyst wall in a multilocular thymic cyst shows simple cuboidal epithelium lining the cyst with focal invaginations into the cyst wall. The wall of the cyst contains dense inflammatory infiltrates mainly composed of small lymphocytes admixed with plasma cells and histiocytes.*

ACQUIRED MULTILOCULAR THYMIC CYST

Fibroepitheliomatous Hyperplasia

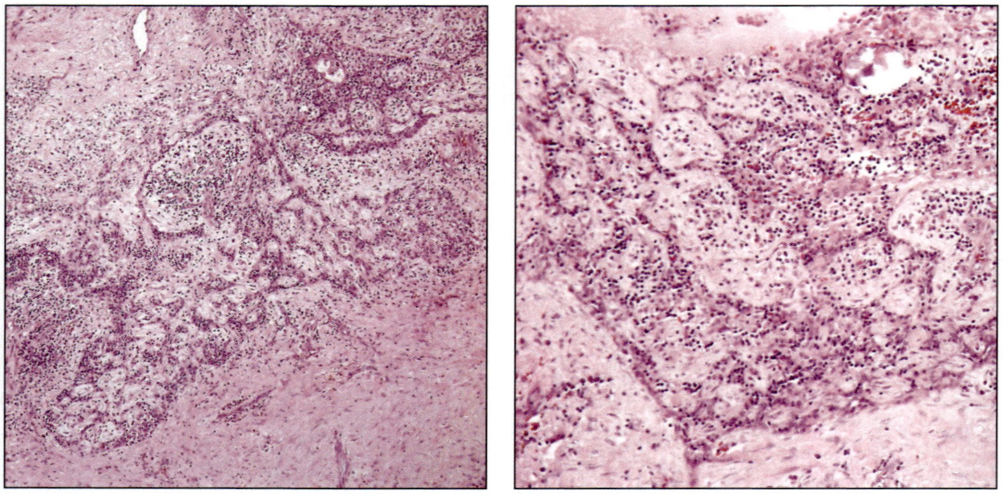

(Left) *Multilocular thymic cyst shows entrapped thymic epithelium within the cyst walls. Note the elongated, branching nature of the strands of thymic epithelium resulting in a complex, fibroepitheliomatous appearance.* ***(Right)*** *A striking fibroepitheliomatous appearance due to strands of residual thymic epithelium located within the cyst wall of a multilocular thymic cyst. The thin strands of epithelium are surrounded by collagenized stroma with abundant lymphocytes.*

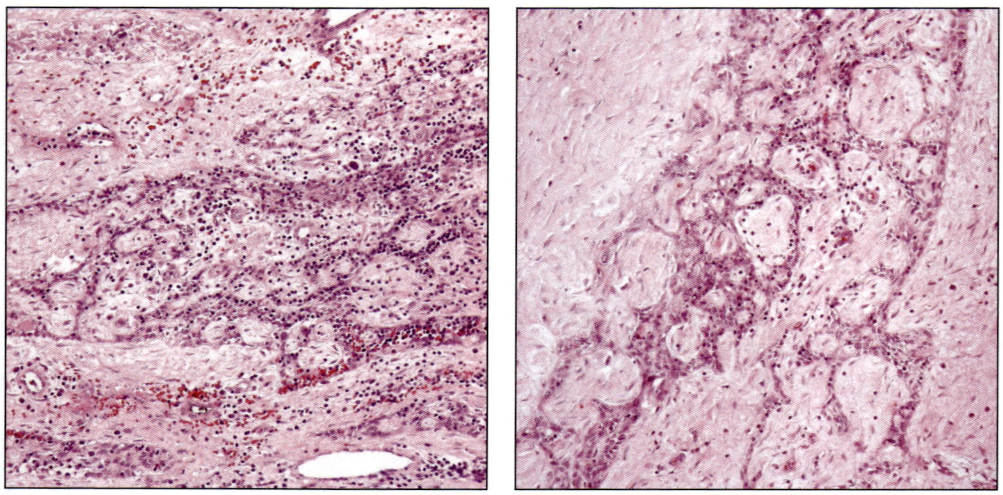

(Left) *Higher magnification of multilocular thymic cyst shows branching strands of residual thymic epithelium entrapped within the walls of the cyst surrounded by mixed inflammatory infiltrate with abundant small lymphocytes.* ***(Right)*** *Striking fibroepitheliomatous appearance is seen in the residual thymic epithelium within the wall of a multilocular thymic cyst. This appearance is quite distinctive for this process and represents a reactive response pattern.*

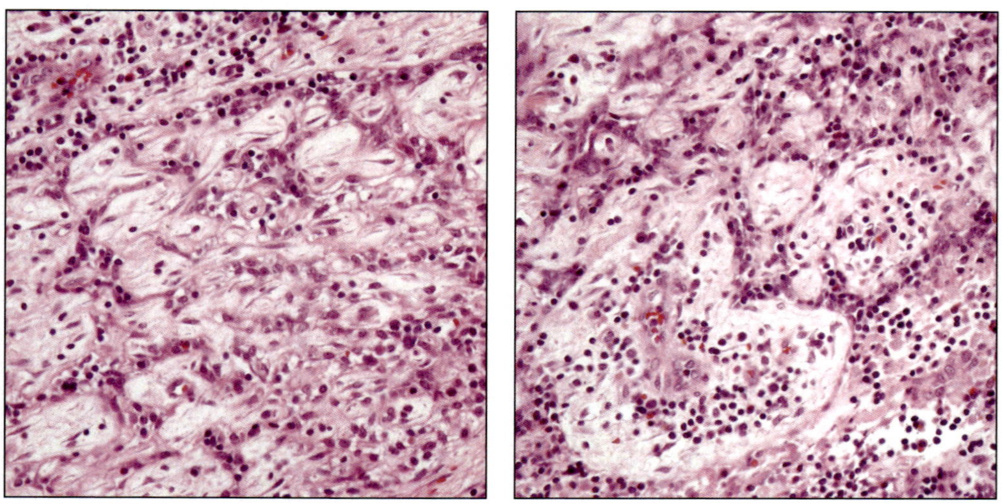

(Left) *High magnification of entrapped thymic epithelial rests within the wall of a multilocular thymic cyst shows a net-like distribution, with thin anastomosing strands of epithelial cells circumscribing areas of collagenized stroma.* ***(Right)*** *High magnification of entrapped thymic epithelium within the wall of a multilocular thymic cyst shows thin interlacing strands of thymic epithelium surrounded by inflammatory infiltrates, including abundant small lymphocytes, eosinophils, and plasma cells.*

Lymphoid Hyperplasia

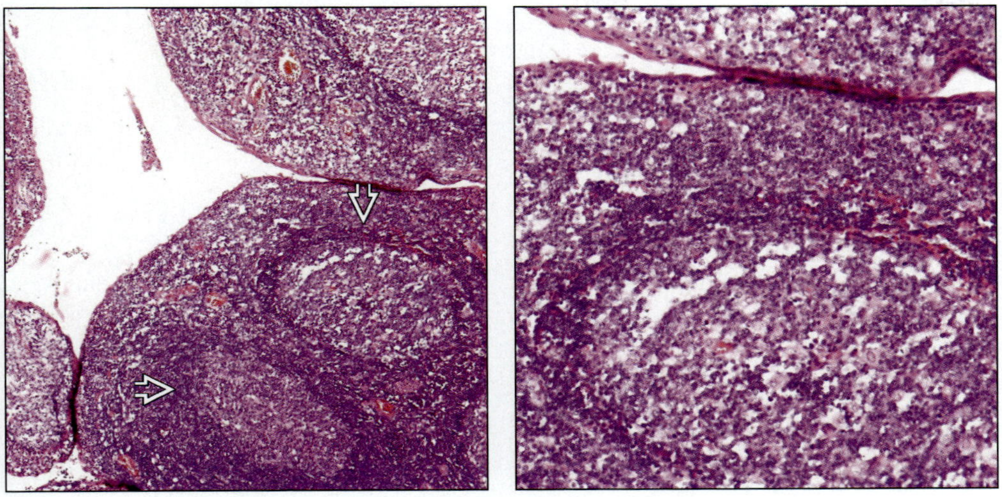

(Left) *Wall of a cyst in a multilocular thymic cyst shows prominent lymphoid follicular hyperplasia* ➡. *Lesions with these features are indistinguishable from lymphoepithelial cysts observed in salivary glands, pancreas, and other secretory organs.* ***(Right)*** *Higher magnification of lymphoid follicle in the wall of a multilocular thymic cyst shows hyperplastic germinal center with tingible-body macrophages. The remainder of the cyst wall also contains a dense lymphoid infiltrate.*

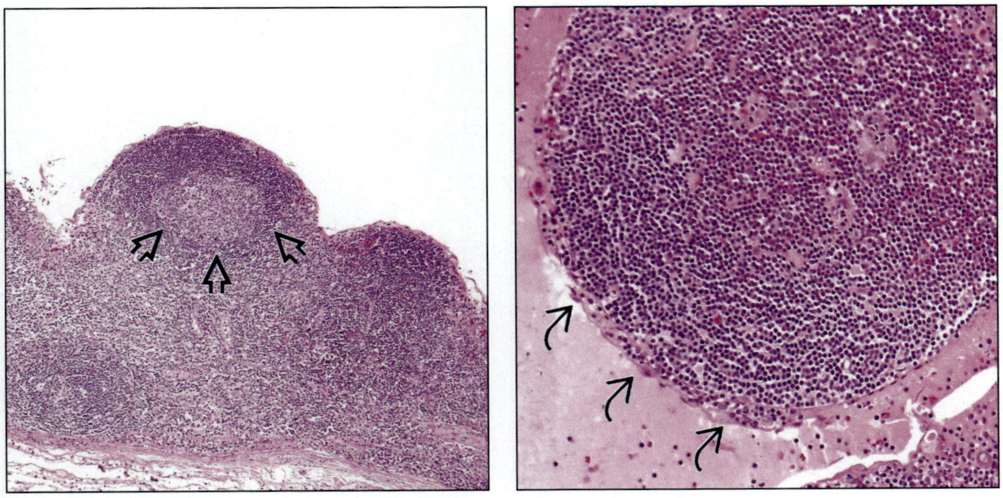

(Left) *Wall of a cyst in a patient with multilocular thymic cyst shows prominent lymphoid follicular hyperplasia. Some of the lymphoid follicles contain prominent germinal centers* ➡. ***(Right)*** *High magnification shows a hyperplastic lymphoid follicle within the wall of a cyst in a patient with multilocular thymic cyst. Note the flattened layer of thymic epithelial cells lining the cyst* ↗.

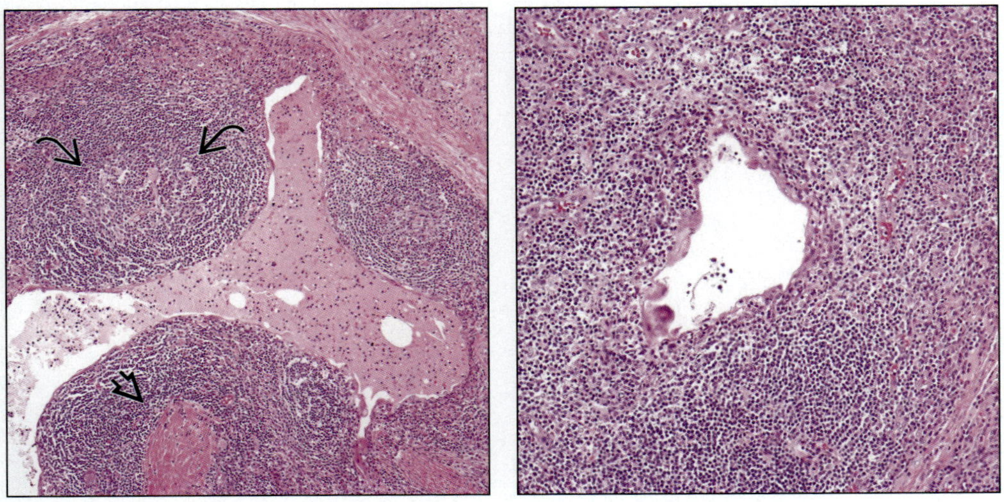

(Left) *Cyst wall in a patient with multilocular thymic cyst shows dense lymphoid infiltrates with lymphoid follicular hyperplasia with expanded germinal centers* ↗*; others show prominent hyalinization* ➡. ***(Right)*** *Higher magnification of multilocular thymic cyst with prominent lymphoid follicular hyperplasia shows early development of a cyst from dilatation of a small, burned-out Hassall corpuscle. This probably represents the earliest stage of the process.*

ACQUIRED MULTILOCULAR THYMIC CYST

Stromal Changes

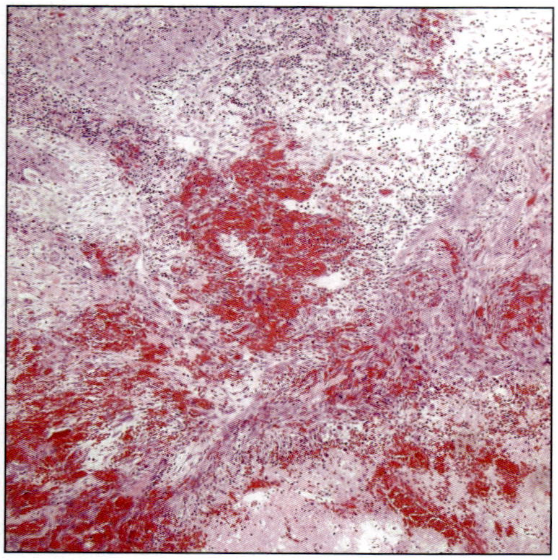
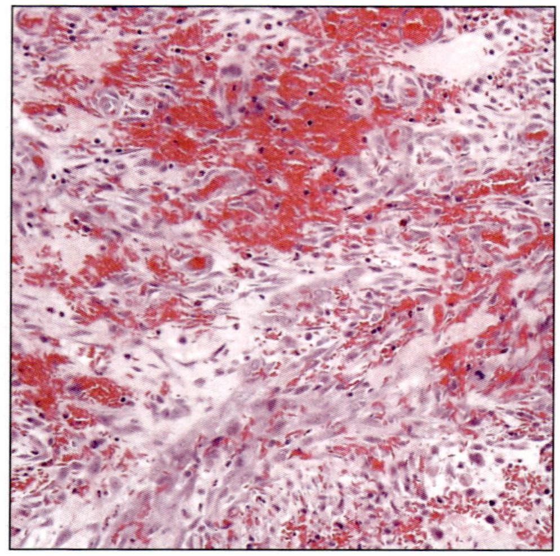

(Left) *Wall of a cyst in a patient with multilocular thymic cyst shows extensive hemorrhage and fibrosis with striking inflammatory changes.* ***(Right)*** *Higher magnification of the wall of a cyst in a patient with multilocular thymic cyst shows fibrosis, inflammation, and stromal hemorrhage. Inflammation and stromal hemorrhage are a prominent component of multilocular thymic cysts. The hemorrhage can sometimes extend into the cystic cavities, filling them with hemorrhagic fluid.*

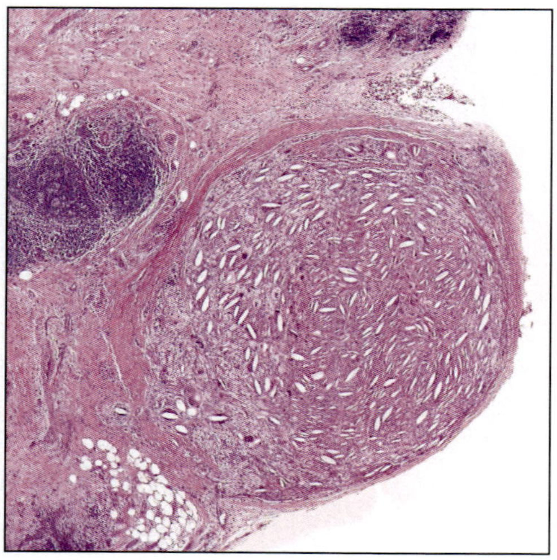
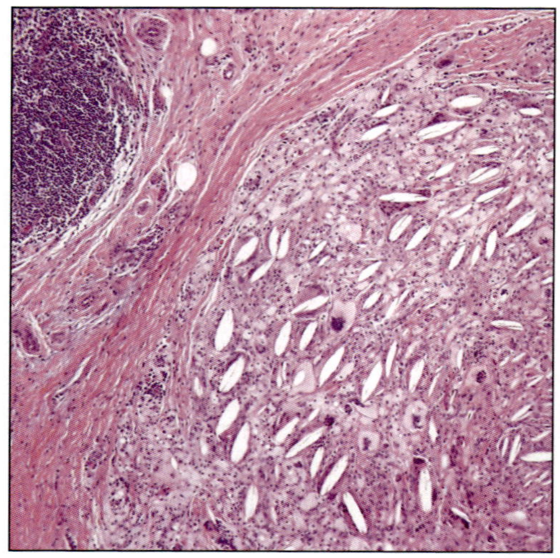

(Left) *Wall of a cyst in a patient with multilocular thymic cyst shows a polypoid protrusion into the lumen by a well-circumscribed nodule containing cholesterol-cleft granuloma.* ***(Right)*** *Wall of a cyst in a patient with a multilocular thymic cyst shows cholesterol-cleft granuloma. Cholesterol-cleft granulomas are a frequent feature seen in multilocular thymic cysts and may result from a reaction to extruded keratin squames or keratinous debris from Hassall corpuscles in the cyst walls.*

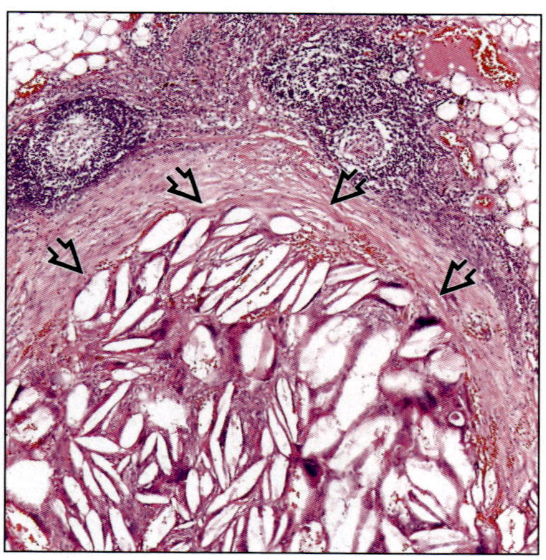
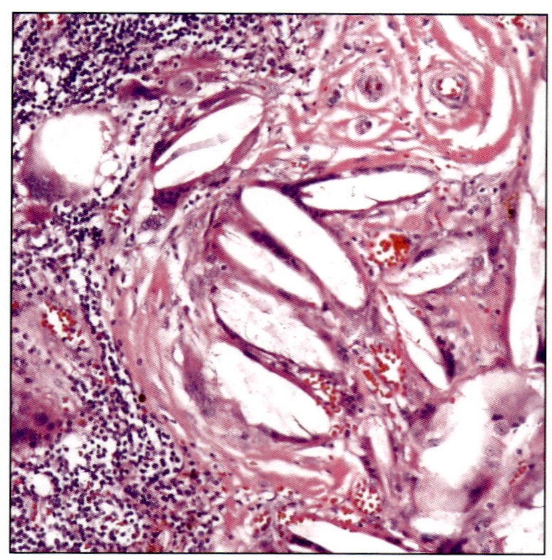

(Left) *Wall of a cyst in a patient with multilocular thymic cyst shows a well-circumscribed area containing cholesterol-cleft granuloma ⇨. Note the well-formed lymphoid follicles surrounding the granuloma at the periphery of the lesion.* ***(Right)*** *High magnification of cholesterol-cleft granuloma within the wall of a multilocular thymic cyst shows cholesterol clefts surrounded by multinucleated giant cells admixed with abundant fibrous stroma.*

ACQUIRED MULTILOCULAR THYMIC CYST

Pseudoepitheliomatous Hyperplasia

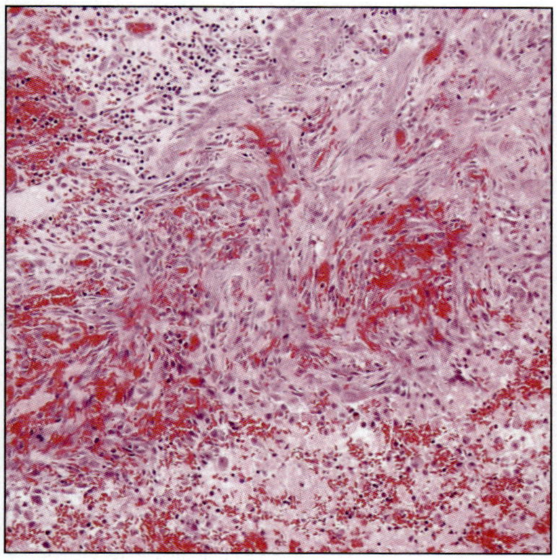

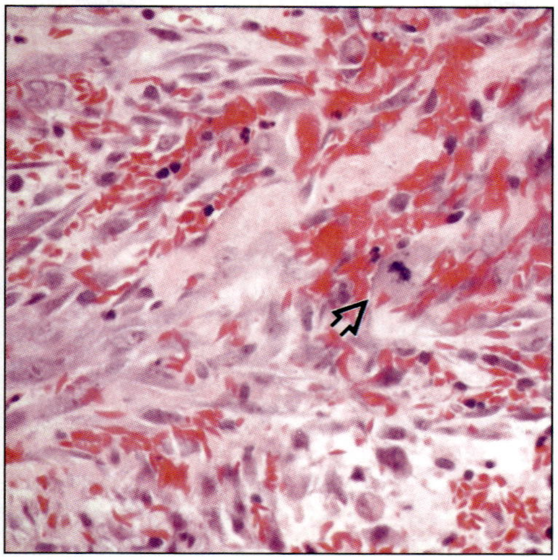

(Left) *Area of cyst wall in a patient with a multilocular thymic cyst shows complex proliferation of squamous epithelium admixed with hemorrhage and inflammation, with focal spindling of the epithelial cells suggestive of an invasive malignant process.* ***(Right)*** *Higher magnification of epithelial proliferation in the wall of a cyst in a patient with multilocular thymic cyst shows spindling of the epithelial cells and occasional scattered mitoses* ⇨.

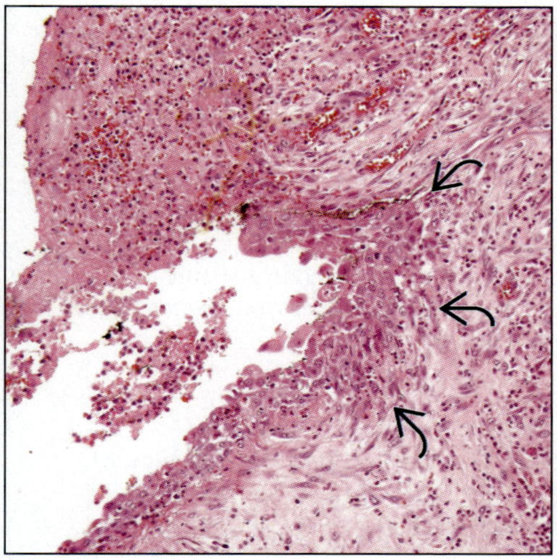

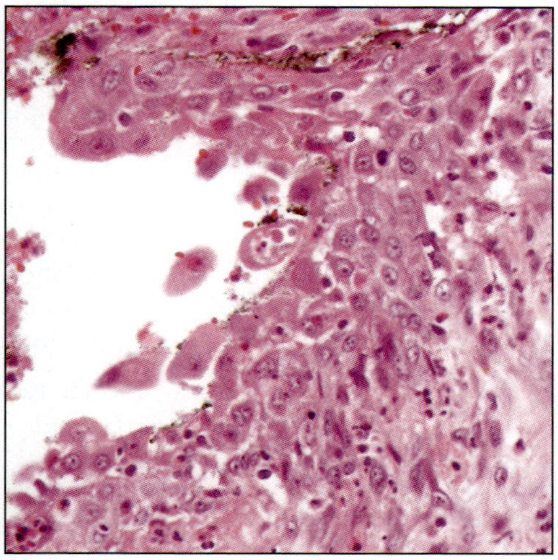

(Left) *Wall of a cyst in a patient with a multilocular thymic cyst shows focus of squamous metaplasia of the lining epithelium with focal invagination of the lining into the wall of the cyst resulting in an appearance of invasion* ↶. ***(Right)*** *Higher magnification shows a focus of squamous metaplasia of the epithelial lining in the wall of a multilocular thymic cyst. Cases showing features of pseudoepitheliomatous hyperplasia can be confused for squamous cell carcinomas arising from the cyst lining.*

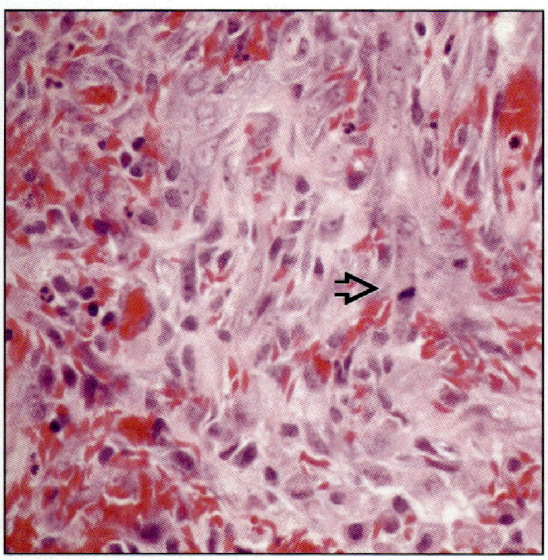

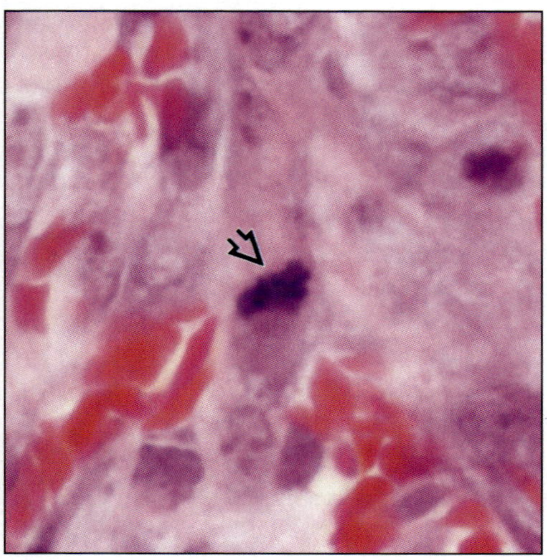

(Left) *Area of pseudoepitheliomatous hyperplasia with cytologic atypia is seen in the wall of a cyst in a patient with multilocular thymic cyst. The epithelial cells show enlarged, hyperchromatic nuclei and scattered mitoses* ⇨ *admixed with granulation tissue.* ***(Right)*** *High magnification from an area of pseudoepitheliomatous hyperplasia in the wall of a cyst in a patient with multilocular thymic cyst shows a mitotic figure* ⇨.

IDIOPATHIC SCLEROSING MEDIASTINITIS

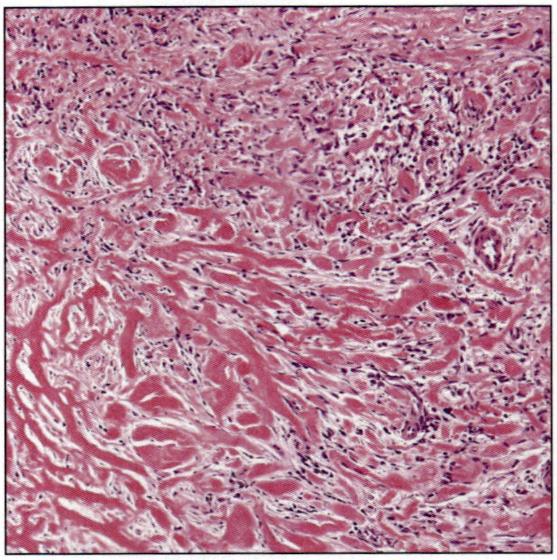

Histologic appearance of idiopathic sclerosing mediastinitis shows thick bands of keloidal collagen arranged in haphazard distribution (bottom) admixed with scattered inflammatory cells.

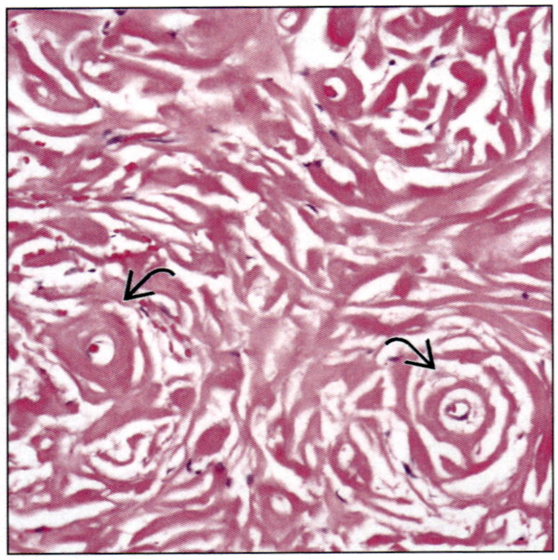

End stage of idiopathic sclerosing mediastinitis shows complex pattern of hyalinization with thick bands of keloidal collagen in concentric arrangement around residual small vessels ➔.

TERMINOLOGY

Abbreviations

- Idiopathic sclerosing mediastinitis (ISM)

Synonyms

- Idiopathic fibroinflammatory lesion
- Sclerosing mediastinitis
- Inflammatory pseudotumor

Definitions

- Chronic condition characterized by fibrous replacement of soft tissues in mediastinum, ± inflammation, of unknown etiology

ETIOLOGY/PATHOGENESIS

Pathogenesis

- Most cases are idiopathic
- May be result of healed infection, such as tuberculosis or toxoplasmosis
- May represent the end stage of burned-out neoplasms, such as Hodgkin lymphoma or seminoma
- May be secondary to autoimmune disorders, sarcoidosis, rheumatic fever, or drugs (e.g., methysergide)
- Some cases thought to represent abnormal immune response due to delayed hypersensitivity reaction to infectious agents in susceptible individuals

CLINICAL ISSUES

Epidemiology

- Age
  - Most often involves young individuals between 20-30 years of age
- Gender
  - Slight female predilection
- Ethnicity
  - Slight increase in African-Americans

Presentation

- Cough
- Shortness of breath
- Fever
- Superior vena cava syndrome in rare instances
- Mediastinal mass or widening of mediastinum on chest x-ray and CT scan
- Can show calcifications on imaging studies
- Location can be in hilum, subcarinal, paratracheal, or anterior mediastinum

Treatment

- Steroids
- Surgery difficult and generally of limited benefit
- Favorable response to antifungal agents has been observed in some cases

Prognosis

- Long protracted course with progressive airway compromise
- Extensive subcarinal involvement most likely to lead to death due to encroachment of vital structures
- Chronic course; may be self-limiting and regress spontaneously or progress to death due to respiratory compromise

IMAGE FINDINGS

General Features

- Focal hilar or mediastinal mass or widening
- No contrast enhancement seen on CT scan

MACROSCOPIC FEATURES

General Features

- Gray-white, homogeneous rubbery tissue

IDIOPATHIC SCLEROSING MEDIASTINITIS

Key Facts

Etiology/Pathogenesis
- Most cases are idiopathic
- May be result of healed infection, such as tuberculosis or toxoplasmosis
- May represent end stage of burned-out neoplasms, such as Hodgkin lymphoma or seminoma
- May be secondary to autoimmune disorders, sarcoidosis, rheumatic fever, or drugs (e.g., methysergide)
- Some cases thought to represent abnormal immune response due to delayed hypersensitivity reaction to infectious agents in susceptible individuals

Clinical Issues
- Mediastinal mass or widening of mediastinum on chest x-ray and CT scan
- Can show calcifications on imaging studies
- Extensive subcarinal involvement most likely to lead to death due to encroachment of vital structures
- Chronic course; may be self-limiting and regress spontaneously or progress to death due to respiratory compromise

Microscopic Pathology
- Stage I: Edematous fibromyxoid tissue with fibroblastic spindle cells, eosinophils, mast cells, lymphocytes, plasma cells, and thin-walled blood vessels
- Stage II: Thick bands of dense collagen haphazardly distributed and containing scattered fibroblastic spindle cells, lymphocytes, and plasma cells
- Stage III: Dense acellular collagen with scattered lymphoid follicles and occasional dystrophic calcifications

- Diffusely infiltrative; permeates surrounding structures including great vessels, nerves, pericardium, etc.
- May contain foci of dystrophic calcifications

MICROSCOPIC PATHOLOGY

Histologic Features
- Stage I: Edematous fibromyxoid tissue with fibroblastic spindle cells, eosinophils, mast cells, lymphocytes, plasma cells, and thin-walled blood vessels
- Stage II: Thick bands of dense collagen haphazardly distributed and containing scattered fibroblastic spindle cells, lymphocytes, and plasma cells
- Stage III: Dense acellular collagen with scattered lymphoid follicles and occasional dystrophic calcifications
- Other features
  - Entrapment of nerve trunks is a common feature
  - Ill-defined or well-formed epithelioid granulomas can also be encountered

Cytologic Features
- Fibroblastic cells show oval nuclei with dense chromatin pattern and indistinct rim of cytoplasm
- No atypical or malignant cells identified
- Special stains for organisms (i.e., GMS, PAS, AFB) should be used to rule out infectious etiology

DIFFERENTIAL DIAGNOSIS

Fibrosis Secondary to Infectious Agents
- Healed or burned-out tuberculosis, histoplasmosis, aspergillosis, mucormycosis, cryptococcosis, atypical mycobacteria, and bacterial infections caused by *Nocardia* and *Actinomyces* species
- Tissue cultures or special stains may help identify organisms
- Clinical history or serologic evidence of infection may help identify cause in some patients

Fibrosis Secondary to Drugs
- History of methysergide or other drug associated with tissue fibrosis favors this diagnosis
- Discontinuation of drug ameliorates progression of disease

Hodgkin Disease
- Often associated with massive sclerosis in mediastinum
- Extensive sampling and diligent search for residual foci of Reed-Sternberg cells

Seminoma with Secondary Fibrosis
- Mediastinal seminoma may be associated with massive sclerosis
- Extensive sampling and diligent search for residual islands of seminoma cells

DIAGNOSTIC CHECKLIST

Clinically Relevant Pathologic Features
- Diffuse fibrosis with variable component of inflammatory cells
- Infiltrating process with entrapment of fat
- Presence of poorly formed granulomas

Pathologic Interpretation Pearls
- Most important role of the pathologist is to rule out infection or a burned-out, sclerotic, malignant neoplasm

SELECTED REFERENCES

1. Flieder DB et al: Idiopathic fibroinflammatory (fibrosing/sclerosing) lesions of the mediastinum: a study of 30 cases with emphasis on morphologic heterogeneity. Mod Pathol. 12(3):257-64, 1999
2. Dehner LP et al: Idiopathic fibrosclerotic disorders and other inflammatory pseudotumors. Semin Diagn Pathol. 15(2):161-73, 1998
3. Flannery MT et al: Hodgkin's disease masquerading as sclerosing mediastinitis. South Med J. 87(9):921-3, 1994

IDIOPATHIC SCLEROSING MEDIASTINITIS

Early and Mid Stages

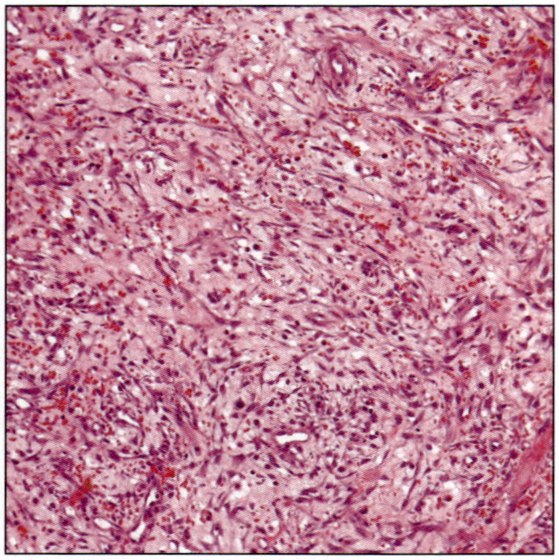
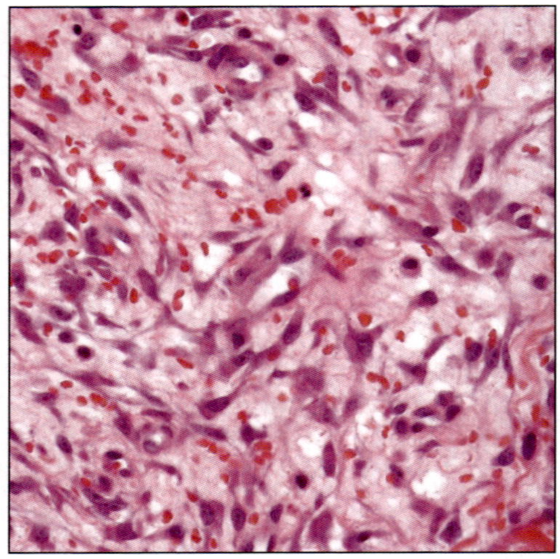

*(**Left**) Scanning magnification of idiopathic sclerosing mediastinitis, early stage, shows cellular proliferation of spindle cells admixed with scattered inflammatory cells, red blood cells, and small vessels set against a myxoid background. (**Right**) Higher magnification of idiopathic sclerosing mediastinitis in early stages shows fibroblastic spindle cells admixed with lymphocytes and small vessels. This appearance is essentially indistinguishable from that of early granulation tissue.*

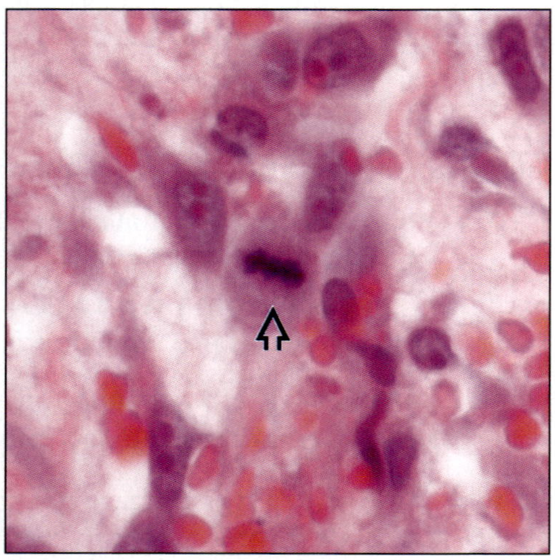
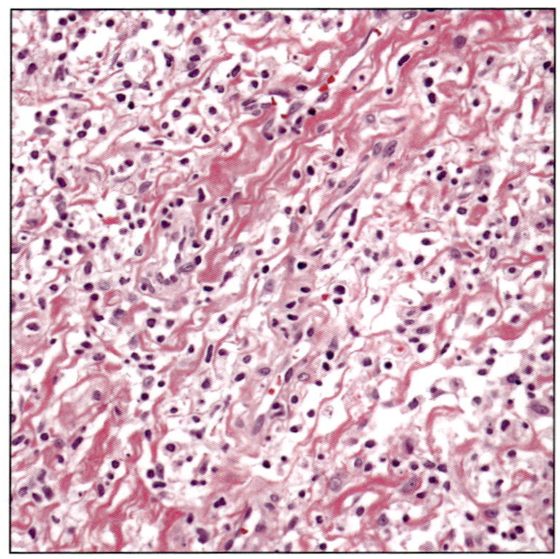

*(**Left**) Higher magnification of idiopathic sclerosing mediastinitis during the early stages shows plump fibroblastic cells admixed with red blood cells. Notice the mitotic figure in the center ⇨. As in granulation tissue, rare scattered mitoses may be present. (**Right**) Idiopathic sclerosing mediastinitis in mid stage shows an equal admixture of inflammatory cells and collagenous stroma. The process becomes more uniform, with more evenly distributed fibrosis in this stage of the process.*

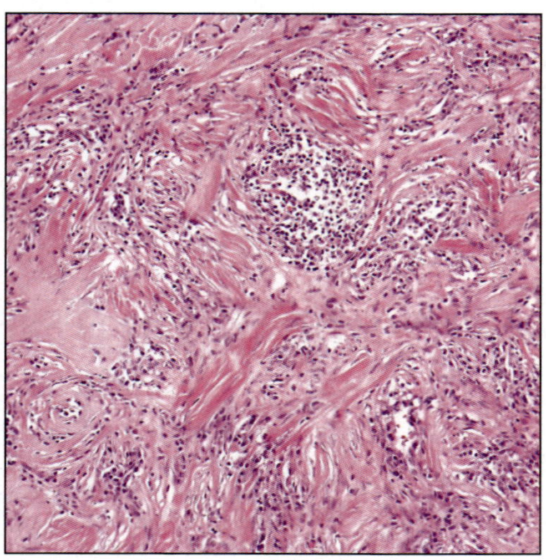
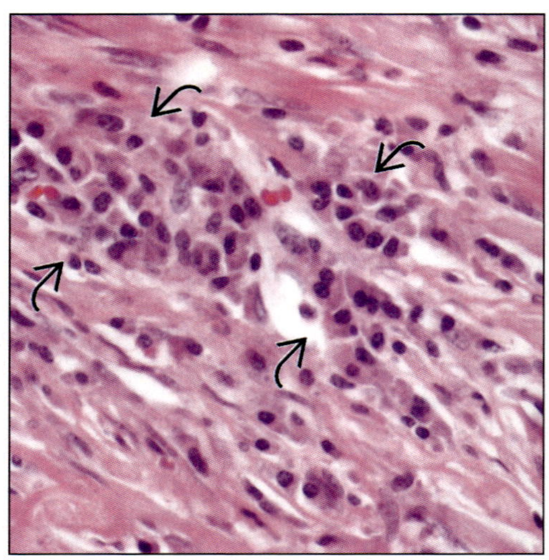

*(**Left**) Mid stage of idiopathic sclerosing mediastinitis shows progression of the fibrosing process, resulting in broad bands of collagen admixed with lymphoid cell aggregates and other inflammatory elements. (**Right**) Higher magnification of idiopathic sclerosing mediastinitis shows clusters of mature plasma cells scattered in the stroma ↪. Lesions with these features can be mistaken for examples of inflammatory myofibroblastic tumors.*

Advanced Stages

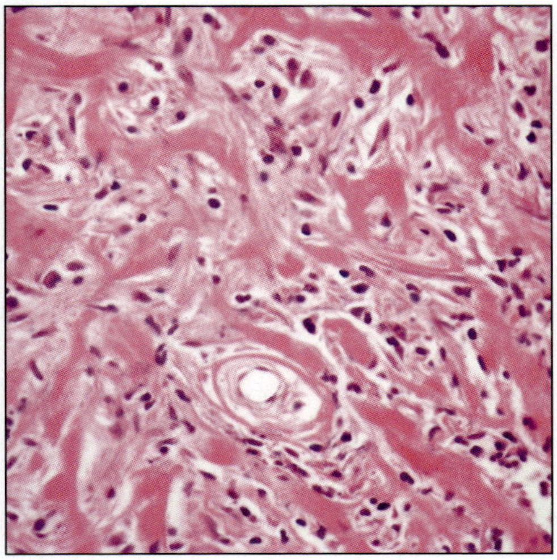

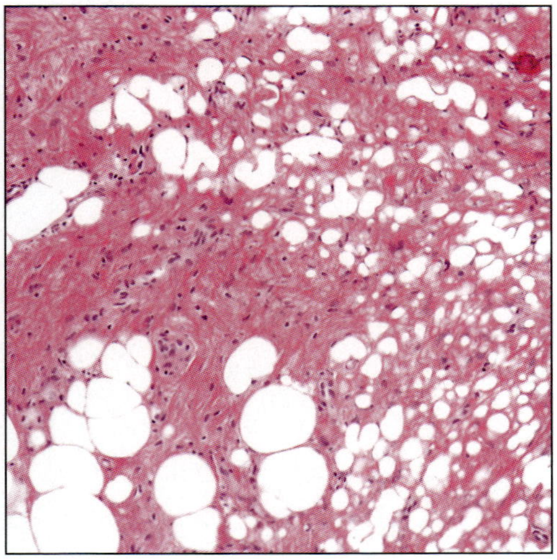

(Left) *More advanced stage of the process in idiopathic sclerosing mediastinitis shows thick bands of keloidal collagen with a few scattered fibroblastic spindle cells admixed with lymphoid cells in the surrounding stroma.* ***(Right)*** *Infiltration of the fat is seen in this case of idiopathic sclerosing mediastinitis. The infiltrative nature of the process makes it very difficult to surgically resect the lesion and may lead to confusion with a malignant neoplasm.*

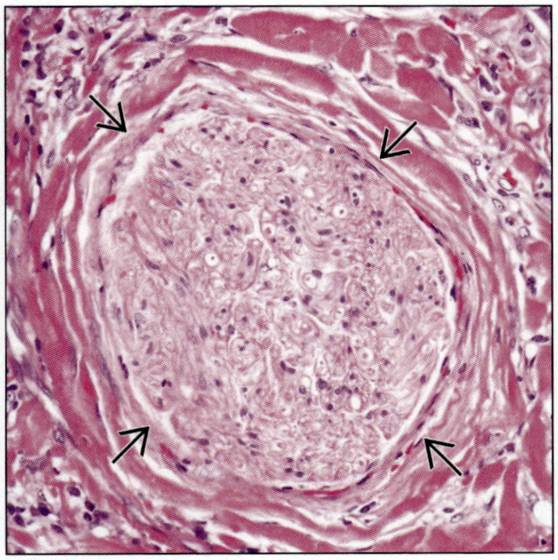

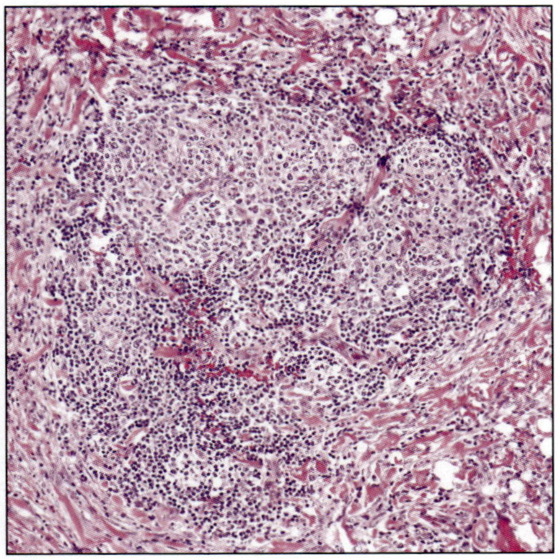

(Left) *Entrapment of large and medium-sized nerve trunks is commonly seen in the late stages of idiopathic sclerosing mediastinitis. Notice the concentric rings of keloidal collagen surrounding the nerve trunk in this lesion* ⇒. ***(Right)*** *An entrapped, residual lymphoid follicle is seen in this example of idiopathic sclerosing mediastinitis. Notice the enlarged germinal center and progressive disappearance of the mantle zone in the follicle. The surrounding stroma is heavily collagenized.*

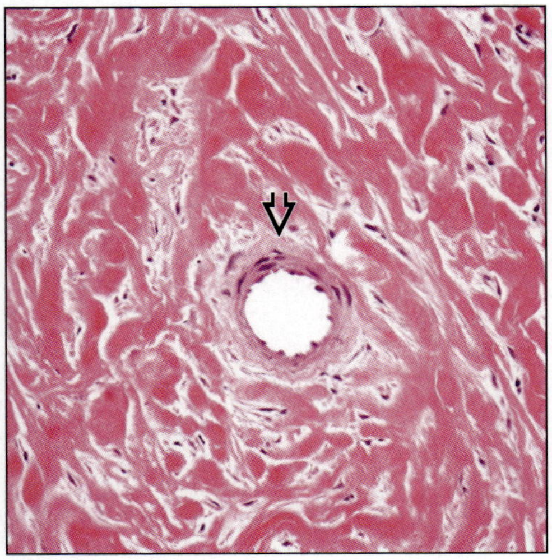

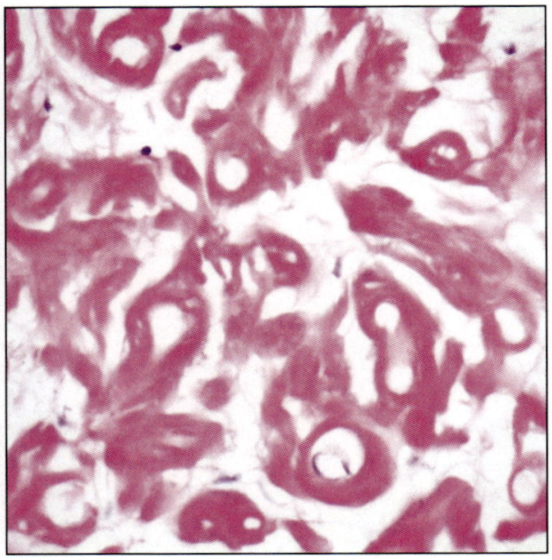

(Left) *Advanced stage of idiopathic sclerosing mediastinitis shows thick bands of keloidal collagen circumscribing a vessel* ⇨*. Lesions with this appearance require extensive sampling to rule out the possibility of a fibrosing neoplasm, such as Hodgkin lymphoma, seminoma, or thymic carcinoma.* ***(Right)*** *Unusual pattern of stromal sclerosis in idiopathic sclerosing mediastinitis shows concentric sclerosis primarily involving the walls of small caliber vessels.*

Antibody Index

ANTIBODY INDEX

Antibodies Discussed

Antibody Name/ Symbol	Antibody Description	Clones/Alternative Names	Chapters
α-fetoprotein	alpha 1 fetoprotein	AFP, Z5A06, clone C3	Choriocarcinoma; Embryonal Carcinoma; Mediastinal Seminoma; Mediastinal Teratoma
κ light chain	kappa light chain	KAPPA	Inflammatory Pseudotumor
λ light chain	lambda light chain	LAMBDA	Diffuse Large Cell Lymphoma of the Mediastinum; Lymphoblastic Lymphoma
35BH11	cytokeratin 8, low molecular weight	CK8, MA-902	Thymic Carcinoma
6F11	estrogen receptor protein	1D5, 6F11, SP1, 15D, H222, TE111, ERP, ER1D5, NCLER611, NCL-ER-LH2 PGP-1A6	Metastatic Carcinoma
ACTH	Adrenocorticotrophic hormone		Neuroendocrine Carcinomas of the Thymus
Actin-HHF-35	muscle-specific actin	MSA, HHF-35	Alveolar Soft Part Sarcoma; Angiosarcoma; Chondrosarcoma; Endobronchial Lipoma; Epithelioid Hemangioendothelioma, Mediastinum; Leiomyosarcoma; Metastatic Sarcoma; Mixed Tumor; Mucoepidermoid Carcinoma of the Pleura; Neurofibroma; Osteosarcoma; Peripheral Nerve Sheath Tumor; Pleomorphic Carcinoma; Pleural Endometriosis; Pulmonary Leiomyosarcoma
Actin-sm	smooth muscle actin	SMA, ASM-1, CGA7, IA4, HUC-1	Adenoid Cystic Carcinoma; Alveolar Adenoma; Calcified Fibrous Tumor; Endobronchial Lipoma; Epi-myoepithelial Carcinoma; Glomus Tumor; Granular Cell Tumor; Inflammatory Pseudotumor; Lymphangioleiomyomatosis; Metastatic Sarcoma; Mixed Tumor; Pulmonary Leiomyosarcoma; Smooth Muscle Tumors of the Pleura; Solitary Fibrous Tumor; Spindle Cell (Sarcomatoid) Carcinoma
AE1/AE3	mixture of 2 anticytokeratin clones that detect a variety of both high and low molecular weight cytokeratins		Alveolar Proteinosis; Atypical Thymoma; Desmoplastic Small Round Cell Tumor; Desquamative Interstitial Pneumonia (DIP); Intrapulmonary Solitary Fibrous Tumor; Intrapulmonary Synovial Sarcoma; Intrapulmonary Thymoma; Large Cell (Anaplastic) Carcinoma; Leiomyosarcoma; Metastatic Carcinoma; Minute Meningothelial-like Nodule; Mucoepidermoid Carcinoma; Neurofibroma; Poorly Differentiated Squamous Carcinoma, Small Cell Variant; Pleural Synovial Sarcoma; Pulmonary BALT Lymphoma; Solitary Fibrous Tumor; Solitary Fibrous Tumor/ Fibrosarcoma; Synovial Sarcoma; Thymic Carcinoma; Thymolipoma; Thymoma; Yolk Sac Tumor
AFP	alpha 1 fetoprotein	Z5A06, clone C3, α-fetoprotein	Yolk Sac Tumor
ALK	anaplastic lymphoma kinase-1	5A4, ALK1, ALKC	Hyalinizing Granuloma; Pulmonary Hodgkin Lymphoma
ALK1	anaplastic lymphoma kinase-1	5A4, ALK1, ALKC	Angiolymphoid Hyperplasia with Eosinophilia; Diffuse Large Cell Lymphoma of the Mediastinum; Embryonal Carcinoma; Inflammatory Pseudotumor; Sclerosing Hemangioma (Pneumocytoma); Signet Ring Cell Carcinoma
AMACR	alpha methylacyl CoA racemase	13H4, P504S	Metastatic Carcinoma
Amylase	salivary gland and pancreatic enzyme		Acinic Cell Carcinoma
Androgen receptor		AR441, F39.4.1, AR-N20, ANDROGEN RE, AR27	Minute Meningothelial-like Nodules; Mucoepidermoid Carcinoma, Pleura

ANTIBODY INDEX

Bcl-2	B-cell CLL lymphoma 2; suppresses apoptosis in a variety of cell systems	ONCL2, BCL2/100/D5, 124, 124.3	Benign Metastasizing Leiomyoma; Calcified Fibrous Tumor; Castleman Disease; Diffuse Large Cell Lymphoma of the Mediastinum; Ganglioneuroma; Hyalinizing Granuloma; Intrapulmonary Solitary Fibrous Tumor; Intrapulmonary Synovial Sarcoma; Intrapulmonary Thymoma; Leiomyosarcoma; Liposarcoma; Lymphoepithelioma-like Carcinoma; Mesenchymal Chondrosarcoma; Metastatic Sarcoma; Neurogenic Sarcoma (Malignant Peripheral Nerve Sheath Tumor); Peripheral Nerve Sheath Tumor; Pulmonary Adenofibroma/Adenomyoma; Pulmonary Amyloidosis; Pulmonary BALT Lymphoma; Pulmonary Leiomyosarcoma; Pulmonary Meningioma; Smooth Muscle Tumors of the Pleura; Solitary Fibrous Tumor; Solitary Fibrous Tumor/Fibrosarcoma; Synovial Sarcoma; Thymic Carcinoma; Thymoma
Bcl-6	B-cell CLL lymphoma 6	LN22, GI191E/A8, N-3, PG-B6P, P1F6, 3FR-1	Diffuse Large Cell Lymphoma of the Mediastinum; MALT Lymphoma of the Thymus; Pulmonary BALT Lymphoma
Bcl-10	B-cell lymphoma 10	151, 331.3	Pulmonary BALT Lymphoma
Beta catenin	involved in regulation of cell adhesion and in signal transduction through Wnt pathway		Smooth Muscle Tumors of the Pleura
Bombesin			Neuroendocrine Carcinoma
CA19-9	tumor marker, cancer antigen 19-9 or sialylated Lewis A antigen	1116NS19-9	Metastatic Carcinoma
Calcitonin	polypeptide hormone released by parafollicular cells (C cells) of the thyroid	CALBINDIN28	Neuroendocrine Carcinomas of the Thymus; Paraganglioma, Lung
Caldesmon	actin interacting and calmodulin binding protein found in smooth muscle and other cell types		Endobronchial Lipoma; Leiomyosarcoma; Pleomorphic Carcinoma; Pulmonary Leiomyosarcoma; Smooth Muscle Tumors of the Pleura; Solitary Fibrous Tumor; Spindle Cell (Sarcomatoid) Carcinoma
Calretinin	calretinin	Calretinin (mesothelial), CALRETININ, DAK-CALRET, 5A5, CAL 3F5, DC8, AB149	Atypical Thymoma; Calcified Fibrous Tumor; Choriocarcinoma; Intrapulmonary Thymoma; Mesothelial Hyperplasia; Pleural Synovial Sarcoma; Pseudomesotheliomatous Adenocarcinoma; Sclerosing Hemangioma (Pneumocytoma); Solitary Fibrous Tumor/Fibrosarcoma; Spindle Cell (Sarcomatoid) Carcinoma; Synovial Sarcoma; Thymic Carcinoma
CAM5.2			Yolk Sac Tumor
Calponin	calponin	N3, 26A11, CALP, CALPONIN	Benign Metastasizing Leiomyoma; Intrapulmonary Solitary Fibrous Tumor; Metastatic Sarcoma; Pleural Synovial Sarcoma; Synovial Sarcoma
Cathespin-B	lysosomal cysteine protease		Clear Cell "Sugar" Tumor; Granular Cell Tumor
CD1a	T-cell surface glycoprotein	JPM30, CD1A, O10, NA1/34	Atypical Thymoma; Clear Cell "Sugar" Tumor (PEComa); Eosinophilic Pneumonia; Erdheim-Chester Disease; Hard Metal Pneumoconiosis Pneumonitis; Intrapulmonary Thymoma; Juvenile Xanthogranuloma; Langerhans Cell Histiocytosis; Lymphoblastic Lymphoma; Paraffinoma (Lipoid Pneumonia) Respiratory Bronchiolitis; Rosai-Dorfman of Lung; Thymoma
CD3	T-cell receptor	F7238, A0452, CD3-P, CD3-M, SP7, PS1	Atypical Thymoma; Diffuse Large Cell Lymphoma; Hodgkin Lymphoma of the Mediastinum; Juvenile Xanthogranuloma; Lymphoblastic Lymphoma; Lymphomatoid

ANTIBODY INDEX

			Granulomatosis; Thymic Carcinoma; Thymoma
CD4	T-cell surface glycoprotein, L3T4	IF6, 1290, 4B12, CD4, 1F6, CD04	Juvenile Xanthogranuloma; Lymphomatoid Granulomatosis; Pneumocystosis
CD5	T-cell surface glycoprotein Leu 1, T1	NCL-CD5, 4C7, 54/B4, 54/F6	Atypical Thymoma; Diffuse Large Cell Lymphoma of the Mediastinum; Embryonal Carcinoma; MALT Lymphoma of the Thymus; Pulmonary BALT Lymphoma; Thymic Carcinoma; Thymoma
CD7	T-cell antigen precursor Leu 9	272, CD7-272	Diffuse Large Cell Lymphoma
CD8	T-cell coreceptor antigen, Leu 2, T-cytotoxic cells	M7103, C8/144, C8/144B	Lymphomatoid Granulomatosis
CD10	neutral endopeptidase	CALLA, neprilysin, NEP	Diffuse Large Cell Lymphoma of the Mediastinum; Lymphoblastic Lymphoma; Malignant Solitary Fibrous Tumor (Fibrosarcoma); Metastatic Sarcoma; Pulmonary BALT Lymphoma
CD15	reacts with Reed-Sternberg cells of Hodgkin disease and with granulocytes	VIM-2,3C4, LEU-M1, TU9, VIM-D5, MY1, CBD1, MMA, 3CD1, C3D1, Lewis x, SSEA-1	Adenocarcinoma; Angiolymphoid Hyperplasia with Eosinophilia; Choriocarcinoma; Diffuse Large Cell Lymphoma of the Mediastinum; Embryonal Carcinoma; Hodgkin Lymphoma; Hodgkin Lymphoma of the Mediastinum; Lymphoepithelioma-like Carcinoma; Lymphomatoid Granulomatosis; Malignant Mesothelioma; Pleural Endometriosis; Pseudomesotheliomatous Adenocarcinoma; Rosai-Dorfman Disease; Signet Ring Cell Carcinoma; Spindle Cell (Sarcomatoid) Carcinoma; Thymic Carcinoma
CD19	B-cell antigen		Diffuse Large Cell Lymphoma of the Mediastinum; Lymphoblastic Lymphoma
CD20	membrane spanning 4 domains of B-lymphocytes	FB1, B1, L26, MS4A1	Angiolymphoid Hyperplasia with Eosinophilia; Diffuse Large Cell Lymphoma; Diffuse Large Cell Lymphoma of the Mediastinum; Embryonal Carcinoma; Hodgkin Lymphoma; Hodgkin Lymphoma of the Mediastinum; Lymphoblastic Lymphoma; Lymphomatoid Granulomatosis; Metastatic Carcinoma; Pulmonary BALT Lymphoma; Pulmonary Plasmocytoma; Thymic Carcinoma; Thymolipoma; Thymoma
CD21	CR2, complement component receptor 2, Epstein-Barr virus receptor	IF8	Diffuse Large Cell Lymphoma of the Mediastinum; Erdheim-Chester Disease; Juvenile Xanthogranuloma; Pulmonary BALT Hyperplasia
CD22	B-cell receptor	FPC1, LEU 14	Diffuse Large Cell Lymphoma of the Mediastinum; Lymphoblastic Lymphoma
CD23	Fc ϵ RII, low-affinity IgE receptor, IGEBF	1B12, MHM6BU38	MALT Lymphoma of the Thymus
CD30	tumor necrosis factor SF8	BER-H2, KI-1, TNFRSF8	Angiolymphoid Hyperplasia with Eosinophilia; Choriocarcinoma; Diffuse Large Cell Lymphoma; Diffuse Large Cell Lymphoma of the Mediastinum; Embryonal Carcinoma; Hodgkin Lymphoma; Hodgkin Lymphoma of the Mediastinum; Lymphomatoid Granulomatosis; Mediastinal Seminoma; Mediastinal Teratoma; Yolk Sac Tumor
CD31	platelet endothelial cell adhesion molecule	JC/70, JC/70A, PECAM-1	Alveolar Adenoma; Angiolymphoid Hyperplasia with Eosinophilia; Angiosarcoma; Angiosarcoma of the Pleura; Carcinosarcoma; Chordoma; Epithelioid Hemangioendothelioma; Epithelioid Hemangioendothelioma, Mediastinum; Hemangioma; Kaposi Sarcoma; Mediastinal Teratoma;

ANTIBODY INDEX

			Metastatic Sarcoma; Pleomorphic Carcinoma; Pulmonary Artery Sarcoma; Sclerosing Hemangioma (Pneumocytoma); Spindle Cell (Sarcomatoid) Carcinoma
CD34	hematopoietic progenitor cell antigen	MY10, IOM34, QBEND10, 8G12, 1309, HPCA-1, NU-4A1, TUK4, clone 581, BI-3c5	Alveolar Adenoma; Angiolymphoid Hyperplasia with Eosinophilia; Angiosarcoma; Angiosarcoma of the Pleura; Bronchial Malignant Melanoma; Calcified Fibrous Tumor; Carcinosarcoma; Cartilaginous Hamartoma; Chondrosarcoma; Clear Cell "Sugar" Tumor; Endobronchial Lipoma; Epithelioid Hemangioendothelioma; Epithelioid Hemangioendothelioma, Mediastinum; Ganglioneuroma; Glomus Tumor; Hyalinizing Granuloma; Intrapulmonary Solitary Fibrous Tumor; Intrapulmonary Synovial Sarcoma; Intrapulmonary Thymoma; Juvenile Xanthogranuloma; Kaposi Sarcoma; Leiomyosarcoma; Liposarcoma; Lymphoblastic Lymphoma; Mediastinal Teratoma; Mesenchymal Chondrosarcoma; Metastatic Sarcoma; Mixed Tumor; Neurofibroma; Peripheral Nerve Sheath Tumor; Placental Transmogrification; Pleural Endometriosis; Pleural Synovial Sarcoma; Pulmonary Adenofibroma/ Adenomyoma; Pulmonary Amyloidosis; Pulmonary Artery Sarcoma; Pulmonary Leiomyosarcoma; Pulmonary Meningioma; Sclerosing Hemangioma (Pneumocytoma); Smooth Muscle Tumors of the Pleura; Solitary Fibrous Tumor; Solitary Fibrous Tumor/ Fibrosarcoma; Synovial Sarcoma
CD35	erythrocyte complement receptor 1, immune adherence receptor, C3b/ C4b receptor	CR1, BER-MAC-DRC, TO5C, E11	Castleman Disease; Juvenile Xanthogranuloma; Pulmonary BALT Lymphoma
CD43	major sialoglycoprotein on surface of human T lymphocytes, monocytes, granulocytes, and some B lymphocytes	LEU-22, DF-T1, L60, MT1, sialophorin, leukosialin, SPN	Lymphoblastic Lymphoma
CD45	leukocyte common antigen	LCA, PD7/26, 1.22/4.14, T29/33, RP2/18, PD7, 2D1, 2B11+PD7/26	Alveolar Proteinosis; Angiolymphoid Hyperplasia with Eosinophilia; Desmoplastic Small Round Cell Tumor; Diffuse Large Cell Lymphoma of the Mediastinum; Hodgkin Lymphoma of the Mediastinum; Juvenile Xanthogranuloma; Lymphoblastic Lymphoma; Pulmonary Plasmocytoma; Thymolipoma
CD45RO	isoform of CD45 located on memory T cells	ICH1-L, low molecular weight isoform LCA	Diffuse Large Cell Lymphoma; Thymolipoma
CD56	NCAM (neutral cellular adhesion molecule)	MAB735, ERIC-1, 25-KD11, 123C3, 24-MB2, BC56C04, 1B6, 14- MAB735, NCC-LU-243, MOC-1, NCAM	Ganglioneuroma; Metastatic Sarcoma; Neuroendocrine Carcinoma; Neuroendocrine Carcinomas of the Thymus; Paraganglioma, Mediastinum; Pulmonary Paraganglioma
CD57	B-1,3-glucuronyltransferase 1 (glucuronosyltransferase P)	LEU-7, NK1, HNK-1, TB01, B3GAT1	Mesenchymal Chondrosarcoma; Metastatic Carcinoma; Neuroendocrine Carcinoma
CD68	cytoplasmic granule protein of monocytes, macrophages	PG-M1, KP-1, LN5	Alveolar Proteinosis; Desquamative Interstitial Pneumonia (DIP); Erdheim-Chester Disease; Juvenile Xanthogranuloma; Pleomorphic Carcinoma; Rosai-Dorfman Disease
CD79-α	immunoglobulin-associated alpha, MB1	MB-1, 11D10, 11E3, CD79A, HM47/ A9, HM57, JCB117	Diffuse Large Cell Lymphoma of the Mediastinum; Lymphomatoid Granulomatosis
CD99	CD 99 (cell surface glycoprotein for migration, T-cell adhesion, MIC2)	CD99-MEMB, CD 99, MIC2, 12E7, HBA71, O13, P30/32MIC2, M3601	Desmoplastic Small Round Cell Tumor; Intrapulmonary Solitary Fibrous Tumor; Intrapulmonary Synovial Sarcoma; Intrapulmonary Thymoma; Kaposi

ANTIBODY INDEX

			Sarcoma; Liposarcoma; Lymphoblastic Lymphoma; Mesenchymal Chondrosarcoma; Metastatic Sarcoma; Neuroblastoma/Ganglioneuroblastoma; Neurogenic Sarcoma (Malignant Peripheral Nerve Sheath Tumor); Pleural Synovial Sarcoma; Rhabdomyosarcoma; Solitary Fibrous Tumor; Solitary Fibrous Tumor/Fibrosarcoma; Synovial Sarcoma; Thymic Carcinoma; Thymoma
CD117	C-kit; tyrosine protein kinase activity	C-19 (C-KIT), 104D2, 2E4, C-KIT, A4502, H300, CMA-767	Intrapulmonary Synovial Sarcoma; Mediastinal Seminoma; Mediastinal Teratoma; Pleural Synovial Sarcoma; Squamous Cell Carcinoma; Thymic Carcinoma; Thymoma
CD138			Pulmonary Plasmocytoma
CD163	macrophage hemoglobin scavenging system	10D6	Rosai-Dorfman Disease
CDK4	Cyclin dependent kinase 4	C-22, DCS-31	Liposarcoma
CDX-2	caudal type homeobox transcription factor 2	AMT28, 7C7/D4, CDX-2-88	Acinic Cell Carcinoma; Adenocarcinoma; Bronchoalveolar Cell Carcinoma; Choriocarcinoma; Metastatic Carcinoma; Mucinous (Colloid) Carcinoma; Mucous Gland Adenoma; Neuroendocrine Carcinoma; Signet Ring Cell Carcinoma
CEA-M	carcinoembryonic antigen, monoclonal	CEA-B18, CEA-D14, CEA-GOLD 1, T84.6, CEA-GOLD 2, CEA 11, CEA-GOLD 3, CEA 27, CEA-GOLD 4, CEA 41, CEA-GOLD 5, T84.1, CEA-M, A5B7, CEJ065, IL-7, T84.66, TF3H8-1, 0062, D14, alpha-7, PARLAM 1, ZC23, CEM010, A115, COL-1, AF4, 12.140.10, 11-7, M773, CEA-M431_31, CEJO65, mCEA	Adenocarcinoma; Angiosarcoma; Bronchial Malignant Melanoma; Bronchoalveolar Cell Carcinoma; Carcinosarcoma; Choriocarcinoma; Embryonal Carcinoma; Endometrioid-like Carcinoma; Ganglioneuroblastoma; Granular Cell Tumor; Malignant Mesothelioma; Mediastinal Seminoma; Mediastinal Teratoma; Mucinous ("Colloid") Carcinoma; Mucoepidermoid Carcinoma; Mucoepidermoid Carcinoma of the Pleura; Mucous Gland Adenoma; Pleural Endometriosis; Pseudomesotheliomatous Adenocarcinoma; Pulmonary Blastoma; Sclerosing Hemangioma (Pneumocytoma); Signet Ring Cell Carcinoma; Spindle Cell (Sarcomatoid) Carcinoma; Yolk Sac Tumor
CEA-P	carcinoembryonic antigen, polyclonal		Metastatic Carcinoma; Metastatic Malignant Melanoma
Chromogranin-A	pituitary secretory protein I	PHE-5, PHE5, E001, DAK-A3, LK2H10, CGA, CHGA, SP1	Neuroendocrine Carcinoma; Alveolar Soft Part Sarcoma; Bronchial Malignant Melanoma; Ectopic Parathyroid Tumors; Ependymoma; Ganglioneuroblastoma; Ganglioneuroma; Glomus Tumor; Granular Cell Tumor; Mediastinal Teratoma; Neuroblastoma/Ganglioneuroblastoma; Neuroendocrine Carcinomas of the Thymus; Paraganglioma, Mediastinum; Pleural Endometriosis; Poorly Differentiated Squamous Carcinoma, Small Cell Variant; Pulmonary Blastoma; Pulmonary Paraganglioma; Spindle Cell (Sarcomatoid) Carcinoma; Squamous Cell Carcinoma; Thymic Carcinoma
Chymotrypsin	serine endopeptidase produced by acinar cells of the pancreas		Acinic Cell Carcinoma; Granular Cell Tumor
CK5	cytokeratin 5	CK 05, XM26, RCK103, 34BEH12	Malignant Mesothelioma
CK5/6	cytokeratin 5/6	CK 05_06, D5/16 B4	Alveolar Soft Part Sarcoma; Atypical Thymoma; Calcified Fibrous Tumor; Carcinosarcoma; Malignant Mesothelioma; Mediastinal Teratoma; Metastatic Carcinoma; Mucoepidermoid Carcinoma; Mucoepidermoid Carcinoma of the Pleura; Pseudomesotheliomatous Adenocarcinoma; Pulmonary Meningioma; Sclerosing Hemangioma (Pneumocytoma); Signet Ring Cell

ANTIBODY INDEX

			Carcinoma; Spindle Cell (Sarcomatoid) Carcinoma; Squamous Cell Carcinoma; Thymic Carcinoma; Thymolipoma
CK7	cytokeratin 7	CK 7, K72.7, KS7.18, OVTL 12/30, LDS-68, CK 07	Acinic Cell Carcinoma; Adenocarcinoma; Bronchoalveolar Cell Carcinoma; Endometrioid-like Carcinoma; Lymphoepithelioma-like Carcinoma; Metastatic Carcinoma; Metastatic Sarcoma; Mucinous ("Colloid") Carcinoma; Mucous Gland Adenoma; Neuroendocrine Carcinoma (Including Small Cell Carcinoma); Poorly Differentiated Squamous Carcinoma, Small Cell Variant; Sclerosing Hemangioma (Pneumocytoma); Signet Ring Cell Carcinoma; Thymic Carcinoma
CK8	cytokeratin 8	K8.8, 4.1.18, TS1, C-51, M20, CK 08, 35BH11, MA-902	Thymic Carcinoma
CK8/18/CAM5.2	cytokeratin 8/18 (CAM 5.2); simple epithelial-type cytokeratins	CAM 5.2, KER 10.11, NCL-5D3, keratin-LMW, cytokeratin 8/18-LMW	Alveolar Soft Part Sarcoma; Chordoma; Choriocarcinoma; Ectopic Parathyroid Tumors; Embryonal Carcinoma; Epithelioid Hemangioendothelioma, Mediastinum; Lymphoepithelioma-like Carcinoma; Mediastinal Seminoma; Signet Ring Cell Carcinoma; Yolk Sac Tumor
CK18	cytokeratin 18	M9, DC-10, CY-90, CK 18, KS18.04	Metastatic Carcinoma; Thymic Carcinoma
CK19	cytokeratin 19	BA17, RCK108, LP2K, B170, A53-BA2, CK 19, KS19.1, 170.2.14	Atypical Thymoma; Thymoma
CD20	cytokeratin 20	CK 20, KS20.8	Acinic Cell Carcinoma; Adenocarcinoma; Bronchoalveolar Cell Carcinoma; Metastatic Carcinoma; Mucinous ("Colloid") Carcinoma; Mucus Gland Adenoma; Signet Ring Cell Carcinoma
CK-HMW-NOS	cytokeratin, high molecular weight, not otherwise specified	keratin-HMW	Neuroendocrine Carcinomas of the Thymus; Paraganglioma, Mediastinum
C-Kit	C-Kit; tyrosine-protein kinase activity	CD117, C-19 (C-KIT), 104D2, 2E4, A4502, H300, CMA-767	Acquired Multilocular Thymic Cyst; Thymic Carcinoma
CK-LMW-NOS	cytokeratin, low molecular weight, not otherwise specified	keratin-LMW	Ganglioneuroma; Mediastinal Seminoma; Mucoepidermoid Carcinoma; Neuroendocrine Carcinomas of the Thymus; Paraganglioma, Mediastinum
CK-PAN	cytokeratin-pan (AE1/AE3/LP34); cocktail of high and low molecular weight cytokeratins	keratin pan, MAK-6, K576, LU-5, KL-1, KC-8, MNF 116, pankeratin, pancytokeratin	Adenocarcinoma; Adenoid Cystic Carcinoma; Alveolar Adenoma; Alveolar Soft Part Sarcoma; Angiolymphoid Hyperplasia with Eosinophilia; Angiosarcoma; Atypical Thymoma; Bronchial Malignant Melanoma; Calcified Fibrous Tumor; Carcinosarcoma; Cartilaginous Hamartoma; Chordoma; Choriocarcinoma; Chondrosarcoma; Clear Cell "Sugar" Tumor (PEComa); Ectopic Parathyroid Tumors; Embryonal Carcinoma; Endobronchial Lipoma; Ependymoma; Epi-myoepithelial Carcinoma; Epithelioid Hemangioendothelioma; Ganglioneuroblastoma; Ganglioneuroma; Glomus Tumor; Granular Cell Tumor; Hyalinizing Granuloma; Inflammatory Pseudotumor; Lymphangioleiomyomatosis; Malignant Mesothelioma; Mediastinal Seminoma; Mediastinal Teratoma; Metastatic Sarcoma; Mixed Tumor; Mucinous (Colloid) Carcinoma; Mucoepidermoid Carcinoma of the Pleura; Mucous Gland Adenoma; Neuroblastoma/ Ganglioneuroblastoma; Osteosarcoma; Paraganglioma, Mediastinum;

ANTIBODY INDEX

			Placental Transmogrification; Pleural Endometriosis; Pseudomesotheliomatous Adenocarcinoma; Pulmonary Adenofibroma/Adenomyoma; Pulmonary Leiomyosarcoma; Pulmonary Meningioma; Sclerosing Hemangioma (Pneumocytoma); Smooth Muscle Tumors of the Pleura; Thymic Carcinoma; Thymolipoma
Clara cell antigen		CC10	Sclerosing Hemangioma (Pneumocytoma)
CMV	cytomegalovirus		Cytomegalovirus
Collagen IV	major constituent of basement membranes along with laminins, proteoglycans, and enactins	CIV22, COL4A [1-5], collagen α-1(IV) chain	Hyalinizing Granuloma
C-reactive protein	acute phase reactant	CRP	Bronchiolitis Obliterans with Organizing Pneumonia (BOOP)
Cyclin-D1			Smooth muscle tumors of the pleura
Cytokeratin			Angiosarcoma of the Pleura; Atypical Thymoma; Chordoma; Desmoplastic Small Round Cell Tumor; Desquamative Interstitial Pneumonia (DIP); Hodgkin Lymphoma of the Mediastinum; Intrapulmonary Solitary Fibrous Tumor; Intrapulmonary Synovial Sarcoma; Intrapulmonary Thymoma; Large Cell (Anaplastic) Carcinoma; Liposarcoma; Malignant Mesothelioma; Malignant Solitary Fibrous Tumor (Fibrosarcoma); Metastatic Carcinoma; Metastatic Sarcoma; Minute Meningothelial-like Nodule; Neurogenic Sarcoma (Malignant Peripheral Nerve Sheath Tumor); Pleural Synovial Sarcoma; Poorly Differentiated Squamous Carcinoma, Small Cell Variant; Pulmonary Paraganglioma Solitary Fibrous Tumor; Solitary Fibrous Tumor/Fibrosarcoma; Synovial Sarcoma; Thymic Carcinoma; Thymoma
D2-40	podoplanin	Podoplanin, D2-40 clone, M2A, PODOPLANIN, gp36, AGGRUS,GLYCOPROTEIN 36 KD, glycoprotein 36, gp 36,GP 38, GP 40, HT1A 1, HT1A1, hT1α1, hT1α2, lung type I cell membrane associated glycoprotein isoform a, OTS 8, PA2.26, PA2.26 antigen,PDPN, T1 α, T1 ALPHA GENE, T1A, TIA 2, TIA2	Alveolar Adenoma
Desmin	desmin	M760, DE-R-11, D33, DE5, DE-U-10, ZC18	Alveolar Soft Part Sarcoma; Angiosarcoma; Calcified Fibrous Tumor; Carcinosarcoma; Cartilaginous Hamartoma; Chondrosarcoma; Desmoplastic Small Round Cell Tumor; Endobronchial Lipoma; Epithelioid Hemangioendothelioma, Mediastinum; Ganglioneuroblastoma; Glomus Tumor; Granular Cell Tumor; Leiomyosarcoma; Liposarcoma; Lymphangioleiomyomatosis; Mediastinal Teratoma; Mesothelial Hyperplasia; Metastatic Sarcoma; Mucoepidermoid Carcinoma of the Pleura; Neuroblastoma/ Ganglioneuroblastoma; Osteosarcoma; Peripheral Nerve Sheath Tumor; Pleomorphic Carcinoma; Pleural Endometriosis; Pulmonary Adenofibroma/Adenomyoma; Pulmonary Artery Sarcoma; Pulmonary Blastoma; Pulmonary Leiomyosarcoma; Rhabdomyosarcoma; Sclerosing Hemangioma (Pneumocytoma); Smooth Muscle Tumors of the Pleura; Solitary Fibrous Tumor/Fibrosarcoma; Spindle Cell (Sarcomatoid) Carcinoma; Thymoma

ANTIBODY INDEX

ANTIBODY INDEX

			Mediastinum; Kaposi Sarcoma; Mediastinal Teratoma
FXIIIA	factor XIIIA (fibrin stabilizing factor)	factor XIIIa	Clear Cell "Sugar" Tumor; Juvenile Xanthogranuloma; Rosai-Dorfman of Lung
GCDFP-15	gross cystic fluid protein 15	SABP, GPIP4, Gp17, 23A3, BRST-2, D6 (GROSS CYSTIC DISEASE FLUID PROTEIN)	Adenocarcinoma; Bronchoalveolar Cell Carcinoma; Mucinous (Colloid) Carcinoma; Signet Ring Cell Carcinoma
GFAP	glial fibrillary acidic protein	6F2, M761, GA-51, GFP-8A	Ependymoma; Granular Cell Tumor; Mediastinal Teratoma; Mixed Tumor; Primary Ganglioneuroblastoma of Lung
HBME-1	mesothelioma antibody		Malignant Mesothelioma; Pleural Synovial Sarcoma
H-caldesmon	h-caldesmon	High molecular weight caldesmon, H-CD, HCAD	Metastatic Sarcoma
HCG	human chorionic gonadotropin		Choriocarcinoma; Mediastinal Seminoma; Mediastinal Teratoma; Yolk Sac Tumor
HCG-α	human chorionic gonadotropin, alpha subunit		Choriocarcinoma
HCG-β	human chorionic gonadotropin, beta subunit		Choriocarcinoma
HER2	v-erb-b2 erythroblastic leukemia viral gene protein, human epidermal growth factor receptor 2	c-erb-B2, HER2/neu, NEU, HER-2, NCL-CBE1, 10A7, 9G6.10, SP3, 4B5, Epidermal Growth Factor Receptor 2, P185, 9G6.20, A0485, C-ERBB-2, CB11, ERBB-2, 3B5, TAB250, HERCEPTEST, E2-4001, HER-2_NEU	Pleural Endometriosis
HHV8	human herpes virus 8	Kaposi sarcoma associated herpes virus, KSHV, HUMAN HERPESVIRUS-8 LATENT NUCLEAR ANTIGEN-1, 13B10, LNA-1	Castleman Disease; Kaposi Sarcoma
HLA-DR	human leukocyte antigen DR	DK22, LN3, TAL.1B5, LK8D3	Diffuse Large Cell Lymphoma of the Mediastinum; Juvenile Xanthogranuloma
HMB-45	antigen present in melanocytic tumors such as melanomas	LB39 AA, CMM1, CMM, DNS, FAMMM, Mart1, Melan-A, MLM, tyrosinase	Bronchial Malignant Melanoma; Clear Cell "Sugar" Tumor (PEComa); Endobronchial Lipoma; Ependymoma; Glomus Tumor; Granular Cell Tumor; Lymphangioleiomyomatosis; Metastatic Malignant Melanoma; Minute Meningothelial-like Nodule; Primary Ganglioneuroblastoma of Lung
HMB-50	antimelanocytic marker		Clear Cell "Sugar" Tumor (PEComa)
HPL	human placental lactogen		Choriocarcinoma; Embryonal Carcinoma; Mediastinal Seminoma
IgA	immunoglobulin A	IGA	MALT Lymphoma of the Thymus
IGF-1	insulin growth factor-like 1	I-5C9	Lymphangioleiomyomatosis
IgG	immunoglobulin G	IGG	Adenovirus; Coccidioidomycosis; Diffuse Large Cell Lymphoma of the Mediastinum; Idiopathic Pulmonary Hemosiderosis; Strongyloidiasis
IgM	immunoglobulin M	IGM	Adenovirus; Coccidioidomycosis; Measles
KI-67	Ki-67 (MIB-1); marker of cell proliferation	MMI, KI88, IVAK-2, MIB1	Atypical Thymoma; Intrapulmonary Solitary Fibrous Tumor; Malignant Solitary Fibrous Tumor (Fibrosarcoma); Mesothelial Hyperplasia; Thymic Carcinoma
Leukocyte common antigen		LCA, PD7/26, 1.22/4.14, T29/33, CD45RB, RP2/18, CD45, PD7, 2D1, 2B11+PD7/26	Diffuse Large Cell Lymphoma of the Mediastinum
Mammaglobin	breast tissue-specific glycoprotein	304-1A5	Adenocarcinoma; Signet Ring Cell Carcinoma
Mart-1	mart-1 clone of Melan A		Bronchial Malignant Melanoma
MDM2	murine double minute oncogene (mdm2)	HDM2, IF2, 2A10, 1B10, SMP14, murine double minute 2	Liposarcoma
Melan-A	melanoma antigen recognized by T cells 1 (MART-1); protein found on melanocytes; melanocyte differentiation antigen	M2-7C10, CK-MM	Granular Cell Tumor; Malignant Solitary Fibrous Tumor (Fibrosarcoma); Metastatic Malignant Melanoma
Melan-A103	clone of Melan-A	A103	Metastatic Malignant Melanoma

ANTIBODY INDEX

Mesothelin	pre-pro-megakaryocyte-potentiating factor	5B2, CAK1, MPF, MSLN, SMR	Malignant Mesothelioma
MMP-1	matrix metalloproteinase 1	41-1E5, F-67, 3B6	Lymphangioleiomyomatosis
MOC-31	lung cancer marker		Adenocarcinoma; Endometrioid-like Carcinoma; Malignant Mesothelioma; Metastatic Carcinoma; Pseudomesotheliomatous Adenocarcinoma; Thymic Carcinoma
MYOD1	myogenic differentiation 1	5.8A, 5.2F	Carcinosarcoma; Chondrosarcoma; Leiomyosarcoma; Mediastinal Teratoma; Osteosarcoma; Pleomorphic Carcinoma; Pulmonary Artery Sarcoma; Rhabdomyosarcoma; Spindle Cell (Sarcomatoid) Carcinoma
Myogenin	myogenic factor 4; class C basic helix-loop-helix protein 3	F5D, MYF3, MYF4, LO26, bHLHc3, cb553, MYF4, MYOG	Liposarcoma; Neurogenic Sarcoma; Osteosarcoma; Rhabdomyosarcoma
Myoglobin	iron and oxygen-building protein found in muscle tissue	MG-1	Alveolar Soft Part Sarcoma; Carcinosarcoma; Ganglioneuroblastoma; Glomus Tumor; Leiomyosarcoma; Mediastinal Teratoma; Osteosarcoma; Pleomorphic Carcinoma; Pulmonary Artery Sarcoma; Pulmonary Blastoma
Nerve growth factor		NGF	Neurogenic Sarcoma
Nerve growth factor receptor		NGFR	Neurogenic Sarcoma
NeuroD1	neurogenic differentiation factor 1	Neuro D	Primary Ganglioneuroblastoma of Lung
NFP	cyclin dependent kinase 4 inhibitor A	Cyclin dependent kinase inhibitor p16 antibody, INK4, INK4a, MLM, MTS1, multiple tumor suppressor 1 antibody, p12, p14, p16, p16 γ, p16 INK4, p16 INK4a, INK4 p19, TP16, P16_INK4A, E6H4, sc1661, JC8, ZJ11, G175-405, F-12, DCS-50, 6H12, 16P07, 16P04	Alveolar Soft Part Sarcoma; Ganglioneuroblastoma; Ganglioneuroma; Granular Cell Tumor; Neurofibroma; Paraganglioma, Mediastinum; Peripheral Nerve Sheath Tumor;
NSE	neuron-specific enolase	BSS/H14	Clear Cell "Sugar" Tumor (PEComa); Embryonal Carcinoma; Ganglioneuroblastoma; Ganglioneuroma; Glomus Tumor; Granular Cell Tumor; Liposarcoma; Mediastinal Teratoma; Mesenchymal Chondrosarcoma; Neuroblastoma/ Ganglioneuroblastoma; Neurofibroma; Paraganglioma, Mediastinum; Peripheral Nerve Sheath Tumor; Poorly Differentiated Squamous Carcinoma, Small Cell Variant; Spindle Cell (Sarcomatoid) Carcinoma; Yolk Sac Tumor
Osteocalcin	bone gamma carboxyglutamate gla protein osteocalcin antibody	OC-1, OC, PMF1, BGLAP, BGP	Mesenchymal Chondrosarcoma
Osteonectin	protein secreted by osteoblasts during bone formation	OST1, NCL-O-NECTIN	Osteosarcoma
Osteopontin		AKm21, NCL-O-PONTIN, LF7, OP3N	Osteosarcoma
p16	cyclin dependent kinase 4 inhibitor 2A	P16_INK4A, E6H4, sc1661, JC8, ZJ11, P16, G175-405, F-12, DCS-50, 6H12, 16P07, 16P04	Metastatic Carcinoma
p21	cyclin dependent kinase inhibitor 1A	WAF1, DCS-60.2, EA10, 6B6, 4D10, SX118, P21, P21_WAF1, WAFT	Pulmonary BALT Hyperplasia
p53	p53 tumor suppressor gene protein	DO7, 21N, BP53-12-1, AB6, CM1, PAB1801, DO1, BP53-11, PAB240, RSP53, MU195, P53	Lymphoepithelioma-like Carcinoma; Malignant Solitary Fibrous Tumor (Fibrosarcoma); Mediastinal Seminoma; Neuroendocrine Carcinomas of the Thymus; Pleomorphic Carcinoma; Pulmonary Blastoma; Solitary Fibrous Tumor
p63	tumor protein p63	P63- P53 HOMOLOGOUS NULCEAR PROTEIN;DELTA-NP63, 4A4, P63, H-137, 7JUL	Atypical Thymoma; Endometrioid-like Carcinoma; Intrapulmonary Thymoma; Mediastinal Teratoma; Metastatic Carcinoma; Mucoepidermoid Carcinoma; Mucoepidermoid Carcinoma of the Pleura; Mucous Gland Adenoma; Poorly Differentiated Squamous Carcinoma, Small Cell Variant; Pseudomesotheliomatous

ANTIBODY INDEX

			Adenocarcinoma; Rhabdomyosarcoma; Signet Ring Cell Carcinoma; Spindle Cell (Sarcomatoid) Carcinoma; Squamous Cell Carcinoma; Synovial Sarcoma; Thymic Carcinoma; Thymoma
p80	anaplastic lymphoma kinase-1	KU	Inflammatory Pseudotumor
PAP	prostatic acid phosphatase	PASE/4LJ, PAP-P	Alveolar Proteinosis
Parathyroid hormone		PTH, Parathyroid	Ectopic parathyroid tumors
pax-5	paired box gene 5	PAX5 (BSAP)	Hodgkin Lymphoma of the Mediastinum; Hodgkin Lymphoma
pax-8	paired box gene 8		Metastatic Carcinoma
PLAP	placental alkaline phosphatase	228M, 8A9, 88B	Choriocarcinoma; Embryonal Carcinoma; Epithelioid Hemangioendothelioma, Mediastinum; Mediastinal Seminoma; Mediastinal Teratoma; Yolk Sac Tumor
PNA	peanut agglutinin		Pneumocystosis
PRP	progesterone receptor protein	PR, 10A9, PGR-1A6, KD68, PGR-ICA, PRP-P, PRI, 1A6, 1AR, HPRA3, PGR-636, 636, PR88, NCL-PGR	Adenocarcinoma; Benign Metastasizing Leiomyoma; Epithelioid Hemangioendothelioma; Metastatic Sarcoma; Signet Ring Cell Carcinoma
PSA	prostate specific antigen	PSA-M, PSA, ER-PR8, PSA-P, F5	Metastatic Carcinoma
PSAP			Metastatic Carcinoma
PTH	parathyroid hormone		Ectopic Parathyroid Tumors; Neuroendocrine Carcinomas of the Thymus; Paraganglioma, Mediastinum
S100	low molecular weight protein normally present in cells derived from neural crest (Schwann cells, melanocytes, and glial cells), chondrocytes, adipocytes, myoepithelial cells, macrophages, Langerhans cells, dendritic cells, and keratinocytes	S-100, A6, 15E2E2, Z311, 4C4.9	Adenoid Cystic Carcinoma; Alveolar Adenoma; Alveolar Proteinosis; Alveolar Soft Part Sarcoma; Angiosarcoma; Benign Metastasizing Leiomyoma; Bronchial Malignant Melanoma; Calcified Fibrous Tumor; Carcinosarcoma; Cartilaginous Hamartoma; Chordoma; Choriocarcinoma; Chondrosarcoma; Clear Cell "Sugar" Tumor (PEComa); Desmoplastic Small Round Cell Tumor; Diffuse Large Cell Lymphoma; Diffuse Large Cell Lymphoma of the Mediastinum; Endobronchial Lipoma; Eosinophilic Pneumonia; Ependymoma; Epi-myoepithelial Carcinoma; Epithelioid Hemangioendothelioma, Mediastinum; Erdheim-Chester Disease; Ganglioneuroblastoma; Ganglioneuroma; Glomus Tumor; Granular Cell Tumor; IgG4 Sclerosing Lung Disease; Intrapulmonary Solitary Fibrous Tumor; Intrapulmonary Synovial Sarcoma; Juvenile Xanthogranuloma; Langerhans Cell Histiocytosis; Liposarcoma; Lymphangioleiomyomatosis; Malakoplakia; Malignant Solitary Fibrous Tumor (Fibrosarcoma); Mediastinal Seminoma; Mediastinal Teratoma; Mesenchymal Chondrosarcoma; Metastatic Malignant Melanoma; Metastatic Sarcoma; Minute Meningothelial-like Nodule; Mixed Tumor; Mucoepidermoid Carcinoma of the Pleura; Neuroendocrine Carcinomas of the Thymus; Neurofibroma; Neurogenic Sarcoma (Malignant Peripheral Nerve Sheath Tumor); Osteosarcoma; Paraganglioma, Mediastinum; Peripheral Nerve Sheath Tumor; Placental Transmogrification; Pleural Endometriosis; Pleural Synovial Sarcoma; Pulmonary Artery Sarcoma; Pulmonary Leiomyosarcoma; Pulmonary Paraganglioma; Rosai-Dorfman Disease; Rhabdomyosarcoma; Sclerosing Hemangioma (Pneumocytoma); Smooth Muscle Tumors of the Pleura;

			Solitary Fibrous Tumor; Solitary Fibrous Tumor/Fibrosarcoma; Spindle Cell (Sarcomatoid) Carcinoma; Synovial Sarcoma; Thymolipoma; Chordoma; Intrapulmonary Synovial Sarcoma; Lipoid Pneumonia (Paraffinoma)
SMAD4	Similar to Mothers Against Decapentaplegic (MAD); mothers against DPP homolog 4	MADR1 JV4-1, DPC4_SMAD4, B-8	Benign Metastasizing Leiomyoma; Metastatic Sarcoma; Neuroblastoma/ Ganglioneuroblastoma; Pulmonary Adenofibroma/Adenomyoma; Solitary Fibrous Tumor; Solitary Fibrous Tumor/ Fibrosarcoma
Somatostatin receptor		SOMATOSTATIN RECEPTOR 2A, SOMATOSTATIN RECEPTOR 3, SOMATOSTATIN RECEPTOR 5, Somatostatin-R	Neuroendocrine Carcinoma
SOX2	SRY (sex-determining region Y)-box 2 protein	SOX2 (AB5603)	Carcinosarcoma; Pulmonary Blastoma
SOX9	SRY (sex-determining region Y)-box 9 protein	CMD1, CMPD1	Calcified Fibrous Tumor; Cartilaginous Hamartoma; Chondrosarcoma; Mesenchymal Chondrosarcoma; Mixed Tumor; Osteosarcoma; Pulmonary Artery Sarcoma
Surfactant	phospholipoprotein formed by type II alveolar cells		Alveolar Adenoma; Pneumocystosis
SV40	simian virus 40		Malignant Mesothelioma
Synaptophysin	major synaptic vesicle protein P38 antibody	SVP38, SY38, SNP-88, SYP, SYPH, Sypl, Syn p38	Alveolar Soft Part Sarcoma; Bronchial Malignant Melanoma; Desmoplastic Small Round Cell Tumor; Ectopic Parathyroid Tumors; Ependymoma; Ganglioneuroma; Mediastinal Teratoma; Minute Meningothelial-like Nodule; Neuroblastoma/Ganglioneuroblastoma; Neuroendocrine Carcinoma (Including Small Cell Carcinoma); Neuroendocrine Carcinomas of the Thymus; Paraganglioma, Mediastinum; Rhabdomyosarcoma; Squamous Cell Carcinoma
TAG72	tumor-associated glycoprotein-72	CC49, B72.3, BRST-3	Endometrioid-like Carcinoma; Pseudomesotheliomatous Adenocarcinoma
TdT	terminal deoxynucleotidyl transferase	SEN 28	Desmoplastic Small Round Cell Tumor; Lymphoblastic Lymphoma; Thymoma
Thrombomodulin	thrombomodulin	1009,15C8	Malignant Mesothelioma
Thyroglobulin	dimetric protein specific to thyroid gland		Adenocarcinoma; Ectopic Thyroid Tumors; Metastatic Carcinoma; Placental Transmogrification
TTF-1	transcription termination factor	8G7G3/1, SPT-24, SC-13040	Acinic Cell Carcinoma; Adenocarcinoma; Alveolar Adenoma; Atypical Adenomatous Hyperplasia; Bronchoalveolar Cell Carcinoma; Choriocarcinoma; Embryonal Carcinoma; Endometrioid-like Carcinoma; Epi-myoepithelial Carcinoma; Lymphoepithelioma-like Carcinoma; Malignant Mesothelioma; Mesothelial Hyperplasia; Metastatic Carcinoma; Metastatic Sarcoma; Mucinous ("Colloid") Carcinoma; Mucous Gland Adenoma; Neuroendocrine Carcinoma (Including Small Cell Carcinoma); Placental Transmogrification; Pseudomesotheliomatous Adenocarcinoma; Pulmonary Blastoma; Pulmonary Meningioma; Sclerosing Hemangioma (Pneumocytoma); Signet Ring Cell Carcinoma; Spindle Cell (Sarcomatoid) Carcinoma; Squamous Cell Carcinoma; Thymic Carcinoma
ULEX-1	Ulex europeaus agglutinin-01	UEA-1 (Ulex Europeaus Agglutinin-1)	Angiosarcoma
Villin		1D2C3	Metastatic Carcinoma

ANTIBODY INDEX

Vimentin		43BE8, 3B4, V10, V9, VIM-3B4, RPN1102	Adenoid Cystic Carcinoma; Angiosarcoma of the Pleura; Calcified Fibrous Tumor; Cartilaginous Hamartoma; Chordoma; Choriocarcinoma; Desmoplastic Small Round Cell Tumor; Diffuse Large Cell Lymphoma of the Mediastinum; Embryonal Carcinoma; Endobronchial Lipoma; Epi-myoepithelial Carcinoma; Epithelioid Hemangioendothelioma, Mediastinum; Glomus Tumor; Granular Cell Tumor; Inflammatory Pseudotumor; Intrapulmonary Solitary Fibrous Tumor; Kaposi Sarcoma; Large Cell (Anaplastic) Carcinoma; Leiomyosarcoma; Malignant Solitary Fibrous Tumor (Fibrosarcoma); Mediastinal Seminoma; Metastatic Carcinoma; Metastatic Malignant Melanoma; Metastatic Sarcoma; Minute Meningothelial-like Nodule; Mixed Tumor; Mucoepidermoid Carcinoma; Mucoepidermoid Carcinoma of the Pleura; Osteosarcoma; Peripheral Nerve Sheath Tumors; Pleomorphic Carcinoma; Pleural Endometriosis; Pulmonary Adenofibroma/ Adenomyoma; Pulmonary Meningioma; Rhabdomyosarcoma; Solitary Fibrous Tumor; Solitary Fibrous Tumor/Fibrosarcoma; Spindle Cell (Sarcomatoid) Carcinoma; Squamous Cell Carcinoma; Synovial Sarcoma; Thymolipoma
WT1	Wilms tumor gene-01	6F-H2, C-19, WT-1	Desmoplastic Small Round Cell Tumor; Endometrioid-like Carcinoma; Malignant Mesothelioma; Metastatic Carcinoma; Pleural Endometriosis; Pleural Synovial Sarcoma
XIAP	sex-linked inhibitor of apoptosis protein	clone 48	Atypical Thymoma

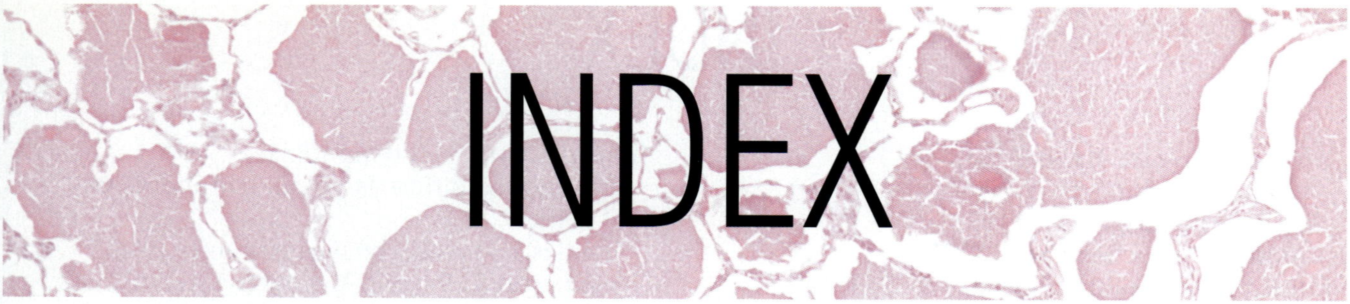

INDEX

A

INDEX

INDEX

INDEX

INDEX

D

INDEX

E

INDEX

F

INDEX

G

INDEX

INDEX

INDEX

INDEX

INDEX

INDEX

M

INDEX

INDEX

N

INDEX

O

P

INDEX

INDEX

INDEX

INDEX

S

INDEX

INDEX

T

INDEX